Management of Trauma

Management of Trauma

PITFALLS AND PRACTICE

SECOND EDITION

Edited by

ROBERT F. WILSON, M.D.

Chief, Department of Surgery
Detroit Receiving Hospital
Wayne State University
Detroit, Michigan

and

ALEXANDER J. WALT, M.B., CH.B.

Distinguished Professor
Department of Surgery
Wayne State University
Detroit, Michigan

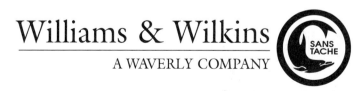

Williams & Wilkins

A WAVERLY COMPANY

BALTIMORE • PHILADELPHIA • LONDON • PARIS • BANGKOK
HONG KONG • MUNICH • SYDNEY • TOKYO • WROCLAW

1996

Editor: Carroll C. Cann
Managing Editor: Tanya Lazar
Production Coordinator: Peter J. Carley
Book Project Editor: Robert D. Magee
Designer: Arlene Puttermann
Illustration Planner: Peter J. Carley
Cover Designer: Arlene Putterman
Typesetter: Clarinda Composition
Printer: Maple Press
Digitized Illustrations: Clarinda Composition
Binder: Maple Press

Accurate indications, adverse reactions and dosage schedules for drugs are
provided in this book, but it is possible that they may change. The reader is
urged to review the package information data of the manufacturers of the
medications mentioned.

Printed in the United States of America

First Edition,

Library of Congress Cataloging-in-Publication Number: 96-28033

*The publishers have made every effort to trace the copyright holders for bor-
rowed material. If they have inadvertently overlooked any, they will be
pleased to make the necessary arrangements at the first opportunity.*

To purchase additional copies of this book, call our customer service department at (800) 638-0672 or fax orders to (800) 447-8438. For other book services, including chapter reprints and large quantity sales, ask for the Special
Sales department.

Canadian customers should call (800) 268-4178, or fax (905) 470-6780. For
all other call originating outside of the United States, please call (410) 528-
4223 or fax us at (410) 528-8550.

Visit Williams & Wilkins on the Internet: http://www.wwilkins.com or contact
our customer service department at custser@wwilkins.com. Williams &
Wilkins customer service representatives are available from 8:30 am to 6:00
pm, EST, Monday through Friday, for telephone access.

96 97 98 99

1 2 3 4 5 6 7 8 9 10

ISBN 0-683-08722-3

9 780683 087222

DEDICATION

Alexander J. Walt, M.B., Ch.B. (1923-1996) dedicated the first edition of this book "To all generations of Wayne State University interns and residents who have served in 'the pits' at Detroit General (Receiving) Hospital with so much private commitment and so little public recognition." We in turn, his students, his residents and colleagues, dedicate this second edition to Doctor Walt who worked at Wayne State University and Detroit Receiving Hospital with such unparalleled commitment and honor form 1961 until his death in 1996.

Born in Cape Town, South Africa in 1923, Doctor Walt received his medical degree from the University of Cape Town in 1948 and completed his training at the Royal College of Surgeons, London, and the Mayo Clinic, Rochester, Minnesota. He edited two books, published more than 150 scientific papers, and held numerous editorial board positions. He was Chairman of the Department of Surgery of Wayne State University from 1966–1988, president of the American Board of Medical Specialties from 1992–1994, and president of the American College of Surgeons from 1994–1995.

Doctor Walt had a remarkable knowledge of classic literature, and some of his favorite quotes were from "Ulysses" by Alfred Lord Tennyson:

"and this...spirit yearning in desire to follow
knowledge like a sinking star beyond the utmost
bounds of human thought."

Even after he retired from the Chairmanship of the Department of Surgery, he noted, as in the last stanza of Ulysses:

"Though much is taken, much abides; and though
we are not now that strength which in old days
Moved earth and heaven; that which we are, we are;
One equal temper of heroic hearts,
Made weak by time and fate, but strong in will
To strive, to seek, to find, and not to yield."

And, as Shakespeare noted:

His life was gentle, and the elements
So mix'd in him that Nature might stand up
And say to all the world, 'This was a man!'

PREFACE

Of the 50 million injuries that occur annually in the United States, over 10 million are disabling, and about 150,000 people die. In the United States, trauma is the leading cause of death and disability up to the age of 44. From the ages of 1 to 34 years, injuries kill more Americans than all diseases combined. If arteriosclerosis is considered as a single entity, trauma is the third leading case of death in all age groups.

In the United States, injuries cause the loss of more working years of life than cancer and heart disease combined. In addition, about 10 to 15% of all hospital admission are due to trauma. Indeed, the cost of accidental injuries to the country is estimated to be 150 to 200 billion dollars annually.

Trauma recognizes no boundaries, customs, or specialty boards. Despite deep interest and extensive experience in the broad field of patient care, we are constantly faced with decisions to which we may have only tentative and often controversial approaches. Even more disturbing, when we analyze these decisions later, it is apparent that frequently there is a need to amend our thinking. The premise that each patient who dies represents something of a defeat or failure is chastening, and it also constantly forces a redefinition of the clinical approach. Recurrent "pitfalls" need to have mental "flags" placed around them. Indeed, certain hallowed traditional concepts may need to be abandoned and new approaches or "axioms" learned. These are our justifications for adding yet another new book to the burgeoning literature on trauma.

No detailed review of all traumatic conditions is possible in a single volume. It has been our purpose to present a broad approach to the management of patients who have suffered major trauma. Some of the more important points in each chapter are highlighted as "axioms" or "pitfalls," and most of these are collected at the end of each chapter as "summary points" for review along with a list of the "most frequent errors." We hope that this approach may be of help to our readers.

Detroit, Michigan   Robert F. Wilson

ACKNOWLEDGMENTS

The editors wish to thank the following people without whose assistance this volume would have never come to be: (1) Bernadette M. Daley-who began this project with us, (typing, revisions, organizing figures and tables), (2) Cora L. Massey (typing, telephone calls), (3) others who typed (Sheryl A. Wier, Sandy L. Roberts, Sonja C. Battle, Valerie M. Klima), gathered data (Karyn M. Warsow, Howard C. Larky, Suzanne R. Wilson, Susan M. Kubinec, Shannon M. Hartwell), and developed tables for DRH data (John L. Heins). To each and everyone, the editors are indeed grateful.

Kenneth J. Abrams, M.D.
Director of Trauma Anesthesia
Department of Anesthesiology
Mount Sinai Medical Center
Box 1010
One Gustave L. Levy Place
New York, New York 10029-6574

Robert D. Allaben, M.D.
1151 South Otsego Avenue
Gaylord, Michigan 49735

Richard L. Arden, M.D.
Chief, Department of Otolaryngology
Detroit Receiving Hospital
4201 St. Antoine
Detroit, Michigan 48201

Chenicheri Balakrishnan, M.D.
Burn Center
Plastic & Reconstructive Surgery
Wayne State University
4201 St. Antoine
Detroit, Michigan 48201

William K. Becker, M.D.
U.S. Army Institute of Surgical Residents
Brooke Army Medical Center
Fort Sam Houston, Texas 78234

Jeffrey S. Bender, M.D.
Department of Surgery
Francis Scott Key Medical Center
4940 Eastern Avenue
Baltimore, Maryland 21224

William A. Berk, M.D.
Department of Emergency Medicine
Detroit Receiving Hospital
4201 St. Antoine
Detroit, Michigan 48201

Stephen C. Bonner, R.N.
3063 Palms Road
Richmond, Michigan 48062

Brooks F. Bock, M.D.
Chief, Emergency Medicine
Detroit Receiving Hospital
4201 St. Antoine
Detroit, Michigan 48201

Christopher W. Bryan-Brown, M.D.
Vice Chairman of Clincial Affairs
Department of Anesthesiology
Montefiore Medical Center
One Gustave L. Levy Place
New York, New York 10029-6574

William G. Cioffi, M.D.
U.S. Army Institute of Surgical Residents
Brooke Army Medical Center
Fort Sam Houston, Texas 78234

Michael Dahn, M.D.
Department of Surgery
Detroit Receiving Hospital
University Health Center
4201 St. Antoine
Detroit, Michigan 48201

Lawrence Diebel,
Department of Surgery
Detroit Receiving Hospital
4201 St. Antoine
Detroit, Michigan 48201

Scott Dulchavsky, M.D.
Department of Surgery
Harper Hospital
3990 John R. Street
Detroit, Michigan 48201

David Fromm, M.D.
Penberthy Professor
Chairman, Department of Surgery
Harper Hospital
3990 John R. Street
Detroit, Michigan 48201

Jennifer Gass, M.D.
53 Lincoln Avenue
Providence, Rhode Island 02906

Gregory M. Georgiadis, M.D.
Department of Orthopaedic Surgery
Medical College of Ohio
P.O. Box 1008
3000 Arlington Avenue
Toledo, Ohio 32699-0008

Daniel R. Guyot, M.D.
Chief, Department of Radiology
Detroit Receiving Hospital
4201 St. Antoine
Detroit, Michigan 48201

Thomas Highland, M.D.
Columbia Orthopaedics Group
Box O
Columbia, Maryland 65205

Michael D. Klein, M.D.
Chief, General Pediatric Surgery
Children Hospital of Michigan
3901 Beaubien
Detroit, Michigan 48201

Geoffrey M. Kwitko, M.D.
Assistant Professor
University of South Florida
508 South Habana Street
Suite 315
Tampa, Florida 33609

Anna M. Ledgerwood, M.D.
Department of Surgery
Detroit Receiving Hospital
4201 St. Antoine
Detroit, Michigan 48201

Julie A. Long, M.D.
South Florida Pediatric Surgeons
Central Medical Plaza
9750 North West 33rd Street; Suite 210
Coral Spring, Florida 33065

Charles E. Lucas, M.D.
Department of Surgery
Detroit Receiving Hospital
4201 St. Antoine
Detroit, Michigan 48201

Eberhard Mammen, M.D.
Mott Center
275 East Hancock
Detroit, Michigan 48204

R. Russell Martin, M.D.
Brooke Army Medical Center
Fort Sam Houston, Texas 78234

Kathleen A. McCarroll, M.D.
Vice Chief, Department of Radiology
Detroit Receiving Hospital
4201 St. Antoine
Detroit, Michigan 48201

Daniel B. Michael, M.D.
Chief, Neurosurgery
Detroit Receiving Hospital
4201 St. Antoine
Detroit, Michigan 48201

Brian J. O'Neil, M.D.
Emergency Medicine
Detroit Receiving Hospital
4201 St. Antoine
Detroit, Michigan 48201

Basil Pruitt, M.D.
U.S. Army Institute of Surgical Residents
Brooke Army Medical Center
Fort Sam Houston, Texas 78234

John M. Ramocki, M.D.
Department of Otholaryngology, ENT
Kresge Eye Institute
4201 St. Antoine
Detroit, Michigan 48201

Irwin K. Rosenberg, M.D., J.D.
RD #2; Box 66A
South Harpswell, Maine 04079

Gino Salciccioli, M.D.
Chief, Department of Orthopaedic Surgery
Hutzel Hospital
4707 St. Antoine
Detroit, Michigan 48201

James B. Smith, M.D.
Department of Urology
Providence Hospital
3900 John R. Street; Suites 1021-1031
Detroit, Michigan 48201

Thomas C. Spoor, M.D.
Department of Otholaryngology, ENT
Kresge Eye Institute
4201 St. Antoine
Detroit, Michigan 48201

Christopher Steffes, M.D.
Department of Surgery
Harper Hospital
3900 John R. Street
Detroit, Michigan 48201

Zwi Steiger, M.D.
Department of Cardiothoracic
Harper Hosital
3900 John R. Street
Detroit, Michigan 48201

Larry Stephenson, M.D.
Harper Hospital
3900 John R. Street
Detroit, Michigan 48201

Walter G. Sullivan, M.D.
Chief, Plastic & Reconstructive Surgery
Harper Hospital
3900 John R. Street
Detroit, Michigan 48201

James Tyburski, M.D.
Department of Surgery
Harper Hospital
3900 John R. Street
Detroit, Michigan 48201

Charles Vincent, M.D.
Department of Gynecology
Riverview Hospital
7815 East Jefferson; Third Floor
Detroit, Michigan 48214

Alexander J. Walt, M.B., Ch.B.
Department of Surgery
Harper Hospital
3900 John R. Street
Detroit, Michigan 48201

Robert F. Wilson, M.D.
Chief, Department of Surgery
Detroit Receiving Hospital
Wayne State University
4201 St. Antoine, 4S-13
Detroit, Michigan 48202

Paul Zidel, M.D.
Park Place Therapeutic Center
301 N.W. 84th Avenue; Suite 306
Plantation, Florida 33324

CONTENTS

Chapter 1 Prehospital Medical Care of the Injured Patient

BROOKS F. BOCK, M.D.

WILLIAM A. BERK, M.D.

STEPHEN C. BONNER, R.N.

ROBERT F. WILSON, M.D.

DEFINITION

Emergency medical services (EMS) refers to prehospital care of acutely ill and injured patients, including providing medical support while transporting the patient to a hospital for definitive care.[1] Such care includes notification of hospital personnel about the incoming emergency case, communication of the condition of the patient to physicians, care at the scene and en route to the hospital under physician supervision by radio control, maintenance or establishment of an airway, cardiac monitoring, intravenous line and medication provision, stabilization of injured and possibly fractured limbs prior to movement, and provision of psychological support to the patient. EMS also includes training and certifying individuals involved in this type of care.

AXIOM The EMS systems must work closely with the emergency department (ED) to assure a continuity of patient care from the time of the incident to discharge from the ED.

Multiple components form the modern EMS system. Medical direction of EMS should be close, consistent, and continuous. Medical control should be the responsibility of a physician with knowledge and experience in the types of emergency care that should be administered to patients who become acutely ill or injured.

The concept behind Regional Trauma Systems is that a restrictive and focused health care system is needed for patients at risk of dying from injury.[2] Effective prehospital care is ensured by appropriate protocols and triage guidelines. Prompt access to the trauma center is provided by communications and transport systems. The hub of a Regional Trauma System is the trauma center, a hospital with specialized capabilities available at all times to provide the highest level of care to victims of serious injury.

INCIDENCE OF TRAUMA

In the United States approximately 160,000 people a year die from injuries.[2,3] Of these, some 50,000 deaths are related to automobile accidents, and approximately 30,000 are due to ballistic weapons, predominately handguns.[3] Injury is the leading cause of loss of productive work years in the United States, surpassing cancer and cardiovascular disease combined.

During the past 10 years, some 50 studies on preventable deaths identified that, on average, 19.3% of injury-related deaths occurring in hospitals are preventable.[2] Thus, approximately 32,000 lives could potentially be saved each year with improved medical care. The most common cause of these preventable deaths is delaying or failing to perform needed emergency surgery. Thus, an appropriately configured and focused acute health care system should substantially reduce the mortality of major injury, as well as the morbidity and expense, which in 1985 exceeded $107 billion.[1]

Approximately 50% of those who die from injuries do so before reaching the hospital.[2] Of those who reach the hospital alive, 60% of the deaths resulting from hemorrhage occur within the first 4 hours.

About 40% of deaths from central nervous system-related injuries also occur within the first 4 hours. Thus, if a measurable reduction in trauma mortality is to be achieved, the necessary intervention should be provided as close to the time of injury as possible.

The number of individuals with severe or life-threatening injuries is small.[2] Where population-based statistics are available, the number of patients with an injury severity score[4] of 15 or more approaches 550 patients per million population per year.[5] However, other patients also may require intensive care secondary to trauma.[6] Although more than 200,000 patients with severe or multiple injuries present for treatment in the United States each year, they represent just over 5% of those who require hospitalization for trauma.[2]

A large proportion (more than 30%) of urban trauma patients are not covered by any health insurance.[2] Thus, hospitals that care for these patients often bear a large financial burden.

HISTORICAL PERSPECTIVE

Organized care of injured patients began with early efforts by military surgeons concerned with treatment of battlefield injuries.[1] EMS had its origins during the time of Dominique Jean Larrey, who was Napoleon's chief surgeon in the late 1700s. Larrey realized that many battlefield deaths could be prevented by early treatment. Consequently, he instituted a system for rapid movement of injured patients to field hospitals behind the lines.[7] His "flying ambulances" were nothing more than a covered cart into which the victim was loaded and transported to the surgeons in the rear. The basic principles that he set forth, including rapid transportation and patient care while en route to the hospital, represent the birth of the concept of EMS.

Improvements in the EMS system came slowly at first, but rapid progress occurred during World War I.[1] Although evacuation time for wounded soldiers still averaged 18 hours, improvements in immediate care were reflected in a decrease in the mortality rates from closed fracture of the femur from 80 to 20%. This was largely due to the simple measure of immobilizing the injured limb with a Thomas ring splint.

Aeromedical evacuation of the injured patient is thought to have originated with the removal from Paris of a number of injured soldiers by hot air balloon during the siege of that city in 1870.[2] The end of World War I found the French adapting some of their planes for the transport of wounded patients.[1] World War II saw the development of better air medical transport systems, and further improvements, particularly with helicopters, were seen in the Korean conflict and Vietnam War.

Until the 1940s, hospitals had admitting offices for patients coming into the hospital, and there were only a few emergency-receiving areas.[1] Because of the success of battalion aid stations during World War II, returning surgeons developed accident rooms to be used largely for the treatment of outpatient fractures. As these areas began to be used to treat an increasing number of patients with other problems, the name was changed to "emergency room." This space used for emergency care continued to expand, and in the 1960s these treatment areas increasingly began to be known as emergency departments or centers.

In September 1966, the National Academy of Sciences National Research Council published a paper entitled "Accidental Death and Disability: the Neglected Disease of Modern Society,"[8] and recommended the following to improve the care of severely injured patients:

1. Extension of basic and advanced first aid to greater numbers of the population. Preparation of teaching material for emergency personnel, including ambulance attendants.
2. Ambulance services should play a defined role in medical care. Traffic safety legislation should provide standards for ambulance design, construction, equipment, supplies, and qualifications of personnel.
3. Development of communication between ambulances and physicians in the hospital. Designation of a standard telephone number for all EMS calls nationwide.
4. Improvement of emergency departments and hospitals and categorization of these units based on their ability to provide trauma care.
5. Expansion of intensive care units for continuity of care.
6. Use of trauma registries, autopsies, and various quality assurance programs to evaluate and improve trauma systems.

Farrington and others, working with the Chicago Fire Department, developed what became, in 1969, the United States Department of Transportation's Manual for Emergency Medical Technician-Ambulance (EMT-A) Training.[1] In his later work with the American Academy of Orthopedic Surgeons, Farrington also helped develop a book for EMT-A instructors. He was a founder, along with Rocco Morando, of the National Registry of Emergency Medical Technicians (NREMT).

It was not, however, until after the Vietnam War that the modern EMS system was developed.[1] Upon return from Vietnam, many corpsmen found themselves without adequate employment and were often enthusiastically received by fire departments who wanted to use their talents in the provision of prehospital care. Prototype systems using paramedics developed in the late 1960s in Seattle, Miami, Los Angeles, Houston, Jacksonville, and Columbus. These programs were closely reviewed for their effect on patient care by the physicians who developed them.

During the 1970s, cities throughout the country recognized the importance of prehospital emergency medical services and, with the help of federal aid, rapidly developed and expanded these services.[1] The Emergency Medical Services System Act of 1973 is particularly noteworthy for having provided government funding for training and equipping EMS personnel throughout the country. However, these funds are no longer available, and it has become the responsibility of each city or county provider to develop its funding sources so that these services can be maintained. Problems with obtaining funding are a major challenge to those responsible for the prehospital management and in-hospital care of critically injured patients.[9]

TRANSPORT VEHICLES

Ground Ambulance

BASIC AMBULANCE

During the past 15 years, the station wagons and hearses that had been converted in the past to serve as basic ambulances were taken out of service because they could not conform to new local, state, and national safety codes. Basic ambulances now had to be equipped with medical devices and equipment to allow the attendants on board to perform basic life support measures.[10,11]

ADVANCED LIFE SUPPORT AMBULANCE

In general, the advanced life support (ALS) ambulance is staffed with EMTs whose skills include advanced airway management, intravenous fluid and medication administration, and defibrillation. In addition to the basic life support equipment, the ALS ambulance usually possesses telemetry, defibrillators, endotracheal intubation equipment,

various resuscitation drugs recommended by the EMS committee of the county or city medical society, and other specialized equipment.[12,13] The United States Department of Transportation reported that the application of EMS care to highway injuries from 1966 through 1981 resulted in 5.1 less deaths per 100 injuries with an additional 1.9 fewer deaths per 100 injuries if ALS was provided.[14] Potter et al reported from Australia that ALS care for trauma patients increased survival during the first 24 hours of hospitalization but had little effect thereafter.[15]

Air Ambulance

HELICOPTER

Because transporting patients rapidly via helicopter to hospitals during the Vietnam War was considered to be a major reason for the improved survival rate of military casualties during that conflict,[16] helicopter use in the United States and other countries has proliferated.[17] In 1982, there were only 55 hospital-based helicopter programs in the United States; by March 1986, 117 programs were operating 136 helicopters.[18] The considerable increase in helicopter use has led to an increase in the number of helicopter accidents.

A report in 1986 noted that hospital-based helicopter programs were experiencing an accident rate three times greater and a fatal accident rate five times greater than that of all general aviation turbine helicopters.[18] Flying in adverse conditions, inadequate consideration of flight safety before lift-off, lack of current pilot instrument rating, and pilot fatigue have been cited as the actual causes of fatal accidents. A recent study found that busier flight programs and those with the ability to fly under instrument controls were significantly less likely to have accidents.[19] The issue of helicopter safety must be addressed[2] by including flight safety as a program component of the transport service.

In addition, several items should be considered by the regional EMS medical director when an air ambulance service is proposed.[2]

1. Will the proposed air ambulance service serve only one hospital, or is it a regional resource?
2. What are the specific medical/surgical criteria for determining when an air ambulance (versus ground ambulance) should be used?
3. What are the realistic time-distance relationships for the region that would justify use of the air ambulance?
4. How many helicopters (and/or competing helicopter services) should be allowed to operate in a geographic catchment area? Each helicopter can effectively transport 600 to 800 patients a year before availability becomes a problem.

Helicopter ambulances are probably best used when the prehospital or hospital-to-hospital ground transport time is expected to be more than 35 minutes or when there is nonavailability of ground ambulances for rural and wilderness rescue.[20-22] Rotorcraft provide the ability to rapidly move a nursing care team, with or without a highly skilled physician, over a far wider geographic area than is possible by land transport. Patients can then be stabilized as appropriate and quickly transported with the on-board medical team providing continuing care. Definitive care at the destination hospital can be prearranged by radio prior to arrival.[22]

Baxt compared mortality figures for 150 consecutive trauma patients treated at the site and transported by ground ambulance with a group treated at the site and transported by air.[24] The mortality figures for the land transport group were similar to those usually seen at major trauma centers; however, there was a 52% reduction in predicted mortality among the air-transported group.

AXIOM A properly run air transport system can save lives that might be lost during a long EMS run.

There seems to be little disagreement that helicopter transfers of critically ill patients from rural hospitals (which have fewer staff and facilities) to a major trauma center is usually beneficial for the patient.

Although rapid helicopter transport of critically injured patients from remote areas may be lifesaving, there is great potential for misuse of this expensive modality. For effective use of helicopter transport: (a) it should be integrated into the regional EMS systems, (b) it should be staffed to provide advanced life support, and (c) flying to the scene of an accident should be based on medical need.

AXIOM   The cost of running a helicopter service, which is at least one million dollars a year, as well as the potential for injury or fatality to the crew from accidents, must be considered by those contemplating helicopter transport of severely injured patients.

Urban systems in the northeastern United States have very little call for helicopters to expedite care for trauma victims.[2] Most of these trauma systems have wide access to tertiary care teaching hospitals that meet level 1 or level 2 American College of Surgeons trauma center standards. In such cities, helicopters should be reserved for: (a) expediting care where access to the site is impeded by traffic or other problems, (b) bringing physicians or critical care nurses to the scene where victims are entrapped or where delayed transport will likely occur, and (c) distributing multiple casualties with severe injuries throughout a number of trauma centers. In other cities where the surface area is large and the concentration of hospitals is generally in one area, helicopters may be necessary to expedite care to distant parts of the city. Houston, with a surface area of over 160 square miles, is a good example of an urban environment where helicopters have proven to be useful.

FIXED WING AIR AMBULANCE
For patient transport distances exceeding 150 miles, a fixed wing aircraft can be very helpful.[1] However, appropriately placed landing strips and airports are required. Furthermore, requisite equipment and personnel are not as well defined as for helicopters and ground ambulances. Long-distance transport of donors, organs, and patients to specialized institutions, such as burn and transplant centers, is an ideal use of fixed wing aircrafts.

EMS ORGANIZATION

Dispatching

Dispatch of prehospital medical personnel has been greatly refined over the last 5 to 10 years.[1] Protocols that allow dispatch operators to gather appropriate information from patients or first responders are used in many locations to determine the priority and level of response which will be assigned to each call into the system. Priority medical dispatching, as it has become known, has advanced even further with the development of prearrival instructions. These allow the dispatcher or emergency operator to give specific instructions to medically untrained bystanders regarding care that can be given to the patient prior to the arrival of EMS personnel. Both of these areas have resulted in improved care and a decrease in mortality and morbidity for injured patients.

AXIOM   Proper communication between all involved individuals is essential for a properly working EMS system.

Effective dispatch implies adequate means of communication between the dispatcher and the EMTs or paramedics.[1] An effective system also allows these individuals to contact the hospital to which they will be transporting the patient. This allows for physician direction of the patient's care and assures that the institution to which the patient is being transported has an opportunity to make necessary preparations.

A community with a well-integrated EMS system will have evaluated each of its receiving facilities and will know their routine capabilities as well as their ability to provide specialty care. This is particularly important in urban areas where transport times are relatively

short. In such circumstances, patient care may by optimized by having ambulances bypass the closest facility so that a critically injured patient may receive definitive care at an institution capable of providing it. In Los Angeles, implementation of a trauma system with an emphasis on transport of seriously injured patients to trauma centers resulted in a significant decrease in mortality.[25]

Staffing Patterns

AXIOM   Making emergency medical services (EMS) personnel and equipment rapidly available to appropriate patients is the first goal of any emergency medical services system.

It is estimated that to achieve a 4- to 6-minute response time in an urban community, one EMS unit is required for each 50,000 population.[1] Therefore, in a city of 600,000 people, approximately 12 units are needed on the street at all times, at a total cost of at least $4.8 million per year.

Current staffing patterns require 10 EMTs per ambulance if they work a 40-hour week and seven EMTs per ambulance if they work a 56-hour week. In addition, based on an average of one true emergency per 10,000 population every 24 hours, one dispatcher/telephone operator is usually required for each 200,000 population on a 24-hour basis.[26]

AXIOM   One of the biggest problems with providing adequate EMS personnel and equipment to all potential patients in the United States is the tremendous maldistribution of resources.

The United States has a land area of 3.6 million square miles and a population of about 250 million, thereby providing a population density of about 70 people per square mile.[27] According to hospital data published in December, 1989, this population is served by 407,177 emergency medical technicians (EMTs), 55,331 paramedics, 43,285 advanced EMTs, and at least 34,789 ambulances.[28,29] Most of these resources are concentrated in urban areas.

Approximately 5,000,000 people reside in rural areas where the population density can be less than one person per square mile. A survey on rural emergency medical services revealed 152 EMS systems, 90 (59%) of which served populations of less than 6,000, and 25 (16%) of which served populations of less than 1,500.[29] Thirty-nine percent of the systems indicated that their average response time was more than 8 minutes, and 7% had a response time of more than 15 minutes. One system reported an average patient transport time of nearly 6 hours.[30] These figures underscore the limitations that geography and demography place on EMS.

Levels of Training for EMTs

AXIOM   Adequate training for EMT, EMT-A, and EMT-P personnel is critical to giving the best care possible while the trauma patient is in the field.

EMT is a generic term that refers to a trained emergency medical (prehospital) technician.[1] Although terminology to designate the various educational and patient care EMT skill levels varies from state to state, three levels of ambulance attendant skills are recognized nationwide. Training for all three levels should include didactic, clinical, and field internship programs. Students should spend adequate time in all three of these areas to function properly. The EMT-A and EMT-P levels are well recognized and quite similar from state to state. However, there are 32 variations of the EMT-I level of prehospital providers throughout the 50 states.

EMERGENCY MEDICAL TECHNICIAN-AMBULANCE (EMT-A)
A certified EMT-A has completed the standard 110-hour course of instruction developed by the United States Department of Transpor-

tation.[31] After completion of the course, the EMT-A takes a written and practical examination provided by either the National Registry of EMTs or the state. The skills used by a technician at this level include CPR, splinting and bandaging, extrication, emergency childbirth, pneumatic antishock garment (PASG) application, and airway management using an oral or nasal airway and bag-valve mask.

EMERGENCY MEDICAL TECHNICIAN-INTERMEDIATE (EMT-I)

The EMT-I has completed the EMT-A course, has competence in the EMT-A skills, and has an additional 150-200 hours of training.[32] The additional training hours are spent on instruction in shock management (including use of intravenous therapy), patient assessment and physiology (especially regarding resuscitation, evaluation, and management of critically injured trauma patients), and in improving airway management skills.

Although the esophageal obturator airway had been the airway of choice in the National Standard Curriculum, use of the endotracheal (ET) tube is now increasingly emphasized at the EMT-I level. The EMT-I is also instructed on the fluids and medications that might be beneficial in trauma patients, as well as the use of nitrous oxide and oxygen for long extrications or difficult transports.

EMERGENCY MEDICAL TECHNICIAN-PARAMEDIC (EMT-P)

The EMT-P is trained in all of the skills identified for the EMT-I and, in addition, in the use of the endotracheal tube.[33,34] The EMT-P is trained to administer a number of medications including epinephrine, bicarbonate, calcium, dopamine, insulin, glucose, naloxone (Narcan), morphine, diazepam, nitrous oxide, meperidine, and furosemide. The major impact of the EMT-P is in resuscitation of patients with severe cardiac and other major medical problems.

Probably the most important skill for the EMT-P is endotracheal intubation, which is an important component of prehospital care of unconscious head-injured patients and those with airway obstruction. Although the skills of the EMT-P can also be beneficial in rural areas, skill deterioration because of infrequent use requires far more continuing education. This is a major cost consideration for systems incorporating this level of training.

NURSES

AXIOM   Due to the education of nurses in pathophysiology and quality assurance, their use in prehospital EMS systems can be of great benefit.

In the EMS system, nurses often play important roles as instructors and quality control proctors.[1] Nurses have a great deal of understanding of patient care and the long-term results of the pathophysiologic processes involved. As EMTs, they can integrate the patient's immediate care with long-term needs. However, registered nurses cannot function in the field until they have been taught certain skills, such as extrication and splinting and bandaging. Furthermore, nurses are not allowed to intubate patients or insert an EOA on the basis of their nursing license alone. In fact, many states do not allow a nurse to use a defibrillator without special training. Thus, a fair amount of additional skills and related knowledge must be gained by nurses before they can function properly as EMTs in the field.

Nevertheless, nurses can perform vital functions in the EMS system by serving either as instructors in training programs or as proctors of patient care in the field and in the ED. These roles are vital in the initial training and continuing education of EMTs. Many EMS services employ nurses as field observers and on-site providers of continuing education. Nurses can give EMTs valuable insights about the pathology of various disease processes and can help provide a smooth integration of the patient's care from the field to the ED. Time spent in the field by nurses and other hospital personnel also contributes toward giving them a better understanding of the difficulties involved in providing prehospital care.

The role of nurses has been expanded into the air evacuation of patients both in fixed wing aircraft and helicopter. The need for physicians in air ambulance services is controversial.

Funding

Based on the initial ambulance placement study done at the Georgia Institute of Technology in the late 1960s and other more recent surveys, it costs an average of about $400,000 (1989 dollars) per year to run one ambulance (equipped with two trained individuals) providing coverage 24 hours per day, 7 days per week.[1] This cost includes support personnel, supervisors, communication personnel and equipment, vehicles, and supplies. Naturally these costs vary somewhat depending on the cost of living in various cities and regions in the United States.

Unfortunately, the majority of federal funding for EMS systems has been eliminated. Creative methods to fund medical direction, audit, and quality assurance activities must be found by communities that wish to have state-of-the-art prehospital care for their citizens.

MEDICAL CONTROL

AXIOM   An EMS system is only as good as its medical control.

Medical control of an effective EMS system is provided by physicians interested in and committed to prehospital care.[1,12] These physicians must spend time in the field observing all aspects of the system in operation. The physician unable or unwilling to dedicate time to this type of effort cannot adequately supervise the system. Lack of such supervision will result in a system that provides substandard patient care.[13] Despite their expertise, physicians are susceptible to making errors in medical control, making quality assurance and continuing medical education important issues for those assuming medical control.[35]

Development of proper medical control of EMS care involves a prospective (preparation) phase, an immediate phase (related to care at the scene), and retrospective (review) phase.

Prospective Phase

AXIOM   The prospective phase of an EMS system includes training personnel and developing treatment protocols.

PROTOCOLS

The development of protocols to address standards of care by EMTs and to identify individual hospital capabilities are important in setting up a properly running EMS system.[1] Included in these protocols are "standing orders," or the steps in patient care that an EMT can perform before contacting the hospital for additional instructions. If radio communication cannot be maintained, the paramedic should follow standard guidelines, such as ACLS procedure and/or county protocols. EMTs functioning without effective protocols and medical control may result not only in substandard care but is the basis for many medical liability cases involving the EMS system and EMTs. Although the effect of standing orders on scene-time is controversial,[36] their importance is clear for prehospital personnel unable to obtain medical control.

AXIOM   Standing orders, when used with proper medical control and quality assurance programs, can significantly reduce prehospital times without reducing the quality of care provided.[37]

Many states now require complete protocols regarding the prehospital care of both ill and injured patients. These protocols specifically define the steps that can be taken by prehospital providers for various symptom presentations and/or disease processes.

AXIOM   An EMS system that is developed without local medical society involvement can suffer from political controversies and lack of medical support in its operation.

LOCAL MEDICAL SOCIETY

Evaluating and maintaining the quality of an EMS system is the responsibility of an organized medical body, often the county medical society. Ideally, the medical society should appoint an EMS committee to help develop protocols and oversee the operation of the system. It is important that the medical director of the EMS system work closely with the EMS committee of the local medical society to provide optimal patient care, considering such issues as public education, financing, and quality assurance.[38]

Immediate Phase

When the EMS unit is on the scene, medical control usually consists of supervision via radio or telephone.[1] It may involve orders provided to the EMTs from a physician at the base hospital (medical command authority) or a supervising physician in constant contact with the system via a portable radio. These orders can be given by the physician or relayed on the radio in the name of the physician by a nurse or an EMT. Even though these orders may be relayed by non-physician personnel, they are the legal orders of the physician, and that physician is medically and legally responsible for the orders as well as for the care rendered in the physician's name.

If a licensed physician on the scene wishes to assume medical control of the patient, that physician becomes responsible for the patient until medical responsibility is assumed by another physician.[1] The physician on the scene may either accompany the patient to the hospital, supervising the medical care en route, or transfer medical control via radio to the physician at the medical command authority.

AXIOM If a physician supervising care at the scene accompanies the patient, the on-scene and en route medical care must still conform to the prehospital care protocols that have been developed and approved by the physicians supervising the EMTs and the local medical society.

Retrospective Phase

In the retrospective phase of an EMS run, the run reports are reviewed to assure that proper prehospital care was rendered.[1] This review comparing each run report to the accepted treatment protocol can be done by the medical director or by a registered nurse or EMT. Any report indicating that care deviated from protocol guidelines is referred to the medical director's attention.

Computers can be designed to review and analyze run reports for conformity to protocol. Inexpensive and readily available computer hardware and software can tabulate basic data on each EMT, generating monthly reports on times in the field, the number of intravenous infusions started, and the number of times drugs were administered and endotracheal tubes were inserted. This type of analysis enables the medical director to gain an overall view of the EMS system. Analysis of individual performance can then be undertaken on a periodic basis. This computer review does not take the place of individual run reviews but does provide a collective analysis of each EMT's overall performance and experience.

AXIOM A combined computer review and individual run report review is probably the best overall system for providing quality control.

The retrospective component of proper medical control also involves the development of continuing education programs to bring new information to the EMTs.[1] Continuing education in trauma care should also include reviews of Prehospital Trauma Life Support (PHTLS) and Basic Trauma Life Support (BTLS). On-going training coordinated by the medical director of the system is essential for all prehospital personnel, including dispatchers, and is necessary for licensure and maintenance of certification.

Audit and quality assurance activities performed on the system should be used to help guide continuing education for prehospital personnel. It is important that all components of the system be evaluated for medical accountability, appropriateness, and cost effectiveness.

PREHOSPITAL CARE IN TRAUMA

Appropriate prehospital care for seriously injured patients is controversial. While some advocate aggressive attempts at resuscitation in the field, others contend that performing procedures in the prehospital setting unduly delays delivery of the traumatized patient to the hospital for definitive surgical care.

Design and implementation of a trauma emergency medical service rests on a rational decision as to how aggressively one should manage severely injured patients in any given setting. Relevant considerations for making such decisions include the local incidence of trauma, average time from scene to hospital, budgetary constraints, and the availability of competent medical control.

Basic Prehospital Trauma Care

Conservative or "basic" prehospital care of acutely traumatized patients includes: (a) competent extrication when required, (b) simple maneuvers to establish airway patency, such as suctioning and assisted ventilation with a bag-mask apparatus, (c) spinal immobilization, (d) splinting, and (e) control of bleeding with direct pressure or tourniquet as appropriate. This level of service can be provided by a "basic" emergency medical technician (EMT-A).

BACKBOARDS

The exponential rise of motor vehicle accidents has resulted in an increasing number of patients with cervical and lumbar spine fractures.[39,40] Approximately 10,000 new spinal cord injuries occur each year in the United States and a proportionate number in Canada. Protecting these patients from additional spinal or spinal cord injury during transport is an essential part of emergency medical care.

Basically, two types of backboards are used in prehospital care: the short backboard and the long backboard. The short backboard is used during extrication and the long backboard is used to transport the patient. A properly constructed and used backboard should immobilize the entire cervical, thoracic, and lumbar spine. Many of the backboards available on the market today are short and immobilize only the cervical and some of the thoracic spine, therefore increasing the risk of complicating an existing spinal injury.

CERVICAL COLLARS

AXIOM The cervical collar can be a useful device as a reminder to a cooperative patient not to move the neck while awaiting definitive evaluation.

Cervical collars are used when the possibility of cervical spine fracture exists, and they are intended to reduce head movement on the cervical spine while the patient is on a rigid backboard. However, by themselves, these rigid collars really do not immobilize the neck very well.[1] Numerous studies have identified that the Philadelphia and other similar hard collars allow approximately 60% of normal rotary and lateral head motion and 40% of normal anterior-posterior cervical spine movement.[41]

PNEUMATIC ANTISHOCK GARMENT (PASG)

History

Experimental observations by Crile in animals in shock led to a suit fabricated to his design by the Goodrich Rubber Company. Later both Crile[42,43] and Gardner[44] used lower body compression during elective surgery to manage hypotension. A similar device has been used in war planes to prevent blackouts while pilots are coming out of a power dive. Military antishock trousers (MAST) and pneumatic antishock garments (PASG) were also used to elevate blood pressure (BP) in hypotensive patients during the Vietnam War and in prehospital emergency care in Miami.[45]

Pathophysiology

Physiologic observations of increased blood pressure, higher level of consciousness, decreased pulse rates, and increased ability to start intravenous infusions have been reported when PASGs have been applied.[45] Initially, the physiologic effect of the PASG was thought to be due to relocation of blood from the lower extremities and abdomen into the central circulation.[46] Further studies by Gaffney et al[47] and others[48-50] revealed that major autotransfusion does not occur, but that increased peripheral vascular resistance is responsible for the increased BP when the PASG is inflated in hypovolemic patients. Well-controlled randomized studies in large and small animals indicate that the PASG may also help control hemorrhage in the abdomen, pelvis, and lower extremities.

Indications, Contraindications, and Complications

Based on present knowledge, the PASG may be used in:

1. Patients with transport times exceeding 10-15 minutes where signs and symptoms of shock include a blood pressure less than 90 mm Hg systolic, tachycardia, and cold, clammy skin.
2. Patients requiring a mechanism of indirect pressure to reduce or control abdominal, pelvic, or lower extremity hemorrhage.
3. Patients requiring stabilization of fractures of the pelvis or femur.

An absolute contraindication to inflation of a PASG is the presence of pulmonary edema. Respiratory difficulty may be a relative contraindication for inflating the abdominal portion of the garment.

With a hypotensive pregnant patient, the abdominal panel should not be inflated except for control of uterine hemorrhage. Complications, such as lower extremity compartment syndrome, have developed when the PASG is left inflated greater than 40-60 mm Hg for more than 2 hours.[51,52]

Many physicians and prehospital providers feel that the PASG is extremely helpful in prehospital care of injured hypotensive patients. They have supported their clinical impressions with many studies of animals and human volunteers.[53] Such studies have demonstrated that the PASG does, in fact, improve blood pressure, help control hemorrhage from injuries in the pelvis and lower extremities, improve carotid and upper body blood flow, improve the ability of prehospital providers to start intravenous lines, and improve survival (particularly short-term) with few prehospital or hospital complications.[54]

These contentions have been challenged by Mattox et al, who performed a randomized prospective study which found that PASGs did not improve the outcome of hypotensive injured patients.[55] Indeed, patients with an inflated PASG actually had worse outcomes than those without such treatment. Clearly, further clinical investigation is necessary to reconcile the differences between this study and the experience of others.

AXIOM   Although there is controversy about the value of raising blood pressure with the PASG in prehospital patients, there is no question that deflating the PASG and allowing an abrupt drop in blood pressure can be very deleterious.

By whatever means the PASG physiologically raises blood pressure, a reverse response would be expected by rapidly deflating the PASG. Therefore, when the PASG is going to be deflated in the operating room or in the ED, it should be done gradually while the patient's blood pressure is monitored closely. With any decrease in blood pressure of 5 mm Hg or more, deflation of the PASG should be stopped and further fluid infused as needed to fill the intravascular space.

If intra-abdominal hemorrhage from trauma is strongly suspected, deflation of the PASG should not be attempted until the anesthetized patient is on the operating table and the surgeon is prepared to immediately open the abdomen. Release of the intra-abdominal tamponade may result in recurrent hemorrhage within the abdominal cavity, thus precipitating hypotension.

ADVANCED LIFE SUPPORT

There is little doubt that the development of trauma systems has profoundly increased the likelihood of survival after major trauma.[56-59] The literature has also shown clearly that the impact on outcome is substantially time dependent.[60-63] Finally, it has also been shown that an ISS of more than 15 is strongly associated with a significant risk of mortality.[64-66] It is this severely injured group that benefits most from rapid evacuation to definitive care.[67]

As sophisticated EMS systems have developed, concern has been raised about the risk of excessive time being spent at the scene in attempts to "stabilize" trauma patients.[68-70] Numerous authors have suggested that a "stay and play" approach to trauma in the field will use precious time that is more appropriately spent rapidly evacuating the victim to definitive care.[68-71] They suggest that the only appropriate on-scene interventions for severely injured patients are extrication, spinal immobilization, external hemorrhage control, and airway management.[60-63,68-71]

Few would argue that ALS care per se is undesirable. In fact, some authors believe that a considerable number of patients die or deteriorate en route to a hospital from physiological abnormalities that could be improved by prehospital ALS care (i.e., intubation, intravenous fluids), giving victims the chance to benefit from "definitive" care.[67,72] Thus, when ALS care is provided to severely injured patients without delaying transport,[73] relatively little controversy would exist regarding the desirability of its use.[71,74] Although much discussion and editorializing has occurred regarding this controversy, data concerning ALS-associated time delays in EMS systems are scant. Some authors have reported significant time delays associated with ALS care,[61,70,75,76] whereas others have found little or no delay.[77-80] In fact, some authors have even reported shorter times associated with ALS care compared with BLS care.

Of particular interest is a retrospective study by Spaite et al[67] of 98 consecutive patients with an injury severity score of more than 15 who were brought to a trauma center by fire department paramedics. Thirty-three patients (33.7%) had successful advanced airway procedures, and 81 (82.7%) had at least one intravenous line started in the field. Analysis of scene time, prehospital procedures, and injury severity parameters revealed that more procedures were performed in the field on the more severely injured cases; however, severely injured patients had a shorter mean scene time of 8.1 minutes. Thus, appropriately short scene times can be attained without foregoing potentially lifesaving advanced life support interventions in an urban EMS system with strong medical control.

Studies that have addressed the question of on-scene ALS interventions have utilized only a historical control group. Converting prehospital trauma care from police vans with "marginally trained personnel and first aid equipment" to paramedic level services in Milwaukee resulted in a decline in mortality from 86 to 50% in victims of intra-abdominal vascular trauma with shock.[81] Analysis of the mortality of 180 victims falling or jumping 50 meters from a single bridge in Seattle over 49 years also revealed a significant improvement following establishment of a paramedic system.[82] However, upgrading of prehospital services was not the only improvement in the management of severely injured patients over the time surveyed by these studies.

Addressing the issue of whether to perform time-consuming procedures at the scene of trauma, a second study in Seattle reviewed 131 trauma patients requiring CPR over 3 years and reported that patients on whom intubation and/or volume repletion had been performed had a significantly higher rate of survival than those who had not. On the other hand, an evaluation in Tucson of patients suffering penetrating cardiac injuries with a 9-minute transport to definitive surgical care found a significant delay in arrival in patients on whom advanced life support procedures were performed.[83] The hospital survival rate of patients receiving advanced life support procedures in the field was only 9%. This was much lower than the 83% survival rate in those on whom "scoop and run" were performed. A factor of particular importance in patients who have sustained cardiac injury for which salvage is possible is the prompt initiation of transfer to an appropriately equipped and staffed trauma facility.[83]

The resolution of these and similar questions is obscured by: (a) The absence of satisfactorily controlled trials,[84] (b) study-to-study variability in the types and severity of injuries, and (c) local variations in patient care. Some truths, however, appear to be self-evident.

AXIOM   If a paramedic system is to be successful and save lives, it must have responsible medical control with active quality assurance programs and protocols that discourage prolonged attempts to perform procedures in the field.

Although trauma patients should generally be brought to the hospital as soon as possible, injured patients with certain types of problems may benefit from field interventions. Examples include endotracheal intubation for patients with severe respiratory insufficiency and volume resuscitation for severely hypotensive patients with hemorrhage that can be controlled by direct pressure.[1] Under special circumstances, such as traumatic amputation, a tourniquet may be needed, but it must be used with special precautions or it can cause more bleeding and/or irreversible ischemia to the extremity.

Trunkey[85] has cited three issues to be considered in planning interventional emergency medical services: (a) decisions on what procedures are likely to benefit different types of patients with particular problems, (b) calculation of the value of time at the scene versus early delivery to definitive care, and (c) the issue of medical control. Surgeons and emergency physicians share the responsibility for competent medical control of prehospital trauma care, including training, development of patient care protocols, quality assurance, and continuing medical education.

AXIOM   Implementation and operation of an emergency medical service with an interventional philosophy requires extensive physician involvement in medical control and quality assurance.

A considerable investment is required not only in training and continuing medical education of personnel but also in acquisition and maintenance of equipment. Systems operating rudimentary "scoop and run" units can utilize "basic" EMTs with about 150 hours of training, whereas interventional systems with advanced life support capabilities require paramedics who have received 400-1000 hours of training.

TRAUMA CARE IN THE FIELD

CPR

Use of the automatic (semiautomatic) defibrillator by basic prehospital providers has become the accepted standard of care in medical cardiac arrest situations. Its usefulness in the trauma patient has yet to be defined. Since the usual cardiac arrest in the trauma patient is related to hypovolemia or airway compromise and is not primarily cardiac in origin, CPR probably will not play a very important role.[86,87] If intracranial damage is sufficient to compromise the respiratory and cardiac systems, the patient is not likely to benefit from CPR.

AXIOM   Transportation of non-breathing patients to a hospital without appropriate airway and ventilatory management constitutes a major failure of prehospital care.

An injured patient with hypovolemic cardiac arrest rarely survives if external cardiac massage and forced ventilation are performed for more than 5 minutes prior to arrival at a hospital.[88] Airway control, intravenous fluid administration, and the PASG have been used in attempts to prevent hypovolemic cardiac arrest.

Prehospital cardiopulmonary resuscitation combined with endotracheal intubation, vigorous fluid resuscitation, and rapid transport can be effective in resuscitating some trauma patients in cardiopulmonary arrest.[89] Once the patient has a cardiac arrest, survival does not correlate with the injury severity score or transport time, but it does correlate with the mechanism of injury, endotracheal intubation, and placement of intravenous lines.[89]

Airway Management

AXIOM   Providing and/or maintaining an adequate airway is the single most important therapy provided to a victim of severe injuries.[2]

Establishing and maintaining an adequate airway require maneuvers to clear the airway and ensure adequate ventilation and oxygenation by using simple techniques such as oral airway, bag-mask techniques, or for the unconscious victim or patient in shock, endotracheal intubation.

Airway management in the field begins with ensuring that the cervical spine is maintained in a neutral position while the airway is opened. The oral and nasopharyngeal airway devices prevent the lax tongue from occluding the oropharynx.[1]

During the past 5-10 years there has been increasing skepticism about the efficacy of the esophageal obturator airway (EOA).[90] This device combines esophageal intubation (to reduce the risk of aspiration of gastric contents) with a mask apparatus for ventilation. Although placement of an EOA may require less skill than endotracheal tube insertion, mask ventilation can be difficult to perform in the field. One of the problems with the EOA is that it is difficult to perform CPR with two rescuers when the EOA is utilized. Effective use of the EOA requires at least two hands, one to maintain the seal and the other to ventilate. The difficulty of adequate ventilation during CPR is increased when the ambulance is in motion.[90]

AXIOM   Use of the EOA for prehospital ventilation is decreasing because of the poor ventilation it provides and the potential complications associated with its use.

In addition to the inadequacy of ventilation with the EOA, the device is not without inherent complications. Potential and documented complications include inadvertent tracheal intubation, inability to intubate the esophagus, inability to ventilate edentulous patients, and esophageal perforation.[91-94]

Poor arterial blood gas results have been reported in several studies evaluating the EOA. Smith et al[90] showed that when the $PaCO_2$ was assessed on arrival with the EOA in place and after ET intubation, there was a marked improvement in ventilation with the ET tube. The mean $PaCO_2$ with the EOA was 93 mm Hg, which promptly fell to a mean of 48 mm Hg with the ET tube.[90] Therefore, it cannot be recommended as a device for definitive airway management. Newer versions, while addressing other problems, do not represent improvements of the basic concept.

The endotracheal tube is a much more effective device and should be the technique of choice by advanced life support providers. If the EOA is used by prehospital providers not trained in the use of ET intubation, ET insertion in the ED should precede esophageal balloon deflation and removal of the EOA. In the spontaneously breathing patient, a nasotracheal tube is an effective way to control the airway. Short-acting paralytic agents can be used in the patient who is uncooperative or has trismus.[95]

Endotracheal intubation was second only to defibrillation in enhancing survival in Seattle, a municipality with extensive experience in advanced life support. Therefore, this procedure should be considered an important part of urban prehospital trauma protocols.

Although some have advocated emergency cricothyroidotomy for severe airway problems and various devices for prehospital treatment of simple or tension pneumothoraces, the efficacy of these modalities in paramedics' hands has not been established and cannot be recommended at this time.

Intravenous Fluids

AXIOM   Transport of injured patients in an urban setting should not be delayed while multiple attempts are made to start an intravenous line.

The use of intravenous lines in resuscitation of a trauma patient in the field is an area that is still under study. Of particular concern has been the association between prehospital procedures, particularly the placement of intravenous lines, and increased on-scene time.[61-63,67,71,96] Although recent studies have shown that intravenous line placement can be done much more rapidly than reported in early investigations,[74,78,97] many authors believe that the clear priority of rapid evacuation to a trauma center remains paramount.[63,68,70,71,85]

Although it has been thought wise to keep the duration and severity of prehospital hypotension to a minimum, it has been increasingly found that aggressive prehospital fluid administration to hypotensive trauma patients does not improve survival and may actually increase mortality rates. For example, in a landmark study by Martin et al[98] in 1991, in 177 patients with a systolic BP less than 90 mm Hg, a mean preoperative fluid resuscitation of 3125 ml (versus 3 ml in the control group) resulted in a fall in survival from a PS of 57% to an OS of 52%. In contrast, the patients with essentially no preoperative fluid resuscitation had a PS of 49% and an OS of 58%. Thus, a trend toward better survival was seen in the patients who were not fluid-resuscitated.

In a follow-up study published in 1992, Martin et al[99] showed that patients with penetrating trauma and a systolic BP ≤ 90 mm Hg did not benefit from intravenous fluid resuscitation begun in the ambulance. The survival rate with immediate resuscitation was 56% (54/96), significantly less than the survival rate of 67% (56/81) (P less than 0.08) in those getting delayed fluid resuscitation.

In urban areas where the transport time is often less than 15 to 30 minutes, the amount of fluid administered prehospital is often only 500-1000 ml. Furthermore, the time for intravenous placement in the field may average 10 to 12 minutes. Thus, it appears that in hemorrhagic shock, early fluid administration may be helpful if the hemorrhage is controlled, but if the blood loss is uncontrolled, giving prehospital fluid will probably increase the loss of blood.

Interestingly, in trauma patients who are severely hypotensive, there may be some advantage to giving some prehospital fluid. Ideally, one would raise the BP to a critical value which improves perfusion of vital organs but does not restart significant bleeding. In some experimental studies it is suggested that critical mean BP is about 40 mm Hg. For example, in a study by Kowalenko et al,[100] 24 immature swine were bled to a mean arterial pressure of 30 mm Hg and the abdominal aorta was then torn with a previously placed wire. The animals were then resuscitated with saline to either a MAP of 40 mm Hg (Group I) or a MAP of 80 mm Hg (Group II); Group III had no resuscitation. The 1-hour survival rates were 88%, 38%, and 13% respectively (P < 0.05).

Increased survival by resuscitation to a mean BP of 40 mm Hg in uncontrolled hemorrhagic shock was also studied by Capone et al.[101] Animals that received no early fluids or were resuscitated to 80 mm Hg mean arterial pressure (MAP) had a survival of only 3% at 3 days. In contrast, of 10 animals with controlled hypotension (resuscitation to a mean BP of 40 mm Hg), six (60%) survived for 3 days. The base deficit was also much less in these animals (−7 ± 2 versus −13 ± 7 mEq/L).

In spite of the concerns that intravenous fluids given before hemorrhage is controlled might be detrimental,[98-102] a detailed computer model by Wears and Winton[103] showed a much improved survival rate when intravenous lines were placed prehospital. Thus, the value of prehospital fluids in hypotensive patients remains controversial. Although increasing the blood pressure by administering intravenous

fluids before controlling the hemorrhage is detrimental, particularly in patients only minutes away from an operating room, giving some intravenous fluids to severely hypotensive trauma patients while en route to the hospital may be helpful, especially if some time will elapse before definitive therapy can be provided; however, intravenous lines should be inserted in the field only while other stabilization procedures are in progress.

TRIAGE

One of the most important functions of EMS is triage of trauma patients to the appropriate hospital or care facility. Regionalized trauma systems have been relatively slow to develop[104,105] mainly because of their high cost. A major determinant of the resources required by a regional trauma system is the number of patients the system will have to manage. This is determined primarily at the prehospital level by triage criteria that identify patients who require care at a trauma center.

Different physiologic or anatomic and mechanistic criteria have been used to form the basis for various scoring systems designed to be predictive of major injury. These scoring systems were found to be predictive by some,[106-108] but not by others.[109,110] The inaccuracy of one system was illustrated in a report that stated that to obtain a sensitivity of 95%, a specificity of 40% had to be accepted.[111] These problems appear to be inherent in all triage systems used to date. Another recent analysis revealed that, although all triage systems could accurately predict death, a sensitivity and specificity of 70% are the best that has been achieved for predicting major injury.[112] These findings were corroborated by another study based on pediatric trauma patients.[113]

In an interesting counterpoint to the trend of scoring patients with potentially serious injuries, one group found no difference between the predictions of mortality by EMTs and the predictions of three scoring systems.[114] The implication is clear: since trauma is a common disease, criteria with a low specificity for identifying patients with major injuries will result in a large number of patients being triaged to trauma centers with a resulting great increase in medical costs.[115,116]

The injury severity score (ISS)[117,118] has been used as the gold standard against which the accuracy of trauma prediction criteria is measured. The ISS defines major injury based on the retrospective analysis of the anatomic injuries patients sustained. However, a lack of complete correlation between the ISS and the resources required by severely injured patients has been reported.[119] Because the proper matching of available treatment resources to patient injury is at the heart of effective prehospital trauma triage, attempts continue to be made to determine what variables could be used to develop more effective triage systems.

For example, Baxt et al[120] developed a trauma decision rule from data obtained from 1,004 injured adult patients using an operational definition of major trauma (Table 1-1 and Table 1-2). The rule, termed the Trauma Triage Rule, defined a major trauma victim as any injured adult whose systolic blood pressure is less than 85 mm Hg; whose motor component of the Glasgow Coma Scale is less than 5; or who has sustained penetrating trauma of the head, neck, or trunk.

The Trauma Triage Rule is simple to use in that no calculations are required and only two variables need to be considered in blunt injuries and three with penetrating injuries. The rule can be applied almost instantly by prehospital personnel. Both systolic blood pressure and the motor component of the Glasgow Coma Scale are documented by virtually all advanced life support systems and by most basic life support systems.

The only other triage rule that has been derived from a resource-based definition of major trauma is the Prehospital Index, which defined major trauma as death or the need for an emergency nonorthopedic operative procedure.[121,122] Unfortunately, this definition was too limited in its scope because it omitted some of the major interventions that severely injured patients may require to sustain life.

Using the operational definition of major trauma, the Trauma Triage Rule had a sensitivity of 92% and a specificity of 92%. This rule could significantly reduce the number of patients incorrectly identified as

TABLE 1-1 Criteria Screened for Association with Major Trauma

Physiologic
  Systolic blood pressure
  Pulse
  Respiratory rate
  Glasgow
    Motor
    Speech
    Eye
  Capillary refill
  Respiratory effort
  Rigid abdomen
  Multiple extremity fractures
Anatomic
  Penetration to head, neck, trunk
  Amputation proximal to ankle or wrist
  Burn (2°/3°) 10%+ body surface area
Mechanistic
  Fall 15+ feet, adult
  Motor vehicle accident with:
    Extrication required
    Space intrusion 1+ feet
    Death of other passenger(s)
    Major vehicle damage
    Pedestrian struck
    Unrestrained occupant
    Rollover
    Motorcycle, no helmet

From: Baxt WG, Jones G, Fortlage D. The trauma triage rule: a new, resource-based approach to the prehospital identification of major trauma victims. Ann Emerg Med 1990;19:1401-1406.

major trauma victims and needlessly transported to trauma centers, with only a slight drop in sensitivity. The approach must be validated prospectively on a large cohort of patients before it can be used.

In some areas, mechanism of injury has been used to activate the trauma team. However, Shatney and Sensaki[123] have recently noted that the patient may have none of the physiologic triggers or anatomic indicators of severe injury. In their study of 2298 such patients, only 15 had an ISS greater than or equal to 16 and none required emergency surgery. The authors noted that a competent trauma center or emergency center physician should be able to safely perform an initial assessment of such patients and summon the surgery trauma team for specific clinical or radiologic indicators.

Prehospital identification of those at risk of dying from their injuries has received inadequate attention. Yet, such identification is critical because it determines the pace and level of care that a trauma victim will receive.[2] The American College of Surgeons has promulgated a set of guidelines that may aid in the early identification of patients at risk of dying from injury. The intent of these guidelines is to identify the 5% of patients with life-threatening injuries. Identifying these patients necessitates hospital-based evaluation of a considerable number of patients.

When Not to Resuscitate and Transport Trauma Victims

There are certain trauma patients on whom resuscitation should not be attempted. Rapid transportation of obviously dead patients endangers the lives of EMTs as well as pedestrians and occupants of other vehicles. Furthermore, the services, equipment, and personnel utilized during such transports could be applied to patients who may otherwise not receive them.

The decision as to whether or not to resuscitate in the field is made via radiotelephone to medical control and is based on information communicated by the EMTs. When one or more of the following conditions exists, resuscitation should not be attempted:

1. Decapitation
2. Decomposition
3. Hemicorporectomy
4. Rigor mortis
5. Lividity
6. Trauma score of 1 for 10 minutes
7. Complete incineration
8. Multiple extremity amputations without signs of life
9. Penetrating cranial injury with extrusion of brain matter and no signs of life
10. Evisceration of the heart

SPECIAL PROBLEMS

Prehospital care of pregnant women, children, and patients with burns and radiation injuries are special situations requiring prior planning and established protocols. Wilderness rescue of traumatized patients is an EMS specialty of particular interest to physicians working in or near mountainous or recreational areas.

Search and Rescue

AXIOM It is important that search and rescue plans be developed prior to their actual need, particularly for disasters.

"Search and rescue" (SAR) systems provide the response for overdue, lost, injured, or stranded people, and people missing in outdoor environments. Search and rescue programs, equipment, and personnel vary geographically in accordance with local needs. Search and rescue is an area that encompasses multiple levels of expertise from the first responders to paramedics to helicopters and fixed wing aircraft. It may involve a great many volunteers with a multitude of skills. The recent eruption of Mt. St. Helens was considered one of our nation's most catastrophic disasters, and also the largest peacetime "search and rescue" operation in the nation's history.[124,125]

There are eight key elements to on-scene direction and control in SAR. These have proven their importance through many documented case histories.

1. All activity and operations in the field must be victim oriented.
2. Identify all hazards.
3. Do efficient reconnaissance (terrain analysis).
4. Protect the access to the search base site.

TABLE 1-2 Demographic Summary of Triage Study

	Minor Trauma Victims	Major Trauma Victims	Student's T Test P
Total	793	211	
Average age	30.66	31.22	
Sex			
Female	374	50	
Male	419	161	
Average systolic blood pressure	122.80	89.58	8.21 < .001
Average pulse	95.04	85.64	3.47 < .001
Average respiratory rate	20.36	18.34	3.01 < .002
Average motor score	5.68	3.96	11.20 < .001
Number with penetrating trauma to the head, neck, or trunk	0	81	
Average P_s	0.87	0.71	5.724 < .001

From: Baxt WG, Jones G, Fortlage D. The trauma triage rule: a new, resource-based approach to the prehospital identification of major trauma victims. Ann Emerg Med 1990;19:1401-1406.

5. Monitor and control communications flow and volume; always have a back-up.
6. Brief and debrief as a matter of routine.
7. Establish victim care as soon as possible.
8. Establish and log each subject's destination and ETA at a medical facility.

PUBLIC EDUCATION

AXIOM The public needs much more education on the proper use of EMS.

An issue which is becoming more and more important in many communities involves public education. It was initially hypothesized that an educated public would learn when to access the EMS system. This unfortunately is not always true. The EMS system is frequently activated for conditions which could be handled in another fashion, and on other occasions, the EMS system is not activated when it should be. Input here is required from physicians, pre-hospital care providers, hospital administrators, and public health officials so that an integrated approach can be developed and the maximal effect by the EMS system can be provided to the general public.

⊘ FREQUENT ERRORS

1. *Poor medical control leading to poor prehospital care.*
2. *Poor management of trauma patient because of inadequate EMS training.*
3. *Failure to promptly recognize and correct esophageal intubation for respiratory distress.*
4. *Delay in delivery of the patient to an appropriate trauma facility because of attempts at resuscitation in the field.*
5. *Failure to have adequate written protocols for prehospital personnel to follow.*
6. *Inadequate backboarding which can lead to more severe spinal injuries.*
7. *Improper use of tourniquets leading to further damage and/or ischemia of the injured limb.*
8. *Inadequate prior planning for wilderness rescues.*

▼▼▼▼▼▼▼▼▼▼▼▼▼▼▼▼▼▼▼▼▼▼▼▼▼▼▼▼▼

SUMMARY POINTS

1. The EMS systems must work closely with the emergency department (ED) to assure a continuity of patient care from the time of the incident to discharge from the ED.

2. A properly run air transport system can save lives that might be lost during a long EMS run.

3. The cost of running a service, which is at least one million dollars a year, as well as the potential for injury or fatality to the crew from helicopter accidents, must be considered by those contemplating helicopter transport of severely injured patients.

4. Proper communication between all involved individuals is essential for a properly working EMS system.

5. Making emergency medical services (EMS) personnel and equipment rapidly available to appropriate patients is the first goal of any emergency medical services system.

6. One of the biggest problems with providing adequate EMS personnel and equipment to all potential patients in the United States is the tremendous maldistribution of resources.

7. Adequate training for EMT, EMT-A, and EMT-P personnel is critical to giving the best care possible while the trauma patient is in the field.

8. Due to the education of nurses in pathophysiology and quality assurance, their use in prehospital EMS systems can be of great benefit.

9. An EMS system is only as good as its medical control.

10. The prospective phase of an EMS system includes training personnel and developing treatment protocols.

11. Standing orders, when used with proper medical control and quality assurance programs, can significantly reduce prehospital times without reducing the quality of care provided.

12. An EMS system that is developed without local medical society involvement can suffer from political controversies and lack of medical support in its operation.

13. If a physician supervising care at the scene accompanies the patient, the on-scene and en route medical care must still conform to the prehospital care protocols that have been developed and approved by the physicians supervising the EMTs and the local medical society.

14. A combined computer review and individual run report review is probably the best overall system for providing quality control.

15. The cervical collar can be a useful device as a reminder to a cooperative patient not to move the neck while awaiting definitive evaluation.

16. Although there is controversy about the value of raising BP with the PASG in prehospital patients, there is no question that deflating the PASG and allowing an abrupt drop in BP can be very deleterious.

17. If a paramedic system is to be successful and save lives, it must have responsible medical control with active quality assurance programs and protocols which discourage prolonged attempts to perform procedures in the field.

18. Implementation and operation of an emergency medical service with an interventional philosophy requires extensive physician involvement in medical control and quality assurance.

19. Transportation of non-breathing patients to a hospital without appropriate airway and ventilatory management constitutes a major failure of prehospital care.

20. Providing and/or maintaining an adequate airway is the single most important therapy provided to a victim of severe injuries.

21. Use of the EOA for prehospital ventilation is decreasing because of the poor ventilation it provides and the potential complications associated with its use.

22. Transport of injured patients in an urban setting should not be delayed while multiple attempts are made to start an intravenous line.

23. It is important that search and rescue plans be developed prior to their actual need, particularly for disasters.

24. The public needs much more education on the proper use of EMS.

▲▲▲▲▲▲▲▲▲▲▲▲▲▲▲▲▲▲▲▲▲▲▲▲▲▲▲▲▲▲▲▲

REFERENCES

1. McSwain NE Jr. Prehospital emergency medical systems and cardiopulmonary resuscitation. In: Moore EE, Mattox KL, Feliciano DV, eds. Trauma. 2nd ed. Norfolk: Appleton and Lange, 1991:99.
2. Champion HR. Organization of trauma care. In: Kreis DJ Jr, Gomez GA, eds. Trauma management. Boston: Little, Brown and Co, 1989:11-27.
3. Accident Facts 1986. Chicago: National Safety Council, 1986.
4. Baker SP, O'Neill B, Haddon W, and Long WB. The injury severity score: a method for describing patients with multiple injuries and evaluating emergency care. J Trauma 1974;14:187.
5. Annual Report of the San Diego Trauma System. San Diego Hospital Association. San Diego: Department of Health Services, 1987.
6. Field categorization of trauma patients. American College of Surgeons Committee on Trauma. Am Coll Surg Bull 1986;71:17-21.
7. Larrey DJ. Memoirs of a military surgeon. Willmott R, trans. Classics of surgery library. Birmingham, AL: Joseph Cushing.
8. Accidental death and disability: the neglected disease of modern society. National Research Council National Academy of Sciences. Rockville, MD: US Department of Health, Education and Welfare, 1966.
9. Position paper on trauma care systems. J Trauma 1992;32:127.
10. Hospital and prehospital resources for optimal care of the injured patient. American College of Surgeons Committee on Trauma. Chicago: American College of Surgeons, February 1987:1.

11. Treatment protocols for prehospital management of the trauma patient. Appendix E to hospital resources document. Chicago: American College of Surgeons Committee on Trauma, 1987.

12. McSwain NE. Medical control of prehospital care. J Trauma 1984; 24:172.

13. McSwain NE. Medical control: what is it? J Am Coll Emerg Phys 1978;7:114.

14. Effectiveness and efficiencies in emergency medical services. National highway traffic safety report. Publication no. DOT HS-806 143. US Department of Transportation, March 1982.

15. Potter D, Goldstein G, Fung SC, et al. A controlled trial of prehospital advanced life support in trauma. Ann Emerg Med 1988;17:582.

16. Neel S. Army aeromedical evacuation procedures in Vietnam. JAMA 1968;204:99.

17. Current listing of hospital-based air ambulance operations. Hosp Aviation, April 4, 1984.

18. Collett HM. Risk management and the aeromedical helicopter. Emerg Care Q 1986;2(3):31.

19. Low RB, Dunne MJ, Blumen IJ, Tagney G. Factors associated with the safety of EMS Helicopters. Am J Emerg Med 1991;9:103-106.

20. Fisher RP, Flynn TC, Miller PW, et al. Urban helicopter response to the scene of injury. J Trauma 1984;24:946.

21. Baxt WG, Moody P. The impact of rotorcraft aeromedical emergency care service on trauma mortality. JAMA 1983;249:3047.

22. Law DK, Law JF, Brennan R, et al. Trauma operating room in conjunction with an air ambulance system: indications and outcomes. J Trauma 1982;22:759.

23. Cowart VS. Helicopter, other "air ambulances": time to assess effectiveness? Medical News. JAMA 1985;253;2469.

24. Baxt WG. Helicopter, other "air ambulances":time to assess effectiveness? Medical News. JAMA 1985;253;2475.

25. Kane G, Wheeler NC, Cook S, Englehardt R, Pavey B, Green K, Clark ON, Cassou J. Impact of the Los Angeles County trauma system on the survival of seriously injured patients. J Trauma 1992;32:576.

26. Blum J. Ambulance placement strategy. Research study. Atlanta Georgia Institute of Technology, 1974.

27. The world almanac and book of facts (1991). New York: 765.

28. Johnson JC. Prehospital care: the future of emergency medical services. Ann Emerg Med 1991;20:426.

29. State and province survey. Emerg Med Serv 1989;18:201.

30. Faulk D, Ryan R. Getting to the heart of rural EMS. Emerg Med Serv 1989;14:54.

31. National standard EMT ambulance curriculum. US Department of Transportation. Washington, DC: US Government Printing Office, 1984.

32. National standard EMT-intermediate curriculum. US Department of Transportation. Washington, DC: US Government Printing Office, 1986.

33. National standard EMT-paramedic curriculum. US Department of Transportation. Washington, DC: US Government Printing Office, 1986.

34. McSwain NE, ed. Prehospital trauma life support. Akron, OH: Educations Directions, 1990. Nat Assoc Emerg Med Tech:170.

35. Holliman CJ, Wuerz RC, Meader SA. Medical command errors in an urban advanced life support system. Ann Emerg Med 1992;71:347.

36. Gratton MC, Bethke RA, Watson WA, Gaddis GM. Effect of standing orders on paramedic scene time for trauma patients. Ann Emerg Med 1991;20:1306.

37. Pointer JE, Osur MA. Effects of standing orders on field times. Ann Emerg Med 1989;18:1119.

38. Eastmen BA, Rice CL, Bishop GS, Richardson JD. An analysis of the critical problem of trauma center reimbursement. J Trauma 1991;31:920.

39. Green BA, Callahan RA, Klose KJ, et al. Acute spinal cord injury: current concepts. C.O.R.R. 1981;150:125.

40. Reid DC, Henderson R, Saboe L, et al. Etiology and clinical course of missed spine fracture. J Trauma 1987;27:980.

41. McSwain NE. Acute management in cervical spine trauma. In: McSwain NE, Martinez JA, Timberlake GA, eds. Cervical spine trauma: evaluation and acute management. New York: Thieme Medical Publishers, 1989:105.

42. Crile GW. Blood pressure in surgery: experimental and clinical research. Philadelphia: Lippincott, 1903:288.

43. Crile GW. Hemorrhage and transfusion: experimental and clinical research. New York: Appleton, 1909:139.

44. Gardner WJ. The antigravity suit (g-suit) in surgery. JAMA 1956;162:274.

45. McSwain NE. Pneumatic trousers and the management of shock. J Trauma 1977;17:719.

46. Ferrario CM, Nadzam G. Effects of pneumatic compression on the cardiovascular dynamics in the dog after hemorrhage. Aerospace Med 1970;41:411.

47. Gaffney FA, Thal ER, Taylor WF, et al. Hemodynamic effects of medical antishock trousers (MAST garment). J Trauma 1981;21:932.

48. Pepe PE. Clinical trials of the pneumatic antishock garment in the urban prehospital setting.

48a. Bass RR, Mattox KL. Ann Emerg Med 1986;15:1407.

49. Kaback KR, Sanders AB, Meislin HW. MAST suit update. JAMA 1984;252:2598.

50. Niemann JT, Stapczynski JS, Rosborough JP, et al. Hemodynamic effects of pneumatic external counterpressure in canine hemorrhagic shock. Ann Emerg Med 1983;12:661.

51. Maull K, Capehart JE, Cardea JA, et al. Limb loss following antishock trousers (MAST) application. J Trauma 1980;21:60.

52. Bass RR, Allison EJ, Reines HD, et al. Tight compartment syndrome without lower extremity trauma following application of PASG trousers. Ann Emerg Med 1983;12:382.

53. McSwain NE. Pneumatic antishock garment: state of the art 1988. Ann Emerg Med 1988;17:506.

54. Mattox KL, Bickell WH, Pepe PE. Prospective MAST study in 911 patients. J Trauma 1989;28:1104.

55. Messick J, Rutledge R, Meyer AA. Advanced life support training is associated with decreased trauma death rates. An analysis of 12,417 trauma deaths. J Trauma 1990;30:1621.

56. Clemmer TP, Orme JF, Thomas FO, et al. Outcome of critically injured patients treated at level 1 trauma centers versus full-service community hospitals. Crit Care Med 1985;13:861-863.

57. Shackford SR, Mackersie RC, Hoyt DB, et al. Impact of a trauma system on outcome of severely injured patients. Arch Surg 1987;122:523-527.

58. West JG, Cales RH, Gazzaniga AB. Impact of regionalization: the Orange County experience. Arch Surg 1983;118:74-744.

59. Smith JS, Martin LF, Young WW, et al. Do trauma centers improve outcome over non-trauma centers? The evaluation of regional trauma care using discharge abstract data and patient management categories. J Trauma 1990;30:1533-1538.

60. Eastman AB, Lewis FR, Champion HR, et al. Regional trauma system design: critical concepts. Am J Surg 1987;154:79-87.

61. Smith P, Bodai B, Hill A, et al. Prehospital stabilization of critically injured patients: a failed concept. J Trauma 1985;25:65-70.

62. Border JR, Lewis FR, Aprahamian C, et al. Panel: prehospital trauma care: stabilize or scoop and run. J Trauma 1983;23:708-711.

63. Gervin AS, Fischer RP. The importance of prompt transport in salvage of patients with penetrating heart wounds. J Trauma 1982;22:443-448.

64. Spaite DW, Criss E, Valenzuela T, et al. Railroad accidents: a metropolitan experience of death and injury. Ann Emerg Med 1988;17:620-625.

65. Long WB, Bachulis BL, Hynes GD. Accuracy and relationship of mechanisms of injury, trauma score, and injury severity score in identifying major trauma. Am J Surg 1986;151:581-584.

66. Smith JS, Bartholemew MJ. Trauma index revisited: a better triage tool. Crit Care Med 1990;18:174-179.

67. Spaite DW, Tse DJ, Valenzuela TD, et al. The impact of injury severity and prehospital procedures on scene time in victims of major trauma. Ann Emerg Med 1991;20:1299-1305.

68. Gold CR. Prehospital advanced life support versus "scoop and run" in trauma management. Ann Emerg Med 1987;16:797-801.

69. Ramenofsky ML, Luteman A, Curreri PW, et al. EMS for pediatrics: optimum treatment or unnecessary delays? J Pediatr Surg 1983;18:498-503.

70. Ivatury RR, Nallathambi MN, Roberge RJ, et al. Penetrating thoracic injuries: in-field stabilization versus prompt transport. J Trauma 1987;27:1066-1073.

71. Blaisdell FW. Myths and magic: the 1984 Fitts Lecture. J Trauma 1985;25:856-863.

72. Durham LA III, Richardson RJ, Wall MJ, Pepe PE, Mattox KL: Emergency center thoracotomy: impact of prehospital resuscitation. J Trauma 1992;32:775.

73. Spaite DW, Tse DJ, Valenzuela TD, Criss EA, Meislin HW, Mahoney M, Ross J. The impact of injury severity and prehospital on scene time in victims of major trauma. Ann Emerg Med 1991;20:1299.

74. O'Gorman M, Trabulsy P, Pilcher DB. Zero-time prehospital IV. J Trauma 1989;29:84-86.

75. Cayten CG, Longmore W, Kuehl A, et al. Prolongation of scene time by advanced life support (ALS) in an urban setting. J Trauma 1985;25:679.

76. Donovan PJ, Cline DM, Whitley TW, et al. Prehospital care by EMTs and EMT-1s in a rural setting: prolongation of scene times by ALS procedures. Ann Emerg Med 1989;18:495-500.

77. Jacobs L, Sinclair A, Beiser A, et al. Prehospital advanced life support: benefits in trauma. J Trauma 1984;24:8-13.

78. Pons PT, Honigman B, Moore EE, et al. Prehospital advanced trauma life support for critical penetrating wounds to the thorax and abdomen. J Trauma 1985;25:828-832.

79. Hedges JR, Ferro S, Moore B, et al. Factors contributing to paramedic on-scene time during evaluation and management of blunt trauma. Am J Emerg Med 1988;6:443-448.

80. Honigman B, Rohweder K, Moore EE, et al. Prehospital advanced trauma for penetrating cardiac wounds. Ann Emerg Med 1990;19:145-150.

81. Aprahamian C, Thompson B, Towne J, et al. The effect of a paramedic system on mortality of major open intra-abdominal vascular trauma. J Trauma 1983;23:687-690.

82. Fortner GS, Oreskovich MR, Copass MK, et al. The effects of prehospital trauma care on survival from a 50-meter fall. J Trauma 1983;23:976-980.

83. Gervin AS, Fischer RP. The importance of prompt transport in salvage of patients and penetrating heart wounds. J Trauma 1982;22:443.

84. Jones SE, Brenneis AT. Study design in prehospital trauma advanced support-basic life support research: a critical review. Ann Emerg Med 1991;20:857.

85. Trunkey D. Is ALS necessary for prehospital trauma care? J Trauma 1984;24:86.

86. Bucka JJ. Automatic defibrillators. Ann Emerg Med 1989;18:1264.

87. Cummins R. From concept to standard of care? Review of the experiences with automated external defibrillators. Ann Emerg Med 1989;18:1269.

88. Mattox KL, Feliciano DV. Role of external cardiac compression in truncal trauma. J Trauma 1982;22:934.

89. Copass MK, Oreskovich MR, Bladergroen MR, et al. Prehospital cardiopulmonary resuscitation of the critically injured patient. J Surg 1984;148:20.

90. Smith JP, Balazs IB, Augourg R, Ward RE. A field evaluation of the esophageal obturator airway. J Trauma 1983;23:317.

91. Bryson TK, Benumof JL, Ward CF. The esophageal obturator airway: a clinical comparison to ventilation with a mask and oropharyngeal airway. Chest 1978;74:537.

92. Carlson WJ, Hunter SW, Bonnabean RC. Esophageal perforation with the obturator airway. JAMA 1979;241:1154

93. Strate RG, Fischer RP. Mid-esophageal perforations by esophageal obturator airways. J Trauma 1976;16:503.

94. Walloch Y, Zer M, Dintsman M, et al. Iatrogenic perforations of the esophagus. Arch Surg 1974;108:357.

95. Phillips TF, Goldstein AS. Airway management In: Mattox KL, Moore EE, Feliciano DV, Eds. Trauma. Norwalk, CT, Appleton and Lange, 1988;125.

96. Lewis FR. Prehospital intravenous fluid therapy: physiologic computer modelling. J Trauma 1986;26:804-811.

97. Cwinn AA, Pons PT, Moore EE, et al. Prehospital advanced trauma life support for critical blunt trauma victims. Ann Emerg Med 1987;16:399-403.

98. Martin RR, Bickell W, Mattox KL, et al. Prospective evaluation of preoperative volume resuscitation in hypotensive patients with penetrating truncal injuries. J Trauma 1991;31:1033.

99. Martin RR, Bickell WH, Pepe PE, et al. Prospective evaluation of preoperative fluid resuscitation in hypotensive patients with penetrating truncal injury. J Trauma 1992;33:354.

100. Kowalenko T, Stern S. Wang X, Dronen S. Improved outcome with "hypotensive" resuscitation of uncontrolled hemorrhagic shock in a swine model. J Trauma 1991;31:1033.

101. Capone A, Safar P, Tisherman S, et al. Treatment of uncontrolled hemorrhagic shock: improved outcome with fluid restriction. J Trauma 1993;35:984.

102. Bickell WH, Shaftan GW, Mattox KL: Intravenous fluid administration and uncontrolled hemorrhage. Trauma 29:409, 1989.

103. Wears RL, Winton CN. Load and go versus stay and play: analysis of prehospital intravenous fluids therapy by computer simulation. Ann Emerg Med February 1990;19(2):163.

104. West JG, Williams MJ, Trunkey DD, et al. Trauma systems: current status—future challenges. JAMA 1988;259:3597-3600.

105. Aprahamian C, Wolferth CC Jr, Darin JC, et al. Status of trauma center designation. J Trauma 1988;29:566-570.

106. Clemmer TP, Orme JF, Thomas F, et al. Prospective analysis of the CRAMS score for major trauma. J Trauma 1985;25:188-191.

107. Clemmer TP, Orme JF, Thomas F, et al. Outcome of critically injured patients treated at level 1 trauma centers versus full-service community hospitals. Crit Care Med 1985;13:861-863.

108. Clemmer TP, Thomas C, Thomas F, et al. Comparison of the trauma score and CRAMS score for trauma triage. Crit Care Med 1986;14:427.

109. Ornato J, Mlinek EJ, Craren EJ, et al. Ineffectiveness of the trauma score and CRAMS scale for acutely triaging patients to trauma centers. Ann Emerg Med 1985;14:1061-1064.

110. Morris JA, Auerbach PS, Marshall GA, et al. The trauma score as a triage tool in the prehospital setting. JAMA 1986;256:1319-1325.

111. Knudson P, Frecerri CA, DeLateur JA. Improving the field triage of major trauma victims. J Trauma 1988;28:602-606.

112. Baxt WG, Berry CC, Epperson MD, et al. The failure of prehospital trauma prediction rules to classify trauma patients accurately. Ann Emerg Med 1989;18:1-8.

113. Eichelberger MR, Gotschall CS, Sacco WJ, et al. A comparison of the trauma score, the revised trauma score, and the pediatric trauma score. Ann Emerg Med 1989;18:1053-1058.

114. Emerman CL, Shade B, Kubincanek J. A comparison of EMT judgement and prehospital triage instruments. J Trauma 1991;31:1369.

115. Cales RH, Anderson PG, Heilig RW. Utilization of medical care in Orange County: the effect of implementation of a regional trauma system. Ann Emerg Med 1985;14:853-858.

116. County of San Diego Annual Trauma System Report. Department of Health Services Division of Emergency Medical Services. San Diego, 1989;1-9

117. Baker SP, O'Neill B, Haddon W Jr, et al. The injury severity score: a method for describing patients with multiple injuries and evaluating emergency care. J Trauma 1974;14:187-196.

118. Baker SP, O'Neill B. The injury severity score: an update. J Trauma 1976;16:882-885.

119. Baxt WG, Upenieks V. The lack of full correlation between the injury severity score and the resource needs of injured patients. Ann Emerg Med 1990;19:1396-1400.

120. Baxt WG, Jones G, Fortlage Dale. The trauma triage rule: a new, resource-based approach to the prehospital identification of major trauma victims. Ann Emerg Med 1990;19:1401-1406.

121. Koehler JJ, Baer LJ, Malafa SA, et al. Prehospital index: a scoring system for field triage of trauma victims. Ann Emerg Med 1986;15:178-182.

122. Koehler JJ, Malafa SA, Hillesland J, et al. A multicenter validation of the prehospital index. Ann Emerg Med 1987;16:380-385.

123. Shatney CH, Sensaki. Trauma team activation for mechanism of injury in blunt trauma victims: time for a change? J Trauma 1994;37:275.

124. LaValla PH, Stoffel RC. Search and rescue. In: Management of wilderness and environmental emergencies. C V Mosby, 1989;321.

125. Bowman WD Jr. Wilderness survival. In: Management of wilderness and environmental emergencies. C V Mosby, 1989:267-288.

Chapter **2** Initial Evaluation and Management of Severely Injured Patients

CHARLES E. LUCAS, M.D.

ANNA M. LEDGERWOOD, M.D.

TRAUMA SYSTEM REQUIREMENTS

Optimal care of the injured patient requires the integrated implementation of multiple, seemingly different, functions into a finely tuned team activity designed for the patient's welfare.[1,2] These multiple functions include a societal effort at prevention of injury, a well-tuned communication system for informing the team members of the injury, a highly skilled emergency medical service trained to provide on-scene care and rapid transportation to the closest appropriate emergency facility, incorporation of well-spaced and well-equipped emergency centers to handle injured patients upon arrival, and highly disciplined teams of physicians designed to provide a well-coordinated and prioritized program of health care delivery.

Like all highly integrated systems, there must be a gauleiter who is able to oversee the total program without emotion and, thereby, able to implement various subsections of the program without regard to petty jealousies or turf battles. This gauleiter assumes responsibility for the yearly maintenance of emergency medical system education and quality assurance. This person also must keep abreast of the new scientific data which is emerging constantly and be able to transmit this information to the appropriate team members by means of frequent conferences designed for that purpose. The system within each hospital must be coordinated with regional hospital systems in order to prevent both underuse and overuse of any one facility. Finally, the program must be implemented in such a manner as to provide the best possible medical care, independent of financial resources within the community and independent of the so-called "wallet biopsy" which has the long range potential of destroying quality care of injured patients.

AXIOM Trauma care in a properly functioning system should be independent of a patient's financial resources.

CARE AT THE SCENE

Once the emergency medical service (EMS) team arrives at the scene of a severely injured patient, it institutes care based upon well-established priorities.[1,2]

AXIOM The priorities of care at the scene of an accident are establishment of the airway, maintenance of adequate ventilation, and control of external bleeding.

Airway

The first priority in the care of trauma victims is to ensure an adequate airway.[1,2] Positional changes which could lead to aspiration of blood or vomitus are avoided. The appropriate use of an oral or nasal airway can often help prevent catastrophes related to soft tissue occlusion of the airway in comatose patients.

Ventilation

After the airway is secured, the team members may provide ventilatory support by either the more simple means of ambu bag and mask or the more controlled techniques of endotracheal intubation. The use of an esophageal oral airway has been associated with an unacceptably high incidence of serious complications. The emergency medical service teams of the future will be adept at nasotracheal and orotracheal airway. Concomitant with providing modalities for supporting airway and ventilation, attention must also be directed toward control of any external bleeding with direct pressure.

Control of External Bleeding

The next priority is control of active external bleeding. This can usually be accomplished by local pressure.[1,3] The appropriate use of a gauze dressing and ace wrap helps control bleeding from most soft tissue injuries and should be applied before splinting. The use of appropriate splints, particularly air inflation splints, will help control bleeding from long bone fractures and extremity soft tissue injuries.[4]

MAST

AXIOM Although MAST can help splint pelvic and lower extremity fractures and reduce associated blood loss, this device has little value in hypotensive patients in an urban setting.

The routine application of military antishock trousers (MAST), a type of pneumatic antishock garment (PASG), to injured hypotensive patients at the scene in an urban setting no longer appears to be warranted. The only controlled studies on the use of MAST for patients with impending or actual hypovolemic shock demonstrate that the time lost in applying the trousers outweighs any minimal benefit that may accrue from acute blood volume expansion.[4,5] This probably reflects the fact that the patient with impending or actual shock already has marked vascular constriction with a decreased blood volume. Consequently, the use of the PASG, which is known to increase the central circulatory volume in normal patients, does not exert the same benefit in patients with diminished blood volume and venous constriction.[6-11] Furthermore, the PASG has the potential for causing compartment syndromes, particularly if applied with high pressures for prolonged periods.[12]

AXIOM When the transit time from the site of injury to the closest skilled emergency center is less than 15-20 minutes, time spent starting intravenous fluids at the scene is usually counterproductive.

Emergency medical service teams should be adept at instituting intravenous therapy for trauma victims en route to the hospital.[3] This is more critical in rural areas than in the urban setting. The type of fluid provided should be a balanced electrolyte solution without supplemental colloid.[1,3,13-17] Hypertonic saline may produce

13

comparable plasma volume expansion with lower infusion volumes, but this effect is short term as total body fluid equilibration ensues.[18-20] The ultimate role of hypertonic saline resuscitation at the scene will be determined after further controlled studies are conducted.

EMERGENCY DEPARTMENT RESUSCITATION

General Principles

Once the patient arrives in the medical center, a highly integrated team needs to bring to the patient the expertise of multiple disciplines in a well-prioritized manner. The priority of care should be established prior to the initiation of treatment to any particular patient. Multidisciplinary conferences designed to identify the priorities, put them into writing, and guide practice of that system of care are essential.[1,2]

Since the scientific foundation of any prioritized trauma care system is always changing, a policy for providing updates on the care system to all disciplines is essential. These timely updates should not reflect any individual desires to enhance experience or profit at the expense of the injured patient, but should be designed to provide optimum care independent of turf battles or individual privileges to do specific procedures.

AXIOM   A team captain is essential for optimal management of the multiply-injured patient.

When questions arise about which of the highly prioritized components of trauma therapy should be implemented on a patient at a particular point in time, these questions need to be resolved promptly by a "team captain" who is the accepted arbiter of any ongoing disagreements. Traditionally, this team captain is a surgeon with a special interest in trauma. Often this surgeon has a general surgical or cardiothoracic surgical background. With the more recent expansion of emergency departments and the development of emergency medicine as a specialty, one recognizes that the specific discipline of the team captain is less important than the dedication of that captain to the needs of the injured patient and maintenance of the team. Consequently, the team captain may be a general or cardiothoracic surgeon, an emergency physician, or even an orthopedic surgeon (as is the practice in some European countries).

AXIOM   Once a team captain is identified, all participants of the trauma care team must respect his position as the final arbiter.

Establishing an Airway

An important aspect of care of the injured patient is flexibility. Usually the patient is lying flat on the cart. Common sense, however, should permit the patient to remain in a sitting position, as needed, to be able to clear his airway of secretions or blood.

AXIOM   One must avoid the temptation to force all trauma patients to lie flat on the cart and restrain those who resist such positioning.

Forcing an unwilling patient to lie supine often leads to a sequence of combativeness, restraints, medications for sedation, and endotracheal intubation, all of which can be very traumatic. This sequence can often be circumvented by simply talking to the patient and recognizing the patient's desire to be able to control his or her own airway. When a patient with this type of airway problem arrives, the emergency room team should be cognizant of this need and arrange to have anesthesia close by. This allows the team to provide appropriate intubation as needed in a more relaxed and controlled setting when the patient is ready for operative intervention.

AXIOM   One should assume that an uncooperative or restless patient is either hypoxic, has a head injury, or is under the influence of drugs or alcohol.

Cooperative patients with stable vital signs may be provided with supplemental oxygen by face mask.[1,3,13] Restless patients not responding to oxygen will require early endotracheal intubation to correct hypoxia, and may need hyperventilation for a head injury.

During intubation, prevention of cervical spine injury by stabilization of the head and neck in a neutral position is essential. Use of the nasotracheal route is also desirable if a cervical spine injury is suspected.[1,2] However, if a cervical spine injury is suspected and the patient is in severe distress from ventilatory insufficiency, one should not delay intubation to obtain x-rays or provide more secure methods of stabilization.

AXIOM   When conflicting priorities exist, one should perform the procedure which provides the best chance for protecting life. One should not withhold critical therapy because of a possible procedure-related complication.

The complexity of care to patients with severe multiple injuries is such that one frequently has to make hard choices about which type of therapy statistically is most apt to help the patient. Consequently, the team should provide treatment which statistically is best for the vast majority of patients, even if it may inadvertently cause injury to an occasional individual.[1,2] In addition to having individuals skilled in orotracheal and nasotracheal intubation, the team may need to provide a coniotomy (cricothyroidotomy) to some patients with active bleeding into the upper airway from severe maxillofacial injuries or in others in whom orotracheal and/or nasotracheal intubation has failed. Upper airway obstruction should be suspected if there are harsh upper airway sounds or intercostal and chest wall retraction with inspiration. Lower airway problems due to hemothorax or tension pneumothorax do not cause chest wall retraction.

The coniotomy tube inserted is usually a 6 mm cuffed tracheotomy or endotracheal tube. This type of airway can be easily occluded by clots or secretions and should be converted to a standard tracheostomy as soon as possible. This allows the surgeon to insert a larger tube, reduce the chances of laryngeal injury, and control any bleeding that may have occurred at the coniotomy site.

Establishing Intravenous Fluid Routes

When the patient presents to the emergency facility with serious injuries and/or hemorrhagic shock, one should rapidly restore the circulatory volume through at least two or three large intravenous catheters. If the patient is not in shock, one has more time to establish intravenous routes by way of percutaneous upper arm venipuncture or basilic or saphenous vein cutdowns.

If the patient presents with severe hypovolemic shock causing venous collapse or if there is a history of previous intravenous narcotic usage, the above techniques often are inadequate for establishing rapid venous access.[1,3] Under such circumstances, percutaneous insertion of subclavian catheters provides rapid and safe venous access in most patients. If the subclavian venipuncture technique is used routinely for the resuscitation of injured patients, a high level of expertise can be attained, thereby minimizing the risk of pneumothorax or vascular injury.

AXIOM   For trauma patients with severe hypovolemia, subclavian veins are often the quickest sites for establishing intravenous access.

Subclavian vein catheters should generally be inserted by making the percutaneous puncture at the junction of the middle and lateral thirds of the clavicle while advancing the needle perpendicular to the median plane and parallel to the floor toward the suprasternal notch.[1,3] This technique generally leads to successful antegrade passage of the catheter into a central vein. Although the distance from the percutaneous puncture site to venipuncture with this technique is increased over other techniques so that the success rate is not as high, this is usually safer than other more direct techniques.

If the patient is unstable, the percutaneous puncture may be placed more medially near the mid-clavicular line, and the catheter is then directed cephalad about 15° and posteriorly about 10°. This leads to quick entrance into the subclavian vein, but the catheter may then pass retrograde up into the internal jugular vein. Regardless of which technique is used, the incidence of successful passage is extremely high; the incidence of complications, such as pneumothorax, is less than 1.5% at the Detroit Receiving Hospital.

Percutaneous catheterization of the internal jugular vein is also an excellent means of rapid large bore catheter venous access, particularly in patients who require immediate operative intervention and are intubated in the operating room at the time additional lines are needed. This technique is best performed with the patient in the Trendelenburg position.[1,3,21] The skin puncture site is about 0.5-1.0 cm above the top of the triangle formed by the sternal and clavicular heads of the sternocleido-mastoid muscle. The needle is directed caudally at the ipsilateral nipple. More medial direction of the catheter may lead to inadvertent puncture of the carotid artery.

Obtaining rapid, large bore intravenous access using an intravenous catheter which is passed through a large bore needle can be hazardous. If the catheter is pulled back within the needle because of poor blood return, the catheter may be sheared off by the sharp needle tip. Despite frequent warnings to all new house officers, this complication continues to occur with regularity, and the sheared off portion of the catheter may embolize centrally into the heart or lungs.

AXIOM   If an intravenous catheter is passed through a needle into a vein, the catheter is never pulled back within the needle.

More recently, the use of venous guide wires and catheter introducers placed over the guide wires have become more popular. However, this technique requires more time, and this can be a disadvantage in patients with severe hemorrhagic shock requiring rapid intravenous access.

AXIOM   Introducers should not be forced over guide wires into veins.

When the introducer technique is used, one should be cautioned to insert the introducer over the guide wire gently and not force the introducer if resistance is encountered. Such forcing can perforate large veins or arteries and could lead to rapid exsanguination and death. Other complications with this technique include: mediastinal hemorrhage, mediastinal infusion of resuscitation fluid, pneumothorax, hemothorax, and occasional arterial injury with thrombosis.

AXIOM   Subclavian catheterization should be performed on the side of injury in patients with chest wounds to reduce the chances of collapse of the uninjured lung.

When one lung may be damaged, iatrogenic injury to the contralateral lung must be avoided.[1,3] Collapse of both lungs, one by injury and the other by resuscitation, could be fatal.

AXIOM   With injuries in the neck or upper chest, at least one venous access should be inserted in a lower extremity. If the injury is in the abdomen, at least one intravenous route should be in a tributary of the superior vena cava.

Patients presenting with hemorrhagic shock associated with upper thoracic wounds may be hemorrhaging from proximal central veins, such as the innominate vein or superior vena cava.[1,3] Such patients

should have at least one large intravenous access line rapidly established in a lower extremity. This can be accomplished with a large bore catheter placed percutaneously or by cutdown in the saphenous vein at the level of the ankle. The physician should remember that the saphenous vein courses just anterior to the medial malleolus at the ankle. Alternatively, rapid access can be achieved in the groin by means of a percutaneous stick with a guide wire and introducer or by means of a direct cutdown and insertion of a large bore catheter into the saphenous vein as it enters the femoral vein. Patients with catheters in the lower extremity have a higher incidence of venous thrombosis and, therefore, these catheters should be removed as soon as possible after correction of the injuries.

Cardiopulmonary Resuscitation

The patient presenting with no signs of life and ECG evidence of asystole or ventricular fibrillation will require cardiopulmonary resuscitation once an airway and intravenous route have been established. If the patient has no truncal trauma and is not hypovolemic, external cardiac compressions can be attempted. Ventilatory support is coordinated with the external chest compressions in order to increase intrathoracic pressure and maximize the benefits of cardiopulmonary resuscitation.[1,3,13]

Both tension pneumothorax and pericardial tamponade can cause severe hypotension and must be corrected or the patient will not respond to cardiopulmonary resuscitation. Both entities may be associated with shock, distant heart tones, and neck vein distension. The initial examination will demonstrate the trachea to be in the midline or slightly to the right in patients with pericardial tamponade, whereas the trachea will usually be clearly shifted to the contralateral side in patients with tension pneumothorax.

AXIOM   If a patient with a cardiac arrest from a penetrating chest wound is not rapidly responding to external chest compressions and/or other resuscitation, an open thoracotomy with internal cardiac massage may be indicated.

Open thoracotomy can be performed as part of the emergency room resuscitation with reasonable expectation for success in patients who have a penetrating wound to the chest and have had a cardiac arrest just before or soon after arrival in the ED.[1,3] However, open cardiac massage in the emergency department is rarely successful in patients with cardiac arrest due to penetrating intra-abdominal injuries or severe blunt trauma to the head or trunk. The emergency thoracotomy allows the surgeon to not only compress the heart more effectively but also to correct underlying lesions, such as tension pneumothorax, pericardial tamponade, or active bleeding from the heart, lungs, great vessels, or chest wall.

Control of External Bleeding

AXIOM   The most urgent priorities in trauma resuscitation are establishment of an airway and adequate ventilation and control of external bleeding.

External bleeding in most patients is best controlled by direct digital pressure. This is particularly true in patients with small deep wounds adjacent to vessels and in patients with neck wounds.[1,3] Attempts to stop external bleeding with clamps placed in the depths of a wound are to be condemned. Such efforts may cause inadvertent and irreparable injury to important vessels or nerves.

PITFALL ⊘

One should not attempt to control major bleeding in an extremity by blindly clamping in the depths of the wound.

If bleeding from a wound cannot be controlled digitally, one may apply a compression dressing reinforced with an ace wrap. If the bleeding persists through the compression dressing, the dressing should be removed and reapplied with careful attention to maintaining uniform compression throughout the length and width of the wound. A repeat careful application of a compressive dressing and ace wrap in this setting will stop refractory bleeding in most extremity wounds.

If bleeding persists despite a second application of a compression dressing, the dressing may be reinforced by a tourniquet; however, one should be careful to apply the tourniquet pressure over the most proximal portion of the wound or even proximal to the wound and to inflate the cuff well above systolic pressure. If the tourniquet pressure is slightly below the systolic pressure, increased venous bleeding results.

AXIOM   If tourniquets are not applied properly, they can increase bleeding and tissue loss.

Pneumatic splints may assist in control of bleeding from soft tissue extremity wounds or in patients with long bone fractures. This technique is especially valuable during transit from the scene of injury to the trauma center.[22,23]

Etiology of Shock After Trauma (Table 2-1)

AXIOM   Continued shock after trauma is usually due to continued bleeding or inadequate resuscitation.

HYPOVOLEMIA
Hemorrhage is the most common cause of shock in injured patients.[1,3] Patients arriving at the hospital in shock after blunt trauma are likely to be bleeding from intraperitoneal injuries, pelvic or long bone fractures, or intrathoracic wounds.[24,25] Internal hemorrhage from fractures and severe muscle contusions is also a frequent, potentially lethal, cause of hypovolemia after trauma.[1,3] Hypovolemic shock following trauma may also occur from translocation of fluids into burned, contused, or contaminated tissues.[20]

AXIOM   The combination of prolonged shock and a severe head injury is lethal.

Hypovolemic shock with consequent cerebral hypoxia is a major factor leading to death in patients with head injury. Damaged brain tissue is particularly sensitive to a decrease in cerebral perfusion or oxygenation.[19]

TABLE 2-1   Etiology of Circulatory Shock in the Injured

Type of Shock	Etiology
Hypovolemic	Blood loss due to hemorrhage
	Plasma loss due to burns, surgery, and/or infections
Cardiogenic	Myocardial contusion
	Myocardial infarction
	Congestive heart failure
	Arrhythmia
Distributive*	Spinal cord injury
	Septic shock
	Intoxication
	Anaphylactic reaction
Obstructive	Pericardial tamponade
	Pulmonary embolism
	Pneumothorax; hemothorax
	Air embolism
	Fat embolism

*(increased venous capacitance and/or decreased vascular resistance)

CHEST TRAUMA
Shock following chest trauma may be due to hemorrhage, tension pneumothorax, pericardial tamponade, arrhythmias, or cardiac failure.[1,3]

EXCESS VASODILATION

PITFALL ⊘

> *One should not assume that persistent shock after a spinal cord injury is due only to spinal shock.*

Hypotension to systolic pressures below 90 torr in patients with spinal cord injuries is primarily due to dilatation of capacitance or resistance vessels.[1,3,26] Intoxication with alcohol or other drugs may accentuate this phenomenon. Other sites of injury, however, must also be anticipated, particularly if the systolic pressure falls below 80 torr. Anaphylactic reactions to various medications, blood transfusions, or toxins can also cause severe vasodilatation and hypotension, but the clinical circumstances should help identify these etiologies. Shock due to sepsis is extremely unusual within 48 hours of the injury unless the patient already had an infected focus, such as a urinary tract infection due to bladder outlet obstruction.[27]

EMBOLI
Fat emboli can cause acute respiratory failure which usually does not become clinically apparent for 12-48 hours after injury.[1,3] Emboli from deep venous thrombosis after crush or compression injuries can cause sudden hypotension, and even cardiac arrest, within 24 hours of severe injury. Air embolism should be suspected in any patient with a lung injury who develops sudden cardiovascular embarrassment or bizarre cerebral changes shortly after being intubated and placed on positive pressure ventilation.[3]

MISCELLANEOUS CAUSES
Chemical or biologic agents such as toxic gases or "biowarfare" agents, and venom stings or bites are rare causes of shock in injured patients. These should be considered in the appropriate clinical settings.

Physiologic Changes in Hemorrhagic Shock
FLUID SPACES
Optimal resuscitation of injured patients with hemorrhagic shock requires an understanding of both the normal and abnormal physiology of the body fluid compartments. The normal 70 kg patient has a total body water content of approximately 60% of the body weight or about 42 liters.[3,14] This total body water content is distributed into an intracellular space of approximately 28 liters and an extracellular fluid space of about 14 liters.[12,13] The intracellular fluid space can be further subdivided into an intravascular portion, the red blood cell mass, which averages about 2 liters with the remainder of the 26 liters of intracellular fluid distributed within muscles and viscera. Likewise, the extracellular fluid space is divided into an intravascular portion or plasma volume of about 3 liters and an extravascular portion or interstitial fluid space of about 11 liters.

FLUID FLUX
The various fluid compartments are in a constant state of flux, but during a steady state, bidirectional fluxes are balanced.[14] One of the main fluid fluxes involves movement of water and electrolytes between the vascular space and the interstitial fluid space.[14,28,29] In the arterial end of the capillary, movement of fluid into the interstitial fluid space is controlled primarily by the hydrostatic pressure difference between the plasma and the interstitial fluid. At the venous end of the capillary, there is a reverse movement of water and electrolytes out of the interstitial space back into the vascular space. This reverse movement is thought to be primarily controlled by the relative difference between the oncotic pressures within the vascular space and the interstitial fluid space.[29]

PROTEIN FLUX

The dynamic movement of protein, especially albumin, between the vascular and interstitial fluid compartments must be appreciated in order to understand its effects on the fluid balance between the intravascular and extravascular compartments.[3,29] Normally, plasma contains approximately 45% of the extracellular albumin with the remaining 55% located in the interstitial fluid space. The rate at which proteins move out of the vascular space into the interstitial fluid space at the capillary level is regulated by the volume of fluid movement and the molecular weight, geometric configuration, and charge of the proteins.[3,14]

Once protein enters the interstitial fluid space, it comes into equilibrium with the sol and gel portions of the interstitial fluid space. Based upon the three-dimensional configuration of the interstitial fluid space matrix, protein, especially albumin, has the capacity to become attached to the interstitial fluid space matrix proteoglycans or to pass through the sol portion of the interstitial fluid space into the lymphatics and then back to the vascular space.[3,29] Consequently, the configuration of the interstitial space matrix, which controls the amount of albumin within the interstitial fluid space, is extremely important in the control of intravascular protein concentrations.

AXIOM The configuration of the interstitial space matrix determines the ratio of the albumin concentrations in the plasma and interstitial fluid.

CHANGES IN THE INTERSTITIAL FLUID SPACE

During severe hemorrhagic shock, the interstitial fluid space contracts because of increased movement of salt and water into the vascular space at the venular end of the capillary.[28,29] The interstitial fluid space contraction also causes increased movement of albumin from the interstitial space into the vascular space through the lymphatic system. This is one of the most important homeostatic responses to shock.

AXIOM Resuscitation of shock in adults and older children should not be done with glucose-containing solutions.

During resuscitation with balanced electrolyte solutions, one should avoid glucose infusions to counter the tendency toward shock induced hyperglycemia.[3,30] Even if no glucose is given, hyperglycemia tends to occur during shock and following trauma because of increased catecholamine, glucagon, cortisol, and growth hormone release. The resultant increased glycogenolysis and gluconeogenesis combined with increased cellular resistance to insulin can cause glucose levels to be very high.[3,14] If exogenous glucose is added to these endogenous events, glucose levels may become extremely high and can lead to inappropriate osmotic diuresis at a time when fluid conservation is critical.[3,14]

The interstitial fluid space and its matrix have a tremendous capacity to adjust to the hemorrhagic insult and thereby protect the environment in which the cells must function.[29] The alterations within the interstitial fluid space allow the pH surrounding the cells to be maintained at relatively constant levels in spite of a rather severe metabolic acidosis as reflected by arterial and mixed venous blood.[3]

THE THREE PHASES OF SHOCK

Most patients with severe injury and hypotension present with large intravascular and extravascular fluid deficits.[14] Patients with hollow viscus perforation can also have significant fluid shifts into the extravascular spaces due to inflammation and/or infection. These fluid shifts continue into the postoperative period. Thus, treatment of hypovolemic shock must be continued beyond the initial restoration of blood volume and vital signs in the emergency room and/or operating room.

AXIOM Significant fluid shifts out of the vascular space can continue for 24-48 hours or longer after bleeding has been controlled.

The body's physiologic responses to hypovolemic shock may be divided into three phases[3,14] (Table 2-2). Although the transition from one phase into the next may be indistinct, the stages themselves are clearly different and each phase has its own characteristics and treatment objectives.

Phase 1

Phase 1 includes the period of shock and active hemorrhage. This phase extends from the beginning of treatment to the completion of the resuscitation and surgery for control of bleeding. Phase 1 in patients with serious injury requiring operative intervention and massive blood transfusions for ongoing hemorrhagic shock averages 7 to 8 hours. The first 30 to 60 minutes includes preoperative management, and the remaining 6 to 7 hours includes the operative time needed to repair multiple injuries.

Phase 2

Phase 2 is the period of extravascular fluid sequestration. It begins after the bleeding is controlled and resuscitation is completed, and extends until the time of maximum weight gain. This fluid sequestration phase averages 24 to 36 hours in patients receiving 15 units of blood during phase 1.[3,14] The extravascular fluid sequestration seen during phase 2 is obligatory; it cannot be safely prevented by limiting fluid infusion. Indeed, fluid restriction in phase 2, particularly in its early stages, can rapidly lead to hypotension, renal failure, and cardiovascular collapse.

PITFALL ⊘

Restricting fluids in the post-traumatic extravascular fluid sequestration phase.

The expansion of the extravascular space following shock and trauma appears to include both the interstitial and intracellular compartments.[3,31-34] The obligatory nature of this "third-space" expansion is comparable to that seen in burn patients, with the mechanism of injury as the prime difference. With burns there is direct tissue damage due to the heat, and with shock the cell damage is due to ischemia.[3,20]

Cell ischemia in severe experimental shock is associated with an increase in the cell membrane potential from -90 mV to about -60 mV.[34,35] This results in the intracellular accumulation of sodium and water as depression of the sodium pump reduces the quantity of these substances that can be removed from the cell.[34] Intracellular swelling after shock has been confirmed in rodents by electron microscopy of both hepatocytes and myocytes.[35]

Studies indicate that during phase 2, the volume of the interstitial space may increase by more than 10 liters, and the total extravascular fluid increase may exceed 20 liters in some patients.[3,14,29] The severity of this obligatory extravascular expansion appears to be directly related to the degree and duration of cellular insult as reflected by the duration of the shock and the number of transfusions needed to restore blood volume.[14]

TABLE 2-2 Three Phases of Shock and Resuscitation

Phase 1	Active hemorrhage and acute hypovolemia
	From admission to end of operation
Phase 2	Extravascular fluid sequestration
	From end of operation until maximal weight gain
Phase 3	Fluid mobilization and diuresis
	From maximal weight gain until restoration of positive fluid balance

Phase 3

Phase 3 is the mobilization and diuretic period. It extends from the time of maximum weight gain until the end of diuresis as reflected by maximal weight loss. Although there is no precise moment when one phase ends and the next begins, most patients appear to reach a steady state of blood pressure and pulse toward the end of phase 2 when only small volumes of fluid are needed to maintain vital signs and urine output. During phase 3, salt and water leave the interstitial and intracellular spaces to enter the lymphatic channels and plasma. This reverse movement is thought to reflect the restoration of cell membrane potential and normal cellular function.[3,28,34] During this time, an increased intravascular volume and other changes may cause hypertension and/or heart failure.[3,14]

Treatment of Hemorrhage

FLUID REPLACEMENT AND THE DEGREE OF HEMORRHAGE

The amount and type of fluid used to treat hemorrhage varies according to its severity which can be divided into four levels or grades.[1,3]

Grade 1 Hemorrhage

A grade 1 hemorrhage is an acute loss of 10 to 15% of the circulating blood volume. This acute reduction of about 750-1000 ml blood in an average 70 kg adult is usually associated with some tachycardia and oliguria, but no apparent decrease in blood pressure or organ function. The central venous pressure will be either normal or slightly low. The acute blood volume deficit will normally be rapidly and easily corrected by movement of fluid from the interstitial fluid space into the vascular space.

> **AXIOM**   Whenever an acute blood volume loss occurs, early administration of three times that amount of a balanced electrolyte solution will usually restore the blood volume to normal.

Patients who present to the emergency department with a grade 1 hemorrhage can usually have their circulatory volume fully restored by the administration of 2-3 liters of a balanced electrolyte solution.[3,14,36,37] Blood transfusions will not be required as long as there is no further blood loss.

Grade 2 Hemorrhage

A moderate or grade 2 blood loss is defined as an acute loss of 20 to 25% of the blood volume or approximately 1250-1750 ml of blood in a 70 kg adult. Such blood loss will usually cause a significant tachycardia, a reduced pulse pressure, and oliguria reflecting renal vasoconstriction with decreased renal blood flow and glomerular filtration rate.

> **AXIOM**   In previously young and healthy individuals, loss of 20 to 25% of the blood volume may be associated with minimal or no arterial hypotension.[23]

The blood pressure response to hemorrhage in patients depends on numerous factors including: (a) the rate, total volume, duration, and site of the blood loss, (b) the patient's age and medical status, and (c) the rate and adequacy of fluid resuscitation. However, stroke volume and cardiac output tend to fall much earlier and much more severely than the blood pressure.[3,38]

> **AXIOM**   A normal arterial blood pressure in a trauma patient may be associated with a significant reduction in extracellular fluid, cardiac output, and stroke volume.

Changes in pulse pressure generally correlate with changes in stroke volume. Many clinicians monitor the changes in pulse pressure along with the systolic and diastolic pressures as an index of the adequacy of fluid resuscitation.[3,14,39] Cullen, however, observed no correlation between stroke volume and pulse pressure in both anesthetized and awake patients.[40]

> **AXIOM**   In most hypovolemic patients, urine output is an important guide to the adequacy of fluid resuscitation.

During hemorrhage, any reduction in cardiac output and renal blood flow will cause a reduced glomerular filtration and increased water and sodium reabsorption which will result in a decreased urine output.[3,41] Careful monitoring of urine output can help guide volume replacement during resuscitation. Increased serum osmolality (such as occurs in diabetic patients, some septic patients, and in those who have received radiocontrast dye) can lead to increased urine output despite a compromised plasma volume.[3,40]

> **AXIOM**   Urine output will not reflect the adequacy of the fluid resuscitation if there are other factors present that can cause a diuresis.

Blood volume restoration in patients with a grade 2 hemorrhage requires the rapid infusion of at least 3-4 liters of balanced electrolyte solution. If the bleeding has stopped, this should restore vital signs, total body perfusion, and urine output to normal without the use of blood or blood products.[3]

Grade 3 Hemorrhage

Patients presenting with a severe acute loss of 30-35% of the blood volume or approximately 2100-2450 ml in a 70 kg adult will present with hypotension, severe tachycardia, and oliguria. The hypotension will be associated with a marked narrowing of the pulse pressure and evidence of a greatly increased catecholamine release as reflected by a cold clammy skin and a very low urine output.[3,36,41] The marked oliguria reflects not only the effects of the circulating catecholamines on the kidneys but also the release by the kidneys of renin which in turn causes angiotensin and aldosterone release.[40,42,43] Complete restoration of the circulating blood volume can usually be achieved by the prompt infusion of 4-5 liters of balanced electrolyte solution along with 1 or 2 units of blood. Although use of whole blood would provide both red blood cell mass and plasma volume, packed red blood cells are usually the only type of bank blood available now.[3]

> **AXIOM**   If there is evidence of continued severe bleeding in a hypotensive patient, blood should be started early.

Our data indicate that patients who receive multiple blood transfusions of packed red cells require approximately 1.6 liters of a balanced electrolyte solution (BES) for each transfusion by the time the operative intervention is completed.[3] This volume of BES will allow the patient to maintain an adequate circulatory volume, vital signs, renal function, and urine output by the end of the surgical procedure.[40] The volume of BES needed to achieve these objectives in patients resuscitated with whole blood is 1.1 liters of BES for each transfusion given during phase 1.

The use of blood alone without BES for resuscitation has long been known to reduce the survival rate from hemorrhagic shock in experimental animals.[3,30-34] Likewise, administration of only Ringer's lactate solution to dogs bled to 40% of their blood volume is associated with a high mortality.

> **AXIOM**   The initial resuscitation of trauma patients with moderate to severe blood loss should utilize both blood and crystalloid solutions.

Grade 4 Hemorrhage

Patients presenting with catastrophic hemorrhage and severe shock will have an acute loss of at least 40-45% of their circulating blood volume or about 3 liters of whole blood loss. This usually causes a precipitous fall in blood pressure, which may not be obtainable by the cuff technique, and a marked catecholamine release causing cold clammy skin, an ashen appearance, and anuria.[3,14,40] Such patients are in danger of dying soon after their arrival in the emergency department (ED). Immediate expansion of the plasma volume with balanced electrolyte solution is essential and, if this does not rapidly restore a palpable pulse and a measurable blood pressure, the addition of type-specific or unmatched type O, Rh-negative blood, depending upon the circumstances, is appropriate.[3]

AXIOM   Severe oliguria during and immediately following traumatic shock is a renal adaptation to the hypotension and should not be treated with diuretics.

COLLOID SUPPLEMENTATION

Starling, in 1896, published the equation that now bears his name.[44] This equation proposes that the flux of water out of the vascular system will be directly related to capillary conductivity (often inappropriately referred to as permeability), multiplied by the capillary surface area and the net forces on the capillary by the plasma hydrostatic pressure, interstitial hydrostatic pressure, plasma oncotic pressure, and interstitial oncotic pressure.[3,44] In effect, the equation also seems to state that the flux of water out of capillaries will be inversely related to capillary oncotic pressure if all of the other factors remain constant. Contrary to popular belief, however, Starling highlighted the inadequacies of this equation when the publication appeared.[3] He pointed out that this equation does not apply to humans since there is a third fluid system, namely the lymphatic system, which drains off fluid from the interstitial space. He further pointed out that this equation is not applicable because there are also dynamic activities occurring between the interstitial and intracellular fluid spaces. Starling also indicated that the other factors in the equation would probably not remain constant and, therefore, one could not assume their constancy when applying this equation.

PITFALL ⊘

A misinterpretation of Starling's equation has created confusion about the forces regulating fluid movement across capillary membranes.

Despite these disclaimers by this great physiologist, some modern critical care physicians have used Starling's equation to justify the routine addition of albumin to resuscitation regimens for hemorrhagic shock and other hypovolemic insults.[45-50] This has caused albumin to be one of the most expensive pharmaceutical items in many countries. When our own retrospective, non-randomized studies suggested that albumin therapy was associated with increased pulmonary dysfunction, we stopped using supplemental albumin.[3,51] This also stimulated a prospective randomized analysis of the effects of albumin supplementation.

During a 2-year period, 94 patients with severe injury and hemorrhagic shock were randomized to receive albumin or no albumin.[3,52-56] The 94 patients had an average systolic pressure below 80 torr for more than 30 minutes and received an average of 15 blood transfusions during phase 1. The non-albumin patients received blood, balanced electrolyte solution, and some plasma for coagulation factor deficiency. The albumin patients received similar fluids plus up to 150 grams of supplemental human serum albumin during phase 1 followed by 150 grams daily for the next 3-5 days. The amount of albumin supplementation was designed to restore serum albumin levels to normal during the postoperative extravascular fluid sequestration phase (phase 2) and was based upon multiple sequential measurements of serum albumin concentration, hourly albumin efflux, and plasma volumes. The serum albumin levels were restored to normal in the albumin-supplemented patients, but they were consistently below 3 gm/dl and often below 2 gm/dl in the non-albumin patients.[29] In spite of the normal serum albumin levels, the capillary oncotic pressure was not restored to a normal 22-24 torr in the albumin patients; indeed, their capillary oncotic pressures averaged only 19.7 torr, but this was higher than the mean capillary oncotic pressure of 14.8 torr in the non-albumin patients.[29]

The patients receiving albumin supplementation had a significant increase in effective renal plasma flow as measured by para-aminohippurate clearance.[55] Despite the increase in renal plasma flow, the albumin-supplemented patients had a decrease in glomerular filtration rate, sodium clearance, osmolar clearance, and urine output.[55]

The mechanisms for this seemingly paradoxical response of increased blood flow to the kidneys with decreased glomerular filtration has been known to renal physiologists for many years.[3,55] Experimentally, the addition of albumin to the resuscitation regimen in animals causes an increase in the oncotic and osmotic pressures within the glomerulus. This leads to salt and water retention within the vascular system and also produces an increase in the oncotic and osmotic pressures within the peritubular vessels perfusing the inner medulla of the kidney.

The only controversy among many renal physiologists has to do with the mechanism by which albumin leads to sodium retention. Our own findings support those physiologists who maintain that the sodium retention following albumin therapy is brought about by a sodium-potassium exchange at a tubular level.[3]

These effects of albumin on renal blood flow and excretion force one to rethink the original purpose of albumin supplementation, which was to exert an oncotic effect within the vascular system to, hopefully, extract extravascular fluid from the pulmonary interstices and deliver this fluid to the kidneys where it can be excreted.[47,50] Unfortunately, the resultant salt and water retention led to increased diuretic therapy, was associated with a higher incidence of renal failure, aggravated the pulmonary insult as reflected by higher central venous pressures, increased physiologic shunting in the lungs, and prolonged ventilatory support.[56,57] These changes also resulted in a significantly increased mortality rate in the albumin-supplemented patients.[3,15,58]

After analyzing the decreases in pulmonary oxygenation, the increased central filling pressures, and the increased need for diuretics after albumin therapy, it became apparent that albumin may also interfere with left ventricular function and exert a negative inotropic effect on the heart.[52,54,57] This possibility was analyzed by noting the ratio of left ventricular work to central filling pressure as monitored by either the calculated left ventricular stroke work index/pulmonary artery wedge pressure ($LVSWI/P_{pw}$) ratio or of left ventricular stroke work index/central venous pressure ratio.[52] All of these ratios were reduced in the albumin patients compared with the non-albumin patients. The compromised left ventricular function in the albumin-treated patients resulted in an increased need for inotropic support of the heart. Twenty-four (52%) of the 46 albumin patients had to be digitalized for congestive heart failure, whereas only 11 (23%) of the 48 non-albumin patients required digitalization.[52]

The mechanisms whereby supplemental albumin might cause ventricular dysfunction are unclear. Myocardial depression has been reported after shock, and a myocardial depressant factor, possibly of pancreatic origin, has been postulated.[52,54] Albumin might potentiate the release of such a factor although no evidence for this phenomenon is available. Alternatively, albumin might impair cardiac function by altering calcium dynamics.[54] The albumin patients had an increase in total serum calcium concentration but a reduction in both the level of ionized calcium and the ratio of ionized to total calcium. The reduced ionized calcium may be one of the reasons that myocardial depression after shock is aggravated by giving human serum albumin.[3,54] Ionic hypocalcemia is also known to decrease the excitability of myocardial cells and to inhibit intracellular enzyme function, including oxidative phosphorylation.

AXIOM   The detrimental effects of albumin on myocardial, renal, and respiratory functions are interrelated and mitigate against its use in hypovolemic shock.

Other potential hazards of albumin administration relate to its effects on immunoglobulins,[59] coagulation factors,[60,61] and the intrahepatic production of needed proteins.[29] The albumin-treated patients had a uniform reduction in all non-albumin proteins.[29] This included decreased levels of immunoglobulins and reduced immunoglobulin activity as judged by the immune response to tetanus toxoid.[59] Albumin-treated patients also had a reduction in coagulation activity as reflected by increased prothrombin times and decreased fibrinogen activity.[60,61] These alterations correlated with an increased need for transfusion after the operation.[3,29] These findings have been confirmed in a canine model of hemorrhagic shock in which one group was resuscitated with shed blood and crystalloid, whereas the other received blood, crystalloid, and albumin.[60] Confirmation of these adverse effects of albumin supplementation in a controlled animal study indicates that the clinical findings were not spurious.

AXIOM   Exogenous albumin administration reduces immunoglobulin and coagulation protein synthesis and/or activity.

In spite of all these findings, controversy still exists regarding the use of albumin versus crystalloids. Proponents of albumin contend that volume resuscitation can be accomplished faster and with much smaller volumes of colloid than of crystalloid solutions.[45-50] Such studies place little emphasis on restoration of function to organs such as the kidneys. Another argument involves the severe reduction of colloid oncotic pressure (COP) and the decreased gradient between COP and P_{pw} (COP-P_{pw}) seen with crystalloids which is said to favor the development of pulmonary edema.[45-50]

Reduction in COP is a common occurrence with large-volume crystalloid resuscitation. Interstitial COP, however, changes with the intravascular COP; thus, the effective oncotic pressure across the capillary membrane is not altered after crystalloid resuscitation.[3,29] Furthermore, it has been shown in both animals and humans that the reduction in COP during crystalloid infusion is not associated with increased pulmonary extravascular lung water.[3,62-64] Indeed, the use of the COP-P_{pw} gradient[68] as an index of pulmonary interstitial water content or as a predictor of pulmonary edema may be erroneous.[3] In addition, since pulmonary artery wedge pressure is not equal to pulmonary capillary pressure, it cannot be used in Starling's equation.[3,44] Furthermore, Starling's equation does not take into account the balance between fluid flux into the interstitium from cells and the evacuation of interstitial fluid by lymphatic vessels. Tranbaugh et al[64] suggested that the primary determinants of pulmonary interstitial fluid accumulation in trauma patients were sepsis and lung contusion and not the type of fluid administered. Crystalloid proponents argue that: (a) the contracted extracellular compartment seen in most types of shock can be expanded more effectively by crystalloid solutions than by albumin,[3,14,57,65,66] (b) an increased P_{pw} is less likely with crystalloids than with albumin because of its rapid equilibration with the interstitial fluid space,[3,57] (c) crystalloid solutions are considerably less expensive than albumin or synthetic colloids,[65,66] (d) better postoperative heart, lung, and kidney function can be maintained with crystalloid solutions than with albumin,[52,54-56,67] and (e) the risk of anaphylactoid reactions is eliminated by the use of crystalloid solutions. In addition, a recent meta-analysis that compared mortality following resuscitation with crystalloid and colloid solutions indicated that the overall mortality of trauma patients treated with crystalloids was 12.3% less than the rate of those treated with colloids.[58]

Although colloids are not needed for resuscitation from hemorrhagic shock, the transfusion of multiple units of packed red blood cells may lead to a coagulation-protein deficiency. There is no clinical or laboratory evidence to support the prophylactic use of fresh frozen plasma in patients requiring less than 10 transfusions for severe injury with hemorrhagic shock. There is, however, anecdotal data supporting the use of fresh frozen plasma replacement in patients requiring more than 10 transfusions. Currently, the authors recommend 1 unit of fresh frozen plasma for every five to six blood transfusions after the initial 10 blood transfusions.[10] The use of platelet supplementation is also controversial. Prophylactic platelet replacement in patients who require less than 10 blood transfusions during their initial resuscitation is not warranted. However, if more than 10 transfusions are required, platelet supplementation should be used if there is

oozing and laboratory documentation of a platelet count of less than 50,000/mm³.[3]

Hemodynamic Effects of the Trendelenburg Position

Head-down positioning of hypovolemic patients has been used since World War I in an attempt to improve central blood volume and cardiac output.[68,69] However, recent studies suggest that even 35° of tilt provides little hemodynamic improvement.[70,71] Using radionuclide scanning techniques, Bivins and coworkers demonstrated that there was only a 1.8% increase in central blood volume in awake normovolemic volunteers who were placed in 15° of the (head down) Trendelenburg position.[21] Other studies found no beneficial hemodynamic effect of this position in either normotensive or hypotensive patients.[70,71] In anesthetized patients with coronary artery disease, Reich et al found that a 20° Trendelenburg position caused a slight (10%) increase in systemic blood pressure, cardiac index, and filling pressures; however, right ventricular dilatation and decreased right ventricular ejection fraction were also noted.[72] This position may decrease cerebral blood flow, probably by increasing the jugular venous pressure and impeding venous drainage.

The hemodynamic effects of the Trendelenburg position in hemorrhagic shock are not known, but these patients probably respond similarly. Greater degrees of head-down tilt (up to 75°) cause a significant reduction in right atrial pressure, probably because of drainage of blood from the heart toward the head.[69] Thus, it appears that the Trendelenburg position offers little, if any, beneficial hemodynamic effect during management of shock. The head-down position may also cause respiratory embarrassment because cephalad displacement of intra-abdominal contents and the resultant elevation of the diaphragm reduces lung volumes. The hemodynamic effects of passive leg raising are similar to those of the Trendelenburg position.[72]

HEMODYNAMIC MONITORING

Class 1 Hemorrhage

Patients with only a class 1 hemorrhage can usually be monitored adequately with observation of the skin, urine output, cuff BP, and heart rate.

Class 2 Hemorrhage

CENTRAL VENOUS PRESSURE (CVP)

Patients presenting with class 2 hemorrhage may have some mild hypotension, but the BP usually stabilizes rapidly with crystalloid resuscitation. They should have two large intravenous lines, one of which can function as a central venous pressure (CVP) monitor. Monitoring of the CVP may be useful in these patients since the CVP reflects the interplay between blood volume, venous capacitance, and cardiac function.[3,39] A low CVP in injured patients with normal hearts and normal reflexes may reflect hypovolemia. An abrupt rise in the CVP during fluid resuscitation suggests that intravascular volume has been adequately restored.[3,40]

By noting the response of the CVP and systemic arterial pressure to a fluid challenge, one obtains added information regarding the patient's overall cardiovascular dynamics.[51,54] For instance, an abrupt increase of the CVP associated with a declining arterial pressure after a fluid challenge points toward cardiac failure. Although the CVP primarily monitors right heart function and will rise as the pulmonary vascular resistance increases, severely injured patients seldom develop isolated left ventricular failure and pulmonary edema with a normal CVP.[3,73] Other factors that may affect the CVP include changes in intrathoracic pressure caused by positive pressure ventilation, coughing, Valsalva maneuvers, or intrathoracic or mediastinal accumulations of air, blood, or fluid.

Although restoration of a normal (4 to 8 torr) or elevated CVP during resuscitation suggests adequate blood volume restoration, a 20 to 30% blood volume deficit may still be present.[73,74] Similar findings have been reported for pulmonary artery wedge pressures during fluid resuscitation.[39]

AXIOM	The CVP is useful in the hemodynamic monitoring of trauma patients but, like all tools, is limited in its application.

INTRA-ARTERIAL PRESSURE

Direct arterial pressure monitoring provides beat-to-beat information, allowing early intervention when hypotension occurs. Furthermore, exaggerated respiratory variations in systolic blood pressure during mechanical ventilation may be an early indication of hypovolemia or pericardial tamponade.[41,42] The difference between the highest and lowest systolic pressures often exceeds 10 mm Hg when the patient is hypovolemic, has a pericardial tamponade, or severe bronchospasm. The difference between the highest and lowest systolic pressures during a ventilatory cycle often correlates well with a plasma volume deficit.[75]

AXIOM	Large respirophasic variations in systolic blood pressure may be an early sign of hypovolemia.

Changes in systolic blood pressure during the ventilatory cycle correspond to alterations in left ventricular output which is affected primarily by the venous return to the left atrium. Systolic blood pressure variations during hypovolemia are due to squeezing of pulmonary capillary blood into the left ventricle, resulting in increased left ventricular preload and thus increased stroke volume during early inspiration.[75,76] This phenomenon does not occur in normovolemic animals since zone 3 conditions ($P_{pa} > P_{LA} > P_{alv}$) predominate, and significant increases in pulmonary outflow do not occur during early inspiration. With fluid resuscitation and restoration of normovolemia, this response disappears.[76]

Arterial pressure tracings may also provide information about myocardial contractility, stroke volume, and the systemic vascular resistance.[75] A steep upstroke of the pressure wave indicates a vigorous left ventricular contraction, the area under the systolic ejection period (from the beginning of the systolic upstroke to the dicrotic notch) correlates with the stroke volume, and the location of the dicrotic notch and the steepness of the downstroke are proportional to the systemic vascular resistance (SVR). A low dicrotic notch and steep downstroke suggest low systemic vascular resistance.[72]

Class 3 Hemorrhage

HEMOGLOBIN AND HEMATOCRIT

During the initial resuscitation and operative procedure, the relative amounts of blood and balanced electrolyte solution needed for patients with a class 3 hemorrhage should be partly guided by serial hemoglobin or hematocrit measurements, by careful observation of the changes in systemic and central pressures, and by urine output.[1,3]

Absolute levels of hemoglobin or hematocrit are not reliable indices of blood loss until the restoration of plasma volume by transcapillary refill and fluid infusion is complete; this may take 12 to 48 hours, or even longer, in some elderly patients.

PULMONARY ARTERY CATHETER

When circumstances permit, a pulmonary artery (PA) catheter may allow one to determine left heart filling pressures, cardiac output, oxygen transport variables, and systemic and pulmonary vascular resistance.[52,53] This catheter may be particularly helpful during prolonged operative procedures, but hypotension in these patients is usually due to inadequate fluid and/or blood replacement.

AXIOM	Hypotension in the seriously injured patient is generally an indication for more blood and fluid replacement.

The major benefits of a pulmonary artery catheter are realized during the postoperative period. The pulmonary artery wedge pressure (P_{pw}) is usually a reliable index of left ventricular end-diastolic pressure. Wedge pressures below 10 torr in injured patients usually indicate hypovolemia, whereas values above 15-18 torr may be seen with hypervolemia or altered left ventricular function. However, interpretation of the P_{pw} may be difficult during hypovolemia, since pulmonary vascular pressure may decrease below alveolar pressure, and thus the P_{pw} may measure alveolar rather than intravascular pressures. Many patients with a P_{pw} greater than 15 mm Hg after resuscitation from severe shock will respond to a fluid challenge with an increased cardiac output and little change in P_{pw}, thus indicating normal left ventricular function. On the other hand, an abrupt rise in the P_{pw} during a fluid challenge without an increase in stroke volume or cardiac output suggests exhaustion of cardiac reserve.[75]

Class 4 Hemorrhage

Patients with class 4 hemorrhage should have invasive monitoring of arterial blood pressure, CVP, pulmonary artery pressure, P_{pw}, and pulmonary artery oxygen saturation (S_vO_2). Periodic determinations of cardiac output, blood gases, and electrolytes may also be necessary.[76] However, placement of pulmonary artery catheters during the initial resuscitation, when venous pressures are low, can be extremely difficult. Furthermore, delaying treatment of a severely hypotensive patient in order to insert a central venous catheter can be counterproductive.

AXIOM	The first 60 minutes after trauma is the golden period for the diagnosis of injuries and aggressive treatment of hypovolemia.

Hypotension in the presence of bleeding is almost always due to hypovolemia; early control of the bleeding plus rapid fluid and blood administration is mandatory. Aggressive resuscitation with Ringer's lactate does not increase an existing lactic acidosis when shock is reversible. Each liter of Ringer's lactate solution contains 28 mEq of lactate, about half of which is metabolized in the liver. The remaining lactate is usually cleared rapidly from the plasma once tissue perfusion is improved by fluid infusion.[76] Thus, the past concerns expressed by some clinicians about giving Ringer's lactate during resuscitation seem to be unwarranted.[33]

PATIENT EXAMINATION

Initial Assessment

A multidisciplinary team approach to the injured patient dictates that an initial assessment be performed simultaneously with establishing an airway, adequate ventilation, and intravenous routes and controlling external bleeding as needed. The patient who is awake should be questioned concerning the mode and mechanism of injury, any loss of consciousness, and any head, neck, chest, abdomen, or extremity complaints. A brief history is also obtained regarding allergies, previous and concurrent illnesses and present medications, use of drugs or alcohol, the time of the last meal or liquids, and the events preceding the injury.[1,3]

The initial physical examination includes palpation of the head, facial bones, and cervical spine. Careful bilateral chest palpation may detect crepitation, and compression may detect tenderness associated with rib fractures. The abdomen is evaluated for distension and tenderness, and the pelvis is compressed laterally and from anterior to posterior to detect pain or instability from fractures. The extremities are assessed for deformity, crepitation, swelling, tenderness, motion, sensation, and the presence or absence of pulses. Lastly, the perineum is assessed for hematoma involving the genitalia or perineum, blood at the urethral meatus, and blood or lack of sphincter tone in the rectum.[1,3]

Secondary Assessment

CHEST

AXIOM The combination of shock and acute respiratory distress is highly lethal unless corrected rapidly.

When a patient presents in acute distress with apprehension, agitation, cyanosis, air hunger, and shock following a penetrating chest wound, one must consider the potential for rapid death from either a pericardiac tamponade, tension pneumothorax, or a massive hemothorax.[1,3] Two of these conditions, cardiac tamponade and tension pneumothorax, may cause hypotension, neck vein distension, and distant heart tones, whereas patients with a massive hemothorax tend to have flat neck veins. In order to distinguish between cardiac tamponade and tension pneumothorax, one should rapidly note the position of the trachea which would be midline with pericardial tamponade and shifted to the contralateral side with tension pneumothorax.

If pericardial tamponade is suspected, rapid beneficial results can often be obtained by a pericardiocentesis, which is usually performed by inserting a long needle just to the left of the xiphoid with the tip of the aspirating needle directed superiorly and to the left. With patients in shock from pericardial tamponade, the removal of as little as 5 or 10 ml of blood from the pericardial sac can often raise the systolic pressure to 90 or 100 torr and give the treating team time to safely transport the patient to the operating room for definitive correction.[1,3]

If the patient is in severe respiratory distress and the trachea is shifted, rapid aspiration of the contralateral pleural cavity with a large needle, three-way stop cock, and a 20 or 50 cc syringe can temporarily relieve a tension pneumothorax while preparations are made to insert a chest tube.

AXIOM Open chest wounds should not be covered or closed until a chest tube is in place.

Some patients with high velocity rifle wounds or severe autopedestrian mishaps present with open chest wounds which have obvious to-and-fro movement of air through the chest wall defect. Although much has been written about the need to cover such wounds in order to improve ventilation of the lungs through the tracheobronchial tree, covering such a wound has the potential to create a tension pneumothorax. Since most of these severe chest wall injuries are associated with tears of the underlying lung, there is ongoing leakage of air from the lung itself, and this air needs to get to the outside lest a tension pneumothorax develop. When such patients present to the hospital, they are best served by the placement of a large chest tube and then the open chest wound can be covered. When the chest wall wound is huge, the patient should be intubated, supported with a ventilator, and preparations made for early thoracotomy with definitive repair of the underlying injuries and closure of the chest wall defect.[1,3]

AXIOM Most life-threatening chest injuries with severe shock are due to massive severe hemorrhage.

The common bleeding sites from penetrating wounds of the chest include the heart, great vessels, lungs, and internal mammary and intercostal arteries. Severe, continuing bleeding from stab wounds is usually from a partially severed intercostal artery or internal mammary artery. In contrast, patients with bleeding gunshot wounds of the chest are more likely to have lung injuries. Both stabs and gunshot wounds can rapidly cause death from bleeding from injuries to the heart or great vessels. Patients presenting with severe hemorrhagic shock and respiratory distress from a penetrating chest wound should have an immediate tube thoracostomy without chest x-ray confirmation of hemothorax or pneumothorax. The decision to proceed with further emergency department resuscitation efforts or to go directly to the operating room is based upon the results of the tube thoracostomy. If the patient's vital signs improve rapidly with intravenous fluid replacement, appropriate diagnostic chest films may be obtained.

If a stable patient has more than 50% of one chest cavity filled with blood, the potential need for a thoracotomy to control the bleeding is significant, even if the patient's vital signs are stable. A difficult decision occurs when a patient has continued bleeding after evacuation of the initial hemothorax. If this continued bleeding exceeds 400 ml during the first hour, 200 ml per hour from hour 2 through hour 6, or 100 ml per hour after hour 6, operative intervention is indicated even though the patient has remained stable.

AXIOM Continued significant bleeding into the chest is an indication for thoracotomy.

When a patient presents with stable vital signs after a penetrating chest wound, chest x-rays are ordered to rule out a hemothorax or pneumothorax.[3] If either one is present, a chest tube should be placed in the mid-axillary line in the fifth or sixth interspace. The skin incision is made over the fifth or sixth rib in the anterior axillary line and the tube is directed posteriorly so that it enters into the chest just above the same rib in the mid-axillary line. This technique gives a long tunnel to reduce the likelihood of inadvertent air leak or recurrent pneumothorax when the chest tube is removed. Repeat chest x-rays are essential after chest tube placement to confirm the position of the tube, the expansion of the lung, and adequate evacuation of the intrathoracic air and blood. Inadequate expansion of the lung and/or a significant amount of retained blood calls for either additional chest tubes if the patient is stable or operative intervention if the patient is unstable.

If the patient becomes unstable while being observed for continuing bleeding, immediate operative intervention is advocated. Patients with penetrating heart wounds do not always develop pericardial tamponade. If there is active bleeding from a heart wound into the pleura cavity, rapid resuscitation and operative intervention are required.

The diagnosis of cardiac injury with pericardial tamponade following blunt thoracic trauma can be quite difficult, but occasionally patients will exhibit a typical triad of hypotension, distended neck veins, and distant heart tones.[1] When questions exist about the presence or absence of a pericardial tamponade in a relatively stable patient, a pulmonary artery catheter may help confirm the diagnosis by showing equalization of the central venous pressure, pulmonary capillary wedge pressure, and right ventricular diastolic pressure. An echocardiogram can also be diagnostic.

ABDOMEN

Intra-abdominal Bleeding

AXIOM The most urgent threat to life in patients with abdominal injury is severe intraperitoneal hemorrhage from injuries to the liver, spleen, or major vessels.

The most important clinical finding in patients with abdominal injury is hypotension that cannot be explained by other injuries.[1,3] Although patients with severe intra-abdominal bleeding often also have abdominal pain, tenderness, and distension, these findings may be inconsistent and unreliable. A four-quadrant diagnostic paracentesis (DPC) can be performed in 30 seconds and will confirm the presence of hemoperitoneum if any blood is aspirated.

The DPC may be performed by aspirating the peritoneal cavity in all four quadrants of the abdomen just lateral to the rectus muscle.[1,3] Aspiration of any amount of non-clotting blood indicates significant hemoperitoneum requiring laparotomy. When the DPC is negative, massive hemoperitoneum causing severe shock is unlikely. However, such a patient is a candidate for diagnostic peritoneal lavage (DPL) which is more time-consuming but more sensitive. If the DPL is also negative, the hypotension is almost always due to other causes. Thus, DPC and DPL can be invaluable in this setting.

For the DPL, the authors prefer a closed or semi-closed technique with the introducer placed through the abdominal wall after careful hemostasis in the skin incision has been achieved. One liter in adults or 10 ml/kg in children of crystalloid solution is infused and then siphoned out. Following blunt abdominal injury, an aspirate that contains 100,000 red cells/mm³, 500 white cells/mm³, bowel content, or particulate matter indicates the presence of significant intraperitoneal injury. A red blood cell count of 100,000/mm³ approximates a 1% hematocrit and impedes the reading of standard newsprint through intravenous extension tubing.

> **AXIOM**   The most common cause for a false negative DPL after blunt trauma is a ruptured diaphragm, and the most common cause for a false positive DPL is a pelvic fracture.

Increased bloody drainage from a chest tube during the DPL suggests diaphragmatic rupture. Patients with severe pelvic fracture will generally not have a life-threatening intraperitoneal bleed unless the DPL aspirate has a hematocrit above 3%.

The definition of a positive DPL after penetrating abdominal injury is variable. Most authors agree that a significant red cell count is much lower with penetrating injury than with blunt trauma, and is probably in the range of 10,000-50,000/mm³. The authors reserve DPL after penetrating wounds for identifying the presence or absence of peritoneal penetration. Penetration is assumed if any blood is visible in the DPL aspirate.

> **AXIOM**   When a stable patient is known to have a gunshot wound that entered the peritoneal cavity, a laparotomy should be performed regardless of the DPL findings.

When a stable patient is known to have a stab wound with penetration, laparotomy is advocated only if the patient develops signs of intraperitoneal injury, is mentally incapacitated from drugs or alcohol, or requires general anesthesia for treatment of other injuries. Hemodynamically stable, awake, and alert patients with peritoneal penetration can be observed, but they should be examined at least every 2 hours for the development of tachycardia or abdominal tenderness.

Hollow Viscus Injuries

Once one rules out intraperitoneal hemorrhage, the next most critical threat to life from abdominal trauma is intraperitoneal hollow viscus rupture.[1,3] In order of sequence after blunt trauma, the most likely intraperitoneal hollow viscus injuries involve the small bowel, stomach, and colon. The clinical features of bowel perforation include early abdominal pain and tenderness due to soilage of the peritoneal cavity with enteric contents. If the perforation goes unrecognized for more than 12 hours, increasing peritoneal infection will produce the typical signs and symptoms of sepsis. Delayed diagnosis beyond this point markedly increases the likelihood of death.

> **AXIOM**   It often takes 12 or more hours for bowel leakage to produce signs and symptoms of peritonitis.

Early roentgenographic findings of hollow viscus perforation may include pneumoperitoneum, especially in patients with blunt gastric rupture. Pneumoperitoneum is less common in patients with small bowel tears and seldom occurs in patients with blunt colon injury. DPC is seldom helpful in the early diagnosis of blunt hollow viscus rupture, but DPL may show an increased white cell count, amylase, or alkaline phosphatase in the aspirate. Abdominal CT scans with oral and intravenous contrast may help with the diagnosis in selected patients in whom less sophisticated techniques have been inconclusive.

Extrahepatic Biliary Tract Injuries

The extrahepatic biliary tract is infrequently injured after blunt trauma to the abdomen. Most blunt gallbladder injuries are associated with a concomitant liver injury so that the diagnosis is usually made at the time of exploratory laparotomy for the signs and symptoms of hemoperitoneum. Rarely, the blunt injury will cause a severe full-thickness contusion of the gallbladder fundus, resulting in transmural ischemia followed by delayed rupture, often after the patient has resumed diet.

The delayed and localized leakage from an injured gallbladder, which may rupture 3 days to several weeks after the trauma, can lead to cryptic findings such as ascites, jaundice, and tenderness. Extrahepatic bile duct rupture after blunt trauma usually occurs at the point where the common bile duct passes posterior to the duodenum.

Occasionally, an isolated blunt rupture of an extrahepatic bile duct will be diagnosed at an exploratory laparotomy that was performed because the patient had signs suggesting peritonitis. Frequently, however, the patient has no associated injuries mandating exploratory laparotomy and has little or no findings during the early postinjury period. Many such patients are resuscitated, examined, and then discharged home only to return to the hospital several days later with bile-stained ascites, jaundice, anorexia, and mild to moderate elevations in the hepatic enzymes. Paracentesis will confirm that the patient has bile ascites, whereas an abdominal CT scan may only show a nonspecific finding of intraperitoneal fluid. The definitive diagnosis, in difficult cases, can be made by performing endoscopic retrograde cholangiopancreatography (ERCP). Once the definitive diagnosis is made, exploratory laparotomy and repair are indicated.

Retroperitoneal Injuries After Blunt Trauma

The next most urgent threats to life after intraperitoneal organ injuries are retroperitoneal injuries to the pancreas, duodenum, or genitourinary system.[1] The types of retroperitoneal pancreatic or duodenal injuries vary with the clinical setting. Injuries occurring in the inner city are usually caused by penetrating wounds, and decisions regarding laparotomy are based upon the same criteria used with intraperitoneal penetrating wounds.

Patients who present with blunt trauma to the retroperitoneal organs usually are involved in automobile mishaps, farm accidents, auto-pedestrian accidents, or muggings. When the patient has multiple injuries, the injury to the duodenum or pancreas is usually made at the time of a laparotomy performed for other reasons. Isolated injuries to the pancreas or duodenum can be extremely difficult to diagnose.

DUODENAL INJURY.   Many patients with blunt injury to the retroperitoneal pancreas or duodenum have no associated intraperitoneal injuries.[1] In such individuals, the usual diagnostic studies (such as abdominal x-rays, laboratory studies, and paracentesis) will usually be negative. However, early diagnosis of blunt duodenal injury can be facilitated by a high index of suspicion plus recognition that the physical findings are often subtle and don't usually become severe until at least 6 to 12 hours after the initial insult. The most common physical findings in patients with duodenal rupture include mild pain and tenderness in the epigastrium and right periumbilical area which gradually become worse over a period of 6-12 hours. Often there is a transient period when the clinical findings are less obvious so that the physician may be lulled into a false sense of security thinking that the injury to the abdomen is only "an abdominal wall contusion." When pain persists or tenderness becomes worse during a 6-hour period of observation, one should assume that serious injury is present and make plans for admission to hospital for continued observation or for a definitive diagnostic laparotomy.

> **AXIOM**   Patients with abdominal trauma should have flat and upright films of the abdomen. This will help identify the retroperitoneal air that is present in many patients with blunt rupture of the retroperitoneal duodenum.

The roentgenographic findings suggestive of retroperitoneal duodenal rupture include decreased visualization of the ipsilateral psoas muscle, scoliosis of the lumbar spine (usually concave to the right), and retroperitoneal air bubbles along the lateral border of the right psoas muscle and around the right kidney. Although blurring of the ipsilateral psoas shadow and scoliosis with retroperitoneal duodenal injury are often readily apparent, the presence of retroperitoneal air is frequently overlooked or is misinterpreted as gas within the hepatic flexure of the colon or within the duodenum.

AXIOM   Retroperitoneal air, scoliosis, and blurring of the right psoas shadow on x-ray can be found soon after the injury in over 50% of patients with blunt retroperitoneal duodenal rupture.

Careful examination of the gas pattern within the right and transverse colon can often help determine whether or not suspected retroperitoneal air is actually outside of the intracolic mixture of feces and gas.[1] Patients with retroperitoneal duodenal rupture will generally not have free intraperitoneal air. Whenever a patient has free intraperitoneal air, it is almost always due to rupture of an intraperitoneal hollow viscus. When the patient has suggestive findings of duodenal rupture as evidenced by scoliosis and decreased visualization of the psoas shadow, an emergency upper gastrointestinal series with a radioiodinated contrast agent will confirm the diagnosis if the dye extravasates into the right gutter and retroperitoneal space.

PANCREATIC INJURY.   The diagnosis of blunt pancreatic injury is suspected clinically on the basis of physical findings and laboratory data. Plain films of the abdomen are usually noncontributory.[1] The physical findings are similar to those seen in patients with duodenal trauma. Often the patient has little pain or tenderness during the initial examination, but 4 to 6 hours later, the pain and tenderness tend to be worse. The tenderness typically is less than that seen in patients with intraperitoneal rupture of either a hollow or solid viscus. Concomitant with the progressive increase in abdominal discomfort and tenderness, the patient often shows a rise in the serum amylase at 6 to 12 hours in comparison to the amylase levels found upon arrival in the emergency department.

AXIOM   Obtaining serial serum amylase measurements following blunt abdominal trauma can facilitate the diagnosis of pancreatic injury by demonstrating a rise in serum amylase levels at 6 or 12 hours, coinciding with increasing abdominal pain and tenderness.

When the diagnosis of pancreatic injury is still in doubt and an intraperitoneal injury has been ruled out, an abdominal CT scan may facilitate the diagnosis of pancreatic disruption by demonstrating edema around the pancreas in the lesser sac and, sometimes, actual division of the mid-portion of the pancreas.[1]

AXIOM   The definitive diagnosis of pancreatic disruption can be made with ERCP.

The abdominal CT scan can be falsely positive in some patients. If the CT scan shows evidence of pancreatic disruption but the ERCP demonstrates complete integrity of the primary, secondary, and tertiary pancreatic radicals, there is no need for operative intervention unless the patient has clinical findings suggesting some other intraabdominal injury.

URINARY TRACT INJURY.   Injury to the urinary tract is often initially suspected on the basis of gross or microscopic hematuria.[1,3] If the patient has hematuria (greater than 5 RBC/hpf) and has other indications for a laparotomy, the genitourinary tract needs to be assessed. This should be done as an emergency procedure in the preoperative period if the patient is stable. If the patient is not hemodynamically stable, it can be done as an emergency procedure during operation after control of other more life-threatening injuries has been completed.

When injury to the genitourinary tract is the only consideration, the emergency workup can be performed by means of a retrograde urethrogram, cystogram, and a pyelogram. A drip infusion pyelogram is obtained by infusing 2.0-2.5 ml/kg of 50% radioiodinated contrast agent over a 5-minute period while serial x-rays are obtained. If the genitourinary evaluation is performed in conjunction with assessment for other organ injuries in a stable patient, the renal evaluation can be achieved by means of an abdominal CT scan with oral and intravenous contrast.

Extremity Injuries and Neurovascular Function

Severe internal and external bleeding can occur with extremity trauma, especially if major vessels are torn. Fractures or severe muscle contusions can cause massive blood loss and extravasation of fluid into injured muscle or associated fascial compartments.

AXIOM   Early complete evaluation of neurovascular function is an important part of the examination of extremity injuries.

Assessment of extremity sensation and movement in injured patients cannot be overemphasized.[1,3] Less experienced house officers may focus on obvious injuries and may not look carefully for lack of extremity movements or impaired sensation during their resuscitation efforts. Furthermore, many patients, even when fully awake and aware of their paralysis, will seldom, if ever, volunteer such information. Sometimes the life-threatening, overwhelming nature of the other injuries distracts the whole team from recognizing an otherwise obvious paraplegia or quadriplegia. Occasionally, postmortem examination reveals a complete severance of the spinal cord in a patient in whom the resuscitation team has failed to recognize any neurological deficit. Such oversights by the treating team can create immense medicolegal problems even if it can be documented that the initial injury caused complete severance of the spinal cord. Comprehensive resuscitation forms filled out by experienced trauma surgeons, hopefully, can prevent such oversights.

Ongoing Assessment and Consultation

During the initial evaluation and resuscitation of the severely injured patient, multiple repeat assessments are necessary.[1] During these assessments, one should quickly examine the different systems as part of a 1- or 2-minute reassessment of the total patient. This must be done in order to be sure that areas which were previously cleared do not develop evidence of an injury with time. Repeat assessment of the cardiovascular system and pulmonary system is also done in conjunction with these repeat examinations. These repeated examinations are done in conjunction with the various specialty physicians who may become involved in the care of a multiply injured patient.

Throughout all of the resuscitation and evaluation period, one should follow guidelines based upon a well-established system of priorities, but one must also use common sense as it relates to doing what is best for the patient at that time. Following such guidelines, will provide the patient with the best chance for successful treatment and outcome.

⊘ FREQUENT ERRORS

In the Initial Evaluation and Management of Severely Injured Patients

1. *Not following the priorities of correction of airway, ventilation, and circulation problems in multiply injured patients.*
2. *Taking time at the scene to start intravenous lines or apply MAST to a hypotensive trauma victim who is just 10-15 minutes from the hospital.*
3. *Not having a designated team captain to oversee management of severely injured patients.*
4. *Forcing all trauma patients to lie flat on a cart even though they can obviously breathe better sitting up.*
5. *Starting an emergency subclavian line on the uninjured side of a patient with chest trauma.*
6. *Performing external cardiac massage in a patient with a cardiac arrest after truncal trauma.*
7. *Assuming that continued hypotension in a trauma patient is due to factors other than persistent severe bleeding or inadequate fluid resuscitation.*

8. *Using diuretics to increase urine output during the fluid-sequestration phase.*
9. *Relying on albumin or other colloids to correct hypovolemia or restore a normal plasma oncotic pressure after trauma.*
10. *Failing to obtain and carefully examine abdominal x-rays in patients who might have blunt duodenal injury.*

▼▼▼▼▼▼▼▼▼▼▼▼▼▼▼▼▼▼▼▼▼▼▼▼▼▼▼▼▼▼▼▼

SUMMARY POINTS

1. Trauma care in a properly functioning system should be independent of a patient's financial resources.
2. The priorities of care at the scene of an accident are establishment of an airway, maintenance of adequate ventilation, and control of external bleeding.
3. Although MAST can help splint lower extremity fractures and reduce associated blood loss, this device has little value in hypotensive patients in an urban setting.
4. When the transit time from the site of injury to the closest skilled emergency center is less than 15-20 minutes, time spent starting intravenous fluids at the scene is usually counterproductive.
5. A team captain is essential for optimal management of multiply injured patients.
6. Once a team captain is identified, all participants of the trauma care team must respect his position as the final arbiter.
7. One must avoid the temptation to force all trauma patients to lie flat on the cart and then restrain those who resist such positioning.
8. One should assume that an uncooperative or restless patient is either hypoxic, has a head injury, or is under the influence of drugs or alcohol.
9. When conflicting priorities exist, one should perform the procedure which provides the best chance for protecting life. One should not withhold critical therapy because of a possible procedure-related complication.
10. For trauma patients with severe hypovolemia, subclavian veins are often the quickest sites for establishing intravenous routes.
11. If an intravenous catheter is passed through a needle into a vein, the catheter is never pulled back within the needle.
12. Introducers should not be forced over guide wires into veins.
13. Subclavian catheterization should be performed on the side of injury in patients with chest wounds to reduce the chances of collapsing an uninjured lung.
14. With injuries in the neck or upper chest, at least one venous access should be inserted in a lower extremity. If the injury is in the abdomen, at least one intravenous route should be placed in a tributary of the superior vena cava.
15. If a patient with a cardiac arrest from a penetrating chest wound is not rapidly responding to external chest compressions and/or other resuscitation, an open thoracotomy with internal cardiac massage may be indicated.
16. The most urgent priorities in trauma resuscitation are establishment of an airway and adequate ventilation and control of external bleeding.
17. If tourniquets are not applied properly, they can increase bleeding and tissue loss.
18. Continued shock after trauma is usually due to continued bleeding or inadequate resuscitation.
19. The combination of prolonged shock and a severe head injury is lethal.
20. The configuration of the interstitial space matrix determines the ratio of the albumin concentrations in the plasma and interstitial fluid.
21. Resuscitation of shock in adults and older children should not be done with glucose containing solutions.
22. Significant fluid shifts out of the vascular space continue for 24-48 hours or longer after bleeding has been controlled.
23. Whenever an acute blood volume loss occurs, early administration of three times that amount of a balanced electrolyte solution will usually restore the blood volume to normal.

24. In previously young and healthy individuals, loss of 20 to 25% of the blood volume may be associated with minimal or no arterial hypotension.
25. A normal arterial blood pressure in a trauma patient may be associated with a significant reduction in extracellular fluid, urine output, cardiac output, and stroke volume.
26. In most hypovolemic patients, urine output is an important guide to the adequacy of fluid resuscitation.
27. Urine output will not reflect the adequacy of the fluid resuscitation if there are other factors present that can cause a diuresis.
28. If there is evidence of continued severe bleeding in a hypotensive patient, blood transfusions should be started early.
29. The initial resuscitation of trauma patients with moderate to severe blood loss should utilize both blood and crystalloid solutions.
30. Severe oliguria during and immediately following traumatic shock is a renal adaptation to the hypotension and should not be treated with diuretics.
31. A misinterpretation of Starling's equation has created confusion about the forces regulating fluid movement across capillary membranes.
32. The detrimental effects of albumin on myocardial, renal, and respiratory functions are interrelated and mitigate against its use in hypovolemic shock.
33. Exogenous albumin administration reduces immunoglobulin and coagulation protein synthesis and/or activity.
34. The CVP is useful in the hemodynamic monitoring of trauma patients but, like all tools, is limited in its application.
35. Large respirophasic variations in systolic blood pressure may be an early sign of hypovolemia.
36. Hypotension in the seriously injured patient is generally an indication for more blood and fluid replacement.
37. The first 60 minutes after trauma is the golden period for the diagnosis of injuries and aggressive treatment of hypovolemia.
38. The combination of shock and acute respiratory distress is highly lethal unless corrected rapidly.
39. Open chest wounds should not be covered or closed until a chest tube is in place.
40. Most life-threatening chest injuries with severe shock are due to massive severe hemorrhage.
41. Continued significant bleeding into the chest is an indication for thoracotomy.
42. The most urgent threat to life in patients with abdominal injury is severe intraperitoneal hemorrhage from injuries to the liver, spleen, or major vessels.
43. The most common cause for a false negative DPL after blunt trauma is a ruptured diaphragm, and the most common cause for a false positive DPL is a pelvic fracture.
44. When a stable patient is known to have a gunshot wound that entered the peritoneal cavity, a laparotomy should be performed regardless of the DPL findings.
45. It often takes 12 or more hours for bowel leakage to produce signs and symptoms of peritonitis.
46. Patients with abdominal trauma should have flat and upright films of the abdomen. This will help identify the retroperitoneal air that is present in many patients with blunt rupture of the retroperitoneal duodenum.
47. Retroperitoneal air, scoliosis, and blurring of the right psoas shadow on x-ray can be found soon after the injury in over 50% of patients with blunt retroperitoneal duodenal rupture.
48. Obtaining serial serum amylase measurements following blunt abdominal trauma can facilitate the diagnosis of pancreatic injury by demonstrating a rise in serum amylase levels at 6 or 12 hours, coinciding with increased abdominal pain and tenderness.
49. The definitive diagnosis of pancreatic disruption can be made with ERCP.
50. Early complete evaluation of neurovascular function is an important part of the examination of extremity injuries.

▲▲▲▲▲▲▲▲▲▲▲▲▲▲▲▲▲▲▲▲▲▲▲▲▲▲▲▲▲▲▲▲

REFERENCES

1. Committee on Trauma, American College of Surgeons. Advanced trauma life support course, instructor's manual. Chicago: American College of Surgeons, 1984:189.
2. Weiner S, Barrett S. Hypovolemic shock and resuscitation. In: Wiener S, Barrett S, eds. Trauma management for civilian and military physicians. Philadelphia: WB Saunders, 1986:37.
3. Lucas CE, Ledgerwood AM. Hemodynamic management of the injured. In: Capan LM, Miller SM, Turndorf H, eds. Trauma anesthesia and intensive care. Philadelphia: J.B. Lippincott, 1991:83.
4. McSwain NE. Pneumatic trousers and the management of shock. J Trauma 1977;17:719.
5. Mattox KL, Bickell W, Pepe P, Mangelsdorff AD. Prospective randomized evaluation of antishock MAST in post-traumatic hypotension. J Trauma 1986;26:779-786.
6. Mattox KL, Bickell W, Pepe P, et al. Prospective MAST study on 911 patients. J Trauma 1989;29:1104-1111.
7. Jennings TJ, Usaf C, Seaworth JF, et al. The effects of inflation of antishock trousers on hemodynamics in normovolemic subjects. J Trauma 1986;26:544.
8. Bellamy RF, DeGuzman LR, Pedersen DC. Immediate hemodynamic consequences of MAST inflation in normal and hypovolemic anesthetized swine. J Trauma 1984;24:889.
9. Burchard KW, Slotman GJ, Jed E, et al. Positive pressure respirators and pneumatic antishock garment application: hemodynamic response. J Trauma 1985;25:83.
10. Holcroft JW, Link DP, Lantz BMT, et al. Venous return and the pneumatic antishock garment in hypovolemic baboons. J Trauma 1984; 24:928.
11. Wangensteen SL, Ludewig RM, Eddy DM. The effect of external counterpressure on the intact circulation. Surg Gynecol Obstet 1968;127:253.
12. Aprahamian C, Gessert G, Banoyk DF, et al. MAST-associated compartment syndromes (MACS): a review. J Trauma 1989;29:549.
13. Carey LD, Lowery BD, Cloutier CT. Hemorrhagic shock. Curr Prob Surg 1971;8:1048.
14. Lucas CE. Resuscitation of the injured patient: the three phases of treatment. Surg Clin North Am 1977;57:3.
15. Moss GS. An argument in favor of electrolyte solution for early resuscitation. Surg Clin North Am 1972;52:3.
16. Shires GT, Canizaro PC, Carrico CJ. Shock. In: Schwartz SI, Shires GT, Spencer FC, Storer EH, eds. Principles of surgery, 4th ed. New York: McGraw-Hill, 1984:116.
17. Shires GT, Carrico CJ, Canizaro PC. Response of the extracellular fluid. In: Shires GT, ed. Shock: major problems in clinical surgery. Philadelphia: WB Saunders, 1973;13:15.
18. Boutros AR, Ruess R, Olson L, et al. Comparison of hemodynamic, pulmonary and renal effects of use of three types of fluids following major surgical procedures on the abdominal aorta. Crit Care Med 1979;7:9.
19. Hekmatpanah J. The management of head trauma. Surg Clin North Am 1973;53:47.
20. Monafo WW, Chuntrasakul C, Ayvazian VH. Hypertonic sodium solutions in the treatment of burn shock. Am J Surg 1973;126:778.
21. Bivins HG, Knopp R, dos Santos PAL. Blood volume distribution in the Trendelenburg position. Ann Emerg Med 1985;14:641.
22. Bickell WH, Pepe PE, Bailey ML, et al. Randomized trial of pneumatic antishock garments in the prehospital management of penetrating abdominal injuries. Ann Emerg Med 1987;16:653.
23. Pelligra R, Sandberg EC. Control of intractable abdominal bleeding by external counterpressure. JAMA 1979;241:708.
24. Lane PL, McLellan BA, Johns PD. Etiology of shock in blunt trauma. Can Med Assoc J 1985;133:199.
25. Pedowitz RA, Shackford SR. Non-cavitary hemorrhage producing shock in trauma patients: incidence and severity. J Trauma 1989;29:219.
26. Wilson RF. Science and shock: a clinical perspective. Ann Emerg Med 1985;14:714.
27. Lucas CE, Ledgerwood AM. The fluid problem in the critically ill. Surg Clin North Am 1983;63:439.
28. Dawson CW, Lucas CE, Ledgerwood AM. Altered interstitial fluid space dynamics and postresuscitation hypertension. Arch Surg 1981;116:657.
29. Lucas CE, Ledgerwood AM, Benishek DJ. Reduced oncotic pressure after shock. Arch Surg 1982;117:675.
30. Saxe JM, Guan ZX, Grabow D, et al. The myth of hyperglycemia-induced plasma volume expansion in shock. Surgical Forum 1988;39:73-74.
31. Cunningham JN, Shires GT, Wagner Y. Cellular transport defects in hemorrhagic shock. Surgery 1971;70:215.
32. Cunningham JN, Shires GT, Wagner Y. Changes in intracellular sodium and potassium content of red blood cells in trauma and shock. Am J Surg 1971;70:215.
33. Day B, Friedman SM. Red cell sodium and potassium in hemorrhagic shock measured by lithium substitution analysis. J Trauma 1980;20:52.
34. Shires T, Cunningham JN, Barke CRE, et al. Alterations in cellular membrane function during hemorrhagic shock. Ann Surg 1972;176:288.
35. Antonenko DR. Early structural changes in mitochondria in response to acute reductions in capillary flow on oxygen transport to tissues. Adv Med Biol 1976;75:165.
36. Smith JAR, Norman JN. The fluid of choice for resuscitation of severe shock. Br J Surg 1982;69:702.
37. McNamara JJ, Suehiro GT, Suehiro A, et al. Resuscitation from hemorrhagic shock. J Trauma 1983;23:552.
38. Hinshaw LB, Peterson M, Huse WM, et al. Regional blood flow in hemorrhagic shock. Am J Surg 1961;102:224.
39. Sheldon CA, Cerra FB, Bohnhoff N. Peripheral postcapillary venous pressure: a new, more sensitive monitor of effective blood volume during hemorrhagic shock and resuscitation. Surgery 1983;94:399.
40. Cullen DJ. Interpretation of blood pressure measurements in anesthesia. Anesthesiology 1974;40:6.
41. Lucas CE. Renal considerations in the injured patient. Surg Clin North Am 1982;62:133.
42. Perel A, Pizov R, Cotev S. Systolic blood pressure variation is a sensitive indicator of hypovolemia in ventilated dogs subjected to graded hemorrhage. Anesthesiology 1987;67:498.
43. Pizov R, Ya'ari Y, Perel A. Systolic pressure variation is greater during hemorrhage than during sodium nitroprusside-induced hypotension in ventilated dogs. Anesth Analg 1988;67:170.
44. Starling EH. On the absorption of fluids from the connective tissue spaces. J Physiol (London) 1896;19:312.
45. Hauser CJ, Shoemaker WC, Turpin I, et al. Oxygen transport responses to colloids and crystalloids in critically ill surgical patients. Surg Gynecol Obstet 1980;150:811.
46. Jelenko C III, Williams JB, Wheeler ML, et al. Studies in shock and resuscitation, I: use of a hypertonic, albumin containing, fluid demand regimen (HALFD) resuscitation. Crit Care Med 1979;7:157.
47. Shoemaker WC, Hauser CJ. Critique of crystalloid versus colloid therapy in shock and shock lung. Crit Care Med 1979;7:117.
48. Shoemaker WC, Schluchter M, Hopkins JA, et al. Comparison of the relative effectiveness of colloids and crystalloids in emergency resuscitation. Am J Surg 1981;142:73.
49. Twigley AJ, Hillman KM. The end of crystalloid era? A new approach to peri-operative fluid administration. Anaesthesia 1985;40:860.
50. Weil MH, Henning RJ, Puri VK. Colloid oncotic pressure: clinical significance. Crit Care Med 1979;7:113.
51. Ledgerwood AM, Lucas CE. Postresuscitation hypertension: etiology, morbidity, and treatment. Arch Surg 1974;108:531.
52. Dahn MS, Lucas CE, Ledgerwood AM. Negative inotropic effect of albumin resuscitation for shock. Surgery 1979;86:235.
53. Johnson SD, Lucas CE, Gerrick SJ, et al. Altered coagulation after albumin supplements for treatment of oligemic shock. Arch Surg 1979; 114:379.
54. Lucas CE, Kovalik, SG, Ledgerwood AM, et al. The cardiac effect of altered calcium homeostasis after albumin resuscitation. J Trauma 1981;21:275.
55. Lucas CE, Ledgerwood AM, Higgins RF. Impaired salt and water excretion after albumin resuscitation for hypovolemic shock. Surgery 1979;86:544.
56. Lucas CE, Ledgerwood AM, Higgins RF, et al. Impaired pulmonary function after albumin resuscitation from shock. J Trauma 1980;20:446.
57. Virgilio RW, Rice CL, Smith DE, et al. Crystalloid versus colloid resuscitation: is one better? Surgery 1979;85:129.
58. Velanovich V. Crystalloid versus colloid fluid resuscitation: a meta-analysis of mortality. Surgery 1989;105:65.
59. Faillace DF, Ledgerwood AM, Lucas CE, et al. Immunoglobulin changes after varied resuscitation regimens. J Trauma 1982;22:1.
60. Leibold W, Lucas CE, Ledgerwood AM, et al. Effect of albumin resuscitation on canine coagulation activity and content. Ann Surg 1983;198:630.
61. Lucas CE, Ledgerwood AM, Mammen EF. Altered coagulation protein content after albumin resuscitation. Ann Surg 1982;196:198.
62. Gallagher TJ, Banner MJ, Barnes P. Large volume crystalloid resuscitation does not increase extravascular lung water. Anesth Analg 1985;64:323.

63. Gallagher JD, Moore RA, Kerns D, et al. Effects of colloid or crystalloid administration on pulmonary extravascular water in the postoperative period after coronary artery bypass grafting. Anesth Analg 1985;64:753.

64. Transbaug RF, Elings VB, Christensen J, et al. Determinants of pulmonary interstitial fluid accumulation after trauma. J Trauma 1982;22:820.

65. Moss GS, Lowe RJ, Jilek J, et al. Colloid or crystalloid in the resuscitation of hemorrhagic shock. Surgery 1981;89:434.

66. Messmer K. Blood substitutes in shock therapy. In: Shires GT III, ed. Clinical surgery international: shock and related problems. Edinburgh: Churchill Livingstone, 1984;9:192.

67. Lower RJ, Moss GS, Jilek J, et al. Crystalloid versus colloid in the etiology of pulmonary failure after trauma: a randomized trial in man. Crit Care Med 1979;7:197.

68. Coonan TJ, Hope CE. Cardiorespiratory effects of change of body position. Can Anaesth Soc J 1983;30:424.

69. Gunteroth WG, Abel FL, Mullins GL. The effect of Trendelenburg's position on blood pressure and carotid flow. Surg Gynecol Obstet 1965;119:345.

70. Sibbald WJ, Paterson NAM, Holliday RL, et al. The Trendelenburg position: hemodynamic effects in hypotensive and normotensive patients. Crit Care Med 1979;7:218.

71. Taylor J, Weil MH. Failure of the Trendelenburg position to improve circulation during clinical shock. Surg Gynecol Obstet 1967;124:1005.

72. Reich DL, Konstadt SN, Raissi S, et al. Trendelenburg position and passive leg raising do not significantly improve cardiopulmonary performance in the anesthetized patient with coronary artery disease. Crit Care Med 1989;17:313.

73. Civetta JM, Gabel JC, Laver MB. Disparate ventricular function in surgical patients. Surg Forum 1971;22:136.

74. Gerber MJ, Hines RL, Barash PG. Arterial waveforms and systemic vascular resistance: is there a correlation? Anesthesiology 1987;66:823.

75. Coyle JP, Teplick RS, Long MC, et al. Respiratory variations in systemic arterial pressure as an indicator of volume status. Anesthesiology 1983;59:A53.

76. Robtham JL, Bell RL, Badke FR, et al. Left ventricular geometry during positive end-expiratory pressure in dogs. Crit Care Med 1985;13:617.

Chapter **3** Cardiopulmonary Resuscitation After Trauma

BRIAN J. O'NEIL, M.D.
ROBERT F. WILSON, M.D.

INTRODUCTION

Cardiac arrest can be defined as a sudden cessation of effective cardiac output. It may be due to asystole, ventricular fibrillation, or other arrhythmias, or any condition that reduces cardiac output to a negligible level.[1,2]

PITFALL ⊘

If a physician, confronted by a patient with a possible cardiac arrest, delays resuscitation because of uncertainty about the diagnosis, the chances for survival with intact neurologic function fall precipitously.

Every physician who may see critically ill or injured patients should have a clear idea of how cardiac arrest is diagnosed and treated.

PREHOSPITAL CARDIAC ARREST IN TRAUMA VICTIMS

Etiology

PREEXISTING DISEASES

Preexisting coronary artery disease may cause an acute myocardial infarction, which can then result in a motor vehicle accident or fall.[2] Various arrhythmias and heart block, such as with a Stokes-Adams attack, can also precipitate vascular collapse followed by trauma.

PITFALL ⊘

If the underlying cause of a cardiac arrest is not recognized and corrected immediately, successful resuscitation is apt to be infrequent and temporary.

Trauma itself can also precipitate an acute myocardial ischemia or infarction due to the related anxiety, pain, or hemorrhage.[2] If the myocardial ischemia is severe enough, it can progress to arrhythmias and cardiac arrest either with or without an antecedent period of shock.

NO PREEXISTING DISEASE

In young, healthy individuals, cardiac arrest usually results from: (a) severe brain injury, (b) exsanguination because of damage to major blood vessels or organs such as the spleen or liver, (c) previously undiagnosed cardiac abnormality, or (d) asphyxia due to damage to the airway, lungs, chest wall, or diaphragm. Occasionally, severe myocardial contusion may also cause a prehospital cardiac arrest.

Prehospital Care

AXIOM Prehospital cardiac arrest is almost uniformly lethal if it persists for more than 5 minutes or is due to problems that cannot be rapidly corrected.

If an out-of-hospital cardiac arrest is due only to airway obstruction or ventilatory insufficiency and it is managed rapidly and correctly in the field, survival rates are high; however, without such therapy these injuries are lethal.

Transportation of non-breathing patients to the hospital without appropriate airway and ventilatory management constitutes a failure of the EMS system.[2] A patient with hypovolemic cardiac arrest rarely survives if external cardiac massage and non-intubated ventilation are performed for more than 5 minutes prior to arrival at the hospital.[3] Prehospital intubation increased the length of successful CPR to 9.4 minutes in this same study.[4] Consequently, airway control, intravenous fluid administration, and in some cases, the PASG should be employed as needed to prevent hypovolemic cardiac arrest.

Prehospital cardiac arrest management should include immediate establishment of an airway and ventilation with 100% oxygen, preferably via an endotracheal tube. External cardiac massage provided to most truncal trauma victims is apt to cause much more harm than good.[5] An exception, of course, would be the trauma victim without significant truncal injury in cardiac arrest.

If possible, while en route to the hospital, Ringer's lactate should be administered via a large bore (14-gauge) peripheral intravenous line. Fluid administered is probably helpful if the patient is in severe shock and has stopped bleeding or has compressible bleeding. Recent studies by Pepe and Mattox[6,7] suggest that aggressive preoperative fluid resuscitation in patients with shock due to major penetrating truncal injuries may increase bleeding and reduce survival. Thus, the benefit of such lines in this patient population may be only to reduce the time in the ED.

Causes of Cardiac Arrest in the ED

In our experience, the most frequent time for a critically ill or injured patient to have a cardiac arrest in the ED is during or shortly after endotracheal intubation. This can occur because of any one of at least seven reasons.

INADEQUATE PRE-INTUBATION OXYGENATION

AXIOM Pre-intubation oxygenation is extremely important in patients in acute respiratory failure after trauma.

It is important to ventilate patients with acute respiratory failure, ideally with an ambu bag and mask and 100% O_2, prior to attempts at endotracheal intubation. This not only reduces the severe hypoxia usually present, but also aids in keeping the oxygen saturation up during intubation. Two to 3 minutes of effective bag-mask ventilation with 100% O_2 can raise the arterial PO_2 of most patients to 200-300 mm Hg. This is usually enough to prevent hypoxemia even if the patient is then apneic for 2-3 minutes.[8]

AXIOM Pulse oximetry should be used in all patients with severe trauma especially during and following emergency intubation.

If a pulse oximeter is attached to all severely injured patients, it will soon become obvious that many of them are quite hypoxemic, even if intubated before arrival at the hospital. The limitations of pulse oximetry in accurately diagnosing hypoxia include anemia, dyshemoglobinemias (such as met or carboxyhemoglobin) intravascular dyes, and poor perfusion at the probe site because of hypotension, vasoconstriction, or hypothermia.[9]

AXIOM   Any manipulations of the upper airway, such as laryngoscopy, are prone to make hypoxemia worse. If this is not recognized and corrected rapidly, morbidity and mortality will increase.

ESOPHAGEAL INTUBATION

During emergency intubations, especially in uncooperative patients, it is easy to unknowingly insert the endotracheal tube into the esophagus. Some ways to help ensure that the tube is in the trachea include: (a) visualizing the tube going between the vocal cords (which can easily be misinterpreted by inexperienced intubators), (b) noting the compliance of the pilot balloon (when the cuff is being inflated, the pressure in the pilot balloon is less if the tube is in the esophagus), (c) noting the compliance of the ventilating bag (it is initially easier to ventilate the stomach than the lungs), (d) palpating the inflated balloon of the endotracheal tube in the trachea in the lower neck just above the sternal notch, (e) looking for breath condensation in the tube (this generally occurs if the tube is in the trachea, but it is not 100% reliable), (f) looking and feeling for anterior and lateral chest wall motion as the ambu bag is squeezed, (g) auscultating both axillas and epigastrium (if the breath sounds in the epigastrium are better than those in the lateral chest, or if gurgling or tympanitic sounds are heard, the tube is in the esophagus), and (h) actually measuring the end-tidal carbon dioxide with a capnograph or disposable $ETCO_2$ detector. The $ETCO_2$ in the esophagus is close to 0.

AXIOM   If there is any suspicion that the endotracheal tube is in the esophagus, it should be replaced.

There is a tendency to immediately pull out an endotracheal tube if one thinks it is in the esophagus. However, insertion of the new endotracheal tube may be much easier with the initial tube still in the esophagus. This will also decrease the incidence of aspiration.

INTUBATION OF A MAIN STEM BRONCHUS

AXIOM   Even if the endotracheal tube is correctly placed, it is easy for it to move down into a main stem bronchus, especially on the right, particularly if the patient is small and agitated.

The tip of the endotracheal tube moves up and down several cm as the head and neck move from complete extension to complete flexion. During CPR, some patients become extubated, and some have the tip of their endotracheal tube end up in the right or left main stem bronchus. Consequently, the chest must be repeatedly auscultated to ensure that the breath sounds are equal and adequate bilaterally.

AXIOM   Not infrequently, poor breath sounds on the left side in an intubated patient with chest trauma are due to a misplaced endotracheal tube rather than a left hemopneumothorax.

EXCESS VENTILATORY PRESSURES

If the patient is hypovolemic, excessive positive pressure ventilation will further reduce venous return, and a critical reduction in the venous return can increase hypotension and cause cardiac arrest. Hypovolemic patients should be ventilated relatively cautiously until the hypovolemia is at least partially corrected and venous return is improved. If the lung has blebs or a penetrating injury, bagging the patient vigorously can either cause or worsen a tension pneumothorax. Even with normal lungs, ventilatory pressures exceeding 60-80 H_2O, can cause interstitial emphysema or pneumothorax, again further reducing venous return.

SYSTEMIC AIR EMBOLISM

AXIOM   Severe hemoptysis after trauma is a relative indication for an emergency thoracotomy, especially if there is evidence of air embolism.

Any patient with a lung injury, particularly if there is hemoptysis, should be considered at risk for developing a systemic air embolus, especially if positive pressure ventilation is used. In addition, patients with hemoptysis are at risk for flooding normal alveoli with blood, which can quickly cause severe hypoxemia.[10]

AXIOM   Any new cardiovascular or neurologic changes occurring during or just after endotracheal intubation and positive pressure ventilation should be considered due to systemic air emboli until proven otherwise.

VASOVAGAL RESPONSES

Vasovagal responses are rare after trauma, but they can occur, especially with gastric insufflation or during insertion of endotracheal, nasogastric, or chest tubes. One should particularly look for this problem if the patient has an inappropriately slow pulse rate. Patients with an inappropriately slow pulse rate after trauma, not secondary to spinal cord injury or medications, have a poor prognosis and must be watched carefully.[11]

AXIOM   Inappropriately slow pulse rates after major trauma can cause several problems because: (a) there is an increased incidence of arrhythmias, (b) the cardiac output is often reduced, and (c) the patients are more prone to have a vasovagal response.

DEVELOPMENT OF SEVERE ALKALOSIS

Patients who have emergency intubation are often hyperventilated very vigorously, and this can drive the PCO_2 down to less than 20 mm Hg. If the plasma bicarbonate levels are normal (24 mEq/L), this degree of hypocarbia will raise the pH to 7.70 or higher. If the plasma bicarbonate is elevated to 30 mEq/L or higher, as it can be in some patients with COPD, the hypocarbia will drive the pH even higher. An arterial pH rise is associated with a shift to the right of the oxyhemoglobin dissociation curve. For each increase of 0.10 pH, there is a 10% decrease in the oxygen available to the tissue, and a pH greater than 7.55 is associated with a poor prognosis.[12]

AXIOM   Sudden severe alkalosis can reduce ionized calcium and magnesium levels by 15 to 24% (5 to 8% decrease for each 0.1 pH rise) which may cause severe arrhythmias.[13]

Cardiac Arrest in the OR

Operating room cardiac arrest in trauma patients is usually due to continued severe hypovolemic shock, and is best treated by open cardiac massage and cross-clamping of the descending thoracic aorta while fluids and blood are rapidly infused. Other correctable etiologies of cardiac arrest, such as pericardial tamponade, tension pneumothorax, hyperkalemia, hypoxia, severe acidosis, hypothermia, and air embolism, must also be ruled out. In severe retrohepatic caval or hepatic vein injuries, iatrogenic occlusion of the inferior vena cava (IVC), in an effort to reduce blood loss, can also cause sudden cardiac arrest secondary to further reduction of preload and cardiac output.

Cardiac Arrest in the ICU or Wards

Cardiac arrest in trauma patients in the ICU or wards should be treated like most other cardiac arrests, except one should be particularly looking for correctable causes such as hypovolemia, pericardial tamponade, pneumothorax, air embolism, or airway obstruction.

PATHOPHYSIOLOGY

The two most frequent types of arrhythmias causing cardiac arrest are ventricular fibrillation and asystole.

Ventricular Fibrillation

Ventricular fibrillation is a random chaotic twitching of the myocardium that produces no functional contractions. After cardiac ischemia, whether secondary to an MI or hypovolemia, there is enhanced automaticity of myocardial cells,[14] leading to ventricular ectopic beats. Re-entrant mechanisms may also be facilitated by biochemical changes at the junction of the ischemic and non-ischemic tissue.[15] Bradycardia, because of the long diastolic intervals, also increases the risk of ventricular escape beats and tachyarrhythmias.

PITFALL ⊘

> *If acid-base balance and arterial blood gases are not monitored closely in patients with traumatic or ischemic myocardial damage, ventricular fibrillation may occur suddenly and prove difficult to reverse.*

The myocardial fibrillation threshold is reduced by increased levels of circulating catecholamines, such as norepinephrine and epinephrine, and this effect is compounded if concurrent hypoxemia or acidosis is present. Drugs which can increase the incidence of ectopic beats and tachyarrhythmias include digitalis and quinidine in toxic doses, diuretics, and beta agonists. The risk of ventricular fibrillation is increased following an acute myocardial infarction and during prolonged severe hypovolemia, hypoxia, or acidosis. These abnormalities may also cause other arrhythmias such as premature ventricular beats, A-V nodal or bundle branch block, ventricular tachycardia, or supraventricular tachyarrhythmia.

Ventricular Asystole

Ventricular asystole after trauma is essentially universally fatal.[16] For ventricular asystole to occur and persist, not only must supraventricular impulse formation and/or conduction pathways fail, but the myocardial insult must be so extensive that normal ventricular escape mechanisms are ineffectual. Occasionally, asystole is preceded by sinus-node dysfunction and varying degrees of A-V nodal or bundle branch blocks. The incidence of asystole is increased by factors such as excessive pain or fear, which can increase vagal·tone.[15]

Other Rhythms

Ventricular tachycardia, electromechanical dissociation (now referred to as pulseless electrical activity), and a number of other arrhythmias may also be associated with ineffective cardiac function.

AXIOM   Ventricular tachycardia without hypotension can often be treated with medications alone, but immediate cardioversion is indicated if associated hypotension or instability (i.e., chest pain, CHF, or signs of end organ hypoperfusion) is present.

DIAGNOSIS

The cardinal signs of cardiac arrest include lack of a palpable pulse or audible heart beat plus loss of cerebral or brain stem function, such as unresponsiveness and apnea. Although generally reliable when considered altogether, taken individually, these signs can be misleading. If the stroke volume is low, it may produce a non-palpable pulse or unresponsiveness. If there is loss of pulses during a trauma resuscitation and the cardioscope reveals a fairly normal rhythm, a true cardiac arrest probably did not occur, but the cardiac output is usually greatly decreased.

If a cardiac arrest is suspected during an operation, the surgeon should immediately palpate the largest vessel in the field. During an abdominal operation, one can palpate either the aorta or the pericardial diaphragm to ascertain whether or not the heart is still beating. There is a significant false positive rate with asystole on the cardioscope, and this is usually due to lead displacement. Therefore, it is imperative to check all the leads if asystole is seen on the ECG monitor.

In some instances, a cardiac arrest is not suspected until severe cyanosis develops and/or the patient becomes apneic. Unfortunately, attempts to breathe or gasp do not always stop immediately after a cardiac arrest, and the patient may continue to have some sort of respiratory effort for 20 to 30 seconds after the heart has stopped. In addition, if the patient is anemic, cyanosis may not develop until blood flow or ventilation has stopped for more than 30 to 60 seconds and the arterial oxygen saturation falls below 50-60%. If the patient is receiving ventilatory assistance or is under general anesthesia and if the end-tidal CO_2 ($P_{ET}CO_2$) is monitored on a capnograph, a sudden drop in the $P_{ET}CO_2$ is diagnostic of either a cardiac arrest, disconnection of the ventilatory tubing, or movement of the endotracheal tube out of the trachea.

PITFALL ⊘

> *If the diagnosis of cardiac arrest is made only after the patient has had a convulsion, brain damage has probably already occurred.*

Not infrequently a cardiac arrest is noticed only after the patient has had a convulsion or regurgitated gastric contents. It is then, often mistakenly, assumed that the convulsion or aspiration actually caused the cardiac arrest. In many instances, it is not possible to determine whether the convulsion was a result of cerebral hypoperfusion or whether the convulsion itself caused the hypoxic cardiac arrest. In general, however, the convulsion is due to the cardiac arrest and not the reverse.

AXIOM   Although regurgitation of gastric contents can be the cause of a cardiac arrest, the reverse is usually true.

Use of a cardiac monitor is the most reliable way, besides direct visualization, of monitoring for cardiac arrest; however, cardioscopic asystole is frequently due to lead displacement. If a suspected cardiac arrest occurs and a cardioscope or ECG is not immediately available, the physician must establish whether a true cardiac arrest has occurred and what the etiology may be. If a cardiac arrest has occurred, immediate aggressive therapy is indicated.

PITFALL ⊘

> *If critically ill or injured patients undergoing surgery or resuscitation are not continuously monitored with a cardioscope, the diagnosis and treatment of a cardiac arrest may be significantly delayed.*

Patients susceptible to developing sudden hypoxia, hypotension, and metabolic or electrolyte abnormalities should be monitored for arrhythmias with a cardioscope. In the trauma patient, these abnormalities and arrhythmias are most likely to be noted during: (a) transport to the hospital, (b) the initial emergency department resuscitation, (c) induction of general anesthesia, or (d) in the immediate postoperative period.

TECHNIQUES OF CARDIOPULMONARY RESUSCITATION

Resuscitation of a cardiac arrest should begin immediately. A mnemonic frequently used in teaching the techniques of cardiopulmonary resuscitation are the letters, A, B, C, D; these can stand for airway, breathing, circulation, defibrillation, drugs, and definitive therapy.

Airway

HISTORY

Since about 1900, endotracheal intermittent positive-pressure ventilation (IPPV) and open-chest manual cardiac massage have been used effectively to treat cardiac arrest in operating rooms.[17,18] Although some of the individual steps of closed-chest CPR and defibrillation had been used in animal research for over half a century, their importance was not recognized nor were these steps combined into an effective system for resuscitation until the 1950s.[17,19]

In 1954, Elam et al[20] published measurements of the effectiveness of mouth-to-mask and mouth-to-tube ventilation in anesthetized adults. These studies proved that exhaled air can be used as a resuscitative gas. Indeed, in 1958, Safar et al[21] proved that direct mouth-to-mouth ventilation in curarized adult human volunteers without an endotracheal tube was superior to the chest-pressure arm-lift methods being taught at that time. Subsequently, Gordon et al[22] confirmed the superiority of mouth-to-mouth techniques over manual chest compression and relaxation methods for ventilating children.

TECHNIQUES FOR PROVIDING AN AIRWAY

A patent airway must be established without delay in patients who are apneic or unable to protect their airways. Since, in trauma, it is nearly impossible to be sure cervical trauma has not occurred, we recommend initially pulling the mandible forward with jaw thrust or chin lift maneuvers, or inserting a nasal or oropharyngeal airway. A plastic oral airway, which should only be used in unconscious patients, can not only hold the tongue forward and allow suction of secretions from the mouth and pharynx, but it can also prevent the patient from clamping his jaws shut.

Although an endotracheal tube provides much better ventilation than mask-to-mouth techniques and can greatly reduce gastric insufflation and subsequent aspiration of gastric contents, a significant amount of expertise is needed to insert it rapidly, especially if the patient has a short "bull" neck, stiff jaws, or excessive pharyngeal and laryngeal secretions.

PITFALL ⊘

If an inexperienced individual attempts to insert an endotracheal tube during cardiopulmonary resuscitation, the prolonged interruption of ventilation and cardiac massage may be fatal.

Unfortunately, it sometimes becomes a matter of pride for an individual to insert an endotracheal tube successfully. However, if the tube cannot be inserted in less than 30 seconds, that attempt at intubation should stop, and the patient should be ventilated by mask with 100% oxygen for 2-3 minutes before attempting again. If the endotracheal tube is soft, a stylet can often be of assistance in angling it anteriorly to reach between the vocal cords.

AXIOM If an adequate airway cannot be rapidly established with an oral airway or endotracheal tube in an apneic patient, an emergency coniotomy (cricothyroidotomy) should be performed.

Ventilation

Ventilation can usually be provided effectively and safely with a bag-mask set-up or a bag-endotracheal tube connection. The chest should rise perceptively with each breath. If the chest does not seem to inflate with bag-mask ventilation, but the abdomen does, the upper airway is probably not open properly, and the position of the head, neck, mandible, and/or oral airway should be adjusted and cricoid pressure (Sellick maneuver) should be applied.

AXIOM Patients with severe trauma are hypermetabolic and often have an oxygen debt requiring a minute ventilation that is at least twice normal.

Maintenance of Circulation

HISTORY

From the early 1900s until 1956, when Zoll et al[23] reported successful use of external countershock for ventricular fibrillation, resuscitation of cardiac arrest was performed primarily as open cardiac massage in the operating room (OR), and defibrillation was only done on an exposed heart.

In 1958, Kouwenhoven and Knickerbocker noted that a significant cardiac output could be generated by intermittent compression of the chest in dogs.[19] By 1961, Jude et al[24] reported on 118 cases of external cardiac massage in patients. In 1961, Safar et al[25] described specific steps to take to ensure adequate ventilation of the lungs during closed chest CPR.

TECHNIQUES AVAILABLE

Once pulselessness has occurred, some form of "artificial circulation" must be rapidly provided to maintain life. Methods of artificial circulation include: (a) multiple variations of "closed chest cardiac massage," which can be performed anywhere by anyone; (b) open-chest cardiac massage, or (c) emergency cardiopulmonary bypass. If exsanguination is the cause of the pulselessness, rapid control of hemorrhage and blood replacement are essential.

External Cardiac Massage

PHYSIOLOGIC POTENTIALS AND LIMITATIONS. Kouwenhoven et al[19] assumed that the arterial blood flow produced by external CPR was the result of direct compression of the heart between the sternum and spine (the so-called "heart-pump" mechanism). However, they also recognized that external chest compressions increased pressures throughout the chest so that the venous pressure peaks were as high as the aortic pressure peaks.

In the 1980s, Weisfeldt et al[26] demonstrated that external chest compressions can produce forward blood flow by increasing overall intrathoracic pressure, like that occurring in cough CPR (the so-called "chest-pump" mechanism), even if the heart itself is not compressed. It is thought that forward blood flow is possible with the "chest-pump" mechanism because veins have valves (even the large veins entering the heart have rudimentary valves).[27]

AXIOM External CPR probably produces vital organ perfusion by a combination of chest-pump and heart-pump mechanisms.

In spite of valves in the internal jugular veins, external CPR increases cerebral venous and intracranial pressures, which can reduce cerebral perfusion pressures and oxygenation.[28] In contrast, direct or open massage of the heart,[17,18] and emergency cardiopulmonary bypass (using veno-arterial pumping with an interposed oxygenator)[29] does not occlude the veins in the chest and, therefore, can provide near-normal aortovenous perfusion pressures.

Experimental and clinical data suggest that, for a successful outcome, CPR should produce at least 20% of the normal cardiac output and a coronary perfusion pressure of at least 20-30 mm Hg in humans.[30] These pressures are more likely to be approached during external CPR if high dose epinephrine (0.1-0.2 mg/kg) is administered to increase systemic vascular resistance (SVR), aortic diastolic pressure (ADP), and coronary perfusion pressure (CPP). Coronary perfusion pressure is aortic diastolic pressure minus right atrial diastolic pressure (CPP = ADP-RADP).[31] Cardiac outputs and cerebral and myocardial blood flows measured in animals and patients during external CPR without drugs have ranged between 0 and 30% of normal. Various modifications of external CPR to improve blood flow have generally proved disappointing, with the possible exception of inter-opposed abdominal and chest compressions, which increased resuscitation and discharged rates when compared with standard CPR in ICU patients.[26]

TECHNICAL CONSIDERATIONS

Importance of a Firm Surface.   It is important that the patient lie on a firm surface while external cardiac massage is applied. It is virtually impossible to compress the chest adequately if the energy of compression is transmitted to an underlying mattress.

Compression of the Chest.   To perform external cardiac massage, the heel of one hand, not the palm, is placed over the lower half of the sternum. The other hand is placed on top of the first hand. In the adult, the sternum is depressed about 3 to 5 cm (1.0-1.5 inches) with each compression. The ideal rate for cardiac massage in adults is about 80 times per minute. Inexperienced personnel tend to massage too rapidly, thereby reducing the time for heart filling between compressions.

PITFALL ⊘

> *If cardiac massage is performed too rapidly or if the pressure on the heart is not released quickly after each compression, the diastolic filling of the heart may be significantly impaired.*

If the pressure on the heart or chest is not released immediately after each compression, diastolic filling of the heart is impaired and the stroke volume will tend to remain extremely low. Other causes of poor ventricular filling include cardiac tamponade, hypovolemia, and pneumothorax.

In the shock unit of the old Detroit General Hospital, patients often had intra-arterial catheters for continuous pressure monitoring, thus the effects of cardiac massage could be directly observed. Most house officers provided a systolic pressure of only about 40 to 60 mm Hg during their initial external chest compressions. However, if they viewed the intra-arterial pressures produced with their efforts, they could usually adjust their technique to increase intra-arterial pressures by 50 to 100%.

Since a significant amount of strength and stamina is needed to depress the sternum 3 to 5 cm at 80 times per minute for more than a few minutes, persons performing external cardiac massage should position themselves properly utilizing the weight of the upper body by bending at the waist. To accomplish this, one can stand on a footstool at the bedside or kneel on one leg next to the patient. If proper help is available, individuals should alternate about every 5 minutes, depending on their strength and endurance. Mechanical devices for performing external massage may be of great value if rapidly applied and closely monitored.

PITFALL ⊘

> *If external cardiac massage is interrupted for more than a few seconds at a time, additional ischemic damage to the brain, heart, and other vital organs may occur.*

Under no circumstance should external cardiac massage be interrupted for more than a few seconds at a time, since it usually provides less than a quarter of the patient's normal cardiac output.[32] Flow to the vital organs is already compromised and further interruptions of myocardial or cerebral blood flow are not well tolerated.

It is our personal observation that, as the individual performing cardiopulmonary resuscitation becomes increasingly tired, he or she seems to spend more time watching the patient's response to each drug and each attempt at defibrillation.

Even if relatively normal electrical activity is restored and some cardiac output is obtained, it is our experience from multiple cardiac surgeries, that cardiac massage should be continued until the patient,

with preload and inotropic support as needed, can achieve a definitely palpable carotid or femoral pulse. If an intra-arterial catheter is in place, the mean arterial pressure should be at least 60 to 70 mm Hg.

Prolonged External Cardiac Massage.   External cardiac compression becomes less effective and myocardial and cerebral blood flow progressively decrease with increased downtime.[33] Of 1,445 patients in eight studies of failed prehospital resuscitation, the discharge survival rate was 0.7% (10 patients) with six of the survivors having a transient pulse in the field.[34]

AXIOM   After 20 minutes of unsuccessful resuscitation, further interventions are likely to be futile, except when cardiac arrest occurs during hypothermia.[35]

Interposed Abdominal Compression.   The use of aortic counterpulsation during cardiopulmonary resuscitation (CPR) was first described by Molokhia et al[36] in an open-chest canine model. They demonstrated that manual aortic compression during open-chest cardiac massage significantly improved coronary sinus blood flow.

The use of interposed abdominal compression (IAC) during closed-chest CPR augments aortic diastolic pressure and improves artificial circulation in animals[37] and humans[38] with cardiac arrest. IAC-CPR has been shown to significantly improve coronary perfusion,[38] cardiac output,[39] and common carotid artery blood flow[40] when compared with standard CPR.

Recently, Sack et al[41] showed increased patient survival with IAC-CPR (Fig. 3-1). In his study of 135 resuscitation attempts in 103 ICU patients, return of spontaneous circulation was significantly greater in the group receiving IAC-CPR than in the group receiving standard CPR (51% versus 27%, P = .007). At hospital discharge, significantly more patients were alive in the IAC group than in the control group (25% versus 7%, P = .02). In addition, eight (17%) of the 48 patients who received IAC during CPR survived and were neurologically intact at discharge, compared with only three (6%) of the 55 patients from the standard CPR group.

AXIOM   The addition of IAC to standard CPR may improve survival following in-hospital cardiac arrest.

COMPLICATIONS OF EXTERNAL CPR.   Serious iatrogenic injuries to thoracic and abdominal structures are not infrequent in autopsy findings following external cardiac compressions in patients with thoracic trauma. The incidence of such iatrogenic injuries range from 10 to

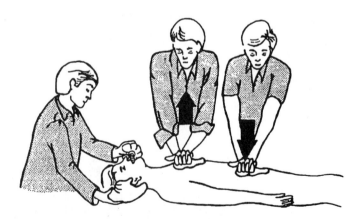

FIGURE 3-1   Interposed abdominal counterpulsation during human cardiopulmonary resuscitation. All patients underwent intubation. The abdominal compression rate was equal to the chest compression rate of 80/min to 100/min. The abdominal compression force was standardized at 100 ± 20 mm Hg. (From: Sack JB, Kesselbrenner MB, Bregman D. JAMA 1992;267:381.)

40%, with about 30% of the victims having rib fractures and almost 20% having sternal fractures.[42,43] One may also find mediastinal and pericardial hemorrhage and cardiac contusion.[43] Less frequent, but potentially lethal complications include lacerations to the heart, large vessels, liver, spleen, or gastroesophageal area. In older individuals with severe emphysema or a rigid chest wall, fractures of the sternum or ribs may be unavoidable if effective compressions are to be administered.

AXIOM Vigorous external cardiac massage can cause internal damage, especially in patients with recent truncal surgery or trauma.

The incidence and severity of injuries with external CPR is increased when less experienced operators perform the compressions. This is usually due to improper positioning of the hands or application of excessive pressure. The incidence of complications also increases with the duration of the resuscitation procedure, especially in the elderly.[43]

Open-chest (Direct) Cardiac Massage

In a review of the historical aspects of cardiac resuscitation, Barber and Wadden[44] pointed out that the first suggestion for open cardiac massage was made by Shiff in 1874 as a resuscitative measure for chloroform induced cardiac arrest. However, the first successful open cardiac resuscitation was not performed until 1889 by Tuffier.[45] In 1901, Ingelsrod resuscitated a postinjury cardiac arrest victim with open cardiac massage.[46]

For the next 50 to 60 years, cardiac arrest in the operating room was treated by open cardiac massage. Claude Beck popularized internal cardiac massage and in 1947[47] he established the precedent of electrical defibrillation in the operating room. In 1953, Stephenson et al[17] reported the clinical outcome of open cardiac massage on 1,200 patients, 29% of whom were successfully resuscitated and discharged alive from the hospital.

In normovolemic cardiac arrest, open cardiac massage has been shown to generate aortic pressures of about 60% of pre-arrest values.[48] Studies have also indicated that reasonable coronary and cerebral perfusion can be maintained for up to 30 minutes during manual open cardiac massage.[32] Since external chest compressions provide only 3-10% of the normal coronary and cerebral perfusion, there is increasing discussion about returning to open cardiac massage for resuscitation.

Although the advantages of open cardiac massage are not generally accepted as an independent indication for thoracotomy in non-traumatic cardiac arrest, the results of emergency department thoracotomies in patients sustaining cardiac arrest after penetrating chest trauma have been promising.[2]

AXIOM If patients with an otherwise good prognosis have a cardiac arrest due to a mechanical problem (such as pericardial tamponade) and do not respond rapidly to closed cardiac massage, open cardiac massage may substantially improve their survival.

In spite of the increased morbidity and mortality of thoracotomy in cardiac arrest patients, one should not hesitate to perform open cardiac massage if the cardiac arrest is secondary to a penetrating chest wound.[49] Prerequisites for performing open cardiac massage include: (a) a physician experienced in performing thoracotomies and direct cardiac massage, and (b) an ED/OR system which can rapidly provide the needed surgical support.

Monitoring Preload

AXIOM Because many patients with a cardiac arrest have a tendency to develop congestive heart failure, a large fluid bolus should not be given unless there is evidence of hypovolemia.

As soon as resources are available, two intravenous catheters at least 18-gauge in size should be inserted percutaneously or by a cutdown. One of the catheters should be long enough to be advanced into a large central vein for monitoring the central venous pressure (CVP) and for administration of drugs centrally.

AXIOM If a patient remains hypotensive after an otherwise successful cardiac resuscitation, insertion of a pulmonary-artery catheter should be considered.

After a cardiac arrest or acute myocardial infarction, severe left ventricular failure may persist, allowing the left atrial pressure to rise rapidly and pulmonary edema to develop in spite of a low CVP.[50] Under such circumstances, pulmonary artery wedge pressures (PAWP) have been thought to reflect left heart filling pressures much better than the CVP. It is increasingly apparent that with changes in ventricular compliance and pulmonary vascular resistance, monitoring of right ventricular end-diastolic volumes may be preferable to PAWP.[51]

Evaluating CPR Effectiveness

To evaluate the effectiveness of the resuscitative efforts during and after CPR, the pulse, blood pressure, spontaneous respirations, skin color, state of consciousness, and electrocardiographic changes should be closely monitored.

PALPABLE PULSES. There is no correlation between a palpable pulse during external CPR and an actual fluid wave; therefore, there is no way to estimate cardiac output by palpating pulses. The deceptiveness of palpable pulses has been highlighted by Weil et al[52] who noted that even with the abdominal aorta completely occluded by an inflated balloon, the pressure waves from the proximal aorta were transmitted to various branches of the aorta distal to the occluding balloon.

INTRA-ARTERIAL PRESSURE MONITORING. Direct intra-arterial pressure monitoring during external CPR in patients has consistently demonstrated that the maximal aortic pressures generated during precordial compression correlates poorly with cardiac output.[32,48,52] Normal or higher systolic pressures are frequently found in spite of cardiac outputs which are substantially less than 50% of pre-arrest levels.

AXIOM Measurement of CVP and both mean and diastolic aortic pressures during cardiac arrest can serve as useful indicators of both systemic and coronary perfusion pressures.[52]

If the right atrial and aortic diastolic pressures are known, one can calculate coronary perfusion pressures. However, placement of arterial and central venous or pulmonary artery catheters during or following CPR may be limited to the intensive care setting or the OR.

ACID-BASE MONITORING

AXIOM Acid-base monitoring during cardiac resuscitation should include arterial and mixed venous blood, lactate levels, and expired CO_2.[52]

Studies in animals and humans during CPR have demonstrated increased systemic venoarterial PCO_2 differences which are directly proportional to the reduced pulmonary blood flow. Normally, arterial blood has a pH which is 0.05-0.06 higher, a bicarbonate which is 1.1 mEq/L lower, and PCO_2 which is 6-8 mm Hg lower than central venous or mixed venous blood.[53] In patients with a very low cardiac output, the PCO_2 differences may be increased two- to fourfold. In one study of 16 patients during cardiac arrest, the arterial pH was 7.41 and the arterial PCO_2 was 31 mm Hg, but the mixed venous gases showed a severe respiratory acidosis (pH = 7.10 and PCO_2 73 mm Hg). If bicarbonate had been given to treat the acidosis, the mixed venous PCO_2 would have risen even higher, causing an increasing cellular acidosis (Fig. 3-2).

CAPNOGRAPHY.   Normally, arterial, alveolar, and end-tidal (ET) PCO_2 measurements are almost identical, measuring about 40 mm Hg. However, if cardiac output falls substantially, the alveolar PCO_2 falls and the end-tidal PCO_2 falls even more. When $P_{ET}CO_2$ has been simultaneously measured during CPR and compared with the cardiac index in experimental animals and patients, the direct linear correlation between them was significant (r = .76)[54]

AXIOM   The $P_{ET}CO_2$ is a relatively good indicator of the quantity of (pulmonary) blood flow generated with closed-chest CPR.

A number of studies have confirmed that the cessation of systemic blood flow after cardiac arrest causes a sharp decrease in $P_{ET}CO_2$ to levels near zero.[52] With chest compression, the increase in $P_{ET}CO_2$ directly correlates with pulmonary blood flow, coronary perfusion pressure (CPP), and cardiac output (CO). When spontaneous circulation is restored, an abrupt further increase in $P_{ET}CO_2$ occurs to levels that transiently exceed pre-arrest values. This is secondary to the washout of the elevated venous CO_2. $P_{ET}CO_2$ can also be used to assess the effectiveness of compressions during CPR. The $P_{ET}CO_2$ is decreased by increased ventilation or administration of epinephrine. Epinephrine increases CPP but also constricts the pulmonary vasculature. $P_{ET}CO_2$ is transiently increased by the administration of bicarbonate.

The $P_{ET}CO_2$, like the coronary perfusion pressure, correlates with resuscitability and, therefore, may serve as a prognostic indicator.[55] If the $P_{ET}CO_2$ stays less then 10 mm Hg during CPR, the likelihood of successful resuscitation is remote (Fig. 3-3).

Definitive Therapy

Once the airway has been opened, adequate ventilation established, and circulation provided by internal or external massage, definitive therapy based on the etiology of the cardiac arrest should be initiated. Specific etiologies of a cardiac arrest include arrhythmias (ventricular fibrillation, ventricular tachycardia, asystole, bradycardia), hypovolemia, hypoxemia, congestive heart failure, massive pulmonary embolus or myocardial infarction, and the more easily treated cardiac tamponade and tension pneumothorax.

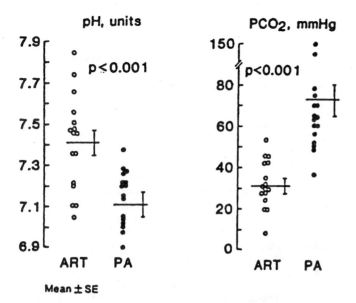

FIGURE 3-2   Arterial (Art) and mixed venous (PA) blood pH and PCO_2 during cardiopulmonary resuscitation in 16 patients. (From: Weil MH, Rackow EC, Trevino R, et al. N Engl J Med 1986;315:153-156.)

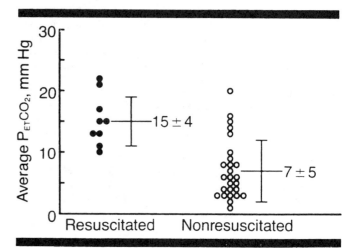

FIGURE 3-3 $P_{ET}CO_2$ during closed-chest cardiac resuscitation. (From: Sanders AB, Kern KB, Otto CW, et al. JAMA 1989;262:1347-1351.)

VENTRICULAR FIBRILLATION

AXIOM   Early defibrillation is the most important determinant of survival from sudden cardiac arrest.[56]

Ventricular fibrillation (V-fibb) is the most common cause of cardiac arrest, especially after an acute myocardial infarction. The most important aspect of survival in out-of-hospital V-fibb is early defibrillation.[56] The probability of successful cardioversion depends largely on the duration of V-fibb, and evidence exists to suggest that defibrillation after prolonged V-fibb leads to an increased incidence of asystole and EMD.

Defibrillation

TECHNIQUES USED

PITFALL ⊘

If there is any delay in defibrillating the heart, the chances of successful resuscitation are reduced.

If a patient suffers a sudden cardiac arrest and a defibrillator without a monitor is present, one should attempt immediate defibrillation, without waiting to ascertain the type of cardiac rhythm present by an ECG or cardioscope. Since ventricular fibrillation causes almost 75% of sudden cardiac arrests, if there is no effective cardiac function, an attempted defibrillation causes few untoward effects, even if ventricular fibrillation is not present. If the defibrillator has the quick-look option, this can be utilized to check the rhythm, while the unit is charging, without significant delay.

The new technology for automatic external defibrillation appears very promising because it enables immediate defibrillation by a wide variety of individuals, including first responders, such as policemen and trained lay persons, and family members of high risk patients.[57]

Virtually all defibrillators used now are of the DC (direct current) type. During defibrillation, one defibrillator paddle is placed over the left lateral chest at about the fifth or sixth intercostal space in the midaxillary lines and the other is placed to the right of the upper sternum below the clavicle. Electrode jelly is applied liberally to each paddle, taking care not to allow a "bridge" of electrode jelly to extend between the two paddles, as this may cause an electrical arc burn. If electrode jelly is not available, saline soaked 4 × 4 dressings can be placed under the paddles. No one should be touching the patient or the bed when the current is applied; however, defibrillators which negate the need for this precaution are now available.

The actual amount of energy required to defibrillate a heart varies greatly between patients. The ACLS starting dose for external defibrillation is 200 joules. If the ventricular fibrillation is not terminated by the first attempt, a second shock should be given immediately at 300 joules, and immediately followed by a third defibrillation at 360 joules if the second is also unsuccessful.

PROBLEMS

Persistent Ventricular Fibrillation

PITFALL ⊘

If severe metabolic acidosis or hypoxemia is allowed to persist, it may be impossible to defibrillate the patient.

One of the most frequent reasons for persistent ventricular fibrillation is a severe metabolic acidosis. If there is essentially no tissue perfusion, it is not unusual, in our experience, for the central venous or pulmonary arterial pH to fall below 7.0 within 4 to 5 minutes of the cardiac arrest.

It is important to emphasize that much of the acidosis of cardiac arrest can be treated with hyperventilation alone and to date no beneficial effect from the use of bicarbonate has been shown.[58] Studies also indicate that the PCO_2 at the coronary sinus can be extremely high even when the arterial PCO_2 is near normal.[58] After return of spontaneous circulation, ABGs should be followed and sodium bicarbonate given as needed for the metabolic acidosis. Under normal circumstances, it takes about 100 to 150 mEq of bicarbonate to raise the arterial pH 0.10. One should also monitor the central and mixed venous PCO_2 because, if the venous PCO_2 is high, giving bicarbonate will tend to make the cellular acidosis worse. This "paradoxical acidosis" is caused by the more rapid diffusion of CO_2 into cells than HCO_3.

Recurrent Fibrillation. If ventricular fibrillation is terminated by an electric shock but quickly recurs, various drugs, which will be covered later in this chapter, may be used to attempt to reduce the irritability of the heart. One should, however, ascertain that the patient is not severely acidotic, alkalotic, hypoxic, or hypothermic.

ASYSTOLE

Studies show that successful resuscitation from out-of-hospital cardiac arrest with asystole is extremely rare, with the prognosis much worse than in ventricular fibrillation.[34] V-fibb can masquerade as asystole in certain leads, consequently, asystole should be confirmed in at least two leads.[59] With asystole, epinephrine is probably the best drug available for stimulating the heart. Atropine can also be used, but lidocaine, procainamide, and quinidine should be avoided.

BRADYCARDIA

Persistent severe bradycardia is often associated with poor myocardial contractions and an increased chance of recurrent cardiac arrest. Suggested therapy includes atropine in 0.5 increments to a total of 3.0 mg (adult dose). Isoproterenol, once one of the mainstays in bradycardia therapy, is now the last line therapy. Isoproterenol, if used, is only to be administered in low doses as to avoid the harmful systemic vasodilatation occurring at higher doses.

If adequate ventilation, effective cardiac massage, and the various drugs are unsuccessful in correcting asymptomatic bradycardia, one should consider trying an external or transcutaneous cardiac pacemaker. Such pacemakers may be especially helpful in cases of heart block or drug toxicity.

If external pacing is unsuccessful or prolonged pacing will be necessary, an internal pacemaker should be placed. One can attempt to pass a transvenous pacemaker blindly into the right ventricle and look for capture on the monitor. Another option is to place the "V" lead of the monitor on the distal electrode of the pacing wire and follow the changes in the P and QRS complexes to sense where the catheter is located. Of note, the surface leads of the monitor need to be in place as usual and the ECG machine switched on the "V" lead. These lines can be placed through a cutdown in an antecubital, cephalic, basilic, or external jugular vein, or percutaneously through an internal jugular or a subclavian vein. If such attempts are unsuccessful, a direct percutaneous puncture of the heart with a needle electrode can be attempted, but it is rarely successful, especially as a last resort.

HYPOTENSION

If a regular cardiac rhythm is restored, but the patient continues to be severely hypotensive, cardiac massage should be continued until a palpable carotid pulse is felt without cardiac massage, with or without inotropic or vasopressor agents. Some of the drugs that may be used to treat hypotension include dopamine, epinephrine, and norepinephrine. The new ACLS guidelines suggest the use of norepinephrine before dopamine for SBP less than 70 mm Hg because the higher doses of dopamine needed at this pressure have a greater dysrhythmogenic effect.[58] In trauma patients, one must always rule out pericardial tamponade, tension pneumothorax, and hypovolemia from exsanguination as causes of continued hypotension.

AXIOM Persistent hypotension in trauma patients is usually due to hypovolemia from continued bleeding.

Corticosteroids in "stress" doses of 100 mg of hydrocortisone intravenously every 8 hours may be of great value for combating hypotension due to known or suspected adrenal insufficiency.

DRUG THERAPY

Types of Drugs

ADRENERGIC AGONISTS

Because cardiac resuscitability is contingent on rapid reversal of myocardial ischemia, interventions which improve myocardial blood flow are associated with improved resuscitation.[52] Agents that increase peripheral vascular resistance tend to increase central aortic blood pressure and favor redistribution of blood flow from less vital organs and tissues to the myocardium and the brain.[60]

When alpha-adrenergic agents, such as epinephrine or phenylephrine, are administered during CPR, the incidence of successful laboratory cardiac resuscitation is increased. In addition, it has been shown that the alpha effects are essential to successful resuscitation. Experiments have shown that alpha-adrenergic blocking agents decrease cardiac resuscitability, but the use of beta-blockers does not.[61] Epinephrine and norepinephrine are more effective at increasing cerebral and myocardial blood flow and resuscitation rates than phenylephrine and methoxamine. This is despite the fact that phenylephrine and methoxamine are almost pure alpha-adrenergic agonists and have little direct effect on cardiac contractility.[62] Some investigators feel that epinephrine and norepinephrine are the most effective alpha agonists for CPR because of their greater alpha$_2$ receptor effect versus the alpha$_1$ receptor effects seen with methoxamine and phenylephrine.[60] The alpha$_2$ receptors are located at the intima of the vasculature and, therefore, are able to respond to circulating catecholamines.[60]

AXIOM Alpha adrenergic agents, such as epinephrine, can increase successful return of spontaneous circulation with CPR by increasing diastolic aortic pressure and coronary perfusion pressure.

Epinephrine has both alpha and beta receptor activity. The powerful alpha vasoconstrictor effect can dramatically increase central aortic pressures and coronary and cerebral blood flow. Its beta$_1$ adrenergic effects increase the contractility and irritability of the heart and may convert asystole to ventricular fibrillation. It can also increase the amplitude of ventricular fibrillation and make it more susceptible to electrical conversion.[52] The increased inotropism and chronotropism of epinephrine also may be of benefit after the return of spontaneous cardiac contractions.

In the clinical setting, epinephrine has been the preferred agent for attempting to restart an arrested heart, particularly after prolonged CPR.[63] However, high doses appear to be required to significantly increase myocardial and cerebral blood flows. This is probably due to the fact that catecholamine levels in cardiac arrest victims are already extremely high.

AXIOM   Epinephrine should be administered in increasing doses if there is no satisfactory response to CPR within 2 to 3 minutes.

The usual initial intravenous or intracardiac dose of epinephrine is 0.01-0.02 mg/kg or 1 mg (10 cc of a 1:10,000 solution) and this may be repeated every 3 to 5 minutes. If this is unsuccessful, multiple other regimens can be tried: (a) intermediate: 1-5 mg every 3-5 minutes, (b) escalating: 1, then 3, then 5 mgs, 3 minutes apart, or (c) high dose: 0.1 mg/kg every 3-5 minutes.

High dose epinephrine (0.1-0.2 mg/kg) is now one of the recommendations during CPR in patients who are responding poorly or have very low aortic pressure with standard or low dose epinephrine. The larger doses cause greater increases in diastolic and coronary perfusion pressures and can increase the initial success rates with CPR; however, incidence of survival with normal neurologic function does not appear to be improved by high dose epinephrine.[64-66] There was, however, a trend toward increased survival in one study if the high dose epinephrine was given to patients with down times less than 10 minutes.[66] Problems with high dose epinephrine include increased myocardial automaticity and increased myocardial oxygen demand resulting in elevated myocardial adenosine triphosphate consumption and lactate production.[67]

For percutaneous intracardiac injections, the ideal needle is 4½ inches long and 18- to 20-gauge in diameter. Spinal needles are often very good for this. The quickest technique is to insert the needle in the fourth intercostal space about an inch lateral to the sternum, directing it medially and posteriorly; however, one must be sure that blood can be aspirated back freely before the epinephrine is injected.

Epinephrine injected into any tissue causes such severe vasoconstriction and ischemia that local tissue necrosis can occur. Such a damaged area in the heart can act as a focus for persistent or recurrent ventricular fibrillation.

PITFALL ⊘

If adrenalin is injected into myocardium rather than the ventricular chamber, it can cause myocardial necrosis and refractory ventricular fibrillation.

Administration of epinephrine via a CVP or pulmonary artery catheter in slightly larger doses is probably as effective as intracardiac adrenalin, and it is certainly much safer. Furthermore, the hazards of injuring the anterior descending coronary artery or anterior myocardium with the intracardiac needle are eliminated.

Isoproterenol (Isuprel)

Isoproterenol is a pure beta-adrenergic agonist and as such it: (a) increases the rate and force of myocardial contraction, (b) causes significant arteriolar vasodilation in skeletal muscles, and (c) causes some constriction of capacitance veins. The increased heart rate and myocardial contractility can greatly increase myocardial oxygen consumption. However, because of its arterial vasodilating properties, isoproterenol tends to cause the systolic and diastolic pressures to fall, in spite of the increased cardiac output. As a consequence, myocardial blood flow may be reduced at a time when myocardial oxygen consumption is increased. Therefore, it decreases resuscitability when compared to drugs with predominant alpha-adrenergic activity.[68]

PITFALL ⊘

There is no indication for the administration of isoproterenol in the presence of a tachycardia or an irritable heart, and if administered under such circumstances, the patient is apt to develop severe tachyarrhythmias and myocardial ischemia.

The only indication for isoproterenol in acute cardiac care is for temporary control of hemodynamically significant atropine-resistant bradyarrhythmias and refractory torsades de pointes.[58] Under such circumstances, 1 ampule (0.2 mg) of isoproterenol is usually diluted in 100 ml of 5% glucose in water. This produces a solution with a concentration of 2 mcg/ml which can be infused at 1 to 2 mcg/min. This may produce a significant increase in cardiac output; however, higher doses may greatly increase cardiac irritability.

Norepinephrine (Levophed)

Norepinephrine (Levophed) is an excellent vasopressor that is essentially devoid of beta$_2$ activity. In fact, it is now recommended as a first line drug in patients with SBP less than 70 mm Hg following CPR because of the increased arrhythmias seen with the higher doses of dopamine needed to treat these pressures. The usual dose of norepinephrine is 4 ampules (16 mg) in 500 ml of 5% glucose in water, producing a solution with a norepinephrine concentration of 32 mcg/ml. Addition of 2 ampules (10 mg) of phentolamine (Regitine) to the same bottle of norepinephrine does not greatly affect the rise in BP, but does reduce the chances of excessive vasoconstriction, decreasing the chance of skin sloughing if extravasation into perivascular tissue occurs.[69] The intravenous drip rate is controlled to keep the systolic BP above 90 mm Hg or whatever level is needed to maintain adequate cerebral, cardiac, and renal function.

AXIOM   Use of norepinephrine in hypovolemic patients can cause such severe vasoconstriction that tissue necrosis occurs.

Norepinephrine can cause such severe vasoconstriction, especially in the presence of hypovolemia, that arterioles can be completely obstructed leading to severe tissue ischemia. Consequently, before or while the patient is placed on a vasopressor, one should make great efforts to provide adequate fluid resuscitation.

AXIOM   Adequate fluid resuscitation should be completed on all patients before the administration of vasopressors.

Dopamine

Dopamine is a naturally-occurring catecholamine that has various dose dependent effects. At 1 to 3 mcg/kg/min, dopamine is predominantly a splanchnic vasodilator causing increased blood flow to the kidneys and other viscera. Dopamine at this dose may cause a significant increase in urine output without an increase in BP or cardiac output.

Dopamine in doses of 5 to 15 mcg/kg/min acts primarily as a positive inotropic agent and, as such, increases cardiac output and blood pressure.[70] Larger doses of dopamine tend to have an increasing alpha effect so that, with doses above 30 to 40 mcg/kg/min, its effects tend to be primarily those of a vasoconstrictor.

Dobutamine

Dobutamine is a synthetic adrenergic-like drug with predominately beta$_1$ effects and therefore is a positive inotrope.[71] Dobutamine also causes some decrease in SVR and PCWP. At doses of 5 to 15 mcg/kg/min, it increases cardiac output and slightly lowers systemic vascular resistance. Blood pressure tends to remain constant or decrease slightly. Dobutamine is less likely to increase pulmonary artery pressure and heart rate than dopamine.[71]

SODIUM BICARBONATE

In the past, sodium bicarbonate was routinely administered during cardiopulmonary resuscitation based on the assumption that a severe metabolic acidosis developed after a cardiac arrest and that correction of the severe metabolic acidosis would favor cardiac resuscitability.[72] Jude, Kouwenhoven, and Knickerbocker,[24] felt that the arterial pH should be maintained within the normal range by administering sodium bicarbonate in amounts of 44 mEq/L (37.5 g) at intervals of 5 to 10 minutes to adults. The intent was to improve cardiac function and responsiveness to vasopressor agents.

More recent observations, both laboratory and clinical, have shown that although bicarbonate levels may decline during CPR, if the patient is hyperventilated, the $PaCO_2$ is usually low enough to maintain arterial pH within a reasonable range during the initial 10 minutes of CPR.[52] However, because the low blood flow to the lung greatly increases pulmonary dead space, the PCO_2 of venous blood may be greatly increased. Consequently, the venous pH, which is a better indicator of cellular pH in shock states, may be decreased to 7.1 or even lower when arterial values are relatively normal.[52,53]

AXIOM Even though the arterial PCO_2 may remain relatively normal in shock states, the mixed venous blood may be quite acidotic due to a high PCO_2.[52]

A PCO_2 as high as 150 mm Hg with corresponding decreases in pH to 6.80 have been observed in coronary venous blood during cardiac arrest in spite of relatively normal arterial PCO_2 levels.[52] With experimental ventricular fibrillation, the myocardial PCO_2 may increase from 50 mm Hg to 400 mm Hg and the myocardial pH may fall from 7.20 to 6.40 within 11 minutes.[73]

AXIOM Bicarbonate should be withheld or given with extreme caution if the arterial or venous PCO_2 levels are elevated.

Venous and myocardial hypercarbia have negative inotropic effects,[74] thereby reducing the resuscitability of the heart. Since CO_2 diffuses much more rapidly into cells than HCO_3 ions,[75] bicarbonate administration can cause a paradoxical intracellular acidosis. Indeed, transient but significant decreases in myocardial contractility have been documented following intracoronary and intra-atrial administration of $NaHCO_3$ in the intact dog heart.[76] Failure of bicarbonate to increase resuscitability of fibrillating canine hearts has also been reported by Guerci et al.[77]

Other potential adverse effects of bicarbonate, which can compromise both myocardial and cerebral function, relate to increases in plasma osmolality and decreased dissociation of oxygen from hemoglobin. Increases in plasma osmolality may also cause neurologic complications[78] and decreased systemic vascular resistance, leading to a drop in aortic diastolic and coronary perfusion pressures.[79] Alkalemia from increased plasma bicarbonate levels shifts the oxyhemoglobin dissociation curve to the left, thereby increasing the affinity of hemoglobin for oxygen and decreasing oxygen release at the tissue level.[80] Alkalosis also increases cerebral vascular resistance and reduces cerebral blood flow.

The American Heart Association no longer recommends sodium bicarbonate during the first 10 minutes of cardiac resuscitation.[58] The current recommendations for acid administration during CPR include hyperkalemia, known severe metabolic acidosis, tricyclic antidepressant overdose, rhabdomyolysis, and some drug overdoses.

Alternative buffer agents, such as the organic buffer tromethamine (THAM), which not only buffers acid, but also takes up CO_2, and the newly developed equimolar mixture of sodium bicarbonate and sodium carbonate (Carbicarb[R]), can increase myocardial contractility in the nonischemic heart.[81] Although these agents can significantly increase the pH and bicarbonate levels in systemic and coronary venous blood, they do not reduce the severe myocardial acidosis that can rapidly develop during ventricular fibrillation and cardiac resuscitation.[82]

CALCIUM

The entry of calcium ions into the myocardial cell during the plateau phase of the action potential is essential for excitation-contraction coupling.[83] Calcium increases the myocardial contractile force and enhances ventricular excitability.[84]

AXIOM Intravenous calcium can have a strong positive inotropic effect in patients with low ionized calcium levels.

During a cardiac arrest, plasma ionized calcium levels may fall abruptly,[85] and some authors have felt that this can cause electromechanical dissociation. It was also previously thought that intravenous calcium might be helpful if the patient has a low-amplitude ventricular fibrillation or a weakly beating heart in regular sinus rhythm. There is, however, no evidence that administration of calcium salts improves outcome in the above states.[86] In fact, increased plasma levels of calcium tend to cause smooth muscle vasoconstriction and impair myocardial relaxation. These circumstances can adversely affect recovery of myocardial and cerebral function.[87] The only time that calcium has been shown to be helpful is in patients with severe hyperkalemia, severe ionic hypocalcemia from multiple rapid blood transfusions, or calcium channel blocker overdoses. However, even in these cases, calcium administration may impair cerebral resuscitation.[88]

Calcium can also cause ventricular ectopic beats and coronary and cerebral vasospasm.[84] Even if calcium is indicated, rapid intravenous injection of 5 ml of 10% calcium chloride or 10 ml of 10% calcium gluconate may transiently increase serum levels of calcium to toxic ranges exceeding 15 mg/dl (3.8 mmol/L) and cause sinus bradycardia or even sinus arrest.[89] Development of hypercalcemia in patients with massive transfusions was almost uniformly fatal.[90]

AXIOM The administration of calcium is not advised during CPR except when cardiac arrest is associated with hyperkalemia, hypocalcemia, or calcium channel blocking drugs.

Some calcium channel blockers are under investigation for potential myocardial and cerebral protective effects during CPR.[91] If calcium channel blockers are given and a cardiac arrest or a decrease in inotropicity occur, administration of calcium chloride or gluconate intravenously can at least partially restore contractility.

Calcium chloride and calcium gluconate are both stocked as 10% solutions in 10 ml ampules. The calcium chloride, however, contains more ionic calcium than calcium gluconate (13.4 mEq versus 4.7 mEq in each 10 ml 10% ampule), and it is more rapidly and completely ionized, especially in shock or hepatic failure.

ATROPINE

Atropine is an anticholinergic agent which has been used during CPR to treat sinus bradycardia, high degree atrioventricular (AV) block, and ventricular asystole.[92] It is particularly indicated in severe bradycardia with hypotension. Atropine may improve resuscitation in ventricular asystole by: (a) abolishing parasympathetic tone, (b) enhancing sinus node discharge, and (c) improving AV conduction.[93] The usual dose is 0.5 to 1.0 mg intravenously with a maximum dose of 0.04 mg/kg (3 mg in a 70 kg person). The pediatric dose is 0.02 mg/kg with a minimum dose of 0.1 mg and maximum dose of 1 mg in children and 2 mg in adolescents. Doses smaller than 0.5 mg in adults and 0.1 mg in children may produce paradoxical bradycardia due to either central vagal stimulation or peripheral parasympathomimetic reflex actions. The dose may have to be doubled to produce the desired effect, which can then last for 24 hours or longer.

Controlled prospective clinical studies in cardiac arrest have failed to demonstrate beneficial effects of atropine, even with bradysystolic cardiac arrest.[94] Atropine, however, may prevent cardiac asystole after intense vagal stimulation during anesthesia or surgical intervention.[95]

If severe bradycardia or electromechanical dissociation are the presenting signs during a witnessed cardiac arrest, the primary cause is likely to be hypoxia. Consequently, adequate ventilation and oxygenation are the most appropriate initial interventions.

AXIOM   Atropine may be used to help prevent asystole in high degree A-V blocks, but it is usually only indicated during symptomatic bradycardia, EMD, or asystole.

Atropine can cause a number of prolonged undesirable anticholinergic side effects, and should be given with caution to patients with glaucoma or bladder-outlet obstruction. Other unfavorable side effects include an excessive tachycardia with resultant increased myocardial oxygen consumption, which can be particularly hazardous to patients with ischemic heart disease.[96]

ANTIARRHYTHMIC AGENTS

Lidocaine (Xylocaine)

Lidocaine has been used for many years to prevent ventricular fibrillation because of its ability to reduce the irritability of the myocardium without significantly reducing contractility. Ventricular tachycardia and unifocal or multifocal premature ventricular contractions may respond dramatically to this drug. The usual dose of lidocaine for dangerous premonitory arrhythmias is 1.0-1.5 mg/kg bolus with 0.5-0.75 mg/kg repeated in 5 to 10 minutes as needed. Once an adequate response has been obtained, lidocaine levels may be maintained by an intravenous infusion of 1 to 4 mg/min. Some investigators and current AHA guidelines[58] state that 4-6 PVCs/min is no longer an indication for lidocaine after an acute myocardial infarction or thrombolysis.

It is not uncommon for critically injured patients to have some degree of hypovolemia which is at least partially compensated for by increased arteriolar and venous constriction. Many drugs, including lidocaine, morphine, and meperidine (Demerol), can produce significant vasodilation, thereby increasing vascular capacity. In hypovolemic patients, the increase in vascular capacity seen with these agents, in conjunction with an already low blood volume, can cause a sharp drop in blood pressure.

PITFALL ⊘

If large amounts of lidocaine are given to a patient who is hypovolemic, significant hypotension may occur.

Most antiarrhythmic drugs decrease the excitability of cardiac muscle and thereby alter both the defibrillatory and fibrillatory thresholds.[52] Babbs et al[97] demonstrated that lidocaine, quinidine, and diphenylhydantoin increase the amount of electrical energy required for ventricular defibrillation in dogs. The increased defibrillatory threshold induced by these antiarrhythmic agents may account, at least in part, for the failure of defibrillation in in-hospital cardiac arrest patients.

AXIOM   Lidocaine may be of benefit for preventing ventricular fibrillation, but once it occurs, lidocaine may make it more difficult for ventricular fibrillation to be cardioverted to a sinus rhythm.

Bretylium

Bretylium tosylate initially releases norepinephrine at adrenergic nerve endings, with the resultant sympathomimetic effects lasting for about 20 to 30 minutes.[98] After the initial increase in arterial resistance, bretylium then prevents synaptic norepinephine release causing a decrease in systemic vascular resistance and tends to cause a mild hypotension.[52] However, the cardiac output is usually unchanged.

Although bretylium, like lidocaine, raises the threshold for ventricular fibrillation to occur,[100] it differs from lidocaine in that the energy requirements for defibrillation are not increased.[101] Bretylium

also has been shown to produce chemical defibrillation in animals,[58] and Holder et al[102] found that bretylium was frequently lifesaving in patients with refractory ventricular fibrillation. However, bretylium has not been shown to be more effective than lidocaine in V-fibb/V-tach in direct comparisons.

AXIOM   Bretylium may be a potent alternative for recurrent ventricular fibrillation/tachycardia that is refractory to lidocaine.

Bretylium's onset of antiarrhythmic action is relatively slow because of its early catecholamine release, which can exacerbate ventricular irritability for 20 to 30 minutes.[99] Because of the side effects and the marked prolongation of the action potential which it causes, it has not replaced lidocaine as a first line antiarrhythmic agent during CPR, and remains the third line agent in both V-tach and V-fibb.

Procainamide (Pronestyl)

Procainamide has a mechanism of action similar to that of lidocaine. However, it is generally reserved for PVCs, V-tach, and wide complex tachyarrhythmias that are resistant to lidocaine.[52] It is a second line agent because it has a greater myocardial depressant effect than lidocaine, and it is more likely to cause severe hypotension. The usual dose of procainamide is 20-30 mg/min IVP until either the arrhythmia is suppressed, the QRS is lengthened by 50%, hypotension occurs, or the patient receives a maximum of 17 mg/kg. If the arrhythmia is suppressed, a drip can then be started at 1-4 mg/min; however, drug levels should be monitored, and the maintenance dose should be lowered in patients with renal failure.

Adenosine

Adenosine is a purine nucleotide that suppresses SA and AV nodal function and is effective in terminating re-entrant supraventricular tachyarrhythmias.[52,58] Adenosine's short half-life of approximately 5 seconds makes it an attractive drug to use in emergencies because, if a side effect occurs, the drug is already gone. The usual dose of adenosine is 6 mg over 1-3 minutes, followed by 12 mg if no response is seen in another 1-2 minutes. Doses may need to be increased in the presence of methylaxanthines (e.g. theophylline), and the dose should be decreased in patients on tegretol. Adenosine is the first line agent in paroxysmal supraventricular tachycardia (PSVT) and a second line agent (behind lidocaine) in the treatment of wide complex tachycardias of uncertain etiology.[58]

Magnesium

Hypomagnesemia may increase the incidence of cardiac arrhythmias, such as refractory V-fibb, and cause sudden death. Magnesium infusion in the LIMIT-2 trial decreased 28 day mortality (8% versus 24%) and decreased left ventricular failure by 25%.[103] Magnesium administration has also been shown to suppress refractory V-tach, V-fibb, and multifocal atrial tachycardia (MAT), and it can reduce post-MI arrhythmias in some patients.[104] Magnesium should be administered in 1-2 gm boluses over 5-60 minutes, depending on the urgency of the situation, and then continue as a maintenance drip at 0.5-1.0 gm/hr for 24 hours. Magnesium is currently recommended by the American Heart Association for use in torsade de pointes and refractory V-fibb/V-tach. Magnesium should also be considered for the treatment of post-MI arrhythmias.

Quinidine

Quinidine is a potent antiarrhythmic drug. The dose is 200 mg every 4 to 8 hours, and it is used primarily to treat atrial tachyarrhythmias after the patient has been digitalized.

Digitalis Preparations

If the patient has rapid atrial fibrillation or flutter following cardiac resuscitation, a digitalis-like drug may be beneficial. The usual total intravenous dose of digoxin is 1.0 to 1.5 mg given in divided doses over 12 to 18 hours; in more urgent situations, 1 mg can be given in divided doses over 1 hour. If the patient is in congestive heart failure, furosemide or morphine sulfate may help reduce the fluid overload.

Other Antiarrhythmics

Dilantin, Digibind (an antibody to digoxin), and magnesium may be useful in managing arrhythmias caused by digitalis toxicity. Low potassium and high calcium levels should also be corrected in digitalis toxicity because they tend to increase cardiac sensitivity to digitalis.

Sites of Drug Administration

Insertion of an intravenous catheter is a high priority during the initial phase of advanced cardiac life support. However, technical difficulties may occasionally preclude rapid venous catheterization, and precious time may be lost in an effort to establish an intravenous route for injection of drugs.

AXIOM If an intravenous line can't be started promptly in a patient with a cardiac arrest, epinephrine can be given via the endotracheal tube.

If an intravenous line is not promptly available for administering drugs during CPR, intratracheal instillation of selected agents may be a practical alternative.[105] Epinephrine, atropine, naloxone, bretylium, propranolol, isoproterenol, and lidocaine may be safely injected into the trachea through an endotracheal tube without producing significant tissue damage or altered lung function. However, the dose should be at least 2 to 2.5 times greater than the intravenous dose, with each dose diluted in 10 ml of normal saline.[106] The absorption of endotracheal drugs is prolonged by approximately 25% when compared to intravenous injection, and a depot effect in some patients may prolong the duration of action by as much as tenfold. Sodium bicarbonate inactivates alveolar surfactant and increases the risk of atelectasis, and therefore should not be administered by the intratracheal route.[105]

AXIOM Sodium bicarbonate should not be administered via the tracheobronchial tree.

SPECIFIC THERAPY

Prehospital Care

If an out-of-hospital cardiac arrest is due only to airway obstruction or ventilatory insufficiency, and they are corrected rapidly in the field, there is a high probability of survival;[107] however, without such therapy, the patient will probably die.

Patients with hypovolemic cardiac arrest rarely survive if external cardiac massage and forced ventilation are performed for more than 5 minutes prior to hospital arrival.[4] Consequently, airway control, ventilation, and intravenous fluid administration should be used as needed in an attempt to prevent hypovolemic cardiac arrest. The use of the PASG has been shown to adversely affect outcome in chest, abdominal, and neck trauma, and therefore generally should not be used in patients with these injuries.[108]

If a patient with a penetrating injury of the chest or extremities has a cardiac arrest in the ambulance, prehospital treatment should include immediate establishment of an airway and ventilation with 100% oxygen, preferably by an ET tube. If there is blood loss from the lower extremities, a tourniquet or PASG can be applied. Although external cardiac massage can be helpful in a trauma victim who has had an acute myocardial infarction, it should probably not be performed on patients with truncal trauma, because it may cause more harm than good.[56]

Although intravenous administration of Ringer's lactate or normal saline while en route to the hospital should theoretically be helpful if the patient is in severe shock and either has stopped bleeding or has easily tamponadable bleeding, recent studies suggest that aggressive preoperative fluid resuscitation in patients with penetrating truncal injuries may increase bleeding and reduce survival.[6,7] Thus, the only benefit of such lines in this scenario may be to reduce the amount of time spent in the ED prior to moving to the OR.

Initial ED Management

A cardiac arrest is often assumed to be present in the patient who has no palpable pulse or blood pressure. However, if a relatively normal ECG rhythm is present, the patient may just be in shock. If external cardiac massage is in progress at the time of the patient's arrival, it should be interrupted temporarily to get a good ECG reading and allow palpation of carotid and femoral pulses. Rapid application of ECG leads or use of the "quick-look" paddles can help determine if a rhythm is actually present. Even if there were no vital signs at the scene, the presence of a fairly normal ECG, especially if at a rapid rate, may indicate that aggressive fluid administration and ventilation with oxygen might be of benefit.

AXIOM If a patient had vital signs in the ambulance and then lost them, open-chest CPR in the ED may be worthwhile for penetrating wounds, especially stab wounds to the chest or extremities.

ED Resuscitative Thoracotomy

Although there has been much enthusiasm for external cardiac massage and defibrillation since the work of Zoll[23] and others,[24] it has become increasingly apparent that closed-chest compressions are not very effective, especially in hypovolemic patients. In addition, publications in 1966 confirmed that penetrating wounds of the heart should be managed primarily by emergency thoracotomy and that thoracotomy should be performed in the ED if the patient had a cardiac arrest just prior to or soon after hospital arrival.[109] It also has been pointed out that cardiac arrest during anesthesia for open-heart surgery and for 72 hours after the cardiotomy are strong indications for open-chest cardiac resuscitation.[110] Relative indications for open-chest cardiac massage, according to Blakeman,[110] include failure of closed-chest massage and severe chest wall deformities where closed-chest massage is apt to be ineffective.

AXIOM Open cardiac massage is more effective than closed-chest compression in patients with chest or abdominal trauma.

Animal research has clearly shown that there is a marked improvement in hemodynamics with open cardiac massage (versus closed-chest compressions), especially if the resuscitation extends beyond 2 minutes.[18,111] Relatively normal electroencephalograms and carotid blood flows have been maintained with open-chest cardiac massage for up to 1 hour. Cardiac output can often be maintained at 50-70% of normal with open-chest cardiac massage (versus 10-20% of normal with closed-chest massage).

INDICATIONS FOR ED RESUSCITATIVE THORACOTOMY

Most surgeons agree that, with the proper personnel and facilities, an ED thoracotomy should be performed on patients who have a cardiac arrest just prior to or soon after arrival in the ED due to a penetrating wound of the chest or extremities.

In one study of 177 patients without signs of life (absent pulse, pupil reactivity, and respirations) at the scene, only one survived with intact neurologic function following an ED thoracotomy.[48] This patient had multiple stab wounds, but the only significant injury was a transected brachial artery which was rapidly controlled by direct pressure at the scene.

> **AXIOM**   The highest salvage rate with CPR via an emergency room thoracotomy occurs in patients with a stab wound to the heart who have a cardiac arrest just before or soon after arrival to the ED.[2,48,49,109]

If blunt trauma to the chest or abdomen is the cause of cardiac arrest in a patient of any age, the chance of salvage by ED thoracotomy is less than 1 to 5%.[112-114] Indeed, a combination of massive head injury and cardiac arrest from blunt injury is a contraindication for ED thoracotomy. Of 175 patients at San Francisco General Hospital who underwent an ED thoracotomy, there was only one survivor (1.7%) among the 63 who had blunt trauma.[112] This patient was agonal upon admission and arrested in the emergency room. The poor prognosis of patients arriving without vital signs following blunt trauma does not, however, imply that ED thoracotomy should never be employed in blunt trauma, because the rare salvage of such patients has been described.[112]

> **AXIOM**   Resuscitative thoracotomy and open cardiac massage will only on rare occasion successfully resuscitate a patient with cardiac arrest secondary to blunt trauma.

BENEFITS OF ED RESUSCITATIVE THORACOTOMY

The objectives of an ED resuscitative thoracotomy are: (a) to release cardiac tamponade, (b) to control intrathoracic bleeding, (c) to treat or prevent air embolism, (d) to redistribute the available blood flow to vital organs (brain and heart) by cross-clamping the descending thoracic aorta, and (e) to optimize cardiac output by performing open cardiac massage.[48,114]

Relief of Pericardial Tamponade

> **AXIOM**   Early recognition and prompt relief of pericardial tamponade is essential to improve survival in patients with cardiac wounds.

Pericardial tamponade is said to be characterized by Beck's triad which includes hypotension, distended neck veins, and muffled heart tones. In the hypovolemic patient, however, distended neck veins may not appear until fluid resuscitation has begun, and even then, Beck's triad is often falsely positive or falsely negative.[109]

The hemodynamic and cardiac perfusion abnormalities seen with a rising intrapericardial pressure can be divided into four phases according to the adequacy of compensatory mechanisms.[48] In the first phase, the increased pericardial pressure restricts ventricular diastolic filling and reduces subendocardial blood flow. The resultant reduction in cardiac output is initially compensated by an accelerated heart rate and increased systemic vascular resistance and central venous pressure. In the second phase of pericardial tamponade, the rising intrapericardial pressure further reduces cardiac output and coronary perfusion, and the resultant increased subendocardial ischemia begins to compromise ventricular ejection.[115] Although systemic blood pressure may be maintained relatively well, signs of impaired perfusion, such as anxiety, diaphoresis, and pallor will become increasingly apparent.

During the third phase, the intrapericardial pressure approaches ventricular filling pressure, and the stroke volume may fall to less than 20-25 ml per beat with a corresponding severe reduction in systemic BP. In the fourth and final phase, intrapericardial pressure exceeds atrial and ventricular diastolic pressures leading to profound coronary hypoperfusion which can result in severe myocardial depression and an unobtainable BP which can rapidly progress to cardiac arrest if uncorrected.

> **AXIOM**   The quickest way (before pericardiocentesis or thoracotomy) to raise the blood pressure in a patient with pericardial tamponade is to give intravenous fluids.

If the bleeding into the pericardium has stopped, volume loading may raise diastolic filling pressures enough to restore a reasonable BP. However, rebleeding into the pericardial cavity may occur as the arterial and central venous pressures rise. If the systemic BP is reasonable, the patient should be brought immediately to the OR for emergency thoracotomy. If the patient is in severe shock in spite of aggressive fluid resuscitation and is apt to have a cardiac arrest before he reaches the OR, an ED thoracotomy should be performed. If a thoracotomy cannot be performed promptly, pericardiocentesis should be attempted.

Control of Intrathoracic Hemorrhage

Life-threatening intrathoracic hemorrhage requiring a thoracotomy occurs in less than 5% of patients following penetrating trauma, and is most frequently due to bleeding from the lung.[49] A hemithorax can rapidly fill with more than one half the total blood volume.[48] In patients with severe hypotension, the injured lung should be clamped at the hilum as soon as the chest is entered rather than making an attempt to repair the injured area of lung.[116] If a major systemic vessel is involved, bleeding should be controlled with proximal and distal clamping. If the aorta is involved, side clamping, digital pressure, or a rapid running suture is used to control the bleeding until an adequate heart beat is obtained.

REQUIREMENTS FOR ED OPEN CARDIAC MASSAGE

Although a successful roadside resuscitative thoracotomy of a man with a stab of the left lower lung has been reported by Wall et al,[117] enthusiasm for the use of emergency room thoracotomy should be tempered by at least two considerations:[114] the ED and hospital resources and the surgical experience of the available physicians.

ED and Hospital Resources

Not all hospitals are set up to perform ED thoracotomies. Special planning and resources are needed to perform thoracotomies outside the OR.[114] However, with the appropriate type of trauma and brief "down times," good results can be achieved in an emergency department where: (a) proper lighting, instrument trays (Table 3-1), and trained personnel are available at all times, and (b) a full-scale operating room is available without delay to provide definitive care. Mazzorana et al[118] have recently reported that their average expenditure per successful ED thoracotomy was $93,000. If thoracotomy was limited to patients with penetrating trauma who demonstrated signs of life, the expenditure per successful thoracotomy was $20,137.

TABLE 3-1   ED Thoracotomy Tray (Modified from Moore et al[48])

Sterile towels ×4	DeBakey's aortic clamp
Laparotomy pads ×10	Long and regular needle holder
Scalpel with No. 10 blade	Kelly clamps ×6
Mayo's scissors - curved	Teflon pledgets - different sizes ×5
Metzenbaum's scissors	2-0 cardiovascular ethibond suture ×2
DeBakey's vascular forceps (long) ×2	2-0 cardiovascular pledgetted ethibond suture ×2
Finchetto's chest retractor	Internal defibrillator paddles
Lebsche's knife and mallet or rib shears	
2-0 silk sutures for "stick-ties"	
Tooth forceps × 2	
Satinsky's vascular clamps (large) ×2	

Surgical Experience

Properly trained individuals with experience in performing ED thoracotomy should be present before one decides to open the chest of a patient with a traumatic cardiac arrest.[114] One must not only be able to make the incision, but also immediately clamp or repair any structure in the chest as needed.

Although the initial incision may be made by a properly trained emergency physician, considerable thoracic trauma experience may be necessary to ensure proper management once the chest is open. Furthermore, ED thoracotomies should not continue to be performed at a particular institution unless their results are periodically reviewed and indicate acceptable rates of salvage.

TECHNIQUES IN RESUSCITATIVE ED THORACOTOMIES

Incision

A left anterolateral thoracotomy incision is the preferred approach for open cardiac massage.[2,48] If needed, the incision can be extended across into the right chest to provide exposure of both pleural spaces, the heart, and virtually all of the anterior mediastinal structures.

AXIOM The initial incision of choice for ED thoracotomy for open CPR is an anterolateral thoracotomy.

The anterolateral thoracotomy is begun in the fourth or fifth intercostal space beginning about 2 cm lateral to the sternum (to avoid transecting the internal mammary vessels which run about 0.5-1.0 cm lateral to the sternum) and extending into the axilla. In women, the breast should be retracted superiorly to gain better access to this interspace. The intercostal muscles are divided initially with a knife and then with heavy scissors. The intercostal incision should avoid the inferior margin of the upper rib in the interspace to reduce the chances of damaging the intercostal neurovascular bundle.

A standard (Fenichetto) rib spreader is inserted with the handle directed inferiorly toward the axilla. Resistance encountered with the rib spreader can be reduced by cutting the intercostal muscle back further laterally and posteriorly and by cutting the costal cartilages medially. If the incision extends too far medially or if the sternum is transected for additional exposure, the internal mammary vessels must be secured, preferably with suture ligatures.

Extension of the incision into the other hemithorax can be accomplished quickly with a Lebsche knife or rib shears. If better exposure of the superior mediastinum is needed, the superior sternum can be split in the midline. This incision can be extended into the right or left neck or supraclavicular fossa as needed for control of more distal injuries to arch vessels.

Pericardiotomy

The pericardial sac is opened for optimal internal cardiac massage, relief of any suspected tamponade, and operative control of any heart wounds. The tight pericardium may be difficult to grasp and cut with a scissors, and one may have to carefully nick the pericardium with a knife to get the incision started. The pericardial incision is then extended cephalad, 1-2 cm anterior to the phrenic nerve, up along the ascending aorta to the top of the pericardium, and then down to the diaphragm. If the pericardial opening still seems too small, the pericardium can also be opened transversely, but should not extend to the phrenic nerves. Blood clots should be rapidly evacuated from the pericardium.

AXIOM At the time of ED thoracotomy, further attempts at resuscitation should cease if there is no cardiac activity, the heart is completely empty, and the patient has had no signs of life for more than 5 minutes.

With penetrating injuries confined to the lung or heart, especially if caused by stab wounds, and any recent signs of life, one can try to rapidly resuscitate the patient by: (a) controlling or repairing the injury, (b) rapid fluid resuscitation, (c) clamping of the descending thoracic aorta, and (d) open cardiac massage for 5 to 10 minutes. Epinephrine, in an intravenous dose of 0.5 to 1.0 mg, repeated every 2 to 4 minutes with open massage and aortic clamping may produce a reasonable proximal aortic BP. Intracardiac injection of 3 to 4 ml of a 1:10,000 adrenal solution may help convert asystole to ventricular fibrillation.

Moore et al[48] noted that of 139 patients with no cardiac activity at thoracotomy, only one eventually survived to hospital discharge. This patient sustained a ventricular laceration with pericardial tamponade and resultant cardiac arrest, which was remedied quickly in the ED.

Cardiorrhaphy

Bleeding sites from the heart can usually be controlled immediately with digital pressure. Sometimes a partially occluding vascular clamp can be used to control bleeding from an atrium or a great vessel. In some instances, bleeding from a ventricle can be controlled by inserting a Foley catheter through the wound into the cardiac chamber, blowing up the balloon, and then pulling the inflated balloon up against the inside of the cardiac wound.

In the beating heart, efforts at cardiorrhaphy should be delayed until the initial resuscitative measures have been completed. In the nonbeating heart, the suturing should be done rapidly prior to defibrillation.

Ventricular wounds are generally closed with 2-0 nonabsorbable horizontal mattress sutures. If available, buttresses with Teflon pledgets reduce the chances of the sutures pulling through the myocardium when they are tied. Lacerations of the atria or large veins can often be repaired with simple running 3-0 nonabsorbable sutures.

Posterior cardiac wounds may be particularly treacherous if the heart has to be lifted up to expose them. Definitive closure of such wounds is best accomplished in the operating room with optimal lighting and equipment. Cardiopulmonary bypass should be considered if there is massive bleeding and/or ventricular fibrillation every time the heart is lifted to view or repair a posterior injury.

AXIOM Difficult cardiac wounds are best repaired under cardiopulmonary bypass.

For massive wounds of the ventricle or inaccessible posterior wounds, one would ideally put the patient on cardiopulmonary bypass to accomplish a proper unhurried closure. If bypass is not rapidly available, one can apply saline ice slush over the heart and temporarily occlude the superior and inferior vena cava to facilitate repair.

If there is a suspicion that cardiac arrest was caused by air embolism from an injured lung, further air embolism is prevented by placing a vascular clamp across the pulmonary hilum proximal to the injured lung. An attempt should then be made to evacuate air from the least dependent portions of the proximal aorta, left atrium, and left ventricular apex while elevating the apex of the heart.

If the heart is arrested, clamping the ascending aorta just proximal to the innominate artery and alternatively squeezing the heart and ascending aorta may help rid the coronary arteries of any air they may contain. Cardiopulmonary bypass can be extremely helpful if coronary air emboli are present.

Internal Cardiac Massage

If no effective cardiac activity is present when the chest is opened, but it seems worthwhile to continue aggressive attempts at resuscitation because of favorable factors, such as young age, short down time, knife injury, full heart, or tamponade, internal cardiac massage should be instituted promptly. If the sternum is intact, we prefer to grasp the sternum with a thumb and squeeze the heart up against the sternum with the other fingers. If the sternum has been transected, two-handed massage is safer. Moore et al[48] specifically describe using a hinged clapping motion with the wrists apposed and with the ventricular compression proceeding from the apex to the base of the heart. Massaging the heart while it is held with the fingers and thumb of one hand increases the risk of myocardial perforation during compressions.

Thoracic Aorta Occlusion

If the heart is completely empty and/or internal defibrillation does not rapidly result in vigorous return of cardiac activity, the descending thoracic aorta should be occluded to maximize coronary and cerebral perfusion. Markison and Trunkey[114] point out that manual occlusion of the descending aorta is simpler and safer than using a clamp.

If the descending aorta is to be clamped, it should be done under direct vision rather than by palpation alone. This usually requires a rather large incision and retraction of the left lung anterior out of the chest by the two hands of an assistant standing on the right side of the patient. Another temporary method is to take the ambu bag off the ET tube to deflate the lungs then push the ET tube into the right main stem bronchus, thus deflating the left lung.

Under direct vision, the thoracic aorta is bluntly separated from the esophagus anteriorly. The prevertebral fascia is then incised posterior to the aorta. Some surgeons feel that the aorta should not be completely encircled because this increases the likelihood of intercostal branches being avulsed.[48] However, if one of the blades of the clamp does not go completely past the posterior border of the aorta, the occlusion is less apt to be complete and the aortic clamp is more likely to slip. When properly exposed, the thoracic aorta can usually be occluded satisfactorily with a large Satinsky or DeBakey vascular clamp.

Temporary occlusion of the descending thoracic aorta cannot only improve blood flow to the heart and brain two- to threefold, but it can also reduce subdiaphragmatic blood loss.[119] Canine studies by Dunn et al[120] demonstrated that left ventricular stroke work index and myocardial contractility increased in response to thoracic aortic occlusion during hypovolemic shock. Although the improvement in myocardial function in the study of Dunn et al[120] occurred without an increase in pulmonary capillary wedge pressure or a significant change in systemic vascular resistance, in our own patients, both of these parameters usually rise rather abruptly after the thoracic aorta is cross-clamped.

Dunn et al[120] felt that the improved coronary perfusion due to the elevated aortic diastolic pressure accounted for the enhanced contractility following aortic cross-clamping. This experimental observation suggests that temporary aortic occlusion may be valuable in the patient with continued shock during or following repair of cardiac or other exsanguinating wounds.

Vasomotor tone below the aortic clamp is partially re-established by increased levels of epinephrine and angiotensin. However, some abdominal vital organ dysfunction is inevitable from prolonged thoracic aortic clamping. Although thoracic aortic occlusion has been tolerated for as long as 75 minutes without spinal cord sequelae,[121] clinical experience with elective thoracic aortic procedures indicates that 30 minutes is generally the safe limit for reversible normothermic spinal cord ischemia.[11,48] Intermittent clamp removal to allow systemic perfusion has not been studied adequately, and theoretically may cause more harm by increasing the production of toxic oxygen metabolites.[48]

> **AXIOM**   Thoracic aortic cross-clamping should be considered a potentially dangerous temporary maneuver designed to keep the patient alive while life-threatening problems are rapidly corrected.

Thoracic aortic cross-clamping may be deleterious in normovolemic patients because of significantly increased myocardial oxygen demands caused by the elevated systemic vascular resistance.[122] Blood flow to the abdominal viscera, spinal cord, and kidneys may be reduced to 10% of normal following thoracic aortic occlusion and femoral systolic blood pressures may fall to less than 10-20 mm Hg. Thus, aortic occlusion can induce a high degree of anaerobic metabolism in the tissues below the clamp, resulting in lactic acidemia and

release of numerous inflammatory mediators, such as thromboxane and other prostanoids.[123]

> **AXIOM**   The BP response to aortic clamping should be monitored very closely.

If the heart begins to beat and if the systolic BP in the proximal aorta is allowed to exceed 160-180 mm Hg, the resultant strain on the left ventricle can cause acute left ventricular distension with resultant failure and pulmonary edema.

The proximal aortic pressure also provides important prognostic information. Moore et al[48] have had no survivors among 180 patients in whom the proximal systolic blood pressure remained less than 70 mm Hg after aortic clamping despite full resuscitative efforts. In the studies of Wiencek et al,[118,123] the critical systolic BP was 90 mm Hg with none of their patients leaving the OR alive unless the proximal systolic BP exceeded 90 mm Hg within 5 minutes of thoracic aortic clamping.

The metabolic penalty of aortic cross-clamping becomes exponential when occlusion time exceeds 30 minutes, especially in patients with multisystem trauma.[48] Consequently, the aortic clamp should be gradually removed as soon as an effective systemic arterial pressure has been achieved.

Optimizing Oxygen Transport

If spontaneous cardiac function resumes, the resuscitation priorities shift to maximizing tissue oxygen delivery (DO_2). The combination of direct cardiac injury, ischemic myocardium, circulating cardiac depressants, and pulmonary hypertension can all adversely impact on postinjury cardiac work. Aortic declamping causes washout of metabolic by-products, inflammatory mediators, and other factors such as myocardial depressant factor from the previously ischemic areas back into the central circulation.[48]

> **AXIOM**   The ultimate metabolic goal of resuscitation from shock is non-delivery dependent oxygen consumption. This is accomplished by raising oxygen delivery (DO_2) until oxygen consumption (VO_2) is above normal and/or will not rise any further with an increased DO_2.

Oxygen delivery is a function of cardiac output and oxygen carrying capacity, which is largely related to the amount of hemoglobin present. To optimize DO_2, the circulating blood volume is increased until the cardiac index (CI) is 4.0-4.5 $L/min/m^2$ or until the cardiac output will not increase with further elevation of the CVP and PAWP with fluid or blood.[124] Oxygen carrying capacity can be maximized by increasing hematocrit levels to 35-40% or higher. If these measures fail to raise the VO_2 to 150 $ml/min/m^2$ or higher within 12 hours of injury, there is an increased incidence of multiple organ failure.[125] Using supranormal CI, DO_2, and VO_2, Fleming et al[126] and Yu et al[127] decreased mortality from 44 to 24% and 56 to 14%, respectively.

CLINICAL RESULTS WITH ED THORACOTOMY

Results of ED thoracotomy vary considerably due to the heterogeneity of the patient populations reported. It is also critical to distinguish between "no vital signs" and "no signs of life."[48] The patient with "no vital signs" is alive, but has no obtainable cuff BP or palpable pulse. "No signs of life" describes the patient who has no vital signs, no movements or reflexes, no pupil reactivity, no corneal reflexes, no respiratory efforts, and no heart sounds. In a review of 11 reports by Moore et al,[48] the survival rate with an ED thoracotomy for trauma was 27% (81/296) for patients in shock, 13% (65/511) for patients with no vital signs, and 2.3% (15/651) for patients with no signs of life. The overall survival rate was 11% (161/1458). Our overall survival rate with ED thoracotomy at Detroit Receiving Hospital was 10% (26/272). The survival rate with stab wounds (20% = 14/69) (Table 3-2) was much better than for gunshot wounds (6% = 12/203) (Table 3-3). If the patients with no signs of life at the scene are excluded, the survival rates were 25% and 8% respectively.

TABLE 3-2 **Survival Rates with ED Thoracotomy Done for Stab Wounds of the Chest at Detroit Receiving Hospital (1980-1993)**

Main Organ Injured	Isolated Injury	Combined Injury	Total
	(42)	(14)	(56)
Heart	24%	14%	21%
	(1)	(10)	(11)
Lung	100%	10%	18%
	(2)	(0)	(2)
Great Vessel	0%	0%	0%
	(75)	(24)	(99)
TOTAL	24%	13%	20%

( ) = number of patients in each group
% = survival rate in each group

In a 1974 report from Houston, a 59% survival rate was achieved in patients with cardiac wounds who were alive and had an obtainable blood pressure.[128] However, patient outcome is dismal if an ED thoracotomy is done either in patients with blunt trauma or in patients arriving without signs of life, regardless of the injury mechanism.

In addition to its selective use in cardiac arrest patients, an ED "resuscitative" thoracotomy may also be indicated in patients who are deteriorating and have a systolic blood pressure less than 60 mm Hg.[48] However, our results with ED thoracotomy for refractory shock at Detroit Receiving Hospital have tended to be worse than thoracotomies performed in the OR for apparently similar injuries.[49]

COMPLICATIONS OF ED THORACOTOMY

Technical complications of ED thoracotomy may involve virtually every intrathoracic structure and have included lacerations of the heart, coronary arteries, aorta, phrenic nerves, esophagus, and lungs, as well as avulsion of intercostal arteries from the aorta during cross-clamping. Adhesions from a previous thoracotomy make emergency ED thoracotomy extremely difficult and represent a relative contraindication to the procedure.[48] However, in such cases, a midsternotomy for heart lesions may still be possible.

AXIOM If the patient has had a remote thoracotomy, open cardiac massage, if indicated, should be performed through a midsternotomy incision.

In individuals who survive an ED thoracotomy, the more frequent postoperative morbidities include atelectasis, pneumonia, recurrent in-

TABLE 3-3 **Survival Rates with ED Thoracotomy Done for Gunshot Wounds of the Chest at Detroit Receiving Hospital (1980-1993)**

Major Organ Injured	Isolated Injury	Combined Injury	Total
	(64)	(44)	(108)
Heart	1.6%	2.3%	1.9%
	(25)	(11)	(36)
Lung	12.0%	9.1%	11.1%
	(17)	(42)	(59)
Great Vessel	11.8%	9.5%	10.2%
	(106)	(97)	(203)
TOTAL	5.7%	6.2%	5.9%

( ) = number of patients in each group
% = survival rate in each group

trathoracic bleeding, empyema, chest wall infections, and postpericardiotomy syndrome.[48]

Temporary mechanical assist devices should also be considered if the cardiac output remains low in spite of optimal fluid loading and maximal inotropic and/or vasoconstrictor/vasodilator support.

Mechanical Cardiac Support

INTRA-AORTIC BALLOON PUMPING

Our experience with the intra-aortic balloon pump (IABP) for cardiac failure or persistent shock after chest trauma has been very disappointing. Apparently, the degree of cardiovascular failure was irreversible by the time IABP was initiated.

CARDIOPULMONARY BYPASS (CPB)

Although the concept of cardiopulmonary support by extracorporeal circulation of oxygenated blood was proposed in 1813 by LeGallios, the first successful use of cardiopulmonary bypass for open cardiac surgery was not reported until 1954 by John Gibbon.[52] Extracorporeal circulation was first utilized for the treatment of cardiac arrest by Fell et al[129] in 1968. These clinicians described a patient who presented with ventricular fibrillation and profound hypothermia. He was refractory to open cardiac massage and internal defibrillation. Following rewarming with the aid of cardiopulmonary bypass, the patient was successfully defibrillated and discharged alive from the hospital.

Partial cardiopulmonary bypass (PCPB) was subsequently used in conjunction with closed-chest CPR in 1972 by Towne et al.[130] Utilizing femoral vein to femoral artery vascular access, a patient with ventricular fibrillation unresponsive to conventional CPR was successfully resuscitated by PCPB and discharged alive from the hospital.

In 1976 Mattox et al[131] reported on 39 moribund patients, of whom six presented with cardiac arrest and were treated with a portable cardiopulmonary bypass system. Three of these six patients were successfully resuscitated, and one was discharged alive from the hospital. When used for management of cardiac arrest, vascular access has been accomplished within 5 minutes without interrupting external massage.[132] The exact role of cardiopulmonary bypass in the management of cardiac arrest is still not clear; however, it may be extremely helpful in patients with massive pulmonary emboli[133] or severe hypothermia[134] with cardiac arrest.

CENTRIFUGAL PUMPS FOR PARTIAL BYPASS

The advent of centrifugal pumps (Biomedicus pump and Sarns centrifugal pump), which when pumping blood from the left atrium or left ventricle to the distal aorta or to a femoral artery allow partial cardiac bypass without an oxygenator and with little or no systemic anticoagulation.[135] This offers another potential mechanism for increasing the salvage of moribund patients.[48] Indeed, this device has revamped the approach to the treatment of torn descending thoracic aorta in some centers, especially in patients with associated myocardial contusion.[136]

EXTRACORPOREAL MEMBRANE OXYGENATION (ECMO)

Adjunctive use of extracorporeal membrane oxygenation (ECMO) with partial or complete cardiopulmonary bypass may also play a role in supporting patients with multiple organ failure.[48] Under optimal conditions, it can sustain myocardial and cerebral blood flow at levels which may prevent irreversible injury even after prolonged periods of cardiac arrest. Extracorporeal pump oxygenators may also extend the time for successful outcome beyond that documented experimentally with open or closed chest cardiac massage.[137]

DIRECT MECHANICAL VENTRICULAR ACTUATION

Direct mechanical ventricular actuation (DMVA) is a biventricular circulatory support device applied to the exterior of the heart.[138] In DMVA, the heart is placed inside a contoured cup and the ventricular myocardium is pneumatically "pushed" into systole and "pulled" out into its diastolic configuration. Recent studies have found DMVA to be superior to closed-chest compressions and open-chest cardiac massage (OCCM).[111] DMVA has also been shown to improve salvage of ischemic myocardium.[139]

MYOCARDIAL ISCHEMIA/REPERFUSION INJURY

The traditional approach to salvage of cardiac muscle and the reduction of peri-infarction mortality has been directed toward optimization of myocardial oxygen supply and demand[48,140] This may be at least partially accomplished by early coronary reperfusion, using coronary vasodilators, beta blockers, and left ventricular afterload reduction. However, such efforts to improve myocardial reperfusion do not uniformly restore or preserve regional wall motion.[141] Continuing abnormalities in myocardial metabolism which may follow transient ischemia include: (a) conversion from glucose to a free fatty acid based metabolism for myocardial energy production, (b) loss of tricarboxylic acid cycle intermediates, and (c) depletion of enzymes with sulfhydryl groups involved in energy production.[142]

Following CPR, production of toxic oxygen metabolites has been associated with tissue injury in the brain, lung, intestine, liver, and heart.[143] Evidence is emerging that controlled reperfusion directed toward restoration of intermediary metabolism, scavenging of toxic oxygen metabolites, suppression of cell membrane lipid peroxidation, and reduced activation of neutrophils can dramatically attenuate the tissue damage associated with post-ischemic reperfusion injury.[143] Indeed, current investigations suggest that muscle injury may be reversible after 3 to 6 hours of local ischemia.[144,145]

CEREBRAL RESUSCITATION

Causes of Cerebral Dysfunction and Damage

ISCHEMIC ANOXIA

In healthy dogs, cerebral ischemic changes after up to 12 minutes of cardiac arrest can be reversed by advanced cardiopulmonary life support, resulting in almost uniform spontaneous normotension and conscious survival.[146] However, 15 minutes of cerebral ischemia seems at present to be the upper limit of experimental conscious survival, usually only when open-chest cardiac massage or cardiopulmonary bypass are utilized. Although reperfusion by cardiopulmonary bypass can result in resumption of a heartbeat, even after a cardiac arrest of 30 minutes, irreversible hemorrhagic cardiac necrosis usually follows.[146]

Within 10-15 seconds after a sudden complete circulatory arrest, brain oxygen stores are exhausted, resulting in unconsciousness, and within 5 minutes brain glucose and adenosine triphosphate (ATP) are depleted.[147] Anaerobic glycolysis causes increasing cerebral lactic acidosis, which is maximal after about 15 minutes;[148] however, brain tissue osmolality and free fatty acid levels from membrane breakdown continue to rise.[149]

> **AXIOM**   Intracellular accumulation of ionized calcium is one of the most important initial factors limiting successful cerebral resuscitation after ischemia anoxia.

With severe ischemia anoxia, the energy-dependent extracellular-to-intracellular gradient of ionized calcium (Ca^{++}), which is normally 10,000:1, is lost and Ca^{++} accumulates in the cytosol.[88] The increased cytosolic Ca^{++} concentrations activate cellular phospholipases and may cause the proteolytic conversion of xanthine dehydrogenase (in brain capillary endothelium) to xanthine oxidase. These events, along with the accumulation of hypoxanthine, a degradation product of ATP and free fatty acids, set the stage for excessive production of superoxide radicals during reoxygenation.[150] Similar intracellular derangements occur in other organs, but the brain appears to be the most vulnerable.

Iron-dependent oxygen free radical reactions could potentially "nick" the DNA by attacking the sugar-PO_4 backbone. This could convert single-strand DNA regions occurring during ischemia to lethal double-strand breaks upon reperfusion. However, after a 20-minute cardiac arrest and 8 hours of reperfusion in dogs, no significant DNA damage could be validated by extremely sensitive assay techniques.[151]

POSTRESUSCITATION SYNDROMES

After reperfusion and reoxygenation, secondary tissue insults, which can prevent complete recovery, occur in all ischemic organs. Animal research has disproved the prevalent concept that irreversible damage in the brain is inevitable whenever complete normothermic circulatory arrest has lasted for more than 5 minutes. Outcome studies in animals[30,145,146] have shown that occasionally, owing to poorly understood mechanisms, normothermic cardiac arrest can be survived with complete neurologic recovery. Evidence also suggests that a period of a complete cerebral ischemia due to exsanguination is less injurious to the brain than an equal period of ischemia secondary to normovolemic ventricular fibrillation. Interestingly, although asphyxia cardiac arrest is more injurious to the brain, the asphyxiated heart can be restarted more easily.[146]

Retinal neurons in vitro can tolerate normothermic anoxia for up to 20 minutes, and some cerebral neurons in vitro can tolerate up to 60 minutes of normothermic anoxia.[152] However, other neurons, such as those in the neocortical layers 3 to 5, the hippocampus region CA 1, and cerebellar Purkinje's cells, are much more vulnerable.[148] For several days after the reperfusion, varying degrees and stages of ischemic neuronal histologic changes can be seen, side-by-side with normal neurons. Ischemic neuronal changes and microinfarcts occur predominately in arterial boundary zones, suggesting a vascular etiology for these changes.

Several hypotheses have been advanced to explain the selective vulnerability of neurons. One theory suggests that excitatory neurotransmitters, such as glutamate, trigger neuronal hyperexcitability, which is accompanied by excessive Ca^{++} entry with its resultant cell damage.[153] Another hypothesis suggests that the neurons are more vulnerable because they are relatively deficient in oxygen radical scavengers, such as glutathione peroxidase and catalase. A final theory postulates that neurons are terminally differentiated and therefore unable to repair the cell membrane damage incurred.

Safar and his colleagues have been studying the hypothesis that the postresuscitation syndrome consists of four interacting secondary derangements that may eventually be either preventable or treatable.[30,154] These include: (a) cerebral and extracerebral (multifocal) perfusion problems that reduce blood supply below demand,[155] (b) reoxygenation injury caused by cascades of necrotizing chemical reactions,[30,150] (c) brain and heart intoxication caused by anoxia,[154] and (d) blood element derangement caused by the abnormal stasis and interactions with endothelium and tissues.[156]

PROBLEMS WITH PERFUSION

After total circulatory arrest of more than 5 minutes, the brain seems to go through three successive phases of postarrest perfusion: (a) transient global hyperemia, lasting 15 to 30 minutes,[155] (b) delayed, prolonged global and multifocal hypoperfusion, lasting 12 to 48 hours,[30,147,157] and finally (c) resolution to either normal reperfusion, continued hypoperfusion, or progression to zero flow and brain death. The myocardium also appears to go through the same hyperemia to hypoperfusion phases, with eventual development of cardiac failure and increased vascular resistance.[154]

The protracted hypoperfusion phase (phase 2) seems to include inhomogeneous areas of trickle flow,[158] which fluctuate over time and are adjacent to normal or high flow areas. This inhomogeneity of flow makes the evaluation of potential treatments unsatisfactory if based on global or only selected unifocal blood flow measurements. Inhomogeneous perfusion failure also seems to occur in the myocardium and remains to be studied in other organs.

Postarrest perfusion failure can occur in spite of normotension. This failure has many possible pathogenic factors, including aggregation of platelets and/or red and white blood cells, vasospasm, and tissue edema.[30,155,156] Reoxygenation injury cascades also contribute factors, such as arachidonate and leukotrienes. Arachidonic acid, which is released after lipid membrane damage, can be oxidatively metabolized to many vasoactive substances such as prostaglandins (prostacyclin and thromboxane) and leukotrienes. Although arachidonate levels return quickly to normal after reperfusion, tissue levels of leukotrienes, which are potent vasoconstrictors, may remain elevated for more than 24 hours.[150] Local development of granulocyte aggregates can be a source of oxygen radicals and cause microvascular obstruction and endothelial damage.[159]

RE-OXYGENATION INJURY

There are a number of partially proven hypotheses regarding the reoxygenation injury cascade[30,147,150] that can be integrated in an attempt to explain the events after complete ischemia and reperfusion. These hypotheses may also help to separate cellular events from those occurring in plasma, blood, endothelium, and vascular smooth muscle.

Iron-dependent Radical Reactions

Polyunsaturated fatty acids (PUFA) in lipid membranes are extensively peroxidized by iron-dependent radical reactions during reperfusion.[30,147,150,159–161] At 8 hours of postischemic brain reperfusion, tissue levels of malondialdehyde, which is a breakdown product of peroxidized PUFA, are increased fivefold, cellular ionic gradients are lost (having been equilibrated with extracellular fluid), and 30% of the tissue unsaturated lipids have been lost. These effects were significantly inhibited by the iron chelator deferoxamine administered during the first 15 minutes of reperfusion; however, neurologic survival in dogs was not improved.[151]

Suppression of Protein Synthesis

Postischemic reperfusion is associated with significant protein synthesis suppression in the selectively vulnerable areas of the brain.[151] Specific brain proteins are gradually lost over several days following reperfusion, presumably secondary to decreased production. The individual components of the transcription-translational pathway have been extensively studied, and the DNA, mRNA, ribosomal RNA, and the ribosomes themselves have not been shown to have fragmentation damage, and more importantly, they appear to function normally in vivo.[151] The translational system is very sensitive to potassium and magnesium concentrations, and the shift in these ions during the postischemic loss of cellular ionic gradients might be directly involved in the in vitro protein suppression.[151]

Terminal Differentiation

Tissues with cell lines that are terminally differentiated and unable to divide without stem cell support, such as glomeruli, myocardial cells, and central nervous system neurons, are quite sensitive to damage and are unable to divide after ischemia and reperfusion. Cell membrane and DNA production are coregulated, so that if you block one, you block the other. Following ischemia-anoxia, there is a 90% decrease in cholesterol synthesis in differentiated neurons, and sterol and phospholipid synthesis during myeloid differentiation are also significantly decreased.[151,162]

Tumor cell lines are less susceptible to lipid peroxidation.[163] A differentiable neuroblastoma cell line in our laboratory showed that differentiated cells were significantly more susceptible to oxygen radical induced insults than undifferentiated cells. Therapies, such as the use of various growth factors which have proto-oncogenic effects and therefore are able to turn on lipid membrane synthesis are currently under investigation.

EXTRACEREBRAL ORGAN FAILURE

Intoxication of the brain and heart following cardiac arrest by a temporary derangement in the function of the liver and kidneys is suggested by evidence showing some benefit achieved with detoxification.[152,155] A deleterious role of extracerebral organ dysfunction is also suggested by improved toleration of longer periods of circulatory arrest to the brain alone as compared to circulatory arrest to the entire organism.[145,146]

Numerous other extracerebral factors pre and post cardiac arrest can also affect cerebral recovery. For example, hyperglycemia at the onset of the cardiac arrest or trickle flow with high blood glucose levels during the arrest both increase cerebral lactic acidosis and the severity of the ultimate brain damage.[147]

Newer Efforts to Improve Cerebral Perfusion

New treatments to improve cerebral and cardiac resuscitation have been suggested by the increasing knowledge of organ changes occurring after ischemic anoxia and reperfusion.[30,147,164] Special treatment studies with long-term outcome animal models[165] have shown that at least six types of treatment might reduce the amount of brain damage developing after experimental circulatory arrest of over 10 minutes.

BRAIN-ORIENTED EXTRACEREBRAL LIFE SUPPORT

Brain-orientated extracerebral life support protocols are designed to reduce postischemic brain damage by maintaining normal BP, blood gas values, blood composition, and other extracerebral variables after restoration of spontaneous cardiac activity.[30,154,165] Their use seems to improve both cerebral and overall cerebral outcome compared with "usual care," in both animals and patients.

BLOOD FLOW PROMOTION[29,145]

Hemodilution and moderate hypertension have improved outcome after 12 minutes of cardiac arrest in dogs.[146] Cardiopulmonary bypass with circuit priming by plasma substitutes also has increased conscious survival rates,[29] possibly due to increased homogeneous reperfusion.

BARBITURATES[30,166,167]

The ability of barbiturates to reduce cerebral oxygen consumption during post-arrest hypoperfusion, along with its other beneficial effects, such as oxygen radical scavenging,[148] provided the rationale to test its usefulness immediately following cardiac arrest. Although initial studies of global brain ischemia in monkeys provided promising data,[167] subsequent studies in other animal models have yielded variable results.[30] In addition, the first randomized clinical study of cardiopulmonary cerebral resuscitation (CPCR), developed by Safar in the late 1970s and published in 1982, showed no significant overall differences between thiopental-loaded patients and control patients with respect to neurologic outcome.[165]

AXIOM Barbiturate loading, which also depresses cardiovascular function, is not recommended for routine use following a cardiac arrest.

CALCIUM ENTRY BLOCKERS[87,146,157]

Following a cardiac arrest, the brain might benefit from the ability of calcium entry blockers to improve cerebral blood flow and reduce the calcium shifts that are a contributing factor in reoxygenation injury.[30,87] Indeed, long term outcome studies using lidoflazine after global brain ischemia in dogs[146] and nimodipine in monkeys[161] have shown beneficial results. However, calcium entry blockers ameliorate some post-ischemic brain damage[147] without improving outcome.[168] Calcium channel blockers may also cause hypotension due to vasodilation and a reduced cardiac output. The Brain Resuscitation Clinical Trial II used lidoflazine postarrest and did not show any improvement in outcome when compared to controls.[28]

FREE RADICAL SCAVENGERS[150,168]

The natural detoxification mechanisms against oxygen radicals, which include superoxide dismutase, catalase, and glutathione peroxidase,[150] are limited, especially in vulnerable neurons, and are overwhelmed during reperfusion. Microhemorrhages which occur during reperfusion may be related to oxygen concentrations and therefore may be reduced by control of free radical reactions.[159]

The use of a cocktail of free radical scavengers has produced a modest, but significant improvement in outcome after asphyxial cardiac arrest in dogs;[169] however, SOD, deferoxamine, or both, administered after global brain ischemia, has shown no effect on survival or neurologic deficit scoring.[169,170] Explanations for the lack of neurologic improvement with this cocktail include: (a) slow or poor movement of deferoxamine[169,170] and SOD[169] across the blood-brain barrier, (b) presence of brain xanthine oxidase only in the capillary endothelium,[169] and (c) the ability of calcium channel blockers to only work on L channels and not on glutamate NMDA receptor calcium channels.[169] Unless free radical scavengers can be modified to penetrate the blood-brain barrier very rapidly, their therapeutic effects will be limited to the microcirculation.

MULTIFACETED TREATMENTS[145,171]
Our present understanding of the multifactorial pathogenesis of the postresuscitation syndrome suggests that multifaceted, etiology-specific combined therapies are certainly needed.[30] Since one treatment component might offset the benefit of another, it will be important to adapt treatments to specific mechanisms and to conduct systematic studies of individual components and combinations.

Special Problems Following CPR

POSTRESUSCITATION PULMONARY EDEMA
A unique syndrome of postresuscitation pulmonary edema occasionally occurs following CPR; however, its mechanism is not well understood.[172] It is still not completely clear whether this represents hydrostatic (high pulmonary capillary pressure) or permeability (normal pulmonary capillary pressure) pulmonary edema, but current data tend to suggest that it is due to increased capillary permeability.

GASTRIC DILATATION
If the initial resuscitative attempts have included mask-to-mouth ventilation, it can be assumed that substantial amounts of air have been forced into the stomach. The resulting gastric dilatation can be especially dangerous if the patient has recently eaten. During the cardiac arrest, the esophageal sphincters and vocal cords tend to relax, and the gastric contents can be easily regurgitated into the mouth, pharynx, larynx, and lungs. Thus, if there is any suspicion that gastric dilatation may be present, the stomach should be emptied of liquid and gas with a nasogastric tube as soon as possible. Gastric dilatation can also cause significant vagal stimulation.

HYPERKALEMIA
If there is evidence of severe hyperkalemia, the emergency treatment includes intravenous calcium gluconate or chloride, sodium bicarbonate, and hypertonic glucose with insulin. One should particularly suspect hyperkalemia in oliguric patients with severe burns or crush syndromes.

WHEN TO STOP ATTEMPTS AT CARDIAC RESUSCITATION

The only definite contraindication to cardiac resuscitation are decapitation, dependent lividity and a terminal disease in which the patient's suffering would only be prolonged. In addition, cardiac resuscitation should not be continued if there are unreconstructable injuries, uncontrollable bleeding, or apparent brain death demonstrated by fixed dilated pupils and absence of all reflexes for more than 20 to 30 minutes without hypothermia. However, even without these injuries or signs, if adequate myocardial function cannot be restored after 30 minutes of effective massage, then this is essentially a lethal injury and further attempts at resuscitation will be futile.

⊘ FREQUENT ERRORS

In Preventing or Treating Cardiac Arrest in Trauma Patients

1. *Any delay in beginning CPR in a patient who apparently has no effective cardiac output.*
2. *Failure to look for and rapidly correct the initial cause of a cardiac arrest.*
3. *Failure to attempt preoxygenation of a "live" patient before attempting endotracheal intubation.*
4. *Not using pulse oximetry to monitor critically injured patients in the ED.*
5. *Failure to promptly check the position of the endotracheal tube after it is inserted.*
6. *Delay in preforming an emergency thoracotomy to control the source of massive hemoptysis in a trauma patient.*
7. *Not recognizing a cardiac arrest until the patient has had a seizure or has regurgitated gastric contents and aspirated.*
8. *Not recognizing that any new cardiovascular or neurologic symptoms after beginning positive pressure ventilation may be due to air emboli.*
9. *Giving bicarbonate for severe acidosis without checking venous gases or end-tidal CO_2 levels.*
10. *Delay in cardioverting ventricular tachycardia if the patient is hypotensive.*
11. *Using external cardiac massage in a patient with severe truncal trauma.*
12. *Not taking advantage of an opportunity to immediately electrically defibrillate a patient who has just had a cardiac arrest.*
13. *Administering calcium during CPR without a good indication.*

▼▼▼▼▼▼▼▼▼▼▼▼▼▼▼▼▼▼▼▼▼▼▼▼▼▼▼▼▼▼▼▼

SUMMARY POINTS

1.   Prehospital cardiac arrest is almost uniformly lethal if it persists for more than 5 minutes or is due to problems which cannot be rapidly corrected.

2.   Pre-intubation oxygenation is extremely important in patients in acute respiratory failure after trauma.

3.   Pulse oximetry should be used in all patients with severe trauma, especially during and following emergency intubation.

4.   Any manipulations of the upper airway, such as laryngoscopy, are prone to make hypoxemia worse. If this is not recognized and corrected rapidly, morbidity and mortality will increase.

5.   If there is any suspicion that the endotracheal tube is in the esophagus, it should be replaced.

6.   Even if the endotracheal tube is correctly placed, it is easy for it to move down into a main stem bronchus, especially on the right, particularly if the patient is small and agitated.

7.   Not infrequently, poor breath sounds on the left side in an intubated patient with chest trauma are due to a misplaced endotracheal tube rather than a left hemopneumothorax.

8.   Severe hemoptysis after trauma is a relative indication for an emergency thoracotomy, especially if there is evidence of air embolism.

9.   Any new cardiovascular or neurologic changes occurring during or just after endotracheal intubation and positive pressure ventilation should be considered due to systemic air emboli until proven otherwise.

10.   Inappropriately slow pulse rates after major trauma can cause severe problems because: (a) there is an increased incidence of arrhythmias, (b) the cardiac output is often reduced, and (c) the patients are more prone to have a vasovagal response.

11.   Sudden severe alkalosis can reduce ionized calcium and magnesium levels by 15 to 24% (5 to 8% decrease for each 0.1 pH rise) which may cause severe arrhythmias.

12. Ventricular tachycardia without hypotension can often be treated with medications alone, but immediate cardioversion is indicated if associated hypotension or instability (i.e., chest pain, CHF, or signs of end organ hypoperfusion) is present.

13. Although regurgitation of gastric contents can be the cause of a cardiac arrest, the reverse is usually true.

14. If an adequate airway cannot be rapidly established with an oral airway or endotracheal tube in an apneic patient, an emergency coniotomy (cricothyroidotomy) should be performed.

15. Patients with severe trauma are hypermetabolic and often have an oxygen debt requiring a minute ventilation that is at least twice normal.

16. External CPR probably produces vital organ perfusion by a combination of chest-pump and heart-pump mechanisms.

17. After 20 minutes of unsuccessful resuscitation, further interventions are likely to be futile, except when cardiac arrest occurs during hypothermia.

18. The addition of IAC to standard CPR may improve survival following in-hospital cardiac arrest.

19. Vigorous external cardiac massage can cause internal damage, especially in patients with recent truncal surgery or trauma.

20. If patients with an otherwise good prognosis have a cardiac arrest due to a mechanical problem (such as pericardial tamponade) and do not respond rapidly to closed cardiac massage, open cardiac massage may substantially improve their survival.

21. Because many patients with a cardiac arrest have a tendency to develop congestive heart failure, a large fluid bolus should not be given unless there is evidence of hypovolemia.

22. If a patient remains hypotensive after an otherwise successful cardiac resuscitation, insertion of a pulmonary-artery catheter should be considered.

23. Measurement of CVP and both mean and diastolic aortic pressures during cardiac arrest can serve as useful indicators of both systemic and coronary perfusion pressures.

24. Acid-base monitoring during cardiac resuscitation should include arterial and mixed venous blood, lactate levels, and expired CO_2.

25. The $P_{ET}CO_2$ is a relatively good indicator of the quantity of (pulmonary) blood flow generated with closed-chest CPR.

26. Early defibrillation is the most important determinant of survival from sudden cardiac arrest.

27. Persistent hypotension in trauma patients is usually due to hypovolemia from continued bleeding.

28. Alpha adrenergic agents, such as epinephrine, can increase successful return of spontaneous circulation with CPR by increasing diastolic aortic pressure and coronary perfusion pressure.

29. Epinephrine should be administered in increasing doses if there is no satisfactory response to CPR within 2 to 3 minutes.

30. Use of norepinephrine in hypovolemic patients can cause such severe vasoconstriction that tissue necrosis occurs.

31. Adequate fluid resuscitation should be completed on all patients prior to the administration of vasopressors.

32. Even though the arterial PCO_2 may remain relatively normal in shock states, the mixed venous blood may be quite acidotic due to a high PCO_2.

33. Bicarbonate should be withheld or given with extreme caution if the arterial or venous PCO_2 levels are elevated.

34. Intravenous calcium can have a strong positive inotropic effect in patients with low ionized calcium levels.

35. The administration of calcium is not advised during CPR except when cardiac arrest is associated with hyperkalemia, hypocalcemia, or calcium channel blocking drugs.

36. Atropine may be used to help prevent asystole in high degree A-V blocks, but it is usually only indicated during symptomatic bradycardia, EMD, or asystole.

37. Lidocaine may be of benefit for preventing ventricular fibrillation, but once it occurs, lidocaine may make it more difficult for ventricular fibrillation to be cardioverted to a sinus rhythm.

38. Bretylium may be a potent alternative for recurrent ventricular fibrillation/tachycardia that is refractory to lidocaine.

39. If an intravenous line can't be started promptly in a patient with a cardiac arrest, epinephrine can be given via the endotracheal tube.

40. Sodium bicarbonate should not be administered via the tracheobronchial tree.

41. If a patient had vital signs in the ambulance and then lost them, open-chest CPR in the ED may be worthwhile for penetrating wounds, especially stab wounds to the chest or extremities.

42. Open cardiac massage is more effective than closed-chest compression in patients with chest or abdominal trauma.

43. The highest salvage rate with CPR via an emergency room thoracotomy occurs in patients with a stab wound to the heart who have a cardiac arrest just before or soon after arrival to the ED.

44. Resuscitative thoracotomy and open cardiac message will only on rare occasion successfully resuscitate a patient with cardiac arrest secondary to blunt trauma.

45. Early recognition and prompt relief of pericardial tamponade is essential to improve survival in patients with cardiac wounds.

46. The quickest way (prior to pericardiocentesis or thoracotomy) to raise the blood pressure in a patient with pericardial tamponade is to give intravenous fluids.

47. The initial incision of choice for ED thoracotomy for open CPR is an anterolateral thoracotomy.

48. At the time of ED thoracotomy, further attempts at resuscitation should cease if there is no cardiac activity, the heart is completely empty, and the patient has had no signs of life for more than 5 minutes.

49. Difficult cardiac wounds are best repaired under cardiopulmonary bypass.

50. Thoracic aortic cross-clamping should be considered a potentially dangerous temporary maneuver designed to keep the patient alive while life-threatening problems are rapidly corrected.

51. The BP response to aortic clamping should be monitored very closely.

52. The ultimate metabolic goal of resuscitation from shock is non-delivery dependent oxygen consumption. This is accomplished by raising oxygen delivery (DO_2) until oxygen consumption (VO_2) is above normal and/or will not rise any further with an increased DO_2.

53. If the patient has had a remote thoracotomy, open cardiac massage, if indicated, should be performed through a midsternotomy incision.

54. Intracellular accumulation of ionized calcium is one of the most important initial factors limiting successful cerebral resuscitation after ischemia anoxia.

55. Barbiturate loading, which also depresses cardiovascular function, is not recommended for routine use following a cardiac arrest.

▲▲▲▲▲▲▲▲▲▲▲▲▲▲▲▲▲▲▲▲▲▲▲▲▲▲▲▲▲▲▲▲▲▲▲

REFERENCES

1. Lemire JG, Johnson AL. Is cardiac resuscitation worthwhile? A decade of experience. N Engl J Med 1972;286:970.
2. Wilson RF, Thoms N, Arbulu A, Steiger Z. Cardiopulmonary resuscitation. In: Walt AJ, Wilson RF, eds. The management of trauma: practice and pitfalls. Philadelphia: Lea & Fibiger, 1975:149-162.
3. Wilson RF. Controversies and problems in the management of penetrating wounds of the chest. In: Najarian JS, Delaney JP, eds. Trauma and critical care. Chicago: Year Book Medical Publishers, 1987:93-106.
4. Durham ' '. Richardson RJ, Wall MS. Emergency center thoracotomy: impact .ehospital care. J of Trauma 1992;32:775.
5. Wilson RF, Steiger Z. Thoracic injuries. In: Tintinalli J, Krome R, eds. Emergency medicine. 2nd ed. A comprehensive study guide, 1988:850.
6. Martin RR, Bickell WH, Pepe PE, et al. Prospective evaluation of preoperative fluid resuscitation in hypotensive patients with penetrating truncal injury: a preliminary report. Trauma 1992;33:354.
7. Mattox KL, Maningas PA, Moore EE, et al. Prehospital hypertonic saline/dextran infusion for post-traumatic hypotension. USA multicenter trial. Ann Surg 1992;213:482.
8. Valentine SJ, Marjot R, Mong CR. Preoxygenation in the elderly: a comparison of the four maximal-breath and three minute techniques. Anesth Analg 1990;71:516.

9. Bowes WA. Pulse oximetry: a review of the theory, accuracy and clinical applications. Obstet Gynecol 1989;74:541.

10. Wilson RF, Soullier GW, Wienck RG. Hemoptysis in trauma. J Trauma 1987;27:1123-1126.

11. Wilson RF. Injury to the heart and great vessels. In: Henning RJ, Grenvik A, eds. Critical care cardiology. New York: Churchill, Livingstone, 1989.

12. Wilson RF, Gibson DB, Percineal AK, et al. Severe alkalosis in critically ill patients. Arch Surg 1972;105:197-203.

13. Wilson RF, Soullier G, Antoneko D. Ionized calcium levels in critically ill surgical patients. Am Surg 1979;45:485-90.

14. Hoffman BF. The genesis of cardiac arrhythmias. Prog Cardiovas Dis 1966;8:319.

15. Han J. Mechanisms of ventricular arrhythmia associated with myocardial infarction. Am J Cardiol 1969;24:800.

16. Lorenz HP, Steinmetz B, Lieberman J, et al. Emergency thoracotomy: survival rates correlate with physiologic status. J Trauma 1992;32:780.

17. Stephenson HE Jr., Reid LC, Hinton JW. Some common denominators in 1200 cases of cardiac arrest. Ann Surg 1953;137:731.

18. Bircher N, Safar N. Manual open-chest cardiopulmonary resuscitation. Ann Emerg Med 1984;13:770.

19. Kouwenhoven WB, Jude JR, Knickerbocker GG. Closed-chest cardiac massage. JAMA 1960;173:1064.

20. Elam JO, Brown ES, Elder JD Jr. Artificial respiration by mouth-to-mask method. A study of the respiratory gas exchange of paralyzed patients ventilated by operator's expired air. N Engl J Med 1954;250:749.

21. Safar P, Escarraga LA, Elam J. A comparison of mouth-to-mouth and mouth-to-airway methods of artificial respiration with the chest-pressure arm-lift methods. N Engl J Med 1958;258:671.

22. Gordon AS, et al. Mouth-to mouth versus manual artificial respiration for children and adults. JAMA 1958;167:320.

23. Zoll PM, Linenthal AJ, Gibson W, et al. Termination of ventricular fibrillation in man by externally placed electric countershock. N Engl J Med 1956;254:727.

24. Jude JR, Kouwenhoven WB, Knickerbocker GG. Cardiac arrest: report of application of external cardiac massage on 188 patients. JAMA 1961;178:1063.

25. Safar P, et al. Ventilation and circulation with closed chest cardiac massage in man. JAMA 1961;176:574.

26. Weisfeldt ML, et al. Mechanisms of perfusion in cardiopulmonary resuscitation. In: Shoemaker WC, Thompson WL, Holbrook PR, eds. Textbook of critical care. Philadelphia: WB Saunders, 1984:31.

27. Fisher J, Vaghaiwalla F, Tsitlik J, et al. Determinants of and clinical significance of jugular venous valve competence. Circulation 1982;65:188.

28. Robers MC, Nugent SK, Stidham GL. Effects of closed-chest cardiac massage on intracranial pressure. Crit Care Med 1979;7:454.

29. Pretto E, Safar P, Saito R, et al. Cardiopulmonary bypass after prolonged cardiac arrest in dogs. Ann Emerg Med 1987;16:611.

30. Paradis NA, Martin GB, Bovell D, et al. Coronary perfusion pressures during CPR are higher in patients with eventual return of spontaneous circulation. Ann Emeg Med 1989;18:478.

31. Ditchey RV, Winkler JV, Rhodes CA. Relative lack of coronary blood flow during closed-chest resuscitation on dogs. Circulation 1982;66:297.

32. DelGuercio LMR, et al. Comparison of blood flow during external and internal cardiac massage in man. Circulation 1964;31:63; 1965;32 (Suppl 1):171.

33. Sharff JA, Pantley G, Noel E. Effect of time on regional organ perfusion during two methods of cardiopulmonary resuscitation. Ann Emerg Med 1984;13:649.

34. Kellerman AL, Staves DR, Hackman BB. In-hospital resuscitation following unsuccessful prehospital advanced life support: "heroic efforts" or an exercise in futility? Ann Emerg Med 1988;17:589.

35. Southwick FS, Dalglish PH Jr. Recovery after prolonged asystolic cardiac arrest in profound hypothermia. A case report and literature review. JAMA 1980;243:1250-1253.

36. Molokhia FA, Ponn RB, Robinson WJ, et al. A method of augmenting coronary perfusion pressure during internal cardiac massage. Chest 1972;62:610-613.

37. Lindner KH, Ahnefeld FW, Bowdler IM. Cardiopulmonary resuscitation with interposed abdominal compression after asphyxial or fibrillatory cardiac arrest in pigs. Anesthesiology 1990;72:675-681.

38. Berryman CR, Phillips GM. Interposed abdominal compression-CPR in human subjects. Ann Emerg Med 1984;13:226-229.

39. Ward KR, Sullivan RJ, Zelenak RR, Summer WR. A comparison of interposed abdominal compression CPR and standard CPR by monitoring end-tidal PCO$_2$. Ann Emerg Med 1989;18:831-837.

40. Einagle V, Bertrand F, Wise RA, et al. Interposed abdominal compressions and carotid blood flow during cardiopulmonary resuscitation: support for a thoracoabdominal unit. Chest 1988;93:1206-1212.

41. Sack JB, Kesselbrenner MB, Bregman D. Survival from in-hospital cardiac arrest with interposed abdominal counterpulsation during cardiopulmonary resuscitation. JAMA 1992;267:381.

42. Bedell SE, Fulton EJ. Unexpected findings and complications at autopsy after cardiopulmonary resuscitation (CPR). Arch Intern Med 1986;146:1725-1728.

43. Krischer JP, Fine EG, Davis JH, et al. Complications of cardiac resuscitation. Chest 1987;92:287-291.

44. Barber RF, Wadden JL. Historical aspects of cardiac resuscitation. Am J Surg 1945;70:135.

45. Hanke TG. Studies on ether and chloroform from Professor Shiff's physiological laboratory. Practitioner 1974;12:241-250.

46. Jackson RE, Freeman SB. Hemodynamics of cardiac massage. Emerg Med Clin North Am 1983;1:501.

47. Beck CS, Pritchard WH, Feil H. Ventricular fibrillation of long duration abolished by electric shock. JAMA 1947;135:985-986.

48. Moore JB, Moore EE, Harken AH. Emergency department thoracotomy. In: Moore EE, Mattox KL, Feliciano DV, eds. Trauma. 2nd ed. Norwalk, CT: Appleton & Lange, 1991:181-193.

49. Washington B, Wilson RF, Steiger Z. Emergency thoracotomy: a four-year review. Ann Thorac Surg 1985;40:188.

50. Wilson RF, Sarver E, Birks R. Central venous pressure and blood volume determinations in clinical shock. Surg Gynecol Obstet 1971;132:631.

51. Diebel LN, Wilson, RF, Tagett MG, Kline RA. End-diastolic volume: a better indicator of preload in the critically ill. Arch Surg 1992;127:817.

52. Weil MH, Gazmuri RJ, Rackow EC. The clinical rationale of cardiac resuscitation. Diseases of the Month 1990;36:431.

53. Weil MH, Rackow EC, Trevino R, et al. Difference in acid-base state between venous and arterial blood during cardiopulmonary resuscitation. N Engl J Med 1986;315:153.

54. Weil MH, Bisera J, Trevino RP, et al. Cardiac output and end-tidal carbon dioxide. Crit Care Med 1985;13:907-909.

55. Sanders AB, Kern KB, Otto CW, et al. End-tidal carbon dioxide monitoring during cardiopulmonary resuscitation: a prognostic indicator of survival. JAMA 1989;262:1347-1351.

56. Eisenberg MS, Copass MD, Hallstrom AP. Treatment of out-of-hospital cardiac arrests with rapid defibrillations by emergency medical technicians. N Engl J Med 1980;302:1379.

57. Cummins RO, Eisenberg MS. Automatic external defibrillators: clinical issues for cardiology. Circulation 1986;73:381.

58. Guidelines for cardiopulmonary resuscitation and emergency cardiac care. JAMA 1992;268:2201.

59. Ewy GA, Dahl CF, Zimmerman M, et al. Ventricular fibrillation masquerading as ventricular standstill. Crit Care Med 1981;9:841.

60. Brown CG, Werman HA. Adrenergic agonists during cardiopulmonary resuscitation. Resuscitation 1990;19:1-16.

61. Yakaitis RW, Otto CW, Blitt CD. Relative importance of alpha and beta adrenergic receptors during resuscitation. Crit Care Med 1979;7:293-296.

62. Redding JS, Pearson JW. Resuscitation from ventricular fibrillation. Drug Therapy. JAMA 1968;203:255-260.

63. Schleien CL, Dean JM, Koehler RC, et al. Effect of epinephrine on cerebral and myocardial perfusion in an infant animal preparation of cardiopulmonary resuscitation. Circulation 1986;73:809-817.

64. Callahan M, Madeu CD, Barton CW, et al. A randomized clinical trial of high-dose epinephrine and nonepinephrine versus standard-dose epinephrine in prehospital cardiac arrest. JAMA 1992;268:266.

65. Steill EG, Herbert DC, Weitzmann BN, et al. High dose epinephrine in adult cardiac arrest. N Engl J Med 1993;327:1045.

66. Brown CG, Martin DR, Pepe PE, et al. A comparison of standard-dose and high-dose epinephrine in cardiac arrest outside the hospital. N Engl J Med 1992;327:1951.

67. Livesay JJ, Follette DM, Fey KH, et al. Optimizing myocardial supply/demand balance with alpha-adrenergic drugs during cardiopulmonary resuscitation. J Thorac Cardiovasc Surg 1978;76:244-251.

68. Redding JS, Pearson JW. Evaluation of drugs for cardiac resuscitation. Anesthesiology 1963;24:203-207.

69. Walt AJ, Wilson RF. The treatment of shock. Adv Surg 1975;9:1-39.

70. Wilson RF, Sibbald WJ, Jaanimagi JL. Hemodynamic effects of dopamine in critically ill septic patients. J Surg Res 1976;20:163-72.

71. DiSea UJ, Gold JA, Shemin RJ, et al. Comparison of dopamine and dobutamine in patients requiring postoperative circulatory support. Clin Cardiol 1986;9:253.

72. Stewart JA. Management of cardiac arrest with special reference to metabolic acidosis. Br Med J 1964;1:476-479.

73. Kette F, Weil MH, Gazmuri RJ, et al. Increases in myocardial PCO$_2$ during CPR correlate inversely with coronary perfusion pressures (CPP) and resuscitability (abstr). Circulation 1989;80:II-494.

74. Tang W, Gaxmuri RJ, Weil MH, et al. Myocardial depressant effect of carbon dioxide in the intact rat heart (abstr). Crit Care Med 1989;17:S14.

75. Jacobs MH. The production of intracellular acidity by neutral and alkaline solutions containing carbon dioxide. Am J Physiol 1920;53:457-463.

76. Bello A, Bianco JA, Velarde H, et al. Effect of sodium bicarbonate on canine left ventricular function. Angiology 1977;28:403-410.

77. Guerci AD, Chandra N, Johnson E, et al. Failure of sodium bicarbonate to improve resuscitation from ventricular fibrillation in dogs. Circulation 1986;74(14):75-79.

78. Mattar JA, Weil MH, Shubin H, et al. Cardiac arrest in the critically ill. II. Hyperosmolal states following cardiac arrest. Am J Med 1974;56:162-168.

79. Kette F, Gazmuri RJ, Weil MH, et al. Hypertonic buffer solutions decrease coronary perfusing pressure during CPR (abstr). Crit Care Med 1989;17:S130.

80. Bureau MA, Begin R, Berthaiume Y, et al. Cerebral hypoxia from bicarbonate infusion in diabetic acidosis. J Pediatr 1980;96:968-973.

81. Gonzalez NC, Cingolani HE, Mattiazzi AR, et al. Mechanism of action of tris(hydroxymethyl)aminomethane on the negative inotropic effect of carbon dioxide. Circ Res 1971;28:74-83.

82. Kette F, Von Planta M, Weil MH, et al. Buffer agents do not reverse intramyocardial acidosis during cardiac resuscitation. Circ 1990;81:1660.

83. Seifen E, Flacke W, Alper MH. Effects of calcium on isolated mammalian heart. Am J Physiol 1964;207:716-720.

84. Reuter H. Exchange of calcium ions in the mammalian myocardium. Mechanisms and physiological significance. Circ Res 1974;34:599-605.

85. Urban P. Scheidegger D, Buchmann B, et al. Cardiac arrest and blood ionized calcium levels. Ann Intern Med 1988;109:110-113.

86. Blecic S, De-Backer D, Huynh CH, et al. Calcium chloride in experimental electromechanical dissociation: a placebo-controlled trial in dogs. Crit Care Med 1987;15:324-327.

87. White BC, Winegar CD, Wilson RF, et al. Possible role of calcium blockers in cerebral resuscitation: a review of the literature and synthesis for future studies. Crit Care Med 1983;11:202-207.

88. White BC, Winegar CD, Wilson RF, Hoehner PJ. Calcium blockers in cerebral resuscitation. J Trauma 1983;23:788.

89. Dembo DH. Calcium in advanced life support. Crit Care Med 1981; 9:358-359.

90. Wilson RF, Binkley LE, Sabo FM, et al. Electrolyte and acid base changes with massive blood transfusions. Am Surg 1992;58:535-44.

91. von Planta M, Weil MH, Gazmuri RJ, et al. Calcium entry blockers during porcine CPR. Clin Science 1990;78:207-213.

92. Brown DC, Lewis AJ, Criley MJ. Asystole and its treatment: the possible role of the parasympathetic system in cardiac arrest. J Am Coll Emerg Physicians 1979;8:448-452.

93. Akhtar M, Damato AN, Caracta AR, et al. Electrophysiologic effects of atropine on atrioventricular conduction studies by His bundle electrogram. Am J Cardiol 1974;33:333-343.

94. Coon GA, Clinton JE, Ruiz E. Use of atropine for brady-asystolic prehospital cardiac arrest. Ann Emerg Med 1981;10:462-467.

95. Sorensen O, Eriksen S, Hommelgaard P, et al. Thiopental-nitrous oxide halothane anesthesia and repeated succinylcholine: comparison of preoperative glycopyrrolate and atropine administration. Anesth Analg 1980;59:686-689.

96. Richman S. Adverse effect of atropine during myocardial infarction. Enhancement of ischemia following intravenously administered atropine. JAMA 1974;228:1414-1416.

97. Babbs CF, Yim GKW, Shistler SJ, et al. Elevation of ventricular defibrillation threshold in dogs by antiarrhythmic drugs. Am Heart J 1979;98:345-350.

98. Markis JE, Koch-Weser J. Characteristics and mechanism of inotropic and chronotropic actions of bretylium tosylate. J Pharmacol Exp Ther 1971;178:94-102.

99. Sasyniuk BI. Symposium on the management of ventricular dysrhythmias. Concept of re-entry versus automaticity. Am J Cardiol 1984;54:1A-6A.

100. Hanyok JJ, Chow MS, Kluger J, et al. Antifibrillatory effects of high dose bretylium and a lidocaine-bretylium combination during cardiopulmonary resuscitation. Crit Care Med 1988;16:691-694.

101. Chow MS, Kluger J, Lawrence R, et al. The effect of lidocaine and bretylium on the defibrillation threshold during cardiac arrest and cardiopulmonary resuscitation. Proc Soc Exp Biol Med 1986;182:63-67.

102. Holder DA, Sniderman AD, Fraser G, et al. Experience with bretylium tosylate by a hospital cardiac arrest team. Circulation 1977;55:541-544.

103. Woods KL, Fletcher S, Raffe C, Haider Y. L I M I T - 2 trial. Lancet 1992;339:1553.

104. Ceremuzynski L, Jurgizil R, Kulakowski P, et al. Threatening arrhythmia and acute myocardial infarction are prevented by IV Mg SO$_4$. Am Heart J 1989;118:1333.

105. Raehl C. Endotracheal drug therapy in cardiopulmonary resuscitation. Clin Pharmacol 1986;5:572-579.

106. Gonzalez ER. Pharmacologic controversies in CPR. Ann E Med 1993;22:317.

107. McSwain NE Jr. Prehospital emergency medical systems and cardiopulmonary resuscitation. In: EE Moore, KL Mattox, DV Feliciano, eds. Trauma. 2nd ed. Norwalk, CT: Appleton & Lange, 1991:99-107.

108. Mattox KL, Bickell W, Pepe PE, et al. Prospective MAST study in 911 patients. J of Trauma 1989;29:1104.

109. Wilson RF, Bassett JS. Penetrating wounds of the pericardium or its contents. JAMA 1966;195:513-518.

110. Blakeman B. Open cardiac massage—a surgeon's viewpoint. Postgraduate Med 1990;87:247.

111. Bartlett RL, Steward NJ, Raymone J, et al. Comparative study of three methods of resuscitation: closed chest, open-chest manual and direct mechanical ventricular assist. Ann Emerg Med 1984;13:773.

112. Baker CC, Thomas AN, Trunkey DD. The role of emergency room thoracotomy in trauma. J Trauma 1980;20:848.

113. Baxter BT, Moore EE, Moore JB. Emergency department thoracotomy following injury: critical determinants for patient salvage. World J Surg 1988;12:671.

114. Markison RE, Trunkey DD. Establishment of care priorities. In: Capan LM, Miller SM, Turndorf H, eds. Trauma: anesthesia and intensive care. Philadelphia: JB Lippincott, 1991:29-42.

115. Wechsler AS, Auerback BJ, Graham TC, et al. Distribution of intramyocardial blood flow during pericardial tamponade. J Thorac Cardiovasc Surg 1974;68:847.

116. Stueven HA, Thompson BM, Aprahamian C, et al. Calcium chloride: reassessment of use in asystole. Ann Emerg Med 1984;13:820-822.

117. Wall MJ, Jr., Pepe PE, Mattox KL. Successful roadside resuscitative thoracotomy: case report and literature review. J Trauma 1994;36:131.

118. Mazzorana V, Smith RS, Morabito DJ, et al. Limited utility of emergency department thoracotomy. Am Surg 1994;60:516.

119. Wiencek RG, Wilson RF. Injuries to the abdominal vascular system: how much does aggressive resuscitation and prelaparotomy thoracotomy really help? Surg 1987;102:731-736.

120. Dunn EL, Moore EE, Moore JB. Hemodynamic effects of aortic occlusion during hemorrhagic shock. Ann Emerg Med 1982;11:238.

121. Katz NM, Blackstone EH, Kirklin JW, et al. Incremental risk factors for spinal cord injury following operation for acute traumatic aortic transection. J Thorac Cardiovasc Surg 1981;81:669.

122. Peng CF, Kane JJ, Jones EM, et al. The adverse effects of systemic hypertension following myocardial reperfusion. J Surg Res 1983; 34:59.

123. Huval WV, Leluck S, Allen PD, et al. Determinants of cardiovascular stability during abdominal aneurysmectomy. Ann Surg 1983;199:216.

124. Shoemaker WC, Appel PL, Kram H et al. Prospective trial of supranormal values of survivors as therapeutic goals in high-risk surgical patients. Chest 1988;94:1176-1186.

125. Moore FA, Haenel JB, Moore EE, et al. Incommensurate oxygen consumption in response to maximal oxygen availability predicts post-injury multiple organ failure. J Trauma 1992;33:58.

126. Fleming A, Bishop M, Shuemaker W, et al. Prospective trial of supranormal values as goals of resuscitation in severe trauma. Arch Surg 1992;127:1175.

127. Yu M, Levy MM, Smith P, et al. Effect of maximizing oxygen delivery on morbidity and mortality rates in critically ill patients: a prospective randomized controlled study. Crit Care Med 1993;21:838.

128. Mattox KL, Beall AC, Jordon GI, et al. Cardiorrhaphy in the emergency center. J Thorac Cardiovasc Surg 1974;68:886.

129. Fell RH, Gunning AJ, Bardhan KD, et al. Severe hypothermia as a result of barbiturate overdose complicated by cardiac arrest. Lancet 1968;1:392.

130. Towne WD, Geiss WP, Vanes HO, et al. Intractable ventricular fibrillation associated with profound accidental hypothermia-successful treatment with partial cardiopulmonary bypass. N Engl J Med 1972; 287:1135-1136.

131. Mattox KL, Beall AC Jr. Resuscitation of the moribund patient using portable cardiopulmonary bypass. Ann Thorac Surg 1976;22:435-442.

132. Phillips SJ, Ballentine B, Slonine D, et al. Percutaneous initiation of cardiopulmonary bypass. Ann Thorac Surg 1983;36:223-225.

133. Mattox KL, Feldman RW, Beall AC Jr, et al. Pulmonary embolectomy for acute massive pulmonary embolism. Ann Surg 1982;195:726.

134. Splittgerber FH, Talbert JG, Sweezer WP, Wilson RF. Partial cardiopulmonary bypass for core rewarming in profound accidental hypothermia. Am Surg 1986;52:407-412.

135. Hess PJ, Howe HR, Bobiesek F. Traumatic tears of the thoracic aorta: improved results using the BioMedicus pump. Ann Thor Surg 1989;48:6.

136. Kim FJ, Moore EE, Moore FA, et al. Trauma surgeons can render operative care for major thoracic injuries. J Trauma 1993;35:165.

137. Gazmuri RJ, Weil MH, von Planta M, et al. Cardiac resuscitation by extracorporeal pump oxygenator (ECPO) after failure of precordial compression (abstr). J Am Coll Cardiol 1989;13:220A.

138. Anstadt MP, Bartlett RL, Malone JP, et al. Direct mechanical ventricular actuation for cardiac arrest in humans. Chest 1991;100:86.

139. Anstadt MP, Malone JP, Brown GR, et al. Direct mechanical ventricular assistance promotes salvage of ischemic myocardium. Trans Am Soc Artif Intern Organs 1987;33:720-725.

140. Braunwald E. The aggressive treatment of acute myocardial infarction. Circulation 1985;71:1087.

141. Lazar HL, Piehn JF, Shick EM, et al. Effects of coronary revascularization on regional wall motion. J Thorac Cardiovasc Surg 1989;98:498.

142. Beyersdorf F, Acar C, Buckberg GD, et al. Studies in prolonged acute regional ischemia. J Thorac Cardiovasc Surg 1989;98:567.

143. Brown JM, Grosso MA, Whitman GH, et al. The coincidence of myocardial reperfusion injury and H$_2$O$_2$ production in the isolated rat heart. Surgery 1989;105:496.

144. Kharazmi A, Andersen LW, Back L, et al. Endotoxemia and enhanced generation of cardiac radicals by neutrophils from patients undergoing cardiopulmonary bypass. J Thorac Cardiovasc Surg 1989;98:381.

145. Beyersdorf F, Acar C, Buckberg GD, et al. Studies of prolonged acute regional ischemia: I. evidence for preserved cellular viability after 6 hours of coronary occlusion. J Thorac Cardiovasc Surg 1989;98:112.

146. Safar P, Stezoski SW, Nemoto EM. Amelioration of brain damage after 12 minutes cardiac arrest in dogs. Arch Neurol 1976;33:91.

147. Vaagenes P, et al. Amelioration of brain damage by lidoflazine after prolonged ventricular fibrillation cardiac arrest in dogs. Crit Care Med 1984;12:846.

148. Siesjo BK. Cell damage in the brain: a speculative synthesis. J Cereb Blood Flow Metab 1981;1:155.

149. Siesjo BK, Wieloch T. Cerebral metabolism in ischemia: neurochemical basis for therapy. Br J Anaesth 1985;57:47.

150. McCord JM. Oxygen-derived free radicals in postischemic tissue injury. N Engl J Med 1985;312:159.

151. White BC, DeGracia DJ, Krause GS, et al. Brain nuclear DNA survives cardiac arrest and reperfusion. J Free Rad Biol Med 1991;10:125-135.

152. Ames A III, Nesbett FB. Pathophysiology of ischemic cell death. I. Time of onset of irreversible damage; importance of the different components of the ischemic insult. Stroke 1983;14:219.

153. Hossmann KA, Kleihues P. Reversibility of ischemic brain damage. Arch Neurol 1973;29:375.

154. Brierley JB, Graham DI. Hypoxia and vascular disorders of the central nervous system. In: Adams JH, Corsellis JAN, Duchen LW, eds. Greenfield's neuropathology. New York: Wiley Medical, 1984: 125-156.

155. Meldrum B, Evans M, Griffiths T, Simon R. Ischemic brain damage: the role of excitatory activity and of calcium entry. Br J Anaesth 1985;57:44.

156. Snyder JV, Nemoto EM, Carroll RG, et al. Global ischemia in dogs: intracranial pressures, brain blood flow and metabolism. Stroke 1975; 6:21.

157. Kochanek PM, Dutka AJ, Hallenbeck JM. Indomethacin, prostacyclin and heparin improve postischemic cerebral blood flow without affecting early postischemic granulocyte accumulation. Stroke 1987;18:634.

158. White BC, Gadzinski DS, Hoehner PJ, Krome C, Hoehner T, et al. Effect of flunarizine on canine cerebral cortical blood flow and vascular resistance post-cardiac arrest. Ann Emerg Med 1982;11:110.

159. Kagstroem E, Smith ML, Siesjo BK. Local cerebral blood flow in the recovery period following complete cerebral ischemia in the rat. J Cereb Blood Flow 1983;Metab 3:170.

160. Safar P. Amelioration of postischemic brain damage with barbiturates. Stroke 1980;15:1.

161. Steen PA, Gisvold SE, Milde JH, et al. Nimodipine improves outcome when given after complete cerebral ischemia in primates. Anesthesiology 1985;62:406.

162. Cooper RA, Ip SHC, Cassileth PA, et al. Inhibition of sterol and phospholipid synthesis in HL-60 promyelocytic leukemia cells by inducers of myeloid differentiation. Cancer Res 1981;41: 1847-1852.

163. O'Neil BJ, Chapman S, White BC. Increased radical induced death after neuronal differentiation. Ann E Med 1993;22:928.

164. White BC, et al. Brain injury by ischemic anoxia—hypothesis extension. A tale of two ions? Ann Emerg Med 1984;13:862.

165. Abramson NS, Safar P, Detre KM, et al. Randomized clinical study of thiopental loading in comatose survivors of cardiac arrest. N Engl J Med 1986;314:397.

166. Gisvold SE, Safar P, Rao G, et al. Multifaceted therapy after global brain ischemia in monkeys. Stroke 1984;15:803.

167. Hossman KA. Treatment of experimental cerebral ischemia. J Cereb Blood Flow Metab 1982;2:275.

168. Sakabe T, Nagai I, Ishikawa T, et al. Nicardipine increases cerebral blood flow but does not improve neurologic recovery in a canine model of complete cerebral ischemia. J Cereb Blood Flow Metab 1986;6:684.

169. Reich HS, Safar P, Angelos M, et al. Failure of a multifaceted anti-reoxygenation injury (anti-free radical) therapy to ameliorate brain damage after ventricular fibrillation cardiac arrest of 20 minutes in dogs. Crit Care Med 1988;16:387.

170. Krause GS, White BC, Aust SD, et al. Brain cell death following ischemia and reperfusion: a proposed biochemical sequence. Crit Care Med 1988;16:714.

171. Safar P. Effects of the postresuscitation syndrome on cerebral recovery from cardiac arrest. Review and hypotheses. Crit Care Med 1985;13:932.

172. Nagel EL, Fine EG, Krischer JP, Davis JH. Complications of CPR. Crit Care Med 1981;9:424.

Chapter 4 Blood Replacement

ROBERT F. WILSON, M.D., FACS

Although prompt correction of severe blood-volume deficits in the critically injured patient may be lifesaving, the blood and fluids used for replacement can, in themselves, cause significant complications, especially if used inappropriately. This chapter will deal primarily with the characteristics of various types of fluids and stored (bank) blood and the complications associated with their use.

CRYSTALLOIDS

Physiological and Pharmacokinetics

Resuscitation from shock is usually begun with balanced electrolyte (crystalloid) solution. The terms "crystalloid" and "colloid" were coined by Thomas Graham in 1861 and refer respectively to solute particles that will or will not pass through semipermeable membranes and are smaller or larger than an arbitrarily determined particle weight, usually taken as 10,000-30,000. The crystalloids generally used in resuscitation are solutions which are isotonic with human plasma, contain sodium as their major osmotically active particle, and have no particles with a molecular weight (MW) greater than 10,000.

Isotonic fluids such as Ringer's lactate and normal saline distribute evenly throughout the extracellular space. In normal healthy adults, equilibration with the extracellular space occurs within 20 to 30 minutes after infusion, and after 1 hour only about a third of the volume infused remains in the intravascular space. Glucose in water, in contrast, equilibrates with the entire body water so that only about one-fifteenth (60 to 70 ml out of a liter) will remain in the vascular space. Although crystalloids can usually restore BP fairly rapidly, in critically ill or injured patients, only 10 to 20% of these solutions will remain in the circulation after 1 to 2 hours.[1]

PITFALL ⊘

If crystalloids alone are used to replace massive blood loss, excessive amounts of fluid may be required, and the risk of cerebral and other tissue edema will increase.

The major pitfall to avoid in resuscitation is inadequate or slow fluid administration. Up to 5 liters of crystalloid may be needed to replenish a 1000 ml blood loss. Adequacy of intravascular volume repletion must be assessed by the usual parameters which indicate adequacy of peripheral perfusion. These include a stable mean arterial pressure of at least 70-80 mm Hg, heart rate falling to less than 100 to 110 beats/min, warm extremities with good capillary refill, adequate CNS function, urine volume of at least 0.5-1.0 ml/kg.hr, absence of lactic acidosis, and core temperature above 35° C. In resuscitation of patients with underlying cardiopulmonary or septic problems, monitoring of pulmonary artery wedge pressure, cardiac output, mixed venous oxygen content, and arteriovenous oxygen concentration differences should supplement these other parameters in guiding fluid administration.

Normal (0.9%) saline and Ringer's lactate are the most frequently used crystalloids for resuscitation and can generally be given interchangeably. The 28 mEq/L of lactate present in Ringer's lactate solution does not usually increase the lactic acidemia associated with shock, unless the patient has severe liver dysfunction. In fact, as circulating blood volume is restored, serum lactate levels tend to fall. The use of Ringer's lactate does not usually alter the reliability of blood lactate measurements,[2] except perhaps in patients with hepatic failure.

The theoretical concern that large volumes of normal saline produce a "dilution acidosis" or hyperchloremic acidosis is seldom a problem clinically. The excess circulating chloride ions are normally excreted by the kidney quite readily. However, in patients with severe or continuing organic acidosis (ketoacidosis or lactic acidosis), hyperchloremic acidosis is seen not infrequently during the postresuscitation period.[3] However, this hyperchloremic acidosis is due more to the loss of bicarbonate with the increased ketones being excreted into the urine than it is to the administered chloride load.

AXIOM Administration of large quantities of saline in patients with continuing inadequate tissue perfusion or ketoacidosis can contribute to the development of a hyperchloremic (non-anion gap) metabolic acidosis.

INDICATIONS

Crystalloid solutions are indicated for plasma volume expansion in the initial resuscitation of almost all shock patients. They are inexpensive, readily available, easily stored, reaction-free, and can readily correct most extracellular volume deficits. In hemorrhagic shock, crystalloids can be used to replace plasma volume immediately and can reduce the amount of blood required for resuscitation. Crystalloids also decrease blood viscosity and thereby further improve capillary blood flow.

SIDE EFFECTS

Although crystalloids can expand the intravascular volume temporarily, they dilute the remaining red cells and protein, reducing the oxygen-carrying capacity, buffering ability, and colloid osmotic pressure of the blood. In disease states such as severe trauma, sepsis or shock, in which the capillaries may have a greatly increased permeability, these solutions may leave the intravascular space so rapidly that only transient volume expansion is provided. Consequently, there is often an increase in extravascular lung water (EVLW) during and after crystalloid resuscitation of severe shock. This may occur not only because of an increased pulmonary capillary pressure but also because of a decrease in plasma colloid pressure.[4] Whether this reduction in plasma proteins and consequent lowering of plasma colloid oncotic pressure with increased EVLW impairs lung function is controversial.[5,6]

AXIOM Crystalloid resuscitation of trauma usually does not impair pulmonary function unless there is coincident direct or indirect lung damage or the patient is thrown into right heart failure.

"Edema safety factors" that limit the tendency for lowered colloid oncotic pressure to increase EVLW include increased lymphatic flow, diminished pulmonary interstitial oncotic pressure, and increased interstitial hydrostatic pressure.[7] When the total crystalloid volume administered is controlled to prevent volume overload, there is usually no difference in lung function in shock patients resuscitated with crystalloids or colloid solutions.

RECOMMENDATIONS FOR USE

The volume of crystalloid is usually at least three times the volume of colloid solution required to reach the same hemodynamic endpoint.[8] Acute blood loss of up to 30% of the blood volume may be adequately replaced with crystalloid alone if given rapidly in quantities equal to three to four times the blood lost.[9]

Nevertheless, in the most critically ill or injured patients, it is our practice to maintain the hemoglobin concentration above 10.0 gm/dl

51

and preferably above 12.0 gm/dl, without giving large amounts of albumin. The serum albumin level should probably be kept above a minimum level of 2.2 gm/dl. Consequently, after the initial 3000 to 4000 ml of crystalloids are given to a critically injured patient, some consideration should be given to administering some colloid as needed to maintain a reasonable colloid osmotic pressure.

PITFALL ⊘

If large quantities of Ringer's lactate are given to patients with severe liver disease, an increasing lactic acidosis may develop.

Because lactate may be metabolized very slowly when liver function or perfusion is severely impaired, we prefer, in patients with advanced cirrhosis, to use normal saline with an ampule of sodium bicarbonate (44.6 mEq) in each liter of fluid.

PRESCRIBING INFORMATION

Normal (0.9%) saline contains 154 mEq/L each of sodium and chloride. Ringer's lactate contains 130 mEq/L sodium, 109 mEq/L chloride, 28 mEq/L lactate, 4 mEq/L potassium, and 3 mEq/L calcium. Half (14 mEq) of the lactate is L-lactate and can undergo hepatic metabolism to bicarbonate to release 14 mEq of free base per liter of solution. The other 14 mEq/L are R-lactate which can be excreted unchanged in the urine. In patients with renal failure, the 4 mEq/L of potassium present may be a problem, and normal saline should be used. Similarly, normal saline is preferred over Ringer's lactate in hypercalcemic, hyperkalemic or hyponatremic states. In the presence of established hyperchloremic metabolic acidosis, Ringer's lactate is preferred because it provides a bicarbonate source and reduces the administered chloride load.

COLLOIDS

Clinically the term "colloid" refers to solutions containing substances of high molecular weight (usually at least 10,000) that cannot readily diffuse through normal capillary membranes. These agents are used primarily to expand intravascular volume and to try to raise colloid osmotic pressure (COP) or oncotic pressure back to normal.[11]

Oncotic pressure is the result of the inward force exerted across the capillary membrane by the intravascular proteins. Plasma oncotic pressure which is normally about 28 mm Hg is an important factor in determining the distribution of fluid across capillary membranes. If other factors are kept constant, a lower plasma colloid osmotic pressure will result in fluid shifting out of the intravascular space into the interstitial space, increasing the tendency to tissue edema. Conversely, a high plasma oncotic pressure tends to "pull" fluid into the capillaries, and this tends to restore intravascular volume and reduce interstitial edema. A profound reduction in COP may reduce left ventricular compliance, increase pulmonary extravascular water, decrease tissue oxygen delivery, and impair wound healing.[10,11]

The ideal colloid for plasma volume expansion should be able to restore plasma oncotic pressure back to normal and have a molecular size and shape similar to albumin.[12] It would remain intravascular for an extended period of time in order to maintain the plasma volume expansion. The ideal colloid also would possess no antigenic, allergenic, or pyrogenic properties. It would not interfere with the typing or cross-matching of blood, nor be capable of causing coagulation defects. It would cause no changes in hepatic, renal, or immunologic function. It would also be inexpensive, easy to sterilize, and pharmacologically inert. Unfortunately, all currently available colloid solutions lack many of these properties and have significant, but relatively infrequent, side effects.

The colloids used most frequently now include albumin, dextran, hydroxyethyl starch, pentastarch, and fresh frozen plasma. Other colloids sometimes used, particularly in other countries, include plasma protein fraction and gelatin.

Albumin

AXIOM   Albumin may be of value for expanding blood volume, especially in severely hypoproteinemic patients, but it is expensive, and excessive amounts can cause cardiac, pulmonary, and renal problems.

Human serum albumin can be very effective in rapidly restoring blood volume, particularly if plasma protein levels are extremely low. However, its clinical indications are controversial, and it costs much more than other plasma expanders. In fact, it costs at least 30 times as much as the crystalloids required to produce an equivalent expansion of blood volume.[13]

PHARMACOLOGY AND PHARMACOKINETICS

Endogenous Albumin

The average molecular weight of endogenous albumin is 65,000. Normally, 12 to 14 grams are made by the liver daily. It is the major oncotically active plasma protein, accounting for about 80% of the plasma colloid oncotic pressure.[10]

An adult has 4 to 5 gm of albumin/kg body weight in the extracellular space, but only about 30-40% of this is present in the intravascular compartment, resulting in a normal serum level of about 3.5 to 5.0 gm/dl. The plasma level varies with the rate of hepatic synthesis, metabolic breakdown and the rate of flow back and forth between the interstitial and intravascular spaces.[7] Much of the endogenous albumin in the interstitial space is tissue-bound and unavailable to the circulation. Unbound or "free" interstitial space albumin returns to the intravascular compartment via lymphatic drainage. The half-life of albumin in the body is approximately 20 to 22 days.[10]

AXIOM   In severe injury or stress, hepatic albumin synthesis decreases acutely, and the liver production of acute phase reactants (such as fibrinogen and C-reactive protein) increases significantly.

Exogenous Albumin

Administered albumin distributes itself throughout the extracellular space. The plasma half-life of exogenous albumin is usually about 12 to 16 hours. However, in severe shock or sepsis, the hourly disappearance rate of exogenous albumin increases from 7 to 8% per hour to over 30% per hour.[14]

Albumin is clinically available as a 5% or 25% solution in isotonic saline. It is prepared by fractionating blood from healthy donors and heating it to 60° C for 10 hours, which inactivates the hepatitis viruses and probably the human immunodeficiency virus (HIV). The 5% solution contains 50 grams of albumin per liter in normal saline and exerts an oncotic pressure of approximately 20 mm Hg. Thus, 1 gram of intravascular albumin can bind about 18 ml of water by its oncotic activity.[6] However, the effects of 5% albumin on plasma volume expansion are not entirely predictable. Reports of plasma volume expansion due to infusion of 500 ml of 5% albumin range anywhere from 250 up to 750 ml.[12] These reported differences may be caused by variability of the volume deficits, initial colloid oncotic pressure, vascular permeability, and the adequacy of the volume resuscitation itself.

The 25% albumin solution contains 12.5 grams of albumin in 50 ml of a buffered solution containing approximately 130 to 160 mEq/l sodium. The oncotic pressure of 25% albumin is approximately 100 mm Hg. When 100 ml of 25% albumin solution (25 g albumin) are infused, intravascular volume increases by about 300 to 600 ml (avg. of 450 ml) over 30-60 minutes.

INDICATIONS

Albumin is generally used in critically ill patients with extremely low protein levels for its oncotic properties. However, it is also used to help resuscitate some patients with an acutely diminished intravascular volume.

Because the 25% albumin solution is quite expensive to prepare, the 5% solution of human serum albumin is what is generally used in the resuscitation of hypovolemic shock.[12] The more concentrated 25% solution is usually reserved for patients in whom the interstitial space is expanded but the plasma volume and albumin concentration are decreased. Postoperative surgical patients, as well as burn patients, after their initial resuscitation may benefit from infusion of 25% albumin by expanding their total plasma volume by transcapillary movement of fluid from the interstitial to the intravascular space. However, albumin administration caused no significant improvement in a canine hind-limb scaled model[15] nor in children with an average burn of 46% TBSA.[16]

In addition to its plasma volume expansion effects, albumin may have other unique properties that make it clinically useful. These include binding and inactivation of toxic products, including proteolytic enzymes, maintenance of microvascular permeability to protein, and scavenging of free radicals.[17]

SIDE EFFECTS
Although albumin generally is a very safe plasma expander, many studies have documented a number of adverse effects.

Pulmonary Edema

PITFALL ⊘

Administration of excessive amounts of albumin can increase the risk of pulmonary edema in susceptible individuals.

Trauma patients with hypovolemia who are resuscitated with albumin may have increased requirements for both total and blood resuscitation volumes and an increased tendency to heart and pulmonary failure.[18] In sepsis, the increased pulmonary capillary permeability may allow increased albumin to enter and remain in the interstitial fluid space. Raising the COP in the pulmonary interstitium contributes to the formation of increased extravascular lung water (EVLW). However, the pulmonary capillary pressure is much more important than the COP.[19] It is also clear that the overall volume of fluid used[20] and the presence or absence of sepsis[21] affect pulmonary function to a far greater extent than does the type of resuscitation fluid.

Renal Dysfunction
Trauma patients resuscitated with large amounts of albumin tend to have lower hourly urine volumes, suggesting that the use of albumin may prolong the renal insult by transiently maintaining the intravascular volume at the expense of the depleted interstitial fluid volume.[17] Another study[22] showed that seriously injured patients receiving supplemental albumin therapy had an effective expansion of plasma volume and renal blood flow but, paradoxically, there was a drop in glomerular filtration rate. This many have been caused by increased oncotic pressure within the tuft and peritubular vessels, causing a decrease in excretion of sodium and water during the early phase of extravascular fluid sequestration.

Depressed Ionized Calcium Levels

PITFALL ⊘

Excessive use of albumin may reduce ionized calcium levels and contribute to myocardial failure or shock.

Each gram of albumin binds about 0.8 mg of calcium and may temporarily lower ionized calcium levels, producing a negative inotropic effect on the myocardium.[23] In one series of trauma patients, resuscitation with large amounts of albumin maintained normal serum albumin levels and high total calcium levels, but significantly depressed the levels of ionized calcium.[17] The ionized calcium level correlated directly with the calculated myocardial work and, thus, albumin, by binding free calcium, appeared to depress myocardial function.[23]

Allergic Phenomena
Because albumin is a constituent of blood, reactions similar to those occurring with blood transfusions may be seen during its administration. However, these allergic reactions are relatively mild and uncommon. The incidence of short-lived urticaria, fever, chills, and nausea ranges between 0.5% and 1.5%;[13] however, changes in blood pressure, heart rate, and respirations are very uncommon. Indeed, many physicians who have used a great deal of albumin have never noted such reactions.

Hepatitis/AIDS Risk
There is no hepatitis risk with albumin.[7] The albumin is heated during processing to 60° C for 10 hours. This is sufficient time to inactivate both the hepatitis and AIDS viruses.

Immunoglobulin Deficiencies

PITFALL ⊘

Excessive use of albumin may contribute to an impaired host defense.

Patients in hypovolemic shock who have been resuscitated with albumin have been shown to have decreased levels of immunoglobulins and a reduced immune response to tetanus toxoid compared with similar patients resuscitated with crystalloid solutions.[24,25] The reduced levels of immunoglobulins may be due to nonspecific binding to the albumin, with a subsequent passive loss as albumin-immunoglobulin complexes extravasate from the intravascular space.

Coagulation Protein Deficiencies
Lucas and Ledgerwood have shown that use of large quantities of albumin can reduce plasma concentrations of various coagulation proteins. The mechanism for this is not clear.[25]

Abnormal Albumin Production
Hepatic albumin production may be regulated by the albumin concentration within the interstitial space of the liver. Exogenously administered albumin may elevate this level, leading to suppression of subsequent endogenous production of albumin.[26]

AXIOM The rapid clearance of exogenous albumin coupled with a delay in the production of endogenous albumin impedes the return of normal oncotic pressure within the vascular space.

RECOMMENDATIONS FOR USE
In 1975 a National Institute of Health task force examined the appropriate use of albumin in the light of its increasing cost and apparent indiscriminate use.[27] It was agreed that for major volume resuscitation (replacement of greater than 30% of the blood volume) colloids such as albumin can be used as part of the resuscitation regimen. The total volume of crystalloid administered, and thus the potential interstitial space fluid distribution, can be limited by using 5% albumin solution as part of the resuscitation. If the patient is edematous, 25% albumin can be used to help mobilize the patient's own interstitial fluid into the vascular space. A COP of ≥20 mm Hg, a serum albumin of ≥2.5 g/dl, or a total serum protein of ≥5.0 g/dl indicates an adequate plasma oncotic activity for most clinical situations.

PRESCRIBING INFORMATION
Albumin can be provided as normal serum albumin (NSA), 5% and 25%, and purified protein fraction (PPF). The protein content of NSA preparations is 96% albumin. There is no such thing now as "salt poor albumin"; the sodium content of all albumin preparations is 145 ± 15 mEq/liter. PPF preparations contain only 83% albumin, with the remainder made up of alpha and beta globulins. Use of PPF is occasionally associated with development of some hypotension, which is

thought to be secondary to kinins or prekallikrein activator activity present in the solution.[28]

Dextran

PHARMACOLOGY AND PHARMACOKINETICS

AXIOM   Dextran 40 and dextran 70 can be effective colloids, but they may cause increased oozing from open wounds, difficulty with type and cross-matching of blood, and occasional anaphylactoid reactions.

Dextran is a glucose polymer with primarily 1,6-glucosidic linkages. This synthetic colloid was originally isolated from sugar beets contaminated with the bacterium *Leuconostoc mesenteroides* which acted on the sucrose present. Lactobacilli are also utilized to convert sucrose to dextran by the action of dextran-sucrase. In its native form, dextran is a branched polysaccharide of about 200,000 glucose units.[7] Partial hydrolysis produces polysaccharides of smaller size, which are available commercially as preparations having average molecular weights of 40,000 Rheomacrodex (dextran 40; D-40) or 70,000 (dextran 70; D-70).

Dextran molecules distribute initially in the intravascular compartment, but quickly equilibrate with the entire extracellular space. The major route of loss of dextran from the intravascular space is through the kidney. D-40 and D-70 contain particles with molecular weights ranging from 10,000 to 80,000 and 40,000 to 100,000, respectively.[29] Particles below 15,000 molecular weight are rapidly filtered by the kidney, and 50 to 75% of these are lost in the urine in 15 to 30 minutes; however, while in the circulation, they exert osmotic activity. Larger particles (MW of 15,000-50,000) are lost more slowly in the urine, but approximately 40% of the dextran with a molecular weight below 50,000 is excreted in the urine within 24 hours.

Up to 60 to 70% of D-40 and 30 to 40% of D-70 is cleared from the plasma into the urine or interstitial fluid space within 12 hours. After 24 hours the particles remaining in the circulation have an average molecular weight of more than 80,000. These particles are taken up by the reticuloendothelial system and enzymatically degraded to glucose at a rate of 70 to 90 mg/kg per day and metabolized to carbon dioxide and water. Some of the larger dextran molecules may also be excreted through the gut.

INDICATIONS FOR USE

Volume Expansion

Dextran has at least two properties of an ideal plasma volume expander: a relatively long dwell time and ultimate biodegradability. In shock, dextran can improve hemodynamic parameters and increase survival rates.[30] Dextran infusion increases the intravascular volume by an amount equal to or greater than the volume infused. A 500-ml bolus of D-40 produces an intravascular volume expansion of 750 ml at 1 hour and 1050 ml at 2 hours.[31] This volume expansion may persist for up to 8 hours in hypovolemic patients, however, the osmotic diuresis limits the duration of the volume expansion. Urine flow may also increase because dextran resuscitation is associated with increased renal plasma flow and a fall in plasma antidiuretic hormone levels.[32]

Promotion of Peripheral Blood Flow

Dextran tends to improve blood flow in the microvasculature by coating endothelial and blood cell surfaces, decreasing viscosity, and preventing red blood cell (RBC) sludging in the microcirculation. It also reduces platelet adherence and degranulation,[33] and may decrease platelet factor III[34]. These changes decrease the activation of the clotting cascade mechanism and limit thrombus formation.[35] Dextran is also reported to copolymerize with fibrin monomers, resulting in a less stable clot that is more susceptible to endogenous lysis.[34] All of these changes increase the likelihood of oozing from raw surfaces.

SIDE EFFECTS

PITFALL ⊘

If dextran is given with multiple blood transfusions, it may be difficult to determine the cause of reactions or increased hemorrhage, and problems with cross-matching may occur.

Anaphylactoid Reactions

Anaphylactoid reactions can be clinically identical to anaphylactic reactions, but they occur with synthetic compounds and do not involve IgE (reagin). In contrast, anaphylactic reactions involve naturally occurring compounds and involve reagin (IgE). The incidence of anaphylactoid reactions to dextran prior to 1977 was between 0.34% and 5.3%.[36] Since that time, however, improved testing methods for the presence of antigens, as well as manufacturing of dextrans with more linear molecules and fewer antigenic properties, have drastically reduced the number of severe allergic reactions. Allergic reactions usually occur within half an hour after the infusion is begun and may include urticaria, rash, nausea, bronchospasm, shock, and death. Dextran is a potent antigen and has cross-reactivity with several bacterial polysaccharide antigens. Gut flora can make endogenous dextran from dextrose, and patients with *Streptococcus pneumoniae* or Salmonella infections are more prone to dextran reactions. Consequently, a small portion of the patient population has never received dextran but has circulating precipitins to the dextran molecule.

Cross-matching Problems

PITFALL ⊘

If the blood bank is not informed of the recent administration of dextran to a patient who requires blood transfusions, it may fail to obtain a proper type and cross-match.

Dextran can interfere with the cross-matching of blood. This problem is handled best by drawing blood prior to dextran infusion and/or notifying the blood bank that the patient is receiving dextran so that the dextran can be washed off the red blood cells prior to the tests.

Increased Bleeding

PITFALL ⊘

If dextran is given to patients with large open wounds, excessive oozing and blood loss may occur.

In addition to a dilutional effect, dextran inhibits erythrocyte aggregation in vivo.[37] It also adheres to vessel walls and cellular elements of the blood, decreases platelet adhesiveness, and can precipitate fibrinogen, factor VIII fibrin monomers, and von Willebrand factor. This can result in prolonged bleeding times and increased incisional bleeding.[38] Such oozing can be a particular problem in patients with large open wounds. However, at doses less than 20 ml/kg/day (1.5 g/kg/day), clinical bleeding is usually not encountered.[39]

Renal Failure

Because dextran particles with molecular weights less than 50,000 are rapidly filtered through the glomerulus, a highly viscous urine may result, and acute renal failure can rapidly develop if unrecognized hypovolemia is present.[40] The risk of acute renal dysfunction by tubular plugging with dextran is therefore particularly great with the use of the lower molecular weight dextran fraction in patients with decreased renal blood flow. The mechanism for the renal failure appears to be tubular obstruction secondary due to concentration and precipitation of dextran in the tubules.[41] Patients receiving dextran, therefore, should be kept well-hydrated by aggressive concomitant administration of crystalloids.[42]

Osmotic Diuresis

Assuming a high urine specific gravity in a patient who has been given LMWD is due to continued hypovolemia.

An osmotic diuresis can occur almost immediately with dextran because the smaller molecules are filtered and not absorbed. The effect is greater with D-40 than with D-70. In the face of this obligate osmotic diuresis, urine volume cannot serve as a guide to the adequacy of intravascular volume repletion. If blood volume is inadequately restored in the patient receiving dextran, the stage is set for producing dextran nephropathy.

Reticuloendothelial Blockade

Because the larger dextran molecules are cleared by the reticuloendothelial system, there is some concern that the larger molecules will adversely affect immune function. Although dextran may temporarily, partially impair reticuloendothelial system function and immune competence, there have been no reports of this in patients.[43]

Biochemical Alterations

Blood glucose levels can be falsely elevated in patients receiving dextran if the glucose measurement is done by an analysis using acid, which converts dextran to dextrose. Dextran may also cause false elevations of the total protein concentration and serum bilirubin levels.[43] However, the total protein measurements can be checked using a refractometer which provides readings within 1.0 gm/dl of the true value. Other adverse effects that may occur with administration of dextran include depression of plasma levels of several important plasma proteins, such as fibrinogen, haptoglobin, C_3, C_4, and the immunoglobulins.[44]

PRESCRIBING INFORMATION

Dextran 40 (Rheomacrodex, low molecular weight dextran) is commercially available as a 10% solution in normal saline or 5% dextrose in water. Dextran 70 (macrodex) is commercially available as a 6% solution in normal saline, 5% dextrose in water, or 10% invert sugar in water.

For restoration of blood volume in shock, approximately 1,000 ml of 10% D-40 (for a 70 kg man) may be given acutely in conjunction with crystalloid, packed red blood cells, and plasma as necessary. To avoid excessive bleeding, the total dosage of D-40 and D-70 should be less than 1.5 gm/kg/day and 2.0 gm/kg/day, respectively.[45]

Gelatin

Gelatin is prepared by hydrolysis of bovine collagen. The solutions prepared for clinical use have a rather wide range of molecular weights, which average under 100,000.[12] Although no gelatin solutions are available for use in the United States now, there are two types of commercially prepared gelatin solutions for intravenous infusion in the United Kingdom. Urea-linked gelatin (Haemaccel) has a tenfold higher content of calcium (6.26 mmol/L) and potassium (5.1 mmol/L) than succinylated gelatin (Gelofusine), in which the concentration of both elements is less than 0.4 mmol/L. Because of its higher calcium content, Haemaccel can cause clotting in the warming coils if it is infused with bank blood.

Although it was originally claimed that the new-generation gelatins were non-antigenic, all types have been associated with allergic reactions. Haemaccel has been associated with over twice the incidence of anaphylactoid reactions (0.146%) as Gelofusine. Histamine release and complement activation may also occur with both types. Gelatins may also cause prolonged depression of plasma fibronectin levels in postoperative patients.[46] Although there is a dose-dependent dilution of clotting factors, the newer gelatins do not impair hemostasis nor do they interfere with blood typing and cross-match reactions.

Hydroxyethyl Starch (Hetastarch, HES)

AXIOM HES is an effective colloid for expanding blood volume, but excessive use can cause increased bleeding.

PHYSIOLOGY AND PHARMACOKINETICS

Hydroxyethyl starch (hetastarch, HES) is a synthetic starch molecule derived from a waxy starch composed almost entirely of amylopectin.[12] Its production involves introduction of hydroxyethyl ether groups into the glucose units of the starch to retard degradation by serum amylase. HES is available for clinical use as a volume expander as a 6% solution in normal saline.

Molecular weights of hydroxyethyl starch are reported as either the number average molecular weight (M_N), the arithmetic mean of all the molecules present, or as the weight average molecular weight (M_W), the sum of the number of hydroxyethyl starch molecules at each molecular weight fraction divided by the total weight of the hydroxyethyl starch molecules. M_N and M_W are measured differently, the former by reducing osmotic pressure and the latter by light scattering techniques allowing determination of mass.[47] Thus, M_W is greatly affected by the number of high molecular weight molecules present, which may be a relatively small percentage of the total population, and the M_W is always greater than the M_N.

The molar substitution ratio, defined as the number of moles of hydroxyethyl groups per mole of glucose, determines the rate of hydrolysis of the polymer by serum alpha amylase. Hydroxyethyl starch subunits that are 50,000 to 70,000 daltons or less are rapidly filtered and excreted by the kidney. Larger subunits persist intravascularly until they are hydrolyzed intravascularly or sequestered extravascularly by reticuloendothelial cells.[48] Hydroxyethyl starch compounds with a lower molar substitution undergo more rapid hydrolysis, resulting in faster elimination. Hydroxyethyl starch compounds with fewer hydroxyethyl groups also undergo more rapid hydrolysis, resulting in faster elimination.[49,50] Thus, M_N is the primary determinant of the rapid phase of elimination by glomerular filtration, whereas M_W and molar substitution influence the later elimination phase regulated by the rate of enzymatic hydrolysis.

After intravenous infusion, there is an almost immediate appearance of smaller particles of HES in the urine. In normal volunteers, an average of 46% of an administered dose is excreted in the urine by 2 days and 64% by 8 days.[51] However, the reported half-life of hetastarch varies from 2 to 65 days, depending on the time and duration of sampling.[12] This variability in half-life is due to the heterogenous molecular weight of the particles found in the commercially available product, as well as the complexity of distribution and degradation within the body. The rate of disappearance of the larger particles of HES from the plasma depends on their absorption by tissues, gradual return to the circulation, uptake by the reticuloendothelial system (RES), and subsequent degradation by the RES to smaller particles which are then cleared into urine and bile.[52]

Although the heterogeneous nature of hetastarch complicates pharmacokinetic modeling, a study in normovolemic volunteers reported terminal elimination half-life of 17 days during the first 42 days after administration, which accounted for elimination of 90% of the total dose.[53] The remaining 10% was eliminated with a half-life of 48 days. Mishler et al[50] reported a small amount (less than 1% of the original dose) in the blood 17 weeks after administration.

The uptake of hetastarch molecules by the cells of the reticuloendothelial system has caused concern that the immune function of the patient could be compromised. However, clinically significant reticuloendothelial system dysfunction has not been demonstrated.[52]

Administering large amounts of hetastarch to patients who already have a coagulopathy.

Administering hetastarch to subjects who are bleeding can cause a number of coagulation and bleeding changes including: (a) reduction in fibrinogen levels because of hemodilution, (b) minor prolongation of partial thromboplastin and bleeding times, (c) shortening of thrombin, reptilase, and urokinase-activated clot lysis times, and (d) a reduction in factor VIII complex concentration to a greater degree than accounted for by hemodilution.[53,54] These findings, suggestive of enhanced fibrinolysis and a direct interaction with factor VIII, may result in varying degrees of subclinical coagulopathy. There is also evidence that hetastarch results in impaired fibrin clot formation.[55] When the daily dose exceeds the recommended maximum (more than 20 ml/kg) and is repeatedly administered, clinically significant coagulopathy has also been reported.[56]

Plasma volume expansion after infusion of hetastarch is approximately 100% to 170% of the infused volume of HES. This is equal to or slightly greater than the volume expansion produced by D-70 or 5% albumin, and HES has a slightly longer plasma retention time, which has been reported to be between 12 and 48 hours.[57] The increase in colloid pressure is similar to that seen with albumin.

SIDE EFFECTS

Coagulopathy

One of the main concerns with hetastarch is its effects on blood coagulation. The exact mechanism of the hemostatic defect is not clear. Although hetastarch precipitates factors I and VIII, fibrin monomer, and von Willebrand factor from plasma, this precipitation appears to vary widely between patients.[58] Platelet coating with hetastarch and dilutional changes in the serum have also been implicated.

AXIOM Although administration of hetastarch can cause multiple coagulation changes, it rarely produces clinically significant bleeding problems if used in doses lower than 20 ml/kg/day.

Platelet counts and fibrinogen levels may decrease transiently after administration of HES, and slight prolongations of prothrombin time and partial thromboplastin time and decreased tensile clot strength are not uncommon; however, multiple studies in varying patient populations have failed to demonstrate clinically significant bleeding or increased requirements for blood transfusion.[58] In one study, the administration of 3600 ml of hetastarch within a 24-hour period to a group of trauma patients did not increase the incidence of local bleeding or systemic coagulopathy.[59]

Anaphylactoid Reactions

Hetastarch is not immunogenic and does not induce histamine release. Consequently, the incidence of anaphylactic reactions to hetastarch is very low (0.0004 to 0.006%) and the incidence of severe reactions, including shock or cardiopulmonary arrest, is even lower.[40] This low incidence of allergic reactions presumably is due to the fact that the starch molecule itself is nonantigenic and has a close structural relationship to liver glycogen. However, a number of miscellaneous adverse effects, including chills, itching, mild temperature elevations, submaxillary and parotid gland enlargement, and erythema multiforme, have been reported.[12]

Hyperamylasemia

Serum amylase levels may rise to values about double normal, reaching a maximum at about 20 hours and persisting for 3 to 5 days following hetastarch administration. This occurs because plasma amylase forms complexes with hetastarch molecules creating large macroamylase particles, which are excreted in the urine at a much slower rate than the usual amylase molecules.[60] There is no alteration of pancreatic function.

AXIOM The elevated plasma amylase levels after hetastarch administration are due to formation of macroamylase molecules and do not reflect any pancreatic problems.

Impaired Reticuloendothelial System (RES) Function

Because the larger molecules of hetastarch are cleared to a large degree by macrophages and other members of the reticuloendothelial system, a theoretical concern over its potential depression of the immune system has been raised.[12] While the uptake of the larger hetastarch molecules may temporarily overload the reticuloendothelial system and make it unable to clear bacteria and other circulating debris, no evidence has been found clinically to confirm this.

RECOMMENDATIONS FOR USE

Hetastarch may be used whenever colloid is required to restore plasma volume.[59] At doses of 1500 ml/day or less, bleeding complications are rare.[59] Nevertheless, hetastarch should be used with extreme caution in the presence of a known bleeding problem.

Adequate monitoring for early detection of volume overload is important. However, the immediate osmotic diuresis associated with its use protects somewhat from this phenomenon.

Hetastarch costs about one-fourth as much as an equivalent amount of 5% albumin. Although hetastarch costs more than dextran, it has fewer side effects.

PRESCRIBING INFORMATION

Hetastarch is available as a 6% solution in 0.9% sodium chloride. The pH is 5.5 and the osmolarity is 310 mOsm/liter. The usual total dosage is 20 ml/kg/day. The total volume may be administered over 1 hour if the clinical situation demands very rapid volume resuscitation.

Pentastarch

PHYSIOLOGY AND PHARMACOKINETICS

Pentastarch is a low molecular weight form of hydroxyethyl starch, with a lower number average molecular weight (M_N) of 63,000 and a lower weight average molecular weight (M_W) of 260,000.[12] Pentastarch is more rapidly and completely degraded by circulating amylase than is hetastarch and, therefore, it is more rapidly and effectively eliminated directly in the urine. Larger particles are phagocytized by the reticuloendothelial system. The volume expansion produced by pentastarch is about 1.5 times the administered volume; however, this effect usually lasts less than 12 hours.[61]

In contrast with hetastarch, the degree of plasma volume expansion with pentastarch is typically equivalent to the infused volume (although variable results have been reported), and the duration of volume expansion is prolonged (24 to 34 hours). Thus, the potential advantages of pentastarch include a greater degree of plasma volume expansion per volume infused, faster onset, and more rapid elimination from blood than hetastarch. London et al[61] also found that 10% pentastarch was as effective as 5% albumin in augmenting and maintaining mean arterial pressure, cardiac index, and cardiac filling pressures. It has also been recently shown by Hakaim et al[62] that HES inhibits ischemia-induced compartment syndrome, supposedly by sealing interendothelial clefts at the capillary level.

SIDE EFFECTS

When administered to normal persons undergoing leukopheresis, it is associated with lengthening of the activated partial thromboplastin time, reduction in fibrinogen and factor VIII levels, and shortening of the thrombin time; however, urokinase-activated clot lysis time and bleeding time are unchanged.[61] Furthermore, the effects on factor VIII levels, urokinase-activated clot lysis time, and bleeding times were of a lesser magnitude (despite a greater degree of hemodilution) than those previously reported from hetastarch.[61] Therefore, the effects of pentastarch on coagulation appear to be proportional to its degree of hemodilution only. The lesser presumed interaction with factor VIII may be related to its smaller average molecular size.

Although clinical data are lacking, it is likely that the incidence of anaphylactoid reactions occurring with pentastarch are similar to that of hetastarch. Comparable groups given pentastarch or albumin have revealed no differences in respiratory, oncotic, or coagulation measurements, no untoward reactions attributable to either colloid, and no differences in total chest tube drainage or blood product usage.

RECOMMENDATIONS FOR USE

Pentastarch has been used very successfully as an adjunct to leukopheresis, but clinical trials have shown that it may also be a useful colloid in fluid resuscitation. Low molecular weight hydroxyethyl starch compounds have been used clinically abroad. Given its favorable elimination profile and lack of clinically significant effects on coagulation, it appears that pentastarch may be safer than hetastarch. If commercially available at a lower cost than albumin, pentastarch would appear to be a reasonable first choice of postoperative plasma volume expansion.

PRESCRIBING INFORMATION

Pentastarch is available for use as a 10% solution in normal saline. Doses of pentastarch up to 2000 ml appear to be well tolerated, and its volume-expanding capability is similar to, or possibly greater than, that of 5% albumin.

Fresh Frozen Plasma

AXIOM Fresh frozen plasma can correct deficiencies in clotting factors (not platelets) and antithrombin, but it can transmit blood-borne diseases, especially hepatitis.

PREPARATION AND PRODUCT DESCRIPTION

Fresh frozen plasma (FFP) is prepared from whole blood by separating and freezing the plasma within 6 hours of phlebotomy. It may be stored for up to 1 year at $-18°$ C or lower. The typical unit has a volume of 200-300 ml. When frozen, the labile clotting factors (V and VIII) deteriorate to a minimal extent.[63]

INDICATIONS AND CONTRAINDICATIONS

The main indication for use of fresh frozen plasma is the presence of multiple coagulation factor problems.[63] Fresh frozen plasma should not be used just to provide volume expansion.

SIDE EFFECTS

Although there is a possibility of fluid overload when using fresh frozen plasma, its main risk is that of transmission of various serious infections. Fresh frozen plasma has a risk of hepatitis and AIDS transmission equal to that of whole blood.[62] Since FFP exposes the recipient to the risks of hepatitis, AIDS, and other transfusion-transmitted diseases, it should not be used when only a volume expander is needed. Allergic reactions and noncardiogenic pulmonary edema may also occur, but are unusual.

AXIOM Fresh frozen plasma should not be used just to expand plasma volume.

DOSE AND ADMINISTRATION

The dose of fresh frozen plasma depends on the clinical situation and the degree of clotting abnormality noted clinically or by measurement of prothrombin time, partial thromboplastin time, or specific factor assay. Fresh frozen plasma takes 20 to 40 minutes to thaw and must be given through a filter. If used within 2 hours of thawing, it contains normal levels of coagulation factors. However, larger delays decrease the coagulation factor activity, especially for factor VII.[62]

AXIOM Compatibility testing for fresh frozen plasma is not required, but it should be ABO-compatible with the patient when possible.

Liquid Plasma

Liquid plasma is a blood component obtained by separating plasma from whole blood at any time up to 5 days after the expiration date of the unit of blood. It contains all the stable coagulation factors, but it has reduced levels of factors V and VIII. The indications for liquid plasma are deficiencies of coagulation factors other than V or VIII. The contraindications and precautions, dosage and administration are the same as for fresh frozen plasma.

Plasma Protein Fraction

Plasma protein fraction (PPF) is a 5% solution of stabilized human plasma proteins in normal saline.[12] It is a mixture of plasma proteins, of which at least 83% is albumin, no more than 17% is alpha and beta globulins, and no more than 1% is gamma globulin. There are no clotting factors in PPF. PPF is prepared from large pools of normal human plasma by fractionation, involving a series of controlled precipitations with cold ethanol. Viral hepatitis and HIV are probably not a hazard because this product is heated to 60° C for 10 hours.

The pharmacologic properties of PPF are very similar to those of its primary constituent, albumin, but the presence of the globulins seems to induce a larger number of side effects, such as hypersensitivity and hypotension. Originally, bradykinin was thought to be the offending substance causing the hypotension seen with rapid infusion of PPF; however, it appears that the primary vasodilator is Hageman factor fragments present in the solution.[3]

CRYSTALLOIDS VERSUS COLLOIDS

AXIOM Successful resuscitation is primarily dependent on the rapidity and adequacy of fluid repletion, not on the composition of the resuscitation fluid.

Controversies over the selection of the type of fluid for resuscitation ("colloid versus crystalloid") center mainly on issues relating to philosophy, side effects, and economics.[64] Proponents of colloids argue that: (a) since the key problem in shock is a loss of circulating blood volume, replacement with colloid is more appropriate and more rapidly effective, (b) crystalloids reduce the colloid osmotic pressure, thus favoring the development of pulmonary edema,[65] and (c) crystalloids, because of their prompt equilibration with extracellular fluid (ECF), must be infused in amounts exceeding estimated losses by at least three to four times. Patients who are older, who have more significant hemodynamic instability, or who require both volume and an increase in plasma colloid osmotic pressure may do better with a colloid resuscitation. In critically ill patients, 1000 ml of a balanced electrolyte solution increases plasma volume by 194 ml, whereas 500 ml of 5% albumin increases plasma volume by 700 ml.[65]

Supporters of crystalloid solutions, on the other hand, argue that: (a) since the main problem in shock is shrinkage of the ECF, replacement with crystalloid is more appropriate, (b) fluid overload causing congestive heart failure and/or pulmonary edema is less likely to occur with crystalloids because of their rapid equilibration with ECF, (c) crystalloids are free from the risk of occasional (less than 0.05%) anaphylactoid reactions which can occur with any colloid solution, especially synthetic colloids, (d) colloids, except possibly for FFP,[66,67] have adverse effects on coagulation either by dilution of the factors or by actually interfering with their production or function, (e) administered colloids may cross the pulmonary capillary membrane in patients with increased microvascular permeability pulling water along with them, (f) all commercially available colloid solutions are capable of supporting bacterial growth and transmitting infection, and (g) fluid resuscitation with colloids is 10 to 100 times more expensive than equivalent blood volume expansion with crystalloid infusions.

Appropriate use of either crystalloids or colloids with comprehensive monitoring will lead to successful resuscitation in most patients.

Careful judgment is often required to provide the rate of fluid administration needed for optimal tissue perfusion without producing fluid overload.

HYPERTONIC SALINE SOLUTIONS

AXIOM Hypertonic saline can rapidly expand blood volume, but it can cause excess vasodilation, and serum sodium levels greater than 165 mEq/L can cause severe side effects.

Hypertonic saline (7.5% NaCl) may be useful in resuscitation from shock because of the small volume required to produce significant hemodynamic improvements. Velasco demonstrated that a single bolus of hypertonic saline (HTS), given in a volume equal to 10% of the shed blood, produced permanent recovery from hemorrhagic shock in anesthetized dogs.[68] Other investigators have shown similar beneficial results with HTS in dogs with endotoxic shock[69] and in swine with hemorrhagic shock.[70]

Hypertonic saline appears to be more effective in resuscitation from shock than other solutions of equal osmolarity.[71] Several mechanisms may contribute to the hemodynamic response seen with HTS resuscitation from hemorrhagic shock. Hyperosmotic solutions increase plasma osmolarity which increases blood volume.[72] In addition, HTS has been demonstrated to transiently increase myocardial contractility and catecholamine levels.[73] Permanent survival after HTS resuscitation in dogs from severe hemorrhagic shock has been reported to involve a pulmonary reflex resulting in selective vasoconstriction.[74] Lung denervation or arterial injection has been shown to prevent permanent resuscitation from hemorrhagic shock with a single injection of HTS.[75] Angiotensin II antagonism has also been shown to block the selective venoconstriction and prevent the long-term hemodynamic improvements.[76] Finally, increased osmolarity may result in release of vasopressin which produces vasoconstriction.[77]

Hypertonic saline solutions (HSS, 1200-2500 mosm/L) has been shown to effectively resuscitate patients with less volume,[77] less edema formation,[79] and better tissue perfusion than normal saline solutions (NSS).[80,81] The increased interstitial fluid that might occur in the heart, the gastrointestinal tract, the cutaneous tissues, or the brain with isotonic solutions can reduce organ function, impair healing, increase risk of infection, and even result in death after an otherwise successful resuscitation.

There is no risk of transmission of infectious agents with hypertonic saline, and the cost is approximately 1 : 100 compared to colloid agents.[82] In addition to pulling intracellular fluid into the extracellular space,[83] hypertonic saline is also reported to exert direct inotropic actions on the myocardium,[84] cause vasodilation,[85] decrease intracranial pressure,[86] and enhance vagally mediated reflex venoconstriction.[85] Dextran, HSS, and HSD, have also been shown to keep the interstitial fluid space contracted for at least 60 minutes in a canine hemorrhagic shock model.[87] Hypertonic crystalloid solutions of varying osmolality have been investigated in hemorrhagic,[83,85] burn,[86] traumatic,[88] and endotoxic shock.[88] Collectively, these studies demonstrate that HSS and HSD provide effective shock resuscitation without significant adverse effects.

In a study that compared several different hypertonic solutions in sheep with moderate hemorrhagic shock, 2400 mOsm NaCl with 6% dextran 70 (HSD) (colloid Osm pressure = 70 mm Hg) produced a higher and more sustained rise in blood pressure and cardiac output than several other hypertonic solutions which included 1.2 M NaHCO$_3$, 0.6 M NaCl with 0.6 M Na acetate, 0.7 M NaCl with 1.0 M mannitol, and 2.4 M glucose.[89] Recently, Runyon et al[90] showed that a saturated salt-dextran solution (25% NaCl in 24% dextran 70) (SDD) could be given intraosseously. He did this successfully to 14 swine in hemorrhagic shock using a volume of fluid only about 1/25 that required with normal saline.

In a recent review of the efficacy and safety of 7.5% NaCl in 6% dextran 70, Dubick and Wade[91] found that, at the proposed therapeutic dose of 4 ml/kg, HSD can be very beneficial and has little risk. In patients with head trauma and shock, it may be advantageous to keep intracranial pressure (ICP) as low as possible. In a recent study in dogs, HSS (2500 mOsm/L) raised the ICP 45% less than Ringer's lactate (RL) for an equivalent resuscitation.[92] Preliminary data also suggest that HSS attenuates the ACTH, cortisol, and aldosterone responses to trauma.[93] There was also suppression of the angiotensin II response in the HSS patients, and this might increase perfusion to the intestines, heart, and kidney.

Although HSS apparently has many benefits, it should not be used in every patient. Most patients, in fact, do very well with isotonic crystalloid resuscitation. However, HSS may be more effective than isotonic crystalloids in reducing third-space losses in selected patients with hypotension and large volume requirements. It may also be very helpful when peripheral or central edema could be very detrimental.

AUTOLOGOUS TRANSFUSION (AUTOTRANSFUSION)

AXIOM Autotransfusion can reduce blood bank needs and reduce the risk of blood-borne diseases, but if used in excess, especially in patients in shock, it can cause coagulopathies.

Auto transfusion involves the collection of shed blood from a body cavity with acute reinfusion into that patient's circulation. The first reported use of autotransfusion was in 1886 when Duncan reinfused blood that he collected during amputation of the crushed legs of a victim of a railway accident.[94] In 1917 Elmendorf successfully reinfused blood that he had collected from a recent hemothorax. In that same year, Lockwood autotransfused blood he collected during a splenectomy for Banti's disease.

Autotransfusion offers many advantages. Blood can be available for administration without delays for a cross-match. Of greater importance to many individuals, however, has been the concern over transmission of disease with bank blood. With autotransfusion, the risk of transmitted disease such as hepatitis, AIDS, malaria, and syphilis is eliminated. Furthermore, no hemolytic, febrile, or allergic reactions have been reported during auto-transfusion.

Autotransfusion practices and devices fall into three main categories. Direct reinfusion of pleural blood was popularized by Symbas,[95] who pointed out that blood drained from the pleural space is usually already defibrinated and requires little or no anticoagulant. The only real problem is that relatively few patients have enough hemothorax to justify setting up for an autotransfusion. Most chest tube placements in trauma result in the collection of less than 500 ml of blood.

The second category is suction collection,[96] such as with a Sorenson apparatus, to recover blood lost at an operation. A collection trap is placed in the suction line, and blood collected there is reinfused using a transfusion filter to catch whatever aggregates; fat particles and debris may have also been collected. The apparatus is simple and easy to set up, and the overall cost is about half as much as bank blood. It is ideal for bleeding inside the chest. In the abdomen, it can be used for bleeding from solid organ or vascular injuries. Although most surgeons feel that an intestinal injury is a contraindication to autotransfusing intra-abdominal blood, some surgeons feel that, even if intestinal contents are present, they can be removed by washing the red blood cells thoroughly, and antibiotics will take care of any residual bacteria.[97]

AXIOM Massive abdominal blood loss contaminated with intestinal contents is not a contraindication to autotransfusion, especially if no other blood is available and the autotransfused red cells are washed well and antibiotics are given in full dose.

Blood collected during operations may or may not be washed, but it must be filtered prior to reinfusion. Although the washing takes some time, it is advantageous because it removes fibrin, cellular debris, free hemoglobin, potassium, and various procoagulants and anticoagulants. Obviously, blood collected by intraoperative salvage cannot be transfused into other patients.

The third category of autotransfusion device is the blood concentrator which uses a special console that is capable of rapidly washing and concentrating the aspirated blood to a hematocrit of about 45%. However, the wash is usually only one pass and cannot clear bacteria reliably. Also, it takes 15 to 30 minutes to set up the blood concentrator, and the set-up pack costs $200. Furthermore, relatively few patients benefit. In one study,[98] the device was set up for 85 trauma patients, but only 22 actually received blood from it, and only 28% of the total blood received was from the autotransfuser. The major reasons for patients not receiving autotransfused blood were inadequate collection (60%), colon contamination (21%), and death before reinfusion (19%). Whether a hospital should spend $40,000 for a blood concentrator and intensively train its personnel for the benefit of a relatively small number of patients is an important question. However, this type of autotransfuser can be appropriate for a major trauma center or for a hospital with a busy cardiac or vascular program.

AXIOM Autotransfusions are safest if used in moderation and the red cells are carefully washed before infusion.

Several disadvantages of autotransfusion have been described. Air embolism is a disastrous complication; however, most reports of air embolism occurred with early autotransfusion systems that are no longer in use. The administration of large volumes of autotransfused blood may also cause thrombocytopenia and decreased levels of coagulation factors. In patients with extensive tissue damage or prolonged shock, this may increase the tendency to disseminated intravascular coagulation and activation of fibrinolytic mechanisms. Increased bleeding due to heparinization of the patients may also occur because of residual heparin that also gets reinfused despite washing of these RBCs. Increased free hemoglobin and the presence of red cell stroma and surgical field debris are of unclear significance.[99]

To minimize complications, autotransfused blood should be reinfused through in-line micropore filters for the removal of debris. For best results, it is generally felt that autotransfused blood should be transfused within 1 to 4 hours of collection.[94] However, if blood is promptly refrigerated after collection, storage for up to 24 hours is probably safe. In general, the amount of autotransfused blood should be limited to 3000 ml or less.[94] If autotransfusion is employed in a trauma victim, it should be considered as an adjunct to the use of cross-matched blood available from the blood bank. Patients who are autotransfused should have serial coagulation studies, which include platelet count, platelet function, PT, PTT, and fibrinolytic activity. Abnormalities should be treated as needed.

BLOOD TRANSFUSIONS

History

In February of 1665, Richard Lower successfully transfused blood from the artery of one dog into the vein of another.[100] Two years later, Denis transfused blood from sheep into four men in an attempt to introduce "ovine (sheep-like) docility" into these agitated individuals. Their reports contain vivid descriptions of hemolytic transfusion reactions with nasal bleeding and dark urine. It was not until 1818 that human blood was used successfully for transfusion by James Blundell in London for postpartum hemorrhage.

Indications for Transfusion

AXIOM Young, healthy individuals can do well with a hemoglobin of 7.0 gm/dl if the patient is hemodynamically stable and the bleeding is controlled.

The main indication for blood transfusions is the restoration of red blood cell (RBC) mass. As a general rule, a hematocrit of 20 to 25% provides adequate oxygen delivery if blood volume and cardiac output are normal or increased and the RBC hemoglobin is at least 90% saturated with oxygen. However, in most critically ill or injured patients, a hematocrit of at least 30 to 35% is generally considered preferable, and in patients with severe sepsis or cardiopulmonary dysfunction, a hematocrit of 35 to 40% is preferred. Nevertheless, hemoglobin levels of 6.0-6.5 gms/dl have been well tolerated in burn patients,[101,102] especially those who only need limited burn excisions.

Blood Products for Transfusion

FRESH AND WHOLE BLOOD

Whole blood that is transfused within 24 hours of drawing contains most of the coagulation factors and active platelets and is thought to be the "ideal" blood for use in trauma victims.[94] However, fresh blood is unavailable to most trauma surgeons today.

PACKED RBCS

Almost all blood transfusions today are packed RBCs. The average volume of a unit of packed RBCs is approximately 250 cc with an average hematocrit between 60 and 80%. Only 10 to 15% of the plasma and less than 30% of the platelets and 10% of the leukocytes remain.[94]

WASHED RBCS

RBCs may be washed by resuspension with saline solution, which can then be removed through centrifugation. Rinsing a unit of blood with 2 L of saline removes 98% of the residual plasma, including the majority of the remaining leukocytes and platelets. However, washing also decreases the red blood cell mass by approximately 15%.[103]

Washed suspensions of red blood cells have potential advantages in that the incidence of reactions is reduced by almost one-half (compared to unwashed blood, 0.21 versus 0.49%) and immunization against leukocytes is decreased.[103] Because of the delays in preparation, washed red cells are of little use in acute resuscitation; however, they may be indicated for transfusion in patients with previous blood reactions or sensitivity to RBC components.

FROZEN RBCS

By 1973 the technique for the glycerol freezing of RBCs had been perfected. After mixing with the glycerol solutions, the RBCs are frozen at $-80°$ C ($-176°$ F), at which temperature they can be maintained indefinitely.[104] When needed, the red cells are thawed by direct immersion into a stirring bath at $37°$ C ($98.6°$ F). The thawed cells are washed, centrifuged to remove the glycerol solution, and resuspended in a saline-glucose solution, producing a final hematocrit of 35 to 55%. The advantages of frozen cells are: (a) no citrate or other additives are required, (b) there are no incompatible antibodies, (c) the risk of hepatitis is reduced, (d) there is less chance of sensitization by plasma proteins, white cells, and platelets, and (e) blood can be stored indefinitely. However, frozen RBCs are of little benefit for acute resuscitation because of delays secondary to preparation and thawing.

Techniques of Red Blood Cell Preservation

Three anticoagulants for blood are currently in use: CPD, CPD A-1, and Adsol. All cause anticoagulation of the blood through calcium chelation by citrate. Adsol, the newest anticoagulant, also contains adenine and mannitol, which allow blood to be stored up to 35 to 49 days before becoming outdated. The volume of anticoagulant in Adsol is greater than in CPD or CPD A-1; hence the viscosity is somewhat less, making this blood easier to administer.

Blood Types

The "safest" type of blood to administer is that which has fully cross-matched, so as to have the lowest risk of major hemolytic reactions. Unfortunately, full cross-matching of blood may take 30-45 minutes or even longer if delays of transportation to and from the blood bank are incurred. Thus, fully cross-matched blood is not rapidly available for emergency resuscitation.

O-NEGATIVE BLOOD

PITFALL ⊘

If a physician uses group-O uncross-matched blood when it might be possible to delay 5-10 minutes by using other fluids or colloids, he greatly increases the risk of complications to the patient.

As the O blood contains no cellular antigens, it is theoretically safe to give to recipients of any blood type with minimal risk of a donor antigen-versus-patient antibody major hemolytic reaction. The major benefit of O-negative blood is that it is available for transfusion without a cross-match. However, because the plasma of O-negative blood does contain anti-A and anti-B antibodies, significant minor transfusion reactions can occur if large volumes are infused.

If more than 4 units of O-negative blood are administered to a patient with a different blood type, admixture situations may occur complicating the subsequent cross-matching of blood. Additionally, if a blood sample is sent upon arrival of a trauma patient with a non-O blood type and the patient then receives large volumes of type O blood, subsequent administration of non-O blood may create a potential for major hemolytic reactions.[105]

TYPE-SPECIFIC BLOOD

Blood of the recipient's type (i.e., type-specific blood) that has not been cross-matched can be administered safely and can usually be released for transfusion within 10 to 15 minutes of arrival. A large civilian study has recently documented the safety of type-specific uncross-matched blood in trauma.[106]

Mortality Rates

Patients who require massive transfusions of 10 or more units of blood within 24 hours have a mortality rate which averages about 50%. In a recent series of 339 of our trauma patients receiving massive transfusions, the mortality rate averaged 47%. In those receiving 10-19 units of blood, the mortality rate was 28% (51/182); in those receiving 20-39 units, the mortality rate rose to 65% (78/121); and in those receiving 40 or more units, the mortality rate was 83% (30/36) (Table 4-1). However, the presence of a systolic blood pressure below 80 mm Hg for 30 minutes or more and the presence of pre-existing disease were also important (Table 4-2). Of 146 patients who had no pre-existing disease, were less than 65 years of age, and had shock for 30 minutes or less, the mortality rate was only 17% (25/146). In contrast, in the patients having any of these problems, the mortality rate rose to 69% (134/193) (P <0.0001).

In examining the acid-base balance in critically ill or injured patients during and after massive transfusions, it was noted that overall the patients who died had a lower mean ($\pm$SD) pH (7.08 $\pm$ 0.15 versus 7.21 $\pm$ 0.15; P <0.001), a lower mean bicarbonate (13.5 $\pm$ 6.5 versus 15.7 $\pm$ 5.2 mEq/L; P <0.001), and a higher mean PCO_2 (47 $\pm$ 16 versus 43 $\pm$ 9 mm Hg; P <0.01). Even more interesting was the progression of these acid-base changes in the 28 trauma patients with the most severe acidosis (Table 4-3). During the first 2 hours in the

TABLE 4-2 Mortality Rates in Trauma Patients Receiving Massive Transfusions and the Importance of Prolonged Shock or Pre-existing Disease

Shock + ≥ 30 mins	Pre-existing Dsx or age ≥65 yrs	Units of Blood in First 24 Hours			
		10-19	20-39	40+	Total
No	No	(94) 9%	(44) 30%	(8) 50%	(146) 17%
Yes	No	(49) 43%	(42) 83%	(22) 93%	(113) 67%
No	Yes	(24) 38%	(21) 81%	(4) 100%	(49) 61%
Yes	Yes	(15) 87%	(14) 93%	(2) 100%	(31) 90%
Total		(182) 28%	(121) 65%	(36) 83%	(339) 47%

( ) = Number of patients in each group.
% = Mortality rate in each group.
* = Systolic BP < 80 mm Hg plus clinical signs of shock.

OR, the mean ($\pm$ SD) pH in those who survived in the OR was actually lower than those who died in the OR (6.92 $\pm$ 0.12 versus 7.03 $\pm$ 0.22; P = 0.11). However, over the next 2 hours, the patients who survived developed a higher pH (7.22 $\pm$ 0.09 versus 7.08 $\pm$ 0.14; P <0.005) and lower PCO_2 (39 $\pm$ 9 versus 54 $\pm$ 10 mm Hg; P <0.0001). Indeed, no massive transfusion patient who maintained a PCO_2 above 40 mm Hg in addition to a metabolic acidosis survived.

Reactions

AXIOM The most severe hemolytic transfusion reactions are generally due to simple clerical errors.

INCOMPATIBILITY REACTIONS

The administration of blood products may produce hemolytic or nonhemolytic reactions. The most frequent type of reactions are nonhemolytic and involve the development of fever, urticaria, hives, or asthma after the administration of blood. The incidence of these reactions is approximately 2 to 10%.[107] They may be related to leukocytes or proteins, and the incidence of these reactions may be reduced by the use of packed RBCs, washed RBCs, or special filters for the removal of leukocytes.[108]

TABLE 4-3 Serial Acid-Base Changes in the 28 Trauma Patients with the Most Severe Acidosis in the Operating Room (X $\pm$ SD)

	pH		
Time* (hours)	Died in OR (n=15)	Survived OR (n=13)	
0-2	7.03 $\pm$ 0.22	6.92 $\pm$ 0.12	NS
2-4	7.08 $\pm$ 0.14	7.22 $\pm$ 0.09	P < 0.005

	PCO_2 (mm Hg)		
Time* (hours)	Died in OR (n=15)	Survived OR (n=13)	
0-2	43 $\pm$ 20	44 $\pm$ 13	NS
2-4	54 $\pm$ 10	39 $\pm$ 9	P < 0.001

*from beginning of massive transfusions

TABLE 4-1 Mortality Rate Correlated with Units of Blood in Trauma Patients

Units of Blood*	Lived	Died	Mortality Rate
10-19	131	51	28%
20-39	43	78	65%
40+	6	30	83%
Total	180	159	47%

P < 0.0001
*given in first 24 hours

Major hemolytic transfusion reactions occur from the interaction of antibodies in the plasma of the recipient with antigens in the red cells of the donor. The incidence of major hemolytic transfusion reactions is unknown, but since 1975, 328 transfusion-related fatalities have been reported.[94] The majority of these (45%) involved simple clerical errors in which mistakes were made in the identification of blood samples or in the administration of appropriately matched blood to an incorrect patient. Most major transfusion reactions in trauma occur in the operating room (40%) and less frequently in the emergency department (20%).

TRANSFUSION REACTIONS

In studies in trauma patients, it has been found that approximately 50% of the fatalities related to transfusion reactions since 1979 have involved type-specific (33%) or O-negative (19%) blood.[94] With O-negative blood, half of the fatal hemolytic reactions resulted from previously unidentified antibodies. In the remaining half, continued administration of type O blood caused non-O patients to develop admixture blood types with difficulty in subsequent cross-matching. Nevertheless, it must be emphasized that virtually all fatal transfusion reactions in patients receiving type-specific uncross-matched blood were due to clerical errors.

RECOGNITION

Although the typical signs and symptoms of a transfusion reaction are usually readily discernible in most patients, they may be extremely difficult to identify in a patient who is anesthetized, especially if he is in shock. Under these conditions, the first sign of a transfusion reaction may be the sudden onset of urticaria, increased oozing from open wounds, or hypotension.

PITFALL ⊘

If the usual signs of incompatibility are watched for only during the first few minutes of a transfusion, recognition of later significant reactions may be missed entirely.

Transfusion reactions seldom declare themselves clinically until at least 50 to 100 ml of blood have been given, and nonhemolytic febrile or allergic reactions may not occur until all units of blood have been infused. Most reactions, such as chills, urticaria, and fever, occur in spite of a satisfactory type and cross-match. Dyspnea, pain, nausea, hematuria, and shock are less common, but are apt to be related to transfusion incompatibilities. In a series of 624 transfusion reactions studied at Detroit General Hospital, only 35 were found to involve a factor that might have been predicted by the cross-matching or prevented with more care. These included a positive Coombs' test in nine patients, bacterial contamination in seven, transfusion with wrong blood in five, incompatible major cross-match in five, and non-specific agglutinins in two.

MANAGEMENT

If a reaction is suspected, the transfusion should be stopped immediately and the remainder of the stored blood, with a sample of the patient's blood, should be sent to the blood bank for repeat cross-match and analysis. Benadryl (50 mg) is given intramuscularly or intravenously immediately and every 6 hours as needed for urticaria, itching, or other allergic phenomena. If the patient is not in danger of being overloaded, intravenous fluids should be administered rapidly with 12.5 to 25.0 gm of mannitol to ensure a copious urine output. One to 2 ampules of sodium bicarbonate may also be added to each IV to alkalize the urine. If shock occurs, adrenalin and hydrocortisone should be administered. If the hypotension is mild, the adrenalin can be given subcutaneously as 0.2 to 0.5 cc of a 1:1000 solution. If severe shock develops, 1.0 cc of 1:1000 adrenalin can be given intravenously in 50 to 100 ml of 5% glucose in water over a 5- to 20-minute period; however, if the pulse is irregular or faster than 120 per minute, adrenalin is usually contraindicated. Hydrocortisone also can be given as a 200 mg intravenous bolus.

Lesions Related to Storage of Blood

Although transfused blood is essential for its oxygen carrying capacity in the bleeding hypovolemic patient, its use, particularly in large quantities, may cause significant problems. The effects of the anticoagulant preservative solution and refrigeration on the physical and chemical properties of the stored blood are sometimes referred to as the "lesion of storage."[109] These changes include reduced RBC viability, increased plasma hemoglobin and potassium concentrations, and reduced red blood cell concentrations of ATP and 2,3-DPG.

DECREASED RED BLOOD CELL VIABILITY

In spite of storage at 4° C, there is a progressive loss in red cell viability and adenosine triphosphate (ATP) and 2,3 diphosphoglycerate (2,3-DPG) content. The ATP content of the red cells is maintained at normal levels for about 3 weeks; however, at 35 days it is only 50% of normal.[109] Lower levels of ATP result in loss of the biconcave disc shape and decreased deformability, thereby interfering with blood flow through capillaries.

AXIOM Blood which has been recently transfused can carry oxygen to the tissues but may not release it.

Levels of 2,3-DPG, although now better maintained than in previously used preservatives, are still only 70% of normal in bank blood at 14 days, 30% at 21 days, and 5% at 35 days. These low levels of 2,3-DPG greatly reduce oxygen availability to the tissues, and may be a critical factor if cardiac output and/or the arterial PO_2 are low. However, regeneration of 2,3-DPG in the patient without shock is rapid following transfusion, and levels usually rise to more than 50% of normal within 4 to 12 hours.

THROMBOCYTOPENIA

After 24 to 48 hours of storage, there are virtually no functioning platelets in bank blood. Trauma patients with massive fluid and transfusion requirements frequently have platelet counts that are significantly decreased immediately postoperatively and continue to fall for 2-3 days.

AXIOM The two most common causes of increased postoperative bleeding in a patient who has received massive transfusions are inadequate surgical hemostasis and thrombocytopenia.

Although it is generally agreed that thrombocytopenia is the most important defect causing excessive bleeding following massive blood transfusions,[110] one must look for surgical causes of bleeding that may have been overlooked while the patient was hypotensive.

In a recent study, the platelet counts averaged about 50,000/mm³ after 20 or more blood transfusions.[111] In more recent data, the mean platelet count fell with the units of blood given from 72,000 to 52,000 to 41,000/mm³ after 10-19, 20-39, and 40 or more transfusions, respectively (Table 4-4). The platelet count tends to fall even further over the next 2-3 days, even when platelets are given. This further decline in the platelet count on the first 2 or 3 postoperative days has been described previously and may reflect a delay in bone marrow production of megakaryocytes and new platelet release.[112]

TABLE 4-4 *Change in Platelet Count, Prothrombin Time (PT), and Accelerated Partial Thromboplastin Times (aPTT) with the Number of Units of Blood (X ± SD)*

	10-19 Units	*20-39 Units*	*40⁺ Units*
Platelets*	72±50 (89)	52±38 (90)	41±70 (27)
PT**	18±10 (89)	21±11 (82)	27±20 (25)
aPTT**	62±47 (89)	89±68 (92)	132±13 (26)

( ) = Number of patients; * X 10³; ** seconds

Although it is often recommended that 6 to 10 units of platelets be given for every 10 units of banked blood to prevent or correct clinical oozing caused by a derangement in primary hemostasis, arbitrary infusion of platelets after some fixed level of transfusions is probably inappropriate. Nevertheless, any patient who is receiving massive blood transfusions and develops diffuse clinical bleeding (i.e., more than that normally associated with the surgical procedure) should be considered for platelet transfusions to raise the platelet count to at least 50,000/mm^3 and preferably to 80,000 to 100,000/mm^3.

During storage of whole blood a marked decrease in coagulation factors occurs. By day 14, approximately 25% of factor VIII and 60% of factor V are lost.[113] In addition by 24 to 72 hours, platelet counts have decreased by 50%, and the remaining platelets are non-functional.

COAGULATION DEFECTS

The changes in the accelerated partial thromboplastin time (aPTT) with massive blood transfusions are often very striking. An aPTT greater than 60 seconds is usually considered evidence of adequate anticoagulation with heparin. In a recent review of our patients, we found that the mean aPTT went from 62 to 89 to 132 seconds as the units of blood given rose from 10-19 to 20-39 to 40 or more within 24 hours (Table 4-4). In another retrospective review of patients receiving more than 10 units of packed red blood cells plus crystalloid within 12 hours, two consecutive patterns of aPTT elevation have been found.[110] The initial rise (at 3 to 4 hours) in aPTT correlates with the amount of crystalloid infused, whereas the later aPTT rise tended to correlate with the number of hours of hypotension. The later rise in aPTT may be due to impaired RBC production, disseminated intravascular coagulation (DIC), and/or dilution due to internal shifts of fluids and/or proteins.

When we reviewed the changes in the prothrombin time (PT) in patients receiving massive transfusions, we found that the mean PT rose from 18 to 21 to 27 seconds as the number of blood transfusions in 24 hours increased from 10-19 to 20-39 and 40 or more, respectively. The mean control PT was 12 seconds (Table 4-4). Hypothermia and increased duration of shock also increased the aPTT (Tables 4-5 and 4-6).

PITFALL ⊘

If excessive operative bleeding in a critically injured patient is assumed to be due to a coagulopathy, the surgeon may not spend the time and effort needed to obtain proper hemostasis.

By far the most frequent cause of excessive bleeding at surgery is inadequate effort by the surgeon in tying, suturing, or coagulating open bleeding vessels. When the bleeding seems to occur from multiple small vessels, especially after a long operation in a poor-risk patient, the surgeon may attribute the bleeding problem to a platelet or clotting defect; therefore, he may attempt to terminate the anesthetic as soon as possible, hoping that hemostatic agents and/or packs will control the bleeding or prevent hematoma formation. Certainly,

TABLE 4-5   Changes in Accelerated Partial Thromboplastin Times (aPTT) Correlated with Core Temperature in Patients Receiving Massive Transfusions*

Core Temp °C	Number of Patients	aPTT (sec) X ± SD
35° C or more	18	48 ± 41
34.0 - 34.9	24	66 ± 54
32.0 - 33.9	43	87 ± 63
Less than 32° C	25	120 ± 79

*≥10 units of blood in 24 hours

TABLE 4-6   Changes in Accelerated Partial Thromboplastin Times (aPTT) Correlated with Duration of Shock* in Patients Receiving Massive Transfusions**

Duration of Shock (min)	Number of Patients	aPTT (sec)
<30	100	58 ± 51
30 - 59	31	101 ± 72
60 or more	27	118 ± 81

* systolic BP <80 mm Hg plus clinical signs of shock
** ≥10 units of blood in 24 hours

if excessive or abnormal bleeding appears to have developed, transfusion reactions and coagulation defects should be considered; under these circumstances, however, there is even greater need for increased effort to obtain complete hemostasis.

If a coagulation problem does develop or is suspected, the physician should have a definite and practical plan of management. We believe that the initial coagulation tests in such a patient should include a platelet count, prothrombin time (PT) and accelerated partial thromboplastin time (aPTT). More sophisticated tests include thrombin times, euglobulin lysis time and direct measurement of fibrinogen and other individual clotting factors. Unfortunately, these may not be readily available to the surgeon, especially on weekends and at night.

AXIOM   If sophisticated clotting studies are not available in a patient who may have a coagulopathy, observation of 2-3 ml of blood placed in a clear test tube for evaluating clotting and lysis may provide invaluable information.

If 2 to 3 ml of blood in a clean test tube clots within 5-10 minutes, it is unlikely that there is a significant deficit of platelets or other clotting factors. If the clot involves all the blood that was present, the fibrinogen level is probably greater than 100 mg/dl. The test tube with the clot should then be taped to the bed or wall so that the clot can be observed for retraction and lysis. If the clot begins to retract within an hour, at least 75,000 platelets/mm^3 are probably present. If the clot lyses rapidly, there is excessive fibrinolytic activity, which can be treated with epsilon-aminocaproic acid (Amicar), but only if DIC can be ruled out.

AXIOM   Blood for clotting studies should not be drawn from an indwelling catheter.

If blood drawn directly from a vein does not clot properly in the test tube, the patient probably has a deficit of platelets or other clotting factors. Blood drawn from a venous or arterial line may have heparin present from flushing solutions.

Bleeding rarely occurs from a platelet deficiency unless the count is below 30,000 to 50,000/mm^3. Occasionally, however, excessive bleeding may occur with larger numbers of aged, damaged, or otherwise ineffective platelets. If there is a platelet deficit, platelet concentrates or fresh warm blood less than 6 hours old should be given. If there is no platelet deficit, the clotting defect may be due to low levels of factor V, factor VIII, or fibrinogen, all of which may be restored with fresh frozen plasma or fresh whole blood.

It must be stressed that the excessive bleeding in acutely injured patients is often attributed to clotting abnormalities; however, it is more likely a result of inadequate or incomplete efforts by the surgeon to control bleeding vessels. Meticulous hemostasis, rapid complete correction of any hypovolemia or impaired tissue perfusion, and keeping the core temperature at 35° C or higher are the best prophylaxis and treatment for coagulation abnormalities during an operation.

In one series, a clinical coagulopathy was thought to be present in 43 (33%) of 128 patients receiving massive transfusion, and 14 (11%) had to be reoperated for continued severe bleeding.[111] However, there was a poor correlation between the laboratory tests and the clinical findings, apparently reflecting an inherent weakness in currently available coagulation tests. Serial examination of the coagulation parameters in these patients showed a gradual correction toward normal on the first few days postoperatively. Interestingly, there was no correlation between the amount of FFP, the resuscitation regimen, and the PT/PTT levels, adding further doubt to the value of "routine" prophylactic use of fresh frozen plasma in patients requiring massive transfusions.

If large quantities of packed RBCs are administered, fresh frozen platelets and platelet packs may be needed, as indicated by clinical or laboratory evidence of bleeding or clotting abnormalities. Fresh frozen plasma, which takes 20 to 40 minutes to thaw, contains normal levels of coagulation factors if administered within 2 hours of thawing; however, with further delays, decreases in coagulation factors, particularly factor VII, are noted.[94]

POTASSIUM ABNORMALITIES

During the storage of whole blood, levels of plasma potassium, ammonia, lactate, and hemoglobin increase while plasma bicarbonate and pH levels decrease. Although potassium levels in the plasma may rise by up to 1 mEq/day, the amount of plasma present is greatly reduced during the preparation of the packed RBCs. Consequently, the actual amount of potassium administered may be only between 5.2 to 6.6 mEq per unit of packed RBCs.[94] Since the mean age for blood administered to trauma patients is 14 days, the actual amount of potassium administered per unit may be only 1 to 3 mEq per unit of packed RBCs.

PITFALL ⊘

> *If it is assumed that all patients who have had recent massive transfusions are hyperkalemic, serious errors in the administration of electrolytes and digitalis preparations can be made.*

In spite of the increased potassium levels in transfused blood, hypokalemia is encountered almost as frequently as hyperkalemia. Of a recent series of 409 of our critically ill or injured patients receiving greater than 10 units of blood, 130 (32%) developed serum potassium levels greater than 5.0 mEq/L,[114] in addition, 19% developed hypokalemia. If the serum potassium levels were corrected for the arterial pH (i.e., reduced 0.5 mEq/L for each 0.10 the pH was less than 7.40), only 5% had a hyperkalemia and 47% had hypokalemia. The causes of this hypokalemia are still unknown but might include: (a) postresuscitation alkalosis due to citrate metabolism to bicarbonate, (b) a tendency for the patients to be hyperventilated, and (c) postresuscitation diuresis. In a recent study, Vanek et al[115] showed that hypokalemia occurred in 50 to 68% of trauma patients during the first 1 to 23 hours. In a multiple regression model, the only significant independent variables to which the hypokalemia was associated were age, arterial pH, and serum epinephrine levels. Nevertheless, with very rapid blood transfusions in patients who are still acidotic, hyperkalemia frequently occurs.

CITRATE TOXICITY

AXIOM   Administration of large quantities of bank blood faster than 1 unit every 5 minutes, especially in patients with shock, cirrhosis, or hypothermia, can cause severe cardiovascular dysfunction due to citrate toxicity and/or ionic hypocalcemia.

Normal plasma contains approximately 1 mg/dl of citrate, as citric acid.[116] Because citrate is the anticoagulant in bank blood, a citrate load is administered during massive transfusion. This is particularly true for CPD anticoagulated blood (29 mg/ml of citrate) and less so for CPD A-1 (approximately 5 mg/ml citrate) or Adsol (2 mg/ml).[62] A healthy, warm, well-perfused adult with adequate hepatic function can tolerate the amount of citrate in 1 unit of blood every 3 to 5 min-

utes without developing symptoms or requiring supplementation with calcium.[117] Nevertheless, in hypothermic and shock patients receiving massive transfusions, plasma citrate levels may reach 60 to 100 mg/dl.[117] As these levels are approached, plasma levels of ionized calcium may fall significantly. This may produce muscle tremors and changes in the ECG, such as prolongation of the QT interval, pulsus alternans, and depression of the P and T waves.[118] Irreversible ventricular fibrillation may follow, particularly if citrate levels of greater than 60 mg/dl are achieved.

Citrate may also have a direct depressant effect on the myocardium separate from its effect on ionized calcium. The administration of sodium citrate in dosages of 2.5 to 12.0 mg/kg/min may decrease cardiac output, stroke volume, left ventricular work, and left ventricular pressure.[119] The presence of hepatic disease, mechanical obstruction to the hepatic circulation, major hepatic trauma, or hypothermia all increase the likelihood of citrate toxicity during massive transfusion.

Citrate toxicity can be prevented or its effects minimized by the administration of calcium. An improved approach to the question of citrate toxicity is the measurement of ionized calcium levels with calcium supplementation as needed.

HYPOCALCEMIA

AXIOM   Calcium does not usually have to be given with blood transfusions unless large amounts (>6-10 units) are given rapidly (more than 1 unit every 5 minutes) and the patient is in heart failure or shock.

Increasing attention has been given to the role of ionized calcium fluxes in severe ischemia-anoxia and their effect on cardiovascular function.[120] It is now clear that ionized calcium levels can fall rapidly during shock because of increased movement of calcium into the cytoplasm of cells which have impaired metabolism. In addition, the citrate in bank blood chelates divalent cations, such as calcium and magnesium, further reducing plasma levels of ionized calcium.[121] In one series, an ionized calcium level of 0.7 or less was associated with a significant increase in mortality. Since plasma ionized calcium levels below 0.85 mmol/L may interfere with cardiovascular function, infusion of calcium may be of some benefit.[122] However, if shock persists, the infused calcium may further increase the already high cytoplasmic calcium levels, causing even more problems.

In a recent series of 116 of our critically ill or injured patients who had 10-19 units of blood within 24 hours, 37 (32%) had very low ionized calcium levels (0.69 mmol/L or less).[114] In 118 patients receiving 20 or more units, 71 (60%) had a very low ionic hypocalcemia. Interestingly, of the patients who were given enough calcium to develop an ionic hypercalcemia, none survived.

Because plasma proteins may also be greatly reduced by blood loss and hemodilution, total calcium levels may fall proportionally much more than the ionized calcium. This is an added reason to obtain serial measurements of ionized calcium in these patients.

HYPOTHERMIA

AXIOM   Coagulation defects, arrhythmias, and impaired cardiovascular function in patients receiving massive transfusions are frequently due to an associated hypothermia (below 32-33° C).

Hypothermia is generally seen during massive blood transfusions in the operating room, no matter how much effort is made to prevent it by warming all fluids and using heating blankets and heated ventilator gases. Since myocardial contractility becomes impaired below temperatures of 32 to 34° C, a vicious cycle of hypothermia and progressively deteriorating cardiovascular function can develop. The hypothermia may also interfere with coagulation mechanisms. Patients maintaining a core temperature below 32° C during massive transfusions have a mortality rate exceeding 85%.[111]

Once bleeding is controlled, every effort should be made to warm the patient to at least 34 to 35° C. This should include warming all infused fluid and blood, warming inhaled gases, and placing the patient on a heating blanket. Irrigating all exposed cavities with warmed fluids also may be necessary.

PULMONARY DYSFUNCTION

Pulmonary dysfunction after massive transfusions has been recognized for many years and is a prominent feature of the postoperative problems in many series, especially in patients who die. It has been suggested that the post-transfusion pulmonary problem is due to trapping of microaggregates from the stored blood in the pulmonary capillaries. One early study showed that when over 5 units of blood were infused through a standard blood filter with a pore diameter of 170 microns, there was a fall in PaO_2 within 48 hours and the decrease in PaO_2 was proportional to the amount of blood transfused.[123] Snyder, on the other hand, found no such correlation.[124] Indeed, a study of patients with ARDS showed that when multiple transfusions were the sole risk factor, this clinical syndrome occurred only in patients receiving over 22 units of blood in 12 hours.[125] Thus, the routine use of microfilters for all blood transfusions cannot be justified by the published data.

AXIOM   One should assume that there will be some degree of pulmonary dysfunction if a patient receives more than 20 units of blood and has been in shock more than 30 minutes.

AMMONIA INTOXICATION

Ammonia levels in fresh blood are about 100 μg/dl plasma. This may increase to 500-900 μg/dl after 21 days of storage. With massive transfusion, the levels of ammonia may be significant, especially if severe hepatic failure is present.[126]

INFECTIOUS COMPLICATIONS

Transfusion-associated Hepatitis

Transfusion-associated hepatitis is the major infectious complication of the therapeutic use of blood and components, affecting 7 to 12% of all recipients and perhaps as many as 20 to 50% of multiply-transfused patients.[127] Currently there are at least four types of hepatitis recognized: type A (infectious), type B (serum), type D (delta hepatitis), and type non-A, non-B. Types A and B have identified and well-characterized viruses as etiologic agents, and sensitive and specific assays for antibodies for these two viruses are now available. The so-called delta agent has been recently identified as the causative agent of hepatitis D, but commercial testing is not available. Hepatitis A virus is a rare cause of post-transfusion hepatitis. In contrast, hepatitis B virus accounts for approximately 10% of transfusion-included cases.

AXIOM   Non-A, non-B hepatitis is one of the biggest threats to life in patients surviving more than a month after massive blood transfusions.

Approximately 85 to 98% of post-transfusion hepatitis is now of the non-A, non-B type.[128] This disease has an incubation period of 8 weeks, compared to 11 weeks for hepatitis B, although clinical symptoms may appear in 10% of patients as early as 2 weeks after transfusion.[129,130] Seventy-five percent of the infected patients are anicteric and relatively asymptomatic with mild elevations of liver enzymes.[130] Forty to fifty percent of all cases of fulminant viral hepatitis are related to non-A, non-B hepatitis, with a mortality rate of 87 to 100%.[131] Additionally, 29% of transfusion-related fatalities involve hepatitis, predominantly non-A, non-B.[132] Non-A, non-B hepatitis also has a higher rate of chronicity (5 to 36%) as compared to the 5 to 10% risk associated with hepatitis B.[133]

At this time, the risk of developing hepatitis is approximately 0.5% per unit, of developing chronic active hepatitis about 0.16% per unit, and of developing clinical cirrhosis 0.03% per unit of blood or blood

products administered. Therefore, the risk of hepatitis is low (i.e., 4% with 5 units or less, 19% with 11 to 20 units, and greater than 42% with 21 units or more). An increased risk of chronic active hepatic disease appears after 25 units.[134]

Jaundice developing after 10 to 14 days is often due to sepsis, but it may also occur in patients who receive halogenated inhalation anesthetics such as halothane or methoxyflurane. With rare exceptions, cytomegalovirus appears to survive only in fresh blood and may cause the splenomegaly, fever, and lymphocytosis which is sometimes referred to as the "postperfusion syndrome."

Acquired Immune Deficiency Syndrome

An estimated 21,000 patients have developed a positive HTLV-3 test from blood transfusions.[135] Today about 1 to 2% of all AIDS cases result from blood transfusion to nonhemophiliac patients.[136] Assuming a 5% outdating of blood units, the risk of developing AIDS is approximately 0.0019 to 0.003% per unit of blood or blood products transfused. The risk of acquiring AIDS is markedly reduced if less than 10 units are administered.[137]

Bacterial Infections

As high as 2.3% of all blood units prepared may be contaminated with bacteria that are capable of using citrate as a carbon source and of growing at low temperatures.[138] From 1976 to 1985, 19% of all fatal transfusion reactions involved blood products with significant contamination.[132] Units contaminated with gram-negative organisms, predominantly *Klebsiella* and *Pseudomonas spp.* accounted for 68% of the reactions. When gram-positive organisms were responsible, staphylococci were most commonly present.

Symptoms such as acute hypotension, fevers of 40° C (104° F) to 40.5° C (105° F), severe abdominal or extremity pain, and a clinical picture of sepsis during transfusion of blood or platelets should suggest a reaction to contaminated products.[94] Symptoms usually appear after a latent period of 30 minutes and may result from transfusion of as little as 50 cc of blood.

The septic reaction to contaminated blood may be difficult to differentiate from a hemolytic transfusion reaction; however, hemolysis does not commonly occur with septic reactions. Thus, septic and transfusion reactions can usually be differentiated by microscopic examination of the blood product for bacteria, determining the presence or absence of hemoglobin in the urine of the patient, and by a review of the transfusion cross-match by the blood bank. Other diseases that can be transmitted through transfusion of blood include malaria, syphilis, brucellosis, cytomegalovirus (CMV), trypanosomiasis, babesiosis, Chagas' disease, toxoplasmosis, leishmaniasis, and infectious mononucleosis.

Increased Tendency to Nosocomial Infections

AXIOM   The majority of patients requiring massive blood transfusions after trauma will develop a nosocomial infection.

Another major problem seen in massive transfusion patients once they become hemodynamically stable is sepsis. All of the survivors in one series of patients requiring 20 or more units of blood developed some type of infection following the massive transfusions.[111] The lungs were the most frequent site of infection, usually by gram-negative organisms. Patients with colon or small bowel injuries frequently developed intra-abdominal abscesses requiring multiple operative procedures. These severe infections significantly delayed discharge from the hospital, and multiple organ failure from persistent sepsis was the most common cause of death in those who survived beyond 48 hours.

The exact cause of the greatly increased tendency to sepsis after massive transfusions in this and other series is not clear. Natural killer cell activity in the peripheral blood of patients receiving blood transfusions tends to be markedly decreased in comparison with that of normal laboratory personnel (P <0.001).[127] In animals, decreased natural killer cell activity has serious consequences, including increased susceptibility to viral infection and tumor engraftment.

ARTIFICIAL BLOOD

Although the primary purpose of the various types of artificial blood is to obviate the need for red blood cell transfusions, they can also expand plasma volume. However, their relative usefulness is limited primarily by their toxic side effects.

Stroma-free Hemoglobin

AXIOM Encapsulated "stroma-free" hemoglobin can carry oxygen, but it can cause cardiovascular and renal problems, and it does not give up its oxygen to tissue very well.

Human hemoglobin solutions have many advantages as an oxygen-delivering blood substitute when compared with plasma expanders and other blood substitutes.[12] Hemoglobin molecules seem to have no antigenicity and minimal allergenic properties, and they do not require typing or cross-matching prior to administration. Solutions prepared with stroma-free hemoglobin have a viscosity lower than that of blood and do not contain microaggregates. Their major disadvantages, which are high oxygen affinity and insufficient intravascular retention time, have been largely overcome by pyridoxylation and polymerization of the crystalline hemoglobin molecule so that the plasma half-life is about 30 hours.

A number of temporary, reversible physiologic alterations in cardiovascular, renal, and coagulation parameters have been reported in healthy volunteers infused with stroma-free hemoglobin solution. These include bradycardia, hypertension, decreased urine output and creatinine clearance, and prolongation of the PTT. By developing improved techniques for the removal of the red cell membrane products produced by lysis (stroma) and by cross-linking the hemoglobin, stroma-free hemoglobin solutions are now available with reduced renal toxicity and a half-life of about 30 hours.

Although highly purified solutions of hemoglobin may now be prepared, questions of safety still remain. Coagulation and renal abnormalities still occur following the administration of the most purified hemoglobin solutions. Finally, only 7 g/dl of free hemoglobin can be administered as a one-to-one replacement for blood without exceeding the normal oncotic pressure of plasma.

Before stroma-free hemoglobin can be considered for clinical trials as a substitute for blood, its effects on immunocompetence, renal function, and coagulation parameters will have to be further defined. As purer and apparently safer hemoglobin preparations have been developed, the biggest remaining problem with SFH had been its very high oxygen affinity. Because of its high oxygen affinity, SFH causes the PO_2 to be low, and only a small fraction of the oxygen transported to the tissues is actually available to the cells. However, recently developed products, including polymerized pyridoxalated hemoglobin (SFH-PLP) with a P_{50} of 20 mm Hg, appear to have overcome this,[139] although further testing is needed.

Encapsulated Hemoglobin

The mixing of phospholipid and cholesterol in the presence of free hemoglobin can form a sphere (liposome) with hemoglobin in the center. The level of hemoglobin that can be achieved in these liposomes approaches that of native blood.[140] Additionally, the functional characteristics of these spheres are remarkably similar to red cells with normal O_2 dissociation curves and P_{50} values of 26 to 28 torr. As they contain no protein, they are apparently free from immune reactions.

However, the half-life of these spheres is only 5 hours, and they are readily removed from circulation.[141] Primary sites of removal are the liver and reticuloendothelial system (RES), and this has created concerns about RES saturation and blockade with subsequent compromise of the immune system.

Diaspirin Cross-linked Hemoglobin Solution

Diaspirin cross-linked hemoglobin (DCLHb) solution is a vasoactive oxygen-carrying solution that has recently received close examination. Cohn and Farrell[142] showed that, in comparison with NSS and HSS in a rat model of hemorrhagic shock, DCLHb more rapidly restored mean BP while at the same time preventing flow dependency and minimizing oxygen debt (base deficit). DCLHb has also been shown to improve tissue perfusion and oxygen delivery without increasing blood loss from injured vessels in rats with uncontrolled hemorrhage.[143,144]

Perfluorocarbons

AXIOM Currently available fluorocarbons can carry oxygen, but they are very toxic and are probably of little value except with very severe anemia (Hb less than 5 g/dl) in patients who will not take blood transfusions.

Perfluorocarbons are large organic compounds in which hydrogen atoms have been replaced by fluoride atoms. Because of their ability to dissolve large amounts of oxygen and carbon dioxide, perfluorochemicals have been studied as possible blood substitutes. Although the main interest in perfluorochemicals has focused on their potential as oxygen-carrying solutions, their favorable effects on the rheologic properties of blood may broaden their use in clinical medicine. Forty to seventy percent oxygen per unit volume can be dissolved in and carried by these compounds-more than three times that of blood. In 1966 Clark and Gollan[145] first demonstrated that these chemicals could provide oxygenation when they reported survival of mice totally submerged in this oxygenated liquid.

The most successful preparation of perfluorochemicals is Fluosol DA, a 20% solution of perfluorotripropylamine and perfluorodecalin. Fluosol was first clinically used in 1979 by Tremper et al[146] in seven severely anemic patients undergoing operative procedures. With administration, patients had increased oxygen arterial contents, and 24% of the oxygen consumed was provided by Fluosol DA.

The use of Fluosol DA as a blood substitute in trauma has several disadvantages. Inspired oxygen concentrations of 80 to 100% are required to raise the arterial oxygen to reasonable levels. This may lead to oxygen toxicity syndromes. Also, Fluosol DA is unstable at room temperature and must be stored frozen, making it unavailable as an initial resuscitation fluid.

When administered at the recommended dose of 20 ml/kg, perfluorochemicals appear to be relatively safe. Early reports of reactions, including systemic hypotension, pulmonary hypertension, hypoxia, and bradycardia, were later found to be attributable to the nonionic emulsifying agent. Replacement of this agent with egg yolk phospholipids may have eliminated some of the problem.

Although the perfluorochemicals are taken up by the reticuloendothelial system, particularly in the liver and spleen, no significant side effects, other than a mild elevation in the aspartate aminotransferase, were reported. Ohnishi and Kitazawa[147] reported substantial morphologic evidence of perfluorocarbon retention at autopsy 4 months later in a patient who had received 4 liters of Fluosol DA over 12 days. Additionally, Fluosol DA may activate the complement system resulting in formation of microaggregates with subsequent pulmonary congestion and hypoxemia.[148]

From 1979 to 1983 a national multicenter study was undertaken to determine the effectiveness of Fluosol DA as a blood substitute for anemic patients undergoing surgery. The unreported results of this study demonstrated increased arterial oxygen in patients undergoing both elective and emergency surgery if hemoglobin levels were between 2.5 and 5.0 gm/dl. No difference was noted between Fluosol DA and lactated Ringer's solutions when hemoglobins were greater than 5. Furthermore, no difference in mortality and morbidity could be demonstrated.

Fluosol-DA 20% (Flusol) has been used to treat life-threatening blood loss in patients who refused blood products for religious reasons. However, in a recent report, all three patients treated at one institution with this agent developed complications of fever, leukocytosis, diffuse pulmonary infiltrates, and hypoxemia.[149]

⊘ FREQUENT ERRORS

In Blood Replacement

1. *Delayed and/or inadequate replacement of extracellular fluid deficits.*
2. *Administration of large amounts of albumin in an effort to raise plasma albumin levels to normal after trauma or during sepsis.*
3. *Giving large amounts of dextran to patients with large open wounds.*
4. *Not notifying the blood bank that the blood for type and cross-matching was drawn after dextran was given.*
5. *Assuming that a high urine specific gravity soon after dextran 40 administration is due to hypovolemia.*
6. *Giving excessive amounts (more than 20 ml/kg/day) of hydroxyethyl starch to patients with a coagulation problem and oozing.*
7. *Using fresh frozen plasma to correct volume deficiencies in a patient with normal coagulation.*
8. *Excessive autotransfusion (more than 6 units) to a patient with a coagulation abnormality.*
9. *Giving uncross-matched type O, Rh-negative blood to a patient who could be treated with crystalloids or colloids for another 5-10 minutes so that type-specific blood could be given.*
10. *Assuming that excessive bleeding during surgery is due to a coagulopathy, without looking for open vessels that can be controlled surgically.*
11. *Not giving calcium to a patient in persistent shock who has been given 6 or more units of blood faster than 1 unit every 5 minutes.*
12. *Assuming a patient is hyperkalemic because he has received massive blood transfusions.*
13. *Giving bicarbonate to a patient who has received massive transfusions and has a severe combined metabolic and respiratory acidosis.*
14. *Giving blood products when not really necessary.*
15. *Not looking closely for nosocomial infections in patients who have been in shock and have received massive transfusions.*

▼▼▼▼▼▼▼▼▼▼▼▼▼▼▼▼▼▼▼▼▼▼▼▼▼▼▼▼

SUMMARY POINTS

1. If crystalloids alone are used to replace massive blood loss, excessive amounts of fluid may be required, and the risk of cerebral and other tissue edema will be increased.
2. Administration of large quantities of saline in patients with continuing inadequate tissue perfusion or ketoacidosis can contribute to the development of a hyperchloremic (non-anion gap) metabolic acidosis.
3. Crystalloid resuscitation of trauma usually does not impair pulmonary function unless there is coincident direct or indirect lung damage or the patient is thrown into right heart failure.
4. If large quantities of Ringers's lactate are given to patients with severe liver disease, a severe lactic acidosis may develop.
5. Albumin may be of value for expanding blood volume, especially in severely hypoproteinemic patients, but it is very expensive, and excessive amounts can cause cardiac, pulmonary, and renal problems.
6. In severe injury or stress, hepatic albumin synthesis falls rapidly, and the liver production of acute phase reactants (such as fibrinogen and C-reactive protein) increases markedly.
7. Administration of excessive amounts of albumin can increase the risk of pulmonary edema in susceptible individuals.

8. Excessive use of albumin may reduce ionized calcium levels and contribute to myocardial failure or shock.
9. Excessive use of albumin may contribute to impaired host defense and/or a hypocoagulable state.
10. The rapid clearance of exogenous albumin coupled with a delay in the production of endogenous albumin impedes the return of normal oncotic pressure within the vascular space.
11. Dextran 40 and dextran 70 can be effective colloids, but they may cause increased oozing from open wounds, difficulty with type and cross-matching of blood, and occasional anaphylactoid reactions.
12. If dextran is given with multiple blood transfusions, it may be difficult to determine the cause of any reactions or increased hemorrhage that may occur.
13. If the blood blank is not informed of the recent administration of dextran to a patient who requires blood transfusion, it may fail to obtain a proper type and cross-match.
14. If dextran is given to patients with large open wounds, excessive oozing and blood loss may occur.
15. Hydroxyethyl starch (HES) is an effective colloid for expanding blood volume, but excessive use can cause increased bleeding.
16. Although administration of hetastarch can cause multiple coagulation changes, it rarely produces clinically significant bleeding problems if used in doses less than 20 ml/kg/day.
17. The elevated plasma amylase levels after hetastarch administration are due to formation of macroamylase molecules and do not reflect pancreatic problems.
18. Fresh frozen plasma can correct deficiencies in clotting factors (not platelets) and antithrombin, but it can transmit blood-borne diseases, especially hepatitis.
19. Fresh frozen plasma should not be used just to expand plasma volume.
20. Compatibility testing for fresh frozen plasma is not required, but it should be ABO-compatible with the patient when possible.
21. Successful resuscitation is primarily dependent on the rapidity and adequacy of fluid repletion, not on the composition of the resuscitation fluid.
22. Hypertonic saline can rapidly expand blood volume, but it can cause excess vasodilation and serum sodium levels greater than 165 mEq/L, which can cause severe side effects.
23. Autotransfusion can reduce blood bank needs and reduce the risk of blood-borne diseases, but if used in excess, especially in patients in shock, it can cause severe coagulopathies.
24. Massive abdominal blood loss contaminated with intestinal contents is not a contraindication to autotransfusion if the red cells are washed well and antibiotics are given in full dose.
25. Autotransfusions are safest if used in moderation and if the red cells are carefully washed before infusion.
26. Young, healthy individuals can do well with a hemoglobin of 7.0 gm/dl if they are hemodynamically stable and the bleeding is controlled.
27. If physicians use group O uncross-matched blood when it might be possible to delay 5-10 minutes by using other fluids or colloids and thereby give type-specific blood, they increase the risk of complications to their patients.
28. The most severe hemolytic transfusion reactions are generally due to simple clerical errors.
29. If the usual signs of incompatibility are watched for only during the first few minutes of a transfusion, recognition of significant delayed reactions may be missed entirely.
30. Blood that has been recently transfused can carry oxygen to the tissue but may not release it.
31. The two most common causes of increased postoperative bleeding in a patient who has received massive transfusions are inadequate surgical hemostasis and thrombocytopenia.
32. If excessive operative bleeding in a critically injured patient is assumed to be due to a coagulopathy, the surgeon may not spend the time and effort needed to obtain proper hemostasis from larger bleeding vessels.
33. If sophisticated clotting studies are not available in a patient

who may have a coagulopathy, observation of 2-3 ml of blood placed in a clear test tube for evaluating clotting and lysis may provide invaluable information.

34. Blood for clotting studies should not be drawn from an indwelling catheter.

35. One should not assume that all patients who have had massive transfusions are hyperkalemic.

36. Administration of large quantities of bank blood faster than 1 unit every 5 minutes, especially in patients with shock, cirrhosis, or hypothermia, can cause severe cardiovascular dysfunction due to citrate toxicity and/or ionic hypocalcemia.

37. Calcium does not usually have to be given with blood transfusions unless large amounts (6-10 units) are given rapidly (more than 1 unit every 5 minutes) and the patient is in heart failure or shock.

38. Coagulation defects, arrhythmias, and impaired cardiovascular function in patients receiving massive transfusions are frequently due to the associated hypothermia (below 32-33° C).

39. One should assume that there will be some degree of pulmonary dysfunction if a patient receives more than 20 units of blood and has been in shock more than 30 minutes.

40. Non-A, non-B hepatitis is one of the biggest threats to life in patients surviving more than a month after massive blood transfusions.

41. The majority of patients requiring massive blood transfusions after trauma will develop a nosocomial infection.

42. Encapsulated "stroma-free" hemoglobin can carry oxygen, but it can cause cardiovascular and renal problems, and it does not give up its oxygen to tissue very well.

43. Currently available fluorocarbons can carry oxygen, but they are toxic and are probably of little value except with very severe anemia (Hb less than 5 gm/dl) in patients who will not take blood transfusions.

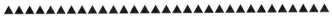

REFERENCES

1. Carey JS, Scharschmidt BF, Culliford AT. Hemodynamic effectiveness of colloid and electrolyte solutions for replacement of simulated operative blood loss. Surg Gynecol Obstet 1970;131:679.
2. Lowery BD, Cloutier CT, Carey LC. Electrolyte solutions in resuscitation in human hemorrhagic shock. Surg Gynecol Obstet 1971;133:273.
3. Oh MS, Carroll HT, Goldstein DA. Hyperchloremic acidosis during the recovery phase of diabetic ketosis. Ann Intern Med 1978;89:925.
4. Haupt MT, Rackow EC. Colloid osmotic pressure and fluid resuscitation with hetastarch, albumin, and saline solutions. Crit Care Med 1982;10:159.
5. Virgilio RW, Smith DE, Zarino DK. Balanced electrolyte solutions: experimental and clinical studies. Crit Care Med 1979;7:98.
6. Hauser CJ, Shoemaker WC, Turpin I. Oxygen transport responses to colloids and crystalloids in critically ill surgical patients. Surg Gynecol Obstet 1980;150:811.
7. Rainey TG, English JF. Pharmacology of colloids and crystalloids. In: Chernow B, ed. The pharmacologic approach to the critically ill patient. Baltimore: Williams & Wilkins, 1983:219.
8. Davidson I, Eriksson B. Statistical evaluations of plasma substitutes based on 10 variables. Crit Care Med 1982;10:653.
9. Virgilio RW, Rice CL, Smith DE. Crystalloid versus colloid resuscitation: is one better? A randomized clinical study. Surgery 1979;85:129.
10. Chan STF, Kapadia CR, Johnson AW, Radcliffe AG, Dudley HAF. Extracellular fluid volume expansion and third space sequestration at the site of small bowel anastomoses. Br. J Surg 1983;70:36-39.
11. Laks H, Standever J, Blair O, Hahn J, Jellinek M, William VL. The effects of cardiopulmonary bypass with crystalloid and colloid hemodilution on myocardial extravascular water. J Thorac Cardiovasc Surg 1977;73:129-138.
12. Nearman HS, Herman ML. Toxic effects of colloids in the intensive care unit. Crit Care Clin 1991;7:713.
13. Rothschild MA, Oratz M, Schreiber SS. Albumin synthesis. N Engl J Med 1972;286:748.
14. Wilson RF, Sarver E, Birks R. Central venous pressure and blood volume determinations in clinical shock. Surg, Gynec & Obstet 1971;132:631.
15. Collins JN, Dyess DL, Ardell JL, et al. The effects of albumin administration on microvascular permeability at the site of burn injury. J Trauma 1994;36:27.
16. Greenhalgh DG, Housinger T, Kagan RJ, et al. Maintenance of serum albumin levels in pediatric burn patients: a prospective, randomized trial. J Trauma 1994;37:153.
17. Emerson TE. Unique features of albumin: a brief review. Crit Care Med 1989;17:690.
18. Ledgerwood AM, Lucas CE. Postresuscitation hypertension, etiology, morbidity and treatment. Arch Surg 1974;108:531.
19. Lewis RT. Albumin: role and discriminative use in surgery, Can J Surg 1980;23:322.
20. Poole GV, Meredity JW, Pernell T, et al. Comparison of colloids and crystalloids in resuscitation from hemorrhagic shock. Surg Gynecol Obstet 1982;154:577.
21. Esrig BC, Fulton RL. Sepsis, resuscitated hemorrhagic shock and "shock lung": an experimental correlation. Ann Surg 1975;182:218.
22. Lucas CE, Ledgerwood AM, Mammen EF. Altered coagulation protein content after albumin resuscitation. Ann Surg 1982;196:198.
23. Kovalik SG, Ledgerwood AM, Lucas CE. The cardiac effect of altered calcium homeostasis after albumin resuscitation. J Trauma 1981;21:275.
24. Faillace D, Ledgerwood AM, Lucas CE, Kithier K. Effects of different resuscitation regimens on immunoglobulins. Surg Forum 1979;30:18.
25. Clift DR, Ledgerwood AM, Lucas CE, et al. The effect of albumin resuscitation for shock on the immune response to tetanus toxoid. J Surg Res 1982;32:449.
26. Rothschild MA, Oratz M, Schreiber SS. Albumin metabolism. Gastroenterology 1973;64:324.
27. Tullis JL. Albumin. I. Background and use. JAMA 1977;237:355.
28. Alving BM, Hojima Y, Pisano JJ. Hypotension associated with prekallikrein activator (Hageman factor fragments) in plasma protein fraction. N Engl J Med 1978;299:66.
29. Data JL, Nies AS. Dextran 40. Ann Intern Med 1974;81:500.
30. Shoemaker WC, Schluchter M, Hopkins JA. Fluid therapy in emergency resuscitation: clinical evaluation of colloid and crystalloid regimens. Crit Care Med 1981;9:367.
31. Thoren L. The dextrans-clinical data. Joint WHO/IABS symposium on the standardization of albumin plasma substitutes and plasmaphoresis. Geneva 1980. Dev Biol Stand 1981;48:157.
32. Shoemaker WC. Comparison of the relative effectiveness of whole blood transfusions and various types of fluid therapy in resuscitation. Crit Care Med 1976;4:71.
33. Aberg M, Hedner V, Bergentz S. Effect of dextran on factor VIII and platelet function. Ann Surg 1979;189:243.
34. Sashahara AA, Sharma GVRK, Parisi AF. New developments in the detection and prevention of venous thromboembolism. Am J. Cardiol 1979;43:1214.
35. Lewis JH, Szetol LF, Beyer WL. Severe hemodilution with hydroxyethyl starch and dextrans. Arch Surg 1966;93:941.
36. Ring J, Messmer K. Incidence and severity of anaphylactoid reactions to colloid volume substitutes. Lancet 1977;1:466.
37. Cohn JN, Luria MH, Daddario RC. Studies in clinical shock and hypotension. V. Hemodynamic effects of dextran. Circulation 1967;35:316.
38. Thompson WL. Rational use of albumin and plasma substitutes. Johns Hopkins Med J 1975;136:220.
39. Alexander B, Odake K, Lawlor J, et al. Coagulation, hemostasis and plasma expanders: a quarter-century enigma. Fed Pro 1975;34:1429.
40. Feest TG. Low molecular weight dextran: a continuing cause of acute renal failure. Br Med J 1976;2:1300.
41. Chinitz JL. Pathophysiology and prevention of dextran 40 induced anuria. J Lab Clin Med 1971;77:76.
42. Bergentz SE, Falkheden T, Olson S. Diuresis and urinary viscosity in dehydrated patients: influence of dextran 40 with and without mannitol. Ann Surg 1965;161:562.
43. Lamke JH, Liljedahl SO. Plasma volume expansion after infusion of 5%, 20%, and 25% albumin solutions in patients. Resuscitation 1976;5:85.
44. Skrede S, Ro JS, Mjolnerod O. Effects of dextrans on the plasma protein changes during the postoperative period. Clin Chim Acta 1973;48:143.
45. Abramowicz M, ed. Med Lett Drugs Ther 1968;10(1):3.
46. Perttila J, Salo M, Peltola O. Effects of different plasma substitutes on plasma fibronectin concentrations in patients undergoing abdominal surgery. Acta Anaesthesiol Scand 1990;34:304.
47. Mishler JM. Pharmacology of hydroxyethyl starch: use in therapy and blood banking. Oxford: Oxford Univesity Press, 1982:1-30.

48. Yacobi A, Stoll RG, Sum CY, Lai CM, Gupta SD, et al. Pharmacokinetics of hydroxyethyl starch in normal subjects. J Clin Pharmacol 1982;22:206.

49. London MJ, Ho SJ, Triedman JK et al. A randomized clinical trial of 10% pentastarch (low molecular weight hydroxyethyl starch) versus 5% albumin for plasma volume expansion after cardiac operations. J Thor Cardiovasc Surg 1989;97:785.

50. Mishler JM, Richetts CR, Parkhouse EJ. Post-transfusion survival of hydroxyethyl starch 450/0.70 in man: a long-term study. J Clin Pathol 1980;33:155.

51. Yacobi A, Stoll RG, Sum CY. Pharmacokinetics of hydroxethyl starch in normal subjects. J Clin Pharmacol 1982;22:206.

52. Lenz G, Hempel V, Jurger H, Worle H. Effect of hydroxyethyl starch, oxypolygelatin and human albumin on the phagocytic function of the reticuloendothelial system in healthy subjects. Anaesthesist 1986;35:423.

53. Strauss RG, Stump DC Henriksen RA, et al. Effects of hydroxyethyl starch on fibrinogen, fibrin clot formation, and fibrinolysis. Transfusion 1985;25:230.

54. Stump DC, Strauss RG, heinriksen RA, et al. Effects of hydroxyethyl starch on blood coagulation, particularly factor VIII. Transfusion 1985;25:349.

55. Sanfelippo MJ, Suberviola PD, Geimer NF. Development of a von Willebrand-like syndrome after prolonged use of hydroxyethyl starch. Am J Clin Pathol 1987;88:653.

56. Damon L, Adams M, Stricker RB, et al. Intracranial bleeding during treatment with hydroxyethyl starch. N Engl J Med 1987;317:964.

57. Lazrove S, Waxman K, Shippy C. Hemodynamic blood volume and oxygen transport responses to albumin and hydroxethyl starch infusions in critically ill post operative patients. Crit Care Med 1980;8:302.

58. Strauss RG, Stump DC, Henrikson RA, Saunders R. Effects of hydroxyethyl starch on fibrinogen, fibrin clot formation and fibrinolysis. Transfusion 1985;25:230.

59. Shatney CH, Deapiha K, Militello PR, Majerus TC, Dawson RB. Efficacy of hetastarch in the resuscitation of patients with multisystem trauma and shock. Arch Surg 1983;118:804.

60. Kohler H, Kirch W, Horstmann HJ. Hydroxyethyl starch induced macroamylasemia. Int J Clin Pharmacol 1977;15:428.

61. London MJ, Ho JS, Triedman JK, et al. A randomized clinical trial of 10% pentastarch (low molecular weight hydroxyethyl starch) versus 5% albumin for plasma volume expansion after cardiac operations. Thorac Cardio 1989;97:785.

62. Hakaim AG, Corsetti R, Cho SI. The pentafraction of hydroxyethyl starch inhibits ischemia-induced compartment syndrome. J Trauma 1994;37:18.

63. Office of Medical Applications of Research, National Institutes of Health. Fresh frozen plasma: indications and risks. JAMA 1985;253:551.

64. Ledingham IM, Ramsey G. Hypovolemic shock. Brit J Anest 1986;8:169.

65. Rackow EC, Falk JL, Fein IA, et al. Fluid resuscitation in circulatory shock. Crit Care Med 1983;11:839.

66. Lucas CE, Martin DJ, Ledgerwood AM, et al. Effect of fresh frozen plasma resuscitation on cardiopulmonary function and serum protein flux. Arch Surg 1986;121:559.

67. Martin DJ, Lucas CE, Ledgerwood AM, et al. Fresh frozen plasma supplement to massive red blood cell transfusion. Ann Surg 1985;202:505.

68. Velasco IT, Pontieri V, Silva MR, et al. Hyperosmotic NaCl and severe hemorrhagic shock. Am J Physiolo 1980;239:H664.

69. Mullins RJ, Hudgens RW. Hypertonic saline resuscitates dogs in endotoxin shock. J Surg Research 1987;43:37.

70. Traverso LW, Bellamy RF, Hollenbaugh SJ, et al. Hypertonic sodium chloride solutions: effect on hemodynamics and survival after hemorrhage in swine. J Trauma 1987;27:32.

71. Silva MR, Velasco IT, Nogueira RI, et al. Hyperosmotic sodium salts reverse severe hemorrhagic shock: other solutes do not. Am J Physiol 1987;253:H751-762.

72. Mazzoni MC, Borgstrom P, Arforse KE, et al. Dynamic fluid redistribution in hyperosmotic resuscitation of hypovolemic hemorrhage. Am J Physiol 1988;255:J629-H637.

73. Liang CS, Hood WB. Mechanism of cardiac output response to hypertonic sodium chloride infusion in dogs. Am J Physiol 1978;235:H18-22.

74. Silva MR, Negraes GA, Soares AM, et al. Hypertonic resuscitation from severe hemorrhagic shock: patterns of regional circulation. Circ Shock 1986;19:165-175.

75. Younes RN, Aun F, Tomida RM, et al. The role of lung innervation in the hemodynamic response to hypertonic sodium chloride solutions in hemorrhagic shock. Surgery 1985;98:900-906.

76. Velasco IT, Baena RC, Rocha E, Silsa M, et al. Central angiotensinergic system and hypertonic resuscitation from severe hemorrhage. Am J Physiol 1990;259:H1752-1758.

77. Wallace AW, Tunin CM, Shoukas AA. Effects of vasopressin on pulmonary and systemic vascular mechanics. Am J Physiol 1989;257: H1228-1234.

78. Holcroft JW, Vassar MJ, Turner JE, et al. 3% NaCl and 7.5% NaCl/dextran 70 in the resuscitation of severely injured patients. Ann Surg 1987;206:279.

79. Bowser BH, Caldwell FT. The effects of resuscitation with hypertonic saline versus colloid on wound and urine fluid and electrolyte losses in severely burned children. J Trauma 1983;23:916.

80. Monafo WW, Haverson JD, Schectman K. The role of concentrated sodium solutions in the resuscitation of patients with severe burns. Surgery 1984;95:129.

81. Shackford SR, Fortlage DA, Peters RM et al. Serum osmolar and electrolyte changes associated with large infusions of hypertonic sodium lactate for intravenous volume expansion of patients undergoing aortic reconstruction. Surg Gynecol Obstet 1987;164:127.

82. Moss GS, Gould SA. Plasma expanders: an update. Am J Surg 1988;155:425.

83. Kramer GC, Perron PR, Lindsey C, et al. Small-volume resuscitation with hypertonic saline-dextran solution. Surgery 1986;100:239.

84. Wildenthal K, Mierzwiak DS, Mitchell JH. Acute effects of increased serum osmolality on left ventricular performance. Am J Physiol 1969;216:898.

85. Nerlick M, Gunther R, Demling RH. Resuscitation from hemorrhagic shock with hypertonic saline or lactated Ringer's: effect on the pulmonary and systemic microcirculations. Circ Shock 1983;10:179.

86. Prough DS, Johnson JC, Stulken EH, et al. Effects on cerebral hemodynamics of resuscitation from endotoxic shock with hypertonic saline versus lactated Ringer's solution. Crit Care Med 1985;13:1040.

87. Saxe JM, Dombi G, Lucas WE, et al. Interstitial matrix reactions to hypertonic saline resuscitation in a canine model. Trauma 1994;37:162.

88. Cross JS, Gruber DP, Burchard KW, et al. Hypertonic saline fluid therapy following surgery: a prospective study. J Trauma 1989;29:817.

89. Prough DD, Johnson JC, Stump DA, et al. Effects of hypertonic saline versus lactated Ringer's solution on cerebral oxygen transport during resuscitation from hemorrhagic shock. J Neurosurg 1986;64:627.

90. Runyon DE, Bruttig SP, Dubick MA, et al. Resuscitation from hypovolemia in swine with intraosseous infusion of a saturated salt-dextran solution. J Trauma 1994;36:11.

91. Dubick MA, Wade CE. A review of the efficacy and safety of 7.5% NaCL/6% dextran 70 in experimental animals and in humans. J Trauma 1994;36:323.

92. Johnston WE, Alford PT, Prough DS, et al. Cardiopulmonary effects of hypertonic saline in canine oleic acid-induced pulmonary edema. Crit Care Med 1985;13:814-817.

93. Armistead CS, Vincent JL, Preiser JC, et al. Hypertonic saline solution-hetastarch for fluid resuscitation in experimental septic shock. Anesth Analg 1989;96:714.

94. Gervin AS. Transfusion, autotransfusion, and blood substitutes. In: Mattox KL, Moore EE, Feliciano DV, eds. Trauma. Norwalk, CT: Appleton & Lange, 1988:159.

95. Symbas PN, Levin JM, Ferrier FL, et al. A study of autotransfusion from hemothorax. South Med J 1969;62:671.

96. Popovsky MA, Devine PA, Taswell HF. Intraoperative autologous transfusion. Mayo Clin Proc 1985;60:125.

97. Glover JL, Smith R, Yaw PB, et al. Autotransfusion of blood contaminated by intestinal contents. J Am Coll Emerg Physicians 1978;7:142.

98. Jurkovich GJ, Moore EE, Medina G. Autotransfusion in trauma: a pragmatic analysis. Am J Surg 1984;148:782.

99. Moore EE, Dunn E, Brestich DJ, et al. Platelet abnormalities associated with massive autotransfusion. J Trauma 1980;20:1052.

100. Hammerschmidt DE, Jacobs H. Adverse pulmonary reactions to transfusions. In: Massive transfusion. Year Book Medical Publisher, Inc., 1982:511.

101. Sittig KM, Deitch ED. Blood transfusions: for the thermally injured or for the doctor. J Trauma 1994;36:369.

102. Mann Roberta, Heimbach DM, Engrav LH, Foy H. Changes in transfusion practices in burn patients. J Trauma 1994;37:220.

103. Goldfinger D, Lowe C. Prevention of adverse reactions to blood transfusions by administration of saline washed red blood cells. Transfusion 1981;21:277.

104. Meryman HT, Hornblower M. A method for freezing and washing red cells using high glycerol concentration. Transfusion 1972;12:145.

105. Barnes A. Transfusions of universal donor and uncross-matched blood. Bibl Haematologica 1980;46:132.
106. Gervin AS, Fisher RP. Resuscitation of trauma patients with type specific uncross-matched blood. J Trauma 1984;27:327.
107. Baker RJ, Moinichen BS, Nyhus LM. Transfusion reaction. Ann Surg 1969;169:684.
108. Gervin AS, Limbird TJ. Puckett CL, et al. Ultrapore hemofiltration: the effects on the coagulation and fibrinolytic mechanisms in fresh and stored blood. Arch Surg 1973;106:333.
109. Sohmer, PR, Scott RL, Metabolic burden of massive transfusion. In: Massive transfusion in surgery and trauma. Alan R. Liss, Inc, 1982:272.
110. Hewson OR, Neale PB, Kumar N, et al. Coagulopathy related to dilution and hypotension during massive transfusion. Crit Care Med 1985;13 (5):387.
111. Wilson RF, Dulchavsky SA, Soullier G, et al. Problems with 20 or more blood transfusions in 24 hours. Am Surg 1987;53:410.
112. Harrington C, Lucas CE, Ledgerwood AM, et al. Serial changes in primary hemostasis after massive transfusion. Surgery 1985;98(4):836.
113. Latham JT, Bove JR, Weirich L. Chemical and hematologic changes in stored CPDA-1 blood. Transfusion 1982;22:158.
114. Wilson RF, Mammen E, Walt AJ. Eight years of experience with massive transfusions. J Trauma 1971;11:275.
115. Vanek VW, Seballos RM, Chong D, Bourguet CC. Serum potassium concentrations in trauma patients. South Med J 1994;87:41.
116. Howland WS, Bellville JW, Zucker MB, et al. Massive blood replacement. Surg Gynecol Obstet 1957;105:529.
117. Mollison PL. Blood transfusion in clinical medicine. 7th ed. London: Blackwell Scientific, 1983:751.
118. Nakasone N, Watkins E, Janeway CA, et al. Experimental studies of circulatory derangement following the massive transfusion of citrated blood. J Lab Clin Med 1954;43:184.
119. Corbascio AN, Smith NT. Hemodynamic effects of experimental hypercitremia. Anesthesiology 1967;28:510.
120. Howland WS, Schweizer O, Carlton GC, et al. The cardiovascular effects of low levels of ionized calcium during massive transfusion. Surg Gynecol Obst 1977;145:581.
121. McLellan, BA, Reid SR, Lane PL. Massive blood transfusion causing hypomagnesemia. Crit Care Med 1984;12(2):146.
122. Bashour TT. Hypocalcemic acute myocardial failure secondary to rapid transfusion of citrated blood. Am Heart J 1984;108:146.
123. McNamara, JJ. Microaggregates in stored blood: physiologic significance. In: Chaplin H, Jaffee ER, Lenfort C, Valeri CR, eds. Preservation of red blood cells. Washington: National Academy of Science, 1972:315.
124. Snyder EL, Bookbinder M. The role of microaggregate blood filtration in clinical medicine. Transfusion 1983;23(6):460.
125. Pepi, PE, Potkin RT, Rheu RH, et al. Clinical predictors of the adult respiratory distress syndrome. Am J Surg 1982;144:124.
126. Spears PW, Sass M, Cincotti JJ. Ammonia levels in transfused blood. J Lab Clin Med 1956;48:702.
127. Alter HJ. Post transfusion hepatitis. In: Dodd RY, Barker LF, eds. Infection immunity and blood transfusion. New York: Alan Liss, 1985:47.
128. Blum HE, Vyas GN. Non-A, non-B hepatitis: a contemporary assessment. Haematologia 1982;15:162.
129. Alter HJ, Purcell RH, Holland PV, et al. Clinical and serological analysis of transfusion-associated hepatitis. Lancet 1975;2:838.
130. Hruby MA, Schauf V. Transfusion-related short-incubation hepatitis in hemophilic patients. JAMA 1978;240:1355.
131. Rakela J, Redeker AG, Edwards VM. Hepatitis A virus infection in fulminant hepatitis and chronic acute hepatitis. Gastroenterology 1978; 74:879.
132. Food and Drug Administration. Records on transfusion fatalities 1979-1985.
133. Jeffers LJ, et al. Post transfusion non-B hepatitis resulting in cirrhosis of the liver. Hepatology 1981;1:521.
134. Knodell RG, Conrad ME, Ishak KG. Development of chronic liver disease after non-A, non-B post-transfusion hepatits. Gastroenterology 77:902, 1977.
135. Sivak SL, Wormser GP. How common is HTLV-III infection in the United States? N Engl J Med 1985;313:1352.
136. Carlson J, Hinrichs S, Levy M. et al. HTLV-III antibody screening of blood bank donors. Lancet 1985;1:523.
137. Hardy AM, Allen JR, Morgan M, et al. Incidence rate of acquired immunodeficiency syndrome in selected populations. JAMA 1985; 253:215.
138. Braude AI, Sanford JP, Bartlett, et al. Effects and clinical significance of bacterial contaminants of transfused blood. J Lab Clin Med 1952;39:902.
139. Devennto F. Hemoglobin solutions as oxygen delivery resuscitation fluids. Crit Care Med 1982;10:238.
140. Djordjevich L, Miller IF. Synthetic erythrocytes from lipid encapsulated hemoglobin. Exp Hematol 1980;8:584.
141. Farmer MC, Garber BP. Encapsulation of hemoglobin in phospholipid vesicles: surrogate red cells in vitro and in vivo. Biophys J 1984;45:201a.
142. Cohn SM, Farrell TJ. Comparison of diaspirin cross-linked hemoglobin (DCLHb) to hypertonic saline in resuscitation of hemorrhagic shock. J Trauma 1994;37:163.
143. Schultz SC, Powell CC, Burris DG, et al. The effects of diaspirin crosslinked hemoglobin solution resuscitation in a model of uncontrolled hemorrhage. J Trauma 1994;37:408.
144. Schultz SC, Powell C, Burris D, et al. Effects of diaspirin crosslinked hemoglobin on blood pressure, blood loss and survival in a model of uncontrolled hemorrhage. J Trauma 1994;37:154.
145. Clark LC, Gollan F. Survival of mammals breathing organic liquids equilibrated with oxgen at atmospheric pressure. Science 1966;152:1755.
146. Tremper KK, Friedman AE, Levine EM, et al. The preoperative treatment of severely anemic patients with a perfluorochemical oxygen-transport fluid, Fluosol-DA. N Engl J Med 1982;307:277.
147. Ohnishi Y, Kitazawa M. Application of perfluorochemicals in human beings. Acta Pathol Jpn 1980;30:489.
148. Vercellotti GM, Hammerschmidt DE, Craddock PR, et al. Activation of plasma complement by perfluorocarbon artificial blood: probable mechanism of adverse pulmonary reactions in treated patients and rationale for corticosteroid prophylaxis. Blood 1982;59:1299.
149. Police AM, Waxman K, Tominaga G. Pulmonary complications after Fluosol administration to patients with life-threatening blood loss. Crit Care Med 1985;13:96.

Chapter 5 General Principles of Wound Care

ROBERT F. WILSON, M.D.

CHENICHERI BALAKRISHNAN, M.D.

Wound healing is a complex dynamic process that results in the restoration of anatomic continuity and function. Understanding the principles of wound healing has important implications in the management of wounds and treating conditions such as keloids and tendon adhesions. Whether a wound occurs as a result of surgical intervention or trauma, adherence to basic tenets of wound care will optimize the long-term results.

STAGES OF WOUND HEALING

A wound may be inflicted by physical trauma, heat, cold, radiation, chemicals, injury, and infection. Healing begins from the moment of injury, and in every wound, the stages of healing are quite similar.[1-5] In open wounds, the stages of healing are usually referred to as inflammation, proliferation, maturation, and remodeling. In wounds that are closed promptly, epithelialization will begin before there is proliferation of collagen. Yet, in many experimental models of wound healing, re-epithelialization has been taken as the end point of healing. These five stages of wound healing overlap in time with each other so that various stages can be seen simultaneously in the wound (Fig. 5-1).

Inflammation

Inflammation is the result of trauma to tissue from any stimulus. Aurelius Cornelius Celsus in the 1st century AD characterized the signs of inflammation as heat (calor), redness (rubor), swelling (tumor), and tenderness (dolor). They remain the cardinal signs of inflammation.

The inflammatory response involves both a vascular and a cellular reaction. The inflammatory phase is important for the phagocytosis and debridement of foreign materials and irreparably damaged tissue. Most wounds result in injury to blood vessels with a hemorrhage. Vasoconstriction occurs almost immediately, followed 5 to 10 minutes later by vasodilation. The initial inflammation lasts up to 3 days. This is followed by and occurs with a destructive phase (for another 2-5 days) in which macrophages remove any unwanted or devitalized material.[3] The inflammatory phase generates a wide variety of soluble mediators which help regulate the subsequent stages of wound healing.

Numerous substances, including histamine, serotonin, kinins, and prostaglandins, participate in increasing the permeability of venules in a wound. Histamine, which is synthesized at the wound site and is also released from stores within mast cells, augments the permeability of arterioles, capillaries, and venules to albumin, globulin, and fibrinogen.[6] This is accomplished, at least in part, by causing the contraction of endothelial cells and increasing the intercellular gaps in the endothelium. Serotonin (hydroxytryptamine) is released from platelets and mast cells. Kinins are polypeptides produced at the site of inflammation from alpha-globulins found in plasma. They not only increase venule permeability, but are also potent vasodilators. Prostaglandins E_1 and E_2 are synthesized at the site of injury. They cause vasodilation by activation of adenyl cyclase and increased production of cyclic adenosine monophosphate (cAMP).[7]

AXIOM Use of drugs to reduce inflammation in wounds may impair healing.

The inflammatory exudate includes fibrin and fibronectins. Fibrin, which is produced in the wound by conversion of circulating plasma fibrinogen, promotes hemostasis, and provides a scaffolding for the ingrowth of cells. Fibronectins constitute a family of high-molecular-weight glycoproteins. They are present in an insoluble form in connective tissue and in a soluble form in plasma and other body fluids. Fibronectins facilitate the attachment of migrating fibroblasts to the fibrin latticework within the wound.[8]

After an incision is made in the skin, blood components extravasate into the wound cavity. Endothelial cells retract and lose their attachments with adjoining cells, thereby exposing the fibrillar collagen to which platelets adhere. These are followed by circulating polymorphonuclear cells and monocytes which adhere quickly to the vascular endothelium in the injured region and traverse the vessel walls through a process of diapedesis. These cells then migrate toward the injured area where they phagocytize bacteria, foreign materials, or necrotic tissue.

The polymorphonuclear and mononuclear cells are present initially at the site of injury in proportions similar to those in the blood. The polymorphonuclear leukocytes are important for controlling any bacterial contamination that may have occurred at the time of wounding. The macrophages remove necrotic tissue and foreign bodies from the wound. More importantly, the macrophages respond to numerous stimuli from the wound and translate these stimuli into chemical signals (cytokines) to a large number of other cells.

The polymorphonuclear cells in the wound are relatively short-lived, and are not needed for the subsequent stages of wound healing. The mononuclear cells become increasingly abundant after 24-72 hours. In addition to aiding in bacterial phagocytosis and tissue debridement, the macrophages have an important function in directing the subsequent course of wound healing. After activation in the wound, the macrophages release proteases, vasoactive peptides, and chemotactic factors for fibroblasts. The macrophages also actively stimulate the proliferation of both fibroblasts and endothelial cells (Fig. 5-2).[9]

AXIOM In the presence of extensive tissue injury or massive bacterial contamination, the inflammatory phase will be prolonged, and wound healing may be greatly delayed.

Chemotaxis refers to the movement of cells in response to various chemicals. Macrophages release chemotactic factors for fibroblasts and endothelial cells. The complement factors C3a and C5a are particularly powerful chemoattractants. The fibroblasts entering the wound become closely associated with the fibronectin lattice laid down in the wound. Migration of fibroblasts into the traumatized area is followed closely by the formation of capillaries and their ingrowth into the wound. Endothelial cells accomplish this by secreting a powerful activator that converts plasminogen to plasmin, which dissolves the fibrin network as the endothelial cells advance.

AXIOM Although many experimental models of wound healing use reepithelialization as the end point of healing, the tensile strength of the wound is inadequate at that time.

INJURY

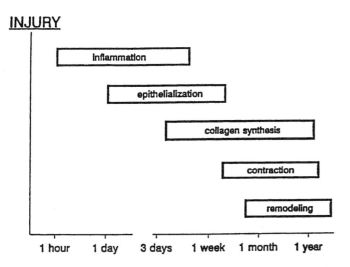

FIGURE 5-1 Sequence of events in wound healing (From: O'Leary, p 100, #4).

Epithelialization

Epithelialization of an incised and sutured wound can occur very quickly. There is relatively little inflammation in a primarily closed wound, and such wounds heal normally with few if any polymorphonuclear cells.[4] The process of epithelialization includes detachment, migration, proliferation and, differentiation.[10] Within 24 hours after injury, basal cells along the wound margins increase their rate of mitoses and detach themselves from the underlying dermis.[1] The cells enlarge, flatten, and begin to migrate across the wound and cover any exposed dermis. The plane of movement of epidermal cells is determined in part by the water content of the wound bed. Hence, open desiccated wounds epithelialize slowly.

Within 24-48 hours, a clean, primarily closed wound is usually covered with epithelial cells. Mitosis is also rapid in the epithelial cells covering the gap. As the epithelium thickens, the older outer cells then go on to mature, differentiate, and keratinize. Unfortunately, regenerated epithelium has relatively few basal cells and the rete pegs of normal epidermis that penetrate into the dermis and attach it there are largely lacking.

AXIOM The smooth epidermal-dermal interface of large re-epithelialized wounds probably accounts for much of their fragility.[4]

Proliferative Phase

The proliferative phase, also known as the cellular phase or phase of fibroplasia, is characterized by the deposition of collagen in the wound. It begins on the third to fifth day and usually lasts at least 21 to 28 days. Fibroblasts are specialized cells that differentiate from resting mesenchymal cells in connective tissue. The differentiation of the mesenchymal cells into fibroblasts is stimulated by substances secreted by platelets, macrophages, and other cells[11] (Table 5-1). The time required for mesenchymal cells to differentiate into fibroblasts and form collagen is also known as the "lag phase" of wound healing.[4] Since the cellular elements responsible for repair are concentrated near the wound margins, a resutured wound will heal faster than the original wound. This phenomenon of more rapid healing with repeat closures of wounds is maximal in the second and third weeks after the initial wounding.[12]

AXIOM Collagen is the most important component supporting the healed wound.

Collagen is a complex protein, and it is unique in that it almost completely lacks the sulfur-containing amino acids cystine and tryptophan. The structure of collagen is characterized by the presence of three peptide chains, each in a right-handed helical formation with the three chains aligned parallel to one another and twisted into a left-handed configuration. The resultant structure, termed tropocollagen, is initially held together by hydrogen bonds. The tropocollagen molecule is very large, having a molecular weight of approximately 300,000 and dimensions of 15 Å in width and 2800 Å in length. As the molecule matures, stronger covalent bonds form between the three peptide chains. The tropocollagen molecules then aggregate to form collagen filaments which join together as collagen fibrils. The collagen fibrils then combine to form collagen fibers.

There are at least six types of collagen, each differing in their amino-acid sequences or in the combination of the basic polypeptide chains making up the tropocollagen.[1] The interstitial or fibrillar collagens, types I, II, and III, are products of separate genes. Type I is the most common type and is found in bone, skin, and tendon. It is low in carbohydrate and hydroxylysine and has broad fibrils. Type II collagen is found primarily in cartilage and contains relatively more hydroxylysines and carbohydrate per chain. Type III collagen contains cysteine, and is relatively high in hydroxyproline and low in hydroxylysine. It was originally believed to be fetal collagen, and it is commonly found in blood vessels, skin, and the parenchyma of internal organs. The collagen of adult skin is 80% type I and 20% type III.

Type IV collagen is high in carbohydrate and very high in hydroxylysine. It also retains procollagen extension peptides. Type IV

TABLE 5-1 Peptide Factors that Affect Wound Healing

Factor	Abbreviation	Source	Functions Regulated
Platelet-derived growth factor	PDGF	Platelets and macrophages	Fibroblast proliferation, chemotaxis, and collagenase production
Transforming growth factor β	TGF-β	Platelets, polymorphonuclear leukocytes, T lymphocytes, and macrophages	Fibroblast proliferation, chemotaxis, collagen metabolism, and action of other growth factors
Transforming growth factor α	TGF-α	Activated macrophages and many tissues	Similar to EGF functions
Interleukin-1	IL-1	Macrophages	Fibroblast proliferation
Tumor necrosis factor	TNF	Macrophages, mast cells, and T lymphocytes	Fibroblast proliferation
Fibroblast growth factor	FGF	Brain, pituitary, macrophages, and many other tissues and cells	Fibroblast proliferation, stimulates collagen deposition and angiogenesis
Epidermal growth factor	EGF	Saliva, urine, milk, and plasma	Stimulates epithelial cell proliferation and granulation tissue formation
Insulin-like growth factor	IGF	Liver, plasma, and fibroblasts	Stimulates synthesis of sulfated proteoglycans, collagen, and cell proliferation
Human growth factor	HGF	Pituitary	Anabolism

From: Greenfield, p 89, Ref #1.

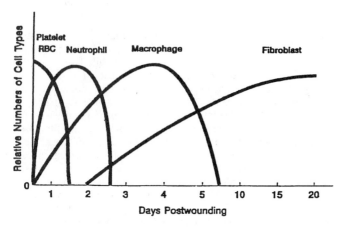

FIGURE 5-2 Cellular phase of wound healing. Relative concentrations of the various cellular components versus wound. RBC, red blood cell (From: O'Leary, p 99, #4).

collagen is found primarily in basement membranes. Type V and VI collagen have a unique molecular formula and are found in essentially all tissues.

The synthesis of collagen occurs through a series of reactions that begin intracellularly, are continued on or near the cell-surface membrane, and are completed in the extracellular space. Collagen can be synthesized by fibroblasts, osteoblasts, smooth muscle cells, chondrocytes, epithelial cells, and endothelial cells. In the cell, the appropriate sequences of amino acids are synthesized into polypeptide chains at the ribosome, and the resulting nonhelical procollagen consists of three initial polypeptide chains aggregated together. Proline and lysine in the polypeptide chains are hydroxylated through the action of the enzymes prolyl hydroxylase and lysyl hydroxylase. Essential cofactors for these reactions are ferrous ions, alpha-ketoglutarate, oxygen and ascorbic acid. After hydroxylation, the polypeptide chains fold into a helical formation. This structure is then excreted from the cell as a procollagen which consists of a collagen molecule with attached nonhelical N-terminal and C-terminal polypeptides. Procollagen peptidase, which is on or near the cell surface, then converts the procollagen into tropocollagen.

The tropocollagen undergoes assembly into collagen filaments, which combine to form collagen fibers. As the collagen matures, the polypeptide chains comprising each tropocollagen unit form strong intramolecular bonds mediated by lysyl amine oxidase. Intermolecular cross-linking among the tropocollagen molecules also occurs and further strengthens the collagen complex. In addition, the water content of the scar decreases, thereby allowing the collagen fibers to lie closer together.

Maturation

At the end of the proliferative phase, the number of active fibroblasts decreases, and the glycoprotein and mucopolysaccharide levels fall. The rate of collagen synthesis and degradation then reach equilibrium. The process of remodeling of collagen and extracellular matrix continues for months after reepithelialization has occurred and is responsible for the changes in the physical properties of the scar.

AXIOM Maturation or remodeling of a wound involves a continuous process of collagen lysis and collagen synthesis for at least 6-12 months.

The breakdown of collagen (collagenolysis) in maturing wounds and in stable scars is caused by collagenase, which is secreted by polymorphonuclear leukocytes, macrophages, and epithelial cells. This degradation of collagen is as important as collagen production. Loss of equilibrium between collagen production and degradation can lead

to excessive deposition of collagen as in hypertrophic scars or to failure to heal and disruption in repaired wounds.

By the end of 2 weeks, most skin wounds have gained only about 12% of their preinjury tensile strength, and by 4 to 6 weeks, only 50% of the preinjury tensile strength has returned.[5] By 10-12 weeks, the tensile strength of the wound is only about 80% of the preinjury value. After 6-12 months, it is still usually only 90% of normal. This increase in wound bursting strength continues even though there is no net increase in the scar collagen content after the third postinjury week.

Healed wounds regain tensile strength slowly over many months through the maturation phase as collagen fibers are degraded, cross-linked, and realigned along the lines of stress. Injured skin, tendons, and fascia never regain their normal or uninjured strength. Type III collagen, which is abundant in the early scar, is gradually replaced by type I collagen. The immature scar is often raised, erythematous, and pruritic; however, as maturation progresses, the ideal scar becomes flat, white, soft, and nonirritating.

AXIOM Scars are usually not considered fully mature until at least 1 year after the injury occurred.

CLOSING OF OPEN WOUNDS

Acute wounds, if closed normally, proceed through an orderly reparative process that results in restoration of anatomic and functional integrity. The typical sequence of biologic events includes control of infection, resolution of inflammation, angiogenesis, regeneration of a functional connective tissue matrix, contraction, resurfacing, and remodeling.[13]

Healing of open wounds progresses through stages similar to those seen in closed wounds. Wound contraction, however, assumes a more important role in open wounds. Contraction occurs by centripetal migration of the surrounding skin and is independent of the epithelialization of the wound. Wound contraction is maximal between 5 and 15 days after wounding and is mediated to a great extent by the myofibroblasts and their specialized connections with the surrounding extracellular matrix.[14] The myofibroblast resembles a fibroblast ultrastructurally, but it also has intracellular smooth muscle elements.

AXIOM Wound contraction can be diminished by skin grafting, and full-thickness grafts impede wound contraction more than split-thickness grafts.[14]

FACTORS AFFECTING WOUND HEALING (Table 5-2)

Infection

The presence of bacteria in a wound (contamination) does not necessarily imply that infection with invasion of the tissues is present.[4] However, if beta-hemolytic streptococci are present or if the bacterial count exceeds 10^5/per gram of tissue, infection is likely to be present. Obviously local infection retards wound healing, but systemic sepsis can also decrease wound healing by causing reduced chemotaxis and phagocytosis of macrophages.[5]

AXIOM Open wounds containing any beta-hemolytic streptococci or more than 10^5 other bacteria per gram of tissue should not be closed, even if they look good clinically.

With all wounds, special efforts should be taken to reduce contamination. Although short-term antibiotics may be of some help if contamination occurs, they are generally not effective in preventing wound infections. Careful tissue techniques and avoidance of any foreign material, devitalized tissue, or dead space in the wound are much more important.

AXIOM	One of the best ways to prevent wound infection in a contaminated case is to leave the skin and subcutaneous tissue open.

Age

It is generally believed that advancing age adversely affects wound healing. The growth rate and multiplication of fibroblasts and the synthesis of collagen may be affected by aging, but the elderly patient suffering from a wound healing problem also often has concurrent lung or cardiovascular disease resulting in reduced local wound oxygen tension and perfusion. Likewise, severe nutritional deficiencies, which are more common in older individuals, can also lead to disturbed wound healing.

Malnutrition

An acute decrease in lean body mass of 15% has been shown to result in decreased strength of healed skin wounds and colon anastomoses.[16,17] Protein depletion is particularly apt to impair healing if it results in edema in the wound or if it is associated with a deficiency of critical amino acids, such as cystine, which is essential for collagen synthesis.[4]

Steroids

Corticosteroids are lysosomal stabilizers and can retard epithelialization and contraction of wounds. They inhibit inflammation, normal fibroplasia, collagen synthesis, and neovascularization. They also increase susceptibility to infection because of their immunosuppressive effects. All of these effects result in slower healing and an increased incidence of wound dehiscence in patients on high dose corticosteroids.

AXIOM	One should look for and make allowances for delayed healing in patients receiving high doses of corticosteroids.

Radiation

Radiation inhibits all aspects of wound healing. The principal mechanisms of radiation injury are the destruction of replicating and differentiating stem cells and the initiation of progressive obliterative endarteritis.

Diabetes Mellitus

A wide variety of problems seen in diabetics, including vascular disease and malnutrition, may cause delay in wound healing. Hyperglycemia causes a delayed response to injury and impaired function of white blood cells.[18] Recent data suggests that endothelial cells in diabetics are also phenotypically different and show decreased adhesion and/or cell growth on non-enzymatically glycosylated laminin.[19] In the absence of essential cystine residues, disulfide bonding cannot occur, and proper alignment of peptide chains into a triple helix is prevented.[20]

AXIOM	Even if distal pulses feel normal, wound healing in patients with diabetes mellitus tends to be impaired, particularly if blood glucose levels are not under good control.

Vitamin A

Retinoic acid (vitamin A) is an important factor in wound healing, although deficiency of this vitamin is rare. Indeed, administration of retinoic acid in high doses (25,000 IU/per day) can reverse the healing retardation caused by cortisone.[21] Topical vitamin A has also been found to be effective for open wounds.[22] However, vitamin A given to an animal not deficient in the vitamin does not increase the normal healing rate. Transforming growth factor B_1 (TGF-B_1) also reverses steroid-induced impairment of wound healing.[23] It has also been suggested from experiments on rats that corticosteroids inhibit TGF-B_1 production in wounds, and retinoic acid antagonizes this effect.[24]

Vitamin C

Vitamin C (ascorbic acid) has long been recognized as important in healing. Scurvy, a disease caused by vitamin C deficiency, is characterized by a failure in collagen synthesis. Specifically, the hydroxylation of proline requires vitamin C as a cofactor. Interestingly, even old healed wounds in scorbutic animals can break down because the collagenolysis continues at a normal rate, but collagen synthesis is retarded.

AXIOM	Chronic severe lack of vitamin C can cause previously well-healed wounds to break down.

Zinc

Zinc is necessary for the activity of DNA and RNA polymerases and transferases. Zinc deficiency can retard epithelialization and fibroblast proliferation. A normal zinc level is essential for healing, although the administration of this element to a patient who is not zinc depleted does not enhance healing and may actually have detrimental effects on inflammation.[12] Ferrous iron and copper are also necessary for normal collagen metabolism.

AXIOM	Zinc, iron, and copper are the most important trace elements in wound healing.

Blood Loss and Anemia

Significant blood loss causing hypovolemia has a detrimental effect on wound healing in animals because of a decreased tissue oxygenation.[4] Severe, chronic anemia is also believed to retard wound healing, although experimental data supporting this hypothesis are difficult to obtain. Healing is generally unaffected if normal blood volume is maintained and hematocrit levels do not fall below 15%.

AXIOM	Giving blood transfusions to normovolemic patients does not improve wound healing.

Oxygen Tension

Oxygen is an essential element in wound healing. It is necessary for cell migration, proliferation, and protein and collagen synthesis.[4] Increasing tissue oxygen tension with hyperbaric oxygen may also further enhance wound healing. Although oxygen tension is low in the wound, anything that interferes with the delivery of oxygen to the wound (e.g., anemia, cardiovascular disease, diabetes, radiation) will have a detrimental effect on wound healing.

AXIOM	Anything reducing oxygen tension below normal can retard healing.

Cancer

Cancer can impair wound healing in a wide variety of ways, including cachexia, anorexia, altered host metabolism, and altered immune factors.[4] The changes in host metabolism in cancer patients includes increased glucose turnover, accelerated protein catabolism, decreased food intake, and limited availability of vitamin C.

EVALUATION OF THE WOUND

AXIOM   There is no substitute for a good history in evaluating traumatic wounds.

History

A good history should elicit the mechanism of injury and indicate the probable amount of contamination of the wound. This can then direct further efforts toward possible debridement of the wound or other prophylactic measures to prevent infection. A good history can also indicate the possibility of foreign bodies in the wound, thereby stimulating efforts to locate and remove them. It can also raise the question of possible deeper injury and result in a more intense, direct physical examination.

AXIOM   The physical examination must include an evaluation of the underlying structures even if the wound appears too superficial to involve these.

Physical Examination

Whether the patient is able to give an adequate history or not, a thorough physical examination is a necessity. Possible involvement of deeper structures must be investigated and the wound should be evaluated for possible foreign bodies or necrotic debris. Finally, an adequate record, including photographs, is invaluable for documenting the extent and severity of the injury.

An examination of facial lacerations should include evaluation of the underlying sensory and motor nerves and their function. The depth of the wound should be carefully visualized and not just palpated to determine if there has been extension into the oral cavity. Lid lacerations must also be carefully examined to determine if the eye is involved. Finally, if a wound is in the area of the parotid gland or duct, these should be carefully examined, possibly using ductograms. Extremity wound examinations should include distal testing of sensation, motor function, capillary refill, and joint mobility to rule out more proximal nerve, arterial, or musculotendinous injuries.

Radiological Studies

The history and physical examination will usually indicate whether or not additional studies may be of benefit. The type and amount of force involved in the trauma determine whether underlying bony structures may have been fractured. The type and amount of force will also indicate whether a body cavity may have been violated.

The possibility of the presence of foreign bodies may require either plain x-rays or xeroradiographs. Ninety percent of all glass fragments are radiopaque. Certainly, bullet fragments are visible on plain x-rays. However, 10% of all glass is not radiopaque, and material such as gravel or wood will not be visible on such x-rays. In this case, a xeroradiograph can often determine whether foreign bodies are present in the depths of the wound.

PITFALL ⊘

> *If it is assumed that a foreign body is not present in a wound because it does not show up on x-ray, a variety of radiolucent foreign bodies may be left behind.*

It is difficult for physicians treating traumatic wounds to exclude with certainty the presence of a foreign body in small, deep punctures or lacerations. Even extensions of the wound may not permit completely satisfactory exploration. If the suspected foreign body is not radiopaque, thorough careful local exploration of the wound is mandatory.

TYPES OF WOUNDS

Puncture Wounds

Punctures have small entrance wounds through which bacteria and foreign bodies can be driven deep into the tissue. Obviously, tissue destruction, bleeding, and contamination can be present deep in a wound in spite of a normal appearing surface. If the history suggests the presence of foreign bodies or increased contamination, these wounds should be explored so that foreign bodies can be removed and the wound cleaned properly.

Lacerations

Superficial or deep lacerations, depending on their orientation the tension lines in the skin, can result in significant spreading of the wound edges, giving one the impression that there has been significant tissue loss. This is more common in children and young adults owing to the elastic quality of their dermis.

Tissue Avulsion

A glancing blow by a sharp object can cause skin and subcutaneous tissues to be detached from the underlying tissues. The layers of dermis, subcutaneous tissue, fascia, and muscle can be seen at various angles in an avulsed flap. These can easily be aligned incorrectly during suturing of the wound.

Crush Injury

Crushes are high pressure injuries that can cause skin to be compressed and split apart. With such injuries, nonviable tissue may be present below deceptively normal appearing skin and dermis and must be debrided prior to closure.

MANAGEMENT OF THE WOUND

Vascular Injuries

Occasionally, vascular trauma can cause significant or even life-threatening hemorrhage. In such a situation, important adjacent structures may not be visible. It must be remembered that nerves and other important structures frequently accompany large vessels. Using clamps or suture ligatures in blind attempts to obtain hemostasis can significantly damage the vessels, causing a need for interposition grafting. Adjacent structures, which were otherwise unharmed, or which could have easily been repaired, can also be damaged by such attempts at hemostasis. Whenever possible, it is preferable to obtain hemostasis using direct pressure with a sterile gauze pad. The patient can then be taken to an operating room so that the entire wound and its contents can be examined carefully.

AXIOM   Hemostasis is generally best obtained by accurately applying direct external pressure.

Although most hemorrhage can be controlled with direct external pressure, bleeding from large arteries may occasionally require a temporary proximal tourniquet, direct ligation, or occlusion with a vascular clamp before repair can be accomplished in the operating room. Tourniquets are seldom needed except above major amputations and, if used incorrectly, can increase bleeding and cause much harm. A tourniquet should ideally be at least 2 to 3 inches wide so that the pressure is evenly distributed (a blood pressure cuff makes an excellent tourniquet). The pressure applied must be high enough to prevent arterial inflow. If the tourniquet pressure is less than arterial, blood will enter the extremity but is prevented from returning to the heart, and the resulting rise in venous pressure distal to the tourniquet causes additional bleeding from open veins. If the tourniquet is applied tightly for too long a period, it can cause irreversible distal ischemic damage.

AXIOM Use of a tourniquet outside the operating room can be extremely dangerous because it can cause irreversible distal ischemia.

CLEANSING OF THE WOUND

AXIOM All traumatic wounds are contaminated.

Since all wounds are contaminated to some extent, efforts must be directed both toward preventing further contamination and controlling that which is already present. In the emergency department, all wounds should immediately be covered with sterile dressings until they can be properly treated.

Prior to examination or repair, the surrounding skin should be carefully scrubbed with a contact antimicrobial agent (preferably povidone-iodine). The povidone-iodine solution, which is bactericidal, should not generally be applied to the wound itself because this agent is also cytotoxic. Full-strength hydrogen peroxide and Dakin's solution are also injurious to tissues.

The wound itself is best cleansed by irrigation with normal saline solution. If this causes pain, appropriate local, regional, or general anesthesia should be provided. After adequate debridement, the wound can be cleansed by irrigating it with a pulsating jet lavage.[25] Indeed, it has been shown that irrigation under pressures as high as 70 pounds per square inch is needed to adequately remove small debris and bacteria. The pulsating jet lavage can remove as much as 100 times greater bacterial load than other methods of irrigation. The decrease in bacterial counts and removal of small foreign bodies and necrotic debris can help prevent wound infection after closure. If the wound is to be primarily repaired, fresh drapes and gloves should be used prior to placing the closing sutures.

PITFALL ⊘

If small wounds are not accorded the same attention as large wounds, an increased incidence of infection will result.

There is sometimes a tendency to handle small wounds less conscientiously than larger, more open wounds; but small wounds may give rise to large infections. In fact, dirt and foreign bodies in small wounds are often more difficult to see and are more apt to be incompletely removed than in larger wounds.

PITFALL ⊘

Relying on wet drapes to keep a wound from becoming contaminated during surgery.

A frequent error in sterile technique during long operations for severe trauma is to continue to use drapes which have become saturated with blood or fluid. Wet drapes are not an effective barrier to bacteria and should be changed.

LOCAL ANESTHESIA

Local anesthesia can provide a good field block. It can be injected slowly using a very small needle (27- or 30-gauge). This will minimize the pressure-pain effect during the injection. The addition of epinephrine can improve hemostasis during the procedure; however, this solution, with its more acidic pH, is more painful. The use of epinephrine is usually thought to be contraindicated in digits and the penis because the vasoconstriction may cause ischemia and further tissue loss.[26]

Individual sensory nerves to specific areas can be blocked with small amounts of local anesthetics precisely placed in the correct location. Excessive local infiltration should be avoided to prevent distortion of anatomic landmarks. If injected into small fascial compartments, it can also cause local ischemia and/or impair venous return.

AXIOM If there is any chance that a local anesthetic may interfere with perfusion of a digit or some other anatomical structure, one should not combine it with epinephrine (adrenalin).

If a digital block is performed, care must be taken to prevent digital artery obstruction from the pressure of the injected anesthetic. Local anesthetics should never be injected into blood vessels. Direct intravenous injection can cause rapid systemic toxicity. If a local anesthetic must be injected near an artery, the syringe should be used to aspirate first. If no blood can be aspirated, then the anesthetic may be carefully injected.

DEBRIDEMENT

Open contaminated wounds will often heal quite well, but closed contaminated wounds are apt to develop severe infections. Meticulous removal of nonviable tissue is essential for uncomplicated wound healing because necrotic tissue is an excellent medium for bacterial growth, and it places excessive phagocytic demands on leukocytes, thereby impairing their bactericidal capacity. Debridement can be carried out using a scalpel and by irrigation with physiological saline. Accidental deposition of pigmented particles in the wound (as in road burns) will result in traumatic tattoos if not removed immediately following injury.

PITFALL ⊘

If a wound is closed without first carefully cleansing it and removing all devitalized tissue and foreign bodies, there is a greatly increased chance of infection.

A wound should not be closed if all apparent devitalized tissue and foreign bodies cannot be removed from it. Occasionally, however, wounds of the face may be closed with tissue of questionable viability because of the excellent blood supply and the better cosmetic result that can be obtained by performing a primary repair. If a wound is excessively contaminated or more than 8 to 12 hours old, it can be converted to a relatively clean, fresh wound by completely excising the wound edges. Although skin and subcutaneous tissues can be left open, bowel, cartilage, tendons, vessels, and bones should be covered with at least one layer of tissue such as peritoneum, fascia, or muscle.

IRRIGATION

AXIOM The solution to pollution is dilution.

The bacterial population in contaminated wounds can be reduced by irrigating the area thoroughly with large amounts of saline under pressure. Antibiotic solutions, such as 1% neomycin or 0.1% Cephazolin, may also help reduce the local bacteria count. Since chemicals such as Merthiolate, Mercurochrome, and alcohol damage cells and interfere with healing, they should not be applied directly to wounds.

AXIOM In general, wounds should not be irrigated with any solution that can cause irritation of the tissue.

Indeed, some surgeons say that one should not irrigate a wound with anything they would not use to irrigate their own eyes. In large contaminated or open wounds associated with fractures, large volumes of irrigant should be used. Pulsating pressure irrigation systems generally produce much better cleansing of such areas than other techniques.

AXIOM Large contaminated wounds should be washed out thoroughly with large volumes of fluid using a pulsating irrigator.

FOREIGN BODIES

In grossly contaminated wounds, not only must debridement be complete, but careful consideration must also be given to keeping the introduction of foreign material, including sutures, to a minimum. Certainly, prosthetic grafts or other materials should not be placed in grossly contaminated wounds. Nonabsorbable sutures such as silk and cotton should be used as little as possible because they may act as foreign bodies and perpetuate infection with resultant chronic draining sinuses. If absorbable sutures are used for tying off small vessels, slowly absorbable varieties are usually preferable to catgut because they cause less local inflammatory response while being absorbed.

HEMATOMAS

A hematoma is an ideal culture medium for bacteria and, acting as a foreign body, it also prevents or inhibits the delivery of phagocytic cells to the area. Meticulous hemostasis is therefore an absolute requirement before closing any deep wound. If all of the oozing cannot be stopped, hematoma formation should be prevented with a pressure dressing and/or closed suction.

> **AXIOM** If complete hemostasis cannot be obtained in a wound, there is an increased risk of wound infection, particularly if a drain is used.

WOUND CLOSURE

When Closure Should Not Be Attempted

One of the first questions that must be asked in attempting to close a traumatic wound is whether or not the wound closure should even be attempted. The history, revealing both the time since injury and the mechanisms by which the wound was produced, will determine whether or not a wound is appropriate for closure. If there is any question regarding the number of bacteria in the wound, the tissue can be biopsied. A small portion of viable tissue (250 mg) can be removed and processed by a rapid slide technique to determine the level of bacterial contamination. If there is greater than 100,000 (10^5) organisms per gram of tissue, bacterial contamination is too great to allow normal wound healing without infection.[27] Such a wound will not allow closure with sutures, skin grafts, or flaps.[28] However, much smaller numbers of beta-hemolytic streptococcus can cause severe infections.

> **AXIOM** The mere presence of any beta-hemolytic streptococci in a wound is a contraindication to closure.[29]

Timing of Wound Closure

There has been much controversy regarding the proper timing of closure of wounds. Often heard are unattributed quotes of "no closure after 24 hours" or "no closure after 12 hours." In a study of bacterial counts in wounds, it was found that the wounds with greater than 10^5 organisms per gram of tissue were, on an average, at least 5 hours old.[30] Indeed, the only wounds that developed infection were those in which bacterial count was 100,000 or greater per gram of tissue. Wounds in areas with greater vascularity tend to have less bacterial proliferation per unit of time. On the other hand, wounds that have a particularly high inoculum of bacteria tend to have more rapid bacterial proliferation. Clearly, the time from wounding is less important than the number of bacteria present in the wound.[30]

> **AXIOM** The number of bacteria in a wound, not its age, determines if it is safe to close at a particular time.

The mechanism of injury may suggest a heavy bacterial contamination. Animal bites contaminated by saliva have a high bacterial

count. Cat saliva contains 10^8 organisms per ml of fluid. Human saliva contains at least 10^6 organism per ml. People with poor dentition may have counts exceeding to 10^{10}/ml. Animals that eat meat tend to incur debris in their mouth and tend to cause more heavily contaminated wounds than non-meat eaters.[31] Some animals, such as the pig, cause a crushing injury as well as lacerations. Such crushing creates a wound with a higher chance of becoming infected.

Delayed Closure

In heavily contaminated wounds or in wounds from which all foreign material or devitalized tissue cannot be satisfactorily removed, delayed closure greatly reduces the risk of serious infection. Some physicians working in emergency departments have been deterred from using the delayed closure techniques because of a false belief by them or the patient that an unsightly scar is more likely to result. In actual practice, the final result often is quite similar to that which would be achieved by a primary closure.

Healing by primary intention occurs when clean full-thickness wounds are approximated shortly after incision. This type of healing requires a fresh clean wound which is free of foreign bodies, nonviable tissue, or bacterial contamination. There should also be an adequate blood supply to the margins.

> **AXIOM** Contaminated wounds that close by secondary intention will generally provide much better cosmetic results than primary closures that become infected.

TECHNIQUES OF WOUND CLOSURE

Wound Configuration

A jagged, irregular wound running perpendicular to the "wrinkle lines" is likely to give a wide unsightly scar. Not only will such a wound have a poor cosmetic result but healing will be retarded and the scar is likely to be painful. Wherever possible, wound edges should be straight, sharp, and parallel to the wrinkle lines (which are not the same as Langer's lines). If the wound must be debrided or lengthened to achieve this, it should be done without hesitation.

Whenever possible, the wound edges should be slightly everted or elevated to compensate for the tendency for the scar to sink in slightly as it heals. This can usually be achieved with fine vertical mattress sutures. A trap door (semicircular) type of laceration will often produce a poor scar as wound contraction will cause lifting of the flap of skin.

> **AXIOM** Whenever possible, wounds should be closed parallel to tension and wrinkle lines and should be slightly everted.

Wound Tension

Wound edges should come together with little or no tension. Relaxing incisions or freeing of more tissues at the level of the superficial fascia may help to bring wound edges together with less tension. There are, however, limits to the amount of undermining that is possible without danger of producing ischemia. Except for the face and scalp, it is generally unwise to undermine skin and subcutaneous tissue for more than 2 to 3 cm from the wound edge. If some tension is needed to pull the wound edges together, it is better to apply the tension to the underlying tissue and leave the skin itself "approximated, but not strangulated."

The best technique for wound closure is one that is as atraumatic as possible. Wound edges should be coapted to permit healing without a step-off. Sutures should not be tied so tightly that the resultant edema causes local ischemia.

The major strength in the skin is in the dermis. The collagen fibers present in the dermis will give the wound most of its tensile strength. Good approximation of the dermis will minimize the step-off between the two edges, and minimize the distance that the scar must bridge. In contrast, sutures placed in fat will tend to cause necrosis of that tissue, which will then serve as a foreign body and a nidus for infection.[32]

AXIOM A large number of sutures placed in subcutaneous tissue to reduce dead space tends to increase the risk of infection.

While fascia has sufficient amount of collagen to permit approximation with sutures and promote collagen formation in the scar, the underlying muscle supports sutures poorly and may even necrose if the edges are tightly approximated. For this reason, the best closure of a wound extending through muscle includes good apposition of the fascia and dermis.

A buried dermal closure will place the suture knots in the depth of the wound and minimize the likelihood of their erosion to the surface of the skin or formation of stitch abscesses. A buried dermal suture performed with absorbable material will be even less likely to eventually erode through the skin.

SUTURE MATERIALS

Suture materials can be classified as either absorbable or nonabsorbable. They may also be single stranded (monofilament) or composed of multiple strands (multifilament). The multifilament sutures are twisted or braided for strength. Nonabsorbable sutures remain in place indefinitely, and absorbable sutures are gradually removed by physiologic processes.

AXIOM Nonabsorbable monofilament sutures generally cause much less tissue reaction than sutures which are absorbable and braided.

Absorbable sutures are useful in providing early strength to a closed wound. They are most frequently placed in an intradermal or subcutaneous position. Catgut suture is produced from bovine intestinal serosa. Chromitization of the catgut sutures prolongs absorption 2 to 6 weeks postoperatively. Newer absorbable sutures (Dexon, Vicryl) are synthesized by polymerization of glycolic acid. They incite less inflammatory response than do the catgut sutures.

Nonabsorbable sutures are most often used for skin closure and in internal sites that require prolonged tissue strength. Examples of nonabsorbable suture materials include silk, nylon, cotton, Prolene, Dacron, and stainless steel. When placed in the skin, a monofilament (Prolene, nylon, and stainless steel) suture invokes a less severe inflammatory reaction than does a multifilament (silk and cotton) suture. Skin staples allow rapid skin wound closure but leave less satisfactory skin marks if applied too tightly or if allowed to remain in the skin longer than 1 week.

AXIOM Foreign bodies, including sutures, increase the risk of infection in wounds.

The increased ease with which infections occur in the presence of foreign bodies has been demonstrated by experiments showing that a single silk suture reduces the minimal pus-forming number of bacteria by a factor of 1/10,000.[33] The infective dose is even further reduced if the suture contains a minute piece of tissue. Consequently, the surgeon should use the finest suture material possible and incorporate the smallest amount of tissue needed to accomplish the suture's purpose.

Chromic or plain gut sutures are degraded by hydrolysis and usually do not remain in the wound long enough to allow good tensile strength to develop in the scar before their effect is lost. Use of these sutures not only increases inflammation but may lead to the widening of the scar because the dermis is no longer tightly approximated.

Polyglycolic suture is enzymatically degraded. This tends to occur on an average of 14 to 28 days after placement. Thus, the suture remains in place long enough to allow a greater tensile strength to occur in the wound. This minimizes the amount of scar widening that will occur as these sutures are degraded.

AXIOM Use of braided sutures leaves more interstices for bacterial adherence and proliferation and tends to result in a higher incidence of wound infections.[34]

DEAD SPACE

During closure of any wound, all tissue should be carefully approximated. Any residual dead space is soon filled with tissue fluid which, like a hematoma, can act as an excellent culture medium for bacteria. In some circumstances, it may be necessary to rotate adjacent muscle into the area to fill the dead space.

AXIOM When all dead space in a wound cannot be obliterated, the wound should be left open or kept evacuated with a closed drainage system.

Following closure of the dermis, the epidermis can usually be approximated with running nonabsorbable sutures, such as nylon, which will more exactly approximate the wound edges and give a polished effect to the eventual scar. These sutures should be removed prior to invasion of collagen bundles into the suture holes to prevent stitch marks. The density of the dermal appendages in the area will determine the optimal timing for suture removal.

Areas such as the face, which has a high density of dermal appendages, should have the epidermal sutures placed only through the depth of the epidermis. If the dermis is included in the suture, suture tracks will occur if these stitches are left in place for as short a period as 4 days.

AXIOM Skin sutures in the face should incorporate as little dermis as possible and should be removed early.

The palmar or plantar surfaces have such a low density of dermal appendages that these sutures may be left in place through both the dermis and epidermis for as long as 3 weeks without suture track formation. In fact, a truly epidermal suture will tend to fall out in 7 to 8 days as the epidermal cells are sloughed.

When the skin sutures are removed, if desired, the surface of the wound may be further splinted for a period of time with steri-strips. Adhesive tape used to primarily close the epidermis will not generally approximate the epidermal edges as well as nylon suture will.

AXIOM Whenever possible, fresh traumatic wounds should be closed primarily without use of complicated reconstruction techniques.

If at all possible, fresh traumatic wounds should be closed primarily; however, allowing wounds which appear unfavorable at the time of injury to close by secondary intention may eventually heal quite well. When there has been a significant loss of skin, treatment will depend on the type and size of the defect, its location, and the expertise of the physician. Furthermore, the use of Z-plasties or other complicated closures in the acute setting may prevent use of such techniques when reconstruction is necessary at a later date. In addition, a Z-plasty actually increases the length of the scar. If there is a true lack of tissue, occasionally the edges may be coapted simply by undermining the adjacent edges of the dermis. When this is insufficient, acute placement of a graft or flap may be necessary to achieve closure.

ABRASIONS

Treatment of partial-thickness skin loss is aimed at protecting the area from infection and mechanical injury. The area must be cleaned thoroughly and all dirt and embedded foreign material should be removed

TABLE 5-2 *Etiologies of Wound Complications*

Pre-existing Factors
  Malnutrition
  Diabetes mellitus
  Liver failure
  Radiation
  Obstructive lung disease
  Uremia
  Obesity
  Age
  Anemia
  Sepsis
  Genetic defects
  Medications
  Immune suppression
  Compliance
Wound Specific Factors
  Size
  Shape
  Location
  Wounding agent
  Contamination
  Oxygen tension
  Perfusion
  Shock
  Assessment
Surgeon and Technique Specific Factors
  Experience
  Duration of surgery
  Hemostasis
  Anatomic dissection
  Wound tension
  Mass ligature
  Electrocautery
  Dead space
  Anastomosis
  Enterotomy
Material Specific Factors
  Suture
  Drains
  Foreign body
  Packing
  Dressing

From: Rhodes; *In* Mattox, p 281, Ref #5).

to prevent tattooing. Bulky dressings may reduce local pain, but they tend to allow exudate to accumulate. Leaving contaminated wounds open reduces the chances of infection, but this may result in more pain initially. Fine mesh gauze impregnated with a water-soluble emollient is probably the best compromise dressing.

FULL-THICKNESS SKIN LOSS

Direct Closure

If tissue loss occurs where the skin is relatively loose, the wound can sometimes be closed by just approximating the skin edges. Wound tension may be at least partially relieved in such circumstances by undermining the adjacent skin and subcutaneous tissue, taking care not to devitalize the tissue. With greater wound tension, healing is impaired and the chances of infection and unsightly scars increase.

AXIOM Wounds should not be closed under tension.

Partial-thickness Skin Grafts

If the tissue loss in a fresh clean wound is too extensive to allow a direct closure, a partial thickness skin graft can be used as either a

temporary or permanent surface repair. The donor site should match the wound area as closely as possible for color and amount of hair. Supraclavicular and postauricular skin are good color matches for the face. For most other parts of the body the nonhairy portion of the thigh is quite satisfactory.

AXIOM Avulsed or surgically removed skin can be an important source of split-thickness grafts in some trauma patients.

During the first 24 hours prior to the establishment of new vascular and lymphatic channels in the graft, skin grafts are nourished by fluid from the host by a process referred to as imbibition. Hence, improper preparation of the host tissue, collections of fluid beneath the graft, movement between the graft and its bed, and infection are the most common causes of autograft failure. The graft should be pressed down firmly to provide uniform complete tissue contact. In concave defects, the fine sutures used to tack the graft down should be left long enough to be tied over a stent as a pressure dressing. If the wound is on an extremity, a splint should be applied to prevent undue motion at the wound site. The skin graft should be examined after 3 days for adherence and puncture or aspiration of any hematomas or seromas.

In certain wounds with questionable devitalized tissue or contamination, one can use autograft, homograft, or heterograft as temporary biologic dressings. Such grafts are often far superior to the wet soaks usually used to clean up these wounds.

AXIOM In large wounds, partial-thickness autografts, homografts, or heterografts can be almost ideal temporary biologic dressings.

Full-thickness Skin Grafts

Full-thickness skin grafts should seldom be used to treat fresh wounds (except for clean wounds of the head and neck by experienced surgeons). Full-thickness grafts vascularize very slowly and require optimal conditions and postoperative care; however, when they do take, the color and function of the graft are usually better than those achieved with split-thickness grafts.

The dermal component of grafted skin appears to exert the main influence on wound contraction. Full-thickness grafts are particularly good in children because the growth potential of split-thickness grafts is limited. Sensation is regained in skin grafts as nerve endings grow into the graft. This is particularly important in areas such as fingertips and the palm of the hand. Full-thickness grafts appear to achieve better sensation than split-thickness grafts.

AXIOM Full-thickness skin grafts do not take as easily as partial-thickness skin grafts, but the cosmetic result and function of a full-thickness graft are usually much better.

Epidermal Cell Grafts

Significant advances in tissue culture techniques have allowed the rapid growth of confluent sheets of epidermal cells suitable for wound coverage. A large surface area of viable epidermal cell grafts can be grown in the laboratory in about 3 weeks. Under ideal conditions, these cultured epidermal autografts adhere to the wound, differentiate to form a stratum corneum barrier, and persist on the surface.[34]

SKIN AVULSIONS

Completely avulsed tissue, except for fingertips, is usually contaminated and too thick to allow adequate revascularization. Amputated portions of a composite structure such as the eyelid, nose, or ear should be placed in a sterile container and saved in case a plastic surgeon may be able to use them later. Partial or complete avulsions on the face and neck usually heal well if the surrounding tissue is healthy. Partial avulsions on extremities, especially if long and narrow or if pedicled distally, are apt to die; therefore, if the partial avulsion is clean, it should be converted to a fat-free partial-thickness graft.

SIMPLE LOCAL FLAPS

Local skin flaps have certain advantages in that they carry their own blood supply and match the color and contour of the surrounding skin much better than free grafts. Although straight advancement flaps with minimal undermining can be utilized readily by most physicians, complicated transposition and rotation of tissue and Z-plasty require much more experience and skill.

MUSCLE FLAPS

Infection in peripheral vascular prostheses continues to be a serious complication in arterial reconstructive surgery. Aggressive debridement and muscle flap coverage is an effective means of treating vascular bypass grafts which are only infected superficially in a localized area. Several studies have shown that transposed muscle improves healing and decreases local wound bacterial counts.[35,36,37]

DRAINS

Whether or not to use drains is a recurrent controversy. While in situ, they encourage the drainage of pus, bile, and leaking intestinal contents, but they also permit the ingress of bacteria, especially if the wound area is carelessly dressed or handled. Hence, drains should not be left in indefinitely.

AXIOM Drains should be used only for specific definable reasons: the obliteration of dead space, uncontrollable oozing, or to provide egress for bile, pancreatic juice, or intestinal contents.

DRESSINGS

A wound dressing serves several important functions. Acutely, it can protect the wound from additional bacterial contamination. Additionally, it may protect the area from further injury. A dressing of absorptive gauze helps to move exudate away from the skin.

Various occlusive dressings that are permeable to oxygen have been developed to maximize the advantages of humid wound healing. Clinical studies have shown that wounds treated with occlusive dressings have less pain, swelling and tenderness, and the cosmetic results of the scars are often superior.[38,39] A grease-containing gauze such as Xeroform, Xeroflo, or Scarlet Red will not stick to the wound when it is removed. However, these gauzes also contain a large amount of grease, and most of this should be removed prior to application to prevent the dressing from becoming occlusive and impermeable to oxygen.

AXIOM Occlusive dressings tend to trap exudate between the dressings and the wound, increasing the tendency to bacterial proliferation and skin maceration.

A wound that is likely to become very edematous, either due to a dependent position or the force of the injury, can be gently compressed with gauze wrappings to minimize the edema formation and the pain. Edema causes pain, slows wound healing, and decreases function of the extremity.

AXIOM Excessive edema in wounds can be painful, and it can slow the healing of the wound and increase the chance of infection.[40]

Some wounds, especially over joints or in highly mobile areas, may benefit from a period of immobilization by a stiff dressing or even a splint or cast. Limiting mobility tends to reduce pain and edema formation and increase the coaptation of wounded structures during the healing period. A well-executed dressing is more aesthetic and gives the patient a better self-image. It may also increase the patient's impression of the craftsmanship involved in his care.

The duration of wound coverage by a dressing is variable. A simple skin incision closed primarily is epithelialized within 24 to 48 hours and, as such, is protected against bacterial invasion. With such a simple wound, the dressing can be removed permanently after 48 hours; however, dressings may be left in place on extremity wounds for many days or weeks to protect them from accidental trauma or rubbing on clothes.

BACTERIAL PROPHYLAXIS

The mechanism of injury and the patient's medical history may provide important clues to a vulnerable situation which could benefit from bacterial prophylaxis (Table 5-3). Patients with penetrating injuries who have not had a tetanus booster inoculation in the last 5 years are more vulnerable to tetanus infection, especially if the wound is deep or if there is a large amount of necrotic tissue; which may facilitate proliferation of anaerobic organisms. Treatment of these wounds should include a tetanus toxoid booster. In patients who are uncertain of the status of their prior tetanus immunization, tetanus immunoglobulin (Hypertet) should also be given.

AXIOM The immunization status of all patients with an open wound should be carefully ascertained. If the history is in doubt, one should assume that the patient is inadequately immunized against tetanus.

Patients whose wounds were inflicted by animals that are prone to rabies infection must be closely questioned whenever possible, so that the animal may be found and observed. If suspicion is sufficiently high, a prophylactic course of rabies immunization should be undertaken.

REMOVAL OF SUTURES

If the underlying tissues are closed properly, sutures on the face can be removed in 3 to 4 days to reduce the chances of permanent stitch marks. Sutures in the skin of the abdomen or chest can usually be removed in 7 days, while sutures on the hands, feet, or legs should often be left in place for 10 to 14 days. If the sutures are in an area that is subject to much movement or if the patient is apt to heal poorly, the sutures may have to be left in place for an additional 1 to 2 weeks. Adhesive strips or tape have been used enthusiastically for several years by a number of physicians and may be particularly useful for closing wounds that will have relatively little tension or movement.

TABLE 5-3 Suggested Guidelines for Use of Prophylactic Antibiotics in Wounds

1. All contaminated or dirty wounds.
2. All surgery or wounds that may allow spillage from organs that may contain bacteria.
3. Patients with clean wounds but in whom infection would be especially dangerous, such as when vital prosthetic materials are implanted.
4. Patients who have a greatly increased chance of infection. This includes those with shock, large areas of traumatized tissue, massive transfusions, hematologic disorders, and immunosuppressive drug therapy.

WOUND INFECTION

Etiology of Wound Infection

The likelihood of an infection depends on the interaction between the patient's host defenses and the dose and virulence of the microorganisms. A wound infection arises when the body's defense mechanisms are inadequate to eradicate the bacteria contaminating the wound and prevent their proliferation and invasion of the tissue.

AXIOM   The three main elements predisposing a patient to the development of wound infection are a susceptible wound, infecting organisms, and a compromised host.

A susceptible wound is one that contains devitalized tissue and/or is inadequately perfused (Table 5-4). Foreign bodies and hematomas retained in a wound can promote bacterial growth. A severely traumatized and poorly debrided wound that is repaired by suturing provides a closed space that is hypoxic, hypercarbic, acidic, and thus very conducive to bacterial proliferation.

Many different organisms are capable of initiating a wound infection. A bacterial strain's ability to survive in tissue is related to its absolute numbers as well as to its capacity to damage tissue with toxins, to propagate, and to spread (i.e., its virulence). Streptococci enter through even minor wounds and can rapidly cause a severe cellulitis. Skin and subcutaneous abscesses often are caused by

TABLE 5-4   Wound Contamination Classification and Infection Risk

Class	Type	Definition	Infection Rate (%)
I	Clean	Elective surgical incisions not involving the alimentary, genitourinary, or respiratory tracts; no breaks in technique; no inflammation encountered; no drains	<1-2%
II	Clean-contaminated	Alimentary or respiratory tract entered during elective surgery, but with minimum spillage (i.e., appendectomy); genitourinary or biliary tract entered, but urine or bile is not infected; minor break in technique	< 5-10%
III	Contaminated	Fresh trauma wounds; nonpurulent inflammation; wounds made in or near contaminated skin; genitourinary or biliary tract entered and urine or bile is infected; gross spillage from gastrointestinal tract; major break in sterile technique	10-20%
IV	Dirty/infected	Wounds heavily contaminated or clinically infected prior to operation (i.e., perforated viscera, abscess); traumatic wound with retained devitalized tissue, acute bacterial inflammation; wounds with purulent exudate	20-40%

staphylococci. Wounds contaminated by gastrointestinal flora tend to become infected by gram-negative aerobes (such as *E. coli*) and anaerobes (such as *Bacteroides fragilis*).

By definition, a compromised host has some local or systemic impairment of resistance to bacterial invasion. Radiation changes or ischemia due to vascular disease are local factors that reduce resistance to infection. Systemic conditions (e.g., diabetes mellitus, administration of corticosteroids, shock, burns, renal disease, cancer, and the use of immunosuppressive agents) also impair host resistance.

Tissue Viability

Predicting tissue viability can be a major challenge for some wounds. Clinical judgment and examination under a Wood's lamp after intravenous administration of fluorescein is a common method used in predicting tissue viability. In areas of impaired circulation, there is delayed uptake as well as delayed clearance of the organic dye fluorescein.

AXIOM   The three final common pathways of host resistance that are most apt to be impaired in patients with wounds are the acute inflammatory response, phagocytic mechanisms, and bacterial killing.

When viewed in the clinical or operating room setting, a wound can be classified as clean, clean-contaminated, contaminated, or infected.[1,6] Knowledge of these wound types helps the surgeon understand and anticipate subsequent wound infections. The clean wound is nontraumatic and free of inflammation. If it is created in the operating room, no break in surgical technique has occurred, and the respiratory, alimentary, and genitourinary tracts have not been violated. A clean-contaminated wound is also nontraumatic but is characterized by a minor break in surgical technique or the involvement of the gastrointestinal, genitourinary, or respiratory tracts without significant spillage of contents. Contaminated wounds by definition include all traumatic wounds and all wounds caused by a dirty source, contaminated with feces, containing a foreign body, or that are devitalized. Wounds receiving delayed treatment are also considered to be contaminated. A surgical wound in which a major break has occurred in surgical technique, gross spillage has occurred from the gastrointestinal tract, or there has been spillage from infected genitourinary or biliary tracts is also considered to be contaminated. The rate of postoperative wound infection ranges from 1% in most clean wounds to over 25% in dirty and infected ones.[16]

A wound infection is suspected if signs of inflammation (warmth, erythema, induration, and pain) or drainage appear at the operative or injured site within the first month after surgery or injury. Cellulitis is characterized by all the signs of inflammation but without a collection of pus. Beta-hemolytic streptococci typically spread through tissues and cause cellulitis without stimulating a purulent exudate. A wound abscess is initially seen as a purulent collection, and is usually accompanied by signs of acute inflammation.

The treatment of a wound infection must be both prompt and appropriate. A sample of any wound discharge is submitted for Gram's staining, aerobic and anaerobic culture, and determination of bacterial sensitivity. Antibiotics to cover the microorganisms most likely to be present are initiated before obtaining the culture results.

AXIOM   The most important aspect of the early management of any infected wounds is adequate drainage; antibiotics are generally not needed.

A wound that is only suspicious for infection can be aspirated using a large bore needle. If pus is returned or if the wound remains questionable, it should be opened and drained. Any abscess discovered is drained as thoroughly as possible, and the wound is dressed with saline-soaked dressings.

AXIOM Delayed primary closure (within 3 days of injury) or secondary closure (3 to 7 days after injury) of contaminated wounds usually produces satisfactory healing and reduces the incidence of infection.

In severely traumatized or contaminated wounds, primary closure greatly increases the risk of subsequent wound infection. Consequently, it is prudent to leave the skin and subcutaneous tissues open or packed lightly with saline-soaked fine mesh gauze. Whether or not healing is occurring without infection is determined by daily wound inspections. If no infection occurs and the wound is granulating well, it can be closed with excision of the margins.

HYPERTROPHIC SCARS AND KELOIDS

Under ideal circumstances, a wound develops into a narrow, flat, white scar causing no functional or significant aesthetic problem. This ideal scar is the product of a balance between collagen deposit and its subsequent maturation and collagenolysis.

AXIOM Alterations in the normal process of wound maturation are most apt to present themselves as hypertrophic scars or keloids.

The hypertrophic scar is characterized by the deposition of excess collagen that remains within the borders of the scar bed. The hypertrophic scar may be seen anywhere on the body and is more common in dark-skinned people and in the young. Keloids also are more common in dark-skinned and younger individuals. In contrast to hypertrophic scars, the keloid exceeds the boundaries of the original wound and has continued growth. Certain wounds will have such a high chance of developing hypertrophic scars or even keloids that adjunctive measures should be begun early to limit their development.[41]

AXIOM Wounds that are perpendicular to the lines of facial expression are more likely to become hypertrophic than those that lie parallel to the wrinkle lines.[42]

Wounds that heal over a very thin layer of remaining dermis, such as a burn, also have a high chance of developing excessive scarring. Hypertrophic scars and keloids are more commonly found in regions of tension (deltoid, parasternal, back), in wounds with retained foreign bodies (ear lobes), in wounds complicated by inflammation or infection, and in families with a history of excessive scarring.

AXIOM Wounds occurring above the clavicles or in the forearms or hands have an increased likelihood of developing keloids.

Once wounds on the hands or face or above the clavicles are sufficiently healed in a patient with a history of abnormal wound healing, external compression can be applied. This may take the form of a compression elastic garment, such as Jobst garment, or an external plastic mold, such as the clear plastic Uvex. These garments must be carefully fitted for the individual patient. They will also need to be refitted or replaced as they stretch out or change configuration so as to maintain pressure greater than the capillary hydrostatic pressure (25 mm Hg). Finally, when the wound has sufficiently matured, the option must be left open for possible future revision.

Numerous techniques have been used in the treatment of hypertrophic scars and keloids. They include surgical excision, pressure, irradiation, silicone gel sheeting, and the administration of corticosteroids. Performance of a surgical excision alone is usually followed by recurrence of the hypertrophic scar or keloid. Pressure in the form of elastic garments can help prevent the formation of hypertrophic burn scars and can cause regression of some established lesions. Maximal benefit is obtained if the patient wears the garment almost constantly for several months. Irradiation and corticosteroids both act

to inhibit collagen synthesis. However, many physicians are reluctant to suggest irradiation since it is irreversible and the long-term effects of even small doses are unknown. Silicone gel sheets have been shown to be effective in preventing hypertrophic scars as well as in reducing and softening established scars when applied directly over the scars.[43,44]

AXIOM Careful surgical excision plus steroid injections and pressure garments can be very useful for treating keloids and hypertrophic scars.

Many chemical compounds have also been used in an attempt to control excess scarring.[45] Beta-aminoproprionitrile irreversibly inhibits lysyl oxidase, preventing aldehyde formation and subsequent collagen cross-linking. Penicillamine inhibits collagen cross-linking by chelating copper and interfering with the formation of aldehyde groups; however, neither of these compounds has been proven safe or effective enough for broad clinical application.

CHRONIC WOUNDS

The basic approach to the treatment of chronic wounds is very similar to that used for acute wounds. The wound must first be cleansed of all necrotic debris. The bacterial count should then be assessed by both qualitative and quantitative analyses. If the bacterial count is greater than 100,000 organisms per gram of tissue or if any beta-hemolytic streptococcus is present, the wound should be treated with topical antimicrobials, such as silver sulfadiazine or mafenide acetate, to decrease the bacterial count and allow for wound healing. The scar tissue around chronic wounds makes these areas relatively ischemic and decreases the ability of systemic antibiotics to penetrate into the edges of the open wound.[46] Chronic wounds eventually heal by contraction and epithelialization.

AXIOM Systemic antibiotics do not penetrate chronic scarred wounds well, but they are indicated if there is surrounding cellulitis or evidence of sepsis.

The underlying cause of the chronic wound should be removed if at all possible. If the wound is a pressure sore, the patient should be placed on a mattress which will reduce its exposure to excessive pressure and ischemia. If the wound is due to venous stasis, the patient should have the leg elevated until the wound is closed either spontaneously or by a skin graft. After the graft has stabilized, at approximately 2 weeks, the patient may be ambulated with support using a compression garment that is made to order for the patient to prevent excessive hydrostatic pressure developing under the graft.

Ischemic ulcers may require an in-flow vascular procedure to improve blood flow to the limb. Ulcers due to a blood dyscrasia will not heal until the underlying hematologic status is improved either through transfusion or treatment of the blood dyscrasia directly. Diabetic ulcerations occur due to both the patient's underlying neuropathy and the tendency toward soft tissue infection caused by hyperglycemia.[47]

AXIOM One should not attempt to close a chronic wound until the local infection is cured and the systemic status of the patient is optimized.

After controlling infection, linear lacerations should be excised and closed whenever possible. Chronic ulcerations must usually be closed with split-thickness skin grafts. Pressure sores that lack tissue in three dimensions usually require flap closure to fill the dead space and allow closure without tension, minimizing the chances of recurrence.

AXIOM Following closure, chronic wounds should be protected until their tensile strength is sufficient to allow mobility or dependency.

A graft on a lower extremity should be externally splinted with compression garments from the time ambulation resumes (2 weeks) until full tensile strength is achieved (6 months). A flap closure for a pressure sore should not be sat upon until the suture line has sufficient tensile strength (3 weeks). Even then, the suture line can only be ischemic for 10-15 minutes without suffering tissue damage. The patient is given a schedule of increasing frequency and duration of weight-bearing to prevent injury to the freshly repaired wound.

SUMMARY

The body's response to wounding allows survival in a harsh, pathogen-contaminated environment. When closed primarily, a wound heals by the simultaneous and interrelated processes of inflammation, epithelialization, cellular production of collagen, maturation, and remodeling. A wound that is left open diminishes in size by contraction while undergoing the same healing phases as its closed counterpart.

The speed and adequacy of healing are directly dependent on the patient's nutrition and local vascularity of the wound. Advanced age, associated illnesses, and various medications have a deleterious effect on healing. Many other factors also determine the appearance of the mature scar. Consequently, special care must be taken in patients who are prone to develop scar hypertrophy or keloids.

The nature and extent of a wound dictates the physician's management of it. After cleansing and debridement, wounds are closed primarily, are covered with a skin graft or flap, or are allowed to heal by secondary intention. In some instances, wound contraction may be utilized to great advantage by the surgeon. Wound infection, should it occur, is treated by incision or reopening of the wound and adequate debridement and drainage. Administration of appropriate local and/or systemic antibiotics should be added as needed. Careful adherence to the principles of wound care will usually result in development of a scar that is satisfactory to both the patient and the physician.

⊘ **FREQUENT ERRORS**

In Wound Management

1. *Not checking tissue bacterial counts in chronic or previously contaminated wounds prior to attempting closure.*
2. *Inadequate attention to local blood flow in older individuals and those with diabetes mellitus.*
3. *Inadequate attention to replenishment of vitamin C and zinc in malnourished individuals who have large or difficult wounds.*
4. *Inadequate attention to possible reductions in wound PO_2 in patients with respiratory problems.*
5. *Assuming a foreign body is not present in a wound because it does not show on x-ray.*
6. *Use of a tourniquet or hemostats to control bleeding from a deep wound on an extremity when direct local pressure might have been adequate.*
7. *Not switching to dry drapes around a clean wound after the drapes have become saturated with fluid.*
8. *Inadequate irrigation of contaminated wounds.*
9. *Irrigating wounds with solutions that may be irritating to the tissue.*
10. *Using multiple subcutaneous closure sutures to eliminate dead space.*
11. *Assuming that skin sutures will provide adequate hemostasis for deep wounds.*
12. *Failing to drain a wound if there is residual dead space and/or oozing.*
13. *Relying on antibiotics rather than adequate incision and drainage to treat a wound infection.*

▼▼▼▼▼▼▼▼▼▼▼▼▼▼▼▼▼▼▼▼▼▼▼▼▼▼▼▼▼▼▼
SUMMARY POINTS

1. Use of drugs to reduce inflammation in wounds may impair healing.
2. In the presence of extensive tissue injury or massive bacterial contamination, inflammation can be greatly prolonged and wound healing may be greatly delayed.
3. The smooth epidermal-dermal interface of large re-epithelialized wounds probably accounts for much of their fragility.
4. Collagen is the most important component supporting the healed wound.
5. Maturation or remodeling of a wound involves a continuous process of collagen lysis and collagen synthesis for at least 6-12 months.
6. Scars are usually not considered fully mature until at least 1 year after the injury.
7. Wound contraction can be diminished by skin grafting, and full-thickness grafts impede wound contraction more than split-thickness grafts.
8. Open wounds containing any beta-hemolytic streptococci or more than 10^5 other bacteria per gram of tissue should not be closed, even if they look good clinically.
9. Even if distal pulses feel normal, wound healing in patients with diabetes mellitus tends to be impaired, particularly if blood glucose levels are not under good control.
10. Chronic severe lack of vitamin C can cause previously well-healed wounds to break down.
11. Giving blood transfusions to normovolemic patients does not improve wound healing.
12. Anything reducing oxygen tension below normal in a wound can retard its healing.
13. There is no substitute for a good history in evaluating traumatic wounds.
14. If it is assumed that a foreign body is not present in a wound because it does not show up on x-ray, retained glass, wood, or plastic may be left behind.
15. Hemostasis is generally best obtained by accurately applying direct external pressure.
16. Use of a tourniquet outside the operating room can be extremely dangerous because this may result in irreversible ischemia of the entire limb.
17. If small wounds are not accorded the same careful attention as large wounds, an increased incidence of infection will result.
18. Do not rely on wet drapes to keep a wound from becoming contaminated during surgery.
19. If there is any chance that a local anesthetic may interfere with perfusion of a digit or some other anatomical structure, one should not combine it with epinephrine (adrenalin).
20. If a wound is closed without first carefully cleansing it and removing all devitalized tissue and foreign bodies, there is an increased chance of infection.
21. In general, wounds should not be irrigated with any solution that can cause tissue irritation.
22. Large contaminated wounds should be washed out thoroughly with large volumes of fluid using a pulsating irrigator.
23. If complete hemostasis is not obtained in a wound, there is an increased risk of wound infection, particularly if a drain is used.
24. The number of bacteria in a wound, not its age, determines if it is safe to close at a particular time.
25. Allowing contaminated wounds to close by secondary intention will generally provide much better cosmetic results than primary closures that are apt to get infected.
26. Whenever possible, wounds should be closed parallel to tension and wrinkle lines and should be slightly everted.
27. A large number of sutures placed in subcutaneous tissue to reduce dead space will tend to increase the risk of infection.

28. Nonabsorbable monofilament sutures cause much less tissue reaction than sutures which are absorbable and braided.

29. Foreign bodies, including sutures, greatly increase the risk of infection in wounds.

30. When all dead space in a wound cannot be obliterated, the wound should be left open or drained.

31. Skin sutures in the face should incorporate as little dermis as possible and should be removed early.

32. Whenever possible, fresh traumatic wounds should be closed primarily, without use of complicated reconstruction techniques.

33. Wounds should generally not be closed under tension.

34. In large open wounds, partial-thickness autografts, homografts, or heterografts are almost ideal temporary biologic dressings.

35. Full-thickness skin grafts do not take as easily as partial-thickness skin grafts, but the cosmetic result and function of a full-thickness graft is usually much better.

36. Drains should be used only for specific definable reasons: the obliteration of dead space, uncontrollable oozing, or to provide egress for bile, pancreatic juice, or intestinal contents.

37. Occlusive dressings tend to trap exudate between the dressing and the wound, allowing bacterial proliferation and skin maceration.

38. Excessive edema in wounds can be painful, and it can slow the healing of the wound and increase the chance of infection.

39. The immunization status of all patients with an open wound should be carefully ascertained. If the history is in doubt, one should assume that the patient is inadequately immunized against tetanus.

40. The three main elements predisposing a patient to the development of a wound infection are a susceptible wound, infecting organisms, and a compromised host.

41. The three final common pathways of host resistance that are most apt to be impaired in patients with wounds are the acute inflammatory response, phagocytic mechanism, and opsonization.

42. The most important aspect of the early management of any infected wound is adequate drainage; antibiotics are generally not needed.

43. Delayed primary closure (within 3 days of injury) or secondary closure (3 to 7 days after injury) of contaminated wounds generally produces satisfactory healing and reduces the incidence of infection.

44. Alterations in the normal process of wound maturation are most apt to present themselves as hypertrophic scars or keloids.

45. Wounds that are perpendicular to the lines of facial expression are less likely to become hypertrophic than those that lie parallel to underlying muscle.

46. Wounds occurring above the clavicles or in the forearms or hands have an increased likelihood of developing keloids.

47. Careful surgical excision plus steroid injections and pressure garments can be very useful in treating keloids and hypertrophic scars.

48. Systemic antibiotics do not penetrate chronic scarred wounds well, but they are indicated if there is an associated cellulitis or evidence of sepsis.

49. One should not attempt to close a chronic wound until the local infection is cured and the general condition of the patient has been optimized.

50. Following closure, chronic wounds should be protected until their tensile strength is sufficient to allow mobility or dependency.

▲▲▲▲▲▲▲▲▲▲▲▲▲▲▲▲▲▲▲▲▲▲▲▲▲▲▲▲▲▲▲▲▲▲▲▲▲

REFERENCES

1. Cohen IK, Diegelmann RF. Wound healing. In: Greenfield LJ, ed. Surgery: scientific principles and practice. Philadelphia: J.B. Lippincott, 1993:86-102.
2. Edington HD. Wound healing. In: Simmons RL, Steed DL, Sanders WB, eds. Basic science review for surgeons. Philadelphia, 1992:41-55.
3. Westaby S. Fundamentals of wound healing. In: Westaby S, Heinemann W, eds. Wound care. London: Medical Books Ltd., 1985:11-21.
4. Peacock JL, Lawrence WT, Peacock EE Jr. Wound healing. In: O'Leary JP, ed. The physiologic basis of surgery. Baltimore: William & Wilkins, 1993:95-111.
5. Rhodes M. Wound healing complications. In: Mattox KL, ed. Complications of trauma. New York: Churchill Livingstone, 1994:279-304.
6. McLean AEM, Ahmed K, Judah JD. Cellular permeability and the reaction to injury. Ann NY Acad Sci 1964;116:986,.
7. Singfelder JR. Prostaglandins: a review. N Eng J Med 1982;307:746.
8. Stevenson TR, Mathes SJ. Wound healing. In: Miller TA, ed. Physiologic basis of modern surgical care. St. Louis: CV Mosby, 1988:1010-1018.
9. Diegelmann RF, Cohen IK, Kaplan AM. The role of macrophages in wound repair: a review. Plast Reconstr Surg 1981;68:107.
10. Johnson FR, McMinn RM. The cytology of wound healing of body surfaces in mammals. Biol Rev 1962;35:364.
11. Ross R, Everett NB, Tyler R. Wound healing and collagen formation, VI. The origin of wound fibroblasts studied in parabiosis. J Cell Biol 1970;44:645.
12. Peacock EE, Jr. Wound healing. In: Peters RM, Peacock EE Jr., Benfield JR, eds. The scientific management of surgical patients. Boston: Little, Brown 1983:27-63.
13. Baran NK, Horton CE. Growth of skin grafts, flaps and scars in young minipigs. Plast Reconstr Surg 1972;50:487.
14. Guber S, Rudolph R. Collective review. The myofibroblast. Surg Gynecol Obstet 1978;146:641.
15. Sawhney CP, Monges HL. Wound contraction in rabbits and the effectiveness of skin grafts in preventing it. Br J Plast Surg 1970;23:318.
16. Daly JM, Vars HM, Dudrick SJ. Effects of protein depletion on strength of colonic anastomoses. Surg Gynecol Obstet 1972;134:15.
17. Ward MW, Danzi M, Lewin MR, et al. The effects of subclinical malnutrition and refeeding on the healing of experimental colonic anastomosis. Br J Surg 1982;69:308.
18. Gocke TM. Infection complicating diabetes mellitus. In: Grieco MH, ed. Infections in the abnormal host. New York: Yorke Medical Books, 1980:585.
19. Subin B, Tuan TL, Cheung D, et al. Cellular and molecular pathogenesis of defective healing in diabetes mellitus. Surg Forum 1994;45:707.
20. Williamson MB, Fromm HJ. Effect of cystine and methionine on healing of experimental wounds. Proc Soc Exp Biol Med 1957;80:623.
21. Ehrlich HP, Hunt TX. Effect of corticosterone and vitamin A on wound healing. Ann Surg 1968;167:324.
22. Hunt TK, Ehrlich HP, Garcia JA, et al. Effects of vitamin A on reversing the inhibitory effects of cortisone on healing of open wounds in animals and man. Ann Surg 1969;170:633.
23. Pierce GF, Musto TA, Lingelbach J, et al. Transforming growth factor beta reverses the glucocorticoid-induced wound healing deficit in rats: possible regulation in rats by platelet-derived growth factor. Proc Nat Acad Sci USA 1989;86:2229.
24. Ulland NE, Gartner MH, Richards JR, et al. Retinoic acid restores transforming growth factor: beta[1] concentrates in a steroid-impaired wound healing model. Surg Forum 1994;45:714.
25. Hamer ML, Robson MC, Krizek TJ, et al. Quantitative bacterial analysis of comparative wound irrigations. Ann Surg 1975;181:819.
26. Robson MC, Raine T, Smith DJ Jr. Wounds and wound healing. In: Lawrence PF, ed. Essentials of general surgery. Baltimore: Williams and Wilkins, 1988:107.
27. Heggers JP, Barnes ST, Robson MC, et al. Microbial flora of orthopaedic war wounds. Milit Med 1969;134:602.
28. Krizek TJ, Robson MC, Kho E. Bacterial growth and skin graft survival. Surg Forum 1967;18:518.
29. Robson MC, Heggers JP. Surgical infection, II. The beta-hemolytic streptococcus. J Surg Res 1969;9:289.
30. Robson MC, Duke WF, Krizek TJ. Rapid bacterial screening in the treatment of civilian wounds. J Surg Res 1973;14:426.
31. Gilmore GT, Boertman JA, Robson MC, et al. The effect of diet on dog's oral bacterial flora. Surg Forum 1987:39.
32. Grabb WC, Smith JW, eds. Plastic surgery: a concise guide to clinical practice. 3rd ed. Boston: Little, Brown, 1973:3.
33. Robson MC, Raine TR, Smith DJ, et al. Principles of wound healing and repair. In: James EC, Corry RJ, Perry JF, eds. Basic surgical practice. Philadelphia: Hanley and Belfus, Inc., 1987:69.
34. Gallico GG, O'Connor NE. Cultured epithelium as a skin substitute. Clinics Plast Surg 1985;12:149.
35. Mixter RC, Turnipseed WD, Smith DJ Jr, et al. Rotational muscle flaps: a new technique for covering infected vascular grafts. J Vasc Surg 1989;9:472.
36. Gomes MN, Spear SL. Pedicled muscle flaps in the management of infected aortofemoral grafts. Cardiovasc Surg 1994;2:70.
37. Meland NB, Arnold PG, Pairolero PC, Lovich SF. Muscle-flap coverage of infected peripheral vascular prosthesis. Plast Reconstr Surg 1994;93:1005.

38. Eaglstein WH. Experiences with biosynthetic dressings. J Am Acad Dermatol 1985;12:434.

39. Eaton AC. A controlled trial to evaluate and compare sutureless skin closure technique (Opsite skin closure) with conventional skin suturing and clipping in abdominal surgery. Br J Surg 1980;67:857.

40. Katz S, Izhar M, Mirelman D. Bacterial adherence to surgical sutures: a possible factor in suture induced infection. Ann Surg 1981;194:35.

41. Ricketts LR, Squire JR, Topley E, Lilly HA. Human skin lipids with particular reference to the self-sterilizing power of the skin. Clin Sci Mod Med 1951;10:89.

42. Robson MC. Difficult wounds: pressure ulcerations and leg ulcers. Clin Plastic Surg 1979;6:537.

43. Perkins K, Davey RB, Wallis KA. Silicone gel: a new treatment for burn scars and contractures. Burns 1982;9:201.

44. Quinn KJ. Silicone gel in scar treatment. Burns 1987;13:33.

45. Peacock EE Jr, Control of wound healing and scar formation in surgical patients. Arch Surgery 1981;116:1325.

46. Robson MC, Edstrom LE, Krizek TJ, et al. The efficacy of systemic antibiotics in the treatment of granulating wounds. J Surg Res 1974;16:299.

47. Krizek TJ, Davis JH. Effect of diabetes in experimental infection. Surg Forum 1964;15:60.

Chapter 6 Anesthesia for the Trauma Patient

KENNETH J. ABRAMS, M.D.

CHRISTOPHER W. BRYAN-BROWN, M.D.

INTRODUCTION

Trauma is the major cause of death in patients under the age of 44. It is not clear how many of these deaths are preventable; however, institutions with well-integrated, multidisciplinary trauma teams have the opportunity to develop better services and make fewer mistakes in this seemingly "neglected epidemic"[1] (Fig. 6-1).

The Risks of Anesthesia

The anesthetic management of acute trauma victims, particularly those with multiple injuries, is one of the toughest challenges taken on by the anesthesiologist. Although anesthetic accidents that result in permanent injury or death in such patients are infrequent, they can also occur in less severely traumatized patients, when the level of vigilance may be lower. The provision of a "little bit of anesthesia" for a relatively minor surgical emergency can easily result in an inadvertent, serious anesthetic complication.

AXIOM Although there is such a thing as "minor surgery," there is no such thing as a "minor anesthetic."

The risks and dangers of administering general anesthesia are ever-present. Patients may vomit, aspirate, asphyxiate, or develop cardiac arrhythmias or circulatory collapse from undiagnosed hypovolemia, whatever the magnitude of the surgical procedure. Severely traumatized patients may be moved very rapidly from the scene of the injury through the emergency center to the operating room. This provides little or no opportunity for a careful preanesthetic evaluation, which must proceed simultaneously with the resuscitative efforts. Critical details about the mechanism of injury, physical status of the patient at the scene, and prehospital therapy can be obtained from paramedical personnel. This information may provide important clues to critical injury patterns.

General patient information, including drug usage patterns, past history, family history, and prior anesthetic problems are not readily available to the trauma anesthesiologist. The normal range of vital signs is unknown, laboratory data are limited, and consultation from other services is usually absent.

The lack of adequate preanesthetic assessment, when combined with surgical uncertainty about the extent of a patient's injuries, leads the trauma-oriented anesthesiologist to be liberal in the use of invasive monitoring and to be extremely judicious in the administration of drugs that depress the circulation.[2]

Trauma Protocols

In most emergency departments and trauma centers, the surgical members of the trauma team will have started resuscitation and formulated a treatment plan by the time the anesthesiologist sees the patient.[3] Although this is not ideal, it may be necessary. In centers with a constant stream of severely injured patients, the anesthesiologist should have a central role in the initial evaluation and resuscitation.[4]

AXIOM The trauma anesthesia/critical care specialist may represent the ultimate life support physician.

Once the anesthesiologist is involved, he takes on a major part of the responsibility for the life support and physiologic maintenance of the patient. His input into the care plan should enable the needed surgical emergency interventions to be carried out without compromising the patient's chances for survival. The trauma anesthesiologist's role often follows a continuum beyond the initial intervention to include postoperative care and pain management[4] (Table 6-1).

AXIOM A well-designed trauma protocol should provide the level of care to injured patients at 2:00 a.m. that is available when the most experienced members of the team are present at 2:00 p.m.

Effective protocols, such as in the ATLS system, are designed to prevent death or disability, particularly from preventable problems. It is the responsibility of all members of the team to see that, whenever possible, the protocol is followed properly. In critical care, the patient's overall benefit from preplanned management far outweighs the occasional harmful misapplication of therapy.[5,6] In one study, it was possible to show that even when the resuscitators were of equivalent training, those who followed a scientifically developed algorithm had only a fraction of the morbidity and mortality of those who used their best efforts in a less structured fashion.[5] The trauma anesthesiologist should be well aware of such protocols, and be responsible for following them properly. The anesthesiologist is particularly concerned with airway management, breathing, and circulatory support. He may also be involved with monitoring and support of patients during transport, CT scanning, angiography or other studies, especially if the patient is ventilated and paralyzed during these procedures.[4]

Communication Between Surgeons and Anesthesiologists

PITFALL ⊘

When the anesthesiologist and the surgeon each "do his own thing" without being aware of the other's problems, the patient's care is not likely to be optimal.[7]

The surgeon and anesthesiologist should both be well-appraised of each other's plans, needs, and concerns. The "fix everything now" approach makes good communication a key to successful outcome. Immediately upon transporting an unstable patient to the operating room for emergency surgery, the surgeon and anesthesiologist must discuss the patient's condition, the nature and severity of the injuries, and the planned operative procedures.[2] Available historic information, positioning, and difficulties with the airway or vascular access should also be discussed at this time.

AXIOM A failure to discuss surgical and anesthetic strategies preoperatively can lead to major intraoperative difficulties for the entire patient care team.

Intraoperatively the surgeon and anesthesiologist should communicate continuously about vital signs, laboratory determinations, and ongoing therapy with blood, fluid, and drugs. Surgical interference

TABLE 6-1 *Potential Roles of the Anesthesiologist in the Care of a Trauma Patient*

Trauma team member
Trauma team leader
Anesthesiologist
Critical care physician
Pain relief physician
Prehospital care physician
Critical care transport physician or director
Disaster planning consultant

From Grande CM, Nolan JP, Oakley PA: Trauma anesthesia the relationship of the anesthesiology department to trauma systems. In Champion HR, editor: *Trauma systems,* Cambridge, Eng. Cambridge University Press, in press.

with ventilation or circulation, such as by compression of the lung or vena cava, should be announced in advance. Clamping or unclamping of the aorta or anticipated maneuvers associated with major blood loss should also be announced well ahead of time. Conversely, the anesthesiologist should notify the surgeon of changes in any physiologic parameters so that the surgeon can help determine whether these changes are related to the surgical activity or the condition of the patient.

AXIOM Operative procedures should be prioritized in the event that the patient's condition deteriorates so badly that surgery must be discontinued.

The surgical plans should be prioritized so that if the patient begins to deteriorate, the most pressing operations will have been done, and the others can be put off until the patient is restored to a better condition. The decision that the patient cannot tolerate more surgery usually originates from the anesthesiologist, and such decisions are usually far better accepted by other members of the team if the parameters for such a decision were spelled out in advance.

PREANESTHETIC MANAGEMENT

The preanesthetic evaluation and management of the multiply injured patient follows the basic ABCs of trauma care.[8] This tends to be a natural chain of events for most anesthesiologists. If an abnormality is detected during the assessment phase, steps should be taken immediately to correct the situation.

Control of the Airway

PRIOR PREPARATIONS

AXIOM All areas of the hospital that are likely to receive acutely compromised patients should be equipped to provide immediate endotracheal intubation.

Control of the airway is critical in determining the patient's outcome during the management of trauma. Equipment needed includes: (a) an adequate source of suction to clear the mouth and pharynx of foreign material, (b) oral and nasal airways, (c) a variety of laryngoscope blades, with at least two handles or other power sources, and (d) a variety of endotracheal tubes and stylets, resuscitation bags, and face masks.[9]

Additional equipment that should be readily available includes mechanical ventilators, instruments for emergency cricothyroidotomy and tracheostomy, and hand-controlled jet ventilators for insufflation of the trachea with oxygen through a transcutaneous needle cricothyrotomy or tracheal cannula.[10]

The advantage of having fiberoptic or rigid bronchoscopes available depends to a large extent on the expertise of the operators.[11] Practice sessions to ensure availability of the equipment and to learn how

it is used need to be organized for everyone likely to be working in the area.

AXIOM Being prepared for an airway emergency is more than half the battle.

PREINTUBATION OXYGENATION

All severely injured patients should be breathing 90 to 100% oxygen soon after entering the emergency system.[3] If the patient is not in control of his ventilation, gaining control of the airway is of paramount importance. Adequate preoxygenation and denitrogenation can prevent hypoxemia for up to 1 to 3 minutes after the patient stops breathing effectively.

INDICATIONS FOR ENDOTRACHEAL INTUBATION

There are many indications for endotracheal intubation of critically injured patients (Table 6-2). However, the most frequent indications include actual or impending airway obstruction, inadequate ventilation, severe coma, class 3 or 4 hemorrhagic shock, and concern about aspiration of gastric or oral contents.

DETERMINANTS OF THE TYPE OF AIRWAY TO BE USED

AXIOM Critically injured patients with impending ventilatory failure should be intubated immediately by the most experienced individual present.

The best method of performing emergency intubation depends on the time available and the skill of the intubator.[12] When emergency airway control is needed, particularly in a hemodynamically unstable, combative, or uncooperative patient, the time for teaching the neophyte is past, and the most skilled member of the team should insert the endotracheal tube.

AXIOM If airway control is the first priority, oral endotracheal intubation is usually the preferred method.

In unstable patients, if the head and neck are stabilized by an assistant (Fig. 6-2) there is almost no risk of spinal cord injury by orotracheal intubation. Nasal intubation or tracheostomy usually takes more time and cannot be done as safely. As one is preparing to intu-

TABLE 6-2 *Indications for Endotracheal Intubation of the Acute Trauma Patient in the ER and OR*

Respiratory System
  Airway obstruction or dyspnea
  Need for positive pressure ventilation
  Paralysis—high spinal cord injury
  Severe bony or soft tissue injury to face or larynx
  Upper airway burns
  Pulmonary Toilet
  Hypoxic hypoxia—$PaO_2 < 60$ mm Hg in spite of facemask oxygen
Central Nervous System
  Coma (Glasgow Coma Score <8)
  Apnea
Cardiovascular System
  Circulatory shock not responding rapidly to fluids
Surgical
  Operation site in the head and neck requiring an unusual patient position
  e.g. prone
Anesthetic
  Emergency surgery
  Avoidance of aspiration—blood or gastric contents
  Need for muscle relaxants or controlled ventilation
  Insufficient manpower to manage airway and other anesthetic
  concerns—e.g. resuscitation

FIGURE 6-1 The trimodal distribution of traumatic disease (From: Brown DL. Trauma management: the anesthesiologist's role. Int Anesthesiol Clin 1987;25:1-18).

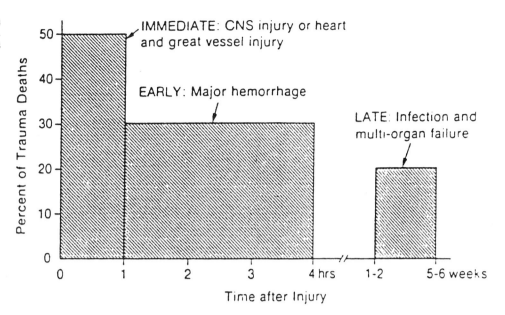

bate the patient, consideration should also be given to the problems likely to be encountered. This can help with prevention and/or management of most major airway surprises and intubation failures.

PITFALL ⊘

Inadequate preintubation assessment and planning increase the likelihood that unnecessary emergencies will develop later.

Problems That Can Occur During Intubation

Multiple problems may develop during intubation of the acute trauma patient (Fig. 6-3). The initial major decision of the anesthesiologist is whether to keep the patient awake (breathing on his own and hopefully cooperative) until the endotracheal tube is passed and then induce anesthesia, or to administer anesthesia and/or a muscle relaxant before intubation. Although the latter option may provide better conditions for intubation, there is the uncertainty of whether or not intubation will be possible.

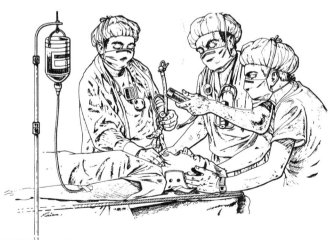

FIGURE 6-2 Technique of oral intubation in the emergency trauma patient using laryngoscopy and "manual in-line axial traction" (From: Stene JK. Anesthesia for the critically ill trauma patient. In: Siegel JH, ed. Trauma: emergency surgery and critical care. New York: Churchill Livingstone, 1987.

FULL STOMACH

AXIOM Aspiration of vomitus or blood into the lungs can occur suddenly any time before surgery, but it is most apt to occur when inducing anesthesia and instrumenting the upper airway.

The majority of acute trauma patients are injured within a few hours of eating a meal, and many have consumed large amounts of alcohol. Trauma tends to cause gastric stasis, so that the stomach is frequently still full of undigested or partially digested food many hours later.

Most general anesthetics and paralytic agents relax the esophagogastric and pharyngoesophageal sphincters. Alcohol and nicotine also reduce the tone of these sphincters, and there is the additional danger that intragastric pressure may be elevated from air swallowing, particularly if mask-to-face artificial ventilation has been used. Thus, the induction of anesthesia can cause the stomach to empty some of its contents into the laryngopharynx and trachea either by active vomiting or passive regurgitation. Aspiration of gastric acid and food particles into the lungs can cause immediate hypoxemia, severe aspiration pneumonitis, and later pulmonary abscesses.

AWAKE INTUBATION

Awake intubation is often a very unpleasant experience for both the patient and the intubator; consequently, there is a tendency to avoid this technique. On the other hand, awake intubation does allow neurological assessment to be continued without interference from anesthetic or sedative medications.

Intubation with the patient awake, with or without sedation, is usually indicated whenever intubation may be difficult. Awake intubation of the uncooperative or combative patient who is intoxicated from drugs or alcohol is hazardous at best, and should be avoided if at all possible. Heavy sedation of such patients is often required, but this places the patient at increased risk of aspiration, airway obstruction, and respiratory arrest.

AXIOM Unless there is significant nasal deformity, patients needing awake intubation can usually tolerate the nasal route better than the oral.

Particular care must be exercised when intubating patients who have sustained severe trauma to the anterior skull or midface. One can easily intubate the cranial vault using a "blind" technique. Similarly, blind intubation of patients with severe injury to the neck or thoracic inlet could cause damage to the larynx, retropharyngeal space, or mediastinum. Skillful awake oral intubation under direct vision or nasal intubation using fiberoptic control is preferred in these patients.

The decision to use direct laryngoscopy on the awake patient is often aided by a quick "look-see" with a warm laryngoscope blade during the preanesthetic assessment. However, it is wise to have a suitable endotracheal tube ready as sometimes the tube can be readily passed at this point.

> **AXIOM** Most patients in severe circulatory shock will tolerate direct laryngoscopy and intubation without too much fighting.

Once the endotracheal tube is in place, the patient can be sedated, if not contraindicated, and given a muscle relaxant to prevent further struggling and inadvertent extubation.

One of the disadvantages of ketamine is a possible adrenergic reaction causing cardiac arrhythmias, especially in cocaine abusers. If this problem is anticipated, other anesthetic agents, such as etomidate (Amidate[R], Abbott) or scopolamine 0.2-0.4 mg intravenously, can help reduce consciousness and produce amnesia.

NASOTRACHEAL INTUBATION

The blind nasal approach to endotracheal intubation, after the application of topical anesthetics and vasoconstrictor drops or spray (e.g., neosynephrine or oxymetazoline [Afrin[R], Shering]) to the nasal mucosa in unstable trauma patients, is a technique that should probably only be used by experts. Topical anesthesia is time-consuming and seldom sufficient to take away all of the considerable discomfort that can accompany passing an endotracheal tube through the nose. The use of transtracheal and translaryngeal nerve blocks in this setting remains controversial.[13,14] In addition, nasal intubation can cause epistaxis, inhibiting visualization of the larynx and aggravating airway compromise should direct or fiberoptic laryngoscopy be required later.

Success with blind nasal intubation seems to be greater if the passage through the nose is gently dilated at least 0.5 mm larger than the intended endotracheal tube with soft nasal airways. The fact that nasotracheal tubes with directable tips (Endotrol[R], Mallinkrodt) are standard in some trauma units is a tribute to their success. O'Brien et al[15] reported a success rate of 95% with blind nasal attempts with 0.5% incidence of epistaxis or nasal mucosal contusion. This success has not been universally experienced.[16]

Intubation over a flexible fiberoptic bronchoscope has been strongly recommended by some.[17] The use of a narrow flexible bronchoscope inside an endotracheal tube will also allow some ventilation of the patient during the intubation. However, the skill and experience of the average physician in the emergency department is generally inadequate for this technique.[11]

CONTROLLED SEQUENCE INDUCTION

If the individual performing the intubation feels that an awake intubation is not necessary, and there is no anatomical bar to direct laryngoscopy and intubation, a controlled (rapid) sequence induction of anesthesia is probably the best alternative.[18,19,20] This is certainly much more comfortable for the patient.

Most anesthesiologists choose a "rapid sequence" induction technique for this group of patients to prevent regurgitation and aspiration of gastric contents.[2] This technique requires preoxygenation and denitrogenation by mask to prevent apnea related hypoxia. Anesthesia is induced with an appropriate intravenous agent, and succinylcholine is given to relax the patient's musculature to facilitate intubation. Alternatively, large doses of non-depolarizing neuromuscular blocking agents may be substituted for succinylcholine. Mask ventilation is not attempted at this point. The trachea is rapidly intubated,

and the cuff is inflated to protect the airway. Proper tube placement is confirmed by auscultation and appropriate levels of exhaled carbon dioxide.

> **AXIOM** During induction of anesthesia on a patient with recent trauma, special efforts are required to prevent regurgitation of gastric contents into the lungs.

During the induction, a skilled assistant provides manual in-line axial stabilization of the head while a second assistant presses backward on the cricoid cartilage to prevent the passage of gastric or esophageal contents in the laryngopharynx (Fig. 6-2). The cricoid pressure is maintained until the cuff on the endotracheal tube has been inflated and proper placement of the tube has been confirmed.

> **AXIOM** "Rapid sequence induction" has the potential of producing either an easy intubation or a catastrophe.

The main disadvantage of rapid sequence induction is that, once anesthesia has been induced, there is no turning back. The patient is rendered apneic at a time when oxygenation is difficult to assure without an endotracheal tube. In addition, if there are facial injuries that do not allow the close application of a face mask, preoxygenation may be impossible or inadequate. There may also be copious foreign material or blood obscuring the view even if the patient has not vomited. Nevertheless, this is the method that most anesthesiologists with extensive trauma experience choose.[9]

The administration of histamine receptor antagonists and nonparticulate antacids has been demonstrated to decrease the severity of the lung changes if aspiration does occur.[2,21] The amount of time available between evaluation and surgery, as well as the nature of the patient's injuries, will determine whether such pharmacologic maneuvers are possible.

Succinylcholine is usually avoided in patients who have sustained a severe eye injury with an "open globe."[2,22] In such circumstances, paralysis for intubation is provided by a large dose of a nondepolarizing relaxant with or without the use of "the priming principle."[23,24,25]

> **AXIOM** The most challenging airway problem in trauma is the patient with an acute, severe airway obstruction.

Respiratory distress associated with trauma to the upper airway or its supporting structures is frequently made worse by blood or gastric contents in the airway and requires prompt action.[2,17] Oxygen administration, although important, may not relieve the hypoxia of airway compromise. Fiberoptic intubation is time-consuming, if not impossible, in the unclean airway. In addition, these patients are often combative because of hypoxia and intolerant of large doses of sedative drugs, making awake intubation extremely difficult. The induction of general anesthesia is frequently accompanied by respiratory standstill, and bag-mask ventilation may be inadequate because of the mechanical airway obstruction that caused the respiratory distress in the first place.

The combination of a technically difficult intubation and airway distress often dictates the establishment of a surgical airway.[26,27] A formal tracheostomy may be possible, but this procedure often takes much longer than expected, especially in agitated patients. A catheter cricothyroidotomy with jet ventilation, however, generally provides sufficient oxygenation to permit the controlled creation of a surgical airway.[10,28,29,30]

CATHETER-GUIDED INTUBATION

Anatomically difficult intubations, in patients who are ventilating adequately, can sometimes be performed over a catheter or wire. A large needle is introduced into the trachea or the cricothyroid membrane, and a long, large-bore vascular catheter or a long "j-wire" is advanced retrograde through the larynx and then into the pharynx.[31,32] The end of the catheter or wire is grasped, and an endotracheal tube is ad-

FIGURE 6-3 Common pitfalls requiring modification of airway management in acute trauma (From: Capan LM. Airway management. In: Capan LM, Miller SM, Turndorf H, eds. Trauma anesthesia and intensive care. New York: JB Lippincott, 1991.

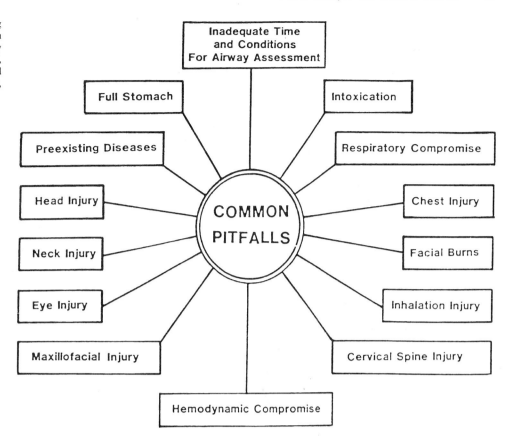

vanced over the guide and through the larynx. Alternatively, the guide wire may be passed through the working channel of a fiberoptic bronchoscope. Intubation then proceeds antegrade over the wire, under direct vision.[31] The catheter is then withdrawn from the trachea, and the endotracheal tube is advanced further down, to a position 3-4 cm above the carina.

Catheter-guided intubations are usually performed with the patient awake, and patient cooperation is mandatory. This technique may also be performed as an emergency measure when, after the induction of anesthesia, the patient is impossible to intubate but can be ventilated. Direct visualization of the catheter end as it emerges retrograde through the vocal cords is necessary, but this may be difficult if blood or vomitus is in the pharynx. Perforation of the esophagus with contamination of the mediastinum is a hazard of this technique.

PITFALL ⊘

Rendering a patient apneic, when endotracheal intubation in that patient is beyond the skill of the operator, may be rapidly fatal.

HEAD INJURY
Endotracheal intubation of a patient with a severe closed head injury is a major concern because intracranial pressure can rise precipitously during the procedure.[33] Even mild drug-induced respiratory depression with its associated hypercapnia can result in a rapid rise in intracranial pressure (ICP). This is of great concern as the patient may already have increased ICP from the trauma or resultant hypercarbia and/or hypoxia.[34]

AXIOM   Systemic vasodilators can be used to correct hypertension, but they may also increase ICP in patients with severe head injuries.

If the patient is hypertensive, beta-blockers have been recommended to control intracranial pressure.[35] Systemic vasodilators, such

as sodium nitroprusside, nitroglycerine, and hydralazine, can lower the systemic blood pressure, but they can also increase cerebral blood flow and intracranial pressure.[36] Consequently, they should not be the first choice for treating hypertension in these patients.[37]

If possible, rapid sequence induction of anesthesia and oral intubation are recommended for patients with head injuries. Oral endotracheal intubation can be performed safely if the head and neck are kept in the neutral position by an assistant during intubation. Nasal intubation is not recommended because it is less expeditious. There is also the danger of passing any nasal tube intracranially if there is an anterior basilar skull fracture.

CERVICAL SPINE INJURY
Although patients with possible cervical spine injury can be intubated asleep or awake according to the preintubation assessment,[38,39,40] the intubation should be done with an assistant maintaining the neck and head in a neutral position[41,42] (Table 6-3).

AXIOM   If intubation is performed before any spine films can be obtained, the patient should be kept in a rigid cervical collar until cervical spine injury has been ruled out.

FACIAL TRAUMA
Severe facial trauma can cause multiple problems with the airway, particularly if there is a need for nasotracheal intubation because the jaws will have to be wired. It may be particularly difficult to oxygenate the patient initially with a mask because of the deformed anatomy, tissue swelling, and blood in the oropharynx and laryngopharynx. A prior "look-see" with a warmed laryngoscope can help determine the optimal course of action. Severe facial injuries may preclude adequate oxygenation before intubation. Consequently, if the probability of a successful intubation is uncertain, but the patient is breathing adequately and skilled assistance is at hand, it may be wiser to go straight to a surgical airway[43] (Table 6-4).

TABLE 6-3   Evaluation of Cervical Spine X-Rays

Alignment
  All seven vertebrae must be seen, including the C-7 to T-1 junction
  Trace the anterior margins of the vertebrae, posterior margins
    spinolaminal line, and the tips of the spinous processes
Bones
  Evaluate bones for fractures and increased density (suggesting a
    compression fracture)
  Look for atlanto-axial dislocation (distance between the posterior aspect
    of C-1 to the anterior odontoid process > 3 mm)
Cartilage and soft tissue spaces
  Evaluate the intervertebral and interspinous process (angulation of the
    space > 11° is abnormal)
  Fanning of the spinous processes suggests posterior ligament disruption
  Evaluate the prevertebral soft-tissue distance (normally < 5 mm at C-3)
  Obliteration of the prevertebral fat stripe suggests a fracture at the same
    level

From Gajraj NM, Pennant JH, Giesecke, AH. Cervical Spine Trauma and Airway
Management. Current Opinion in Anaesthesiology 6:369,1993.

FAILED INTUBATION

AXIOM   Before one attempts endotracheal intubation, particularly
on an unstable trauma patient, an alternate technique for
rapidly providing an airway should be immediately available.

Failure of endotracheal intubation in a critically injured patient
who has been rendered apneic can be terrifying, especially if one
has not planned for that contingency. In an effort to prevent such
problems the Task Force on Guidelines for Management of the
Difficult Airway of the American Society of Anesthesiologists
published Practice Guidelines for Management of the Difficult
Airway[44] (Fig. 6-4 and Table 6-5).

If, in spite of following these guidelines, an airway has not been
established, a cricothyroidotomy can usually be performed within a
few seconds, providing the anterior neck anatomy is normal.[45] If
this is not possible, a 14-gauge intravenous cannula can be passed
through the cricothyroid membrane or anterior upper trachea,
attached to wall or tank oxygen (50 psi), and flushed about 20 times
a minute.[46] Great care should be taken to ensure that the cannula is
in the trachea as mediastinal insufflation of large quantities of
oxygen under pressure can be catastrophic. Although a properly
placed catheter intermittently flushed with wall O_2 can usually keep
the patient oxygenated for at least 20 to 30 minutes, CO_2 retention
can be a problem if the catheter technique is continued for longer
periods.

Occasionally, one can use a semirigid endotracheal tube changer
as an aid to intubation. Since it is smaller and easier to pass into the
trachea than an endotracheal tube, it can be used as a guide over which
to pass the endotracheal tube.

**TABLE 6-4   Indications for Tracheostomy
in Maxillofacial Injuries**

Combined bilateral mandibular fractures and LeFort fractures of the maxilla
Extensive lacerations and/or hematoma of the tongue and floor of the mouth
Gross posterior displacement of the maxilla with split palate and profuse
  bleeding from the nasopharynx
Gunshot and close-range shotgun injuries of the face
Crush-type injuries of the face
Extensive facial burns
Associated head and cervical spine injuries

From Capan LM, Miller SM, Glickman R. Management of Facial Injuries. In Capan
LM, Miller SM, Turndorf H. Trauma Anesthesia and Intensive Care. J.B. Lippincott
NY 1991, p 403.

The laryngeal mask airway (LMA) and esophageal-tracheal combitube have recently emerged as alternatives to transtracheal jet ventilation for providing emergency non-surgical airway ventilation.[47]

SEDATING THE INTUBATED PATIENT

AXIOM   Muscle relaxants are not anesthetics.

Once the endotracheal tube has been passed, the awake patient
should be obtunded or made comfortable with small doses of intravenous anesthetics or narcotics, unless full anesthesia is to be induced
for surgery. The experience of being paralyzed and awake is very dis-
tressing.[48,49] Consequently, sedation is necessary if the patient is to
be kept paralyzed following intubation.

AXIOM   Being awake and paralyzed can be a very terrifying experience for the patient.

Intravascular Access

LOCATIONS FOR VENOUS CATHETERS
Intravascular access in trauma patients is required for both fluid administration and monitoring. The ATLS guidelines recommend that
at least two large bore (16-gauge or larger) cannulas be placed, preferably one in a vein draining into the superior cava and another in a
vein draining into the inferior cava.[3] This will usually provide adequate intravenous access, even if the venous circulation from either
the upper or lower body is interrupted.

NEED FOR LARGE INTRAVENOUS CATHETERS
In an actively bleeding trauma patient, even a 14-gauge catheter may
be "small" when it comes to the high volume blood replacement that
may be needed during resuscitation. A variety of wide bore intravenous devices, up to 9 French, can be extremely effective for emergency high volume infusions, especially when used with a wide bore
administration set.[50] These catheters (e.g., EID Catheter, Arrow[R] International) are passed by a Seldinger technique. Any intravenous
catheter considered inadequate for the purposes of resuscitation can
be used as a conduit for the passage of a wire, over which to pass a

TABLE 6-5   Techniques for Difficult Airway Management

IMPORTANT: This table displays commonly cited techniques. It is not a
  comprehensive list. The order of presentation is alphabetical and does not
  imply preference for a given technique or sequence of use. Combinations
  of techniques may be employed. The techniques chosen by the
  practitioner in a particular case will depend upon specific needs,
  preferences, skills, and clinical constraints.
I. **Techniques for difficult intubation**
  Alternative laryngoscope blades
  Awake intubation
  Blind intubation (oral or nasal)
  Fiberoptic intubation
  Intubating stylet/tube changer
  Light wand
  Retrograde intubation
  Surgical airway access
II. **Techniques for difficult ventilation**
  Esophageal-tracheal combitube
  Intratracheal jet stylet
  Laryngeal mask
  Oral and nasopharyngeal airways
  Rigid ventilating bronchoscope
  Surgical airway access
  Transtracheal jet ventilation
  Two-person mask ventilation

From Practice Guidelines for Management of the Difficult Airway. Anesthesiology
73:3:597, 1993.

FIGURE 6-4 Difficult airway algorithm (From: Practice guidelines for management of the difficult airway. Anesthesiology 1993; 73:597).

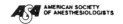

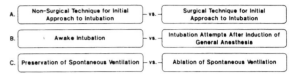

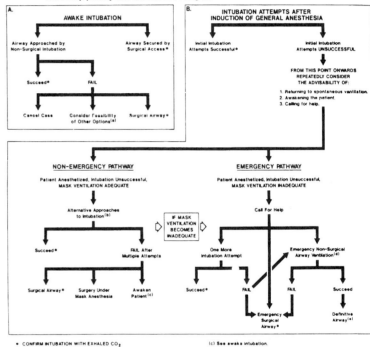

larger catheter (e.g., Rapid Infusion Catheter, Arrow International), provided the vein is of sufficient caliber.

Blood products and crystalloid solutions are available in flexible containers suitable for external compression by an inflatable bladder system. Such compression will provide much higher infusion rates than gravity alone; however, it is essential to have an automated system for compressing these fluid containers. Pipeline gas in the operating room provides a convenient power source for automatic bladder inflation when used in conjunction with a continuous flow stepdown pressure regulator.

DANGERS OF DISCONNECTION OF LARGE CENTRAL INTRAVENOUS CATHETERS

AXIOM   One should make special efforts to ensure that intravenous tubing cannot disconnect from large central intravenous catheters.

If a large bore cannula is passed centrally into a subclavian or jugular vein, massive fatal air embolization can occur during acci-

dental disconnection from the infusion set. When air enters the pulmonary circulation, a "gasp" reflex is initiated that sucks further air in through the cannula, making the situation even worse. Because trauma patients are frequently transported after intravenous cannulation to other areas of the hospital, disconnection of an intravenous catheter from the infusion set can be a particularly dangerous problem. Although many trauma centers have had such experiences, it is seldom reported.

PITFALL ⊘

If a large bore central venous cannula accidentally disconnects, air embolism can be rapidly fatal.

If a central intravenous catheter becomes disconnected, a syringe should be attached to it immediately and an attempt made to aspirate air from the catheter and the vein into which it is inserted. The patient should also be turned on his left side, the head lowered, and legs raised (Durant position) to reduce the tendency for an air lock in the outflow tract of the right ventricle and to reduce the chances for any systemic arterial air to get to the brain.

VASCULAR LINES FOR MONITORING

Most trauma patients are relatively young and without previous cardiovascular disease, and there is usually little need for central venous or pulmonary artery monitoring catheters. However, radial artery cannulation can be very useful for blood pressure measurement and for obtaining repeated blood samples for analysis.

> **AXIOM**   Failure of the patient to respond appropriately to what should be adequate resuscitative fluid is an indication for CVP or PAWP monitoring.

There are multiple reasons for inserting central venous pressure catheters (Table 6-6), but they can be particularly helpful for evaluating preload when there are questions about the patient's fluid status. They can also help in the diagnosis of pericardial tamponade[51] and detection of changes in the circulation from clamping the aorta or using a pneumatic antishock garment (PASG).[52] In addition, central venous oxygen saturations can be reflective of the overall adequacy of tissue oxygenation.[53,54]

Preoperative Analgesia and Sedation

DISCREPANCIES BETWEEN NEED AND TOLERANCE OF MEDICATIONS

Because of the frequent association of trauma with alcohol or drug ingestion, special attention must be focused on possible drug interactions when choosing the type and dosage of premedications and anesthetic agents.[55] If any doubt exists about the adequacy of the patient's circulatory or respiratory function, premedication is omitted.

> **AXIOM**   Premedication designed to reduce patient anxiety is contraindicated for most trauma victims, especially if they are hemodynamically unstable.

Anxiety may be an early manifestation of circulatory inadequacy or hypoxemia, and attempts at controlling it pharmacologically may result in cardiovascular or respiratory collapse.[2] Nevertheless, if a stable patient is extremely frightened, intravenous agents such as the short-acting narcotic fentanyl or the short-acting benzodiazepine, midazolam, may be cautiously titrated to effect. However, combining these drugs can result in severe respiratory depression or cardiovascular collapse.

> **AXIOM**   Titrated small doses of intravenous narcotics are generally the safest premedication for anesthesia.

Premedication designed to reduce pain can also result in cardiovascular or respiratory collapse; however, judicious intravenous administration of narcotics to an injured patient can make the transfer from a stretcher to an x-ray or operating room table much more tolerable. Because inadvertent narcotic overdose resulting in hypotension, respiratory depression, or excessive somnolence can be easily

TABLE 6-6   Indications for Central Venous Cannulation in the Acute Trauma Patient

1. No suitable peripheral veins for percutaneous cannulation in an emergency
2. Central venous pressure monitoring
3. Central venous blood sampling for O_2 tension or saturation
4. Rapid fluid resuscitation (no suitable peripheral cannula available)
5. Drug administration during resuscitation (e.g. anesthetic agents, inotropes, vasoactive drugs, etc.)
6. Aspirating air
7. Access for inserting a pulmonary artery catheter or pacemaker electrode.

antagonized with intravenous naloxone, intravenous narcotics are the first choice for premedication. Flumazenil (Romazicon[R]), an effective pharmacologic antagonist for benzodiazepines, is available. However, because the sympathetic response to naloxone and flumazenil can be dramatic, these agents should be used with extreme caution.

> **AXIOM**   Although pain from trauma may be of a magnitude demanding larger than normal amounts of narcotic analgesics, the sensitivity of the patient to these agents may be considerably increased.

The peripheral, splanchnic, and renal vasoconstriction caused by pain and hypovolemia not only reduce the size of the faster compartments of the volume of distribution, but they also decrease the rate of drug elimination by the liver and kidneys. If hypothermia is present, drug elimination will be further retarded. The patient may also have recently taken other drugs that may have an additive effect. For example, at least 50% of trauma patients are intoxicated to some degree with alcohol.[56]

USE OF THE INTRAVENOUS ROUTE FOR ALL MEDICATIONS

Peripheral vasoconstriction prevents the subcutaneous and intramuscular routes of administration from working reliably. Poor perfusion of muscle and fat also allows a reservoir of the drug to lie in the tissues from which it can be mobilized when the integrity of the circulation is restored, producing a possible overdose in the patient.

Independent of which agents are chosen for premedication, the intravenous route provides prompt patient response and avoids the difficulties associated with the unpredictable uptake of agents given subcutaneously (SQ) or intramuscularly (IM).

> **PITFALL** ⊘
>
> *Patients in traumatic or hemorrhagic shock are often acutely insensitive to SQ or IM drugs and oversensitive to intravenous agents.*

USE OF MULTIPLE SMALL INTRAVENOUS DOSES

The safest method for providing analgesia after severe trauma is to give small frequent intravenous doses until the patient is no longer severely distressed by the pain. Complete relief of all pain sensation may require much larger doses of analgesics. The intermittent doses should be spaced far enough apart to allow time for each dose to exert its effect. This can be 5 to 7 minutes in the case of morphine, and 2 to 3 minutes with fentanyl. Patients with severe second-degree burns may require double or triple the normal dose of analgesics. Whenever this type of therapy is used, the risk of respiratory depression is sufficiently great to require the immediate presence of whatever apparatus and personnel are necessary to provide emergency endotracheal intubation and ventilation.

UNCOOPERATIVE PATIENTS

> **AXIOM**   If patients cannot be made aware of the danger their lack of cooperation is causing, cautious sedation or general anesthesia should be used, as needed, to provide lifesaving treatment.

Sedation, other than that produced by analgesics for severe pain, is seldom indicated preoperatively unless the patient is unruly and physically resisting attempts to provide treatment. Sometimes such restlessness may be due to hypoxia, but if such behavior is sufficiently self-destructive to endanger the patient's life, the use of sedation and muscle relaxants along with mechanical ventilation and oxygen can be justified to bring an impossible situation under control.[57] However, anyone using this form of management must recognize the dangers that can occur if the airway and/or adequate spontaneous ventilation is lost.

HEAD INJURY

AXIOM   Before an analgesic or sedative is given to a head-injured patient, that patient should be examined by the neurosurgeon or whoever will be responsible for definitive care.

Head injury provides one of the most difficult areas for the use of analgesics and sedatives. A thorough neurological examination should precede administration of these agents and may even preclude it. If a patient's neurological status deteriorates following a medication, it can be extremely difficult to determine if it is due to the drug or the underlying brain injury. However, the development of any lateralizing signs or reduction of the Glasgow Coma Scale (GCS) by more than 2 points, regardless of the medication administered, requires prompt repeat neurosurgical evaluation and CT-scanning of the brain. It is inappropriate to attribute a change in mental status to drugs or alcohol, until all metabolic causes and central nervous system pathology have been excluded.

ALTERNATIVE WAYS TO RELIEVE PAIN

AXIOM   Much of the discomfort of a trauma patient can be reduced or corrected without using drugs.

Pain from unstable fractures can usually be managed quite well by proper immobilization with splints. Restlessness can sometimes be prevented or corrected by emptying a full bladder or moving the patient off a hard stretcher. Some patients also are more comfortable with a pillow (after cervical spine fractures have been ruled out). Many patients are restless because they are cold, and such patients can be helped a great deal by covering them with warmed blankets.

Trauma patients who are awake and frightened will usually benefit greatly from calm reassurance by knowledgeable physicians or nurses using straightforward explanations, comforting words, and gentle physical handling.

AXIOM   One of the best treatments for anxiety is reassurance and explanations by a calm, considerate individual.

Transportation and Care Outside the OR

PROTOCOL

AXIOM   Hospital protocols outlining the equipment and personnel involved in monitoring and caring for trauma patients during transport should be worked out in advance.

Whenever possible, issues concerning equipment and personnel required during transport should have been worked out beforehand. Such protocols help ensure that when an acute trauma patient is outside the emergency department or operating suite, adequate staff and apparatus are available. The issues should not be the subject of debate or negotiation with individual patients.

Most radiologists are pleased to have additional personnel with monitoring and resuscitation skills at hand when radiologic procedures are performed on potentially unstable patients. However, even if the anesthesiologist is not directly responsible for the patient's care outside the OR, it is in his or her and the patient's best interest to see that the patient is not jeopardized by suboptimal care before and after surgery.

EQUIPMENT

Small portable monitors capable of displaying the ECG, noninvasive blood pressure, at least one pressure channel, and pulse oximetry should be available and designed for easy attachment to the patient's cart during transport. Compact compressed gas-driven ventilators, an oxygen supply to last for over an hour, and adequate equipment for CPR and defibrillation should also be carried on the special transport stretchers. Similar transporters are often used for moving patients from the OR to the ICU following open-heart surgery.

AXIOM   The caliber of a trauma service is inversely related to the number of cardiac arrests that take place outside the emergency department and operating room.

PREANESTHETIC ASSESSMENT

If a patient is acutely unstable and in need of immediate lifesaving surgical intervention, the preanesthetic assessment should proceed simultaneously with airway control and intravenous access for rapid fluid resuscitation.[8] This may involve a series of spot judgments as the patient is being wheeled into the OR. All of this is accomplished much easier if the trauma team is well-coordinated and all members know beforehand what their roles and special responsibilities are.

History

The salient points in a preanesthetic history include: (a) past or intercurrent cardiovascular, respiratory, renal, or endocrine disease, (b) current medications, (c) allergies or untoward reactions to previous medications, (d) previous use of drugs such as cocaine and opiates, and (e) the time of the patient's last food or drink in relation to the injuries (Table 6-7).

Patients with congestive heart failure, coronary artery disease with angina or a recent myocardial infarction, and/or severe hypertension carry a high anesthetic risk, even without trauma, and may make pulmonary arterial monitoring a high priority. Antihypertensive medications, such as beta-blocking agents, may confuse the assessment by causing an unexpectedly slow pulse rate and an inadequate response to fluid resuscitation. On the other hand, shorter acting agents, such as clonidine (Catapres^R, Boehringer Ingelheim), may wear off during resuscitation and give rise to sudden and severe hypertension.

Asthmatic patients, particularly if they have had a recent attack, have a strong tendency to develop bronchospasm during endotracheal intubation and with the use of some anesthetic drugs. Some asthmatics have been on corticosteroid medications and will need cortisol coverage during surgical procedures. The patient may be particularly at risk during emergence from anesthesia. Chronic lung disease may also be a cause of severe hypoxia and should be considered in any treatment programs, especially if pulmonary contusion or a flail chest is present.

TABLE 6-7   Sample Preanesthetic Assessment

History
AMPLE: *A*llergies, *m*edications, *p*ast medical history, *l*ast ingestion, *e*vents of injury
Mechanisms of injury
Preadmission (EMT field) management (Glasgow Coma Scale, Trauma Score, vital signs, therapy)
Physical examination
Primary survey
ABCDEs: *a*irway, *b*reathing, *c*irculation, *d*isability, *e*xposure
Vital signs
Detailed examination
Revised Trauma Score
Supporting data
Radiographic evaluation: chest and pelvic radiographs, cervical spine radiographic series
Hematologic evaluations: hematocrit level; blood typing, cross-matching, and chemistry studies
Arterial blood gas studies
Electrocardiography
Additional studies as indicated (e.g., angiography)

From Abrams KJ. Preanesthetic Evaluation. In Grande CM. Textbook of Trauma Anesthesia & Critical Care. Mosby Yearbook St. Louis, 1993 p. 422.

Acute or chronic renal failure cannot only make fluid management extremely difficult, but it also increases the hazard of decreased elimination of many drugs. Furthermore, the hourly urine output may be lost as a monitor of the adequacy of fluid resuscitation. Consequently early invasive monitoring may be required.

The most frequent endocrine disorder of concern to anesthesiologists is insulin-dependent diabetes mellitus. Trauma itself tends to cause hyperglycemia in previously normal individuals. This "diabetes of trauma" is caused by reduced insulin secretion and increased insulin resistance because of increased catecholamines, glucagon, and cortisol secretion in stress. In diabetics, this can cause severe keto-acidosis and an osmotic diuresis.

Recent cocaine use is associated with increased ventricular irritability and personality changes, and opiate addiction can lead to severe withdrawal symptoms and the need for much larger doses of morphine or fentanyl. An acute withdrawal reaction can also be precipitated by opiate antagonists (e.g., naloxone [Narcan^R, DuPont]). Tricyclic antidepressants (e.g., amitriptyline [Elavil^R, MSD, Limbitrol^R, Roche] or imipraime [Tofranil^R, Geigy]) are associated with increased myocardial irritability and sensitivity to adrenergic agents.

Monoamine oxidase inhibitors (such as isocarboxazid [Marplan^R, Roche], tranylcypromine [Parnate^R, SKF], pargyline [Eutron^R, Abbott]) have recently made a comeback in the treatment of refractory depression, but they can cause life-threatening hypertensive crises, often associated with hyperthermia. Atropine-like agents, meperidine, and sympathomimetic drugs can be particularly dangerous in such individuals and should be avoided.

Examination of the Airway

The preanesthetic evaluation of trauma patients, no matter how abbreviated, includes an examination of the airway.[2,8] Some questions that must be answered during that examination include: Does the patient have an adequate range of motion in the neck? Can the head be extended? Does the patient's mouth open widely? Is the submandibular space large enough and the tissues filling it pliable enough to permit displacement of the base of the tongue during direct laryngoscopy? If the answers to these questions are all affirmative and there are no associated airway, craniofacial, or cervical injuries, intubation during rapid sequence induction is the preferred technique.

PITFALL ⊘

> **Assuming a trauma patient has an empty stomach because he or she has supposedly not eaten for 6 hours.**

If a patient is injured more than 4 to 6 hours after eating solid food, it is unlikely that there will be much solid material in the upper gastrointestinal tract. However, patient histories are not always reliable, and the gastric stasis that occurs after trauma obligates the anesthesiologist to treat all patients as though they have a full stomach. In this regard, the interval between the time of the last food intake and the time of the injury is a more accurate predictor of the amount of food in the stomach than the interval between eating or drinking and intubation.[9]

Intubation of most traumatized patients is performed with the patient unconscious and paralyzed.[58] The larynx is visualized directly, the tip of the endotracheal tube is observed to pass into the larynx between the vocal cords, and the chest is auscultated for bilateral breath sounds. Levels of carbon dioxide in the end-tidal gas similar to those expected in arterial blood can help confirm that the endotracheal tube is properly positioned. Another confirmatory test of proper endotracheal positioning is to palpate the inflated cuff of the tube in the suprasternal notch.

Preoperative Investigations

In the emergency situation, the anesthesiologist must use whatever information is available, and make a cautious educated guess as to what additional laboratory data would show if it were available. Even with minimal data, however, previously developed management protocols to help guide less experienced practitioners can usually improve patient outcome.

X-RAYS

Whenever possible, one should know the status of the cervical spine before endotracheal intubation. If such information is not available, one should assume that the cervical spine is fractured and unstable. Preoperative chest radiographs can also be extremely helpful and may help rule out a hemopneumothorax, enlarged heart, widened mediastinum, or other conditions likely to increase the anesthetic risk.

LABORATORY STUDIES

Blood should be drawn for typing and cross-matching, and the status of blood availability (cross-matched, type specific or type O Rh-negative) should be known as rapidly as possible. Specific laboratory investigations, such as a complete blood count (CBC), urinalysis, blood urea nitrogen (BUN), serum creatinine, and electrolytes, should be performed as rapidly as possible, even if they are not available at the beginning of anesthesia.

Hemoglobin/Hematocrit

The hemoglobin concentration (Hgb) or hematocrit (Hct) needed in a patient for safe anesthesia is a matter of considerable meta-analytical opinion.[59,60] The efficiency of oxygen transport and uptake in the tissues does not seem to deteriorate until the Hct is below 30%, unless the patient has severe cardiac or pulmonary disease. However, survival in postoperative critically ill patients may decrease when the hematocrit falls below 32%.[61]

Experimental evidence suggests that the oxygen supply to the vital organs remains fairly constant in hematocrit ranges of 30 to 55% if the blood volume is normal.[62] In critically ill or injured patients, especially if they have had variable amounts of fluid resuscitation, the hemoglobin level bears no clinically applicable relationship to the blood volume or red blood cell mass.[63] Even with normal vital signs and a normal hemoglobin level, the red blood cell mass may be 40% lower than normal for up to 8 weeks following severe trauma.[64] In this regard, the use of oxygen transport variables, as obtained from invasive monitoring, is increasingly used to guide resuscitation.[53,54,65]

A normal hemoglobin level in a stable postinjury patient may mislead the surgeon and anesthesiologist into thinking that there is no need for increasing blood volume. However, if the patient is hypovolemic, circulatory collapse is apt to occur when sympathetic tone is reduced by the induction of anesthesia.

AXIOM Many patients, especially the elderly, can have significant, but inapparent, red blood cell and blood volume deficits after trauma.

A particularly high risk group after trauma are the elderly who may have a chronic fluid depleted state because they are being treated for heart failure with diuretics and sodium restriction. If they sustain a hip fracture, even though significant concealed blood loss may occur at the site of injury, the hemoglobin will often not decrease acutely. Consequently, such patients have a reputation for "crashing" following anesthetic induction. Therefore, careful fluid loading before induction is probably a wise precaution, particularly if there is a history of a cardiac problem.

PITFALL ⊘

> **Assuming that normal hemoglobin and hematocrit levels in a trauma patient indicate that the blood volume and red blood cell mass are also normal.**

Biochemical Studies

Important electrolyte abnormalities should be ruled out by appropriate preoperative studies. With blunt chest trauma, an elevated MB fraction of the creatinine phosphokinase (CPK) may help diagnose myocardial injury; however, severe head injury in the absence of myocardial contusion can also give rise to elevated CPK-MB levels, but the elevation with head injury is usually more prolonged.[66]

Serum creatinine and blood urea nitrogen (BUN) levels may provide a clue to clinically unsuspected acute or chronic renal failure. When these values and the blood glucose are known, one can also calculate plasma osmolality. If the measured osmolality is more than 10 mOsm/kg higher than the calculated osmolality, the resultant osmolal gap can be used to estimate blood alcohol levels because each excess mOsm/kg is equal to 4.6 mg/dl ethanol. Thus, if the calculated osmolality is 290 mOsm/kg and the measured value is 350 mOsm/kg, the blood alcohol level may be $(50) \times (4.6) = 230$ mg/dl.

> **AXIOM** Hypoglycemia may occur in some patients with severe alcoholism or cirrhosis, but the great majority of acute trauma patients are hyperglycemic due to the stress hormone response.

Coagulation Studies

Preanesthetic coagulation workups are not routinely indicated, unless major orthopedic surgery or massive blood loss is anticipated. In such instances, a platelet count, prothrombin time (PT), and accelerated partial thromboplastin time (aPTT) may provide useful information. If a coagulopathy is suspected, additional tests should include bleeding time, thrombin time, and fibrinogen levels.

ANESTHETIC MANAGEMENT

Preparedness

Hospitals frequently dealing with severe trauma should have one or more operating rooms always set up and ready to provide emergency surgery.[7] The anesthesia machines, ventilators, intubation apparatus, suction, and monitors should all be checked at routine intervals and be ready for use. The drugs apt to be needed should be drawn up in labeled and dated syringes, and at least one rapid infusion device should be primed for action. Transducers for measuring intravascular pressures should be calibrated, and apparatus for inserting monitoring and intravenous access catheters should be available.

> **AXIOM** Every effort should be made to prevent or rapidly correct hypothermia in patients with severe trauma undergoing major surgery.

A heated, humidified, breathing circuit and warming blankets should be set up to prevent hypothermia and help warm the patient. Rapid infusion devices that can warm fluids to 40-42° C, almost regardless of the rate of fluid and blood administration, should be primed, and the intravenous fluids should be prewarmed.

Until the patient is anesthetized and draped, the operating room temperature should be kept at 75° F (23° C). After the patient is draped, if blood loss is controlled and the core temperature is above 35° C, it is safe to cool the room to normal levels.

Monitoring

During general anesthesia, the monitoring of trauma victims should minimally include an electrocardiogram, urine output via an indwelling Foley catheter, BP (arterial line or cuff), core temperature probe, and oxygen saturation (pulse oximeter). One should also have the endotracheal tube connected to a capnography machine to monitor exhaled CO_2 concentrations. For severely injured patients, additional monitoring may be appropriate (Table 6-8).

> **AXIOM** General anesthesia is usually the technique of choice for unstable trauma patients because the principles of airway management and respiratory and circulatory support common to all general anesthetics are the basic ingredients of cardiopulmonary resuscitation.

The choice of anesthetic techniques suitable for unstable trauma patients requiring emergency surgery is limited. General anesthesia is the most popular technique for trauma patients, and it has many advantages. It allows the surgical team to switch freely from one part of the patient to another, and it ensures that patients with multiple injuries and/or anxiety are pain-free and amnesic for the procedure. Uncooperative or violent patients are easily controlled, and the patient can be positioned to provide optimal surgical exposure with no

TABLE 6-8 *Monitoring Priorities for an Acute Multiple Trauma Patient Undergoing Anesthesia*

Need	Monitor	Indication/Comment
Standard	Electrocardiograph	
	Cuff blood pressure—automatic—manual	Automatic blood pressure apparatus may not function properly in severe hypovolemia or hypotension
	Pulse oximeter	Unreliable or will not function with low peripheral pulse pressure
	Inspired oxygen fraction	
	End-tidal carbon dioxide	Indicates correct endotracheal tube placement. Will fall with very low cadiac output and PE*
	Temperature probe	Esophageal and tympanic more reliable than rectal or bladder
	Anesthetic vapor conc[n]	To verify low vapor concentrations.
High	Arterial catheter	Continuous blood pressure
		Pulse height variation with respiration
		Indicates cardiac failure or hypovolemia
		Blood sampling
High	Blood catheter	Circulatory and renal function
High/Mod	Central venous pressure	Central venous pressure
		Central venous blood gases
		Access for pulmonary arterial catheter
		Reliable administration of active drugs
Moderate	Pulmonary artery catheter	Patient does not respond to resuscitation. Hemodynamic, oxygen and temperature monitoring

*PE = pulmonary embolus—blood clot or air.

added discomfort. The airway is protected, ventilation is assured, and respiratory support techniques, such as PEEP or endobronchial ventilation, can be applied.

AXIOM   General anesthesia for trauma victims should be induced with the minimum amount of agent that will obtund consciousness and provide needed relaxation.

If the patient is hypovolemic, depression of sympathetic tone by a normal dose of anesthetic may cause sudden severe cardiovascular collapse. Consequently, these patients have an increased risk of waking up and moving during the surgery because of excessively light anesthesia or because the anesthetic is turned off during a period of hypotension.[67]

Even in extreme hypovolemia, the cerebral circulation tends to be maintained; however, one can use small doses of scopolamine, ketamine, or midazolam (Versed[R], Roche) to prevent recall if the patient is thought to be almost awake. Larger doses of benzodiazepines should be avoided because they may reduce sympathetic tone and cause hypotension.

PITFALL ⊘

If the depth of anesthesia is reduced to maintain an adequate blood pressure, patients may become aware that they are having a surgical procedure and have severe pain and anxiety without being able to show it.

INDUCTION

The most severely injured patients tend to arrive in the operating room intubated and ventilated. During the anesthetic induction, these patients require paralysis, controlled ventilation, and monitoring. Rapid volume resuscitation may also be required. Patients who have undergone emergency department thoracotomy, either for direct cardiac repair or to permit cross-clamping of the descending thoracic aorta, require little or no anesthetic agent. The agents administered under such circumstances are given to maintain circulatory stability and not for central nervous system (CNS) depression.

Hypotensive, unintubated patients require rapid induction and endotracheal intubation.[5,68] The selection of agents and their doses depends upon the degree of hemodynamic instability and the level of consciousness of the patient. Reduced doses of ketamine, etomidate, thiopental, or other induction agents are supplemented with large doses of muscle relaxants to allow rapid intubation.

AXIOM   Hypertension must be prevented or rapidly corrected if a traumatic rupture of the thoracic aorta is suspected.

In patients with known or suspected traumatic rupture of the thoracic aorta, every effort should be made to avoid a precipitous rise in systemic blood pressure. Vasodilator drugs are prepared in advance of induction to rapidly correct any such tendency. The usual minimal depressant drug technique chosen for the severely injured patient is abandoned in favor of careful control of the BP before surgical control of the injured vessel. The administration of the short-acting beta-blocker, esmolol, can facilitate the management of tachycardia and/or hypertension associated with the stress of intubation.

Thiamylal (Surital[R], Parke-Davis) or thiopental (Pentothal[R], Abbott) are generally the best drugs to induce anesthesia in stable, well-resuscitated patients. If small doses are used, the loss of vasomotor tone and myocardial contractility is minimal and should not be a major risk to the patient.

Currently, the choice of induction agent for unstable hypovolemic patients is very small doses of ketamine or etomidate (Amidate[R], Abbott); however, ketamine has the theoretical disadvantage of being a sympathetic stimulant, which could cause even more vasoconstriction and further reduce blood flow in hypovolemic patients. It is also a direct myocardial depressant, and it may decrease myocardial contractility in a patient who already has a low ejection fraction.[69] Eto-

midate seems to maintain circulatory integrity, but even a single dose has been shown to cause temporary adrenocortical suppression.[70] This could lead to a need for steroid supplementation if the patient has a stressful postoperative period.

The presence of an intracranial injury requires modification of the anesthetic management. An isolated injury to the brain with a possible elevation in intracranial pressure (ICP) is usually managed with large doses of barbiturates or etomidate, hyperventilation, careful positioning, and dehydration of the intracranial contents. However, these ICP control procedures can significantly reduce blood pressure, especially in volume-deficient multiple trauma victims.[71]

AXIOM   Even if the ICP is elevated in patients with brain injury, adequate fluid must be given to maintain a normal or slightly increased BP.

Cerebrospinal fluid (CSF) may be removed by the neurosurgeon during intracranial manipulations if the need arises to quickly reduce the ICP. During extracranial procedures performed on patients with associated closed-head injuries, a cerebral ventricular catheter allows the anesthesiologist to monitor intracranial pressure and adjust therapy to maximize cerebral perfusion. Direct drainage of CSF can also reduce intracranial pressure.

AXIOM   An intracranial ventricular catheter in patients with severe brain injury allows one to monitor the ICP and reduce it as needed by withdrawing CSF.

ASPIRATION

The trauma victim is at risk for aspiration from the time of the injury until after the trachea is intubated. Hypotension, alcohol, recreational drugs, and induction of anesthesia have all been implicated in increasing the risk of aspiration. Intubation of unstable patients at the scene or upon arrival in the emergency center can help prevent continued silent aspiration of gastric or pharyngeal contents into the lungs. Also, sedative or analgesic drugs should be carefully titrated to avoid excessive depression of airway protection reflexes. Care must also be taken in the immediate postoperative period as the trauma victim may continue to have delayed gastric emptying due to an ileus or administration of narcotics.

If aspiration does occur, the tracheobronchial tree should be promptly suctioned clear, and bronchoscopy should be performed to remove any remaining large particulate matter. Supportive therapy with PEEP, oxygen, and controlled ventilation should be provided as needed, based upon serial blood gas analyses.

AXIOM   If aspiration of gastric contents into the lungs is suspected, bronchoscopy should be performed as soon as possible to confirm the diagnosis and to remove any accessible food particles or foreign bodies.

MAINTENANCE OF GENERAL ANESTHESIA

Initial maintenance of general anesthesia is usually safest with low concentrations of a volatile inhalation anesthetic carried in 100% oxygen. Until the patient is fully resuscitated and stable, it is probably wise to avoid nitrous oxide which precludes the use of high inspired oxygen tensions (FiO_2). Nitrous oxide also has the potential to increase the size of a pneumothorax, bowel gas, and air bubbles in the circulation.[72] Blunt trauma patients may also have compromised lung function due to pulmonary contusion, making an elevated FiO_2 even more desirable. In prolonged surgical procedures, the FiO_2 is adjusted by blood gas analyses and oxygen transport variables.

AXIOM   Nitrous oxide should generally be avoided in patients with severe chest or abdominal trauma.

Small doses of narcotic analgesics should be titrated cautiously into the patient while resuscitation is in progress because there may be little or no response while the patient is hypovolemic, but a delayed and exaggerated response may occur after perfusion has been restored. Muscle relaxants are generally given as needed except when patient movement might seriously endanger the procedure (e.g., during a craniotomy). As resuscitation becomes more complete, the depth of anesthesia can usually be increased to a more secure level, and the choice of agents is less critical.

PREGNANCY

AXIOM Displacement of the uterus to the left, off the inferior vena cava, and fetal monitoring are important aspects of anesthetic management in pregnant trauma patients.

The trauma team must be aware of the physiologic changes seen in pregnancy and take these changes into account when planning surgical and anesthetic management.[72] Continuous fetal monitoring, if the surgical site permits, can provide ongoing evidence of the adequacy of the fetal and maternal circulation. After 3 to 4 months of pregnancy, turning the patient 10-15° to the left may alleviate maternal hypotension from aortocaval compression by the uterus. Hypotension unresponsive to rapid, adequate volume replacement is best treated with an indirect vasopressor, such as ephedrine, that also has significant beta-adrenergic activity.[74] Postoperatively, fetal monitoring and left uterine displacement should be continued (Table 6-9).

LOCAL ANESTHESIA
Local anesthesia has a definite role in elective surgical procedures performed on carefully evaluated, motivated, and cooperative patients.[2] In the trauma setting, local anesthesia is rarely chosen, except for the repair of superficial lacerations, the placement of thoracostomy tubes, or the placement of catheters for vascular access. Because of the tissue acidosis that may occur in trauma patients, local anesthetics can be less effective, and the likelihood of a systemic toxic episode is increased. Patient discomfort after the procedure may also increase so that the patient may require large doses of sedative or analgesic drugs.

Local anesthesia administered intraoperatively with the patient anesthetized, resuscitated, and at a normal pH can provide significant postoperative analgesia. A direct intrathoracic block of intercostal nerves with local anesthesia at the termination of a thoracotomy is a useful technique that can facilitate early weaning from mechanical ventilation. Other field blocks, using one of the longer acting local anesthetics, may be performed as required by the operative site and type of injury.

Whenever a field block is performed, communication between the surgeon and the anesthesiologist is mandatory. The combined effects of locally produced analgesia and the systemic effects of large doses of local anesthetic agents can result in a significant decrease in general anesthetic requirements. Failure to anticipate this reduction may result in systemic hypotension.

REGIONAL ANESTHESIA
Regional anesthetic techniques can be useful for single limb injuries, and they will usually not interfere with systemic sympathetic tone. Regional techniques also allow one to check the patient's level of consciousness or mental status following blunt head injury. However, if more extensive surgery than originally anticipated needs to be performed, the required amount of local anesthetic agent may exceed safe levels. The danger of toxicity is also increased in hypovolemic patients because the reduced hepatic and renal blood decrease the patient's ability to metabolize drugs.

Intravenous perfusion (Bier) blocks require little patient cooperation and can be performed on upper or lower extremities with equal success; however, care must be taken to choose a correctly sized tourniquet for the lower extremity. Almost any nonvascular extremity case can be performed under perfusion block, provided the surgeon allows the tourniquet to remain inflated for the entire procedure. When a heparin-locked catheter is used for the primary injection, a follow-up injection can be made intraoperatively if the surgical procedure takes longer than expected.[75]

Formal nerve blocks in an upper or lower extremity require more cooperation from the patient than local anesthesia because the elicitation of paresthesias may be required or unavoidable; however, extended analgesia and sympathetic blockade of the extremity can be attained. In the upper extremity, placing a catheter in the axillary sheath usually provides excellent anesthesia for limb or digit replantations.

AXIOM The main disadvantage of regional anesthesia is that the amount of anesthetic required usually limits the anesthetic technique to only one extremity.

SPINAL OR EPIDURAL ANESTHESIA
The use of spinal or epidural anesthesia in acute trauma patients is a debatable issue (Table 6-10). For cooperative, stable patients, they can provide a safe, comfortable, and non-stressful method for performing surgical procedures on the lower limbs. In addition, epidural techniques can be continued into the postoperative period, when they can provide superb analgesia. Epidural analgesia can also provide other benefits, such as decreases in the stress response, postoperative complications, and overall hospital stay.[76,77]

TABLE 6-9 Guidelines for Anesthetic Management of Pregnant Trauma Patients

1. If possible, delay surgery until second trimester.
2. Note that emergency surgery is best done with regional anesthesia.
3. Visit the patient before surgery to relieve anxiety.
4. Use barbiturates or narcotics instead of benzodiazepines for premedication.
5. Use glycopyrrolate instead of atropine.
6. Empty stomach before induction of anesthesia.
7. Provide left uterine displacement.
8. With general anesthesia, use rapid-sequence induction.
9. Keep nitrous oxide at less than 50%.
10. With regional anesthesia, treat hypotension aggressively.
11. Monitor fetal heart rate if gestational age later than 16 weeks.
12. Record uterine activity and treat preterm labor both intraoperatively and postoperatively.

From Prentice-Berkseth RL, Weinberg RM, Ramanathan S. Anesthesia for Obstetric Trauma patients. In Grande CM. Textbook of Trauma Anesthesia & Critical Care. Mosby Yearbook, St. Louis 1993 p. 640.

TABLE 6-10 Indications and Contraindications for Spinal and Epidural Anesthesia in the Trauma Patient

Indications	Contraindications
Cooperative patient	Uncooperative patient
Agreement by surgeon	Acute central nervous system trauma
	Need for PRN neurological assessment
	Vertebral fracture
	Previous back surgery or injury
Cardiovascular stability	Hemorrhagic shock
	Hypovolemia
	Uncontrolled hemorrhage
	Hypotension
Compromised upper airway	Exploratory laparotomy
"Full stomach"	
Postoperative and injury analgesia	Inadequate facilities for postoperative epidural analgesia management
Fractured ribs	
Laparotomy	
Lower limb surgery or injury	

Although spinal or epidural anesthesia is often safer when there is an upper airway problem or there is a possibility of a full stomach, an accidental "total spinal" anesthetic through an intrathecally placed epidural catheter or an inadvertently high spinal anesthetic can embarrass ventilation.

AXIOM	One should take every precaution to not allow an epidural or low spinal anesthetic to become a total spinal anesthetic with resultant inadequate spontaneous ventilation.

If high spinal anesthesia occurs, the patient's ability to ventilate spontaneously or cough adequately is compromised. Under such circumstances, emergency endotracheal intubation can be extremely difficult. Two other problems associated with spinal or epidural anesthesia also reduce the frequency with which they are chosen for trauma patients. First, the patient must be positioned with the back exposed and then retained in the lateral decubitus, sitting, or prone position for at least 10 to 30 minutes to allow placement of the needle and/or catheter after skin preparation, local anesthesia, and draping of the patient. The traumatized patient with multiple injuries frequently cannot tolerate these positions because of pain or circulatory or respiratory compromise.

Another problem is the sympathetic block accompanying the sensory analgesia and motor paralysis of a neuraxis block.[78] The extent of the sympathetic block correlates with the extent of sensory anesthesia so that a patient who is anesthetized enough to permit a thorough intra-abdominal examination will generally also have an extensive sympathetic block.

AXIOM	One must be sure to prevent or rapidly correct hypovolemia in patients receiving spinal or epidural anesthesia.

The induction of a sympathetic block in a patient with reduced circulating blood volume may cause severe refractory hypotension.[78] This is especially likely to occur if conduction anesthesia is chosen for patients with pelvic or lower extremity fractures in which patients can lose 1 to 2 liters of blood without external manifestations. A stable patient under spinal anesthesia in whom rapid bleeding develops intraoperatively is more difficult to manage than a similar patient under general anesthesia.

AXIOM	Spinal or epidural techniques should be avoided if there may be pre-existing hypovolemia or if there is any expectation of significant intraoperative bleeding.

Exploratory laparotomy for trauma is usually too big an operation for spinal or epidural techniques, particularly if there is any likelihood for the procedure to extend into the upper abdomen. The lower surface of the diaphragm is innervated by the fourth cervical segment via the phrenic nerves, and it will remain sensitive even when the rest of the abdomen is adequately blocked.

Monitoring and Vascular Access

ADDITIONAL MONITORING AND INTRAVENOUS LINES
Once the airway is secured and the patient is well-oxygenated and anesthetized, consideration should be given to inserting catheters as needed for further resuscitation and monitoring, especially if the patient is unstable or may develop severe bleeding. If not already in use, ECG leads, pulse oximeter, and an esophageal temperature probe can be placed. Additional intravenous lines, preferably wide-bore venous cannulas, may also be needed and may have to be inserted by cutdown.

AXIOM	A single large intravenous cannula with a fast infusion device is safer and easier to control than 2-3 smaller intravenous lines with "pumpers."

Fluid resuscitation via inadequate intravenous cannulas leads to the wasteful and tedious necessity of using a team of "pumpers" to force in adequate fluid to keep up with surgical and traumatic hemorrhage. A single fast infusion device, with a wide-bore cannula, usually enables a single anesthesiologist to manage the fluid administration and the anesthetic with just the aid of someone to help change the bags of fluid.

INTRAVASCULAR MONITORING CATHETERS
The next priority is likely to be an arterial catheter for blood pressure monitoring and for frequent blood sampling. If the patient is still not stable, a central venous catheter should be inserted. This will allow the more certain administration of intravenous medications, central venous pressure measurement and sampling, and access for a pulmonary artery catheter if the patient's status does not improve.

AXIOM	Continued need for circulatory support, even in the face of massive fluid resuscitation, generally is due to continued bleeding and hypovolemia.

DIFFERENTIAL DIAGNOSIS OF CONTINUED HYPOTENSION
If hypovolemia has somehow been ruled out as a cause of continued hypotension, other diagnoses, such as tension pneumothorax or pericardial tamponade, should be considered. Tension pneumothorax, in particular, is easily overlooked until the patient has nearly arrested.

AXIOM	In the trauma patient with continuing hypotension, one should always be looking for continued hypovolemia, cardiac tamponade, and tension pneumothorax.

MONITORING PRELOAD
Measurement of left and right ventricular preload (via PAWP and CVP catheters), airway pressure, and cardiac output, particularly in relation to a fluid challenge, will often help sort out the differential diagnosis of an inadequate blood pressure. Central venous pressure is a good guide to the adequacy of volume resuscitation in patients without significant pre-existing cardiac disease. Pulmonary artery catheterization, possibly with a fiberoptic oxygen saturation measuring device, is useful in patients with a history of pulmonary disease, cardiac failure, or prior myocardial infarction. It can also be useful if large doses of barbiturates are needed to lower the ICP.[80] These drugs can cause significant circulatory depression, making the measurement of pulmonary artery wedge pressures helpful.

Recent evidence suggests that there is a large component of right ventricular failure in trauma patients who die later.[2] The availability of balloon-directed pulmonary artery catheters that can be used to measure right ventricular performance will bring such determinations within reach of most clinicians. Whether such interventions will modify survival rates in trauma victims experiencing right ventricular dysfunction has yet to be determined.

URINE OUTPUT
Urine output can be a useful measurement of circulatory function, provided the patient does not have to excrete an osmotic load (e.g., radiographic contrast media, mannitol, or glucose) or has not received diuretics. After severe trauma, there may be a lag of up to 2 hours following adequate crystalloid resuscitation before antidiuretic hormone levels are low enough to allow the kidneys to open up and produce an adequate urine output of at least 0.5-1.0 ml/kg/hr.

AIR EMBOLISM
Air embolism, traditionally associated with neurosurgical operations with the head elevated, has also become recognized as an ever-present danger during other procedures. This is true whenever there is any surgery in which the affected part is elevated in relation to the heart and the central venous pressure.[79] A low venous pressure during a hypovolemic episode increases the risk of air embolism. The use of

nitrous oxide, which can increase the size of air bubbles in the circulation, also increases the risk. Whenever air embolism is suspected, nitrous oxide must be discontinued and the patient ventilated with 100% oxygen.[2] Placing the patient on the left side with the operating table tipped head down will help alleviate the effects of air trapped in the right ventricular outflow tract.

Detection of air embolism in the trauma patient under anesthesia may be difficult. The warning signs of hypotension and changes in the central venous pressure are common and easily attributed to other causes. The classic mill-wheel murmur may not be heard in a noisy operating room; however, a sudden rise in end-tidal nitrogen concentration is diagnostic. The increasing availability of mass spectrometry should facilitate this diagnosis in the future.

AXIOM Mass spectrometric monitoring of exhaled gases can help make an early diagnosis of intraoperative complications, especially air embolism.

Venous air embolism is a common accompaniment of pulmonary injury.[2] The anesthesiologist should make every effort to reduce peak airway pressures in the injured lung or even to eliminate ventilation on the injured side with an elective one-lung endobronchial intubation. This can be accomplished with a smaller endotracheal tube or, preferably, with a specially designed double lumen tube.

AXIOM If air embolism from an injured lung is suspected, emergency thoracotomy with surgical occlusion of the vascular structures at the pulmonary hilum and aspiration of cardiac chambers and the aorta will help prevent it from continuing.

Advanced Monitoring and Intraoperative Investigations

AXIOM Monitoring is not an end in itself. Without an appropriate reaction to data, the system is useless.

The traditional "vital signs" of blood pressure, heart rate and respiratory rate, and even more sophisticated intravascular pressures can all be in the normal range, but have little relationship either to prognosis or blood volume.[63] In one prospective clinical study of patients who were bleeding, half of the patients who subsequently developed renal failure had no documented episode of hypotension.[80]

OXYGEN DELIVERY AND CONSUMPTION

If resuscitation from hemorrhage or trauma is not rapidly achieved, the parameters of oxygen delivery (DO_2) and uptake (VO_2) have important prognostic significance and should be calculated. Such calculations involve determining cardiac output, and obtaining arterial and venous blood gases or oxygen saturations. Even though the patient is anesthetized, he or she should have a normal VO_2 (120-160 ml/min/m²) or higher. Patients recovering from a general anesthetic should be hypermetabolic,[81] with values at least 20% higher than normal.[65,82,83]

INCREASING OXYGEN DELIVERY

The first goal in treating a low VO_2 is to increase the DO_2 enough to satisfy the oxygen needs of the tissues. The initial efforts to increase DO_2 are to increase cardiac output by restoring or expanding the blood volume with aggressive fluid resuscitation. This should not only increase VO_2, but it should also reduce plasma lactate levels if they are elevated.[84]

When data indicate that fluid and blood resuscitation are not increasing DO_2 sufficiently to achieve an adequate VO_2, inotropic pharmacological support can be helpful.[85] If a pulmonary artery catheter is not in place, data derived from central venous blood gases may be used.[86]

LABORATORY STUDIES

To back up the invasive approach to monitoring, one needs an efficient stat laboratory service. Most of the measurements should only take a few seconds (e.g., automatic counter platelet count or CBC) or a few minutes (e.g., blood gases, hematocrit, electrolytes, glucose, urea). Even coagulation profiles should take as little as 20 minutes. Any delays beyond these and the obvious transport times of the blood to the laboratory need administrative attention.[87]

AXIOM A rapidly responsive laboratory and blood bank can remove much of the hassle in anesthetic management and emergency care of trauma victims.

Fluid Management and Blood Products

URINE OUTPUT AND HEMATOCRIT GOALS

The initial approach to fluid resuscitation during anesthesia is to give enough warmed crystalloid, colloid, and/or blood to maintain a mean blood pressure of at least 60 mm Hg (to maintain normal cerebral perfusion) and a urine output greater than 0.5 ml/kg/h. At the same time, the hematocrit should be kept above 20 to 25% in the previously fit patient, and 27 to 32% in patients with pre-existing cardiopulmonary disease.[58-61]

AUTOTRANSFUSION

The use of autotransfusion devices, when the patient is losing blood that can be retrieved into a suction system, may reduce the requirements for banked blood.[88,89] The reluctance of some anesthesiologists to use this technology may partly be based on manpower considerations and the frequent inability to provide the washed red cells in time to be useful during torrential hemorrhage.

CLUES TO HYPOVOLEMIA

Clues to hypovolemia in the anesthetized patient are low blood pressure, low ventricular filling pressures, low urine output, variations in pulse pressure during the mechanical ventilator cycle, and low arterial pH. If more advanced monitoring data are available, hypovolemia may be indicated by a low cardiac output with high systemic vascular resistance.

FRESH FROZEN PLASMA AND PLATELET CONCENTRATES

The use of fresh frozen plasma and platelet concentrates should be based on data indicating a coagulopathy, rather than formulas related to the amount of blood transfused. The blind prophylactic administration of these substances to patients receiving massive transfusions is inappropriate and wasteful.[90] In massive blood replacement, when coagulation laboratory backup is insufficient, thromboelastography may be a useful indicator of the need for component therapy.[91]

Core Temperature

CAUSES OF HYPOTHERMIA

The prevention of hypothermia in the acute trauma victim is one of the most difficult tasks assigned to the anesthesiologist. However, anesthesia with the associated loss of sympathetic tone results in increased cutaneous and peripheral blood flow, so that the surface-to-core temperature gradient is decreased. In addition, the hypothalamic responses that are triggered at lower temperatures are also impaired.[92]

The acute trauma patient is frequently chilled before surgery by exposure to a cool environment while poorly clad, by vasodilation with alcohol, by unwarmed intravenous infusions, and by hypovolemia. When body cavities are opened, heat loss increases from evaporation of large volumes of fluid off the surfaces of exposed viscera. As resuscitation proceeds, the circulation improves in the cold periphery, returning cold blood to the core. This can cause a paradoxical further decrease in rectal and bladder temperatures. If relaxant drugs are given, the patient cannot generate heat by shivering.

PHYSIOLOGICAL CHANGES WITH HYPOTHERMIA

The immediate complications of hypothermia are mainly cardiac and hematologic. By the time core temperature has dropped from 37° C to 28° C, the cardiac output is about half normal, blood viscosity has doubled (if the hematocrit is unchanged), and autoregulation and distribution mechanisms are passive. Below this level the heart has an increasing tendency to ventricular fibrillation.[107,108]

Moderate hypothermia (down to 31° C) may slow down a partially depleted coagulation cascade enough to promote severe bleeding. This can occur in spite of seemingly adequate coagulation profiles, which are measured in the laboratory at 37° C.

PREVENTION AND TREATMENT OF HYPOTHERMIA

AXIOM   The best way to keep a patient warm is not to let him get cold!

In the operating room, heated humidified gases (up to 42° C) can transfer quite large quantities of heat to the patient. Keeping the patient covered with forced air, warming blankets, or reflective wrappings and in a warm room also helps to maintain the body temperature. When possible, uninjured extremities as well as the patient's head should be wrapped in plastic to preserve body heat. Forced hot air warming devices (e.g., Bair Hugger, Augustine Medical, Minn.) have blankets designed for intraoperative use and can provide regional warming during surgery.

At the end of surgery, as the anesthetic wears off, thermoregulation becomes reinforced, and the patient may shiver if not narcotized or paralyzed. Shivering greatly increases VO_2, and this can severely lower venous oxygen saturation in patients unable to compensate by increasing cardiac output.[94]

Patients whose temperatures are above 34° C can usually be rewarmed by surface techniques. However, if the patient has a core temperature below 32° C, active rewarming methods should be used. During recovery from hypothermia, as the circulation begins to open up, there is generally need for additional fluid resuscitation.

AXIOM   A curious feature of warming after hypothermia is an increased sensitivity to non-depolarizing muscle relaxants, probably due to increased cholinesterase activity.

Adjuncture Maneuvers

MAINTENANCE OF NORMOXIA DURING MASSIVE TRANSFUSION

The maintenance of an adequate PaO_2 during massive transfusion depends on avoiding or treating the pulmonary edema that often causes the hypoxia. The tendency to pulmonary edema may be reduced somewhat by maintaining the colloid osmotic pressure in a relatively normal range with colloid solutions. Hetastarch is useful and cost-effective in this regard, although large doses have been implicated in coagulation failure. Pentastarch, because it has a lower molecular weight than hetastarch, has a shorter plasma half-life. There is also no evidence of coagulation dysfunction after intravenous administration of large volumes of this colloid volume expander. In the future, this volume expander may have a greater role in the resuscitation of hypovolemic trauma victims.

If hypoxia occurs, treatment is usually by ventilation with 100% oxygen. Maintenance of the cardiac output in the normal or high range and elevation of the hematocrit will help maintain adequate delivery of available oxygen.[95]

A progressive prolongation of the Q-T interval as seen on the ECG, particularly in individuals with heart failure or shock, is an indication for calcium administration. In persistently hypotensive patients with adequate fluid loading, pharmacologic maneuvers may be needed to increase cardiac output and peripheral resistance.[96] A continuous infusion of dopamine and/or dobutamine in doses of 5-20 ug/kg/min may be helpful. However, if the patient is acidotic, epinephrine may be more effective.[2] Care must be exercised when administering these agents to patients who are cold and acidotic, as the likelihood of producing a serious dysrhythmia is increased.

CONTROL OF ACIDOSIS DURING PROLONGED HYPOTENSION

Sodium bicarbonate may be required for the treatment of persistent severe metabolic acidosis (pH below 7.10) not responsive to other therapy. However, one must carefully monitor arterial and venous pH and PCO_2 and not allow the PCO_2 to rise above normal because it will increase the mortality rate. When the pH rises above 7.20, bicarbonate administration should be discontinued to prevent development of an "overshoot alkalosis."

The release of acid metabolites must be anticipated, and bicarbonate administered prophylactically whenever a portion of the patient's body is reperfused, particularly after prolonged ischemia. The largest acid load results from releasing the cross-clamp on the descending thoracic or supraceliac abdominal aorta.

POSTOPERATIVE MANAGEMENT

After surgery is completed, recovery from anesthesia may prove to be another difficult period for the anesthesiologist. The patient may be cold, in pain, not fully rousable, very restless, and shivering. The full stomach precaution of endotracheal intubation should be continued until the patient is awake and responsive enough to have intact protective airway reflexes.

PITFALL ⊘

Aspiration of gastric contents can occur in the post-anesthesia care unit, and special precautions must be taken until the patient is awake enough to have intact protective airway reflexes.

Early Recovery Room and ICU Care

Transfer to the PACU or SICU is as demanding of attention by the anesthesiologist as the period of intraoperative resuscitation.[2] Respiratory support with controlled ventilation, PEEP, and high concentrations of oxygen should be maintained at the same level as provided intraoperatively. A battery-powered pulse oximeter allows continuous measurement of arterial oxygen saturation during transport. The ECG and intra-arterial pressure should also be monitored electronically enroute to the recovery room or ICU. Small, lightweight, battery-powered infusion devices make continuous drug infusions during transport quite safe and convenient. Finally, adequate personnel to physically move the patient's bed, ventilator, and other equipment should be available so that the anesthesiologist can concentrate on monitoring and ventilation.

Excessive Adrenergic Activity

The patient waking from a general anesthetic will often have a period of severe sympathetic overactivity. This may be demonstrated by hypertension and/or tachycardia that may reach levels requiring immediate treatment. The question that must be answered is whether to sedate and mechanically ventilate the patient, or to extubate him so that he can be made more comfortable.

The blood pressure can usually be brought under control with a short-acting beta-blocker (e.g., esmolol, Brevibloc[R], Dupont). Sodium nitroprusside infusions are rarely needed. However, it is important to keep the patient as comfortable as possible and in warm surroundings.

Renarcotization

The patient, in the absence of painful surgical stimuli, may "renarcotize" himself when the blood levels of opiate medications mobilized from extravascular tissue become higher than needed. If there have been acid-base and electrolyte abnormalities, the reversal of muscle relaxants may also have been inadequate during the surgery. In addition, fluid shifts and continued bleeding may unmask an unsuspected hypovolemia.

Continued Monitoring

The monitoring and vigilance of the operating room has to be continued into the postoperative period, preferably in a critical care area. The handing-over process should be standardized, so that the patient does not get into difficulties through a lack of continuity of care.

AXIOM Lack of adequate communication between anesthesia and intensive care unit personnel is one of the major causes of suboptimal ICU care immediately following surgery.

⊘ FREQUENT ERRORS

In the Anesthetic Management of Critically Injured Patients

1. *Failing to take full advantage of whatever time is available to evaluate the patient before providing anesthesia.*
2. *Delaying surgery for diagnostic studies that are not immediately necessary for providing a safe, effective anesthetic.*
3. *Failing to have an emergency drug and equipment setup ready on a 24-hour basis.*
4. *Allowing oneself to be rushed into a method of anesthetic management that, on reflection, one would not ordinarily choose.*
5. *Failing to anesthetize the patient adequately before starting endotracheal intubation.*
6. *Beginning a general anesthetic without adequate routes of intravenous administration and without adequate blood products or substitutes immediately available.*
7. *Giving too much medication to patients scheduled for imminent operation, particularly during the induction phase of anesthetic management.*
8. *Failing to anticipate and be prepared for the possibility of regurgitation and resultant aspiration during endotracheal intubation.*
9. *Failing to have an adequate plan and necessary equipment to manage a failed intubation.*
10. *Failing to anticipate anesthetic problems based on the patient's mechanism of injury.*
11. *Failing to communicate with others involved in the anesthetic-surgical management of the patient.*
12. *Failing to maintain vigilance immediately after surgery and during transfer to the recovery room or ICU.*

▼▼▼▼▼▼▼▼▼▼▼▼▼▼▼▼▼▼▼▼▼▼▼▼▼▼▼▼▼▼▼

SUMMARY POINTS

1. Although there is such a thing as "minor surgery," there is no such thing as a "minor anesthetic."
2. The trauma anesthesia/critical care specialist may represent the ultimate life support physician.
3. A well-designed trauma protocol should provide the level of care to injured patients at 2:00 a.m. that is available when the most experienced members of the team are present at 2:00 p.m.
4. When the anesthesiologist and the surgeon each "do his own thing" without being aware of the other's problems, the patient's care is not likely to be optimal.
5. Operative procedures should be prioritized in the event that the patient's condition deteriorates so badly that surgery must be discontinued.
6. All areas of the hospital that are likely to receive acutely com-

promised patients should be equipped to provide immediate endotracheal intubation.
7. Being prepared for an airway emergency is more than half the battle.
8. Critically injured patients with impending ventilatory failure should be intubated immediately by the most experienced individual present.
9. If airway control is the first priority, oral endotracheal intubation is usually the preferred method.
10. Inadequate preintubation assessment and planning increases the likelihood that unnecessary emergencies will develop later.
11. Aspiration of vomitus or blood into the lungs can occur suddenly any time before surgery, but it is most apt to occur when inducing anesthesia and instrumenting the upper airway.
12. Unless there is significant nasal deformity, patients needing awake intubation will usually tolerate the nasal route better than the oral.
13. Most patients in severe circulatory shock will tolerate direct laryngoscopy and intubation without too much fighting.
14. During induction of anesthesia on a patient with recent trauma, special efforts are required to prevent regurgitation of gastric contents into the lungs.
15. The most challenging airway problem in trauma is the patient with an acute, severe airway obstruction.
16. Rendering a patient apneic, when endotracheal intubation in that patient is beyond the skill of the operator, may be rapidly fatal.
17. Systemic vasodilators can be used to correct hypertension, but they may also increase ICP in patients with severe head injuries.
18. If intubation is performed before any spine films can be obtained, the patient should be kept in a rigid cervical collar until cervical spine injury has been ruled out.
19. Before one attempts endotracheal intubation, particularly on an unstable trauma patient, an alternate technique for rapidly providing an airway should be immediately available.
20. Muscle relaxants are not anesthetics.
21. Being awake and paralyzed can be a very terrifying experience for the patient.
22. One should make a special effort to ensure that intravenous tubing cannot disconnect from large central intravenous catheters.
23. If a large bore central venous cannula accidently disconnects, air embolism can be rapidly fatal.
24. Failure of the patient to respond appropriately to what should be adequate resuscitative fluid is an indication for CVP or PAWP monitoring.
25. Premedication designed to reduce patient anxiety is contraindicated for most trauma victims, especially if they are hemodynamically unstable.
26. Titrated small doses of intravenous narcotics are generally the safest premedication for anesthesia.
27. Although pain from trauma may be of a magnitude demanding larger than normal amounts of narcotic analgesics, the sensitivity of the patient to these agents may be considerably increased.
28. Patients in traumatic or hemorrhagic shock are often acutely insensitive to SQ or IM drugs and oversensitive to intravenous agents.
29. If patients cannot be made aware of the danger their lack of cooperation is causing, cautious sedation or general anesthesia should be used, as needed, to provide lifesaving treatment.
30. Before an analgesic or sedative is given to a head-injured patient, that patient should be examined by the neurosurgeon or whoever will be responsible for the definitive care.
31. Much of the discomforts of a trauma patient can be reduced or corrected without using drugs.
32. One of the best treatments for anxiety is reassurance and explanations by a calm, considerate individual.
33. Hospital protocols outlining the equipment and personnel involved in monitoring and caring for trauma patients during transport should be worked out in advance.
34. The caliber of a trauma service is inversely related to the num-

ber of cardiac arrests that take place outside the emergency department and operating room.

35. One should not assume that a trauma patient has an empty stomach because he or she has supposedly not eaten for 6 or more hours.

36. Many patients, especially the elderly, can have significant, but inapparent, red blood cell and blood volume deficits after trauma.

37. One should not assume that normal hemoglobin and hematocrit levels in a trauma patient indicate that the blood volume and red blood cell mass are also normal.

38. Hypoglycemia may occur in some patients with severe alcoholism or cirrhosis, but the great majority of acute trauma patients are hyperglycemic due to the stress hormone response.

39. Every effort should be made to prevent or rapidly correct hypothermia in patients with severe trauma undergoing major surgery.

40. General anesthesia is usually the technique of choice for unstable trauma patients because the principles of airway management and respiratory and circulatory support common to all general anesthetics are the basic ingredients of cardiopulmonary resuscitation.

41. General anesthesia for trauma victims should be induced with the minimum amount of agent that will obtund consciousness and provide needed relaxation.

42. If the depth of anesthesia is reduced to maintain an adequate blood pressure, patients may become aware that they are having a surgical procedure and have severe pain and anxiety without being able to show it.

43. Hypertension must be prevented or rapidly corrected if a traumatic rupture of the thoracic aorta is suspected.

44. Even if the ICP is elevated in patients with brain injury, adequate fluid must be given to maintain a normal or slightly increased BP.

45. An intracranial ventricular catheter in patients with severe brain injury allows one to monitor the ICP and reduce it as needed by withdrawing CSF.

46. If aspiration of gastric contents into the lungs is suspected, bronchoscopy should be performed as soon as possible to confirm the diagnosis and remove any accessible food particles or foreign bodies.

47. Nitrous oxide should generally be avoided in patients with severe chest or abdominal trauma.

48. Displacement of the uterus to the left, off the inferior vena cava, and fetal monitoring are important aspects of anesthetic management in pregnant trauma patients.

49. The main disadvantage of regional anesthesia is that the amount of anesthetic required usually limits the anesthetic technique to only one extremity.

50. One should take every precaution to not allow an epidural or low spinal anesthetic to become a total spinal anesthetic with resultant inadequate spontaneous ventilation.

51. One must be sure to prevent or rapidly correct hypovolemia in patients receiving spinal or epidural anesthesia.

52. Spinal or epidural techniques should be avoided if there may be pre-existing hypovolemia or if there is any expectation of significant intraoperative bleeding.

53. A single large intravenous cannula with a fast infusion device is safer and easier to control than 2-3 smaller intravenous lines with "pumpers."

54. Continued need for circulatory support, even in the face of massive fluid resuscitation, generally is due to continued bleeding and hypovolemia.

55. In the trauma patient with continuing hypotension, one should always be looking for continued hypovolemia, cardiac tamponade, and tension pneumothorax.

56. Mass spectrometic monitoring of exhaled gases can help make an early diagnosis of intraoperative complications, especially air embolism.

57. If air embolism from an injured lung is suspected, emergency thoracotomy with surgical occlusion of the vascular structures at the pulmonary hilum and aspiration of cardiac chambers and the aorta can help prevent it from continuing.

58. Monitoring is not an end in itself. Without an appropriate reaction to data, the system is useless.

59. A rapidly responsive laboratory and blood bank can remove much of the hassle in anesthetic management and emergency care of trauma victims.

60. The best way to keep a patient warm is not to let him get cold!

61. A curious feature of warming after hypothermia is increased sensitivity to non-depolarizing muscle relaxants, probably due to increased cholinesterase activity.

62. Aspiration of gastric contents can occur in the post-anesthesia care unit, and special precautions must be taken until the patient is awake enough to have intact protective airway reflexes.

63. Lack of adequate communication between anesthesia and intensive care unit personnel is one of the major causes of suboptimal ICU care immediately following surgery.

▲▲▲▲▲▲▲▲▲▲▲▲▲▲▲▲▲▲▲▲▲▲▲▲▲▲▲▲▲▲▲▲▲▲▲▲

REFERENCES

1. Baker SP. Injuries: the neglected epidemic. J Trauma 1987;27:343.
2. Coveler LA. Anesthesia. In: Moore EE, Mattox KL, Feliciano DV, eds. Trauma. 2nd ed. Norwalk, CT: Appleton & Lange, 1991:219-229.
3. American College of Surgeons Committee on Trauma. Advanced Trauma Life Support Course for Physicians. Chicago, 1988.
4. Grande CM. The trauma anesthesia/critical care specialist. In: Grande CM, ed. Textbook of trauma anesthesia and critical care. St. Louis: Mosby, 1993:93.
5. Hopkins JA, Shoemaker WC, Chang PC, et al. Clinical trial of an emergency resuscitation algorithm. Crit Care Med 1983;11:621.
6. Shoemaker WC, Hopkins JA. Clinical aspects of resuscitation with or without an algorithm: relative importance of various decisions. Crit Care Med 1983;11:630.
7. Optimal Resources for the Care of the Injured Patient. American College of Surgeons Committee on Trauma.
8. Abrams KJ. Preanesthetic evaluation. In: Grande CM, ed. Textbook of trauma anesthesia and critical care. St. Louis: Mosby, 1993:421.
9. Cicala RS, Grande CM, Stene JR, et al. Emergency and elective airway management for trauma patients. In: Grande CM, ed. Textbook of trauma anesthesia and critical care. St. Louis: Mosby, 1993:344.
10. Benunof JL, Schiller MS. The importance of transtracheal jet ventilation in the management of the difficult airway. Anesthesiology 1989; 71:769.
11. Grande CM. Airway management of the trauma patient in the resuscitation area of the trauma center. Trauma Quarterly 1983;5:30.
12. Wright SW, Robinson GG, Wright MB. Cervical spine injuries in blunt trauma patients requiring emergent endotracheal intubation. Am J Emerg Med 1992;10:104.
13. Gotta AW, Sullivan, CA. Anesthesia of the upper airway using topical anesthetic and superior laryngeal nerve block. Br J Anaesth 1981;53:1055.
14. Danzl DF, Thomas DM. Nasotracheal intubation in the emergency department. Crit Care Med 1980;8:677.
15. O'Brien DJ, Danzl DF, Souers B, et al. Airway management of aeromedically transported trauma patients. J Emerg Med 1988;6:49.
16. Dronen SC, Merigan KS, Hoekjtra JW, et al. A comparison of blind nasotracheal and succinylcholine assisted intubation in the poisoned patient. Ann Emerg Med 1987;16:650.
17. Bogdunoff DL, Stone DJ. Emergency management of the airway outside of the operating room. Can J Anesth 1992;39:1069.
18. Wall RM. Airway management. Emerg Med Clinics NA 1993;11:53.
19. Holley J, Jordand RC. Airway management in patients with unstable cervical spine fractures. Am J Emerg Med 1989;18:151.
20. Rhee KJ, Green W, Holocroft JW, et al. Oral intubation in the multiply injured patient: the risk of exacerbating spinal cord damage. Ann Emerg Med 1990;19:511.
21. Joyce TH III. Prophylaxis for pulmonary acid aspiration. Am J Med 1987;83:46.
22. Libomatti MM, Leaky JJ, Ellison N. The use of succinylcholine in open eye surgery. Anesthesiology 1985;62:637.
23. Foldes F. Rapid tracheal intubation with nondepolarizing neuromuscular blocking drugs: the priming principle. Br J Anesth 1984;56:663.
24. Gergis SD, Sokoll MD, Mehta M, et al. Intubation conditions after atracurium and suxemethonium. Br J Anaesth 1983;55(Suppl):83S.

25. Lennon RL, Olson RA, Gronert GA. Atracurium or vecuronium for rapid response endotracheal intubation. Anesthesiology 1926;64:510.
26. Schecter WP, Wilson RS. Management of upper airway obstruction in the ICU. Crit Care Med 1981;9:577-9.
27. Salvino CK, Dries D, Gamelli R, et al. Emergency cricothyroidotomy in trauma victims. J Trauma 1993;34:503.
28. Spoerel WE, Narayann PS, Singh NP. Transtracheal ventilation. Br J Anaesth 1971;43:932.
29. Smith RB, Schaer WB, Pfaeffle H. Percutaneous transtracheal ventilation for anaesthesia and resuscitation: a review and report of complications. Can Anaesth Soc J 1975;22:607.
30. Gaughan S, Ozaki G, Benemol JL. Can anesthesia machine flush valves provide effective jet ventilation. Anesthesiology 1991;75:A130.
31. Lechman MJ, Donahoo JS, MacVauch H III. Endotracheal intubation using percutaneous guide wire insertion followed by antegrade fiberoptic bronchoscopy. Crit Care Med 1986;14:589.
32. King, HR, Wang LF, Khan AK, Wooton OJ. Translaryngeal guided intubation for difficult intubation. Crit Care Med 1987;15:869.
33. Orshaker JS, Whye DW. Head trauma. Emerg Med Clin NA 1993;11:165.
34. Pfenninger E, Ahnefeld FM, et al. Blood gases at the scene of the accident and on admission to hospital following craniocerebral trauma. Anaesthetist 1987;36:570-576.
35. Leeman M, Naeye R, Degaulte JP, et al. Acute central and renal hemodynamic responses to tertatolol and propranolol in patients with arterial hypertension following head injury. J Hypertension 1986;4:581.
36. Gupta B, Cottrell JE. Nitroprusside and nitroglycerine induced intracranial pressure changes. In: Shulman K, Marmarou A, Miller JD, et al, eds. Intracranial pressure IV. Berlin: Springer-Verlag, 1980:613.
37. Cottrell J, Patel K, Ransohoff J, et al. Intracranial pressure changes induced by sodium nitroprusside in patients with intracranial mass lesions. J Neurosurg 1978;48:329.
38. Hastings RH, Marks JD. Airway management for trauma patients with potential cervical spine injuries. Anesth Analg 1991;73:471.
39. Meschino A, Devitt JH, Koch JP, et al. The safety of awake tracheal intubation in cervical spine injury. Can J Anesth 1992;39:114.
40. Walls RM. Airway management in the blunt trauma patient: how important is the cervical spine? Can J Surg 1992;35:27.
41. Gajraj NM, Pennant JH, Giesecke AH. Cervical spine trauma and airway management. Current Opinion in Anesth 1993;6:369.
42. Grande CM, Barton CR, Stene JK. Appropriate techniques for airway management of emergency patients with suspected spinal cord injury. Anesth Analg 1988;67:714.
43. Capan LM, Miller SM, Glickman R. Management of facial injuries. In: Capan LM, Miller MM, Turndorf H, eds. Trauma anesthesia and intensive care. New York: JB Lippincott, 1991:385.
44. ASA Task Force on Management of the Difficult Airway. Practice guidelines for management of the difficult airway. Anesthesiology 1993;78:597.
45. Spoerel WE, Nayaranan PS, Singh NP. Transtracheal cricothyroidotomy in trauma victims. J Trauma 1993;34:503.
46. Klain M, Keszler H, Brader E. High frequency jet ventilation in CPR. Crit Care Med 1981;9:421.
47. Pennant JH, Walker MB. Comparison of the endotracheal tube and laryngeal mask in airway management by paramedical personnel. Anesth Analg 1992;74:531.
48. Editorial: paralyzed with fear. Lancet 1981;1:427.
49. Vitello-Cicciu JM. Recalled perceptions of patients administered pancuronium bromide. Focus on Crit Care 1984;11:28.
50. Landow L, Shahnarian A. Efficacy of large-bore fluid administration sets designed for rapid volume resuscitation. Crit Care Med 1990;18:540.
51. Shoemaker WC. Pericardial tamponade. In: Shoemaker WC, Ayres SM, Grenvik A, et al, eds. Textbook of critical care. Philadelphia: WB Saunders, 1989:440.
52. Mattox KL, Bickell WHO, Pepe PE, Mangelskdorff AD. Prospective randomized evaluation of antishock MAST in post-traumatic hypotension. J Trauma 1986;26:779.
53. Scalea TM, Houman M, Fuortes M, et al. Central venous blood oxygen saturation. An early accurate measurement of volume during hemorrhage. J Trauma 1988;28:725.
54. Rady MY, Rivers E, Martin GB, et al. Continuous central venous oximetry and shock index in the emergency department: use in the evaluation of clinical shock. Am J Emerg Med 1992;10:538.
55. Grande CM, Tissot M, Bhott VP, et al. Pre-existing compromising conditions. In: Capan LM, Miller SM, Turndorf H, eds. Trauma anesthesia and intensive care. New York: JB Lippincott, 1991:219.
56. Soderstrom CA, Cowley RA. A National Alcohol and Trauma Center survey. Arch Surg 1987;122:1067.
57. Stene JK. Anesthesia for trauma. In: Miller RD, ed. Anesthesia. 3rd ed. New York: Churchill Livingstone, 1990.
58. Abrams KJ, Nolan JP, Grande CM. Trauma anesthesia: anesthesiology's oldest specialty reborn. Crit Care Clin NA 1991;9:2;393.
59. Messmer K. Acute preoperative hemodilution: physiological basis and clinical application. In: Tuma RF, White JV, Messmer K, eds. The role of hemodilution in optimal patient care. Munchen: W. Zuckswerdt, 1989: 54-73.
60. Bryan-Brown CW. Systemic oxygen transport. In: Kaplan JA, ed. Thoracic anesthesia. 2nd ed. New York: Churchill Livingston, 1991:143-164.
61. Czer LSC, Shoemaker WC. Optimal hematocrit value in critically ill postoperative patients. Surg Gynecol Obstet 1978;147:363.
62. Fan FC, Chen RYZ, Schuessler GB, et al. Effects of hematocrit variations on regional hemodynamics and oxygen transport in the dog. Am J Physiol 1980;238 (Heart Circ Physiol 7:H545.
63. Shippy R, Appel PL, Shoemarker WC. Reliability of clinical monitoring to assess blood volume in critically ill patients. Crit Care Med 1984; 12:107.
64. Biron PE, Howard J, Altschule MD, et al. Chronic deficits in red-cell mass in patients with orthopaedic injuries (stress anemia). J Bone Joint Surg 1972;54-A:1001.
65. Shoemaker WC, Appel PL, Krom HB, et al. Prospective trial of supranormal values of survivors as therapeutic goals in high risk surgical patients. Chest 1988;94:1176.
66. Hackenberry LE, Miner ME, Rea GL, et al. Biochemical evidence of myocardial injury after severe head trauma. Crit Care Med 1982;10:641.
67. Bogetz MS, Katz JA. Recall of surgery for major trauma. Anesthesiology 1984;61:6.
68. Cicala RS, Stewart RM, Fabian T. Multisystem trauma priorities. In: Grande CM, ed. Textbook of trauma anesthesia and critical care. St. Louis: Mosby, 1993;502.
69. Lippman M, Appel PL, Mok MS, et al. Sequential cardiorespiratory patterns of anesthetic induction with ketamine in critically ill patients. Crit Care Med 1983;11:730.
70. Wagner RL, White PF. Etomidate inhibits adrenocortical function in surgical patients. Anesthesiology 1984;61:647.
71. Traeger SM, Henning RJ, Dobkin W, et al. Hemodynamic effects of pentobarbital therapy for intracranial hypertension. Crit Care Med 1983; 9:697.
72. Eger EI II, Saidman LJ. Hazards of nitrous oxide in bowel obstruction and pneumothorax. Anesthesiology 1965;26:61.
73. Skerman JH. Anesthetic management of the pregnant trauma patient. Semin Anes 1989;8:353.
74. Prentic-Berkwith RL, Weinberg RM, Ramanathan S. Anesthesia for obstretic trauma patients. In: Grande CM, ed. Textbook of trauma anesthesia and critical care. St. Louis: Mosby, 1993;628.
75. Murphy TM. Nerve blocks. In: Anesthesia. Miller RE, ed. New York: Churchill Livingstone, 1981;593.
76. Cuschieri RJ, Moran CG, Howie JC, et al. Postoperative pain and pulmonary complications: comparison of three analgesic regimens. Br J Surg 1985;72:495.
77. El-Baz N, Goldin M. Continuous epidural infusion of morphine for pain relief after cardiac operations. J Thorac Cardiovasc Surg 1987;93:878.
78. Dow AC. Regional anesthesia. In: Grande CM, ed. Textbook of trauma anesthesia and critical care. St. Louis: Mosby, 1993.
79. Spiess BD, Sloan MS, McCarthy RJ, et al. The incidence of air embolism during total hip arthroplasty. J Clin Anesth 1988;1:25.
80. Hou SH, Bushinsky DA, Wish JB, et al. Hospital acquired renal insufficiency: a prospective study. Am J Med 1983;74:243-248.
81. Kinney JM, Duke JH, Long CL, et al. Tissue fuel and weight loss after injury. J Clin Pathol 1970;23(Suppl 4):65.
82. Bland RD, Shoemaker WC, Abraham E, et al. Hemodynamic and oxygen transport patterns in surviving and non-surviving postoperative patients. Crit Care Med 1984;13:85.
83. Shoemaker WC, Appel PL, Kram HB. Tissue oxygen debt as a determinant of lethal and nonlethal postoperative organ failure. Crit Care Med 1988;16:1117.
84. Haupt MT, Gilbert EM, Carlson RW. Fluid loading increases oxygen consumption in septic patients with lactic acidosis. Am Rev Respir Dis 1985;131:912.
85. Shoemaker WC, Appel PL, Kram HB. Hemodynamic and oxygen transport effects of dobutamine in critically ill general surgical patients. Crit Care Med 1986;14:1032.

86. Reinhart K, Budolph T, Bredle DL, et al. Comparison of central-venous to mixed-venous oxygen saturation during changes in oxygen supply/demand. Chest 1989;95:1216.

87. Bryan-Brown CW, Bracey AW, Lorimor KK. Intraoperative monitoring of the liver transplant patient. Acute Care 1984;10:207.

88. Huth VF, Maier RV, Pavlin EG, Carrico CJ. Utilization of blood recycling in nonelective surgery. Arch Surg 1983;118:626.

89. Isbister JP. Autotransfusion: an impossible dream. Anaesth Intens Care 1984;12:236.

90. Reed LR II, Heimbach DM, Counts RB. Prophylactic platelet administration during massive transfusion. Ann Surg 1986;203:40.

91. Kang YG, Martin D, Marquez J, et al. Intraoperative changes in blood coagulation and thromboelastographic monitoring in liver transplantation. Anesth Analg 1985;64:888.

92. Hammel HT. Anesthetics and body temperature regulation. Anesthesiology 1988;68:833.

93. White JD. Cardiac arrest in hypothermia. JAMA 1980;244:2262.

94. Kaplan JA, Guffin AV. Shivering and changes in mixed venous oxygen saturation after cardiac surgery (abstract). Anesth Analg 1985;64:235.

95. Finch CA, Lenfant C. Oxygen transport in man. N Engl J Med 1972;286:407.

96. Denlinger JK, Nahrwold ML, Gibbs PS, et al. Hypocalcemia during rapid blood transfusion in anaesthetized man. Br J Anaesth 1976;48:995.

Chapter 7 Diagnostic and Interventional Radiology in Trauma

DANIEL R. GUYOT, M.D.

KATHLEEN A. McCARROLL, M.D.

ROBERT F. WILSON, M.D.

FACILITIES

During the 10-year period ending July 1990, more than 150,000 acute adult trauma victims have had x-ray examinations performed at Detroit Receiving Hospital. The experience with these patients forms the basis for most of the observations noted in this chapter.

X-ray examinations of traumatized patients are expedited by radiological facilities that are immediately adjacent to the emergency department (ED). While ambulatory patients can walk to a nearby radiology waiting room for their x-rays, severely injured patients are kept in the trauma resuscitation room (TRR) where they can be closely monitored and the x-ray department comes to them. An overhead mounted x-ray tube in the resuscitation room can be moved so that stat x-rays can be taken of patients on any of the stretchers in that area (Fig. 7-1). This overhead equipment is predominantly used to rapidly obtain supine chest and lateral cervical spine x-rays (Fig. 7-2) while resuscitation is still in progress.

Diagnostic radiology in hemodynamically unstable trauma patients is usually restricted to survey films of the cervical spine, chest, and pelvis. Patients who need emergency surgery do not have time for multiple films, and those who must undergo further examination should be examined in the radiology department. Installation of complex radiographic equipment in the ED encourages unnecessary examinations that may not be in the best interest of the patient.[1]

Patients who are stable but not ambulatory are able to travel on a stretcher to the x-ray department. These patients are kept in the ED until an x-ray examination room is available. Leaving patients unattended in the hall outside the x-ray rooms while waiting for their radiological examinations does not provide for optimal observation and monitoring of the injured patient. Proper diagnosis and management of injuries to the head,[2,3] neck, and torso[4-6] often demand early investigation by computed tomography (CT). This calls for installation in the hospital of at least one CT unit in proximity to the ED. An angiographic suite should also be readily available to the ED. Orthopedic radiology equipment should either be part of or adjacent to the fracture treatment unit.

In addition to the equipment that is usually available for operating room radiography, major trauma centers should give some consideration to a combined angiography-surgery room in which angiography, embolization, and surgery can be done simultaneously or in tandem. There is increasing use of interventional radiology in the acute management of hemorrhage, especially in pelvic fractures.[7-10]

RADIOLOGICAL DIAGNOSTIC MODALITIES IN ACUTE TRAUMA

Plain Film Radiography

Plain film radiography is still the best way to visualize the skeleton during the initial examination; however, it has only modest value in the assessment of anatomically complex regions, such as the pelvis, face, and the base of the skull, where it has been replaced or greatly supplemented by CT.

Plain film radiography for the diagnosis of soft-tissue injuries is inferior. Although plain films can offer partial and indirect evidence of wounding, they do not permit precise characterization of injuries, and they have high rates of false-positive and false-negative findings.

Contrast Studies and Fluoroscopy

The diagnosis of certain injuries is helped by the addition of fluoroscopy and contrast media to the plain film. This includes administration of contrast, as in esophagography, cystourethrography, or sinography, under direct visualization as well as injections of contrast medium, such as with intravenous pyelography (IVP).

The IVP has been the most commonly performed emergency study in suspected urologic trauma. However, CT scanning provides much better detail. Nevertheless, when properly done, a normal IVP can be accepted with only a slight risk of missing a major injury. When an IVP is done as a rapid preoperative test, its usefulness is limited to the determination of presence or absence of renal function in both kidneys. In patients who have suffered blunt abdominal trauma, one must often investigate all abdominal and extraperitoneal organs simultaneously. This creates a strong indication for CT and makes an IVP unnecessary. The urethra and bladder can also be reliably evaluated by CT.

Radionuclide Imaging

Radionuclide imaging (RN) has had extensive use in pediatric abdominal trauma; however, it has only limited application now that CT scans are available. Nevertheless, spleen scans may confirm a diagnosis of subcapsular hemorrhage. Liver scans are seldom indicated in the initial study of hepatic injury, but they can be helpful later when evaluating the patient for a possible hepatic hematoma or abscess or subphrenic collections. Hematobilia can also be evaluated using radioactive materials.

Scanning of the lungs can be helpful in the diagnosis of pulmonary embolism or other causes of reduced circulation to the lungs. Radionuclide pyrophosphate scans have been used in assessment of myocardial contusion but with mediocre success.[11] With continued technologic progress in this field, further application may be forthcoming.

Ultrasound

A number of applications of ultrasound are available to the acutely injured patient. Collections of fluid, particularly in the pericardium but also in the abdomen and retroperitoneum, may be studied noninvasively using this technique. Both ultrasonography and radionuclide imaging suffer from inherently low resolution. Even in skilled hands, ultrasound is not reliable for diagnosis of solid organ injury,

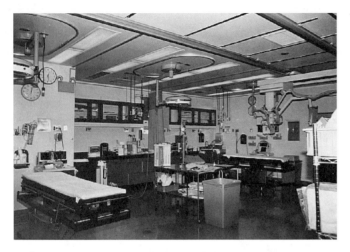

FIGURE 7-1   An overhead x-ray tube should be mounted in the trauma resuscitation room so that stat x-rays can be taken of patients on any of the stretchers in that area.

and it cannot differentiate intraperitoneal hemorrhage from other causes of intraperitoneal fluid, such as ascites.

Soft-tissue foreign bodies are a common clinical problem. Traditionally, radiographs have been used to identify radiopaque foreign bodies, and fluoroscopy has been used for guidance during surgical removal. Recently, however, sonography has been used in the detection, preoperative localization, and confirmation of surgical retrieval of foreign bodies in the distal extremities. In a recent report by Shields et al,[12] 20 localization procedures were performed in 19 patients with 21 foreign bodies including wood, glass, stone, metal, and pencil lead. The foreign bodies were visualized as hyperechoic foci with acoustic shadows that were partial or complete depending on the angle of insonation and foreign body composition. Hyperechoic comet-tail artifacts (reverberation artifacts) were seen with six metallic foreign bodies and one glass fragment. Nine foreign bodies were surrounded by hypoechoic halos caused by edema, abscess, or granulation tissue. A slow meticulous scanning technique and high-frequency transducer helped in detection of small foreign bodies. Sonographically guided removal of the foreign body was successful in all four patients in whom it was attempted. Scanning with the ultrasound beam parallel to the long axis of the hemostat and the foreign body was the fastest way to guide the hemostat to the tip of a foreign body.

Computerized Tomography

Of the various modalities of radiological imaging, computerized tomography (CT) is of the highest value to the traumatologist. CT combines high image resolution with the capacity to demonstrate soft-tissue and skeletal injuries simultaneously. It also differentiates between normal and abnormal soft tissue, delineates the extent of hematomas, detects intraperitoneal blood, and differentiates blood from ascitic and DPL fluid. In addition, it is unsurpassed in assessment and follow-up of head injuries, and it is being increasingly used for the diagnosis of penetrating abdominal trauma and vascular injuries.

Magnetic Resonance Imaging

Magnetic resonance imaging (MRI) will become an increasingly important diagnostic tool in trauma. Its ability to detect soft-tissue abnormalities, including changes in blood flow, is very promising. MRI may replace most methods of detecting abnormalities that hinge on metabolic changes, such as in cardiac contusion. It is currently the choice for evaluation of thoracic aortic dissection.

A major limitation of MRI is the length of time necessary to complete studies. In addition, life-support equipment containing ferromagnetic alloys cannot be allowed near the magnet. Equipment made of

nonferromagnetic materials and improvements in future generations of magnets should shorten the duration of studies and should also permit support personnel to stay with the patient.

Angiography

STANDARD TECHNIQUES

Angiography continues to be the most reliable, nonsurgical, direct diagnostic procedure for detection of vascular injury. Angiography should be performed whenever vascular injury is suspected and immediate surgery is not required. Examination of the abdominal and pelvic arteries is substantially more complex than peripheral arteriography and requires insertion of an intra-arterial catheter, fluoroscopic control, and serial filming. An intra-arterial catheter can usually be placed using the percutaneous Seldinger technique.

THERAPEUTIC ANGIOGRAPHY

Angiography should be done as a formal catheter study using film or digital matrix to record the study. Each angiogram, as with all radiographs, should be done in two views and should include a complete series of images or films showing the arterial, capillary, and venous phases.

Therapeutic angiography is also indicated in certain cases of arterial injury and hemorrhage and when hemostasis can be attained by the angiographer. Indeed, in an increasing number of cases, the radiologist can induce angiographic hemostasis with greater safety and speed and with far less mortality or morbidity than the surgeon. This is especially rewarding if the surgical approach is extremely hazardous (e.g., pelvic ring disruption)[10,13] or technically difficult (e.g., the vertebral artery).[8,15,16] The efficacy of transcatheter embolization to control postoperative hemorrhage has also been well-established.[8]

SINGLE-STICK ARTERIOGRAM

If there is inadequate time to obtain a formal arteriogram, a "single-stick" arteriogram can sometimes be very helpful. The procedure involves insertion of a needle into the femoral or axillary artery, hand injection of radiopaque contrast, and plain film radiography. Although serial rapid filming is preferable, adequate examinations can often be obtained by using a single film with the understanding that repeat injections may be necessary to demonstrate the anatomy. This method carries a higher risk of missing an injury than does a formal arteriogram, and a second view may be desirable if the first film does not reveal an injury. Despite these limitations, percutaneous angiography in the emergency center is highly accurate and cost-effective in the hands of experienced individuals.[17]

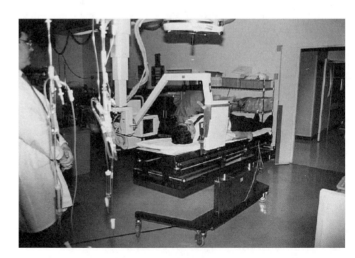

FIGURE 7-2   Properly positioned overhead radiologic equipment can rapidly obtain supine chest and lateral cervical spine x-rays while resuscitation is still in progress.

DIGITAL SUBTRACTION ANGIOGRAPHY

Digital subtraction angiography (DSA) is another way of recording the x-ray image. By virtue of computerized subtraction and enhancement of the image, it creates high quality images with less contrast medium. Real-time projection of the study on the screen at the time of injection allows immediate diagnosis of major injuries without waiting for film processing. Intravenous DSA (IV-DSA) is not recommended except when an arterial approach is impossible. The amount of contrast used for IV-DSA is greater than for intra-arterial DSA (IA-DSA), and the images are often of inferior quality. However, when personnel availability or patient factors necessitate, IV-DSA is of adequate diagnostic quality in the emergency setting. Therapeutic transcatheter embolization cannot be performed via the intravenous route, but IV-DSA serves an important diagnostic role. Further, formal angiography and embolization can easily follow a positive screening IV-DSA.

COST AND COMPLICATIONS

Although most angiographers believe that angiography is extremely safe, these studies can be time-consuming and require costly equipment and highly skilled personnel. In addition, they carry certain inherent risks of their own. Complications of the catheterization procedure can include laceration or thrombosis of the vessel used for the study, hematoma at the puncture site, and intimal damage by the catheter tip as it is manipulated under fluoroscopy. Arterial dissection, with or without occlusion, can be caused by the catheter or by subintimal injection of contrast medium. Allergic reactions to the contrast materials are well known, although not fully understood, and can cause shock or death.

PERSONNEL

Even more important than the required space and equipment for proper radiological studies is the need for technologists and other trained radiology personnel. The emergency radiology facility must be staffed on a 24-hour basis, every day of the year, and an attending or resident radiologist must be available for consultation at all times.

PLANNING FOR X-RAYS

Clinical Indications for Radiological Studies

When it is perfectly clear that an injury is superficial and does not involve bones or viscera, an x-ray examination is generally wasteful and undesirable. At the other extreme, some patients are so severely injured that roentgenographic examinations may waste time which is vitally needed for resuscitation and treatment, and may in fact be harmful if much movement of the patient is involved.

Medicolegal Aspects of Radiology

In these litigious times, increasing numbers of lawsuits are being filed against physicians. In cases of trauma, it has been considered negligent not to have had x-rays made of any injured area, even if the physician believed such examinations were unnecessary. From a strictly medical standpoint, if treatment is the same and outcome identical regardless of the x-ray, the radiologic examination is not needed. Careful clinical notes, with appropriate instruction given to the patient to return if symptoms persist, should eliminate a large percentage of unnecessary x-ray examinations without prejudicing the patient's well-being or jeopardizing the physician. In practice, however, many clinicians feel forced, for their own protection, to request what might otherwise be unnecessary radiologic examinations. At the same time, physicians are held accountable for the rising costs of medical care. This is a dilemma for which no solution is readily available.

Prerequisites for Effective Examinations

HISTORY AND PHYSICAL EXAMINATION

An important prerequisite to an accurate and useful roentgenologic examination is a careful history and physical examination. The x-rays should not be used as a triage tool nor should they be ordered prior to complete evaluation of the patient by a physician. The examining physicians generally have the best information for determining which x-rays to order. Pertinent clinical information on the x-ray requisition slips results in better ordering and interpretation of x-rays.

ANCILLARY INFORMATION

The personnel in the x-ray department routinely should be given the following information on each case:

1. The location of the patient
2. The mode of transportation
3. The precautions to be observed
4. The actual or provisional diagnoses
5. The areas or systems to be examined

If there is any question about which x-rays should be ordered, one should consult with the radiologist.

AXIOM In most instances, the amount of information that a radiologist can provide from reading x-rays is directly proportional to the information supplied to him by the clinician.

In dealing with possible fractures, it is particularly helpful to know the exact site of tenderness when trying to evaluate a shadow which could be a normal variant or the result of an old injury. Statements such as "bruised left shoulder with crepitus," "marked swelling of face and left eyelid," or "board-like abdomen with no bowel sounds" can be very helpful to the radiologist.

CONSULTATION AND PREPARATION

Radiologists can be of greatest help to a clinician if they are properly used as consultants. Once the radiologist knows the information that the clinician wants and the most pertinent facts from the clinical examination, he or she can intelligently direct the technicians to obtain the most rewarding examinations. Limitations of methods, and possible rewards, are best understood through a dialogue between clinician and radiologist.

Not only does careful planning save time, but it also decreases the chances of serious complications developing unnoticed while the patient is being x-rayed. Some of the important aspects of planning are:

1. Performing a thorough physical examination.
2. Evaluating the complete radiologic needs of the patient to avoid repeated trips to the x-ray facility.
3. Communicating the urgency and the amount of time available for getting the studies.
4. Assessing the technical considerations, including the time and number of exposures required, safe positioning of the patient, and the potential need for special investigations, such as arteriography.
5. Making sure that appropriate medical or nursing personnel are on hand to supervise the airway, monitor intravenous fluids, and prevent undesirable movement of the patient while he is being x-rayed.

NEED FOR ANESTHESIA

Children, combative individuals, and patients with widespread injuries may require sedation or anesthesia before and/or during angiography or CT. The duration of most examinations can be shortened and their quality dramatically improved if the patient is not moving. Angiography and embolotherapy are virtually impossible in the uncooperative patient.

X-RAY REPORTS

It should be understood that a record of the radiologic report and diagnosis, typed if possible, should be made available rapidly and included in the patient's chart. Rapid reporting is important to physicians and nurses for guiding and accelerating therapy and for ensuring completeness of the record. Computer systems allow radiological reports to be available instantly throughout the hospital.

Films must be processed and interpreted rapidly so that repeat examinations, when needed, can be obtained without moving the patient unnecessarily. In addition, all films should be reviewed by the clinician, and discrepancies between the clinical picture and the initial radiologic interpretation should be discussed with the radiologist.

AXIOM   Always cross-check the x-rays with the patient's identification and clinical features. In a busy emergency department, it is easy to attach incorrect identification to radiographs.

GENERAL CONSIDERATIONS ON RADIOLOGIC EXAMINATIONS AND FINDINGS

Negative or Normal X-rays

Negative or normal x-rays do not mean that a fracture or injury is not present. Some fractures are not visible on the initial x-rays even with examinations of the highest quality. Generally this is not important as long as both the physician and patient understand this possibility. Patients with suspected fracture of nonweight-bearing bones can be given a splint or sling, and instructions to return if symptoms persist. However, in certain other fractures, this pitfall has special relevance.

When clinical evidence suggests the possibility of a fracture of the femoral neck, the patient should be kept at bed rest despite the absence of an immediately demonstrable fracture. Occasionally, as little as one day can be sufficient time to permit visualization of a fracture line on x-ray. Plain film tomography and CT scans are usually diagnostic. The equivocal cases may need a nuclear bone scan or MRI.

One of the easiest fractures to miss on the original x-rays is one involving the carpal navicular. If such a fracture is suspected but the original films are negative, a cast or splint should be applied to the forearm and hand and the x-rays repeated in a week or two. Radionuclide bone scan can also reliably detect fractures 24 hours after the injury if a definitive diagnosis is necessary.

Children often require x-rays of both the injured and normal extremities. Since the ends of the long bones in children are partially uncalcified cartilage, severe disruptions at the epiphyses can occur with relatively little radiologic change. X-rays of the opposite uninjured extremity may be compared in anyone under the age of 12. Sometimes it is only in this manner that normal anatomic variations of the growing skeleton can be differentiated from changes due to trauma.

Fractures following trauma may be due to underlying disease. It is not uncommon for pathologic fractures to occur through preexisting lesions of bone, especially tumors, cysts, or osteoporosis. These conditions may not be readily apparent radiologically but should be suspected whenever a fracture occurs after relatively mild trauma.

Traumatic Etiologies and Their Wounding Patterns

A mechanism of injury is often reflected in the type, distribution, and severity of the injuries it causes.[18] Various wounding patterns are important because they can provide a mental checklist of injuries that one might expect to find. It is a well-known fact, for example, that steering wheel injuries may cause rupture of the aortic isthmus. It is less well known that rupture of the thoracic aorta is a part of the wounding pattern of broadside impacts.[19] The aortic laceration in this

event tends to be smaller and is often accompanied by only a minimal hematoma. In fact, the accident may not appear to have been very serious.

Proximity Injury in Penetrating Trauma

The concept of proximity wounding by high velocity missiles is very important up to several centimeters from the tract of the missile. It is in the assessment of proximity wounding in the arms and legs that angiographic exploration, or sometimes a CT scan, is superior to surgical exploration. Doppler ultrasound presently is under evaluation for its use in the diagnosis of vascular injuries.

The concept of proximity wounding should also be applied to stabbing and impalement injuries. The wound tract of a knife is not as wide as that of a bullet, but very often there is no clue as to the direction of penetration or its depth. Such a wound may require angiography or surgical exploration to determine if the knife has reached a blood vessel of any significant caliber.

RADIOLOGICAL EXAMINATION OF SPECIFIC AREAS

Skull

There continues to be controversy about when skull x-rays should be ordered on patients with head trauma.[20] Although it is often said that a skull fracture is not very important in determining patient management, patients with a skull fracture have a greatly increased chance of developing a lesion that needs neurosurgical intervention. However, a significant number of patients do not have a skull fracture and are initially clinically alert, but later deteriorate and need neurosurgical intervention.

AXIOM   A normal skull x-ray does not rule out an intracranial injury that may be fatal or require surgery; patients with suspected head injuries should have a CT scan.

As a general rule, a skull x-ray is needed only if a depressed skull fracture is suspected. If skull x-rays are obtained, it is an error to assume that no skull fracture is present (especially in the basilar area) because no fracture line is readily visible on a skull x-ray or on CT scans of the head; thin section CT of the skull base is needed to reliably exclude this diagnosis.

Although fractures of the cranial vault are usually easy to recognize, basilar skull fractures are often impossible to see, even in retrospect. The examination of choice for suspected basilar fracture is thin section CT of the temporal bones.

Brain

Injuries to the brain are the cause of death in at least 25% of patients who die following trauma. The best procedure for evaluating a patient with a possible significant intracranial injury is a nonenhanced CT scan of the brain. With penetrating injuries it can provide excellent data concerning the wound tract and the extent of damage in the area affected by the temporary cavity throughout the projectile's course. Hematomas, pneumocephalus, tissue loss, contusion, the exact location of foreign bodies and bone fragments, and remote intracranial effects of the injury can all be visualized. CT is critical in the selection of patients for surgical decompression.

It has been recommended that a head CT scan be obtained on all patients with Glasgow Coma Scale scores of less than 15, abnormal mental status, or hemispheric neurological deficits. If no operative lesion is found on the CT scan, the patient should be admitted for observation because there is still a risk of deterioration. Those with a Glasgow Coma Scale score of 15, a normal mental status, and no hemispheric neurological deficit may be discharged to be observed at home despite basilar or calvarial skull fracture, loss of consciousness, or cranial nerve deficit. No benefit is gained from skull radiography in any of these groups.[20]

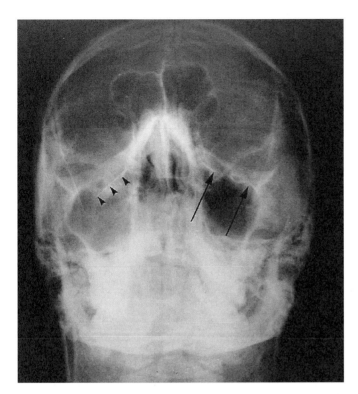

FIGURE 7-3 If one maxillary sinus seems more opaque than the other, this can be caused by overlying soft tissue swelling and/or fluid or blood within the sinus. One should also look for a depressed fracture of the orbital floor.

AXIOM Plain films of the skull should be discouraged if a CT scan will be performed because plain films generally cannot predict the presence of injury to the brain.[3,20]

In comparing the sensitivity and specificity of CT scan and MRI in 107 ED patients with inspected acute brain injury, Orrison et al[21] found that the sensitivity of MRI was significantly higher than that of CT for detection of contusion, shearing injury, subdural and epidural hematomas, and sinus involvement; however, the sensitivity of CT was significantly higher than that of MRI for locating fractures. The sensitivities of MRI and CT were statistically equivalent for the detection of superficial soft-tissue injury. The overall sensitivity of MRI for the detection of abnormalities in acute head trauma was 96%, and 63% for CT.

Face

Unfortunately, there is often an excessive sense of urgency about the need for facial radiography in acutely injured patients. This can cause grave risk to multitrauma patients and should be resisted;[22] however, if such studies will not delay resuscitation or emergency surgery, they can be pursued during the initial exam.

Preliminary plain films are not very helpful in assessment of facial injuries. Fractures of the paranasal sinuses and orbits are frequently difficult to recognize on plain films, but these injuries are of great importance because of the potential consequences of failing to diagnose and treat them. The presence of an air-fluid level in a sinus following injury may be a clue to recognition of an otherwise inapparent fracture, but significant fractures may be present without these changes.

If one maxillary sinus seems more opaque than the other, this can be caused by overlying soft tissue swelling and/or fluid or blood within the sinus (Fig. 7-3). One should also look for a depressed fracture of the orbital floor. Laminography or CT scan often confirms these findings, and they will also often identify other fractures not

seen on plain films. If a facial fracture is suspected, but no definite bone fragments are identified because the area in question is obscured by overlying structures, a tomogram may be helpful (Fig. 7-4). However, CT scans in both the axial and coronal planes have largely replaced tomography for radiological examination of these areas.

If there is no apparent orbital floor fracture, but there is loss of definition of the medial orbital wall, a fracture is suspected (Fig. 7-5). The bony detail of the thin medial wall of the orbit, the globe, optic nerve, and muscles are much better shown by CT than tomography (Fig. 7-6).

CT can provide exquisite delineation of the orbit's complex anatomy and its spatial relationship to the path of a wounding agent as well as the location of residual fragments.

Angiography of trauma to the head and face is limited to diagnosis of major vascular injuries and to an occasional treatment by embolization of a bleeding artery in an area that is very difficult for the surgeon to approach. When injury is confined to the orbit, transorbital ultrasonography may be used in some instances for localization of intraorbital foreign bodies.

Spine

GENERAL CONSIDERATIONS

AXIOM The best way to ensure that a patient's injury is not aggravated by motion during radiological studies is proper immobilization.

One should not send patients to the x-ray department without proper immobilization. While most physicians remember to immobilize extremities and a cervical spine that may be fractured, some for-

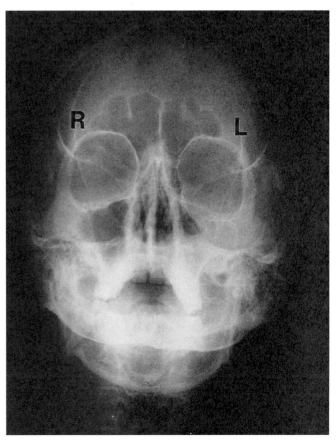

FIGURE 7-4 If a facial fracture is suspected, but the area in question is obscured by overlying structures, a tomogram may diminish the effect of the overlying structures.

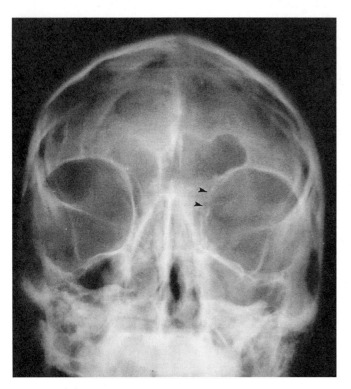

FIGURE 7-5 Even if there is no apparent orbital floor fracture, loss of definition of the medial orbital wall should make one suspicious of a fracture.

get that an unstable lumbar or thoracic spine also needs immobilization.

Plain film is the first and often only method for initial assessment of spinal trauma.[23-25] Recognition of these injuries is of utmost importance, as up to 10% of spinal cord injuries occur when patients with unstable spine fractures are moved.[24]

Many of our trauma patients are brought to the ED with a cervical collar in place. With the collar left in place, a cross-table lateral view of the cervical spine is obtained as soon as possible. If this film is normal and the patient cooperates, we can also obtain open mouth

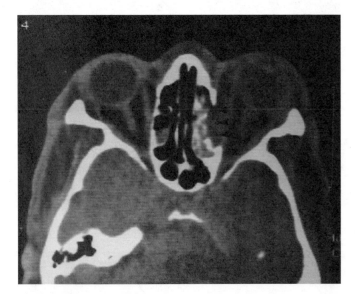

FIGURE 7-6 The bony detail of the thin medial wall of the orbit is much better shown on CT than on tomography. The delineation of the globes, optic nerves, and muscles is also much clearer on CT examinations.

(OM) and anteroposterior (AP) views. If these views are also negative and the patient has a normal neurological exam, the collar is removed, and oblique views can be obtained. The cervical spine may be cleared in MVA patients by lateral cervical spine plus OM and AP views with a risk of missing significant fractures in less than 1% of patients examined.[26]

Physicians reading cervical spine films should be familiar with four radiologic signs that can occur with unstable spinal fractures: (a) displacement of vertebrae, (b) widened interspinous space, (c) widened apophyseal joints, and (d) widened vertebral canal.[24] In addition, most significant cervical spine injuries are accompanied by abnormal prevertebral soft-tissue shadows.

Because excessive overlying tissue and spasm may be present, injuries to the lower cervical and upper thoracic spine can be especially hard to visualize. The ATLS manual emphasizes the importance of visualizing the C7-T1 interspace, which is injured in 3 to 9% of cervical spine injured patients.[27] Not uncommonly, several x-rays of this area must be taken, including swimmer's views, before the seventh cervical and the top of the first thoracic vertebra can be seen clearly. In more than a few patients, laminography or CT scans are required to adequately visualize the entire cervical spine, particularly if there is concern about the lower cervical vertebrae or the odontoid process.

CONDITIONS THAT MIMIC CERVICAL SPINE TRAUMA

If there is any clinical doubt, one should assume that a cervical spine injury is present. However, there are a few conditions that mimic trauma on the lateral view of the cervical spine. For example, the anterior border of the vertebral body of C2 may appear to be 2 to 3 mm anterior to the vertebral body of C3 (Fig. 7-7). Ordinarily, this would be adequate to diagnose a subluxation of the vertebral body of

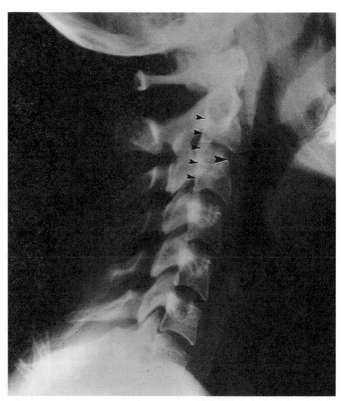

FIGURE 7-7 The patient on whom this study was performed was admitted with tenderness over the upper cervical spine following a motor vehicle accident. Since the anterior border of the vertebral body of C2 was 2-3 mm anterior to the vertebral body of C3 (large arrows), it was thought that subluxation of the vertebral body of C2 on C3 was present. However, the posterior borders of C2 and C3 (small arrowheads) are in good alignment.

C2 on C3. However, if the posterior borders of C2 and C3 are in good alignment, the apparent vertebral body offset anteriorly may just be caused by elongation ("beaking") of the anteroinferior vertebral body border. This "beaking" often becomes more prominent with age and can mimic a subluxation.

If the cervical spine x-ray shows a black line across the inferior third of the vertebral body, a diagnosis of fractured cervical spine is apt to be made (Fig. 7-8A). However, if tomographic studies show no fracture (Fig. 7-8B), such lines may be due to an uncovertebral process. The uncovertebral process is a normal continuation of the intervertebral joint and it is usually orientated at an angle of about 45° to the disc space. A degenerated uncovertebral joint may be oriented horizontally so that it is parallel to and slightly higher than the disc space. This allows its shadow to appear slightly above the inferior vertebral body border on a lateral view. If the uncovertebral process is sclerotic, it will be more prominent because the surrounding sclerosis will form a white border around the black joint space.

Occasionally, a patient is admitted for what is thought to be a small fracture of the anteroinferior aspect of a vertebral body but is actually an arthritic spur. The lower cervical spine commonly develops spurs that may not be connected to the adjacent vertebral bodies (Fig.

7-9). If there is intact white cortical bone surrounding not only the vertebral body but also the spur, it is unlikely that there has been a recent fracture.

With any type of spinal trauma, CT or MRI is the best way to assess the integrity of the spinal canal, its possible compromise by bone fragments, and the craniovertebral junction.[24,25] With penetrating wounds of the spine, CT can also localize foreign bodies and bone fragments.

Recently, Borock et al[28] described their use of CT scanning as an adjunct to plain films of the cervical spine in 179 acutely injured blunt trauma patients. CT scanning of the cervical spine was performed for patients whose x-ray findings were positive, for patients with plain x-ray films suggestive of a pathologic condition, for patients with plain x-ray films that did not reveal all of the cervical vertebrae, and for patients who had persistent pain or neurologic deficits despite normal plain x-ray films. Of 123 patients not able to have their cervical spine cleared by normal roentgenograms, 93% were cleared by CT scans within 24 hours of admission. There were no missed injuries in this setting. A false-positive rate of 28% and a false-negative rate of 1.5% were found for plain roentgenograms. Computed tomographic scans detected 98% of the injuries, and when combined with a three-view plain x-ray series of the cervical spine, 100% of cervical spine injuries were detected.

Assessment of mass effect on the cord is aided significantly by intrathecal contrast media or MRI. Multiplanar reconstruction of the CT images allows intensive study of the spine and soft tissues with

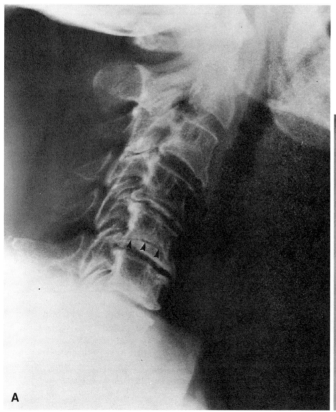

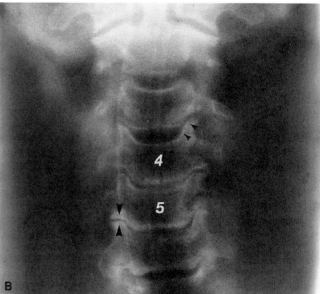

FIGURE 7-8 If the cervical spine x-ray shows a black line across the inferior third of the vertebral body, a diagnosis of fractured cervical spine is apt to be made (Fig. 7-8A). However, if tomographic studies show no fracture (Fig. 7-8B), such lines may be due to an uncovertebral process. The uncovertebral process is a normal continuation of the intervertebral joint and it is usually orientated at an angle of about 45° to the disc space.

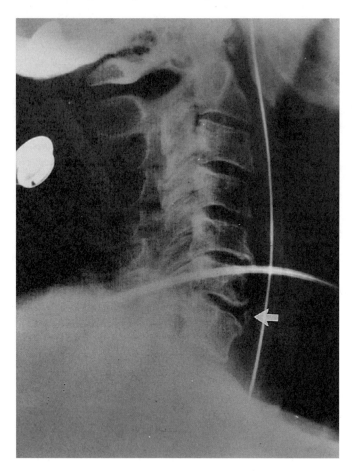

FIGURE 7-9 Occasionally, a patient is admitted for what is thought to be a small fracture of the anteroinferior aspect of a vertebral body but is actually an arthritic spur. If there is intact white cortical bone surrounding the vertebral body and the spur, it is unlikely that there has been a recent fracture.

out unnecessary manipulation of the patient. Currently, MRI is the procedure of choice for evaluation of the spinal cord and surrounding tissues.

Neck

PLAIN FILMS
With penetrating wounds of the neck, laceration of the upper airway or esophagus may be suspected radiologically by the presence of air in the soft tissues of the neck and mediastinum and particularly in the retropharyngeal space. This space is best seen in a lateral view of the neck. If the space between the pharynx and cervical spine is more than 0.5 cm at C3, an abnormal fluid collection should be suspected. At C5, the prevertebral soft tissue may normally be as thick as the body of the C5 vertebra. However, injuries to the esophagus, pharynx, or trachea can occur with little or no evidence on routine chest or neck films. Although abnormal collections of air or fluid in the mediastinum or pleural spaces suggest a pharyngeal or esophageal injury, contrast studies under fluoroscopy are generally needed for confirmation. Even these examinations, however, are not absolutely definitive because the defect in the wall may be occluded by clot, fibrin, or food.

ANGIOGRAPHY
In the neck, selective surgical management of penetrating wounds has gained increasing popularity by virtue of its safety and cost-effectiveness.[29,30] To a great extent, this change was made possible by liberal use of angiography. Angiography is of particular value in assessing penetrating injuries high in the neck between the angle of

the mandible and the base of the skull,[16,29] especially if the vertebral arteries may be involved.[31]

Meier et al[31] reported that routine angiographic assessment of penetrating neck wounds in their institute increased the number of diagnosed vertebral artery injuries from 2.3% between 1957 and 1973 to 19.4% for the years 1978 to 1980. In addition, the rich network of veins in the neck increases the likelihood of a traumatic vertebral arteriovenous fistula (AVF), which is usually best handled by an interventional radiologist. Vascular injuries accompanying an unstable cervical spine fracture in neurologically intact patients should be managed by angiography to eliminate the risk of iatrogenic quadriplegia.[8]

With penetrating injury, CT of the neck is usually limited to localization of small foreign bodies and to assessment of the integrity of the larynx.

Chest

Patients in deep hemorrhagic shock after penetrating truncal trauma have no time for sophisticated imaging prior to emergency surgery. Plain films to indicate the presence of a hemopneumothorax and possibly an abdominal film to record markers that have been over external wounds of the abdomen and to locate missiles is all that is necessary. A repeat chest film may also be needed to determine if a hemopneumothorax has been adequately drained with chest tubes. Subtle signs of a ruptured hemidiaphragm may be seen and targeted for further assessment. The mediastinum must also be evaluated to rule out possible injury to the aorta or its major branches.

CHEST WALL
Rib fractures are common with blunt chest trauma, but it is usually the underlying lung and pleural pathology that is most important. Injuries to the anterior noncalcified cartilaginous ends of the ribs are seldom detectable. In addition, many fractures of the lateral and posterior osseous portions of the rib are invisible on the initial radiologic examinations of the chest, even in retrospect. The diagnostic yield of a search for rib fractures on chest films, rather than rib studies, is quite poor.

> **AXIOM**   Do not assume that the thoracic cage is intact because no fracture is visible, even on routine rib films.

Certain rib fractures are important because of likely associated injuries. Fractures of ribs 1 and/or 2 should make one suspect major bronchial or cardiovascular injury while fractures of ribs 9, 10, and 11 should make one suspect injuries to the liver or spleen. In evaluating the sternum and sternoclavicular joints, laminography or CT may be needed.

PNEUMOTHORAX
In some patients it may be difficult to detect a pneumothorax. This may be a particular problem in patients who are dyspneic. Although failure to insert a needed chest tube may increase the risk of sudden severe cardiopulmonary deterioration, insertion of an unnecessary chest tube can cause significant morbidity.

Absent Lung Markings
A frequently used criterion for diagnosis of a pneumothorax on chest x-ray is the absence of pulmonary markings. This sign can be a good one, but it is limited because other conditions, such as bullae or blebs, may also cause absent lung markings. If a prior chest x-ray is available, it may be clear that the absence of lung marking is not a new finding (Fig. 7-10A and 7-10B). Such areas often represent blebs or bullae, which are often bilateral. Such patients are apt to get much worse if a chest tube is inserted because puncture of a bleb with a chest tube can result in a large air leak.

> **AXIOM**   Comparing current and old x-rays is an inexpensive and reliable method for improving the accuracy of x-ray interpretation.

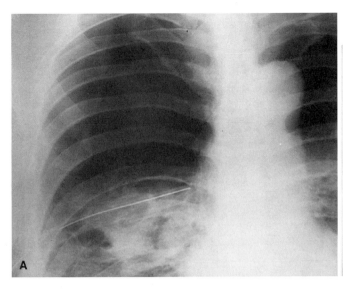

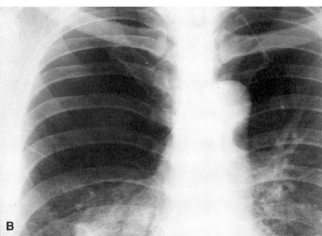

FIGURE 7-10 The patient in Figure 7-10A was thought to have a pneumothorax unresponsive to chest tube therapy. Although there are no lung markings over the right upper lung field, a chest x-ray (Fig. 7-10B) made about 3 months prior to the present admission was retrieved from the files. Notice that there was an absence of lung markings over the right and left upper lung fields at that time. These areas represent blebs and bullae which are often bilateral.

"Thin White Line" Sign

Another criterion, the "thin white line" sign made by visualization of the visceral pleura when air is present in the pleural cavity, is the most diagnostic finding of pneumothorax on a chest radiograph. Normally, the lung with its visceral pleura is in direct contact with the parietal pleura of the inner chest wall. Therefore, the visceral pleura is not visible on the usual chest x-ray. When air is introduced into the pleural space, the visceral pleura seen tangentially is outlined by air within the lung on one side and pneumothorax air on

the other side (Fig. 7-11), producing a "thin white line." Obviously, this line should conform to the anticipated position of a partially collapsed lung. In addition, the thin white line of the visceral pleura in a patient with a pneumothorax has two dimensions and is about 1 millimeter thick. However, the visceral pleura will only be visible with a pneumothorax if there is enough air in the lung to outline it. In situations in which there is major atelectasis or consolidation and there is no air within the collapsed lung, the line will not be seen (Fig. 7-12).

AXIOM The "thin white line" sign is valid only for small to medium-sized pneumothoraces.

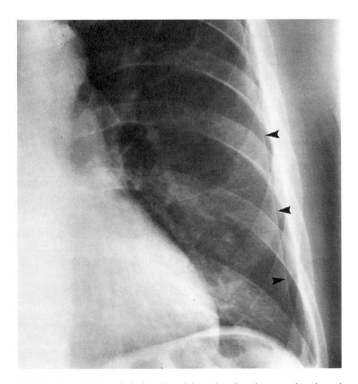

FIGURE 7-11 When air is introduced into the pleural space, the visceral pleura is outlined by air within the lung on one side and by pneumothorax air on the other side, producing a "thin white line" sign that is formed by visceral pleura seen tangentially. This line should conform to the anticipated position of a collapsing lung.

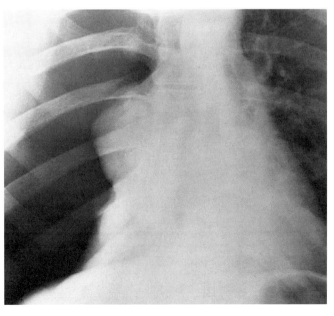

FIGURE 7-12 In situations where there is a pneumothorax and major atelectasis or consolidation, there is no air within the collapsed lung, and consequently the white line will not be seen.

Skin Folds

A skin fold overlying the chest may mimic a pneumothorax, especially when the x-ray is taken with the patient in a supine position (Fig. 7-13). However, the only dimension that a skin fold line has is length. It is not a white line of about 1 millimeter in width. The breast is a relatively frequent cause of skin folds overlying the lung fields. The air on the x-ray appears darker, and the tissue fold appears lighter. Where the two have an interface, there is a density change producing a one-dimensional line. The line does not have the thickness seen when the visceral pleura is outlined by air on both sides.

In some patients there may be an anterior skin fold from the breast and a posterior skin fold from the back. When a portable chest x-ray is taken following severe trauma, the patient is often supine and the cassette is placed under the patient. As a consequence, the skin and subcutaneous tissues over the patient's back are often wrinkled, and wherever air meets skin, a skin fold line may appear. In general, skin fold lines from the patient's back terminate abruptly or gradually fade away, while the thin white line of a pneumothorax follows the course of a partially collapsed lung. Another skin fold that may mimic a pneumothorax can be formed by the patient's arm overlapping the lower chest wall (Fig. 7-14).

AXIOM Not all lines lying over the lung fields indicate a pneumothorax.

It must be emphasized that skin folds are one-dimensional and the fine white line formed by the visceral pleura in a patient with a pneumothorax is two-dimensional.

AXIOM All two-dimensional white lines are not caused by pneumothoraces.

Scapula

Another line that can easily be mistaken for a pneumothorax is the edge of the scapula. This can produce a two-dimensional line projecting over the lung apex. However, the curve of the line is opposite from the expected contour of a partially collapsed lung. Also, if one

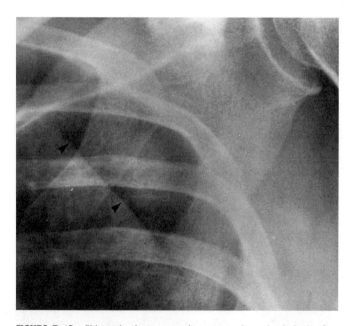

FIGURE 7-13 Skin and subcutaneous tissues over the patient's back often have folds when the patient is supine. In general, skin fold lines from the patient's back terminate abruptly or gradually fade away while the thin white line of a pneumothorax follows the expected course of a partially collapsed lung.

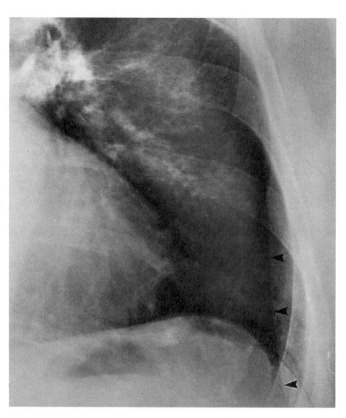

FIGURE 7-14 A skin fold that mimics a pneumothorax can be formed by the patient's arm overlapping the lower chest wall.

follows the line in both directions, it will usually be quite clear that it is the bony edge of the scapula.

Dressings and Tubes

Another two-dimensional white line that may resemble a pneumothorax is the edge of a dressing attached to the chest. As with all other white lines not due to a pneumothorax, it will not follow the expected course of a partially collapsed lung and the line may extend outside the chest.

HEMOPNEUMOTHORAX

Patient Position

AXIOM Large quantities of fluid may not be easily visible on routine x-rays of the chest in a supine patient.

Pleural fluid is not seen well when x-rays are taken on supine patients. Although large amounts of pleural fluid on one side can be suspected on recumbent films because of the increased density of the hemithorax, upright and decubitus views are often necessary to see smaller collections. If even slight blunting of the costophrenic angle is seen on an upright film, it can usually be assumed that at least 200 to 300 ml of fluid are present. However, fairly large quantities of fluid can sometimes remain in a subpulmonic position between the diaphragm and the base of the lung and may be undetected except on decubitus films. A subpulmonic pleural effusion should be strongly suspected on an upright chest x-ray if the dome of the diaphragm is shifted laterally rather than located in the middle of the hemithorax.

AXIOM When a small pleural effusion is suspected or difficult to see on routine chest x-rays, decubitus views may be helpful.

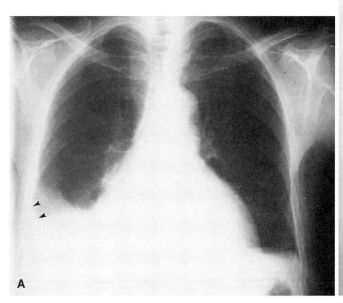

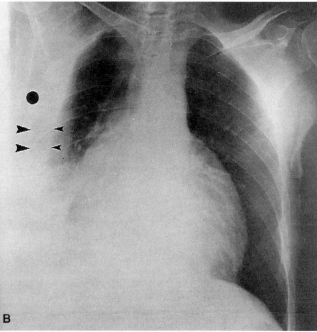

FIGURE 7-15 The patient in Figure 7-15A has a moderate amount of right pleural fluid. The right hemidiaphragm is obscured by a density that forms a meniscus (arrowheads) along the lateral chest wall. Other problems may cause similar patterns, but the use of a right lateral decubitus, in which the patient lies on his or her right side (Fig. 7-15B), will confirm that the density moves along the right lateral chest wall. The large arrowheads represent the inner border of the ribs and the smaller arrowheads represent the edge of the layered fluid.

A moderately large pleural effusion may obscure the diaphragm and form a meniscus along the lateral chest wall (Fig. 7-15A). However, other shadows may cause similar patterns and the use of a right or left lateral decubitus film with the patient lying on his right or left side will confirm that the density moves along the right or left lateral chest wall (Fig. 7-15B). This can also confirm that mobile fluid is present as opposed to loculated fluid, a mass, atelectasis, or pleural thickening or scarring.

Atelectasis

If a chest tube is inserted to drain a pleural effusion, but the x-ray does not improve, one should suspect atelectasis (Fig. 7-16) or an incorrectly placed chest tube. It may occasionally be difficult to differentiate between a large pleural effusion and atelectasis producing a large area of whited-out lung field. As a general rule, however, the heart or mediastinum is usually shifted toward the side of the atelectasis. In contrast, a large pleural effusion will tend to shift the mediastinum away from the area of opacification.

Endobronchial Endotracheal Tube

In some instances, an area of opacification representing atelectasis may be due to an endotracheal tube which is inserted so far down that it lies in the contralateral mainstem bronchus, usually the right. This can occlude the left mainstem bronchus and produce atelectasis of the entire left lung.

Gastric Fundus-Diaphragm Distance

Increased distance between air within the gastric fundus and the top of the left hemidiaphragm on an upright film may also indicate the presence of a pleural effusion or a subdiaphragmatic fluid collection. Air within the fundus of the stomach is usually within 0.5 to 1.0 cm of the top of the left diaphragm on an upright chest x-ray. If the distance is greater, it is likely that subpulmonic pleural fluid is present and mimicking the outline of the diaphragm. Decubitus films will confirm this suspicion.

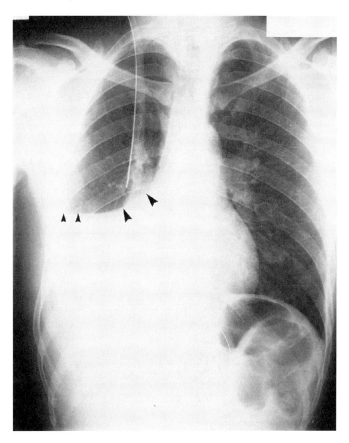

FIGURE 7-16 This illustrates a patient thought to have a right pleural effusion. Notice that although the medial border of the alleged effusion has a meniscus sign (large arrowheads), the lateral border of the alleged pleural effusion (small arrowheads) does not.

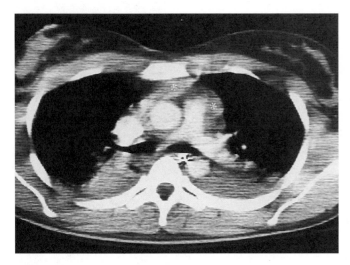

FIGURE 7-17   An extensive mediastinal hematoma is identified by the asterisks. Notice that the normal dark mediastinal fat has been replaced with material that has a density similar to the muscle of the chest wall and back.

Medial and Lateral Meniscus Signs

The meniscus sign may be very helpful for diagnosing a pleural effusion, but it can also be deceptive. If the medial border of the alleged effusion has a meniscus sign, but the lateral border of the alleged pleural effusion does not also have a meniscus sign, the opacification may be due to atelectasis. An additional clue may be the position of the heart. If the heart is not pushed away by a large opacity, some atelectasis is probably present. When there is doubt, lateral decubitus views should be obtained. If the patient cannot assume the decubitus position, a supine film can be helpful. If the upper lung field remains clear, it is unlikely that the density is free fluid that should have gravitated to upward. The layering fluid may also add density to the side of the chest with the effusion.

Pneumatocele

Contusion of the lung produces transudation of fluid and blood into and around the bronchioles and alveoli, increasing the density of the involved area. These changes may progress rapidly to a superimposed atelectasis and infection. Later, necrosis and infection in some of these contused areas may result in abscess formation with an air-fluid level or a pneumatocele. Lacerations of the lung may show more irregular opacification of lung parenchyma and early air-fluid levels.

Pneumatoceles may develop soon after injury and persist as radiolucent "holes" in the lung. Occasionally, however, they may initially fill with blood and appear to be solid. These spherical defects can persist and are sometimes removed in later years as a "solitary nodule" if their etiology is not apparent.

RUPTURED BRONCHUS

Although fracture of a bronchus usually results in massive pneumothorax, the initial x-ray is occasionally normal. Although minimal amounts of subcutaneous emphysema can be expected with any penetrating injury, larger amounts, particularly if they occur after blunt trauma, suggest damage to the trachea or large bronchi. If a bronchial fracture is suspected but is not found on bronchoscopy, a bronchogram may outline the defect clearly. The diagnosis may also be suspected initially by a persistent pneumothorax and later by a persistent atelectasis.

HEART

Occasionally, changes in the size or configuration of the cardiac shadow may help diagnose pericardial tamponade. If the normal pericardial cavity rapidly fills with more than 200 to 300 ml of blood or fluid, tamponade usually occurs. Although this amount of fluid can cause severe hypotension, the enlargement of the heart

shadow it produces may be so slight that it can be easily overlooked.

Echocardiogram has been increasingly suggested for the workup of precordial trauma. Similar experience has been reported for blunt trauma,[32,33] and use of ECHO in penetrating trauma has been limited to isolated case reports or evaluation of delayed complications following cardiorrhaphy.[34-36] ECHO can also be particularly useful for demonstrating septal defects and valvular damage.

In a report by Freshman et al,[37] 36 hemodynamically stable patients had emergent ECHO performed to rule out cardiac injury. Four of the 36 patients had pericardial effusions for a positive rate of 11%. There were no false-negative studies in the 32 patients in whom no pericardial effusion was found, and these patients were safely triaged to a ward bed. None of these patients developed evidence of a missed cardiac injury later, but 5 to 10% false-negatives have been reported.

Although CT scans of the chest following trauma often focus upon evaluation of the superior mediastinum and the great vessels, several other lesions should also be looked for on this study. These include fractures or dislocations of ribs, clavicles, sternum or scapula, hemothorax, pneumothorax, pneumomediastinum, pulmonary contusion/laceration, hemopericardium, and mediastinal hematoma (Fig. 7-17). For example, if a patient had tachycardia, hypotension, and distended neck veins, the CT should be closely examined for increased pericardial fluid (Fig. 7-18). In some instances, the first evidence of a tamponade may be found on a CT scan.

AXIOM   Reassessment of any radiological study with a focused history may identify a previously overlooked lesion. Furthermore, a consistent, thorough routine must be followed in interpretation of all films even after one lesion has been found.

GREAT VESSELS

Any of the thoracic great vessels can be injured by blunt or penetrating trauma resulting in a mediastinal hematoma or extrapleural or intrapleural bleeding. Of particular interest are deceleration injuries of the aorta resulting in false aneurysms, usually of the aortic isthmus just distal to the left subclavian artery.

Plain Films

Plain chest radiography is limited in its ability to accurately screen for major vascular lesions. Large mediastinal hematomas are readily recognized, as they can widen the superior mediastinum, displace midline structures (trachea and nasogastric tube) to the left, depress the left main bronchus, and obliterate normal tissue interfaces.[38] Me-

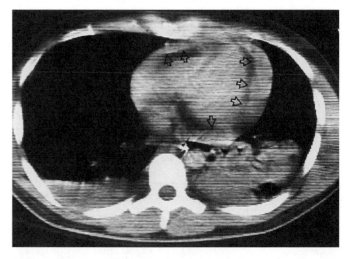

FIGURE 7-18   The soft-tissue density material within the pericardial sac (arrows) is compatible with the diagnosis of hemopericardium and pericardial tamponade.

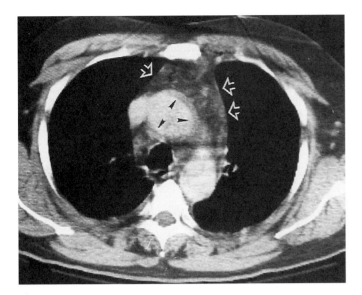

FIGURE 7-19 Extensive mediastinal fat (open arrows) can cause an abnormal mediastinum on chest x-ray. The ascending aorta here is surrounded by circumferential low density material (arrowheads) that may represent thrombus, false lumen, or, in this case, artifact.

diastinal width, whether absolute or as a percentage of thoracic diameter, has proved only moderately sensitive and poorly specific for traumatic rupture of the aorta. Identification of abnormal mediastinal contours has proved considerably more accurate in identification of underlying mediastinal pathology. However, smaller hematomas may not be recognized at all if the chest x-ray is not subjected to meticulous inspection by an experienced radiologist. In a still worse but ever so common scenario, a small mediastinal hematoma is seen but then dismissed as "not enough" to warrant suspicion of a major vascular injury.

CT Scan

If the mediastinal contours are clearly abnormal on the plain chest x-ray, the likelihood of a mediastinal hematoma is high, and arteriography should be performed as soon as possible. However, in a large number of plain chest x-rays, there remains a reasonable question of great vessel injury. It is here that CT provides its greatest benefit. CT is an excellent study to perform in the patient with an equivocal chest radiograph. It is also an excellent study if the individuals reading the chest x-ray are not skilled in evaluation of the subtleties of the mediastinum. Occasionally, the presence of clinically unsuspected hypovolemia may be evident from a collapsed inferior vena cava seen on CT.

Although plain chest films can be very helpful, a large number of patients sent for CT of the mediastinum may have an abnormal appearing chest x-ray on the basis of either technical factors (e.g., rotation, motion, or poor inspiration) or inherent anatomic factors (e.g., tortuosity of the great vessels, vascular engorgement, mediastinal lipomatosis, upper lobe atelectasis, or pleural effusion). The major benefit of CT lies in distinguishing the above causes of mediastinal widening from hematoma; however, such determinations require a high quality film and a cooperative patient. If the patient will not hold still, even with sedatives, no radiologic study can be of optimal quality.

AXIOM If the patient cannot cooperate for a plain chest film, there is only a small likelihood of obtaining a CT of diagnostic quality.

On the CT scan, the presence of soft-tissue density material around the aorta or one of its branches may represent hematoma or mediastinal fat (Fig. 7-19). If the normal dark mediastinal fat is displaced or

infiltrated, it is possible that a hematoma is adjacent to a major vessel, and an arteriogram is needed.

On CT, one will sometimes see lucent lines running through the ascending and descending thoracic aorta, raising the question of an intimal flap (Fig. 7-20). However, if the orientation of these lines changes on adjacent scans, it indicates that they are motion artifact streaks. Thus, evaluation of the lumen of the aorta on CT is fraught with difficulty. Additionally, CT identification of extension of the aortic injury into a major vessel of the neck is extremely difficult; however, rapid spiral CT techniques have significantly improved CT evaluation of vascular structures.[39]

AXIOM Any true finding on CT scan will be present on adjacent cuts or more than one view. Artifacts are not usually consistent from film to film.

In most cases of mediastinal hematoma identified on CT, no major vascular injury is identified. It is now clear that most mediastinal hematomas are produced by injury to venous or small arterial structures. Nevertheless, if the CT demonstrates mediastinal hemorrhage, aortography is warranted.

The potential value of CT in screening for traumatic rupture of the aorta is quite controversial. Fenner et al[40] in 1990 reported that CT and arteriography had comparable specificity (CT 96%, arteriography 92%) and false-positive rates (CT 3.8%, arteriography 7.7%) when CT was used as a screening tool for aortic rupture. Madayag et al[41] used dynamic CT to screen for aortic injury in patients with blunt chest trauma who had normal initial chest x-ray findings. They concluded that emergent aortography should be performed only if there are abnormal chest x-ray or CT findings.

Miller et al[42] in a series of 104 patients who had a CT scan of the chest and an aortogram had five patients with TRA. Three were interpreted as having a mediastinal hematoma seen on CT scan, but one was apparently performed without intravenous contrast and one was misread by a radiology resident. Three aortic branch injuries were also missed.

In another study comparing CT scans of the chest with aortography in 144 stable patients with suspected blunt aortic injury, Durham et al[43] reported that six aortic injuries were detected by aortography, but only four had positive CT scans for a sensitivity of only 67%. There was, however, some inter-reader variation, and the quality of the CT scans is not really known.

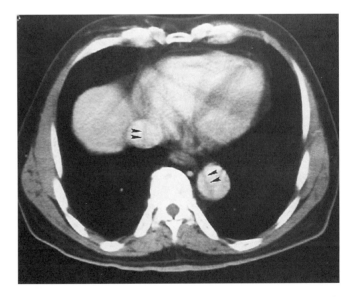

FIGURE 7-20 Lucent lines through the ascending and descending thoracic aorta (arrowheads) may simulate a long intimal flap; however, if the orientation of these lines changes on adjacent scans, this indicates that they represent motion artifact streaks. Evaluation of any lumen (aorta or gut) on CT is fraught with difficulty.

In a recent review and commentary, Raptopoulos[44] has indicated that normal findings on chest CT scans exclude aortic injury rather well. Fisher et al[45] found that CT was at least as good as aortography for excluding aortic injury. Of 579 patients who had normal results on CT in eight studies, only five (0.7%) were found to have abnormalities on aortography. One or two additional case reports describe similar findings. These results are similar to those for chest radiography: of 352 patients with normal radiographic findings in the same eight studies, findings on aortograms were abnormal in three (0.9%).

In a report by Agee et al,[46] no TRA was missed on CT scans. Fisher et al[45] agree that chest CT scans with normal findings exclude aortic/brachiocephalic injury, but only 25% of their patients had unequivocally normal CT findings. Of three patients with aortic injuries, one had only suggestive and two had subtly positive CT findings.

Patients who are hemodynamically unstable or whose mechanism of injury or clinical examination strongly suggests aortic injury should have immediate aortography or surgery. In the absence of these criteria, Raptopoulos[44] feels that overwhelming evidence suggests that CT can be used for screening patients with suspected aortic transection, especially those who are hemodynamically stable and are undergoing CT for other injuries. This additional examination, which may increase the workup time no more than 10 minutes, requires one technologist and one resident, all in house. Usually one physician, one technologist, and one nurse are called in for aortography. This may necessitate up to a 45-minute delay, during which a CT scan can be done.

Tomiak et al,[47] however, are not convinced that normal CT scan excludes the possibility of significant vascular injury in the chest. This is primarily due to the possibility of axial scanning techniques missing transversely oriented injuries. In stable patients with equivocal chest radiographs but with low clinical suspicion of vascular injury, CT can differentiate mediastinal hematoma from other causes of mediastinal widening. CT also often shows additional unsuspected findings, such as sternal or vertebral fractures, that could implicate a greater severity of injury than initially believed and provide an indication for arteriography. Finally, in cases in which aortography is unclear, as in ductus diverticulum, acute dissection, or atherosclerotic aneurysm, CT may help elucidate confusing arteriographic findings.

We and others[48] have yet to see a TRA without a mediastinal hematoma in practice. One of us (RFW), however, has had two patients with a false-negative aortogram and knows of two others. Nevertheless, if there is a reasonable suspicion of a TRA because of the mechanism of injury, physical findings, or the chest x-ray, an aortogram or TEE should be performed promptly. If there is only mild to moderate suspicion of TRA, a CT of the chest can be performed. If there is no evidence of a mediastinal hematoma, there is usually no need for further study. It is important, however, while waiting for these tests in patients with severe blunt chest trauma, to keep the systolic BP below 120 mm Hg to prevent the possibly injured aorta from completely rupturing.

Aortography

Many clinicians and radiologists feel that the only reliable diagnostic tool for evaluating great vessel injury is the aortogram, which must be used liberally on the basis of the slightest abnormality on the chest film and with strong reliance on a history of violent trauma[17,38,49] (Fig. 7-21A and 7-21B). Although arch arteriography remains the standard for identification of great vessel injury, cost and inherent risk

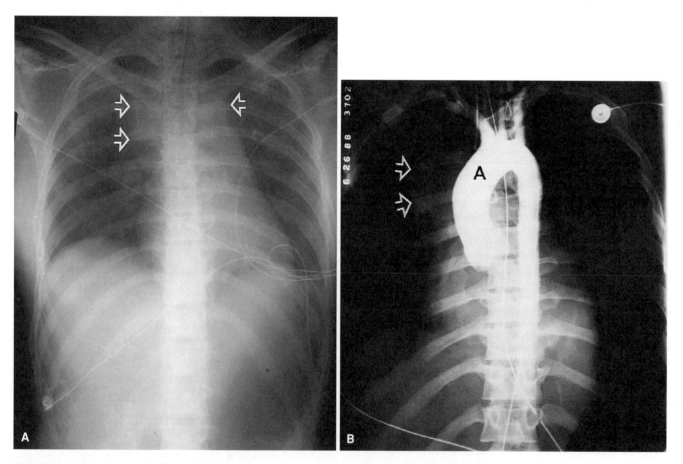

FIGURE 7-21 The chest x-ray in Figure 7-21A demonstrates a wide superior mediastinum (arrowheads). This finding is generally an indication for aortography. However, the aortogram (Fig. 7-21B) demonstrates a normal thoracic aorta within the widened mediastinum.

make it undesirable as a screening examination in spite of its high sensitivity and specificity. MRI is increasingly used to evaluate great vessels for injury or dissection.

Aortography should be done with a transfemoral arterial catheter, with serial images recorded on film or on digital matrix. The latter is more appealing in view of the speed of diagnosis, the low volume of contrast medium required, and the ability to diagnose potential injury to the superior vena cava and the innominate veins on the venous phase of the same series. A single series is sufficient when positive, but a second projection must be made if the first run was normal. Also, it is always useful to do a "pull-out" abdominal aortogram to rule out major vascular or solid organ injuries in the abdomen. An experienced angiographic team should be able to add this information with little additional time.

DIAPHRAGM

AXIOM Traumatic diaphragmatic hernias can be very difficult to recognize on the initial x-rays of the chest.

Many diaphragmatic injuries can be difficult or impossible to diagnose on the initial plain films of the chest or abdomen; however, this problem should always be suspected: (a) when the diaphragm is elevated, (b) when it moves abnormally on fluoroscopy, or (c) if unusual gas shadows are seen above the diaphragm, especially on the left. Not uncommonly, the walls of abdominal viscera which have herniated in the chest are compressed and are mistaken for a high diaphragm.

The diagnosis of diaphragmatic injury is sometimes first made when the end of a radiopaque nasogastric tube is noted to pass from the abdomen into the left chest. Decubitus views and studies with opaque contrast agents may help to confirm the diagnosis. Occasionally, insufflation of 200 to 300 ml of air into the stomach through a nasogastric tube may outline the stomach or intestine in the chest.

Herniation of the bowel into the chest is often better seen with the patient supine, since intrathoracic abdominal contents may slide back below the diaphragm when the patient is upright.

Abdomen

A multitude of intra-abdominal injuries may not be evident from the initial history, physical examination, and laboratory workup. Several possible radiologic studies can aid in the management of such injuries, but deciding which tests to use and when and how to use them can be difficult.

THE UNSTABLE PATIENT

The unstable patient often only has enough time before surgery for a portable plain film of the abdomen and/or pelvis. This is obviously a limited diagnostic study, but occasionally it can be helpful by demonstrating fractures, large hematomas, major organ displacement, pneumoperitoneum, foreign bodies, or evidence of previous surgery. It is also an easy and inexpensive test and virtually without risk; however, unstable patients should not be sent for CT scans except for a rapid screening CT scan of the brain in an individual strongly suspected of having a life-threatening intracranial hematoma that must be drained almost immediately.

AXIOM In general, hemodynamically unstable patients should not be sent to the radiology department for CT scans.

BLUNT ABDOMINAL TRAUMA

In patients with severe blunt abdominal trauma, such as from an MVA, an initial period of hypotension may be rapidly corrected with fluid so that a more extensive radiological investigation may be undertaken to identify the site of blood loss. When the patient is stable and can be moved, radiological investigation of the patient with blunt abdominal trauma should begin with a CT examination; however, if that is

not available, supine and upright or left lateral decubitus films of the abdomen can be helpful.

CT SCAN

The most reliable study for assessment of blunt abdominal trauma is computed tomography. However, accurate CT interpretation is also strongly dependent upon a knowledge of the cross-sectional anatomy and anatomic variants that simulate disease. In addition, there are a multitude of computer and patient-generated artifacts which can cause errors in diagnosis.

CT scans of the abdomen stop above the pelvis unless a pelvic CT is specifically ordered. This is important because large pelvic hematomas may exist with little clinical evidence of their presence and with only minimal amounts of blood in the upper abdomen on the CT. The benefits of abdominal-pelvic CT scans include the ability to evaluate multiple intraperitoneal and retroperitoneal organs simultaneously. The amount and likely sites of hemorrhage can be assessed, and some of the lesions that cause hemoperitoneum that are small enough to treat non-surgically can also be identified. This is particularly true with injuries to the liver or spleen (Fig. 7-22). Conversely, large lesions can be studied and the patient reassessed noninvasively as the clinical condition warrants.

Additional benefits to the multiply injured patient evaluated by CT include significantly increased sensitivity in the detection of unsuspected pneumothorax and pneumoperitoneum. At the time of abdominal imaging, a limited screening examination of the chest can also be performed within minutes to identify or rule out mediastinal hematomas. However, one must also be aware that lap-belt injuries of the lumbar spine may be subtle and can be a pitfall in diagnosis.[50]

AXIOM CT should not be utilized to diagnose skeletal injuries, but if it is used with appropriate techniques, it can be an excellent screen.

Contrast administration is a key but controversial issue in performing CT scans of the abdomen. Many radiologists believe that the quality of the CT scan diagnosis is in direct proportion to the quantity of oral and intravenous contrast administered. Pathological and normal fluid collections may have the same appearance on CT, and accurate interpretation may depend upon opacification of the normal structures with intravenous or oral contrast. Indeed, the injuries most likely to be missed on CT scan are those involving the intestine.[51] Other injuries likely to be missed are mesentery, diaphragm, and pancreas.[53] Nevertheless, careful evaluation of a well-performed CT by an experienced radiologist should result in a high sensitivity for these injuries. A preceding DPL, however, generally precludes making a CT diagnosis of intestinal or mesenteric injuries.

The oral contrast consists of water-soluble iodinated material diluted in water to an approximately 2% concentration. Ideally, 300 to 600 cc of this oral contrast solution is administered via nasogastric tube within 30 minutes of the onset of the study, and the nasogastric tube is withdrawn into the esophagus to decrease streak artifact. If possible, diagnostic peritoneal lavage should be performed after, rather than before, the CT scan because any residual DPL fluid seen on CT could confuse the interpretation for hemoperitoneum. The intravenous contrast, usually 100 ml of a 50 to 60% iodinated substance, is given after an initial scan is performed.

AXIOM In general, the better the intravenous and oral contrast administration, the more likely it is that normal structures and pathology can be reliably differentiated by CT.

Some experienced radiologists have said, relative to CT scanning of the chest and abdomen, "No contrast, no diagnosis." However, Kinnunen et al[51] recently noted in 18 trauma patients undergoing an emergency laparotomy after an abdominal CT scan without oral contrast that omission of the oral contrast medium did not jeopardize the essential diagnoses, and it did save time.

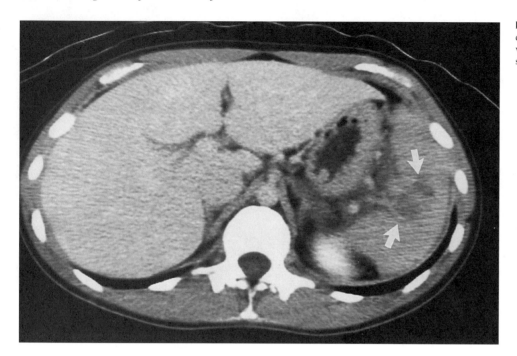

FIGURE 7-22   In this CT scan, the low-density material surrounding the splenic vessels (arrowheads) represents intravasated hemorrhage.

PENETRATING ABDOMINAL TRAUMA

Penetrating abdominal trauma is frequently evaluated by plain film radiography. Such films can be helpful for documentation of entrance and exit wounds and foreign body location. If the amount of free air is substantial, it can often be detected on supine plain films of the abdomen. However, the presence or absence of a small pneumoperitoneum may only be seen with horizontal beam films, such as upright or left lateral decubitus views.

Although a preoperative CT is rarely necessary with penetrating abdominal trauma, there are a few instances when a high quality CT can be helpful. For example, a CT scan with colon contrast can help determine the need for laparotomy in patients who have been stabbed in the flank or back.

Although the diagnostic specificity of CT is far superior to that of peritoneal lavage,[1,2] it is not as sensitive, and opinions differ as to its diagnostic value.[1,52-54] When used judiciously, alone or in combination with DPL, CT can help prevent unnecessary laparotomies in patients with splenic or hepatic injuries that have ceased bleeding. CT scans may also help detect silent injuries of intestine that need urgent attention.

INJURY TO HOLLOW VISCERA

The incidence of free air in the abdomen after penetration of the stomach or colon by a knife or bullet is surprisingly low. The small intestine is generally collapsed or filled with fluid, so that even multiple perforations may not result in visible free air. In the stomach or colon, the penetrating wound may be temporarily self-sealing, thereby limiting the quantity of gas released into the peritoneum.

Although as little as 5 cc of air may be visualized with good radiographic technique in an upright patient, the diagnosis of free air on films made with the patient recumbent is generally possible only if a large amount of air is present. Therefore, in any proper attempt to recognize free air, films of the abdomen should be taken with the patient in the upright or left lateral decubitus positions. In addition, upright PA and lateral projections of the chest are desirable, not only to evaluate the chest but also to allow small collections of free air to be demonstrated below the diaphragm. If possible, the patient should be kept in the upright or decubitus position for at least 5 to 10 minutes before the x-rays are taken. With a patient who is too ill for this, a cross-table lateral can supplement the lateral decubitus view; however, small amounts of pneumoperitoneum can be extremely difficult to identify in this projection. Although it is generally wise to explore

the patient in the operating room if perforation of a hollow viscus is suspected, in high-risk patients normal contrast studies can obviate such surgery. CT is sensitive for detection of pneumoperitoneum, especially when the reviewer specifically searches for its presence.

"Double Wall" Sign

Although most physicians can recognize intraperitoneal air on upright films, it is much more difficult on supine films. However, a "double wall" sign can help make this diagnosis. On a standard supine film of the abdomen, air located within the bowel lumen outlines only the intraluminal side of the bowel (Fig. 7-23). In patients with a ruptured

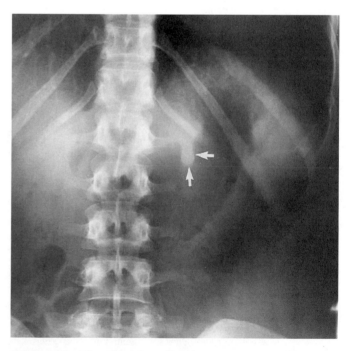

FIGURE 7-23   Normally, air located within the bowel only outlines the intraluminal side of the bowel (arrowheads); however, if there are adjacent loops of intestine, the serosal side of the bowel may be visualized.

viscus, air may outline both the mucosal and serosal sides of the bowel wall, producing a positive double wall sign (Fig. 7-24) conceptually identical to the thin white line produced by air on both sides of the visceral pleura in pneumothorax.

There are a few conditions that can mimic the double wall sign. For example, two adjacent loops of bowel will show both intraluminal walls and this may appear to represent the inside and outside of the same loop. In questionable cases (Fig. 7-25A), a left lateral decubitus film or upright lateral chest x-ray (Fig. 7-25B) may show that all of the air is intraluminal and that the false-positive double wall sign is caused by overlapping bowel loops.

In some instances, an apparent double wall sign can be ruled out by upright lateral chest film obtained at the same time. This often shows the multiple overlapping small bowel loops, the air within the stomach, and the lack of free intraperitoneal air more clearly.

AXIOM When checking for the double wall sign of free intraperitoneal air on a supine film, one should find an isolated portion of bowel that has no overlapping loops.

Occasionally, on a supine abdominal film, a large collection of air due to an abdominal abscess will be seen outside of the areas where bowel might be expected. In such instances, a decubitus view may show that the air is located outside the bowel. The absence of a double wall sign should be an indication that air located outside bowel lumen may not represent pneumoperitoneum.

AXIOM With free intra-abdominal air, the lack of a double wall sign may indicate gas within an abscess.

Occasionally, a patient with excess fat in the mesentery or retroperitoneal area will demonstrate a pseudo double wall sign because the density of fat is similar to air on plain x-rays.

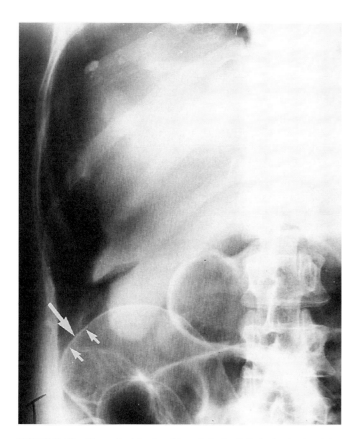

FIGURE 7-24 The patient having this radiologic study had a tender abdomen, and since the serosal side of the bowel (big arrow) is visualized so well, there must be free intraperitoneal air.

Duodenum

The possibility of rupture of the descending or retroperitoneal portion of the duodenum after blunt trauma to the abdomen merits special attention. Both the radiologic and clinical pictures may be subtle, and any delay in treatment greatly increases morbidity and mortality. Roentgenologically, this lesion is characterized by obliteration of the right psoas shadow, with bubbles of air in the right upper quadrant, in the right perinephric space, and/or along the borders of the psoas muscle.

Injury to the duodenum can also produce a large intramural hematoma involving the retroperitoneal portion of the duodenum, producing the picture of a high small bowel obstruction. Radiologically, this entity can be identified by the presence of a duodenal mass following trauma. CT has proved effective in making the diagnosis of intramural duodenal hematoma.

LIVER AND SPLEEN

When the clinical picture is unclear, radiologic techniques can help determine whether or not the liver or spleen has been injured. Although arteriography and CT scans are more precise methods for evaluating such injuries, a number of indirect signs seen on plain films can be helpful. For example, fractures of the lower ribs are often associated with blunt trauma to the liver or spleen, and a visible mass in the region of these organs is suspicious for blood or hematoma. In some instances, the injured organ is not as sharply defined as it normally is. There may also be a pleural effusion on the involved side. With some splenic injuries, the gastric air bubble may be displaced to the right or the splenic flexure may be depressed. Gastric rugae along the greater curvature may also be thicker than normal because the adjacent blood can act as an irritant, producing submucosal edema. Occasionally, the use of radioactive materials can demonstrate hematobilia, subcapsular hematoma, or abscess of the spleen or liver.

The increasing use of CT scanning, with its improved detection of splenic abnormalities and other intra-abdominal findings, has encouraged the development of grading systems for splenic trauma based upon CT findings.[55,56] Although some authors have claimed that the outcome of nonsurgical management of splenic injury can be predicted by the patient's initial CT scan,[57,58] others disagree.[59-61] Kohn et al,[62] in a recent study of 70 patients selected for non-surgical management of a spleen injury, found that properly selected patients can be safely observed regardless of the magnitude of the splenic injury. Indeed, of the ten patients with the worst spleen injuries on CT scan, nine were successfully managed non-operatively.

ANGIOGRAPHY

As previously noted, it is a good rule to finish all thoracic aortograms for blunt trauma with an abdominal angiogram. Abdominal angiography may be an alternative to lavage and/or laparotomy in patients with disruptions of the pelvic ring. Similarly, transcatheter embolization may be a viable alternative to surgery when an operation is designed only for control of hemorrhage, especially in poor-risk patients and in those with pelvic or retroperitoneal bleeding sites.

Pelvis

Hemorrhage is the most common cause of death in patients with disruptions of the pelvic ring. In massively injured patients, the fractures are frequently complex and are usually accompanied by injuries in other areas, resulting in mortality rates that are high, even without associated head injuries.[1,63,64] Precise, rapid localization of hemorrhage in a patient with a pelvic fracture can be a matter of extreme urgency. It is also a serious challenge because the pelvic hemorrhage may come from arteries, veins, or fractured bone.

In patients with pelvic fractures who have a diagnostic peritoneal lavage (DPL), there is a fairly high incidence of RBC counts exceeding $100,000/mm^3$ without any organ injury. However, if gross blood is obtained on DPL, there is at least a 40% chance that a lesion requiring surgery is present. Thus, relying on a positive microscopic exam with DPL could lead to unnecessary exploratory laparotomies.[13]

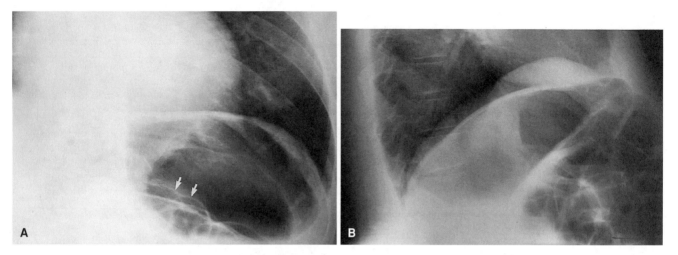

FIGURE 7-25   The patient in these upright chest and supine abdomen films had a tender abdomen. Air in the left upper quadrant (arrowheads) was thought to be outside of normal bowel (Fig. 7-25A); however, the lateral upright chest film showed that the air outside the bowel was due to overlapping loops of intestine.

In contrast, angiography can provide fast, conclusive localization of almost all active sources of arterial and parenchymal hemorrhage.[13]

Venous and osseous pelvic bleeding can generally be controlled by orthopedic reduction and fixation of the pelvic fracture. Arterial pelvic hemorrhage, almost invariably from branches of an internal iliac artery, rarely requires surgery. Surgical ligation of the internal iliac arteries via laparotomy is generally ineffective and should be abandoned in favor of angiographic hemostasis.[10,11,13]

Angiographic hemostasis can also be used instead of surgery to control hemorrhage from arterial or solid intra-abdominal organs.[65–68] It may also be used postoperatively to avoid reoperation for bleeding. Transcatheter embolization is especially effective in organ preservation for the spleen[68] and kidney, as well as in treatment of posterior retroperitoneal injuries, such as lumbar arterial hemorrhage or lumbar/caval arteriovenous fistulas.[69]

IVP and cystourethrography should not be done before angiography for pelvic bleeding. They are unnecessary to save life, and, if positive, the extravasated contrast medium can interfere with later diagnosis of arterial hemorrhage.

It must be understood that angiography and embolization are but one phase of management. Operative stabilization of the pelvic fractures may help prevent rebleeding, but coagulopathy and hypothermia can nullify the benefits of the embolization because hemorrhage can quickly restart via retrograde collaterals. The patient should also be treated supportively in an environment that allows restoration of normal body temperature and clotting activity. Platelets and fresh frozen plasma or cryoprecipitate should be given as needed to restore clotting activity to normal.

Urinary Tract

The roentgenologic evaluation of trauma to the urinary tract requires opacification procedures of one sort or another. Although excretory urography (IVP) is relatively convenient and a potentially important aid in the study of renal trauma, its accuracy is low, and there are many false-positive and false-negative results. CT scans and selective renal arteriography are the most reliable methods for determining the extent of renal injury.

Patients who require an urgent laparotomy for penetrating abdominal wounds and have a possible renal injury should have a rapid, high-dose IVP. The purpose of this IVP is to document the number and position of functioning kidneys and to hopefully identify any gross urologic trauma. An IVP should not be done on patients for whom

angiography or CT is planned. Additionally, if CT is performed primarily for urinary tract diagnosis, administration of oral contrast is unnecessary, and therefore, can be performed with greater speed, less movement, and more accuracy than an IVP.

The excretory urogram can be performed immediately, without prior preparation, by bolus administration of 50 to 60% contrast medium in a relatively high dose of about 1.0 ml/lb, up to 150 ml. Damage to the renal artery is suggested when one kidney is not visualized. Renal vein injuries can produce a swollen non-visualized kidney. Parenchymal injuries can be manifested by distortion of the collecting system or extravasated contrast material. Injuries of the renal pelvis, parenchyma, and ureters are best evaluated by dynamic CT studies.

Injuries to the urinary bladder are best evaluated by retrograde cystography.

Extremities

FOREARM AND LOWER LEG

The forearm and lower leg both have two bones. If either one of the two bones is fractured, the transmitted force frequently fractures or dislocates the other bone, often at the end remote from the injury. If only the injured distal forearm or wrist is examined radiologically, the obvious fracture of the distal ulna would be seen, but an anterior dislocation of the proximal radius would be missed. A similar problem may occur in the lower leg in which fractures of the distal tibia may be associated with proximal fractures of the fibula.

AXIOM   With any suspected fracture, the radiological examination should include the proximal and distal joints.

WRIST

After falling on an outstretched hand, persistent wrist pain with no fracture showing on x-rays of the hand, wrist, and forearm indicates a possible fracture of the navicular. If there are findings suggestive of navicular fracture, tailored navicular views may increase diagnostic accuracy.

FEMORAL NECK

Undisplaced fractures of the femoral neck can be very difficult to diagnose radiologically at times. The difficulty is even greater when the patient has demineralized bones. Unfortunately, falls and demin-

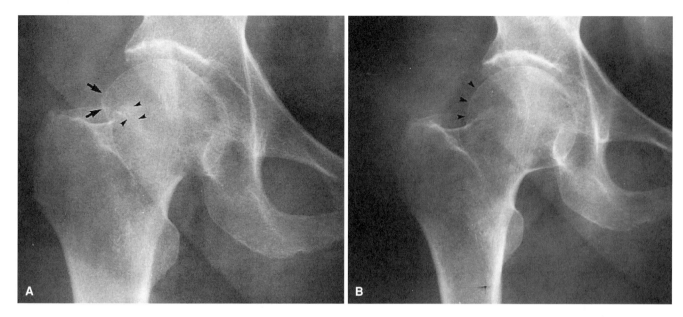

FIGURE 7-26 The patient depicted here was a 63-year-old female who fell off a stool and was tender over her right hip. There are two radiologic findings that suggest a fracture on Figure 7-26A. The first one is an area of increased bony density over the neck of the femur (arrowheads) due to impacted bone. The second finding is an abrupt change in the gentle sloping curve of the lateral aspect. Figure 7-26B is an x-ray of the hip in the same patient two years earlier. Notice that on the older x-ray, there is a gentle sloping curve at the femoral head and neck junction (arrowheads).

the lateral aspect of the femoral head as it joins the femoral neck (Fig. 7-26A). It is easier to appreciate both of these findings if one compares the x-rays to films of the other side or of the same side on a previous x-ray (Fig. 7-26B). If an earlier x-ray of the patient's hip showed a gently sloping curve at the junction of the femoral head and neck, the diagnosis is much easier to make. Conventional plain film tomography, CT, radionuclide bone scans, and MRI are also useful for definitive diagnosis, but at progressively increased cost.

KNEE

Non-displaced fractures of the knee can sometimes be very difficult to detect on x-ray examination. However, fractures of the knee are frequently associated with an accumulation of fat and blood in the knee joint. This condition, lipohemarthrosis, can easily be detected on a cross-table lateral view of the knee. Fat and blood do not mix well and tend to form a fat-fluid interface on a cross-table x-ray (Fig. 7-27). The density of fat is lower than the surrounding fluid and will resemble air on an x-ray. This suggests a fracture involving the knee.

ANKLE

Not infrequently, patients will come to the ED with ankle pain after a misstep off a curb. If only ankle x-rays are ordered, one can miss a fracture of the base of the fifth metatarsal (Fig. 7-28). One must remember that referred pain from a fractured fifth metatarsal will often mimic an injured ankle. Consequently, one must look at the metatarsal bones on all ankle films.

VASCULAR INJURIES

Vascular injuries occur with varying frequency in association with fractures and dislocations. Angiography is recommended whenever the probability of vascular injury is relatively high. For example, injury to the popliteal artery is common with dislocations of the knee,[70,71] as is trauma to the axillary or brachial arteries in conjunction with lateral fractures of the scapula.[70] Positive study results were recorded in 22.9% of calf injuries, 20% of forearm and antecubital injuries, 9.5% of popliteal fossa injuries, 9.0% of

medial and posterior thigh injuries, and 8.3% of medial and posterior upper arm injuries. We recommend arteriography for penetrating injuries to these high-risk areas. However, clinical evaluation alone is accurate for identification of arterial trauma with lateral thigh or upper arm wounds and stab wounds to the extremities.[70]

When an extremity is pulseless after having sustained several fractures, any or all of which have the capacity to cause vascular occlusion, preoperative angiography is important. If an extremity continues to have a diminished pulse after reduction of a fracture

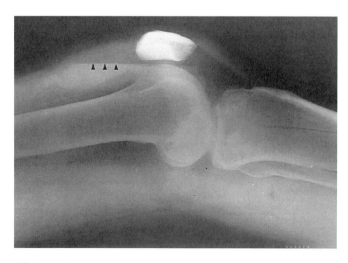

FIGURE 7-27 Fractures of the knee are often associated with an accumulation of fat and blood in the knee joint. This condition, lipohemearthrosis, can easily be detected on x-ray if one takes a cross-table lateral view of the knee as part of the examination for trauma. Fat and synovial fluid do not mix well and form an interface on the cross beam x-ray. The density of fat is lower than the surrounding fluid and will resemble air on the x-ray.

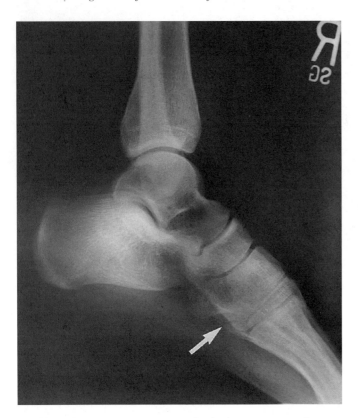

FIGURE 7-28 A common occurrence in the emergency room is a patient complaining of a tender ankle after a fall. If one only looks at the ankle on the x-ray, a fracture of the base of the fifth metatarsal is easily missed.

or a dislocation, early use of angiography is mandatory. It is advisable to do the angiogram before any orthopedic surgery begins to avoid lengthy delays in diagnosis of vascular injuries. Such delays may result in permanent disability or loss of the extremity.[70,71]

In the extremities, vascular injuries after penetrating trauma are often asymptomatic.[17,72,73] However, if overlooked, an ensuing traumatic aneurysm may produce secondary neurologic injury and result in permanent disability.[74,75] In children with vascular injuries of the extremities, there is the additional risk of growth retardation. Although children readily develop collaterals around a segmental occlusion of a main artery, the collateral circulation almost never equals the blood flow in the native artery, and the reduced blood flow may slow the rate of growth of the extremity.[76] Although the vessels in children may be much smaller, angiography is still a relatively safe procedure and should be used under essentially the same guidelines as in adults, but optimally by angiographers with extensive experience in pediatric radiology.

In both neck and extremities, angiographic control of hemorrhage has been highly successful. The radiologist's ability to approach the injury via a remote artery is usually much easier than a standard surgical approach through an area of hemorrhage. Sclafani et al[77] have also used interventional radiology to prevent central migration of a bullet in a large vein before surgery.

FAILURE OF DIAGNOSIS

Among the many causes for delay or failure of a radiologic diagnosis is the absence of a dedicated radiologist in the emergency department. To increase the effectiveness of the radiology of acute trauma, one should attempt to eliminate all unnecessary radiologic procedures from the emergency department.

RADIOLOGY DURING RECOVERY FROM TRAUMA

After initial resuscitation, radiology may have the following objectives: (a) completion of the initial investigation, (b) follow-up of healing and planning of later reconstructive surgery, and (c) diagnosis and management of late sequelae. Angiographic hemostasis is often a far better choice than reoperation for postoperative hemorrhage.[13]

Postoperative abdominal complications are often best diagnosed by CT. CT is especially important in diagnosing and localizing intra-abdominal abscesses, which may be multiple in up to 45% of infected patients.[9,78] CT can clearly define most of these abscesses and their relationship to adjacent or interposed organs. Treatment of posttraumatic and postoperative abscesses is increasingly performed radiologically. In addition, radiologists are becoming more active in postoperative management of complications of biliary and urinary tract trauma.[79]

RECOGNIZING CHILD ABUSE

In 1946 John Caffey described a syndrome in which subdural hematoma was associated with fractures of long bones, often multiple or repetitive, and in varying stages of repair.[80] The problem of unexplained fractures in infancy has received widespread attention but difficulties remain when guardians vehemently deny injuring their child.

The role of the radiologist is to:

1. Differentiate pathology from the borderlands of normality.
2. Define all radiological abnormalities.
3. Offer a differential diagnosis.
4. Suggest the etiology of any fractures that are noted and decide if that is consistent with the explanation offered by the guardians.
5. Date the injuries.

Reports of the frequency of fractures in cases of abuse vary from 11 to 55%. Metaphyseal fractures and posterior rib fractures are highly specific for abuse. In infants and young children, fractures in unusual locations also have a high specificity for abuse. Fractures that may suggest abuse include scapular fractures, fractures involving the small bones of the hands and feet, lateral clavicular fractures, and sternal and spinal fractures. It should also be remembered that lesions that have a low specificity for abuse (e.g., long bone fractures) achieve a higher specificity when a history of trauma is absent or inconsistent with the injuries.[81,82]

RADIOLOGICAL COST-EFFECTIVENESS

Cost-effectiveness is not necessarily synonymous with inexpensive radiography. Plain films offer little or no information on soft-tissue trauma. Repeating them at regular intervals and from different angles will usually provide no more information and may actually be detrimental to the patient.[5] Surgeons and radiologists should work together to determine which studies are best suited for rapid, precise diagnosis of specific injuries. In isolation, CT and angiography are expensive procedures; however, by contributing toward shorter hospitalizations, they can more than offset their cost. Furthermore, the benefits of these expensive procedures can be assessed only in the light of the alternatives their absence might create. Indeed, the cost of permanent disabilities is so high that the cost of CT and angiography, which might provide early diagnosis and guide potentially preventive therapy, is relatively insignificant. The overall cost (in money alone) of one preventable amputation can finance at least 300 angiograms.[1]

SUMMARY

High-quality studies are absolutely necessary if radiological results are to be reliable. Appropriate equipment, space, and well-trained people accustomed to dealing with injured patients are required for proper examinations. A careful and complete history and physical examination and close communication between the clinician and radiologist are essential if the radiology of trauma is to be as rewarding as it can be, not only for the patients, but also for the physicians charged with their care.

⊘ FREQUENT ERRORS

In the Radiological Examination of Injured Patients[82]

1. *Not having the proper organization, people, and equipment to perform the needed radiological studies rapidly and accurately.*
2. *Not providing the appropriate clinical information to the radiologist and x-ray technicians.*
3. *Being satisfied with inferior radiologic examinations.*
4. *Forgetting that all injuries or illnesses cannot be recognized radiologically, particularly at the time of the initial examination.*
5. *Forgetting that associated soft-tissue abnormalities can be more important than skeletal fractures or dislocations.*
6. *Forgetting that clinical considerations must override apparently normal radiological studies.*
7. *Sending an uncooperative patient to the radiologist to get CT scans of the head, chest, or abdomen.*
8. *Delaying a head CT on a patient with a severe head injury to get a skull x-ray.*
9. *Not comparing current films with old x-rays if they are available.*
10. *Diagnosing a pneumothorax without a "thin white line."*
11. *Delaying a CT of the abdomen to get an IVP.*
12. *Not getting x-rays of the joints proximal and distal to a suspected fracture.*
13. *Not obtaining x-rays of the uninjured arm or leg in a child if the bones and their growth centers in the injured side are confusing.*

▼▼▼▼▼▼▼▼▼▼▼▼▼▼▼▼▼▼▼▼▼▼▼▼▼▼▼▼▼▼

SUMMARY POINTS

1. In most instances, the amount of information that a radiologist can provide from reading x-rays is directly proportional to the information supplied to him by the clinician.
2. One should always cross-check the x-rays with the patient's identification and clinical features. In a busy emergency department, it is easy to attach incorrect identification to a radiograph.
3. A normal skull x-ray does not rule out an intracranial injury that may be fatal or require surgery.
4. Plain films of the skull should be discouraged if a CT scan will be performed because plain skull films generally cannot predict the presence of injury to the brain.
5. The best way to ensure that a patient's injury is not aggravated by motion during radiological studies is proper immobilization.
6. When considering vertebral body alignment, the posterior borders are more reliable guidelines than the anterior borders.
7. A moderately degenerated uncovertebral joint superimposed on its vertebral body can mimic a fracture on lateral cervical spine x-rays.
8. If a recent fracture has occurred, cortical bone should be interrupted.

9. Do not assume that the thoracic cage is intact because no fracture is visible, even on routine rib films.
10. Comparing current and old x-rays is an inexpensive and reliable method for improving the accuracy of x-ray interpretation.
11. The "thin white line" sign is valid only for small to medium-sized pneumothoraces.
12. Not all lines lying over the lung fields indicate a pneumothorax.
13. All two-dimensional white lines are not caused by pneumothoraces.
14. Large quantities of fluid may not be easily visible on routine x-rays of the chest in a supine patient.
15. When a small pleural effusion is suspected or difficult to see on routine chest x-rays, decubitus views may be helpful.
16. Reassessment of any radiological study with a focused history may identify a previously overlooked lesion. Furthermore, a consistent, thorough routine must be followed in interpretation of all films even after one lesion has been found.
17. If the patient cannot cooperate for a plain chest film, there is only a small likelihood of obtaining a CT of diagnostic quality.
18. Any true finding on CT scan will be present on adjacent cuts or more than one view. Artifacts are not usually consistent from film to film.
19. Traumatic diaphragmatic hernias can be difficult to recognize on the initial x-rays of the chest.
20. In general, hemodynamically unstable patients should not be sent to the radiology department for CT scans.
21. CT should not be used to diagnose skeletal injuries, but with appropriate techniques, it can be an excellent screen.
22. In general, the better the intravenous and oral contrast administration, the more likely it is that normal abdominal structures and pathology can be reliably differentiated by CT.
23. When checking for the double wall sign of free intraperitoneal air on a supine film, one should find an isolated portion of bowel that has no overlapping loops.
24. With free intra-abdominal air, the lack of a double wall sign may indicate gas within an abscess.
25. With any suspected fracture, the radiological examination should include the joints proximal and distal to the injury.

▲▲▲▲▲▲▲▲▲▲▲▲▲▲▲▲▲▲▲▲▲▲▲▲▲▲▲▲▲▲

REFERENCES

1. Ben-Menachem Y, Fisher RA. Diagnostic and interventional radiology in trauma. In: Mattox KL, Moore EE, Feliciano DV, eds. Trauma. Norwalk, CT: Appleton & Lange, 1988:187.
2. Shalen PR, Handel SR. Diagnostic challenges in closed head trauma. Radiol Clin North Am 1981;19:53.
3. Zimmerman RA, Bilaniuk LT. Head trauma. In: Dalinka MK, Kaye JJ, eds. Radiology in emergency medicine. New York: Churchill Livingstone, 1984:119.
4. Trunkey D, Federle MP. Computed tomography in perspective. J Trauma 1986;26:660.
5. Goldstein AS, Sclafani SJA, Jupperstein NH, et al. The diagnostic superiority of computerized tomography. J Trauma 1985;25:938.
6. Wing VW, Federle MP, Morris JA Jr, et al. The clinical impact of CT for blunt abdominal trauma. AJR 1985;145:1191.
7. Ben-Menachem Y, Handel SF, Ray RD, et al. Embolization procedures in trauma: a matter of urgency. Semin Intervent Radiol 1985;2:107.
8. Ben-Menachem Y, Handel SF, Thaggard A III, et al. Therapeutic arterial embolization in trauma. J Trauma 1979;19:944.
9. Sclafani SJA, Goldstein AS, Shaftan GW. Interventional radiology: an alternative to operative drainage of post-traumatic abscesses. J Trauma 1984;24:299.
10. Peltier LF, Mucha P Jr, Farrell MB. Analysis of pelvic fracture management. J Trauma 1984;24:379.
11. Tenzer ML. The spectrum of myocardial contusion: a review. J Trauma 1985;25:620.
12. Shields WE, Babcock DS, Wilson JL, et al. Localization and guided

removal of soft-tissue foreign bodies with sonography. AJR 1990; 155:1277.

13. Ben-Menachem Y, Handel SF, Ray RD, et al. Embolization procedures in trauma: the pelvis. Semin Intervent Radiol 1985;2:158.

14. Mucha P Jr, Farnell MB. Analysis of pelvic fracture management. J Trauma 1984;24:379.

15. Sclafani SJA. Transcatheter control of arterial bleeding in the neck, mediastinum, and chest. Semin Intervent Radiol 1985;2:130.

16. Sclafani SJA, Panetta T, Goldstein AS, et al. The management of arterial injuries caused by penetration of zone III of the neck. J Trauma 1985;25:871.

17. O'Gorman RB, Feliciano DV, Bitondo CG, et al. Emergency center arteriography in the evaluation of suspected peripheral vascular injuries. Arch Surg 1984;119:568.

18. Ben-Menchem Y. Logic and logistics of radiography, angiography, and angiographic intervention in massive blunt trauma. Radiol Clin North Am 1981;19:9.

19. Eckert WG. Crash injuries on the road. In: Tedeschi CG, Eckert WG, Tedeschi LG, eds. Forensic medicine. Philadelphia: Saunders Publishing, 1977;2:853.

20. Feuerman T, Wackym PA, Gade GF, et al. Value of skull radiography, head computed tomographic scanning, and admission for observation in cases of minor head injury. Neurosurgery 1988;22:449.

21. Orrison WW, Gentry LR, Stimac GK, et al. Blinded comparison of cranial CT and MR in closed head injury evaluation. Am J Neuroradio 1994;15:351-6.

22. Georgiadis G, Riefkohl R, Serafin D, et al. A silent but lethal injury associated with facial trauma. Plast Reconstr Surg 1981;67:665.

23. Handel SF, Lee YY. Computed tomography of spinal fractures. Radiol Clin North Am 1981;19:69.

24. Rogers LF, Lee C. Cervical spine trauma. In: Dalinka MK, Kay JJ, eds. Radiology in emergency medicine. New York: Churchill Livingstone, 1984:275.

25. Daffner RH. Injuries of the thoracolumbar vertebral column. In: Dalinka MK, Kay JJ, eds. Radiology in emergency medicine. New York: Churchill Livingstone, 1984:317.

26. MacDonald RL, Schwartz ML, Mirich D, et al. Diagnosis of cervical spine injury in motor vehicle crash victims: how many x-rays are enough? J Trauma 1990;30:392.

27. Van den Hoek T, Propp D. Cervicothoracic junction injury. AJEM 1990;8:30.

28. Borock EC, Gabram SGA, Jacobs LM, et al. A prospective analysis of a two-year experience using computed tomography as a adjunct for cervical spine clearance. J Trauma 1991;31:1001.

29. Ordog GJ, Albin D, Wesserberger J, et al. 110 bullet wounds to the neck. J Trauma 1985;25:238.

30. Rao PM, Bhatti MFK, Gaudino J, et al. Penetrating injuries of the neck: criteria for exploration. J Trauma 1983;23:47.

31. Meier DE, Brink BE, Fry WJ. Vertebral artery trauma. Arch Surg 1981;116:236.

32. Frazee RC, Mucha P Jr, Farnell MB, et al. Objective evaluation of blunt cardiac trauma. J Trauma 1986;26:510.

33. Beggs CW, Helling TS, Evans LL, et al. Early evaluation of cardiac injury by two-dimensional echocardiography in patients suffering blunt cardiac trauma. Ann Emerg Med 1987;16:542.

34. Phillips TF, Rodriguez A, Cowley RA. Right ventricular outflow obstruction secondary to right-sided tamponade following myocardial trauma. Ann Thorac Surg 1983;36:353.

35. Mattox KL, Limacher MC, Feliciano DV, et al. Cardiac evaluation following heart injury. J Trauma 1985;25:758.

36. Miller JT, Richards KL, Miller JF, et al. Doppler echocardiographic determination of the cause of a systolic murmur following penetrating chest trauma. Am Heart J 1986;111:988.

37. Freshman SP, Wisner DH, Weber, CJ. 2-D echocardiography: emergent use in the evaluation of penetrating precordial trauma. J Trauma 1991;31:902.

38. Fisher RG, Hadlock F, Ben-Menachem Y. Laceration of the thoracic aorta and brachiocephalic arteries by blunt trauma. Radiol Clin North Am 1981;19:91.

39. Costello, P. Spiral CT of the thorax. Semin ultrasound CT MR 1994;15:90-106.

40. Fenner MN, Fisher KS, Sergel NL, et al. Evaluation of possible traumatic thoracic aortic injury using aortography and CT. Am Surg 1990;56:497-9.

41. Madayag MA, Kirsenbaum KJ, Nadimpalli SR, et al. Thoracic aortic trauma: role of dynamic CT. Radiology 1991;179:853-855.

42. Miller FB, Richardson JD, Thomas HA, et al. Role of CT in diagnosis of major arterial injury after blunt thoracic trauma. Surgery 1989; 106:596.

43. Durham RM, Zuckerman D, Wolverson M, et al. Computed tomography as a screening exam in patients with suspected blunt aortic injury. J Trauma 1994;35:161.

44. Raptopoulos V. Chest CT for aortic injury: maybe not for everyone. Am J Roentgenol 1994;162:1053.

45. Fisher RG, Chasen MH, Lamki N. Diagnosis of injuries of the aorta and brachiocephalic arteries caused by blunt chest trauma: CT versus aortography. Am J Roentgenol 1994;162:1047-52.

46. Agee CK, Metzler MH, Churchill RJ, et al. Computed tomographic evaluation to exclude traumatic aortic disruption. J Trauma 1992;33:876-81.

47. Tomiak MM, Rosenblum JD, Messersmith RN, et al. Use of CT for diagnosis of traumatic rupture of the thoracic aorta. Ann Vasc Surg 1993;7:130-9.

48. Wilson D, Voystock JF, Sariego J, et al. Role of computed tomography scan in evaluating the widened mediastinum. Am Surg 1994;60:421-3.

49. Gundry SR, Burney RE, MacKenzie JR, et al. Assessment of mediastinal widening associated with traumatic rupture of the aorta. J Trauma 1983;23:293.

50. Taylor GA, Eggli KD. Lap-belt injuries of the lumbar spine in children: a pitfall in CT diagnosis. AJR 1988;150:1355.

51. Kinnunen J, Kivioja A, Poussa K, et al. Emergency CT in blunt abdominal trauma of multiple injury patients. Acta Radio 1994;35:319-22.

52. Sherck JP, Oakes DD. Intestinal injuries missed by computed tomography. J Trauma 1990;30:1.

53. Matsubara TK, Fong HMT, Burns CM. Computed tomography of abdomen (CTA) in management of blunt abdominal trauma. J Trauma 1990;30:410.

54. Marx JA, Moore EE, Jorden RC, et al. Limitations of computed tomography in the evaluation of acute abdominal trauma: a prospective comparison with diagnostic peritoneal lavage. J Trauma 1985; 26:933.

55. Resciniti A, Fink MP, Raptopoulos V, et al. Nonoperative treatment of adult splenic trauma: development of a computed tomographic scoring system that detects appropriate candidates for expectant management. J Trauma 1988;28:828.

56. Moore EE, Shackford SR, Pachter HL, et al. Organ injury scaling: spleen, liver, and kidney. J Trauma 1989;29:1664.

57. Malangoni MA, Cue JI, Fallat ME, et al. Evaluation of splenic trauma by computed tomography and its impact on treatment. Ann Surg 1990;211:592.

58. Raptopoulos V, Fink MP. CT grading of splenic trauma in adults: how the same statistics can be interpreted differently. Radiology 1991;180:309.

59. Mirvis SE, Whitley NO, Gens DR. Blunt splenic trauma in adults: CT-based classification and correlation with prognosis and treatment. Radiology 1989;171:33.

60. Umlas S, Cronan JJ. Splenic trauma: can CT grading systems enable prediction of successful nonsurgical treatment? Radiology 1991;178:481.

61. Umlas S, Cronan JJ. Reply. Radiology 1991;180:310.

62. Kohn JS, Clark DE, Isler RJ, et al. Is computed tomographic grading of splenic injury useful in the nonsurgical management of blunt trauma? J Trauma 1994;36:385.

63. Cook DE, Walsh JW, Vick CW, et al. Upper abdominal trauma: pitfalls in CT diagnosis. Radiology 1986;159:65.

64. Fabian TC, Mangiante EC, White TJ, et al. A prospective study of 91 patients undergoing both computed tomography and peritoneal lavage following blunt abdominal trauma. J Trauma 1986;26:602.

65. Gilliland MG, Ward RE, Flynn TC, et al. Peritoneal lavage and angiography in the management of patients with pelvic fractures. Am J Surg 1982;144:744.

66. Rothenberger D, Velasco R. Strate R, et al. Open pelvic fracture: a lethal injury. J Trauma 1978;18:184.

67. Grieco JG, Perry JF Jr. Retroperitoneal hematoma following trauma: its clinical importance. J Trauma 1980;20:733.

68. Sclafani SJA. Angiographic control of intraperitoneal hemorrhage caused by injuries to the liver and spleen. Semin Intervent Radiol 1985;2:139.

69. Fisher RG, Ben-Menachem Y. Embolization procedures in trauma: the abdomen-extraperitoneal. Semin Intervent Radiol 1985;2:148.

70. Ben-Menachem Y. Vascular injuries of the extremities: hazards of unnecessary delays in diagnosis. Orthopedics 1986;9:333.

71. Welling RE, Kakkesseril J, Cranley JJ. Complete dislocations of the knee with popliteal vascular injury. J Trauma 1981;21:450.

72. Anderson RJ, Hobson RW, Padberg FT, et al. Penetrating extremity trauma: identification of patients at high risk requiring arteriography. J Vasc Surg 1990;11:544.

73. Feliciano DV. Pitfalls in the management of peripheral vascular injuries. Probl Gen Surg 1986;3:101.

74. Gallen J, Wiss DA, Cantelmo N, et al. Traumatic pseudoaneurysm of the axillary artery: report of three cases and literature review. J Trauma 1984;24:350.

75. Raju S, Carner DV. Brachial plexus compression: complication of delayed recognition of injuries of shoulder girdle. Arch Surg 1981;116:175.

76. Valentine J, Blocker S, Chang JHT. Gunshot injuries in children. J Trauma 1984;24:952.

77. Scalfani SJA, Shatzkes D, Scalea T. The removal of intravascular bullets by interventional radiology: the prevention of central migration by balloon occlusion. J Trauma 1991;31:1423.

78. Sclafani SJA. Radiologic intervention for post-traumatic abscesses. Semin Intervent Radiol 1985;2:182.

79. Sclafani SJA, Goldstein AS, Lipkowitz GS. Radiologic management of a disrupted ureteral anastomosis and infected urinoma after gunshot wound. J Trauma 1984;24:1060.

80. Caffey, J. Multiple fractures in long bones: infants suffering from chronic subdural hematoma. Am J Roentgenology 1946;56:163.

81. Chapman S. Radiological aspects of non-accidental injury. J Royal Soc Med 1990;83:67.

82. Kurtzman R. Radiologic considerations in trauma. In: Walt AJ, Wilson RF, eds. Management of trauma: pitfalls and practice. Philadelphia: Lee & Febiger, 1975:182-183.

Chapter **8** Trauma in Infants and Children

JULIE A. LONG, M.D.

MICHAEL D. KLEIN, M.D.

INTRODUCTION

History

AXIOM Children are a special, different, and important part of society.

The concept that children are a special, different, and important part of society is recent.[1] For most of history, children were of relatively little value. They had no rights and were often considered expendable. In the 19th century, along with the reform movements that accompanied rapid industrialization, pediatrics developed as a specialty, as did children's hospitals; however, it was not until the 20th century that society considered children important.

Medicine, as part of society, has followed society's lead in developing specialties to deal with children's problems. Physicians devoted to the care of children have promoted the concept that children are special people with rights, who need protection and special care.[1] As in other areas of medical specialization, trauma is frequently different in children. There are different pitfalls to avoid in some, although certainly not all, areas. In this chapter we shall focus on what is different about trauma in children.

Recent Trends

The major health and economic impact of trauma, reviewed in 1985 by the National Academy of Science in *Injury in America*, delineated the problem and offered some solutions.[2] Regional pediatric trauma centers, in addition to improving care for trauma victims, are beginning to provide the epidemiologic and educational information found deficient in this report.[3,4]

AXIOM The patterns of injury, as well as the treatment and rehabilitation needs of children, are different from those of adults.

The American Pediatric Surgical Association and the American Academy of Pediatrics are strong advocates of pediatric trauma centers as the ideal place for the injured child. To increase knowledge and facilitate planning, a national pediatric trauma registry was begun in 1985.[5] To date, more than 37,000 children have been entered in the registry. The focus is on functional outcome, as opposed to mortality, since the mortality of pediatric trauma is relatively low, while morbidity from both a personal and social perspective is high.

PITFALL ⊘

The most common pitfall with injured children is to assume that they are small adults and treat them accordingly.

MECHANISMS OF INJURY

Trauma is an extremely important cause of mortality and morbidity in children.[6] It accounts for more deaths than all other causes combined, and results in more than two-thirds of the deaths in young boys.

Patterns and mechanisms of injury differ in children and adults. Furthermore, when pediatric trauma is analyzed epidemiologically, it becomes apparent that children tend to sustain characteristic injuries at different levels of growth and development[7-12] (Table 8-1). The infant explores with the mouth and therefore is susceptible to choking or poisoning. During the first 6 years of life, falls are the predominant form of injury. In the elementary school years, bicycle accidents and automobile-pedestrian injuries predominate. As the child grows older, personality factors, such as attitude and activity, determine the types of injuries.

AXIOM Over 80% of the injuries in childhood are due to blunt trauma and most of these occur in boys.[13]

Children who have three or more separate injuries between birth and 5 years are at increased risk of injury in the next 5 years of their life.[14] As children enter the midadolescent years, high-speed motor vehicle accidents and wounds associated with violent crime become the primary sources of trauma, much as in adults.

Penetrating wounds, which account for only about 10% of traumatic injuries in children, even in an urban environment, are more common after age 13. Also, the predominance of males as victims increases in adolescence.[15]

Children have a higher incidence of head trauma, partly because the head represents a larger proportion of their surface area than it does in adults. Children are more likely than adults to sustain injury from a fall or from a slow moving automobile. They are more likely to suffer multiple organ injury, such as a femur fracture and cerebral concussion, with or without abdominal injury.

AXIOM When trauma occurs, the child's relatively compliant body may have little external evidence of serious internal damage.

Isolated head injury accounts for 19% of pediatric trauma deaths, and head injury combined with another body part injury accounts for 70% of these mortalities.[16,17] Toys, such as lawn darts and air guns, frequently cause childhood injury.[18-20] Children ingest and aspirate far more foreign bodies, including poisons and caustics, than do adults.[21]

AXIOM Almost 30% of childhood traumatic deaths could be prevented by a dozen simple measures.[22]

A child's natural curiosity will lead to many injuries in an unsupervised or "not childproof" setting. Brightly colored, disposable lighters and guns have a particular fascination for children.

Statistics

AXIOM Injury is the most important health problem affecting children and adolescents in the United States.

Half of the patients presenting to emergency rooms in this country are under 14.[15] One-fourth of these are a result of trauma. Each year in the United States, almost 19 million children (3 of every 10) are injured severely enough to seek medical care or to restrict their usual activity.[7,8,9] Although most of these injuries are minor and with-

TABLE 8-1   Injury Deaths (United States, 1980)*

Injury Type	<1 Yr	1-4 Yrs	5-14 Yrs	15-19 Yrs	Total
Motor vehicle					
Occupant	218	493	1122	7246	9079
Pedestrian	13	435	1005	757	2210
Motorcycle	1	8	120	788	917
Pedal cycle	0	16	387	159	562
Other	20	264	285	480	1049
Total	252	1216	2919	9430	13,918
Bicycle	0	4	25	10	39
Burn	177	735	535	348	1795
Drowning	91	693	795	1012	2951
Choking/suffocation	439	214	205	131	989
Foreign body	1	4	2	2	9
Poison	22	83	52	293	450
Falls	44	111	89	209	453
Other	140	253	602	824	1819
Total	1116	3313	5224	12,259	21,962

*Data from National Center for Health Statistics.
From: Pasucci R, Walsh J. In: Capan LM, ed. Trauma anesthesia and intensive care. Philadelphia: JB Lippincott Co, 1991:568.

out serious morbidity, accidents remain the leading cause of death in children and young adults (Table 8-2).

> **AXIOM**   For all ages, accidents are the third most common cause of death, but in children they account for over 50% of all deaths.

Trauma is the leading cause of death for children more than 1 year, with nearly 15,000 children dying from trauma annually.[22] The mortality from major injury during the Vietnam War was 2%, in the multiply injured child it is 6%.

Death, however, is only a portion of the loss that pediatric patients and their families suffer as a result of injury.[15] For each death, there are another 40 to 50 nonlethal injuries requiring hospital admission.[23] These admissions constitute a significant portion of total hospitalization for children.[25]

In addition, every year 2 million children are temporarily disabled, and 100,000 are permanently crippled. In 1982 the National Safety Council estimated that the cost of injuries to children between birth and 16 years exceeded 15 billion dollars annually.[22]

STABILIZATION

Transport

> **AXIOM**   Prehospital invasive procedures should be performed rapidly by personnel with pediatric experience; emphasis should be given to rapid transport to an appropriate hospital.

In small children, invasive procedures are often more difficult, and they are more safely and efficiently performed in the hospital. Vital time may be lost by attempting intravenous access before transport to the hospital. In the youngest children, it may actually be better to "snatch and run" than to attempt any stabilization at the scene, unless the child is not breathing or the transport personnel are expert in their care.

> **PITFALL** ⊘
>
> *Attempting difficult procedures on a child without specific training or experience because they are routine in adults.*

It is important for transport personnel to be able to identify the closest facility capable of properly treating acutely injured children. Much time can be wasted transporting a child to one facility only to have a CT scan, and then transport to another facility.

Pediatric Trauma Score

The pediatric trauma score (PTS) was devised and tested as a triage tool to identify those children who might require care in a pediatric trauma center (Table 8-3).[15,26,27] This is the only trauma score specifically devised for children. Nearly 25% of injured children will present with moderate or severe injuries and require specialized trauma care as expeditiously as possible.[15] The remaining 75-80% of injured children have relatively minor trauma and do not need the expensive and limited resources of a sophisticated trauma unit.

The PTS is relatively simple and quickly calculated, yet it has shown excellent correlation between its users, including physicians and paramedics.[15,26] It has six components which can be scored as +2 (least severe problem), +1 (moderate problem), or −1 (most severe problem). The components include size of the child (more than 20 kg, 10-20 kg, less than 10 kg), airway (normal, maintainable, unmaintainable), CNS (awake, obtunded, comatose), systolic BP (above 90, 50-90, below 50 mm Hg), open wounds (none, minor, major), and fractures (none, one closed, open or multiple).

Three classes of severity of pediatric injury are recognized when analyzing the mortality of PTS scores. Children with a PTS above 8 rarely die, whereas those with a PTS of 0 or less have a mortality approaching 100%.[15,25,26] With scores between 0 and 8, a linear relationship was found between decreasing PTS and increasing potential for death.[27] Thus, any injured child whose PTS in the field is 8 or less should be transported to the highest level trauma care facility in the area.

TABLE 8-2   Major Causes of Death in Pediatric Patients (1980)

	<1 Yr	1-4 Yrs	5-14 Yrs
All causes	1,283.3	63.9	30.6
Malignant neoplasm	3.2	4.5	4.3
Major cardiovascular disease	27.8	3.2	1.3
Respiratory diseases	32.7	2.8	0.8
Congenital abnormalities	260.9	8.0	1.6
Accidents	33.0	25.9	15.0
Homicide	5.9	2.5	1.2
All other	924.8	17.9	6.4

*Data from National Center for Health Statistics. Rates per 100,000 population in specified group.
From: Pasucci R, Walsh J. In: Capan LM, ed. Trauma anesthesia and intensive care. Philadelphia: JB Lippincott Co, 1991:568.

TABLE 8-3   *Pediatric Trauma Score*

Component	+2	+1	−1
Size	>20 kg	10-20 kg	<10 kg
Airway	Normal	Maintainable	Unmaintainable
CNS	Awake	Obtunded	Comatose
Systolic BP	<90 mm Hg	90-50 mm Hg	<50 mm Hg
Open wounds	None	Minor	Major or penetrating
Skeletal	None	Closed fracture	Open/multiple fractures

PEDIATRIC TRAUMA CENTERS

The survival of children who sustain life-threatening trauma depends on prehospital care, appropriate triage, resuscitation, and emergent surgery by teams of specially trained surgeons, nurses, and hospital personnel who can carry out established pediatric trauma protocols rapidly and accurately.[28-31]

The trauma team leader is the surgeon. Since over 25% of injured children requiring hospitalization will need operative care, each step between injury and the operating room can be a potential threat to the patient.[32] The addition of another layer of care, such as triage by a nonoperating physician, in an already complex system, risks delaying definitive care and increases the potential for catastrophe.

AXIOM   Any delay in providing needed surgical care to an injured child can be catastrophic.

RESUSCITATION

Early Measures

In general, one should treat shock and airway or ventilatory impairment and then make a diagnosis. Although the incidence of cervical spine injuries is lower in children than in adults, neck immobilization is important until appropriate radiologic studies have ruled out this injury. Sand bags with proper taping may be used when appropriate size collars are not available.

Children can lose heat quickly. Their surface area is large compared to both their mass and blood volume. In addition, they have less insulating fat and thinner skin than adults. They cannot tolerate the usual 30 to 60 minutes of nakedness at room temperature that often accompanies resuscitation in adults. A trauma room for children should be equipped with both a room thermostat and overhead warmers. All blood and other intravenous fluid infused should be warmed to 40-42° C.

PITFALL ⊘

> *Allowing the child to lose heat by exposure to room temperature air and intravenous solutions.*

Ileus is more common in children than in adults, and early nasogastric intubation to prevent severe gastric distension with vomiting and aspiration is worthwhile. If there is any midfacial or anterior head trauma making one suspicious of a cribriform plate injury, the gastric tube should be placed through the mouth and not the nose. Massive pneumoperitoneum can occur in small children with gastric perforation or serious chest injuries. This can cause significant impairment of ventilation and requires prompt decompression.

AXIOM   Early decompression of the stomach is extremely important in severely injured children.

Airway

Hypoxia is the greatest single threat to the child's life. Children are fearful and anxious following injury, especially when surrounded by strangers. Hypoxia causes anxiety, fear, and agitation. It is easily treated, but if untreated, has disastrous consequences.

AXIOM   Restlessness or any change in mental status in an injured child should be attributed to hypoxia until proven otherwise.

Establishment of an airway by pulling the mandible and tongue forward in a child is most easily done with a chin lift maneuver which avoids neck extension.[15] Despite the flexibility of a child's neck, one must still be certain to stabilize the neck during any airway manipulation until the presence of a cervical spine fracture has been eliminated.

Most children can be adequately ventilated with a bag and mask, but intubation is required for severe head or thoracic trauma and is certainly convenient in many cases. In the acute situation, oral intubation is recommended over nasal. Tracheotomy is rarely indicated and can be difficult to perform in a child. If the airway is unstable and the patient cannot be intubated, a temporary needle catheter cricothyroidotomy can be performed.

AXIOM   Since infants are obligatory nasal breathers, occlusion of the nose by injuries or foreign bodies, such as nasogastric tubes; may severely impair ventilation.

If an infant needs gastric decompression, the tube should be inserted through the mouth to avoid occlusion of the nasal passage. If the nasal passages cannot be cleared, an oral airway or endotracheal tube must be inserted. The proper size endotracheal tube to use in a child may be estimated from the size of the child's external nares or little finger[33] (Table 8-4). The formula for calculating the internal diameter of the endotracheal tube ([16 + age in years] ÷ 4) is also useful.[34]

Because of variations in the size of the upper airway, the endotracheal tubes kept immediately available for insertion in a particular child during exposure of the vocal cords should include the estimated tube size plus one that is a size larger and one that is a size smaller. The endotracheal tubes used in children should be uncuffed and allow some leakage of air to prevent laryngotracheal trauma which can cause subglottic edema, ulceration, and eventual stenosis.

AXIOM   Lack of familiarity with pediatric upper airway anatomy can make endotracheal intubation extremely difficult.

It should be noted that the size of the child's tongue in relation to the oral cavity is much larger than in an adult, and the relationship of the tongue, the hyoid bone, and the epiglottis can make exposure of the glottis difficult. The infant's larynx and glottis are also more

TABLE 8-4   *Average Size of Endotracheal Tubes for Age*

Age of Patient	Internal Diameter (ID)[a] (mm)	Minimum Length, Oral Tube[b] (cm)
Preterm	2.0-2.5	10-11
0-3 months	3.0	11-12
3-7 months	3.5	13
7-15 months	4.0	14
15-24 months	4.5	15
2-10 years	$\dfrac{Age + 16}{4}$	15-21
10-15 years	6.0-7.5 cuffed	21-23
Adult	7.5-9.0 cuffed	24-26

[a]Occasionally a size 0.5 ID smaller or larger is required.
[b]For nasal tubes, add 2 to 3 cm.
(Modified from American Standards Institute, New York. Lee KW, et al. American Academy of Pediatrics Meeting. Las Vegas, Nevada, 1980. Betts EK, Downes JJ. Anesthesia, Pediatric Surgery, Yearbook Med, 1986).

cephalad, making endotracheal intubation more difficult if this peculiar anatomy of the infant is not recognized. Finally, because of the infant's large occiput, the neck is already flexed and the head slightly extended when the child is lying in a supine position.

AXIOM There is little distance in an infant between the position of an endotracheal tube that is down too far and one that is not in far enough.

The trachea in a newborn, extending from just below the vocal cords to the carina, is approximately 5 cm in length; however, it grows rapidly so that by 15 months it is approximately 7 cm long.[15,35] Failure to appreciate this short length can easily result in bronchial, rather than tracheal, intubation with resulting atelectasis of one lung. In addition, failure to secure the tube properly in the infant and to prevent excessive movement of the neck can result in bronchial intubation or accidental extubation.

Care must be taken to pass the endotracheal tube only 2 to 3 cm below the cords, and the tube should be marked at this point. Palpation of the tip of the tube in the trachea at the point between the clavicular heads is a reliable method of positioning the tube in the midtrachea of infants; however, the position of the tube should also be checked by listening for breath sounds over both lung fields before securing the tube. As in adults, the tube is anchored in the appropriate position using adhesive tape and benzoin applied to the cheek and upper lip.

AXIOM In infants, breath sounds can be easily transmitted to both sides of the chest despite lack of ventilation of one lung.

Because of the inaccuracy of checking endotracheal tube position by physical examination, a chest roentgenogram is always obtained to ascertain endotracheal tube position as soon as it has been secured.

In a child with acute obstruction of the upper airway, a large-bore needle (14- to 18-gauge) may be placed directly into the trachea through the cricothyroid membrane.[15,36] As in adults, wall oxygen can be attached to the needle and a hole cut in the tubing occluded intermittently to ventilate the child as a temporizing maneuver. Surgical cricothyroidotomy is rarely, if ever, indicated in infants or children because it can cause severe upper airway problems and has been associated with later subglottic stenosis.

AXIOM If ventilation of an infant or child cannot be promptly provided with an endotracheal tube, a large needle inserted into the trachea and attached to intermittent wall oxygen can be lifesaving.

Infants ventilate primarily with their diaphragms.[15] The rib cage of the infant and the child lacks the bucket handle mechanism present in the adult. As a consequence, any compromise of diaphragmatic excursion severely limits the child's ability to ventilate.

AXIOM Anything pressing on or irritating the diaphragm can greatly reduce the ability of a child to ventilate adequately.

Some of the abdominal problems that can severely compromise an infant's or child's ability to breathe include direct injury to the diaphragm, intra-abdominal injuries with limitation of diaphragmatic excursion, and, most commonly, gastric distension. In addition, frightened children swallow large amounts of air when they cry and the resultant gastric distension and discomfort can closely simulate an intra-abdominal injury. This is another reason to provide gastric decompression.

AXIOM Gastric dilatation can seriously interfere with ventilation and with the abdominal evaluation of critically injured children.

A full-term infant's nose will accept a 10-French nasal tube; however, if there is any local injury or difficulty passing the tube, an oro-

gastric tube can be used.[15] Smaller tubes do not function well because of the thick nature of gastric aspirate. Tube placement should be followed by radiographic evaluation to ensure proper positioning of the tube in the stomach, especially since insufflation of air into the esophagus to try to check the tube's position can easily be confused with insufflation of the stomach.

The mediastinum of infants, particularly those less than 6 months, is very mobile and does not protect the opposite lung from compression by a space-occupying process in the contralateral hemithorax.[15] Mediastinal structures can shift into the contralateral hemithorax when a simple pneumothorax, hemothorax, tension pneumothorax, or ruptured diaphragm is present. All of these will cause compression of both the ipsilateral and the contralateral lung and may result in respiratory failure.

AXIOM The mediastinum shifts easily in children, consequently any problem in one hemithorax can severely impair ventilation and venous return.

The to-and-fro movement of the mediastinum is aggravated by either injury to the phrenic nerve (leading to paradoxical movement of the diaphragm) or by a flail chest (causing paradoxical movement of the chest wall). Infants with these conditions are usually best treated by endotracheal intubation and mechanical ventilation.

After a patent airway has been established, the child's breathing should be observed carefully. If the exchange of air is inadequate or if apnea occurs, mechanical ventilation with oxygen should be instituted immediately via a mask and bag or via endotracheal intubation and then bag or ventilator support.[15] If the exchange of air is still inadequate because of a pneumothorax or hemothorax, this should be treated promptly.

AXIOM Supplemental oxygen should be given to all seriously injured children initially, even if they have no obvious difficulty with the airway or ventilation.

Although the newborn has much smaller lungs than an adult in terms of total lung capacity (63 versus 86 ml/kg) and vital capacity (35 versus 70 ml/kg), the minute ventilation (210 versus 90 ml/min/kg) and oxygen consumption (6.4 versus 3.5 ml/min/kg) are much greater (Table 8-5).[15,37] This must be taken into account when managing acute respiratory problems in the infant and young child.

SHOCK AND VASCULAR ACCESS

Circulation

Shock must be recognized and treated promptly in pediatric patients. Pediatric patients in shock can have a normal systolic blood pressure (BP) because of their ability to increase heart rate and to vasocon-

TABLE 8-5 *Normal Physiologic Data in Infants*

Pulmonary Function	*Newborn*	*Adult*
Alveolar ventilation (ml/kg/min)	130.0	60.0
Oxygen consumption (ml/kg/min)	6.4	3.5
CO_2 production (ml/kg/min)	6.0	3.0
Expired minute volume (ml/kg/min)	210.0	90.0
Respiratory rate (breaths/min)	35.0	15.0
Tidal volume (ml/kg)	6.0	6.0
Total lung capacity (ml/kg)	63.0	86.0
Vital capacity (ml/kg)	35.0	70.0

(From: Searpelle EM. Pulmonary physiology in the fetus, newborn, and child. Philadelphia: Lea & Febiger, 1975:168).

strict while in the supine position as compensation for blood losses in excess of 15% to 20%.[15] Thus, inadequate tissue perfusion in young children should be diagnosed primarily by tachycardia, tachypnea, decreased responsiveness, and decreased urine output.

AXIOM   In the non-crying child, the systolic BP should be at least 80 plus twice the age in years, while the diastolic pressure should be two-thirds the calculated systolic pressure[15,38] (Table 8-6).

Since infants have a relatively fixed stroke volume, they increase their cardiac output primarily by increasing their heart rate. For this reason, any pathologic process or drug that decreases heart rate will also decrease cardiac output, and this must be avoided in infants with shock from significant blood loss.

AXIOM   Any process that reduces pulse rate in young children can reduce their ability to sustain an adequate cardiac output.

In children, shock is generally caused by blood loss. Such hypovolemia is best treated by keeping the patient warm and rapidly administering 20 ml/kg lactated Ringer's solution as a bolus in 10 minutes or less. If there is no response, a second bolus is given rapidly. If there is still no response, type specific or O-negative blood is rapidly given along with further crystalloid.

Whenever time permits, compatibility testing should be performed before beginning blood transfusions.[15] Maternal serum can be used for cross-matching infants less than 1 week old, since IgG blood group antibodies are passively transferred from the mother to the infant during gestation.[39] For older infants and children, samples for compatibility testing are obtained from the patient. However, infants less than 4 months old rarely produce antibodies against blood group antigens. Therefore, patients within this age group do not require repeated compatibility testing, even if different donors are used, unless plasma-containing components, such as whole blood, have been transfused.[39]

AXIOM   Young children do not increase the 2,3-DPG in transfused red cells blood as rapidly as adults.

Blood used for transfusion should have adequate amounts of 2,3-diphosphoglycerate (DPG) to ensure optimal usage of oxygen by the tissues.[15] Although the 2,3-DPG levels in transfused red cells may return to normal within a few hours in adults, there is often a much longer delay in young children. For this reason, blood less than 5 days old should be selected for transfusion in this group.[39] Blood that is less than 5 days old also has relatively lower plasma potassium levels.

The rules for estimating acute blood loss in children are similar to those in the adult[15] and the "three-for-one" rule used for estimating crystalloid replacement for blood loss applies (Table 8-7).[40-43] During operative intervention, third-space requirements of lactated Ringer's are similar to those in adults at about 3-10 ml/kg/hr depending on the operative site.[44] If the hematocrit is equal to or greater than 40% in the newborn or greater than 30% in the older infant or child, colloid may be given for intravascular volume replacement in lieu of blood. This can be given as 5% albumin in lactated Ringer's in doses of 10-20 ml/kg over a 2 to 3 hour period in addition to maintenance fluid.

TABLE 8-6   Pediatric Vital Signs

Age (Yrs)	Heart Rate (/min)	Systolic Blood Pressure (mm Hg)	Respiratory Rate (/min)	Urine Output (ml/kg/hr)
0-1	120	80	40	2
1-5	100	100	30	1
5-10	80	120	20	1

(From: American College of Surgeons Committee on Trauma. Chicago: American College of Surgeons, 1985:293).

TABLE 8-7   Fluid and Blood Management

Maintenance Fluid	5% dextrose in 0.2% saline
<10 kg	100 ml/kg/24 hr
10-20 kg	1000 ml plus 50 ml/kg over 10 kg/24 hr
>20 kg	1500 ml plus 20 ml/kg over 20 kg/24 hr

Neonates may require 10% dextrose in 0.2% saline due to risk of hypoglycemia.

Blood Replacement
Replace blood loss ≤10 ml/kg with lactated Ringer's. "Three-for-one rule" applies to children as in adults.
Replace blood loss 10-20 ml/kg with 5% albumin in lactated Ringer's.
Replace blood loss >20 ml/kg with blood and 5% albumin in lactated Ringer's to maintain hematocrit at 40% in neonates and at 30-35% in older infants and children.

Hematocrit (vol %); Birth, 55%, 1-24 mo, 35%

Estimated Blood Volume

90-100 ml/kg	Premature newborn
90 ml/kg	Newborn
70 ml/kg	Child, adult male
65 ml/kg	Adult female

(From: Holliday MA, Segar WE. Pediatrics 1957;19:823. Furman EB. Int Anesthesiol Clin 1975;13:133. Gross JB. Anesthesiology 1973;58:277.)

Blood replacement can be calculated based on the estimated blood loss. If the estimated blood loss is equal to or less than 20 ml/kg, adequate replacement can usually be provided by "three-for-one" lactated Ringer's. Blood losses greater than 40 ml/kg should be at least partially replaced with packed red blood cells to maintain the hematocrit above 30-40%.

AXIOM   One should not use a scalp vein for intravenous access when rapid fluid administration may be required.

Although the ideal vascular access in severely injured children, as in adults, is one or two large bore upper extremity lines, this may not always be possible. A saphenous vein cutdown at the ankle is safe and efficient. It also keeps the person who is obtaining vascular access out of the way of the person who is securing the airway or placing a chest tube.

Percutaneous, as well as cutdown, approaches to veins in the groin and antecubital fossa are associated with complications. Some of these complications, such as venous thrombosis or nerve injury, may not be appreciated during the initial hospitalization.

Internal jugular vein and subclavian vein catheterization are possible even in the smallest child by trained and experienced personnel. It is important to remember that the anatomy in children is somewhat different than that in adults.[45] Inserting these catheters in an awake child is associated with a higher incidence of pneumothorax and arterial puncture than in adults.[46]

AXIOM   If no vascular access is available, nearly all resuscitation drugs, except NaHCO₃, can be given to children via an endotracheal tube.

Most drugs needed for resuscitation, including epinephrine and atropine, can be given through an endotracheal tube. The rich alveolar blood supply and short bronchi in young children ensure that a significant portion of the agents administered in this manner will rapidly enter the blood stream.

INTRAOSSEOUS INFUSIONS

AXIOM   If adequate vascular access cannot be obtained in a reasonable period of time for resuscitation of a hemodynamically unstable child, the intraosseous route should be considered.

In infants, fluids and drugs may be infused intraosseously. An intraosseous needle or spinal needle can be placed relatively easily into the marrow cavity of the proximal tibial plateau. The distal femur, distal tibia, sternum, clavicle, and humerus may also be used.[15] Sterile technique with a good skin prep is important, and local anesthesia should be injected into the skin and periosteum before placement of the needle. For tibial infusions, the needle should be placed 2 or 3 cm distal to the level of the tibial tuberosity on the anterior medial surface of the proximal tibia.

The needle is inserted perpendicular to the bone or pointing 60° inferiorly with the bevel directed up. Pressure and a rotary motion are used until a decrease in resistance is noted, indicating that the medullary cavity has been entered. It is not always possible to aspirate marrow, but the fluid should run easily without a pump.

> **AXIOM** Provision of adequate ventilation, oxygen, and blood volume are the most important priorities in pediatric trauma resuscitation; drugs may confuse the clinical picture.

Intraosseous infusions have included saline, glucose, blood, sodium bicarbonate, atropine, dopamine, epinephrine, diazepam, antibiotics, phenytoin, and succinylcholine.[15,47] However, use of such medications should be minimal.

Reported complications with intraosseous infusions, such as cellulitis, osteomyelitis, extravasation, and hematoma, are relatively uncommon.[48,49] If there is a nearby fracture or open wound which may be contaminated, that particular site cannot be used. Multiple attempts to place the needle in the medullary cavity should be avoided since the other holes in the bone can allow leakage of fluid into adjacent soft tissue.

> **AXIOM** Intraosseous infusions should be limited to emergency resuscitation and used only until other venous access is obtained.

Maintenance fluid is administered on a ml/kg body weight basis as 5% dextrose solution in 0.2% normal saline (NS) plus 2 mEq potassium chloride (KCL) per 100 ml of intravenous fluid. Because premature infants and stressed full-term infants may have a depletion of liver glycogen, they are prone to develop severe hypoglycemia following injury. Consequently, they should be maintained on a 10% dextrose solution in 0.2% NS and the serum glucose levels followed at regular intervals at the bedside.

> **AXIOM** Severe hypoglycemia can develop rapidly in infants unless some glucose is given in their intravenous maintenance fluids.

URINE OUTPUT

Renal function of the neonate is characterized by an ability to dilute, but not concentrate, urine.[15] The glomerular filtration rate of a term baby is only 25% of that in adults, but it rises to 70% of adult levels by 2 weeks of age.[50] It then slowly rises to normal adult levels by 1 ½ to 2 years of age. Dehydration in these children can rapidly lead to renal impairment.

> **AXIOM** Diuretics or dopamine should not be used to increase urine output when a child is hypovolemic.

A full-term infant, in response to water deprivation, can increase urine osmolality to only 500 to 600 mOsm/kg, while an adult can concentrate to levels of 1200 to 1400 mOsm/kg.[51] Consequently, the needed urine output for a low-birth-weight infant to excrete its solute load may be as high as 4 ml/kg/hr, for a newborn it is 1.5-2.0 ml/kg/hr and, for a child, 0.5-1.0 ml/kg/hr is usually adequate.

In situations in which there is an increase in protein catabolism, such as following trauma, the solute load may be significantly higher,

and a much higher urine output may be required. A urinary osmolality of 600 in the neonate may indicate that the infant is quite dehydrated; in contrast, the same osmolality in an adult usually indicates normal hydration.[52]

> **AXIOM** A urine osmolality of 600 mOsm/kg in a newborn usually indicates hypovolemia.

HYPOTHERMIA

Hypothermic stress is a significant problem in injured infants and children.[15] Hypothermia has been shown to stimulate the secretion of catecholamines and muscle shivering, and this can cause severe metabolic acidosis, especially if tissue perfusion is impaired.[53] The infant who is hypothermic may be refractory to therapy for shock, may develop bleeding disorders, and may have a prolonged effect from anesthetic agents.[54]

> **AXIOM** Severe hypothermia can develop rapidly in young traumatized children and can cause severe physiological derangements.

The high ratio of body surface area to body mass, the small glycogen stores in the liver, the lack of substantial subcutaneous tissue, and the thin skin with increased conductive heat loss all greatly affect a child's ability to regulate core temperature. The range of thermal neutrality, the temperature at which the metabolic activity keeps caloric production at a basal level, is much higher for the newborn and infant than for an adult.[55]

> **AXIOM** Injured infants should be treated in an environment maintained between 24°-27° C (75°-80° F).

In the neonatal nursery, babies are kept warm by using such techniques as radiant warmers, cellophane wraps to decrease convection losses, and warming of inspired gases. The temperature of the operating room should also be kept at 24°-27° C.[15] Attempts should be made to decrease the amount of heat loss due to evaporation of fluid from the baby's skin surface as well as from opened surgical wounds.

Fluids for preparation of the skin and irrigation of body cavities should be warm and should not be allowed to soak the infant's skin and back, resulting in evaporative heat loss.[15] Placement of eviscerated intestine in a plastic bag or maintaining it within the abdominal cavity is also helpful in decreasing the amount of evaporative heat and water loss during celiotomy.[56]

The insertion of intravenous catheters and the induction of anesthesia should begin with the baby under a radiant heater; however, once the baby is covered by the sterile sheets, the radiant warmer is no longer effective, and a heating blanket and extremity wraps must be used.

> **AXIOM** All intravenous solutions, including blood, given to an injured child should be warmed to 40°-42° C.

Only intravenous fluids that have been kept in a warmer should be used. When large volumes of intravenous fluid are needed, the administered blood and fluid should be passed through a warming coil.[15]

PROCEDURES IN THE ED

With the exception of select, penetrating thoracic injuries, there is no place for open procedures in the chest or abdomen in the emergency department during the resuscitative phase. Ventilation and circulation should be established and the patient moved to the operating room for further resuscitation, continued evaluation, or surgery as needed. An exception to this practice would be a child with a penetrating thoracic injury who loses his or her vital signs immediately before or while in the emergency department.

CARDIAC ARREST AND DRUGS

AXIOM Children who experience a cardiac arrest after trauma need oxygen, fluid, and blood rather than multiple drugs or electric shocks.

Attempts to defibrillate hypoxemic and hypovolemic children are generally futile.[57] Nevertheless, if cardiac arrest or hypotension persists after adequate oxygen has been provided and blood volume has been restored, some drugs may be helpful (Table 8-8). Asystole and bradyarrhythmias are responsible for 90% of the rhythms seen in pediatric cardiac arrests. If ventricular fibrillation occurs, children can usually be defibrillated promptly with only a 2 to 4 watt-second (joules)/kg shock.

MONITORING

Vital Signs

It is crucial that all members of the team caring for seriously injured children know the range of normal values for the vital signs in infants and young children (Table 8-3). Thus, a systolic BP of 80, heart rate of 120/min, and respiratory rate of 40/min might be normal in an infant, but it would be evidence of shock and/or acute respiratory distress in an older child.

PITFALL ⊘

Assuming that normal vital signs in an infant or young child are the same as in an adult.

In small children, the stroke volume is relatively fixed, and therefore cardiac output is much more dependent on heart rate than it is in older children and adults. Hypotension and/or severe trauma with a heart rate less than 100 in an injured child is a sign of impending vascular collapse.

AXIOM Bradycardia in an injured child can be an ominous sign.

TABLE 8-8 *Pediatric Doses of Resuscitation Drugs*

Drugs	Dose	Purpose
NaHCO$_3$	1 mEq/kg (1 ml/kg of an 8.4% solution 0.5 mEq/kg in neonates (also in neonates dilute in an equal volume of D5W)	Correction of metabolic acidosis
Atropine	0.02 mg/kg up to 1 mg	Increase heart rate (in children cardiac output is often rate dependent)
Epinephrine	0.01 mg/kg 0.1 ml/kg of a 1:10,000 solution	Chronotropic and inotropic
Isoproterenol	0.1 to 1.0 μg/kg/min 0.6 × kg = mg to add to 100 ml; then 1 ml/hr delivers 0.1 μg/kg/min	Continuing chronotropic and inotropic Bradycardia
Dopamine	5-20 μ/kg/min 6 × kg = mg to add to 100 ml; then 1 ml/hr delivers 1 μg/kg/min	Low dose increases renal perfusion Higher doses are pressor
Dobutamine	5-15 μg/kg/min 6 × kg = mg to add to 100 ml; then 1 ml/hr delivers 1 μg/kg/min	Inotropic and pressor
Lidocaine	1 mg/kg, then 20-50 mg/kg/min	Treatment of ventricular tachyarrhythmias
Bretylium	5 mg/kg	Treatment of ventricular tachyarrhythmias

Most evaluations of injured children will be directed by their "stability." Children who have normal vital signs, or who achieve normal vital signs after receiving 20 ml/kg of fluid, are considered stable. At this point, the patients can undergo further diagnostic evaluation, including radiographic examination of the cervical spine, chest, abdomen, and pelvis, as needed.

NONINVASIVE MONITORING

AXIOM Oxygen saturation monitors usually will show oxygen desaturation before bradycardia develops, allowing time to correct the developing pulmonary or cardiovascular problem before it becomes serious and difficult to reverse.

Monitoring of children who may have had significant injuries should include ECG, blood pressure, pulse oximetry, and urine output. The patient should be hemodynamically stable, and these monitoring devices should be in place before transport to radiology. Monitoring is futile if the child is not constantly attended by at least one knowledgeable member of the trauma team.

PITFALL ⊘

If all injuries in infants and young children are not taken seriously, what appears to be anxiety or fear can rapidly become life-threatening hypoxia, and what appear to be normal vital signs with some tachycardia can rapidly become total cardiovascular collapse.

The most valuable noninvasive monitor is serial physical examination by a concerned and well-trained physician. The most helpful blood test is the serial hematocrit.

INVASIVE MONITORING

Children with a score of 8 or less on the Glasgow Coma Scale (GCS) or other evidence of a severe head injury are treated with hyperventilation, judicious use of fluids, and possibly intracranial pressure monitoring. For children who are less than 6 years of age, the children's coma score (CCS), which has a maximum score of 11, should be used rather than the Glasgow Coma Scale[58,59] (Table 8-9). Furthermore, a CCS of 5 or less is equivalent to a GCS of 3 in an adult (Table 8-10). Indeed, below 1 year of age, spontaneous motor movements may be misinterpreted as responses to the examiner causing the infant to be inappropriately placed in a less severe injury category.

Patients with severe head trauma or multisystem injury should have arterial and central venous lines. Swan-Ganz catheters are seldom used in children, and should be limited to patients who are more than 2 years of age or weigh more than 8 kilograms and who have cardiac or pulmonary disease that might limit the value of CVP monitoring.

EVALUATION

History and Physical Examination

One member of the team should obtain details of the events surrounding the injury from whomever transported the child. These should include the time of the accident, mechanism of injury, position of the child when discovered, speed of any vehicles involved, other people injured, mental state of the victim, type of transport, and any changes in the clinical status before or during transport. Efforts should be made to find a parent or relative who can give past medical history, including immunizations, previous hospitalizations, possible congenital anomalies, and allergies.

A history of minor trauma resulting in significant injury should make one suspicious of child abuse or an underlying congenital anomaly. Hematuria following minor abdominal trauma, for example, may be the presenting sign of congenital hydronephrosis or Wilms' tumor. Pathologic fractures may occur at the site of bone tumors, and excessive bruising may be a presenting feature of leukemia.

TABLE 8-9 **Coma Scoring Systems: Glasgow and Children's**

GCS		CCS	
Eye Opening		Ocular Response (O)	
4	Spontaneous	4	Pursuit
3	Speech	3	Extraocular muscles (EOM)
2	Pain		intact, reactive pupils
1	None		fixed pupils or EOM
			impaired
		2	Fixed pupils and EOM
			paralyzed
		1	
Verbal Response		Verbal Response (V)	
5	Oriented	3	Cries
4	Confused	2	Spontaneous respirations
3	Inappropriate		apneic
2	Incomprehensible	1	
1	None		
Motor Response		Motor Response (M)	
6	Obey command	4	Flexes and extends
5	Localize pain	3	Withdraw from painful
4	Flexor withdrawal		stimuli hypertonic
3	Flex-abnormal	2	Flaccid
2	Extension	1	
1	None		

AXIOM As in adults, careful, repeated physical examination is the most valuable tool for assessing the injured child.

CHILD ABUSE AND NEGLECT

When society had not yet accorded children full rights as people, the concept of child abuse did not exist. For centuries, the flogging of children and even infanticide were tolerated by society. As measures were taken to protect children in the 19th and 20th centuries, it was as if the medical profession had assumed no one would any longer intentionally abuse a child. Yet it was not until the reports of Caffey,[60] and later Wooley and Evans,[61] and Kempe et al,[62] that the widespread problem of child abuse became common knowledge, adding it to the differential diagnoses for many of the presenting signs and symptoms in injured children.

AXIOM Child abuse is common and can have dire consequences if not recognized and treated early.

Child abuse is a growing problem. Approximately one million children are abused in the United States every year, and it is estimated that between 2000 and 5000 children die annually as a result of this type of trauma, usually from major head and abdominal injuries.[60-62]

AXIOM Child neglect may be just as dangerous as child abuse and should be reported as soon as it is suspected.

Shaking, punching, whipping, or burning a child is abuse.[63] Locking a child in a car on a hot summer day, or in a room with poisons and matches, may be more neglect than abuse, but can lead to just as severe an injury.[7] Lack of immunizations, unusual prior hospitalizations, and a mechanism of injury inconsistent with the examination should raise suspicion. A Polaroid camera is an extremely useful tool in the emergency room to record evidence of child abuse such as bruises, cigarette burns, and electrical cord whip marks.

AXIOM The possibility of abuse or neglect should be strongly suspected if the injuries or the child's or parent's behavior are unusual.

LABORATORY EVALUATION

As soon as an intravenous route is established, blood should be drawn for a type and cross-match and for measuring hemoglobin and hematocrit. Other useful, but less urgent, blood tests include liver enzymes, amylase, and blood gases.[64] If the patient can void, the urine can be evaluated with a dipstick. Recent studies indicate that gross hematuria, microscopic hematuria with 50 RBC/HPF or higher, or any microscopic hematuria persisting beyond 24 hours indicates a need for an IVP or CT scan with intravenous contrast.[65-67] Microscopic hematuria below 50 RBC/HPF does not usually demand urgent study. Most urine dipsticks are positive for blood at 10 RBC/HPF or higher, so they are a satisfactory screening device for serious urinary tract injury.

Roentgenograms

Plain films of the neck, chest, and pelvis are usually done as part of the resuscitation protocol for severely injured children. Radiographic evaluation of extremity fractures can wait until resuscitation is completed, but they should not be overlooked. Long-standing disability can occur from an arm fracture if any associated neural or vascular compromise is not given prompt, appropriate therapy, even though it may appear to be a minor problem at the time.

PITFALL ⊘

Failure to assess the neurovascular status of the extremities early and completely, especially if there is any suspicion of a fracture or dislocation.

Skull films are useful when there is a cranial hematoma, palpable fracture, or other evidence of a significant head injury. They are not, however, necessary in all patients with a history of head trauma.[68]

CT Scan

When a CT scan is done for abdominal trauma, both oral and intravenous contrast should be used. The intravenous contrast may dem

TABLE 8-10 **Coma Scoring Systems and Highest Level of Brain Function**

Highest Level of Brain Function	GCS	CCS
Cerebral Cortex	15	
	14	
	13	
	12	11
	11	
	10	
	9	
Subcortical	8	10
	7	
	6	
	5	9
		8
	4	7
		6
Brainstem		5
		4
	3	3

onstrate bleeding sites and distinguish between hematomas and blood vessels. They generally also provide a much better evaluation of both kidneys than a standard IVP. If the duodenum is obstructed by an intramural hematoma or laceration, an oral contrast study will usually be diagnostic.

AXIOM Bowel perforation is less frequent with blunt trauma in children than in adults. Consequently, blunt trauma to the abdomen in a stable child is less apt to need exploration than in an adult.[69]

The CT scan has a very important role in the evaluation of head trauma. At the Children's Hospital of Michigan, children with a history of loss of consciousness, but improving levels of consciousness, are admitted for observation, and do not routinely have a CT scan of the head. However, head CT scans are obtained on children with any persistent alteration in the level of consciousness, any focal neurologic signs, or any acute deterioration.[70]

Although children with severe head trauma who respond to pain can be followed by serial abdominal examinations, it is our policy to perform abdominal CT scans in all patients with an equivocal abdominal examination, abnormal vital signs, or abnormal laboratory evaluation. In addition, if the trauma includes a pelvic or femoral fracture, an abdominal CT scan can help differentiate blood loss into the abdomen from that into and around the fracture sites.

Arteriography

AXIOM Although arteriography in small children is often more hazardous than in adults because of the small size of the vessels and the frequent need for sedation or even general anesthesia, diagnosis of aortic or arterial injury may be impossible without it.

Arteriography should be performed on any extremity with a fracture or dislocation associated with abnormal pulses in conjunction with orthopedic evaluation. Angiography should also be performed for all dislocations of the knee or any fractures of the knee with severe displacement. The presence of an audible doppler pulse does not rule out vascular injury in a child. Even though biphasic pulses can sometimes be heard distal to a completely obstructed artery, it is unlikely that triphasic sounds will be found.

TREATMENT

General

Children have a much higher metabolic rate than adults and require even more calories/kg/day following trauma. Also, their free-water clearance is less efficient so they tend to develop more edema with resuscitation fluids. The diuretic phase usually occurs later than in adults. Consequently, the presence of peripheral edema alone should not cause one to withhold fluid that may be necessary to maintain an adequate intravascular volume and tissue perfusion.

AXIOM Injured children can develop peripheral edema even when they are still hypovolemic.

Head Injuries

Scalp injuries in adults may bleed excessively but seldom cause shock; however, in small children, the blood loss is relatively much greater, and consequently, scalp lacerations should be sutured promptly to control hemorrhage.

AXIOM Many physicians worry that aggressive crystalloid resuscitation can worsen brain edema; however, failure to promptly restore an adequate cerebral perfusion is far more detrimental.

After an adequate resuscitation, volume restriction and/or the judicious use of mannitol (while still maintaining an adequate cerebral perfusion) may help control elevated intracranial pressure. Consequently, if there is a significant head injury and if the intracranial pressure is elevated, monitoring of central venous pressure and arterial blood gases (ABGs) is indicated.

AXIOM Maintenance of optimal tissue perfusion is extremely important and should not be restricted because of concerns about increasing ICP in children with head injury.

The psychological aspects of the child with an acute and painful injury, in a strange and frightening environment, should be considered, but they should not be used to explain symptoms that may also be caused by hypoxia, hypothermia, or hypovolemia. Most children with severe trauma will regress to an earlier stage of development. Children who are walking may no longer be able to do so after the injury even if there is no apparent physical problem that should interfere with that activity. Those who were toilet trained may need diapers again. Hostility is common. The response to pain may be delirium, but is as likely to be expressionless withdrawal. The latter is especially true in children who have been chronically abused.

AXIOM Expressionless withdrawal in an injured child should make one suspect child abuse.

Neck Injuries

As in adults, most neck injuries can be managed nonoperatively. When indicated by physical examination and history, esophogram, esophagoscopy, laryngoscopy, and bronchoscopy can be useful. If there is suspicion of a vascular injury in the neck, arteriography should be done, and this is generally performed using a Seldinger technique via a femoral artery under general anesthesia preceding endoscopy.

Chest Injuries

The epidemiology of thoracic trauma and the pattern of injuries in children may be quite different from those seen in older teenagers and adults.[71] While penetrating injuries to the chest occur frequently in adults, they are extremely rare in children.[72-75] When they do occur in young children, they are frequently the result of fractured ribs or clavicles and not from external missiles.[72]

A major difference between children and adults is the compliance of the thorax.[15] The bony and cartilaginous structures of young children are extremely flexible. While fractured ribs are often seen in teenagers and adults who have severe blunt chest trauma, simple fractures and flail chest are uncommon in younger children; however, because of the elasticity of the chest wall, the force of the trauma can be transferred directly to the underlying pulmonary parenchyma, resulting in a pulmonary contusion in nearly 60% of severe thoracic injuries.[76]

Aspiration of gastric contents often occurs with severe chest trauma, and this may result in severe aggravation of the pulmonary injury. Respiratory distress syndrome is relatively infrequent in children, but it is treated in a manner similar to that described for adults.

An open pneumothorax resulting from penetrating trauma occurs only rarely in children.[15] Of more than 1000 children admitted with life-threatening trauma to Johns Hopkins' Regional Trauma Center for Children, none had a sucking chest wound.[77] In the same series, only one patient had a ruptured diaphragm; however, because the mediastinum of the child is very mobile, a pneumothorax can easily dislocate the heart and cause angulation of the great vessels (reducing venous return) and compression of the lung and trachea (reducing minute ventilation). Consequently, early chest tube decompression is important. The small pericardial sac also means that small amounts of fluid can cause pericardial tamponade and must be removed promptly.

While blunt trauma accounts for 90% of thoracic injuries in children, these injuries are typically less severe than in adults.[78] Partial or impending aortic rupture is also rare in young children, probably because the forces of injury are less and the aorta is very elastic and without atheromata. Nevertheless, Smyth[76] reported 97 children with severe thoracic injuries and documented a mortality of 14%; moreover, in children younger than 5 years of age, the mortality was 23%. Thoracic injuries have also been noted in 28% of children who died before receiving medical therapy.

Severe thoracic trauma may rapidly cause hypoxemia and hypotension, which allows little time for deliberation or consultation, as the child's oxygen demand is relatively greater and the respiratory reserve less than in adults.[78] Consequently, immediate correction of the functional defect is often required before anything can be learned about the mechanism of injury or the child's prior physical condition.

When a chest tube is required to drain a significant hemothorax or pneumothorax, it should be inserted no lower than the fifth intercostal space at the mid or anterior axillary line.[15] Chest tubes are not inserted low in the chest as the diaphragm in a child may be quite high because of intra-abdominal injury, gastric distension, or respiratory effort. Pediatric chest tubes start at size 10-French. Trocars are used more often in children than adults since it is frequently difficult to place a finger or even a clamp into the pleural space through the narrow intercostal space. However, chest tubes must be inserted with great caution in children because the greater chest wall compliance increases the chance of iatrogenic injury to underlying structures.

Abdominal Injuries

Intraoperative treatment of specific injuries has evolved in the past 30 years, but the main controversy is the proper evaluation and selection of patients for nonoperative management of abdominal injuries. Before Shaftan's classic paper in 1960,[79] optimal management of significant penetrating or blunt abdominal trauma was routine laparotomy. Prompted by Lowe's report of 1.6% mortality, 19% morbidity, and 3% readmission for adhesive bowel obstruction after negative laparotomies, a selective nonoperative approach has been developed to minimize unnecessary laparotomies.[80] The increased incidence of postsplenectomy sepsis noted by pediatricians and pediatric surgeons provided further impetus for selective nonoperative management of trauma.[81,82]

AXIOM   Whenever possible, injuries to the liver or spleen in hemodynamically stable children should be treated nonoperatively.

Successful management of a child who sustains abdominal trauma requires avoidance of certain pitfalls.[83,84] Physical examination of the abdomen for peritoneal irritation is difficult and can be misleading in children with either lower rib fractures, contusions of the abdominal wall, pelvic fractures, or gastric dilatation.[15]

The usual response of a child to injury is aerophagia, which can rapidly result in massive gastric distension, and may be made worse by reflex ileus, mask-assisted ventilation, or inadvertent esophageal intubation during airway management. For these reasons, early insertion of a nasogastric tube to decompress the stomach is extremely important. This may prevent respiratory insufficiency, decrease the likelihood of aspiration, minimize the potential for gastric rupture, and facilitate physical examination of the abdomen.

AXIOM   The majority of children with abdominal trauma can be treated nonoperatively, but they must be observed carefully.

Children with transient hemodynamic instability, falling hematocrit, or questionable abdominal exams warrant further careful evaluation. Any child who fails to stabilize with resuscitation or who destabilizes (criteria here vary depending on the clinical situation) requires laparotomy.[15] Laparotomy is also required in all children with gunshot wounds to their abdomen, peritoneal signs, or free air.

The presence of omental evisceration is also considered an indication for laparotomy for two reasons: the high rate of associated intra-abdominal injuries, and the difficulty in reducing an omental evisceration in an awake child.[85]

A CT scan with intravenous and oral contrast can be especially helpful in the evaluation of abdominal trauma in children.[15,86] Some of the indications for CT scanning in injured children with stable vital signs include: (a) suspected intra-abdominal injury, (b) slowly declining hematocrit or requirement for persistent fluid resuscitation, (c) head injuries with altered consciousness, (d) multiply injured patients requiring general anesthesia, and (e) urine with greater than 50 RBC/HPF.

One of the main disadvantages of routine CT scanning of the abdomen and pelvis after trauma includes the amount of time required to do the study and the expense.[15] Nevertheless, CT scans of the abdomen and pelvis are effective in documenting not only specific hepatic and splenic injuries but also other associated intra-abdominal injuries.[87,88] While CT scans will provide an explanation for the clinical situation, it rarely provides information necessitating a laparotomy; such decisions are usually based on clinical information, such as hemodynamic stability and/or evidence of peritonitis, rather than specific laboratory or radiologic findings.

AXIOM   The decision to perform a laparotomy after trauma is primarily based on clinical findings.

Diagnostic peritoneal lavage (DPL) can be used to exclude abdominal injury in children presenting with life-threatening extra-abdominal injury who require operations for those problems. It may also be useful to evaluate peritoneal injury in selected patients with abdominal stab wounds.

When performed in children, DPL is generally performed by the Seldinger technique developed by Lazarus and Nelson because this has far fewer complications in children than the mini-laparotomy procedure often used in adults.[89] Although it is a highly sensitive test for peritoneal injury, presence of intraperitoneal blood is not considered an indication for laparotomy in a child. Powell et al[90] found that nearly a third of children operated on because of increased red cells on DPL had injuries that did not require surgical intervention. For this reason, a strongly positive lavage in hemodynamically stable patients no longer mandates immediate exploratory celiotomy.

AXIOM   Peritoneal lavage is indicated in injured children who require immediate surgical intervention for extrabdominal injuries or who have suspected abdominal injuries causing hemodynamic instability.

Neurological injury, obtundation, or other injuries requiring urgent correction render repeated physical examinations unreliable.[15] Diagnostic peritoneal lavage may be negative in the face of retroperitoneal injuries, including those involving the duodenum and pancreas, and it may be "falsely positive" with pelvic fractures. Nevertheless, it may be useful to reassess the abdomen in multisystem injured children who have a changing abdominal exam 24-48 hours after admission to the intensive care unit.

Splenic Injuries

The spleen is the most commonly injured intra-abdominal organ during childhood.[91] The mechanism of injury and the clinical presentation are similar for children and adults; however, fractures of the overlying ribs are infrequent in young children because of the elasticity of their chest wall.

Several special considerations have led to a more conservative, nonoperative approach to splenic injuries during childhood.[15,92,93] First has been the realization that the incidence of overwhelming sepsis after splenectomy for trauma is more than 85 times the rate in the normal population. Furthermore, the mortality rate in those developing this syndrome is close to 50%.[94] While sepsis may occur any time after splenectomy, the risk is greatest during the first 2 years after splenectomy and occurs most frequently in children less than 5 years of age.[95]

The spleen produces several substances, such as immunoglobulins and tuftsin, that are important in the body's defense against certain infections. Tuftsin is an opsonin-like substance that enhances neutrophil phagocytosis of encapsulated organisms such as the pneumococcus, *Hemophilus influenzae,* and meningococcus.[96]

Second, the splenic capsule and splenic tissue of children hold sutures well and repair more readily than in adults.[15,97] Thus, persistent hemodynamic instability in patients with splenic injuries indicates exploratory laparotomy, but the splenic injury can often be repaired. Even if the injury cannot be repaired, at least part of the spleen can often be salvaged. Ligation of hilar vessels, repair of lacerations with chromic catgut sutures or Vicryl mesh, and application of hemostatic agents such as Gelfoam, Surgicel, Avitene, or fibrin glue to torn parenchyma can control most splenic hemorrhage.[15]

Third, the spleen of the child will often stop bleeding spontaneously; therefore, the vast majority of splenic injuries will respond to nonoperative management.[15,98] The surgical team at Children's Hospital National Medical Center in Washington DC treated 42 children with proven splenic injuries over a 4-year period, and nonoperative management was possible in 37 (88%).[95] An additional three patients underwent splenorrhaphy, and only two required total splenectomy. This is a splenic conservation rate of 95%.

AXIOM   The majority of children with splenic injuries can be safely treated nonoperatively.

In patients with suspected splenic injury, the site and extent of the injury should be defined by CT scan.[15] If the site of bleeding is confirmed to be the spleen, the child may then be treated nonoperatively, provided several prerequisites are fulfilled.[96]

1. The patient must be monitored continuously for at least 48 hours.
2. The surgical team must follow the patient closely and be prepared to intervene at any time.
3. Adequate support from anesthesia and transfusion services must be constantly available.

Patients with massive bleeding should be operated on promptly. In general, patients who require replacement of more than half their blood volume (i.e., more than 40 ml/kg of blood replacement) within the first 24 hours after injury require operative intervention.[99] Those with less bleeding may be treated nonoperatively, but this is a clinical surgical decision.

Sufficient experience with nonoperative management of splenic injuries has shown that these children do well and have decreased transfusion requirements, shorter hospitalizations, and fewer complications compared to children treated surgically.[100] The decision to perform repeat CT scans is based on the extent of the initial injury and the practice at the individual institution. Repeat scans usually show dramatic improvement in 7–10 days, corresponding to the time when most pediatric surgeons allow increased activity. Children can resume complete activity in 2 months, providing other injuries are not present.

Liver Injuries

The liver is the second most frequently injured intra-abdominal organ during childhood.[15] An isolated injury of the liver without involvement of its associated large vessels (portal vein, hepatic veins, or suprarenal inferior vena cava) is like a splenic injury and the majority can be treated nonoperatively.[103]

More frequent CT scanning of children with abdominal trauma has increased diagnoses of small or insignificant hepatic injuries.[15] In addition, many patients with extensive liver injuries seen on CT scan remain hemodynamically stable and can avoid surgical intervention.[101] The same criteria for selecting nonoperative or operative treatment for patients with splenic injury are now used for patients with documented hepatic injuries.[102] The child who is not hemodynami-

cally stable is not a candidate for nonoperative management. The treatment of massive liver injuries with life-threatening hemorrhage in children is similar to that described for adults.[103]

At Children's Hospital National Medical Center seven patients with severe hepatic injuries were treated nonoperatively.[15,104] Although all seven had resolution of their injury without mortality, significant morbidity occurred in five of the seven patients in the form of hemobilia, fever, and sepsis, requiring prolonged hospitalization. Several other centers, however, have reported a favorable outcome and minimal morbidity with nonoperative treatment of hepatic injuries in stable children.[102,104,105]

Stomach Injuries

Blunt injuries to the stomach are more frequent in children than in adults.[15] The injury is usually a blowout or perforation on the greater curvature.[106] It typically occurs in children who are struck by an automobile or who fall across bicycle handlebars shortly after eating.[107,108]

The diagnosis should be suspected in patients who have immediate peritoneal signs and have bloody drainage from the nasogastric tube. Pneumoperitoneum is present on abdominal x-ray. If the patient is comatose, peritoneal lavage may be a useful diagnostic technique. At surgery, the edges of the perforation should be debrided and closed in two layers. The stomach should then be decompressed with a nasogastric tube for several days.

Duodenal Injuries

Duodenal perforation is an uncommon injury in children.[15] During a 12-year period at the Ben Taub General Hospital in Houston, 313 patients were treated for duodenal lacerations and only 2% of these occurred in children less than 13 years of age.[109]

AXIOM   In children, duodenal perforation from trauma is much less frequent than duodenal obstruction by an intramural hematoma.

Duodenal hematomas are relatively common in children, and frequently occur after falling on the handlebars of a bicycle.[15] Vomiting or high nasogastric tube output 24 hours after injury should arouse suspicion of this problem and is an indication for an upper gastrointestinal series. The diagnosis can also be made by ultrasound. The diagnosis is confirmed by a "coiled-spring sign" and cutoff in the duodenum, usually in the second portion, on an upper GI contrast study.[110]

Treatment includes decompression of the child's stomach with a nasogastric tube plus metabolic support with total parenteral nutrition.[15,111] These patients are followed by the daily amount of nasogastric drainage and by sonography to assess for resolution of the hematoma. While the majority of duodenal hematomas will resolve within 10 days of injury, complete resolution of the obstruction may take up to 3 weeks in certain individuals.[112] Large hematomas discovered at operations done for other reasons, or those not resolving after 14 days, should be treated by surgical evacuation of the hematoma via a serosal incision which is then closed.

Small Intestinal Injuries

The small bowel of children is subject to the same types of injuries seen in adults, including penetrating injuries and ruptures from seatbelts or deceleration.[15] Also, abused children suffering direct blows to the abdomen can develop mesenteric hematomas associated with antimesenteric perforations and present with acute abdominal pain and a sketchy history. As in adults, the typical injury often occurs in the areas of retroperitoneal fixation at the ligament of Treitz or ileocecal valve.[113] Compression and transection of the bowel across the spine may also occur.

AXIOM Diagnosis of small bowel perforation is often delayed in children because peritoneal signs develop slowly, and the clinical history may be lacking.

The early diagnosis of small bowel injuries in children may be difficult, and peritoneal signs may not develop until more than 24 hours after the injury.[114] Furthermore, because of the early development of ileus, there may be minimal free intraperitoneal air.[115]

Colon and Rectal Injuries

The diagnosis and treatment of colorectal injuries in children is basically the same as for adults. Since rectal injuries may be very painful and since the child cannot cooperate, proper examination may not be possible except under general anesthesia.[116] Except for straddle injuries, most of the isolated rectal injuries in children are caused by child abuse or deviant sexual activity.[117]

AXIOM One should suspect abuse as a cause of isolated rectal injury in children.

Because the perineum is the source of urine and feces, which can soil clothes and greatly increase the work of parents or caretakers, it is frequently the target of abuse by adults particularly during the toilet training period.[15] During the 2-year period from 1979 to 1980, 16 children (10 male, 6 female) were seen at the Ben Taub General Hospital for rectal trauma.[117] Thirteen (81%) of these patients were the victims of abuse.

Treatment of rectal injuries is relatively standard.[15,118] Mucosal or superficial anal injuries usually resolve with conservative treatment. Full-thickness injuries below the internal sphincter usually do well following a primary repair. Injury above the level of the internal sphincter should be protected by a sigmoid colostomy and presacral drainage. One should look for an intraabdominal perforation at the time of the colostomy, and if such an injury is found, it should be repaired and protected by a proximal colostomy.[119]

Pancreatic Injuries

In teenagers, as in adults, pancreatic injuries are most often the result of penetrating trauma.[15] At the Ben Taub General Hospital, 68% of children between the ages of 13 and 16 years with pancreatic injuries had penetrating wounds.[120] In contrast, 92% (24/26) of the pancreatic damage in children less than 13 years of age was due to blunt trauma.

The operative indications and procedures for pancreatic trauma in children are similar to those for adults.[15,121] The key to treatment of any pancreatic injury is adequate debridement and drainage.

AXIOM With a torn pancreas in a child, the distal pancreas is preserved if at all possible so that a splenectomy can be avoided.

Of particular concern in children is a complete pancreatic transection for which adults are often treated with a distal pancreatic resection. This should be avoided in children, if possible, because a distal pancreatic resection frequently necessitates splenectomy. Consequently, efforts should be made to preserve the distal pancreas. This is generally done by anastomosing the injured end of the distal pancreas to a Roux-en-Y loop of jejunum. The injured portion of the proximal pancreas can then be stapled or oversewn and drained. Thus, viable pancreatic tissue is conserved in the growing child. Since children tolerate 75% distal pancreatectomies for other conditions very well and usually have normal subsequent growth and development, questionably viable distal pancreatic tissue should be excised, but the spleen should be preserved if possible.

Urinary Tract Injuries

Perineal trauma usually occurs after straddle injuries. Sexual abuse must also be considered, and in these cases, cultures and specimens should be obtained from the vagina, rectum, and mouth. When there has been significant perineal injury, evaluation under anesthesia is required.

Whenever possible, a spontaneously voided urine specimen should be obtained and analyzed on all severely injured patients, particularly for red blood cells. After the child with severe trauma has voided, a urethral catheter may be placed to monitor urine output; however, any suspicion of a urethral injury, especially in boys, warrants a retrograde urethrogram prior to insertion of a Foley catheter.

If a bladder injury is suspected, cystography, with oblique views and postevacuation films are obtained.[122] Intraperitoneal injuries must be repaired at surgery, but small extraperitoneal bladder ruptures can often be managed with catheter drainage alone.

Renal injuries seldom require emergency operation.[123] Injuries with a mild extravasation of urine on CT or IVP may be observed after careful evaluation; however, delayed operative intervention may be required for enlarging retroperitoneal hematomas or fluid collections.[124]

Musculoskeletal Injuries

The skeletal immaturity of children is responsible for most of the differences in the treatment of pediatric orthopedic injuries compared to adults. The Salter and Harris classification of physeal and epiphyseal injury, widely used to describe fracture patterns around growth plates, is quite reliable and clinically useful.[125]

Although most fractures in children can be treated by closed reduction, internal fixation may be indicated in the presence of multiple trauma or for specific fractures.[126] Spinal injuries are infrequent in children and may be difficult to diagnose because of normal differences in the radiographic appearance compared to adults. Children can have spine injury without radiologic abnormality (SCIWORA) and therefore thorough physical examination supplemented with CT scan is necessary in suspected cases.[127] This and immobilization maintained until the patient and x-rays are examined by an orthopedist are essential. The potential for recovery of function in fractured extremities in children is much greater than adults. Consequently, all orthopedic injuries in children should be treated acutely to minimize long-term morbidity, even in the face of coma and severe multisystem trauma.

AXIOM Children with fractures through growth centers must be followed carefully because of the serious effects such injuries can have on long-term growth and function.

Any fracture through a growth center can result in reduced or distorted growth of that extremity. The patient and family must be warned of this possibility, and the need for prolonged follow-up must be emphasized.

Vascular Injuries

Vascular injuries in children require early diagnosis and aggressive operative management to prevent serious sequelae.[15] For example, an injury to a major artery in a child's extremity resulting in ischemia can cause growth retardation of that limb.[128] Conversely, if an arteriovenous fistula results from an injury to an adjacent artery and vein, the increased blood flow to the area of the bone may result in overgrowth and an inequality of the length of the extremities.

AXIOM Most vascular injuries in children are due to penetrating accidental or iatrogenic trauma.

Although the mechanisms of vascular trauma in children are similar to those in adults, some injuries are unique to the pediatric group. Most common among these are damage to blood vessels from needles used for therapeutic or diagnostic purposes;[129-131] however, vascular injuries are occasionally caused by long-bone fractures. In a combined study of 110 children with major vascular injuries treated at Johns Hopkins Hospital and Vanderbilt University Hospital over a 10-year period, more than 50% of the injuries resulted from invasive diagnostic vascular procedures.[128] Of the remaining injuries, three-fourths were due to penetrating trauma.

The diagnosis of vascular injuries in children, as in adults, is usually only first suspected when there is an absence or marked diminution of distal pulses, but 15 to 25% of children with major arterial injuries in their extremities have distal pulses.

AXIOM   The presence of distal pulses does not rule out a significant arterial injury.[124]

Coolness of the involved extremity associated with sluggish capillary filling are important but relatively late objective signs of inadequate circulation beyond a vascular injury.[15] Ischemia to adjacent nerves may result in pain, paresthesias, hyperesthesia, and even anesthesia within a few hours of injury, but these may be difficult signs to elicit in infants and young children.[132] Petechial hemorrhages, blister formation, and muscle rigidity are late signs of severe skin and muscle ischemia.

If vascular injury is suspected, objective studies such as Doppler pressure measurements or flow wave analysis and/or arteriography may be required.[15] Unfortunately, arteriography has its own inherent risks in small children and infants and should be done by someone experienced in the technique and only if the vessel would be repaired if an injury were found.

The most important differential diagnosis is between partial occlusion and spasm of an injured vessel.[15] Vascular spasm is often due to damage to adjacent soft tissue, hemorrhage into surrounding tissue, or trauma to the vessel wall. Nevertheless, arterial spasm as the only cause of impaired distal flow is uncommon and will usually disappear within 3 hours. If impaired perfusion of the extremity persists beyond 3 hours, vascular damage is likely; if there is poor perfusion or absent pulses longer than 6 hours, thrombosis or transection of the vessel is almost certain. At this point, the diagnosis of major vascular injury should be confirmed. This can be done by immediate arteriography, but direct operative exploration without a prior arteriogram is often preferred in small children.

AXIOM   With major arterial trauma, blood flow to an extremity may be adequate to maintain viability of the limb but still be inadequate for normal growth.

While it is true that the distal extremity may remain viable without pulsatile flow, the possibility of growth retardation associated with relative ischemia to the extremity is an important factor in the decision to explore the site of major vascular injury in children.[15]

Vascular injuries associated with long-bone fractures, especially supracondylar fractures, are seen commonly in older children and teenagers.[15] Following reduction of long-bone fractures, care must be taken to document distal pulses. Severe prolonged ischemia to the forearm because of brachial artery occlusion can result in Volkmann's ischemic contracture and severe long-term disability. If the circulation to an extremity is questionable or marginal for more than 3 hours, arteriography is indicated to rule out a vascular injury.

Burns

Children are particularly susceptible to accidental burns, most of which are due to hot water and cover less than 20% of the total body surface area. These are generally partial-thickness injuries that can be adequately treated by initial debridement of large blisters and topical closed antibiotic dressings using silver sulfadiazine or mafenide. Most face burns are treated open with Bacitracin ointment.

AXIOM   Burns in children are due to abuse or neglect until proven otherwise.

Many burns are due to either child abuse or neglect, and social service vigilance is important. Partly for this reason, Children's Hospital of Michigan has liberal policies for admission to the burn unit. We admit patients with any size burn to the hands, face, feet, or genitalia as well as any partial-thickness injury more than 8% BSA or full-thickness injury more than 3% BSA. For children less than 1 year of age, these criteria are halved. Children with infected burns or with suspicion of abuse or neglect are also admitted.

When calculating the surface area of a burn, one must consider the age differences in body proportions, particularly the larger surface area of the head and smaller surface area of the lower extremities in infants (Fig. 8-1).

With small superficial burns in non-critical areas, the parents can be taught how to change the dressings, and the child can be discharged early, provided social services can find no evidence of abuse or neglect. If the burns appear particularly deep, early excision and grafting are carried out, keeping in mind that skin grafts add to the total percentage of the body surface area that has a partial-thickness injury.

Children with 10% or higher BSA burn will usually require intravenous support. If the burn is 20% or higher BSA, or if the genitalia are involved, a urethral catheter is necessary. NG tubes are used frequently for prevention of ileus and vomiting and later for enteral feedings. Oral intake is usually inadequate for at least several days following severe burns. Providing adequate intravenous fluids to severely burned children for the initial 24-48 hours is extremely important. Many burn fluid formulas are available for guiding such fluid therapy. The formula used at the Children's Hospital of Michigan, in addition to maintenance fluid, is:

$$\% \text{ BSA} \times \text{weight (kg)} \times 2 = \text{ml lactated Ringer's (1st 24 hrs)}$$

This amount (given as D_5LR) is added to the patient's maintenance fluid requirements. Fluid maintenance can be estimated as 100 ml/kg for each of the first 10 kg of body weight, 50 ml/kg for each kg body weight from 10 to 19 kg, and 20 ml/kg for each kg of body weight above 20 kg. Half of the estimated first day's total fluids is given in the first 8 hours and the remainder in the next 16 hours. In practice, the formula is altered as needed to maintain an adequate urine output (0.5-1.0 ml/kg/hr) and vital signs. Blood is transfused as needed to maintain a hematocrit above 30%.

As in other areas of pediatric trauma, burn treatment should focus on obtaining an optimal functional outcome with minimal psychological trauma and reduced long-term morbidity. This requires use of numerous specialties and supportive services. Physical therapy and occupational therapy provide range-of-motion exercises, splinting, and help with activities of daily living. Recreational therapy provides diversion from a painful routine. Compressive garments are useful to minimize hypertrophic scarring. For children with prolonged hospitalization for burns or other traumatic injuries, social services can help develop coping skills for the child and family, arrange communication with schools, anticipate a wide range of problems, and provide referrals as needed.

RECOMMENDATIONS

Pediatric trauma centers and trauma registries are accumulating valuable experience and data on childhood trauma that can direct prevention strategies on individual, community, and societal levels.[133] Parents and children need to be taught the effectiveness of car restraints and bike helmets on reducing the morbidity of accidents.[134,135] As a society, we need to examine strategies for reducing injuries that have proven effective in other countries.[136]

Children's Hospital of Michigan
DETROIT   MICHIGAN

BURN SHEET

BURN RECORD. AGES — BIRTH - 7½

DATE OF OBSERVATION _____

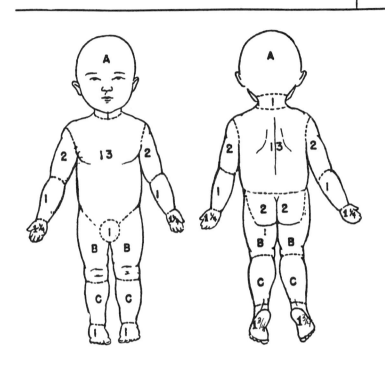

% BURN BY AREAS		
AREA	% 2°	% 3°
HEAD		
NECK		
UPPER ARM		
FOREARM		
ANTERIOR TRUNK		
POSTERIOR TRUNK		
GENITALS		
BUTTOCKS		
THIGHS		
LEGS		
FEET		
HANDS		
TOTAL		

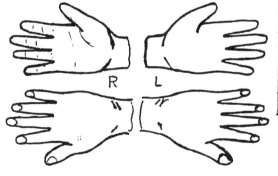

RELATIVE PERCENTAGES OF AREAS AFFECTED BY GROWTH			
AREA	AGE 0	1	5
A = 1/2 of Head	9 1/2	8 1/2	6 1/2
B = 1/2 of One Thigh	2 3/4	3 1/4	4
C = 1/2 of One Leg	2 1/2	2 1/2	2 3/4

WEIGHT_____   HEIGHT_____

SURFACE AREA_____

TYPE OF BURN_____

COMMENT _____

_____

_____ M.D.

⊘ *FREQUENT ERRORS*

1. *Treating injured children as if they were small adults.*
2. *Not appreciating the fact that severe internal injuries may be present in children with little external evidence of trauma.*
3. *Inadequate concern about the patency of the nasal passages in infants.*
4. *Delay in decompressing the stomach in infants with major trauma.*
5. *Delay in diagnosing or relieving a pneumothorax or hemothorax in a child.*
6. *Interpreting and treating agitation as anxiety when it is actually due to hypoxia.*
7. *Failing to give glucose during fluid resuscitation of infants and small children.*
8. *Giving a diuretic to increase urine output when the oliguria may be due to inadequate fluid resuscitation.*
9. *Inadequate efforts to prevent and correct hypothermia.*
10. *Assuming that vital signs in children are the same as in adults.*
11. *Failing to consider abuse or neglect in the etiology of a child's injury.*
12. *Assuming that an edematous injured child cannot be hypovolemic.*
13. *Performing diagnostic peritoneal lavage (DPL) on all suspected abdominal injuries and/or operating just because the DPL is positive.*
14. *Operating for isolated liver or spleen injuries if the child is hemodynamically stable.*
15. *Not making every effort to preserve at least part of a badly injured spleen.*
16. *Inadequate attention to the neurovascular status of an extremity before and after reduction of fractures and dislocations.*

▼▼▼▼▼▼▼▼▼▼▼▼▼▼▼▼▼▼▼▼▼▼▼▼▼▼▼▼▼▼▼

SUMMARY POINTS

1. Children are a special, different, and important part of society.
2. The patterns of injury, as well as the treatment and rehabilitation needs of children, are different from those of adults.
3. The most common pitfall with injured children is to assume that they are small adults and treat them accordingly.
4. Over 80% of the injuries in childhood are due to blunt trauma, and most of these occur in boys.
5. When trauma occurs, the child's relatively compliant body may have little eternal evidence of serious internal damage.
6. Almost 30% of childhood traumatic deaths could be prevented by a dozen simple measures.
7. Injury is the most important health problem affecting children and adolescents in the United States.
8. For all ages, accidents are the third most common cause of death, but in children they account for over 50% of all deaths.
9. Prehospital invasive procedures should be performed rapidly by personnel with pediatric experience.
10. Difficult procedures should not be attempted on a child without specific training or experience, just because they are routine in adults.
11. Any delay in providing needed surgical care to an injured child can be catastrophic.
12. In children it is important to prevent the heat loss that can occur rapidly with exposure to room temperature air and intravenous solutions.
13. Early decompression of the stomach is extremely important in severely injured children.
14. Restlessness or any change in mental status in an injured child should be attributed to hypoxia until proven otherwise.
15. Since infants are obligatory nasal breathers, occlusion of the nose by injuries or foreign bodies, such as nasogastric tubes, may severely impair ventilation.

16. Lack of familiarity with pediatric upper airway anatomy can make endotracheal intubation extremely difficult.
17. There is little distance in an infant between the position of an endotracheal tube that is down too far and one that is not in far enough.
18. In infants, breath sounds can be easily transmitted to both sides of the chest despite lack of ventilation of one lung.
19. If ventilation of an infant or child cannot be promptly provided with an endotracheal tube, a large needle inserted into the trachea and attached to intermittent wall oxygen can be lifesaving.
20. Anything pressing on or irritating the diaphragm can greatly reduce the ability of a child to ventilate adequately.
21. Gastric dilatation can seriously interfere with ventilation and with the abdominal evaluation of critically injured children.
22. The mediastinum shifts easily in children, consequently any problem in one hemithorax can severely impair ventilation and venous return.
23. Supplemental oxygen should be given to all seriously injured children initially, even if they have no obvious difficulty with their airway or ventilation.
24. In the non-crying child, the systolic BP should be at least 80 plus twice the age in years, while the diastolic pressure should be two-thirds the calculated systolic pressure.
25. Any process that reduces pulse rate in young children can reduce their ability to sustain an adequate cardiac output.
26. Young children do not increase the 2,3-DPG in transfused red blood cells as rapidly as adults.
27. One should not use a scalp vein for intravenous access when rapid fluid administration may be required.
28. If no vascular access is available, nearly all resuscitation drugs, except $NaHCO_3$, can be given to children via an endotracheal tube.
29. If adequate vascular access cannot be obtained in a reasonable period of time for resuscitation of a hemodynamically unstable child, the intraosseous route should be considered.
30. Provision of adequate ventilation, oxygen, and blood volume are the most important priorities in pediatric trauma resuscitation; drugs may confuse the clinical picture.
31. Intraosseous infusions should be limited to emergency resuscitation and used only until other venous access is obtained.
32. Severe hypoglycemia can develop rapidly in infants unless some glucose is given in their intravenous maintenance fluids.
33. Diuretics or dopamine should not be used to increase urine output while a child is hypovolemic.
34. A urine osmolality of 600 mOsm/kg in a newborn usually indicates hypovolemia.
35. Severe hypothermia can develop rapidly in young traumatized children and cause severe physiological derangements.
36. Injured infants should be treated in an environment maintained between 24°-27° C (75°-80° F).
37. All intravenous solutions, including blood, given to an injured child should be warmed to 40°-42° C.
38. Children who experience a cardiac arrest following trauma need oxygen, fluid, and blood rather than multiple drugs or electric shocks.
39. One should not assume that normal vital signs in an infant or young child are the same as in an adult.
40. Bradycardia in an injured child can be an ominous sign.
41. Oxygen saturation monitors will often show oxygen desaturation before bradycardia develops, allowing time to correct the developing pulmonary or cardiovascular problem before it becomes serious and difficult to reverse.
42. If all injuries in infants and young children are not taken seriously, what appears to be anxiety or fear, can rapidly become life-threatening hypoxia, and what appear to be normal vital signs with some tachycardia, can rapidly become total cardiovascular collapse.
43. As in adults, careful, repeated physical examination is the most valuable tool for assessing injured children.
44. Child abuse is common and can have dire consequences if not recognized and treated early.

45. Child neglect may be just as dangerous as child abuse and should be reported as soon as it is suspected.

46. The possibility of abuse or neglect should be strongly suspected if the injuries or the child's or parent's behavior are unusual.

47. One must not fail to assess the neurovascular status of the extremities early and completely, especially if there is any suspicion of a fracture or dislocation.

48. Bowel perforation is less frequent with blunt trauma in children than in adults. Consequently, blunt injury to the abdomen in a stable child is less apt to need exploration than in an adult.

49. Although arteriography in small children is often more hazardous than in adults because of the small size of the vessels and the frequent need for sedation or even general anesthesia, diagnosis of aortic or arterial injury may be impossible without it.

50. Injured children can develop peripheral edema even when they are still hypovolemic.

51. Many physicians worry that aggressive crystalloid resuscitation can worsen brain edema; however, failure to promptly restore an adequate cerebral perfusion is far more detrimental.

52. Maintenance of optimal tissue perfusion is extremely important and should not be restricted because of concerns about increasing ICP in children with head injury.

53. Expressionless withdrawal in an injured child should make one suspect child abuse.

54. The majority of children with abdominal trauma can be treated nonoperatively, but they must be observed carefully.

55. Whenever possible, injuries to the liver or spleen in hemodynamically stable children should be treated nonoperatively.

56. The decision to perform a laparotomy after trauma is primarily based on clinical findings.

57. Peritoneal lavage is indicated in injured children who require immediate surgical intervention for extraabdominal or suspected abdominal injuries causing hemodynamic instability.

58. The majority of children with splenic injuries can be safely treated nonoperatively.

59. In children, duodenal perforation from trauma is much less frequent than obstruction by a duodenal hematoma.

60. Diagnosis of small bowel perforation is often delayed in children because peritoneal signs develop slowly and the clinical history may be lacking.

61. One should suspect abuse as a cause of isolated rectal injury in children.

62. With a torn pancreas in a child, the distal pancreas is preserved if at all possible so that a splenectomy can be avoided.

63. Children with fractures through growth centers must be followed carefully because of the serious effects such injuries can have on long-term growth and function.

64. Most vascular injuries in children are due to penetrating accidental or iatrogenic trauma.

65. The presence of distal pulses does not rule out a significant arterial injury.

66. With major arterial trauma, blood flow to an extremity may be adequate to maintain viability of the limb but still be inadequate for normal growth.

67. Burns in children are due to abuse or neglect until proven otherwise.

▲▲▲▲▲▲▲▲▲▲▲▲▲▲▲▲▲▲▲▲▲▲▲▲▲▲▲▲▲▲▲▲

REFERENCES

1. Garland M. The changing face of childhood. New York, Octoberhaus, 1965.
2. National Academy of Sciences. Injury in America. Washington, DC, 1985.
3. Haller JA Jr, et al. Organization and function of a regional pediatric trauma center: does a system of management improve outcome? J Trauma 1983;23:691-696.
4. Colombani PM, et al. One-year experience in a regional pediatric trauma center. J Pediatr Surg 1985;20:8-13.
5. National Pediatric Trauma Registry, National Institute of Handicapped Research, New England Medical Center Hospital, 750 Washington St., Boston, MA 02111.
6. Rouse TM, Eichelberger MR. Trends in pediatric trauma management. Surg Clin North Am 1992;72:1347.
7. Pascucci R, Walsh J. Evaluation and management of the injured child. In: Capan LM, Miller SM, Turndorf H, eds. Trauma: anesthesia and intensive care. Philadelphia: JB Lippincott, 1991:567-598.
8. Gratz IR. Accidental injury in childhood: a literature review on pediatric trauma. J Trauma 1979;19:551.
9. Lovejoy FH, Chaffee-Bahamon C. The physician's role in accident prevention. Pediatr Rev 1982;4:53.
10. Meller JL, Shermeta DW. Falls in urban children. Am J Dis Child 1987;141:1271.
11. Bijur PE, Golding J, Haslum M, Kurzon M. Behavioral predictors of injury in school-age children. Am J Dis Child 1988;142:1307.
12. McCue Horwitz S, Morgenstern H, DiPietro L, Morrison CL. Determinants of pediatric injuries. Am J Dis Child 1988;142:605.
13. Baker CC, Oppenheimer L, Stephens B, et al. Epidemiology of traumatic deaths. Am J Surg 1980;140:144.
14. Bijur PE, Golding J, Haslum M. Persistence of occurrence of injury: can injuries of preschool children predict injuries of school-aged children? Pediatrics 1988;82:707.
15. Pokorny WL, Haller JA. Pediatric trauma. In: Moore EE, Mattox KL, Felicano DV, eds. Trauma. 2nd ed. Norwalk, CT: Appleton & Lange, 1991.
16. Accident facts. Chicago: National Safety Council, 1979.
17. Leschoier I, DiScala C. Blunt trauma in children: causes and outcome of head versus extracranial injury. Pediatrics 1993;91: 721.
18. Hanigan WC, et al. Lawn dart injury in children: report of two cases. Pediatric Emerg Care 1986;2:247-249.
19. Harris W, et al. BB and pellet guns: toys or deadly weapons? J Trauma 1983;23:566-569.
20. Blocker S, et al. Serious air rifle injuries in children. Pediatrics 1982;69:751-754.
21. Johnson DG. Esophagoscopy. In: Pediatric surgery. Chicago: Year Book Medical Publishers, 1986.
22. Accident facts. Chicago: National Safety Council, 1982.
23. Guyer B, Gallagher SS. An approach to the epidemiology of childhood injuries. Pediatr Clin North Am 1985;32:5.
24. Gallagher SS, Guyer B, Kotelchuck M, et al. A strategy for the reduction of childhood injuries in Massachusetts: SCIPP. N Engl J Med 1982;307:1015.
25. Tepas JJ, et al. The pediatric trauma score as a predictor of injury severity in the injured child. J Pediatr Surg 1987;22:14-18.
26. Ramenofksy ML, Ramenofsky MB, Jurkovich GJ, et al. The predictive validity of the pediatric trauma score. J Trauma 1988;28:1038-1042.
27. Tepas JJ, Ramenofsky ML, Mollitt DL, et al. The pediatric trauma score as a predictor of injury severity: an objective assessment. J Trauma 1988;28:425.
28. Harris BH, Latchaw LA, Murphy RE, Schwaitzberg SD. A protocol for pediatric trauma receiving units. J Pediatr Surg 1989;24:419.
29. Eichelberger MR, Zwick HA, Pratsch GL, et al. Pediatric trauma protocol: a team approach. In: Eichelberger MR, Pratsch GL, eds. Pediatric trauma care. Rockville, MD: Aspen Publishers, 1988:11.
30. Rutledge R, Smith CY, Azizkhan RG. A population-based multivariate analysis of the association of county demographic and medical system factors with per capita pediatric trauma death rates in North Carolina. Ann Surg 1994;219:205.
31. Cooper A, Barlow B, DiScala C, et al. Efficacy of pediatric trauma care: results of a population-based study. J Pediatr Surg 1993;28: 299.
32. Kaufman CR, Rivara FP, Maier RV. Pediatric trauma: need for surgical management. J Trauma 1989;29:1120.
33. O'Neill JA. Special pediatric emergencies. In: Boswick JA, ed. Emergency care. Philadelphia: WB Saunders, 1981:137.
34. Kettrick RG, Lidwig S. Resuscitation: pediatric basic and advance life support. In: Fleisher G, Ludwig S, eds. Textbook of pediatric emergency medicine. Baltimore: Williams & Wilkins, 1983:138.
35. Coldiron JS. Estimation of nasotracheal tube length in neonates. Pediatrics 1968;41:823.
36. Spoerel WE, Narayanan PS, Singh NP. Transtracheal ventilation. Br J Anaesth 1971;43:932.
37. Searpelle EM, ed. Pulmonary physiology in the fetus, newborn and child. Philadelphia: Lea & Febiger, 1975:168.
38. American College of Surgeons Committee on Trauma. Advanced trauma

life support course: instructor manual. Chicago: American College of Surgeons, 1984:293.

39. Pediatric transfusions practice. In: Snyder EL, ed. Blood transfusion therapy. Arlington, VA: American Association of Blood Banks, 1983:49.

40. Holliday MA, Segar WE. Maintenance need for water in parenteral fluid therapy. Pediatrics 1957;19:823.

41. Furman EB. Intraoperative fluid therapy. Int Anesth Clin 1975;13:133.

42. Gross JB. Estimating allowable blood loss. Corrected for dilution. Anesthesiology 1973;58:277.

43. Carrico CJ, Canizaro PC, Shires GT. Fluid resuscitation following injury: rationale for the use of balanced salt solutions. Crit Care Med 1976;4:46.

44. Goldberg AI. Anesthesia and intensive care. In: Touloukian RJ, ed. Pediatric trauma. New York: Wiley, 1978:105.

45. Filston HC, Grant JP. A safer system for percutaneous subclavian venous catheterization in newborn infants. J Pediatr Surg 1979;14:564-570.

46. Groff, DB, Ahmed N. Subclavian vein catheterization in the infant. J Pediatr Surg 1974;9:171-174.

47. Glaeser PW, Losek JD. Emergency intraosseous infusions in children. Am J Emerg Med 1986;4:34.

48. Rosetti VA, Thompson BM, Miller J, et al. Intraosseous infusion: an alternative route of pediatric intravascular access. Ann Emerg Med 1985;14:885.

49. Guy J, Haley K, Zuspan SJ. Use of intraosseous infusion in the pediatric trauma patient. J Pediatr Surg 1993;28: 158.

50. McAleer IM, Kaplan GW, Scherz HC, et al. Clinical presentation and radiographic identification of small bowel rupture following blunt trauma in children. Pediatr Emerg Care 1993;9:139.

51. Aperia A, Broberger O, Thodenius K, et al. Renal control of sodium and fluid balance in newborn infants during maintenance therapy. Acta Pediatr Scand 1975;64:725.

52. Rowe MI. Preoperative and postoperative management: the physiologic approach. In: Ravitch MM, Welch KJ, Benson CD, et al, eds. Pediatric surgery. Chicago: Year Book, 1979:39.

53. Stern L, Lees MH, Leduc J. Environmental temperature, oxygen consumption, and catecholamine excretion in newborn infants. Pediatrics 1965;36:367.

54. Roe CF, Santulli TV, Blair CS. Heat loss in infants during general anesthesia and operations. J Pediatr Surg 1966;1:266.

55. Hey EN, Katz G. The optimum thermal environment for naked babies. Arch Dis Child 1970;45:328.

56. Rowe MI, Taylor M. Transepidermal water loss in the infant surgical patient. J Pediatr Surg 1981;16:878.

57. Hazinski MF, Chahine AA, Holcomb GW III, et al. Outcome of cardiovascular collapse in pediatric blunt trauma. Ann Emerg Med 1994;23:1229.

58. Teasdale G, Jennett B. Assessment of coma and impaired unconsciousness: a practical scale. Lancet 1974;2:82-84.

59. Raimondi AS, Hirschauer J. Head injury in the infant and toddler: coma scoring and outcome scale. Child's Brain 1984;11:12-35.

60. Caffey J. Multiple fractures in the long bones of infants suffering from chronic subdural hematoma. Am J Roetgenol 1946;56:163-173.

61. Woolley PV Jr, Evans WA Jr. Significance of skeletal lesions in infants resembling those of traumatic origin. JAMA 1955;158:539-547.

62. Kempe CH, et al. Battered child syndrome. JAMA 1962;181:17-24.

63. American Academy of Pediatrics Committee on Child Abuse and Neglect. Shaken baby syndrome: inflicted cerebral trauma. Pediatrics 1993;92: 872.

64. Isaacman DJ, Scarfone RJ, Kost SI, et al. Utility of routine laboratory testing for detecting intra-abdominal injury in the pediatric trauma patient. Pediatrics 1993;92: 692.

65. Guice K, et al. Hematuria after blunt trauma: when is pyelography useful? J Trauma 1983;23:305-311.

66. Kisa E, Schenk WG. Indications for emergency intravenous pyelography (IVP) in blunt abdominal trauma: a reappraisal. J Trauma 1986;26:1086-1089.

67. Lieu TA, et al. Hematuria and clinical findings as indications for intravenous pyelography in pediatric blunt renal trauma. Pediatrics 1988;82:216-222.

68. Masters SJ, et al. Skull x-ray examination after head trauma: recommendations by a multidisciplinary panel and validation study. N Engl J Med 1987;316:84-91.

69. Fischer JT. Gastrointestinal disruption: the hazard of nonoperative management in adults with blunt abdominal injury. J Trauma 1988;28:1445-1449.

70. Costeff N, Grosswasser Z, Goldstein R. Long-term follow-up review of 113 children with severe closed head trauma. J Neurosurg 1990;73:684.

71. Rielly JP, Brandt ML, Mattox KL, et al. Thoracic trauma in children. J Trauma 1993;34:329.

72. Bellinger SB. Penetrating chest injuries in children. Ann Throac Surg 1972;14:635.

73. Meller JL, Little AG, Shermeta DW. Thoracic trauma in children. Pediatrics 1984;74:813.

74. Randolph H, Melick DW, Grant AR. Perforation of the esophagus from external trauma or blast injuries. Dis Chest 1967;51:121.

75. Sinclair MC, Moore TC. Major surgery for abdominal and thoracic trauma in childhood and adolescence. J Pediatr Surg 1974;9:155.

76. Smyth BT. Chest trauma in children. J Pediatr Surg 1979;14:41.

77. Haller JA Jr. Thoracic injuries. In: Welch KJ, Randolph JG, Ravitch, et al, eds. Pediatric surgery. 4th ed. Chicago: Year Book, 1986:143.

78. Haller JA, Shermeta DW. Major thoracic trauma in children. Pediatr Clin North Am 1975;22:341.

79. Shaftan GW. Indications for operation in abdominal trauma. Am J Surg 1960;99:657-664.

80. Lowe RJ, et al. The negative laparotomy for abdominal trauma. J Trauma 1972;12:853-861.

81. Horan M, Colebatch JR. Relation between splenectomy and subsequent infection: a clinical study. Arch Dis Child 1962;37:398-412.

82. Eraklis AJ, Filler RM. Splenectomy in childhood: a review of 1413 cases. J Pediatr Surg 1972;7:382.

83. Eichelberger MR, Randolph JG. Complications of pediatric surgery and trauma. In: Greenfield L, ed. Complications in surgery and trauma. Philadelphia: Lippincott, 1984:485.

84. Eichelberger MR, Randolph JG. Pediatric trauma: initial resuscitation. In: Moore EE, Eiseman B, Van Way CT, eds. Critical decision in trauma. St. Louis: Mosby, 1984:344.

85. Burnweit CA, Thai ER. Significance of omental evisceration in abdominal stab wounds. Am J Surg 1986;152:670-673.

86. Taylor GA, Kaufman RA, Sivit CJ. Active hemorrhage in children after thoracoabdominal trauma: clincal and CT features. Am J Roentgenol 1994;162:401.

87. Karp MP, Cooney DR, Berger PE, et al. The role of computed tomography in the evaluation of blunt abdominal trauma in children. J Pediatr Surg 1981;16:316.

88. Meyer DM, Thal ER, Coln D, et al. Computed tomography in the evaluation of children with blunt abdominal trauma. Ann Surg 1993;217: 272.

89. Lazarus HM, Nelson JA. The surgeon at work: a technique for peritoneal lavage without risk or complication. Surg Gynecol Obstet 1979;149:889-892.

90. Powell RW, Green JB, Ochsner MG, et al. Peritoneal lavage in pediatric patients sustaining blunt abdominal trauma: a reappraisal. J Trauma 1987;27:6.

91. Wilson RH, Moorehead RJ. Management of splenic trauma. Injury 1992;23:5.

92. Velanovich V, Tapper D. Decision analysis in children with blunt splenic trauma: the effects of observation, splenorrhaphy, or splenectomy on quality-adjusted life expectancy. J Pediatr Surg 1993;28:179.

93. Ein SH, Shandling B, Simpson JS, et al. Nonoperative management of traumatized spleen in children: how and why. J Pediatr Surg 1978;13:117.

94. Francke EL, Neu HC. Postsplenectomy infection. Surg Clin North Am 1981;61:135.

95. Eichelberger MR, Randolph JG. Abdominal trauma. In: Welch KG, Randolph JG, Ravitch MM, et al, eds. Pediatric surgery. 6th ed. Chicago: Year Book, 1986:154.

96. Philippart AI, Hight DW. Splenectomy in childhood: altered concepts of management. Am J Pediatr Hematol Oncol 1980;2:61.

97. Raffensperger JG, Pokorny WJ. Abdominal trauma. In: Raffensperger JG, ed. Swenson's pediatric surgery. 4th ed. New York: Appleton-Century-Crofts, 1980:238.

98. Morse MA, Garcia VF. Selective nonoperative management of pediatric blunt splenic trauma: risk for missed associated injuries. J Pediatr Surg 1994;29:23.

99. Wesson DE, Filler RM, Ein SH, et al. Ruptured spleen: When to operate. J Pediatr Surg 1981;16:324.

100. Schwartz MZ, Kangah R. Splenic injury in children after blunt trauma: blood transfusion requirement and length of hospitalization for laparotomy versus observation. J Pediatr Surg 1994;29:596.

101. Bulas DI, Eichelberger MR, Sivit CJ, et al. Hepatic injury from blunt trauma in children: follow-up evaluation with CT. Am J Roentgenl 1993;160:347.

102. Karp MP, Cooney DR, Pros GA, et al. The nonoperative management of pediatric hepatic trauma. J Pediatr Surg 1983;18:512.
103. Cooney DR. Splenic and hepatic trauma in children. Surg Clin North Am 1981;61:1165.
104. Bass BL, Eichelberger MR, Schisgall R, et al. Hazards of nonoperative therapy of hepatic injury in children. J Trauma 1984;24:978.
105. Geis WP, Schultz KA, et al. The fate of unruptured intrahepatic hematomas. Surgery 1981;90:689.
106. Vassy LE, Klecker RL, Koch E, et al. Traumatic gastric perforation in children from blunt trauma. J Trauma 1975;15:184.
107. Siemens RA, Fulton RL. Gastric rupture as a result of blunt trauma. Am Surg 1977;43:229.
108. Asch MJ, Coran AG, Johnson PW. Gastric perforation secondary to blunt trauma in children. J Trauma 1975;15:187.
109. Martin TD, Feliciano DV, Mattox KL, et al. Severe duodenal injuries: treatment with pyloric exclusion and gastrojejunostomy. Arch Surg 1983;118:631.
110. Felson B, Levin EJ. Intramural hematoma of the duodenum. Radiology 1954;63:823.
111. Holgerson LO, Bishop HC. Nonoperative treatment of duodenal hematoma in children. J Pediatr Surg 1977;12(1):11.
112. Touloukian RJ. Protocol for the nonoperative treatment of obstructing intramural duodenal hematoma during childhood. Am J Surg 1983;145:330.
113. Schenk WG, Lonchyna V, Moylan JA. Perforation of the jejunum from blunt abdominal trauma. J Trauma 1983;23:54.
114. Ford EG, Senac MO Jr. Clinical presentation and radiographic identification of small bowel rupture following blunt trauma in children. Pediatr Emerg Care 1993;9:139-42.
115. Kakos GS, Grosfeld JL, Morse TS. Small bowel injuries in children after blunt abdominal trauma. Ann Surg 1971;174:238.
116. Pokorny WJ, Pokorny SF, Gonzales ET Jr, et al. Perineal injuries in infants and children. In: Brooks BF, ed. The injured child. Austin, TX: University of Texas Press, 1985:85.
117. Black CT, Pokorny WJ, McGill CW, et al. Anorectal trauma in children. J Pediatr Surg 1982;17:501.
118. Robertson HD, Ray JE, Ferrari BT, et al. Management of rectal trauma. Surg Gynecol Obstet 1982;154:161.
119. Slim MS, Makaroun M, Shamma AR. Primary repair of colorectal injuries in children. J Pediatr Surg 1981;16:1008.
120. Graham JM, Pokorny WJ, Mattox KL, et al. Surgical management of acute pancreatic injuries in children. J Pediatr Surg 1978;13:693.
121. Graham JM, Mattox KL, Vaughn GD, et al. Combined pancreatoduodenal injuries. J Trauma 1979;19:340.
122. Mcaleer IM, Kaplan GW, Scherz HC, et al. Genitourinary trauma in the pediatric patient. Urology 1993;42:563.
123. Smith EM, Elder JS, Spirnak JP. Major blunt renal trauma in the pediatric population: is a nonoperative approach indicated? J Urol 1993;149:546.
124. Levy JB, Baskin LS, Ewalt DH, et al. Nonoperative management of blunt pediatric major renal trauma. Urology 1993;42:418.
125. Salter RB, Harris WR. Injuries involving the eiphyseal plate. J Bone Joint Surg 1963;45A:587-622.
126. Thompson GH, et al. Fracture management of the multiply injured child. In: Trauma in children. Rockville, MD: Aspen Publishers, Inc., 1986.
127. Pang D, Pollack IF. Spinal cord injury without radiographic abnormality in children: the SCIWORA syndrome. J Trauma 1989;29:654.
128. Haller JA. Vascular injuries. In: Touloukian RJ, ed. Pediatric trauma. New York: Wiley, 1978:369.
129. Miller DS, Sebeck R. Gangrene of the extremities in infants subsequent to intravenous therapy. Am J Dis Child 1955;90:153.
130. Polesky RE, Harvey JP Jr. Gangrene of the extremity following femoral venipuncture: a report of two cases. Pediatrics 1968;42:676.
131. Klein MD, Coran AG, Whitehouse WM Jr, et al. Management of iatrogenic arterial injuries in infants and children. J Pediatr Surg 1982;17:933.
132. Spencer AD. The reliability of signs of peripheral vascular injury. Surg Gynecol Obstet 1962;114:490.
133. Gratz RR. Accidental injury in childhood: a literature review on pediatric trauma. J Trauma 1979;19:551.
134. Johnston C, Rivara FT, Soderberg R. Children in car crashes: analysis of data for injury and use of restraints. Pediatrics 1994;93:960.
135. Thompson RS, Rivara FP, Thompson DC. A case-controlled study of the effectiveness of bicycle safety helmets. NEJM 1989;320:361.
136. Bergman AB, Rivara FP. Sweden's experience in reducing childhood injuries. Pediatrics 1991;88:69.

Chapter 9A Special Problems of Trauma in the Aged

ROBERT F. WILSON, M.D.

JEFFREY S. BENDER, M.D.

JENNIFER GASS, M.D.

Years, indeed, taken alone are a very fallacious mode of reckoning age: it is not the time but the quality of a man's past life that we have to reckon. . . .

—*Sir James Paget (1877)*

INTRODUCTION

Trauma affects all members of society, but can be especially devastating to those who are aged. These individuals lack resiliency; consequently, care of these patients provides much less margin for error.

The Number of Elderly People

AXIOM The elderly (65 years or older) are the fastest growing segment of our population.

Our population continues to age. In 1960, only 9.2% of the population was 65 years of age or older and consisted of 16,560,000 individuals. In 1990, there were almost 32,000,000 of these individuals and they made up 12.7% of the population. By the year 2020, this age group will have almost doubled to a total of about 51 million and will constitute more than 20% of the total population.[1-5]

Incidence of Trauma and Prognosis in the Elderly

Trauma in the elderly is different in many respects than in the young. Not only do the elderly tend to suffer different types of injuries, but their responses and ultimate outcome reflect the effects of underlying diseases and changes that occur in organ function with time.[1,2]

AXIOM Trauma in the elderly is more apt to be fatal than in younger individuals.

In 1984, unintentional injury accounted for almost 24,500 deaths of persons age 65 and older. This death rate of 86 per 100,000 population was more than twice the accidental death rate of all ages (39/100,000) and for those 25 to 44 years (35/100,000).[6] Although the elderly make up only about an eighth of the population, they account for a fourth of all trauma fatalities.[7] In fact, injuries are the sixth leading cause of death in the elderly.[8]

That elderly patients will do less well than younger ones with similar injuries seems self-evident, and several studies have confirmed this fact.[9-11] The age at which the prognosis following trauma begins to fall significantly is not clear, and this varies with the type of trauma. For example, in a series of patients admitted to Detroit Receiving Hospital with chest trauma, no one past the age of 43 survived the combination of shock (BP below 80 mm Hg) and acute respiratory distress requiring almost immediate intubation.[9] Available data also indicate that elderly trauma patients have a poor long-term prognosis with up to 88% of survivors requiring nursing home placement or full-time in-home assistance.[8]

Interestingly, the trauma score was originally designed to predict outcome in injured individuals under the age of 60.[10] Later, the decision was made to use 55 years as the dividing line.[11] No scientific

reason was given for changing the age recommendation, but one author stated that the change was because of the increased risk above that age.[12] Most series use 65 years of age or older to define elderly, either because it is the usual age of retirement or because the government uses that age for Medicare purposes.[13]

AXIOM The relationship between the condition of a car (or patient) and its age is not as important as how well it was made (genetics), the miles that it has been driven, and the care and maintenance that it has received.

Medical Care Required

In 1986, 816,000 persons age 65 and older were discharged from acute hospital care with a diagnoses of injury or poisoning.[14] Their average hospital stay was 9.8 days, and the total number of hospital days exceeded 7.9 million. This represented 38% of the hospital days for all patients in whom injury was the primary reason for admission.[14,15]

AXIOM Elderly patients who die as a result of trauma often have a long, lingering complicated hospital course prior to death, further increasing the cost of their medical care.

Champion et al[15] found that elderly trauma patients who died had significantly more hospital days (9.9 versus 4.2) and more ICU days (6.0 versus 3.1) than those who were younger.[15] In 1986, hospital expenses for the elderly exceeded $4.4 billion.[16,17] Thus, although the elderly are less numerous than younger individuals and are injured only half as often, they consume much more of our medical resources.[18-20] The outcome of elderly people after falls is particularly interesting. Rubenstein et al[21] noted that, of elderly patients who have a fall requiring care in a hospital, about half will die within a year.

Life Expectancy

The tendency to treat old patients less vigorously because of a projected short life expectancy or an inability to withstand major operation should be avoided.[22]

PITFALL ⊘

Not performing needed surgery on patients just because they are elderly.

The life expectancy of individuals above the age of 60 is greater than many physicians recognize.[23] In 1989, the average 65 year old could expect 17 additional years of life.[25] The average life expectancy for a 75 year old was 11 years, and for the average 85 year old it was 6 years. The rate of increase in the number of people over the age of 74 (about 3% per year) is three times greater than that of the total population.

Manton et al[28] in 1993 not only pointed out the life expectancy of elderly individuals, but also estimated how much of that would be an active existence and how much time would occur with various levels of disability. Although a 95-year-old female has a life expectancy

TABLE 9A-1 Age Specific Disaggregation of Male and Female Life Expectancy

		Life Expectancy for Profile							
		1	*2*	*3*	*4*	*5*	*6*		*7*
Age	*Total Life Expectancy*	*Active*	*Mild Cognitive Impairment*	*Moderate IADL*	*Physical Impairment*	*Frail*	*Highly Frail*	*Nonrespondent*	*Institutional*
					Males				
65	14.44	11.87	0.34	0.27	0.16	0.35	0.39	0.52	0.54
75	8.97	6.44	0.37	0.22	0.14	0.33	0.39	0.43	0.65
85	5.15	2.55	0.39	0.19	0.11	0.30	0.37	0.40	0.84
95	3.22	0.64	0.29	0.11	0.09	0.21	0.38	0.45	1.06
					Females				
65	18.57	13.61	0.48	0.59	0.39	0.72	0.61	0.81	1.36
75	11.70	6.97	0.47	0.48	0.33	0.66	0.58	0.70	1.51
85	6.44	2.25	0.39	0.32	0.22	0.46	0.53	0.58	1.69
95	3.65	0.35	0.21	0.14	0.09	0.20	0.38	0.56	1.73

From: Manton KG, Stallard E, Liu K. Forecasts of active life expectancy: policy and fiscal implications. J Gerontol 1993;48:11.

of 3.65 years, about 40% (1.73 years) will be spent as an institutionalized individual (Table 9A-1).

> **AXIOM** While old age in itself is not a contraindication to surgery, operations in older patients are usually associated with an increased mortality and morbidity.

The higher mortality rate with surgery in the elderly is directly related to deterioration of specific organ systems and, in some cases, to the presence of superimposed chronic diseases. This fact is essential in evaluating the traumatized aged patient. However, since old age may bias physicians against aggressive treatment, the prediction of a poor outcome in these individuals is likely to be fulfilled.[26,27]

CAUSES OF TRAUMA IN THE ELDERLY

The causes of injury resulting in death in the elderly are similar to those for younger individuals, but in different proportions.[29] Falls are the leading cause of injury and the second cause of elderly trauma deaths.[15] Motor vehicle accidents account for 25-50% of trauma deaths in the elderly (Table 9A-2).

Falls

Falls are an enormous problem for the elderly and cause about 7 million injuries and 10,000 deaths per year.[21] As many as one-third of

the elderly have a serious fall (requiring treatment at a hospital) one or more times each year. Although falls that are bad enough to hospitalize a patient are often the final symptom of one or more progressively debilitating diseases, the fall is frequently listed as the cause of death.

> **AXIOM** Most falls in the elderly are the result of their accumulated defects and diseases.[1]

Older people are less coordinated and have less stable gaits. Impairments in vision, hearing, and memory can make any environment dangerous. Drugs, especially sedatives, antihypertensives, diuretics, hypoglycemic agents, and alcohol, can also be contributing factors. Medical problems, such as vertigo, cardiac dysrhythmias, anemia, transient ischemic attacks, unstable joints, spontaneous fractures, epilepsy, and electrolyte imbalances, also contribute to an increased tendency to fall.

Motor Vehicle Accidents

In 1989 in the United States, approximately 5,170 elderly (65 years or older) individuals were killed as drivers or passengers in motor vehicle accidents, and an additional 7,200 were killed as pedestrians.[29] The per capita incidence of accidents is unaffected by age; however, because the elderly drive less, their crash experiences per mile driven are substantially higher than for middle-aged drivers.[30,31]

TABLE 9A-2 Mechanism of Injury, Relative Frequency, and Case Fatality Rate

	Ages ≥65		*Ages < 65*	
Mechanism of Injury	*% Relative Frequency (N:3, 833)*	*% Case Fatality Rate*	*% Relative Frequency (N:42, 944)*	*% Case Fatality Rate*
Fall	40.6	11.7	11.0	6.0
Motor vehicle accident	28.2	20.7	33.5	9.6
Pedestrian hit	10.0	32.6	7.9	13.5
Stab wound	2.6	17.3	11.9	4.7
Gunshot wound	5.5	52.1	13.0	19.5
Motorcycle	0.4	11.8	7.7	11.5
Other	7.0	13.8	14.0	5.4
Unknown	0.3	19.0	0.1	9.8
Total	100	—	100	—

From: Champion HR, Copes WS, Buyer D, et al. Major trauma in geriatric patients. Am J Public Health 1989;79:1278.

Furthermore, although younger drivers are more likely to be involved in serious single vehicle crashes, accidents with elderly drivers are more likely to involve a second vehicle, often at an intersection.[32,33]

AXIOM Elderly pedestrians struck by motor vehicles have the highest mortality rate of all injury victims.

Elderly pedestrian trauma victims have an extremely high mortality rate. Sklar et al[34] found that, although the mean ISS was the same for the young, the elderly died much more frequently. Champion et al[15] found that the death rate for pedestrian accidents in the 65 years or older group (32.6%) was about two and half times that of younger individuals (13.5%)

Burns

AXIOM Burns are relatively common in the elderly and have a high mortality rate.

In some burn units, the elderly may constitute as much as 20% of the admissions,[35] and in some series, burns are the third leading cause of trauma death in the elderly.[29] Indeed, it was not until the 1970s that elderly persons were reported to survive burns greater than 30% body surface area.[36] Even today, mortality rates for unselected elderly patients with greater than 15% burns can be expected to be 80% or more.[37]

Pneumonia in elderly burn victims has been reported as almost uniformly fatal regardless of the organism involved.[37,38] Because of the high mortality rate with operative treatment of burn victims, some burn centers are pursuing a wait-and-see approach that allows as much spontaneous healing as possible.[38]

Suicide

Until recently, little attention has been paid to suicide, the rate of which climbs steadily with ages greater than 40 years. Abuse of the elderly and hidden alcoholism may be important cofactors in this problem.[13]

IMPAIRED ORGAN FUNCTION IN THE ELDERLY

AXIOM It can be difficult to differentiate between the physiological effects of aging and the presence of underlying disease.

Much of the "fragility" of elderly patients who are injured or who have surgery is thought to be related to a loss of "physiological reserve" in multiple organ systems.[39,40] As a result, a fine balance may exist between "normal function" in an older person and what would

TABLE 9A-3 Incidence of Various Preexisting Diseases Correlated with Age in 6392 Trauma Patients Admitted to Detroit Receiving Hospital (1991-1992)

Age (yrs)	N	DAA	HTN	CDZ	DM	COPD
15-49	5192	12.0%	4.7%	5.2%	1.4%	1.6%
50-59	404	21.8%	25.0%	13.9%	8.2%	4.0%
60-69	382	17.6%	31.7%	27.2%	15.2%	8.9%
70-79	233	10.3%	42.1%	39.1%	15.9%	12.9%
80+	181	2.2%	34.8%	47.0%	11.7%	6.7%

% = incidence in each age and disease category
Abbreviations: DAA = Drug or alcohol abuse, HTN = Hypertension, CDZ = Cardiac disease, DM = Diabetes mellitus, COPD = Chronic obstructive pulmonary disease.

TABLE 9A-4 Mortality Rate Correlated with Age and Preexisting Diseases in 6392 Trauma Patients Admitted to Detroit Receiving Hospital (1991-1992)

Age (yrs)	DAA	HTN	CDZ	DM	COPD	All Pts.
15-49	2.0%	1.2%	10.7%	1.3%	1.2%	3.0%
50-59	4.5%	1.0%	12.5%	0	12.5%	6.4%
60-69	0	1.7%	10.6%	6.9%	8.8%	4.2%
70-79	4.2%	4.1%	12.1%	2.7%	3.3%	5.6%
80+	0	3.2%	11.8%	0	0	7.1%
Total	2.2%	1.9%	11.2%	2.7%	4.0%	3.5%

% = mortality rate in each age and disease category
Abbreviations: DAA = Drug or alcohol abuse, HTN = Hypertension, CDZ = Cardiac disease, DM = Diabetes mellitus, COPD = Chronic obstructive pulmonary disease.

be considered disease in a younger patient.[13] The likelihood of preexisting undiscovered chronic disease in the elderly is great and,[41] as a consequence, an injury that might result in only a short-term disability for a young person may lead to morbidity or death in the elderly.[13]

To study the effects of preexisting conditions and older age on outcome from trauma, the records of 6392 traumatized adults admitted to Detroit Receiving Hospital in 1990 and 1991 were reviewed. The incidence of drug or alcohol addiction, hypertension, cardiac disease, diabetes mellitus, and chronic obstructive lung disease were tabulated according to the age of the patients.

The incidence of drug or alcohol abuse (17.6-21.8%) was highest in patients 50-69 years of age, but was present in only 2.2% of the patients who were 80 years of age or older (Table 9A-3). The incidence of hypertension and cardiac disease increased significantly in patients who were 50 years of age or older. The mortality rate increased with age reaching a maximum of 12.9% in patients 70-79 years of age (Table 9A-4). If the patients with cardiac disease at each age group were excluded, the mortality rate was relatively constant at about 1 to 2% in all age groups.

The incidence of preexisting medical conditions (PEMC) increases with age. MacKenzie et al[42] showed that at 45-54 years of age, the incidence of PEMC is 17%, but in individuals over 65 years of age, it is 36-40% (Table 9A-5). The number of preexisting medical conditions had a striking effect on the mortality rate after trauma. In individuals with no preexisting medical conditions, the mortality rate was about 3%, but if more than two medical problems were present, the mortality rate was 25%[43,44] (Table 9A-6).

Central Nervous System

Aging brings about changes in cognitive, sensory, motor, and autonomic nervous functions. Cerebral perfusion pressure and oxygen consumption are decreased. Cerebral autoregulation is often also altered in the elderly, exposing them to an increased risk of cerebral ischemia during hypotension.

TABLE 9A-5 Frequency of Preexisting Medical Conditions by Age

Age (yr)	Frequency (%)
45-54	17
55-64	25
65-74	36
>75	41

Data from MacKenzie et al.[42]

TABLE 9A-6 Frequency of Preexisting Medical Conditions on Mortality

Preexisting Conditions (number)	Mortality Rate (%)
0	3
1	9
2	16
>2	25

Data from Milzman et al.[44]

PITFALL ⊘

If it is assumed that confusion in an elderly patient is due to senile brain changes, easily correctable hypoxia or respiratory dysfunction may be missed.

One should not assume that restlessness and disorientation in elderly patients is due to senile brain changes when in fact they may be caused by hypoxia.[13] Every patient who demonstrates cerebral dysfunction should be treated as if those changes were correctable. For example, transient nocturnal confusion can often be successfully treated with reassurance and a light within the room.

AXIOM Tranquilizers and barbiturates should be used with special care in elderly patients, since they can cause or potentiate confusion.

Cardiovascular System

In the absence of specific disease, the heart undergoes relatively little anatomic change with aging.[44] However, myocardial function progressively decreases with time. The causes of this diminution are multifactorial and include increasing ventricular hypertrophy and stiffness, slowed conduction, and reduced blood supply.[45,46] Cardiac output, stroke volume, and maximum heart rate decrease about 0.5-1.0% per year after the age of 20.[39,47] Myocardial conduction is slowed, and contraction times are prolonged. This predisposes the heart to reentry dysrhythmias and limits the heart's ability to increase its rate in response to added work loads. Since systemic vascular resistance also tends to rise in elderly patients, the cardiovascular system is particularly susceptible to pump failure in response to the increased stress of trauma.

AXIOM Cardiac complications are the most common cause of postoperative death in the elderly.

Since older patients frequently have significant narrowing of important nutrient vessels, arterial flow may be very pressure dependent. Consequently, the likelihood of cerebral or myocardial infarction increases markedly if significant hypotension occurs.

PITFALL ⊘

If serial ECGS and enzyme studies are not obtained in elderly patients who have been hypotensive, many silent myocardial infarctions will be missed.

Arteriosclerotic changes in the arteries in elderly patients alter their ability to compensate for blood loss.[1] Other important cardiovascular factors contributing to an increased risk of death after trauma include angina pectoris (especially if it is "unstable"), recent myocardial infarction, cardiac arrhythmias, and unstable hypertension.[1] A myocardial infarction during the previous 6 months significantly increases the risk of operation.[48] This risk, however, can be reduced to some extent by careful monitoring.[49]

AXIOM Elderly patients with cardiac disease tend to have a small margin of safety between a preload that prevents hypotension and one that causes overt heart failure.

Fluid overload is a constant hazard in patients with chronic heart failure.[1] In addition, patients with chronic cardiac failure have usually been treated with a low salt diet and diuretics for some time, and can have severe deficiencies in sodium, potassium, chloride, magnesium, and calcium. These electrolyte abnormalities may be manifested clinically by weakness, decreased tolerance of blood loss, lethargy, hypotension, and abnormal responses to many drugs, especially anesthetics.

Massive blood transfusions, persistent hypotension, and impaired ventilation can all cause severe acidosis. This can alter not only the excitability of the myocardium and its conducting system but also the patient's response to many drugs. If hypothermia develops, it further impairs cardiac performance and increases the tendency to arrhythmias. Patients with a long history of hypertension may require arterial pressures much higher than normal to maintain adequate perfusion of vital organs, especially the kidneys.

AXIOM Elderly patients who have cardiovascular disease should have their PAWP, cardiac output, oxygen delivery, and oxygen consumption optimized preoperatively, intraoperatively, and postoperatively, for at least 24-48 hours.

In patients with cardiovascular disease, general anesthesia and blood loss tend to produce hypotension. Indeed, even in stable and normovolemic patients, general anesthesia often reduces cardiac output by more than 20 to 30%.

In a study of 100 traumatized elderly patients, Osler et al[2] found no patient with a trauma score less than 7 or injury severity score greater than 50 who survived long enough to reach the hospital. They hypothesized that this was due in part to the inability of the heart to function during the acute phase of injury.

Lungs

With aging, an increase in anterior-posterior diameter of the thoracic cage is common, and this, together with a tendency to kyphosis, can cause a severe loss of intrathoracic volume and thoracic cage compliance.[50] The aging lung also loses much of its elasticity because of decreased elastin and continued cross-linkage between subunits of collagen. Even though total lung capacity (TLC) tends to remain constant with age, residual volume tends to increase from a normal of 20-25% in young adults to 35-45% of the TLC in the elderly, with a corresponding decrease in expiratory and inspiratory reserve volumes and vital capacity.[24,51,52]

Aging causes alveolar ducts to dilate and many interalveolar septa to disappear, thereby further reducing functional alveolar volume.

Because of a reduced stability of the pulmonary "skeleton," the terminal bronchioles collapse earlier in expiration, increasing the "closing volume" of the lungs.[51] Thus, the fraction of tidal ventilation that occurs below the closing volume increases, predisposing the patient to the development of atelectasis. The ratio of the one second forced expiratory volume ($FEV_{1.0}$) to the FVC in young patients is often 0.85 to 0.95, but in elderly patients the gradual increase in airway resistance often reduces the $FEV_{1.0}$/FVC ratio below 0.6 to 0.7.[24]

Because of all these changes and a decreased diffusion capacity, there is an almost linear decline in the arterial PO_2 of 2-3 mm Hg per decade after the age of 20. Little change is noted in the P_aCO_2 in normal subjects as a result of aging; however, if the patient has severe COPD, the P_aCO_2 may rise to levels exceeding 55 to 60 mm Hg. At these $PaCO_2$ levels, hypoxia is the main drive to ventilation.

PITFALL ⊘

> *The use of oxygen on an emphysematous patient with chronic severe hypercarbia can lead to severe respiratory acidosis and/or respiratory arrest.*

The arterial pH in patients with severe chronic obstructive pulmonary disease (COPD) and hypercarbia is usually maintained at a pH of about 7.35 by a compensatory rise in the plasma bicarbonate levels. Under ordinary circumstances, bicarbonate levels change much more slowly than PCO_2. Thus, if the PCO_2 is rapidly reduced by putting such patients on a ventilator with an increased minute ventilation (V_E), the bicarbonate/carbonic acid ratio and pH will rise abruptly. This sudden combined alkalosis can reduce ionized calcium levels abruptly and cause dangerous arrhythmias. As a general rule, the $PaCO_2$ should not be reduced by more than 5.0 mm Hg per hour.

PITFALL ⊘

> *In patients with chronic hypercarbia, the $PaCO_2$ should not be reduced by more than 5.0 mm Hg per hour.*

The efficacy of protective airway reflexes decreases in the elderly,[45,52] increasing the likelihood of preoperative aspiration of foreign bodies or oropharyngeal secretions. Large doses of sedatives or narcotic agents may further interfere with the function of the protective airway reflexes. Thus, avoidance of heavy sedation and protection of the lungs with an endotracheal tube until the return of adequate airway reflexes after surgery are important considerations in the elderly.[52]

Characteristically, elderly patients are poor coughers after surgery or trauma. Increased disorders of swallowing and of the lower esophageal sphincter in the elderly also predispose them to aspiration of oral or gastric secretions. All this, together with preexisting emphysema or bronchitis, not only interferes with gas exchange but also increases the chances of elderly patients developing postoperative atelectasis and pneumonia.

AXIOM   At least 50% of elderly patients undergoing thoracic or abdominal surgery develop postoperative complications, and of these, two-thirds are pulmonary.[2,53,54]

Kidneys

After the age of 30, there is an average 1.5% reduction per year in renal mass, the number of glomeruli, and the filtration rates, and this occurs with increasing rapidity after the age of 50.[55,56] The loss of renal mass involves entire nephrons and, as a consequence, the reductions in renal perfusion and glomerular filtration are the most significant, especially after 60 years of age. Effective renal blood flow and glomerular filtration rate decrease by almost 50% between the third and tenth decade.[57] By 90 years of age, the number of glomeruli and the overall filtration rate will be decreased by 46%.

AXIOM   Renal plasma flow (RPF), glomerular filtration rate (GFR), and the concentrating ability of the kidneys significantly decrease in the elderly.

As the muscle mass of geriatric patients decreases, creatinine production also progressively decreases. Thus, serum creatinine levels in the elderly may remain relatively normal in spite of significantly reduced renal function. Creatinine clearance is a far more reliable index of renal function than the BUN and serum creatinine levels and may be as low as 33% of normal by 70 years of age. Similarly, an elevated serum creatinine level in an older patient usually indicates a much more serious degree of renal impairment that it would in a younger patient.

AXIOM   Significant renal impairment may exist in elderly patients in spite of "normal" serum creatinine and BUN levels.

In spite of the changes with aging, the kidneys in older individuals are capable of maintaining normal acid-base balance as long as adequate perfusion is maintained and the metabolic load is not excessive.[57,58]

The osmolality of urine is determined by the composition of the plasma, the integrity of the renal tubules, and the adequacy of renal perfusion. In healthy, young individuals, the kidneys can concentrate to a specific gravity of 1.035 and a maximum osmolality of about 1400 mOsm/kg. Because of changes in the structure of the renal medulla and reduced renal perfusion, specific gravities greater than 1.024 and urine osmolalities greater than 750 are rarely achieved after the age of 70.[23] As a result, older individuals usually need a larger urine volume to maintain adequate excretion of non-volatile acid and various metabolites.

The decreased renal function that occurs with aging, in conjunction with a loss of cardiac reserve, causes elderly traumatized patients to require increased amounts of fluids to maintain an adequate urinary output at a time when even minimal overloading may cause severe heart failure.

AXIOM   Although large amounts of fluid may be required to maintain an adequate renal perfusion in the elderly, great care must be taken not to overload the heart.

Liver

A gradual decline in hepatic function is observed in patients over the age of 50, particularly regarding the capacity of the liver to conjugate lipid-soluble drugs.[59] This can result in prolonged high serum concentrations and reduced dosage requirements of such drugs.[60] Even if there is no evidence of hepatic, renal, or cardiac disease, plasma concentrations of propranolol, which is eliminated almost entirely by the liver, may be five times higher in the elderly than in younger patients.[61] Diazepam elimination is also greatly prolonged in the elderly because of altered hepatic biodegradation.[61]

Bone

Osteoporosis, characterized by a decrease in the mass of histologically normal bone and consequent loss of strength and resistance to fractures, causes clinical problems in almost half of all elderly people.[1] Causes of osteoporosis include reduced secretion of estrogen, decreased physical activity, and/or inadequate consumption of calcium.

AXIOM   The osteoporosis and reduced activity of advanced age combine to increase bone fragility and the incidence and severity of fractures.

Osteoporosis greatly increases the incidence of spontaneous vertebral compression fractures which, although seldom life-threatening, can be a source of considerable morbidity. Osteoporosis also probably accounts for much of the high incidence of hip fractures in the elderly, which increases about 1% per year for men and 2% per year for women.[62]

Metabolism

Metabolic changes in the elderly include the development of an abnormal glucose tolerance in 50% of patients over 70 years of age.[63] It is not clear whether this should be considered just a physiologic change of aging or actual diabetes mellitus, but it can occasionally cause severe problems, especially during intravenous hyperalimentation after trauma.

The caloric needs of men and women decline about 1% per year after age 30 as lean body mass and metabolic rate gradually decrease.[45] However, protein requirements may actually increase, probably as a result of inefficient utilization. The current recommended daily allowance for protein of 0.8 g/kg/day is probably inadequate for elderly patients, particularly those who are traumatized.[64]

> **AXIOM** Many elderly individuals, even those who are obese, suffer from subclinical malnutrition.

The results of a good surgical procedure can be compromised by poor nutrition.[64] Consequently, adequate nutritional support should be started as soon as the patient is hemodynamically stable. If the gastrointestinal tract is not usable, nutrition can be started intravenously.

Since serum protein levels are decreased in the elderly, and the affinity of some drugs for these proteins is also reduced, more free drug is apt to be available in the serum, increasing its clinical effects.[45] The effects of thiopental and etomidate are augmented by this mechanism, whereas the binding of other drugs, such as midazolam, lidocaine, propranolol, and meperidine, is unaltered.[65] Because of a decrease in total body water, lean body mass, cardiac output, and renal and hepatic function, the incidence of adverse drug reactions is increased in the elderly[66] (Table 9A-7).

> **AXIOM** Close attention to drug dosing is extremely important in the elderly if toxicity and prolonged effects are to be avoided.

Gastrointestinal Tract

Elderly patients with decreased gastrointestinal motility are often dependent on cathartics and are prone to develop a prolonged postoperative ileus.[13] Fecal impaction, which often manifests as diarrhea, is frequent in hospitalized elderly patients.

> **PITFALL** ⊘
>
> *Diarrhea in an elderly bed-ridden patient is due to a fecal impaction until proven otherwise.*

Immune System

Immune impairment in the elderly includes decreased cell-mediated and humoral immune responses to foreign antigens.[67] However, the response to autologous antigens is often increased, so that substantial numbers of elderly patients are allergic to many skin antigens. Because of these changes, the mortality rate of most infections increases in the elderly.[68,69]

Endocrine System

Although several laboratory studies of the steroid response to stress have shown that the adrenal glands in the aged respond normally,[70,71] many elderly patients act clinically as if they have some adrenal insufficiency.[72]

TABLE 9A-7 *Geriatric Physiologic Changes That Contribute to Adverse Drug Reactions*

Physiologic Changes	Adverse Drug Reactions
10-15% decrease in total body water	Reduced half-life and distribution of water soluble drugs
Increased body fat (18-30% in men and 30-45% in women)	Increased half-life and distribution of fat soluble drugs
20-30% decrease in lean body mass	Higher weight corrected dosage
30% reduction in functional glomeruli	Reduced renal excretion
40-45% decrease in hepatic blood flow	Decrease in metabolic excretion and oxidation
Decrease in cardiac output	

Data from Hartford CE and Kealey GP.[66]

There is a precipitous decline in estrogen levels in females after menopause, and a more gradual decrease in testosterone in older males. Significant decreases in androgen production with aging, as measured by urinary 11-deoxy-17-ketosteroids, probably reflect a decrease not only in gonadal but also in adrenal function.[70] This can result in a precarious anabolic-catabolic balance which may be easily tipped to severe catabolism by trauma or surgery.

PHYSIOLOGIC DISTURBANCES PRODUCED BY INJURY IN THE ELDERLY

Pulmonary Dysfunction

The reduction of PaO_2 in elderly patients with hip fractures is often significant.[45,73,74] This decrease in PaO_2 may be related to: (a) atelectasis and pneumonia resulting from prolonged perioperative supine positioning, (b) subclinical fat emboli or other posttraumatic microthromboemboli, or (c) deep venous thrombosis and pulmonary embolism.

> **AXIOM** The combination of aging and the direct and indirect effects of trauma greatly increase the tendency to posttraumatic pulmonary dysfunction.

Pulmonary fat emboli can be found in 80-90% of patients with long bone fractures, especially after prolonged immobilization; however, clinically apparent fat emboli occur in only about 1% of these patients.[75-77] In fact, 89% of these patients demonstrated an increased V_d/V_t (dead space/tidal volume) ratio lasting up to 5 days after injury.[73] Platelets activated by the trauma aggregate and accumulate in the pulmonary vascular bed. However, patients with hip fractures treated with aprotinin, a platelet aggregation inhibitor, failed to have an improved PaO_2 despite increased blood platelet counts.[74]

Plasma levels of fibrinogen, an acute phase protein, can increase significantly for 5-10 days after injury and can produce a hypercoagulable state.[78] Stasis and damage to vessel walls can also occur from the trauma.[79] Clinical signs and routine coagulation tests are of little value as early indicators of DVT, but increased levels of factor VIII-related antigen (F VIII:Ag) and factor VIII procoagulant activity (F VIII:C) are useful indicators of hypercoagulability and intravascular coagulation,[80] especially in patients developing DVT.[81]

INITIAL EVALUATION AND MANAGEMENT

History and Physical Exam

> **AXIOM** Elderly patients should be examined as if some degree of trauma or dysfunction is present in all organ systems and it is our job to detect it and quantify it.

Following adequate resuscitation, a complete history and physical exam should be obtained. The past history should include concurrent illnesses, past surgeries, current medications, allergies, immunization status, and the time of the patient's last meal. If the patient is unable to give a clear history, special attempts must be made to elicit the pertinent data from friends or family.

Radiologic Studies

Radiologic studies are essential to the evaluation of many traumatized patients, especially the elderly. X-rays of the chest and all injured areas may reveal preexisting cardiopulmonary disease and/or subclinical fractures.

Initial Fluid Therapy

> **AXIOM** Resuscitation of elderly trauma victims should generally be more aggressive than in younger individuals.

Hypotension and impaired tissue perfusion should be corrected by aggressive fluid therapy without overloading the cardiovascular system. If the patient is bleeding heavily, the hemorrhage should be controlled before large amounts of fluids and/or blood are given.

Although normal saline is satisfactory for many conditions, it has the potential for producing hyperchloremic acidosis when used in large volumes, especially in patients with impaired renal function.[1] This may be an important consideration in some elderly patients.

AXIOM The best guide to continued fluid therapy is the response to the previous fluid bolus.

Patients who respond rapidly to the initial 1-2 liters of fluid resuscitation and then remain stable have usually lost less than 25% of their blood volume and no further boluses of fluid or blood are likely to be necessary.[1] However, continued careful observation is necessary, and blood should be readily available if needed later.

If the patient responds initially to aggressive fluid resuscitation but deteriorates later, the cause of the hypotension must be rapidly determined. Although this is usually due to continued bleeding, one must also look for tension pneumothorax, pericardial tamponade, myocardial contusion, or cardiac disease.

Patients with a transient or minimal response to fluid resuscitation usually have ongoing blood loss and require prompt surgical intervention.

AXIOM The elderly are intolerant of over-resuscitation, but they are extremely intolerant of continued hypovolemic hypotension.

Preoperative Assessment

The preoperative assessment should be as thorough as possible under the circumstances of the initial evaluation.[1] This evaluation should lead to critical decisions on the need for further fluid administration, special monitoring, or use of various drugs to increase cardiac output or BP before surgery.

INJURIES IN THE ELDERLY

Head Injuries

With increasing age, the dura becomes tightly adherent to the skull, making the development of epidural hematomas relatively uncommon in the elderly.[1] The brain also undergoes a progressive loss of volume with age. This resultant increased space around the brain serves to protect it from contusion, but also makes subdural hematomas more likely to occur.[82]

AXIOM One must have a high index of suspicion for subdural hematomas in elderly patients with head trauma.

Subdural hematomas are three times more common in the elderly than in younger patients, and because there is an increased subdural space, the symptoms may be delayed and/or atypical. In some elderly patients, the only symptom of large or increasing subdural hematomas may be a gradual neurologic decline.

The overall outcome of head-injured patients is discouraging regardless of their age.[1] In a recent survey of 545 injured patients, 31% of those sustaining a major head injury (Glasgow Coma Score less than 8) subsequently died. The prognosis can be expected to be even worse in the elderly. Osler et al,[2] in a review of 100 traumatized elderly patients, found that neurotrauma was second only to shock as a predictor of fatal outcome.[2]

Chest Trauma

AXIOM It is probably wise to consider all elderly patients with chest trauma to have rib fractures and/or pulmonary contusions even if it is not apparent on the initial chest x-rays.

Because of the rigid chest wall and osteoporosis, blunt chest trauma to the elderly frequently results in rib fractures.[1] Even a relatively mild injury with a few fractured ribs or a small lung contusion may make it necessary for an elderly patient to receive ventilatory support for several days.

The loss of respiratory reserve from aging or from chronic disease makes careful monitoring of the pulmonary status of elderly patients imperative.[1] A pulse oximeter should be used to continuously monitor arterial oxygen saturation. Early arterial blood gas evaluation is also important because it may reveal an unexpected metabolic or respiratory acidosis.

Except for occasional severe COPD patients with severe hypercarbia who depend on hypoxia to sustain their respiratory drive, administration of oxygen is usually very beneficial. Although some feel that endotracheal intubation is hazardous for the elderly and may increase the risk of a fatal pneumonia, it should be performed promptly if there is inadequate ventilation that cannot be rapidly improved by other techniques, such as an epidural block for fractured ribs.

Abdominal Trauma

AXIOM Elderly patients do not tolerate continued intra-abdominal bleeding or peritoneal contamination.

Elderly patients may not tolerate an unnecessary laparotomy very well, but persistent bleeding or a bowel leak in the abdomen is apt to be lethal. Therefore, prompt and accurate diagnosis of intra-abdominal injuries that require an operation is imperative.

AXIOM The diagnostic approach to abdominal trauma in the elderly is similar to that used in younger patients; however, there is a greater need for an early accurate diagnosis in the elderly.

Musculoskeletal Injuries

Osteoporosis in the elderly predisposes them to fractures from relatively mild trauma.[1] Consequently, elderly injured patients should have a very careful physical examination and then x-rays should be obtained on any bone which may be fractured. Fractures that are particularly apt to occur in the elderly include Colle's fractures, hip fractures, and fractures of the head of the humerus.

Abuse of the Elderly

Abuse can been defined as any willful infliction of injury, unreasonable confinement, intimidation, or cruel punishment with resulting physical harm, pain, or mental anguish.

The incidence of abuse to elderly individuals is estimated to be at least 10%, with 40% of these defined as victims of moderate to severe abuse. Such abuse has been linked to recent changes in family structure, frustration, cognitive deficits in the aged, failing physical health, financial difficulties, and inadequate community support.[83]

AXIOM If one does not look for abuse in elderly trauma victims, it will generally not be detected and/or prevented from recurring.

In 1980, the United States Senate Special Committee on Elder Abuse reported that there are up to 2,500,000 cases of geriatric abuse, neglect, or mistreatment each year in the U.S.[1] The United States

House of Representatives Select Committee on Aging did a survey estimating that 4% of the nation's elderly population, or approximately 1 million persons, are victims of abuse. Many of these cases have only subtle findings, such as poor hygiene or dehydration, and have a great potential to pass undetected[83] (Table 9A-8). Consequently, it is estimated that only one in six cases of geriatric abuse comes to the attention of authorities.[83,84]

INDICATIONS FOR WITHHOLDING THERAPY IN THE ELDERLY

Certainly there are circumstances in which it may be wise to withhold certain types of therapy from elderly patients. This decision is particularly clear when, as with massive burns, the injury is unsurvivable, and any treatment beyond comfort measures will only prolong a painful death.[85]

Although there are many other circumstances in which survival is impossible, the clinician is usually faced with poorly defined probabilities. Certainly, if all of the physicians involved feel that the patient has no chance of recovery, the continued discomfort of a prolonged ICU stay serves no purpose.

> **AXIOM** Care should not be withheld from elderly patients unless it will only prolong dying.

While the specifics of decision-making are often on an individual basis, one caveat of trauma care in the elderly is that the patient, family, and surgeon often must accept less than optimum results to keep morbidity and/or mortality to a minimum.[13] One example is accepting the deformity of a Colles' fracture to provide early mobilization to maintain wrist and hand function. Another example might be leaving a colostomy in place in high-risk elderly patients who are bedridden rather than risk reoperative bowel surgery.

Frank discussions with patients and/or their families can be a great help and comfort to all concerned.[1] If the patient is unable to participate in these discussions, a "living will" has occasionally been a useful adjunct. Input from the nursing staff and the hospital's ethics committee may also be helpful.

While no absolute generic guidelines can be given, the following observations may be helpful: (a) the patient's right to self-determination is paramount, (b) medical intervention is only appropriate when it is in the patient's best interest, and (c) medical therapy is only appropriate when its likely benefits outweigh its likely adverse consequences.[1]

SPECIAL CONSIDERATION FOR TRAUMA SURGERY IN THE ELDERLY

> **PITFALL** ⊘
>
> *Failure to aggressively treat elderly trauma patients because of a presumed "frail" condition will almost invariably lead to a worse long-term outcome.*

TABLE 9A-8 *Conditions in Which Abuse of the Elderly Should Be Suspected*

Fearful behavior
Family members' or care-giver's attitudes, feeling of being burdened, lack of interest, aggressive behavior
Signs of physical abuse, including bruises, welts, burns, injuries to head and hair
Signs of confinement, such as locks on rooms, telephones, and refrigerator
Neglected wounds and injuries, especially fractures and infections
Unexplained malnutrition or dehydration

From: Rathbone-McCuan E, Voyles B. Case detection of abused elderly patients. Am J Psychiatry 1982;139:189.

Preoperative Workup

In a detailed survey of elderly females with hip fractures, significant dysfunction of at least one organ was found in 92%.[86] This included cardiovascular disease in 78%, mental abnormalities in 39%, pulmonary diseases in 14%, endocrinopathies in 12%, and neurologic disturbances in 10%.[86] Many suffered from dysfunction of more than one organ, a situation confirmed by other surveys of geriatric patients.

> **AXIOM** The preoperative workup of elderly trauma patients should be designed to discover the presence and severity of all major organ dysfunctions.

Many elderly patients are on multiple medications before their injury. In the series of Heljamae et al,[86] 87% of the patients were receiving medication for a variety of problems before their hip fracture. Digitalis preparations, beta-blockers, calcium channel blockers, and antihypertensives were the most common medications. Obviously, such polypharmacy increases the risk of perioperative drug interactions. Alcohol, sedatives, and psychotropic drugs may be a particular problem.

Timing of Trauma Surgery in the Elderly

The modern concept is to perform surgery immediately after adequate optimization of coexisting medical problems. Evaluations of some diseases, such as myocardial ischemia, may require more extensive tests that may not be immediately available.

> **AXIOM** Urgent surgery on elderly trauma patients should be performed as soon as their organ function can be optimized.

The preoperative approach described by Schultz et al[87] involves transfer of the patient, after an admission workup, to a special care unit where a pulmonary artery catheter is introduced to allow optimization of cardiac function and oxygen delivery. If medical problems are found during this period, appropriate therapy is instituted. Surgery is performed as soon as any underlying abnormalities are corrected and cardiopulmonary function has been optimized. The physiologic surveillance of the patient is continued throughout the postoperative period.

Using this approach of early careful monitoring, Schultz et al[87] modified the widespread feeling by many orthopedic surgeons that patients should undergo reduction and fixation of major extremity fractures within 24 hours. Indeed, the "appropriate time for surgery should be accurately determined and chosen on the basis of optimal physiologic balance." The mortality rate in their monitored group was 2.9%, as opposed to 29% in a similar but unmonitored group, even though the mean interval between admission and operation in the monitored group was 3.7 days.

Choice of Anesthesia

Many surgeons and anesthesiologists feel that surgery in the elderly should be performed under regional, rather than general, anesthesia whenever possible because it probably has a less suppressive effect on most organ systems, especially the heart and the lungs. Some authors also claim that regional anesthesia is more effective than general anesthesia in reducing postoperative confusion and maintaining mental function in the elderly.[88] However, the incidence of postoperative confusion in one series of elderly patients with femoral neck fractures was 44%, and the rate of this complication was not reduced by regional anesthesia. It correlated most closely with a history of preexisting mental depression and use of drugs with anticholinergic effects.

> **AXIOM** Preoperative and intraoperative optimization of cardiac and pulmonary function is much more important than the type of anesthetic used.

Despite the apparent advantages of regional anesthesia, postoperative mortality is affected little by the choice of anesthetic technique.[45] Between 1977 and 1984, seven prospective randomized trials compared the mortality rate of hip fracture surgery under general or regional anesthesia. In only one of these trials could a significant reduction in both short-term and long-term mortality be demonstrated with regional anesthesia,[89] and one other study showed a reduction in mortality, but only on a short-term basis.[90] In the remaining five studies, neither short-term nor long-term mortality was significantly reduced, but there was a tendency to a lower death rate when regional anesthesia was employed.[45]

Two more recent prospective trials, each comparing postoperative mortality of more than 500 elderly hip fracture victims after spinal and general anesthesia, concluded that the type of anesthesia had no effect on short-term or long-term mortality of these patients.[91,92]

Fluid Requirements During Surgery

Fluid requirements in the geriatric trauma patient, once corrected for the smaller amount of lean body mass that is present with aging, are similar to those of younger patients;[1] however, one should remember that elderly hypertensive patients on chronic diuretic therapy tend to have a chronically contracted blood volume, a total body potassium deficit, and a reduced ability to concentrate their urine.

AXIOM   The optimal hematocrit in elderly trauma patients is probably higher than in younger individuals, but this is best determined by attempts to optimize oxygen delivery and consumption.

The optimal hematocrit for seriously injured elderly patients is still a debated issue, and this problem is made more complex by concerns about infections and immunosuppression caused by bank blood.[1] Our tendency has been to keep elderly patients at a higher hematocrit (above 35%) than younger individuals. Our experience agrees with that of Horst et al[93] who found that elderly trauma survivors tended to have higher hemoglobins than non-survivors (12.1 versus 10.5 gm/dl).

AXIOM   If vascular disease limits blood flow to an organ, a higher hematocrit may be necessary to provide adequate oxygen delivery.

Intraoperative Monitoring

Monitoring of core temperature is particularly important in the elderly. Some of the factors reducing the ability of elderly patients to maintain an adequate core temperature include: (a) slowed basal metabolism, (b) reduced ability to shiver under anesthesia, and (c) reduced delivery of oxygen and glucose to the tissues.

Arterial pressure monitors, central venous pressure lines, and Swan-Ganz catheters are often employed to monitor pulmonary and hemodynamic function in severely injured patients, even if they are young, because the organ systems may not perform normally. Such monitoring is particularly important in older patients whose pulmonary and cardiac reserves are limited.[1]

AXIOM   The response of the pulmonary artery wedge pressure or central venus pressure to a fluid challenge, particularly in elderly patients, is far more revealing than isolated readings.

Preventing Hypothermia

The reduced basal metabolic rate in the elderly not only slows the degradation of anesthetic drugs, but it also induces more frequent and prolonged interoperative and postoperative hypothermia.[45] Although perioperative hypothermia in these patients is largely a result of decreased heat production and altered thermoregulation caused by gen-

eral anesthesia, it is not uncommon for elderly patients to also develop moderate hypothermia under spinal anesthesia.[61]

AXIOM   Hypothermia can occur quickly and easily in the elderly, and the hypermetabolism to correct it can put great stress on the cardiovascular system.

A drop in rectal or esophageal temperature to less than 95° F can lead to coagulopathies, prolonged stuporous states, and prolonged discomfort.[94,95] This in turn can lead to increased catabolic hormone and interleukin release. How much such problems affect overall outcome in traumatized elderly patients is not certain, but morbidity and mortality are reduced when hypothermia is prevented in burned elderly patients.[95]

Heating pads, coverage of unused body parts with "space blankets," warm intravenous fluids, room temperatures of 85° F or more, and incandescent heating lamps can all be important.[13] If possible, nonoperated areas of the body should be kept dry and covered to reduce insensible heat loss from evaporation.

Shivering postoperatively in hypothermic patients can increase oxygen consumption by more than 400%. If pulmonary and myocardial reserves are limited, hypothermia tends to cause myocardial ischemia, hypoxemia, increased systemic vascular resistance, anaerobic metabolism, and lactic acidosis.[96]

Length of Operation

AXIOM   Operations in the elderly should be as short as possible, but one should try to prevent the need for further surgery if at all possible.

As with all operations, morbidity and mortality in trauma surgery are often directly related to the duration of the surgical procedure.[1] Keeping operative time to a minimum should not only help prevent intraoperative complications such as hypothermia and its attendant complications of coagulopathy and dysrhythmia, but it should also help to minimize the incidence of postoperative complications, such as wound infections.

AXIOM   As with all surgery, the best procedure addresses all of the patient's problems and takes the least time.

Although it is generally felt that splenorrhaphy is preferable to splenectomy, it is probably safer to perform a rapid splenectomy in an elderly person with a badly injured but salvageable spleen even if there are no other injuries.[13] The risk-benefit ratio of trying to repair the spleen may be too high because of the time constraints and the possibility that continued bleeding might require a reoperation. In like manner, with right colon injuries, it is also reasonable to perform an ileostomy rather than an ileocolic anastomosis to save time and obviate the risk of a later leaking anastomosis. Elderly poor-risk patients can often tolerate one long operation much better than two or three shorter procedures, especially if performed under general anesthesia.

AXIOM   Repeat operations in elderly patients should be avoided whenever possible.

POSTOPERATIVE MANAGEMENT OF THE ELDERLY

Management in an Intensive Care Unit

With the advent of more complex postoperative monitoring, the use of the intensive care unit for immediate postoperative care has gained widespread acceptance.[1] The sophisticated monitoring possible in an ICU allows close evaluation of the status of multiple organ systems on a minute-to-minute basis and has improved patient outcomes. Scalea et al,[97] prospectively evaluating multiply injured geriatric patients in an intensive care unit, showed that survival could be improved from 7 to 53% by early admission to the ICU and placement of a Swan-Ganz catheter to optimize cardiac status.

Unfortunately, the cost of ICU care for the elderly can be extremely high. In a two-year study by Campion et al,[98] 44% of the admissions to their intensive care units were patients over 65 years of age, and 21% were patients more than 75 years of age. Major therapeutic interventions, such as intubation and mechanical ventilation, were more likely to occur in the elderly and occurred more frequently as age increased. Furthermore, the one-year accumulated mortality for patients over 75 years of age was 44%.

Nutrition

Over the past 20 years, early provision of adequate carbohydrates, proteins, lipids, vitamins, and trace elements has been associated with an overall reduction in mortality and in complications in geriatric trauma patients.[1]

AXIOM Nutrition in the elderly should be monitored closely to provide adequate protein, but not excessive calories.

The increased energy expenditure after trauma is largely driven by humoral changes that serve not only as mediators of the stress response but also help direct the flow of energy and protein substrate to vital organs and wounded tissue.[1]

As a general rule, parenteral nutrition should be started as soon as the patient is hemodynamically stable. Enteral nutrition, preferably through a tube in the small bowel beyond the ligament of Treitz, should probably also be begun early.

Mobility

There is no question that early mobilization of patients after trauma is of major importance in reducing the risk of atelectasis, pneumonia, and pulmonary embolus.[1] It also helps to prevent skin breakdown and development of decubiti.

One of the greatest benefits of early mobilization is the psychologic lift it provides. The fact that the patient is out of bed reinforces the idea that he or she is recovering and moving toward normal patterns of daily activity.

OUTCOME

Mortality

Surgery in the elderly is associated with an increased mortality rate, particularly in patients with multiple preexisting diseases.[40] The risk of dying is particularly high in patients requiring emergency surgery. In unselected groups of trauma victims, Osler et al[2] found that the elderly died six times as frequently as younger individuals, even when controlled for degree of injury.

In the series by Oreskovich et al,[53] the overall mortality rate in elderly trauma patients was 15%, and this was quite similar to the results of a study by Champion et al[15] in which the mortality rate of injured patients more than 65 years of age was 19.0%. That mortality rate, however, was almost twice as high as the mortality rate of 9.8% in individuals less than 65 years of age, even though the injury severity score and revised trauma score were not significantly different.[15] Even when the data was controlled for the area of the body involved and the severity of the injuries in each area, the elderly did much worse. Differences were especially significant for abdominal injuries with mortality rates of 11.5 versus 29.5 percent.

An impaired cardiopulmonary response to stress is often cited as the major cause of death in the elderly;[93,99,100] however, Steinberg found that when elderly individuals were stressed during exercise, their cardiovascular responses were similar to those of younger patients, but of a different magnitude.[101]

In a study of elderly trauma patients by Horst et al,[93] there were no significant differences between survivors and nonsurvivors in terms of preexisting disease, type of trauma, presence of shock, trauma score, injury severity score, and acute physiology score. However, they did find that elderly survivors had higher hemoglobin levels (12.1 ± 2.0 versus 10.5 ± 1.0 gm/dl), lower systemic vascular resistance (1098 versus 1430 dyne · sec · cm · ^{5}/m^2), and higher oxygen delivery (603 ± 168 versus 483 ± 210 ml/min/m^2) than those who died. The differences in these variables were thought to be primarily a result of differences in resuscitation rather than differences in the cardiopulmonary response to injury. They also found that oxygen delivery could be improved by giving more blood, and that the increased preload tended to increase cardiac output and decrease systemic vascular resistance.

AXIOM The adequacy of the initial resuscitation in restoring an optimal red cell mass appears to be an important prognostic factor in traumatized elderly patients.

Complications

Elderly patients who die after trauma often succumb to complications rather than the injury per se, and such complications can be difficult to foresee at the time of the patient's initial presentation.[1] However, Osler et al[2] found that the presence of shock or head injury at the time of admission was a particularly grave prognostic sign in elderly trauma patients.

In the study of Champion et al,[15] the incidence of complications in older patients was much higher (33.4% versus 19.4%). The difference in the incidence of complications in elderly patients was particularly more frequent at the lower ISS scores.

PULMONARY COMPLICATIONS

Pulmonary complications are the most common posttraumatic problems experienced by geriatric patients, particularly in individuals with preexisting chronic bronchitis or emphysema and heavy tobacco use.[1] The incidence and severity of such complications can be reduced by early mobilization, chest physiotherapy, encouraged coughing and deep breathing, and incentive spirometry. An early sputum smear and culture can give a clue that the patient has an impending pneumonia and may serve as a guide to future antibiotic therapy. Judicious use of narcotics and maintenance of effective nasogastric decompression can also help reduce pulmonary complications.

CARDIOVASCULAR COMPLICATIONS

AXIOM Myocardial ischemia is best prevented by keeping hypotension, hypertension, and tachycardia to a minimum.

Patients with preexisting coronary artery disease and angina are particularly prone to develop myocardial ischemia if any hypotension develops. Patients with preexisting cardiac failure almost invariably get worse after trauma as a result of the increased stress and demands on the heart. Careful monitoring of PAWP can be helpful, at least for preventing fluid overload. Dahn et al[102] found that verapamil could reduce systolic BP and heart rate following aortic surgery, thereby reducing the factors apt to result in an increased myocardial oxygen consumption.

DEEP VENOUS THROMBOSIS

Many factors predispose elderly trauma patients to the development of venous thrombosis including: (a) reduction of venous flow rate because of bed rest, congestive heart failure, hypovolemia, and venous congestion, (b) direct injury to blood vessels, and (c) hypercoagulable states. Although superficial thrombophlebitis is relatively easy to diagnose, less than 20-30% of patients with deep venous thrombosis (DVT) in their legs will have any local signs or symptoms of that problem.

A sudden onset of tachypnea, tachycardia, and hypoxemia should make one suspect an acute pulmonary embolus. If the chest x-ray is normal, a ventilation-perfusion (V/Q) scan can be helpful, especially if it shows several segments or a single large area of impaired perfusion without impaired ventilation. If the V/Q scan is perfectly normal, a pulmonary embolus (PE) of any significance is very unlikely. Confirmation of the presence of a PE is best obtained with a pulmonary arteriogram.

AXIOM   One should use as many techniques as possible to prevent deep venous thrombosis in the legs of all non-ambulating trauma patients.

Deep venous thrombosis is classically prevented by early mobilization, elevation of the lower extremities, and active and passive leg exercises. The use of graduated pressure stockings extending above the knee has not been beneficial in preventing this problem.[1] Low-dose heparin is also of relatively little value in patients with severe trauma, especially extensive fractures. External pneumatic compression stockings, however, by providing rhythmic compression of the legs, appear to reduce the risk of deep venous thrombosis. Even if the pneumatic stockings are only applied to the arms, they can provide some protection by increasing plasma levels of fibrinolysins.

Acute management of DVT and pulmonary embolism generally includes systemic heparinization, usually with an initial bolus of 5,000 units intravenously and then 800-1300 units per hour by "continuous" infusion. If there is a risk to heparinizing a patient with iliofemoral DVT or a pulmonary embolus, a Greenfield or similar filter can be inserted in the inferior vena cava below the renal veins.

ACUTE RENAL FAILURE

The incidence of acute renal failure in the elderly is particularly high in patients with preexisting renal disease who have hypotension, myoglobinuria, or hemoglobinuria. Administration of radiographic contrast and nephrotoxic antibiotics, especially the aminoglycosides, further increases the risk of renal failure after trauma in the elderly.

AXIOM   Acute oliguric renal failure is probably best prevented by maintaining as high a urine output as possible without using diuretics or overloading the patient with fluids.

SEPSIS

Postoperative sepsis in elderly patients can carry an extremely high mortality. Optimal management in addition to preventive efforts include: (a) prompt detection and drainage or debridement of any collections of pus or necrotic tissue, (b) vigorous fluid resuscitation, and (c) appropriate use of antibiotics. Many of these patients have impaired immunity and, therefore, are at double jeopardy. Not only are they much more likely to develop infections, but they are also less likely to show the typical fever, leukocytosis, and local signs and symptoms that can help provide an early diagnosis.

AXIOM   Not infrequently, sepsis is not recognized in the elderly until multiple organ failure begins to develop, and then it is often too late to save the patient.

It can be very difficult to find the source of infection in elderly posttrauma patients who appear to be septic.[1] In these circumstances, the empiric removal of indwelling intravenous catheters and culture of the tip and intracutaneous portion of the catheter can help provide a diagnosis. In patients who are deteriorating after abdominal surgery or trauma and have no evidence of infection clinically or radiologically, a "blind laparotomy" may be indicated; however, for eradication of any localized collections of pus to improve survival rate, it must be done before multiple organ failure develops.

POSTOPERATIVE DELIRIUM

AXIOM   Restlessness is due to hypoxemia until proven otherwise.

Several factors are known to contribute to the development of postoperative delirium in elderly patients.[1] These include hypoxemia, hypotension, reduced cardiac output, fluid and electrolyte abnormalities, various medications, unfamiliar environments, sleep deprivation, excessive stress responses, and sepsis. It is important to look carefully for etiology of any posttraumatic confusion and to realize that, in general, with recovery from the acute stress and transfer from an intensive care environment, the majority of patients will recover their preinjury mental status.

REHABILITATION

AXIOM   Optimal rehabilitation begins when the patient is first seen.[13,22]

Rehabilitation of the elderly can be a long and tedious process, but the sooner it is started, the shorter and more effective it will be. One study of injured patients over 70 years of age showed that although 96% of the patients were independent prior to injury, following the trauma, 72% required care in a nursing home, and another 20% needed prolonged medical assistance.[53]

More recently, however, DeMaria et al[103] found that with aggressive treatment, 89% of elderly survivors of trauma returned home, and 57% returned to living independently. Thus, "when elderly impaired trauma victims receive specific rehabilitation therapy with realistic geriatric goals, they often respond dramatically."[104]

AXIOM   Home care should be provided as soon as services that can only be provided in a hospital are no longer necessary.

Not all elderly trauma patients can be cared for at home, but far greater numbers of patients could receive home health care services than is currently the case.[1] Services that can be provided under a plan of home care may include medical care, dental care, nursing care, physical therapy, speech therapy, occupational therapy, social work, nutrition, home making, home health aid, transportation, laboratory service, and medical equipment and supplies.

Some of the primary objectives of home care programs are:

1. To provide more individualized and more consistent care than could be provided in a hospital or extended care facility.
2. To expedite recovery, to prevent or postpone disability, and to maintain personal dignity by restoring patients to normal family life and to useful functional activity.
3. To complete whatever comprehensive care was begun in the hospital but at greatly reduced costs.
4. To shorten the length of hospital stay and to prevent rehospitalization.
5. To improve the use of existing hospital beds and to reduce the need for additional inpatient facilities.
6. To provide for the needs of ill patients who can be adequately treated in the home rather than in an institutional setting.

⊘ FREQUENT ERRORS

In the Management of Elderly Trauma Patients

1. *Delaying or avoiding needed surgery in elderly patients because of their increased risk.*
2. *Liberal use of tranquilizers and barbiturates to control restlessness in elderly patients.*
3. *Deliberately keeping preload low to not risk overloading an elderly patient who has a relatively low cardiac output.*
4. *Failing to optimize PAWP and O_2 delivery in elderly, high-risk patients who need a general anesthetic.*
5. *Relying on certain levels of CVP and/or PAWP to determine the amount of fluid-loading an elderly patient will receive.*

6. *Rapid correction of chronic acid-base and fluid and electrolyte problems in elderly patients.*
7. *Delay and/or reluctance to provide nasotracheal suction or bronchoscopy for pulmonary toilet in elderly patients who will not breathe and cough adequately.*
8. *Assuming that renal function in an elderly patient is normal because the urine output is good and the BUN and serum creatinine are "within normal limits."*
9. *Assuming that an elderly patient who is still awake after head trauma cannot have a large subdural hematoma.*
10. *Attempting to obtain optimal reduction of fractures, especially in the upper extremities, at the expense of mobility.*
11. *Not looking for evidence of abuse in elderly patients with repeated trauma.*
12. *Relying on a relatively low hematocrit to maintain an adequate O_2 delivery in patients with significant cardiac and/or pulmonary dysfunction.*
13. *Using multiple operations to correct a problem in the elderly rather than relying on one larger operation to correct all the problems.*
14. *Delaying rehabilitation efforts in elderly trauma victims.*

▼▼▼▼▼▼▼▼▼▼▼▼▼▼▼▼▼▼▼▼▼▼▼▼▼▼▼▼▼▼▼▼

SUMMARY POINTS

1. The elderly (more than 65 years) are the fastest growing segment of our population.
2. Trauma in the elderly is more apt to be fatal than in younger individuals.
3. The relationship between the condition of a car (or patient) and its age is not as important as how well it was made (genetics), the miles that it has been driven, and the care and maintenance that it has received.
4. Elderly patients who die as a result of trauma often have a long, lingering complicated hospital course prior to death, further increasing the cost of their medical care.
5. While old age in itself is not a contraindication to surgery, operations in older patients are definitely associated with an increased mortality and morbidity.
6. Most falls in the elderly are the result of their accumulated defects and diseases.
7. Elderly pedestrians struck by motor vehicles have the highest mortality rate of all injury victims.
8. Burns are relatively common in the elderly and can have a very high mortality rate.
9. It can be very difficult at times to differentiate between the physiological effects of aging and the presence of disease.
10. If it is assumed that confusion in an elderly patient is due to senile brain changes, easily correctable hypoxia or respiratory dysfunction may be missed.
11. Tranquilizers and barbiturates should be used with special care in elderly patients, since their effects can cause or potentiate confusion.
12. Cardiac complications are the most common cause of postoperative death in the elderly.
13. Elderly patients with cardiac disease tend to have a small margin of safety between a preload that prevents hypotension and one that causes overt heart failure.
14. Elderly patients who have cardiovascular disease should have their PAWP, cardiac output, oxygen delivery, and oxygen consumption optimized preoperatively, intraoperatively, and for at least 24-48 hours postoperatively.
15. At least 50% of elderly patients undergoing thoracic or abdominal surgery develop postoperative complications, and of these, over two-thirds are pulmonary.
16. The RPF, GFR, and concentrating ability of the kidneys are significantly decreased in the elderly.
17. Significant renal impairment may exist in elderly patients in spite of normal serum creatinine and BUN levels.
18. Although large amounts of fluid may be required to maintain an adequate renal perfusion in the elderly, great care must be taken not to overload the heart.
19. The osteoporosis and reduced activity of advanced age combine to increase bone fragility and the incidence and severity of fractures.
20. Many elderly individuals, even those who are obese, suffer from subclinical malnutrition.
21. The combination of aging and the direct and indirect effects of trauma greatly increase the tendency to post-traumatic pulmonary dysfunction.
22. Elderly patients should be examined as if some degree of trauma or dysfunction is present in all organ systems and it is our job to detect it and quantify it.
23. Resuscitation of elderly trauma victims should generally be more aggressive than in younger individuals.
24. The best guide to continued fluid therapy is the response to the previous fluid bolus.
25. The elderly are intolerant of over-resuscitation, but they are even more intolerant of continued hypovolemia.
26. One must have a high index of suspicion for subdural hematomas in elderly patients with head trauma.
27. It is probably wise to consider all elderly patients with chest trauma to have rib fractures and/or pulmonary contusion even if it is not apparent on the initial chest x-ray.
28. Elderly patients do not tolerate continued intra-abdominal bleeding or peritoneal contamination.
29. The diagnostic approach to abdominal trauma in the elderly is similar to that used in younger patients; however, there is a greater need for early accurate diagnosis in the elderly.
30. If one does not look for abuse in elderly trauma victims, it will generally not be detected and/or prevented from recurring.
31. Care should not be withheld from elderly patients unless it will only prolong dying.
32. The preoperative workup of elderly trauma patients should be designed to discover the presence and severity of all major organ dysfunctions.
33. Urgent surgery on elderly trauma patients should be performed as soon as their organ function can be optimized.
34. Preoperative and intraoperative optimization of cardiac and pulmonary function is much more important than the type of anesthetic used.
35. The optimal hematocrit in elderly trauma patients is probably higher than in younger individuals, and this is best determined by attempts to optimize oxygen delivery and consumption.
36. If vascular disease limits blood flow to an organ, a higher hematocrit may be necessary to provide adequate oxygen delivery.
37. The response of the pulmonary artery wedge pressure or central venus pressure to a fluid challenge, particularly in elderly patients, is far more revealing than isolated readings.
38. Hypothermia can occur quickly and easily in the elderly, and the hypermetabolism attempts to correct it can put great stress on the cardiovascular system.
39. Operations in the elderly should be as short as possible, but they should try to prevent need for further surgery if at all possible.
40. As with all surgery, the best procedure addresses all of the patient's problems and takes the least time.
41. Repeat operations in elderly patients should be avoided whenever possible.
42. Nutrition in the elderly should be monitored closely to provide adequate protein, but not excessive calories.
43. The adequacy of initial resuscitation in restoring an optimal red cell mass appears to be an important prognostic factor in traumatized elderly patients.
44. Myocardial ischemia is best prevented by keeping hypotension, hypertension, and tachycardia to the minimum.
45. One should use as many techniques as possible to prevent deep venous thrombosis in the legs of all non-ambulating trauma patients.
46. Acute oliguric renal failure is probably best prevented by maintaining as high a urine output as possible without using diuretics or overloading the patient with fluids.

47. Not infrequently, sepsis is not recognized in the elderly until multiple organ failure begins to develop, and then it is often too late to save the patient.

48. Optimal rehabilitation begins when the patient is first seen.

49. Home care should be provided as soon as the services that can only be provided in a hospital are no longer necessary.

▲▲▲▲▲▲▲▲▲▲▲▲▲▲▲▲▲▲▲▲▲▲▲▲▲▲▲▲▲▲▲▲▲▲

REFERENCES

1. Osler TM, Demarest GV. Geriatric trauma. In: Moore EM, Mattox KL, Feliciano DV, eds. Trauma. 2nd ed. Norwalk, CT: Appleton & Lange, 1991:703-714.
2. Osler T, Hales K, Baack B, et al. Trauma in the elderly. Am J Surg 1988;156:537.
3. Projection of the population of the United States by age, sex and race 1983 to 2080. Current Population Reports. US Bureau of the Census.
4. Anderson B, and Ostberg J. Long-term prognosis in geriatric surgery:2-17 year follow-up of 7922 patients. J Am Geriatr Soc 1972; 20:255.
5. Taeuber C. America in transition: an aging society. Current Population Reports, Special Studies Series P-23, No 128. US Bureau of the Census. Washington, DC: US Department of Commerce.
6. Accident facts. Chicago: National Safety Council, 1986.
7. Waller J. Injury in the aged. NY State J Med 1974;74:2200.
8. Baker SP, Harvey AH. Fall injuries in the elderly. Clin Geriatr Med 1985;1:501.
9. Wilson RF, Antonenko D, Gibson DB. Shock and acute respiratory failure after chest trauma. J. Trauma 1977;17:697.
10. Sacco WJ, Champion HR, Carnazzo AJ, et al. Trauma score. Crit Care Med 1981;9:672.
11. Committee on Trauma of the American College of Surgeons. Appendix F to the hospital resources. Field categorization of trauma patients (field triage). ACS Bull 1986;71:17.
12. Aprahamian, C. Personal communication (1988). Boyd CR, Tolson MA, Capes WS, eds. The TRISS method. J Trauma 1987;27:370.
13. Watkins GM. Trauma and the geriatric patient. In: Kreis DJ Jr, Gomez GA, eds. Trauma management. Boston: Little, Brown & Co., 1989:409-416.
14. Vital and Health Statistics of the National Center for Health Statistics. 1986 Summary. National Hospital Discharge Surgery. Number 145. Hyattsville, MD: NCHS, September 30, 1987.
15. Champion HR, Copes WS, Buyer D, et al. Major trauma in geriatric patients. Am J Public Health 1989;79:1278.
16. American Hospital Association. Hospital Statistics. Chicago: AHA, 1986.
17. Office of Technology Assessment, US Congress. Intensive care units clinical outcomes, decision making and costs. Washington, DC: OTA, 1984.
18. Companion EW, Mulley AG, Goldstein RL, et al. Medical intensive care for the elderly: a study of current use, costs and outcomes. JAMA 1981;246:2052.
19. Gerson LW, Skvarch L. Emergency medical service utilization by the elderly. Ann Emerg Med 1982;11:610.
20. Mueller MS, Gibson RM. Age difference in health care spending. Soc Secur Bull 1976;36:18.
21. Rubenstein LZ. Falls in the elderly: a clinical approach. Topics Primary Care Med 1983;138:273.
22. Kirkpatrick JR, Krome RL, Walt AJ, et al. Special problems in the aged, addicted and alcoholic. In: Walt AJ, Wilson RF, eds. Management of trauma: pitfalls and practice. Philadelphia: Lea & Febiger, 1975:76-91.
23. Lindeman RD, et al. Influence of age, renal disease, hypertension, diuretics and calcium on the antidiuretic response to suboptimal infusions of vasopressin. J Lab Clin Med 1966;68:206.
24. Mithoefer JC, Karetzky MS. The cardiopulmonary system in the aged. In: Powers JD, ed. Surgery of the aged and debilitated patient. Philadelphia: WB Saunders, 1968.
25. Vital statistics of the United States. US National Center for Health Statistics, 1989:74.
26. Wetle T. Age as a risk factor for inadequate treatment. JAMA 1987;258:516.
27. Midgett MC. Social and emotional needs for geriatric patients. Soc Work Health Care 1981;6:69.
28. Manton KG, Stallard E, Liu K. Forecasts of active life expectancy: policy and fiscal implications. J Gerontol 1993;48:11.
29. Fife DD, Barancik JI, Chatterjee MS. Northeastern Ohio trauma study: injury rates by age, sex, and cause. Am J Public Health 1984; 74:473.
30. Lauer AR. Age and sex in relation to accidents. Traffic Safety Res Rev 1959;3:21.
31. McFarland RA, Tune GS, Wellford AT. On the driving of automobiles by older people. J Gerontol 1964;19:190.
32. Waller JA, Goo JT. Highway crash and citation patterns and chronic medical conditions. J Safety Res 1969;1:13.
33. Baker SP, Spitz WV. Age effects and autopsy evidence of disease in fatally injured drivers. JAMA 1970;214:1079.
34. Sklar DP, Demarest GB, McFeeley P. Increased pedestrian mortality among the elderly. Am J Emerg Med 1989;7:387.
35. Slater H, Gaisford JC. Burns in older patients. J Am Geriat Soc 1981;29:74.
36. Ziffren SE. Management of the burned elderly patient. J Am Geriat Soc 1955;3:36.
37. Anous MM, Heimbach DM. Causes of death and predictors in burned patients more than 60 years of age. J Trauma 1986;26:135.
38. Housinger T, Saffle J, Ward S, et al. Conservative approach to the elderly patient with burns. Am J Surg 1984;148:817.
39. Timeras PS. Developmental physiology and aging. New York: MacMillan, 1977.
40. Ziffren SE, Hartford CE. Comparative mortality for various surgical operations in older versus younger age groups. J Am Geriat Soc 1972;20:485.
41. De Guercio LR. Monitoring operative risk in the elderly. JAMA 1980;243:1350.
42. MacKenzie EJ, Morris JA, Edelstein SL. Effect of preexisting disease on length of hospital stay in trauma patients. J Trauma 1989;29:757.
43. Mitchell FL, Metzler MH. Geriatric complications. In: Mattox KL, ed. Complications of trauma. Churchill-Livingston, 1994:183-197.
44. Milzman DP, Boulanger BR, Rodriguez A, et al. Preexisting disease in trauma patients: a predictor of fate independent of age and injury severity score. J Trauma 1992;32:236.
45. Patel KP, Capan LM, Grant GJ, Miller SM. Musculoskeletal injuries. In: Capan LM, Miller SM, Turndorf H, eds. Trauma: anesthesia and intensive care. Philadelphia: JB Lippincott, 1991:511-546.
46. Harris R. Cardiovascular diseases in the elderly. Med Clin North Am 1983;67:379.
47. Fairman R, Rombeau JL. Physiologic problems in the elderly surgical patient. In: Miller A, ed. Rowlands J, contrib ed. Physiologic basis of modern surgical care. Washington, DC: Mosby, 1988:1108.
48. Tarhan S, Moffit EA, Taylor WF, et al. Myocardial infarction after general anesthesia. JAMA 1972;220:1451.
49. Rao TLK, Jacobs KH, El-Etr AA. Reinfarction following anesthesia in patients with myocardial infarction. Anesthesiology 1983;59:499.
50. Brandstetter RD, Kazemi H. Aging and the respiratory system. Med Clin North Am 1983;67:419.
51. Pontoppidan H, Geffins B, Lowenstein A. Acute respiratory failure in the adult. N Engl J Med 1972;287:690.
52. Pontoppidan H, Beecher HK. Progressive loss of protective reflexes in the airway with the advance of age. JAMA 1960;174:2209.
53. Oreskovich MR, Howard JD, Copass MK, et al. Geriatric trauma: injury patterns and outcome. J Trauma 1984;24:565.
54. Niesenbaum, L. Problems of pulmonary disease in the aged. Geriatrics 1968;23:127.
55. Calloway NO, Foley CF, Lagerbloo PJ. Uncertainties in geriatric data II. Organ size. J Am Geriat Soc 1965;13:20.
56. Miller JH, McDonald RU, Shock NW. Age changes in maximum rate of renal tubular resorption of glucose. J Gerontol 1952;7:196.
57. Miller JH, McDonald RK, and Shock NW. Age changes in the maximal rate of renal tubular reabsorption of glucose. J Geront 1952;7:196.
58. Adler S, et al. Effect of acute acid loading on urinary acid excretion by the aging human kidney J. Lab Clin Med 1968;72:278.
59. Thompson EN, Williams R. Effect of age on liver function with particular reference to bromosulphalein excretion. Gut 1965;6:266.
60. Christensen JH, Andreasen F. Individual variation in response to thiopental. Acta Anaesthesiol Scand 1978;22:303.
61. McLeskey CH. Anesthesia for the geriatric patient. Adv Anesth 1985;2:32.
62. Knowelden J, Buhr AJ, Dunbar O. Incidence of fractures in persons over 35 years of age. Br J Prev Soc Med 1981;18;130.
63. Andres R. Diabetes and aging. Hosp Pract 1967;2:63.
64. Young EA. Nutrition, aging, and the aged. Med Clin North Am 1983;67:295.

65. Wood M. Plasma drug binding: implications for the anesthesiologist. Anesth Analg 1986;65:786.
66. Hartford CE, Kealey GP. Pharmacokinetics in surgical practice. In: American College of Surgeons. Care of the surgical patient. Vol. 1. New York: Scientific American, 1988;XI:4:11.
67. Weksler E. Senescence of the immune system. Med Clin North Am 1983;76:263.
68. Kohn RR. Principles of mammalian aging. Englewood Cliffs, NJ: Prentice-Hall, 1971.
69. Roberts-Thomas IC, Whittingham S, Youngchaiyud U, et al. Aging, immune response and mortality. Lancet 1974;2:368.
70. Solomon DH, Shock NW. Studies of adrenal cortical and anterior pituitary function in elderly men. J Geront 1950;5:302.
71. Duncan LE Jr, et al. The metabolic and hematologic effects of the chronic administration of ACTH to young and old men. J Geront 1952;7:351.
72. Sibbald WJ, Short A, Cohen MP, Wilson RF. Variations in adrenocortical responsiveness during severe bacterial infections. Unrecognized adrenocortical insufficiency in bacterial infections. Ann Surg 1977;186:29.
73. Martin VC. Hypoxemia in elderly patients suffering from fractured neck of femur. Anaesthesia 1977;32:852.
74. Sari A, Miyauchi Y, Yamashita SH, et al. The magnitude of hypoxemia in elderly patients with fracture of the femoral neck. Anesth Analg 1986;65:892.
75. Sevitt S. The significance of fat embolism. Br J Hosp Med 1973;9:784.
76. Sevitt S. The significance and pathology of fat embolism. Ann Clin Res 1977;9:173.
77. Wilson RF, McCarthy B, LeBlanc LP, Mammen E. Respiratory and coagulation changes after uncomplicated fractures. Arch of Surg 1973;106:395.
78. Hirsh J. Hypercoagulability. Semin Hematol 1977;14:409.
79. Stamatakis JD, Kakker VV, Sagar S, et al. Femoral vein thrombosis and total hip replacement. Br Med J 1977;2:223.
80. Rossi EC, Green D, Rosen JS, et al. Sequential change in factor VIII and platelets proceeding deep vein thrombosis in patients with spinal cord injury. Br J Haematol 1980;45:143.
81. Myllynen P, Kammonen M, Rokkanen P. The blood F VIII: Ag/F VIII:C ratio-traumatic immobilization. J Trauma 1987;27:287.
82. Kirkpatrick JB, Pearson J. Fatal cerebral injury in the elderly. J Am Geriat Soc 1978;27:489.
83. Rathbone-McCuan E, Voyles B. Case detection of abused elderly patients. Am J Psychiatry 1982;139:189.
84. Jones J, Dougherty J, Schelble D, et al. Emergency department protocol for the diagnosis and evaluation of geriatric abuse. Ann Emerg Med 1988;17:1006.
85. Imbus SH, Zawacki BE. Autonomy for burned patients when survival is unprecedented. N Engl J Med 1977;297:308.
86. Haljamae H, Stefansson T, Wickstrom I. Preanesthetic evaluation of the female geriatric patient with hip fracture. Acta Anesth Scand 1982;26:393.
87. Schultz RJ, Whitfield GF, LaMura JJ, et al. The role of physiologic monitoring in patients with fractures of the hip. J Trauma 1985;25:309.
88. Chung F, Meier R, Lautenschlager E, et al. General or spinal anesthesia: which is better in the elderly? anesthesiology 1987;67:422.
89. McLaren AD, Stockwell MC, Reid VC. Anaesthetic techniques for surgical correction of fractured neck of femur. Anaesthesia 1978;33:10.
90. McKenzie PJ, Washart HY, Smith G. Long-term outcome after repair of fractured neck of femur. Br J Anaesth 1984;56:581.
91. Davis FM, Laurenson VG, Lewis J, et al. Metabolic response to total hip arthroplasty under hypobaric subarachnoid or general anaesthesia. Br J Anaesth 1987;59:725.
92. Valentin N, Lomholt B, Jensen JS, et al. Spinal or general anaesthesia for surgery of the fractured hip. Br J Anaesth 1986;58:284.
93. Horst HM, Obeid FN, Sorensen VJ, et al. Factors influencing survival of elderly trauma patients. Crit Care Med 1986;14:681.
94. Watkins, GM. Care of the geriatric individual who is burned. *In:* Meakins, MacLarin, eds. Surgical Care of the Elderly. Chicago: Year Book, 1988;455.
95. Watkins GM. Burns in the aged, in pre- and postoperative care. The Biology of Aging—Implications for the Surgeon, Vol. I. Chicago, American College of Surgeons, 1984.
96. MacIntyre PE, Pavilion EG, Dwersteg JR. Effect of meperidine on oxygen consumption, carbon-dioxide production, and respiratory gas exchange in postanesthesia shivering. Anesth Analg 1987;66:751.
97. Scalea TM, Simeon HM, Duncan AO. Geriatric blunt trauma: improved survival with early invasive monitoring. J Trauma 1990;30:129.
98. Campion EW, Mulley AG, Goldstin RL, et al. Medical intensive care for the elderly. JAMA 1981;246:2052.
99. Mason JH, Gau FC, Byrne MP. General surgery. In: Steinberg FV, ed. Care of the geriatric patient. St. Louis: CV Mosby Co., 1983:299-326.
100. Lakatta EG. Age-related alterations in the cardiovascular response to adrenergic mediated stress. Fed Proc 1980;39:3173.
101. Steinberg FV. The aging of organs and organ systems. In: Steinberg FV, ed. Care of the geriatric patient. St. Louis: CV Mosby Co., 1983:3-18.
102. Dahn MS, Wilson RF, Lange MP, et al. Hemodynamic benefits of verapamil after aortic reconstruction. J Vasc Surg 1989;9:806-811.
103. DeMaria EJ, Kenney PR, Merriam MA, et al. Aggressive trauma care benefits the elderly. J Trauma 1987;27:1200.
104. Rubinstein RZ. Geriatric evaluation units. N Engl J Med 1981;311:664.

Chapter 9B Special Problems of Trauma in Addicted Patients

ROBERT F. WILSON, M.D.,

JEFFREY S. BENDER, M.D.,

JENNIFER GASS, M.D.

INTRODUCTION

Drug addiction remains a major problem in trauma with studies showing evidence of marijuana in 26 to 37% and cocaine in 9 to 54% of trauma victims, respectively.[1-5] In addition, more than 80% of violent crime may be associated with the use of illegal drugs. The most common causes of death in the 18 to 35 age group in New York City are drug-related.[6] A number of studies have also shown the relationship between abuse of illicit drugs and deaths from vehicular crashes[7-11] and those treated in trauma centers.[1-5,12] Physicians need to recognize the symptoms of illicit drug use to deal effectively with the problems caused directly or indirectly by them.[13] Unfortunately, despite available resources and repeated recommendations by the American College of Surgeons, measurements of blood alcohol and drug screens are routine in only 64% of level I and 40% of level II trauma centers.[14]

AXIOM Failure to manage trauma patients' addictions as well as their injuries may precipitate serious problems.

Illicit drug use can produce difficulties from either "too little" or "too much."[1] "Too little" can produce severe withdrawal symptoms, whereas "too much" can cause severe physiologic changes related to the side effects of the drug. Associated problems such as infection and thrombosis at sites of injection must also be considered.

DIAGNOSIS

Early diagnosis of drug abuse can establish whether the agents involved may be synergistic, antagonistic, or additive to other drugs needed to maintain homeostasis. Many of the signs and symptoms produced by addiction or withdrawal can be confused with those resulting from various injuries.

PITFALL ⊘

If the diagnosis of drug use is overlooked preoperatively, withdrawal may occur under anesthesia when it is much more dangerous and difficult to treat.

History

Not infrequently, it is difficult to obtain an accurate history from addicted patients after trauma, particularly if the patient is already under the influence of drugs, has organic brain damage, or is in shock.[1] Failure to elicit a history of current drug addiction or to obtain laboratory evidence confirming such use can lead to disastrous results. It is also important to interview any friends or family who accompany the patient to the emergency department; however, they may also be reluctant to provide accurate information.

Physical Examination

Confirmation of drug use can be very difficult to obtain on physical examination.[13] Nevertheless, the physician should check specifically for "needle tracks" (indicative of repeated intravenous injections), nasal ulceration (seen with intranasal cocaine and heroin use), or cardiac murmurs.

Unexplained respiratory difficulty should make the physician suspicious of a narcotic or barbiturate overdose.[14,15] Although a rapid pulse rate after trauma is usually indicative of hypovolemia, tachycardia associated with a normal or elevated blood pressure may be an early clue to the presence of amphetamines or hallucinogens. In contrast, patients with bradycardia and hypotension may have taken large doses of depressants, such as narcotics, barbiturates, or tranquilizers. Patients with sluggish but widely dilated pupils and with no evidence of head injury should be suspected of having taken excessive doses of barbiturates or tranquilizers.

PITFALL ⊘

If impaired consciousness is attributed to the ingestion of a drug, significant head injuries may be overlooked.

Changes in the mental status of a trauma patient should not be considered as drug-related until all other causes (subdural hematomas, skull fractures, and contusion) have been excluded and the diagnosis of drug use is firmly established.[1] Every trauma patient must have a thorough neurologic examination that includes palpation of the scalp for penetrating wounds.

AXIOM Small penetrating wounds of the skull are easily overlooked, especially in addicted patients, and their significance is often underestimated.

Although vague, generalized signs or symptoms are often caused by drugs, unconsciousness associated with localizing signs is more apt to be a result of head injury. X-rays and blood glucose, barbiturate, salicylate, and alcohol levels should also be obtained to aid in the differentiation of traumatic and drug-induced coma.

TYPES OF DRUG ADDICTION

For practical purposes, the various narcotic drugs, including heroin, morphine, Demerol, and codeine, can be considered one group.[1] Paregoric and elixir terpin hydrate with codeine can be grouped with the narcotics, but they also contain a relatively large amount of alcohol. Barbiturates and tranquilizers produce similar symptoms of addiction and withdrawal and can be placed in a second category. Hallucinogens, the third important category of drugs, include LSD, mescaline, and peyote. The final group are the adulterants, i.e., the various agents and inert substances frequently mixed with "street drugs" either to potentiate or dilute the effect of the primary drug. Strychnine, atropine, belladonna, talcum powder, quinine, and sugar are major members of this group. Specific symptom complexes and addiction management vary with each of these agents; however, general guidelines are available for each major category.

Narcotics

AXIOM Narcotic addiction is now recognized as one of the most important causes of violent or unusual behavior.[1]

Antisocial or destructive behavior is not uncommon in individuals who are taking narcotics. In addition, the addict's attempts to procure funds to support his habit can result in a wide variety of crime and violent behavior, including gunshot wounds, stabbings, and blunt injuries. Other problems attributed to drugs or their method of administration include abscesses, septicemia, hepatitis, endocarditis, and pneumothorax. Knowing that there is an increased incidence of these problems among addicts may help the physician to recognize the coincident drug problem. As a corollary, the physician should look for the presence or development of such problems in addicted patients.

COCAINE

Cocaine is a naturally occurring alkaloid derived from the South American shrub *Erythroxylon coca.* By 1988, the National Institute on Drug Abuse (NIDA) estimated that over 21 million Americans had tried cocaine at some time, and at least 3 million Americans were using cocaine on a regular basis.[16]

Methods of Administration

Cocaine is usually sniffed or inhaled, but it can also be injected. There is, however, a growing fear of injecting cocaine because of the high incidence of acquired immunodeficiency syndrome (AIDS) in drug abusers.

Cocaine inhalation can be done in several different ways. The cocaine alkaloid can be dissolved in acetone or alcohol and then purified to a more potent form that can be smoked as "freebase." This may cause injury from fire or explosion of the flammable solvent. The alkaloid form can also be dissolved in hydrochloric acid to form a water soluble salt, available as a crystalline granular powder, that may be inhaled or smoked with a flammable vehicle. "Crack" cocaine is a neutral form of the drug, like freebase, that is made without solvent extraction. In making crack, an alkali is added to an aqueous solution of cocaine hydrochloride, and the resulting alkaloid precipitates from the supernatant.

Cocaine absorption via inhalation is enhanced by use of a Valsalva's maneuver that increases airway pressure.[8] A modified Valsalva's maneuver can be performed when two individuals share a pipe that has a hole on each end, thereby permitting one individual to exhale under force into the other person's airway. Using either technique, one may develop interstitial pulmonary emphysema that may progress to mediastinal emphysema. This can cause a sudden onset of midthoracic pain with or without shortness of breath. Usually, the air is confined to the mediastinum; however, it may also dissect into the neck, pleural spaces, pericardium, and the subdiaphragmatic space.

On physical examination, a "Hamman's crunch," resulting from cardiac contraction adjacent to mediastinal air, may be heard during systole. This is heard best with the patient in the left lateral decubitus position. Cocaine-induced pneumomediastinum is usually treated with observation until the symptoms abate and x-rays show resolution of the abnormal collections of air.

On occasion, patients inhaling cocaine will require a tube thoracostomy for a pneumothorax.[16,17] However, few patients have prolonged or severe adverse affects from these pneumothoraces. Very rarely, the air may dissect centrally into the pulmonary circulation. If air gets into a pulmonary vein it will enter the left heart, from which very small amounts of air can enter a coronary or cerebral artery and cause arrhythmias, shock, cardiac arrest, or strokes.

The increasing popularity of crack is due to its low initial cost and easy preparation without need for a solvent.[16] Crack can be used in pipes, cigarettes, or other homemade contrivances through which deep inhalation can provide a much more rapid rise in the plasma levels of cocaine. The resulting intense euphoria may last several minutes.

AXIOM The intense "high" of cocaine plus the central stimulatory properties can lead to rapid addiction, even with only one or two uses.

Physiologic Effects

Cocaine has both local anesthetic and sympathomimetic actions, and it affects multiple organs throughout the body. When present in the synaptic cleft of neurons, it blocks presynaptic reuptake of the neurotransmitters norepinephrine and dopamine. This greatly potentiates the effects of both circulating catecholamines and direct sympathetic stimulation.

AXIOM Excessive stimulation of the cardiovascular system is probably the most frequent manifestation of severe cocaine toxicity.

The cardiovascular effects of cocaine include dose-dependent increases of mean arterial pressure (MAP), heart rate, and myocardial oxygen consumption (MVO_2). It is also postulated that cocaine can cause vasospasm of the coronary arteries which can lead to acute myocardial ischemia and infarction, even in young adults. Even small doses of cocaine may elicit clinically significant cardiac ischemia without underlying heart disease.[18] Cardiac arrhythmias may also be precipitated by cocaine, and this can cause sudden cardiovascular collapse and death. Prolonged cocaine use may also lead to myocardial lesions similar to those seen after chronic sympathetic stimulation from a pheochromocytoma.

PITFALL ⊘

Cocaine use predisposes the trauma patient to adverse interactions with certain anesthetic agents.

Many trauma patients are unwilling to give a history of illicit drug use. Such knowledge can be very important, however, if a general anesthetic is needed. In particular, cocaine can adversely interact with a number of agents, such as halothane, so that the myocardium is greatly sensitized to the effects of catecholamines.[19]

Development of sudden cardiac arrhythmias or unexplained myocardial decompensation in the midst of massive blood and fluid replacement after severe injury is thought to be more frequent in patients on cocaine.[18] Therefore, careful monitoring of habitual users is mandatory throughout resuscitation.

AXIOM Strokes and acute myocardial infarctions in young drug users should be attributed to cocaine until proven otherwise.

The sudden, severe elevation of blood pressure caused by an acute ingestion of cocaine can result in a hypertensive crisis, and cocaine is the primary cause of stroke in young patients.[8] Cocaine may also induce acute aortic dissection. While the effects of the vascular responses to cocaine on patients without head injuries are largely unknown, patients with brain trauma may be at a much greater risk for intracranial hemorrhage.[20]

The pulmonary effects of cocaine include pulmonary edema, bronchospasm, and transient pulmonary infiltrates with fever.[21] These changes may be difficult to differentiate from direct trauma or the pulmonary response to hypovolemic shock and massive blood replacement.

Cocaine may also cause rhabdomyolysis and acute myoglobinuric renal failure. The exact mechanisms are unknown, but they may be mediated by intense vasoconstriction with hyperpyrexia. A great increase in motor activity probably also contributes to the myonecrosis and acute renal failure.[22]

Gastrointestinal ischemic syndromes, including perforation, have been noted in conjunction with cocaine use.[23] The acute abdominal pain caused by cocaine-induced vascular spasm can interfere greatly with accurate assessment of patients with possible abdominal injuries.

> **AXIOM**   Acute psychotic behavior may be a result of cocaine, but CNS injury or hypoxia must be ruled out.

High doses of cocaine, as with other stimulants, can cause impaired judgment, disinhibition, impulsiveness, compulsively repeated actions, paranoia, and extreme psychomotor agitation.[16] Panic attacks, paranoid ideation, and psychotic behavior may be associated with violence, sometimes with homicidal intent, and drug-related injuries are common during this phase.[24]

Treatment

Treatment of patients suffering from cocaine overdose is primarily supportive. The cardiovascular and pulmonary problems are probably best handled by providing ventilatory support and normalizing hemodynamic function as determined with a Swan-Ganz catheter.

HEROIN

Heroin, a member of the opiate family, is derived from morphine, the principal product of the poppy *Papaver somniferum*.[16] Heroin's effects are mediated by interacting with endogenous opiate receptors that function as neurotransmitters, neurohormones, and modulators of neurotransmission throughout the CNS.

During the past several years, cocaine use in injured patients has risen, but heroin use has declined.[16] Drug-related injuries from heroin include overdose, mycotic aneurysms, and a myriad of infectious complications that impair recovery after injury. Heroin overdose-related injuries or deaths usually reflect user ignorance regarding the strength of a particular injection.

Heroin is distributed in various levels of purity on the street, but pure or almost pure heroin is quite strong, and it may cause sudden unexpected death if a patient thinks the drug has been diluted by various agents.

> **AXIOM**   One of the main problems with heroin is the unpredictable quantity of active drug, toxic additives, and contamination in each dose.

When several agents are used to dilute heroin, the resulting mixture is often called "mixed jive."[16] These additives typically include quinine, strychnine, lidocaine, various sugars, talcum, and starch. Since the dilution is uncontrolled, there is frequent bacterial contamination of the mixture.

> **AXIOM**   Heroin-related problems may be caused by various additives, its inherent pharmacologic toxicity, local infection, or direct injury to the lungs.

The patient with a heroin overdose will usually be somnolent, stuporous, or in a profound coma.[16] The breathing pattern tends to be slow and shallow, resulting in a significantly reduced minute ventilation. Heroin and other opiate agonists cause a reduction in the responsiveness of the brain stem to increases in CO_2 tension, and they also depress the pontine and medullary centers involved in regulating respiratory rhythmicity.[25] Hence, deaths from opiate overdose are usually a result of profound respiratory depression.

> **AXIOM**   Narcotic overdose should be part of the differential diagnosis in somnolent patients with depressed ventilation, pulmonary congestion, vasodilation, and/or hypotension.

Like morphine, heroin induces peripheral vasodilation and a decrease in systemic vascular resistance (SVR) that is augmented by a concomitant release of histamine.[16] Therefore, opiate-intoxicated patients can have severe hypotension with relatively mild degrees of hypovolemia.

Occasionally, young heroin addicts exhibit a bizarre cardiac and respiratory difficulty characterized by mental confusion, x-ray evidence of pulmonary congestion, and progressive cardiac failure.[1] This type of cardiac failure is generally resistant to the usual forms of

therapy. At autopsy, these patients frequently have edematous, congested "wet lungs." Patients with this difficulty should be given narcotic antagonists, but these must be administered cautiously and in small doses with close scrutiny of the pupillary reflexes, the level of consciousness, and respiration.

Therapeutic measures for heroin overdose with cardiac failure include providing ventilatory support as needed and administering naloxone hydrochloride, a specific opiate receptor antagonist. Naloxone, given in intravenous doses of 0.4 mg, repeated every few minutes as necessary, can cause a dramatic reversal of the respiratory depression and peripheral vasodilation resulting from opiate toxicity. However, excessive naloxone can precipitate opiate withdrawal, thereby greatly complicating therapy. Because the effective half-life of naloxone is shorter than that of most opiates, redosing of naloxone every several hours may be necessary until the circulating opiate is excreted.

OTHER NARCOTIC PROBLEMS

> **AXIOM**   Narcotic overdose should be suspected in patients who have a depressed sensorium with no evidence of trauma.

After ventilatory support has been provided in a suspected case of narcotic overdose, a small dose (0.1-0.2 mg) of naloxone should be injected while the pupillary and respiratory changes are closely observed.[1] Too rapid or too large a dose of naloxone may potentiate the depressant effect of the narcotic. If there is no response, a full 0.4 mg dose can be given, but if there is still no response and if serum levels for barbiturates, salicylates, alcohol, and glucose are within normal limits, one can usually assume that this patient's obtunded state is not related to a drug overdose. Consequently, further efforts must be taken to look for an organic cause.

Withdrawal from narcotic addiction can be a frightening experience for both physicians and patients, especially if it occurs during the postoperative period.[1] It is important to realize that rarely, if ever, is death a result of the cardio-respiratory effects of withdrawal alone. The withdrawal syndrome (rhinorrhea, lacrimation, confusion, sweating, cramping, and diarrhea) can, however, produce severe fluid and electrolyte problems.

> **AXIOM**   Narcotic withdrawal during a general anesthetic can provide an extremely confusing clinical picture and can be difficult to treat.

With the current popularity of methadone, the physician should be aware that signs and symptoms of withdrawal can also occur if methadone is not continued, but there may be no clinical changes until 24 hours after the last dose.[1] The physiologic changes of methadone withdrawal can be dangerous in hypovolemic patients under general anesthesia. At least one instance of hypotension and death has been reported in a patient withdrawing from large doses of methadone while undergoing general anesthesia. Talwin should not be administered to narcotic addicts during withdrawal since it is a mild narcotic antagonist and can potentiate the effects of nalorphine.

Whenever possible, narcotic addicts should be stabilized relative to their drug dependence before surgery.[26] If the patient has not previously taken methadone, it can be given orally or intramuscularly in doses of approximately 10 mg every 4 to 6 hours unless signs of an overdose (nystagmus, pinpoint pupils, or drowsiness) appear. Similar doses are given during the second 24 hours. The daily dose can then be reduced by 5 to 10 mg every second or third day so that the patient is kept comfortable. Trauma patients who had been receiving oral methadone from treatment programs should maintain their usual doses.

Methadone is rapidly absorbed from the stomach and small intestine and may be given by mouth even if a nasogastric tube is in place, provided the tube is clamped for 30 minutes after ingestion. It may be prudent to delay surgery for an hour or so after oral methadone administration so that absorption is complete and the patient can be protected from withdrawal.

AXIOM The trauma patient who is in shock and is immediately taken to the operating room will often not manifest narcotic withdrawal symptoms until under anesthesia or postoperatively.

During the operative period, known narcotic addicts should probably be started or continued on methadone.[1] As long as it does not complicate his treatment, the drug may be given orally.

The use of tranquilizers or barbiturates to aid in the treatment of narcotic withdrawal is usually not necessary if the patient can be maintained on a reasonable dose of narcotic or methadone; however, if additional medication is required for comfort or sleep, antihistamines, such as Benadryl, are preferred over barbiturates.[1] If narcotic withdrawal symptoms are managed without methadone, it may be necessary to rely on antiemetics (such as Tigan) and antispasmodics (such as Donnatal) for relief of the gastrointestinal symptoms.

PITFALL ⊘

If the physician fails to care for the addict's narcotic needs while he is in the hospital, the addict may seek drugs from non-medical sources, and this can lead to sudden unexplained cardiorespiratory difficulties and/or death.

Sudden deterioration of an addict's condition in the hospital without explanation should alert the physician to the possibility that the patient has been given heroin by friends or family.[1] Illicit narcotics are readily available to patients in most urban hospitals. On several occasions, visitors have injected heroin into the intravenous lines of critically ill patients causing otherwise unexplained deaths.

Barbiturates and Tranquilizers

Overdoses of barbiturates and tranquilizers tend to depress the central nervous system producing lethargy, slurred speech, inability to solve simple mental problems, and confusion.[1] Severe overdoses may also produce bradycardia and hypotension.

Treatment of barbiturate or tranquilizer intoxication varies with the severity of the symptoms and CNS depression.[1] Gastric lavage, if feasible, should be carried out as soon as possible with a large 40 to 50 French Ewald tube to remove any drug still retained in the stomach. If the patient is reasonably alert and unlikely to aspirate, the stomach can be filled with warm saline and the patient encouraged to vomit. It may take 2 or more liters of saline to clear the stomach adequately.

If little or no drug is obtained, administration of activated charcoal may reduce the absorption of any residual agent in the intestines.[1] If there is severe respiratory depression, an endotracheal tube should be inserted and a ventilator used to maintain adequate blood gases. If the patient becomes hypotensive, large volumes of fluid may be needed to fill the dilated vascular space and provide an adequate cardiac output. Occasionally, inotropic drugs and/or vasoconstrictors may be needed to maintain a satisfactory blood pressure and tissue perfusion.

AXIOM Treatment of barbiturate overdoses involves decreasing drug absorption with charcoal and support of pulmonary, cardiac, and renal function.

Short-acting barbiturates, such as Nembutal and Pentothal, are metabolized primarily by the liver. Long-acting barbiturates, such as phenobarbital, are excreted with little or no change by the kidneys.[1] Since the excretion of both types of barbiturates is increased by alkalinizing the serum and urine and maintaining a high urine output, large volumes of intravenous fluid and bicarbonate should be given. Diuretics in small amounts can also be administered as needed to maintain a urinary output of at least 100 to 200 ml/hr. If treatment is begun within a reasonable period of time, hemodialysis or peritoneal dialysis is rarely required.

Barbiturate withdrawal may produce a variety of symptoms and signs, including seizures, delirium, hyperpyrexia, tachycardia, and coma.[1] The pathophysiologic changes of barbiturate withdrawal occurring in the postoperative period may be especially severe and can cause death.

AXIOM Of all the drugs that may be abused, barbiturates are the most likely to cause death as a result of acute withdrawal.

The problems with barbiturates or tranquilizers during anesthesia may be especially great.[1] If Pentothal is used to induce anesthesia, the barbiturate addict may have a repeat respiratory crisis. Then, when the anesthetic wears off, the patient may develop withdrawal. Barbiturate withdrawal in the postoperative period requires intramuscular injections of short-acting barbiturates, repeated in doses up to 100 mg every hour, until the patient appears to be intoxicated. This dose is then reduced over a period of several weeks at a rate of no more than 100 mg each day.

Hallucinogens

AXIOM Bizarre suicide attempts should make one suspect hallucinogen intoxication.

Patients under the influence of hallucinogens often have wild visual and, rarely, auditory images.[1] Hallucinations may precipitate self-inflicted wounds and suicidal gestures. This type of addiction should always be suspected when the physician is confronted with a bizarre suicide attempt.

A "good trip" can cause a euphoric state, tranquility, or mere vagueness. A "bad trip" can cause excitability, disorientation, inappropriate verbiage, and occasional fits of rage. Overdoses can produce death, seizures, or unconsciousness. Indeed, the psychiatric effects of hallucinogens are often more dangerous than the trauma itself. Physical findings can include mydriasis, hyperthermia, piloerection, hyperglycemia, and bradycardia.

AXIOM The physician should not rely on the patient's history unless he can document that the reported drug is, in fact, the same as the patient thinks he has taken.

Preoperative medication for a patient suspected of taking hallucinogens should not include atropine-like drugs because these may potentiate the anticholinergic effects of hallucinogens.[1] Generally, the safest drug for control of hallucinogenic effects is intramuscular diazepam (Valium) in doses of 5 to 10 mg every 2 to 4 hours as needed. Since these patients often are experiencing active hallucinations and are very susceptible to visual and auditory stimuli, they should be placed in a quiet room and managed by either a physician or a nurse who understands the subjective sensations experienced by the patient.

Adulterants

The most important adulterants mixed with street drugs include lidocaine, atropine, strychnine, and quinine.[1] Any of these drugs may produce symptoms more lethal and incapacitating than the primary narcotic with which they are mixed.

LIDOCAINE
Some of the clinical toxicities of heroin diluents include those associated with local anesthetics, such as lidocaine or tetracaine, which can cause CNS stimulation with tremors, agitation, or seizures, especially after chronic exposure.

ATROPINE
Classic signs of atropine toxicity include tachycardia, fever, cutaneous flushing, dilated pupils, and extreme dryness of the skin and mucous membranes.[1] Recognition is vital, especially when determining

which preoperative medications are to be given. Atropine toxicity is an obvious contraindication to the use of anticholinergic drugs.[1] If the toxicity is mild, no special treatment is required. Severe overdoses, however, should be managed with short-acting barbiturates, hypothermia, and intravenous fluids. Eye patches should be applied to prevent blinding from the excessive light that might otherwise reach the retina through dilated pupils.

Cholinergic drugs such as methacholine and urecholine are of no therapeutic value, but may be useful in substantiating the diagnosis of atropine toxicity.[1] Administration of 10 to 20 mg of methacholine subcutaneously will produce rhinorrhea, lacrimation, salivation, sweating, and cramps in a normal person. Since atropine will prevent these symptoms, a negative response to methacholine stimulation is diagnostic of atropine toxicity.

STRYCHNINE

Strychnine is a popular adulterant and many compounds contain it as an active ingredient.[1] Strychnine, which is a competitive antagonist of the CNS inhibitory neurotransmitter, glycine, tends to cause CNS stimulation. This can result in apprehension, nausea, and muscle twitching, followed by spasms of extensor muscles, opisthotonos, and frank seizures. Strychnine may also cause rhabdomyolysis and myoglobinuric acute renal failure.

Although strychnine toxicity is easily recognized when it is far advanced, early changes may include nothing more than reflex hyperexcitability. The chronic user does not develop tolerance or manifest cumulative effects. Sudden overdosage can produce muscle spasms that can progress to seizures and true opisthotonos. Abdominal cramps and constricted facial muscles are diagnostic of acute toxicity. Treatment is directed primarily towards ventilatory support. Control of seizures can generally be managed with short-acting barbiturates, but occasionally paralysis with curare is required.

QUININE

Quinine has toxic effects on the heart, CNS, and kidneys, and high levels may lead to cardiac dysfunction with conduction delays, arrhythmias, or hypotension.[17] Quinine overdosage is difficult to distinguish from salicylate poisoning.[1] Early symptoms can include tinnitus, headache, nausea, and blurred vision. Either chronic poisoning or acute toxicity can produce photophobia, dyslogia (impairment of reasoning), blindness, cramps, vomiting, and a characteristic papular scarlatina-like rash. Death can occur from respiratory failure. A clue to identifying a chronic user of quinine is the presence of an unexplained hemolytic anemia. Treatment is symptomatic, and survival after 24 hours is usually assurance of complete recovery.

VIRAL DISEASES ASSOCIATED WITH ADDICTION

Hepatitis

Care of addicted patients, particularly intravenous drug abusers, increases risks to health care practitioners. Intravenous drug abusers are frequently carriers of chronic hepatitis. Indeed, the total number of hepatitis infected individuals from all sources, along with its relative ease of transmissibility, makes this disease a much greater overall risk to the surgeon than the more publicized human immunodeficiency virus (HIV). Approximately 25% of practicing surgeons in this country carry antibody to the hepatitis antigen.[27] Two to three hundred health care personnel a year die of occupationally acquired hepatitis, which is several orders of magnitude greater than the worst case scenario postulated for AIDS. Even more tragically, many of these deaths could have been prevented by the use of the hepatitis vaccine.

A high rate of hepatitis B infection exists among intravenous drug users. Estroff et al[28] noted 85% seropositivity for hepatitis B in intravenous heroin and cocaine addicts as compared to a 7% incidence in patients who are not intravenous drug users.

AIDS

An increasing problem in drug addicts presenting with severe injury is the high incidence of AIDS.[29] Since first reported in 1981, the epidemic has escalated to more than 88,000 reported cases. Estimates in 1989 place the number of HIV-infected individuals in this country at 1,500,000 to 2,000,000.[30] At least 4% of the injured patients treated at the Detroit Receiving Hospital are HIV-positive.[16] The Johns Hopkins Hospital has also noted a 4% HIV seropositivity in all patients seen in their emergency department.[29] A subgroup of 126 patients requiring critical care had a 7.8% positivity rate, while trauma patients had a 10.4% positivity rate. Penetrating trauma was associated with the highest HIV-seropositive rate (14.6%), and the incidence is rising.

At the Maryland Institute for Emergency Medical Services Systems, which is in the same city as Johns Hopkins, but serves a predominantly non-urban population, the overall HIV-positivity rate was 1.7%.[31] In their blunt trauma patients, however, the rate was still 1.1%, which is not much different than the Johns Hopkins rate for similar injuries. There are exceptions to these guidelines. Aprahamian et al[32] in 1988 reported no cases of HIV infections in their center in Milwaukee despite high risk behavior in 52% of their patients.

> **AXIOM** All new trauma patients should be considered HIV-positive until proven otherwise.

Intravenous drug users account for most new cases of AIDS in the United States.[16] The trading of sex for drugs, which is almost pandemic among female users of crack cocaine, represents another source of infection.[33]

More rapid identification of HIV-positive patients could be helpful to the trauma team.[16] Although the currently recommended "universal precautions" may be effective, they are not carefully followed in many trauma centers when busy. In Detroit, partly because of the AIDS risk, many addicts have shifted from using heroin with shared jive injection equipment to the inhalation of cocaine.

While the actual risk to surgical personnel caring for HIV-infected individuals is extremely low, certain precautions should reduce this risk even further. Hammond et al[34] observed 81 trauma resuscitations at Jackson Memorial Medical Center in Miami and found only a 16% compliance with strict universal precautions. This rate was improved to 62% by placement of universal precaution packs in all resuscitation rooms and emphasizing their routine use.

Gerberding et al[35] at San Francisco General Hospital observed 130 consecutive surgical procedures to determine the risk of accidental exposure to blood. Parenteral exposure to blood occurred in 1.7% of the cases while cutaneous exposure occurred in an additional 4.7%. Most of the cutaneous exposures could have been prevented by appropriate techniques such as double gloving and wearing impermeable garments. The risk of blood exposure was highest during trauma surgery with 25 exposures (including two parenteral) occurring in 105 cases. Using these figures, along with a seroconversion rate for needlesticks of 0.005, they calculated a theoretical risk of occupationally acquired HIV infections in their surgical personnel of 0.125 per year. While one case every 8 years in a busy trauma center may not seem like a large number in view of the volume of procedures performed, the risk is real to anyone who becomes HIV-positive.

This is particularly true when these results are extrapolated to the whole country. While the risk of acquiring HIV during any single case is almost vanishingly small (with estimates as low as 1 per 450,000 to 1 per 1,300,000,000), the lifetime risk is much higher. Howard[36] has calculated that five exposures per year with an HIV seroprevalence of 0.35% (the least likely rate) would give a risk of seroconversion of 0.0026 in a 30-year period. This would mean that 47 of the current 18,000 Fellows of the American College of Surgeons could anticipate becoming infected during their career.

Surgery may also be hazardous to the HIV-infected patient because of preexisting leukopenia or thrombocytopenia. One study in AIDS patients undergoing laparotomy for non-traumatic indications shows an increased morbidity and mortality rate. This was related primarily to progression of AIDS.[37] Surprisingly, there were no increased problems with wound infection, wound healing, or bleeding.

Standard tests for HIV are too time-consuming to be of use in the emergency setting. There are, however, several findings that may serve to alert the surgeon that his patient is infected. Preoperatively, an abnormally low white count or unexpected thrombocytopenia should serve as a clue. Intra-operatively, splenomegaly and retroperitoneal lymph node enlargement are common findings, as are gastrointestinal lymphomas. With gastrointestinal lymphomas nothing should be done at the initial laparotomy unless obstruction or perforation seems imminent. Enlarged nodes should be biopsied if time permits and sent for culture as well as histologic analysis. The presence of cytomegalovirus or an atypical mycobacterium is virtually diagnostic of AIDS.

⊘ **FREQUENT ERRORS**

In the Management of Trauma in Drug-Addicted Patients

1. *Ignoring a patient's drug addiction and considering only the medical problems caused by trauma.*
2. *Failing to consider drug withdrawal as a cause for unusual behavior during or after a general anesthetic.*
3. *Assuming that unusual behavior in an injured drug addict is due to the drug and not the trauma or a correctable metabolic problem.*
4. *Forgetting that hypertension in a cocaine overdose may hide an underlying hypovolemia.*
5. *Forgetting that cocaine can cause acute cerebrovascular accidents and myocardial infarctions in young drug users.*
6. *Inadequate monitoring of patients who appear to be young and healthy but who may have severe physiologic changes as a result of drug overdose or withdrawal.*
7. *Not appreciating that unusual behavior responses during or following surgery may be a result of drug withdrawal.*
8. *Not following universal precautions completely when operating on a patient who may be a drug addict.*

▼▼▼▼▼▼▼▼▼▼▼▼▼▼▼▼▼▼▼▼▼▼▼▼▼▼▼▼▼▼▼▼

SUMMARY POINTS

1. Failure to manage patients' addictions as well as their injuries may precipitate serious problems.

2. Small penetrating wounds of the skull are easily overlooked, especially in addicted patients, and their significance is often underestimated.

3. Narcotic addiction is now recognized as one of the most important causes of violent or unusual behavior.

4. The intense "high" of cocaine plus the central stimulatory properties can lead to rapid addiction, even with only one or two uses.

5. Excessive stimulation of the cardiovascular system is probably the most frequent manifestation of severe cocaine toxicity.

6. Strokes and acute myocardial infarctions in young drug users should be attributed to cocaine until proven otherwise.

7. Acute psychotic behavior may be a result of cocaine, but CNS injury and hypoxia must be ruled out.

8. One of the main problems with heroin is the unpredictable quantity of active drug, toxic additives, and contamination in each dose.

9. Heroin-related problems may be caused by infection, various additives, its inherent pharmacologic toxicity, or direct injury to the lungs.

10. Narcotic overdose should be part of the differential diagnosis in somnolent patients with depressed ventilation, pulmonary congestion, vasodilation, and/or hypotension.

11. Narcotic overdose should be suspected in patients who have a depressed sensorium with no evidence of trauma.

12. Narcotic withdrawal during a general anesthetic can provide an extremely confusing clinical picture and can be difficult to treat.

13. The trauma patient who is in shock and is immediately taken to the operating room will often not manifest narcotic withdrawal symptoms until under anesthesia or postoperatively.

14. Treatment of barbiturate overdoses involves decreasing drug absorption with charcoal and support of pulmonary, cardiac, and renal function.

15. Of all the drugs that may be abused, barbiturates are the most likely to cause death as a result of acute withdrawal.

16. Bizarre suicide attempts should make one suspect hallucinogen intoxication.

17. The physician should not rely on the patient's history unless he can document that the reported drug is, in fact, the same as the patient thinks he has taken.

18. All new trauma patients should be considered HIV-positive until proven otherwise.

▲▲▲▲▲▲▲▲▲▲▲▲▲▲▲▲▲▲▲▲▲▲▲▲▲▲▲▲▲▲▲▲

REFERENCES

1. Kirkpatrick JR, Krome RL, Walt AJ, et al. Special problems of trauma in the aged, addicted, and alcoholic. In: Walt AJ, Wilson RF, eds. Management of trauma: pitfalls and practice. Philadelphia: Lea & Febiger, 1975:76-91.
2. Lindenbaum GA, Carroll SF, Daskal I, Kapusnick R. Patterns of alcohol and drug abuse in an urban trauma center: the increasing role of cocaine abuse. J Trauma 1989;29:1654.
3. Sloan EP, Zalenski RJ, Smith RF, et al. Toxicology screening in urban trauma patients: drug prevalence and its relationship to trauma severity and management. J Trauma 1989;29:1647.
4. Soderstrom CA, Trifillis AL, Shankar BS, et al. Marijuana and alcohol use among 1023 trauma patients: a prospective study. Arch Surg 1988; 123:733.
5. Rivara FP, Mueller BA, Flinger CL, et al. Drug use in trauma victims. J Trauma 1989;29:462.
6. Richter RW, Baden MN, Pearson J. Medical news. JAMA 1970;212:967.
7. Cimbura G, Lucas DM, Bennett RC, et al. Incidence and toxicologic aspects of drugs detected in 484 fatally injured drivers and pedestrians in Ontario. J Forensic Sci 1982;27:855.
8. Mason AP, McBray AJ. Ethanol, marijuana, and other drug use in 600 drivers killed in single-vehicle crashes in North Carolina, 1978-1981. J Forensic Sci 1984;29:987.
9. Williams AF, Peat MA, Crouch DJ, et al. Drugs in fatally injured male drivers. Public Health Reports 1985;10:19.
10. Budd RD, Muto JJ, Wong JK. Drugs of abuse found in fatally injured drivers in Los Angeles County. Drug Alcohol Depend 1989;23:153.
11. Marzuk PM, Tardiff K, Leon AC, et al. Prevalence of recent cocaine use among motor vehicle fatalities in New York City. JAMA 1990;263:250.
12. McLellan BA, Vingilis E, Liban CB, et al. Blood alcohol testing of motor vehicle crash admission at a regional trauma unit. J Trauma 1990; 30:418.
13. Kirkpatrick JR, Krome RL. Surgical manifestations of heroin addiction. JACEP 1973;2:24.
14. Soderstrom CA, Dailey JT, Kerns TJ. Alcohol and other drugs: an assessment of testing and clinical practices in U.S. trauma centers. J Trauma 1994;36:68.
15. Brill H. Death and disability in drug addiction and abuse. Ann Intern Med 1967;67:205.
16. Lucas CE, Joseph AJ, Ledgerwood AM. Alcohol and drugs. In: Moore EE, Mattox KL, Feliciano DV, eds. Trauma. 2nd ed. Norwalk, CT: Appleton & Lange, 1991:677-687.
17. Sands DE, Ledgerwood AM, Lucas CE. Pneumomediastinum on a surgical service. Am Surg 1988;54:434.
18. Frishman WH, Karpenos A, Molloy TJ. Cocaine induced coronary artery disease. Med Clin North Am 1989;73:475.
19. Barash PG, Koprieva CJ, Langou R, et al. Is cocaine a sympathetic stimulant during general anaesthesia? JAMA 1980;243:1437.
20. Levine SR, Brust JCM, Futrill N, et al. Cerebral vascular complications of the use of the "crack" form of alkaloidal cocaine. N Engl J Med 1990;323:699.

21. Kissner DG, Lawrence WD, Selis JE, et al. Crack lung: pulmonary disease caused by cocaine abuse. Am Rev Respir Dis 1987;136:1250.

22. Herzlich BC, Arsura EL, Pagala M, et al. Rhabdomyolysis related to cocaine abuse. Ann Intern Med 1988;109:335.

23. Lee HS, LaMaute HR, Pizzi WF, et al. Acute gastroduodenal perforations associated with use of crack. Ann Surg 1990;211:15.

24. Gawin FH, Ellinwood EH. Cocaine and other stimulants: actions, abuse, and treatment. N Engl J Med 1988;318:1173.

25. Jaffe JH, Martin WR. Opioid analgesics and antagonists. In: Gilman AG, Goodman LS, Rall TW, et al, eds. The pharmacological basis of therapeutics. 7th ed. New York: MacMillan, 1985:491.

26. Mark LC, et al. Hypotension during anesthesia in narcotic addicts. NY State J Med 1966;66:2685.

27. West DJ. The risk of hepatitis B infection among health professionals in the United States: a review. Am J Med Sci 1984;287:26.

28. Estroff TW, Extein IL, Malaspina R, et al. Hepatitis in 101 consecutive suburban cocaine and opiate users. Int J Psychiatr Med 1986;16:237.

29. Kelen GR, Fritz S, Qaguish B, et al. Substantial increase in human immunodeficiency virus infection in critically ill emergency patients: 1986 and 1987 compared. Ann Emerg Med 1989;18:378.

30. Centers for Disease Control. AIDS and human immunodeficiency virus infection in the United States: 1988 update. MMWR 1989;38:1.

31. Soderstrom CA, Trifillis AL, Shankar BS, et al. HIV infection rates in a trauma center treating predominantly rural blunt trauma victims. J Trauma 1989;29:1526.

32. Aprahamian C, Olsen D, Gottschall JL, Turner P. Potential risks of human immunodeficiency virus in critically injured patients. J Trauma 1988;28:1081.

33. Sterk C. Cocaine and HIV seropositivity. Lancet 1988;1:1052.

34. Hammond JS, Eckes JM, Gomez GA, Cunningham DN. HIV, trauma, and infection control: universal precautions are universally ignored. J Trauma 1990;30:555.

35. Gerberding JL, Littell C, Tarkington A, et al. Risk of exposure of surgical personnel to patients' blood during survey at San Francisco General Hospital. N Eng J Med 1990;322:1788.

36. Howard RJ. Human immunodeficiency virus testing and the risk to the surgeon of acquiring HIV. Surg Gynecol Obst 1990;171:22.

37. Wilson SE. Acquired immune deficiency syndrome (AIDS): indications for abdominal surgery, pathology, and outcome. Ann Surg 1989;210:428.

Chapter 9C Special Problems of Trauma in Alcoholics

ROBERT F. WILSON, M.D.

JEFFREY S. BENDER, M.D.

JENNIFER GASS, M.D.

INCIDENCE

On the basis of various governmental studies from 1987, 1990, and 1991, McGinnis and Foerge[1] reported that an estimated 18,000,000 United States residents suffer from alcohol dependence, and 76,000,000 are affected by alcohol abuse at some time. Motor vehicle accidents are the leading cause of death of people between the ages of 5 and 34, and of these 50,000 deaths, more than 50% are alcohol-related.[4] Two of every five Americans will be in an alcohol-related motor vehicle accident (MVA) sometime during their lifetime.[5] It can also be estimated that one alcohol-related MVA fatality occurs every 22 minutes, and one injury occurs every minute. MVAs cost the nation at least $70 billion in 1988, and at least $35 billion of that can be blamed on alcohol. Alcohol also contributes to 16-67% of home injuries, drownings, fire fatalities, and job injuries.[1,2,6]

> **AXIOM** Alcohol is a major cause of accidental trauma of all types, especially MVAs.

Kamerow et al[7] have estimated that societal costs attributed to alcohol abuse were $116.7 billion and included over 69,000 deaths.

The combination of alcoholism and severe trauma provides the surgeon and emergency physician with some of their most difficult problems. The usual medical difficulties produced by alcohol result from acute alcoholic intoxication; however, one must also be prepared to contend with complications of acute alcoholic withdrawal and/or chronic alcoholism, usually in the form of cirrhosis.

ACUTE ALCOHOLISM

Acute Intoxication

> **AXIOM** The main problems in treating acutely intoxicated trauma victims are the increased incidence of diagnostic errors and respiratory complications.

Not uncommonly, acutely intoxicated patients have a relatively slow pulse, slow respiratory rate, and orthostatic hypotension which may be completely unrelated to the trauma.

Acute alcoholic intoxication is often manifested by a change in mental state, nystagmus, slurred speech, and a staggering gait.[8] Many of these patients are uncooperative, and some are extremely loud and belligerent. Not infrequently, those with small injuries will loudly insist on extensive care, while those with severe trauma often cannot be made to fully appreciate the seriousness of their injuries and will want to leave without definitive care.

> **PITFALL** ⊘
>
> *If it is not appreciated that acute alcoholic intoxication can seriously impair a patient's judgment, critically injured, uncooperative patients may be allowed to leave the hospital without adequate care.[8]*

While the desire to "treat and street" disruptive alcoholic patients is very high, especially if they are "repeaters," such an attitude should be avoided until there is near certainty that no serious problem exists or that a responsible and sober individual will watch over them. These patients will not reliably follow discharge instructions, and they may lapse into unconsciousness following discharge. Our courts have dictated that such patients cannot properly judge the need for medical care while in an intoxicated state. Instead, the burden lies on the attending physician. Rapidly available psychiatric or social workers' help can aid in the management of these patients.

MISTAKEN DIAGNOSES

Because of an absent or unreliable history and a physical examination that is often incomplete because of poor patient cooperation, mistaken or delayed diagnoses in acutely intoxicated patients are not infrequent.[8]

> **PITFALL** ⊘
>
> *If alcoholics are not roused and checked frequently after they have fallen asleep, serious neurologic lesions may not be revealed until too late.*

Although many intoxicated patients are initially hyperactive and may even have to be restrained, later they tend to fall asleep, and they can be extremely difficult to arouse.[8] Under these circumstances, a significant intracranial hematoma can easily be missed unless the patient is carefully examined at least every 30 minutes.

Although significant neurologic lesions in the acutely intoxicated patient can easily be overlooked, the opposite is also true and the stupor of intoxication will occasionally mimic an intracranial lesion and lead to overtreatment.[8] These unfortunate errors can be reduced somewhat by following certain basic rules with all acutely intoxicated patients who have had head trauma or are unconscious:

1. One should obtain complete vital signs at least every 30 minutes.
2. While the patient is "sleeping," he or she should be aroused at least every 30 minutes for a neurologic examination, which includes pupillary size and reaction and deep tendon reflexes.
3. One should obtain CT scans of the brain on all alcoholics with head trauma who do not "wake up" within 4-6 hours or have any lateralizing signs.
4. One should not accept alcoholism as a cause of unconsciousness if the blood level of alcohol is less than 150 mg/dl.

Injuries to the chest or abdomen in unconscious patients are best diagnosed by objective means such as x-rays, CT scans, or peritoneal lavage.

> **AXIOM** Alcoholism should not be accepted as a cause for unstable vital signs, and a careful search should be made for possible sources of bleeding.

Mistakes in diagnosis can be avoided if it is appreciated that the history and physical examination in acutely intoxicated patients may be completely unreliable. Lack of pain or tenderness in such individuals has little significance.

RESPIRATORY COMPLICATIONS

Almost all severely intoxicated patients who are lying down tend to "snore" because of the partial airway obstruction caused by a flaccid, overly lax tongue falling into the pharynx.[8] If the cervical spine x-rays are negative and if it does not appear that turning the patient on his side will aggravate any other injuries, this position can readily solve this problem. Alternatively, an oral airway may be necessary. Occasionally the respiratory depression is so severe that an endotracheal tube and ventilatory assistance are required.

AXIOM Acutely intoxicated patients are prone to aspirate and/or develop severe pulmonary infections.

Chronic smoking very frequently accompanies alcoholism and the resultant chronic bronchitis and emphysema can greatly increase the risk of respiratory complications after trauma. Alcoholics are also prone to aspirate their oral or gastric secretions, and this can cause severe acute respiratory infections, including lung abscesses. Evidence of aspiration should be looked for carefully and treated vigorously with bronchoscopy and ventilatory assistance as needed.

Hemodynamic Effects of Alcohol

EXPERIMENTAL STUDIES

AXIOM The detrimental effects of alcohol on hemorrhagic shock have been observed in both humans and experimental animals.

Gettler and Allbritten[9] compared the effects of hemorrhagic shock on control dogs and dogs given ethanol. After a 35% reduction in blood volume, a metabolic acidosis was produced. In the control animals there was a compensatory increase in respiratory rate, but in the intoxicated dogs, a marked respiratory depression occurred. In addition, the mean arterial pressure (MAP) response was significantly lower in the intoxicated animals. As a result, the mortality rate was 30% in the intoxicated group versus 0% in the controls.

AXIOM Alcohol tends to blunt the ventilatory response to shock.

Malt and Baue[10] studied the effects of alcohol on ventilation and circulation in an awake canine model. They found a marked depression of the normal ventilatory response to shock in inebriated dogs and a significant decrease in the amount of blood loss necessary to induce shock. They also found that increased myocardial irritability, as demonstrated by arrhythmias, was much greater in the dogs that had ethanol administration before the bleeding. These responses were also associated with a higher mortality rate after ethanol.

AXIOM Chronic alcoholics tend to have an increased incidence of arrhythmias after trauma.

Animal studies of nonpenetrating cardiac trauma also show an increased incidence of arrhythmias and death in intoxicated canines versus controls.[11] Using incremental doses of alcohol administered via a gastric tube, Disiderio[13] demonstrated a dose-dependent mortality rate after blunt cardiac trauma. Although no dogs died after blunt injury alone, mortality rates of 17%, 50%, and 71% were found after inducing blood alcohol concentrations of 60, 120, and 180 mg/dl just before the trauma.

CLINICAL STUDIES

Presumably, the same increased mortality rate from hypovolemic shock occurs in intoxicated humans, but this observation is camouflaged by the fact that a patient who dies in the field does not enter into the system for resuscitation and no assessment is made of the trauma score (TS) or injury severity score (ISS) within a hospital setting. Nevertheless, alcohol is known to increase the incidence of arrhythmias in humans and may be part of the cause of the increased mortality rate from hemorrhagic shock in inebriated patients.[12] In addition to the increased incidence of arrhythmias, chronic alcoholics often also have evidence of cardiomyopathy.

AXIOM Ethanol tends to cause vasodilation, and this can increase the amount of hypotension that occurs with blood loss.

Ethanol causes vasodilation which reduces systemic vascular resistance (SVR).[6] Concomitantly it causes a diuresis with increased salt and water excretion. At lower levels, alcohol also promotes the release of catecholamines from sympathetic nerve endings, but this has little effect on cardiac output (CO) or mean arterial pressure (MAP);[13] however, at higher levels, it has a negative inotropic effect. With severe intoxication, the negative inotropic effect combined with a decreased SVR can cause a reduction in MAP far out of proportion to the actual volume of blood loss.[14] Consequently, many injured, intoxicated patients present with severe hypotension even though the volume of blood loss is relatively small. Such patients can usually be resuscitated to a normal MAP with less fluid and blood than injured, nonintoxicated patients with a similar MAP.

Methanol Ingestion

An occasional complication of acute alcoholism, usually occurring in severe chronic alcoholics, is ingestion of methyl alcohol. This can cause acute pulmonary distress associated with severe metabolic acidosis with an arterial pH approaching 7.0 or less without evidence of shock or airway obstruction. Hyperventilation is an attempt to compensate for the severe metabolic acidosis.

AXIOM Severe metabolic acidosis in a chronic alcoholic without evidence of shock or tissue ischemia may be a result of methanol ingestion.

Acute Withdrawal (Delirium Tremens)

The most common and most feared alcohol-related metabolic problem following operation is delirium tremens (DTs).[6] Approximately 30% of patients experiencing seizures from alcohol withdrawal will progress into DTs.[14] DTs may be fatal in up to 10 to 15% of cases.[8] The usual patient with DTs has been recently and acutely deprived of alcohol after having been an excessive and steady drinker for many years. Trauma is a common mechanism by which this deprivation occurs, and DTs under these circumstances are especially lethal.

The full-blown syndrome in the trauma patient usually does not manifest for at least 24 to 48 hours, and in some instances, it may be delayed for 4 to 5 days or longer.[8] During the early phase of DTs, the patient's metabolic rate is increased, and the patient's behavior becomes increasingly disruptive.[6]

The severity of the DTs during this phase can be classified according to the altered neurologic activity. Patients with confusion but without hallucinations are classified as having mild or class I DTs. Class II includes patients with auditory hallucinations, and class III describes patients with visual hallucinations. Class IV patients have all of the above plus total body tremulousness and/or generalized convulsions.

AXIOM Acute restlessness in alcoholics should not be considered a result of alcohol withdrawal until hypoxia, head trauma, sepsis, hypoglycemia, and electrolyte abnormalities have been ruled out.

The first indications of an impending attack of DTs are restlessness and mental irritability.[8] The patient becomes "shaky," and anorexic and has a strong desire for alcohol. In its severe untreated form, DTs are characterized by a disoriented, disheveled patient who is constantly moving, rearranging bedclothes, tugging at his restraints, and often incontinent. The obvious tremor is so grossly disorganized that even simple chores become impossible. The patient actively hallucinates and characteristically engages in imagined conversations. He may shout or scream in anguish to ward off the people or animals who threaten him. Vomiting, dehydration, hyperthermia, hypovolemia, severe electrolyte imbalances and aspiration pneumonitis occur frequently and can progress rapidly to death unless treated aggressively.

PITFALL ⊘

> **Confusing the early manifestations of hypoxia or sepsis with delirium tremens.**

While withdrawal is the most common cause of seizures in the alcoholic patient, the differential diagnosis also includes craniocerebral trauma and alcohol-induced seizures or idiopathic epilepsy.[6] Approximately 10% of patients with symptoms of acute alcohol withdrawal will experience seizures. Ninety percent of these seizures occur between 7 and 48 hours after cessation of drinking, with a peak incidence between 12 and 24 hours. Withdrawal seizures have an abrupt onset, tend to be generalized tonicoclonic in nature, and are usually associated with a loss of consciousness. In contrast, focal seizures imply focal cerebral disease and craniocerebral trauma must be suspected.[15]

AXIOM Focal seizures during alcohol withdrawal are a result of head trauma until proven otherwise.

The most frequent cause of death after operation in injured patients with DTs is an arrhythmia with cardiac arrest that is often related to hypokalemia or hypomagnesemia.[6] For unknown reasons, serum potassium levels often decline below 3.0 mEq/liter during alcohol withdrawal and remain low despite intravenous replacement. Consequently, patients with alcohol-induced injuries must be watched carefully for signs and symptoms of alcohol withdrawal, and if signs of DTs develop, the electrolytes should be checked at least once or twice a day. Hyponatremia, hypophosphatemia, and hypomagnesemia are also frequently encountered during alcohol withdrawal or DTs and need to be addressed.[6]

AXIOM Serum levels of potassium, magnesium, phosphorus, and sodium should be watched carefully during DTs or alcohol withdrawal.

Efforts should be begun to prevent DTs in all patients deprived of alcohol.[8] These patients should be well hydrated with balanced electrolyte solutions administered intravenously. If given oral fluids, the patient is apt to vomit and aspirate.

Trace elements and vitamins, especially magnesium, calcium, thiamine, and nicotinic acid, should be routinely added to the IVs of patients apt to go into alcohol withdrawal.[8] Isolation or restraint of the patient should be avoided if possible at this point, as these measures only increase anxiety and metabolic demands. Sedation is mandatory, but oversedation is injurious and greatly increases the likelihood of aspiration, atelectasis, and pneumonia.

Various drugs have been used to sedate acute alcoholics, including tranquilizers such as Librium, Thorazine, and Valium.[8] Valium is generally a safe, reliable drug, and it has the advantage that it can be given orally, intramuscularly, or intravenously with a fairly wide margin of safety. Large quantities of sedatives or tranquilizers, in addition to restraints and a reasonably quiet environment, are often required to control agitation. Such sedation, however, may be a problem in patients being observed for a head injury. If there is fever, it should be treated by a hypothermia blanket rather than aspirin.

AXIOM Chronic alcoholics can have rather severe total body magnesium deficits even though serum magnesium levels are normal.

If the patient develops full-blown delirium tremens, treatment must be intense.[14] It is vital to closely monitor vital signs, fluid intake and output, and serum electrolytes. The patient may need 6 to 8 or more liters of balanced electrolyte solution per day with added potassium, magnesium, and phosphorous to reverse the tendency to dehydration and electrolyte imbalance. If vomiting occurs, nasogastric suction should be begun.

Many patients with delirium tremens or acute alcohol withdrawal develop seizures, gastrointestinal bleeding, or pneumonia.[8] Convulsions should be controlled or prevented with intravenous or intramuscular Valium or Dilantin, but hypoglycemia should be eliminated as a possible etiologic factor. When boluses of glucose are given, they should be preceded by 100 mg of thiamine every 12 hours to help prevent Wernicke's encephalopathy.[17,18]

CHRONIC ALCOHOLISM

In general, the liver is the organ most obviously damaged by chronic alcoholism, and chronic alcoholism is the most frequent cause of cirrhosis in the United States.[8] In addition, chronic alcoholism causes damage to a wide variety of other organ systems, all of which must be evaluated and monitored in the alcoholic patient with multiple trauma.

Neurologic Changes

AXIOM One should never completely rely on a history provided by a chronic alcoholic patient.

The neurologic changes of chronic alcoholism can make it extremely difficult to obtain a reliable history and to determine if significant head trauma has occurred.[8] Korsakoff's syndrome or similar problems can result in medical histories that are extremely misleading. Wernicke's syndrome, characterized by ophthalmoplegia, nystagmus, pupillary alterations, and ataxia with tremors, can cause severe central neurologic changes that, unfortunately, are not usually localized. The peripheral neuropathy may cause the patient to lose peripheral sensation, coordination, and strength.

Cardiovascular Problems

The cardiovascular changes of advanced cirrhosis include a reduced ability to tolerate hypotension and an increased tendency to congestive heart failure.[8] These patients rely on hepatic artery blood flow to nourish the liver, and shock in these patients is associated with an extremely high incidence of liver failure and death. Cardiomyopathies are common so there is minimal tolerance between hypovolemic hypotension and fluid overloading.

AXIOM Cardiac filling pressures must be monitored closely in chronic alcoholics because of the small margin of safety between hypovolemic hypotension and overt cardiac failure.

In the past, it was thought that most cardiac problems in chronic alcoholics resulted from a thiamine deficiency and were identical to those seen in beriberi heart disease.[8] Many of these patients, however, respond only partially to large doses of thiamine. Furthermore, the lesions make the patient overly sensitive to digitalis, especially if acidosis and hypotension are also present. Since the resultant cardiac failure is difficult to manage, extra care must be taken to avoid fluid overload. Conversely, even though severe uncorrected ascites may produce some respiratory distress, complete removal of the fluid at laparotomy can cause severe hypovolemia and hypotension to develop unless adequate fluids and protein are administered as the ascitic fluid reaccumulates.

AXIOM Reaccumulation of ascitic fluid after laparotomy in a cirrhotic patient can cause delayed shock.

Gastrointestinal bleeding in chronic alcoholics often can be controlled with iced saline gastric lavage; however, endoscopic examination and, rarely, surgical intervention is required.[8] Bleeding from esophageal varices is fraught with an appalling mortality if the patient has concurrent delirium tremens, regardless of the mode of therapy. Administration of Pitressin at 0.2-0.4 units/min into the superior mesenteric artery or through a peripheral vein is often quite effective for controlling variceal hemorrhage. Accurate diagnosis of the cause of the gastrointestinal bleeding is paramount and is best done endoscopically.

Coagulation Problems

Severe coagulation problems, especially prothrombin deficiencies, can be encountered in chronic alcoholics.[8] The injection of vitamin K is mandatory before surgery. If transfusions are needed, fresh frozen plasma should also be given rather liberally. If possible, surgery should be delayed until the prothrombin time is within 3 seconds of the normal (control) values.

AXIOM   Chronic alcoholics can have all of the coagulation abnormalities seen in liver failure.

Anesthetic Considerations

After the initial resuscitation of traumatized cirrhotic patients and attempted correction of coagulation defects, one must decide on the type of anesthetic to use if surgery is required.[8] In general, one should choose agents that do not require detoxification by the liver, such as ether or nitrous oxide. Fluothane is avoided. It is probably more important, however, to keep the patient normotensive and well-oxygenated than to argue the merits of any particular agent, as long as the agent is not primarily hepatotoxic.

AXIOM   Avoid giving chronic alcoholics anesthetic agents that are metabolized by the liver.

Problems During Surgery

During surgery, especially in the abdomen, excessive bleeding must be anticipated in direct proportion to the degree of portal hypertension and coagulation abnormalities.[8] Although bleeding may be extensive and hypotension is common, care must be taken not to overhydrate the patient.

The intra-abdominal organ most commonly injured by long-standing alcohol abuse is the liver, and patients with alcoholic cirrhosis and either blunt or penetrating hepatic injuries can be difficult to treat.[5,15] Some of the difficulties with successful liver hemostasis are related to the intrahepatic fibrosis that impedes contraction and retraction of severed intraparenchymal vessels. Intrahepatic fibrosis can also make it difficult to compress bleeding sites with sutures. Because of the portal hypertension, minor tears and lacerations may bleed profusely. Sutures may not hold well, and exposure is often difficult. In cases like these, consider early placement of intra-abdominal packs and re-exploring the patient in 48 to 72 hours. Packing with omentum and use of fibrin glue also may be helpful.[8]

AXIOM   Cirrhotic patients with portal hypertension can have severe hemorrhage from injuries to any segment of the splanchnic system, and salvage of an injured spleen is rare in patients with severe cirrhosis.[5]

Postoperative Resuscitation

Postoperative management of the chronic alcoholic is often extremely demanding.[8] Some general rules include: (a) liberally supply glucose, trace elements, and vitamins, (b) transfuse as needed, (c) avoid excess water and salt, (d) administer salt-poor albumin as needed,

(e) control ascites with diuretics, particularly aldactone, (f) avoid ammonia intoxication by cleansing the gastrointestinal tract of blood, and (g) administer intestinal neomycin in selected cases.

The most important postoperative problems in cirrhotics include bleeding, ascites, heart failure, respiratory failure, ammonia intoxication, gastritis, and impaired wound healing.[8]

BLEEDING
Continued postoperative bleeding often is assumed to be caused by coagulation abnormalities. However, such bleeding often occurs from open vessels that must be controlled directly at surgery.

AXIOM   Continued or recurrent postoperative bleeding in cirrhotics should be controlled surgically as soon as possible.

ASCITES AND HYPOVOLEMIA
Although reduction of the rate and amount of ascites formation with salt restriction and diuretics is important, overzealous efforts to retard the formation of ascitic fluid can cause severe hypotension and increased liver failure.[8] However, aggressive attempts to correct the hypovolemia caused by continued bleeding and ascites formation may rebound and result in congestive failure. Consequently, carefully monitoring of all vital signs, including CVP and/or PAWP, is essential.

ATELECTASIS AND PNEUMONIA
General debility, poor resistance to infection, an increased tendency to aspiration, and elevation of the diaphragm by ascites all increase the chances of postoperative pneumonitis and respiratory failure.[8] Complete gastrointestinal decompression, early respirator assistance, and vigorous bronchial toilet are mandatory.

AMMONIA INTOXICATION AND LIVER FAILURE
The incidence of ammonia intoxication is greatly increased in cirrhotic patients with trauma.[4] Impaired liver function coupled with an increased protein load to the liver, resulting from blood transfusions, absorption of blood from the gastrointestinal tract and peritoneal cavity, and tissue damage, sets the stage for hepatic encephalopathy. Cleansing of the gastrointestinal tract of blood with enemas and cathartics as soon as possible and the use of parenteral and intestinal antibiotics may help reduce the formation of ammonia by intestinal bacteria. Upper gastrointestinal bleeding may also increase because of portal hypertension and impaired mucus production. H_2 blockers and/or antacids should be begun immediately postoperatively and increased as needed if any blood is seen in the nasogastric aspirate.

Wound Healing

AXIOM   Special efforts must be taken when closing abdominal incisions in chronic alcoholics, and such closures should probably be performed with nonabsorbable sutures.

Alcoholics tend to have poor wound healing and an increased incidence of wound dehiscence.[8] These problems are often attributed to multiple dietary deficiencies, hypoproteinemia, and cirrhosis. Many chronic alcoholics, even those without documented cirrhosis, will manifest similar metabolic derangements, including magnesium, zinc, and vitamin deficiencies, hypoproteinemia, salt retention, and failure to metabolize adrenal steroids properly. Thus, it is extremely important to supply increased quantities of glucose, vitamins, and trace metals.

OUTCOME

Controversy exists regarding the effect that prior alcohol ingestion can have on the severity of injury to various organs and the outcome of the patient.[5] Luna et al[19] suggest that the severity of an intracranial injury in an intoxicated patient after a motorcycle accident is greater following the ingestion of alcohol. The Seattle study also noted an increased risk of severe intracranial injuries in intoxicated cyclists. Both the incidence and mortality rate were doubled compared to the nonintoxicated patients with comparable injuries. Indeed, the presence of alcohol intoxication appeared to negate the protective effect of helmet use. The incidence of severe intracranial injury in nonintoxicated patients without helmets was 25%. In contrast, intoxicated patients with alcohol levels of 100 mg/dl or more had a 75% incidence of severe intracranial injury with helmets and a 74% incidence without helmets.

The same controversy exists with regard to outcome. Ward et al[20] reviewed the records of 1198 injured patients including 386 patients with alcohol in their blood at the time of admission. The alcohol-positive patients had a significantly greater incidence of penetrating trauma. Interestingly, however, when ISSs were compared, the mortality rate was significantly lower in the drinking patients versus the nondrinking patients; however, length of stay (LOS) and number of days in the ICU were equivalent in the two groups.

AXIOM Chronic alcoholics are more prone to have trauma, but they may do relatively well with what appears to be comparable degrees of injury as long as there is not significant blood loss.

Two studies of 182 drivers involved in motor vehicle accidents by Huth et al[21] and 615 consecutive admissions to a trauma service by Thal et al[22] failed to show discernible differences in degree of injury, TS, ISS, mortality, LOS, or complications between intoxicated and nondrinking patients.

Jagger et al[23] demonstrated that intoxicated patients have a GCS that reflects both the injury and the depressant effects of alcohol. In comparison with "matched" controls, inebriated patients appeared to have a more rapid and more complete recovery. Thus, a pseudoprotective effect of alcohol might be assumed by the uncritical observer. However, the alcohol may have artificially made the GSC, TS, and ISS seem worse than they really were.

AXIOM Overall, intoxicated drivers in MVAs tend to have higher morbidity and mortality rates than sober drivers.

One well-designed study of the effect of alcohol on victims of motor vehicle accidents has clearly shown increased morbidity and mortality in the intoxicated group.[6] Using data collected over 5 years on more than a million drivers, Waller et al[24] created a model analyzing the probability of injury as a function of alcohol use. Matching other injury-related variables such as use of a safety belt, vehicular weight, vehicular speed and deformation, and driver age, these investigators showed a consistently greater morbidity and mortality in drinking drivers versus the nondrinking drivers. Alcohol-involved drivers had serious and fatal injuries 1.7 to 2.1 times as often as their sober counterparts with matched collisions.

McClellan et al[25] have noted that drivers in motor vehicle crashes with a positive blood alcohol level differed significantly from blood alcohol negative drivers on the following variables: less driver education (P less than 0.01), increased license suspension 2 years or less before admission, and increased frequency of self-reported intoxication in the month before the motor vehicle accident.

Tinkoff et al[26] found that the mortality rate was 30% in 40 cirrhotic trauma victims admitted to two Pennsylvania hospitals. This was significantly higher than the 7% that could have been predicted by TRISS methodology. Most deaths were due to sepsis and multisystem organ failure. Predictors of poor outcome on admission included ascites, elevated prothrombin time, hyperbilirubinemia, and the need for a laparotomy. Six out of nine cirrhotic patients requiring intra-abdominal surgery died; another cirrhotic who was only observed also died.

Referral to an alcoholism counselor of all patients with an elevated blood alcohol level at the time of admission is increasingly advocated.

Whether one or two visits by a counselor will have any long-term effect on a patient's drinking habits is extremely debatable. Despite repeated recommendations by the American College of Surgeons, measurements of blood alcohol levels and drug screens are routine in only 64% of level I and 40% of level II trauma centers.[27] In addition, less than a third of all trauma centers routinely employ alcoholism counselors.[28] Maio et al[29] noted that only 34% of adolescents with alcohol-related trauma were referred for alcohol and psychiatric assessment.

⊘ FREQUENT ERRORS

In the Management of Trauma in Alcoholic Patients

1. *Failure to look carefully for alcoholic intoxication in MVA victims, especially those with an altered state of consciousness.*
2. *Attributing a tendency to be uncooperative and sleepy only to alcohol.*
3. *Considering CNS changes a result of acute alcoholic intoxication even after 4-6 hours of observation.*
4. *Failure to look for other drugs in patients who are obviously intoxicated.*
5. *Assuming that focal seizures in an alcoholic are a result of alcohol withdrawal.*
6. *Failure to monitor serum electrolytes, especially magnesium, closely enough in alcoholic patients.*
7. *Assuming that total body magnesium levels are normal if serum levels are normal, and thereby failing to provide adequate magnesium to chronic alcoholic patients.*
8. *Failure to monitor cardiac filling pressures closely while correcting hypotension in alcoholic patients.*
9. *Failure to provide adequate fluid postoperatively to cirrhotic patients to make up for reaccumulating ascitic fluid.*
10. *Assuming that excess bleeding intraoperatively or postoperatively is due to a coagulation abnormality and that it doesn't require urgent surgical control.*

▼▼▼▼▼▼▼▼▼▼▼▼▼▼▼▼▼▼▼▼▼▼▼▼▼▼▼▼▼▼

SUMMARY POINTS

1. Alcohol is a major cause of accidental trauma of all types, especially MVAs.

2. The main problems in treating acutely intoxicated trauma victims are the increased incidence of diagnostic errors and respiratory complications.

3. Alcoholism should not be accepted as a cause for unstable vital signs, and a careful search should be made for possible sources of bleeding.

4. Acutely intoxicated patients are prone to aspirate and/or develop severe pulmonary infections.

5. The detrimental effects of alcohol on hemorrhagic shock have been observed in both humans and experimental animals.

6. Alcohol tends to blunt the ventilatory response to shock.

7. Chronic alcoholics tend to have an increased incidence of arrhythmias after trauma.

8. Ethanol tends to cause vasodilation, and this can increase the amount of hypotension that occurs with blood loss.

9. Severe metabolic acidosis in a chronic alcoholic without evidence of shock or tissue ischemia may be a result of methanol ingestion.

10. Acute restlessness in alcoholics should not be considered a result of alcohol withdrawal until hypoxia, head trauma, sepsis, hypoglycemia, and electrolyte abnormalities have been ruled out.

11. Focal seizures during alcohol withdrawal are a result of head trauma until proven otherwise.

12. Serum levels of potassium, magnesium, phosphorus, and sodium should be watched carefully during alcohol withdrawal.

13. Chronic alcoholics can have rather severe total body magnesium deficits even though serum magnesium levels are normal.

14. One should never completely rely on a history provided by a chronic alcoholic patient.

15. Cardiac filling pressures must be monitored closely in chronic alcoholics because of the small margin of safety between hypovolemic hypotension and overt cardiac failure.

16. Reaccumulation of ascitic fluid after laparotomy in a cirrhotic patient can cause delayed shock.

17. Chronic alcoholics can have all of the coagulation abnormalities seen in liver failure.

18. Avoid giving chronic alcoholics anesthetic agents that are metabolized by the liver.

19. Cirrhotic patients with portal hypertension can have severe hemorrhage from injuries to any segment of the splanchnic system, and salvage of an injured spleen is rare in patients with severe cirrhosis.

20. Continued or recurrent postoperative bleeding in cirrhotics should be controlled surgically as soon as possible.

21. Special efforts must be taken when closing abdominal incisions in alcoholics, and such closures should probably be done with nonabsorbable sutures.

22. Chronic alcoholics are more prone to have trauma, but they may do relatively well with what appears to be comparable degrees of injury as long as there is not significant blood loss.

23. Overall, intoxicated drivers in MVAs tend to have higher morbidity and mortality rates than sober drivers.

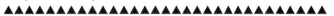

REFERENCES

1. McGinnis JM, Foege WH. Actual causes of death in the United States. JAMA 1993;270:2207.
2. West LJ, Maxwell DS, Noble EP, Solomon DH. Alcoholism. Ann Intern Med 1984;100:405.
3. McCoy GF, Johnstone RA, Nelson IW, Duthie RB. A review of fatal road accidents in Oxfordshire over a 2-year period. Injury 1989;20:65.
4. Maull KI. Alcohol abuse: its implications in trauma care. South Med J 1982;75:794.
5. Lucas CE, Joseph AJ, Ledgerwood AM. Alcohol and drugs. In: Moore EE, Mattox KL, Feliciano DV, eds. Trauma. 2nd ed. Norwalk, CT: Appleton & Lange, 1991:677-687.
6. Smith GS, Falk H. Unintentional injuries. Am J Prev Med 1987;3:143.
7. Kamerow DB, Pincus HA, MacDonal DI. Alcohol abuse, other drug abuse, and metabolic disorders in medical practice. JAMA 1986;255:2054.
8. Kirkpatrick JR, Krome RL, Walt AJ, et al. Special problems of trauma in the aged, addicted, and alcoholic. In: Walt AJ, Wilson RF, eds. Management of trauma: pitfalls and practice. Philadelphia: Lea & Febiger, 1975:76-91.
9. Gettler DT, Allbritten FF. Effect of alcohol intoxication and the respiratory exchange and mortality rate associated with acute hemorrhage in anesthetized dogs. Ann Surg 1963;158:151.
10. Malt SH, Baue AE. The effects of ethanol as related to trauma in the awake dog. J Trauma 1971;11:76.
11. Stein PD, Sabbah HN, Przybylski J, et al. Effect of alcohol upon arrhythmias following nonpenetrating cardiac impact. J Trauma 1988;28:465.
12. Gleenspon AJ, Schaal SF. The "holiday heart": electrophysiologic studies of alcohol effects in alcoholics. Ann Intern Med 1983;98:135.
13. Desiderio, MA. The effects of acute, oral ethanol on cardiovascular performance before and after blunt cardiac trauma. J Trauma 1987;27:267.
14. Morris JC, Victor M. Alcohol withdrawal seizures. Emerg Med Clin North Am 1987;5:827.
15. Swan KJ, Vidaver RM, Lavingne JE, et al. Acute alcoholism, minor trauma and "shock." J Trauma 1977;17:215.
16. Becker CE. The alcoholic patient as a toxic emergency. Em Med Clin N Am 1984;2:47.
17. Massey EW, Coffey CE. Delirium: diagnosis and treatment. South Med J 1983;76:1147.
18. Goulinger RC. Delirium in the surgical patient. Am Surg 1989;55:549.
19. Luna GK, Maier RV, Sowder L, et al. The influence of ethanol intoxication on outcome of injured motorcyclists. J Trauma 1984;24:695.
20. Ward RE, Flynn TC, Miller PW, et al. Effects of ethanol ingestion on the severity and outcome of trauma. Am J Surg 1982;144:153.
21. Huth JR, Maier RV, Simonowitz DA, et al. Effect of acute ethanolism on the hospital course and outcome of injured automobile drivers. J Trauma 1983;23:494.
22. Thal ER, Bost RO, Anderson RJ. Effect of alcohol and other drugs on traumatized patients. Arch Surg 1985;120:708.
23. Jagger J, Fife D, Vernberg K, et al. Effect of alcohol intoxication on the diagnosis and apparent severity of brain injury. Neurosurgery 1984;15:303.
24. Waller PF, Stewart JR, Hansen AR, et al. The potentiating effects of alcohol on driver injury. JAMA 1986;256:1461.
25. McLellan BA, Vingilis E, Larkin E, et al. Psychosocial characteristics and follow-up of drinking and non-drinking drivers in motor vehicle crashes. J Trauma 1993;35:24.
26. Tinkoff G, Rhodes M, Diamond D, et al. Cirrhosis in the trauma victim. Ann Surg 1990;211:172.
27. Soderstrom CA, Dailey JT, Kerns TJ. Alcohol and other drugs: an assessment of testing and clinical practices in U.S. trauma centers. J Trauma 1994;36:68.
28. Soderstrom CA, Cowley RA. A national alcohol and trauma center survey. Arch Surg 1987;122:1067.
29. Maio RF, Portnoy J, Blow FC, Hill EM. Injury type, injury severity, and repeat occurrence of alcohol-related trauma in adolescents. Alcohol Clin Exp Res 1994;18:261.

Chapter **10** Head Injuries

DANIEL B. MICHAEL, M.D., PH.D.

ROBERT F. WILSON, M.D.

INTRODUCTION

Incidence

AXIOM　Head injury is the leading cause of mortality and morbidity after trauma.

Each year in the United States, 350,000 to 500,000 patients suffer a head injury severe enough to be hospitalized.[1-3] At least 50,000 of these patients die because of their head trauma, and another 50,000 to 60,000 are severely disabled. In some series, almost half of all trauma deaths result from head injury.[4] Most head injuries requiring hospitalization occur in young persons between the ages of 15 and 24.[4] Thus, the patients at greatest risk of sustaining a fatal or disabling head injury are individuals just beginning their productive years. The direct and indirect financial losses to society are staggering. One estimate for the year 1977 placed the lost income from head injury deaths alone at about $22 billion.[4] This is equivalent to at least $65 billion in 1993 dollars.

In an average year, the neurosurgical department of Detroit Receiving Hospital sees more than a thousand adult patients with head injuries. During a 2-year period (1992-1993), we admitted 1050 patients with head injuries. Of these, 69% were mild (GCS of 13-15), 10% were moderate (GCS of 9-12), and 21% were severe (GCS of 3-8) (Table 10-1). The in-hospital mortality rates with these three groups were 2%, 7%, and 46%, respectively. About a half of these injuries were accidental and a half were the result of intentional trauma. Alcohol and/or illicit drugs were not only etiologic factors in almost 70% of these injuries, but they also made examination and evaluation more difficult.

History

Skulls showing evidence of craniotomy that may have been done for trauma were discovered in neolithic burial sites in Europe and pre-Columbian sites in Peru.[4] Some of these patients survived both the injury and surgery because there is evidence of healing around the fracture sites and craniotomy wounds.[5]

One of the oldest surviving medical documents, the Edwin Smith papyrus, originally written about 2400 to 2500 BC, describes the symptoms, diagnosis, therapy, and prognosis of 27 cases of head injury.[5] Hippocrates (3rd-4th century BC) and Galen (2nd century AD) established treatment criteria, including trephination, for head trauma that have remained relatively unchanged for about 2000 years.

Anesthesia, asepsis, and localization of intracranial hematomas have progressively improved survival for head injury patients.[5] Clinical indications developed by Cushing for surgery in patients with head injuries remained fairly standard until recent years, when the development of angiography and then computed tomography (CT) scanning made most exploratory intracranial surgery unnecessary.[6]

PATHOLOGY AND PATHOPHYSIOLOGY OF HEAD INJURY

Blunt Injuries

GROSS CHANGES

Primary versus Secondary Brain Injury

Brain damage from head trauma may result from primary or secondary injuries. Primary injury is the damage produced directly by the original mechanical forces.[7] Secondary injury occurs after the initial trauma. Ischemic and hypoxic damage resulting from local factors inside the skull or systemic extracranial problems may contribute to secondary injury.

AXIOM　Although there is usually no specific treatment for primary brain injury, at least some secondary injury is preventable or treatable.

Mechanisms of Primary Brain Injury

The three mechanisms that account for most of the primary injury resulting from head trauma include concussion-compression, sudden deceleration, and rotational acceleration.[3]

CONCUSSION-COMPRESSION.　Concussion-compression forces result directly from the localized impact.[3] Although the scalp provides some cushioning, much of the force is transmitted to the skull. If the compressive force exceeds the elasticity of the bone, the skull will fracture.[1] The initial force is also transmitted to the cranial contents, resulting in varying degrees of local tissue damage.

SUDDEN DECELERATION.　Another mechanism of injury is abrupt deceleration with the rapidly moving head brought to a sudden halt, causing the brain to collide with the inner surface of the skull.[6] Shearing forces result from the differential acceleration and rebound, and contusions or lacerations may occur as the brain comes up against the more irregular contours of the skull (such as the lesser sphenoid wing) or the edges of the dura (such as the undersurface of the falx cerebri).[6]

As the brain moves away from the cranial vault on the side opposite the area of impact, tearing of bridging veins may occur, resulting in a subdural hematoma.[8] The rebound of the brain may also result in contusion or hematoma in the area of brain striking the inner surface of the skull opposite the site of impact. This is referred to as a contrecoup injury.

ROTATIONAL ACCELERATION.　Rotational acceleration is by far the most important factor in generating parenchymal tears.[8] The usual spectrum of injury includes axonal disruption, hemorrhage, and brain edema. This soft tissue shear-strain damage tends to occur in axons at the interface of gray and white matter, primarily in the frontal and temporal lobes and in the corpus callosum.

Shear-strain damage is not seen easily on CT scans; however, magnetic resonance imaging (MRI) can identify many of these nonhemorrhagic lesions. About 10 to 15% of patients with positive MRIs display shear-strain lesions in the brain stem, and patients who sustain these lesions in both the corpus callosum and the brain stem have the highest incidence of permanent vegetative coma.[9]

Hemorrhage in these cases may occur in either the soft tissue at the sites of shear-strain injury or in the subdural or subarachnoid spaces. Simultaneous CAT and MRI studies reveal that about 20% of axonal shear-strain injuries identified by MRI also have microhemorrhages.[10] Many of these microhemorrhages do not become apparent for as long as 4 days, indicating that they probably develop as brain damage progresses.

TABLE 10-1 Outcome Correlated with GCS in 1050 Head Injury Patients Admitted to Detroit Receiving Hospital (1992-1993)

GCS	Expired	Rehab Facility	Home	Total	MR
3-8	101	90	30	221	46%
9-12	7	48	50	105	7%
13-15	16	134	574	724	2%
Total	124	272	654	1050	12%

AXIOM Brain edema of sufficient magnitude to significantly alter intracranial pressure is virtually never observed in patients in the absence of either focal shear-strain injuries or hemorrhage.[10]

Secondary Traumatic Brain Injury

Secondary injuries or insults to the brain are physiologic events occurring within minutes, hours, or days after the primary injury and lead to further damage of nervous tissue. The effects of secondary brain damage are epitomized by the so-called "talk and deteriorate" patients who are able to talk after their initial injury but ultimately die, clearly demonstrating that the primary mechanical injury is not the sole determinant of outcome.[11] Rose et al[12] found that nearly one-third of their head-injured patients who died were in the "talk and deteriorate" category and identified the presence of an avoidable secondary insult in almost 75% of this group. Hypotension and hypoxia are particularly important and have been associated with a doubling of mortality after head trauma.[13]

AXIOM Hypoxemia and hypotension are the most frequent systemic insults causing secondary brain injury.

SYSTEMIC INSULTS. Arterial hypoxemia is commonly seen when the patient arrives in the ED and is usually due to hypoventilation. Brain stem movement at the moment of impact has been thought to be responsible for the loss of consciousness that commonly occurs after significant head trauma.[14] Because the brain stem controls respiration, hypoventilation is also apt to occur. Other causes of hypoxemia, especially in patients with multiple injuries, may include upper airway obstruction, flail chest, hemothorax, pneumothorax, and/or pulmonary contusion.

Hypotension (systolic blood pressure less than 90 mm Hg) accompanies head trauma in about 35% of severely injured patients and increases mortality from 27 to 50%.[13] Compounding the reduction in cerebral perfusion caused by the hypotension is the impairment of cerebral autoregulation that often occurs after severe brain injury.[15] With normal autoregulation, cerebral blood flow remains rather constant despite fluctuations in mean arterial pressure between 60 and 180 mm Hg. However, when cerebral autoregulation is impaired, cerebral blood flow changes directly with the systemic arterial pressure.[15] Consequently, it is not uncommon for head-injured patients to have significant neurologic improvement after the arterial blood pressure is restored to normal levels.

A hematocrit of less than 30% leads to reduced blood oxygen carrying capacity and can make cerebral ischemia much worse. This anemia is likely in patients who have multiple injuries, and it is often associated with arterial hypotension. Miller and Becker[13] found a mortality rate of 52% when anemia accompanied head injury. Less frequent but important systemic causes of secondary brain injury include electrolyte disturbances, hypoglycemia or hyperglycemia, and hyperthermia.

INTRACRANIAL INSULTS. In patients with acute subdural hematomas, Seelig et al[16] found a 90% mortality rate when the operation occurred more than 4 hours after injury, compared with a mortality rate of only 30% in those who had surgery within 4 hours of injury.

AXIOM Unless large intracranial hematomas are removal promptly, intracranial pressure can rise rapidly because of further bleeding or edema formation.

The cause of cerebral deterioration in patients who come to the hospital talking, in approximately 70 to 80% of cases, is an expanding intracranial mass lesion, usually a subdural or epidural hematoma.[17,18] Intracerebral hematomas are relatively infrequent within the first 6 hours after head trauma in these patients.[18] Cerebral deterioration from cerebral contusions with local hemorrhage tends to occur in a more delayed fashion.[19]

Prolonged elevations of intracranial pressure are associated with a poor outcome, and a report from the Traumatic Coma Data Bank of 428 patients with severe head injury demonstrated a strong association between the duration of intracranial hypertension (intracranial pressure of more than 20 mm Hg) and outcome.[20]

Patients can deteriorate from causes other than mass lesions. Most head injuries are associated with transient hyperemia, and this may be particularly prominent in children. Diffuse cerebral edema can also result in rapid deterioration.[21] Cerebral hypoxia for any reason also increases the risk of developing delayed cerebral hematomas.[21]

Cerebral vasospasm is often associated with the presence of subarachnoid blood. Martin et al,[22] using transcranial Doppler ultrasonography, found the incidence of post-traumatic vasospasm to be about 30%. This arterial narrowing tends to be associated with decreased cerebral blood flow and a worse neurologic outcome.

AXIOM If subarachnoid hemorrhage is seen on the CT scan, there is an increased likelihood of the patient developing cerebral vasospasm.

CEREBRAL ISCHEMIA-REPERFUSION INJURY. The molecular events leading to further vascular and neuronal damage after traumatic brain injury may be similar to those seen with reperfusion injury and subarachnoid hemorrhage.[23] These changes may include transmembrane shifts of sodium and calcium into cells and potassium out, oxygen radical formation, and lipid peroxidation.[23,24] The hypoxanthine-xanthine pathway triggered by adenosine release is particularly important for generating toxic free radicals in reperfusion injuries.[25] Although histologic evidence for ischemia and reperfusion injury has been found in more than 50% of patients dying from severe head trauma,[26,27] much of this apparently occurs within a few hours of injury.

HISTOLOGIC AND BIOCHEMICAL CHANGES

Structural Evidence of Injury Progression

Experimental studies of axonal and vascular changes after moderate-severe brain injury indicate that the axonal transection does not occur at the time of initial impact.[11] Instead, there is a focal perturbation that progresses to separation of the proximal axon from its distal segment over a 12- to 24-hour period.

Shapiro et al[28] observed that the appearance of microhemorrhages in experimental animals and in patients is often delayed 12 to 18 hours after brain injury. In ischemic models of brain injury, the incidence and severity of microhemorrhages have been linked to increased oxygen concentrations during postischemic reperfusion, and these are inhibited by early treatment with deferoxamine.[29] This apparently works by suppressing iron-dependent oxygen radical-mediated peroxidation of polyunsaturated fatty acids in the cell membrane.[30]

Abnormalities of Calcium Hemostasis

AXIOM Increased intracellular calcium can cause a number of reactions that can directly or indirectly increase secondary brain damage.

Seisjo[31] believes that an important final common pathway to cell death after trauma or ischemia is loss of calcium homeostasis and enhanced production of free radicals. The biochemical changes in traumatic brain injury include loss of cellular Ca^{++} homeostasis, acidosis, and enhanced free radical production.[32] The cytosolic concentration of ionized calcium (Ca^{++}_i) reflects the balance between the inward flux and the rate of Ca^{++} extrusion. Ca^{++}_i tends to rise after head injury because its influx and/or release from storage is enhanced, even if extrusion pump function is not compromised.

Release of a variety of excitotoxic amino acids has been observed after severe head trauma.[33] Under such circumstances, even mild-moderate reductions in the cellular capacity to generate ATP might allow increased Ca^{++} movement into cells. A rise in endothelial Ca^{++}_i could lead to an increased synthesis of nitric oxide (NO), conversion of XDH to XO, and stimulation of phospholipase A_2. These events, in turn, would be expected to lead to the formation of platelet-activating factor and free radicals.

Even if Ca^{++}-mediated damage does not occur in microvascular tissues, cells in these tissues may be damaged by free radicals diffusing through the extracellular space.[31,34] Indeed, there is increasing evidence that free radicals are responsible for much of the microvascular dysfunction that occurs after trauma.[32]

Ionic Shifts and Cellular Depolarization Accompanying Injury

There is increasing evidence that both the head injury itself and intraparenchymal hemorrhage can initiate massive cellular depolarization with extracellular accumulation of K^+ and intracellular accumulation of Ca^{++}.[35] The intracellular accumulation of Ca^{++} is generally accompanied by a loss of free intracellular Mg^{++} into the extracellular fluid, and these shifts of divalent cations may be directly related to the extent of the ultimate cellular damage.[27]

Free Radical Reactions

Free radicals are compounds with an unpaired electron in the outer orbit. Superoxide ($\cdot O_2^-$), hydrogen peroxide (H_2O_2), and hydroxyl ($\cdot OH$), are produced in small amounts during normal cellular metabolism; however, after trauma, they can be produced in large amounts through several different pathways. Furthermore, once superoxides are formed, they can generate additional oxygen radicals.

Wei et al[36] have shown that immediately after brain injury there is an increase in phospholipase C activity, which can release arachidonic acid in tissue and start the production of oxygen radicals. More direct evidence for oxygen radical formation after experimental brain injury was provided by Kontos and Wei[37] who showed that these radicals are produced not only in cerebral blood vessel walls but also by leukocytes and macrophages that accumulate in the brain starting 3 to 4 hours and peaking 24 hours after experimental injury. Interestingly, oxygen free radicals will not react in vivo with biologic macromolecules in the absence of a transition metal catalyst, and iron is particularly important in this regard.[38,39]

AXIOM Free radical damage of brain tissue may be decreased by making iron unavailable.

Free radical damage to microvascular tissue can compromise the capillary circulation by progressive vasogenic edema and by preventing normal autoregulation of the microcirculation. Loss of autoregulation, in turn, can cause inappropriate shunting of blood and resultant ischemia.[31]

Although the generation of superoxide radicals by damaged brain after blunt trauma has been shown directly,[40] much of the evidence of radical-mediated lipid peroxidation after traumatic brain injury is indirect. The most straightforward evidence is from a study of U-74006F (a 21-aminosteroid that can terminate free radical chain reactions), which was shown to inhibit progressive brain lipid peroxidation and to improve neurologic outcome after experimental head trauma.[30]

If hemorrhage is also present, the extravasated blood can initiate (probably by autoxidation of erythrocyte membranes) massive and prolonged peroxidation of brain lipids. This is associated with blood brain barrier damage and tissue edema, both of which are inhibited by U-74006F.

Excitatory Amino Acids

Of the mechanisms underlying delayed tissue injury, the neurochemical changes associated with excessive neurotransmitter release are receiving increasing attention as a cause of delayed neuronal damage from trauma.[41] The effects of excessive neurotransmitters include deregulation of ion homeostasis and synthesis of several "autodestructive" neurochemical factors.

AXIOM Excessive release of excitatory amino acids after head trauma can greatly aggravate secondary brain injury.

Early experiments demonstrated that the excitatory amino acid neurotransmitters, glutamate (Glu) and aspartate (Asp), can produce cell swelling, vacuolization, and eventual cell death when applied directly to neurons.[42] They can also cause seizures and general central nervous system neuronal destruction when administered in vivo.[43] It has been hypothesized that glutamate-induced neurotoxicity may be mediated by two processes, including an early extracellular Na^+-dependent and a later Cl^--dependent neuronal disintegration.[44] Although either component can lead to irreversible neuronal injury, in vitro studies suggest that toxicity from the transmembrane influx of Ca^{++} predominates at lower glutamate concentrations.

Microdialysis techniques have demonstrated increases in many extracellular excitatory amino acid neurotransmitters after experimental brain injury.[33] Experiments on receptor subtypes after experimental brain injury have demonstrated that the excitatory amino acid agonist-receptor communication occurs predominately at NMDA-receptor subtypes.[45] In addition, injection of excitatory amino acid agonists, such as NMDA, can cause cell death by increasing Ca^{++} influx and/or free radical production.[46] Of the agents that can block the effect of excitatory amino acid neurotransmitters, the noncompetitive NMDA-receptor antagonists (e.g., phencyclidine, ketamine, dextrophan, and MK-801) have some advantages because they are more lipophilic and readily penetrate the central nervous system.[47]

Magnesium Alterations

In vivo phosphorous nuclear magnetic resonance techniques have demonstrated immediate and significant declines in intracellular free Mg^{++} concentrations after traumatic brain injury. This magnesium depletion is maximal at the site of injury and correlates directly with the severity of trauma.[48]

AXIOM Magnesium deficiencies can contribute to the severity of secondary brain injury.

Decreases in free Mg^{++} concentration can contribute to secondary injury by disruption of membrane integrity, normal cellular respiration, transcription by messenger RNA, protein synthesis, and proper glucose utilization.[49] Decreases in Mg^{++} availability could, therefore, at least partially explain the reductions in high-energy phosphate metabolism and resultant tissue acidosis after experimental brain injury.[41,49]

At normal extracellular concentrations, Mg^{++} can directly block the NMDA-receptor subtype of excitatory amino acid neurotransmitter ion channel within the brain. With Mg^{++} depletion, neuronal cells are not protected from the toxic effects of the excitatory amino acids.[49] Increased Mg^{++} concentrations, however, can block glutamate-mediated neurotoxicity in cortical cell cultures.[44]

Rats fed a magnesium-deficient diet (resulting in a 15% decrease in brain free Mg^{++} concentrations) were subjected to a standard fluid-percussion brain injury and found to have significantly worse posttraumatic neurologic dysfunction and an increased mortality.[50] Furthermore, pretreatment with Mg^{++} improved cellular function and neurologic outcome. Administration of $MgCl_2$ 30 minutes after the injury also improved post-traumatic motor and cognitive function.[51]

Gunshot Wounds of the Brain

The energy dissipated in the brain by a bullet is proportional to the square of its impact velocity.[52] The most severe wounds are produced by rifles whose bullets have an initial velocity exceeding 2000-3000 ft/sec (750m/sec). Shell fragments and bullets from handguns with a muzzle velocity of less than 1000 ft/sec (300 m/sec) produce much less destructive wounds. In considering the severe damage caused by high velocity missiles, Crockard et al[52] concluded that it must be attributed to explosively increased intracranial pressure. In his experimental primate model, the ICP peaked as high as 200 mm Hg and produced direct brain stem damage.

PRIMARY INJURIES

Scalp Injuries

Trauma to the scalp can range from mild contusions to complete avulsion from the skull. Because of its rich blood supply, a major laceration can cause hemorrhagic shock, especially in children. An apparently trivial scalp injury may also overlie a wound which has penetrated the skull and has the potential of causing severe bacterial meningitis or a brain abscess.

Skull Fractures

Most skull fractures are linear. Severe impact can produce subsidiary fracturing, resulting in a stellate pattern. If the force is great enough over a limited area, a depressed fracture can result.

AXIOM Skull fractures greatly increase the likelihood of underlying brain injury.

Linear skull fractures may correspond to an underlying brain contusion or intracranial hematoma. Linear fractures that cross the middle meningeal artery or a dural sinus can be particularly dangerous because they may be associated with development of an epidural hematoma.[5]

Depressed skull fractures are usually more serious than linear fractures because of the increased incidence of injury to underlying dural sinuses and brain tissue. Depressed fractures are particularly important if the depression is greater than the thickness of the skull. Emergency surgical intervention may be necessary if the fracture is compound, if

the dura is torn, or if intracranial vessels are ruptured.[6,53] A matter of controversy is whether or not depressed skull fractures, particularly over the motor strip of the cerebral cortex, increase the risk of seizures.

Basilar skull fractures can injure cranial nerves and blood vessels traversing the foramina at the skull base. If a fracture extends into the paranasal sinuses or mastoid air cells, it can cause a cerebrospinal fluid (CSF) leak and subsequent infection.[1]

Penetrating Injuries

Patients sustaining penetrating injuries of the brain are always at risk to develop meningitis or a brain abscess. Stab wounds about the orbits or nasal cavities are particularly prone to enter the cranium through the thin floor of the anterior fossa and cause vascular injuries and neurologic deficits[7] (Fig. 10-1).

Lacerations

Lacerations of various parts of the brain, especially the brain stem, have been reported after severe blunt head trauma. One of the areas particularly apt to tear is the pontomedullary junction, and this is most likely to occur with extreme hyperextension of the head on the neck.[54]

Concussions

Concussion refers to a transient loss of consciousness that may result from temporary dysfunction of either cortical hemispheric neurons bilaterally or the reticular activating system (RAS).[1] There is little or no apparent tissue damage with concussions; however, there is often some amnesia for events occurring just before and during the injury.

In experimental animals, mild-moderate closed-head injury designed to simulate concussion is characterized by a period of unconsciousness averaging 4 to 6 minutes, absence of skull fractures or brain contusions, and no apparent acute neurologic effects.[55] Blood flow in multiple areas of the brain; however, is depressed by an average of 25% at 45 minutes and 12% at 2 hours.

AXIOM Although cerebral concussions are generally considered mild head injuries, extensive subclinical damage may be present.

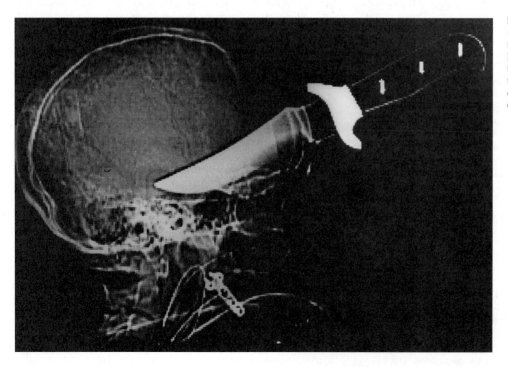

FIGURE 10-1 Low velocity penetrating injury. A hunting knife was embedded in the skull of a woman by her boyfriend. The knife was removed from the patient's frontal lobe in the OR. Subsequently the patient was found to have a pseudoaneurysm of the supraclinoid carotid artery that required clipping.

After concussion, permeability coefficient-capillary surface area products for ^{14}C sucrose, a diffusion limited tracer, are increased by 25% at 45 minutes and 32% at 2 hours, but are back to normal by 24 hours.[55] Intracranial pressure is slightly, but not significantly, elevated during the initial 6 to 8 hours; however, by 24 to 30 hours it may rise to more than 30 mm Hg. The ICP remains elevated for an additional 48 hours, and then returns to normal by 120 hours. At the time of the maximally elevated intracranial pressure, locomotor activity is also decreased. By 72 to 96 hours after trauma, cortical cellular abnormalities and fiber degeneration have also been observed.[55] The severity of the pathologic and histologic changes appears to be related to the length of unconsciousness, particularly in animals that are unconscious for more than 6 minutes.

Contusions (Fig. 10-2)

Cerebral contusions, as contrasted with concussions, imply some tissue injury with capillary damage and interstitial hemorrhage. Contusions have traditionally been labeled as coup, intermediate, or contrecoup and tend to occur in characteristic locations over the inferior frontal and temporal regions.[7] Contusions of the parietal lobe, occipital lobe, or cerebellum usually only occur with overlying fractures. Although contusions can produce some neurologic deficit, they usually exert their major effect as a nidus for hemorrhage, swelling, or post-traumatic epilepsy.[7]

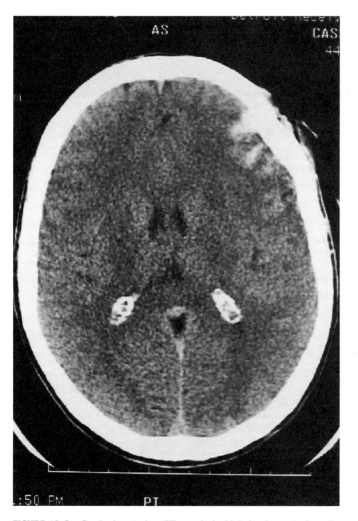

FIGURE 10-2 Cerebral contusion. CT reveals the high density contusion subjacent to a minimally depressed frontal bone fracture. The patient was managed nonoperatively and made a satisfactory recovery.

Diffuse Axonal Injury

Diffuse axonal injury (DAI) in brain-injured humans was initially characterized as a triad of damage involving: (a) the corpus callosum, (b) the dorsal lateral quadrant of the midbrain, and (c) microscopic axonal damage within subcortical white matter.[56,57]

AXIOM The magnitude and distribution of diffuse axonal injury ultimately reflect the morbidity of the head injury, particularly in patients who do not have a mass lesion.

Despite the general belief that DAI is a consistent and important feature of traumatic brain injury, there is some controversy regarding its pathogenesis. Initially it was thought that the axons tore at the moment of injury, causing the mechanically severed axon to extrude a ball of axoplasm called a "retraction ball."[57] Increasing numbers of investigators now assert that the axons are not torn at the moment of injury but rather are "perturbed," setting the stage for progressive intra-axonal changes, eventually leading to axonal disconnection.[58] There is also controversy as to whether the initial intra-axonal perturbation is related to stretching of the axolemma with an increased influx of calcium, or a focal intra-axonal cytoskeletal change.[59]

Studies by Povlishock[62] have shown that, over a course of several hours after injury, there is a discrete focal impairment of anterograde axoplasmic transport that contributes to local axonal swelling and lobulation, progressing to axonal disconnection. The swollen segment in continuity with the sustaining cell body continues to expand as a result of the continued delivery of materials via anterograde transport, and at 12-24 hours, this results in the reactive swelling of the classic "retraction balls."

In all animals analyzed, the discrete intra-axonal locus of impaired anterograde transport is always found in an axon at the point it changes its anatomic course to turn over a blood vessel, decussate, or turn to reach its target nucleus.[56] In all cases, damaged axons are found intermingled with fibers showing no morphological abnormality. With most head injuries, damaged axons can be found adjacent to foci of petechial hemorrhage; however, such vascular abnormalities do not appear to exert any influence on the overall pathogenesis of axonal swelling and disconnection.[56]

Within minutes of the traumatic event, the axons that go on to show progressive reactive change demonstrate complex infolding of the axolemma, suggesting that the axons were stretched maximally at the moment of injury and then allowed to collapse on themselves in an accordion-like fashion.[56] This stretching of the axon alters the axolemma and/or induces other biophysical changes that result in altered intra-axonal chemical function.

Intracranial Hematomas

The most frequent indication for a craniotomy after head injury is the need to evacuate an intracranial hematoma.[1] Such hematomas may occur within the brain substance (intracerebral), beneath the dura (subdural), or between the dura and the skull (epidural).

TYPES OF INTRACRANIAL HEMATOMAS

Intracerebral Hematomas (Fig. 10-3A and 10-3B)

With increasing use of CT scans, it is now recognized that intracerebral hematomas may occur in up to 23% of patients with severe head injuries.[5,7] Symptoms and signs caused by intracerebral hematomas are highly variable and depend on their size and location. Small intracerebral hematomas are best treated non-surgically by improving cerebral oxygen delivery and by keeping the ICP at normal levels; however, this can be difficult, and large accessible hematomas in severely impaired or deteriorating patients should have prompt surgical evacuation.

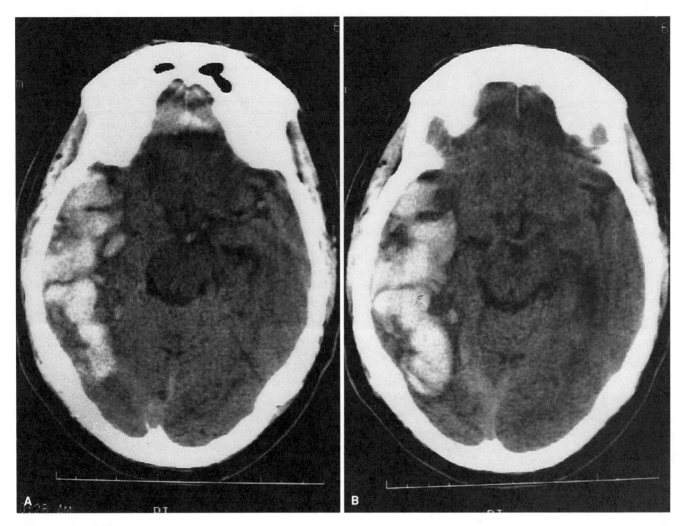

FIGURE 10-3A AND 10-3B Intracerebral hematoma. Two adjacent CT slices show high densities in the temporal lobe of this assault victim. The brain stem is not compromised, as evidenced by the preservation of the quadrigeminal plate cisterns. The patient was managed in the neuro ICU and did not require evacuation of this "pulped" tissue.

Subdural Hematomas

Subdural hematomas may be acute (presenting within 24 hours of injury) (Fig. 10-4A and 10-4B), subacute (presenting between 24 hours and 10 days), or chronic (presenting after 10 days) (Fig. 10-5A and 10-5B).[5] They are most commonly the result of rupture of veins that bridge the space between the brain and the dura. Clinical signs are variable, depending on the size and location of the hematoma and the severity of the injury to the underlying brain.

AXIOM   Much of the relatively poor prognosis associated with acute subdural hematomas is due to the underlying brain damage.

Except for small asymptomatic collections, acute subdural hematomas are best treated by prompt craniotomy and evacuation.[6] The preoperative increased ICP and midline shift may persist after evacuation of the hematoma. Consequently, intensive medical treatment must continue into the postoperative period.[6]

Chronic subdural hematomas and subacute hematomas which have liquified and develop more than a week following injury can often be treated by evacuation and continuing drainage through burr holes rather than through the large bone flap which is often required for drainage of acute collections.[60]

Epidural Hematomas (Fig. 10-6)

AXIOM   Epidural hematomas are uncommon, but with prompt surgical evacuation, usually have a good prognosis.

Epidural hematomas are relatively uncommon, occuring in only about 3% of patients with severe head trauma.[5] They result from stripping of the dura from the skull, and are usually associated with temporal bone fractures with resultant laceration of the middle meningeal artery. Expansion of the hematoma causes further dural separation. The classic clinical course includes an initial period of unconsciousness from the primary insult (concussion), then neurologic recovery ("lucid interval"), followed over several hours by headache, loss of consciousness, and progressive neurologic deterioration.

AXIOM   A lucid interval should warrant special efforts to rule out an acute epidural hematoma.

Unfortunately, only a minority of patients with epidural hematomas show the classic picture.[5] Alcoholic patients with a chronically shrunken brain and an acute subdural hematoma may have a lucid interval. About a third of the patients with epidural hematomas never regain consciousness, and about a third never lose it. Unfortunately, once a patient with an epidural hematoma loses consciousness, neu-

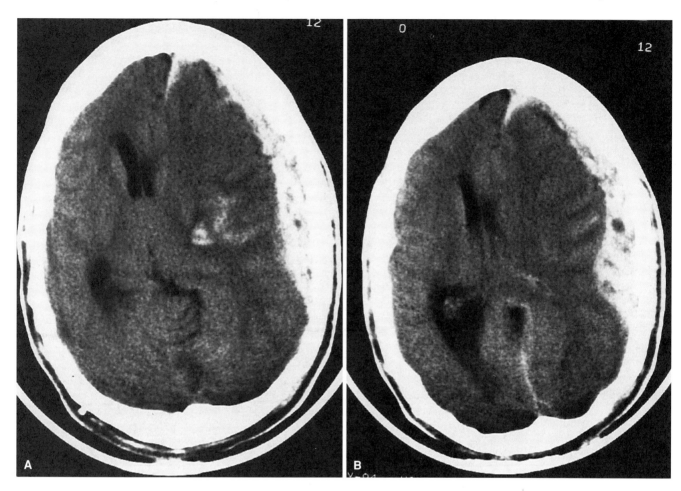

FIGURE 10-4A AND 10-4B Acute subdural hematomas. Two adjacent CT slices demonstrate the crescent density of a large acute subdural hematoma. Massive shift of the midline structures and hemorrhage in the subjacent white matter is present.

rological deterioration may progress rapidly. As with other symptomatic intracranial hematomas, treatment is emergency surgical evacuation. If symptoms are progressing rapidly, intravenous mannitol (50-100 g) and hyperventilation to a PCO_2 of 25-30 mm Hg may gain some time while the patient is rushed to the operating room.[61]

CEREBRAL BLOOD FLOW

Normal Cerebral Blood Flow

Normal cerebral blood flow (CBF) is approximately 50-65 ml/100 g /min.[26] Changes in the EEG occur if the blood flow falls below 25 ml/ 100 g/min, and the threshold for infarction is about 18 ml/100 g/min. Under normal circumstances, if the arterial blood contains 12 ml of oxygen per 100 ml blood (12 vol%), the blood in the jugular bulb will contain 6 vol%. This arteriovenous oxygen difference of 6 vol% or less generally indicates a cerebral oxygen consumption of at least 30 ml/100 gm brain tissue/min.

Local cerebral blood flow is regulated by several factors, including $PaCO_2$, PaO_2, blood pressure, and cerebrovascular resistance (CVR). For every 1 mm Hg decrease in $PaCO_2$ (between 20 and 60 mm Hg), cerebral blood flow decreases 2% to 3%.[62] Thus, a $PaCO_2$ less than 20-25 mm Hg may cause cerebral blood flow to be less than half normal. Hypoxia has little effect on cerebral blood flow until the PO_2 is less than 50 mm Hg, but a decline in the PaO_2 from 50 to 30 mm Hg will usually double cerebral blood flow.

Cerebral perfusion pressure (CPP), defined as the difference between mean systemic arterial pressure and the intracranial pressure, is the pressure gradient across the brain that drives cerebral blood flow.[63] The CPP is also equal to the product of the CBF and CVR (i.e., CPP=CBF x CVR). In the basal state, there is a dynamic interplay of vasoconstriction and vasodilation in the cerebral vascular bed that allows coupling of cerebral blood flow to its metabolic needs over a wide range of CPP. This autoregulation generally is lost if the CPP decreases to less than 50 mm Hg.[63]

When cerebral blood flow is reduced, the brain may extract up to 67% of the oxygen from the blood to maintain cerebral metabolism, decreasing jugular bulb oxygen saturation to about 30-33%.[64] In patients with a Hb of 15.0 gm/dl and arterial O_2 saturation of 98%, the arterial O_2 content will be 20 vol%. If the jugular bulb oxygen saturation is 48%, then 10 vol% oxygen is being extracted, indicating the presence of cerebral ischemia.

AXIOM It is now generally felt that an arteriovenous oxygen difference of 8 ml/dl or more or a jugular bulb oxygen saturation less than 50% is an indication of cerebral ischemia after severe head injury.[23,64]

Cerebral Blood Flow After Head Injury

A number of factors can alter cerebral blood flow (CBF) after head injury.[65] The normal relationship between cerebral blood flow, mean

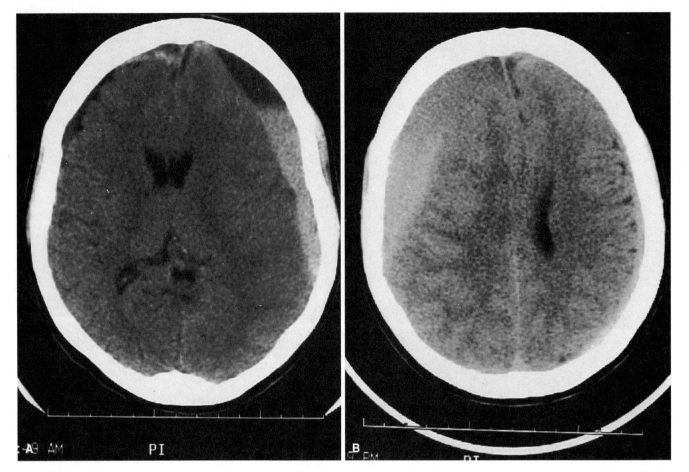

FIGURE 10-5A AND 10-5B Chronic subdural hematomas. Figure 10-5A: The CT shows an extra axial collection with a "hematocrit" density. The patient, a woman with Huntington's disease (note enlarged frontal horns), did well following trephination. Figure 10-5B: The same patient returned several weeks later with a second chronic subdural on the opposite side that required a second operation.

arterial blood pressure, intracranial pressure, and cerebral perfusion pressure may be disturbed in patients with brain injury, particularly if intracranial pressure is increased.[65,66] Because of disturbances in autoregulation, significant decreases in mean arterial blood pressure tend to cause corresponding decreases in cerebral blood flow. Similarly, increases in mean arterial blood pressure may increase cerebral blood flow, but intracranial pressure also tends to increase.[65,66]

Even after cerebral autoregulation has been lost, sensitivity to PCO_2 may remain, and the effect of hypocarbia in lowering intracranial pressure may persist.[65,66] Loss of this response renders the injured brain particularly susceptible to damage from further elevations in intracranial pressure.

> **AXIOM** Even in the absence of increased intracranial pressure, hypercarbia, or hypoxemia, endotracheal intubation of patients with severe head injury is generally indicated for prevention of secondary hypoxic brain damage.[67]

An increasing number of studies show that injured brain tissue has a reduced cerebral blood flow. Yoshino et al[68] performed dynamic computed tomography scanning on 42 patients within 6 to 12 hours of severe head injury and found that 68% (17/25) of the fatally injured patients were severely ischemic. Nonfatal injuries were more aptly associated with a hyperemic brain.

> **AXIOM** Although cerebral blood flow does not correlate with outcome in all head injuries, it appears to be a significant factor in patients with severe injury.[69]

Using xenon Xe 133 to measure cerebral blood flow, Muizelaar[23] found that of 186 patients with head trauma and a GCS of 8 or less, 24 (13%) had global cerebral ischemia (CBF of 18 ml/100 gm/min or less). These low flows were most frequent in the first 6 hours after trauma and were associated with a higher mortality rate and poorer neurologic outcome. Of the 24 patients with cerebral ischemia, 15 (63%) continued to be vegetative or died. Of the other 160 patients with severe cerebral injury who were not ischemic, only 59 (37%) had a similar poor outcome (P below 0.04).

In a similar study of 62 patients with severe head trauma, 12 (19%) had evidence of regional ischemia, and of these 12 patients, 9 (75%) died. Of 50 other patients with no evidence of regional brain ischemia, none died (P below 0.001).

Cerebral Blood Flow in the Presence of Mass Lesions

Intracranial mass lesions are tolerated better in the presence of adequate cerebral perfusion.[70] As intracranial pressure rises, the cerebral vasculature attempts to compensate by vasodilating in an attempt to maintain cerebral blood flow.[70]

In patients with severe head injury (GCS of 7 or less), Rosner and Coley[71] noted that patients with a CPP of 70 mm Hg or higher had

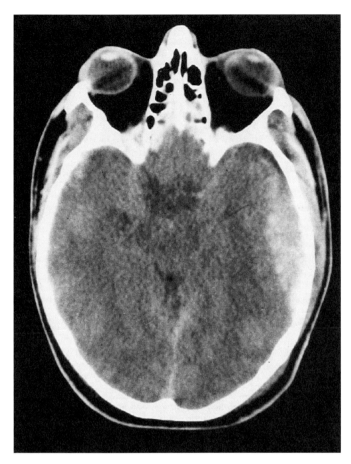

FIGURE 10-6 Epidural hematoma. CT shows a biconvex density in the middle cranial fossa. The patient, an assault victim, made a good recovery after emergency craniotomy.

lower intracranial pressures (26 ± 3 versus 34 ± 4 mm Hg), higher systolic arterial blood pressures (107 ± 4 versus 83 ± 5 mm Hg), and higher central venous pressures (7 ± 1.4 versus 5 ± 1.7 mm Hg).[71]

After a mannitol infusion, patients in the low cerebral perfusion pressure group showed a 60% decline in intracranial pressure and a 50 to 60% increase in cerebral perfusion pressure.[71] Thus, they hypothesized that the mannitol bolus resulted in a beneficial autoregulatory response by the cerebral vasculature that improved oxygen delivery.[63,71]

Managing Cerebral Blood Flow in the Head-Injured Patient

MANNITOL
The initial management of head-injured patients with increased intracranial pressure typically includes intubation, hyperventilation, and mannitol infusion. When given as a bolus, mannitol augments intravascular volume, resulting in a transient increase in blood volume, systolic arterial blood pressure, and cerebral perfusion pressure.[63,71] In the presence of intact autoregulation, mannitol causes reflex cerebral vasoconstriction and an immediate decline in intracranial pressure by much as 27% with a corresponding improvement in cerebral perfusion pressure.[72,73] In patients with impaired autoregulation, mannitol infusion will only decrease intracranial pressure by about 5%, but cerebral blood flow may increase by as much as 17%.[72,73] Thus, vasoconstriction enhances the dehydrating effects of mannitol in patients with intact autoregulatory responses, whereas with altered autoregulation, mannitol increases cerebral blood flow, and this appears to attenuate its osmotic effects.[73]

The osmotic effects of mannitol typically occur 10 to 20 minutes after administration, which is in contrast to the hemodynamic effects that are manifested almost immediately.[71] Mannitol also improves microcirculatory blood flow.[73] The hemodilution caused by the mannitol decreases blood viscosity, and this improves cerebral blood flow and decreases red blood cell aggregation at the capillary level. However, mannitol, if given very rapidly in large doses, can cause a transient hypotension by dilating skeletal muscle vessels. The degree of hypotension is related to the dose and rate of administration of mannitol.[74] In patients with marginal cerebral blood flow and impaired cerebral autoregulation, such hypotension could be a problem.

DIMETHYL SULFOXIDE
Resuscitation with dimethyl sulfoxide in saline can decrease intracranial pressure and increase cerebral oxygen delivery.[75] This agent also has other numerous potential benefits including free radical scavenging, diuresis, improved cerebral perfusion pressure, and decreased platelet aggregation; however, its use is still primarily experimental.

HYPERTONIC SALINE
Hypertonic saline improves cerebral perfusion pressure by augmenting intravascular volume, but its improvement of oxygen delivery at the microcirculatory level may be independent of its effects on intravascular volume.[76] Hypertonic saline may also reduce the tendency to cerebral edema, but it is not routinely used in the management of head injury.

HYPERVENTILATION
Hyperventilation reduces intracranial pressure by constricting pial and cerebral arterioles.[77] Several studies, however, have shown that hyperventilation provides only a temporary reduction in cerebral blood vessel diameter because of rapid return of the brain interstitial pH to normal levels.[78] Prolonged hyperventilation also increases vessel reactivity to changes in PaO_2 so that any hypoxemia can rapidly cause severe damage.[79] In addition, the alkalosis of prolonged hyperventilation shifts the oxygen hemoglobin dissociation curve to the left, thereby reducing the amount of oxygen available to the tissues.[77]

INCREASED INTRACRANIAL PRESSURE

Traumatic Cerebral Swelling

Most traumatic cerebral edema is vasogenic, resulting from increased leakage of plasma ultrafiltrate through hyperpermeable capillary membranes into the extracellular space. However, there is also some cytotoxic edema as a result of cellular injury from the trauma itself and from hypoxic or ischemic insults. The cytotoxic edema from hypoxia or ischemia primarily affects astrocytes in the gray matter.

Cerebral hyperemia after trauma is thought to result from cerebrovascular autoregulation, and it may be regional or involve the entire brain.[7] Hyperemia involving only one hemisphere generally occurs after evacuation of a unilateral acute subdural hematoma. Diffuse, severe cerebral engorgement was initially thought to be more frequent in children and adolescents. However, it is now clear that diffuse cerebral hyperemia causing elevated intracranial pressure may also occur in adults.

Factors Affecting Intracranial Pressure

Intracranial pressure (ICP) changes are related to the interaction of the cranial contents (brain tissue, blood, and CSF) within their rigid container of dura and calvarium.[6] The observation that variations in intracranial pressure may influence survival after head trauma goes back over 200 years. In 1783 Alexander Monro (Secundus), a Scottish surgeon who like his father and son held the Chair of Anatomy at Edinburgh, published his famous article[80] in which he described a relationship between the volume of the contents (brain and blood) and the pressure within the skull. George Kellie wrote a paper[81] in 1824 that supported Monro's thesis, and Burrows in 1846[82] modified the Monro-Kellie hypothesis by identifying three intracranial components: blood, brain, and CSF. He believed that a change in any one of the components would cause a change in the others in reciprocal fashion, so that the intracranial volume remained constant, otherwise the intracranial pressure would rise.

The average intracranial volume in adult humans is approximately 1600 ml. Of this, about 80% is brain, 10% is blood, and 10% is CSF.[83] If the brain swells or there is an intracranial hematoma, the CSF is displaced into the spinal subarachnoid space and blood is displaced into extracranial veins. As long as there is displaceable blood or CSF, an increase in intracranial volume causes only a small rise in ICP. Once there is no more blood or CSF to displace, the ICP rises rapidly with any further increase in intracranial volume (Fig. 10-7).

With increasing brain edema or an intracranial hematoma, CSF decreases to maintain a constant intracranial volume. As ICP rises, the absorption of CSF increases logarithmically until an equilibrium is reached, generally at a higher than normal ICP.[84] Marmarou et al[84] have determined that vascular mechanisms account for about two-thirds of the intracranial volume adjustments in head-injured patients, whereas CSF changes are responsible for about a third.

> **AXIOM** After head injury, the ability of the brain to reduce CSF in response to a rising ICP can be severely limited.

The compensatory decrease in CSF with an increased ICP is lost if the expansion of an intracranial hematoma is so rapid that it causes brain herniation into the tentorium or foramen magnum blocking the CSF exit into the spinal subarachnoid space.[5] Under such circumstances, decompensation may occur at a relatively low ICP.

Intracranial resistance ($\Delta P/\Delta V$), the reciprocal of intracranial compliance, is determined relatively easily in patients with a ventricular catheter or subarachnoid bolt.[5] One can either rapidly add or withdraw 1.0 ml from the CSF and measure the pressure response. The

pressure-volume curve from this maneuver can be estimated by the formula:[85]

$$PVI = \frac{\Delta V}{\log_{10} \dfrac{P_1}{P_2}}$$

The pressure-volume index (PVI) is the volume of fluid required to increase ICP by a factor of 10. It is normally about 25 ml. It decreases soon after brain injury, and the decline in PVI may precede and predict the severity of a subsequent rise in ICP.[86] A declining PVI can provide an early warning of impending herniation, and a severely reduced PVI (10 ml or less) is generally seen in patients who subsequently develop uncontrolled intracranial hypertension.

> **AXIOM** A declining PVI may be an early warning of an impending dangerous rise in ICP.

The significance of an elevated ICP is not completely understood.[5] Most of the clinical signs attributed to an elevated ICP in brain trauma are actually produced by changes in the brain or cerebral circulation that cause the same processes that elevate the ICP. An increased ICP by itself, as in pseudotumor cerebri, can cause papilledema, but it is usually associated with only mild clinical changes such as headache, vomiting, and drowsiness, even at pressures as high as 90 mm Hg. However, in head-injured patients with an elevated ICP, the rapid brain damage or distortion from intracranial hematomas is more serious and can cause severe reflex cardiovascular and respiratory changes.

> **AXIOM** Regardless of the cause of an elevated ICP in head trauma, inability to promptly reduce it to less than 20 mm Hg is generally indicative of a poor prognosis.

Most therapeutic measures in patients with severe head injuries are directed at preventing or reducing an elevated ICP.[5] Indeed, there is a strong correlation between ICP level and outcome.[87] According to the generally accepted criteria, a normal ICP is 10 mm Hg or less. An ICP of 10 to 20 mm Hg requires careful observation, and any ICP above 20 mm Hg should be treated urgently. Indeed, the prognosis of patients with persistent or irreversible high ICP (more than 30-50 mm Hg) is very poor.

Intracranial Pressure Monitoring

INTRODUCTION

Intracranial pressure (ICP) monitoring with intraventricular catheters was begun by Guillaume and Janny in 1951,[88] and its value was emphasized by Lundberg[89] in 1960. Because of the need for a less invasive method, the subarachnoid bolt was developed,[90] and then described by Vries in 1979. Subsequently, fiberoptic catheters were developed to provide monitoring that was even less invasive.

Ward emphasizes several fundamental points about ICP monitoring.[91] First, the information obtained is only as reliable as the system providing the information. If the monitor is not properly inserted or if the system is not properly calibrated, the information may be meaningless. Second, ICP monitoring provides information about only one aspect of the patient's condition. The ICP is of little value without knowledge of the disease being treated, the overall clinical condition of the patient, and the ICP dynamics.[91]

INDICATIONS

> **AXIOM** ICP monitoring is indicated in patients who have severe head injuries (i.e., GCS of 8 or less) after adequate resuscitation.

The main indications for ICP monitoring in trauma are: (a) when it is important to determine if the ICP is elevated, (b) if there is a

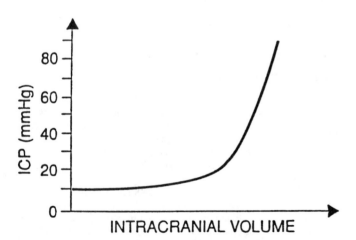

FIGURE 10-7 Relationship between intracranial volume (IVC) and intracranial pressure (ICP). As the volume of one compartment (tissue, cerebrospinal fluid, intravascular blood, or hematoma) increases, the initial compensation by reducing the other compartment volumes is adequate; however, once a critical intracranial volume is obtained, intracranial pressure rises rapidly.

reasonable chance that the ICP is significantly elevated, (c) when treatment is to be undertaken for an elevated ICP, and/or (d) when frequent, accurate assessment of neurologic status is not possible.

ICP MONITORING DEVICES

Several methods of ICP measurement are available.[91] A ventricular catheter connected to a standard strain gauge transducer not only allows continuous ICP monitoring, but also permits withdrawal of CSF as needed or desired to control an elevated ICP. However, it may be difficult to insert such a catheter when hematoma or diffuse brain swelling distorts and/or decreases the size of the lateral ventricles.

Although a subarachnoid bolt is easily inserted under almost any circumstances, it may provide erroneous readings, depending on its placement relative to the site of injury.[91] Epidural bolts have the lowest risk of complications, but they are less accurate than ventricular catheters or subarachnoid bolts and do not permit withdrawal of CSF.

Many centers now monitor the ICP using an intracerebral fiberoptic sensor (Camino Labs, San Diego, CA) that is easy to place and can provide accurate information.[5] The choice of methods is best left to the judgment and experience of the neurosurgeon. If facilities for ICP monitoring are not available, one should assume that the ICP is elevated if the GCS is 7 or less and begin appropriate therapy.

Complications of Increased ICP

CEREBRAL BLOOD FLOW

At any given mean BP, a rise in ICP will reduce the CPP, which should be maintained around 70 to 110 mm Hg to ensure adequate blood supply to the brain.

AXIOM Although a moderate rise in arterial pressure may help maintain the CPP, an exaggerated effect may be harmful.

As part of the Cushing response to an increased ICP, about 20% of patients will develop significant systemic hypertension. Although some rise in BP may produce a beneficial rise in CPP, severe systemic hypertension, by increasing capillary filtration pressures and transcapillary fluid movement into damaged areas, may increase brain swelling and cause further elevation of ICP and ischemia.[92]

AXIOM The management of blood pressure in patients with head injury must tread the fine line between maintenance of adequate cerebral perfusion and exacerbation of cerebral edema.

Maintenance of an adequate CBF in areas of brain injury can be extremely difficult, particularly with loss of cerebral autoregulation.[5] Alterations in the arterial blood gases may further complicate maintenance of an adequate cerebral perfusion, especially in the area of injury.

At $PaCO_2$ levels between 20 and 80 mm Hg, a $PaCO_2$ increase of 1.0 mm Hg will increase CBF by approximately 1.0 to 1.5 ml/100 g/min (i.e., about 2-3%). If the $PaCO_2$ falls below 20-25 mm Hg, CBF may fall to levels that can cause cerebral ischemia, especially in areas of trauma.

AXIOM An arterial $PaCO_2$ less than 25 mm Hg may significantly impair cerebral perfusion.

Arterial oxygen tension has minimal effect on CBF until it falls below 50 mm Hg, at which point, the CBF rises rapidly with further hypoxemia (Fig. 10-8).[93] This effect may be lost, at least partially, in areas of brain injury as a result of local increases in lactic acid.[94]

It is generally accepted that blood gas changes have their greatest effects in undamaged brain.[95] Thus, production of cerebral vasoconstriction (caused by a decreased $PaCO_2$) in uninjured areas of the

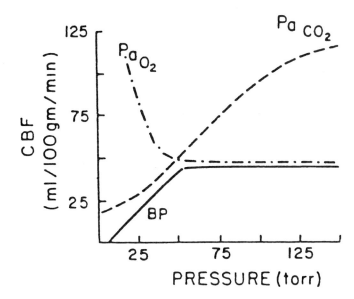

FIGURE 10-8 Cerebral blood flow. Response to changes in PaO_2, $PaCO_2$, and mean arterial blood pressure. (From: Shapiro HM. Intracranial hypertension: therapeutic and anesthetic considerations. Anesthesiology 1975;43:445.)

brain may shunt blood to the damaged area producing an "inverse steal" phenomenon. However, if extensive intravascular coagulation or severe perivascular exudation has occurred, circulation in the area of injury may remain extremely low regardless of what is done.[96]

Although studies have shown no significant correlation between isolated measurements of CBF and the severity of injury or prognosis, an increasing CBF is usually associated with improvement, whereas a decreasing CBF tends to indicate a poor outcome.[5] In general, a CBF of at least 18-20 ml/100 g of brain/min is regarded as the minimal amount needed to maintain cerebral viability under normal circumstances.[23,26] However, considerably higher flows are probably needed in areas of injury to control the accumulation of lactic acid and to prevent secondary injury.

Since there is only one (occasionally incompetent) valve in each internal jugular vein[97] and no valves in the vertebral veins, the ICP will vary somewhat with the CVP and the degree of head elevation. Thus, increased intrathoracic pressure, as from controlled ventilation, coughing, or straining, hypervolemia, jugular venous obstruction, or a head-down position, can all increase cerebral venous pressure and ICP.

BRAIN HERNIATION

As a result of supratentorial swelling and/or hematoma, the brain may herniate through the dural hiatuses or the foramen magnum.[75] Herniation of the medial portion of the temporal lobe through the tentorial hiatus causes midbrain compression, which can result in loss of consciousness and decerebrate rigidity. Compression of the oculomotor nerve on the tentorium results in dilatation of the ipsilateral pupil. At the same time, there is often a herniation of the cingulate gyrus under the falx cerebri (pericallosal herniation). This may be severe enough to compress the anterior cerebral artery and produce weakness of the contralateral lower extremity.

AXIOM If, after head trauma, a decompressive craniotomy is not performed before herniation occurs, a successful outcome is very unlikely.

Axial herniation of the brain stem through the foramen magnum can greatly reduce arterial blood flow to the central medulla.[5,7] This can cause the Cushing response which includes systemic hypertension, bradycardia, and respiratory irregularities. If the cerebellar tonsils also herniate through the foramen magnum, the increased direct brain stem compression can cause even more medullary ischemia and symptoms.

Although the process of herniation initially progresses rather slowly, an abrupt progression may finally occur, producing sudden apnea because of axial herniation of the medulla through the foramen magnum. Bilateral decerebrate rigidity may also develop abruptly because of cerebellar herniation upward through the tentorial hiatus. This process may be precipitated by release of fluid from the lateral ventricles.

ISCHEMIC BRAIN INJURY

Hemorrhagic necrosis of the medial temporal lobes and brain stem tegmentum (Duret's hemorrhages), as well as infarctions in the distribution of the posterior cerebral artery, may result from transtentorial herniation.[7] Focal ischemic lesions in arterial watershed regions, as well as diffuse pseudolaminar necrosis and homogenizing necrosis of cortical neurons, have also been described.[54] Episodes of hypoxia, systemic hypotension, and intracranial hypertension are frequent in such patients. Cerebral vasospasm, which may decrease cerebral blood flow, has also been demonstrated angiographically in some of these head-injured patients.[71,98]

DIAGNOSIS

History

Efforts should be made to learn the details of the accident. It is particularly important to obtain information about any changes in the level of consciousness or other neurologic function occurring before the initial examination in the hospital. One should also try to determine the presence or absence of a period of unconsciousness; however, it may be difficult at times to differentiate between a dazed state and true unconsciousness. The presence of amnesia can be indicative in this regard.

AXIOM   In general, marked and prolonged retrograde amnesia indicates a more serious head injury and more prolonged period of initial unconsciousness.

If the period of unconsciousness was short (i.e., less than 5 minutes), patients with a completely normal neurological examination should still be carefully observed for at least 6 to 12 hours.[1,5,7] Frequently this can be done in the emergency department. Patients with periods of unconsciousness lasting more than 5 minutes, even with no neurological changes, should be observed closely for at least 24 hours. Such observation may require admission to a special neurosurgical unit.

The past medical history should be pursued, with particular reference to seizure disorders, anticoagulant therapy, bleeding problems, hypertension, heart disease, previous neurologic disorders, and drug or alcohol use.

Physical Examination

PITFALL ⊘

Failure to look carefully beyond the obvious head injury in patients with blunt trauma.

An important complicating factor in patients with head injuries is the high incidence of associated injuries. At least one in four patients with blunt head injury has associated injuries of other parts of the body, with the greatest number of problems involving the extremities, face, and chest.[1] Up to 6% of head-injured patients were found to have coincident cervical spine injuries, and 26% of cervical-spinal injured patients were found to have head injuries.[99]

AXIOM   Any tendency to hypoxemia or hypotension should be corrected before performing a complete neurologic examination.

The patient's head is examined carefully for injury, including signs of basilar skull fracture. These include periorbital ecchymoses (raccoon's eyes), subscleral hemorrhage, retroauricular hematoma (Battle's sign), hemotympanum, and CSF rhinorrhea or otorrhea. The carotid arteries in the neck are palpated and auscultated, and the presence of ecchymosis or hematomas overlying them is noted.

NEUROLOGIC EVALUATION

AXIOM   All patients with major trauma should be assumed to have a head injury and cervical spine fracture until proven otherwise.

As soon as possible, a complete neurologic evaluation should be performed on all seriously injured patients. This may not be possible initially in unstable patients; however, as part of a minineurological examination, one should evaluate and record the level of consciousness and pupillary and motor responses.

AXIOM   The sine qua non of head-injury management is repetitive careful neurological examinations and timely intervention.

Mental Status

The mental status and state of consciousness usually provide the most sensitive indication of the amount of brain injury and any tendency to deteriorate.[1] The ability to speak and follow commands after trauma is key. Patients who are unable to do so have a much higher incidence of serious brain injury and a much poorer prognosis. To qualify these findings, the Glasgow Coma score should be recorded at least every 15 to 30 minutes during the early stages of injury (Table 10-2). Since one-third of the Glasgow Coma score is based on verbal response, allowance must be made for this in patients who are intubated. For example, an intubated patient who opens his eyes to pain and withdraws an extremity from pain has a Glasgow Coma score of 6/10. The presence of drugs, alcohol, or severe hypotension or hypoxemia can greatly affect the state of consciousness and should also be noted.

AXIOM   One cannot rely on neurologic assessments until adequate perfusion and oxygenation has been obtained.

Severe hypotension, even without a brain injury, can cause a patient to be comatose. For example, pupils that are fixed and dilated during a cardiac arrest often become small and reactive if cerebral perfusion is rapidly re-established.

A small, but important, subgroup of patients with brain injury are those who "talk and deteriorate."[17,100] They are patients who utter

---

TABLE 10-2 Glasgow Coma Scale

1. Eye Opening	
Spontaneous	4
To Voice	3
To Pain	2
None	1
2. Verbal Response	
Oriented	5
Confused	4
Inappropriate Words	3
Incomprehensible Words	2
None	1
3. Motor Response	
Obeys Command	6
Purposeful Movement (pain)	5
Withdraw (pain)	4
Flexion (pain)	3
Extension (pain)	2
None	1
Total GCS Points (1 + 2 + 3)	3 - 16

recognizable words at some time after the injury and then deteriorate to a GCS of 8 or less. Patients who talk and deteriorate comprise only 1 to 2% of all patients sustaining closed-head injury,[27,109] but they represent approximately 10 to 20% of all patients sustaining severe head injury.

Pupillary Response

AXIOM Any change in the size, shape, or reactivity of a pupil after head trauma may indicate early herniation.

The size, shape, and reactivity of the pupils to light allow evaluation of the integrity of the second and third cranial nerves and the midbrain.[7] Marshall et al[101] emphasized the importance of an oval pupil as a sign of impending transtentorial herniation. Not infrequently, a unilateral dilating pupil that is still reactive to light may be the first sign of an expanding mass in the temporal lobe or an epidural hematoma in the middle fossa. The reaction of the pupils to light, the extraocular movements, and the visual fields should also be carefully checked, if possible.

AXIOM Although a dilated or fixed pupil in an injured patient is usually due to an intracranial hematoma and/or brain damage, it may also be caused by expanding intracranial aneurysms, hypoxia, hypotension, seizures, eye trauma, direct injury to the third cranial nerve, and various drugs.

Eye Movements

The examiner may evaluate extraocular movements by noting spontaneous eye movements and, where appropriate, by performing oculocephalic or oculo-vestibular maneuvers.[7] These reflex eye movements can be elicited by turning the patient's head (if the cervical spine has been cleared), and thus, stimulating the vestibular apparatus (oculocephalic or doll's eye response) or by irrigating the external auditory canal with cold or warm water (oculovestibular or caloric response).

The oculocephalic reflex is elicited by holding the patient's eyes open and rotating the head sharply from neutral to the right and from neutral to the left.[7] If the oculocephalic reflex is normal, the patient's eyes will lag behind the head, but catch up to the position of neutrality shortly. If the eye moves with the moving head, the oculocephalic reflex is abnormal and it indicates that there is injury within the brain stem.

With caloric testing, the patient lies supine with his head elevated 30°.[7] The integrity of the tympanic membrane should be ascertained by direct inspection before irrigating the ear. Using a tuberculin syringe, 0.2 cc of ice water is instilled deep into the external ear canal. The nystagmus (fast component) is normally toward the opposite ear in an awake patient and to the same side in a comatose patient. It is important to note the symmetry or the response in each ear. This response should last about a minute. The caloric response is the most sensitive of the eye movement tests and is the obvious choice in patients with possible cervical spine injury.

These responses test the third, sixth, and eighth cranial nerves and nuclei as well as the ascending brain stem pathways from the pontomedullary junction to the mesencephalon.[7] Obviously, injury to the vestibular apparatus or its nerve can also impair these reflexes.

Motor Responses

AXIOM A new focal motor deficit is an important sign that the patient needs immediate, aggressive care.

The patient's movements in response to various stimuli should be noted. Purposeful movement indicates intact motor pathways from the cortex on down, whereas abnormal flexor and extensor posturing are generally signs of severe neurological impairment.[7] Deep tendon reflexes and passive muscle tone in the extremities should be assessed

for symmetry. Sensory examinations in serious head injury are usually limited to the response to various noxious stimuli.

Other Cranial Nerves

After trauma, it can be helpful to note the function of the first cranial nerve.[1] Simple solutions with a distinctive odor (methylsalicylate, rose water, tincture of benzoin, etc.) can be used to determine the presence or absence of the function of smell.

The sensory function of the fifth cranial nerve and the motor function of the seventh cranial nerve can be checked by examination of the corneal reflexes.[1]

Gross examination of hearing should be carried out, and the external ear canals should be carefully examined for CSF drainage and for bleeding through or behind the tympanic membranes.

The functions of the lower cranial nerves 10 and 12 should not be overlooked. These may be evaluated by observing the patient's ability to swallow and the function of the palate and tongue during that process.

Other Tests

The ability to perform rapid alternating movements, finger-to-nose and finger-to-finger pursuits, and movement of the heel down the shin can screen for slight degrees of weakness and for cerebellar dysfunction in patients who are fairly well awake.[1] One should also carefully examine station and gait.

REPEATED NEUROLOGIC EXAMINATIONS

AXIOM Proper observation of a head-injury patient means repeated careful neurological examinations.

Repeated neurological examination is the key to the proper evaluation and management of patients with possible neurosurgical problems. The state of consciousness and other neurologic functions in patients who require neurosurgical intervention are seldom constant except in the terminal irreversible stages.

VENTILATORY PATTERNS

AXIOM A significant deterioration in the state of consciousness is almost invariably associated with an alteration of the ventilatory pattern.[3]

Although central neurogenic hyperventilation is common after head injury, many of these patients exhibit some degree of respiratory depression. Consequently, the airway should be cleared and intubation performed at the first suspicion of inadequate ventilatory effort or of depressed gag or cough reflexes.

Early ventilatory support is important in patients with severe head injury. Although "adequate" ventilation in a non-head injury patient may provide a $PaCO_2$ of about 40 mm Hg, if a severe head injury is present, the patient should usually be ventilated enough to maintain the $PaCO_2$ between 35 and 40 mm Hg with a PaO_2 of 80-100 mm Hg.

A normal ventilatory pattern in an easily arousable patient generally indicates a mild, unilateral injury. Moderate-severe brain injuries are usually associated with some degree of ventilatory depression. More severe injuries may be associated with several types of abnormal ventilatory patterns,[102] including central neurogenic hyperventilation and various types of phasic respiration.

Central Neurogenic Hyperventilation

AXIOM Central neurogenic hyperventilation is the most frequent type of abnormal breathing in patients with moderate-severe head-injuries.

Central neurogenic hyperventilation is usually associated with severe cerebral acidosis and/or localized hypoxia, pontine damage, or tentorial herniation.[103] It may also be a reflection of a marked increase in metabolism. Although the resultant hypocapnia is usually mild-moderate, excessive hyperventilation may occasionally lower the $PaCO_2$ so far that the resultant severe vasoconstriction may produce further cerebral ischemia.

Phasic Respiratory Patterns

There are three types of phasic respiration seen with CNS problems.[6] Some patients exhibit a Cheyne-Strokes variant, which is a regular, cyclic variation in respiratory depth from hyperventilation to hypoventilation without apneic periods. This pattern is generally associated with a rather mild degree of coma.

True Cheyne-Strokes respiration consists of regular cycles of hyperventilation followed by apnea.[5] It probably results from an exaggerated ventilatory response to increasing $PaCO_2$. This hyperpnea then lowers the $PaCO_2$ to the point at which the respiratory drive is abolished until reaccumulation of CO_2 again stimulates hyperventilation. True Cheyne-Strokes respiration is usually associated with deep coma and generally indicates severe brain injury.

Ataxic ventilation is characterized by inspiratory and expiratory phases that are irregular in both rate and amplitude, with intervening periods of apnea.[5] This pattern is also described as gasping or cluster breathing with expiratory pauses. The respiratory rate is usually slow, and the minute ventilation is significantly decreased. This is generally an indicator of brain stem damage and is almost always a terminal sign.

HEMODYNAMIC CHANGES

Hypertension is common after severe brain injury, probably as a result of central sympathetic stimulation. Although there is a tendency to rapidly begin treatment of such hypertension, it is best not to do so until the extent of injury, the presence of mass lesions, and the ICP and CPP have been determined.[5]

AXIOM Hypotension is extremely dangerous in patients with head injury and must be corrected as soon as possible.

Even with a normal aortic pressure, the cerebral circulation, especially in injured areas, is usually decreased in patients with head trauma.[96] Since cerebral autoregulation is also impaired, hypotension can be extremely dangerous.

In most trauma patients, hypotension results from bleeding or high spinal cord damage. An associated spinal cord injury is seen in approximately 6% of head-injured patients admitted to the hospital.[99,102] If hypotension is a result of high spinal cord damage, the skin is usually warm and the pulse rate is relatively slow. If the hypotension is a result of hypovolemia, the skin tends to be cool and clammy, and the pulse rate is relatively fast. In patients with isolated brain injury, hypotension does not usually occur until there is terminal medullary failure, and this is usually associated with other terminal signs including bradycardia, pupillary dilatation, and agonal or absent respirations.[103]

AXIOM Hypotension in a patient with adequate or increased ventilation generally results from associated non-cerebral injuries.

If the patient is hypotensive, large-bore peripheral intravenous lines are started, and crystalloids, colloids, and/or blood are given as needed to promptly restore an adequate blood volume and tissue perfusion. Vasopressors should generally be avoided because their effects on the cerebral circulation, particularly in injured brain tissue, are uncertain.

If severe associated injuries are present and the vital signs cannot be adequately stabilized by volume replacement, prompt control of the bleeding sites is needed. Such efforts should not be delayed by attempts to further define the patient's neurological condition. Although prompt decompression of intracranial mass lesions is important, correction of hypotension and hypoxemia have even greater priority. Occasionally, simultaneous surgical intervention can be considered, but neurosurgical intervention without appropriate preoperative studies can be hazardous.

LABORATORY ASSESSMENT

AXIOM The presence of alcohol or illicit drugs should be checked in all patients with a head injury.

Victims of severe brain injury should have arterial blood gas determinations, and venous blood should be sent for complete blood count (CBC), platelet count, coagulation profile, electrolytes, illicit drugs and blood alcohol levels, and type and cross-match.[7] Urine should be sent for standard chemical and microscopic analysis and for toxicologic screening. In addition to arterial blood gas analyses, it is wise to monitor the patient's tissue oxygenation constantly with a pulse oximeter.

RADIOLOGIC STUDIES

Plain Radiography of the Skull and Cervical Spine

AXIOM Although skull fractures do not generally require treatment, they indicate a much greater likelihood of severe underlying brain damage (Fig. 10-9).

There is much controversy about the wisdom or necessity of obtaining skull x-rays in patients with head injuries. However, if they are quickly and easily obtained, they can provide useful information.[7] Skull x-rays are generally indicated if: (a) there has been a loss of consciousness for more than a few seconds, (b) there is a scalp laceration that, either on inspection or palpation, appears to be associated with a fractured skull, or (c) the patient has clinical evidence of a basilar skull fracture.

Occasionally, an air-fluid level in the sphenoid sinus is the only evidence of a basilar skull fracture. In addition, linear skull fractures are often best delineated and the margins of a depressed fracture most clearly defined on plain skull radiographs.

AXIOM One should assume that all head-injured patients have associated cervical spine fractures until ruled out by complete clinical and radiologic examinations.

Cervical spine x-rays should be obtained on anyone with severe blunt trauma above the clavicles. As a general rule, 3-6% of patients with significant head trauma will have associated cervical spine injuries.[99,102]

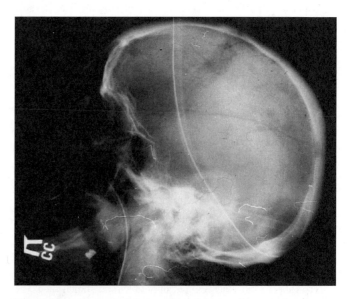

FIGURE 10-9 Linear skull fracture. Note the lucent line traversing the temporal and parietal region. The patient, a pedestrian struck by a car, also sustained a coincident type 3 odontoid fracture (see Michael et al).

CT Scan

Early and appropriate use of computed tomographic (CT) scanning is helpful for detecting significant intracranial lesions before there is severe clinical neurologic deterioration. Altered mental status and focal hemispheric deficits are the best clinical predictors of the presence of an operative hematoma, and indicate a need for CT scanning regardless of the GCS score.[104]

AXIOM CT scanning is the most accurate method to localize and quantify intracranial mass lesions.

A minimum of four axial cuts demonstrating the parasagittal sulci, lateral ventricles, middle fossae, and posterior fossa are usually obtained with CT scans of brain-injured patients.[7] If a patient is rapidly deteriorating, a single CT axial cut at the level of the lateral ventricles will detect the majority of surgical mass lesions requiring immediate craniotomy. Although this test is usually done with intravenous contrast, noncontrast CT scanning is adequate in most cases.[7]

AXIOM Patients who are admitted with signs of cerebral herniation or who deteriorate during their initial evaluation should receive mannitol (1.0 to 1.5 g/kg) by rapid intravenous infusion while attempting to obtain at least a limited CT scan through the cerebral hemispheres before surgery.[7]

In patients who have high-speed deceleration (MVA) injuries but are hemodynamically stable, one should rapidly obtain CT scans of the chest and abdomen at the same time as the head CT to rule out clinically-inapparent associated injuries.[7] Intravenous contrast can provide more detail with the chest CT scan, and a combination of intravenous and enteric contrast can provide much better detail for the abdominal CT scan. One should not, however, wait for the enteric contrast to get the CT of the head; the enteric contrast can be given while the CT of the head is being obtained.

Nuclear Magnetic Resonance Imaging

Data on the use of nuclear magnetic resonance imaging (MRI) in head trauma is just becoming available.[105] However, the time required for the examination, problems with motion artifact, and the inability to have metallic objects (e.g., a ventilator) in proximity to the MRI magnetic field limit the usefulness of this procedure in patients with acute severe trauma.

INTRACRANIAL PRESSURE MONITORING

Marshall and Bowers[106] recommend monitoring of ICP in any patient whose Glasgow Coma score after resuscitation is 7 or less. According to Narayan et al,[107] an exception may be made if there is no mass lesion on CT scan, the patient's age is under 40, the systolic blood pressure is above 90 mm Hg, and there is no motor posturing. In patients who have two or more of the latter three criteria, the incidence of an elevated ICP (7%) is virtually the same as the risk of complications from an intraventricular catheter.[107]

LUMBAR PUNCTURE

Lumbar puncture is usually contraindicated in patients with acute head injuries because it may precipitate cerebral herniation in patients with an elevated ICP.[7]

ANGIOGRAPHY

Cerebral angiography is done rarely for head injuries now, but it can play an important role in the detection of traumatic aneurysms, arteriovenous fistulas, and carotid or vertebral arterial injuries.[7] In addition, isodense subdural collections can at times be difficult to define by CT, but they are generally delineated quite well by cerebral angiography.

AXIOM Cerebral angiography may be the only readily available means of diagnosing traumatic intracranial mass lesions if CT scanning is unavailable.

EXPLORATORY EMERGENCY TREPHINATION

Very rarely in situations in which CT scanning facilities are not readily available and/or the patient's neurological status is deteriorating so rapidly that taking time to perform a CT scan seems unwise, an emergency exploratory trephination may be required. Such emergency trephinations can usually be performed with just local anesthesia; however, an anesthesiologist should be present to monitor the patient's condition and to control the patient's ventilation and hemodynamic function.[108]

CLINICALLY USABLE BIOCHEMICAL AND ELECTROPHYSIOLOGIC MARKERS OF INJURY

CSF Creatine Kinase Isoenzyme

Brain-specific creatine kinase isoenzyme (CK-BB) obtained from cerebral spinal fluid currently is a promising marker of neurotrauma and correlates well with the Glasgow Coma Scale and ultimate neurologic outcome.[109] CK-BB is present in cerebral spinal fluid immediately after trauma, but it does not peak until 6 to 24 hours later. Peak CK-BB levels of more than 200 IU/L predict a 100% mortality or vegetative outcome. After peak CK-BB levels are reached, the enzyme levels demonstrate a half-life of about 10 hours.[110]

Cerebrospinal Fluid Lactate

In head-injured patients, cerebrospinal fluid (CSF) lactate concentrations continue to rise over several days in patients who ultimately develop major permanent neurologic deficits.[110] Rabow et al[110] have noted that increased lactate in ventricular CSF is not a direct consequence of the trauma, but is a result of ongoing metabolic disturbances.

Electrophysiologic Monitoring

Electrophysiologic monitoring has the ability to directly examine brain function; however, there is no consensus on its usefulness. Although Narayan et al[111] found that the predictive value of evoked potentials alone was no better than that of the GCS, Judson et al[112] showed that absence of the cortical potentials within the first 24 hours was an important prognostic sign. In 100 intubated closed-head injury patients with an initial GCS of 9 or less, absence of somatosensory-evoked cortical potentials on one or both sides during the first day after injury predicted death or major disability with a specificity of 95%. Prolonged cortical conduction time did not predict a poor outcome if cortical potentials were present bilaterally.[111]

INITIAL MANAGEMENT

Initial management of the patient with a severe head injury has two primary goals.[113] The first is the immediate diagnosis of potentially treatable surgical lesions such as subdural, epidural, or intraparenchymal hematomas. The second objective is the recognition and prevention of conditions known to cause secondary brain injury. Ideally, efforts to minimize secondary brain injury should be initiated at the scene of the accident. These include maintenance of adequate ventilation, oxygenation, and tissue perfusion.

AXIOM Although not all patients with head injury require neurosurgical consultation, they all require prompt, frequent, and careful neurological assessment.

Prehospital Management

After the cervical spine is stabilized appropriately, the patient is transported to the nearest trauma center capable of providing general surgical and neurosurgical care.[7] During such transport, every effort must be made to prevent or rapidly correct hypotension or hypoxemia. In addition, patients with rapidly progressing CNS dysfunction may benefit from early administration of mannitol. Radio communication en route between a physician and the emergency personnel may allow this therapy to be provided in the field for selected patients.

Initial Management

VENTILATORY SUPPORT

Indications

AXIOM Assisted or controlled ventilation should be provided to severely head-injured patients to ensure adequate oxygenation and a PCO_2 of 35-40 mm Hg for the first 2-3 days.

Early intubation with controlled ventilation in patients with moderate-severe head injury can provide airway maintenance, adequate oxygenation, and reduction of intracranial pressure through induced hypocarbia.

Although the indications for mechanical ventilation in head injury patients are controversial, many neurosurgeons agree with the following criteria for ventilatory assistance:[5,71,114]

1. Clinical respiratory distress, a rate above 30/min or below 10/min, or an abnormal ventilatory pattern
2. Motor posturing or absence of a motor response to pain
3. Abnormal or deteriorating arterial blood gases
4. Repeated convulsions
5. Signs of aspiration, pneumonitis, or pulmonary edema
6. Rising or high ICP
7. Requirement for potent analgesics or sedatives to control pain, restlessness, or posturing
8. Concurrent severe pulmonary, cardiac, or upper abdominal injury.

Ventilatory Goals

The arterial PO_2 in patients with acute severe head injury should be maintained at 80 mm Hg or higher (95% oxyhemoglobin saturation), and the minute volume should be adjusted to provide arterial PCO_2 levels between 35 and 40 mm Hg. Lower levels of positive end-expiratory pressure (PEEP) do not appear to increase intracranial pressure if the head is elevated 30°.

A $PaCO_2$ of 30 to 35 mm Hg will often result in a decrease of ICP to normal or near-normal levels.[5] In extreme cases, the $PaCO_2$ may be lowered to 20 mm Hg, but this should be done with great care. The extreme vasoconstriction that results from $PaCO_2$ levels below 20 mm Hg may cause inadequate cerebral blood flow and greatly increase secondary brain damage.

INTUBATION

Rapid-sequence intubation is preferable to awake, blind nasotracheal intubation in head-injured patients. Apart from the direct stimulation of elevation in intracranial pressure caused by nasotracheal intubation, the procedure usually is more time-consuming, has a higher complication rate,[115] and can result in a significant elevation of the PCO_2.[116]

Premedication

A number of pharmacologic agents have been used in an effort to attenuate adverse hemodynamic and ICP responses to rapid-sequence induction and intubation.

BETA-ADRENERGIC BLOCKERS. Administration of a single bolus dose of the beta-adrenergic blockers esmolol[117] or labetalol[118] has been shown to effectively blunt the rise in heart rate and mean arterial blood pressure that would otherwise occur in response to intubation. Synthetic opioids, such as fentanyl, are also effective in blunting the rise in heart rate and mean arterial blood pressure usually seen with intubation.[119] It is administered intravenously in a dose of 3 to 5 µg/kg about 1 to 3 minutes before intubation. Administration of larger doses may lead to hypoventilation and hypercarbia in spontaneously breathing patients.

AXIOM Although emergency intubation of head-injured patients without appropriate premedication can cause an abrupt rise in ICP, there is not always time for such medications.

Intravenous Lidocaine. Intravenous lidocaine (1.5 mg/kg), given 2-3 minutes before intubation, can often prevent a rise in ICP and may have a directly beneficial effect on the injured brain.[120]

Barbiturates. Barbiturates have been shown to attenuate intracranial pressure responses to intubation, and decrease the cerebral demand for oxygen.[121] Thiopental is an ultrashort-acting barbiturate that has extremely rapid onset and a duration of action similar to that of succinylcholine; however, in induction doses (3 to 5 mg/kg), it can also be a potent cardiovascular depressant. Therefore, in hemodynamically compromised patients, one should either reduce the dose to 0.5 to 1.0 mg/kg or use another agent, such as fentanyl or etomidate.

Etomidate. Etomidate can attenuate the rise in intracranial pressure often seen during intubation, and it causes less cardiovascular depression than barbiturates; however, it has an unfortunate tendency to suppress the synthesis of cortisol, even after a single dose.[122]

CHOICE OF NEUROMUSCULAR BLOCKING AGENTS

Succinylcholine. Because of its rapid onset, complete reliability, and short duration of action, succinylcholine (100 mg intravenous push) has been the principal agent used for neuromuscular blockade in rapid-sequence intubation. Although succinylcholine can cause a further rise in elevated intracranial pressure, it has been shown that prior competitive neuromuscular blockade prevents the intracranial pressure response to succinylcholine.[123]

Vecuronium. Competitive neuromuscular blocking agents, especially vecuronium, have been widely studied in rapid-sequence intubation models.[124] Two alternative approaches have been advocated. A small "priming" dose of vecuronium (0.01 mg/kg) can be administered 3 to 5 minutes before a generous paralyzing dose (0.15 mg/kg). Unfortunately, adequate neuromuscular blockade with vecuronium used in this manner is not achieved as uniformly and rapidly as with succinylcholine. Alternatively, high-dose vecuronium administration (0.3 mg/kg) results in attainment of intubating conditions in approximately 100 seconds;[124] however, this remains slower than succinylcholine, and this high dose of vecuronium results in a complete motor paralysis for approximately 2 hours.

Cardiovascular Status

PREVENTING HYPOTENSION

Blood pressure should be controlled in head-injured patients to maintain a CPP of at least 70 and preferably 90 to 110 mm Hg.[5] A systolic blood pressure of less than 80 mm Hg and an intracranial pressure of more than 20 mm Hg significantly decrease the chance of good recovery in head-injured patients. Hypotension may result in severe regional or global ischemia.[11] It may also trigger reflex cerebral vasodilation which can, in turn, cause an abrupt rise in the ICP.[125]

AXIOM Even if the ICP is elevated, hypotension in head-injured patients is still usually best treated by administering fluids.[4]

It may seem paradoxic to give fluids to correct hypotension in a patient receiving diuretics to reduce the ICP, but the purpose of mannitol therapy is to dehydrate the brain, not to reduce the blood volume.[5,7] A normal blood volume with slightly hyperosmolar plasma (300-320 mOsm/L) is the desired therapeutic aim. Thus, fluid losses should be monitored and carefully replaced. If a vasopressor is needed, 5-10 mcg/kg/min of dopamine, with its inotropic action and tendency to raise the systemic BP, is the best choice.

AXIOM Vasopressors should be used cautiously, if at all, in head-injured patients, because their effect on CBF is not well-defined.

PREVENTING HYPERTENSION

Recent data suggest that, although manipulation of systemic blood pressure may not alter cerebral oxygen utilization, a positive correlation has been found between cerebral perfusion pressure and the intracranial pressure-volume index in patients with intact autoregulation;[72] however, available data does not necessarily argue in favor of induced hypertension, which some investigators have advocated.[63]

Severe hypertension can be deleterious to an injured brain and can also cause cerebral hyperemia and increased vasogenic edema with a resultant rise in ICP.[5] Hypertension associated with head injury is usually in response to an increased ICP. Such hypertension is characterized by increased cardiac output, tachycardia, and increased systemic and pulmonary vascular resistance.[126]

> **AXIOM** The treatment of hypertension in a head-injured patient should be directed primarily at reducing ICP and/or evacuating intracranial hematomas.

Controlling the ICP

In addition to keeping the CVP as low as possible and hyperventilating the patient to an arterial PCO_2 of 35-40 mm Hg, one can use head elevation, mannitol, and furosemide to keep the ICP less than 20 mm Hg.

HEAD ELEVATION

Head-of-bed elevation traditionally has been used to decrease intracranial pressure. Indeed, Feldman et al[127] have shown that head-of-bed elevation from 0 to 30° results in a decreased ICP without a statistically significant decrease in cerebral perfusion pressure, cerebral blood flow, cerebral metabolic rate, or cerebral vascular resistance.

MANNITOL

Osmotic diuretics exert their beneficial effects in head trauma primarily on the uninjured areas of the brain because disruption of the blood-brain barrier in the injured area prevents the development of an osmotic gradient there.[93,106] Mannitol is the most commonly used of these agents. Urea, a smaller molecule, is effective in smaller doses, and may be useful in patients who cannot tolerate the volume load required in mannitol therapy.

In brain-injured patients, mannitol may have three effects: dehydration of the normal brain, increase in CBF and cardiac output (probably by decreasing blood viscosity),[73] and constriction of cerebral vessels.[71] It should be noted that the patient's clinical status often improves before, and to a greater degree than, the actual decrease in ICP.[5] Osmotic diuretics, however, are not recommended if serum osmolarity is above 320 mOsm/L since this degree of hyperosmolarity may produce acute renal failure and electrolyte disturbances.

> **AXIOM** Serum osmolarity should be monitored and kept less than 320 mOsm/L during mannitol therapy.

The standard dose of mannitol is 1.0 to 1.5 g/kg.[5] However, Marshall et al[128] have shown that doses as small as 0.25 g/kg may be as effective as the larger doses, although for a somewhat shorter time. They demonstrated that a rise in serum osmolarity of 10 mOsm/L or more is sufficient to lower the ICP to normal levels in most patients. The lower dose permits prolonged use of mannitol to maintain the decrease in ICP. The recommended dosage schedules for continued mannitol therapy are 0.25 g/kg every 4 hours on a fixed schedule or 20 g as needed, titrated to the patient's ICP.[128]

FUROSEMIDE

Use of the loop diuretics, furosemide and ethacrynic acid, is somewhat controversial. Although they do not reliably lower ICP, they can help reduce the extent of secondary brain injury by decreasing glial swelling. Indeed, some early studies[129] showed an increased survival in patients treated with ethacrynic acid, but controlled clinical trials have not yet been performed.[5] Administering loop diuretics before beginning mannitol therapy may help prevent the initial hypervolemia and pulmonary congestion that is seen not infrequently when mannitol therapy is begun.[61] They may also potentiate the rate and duration of the ICP reduction produced by mannitol.

Control of Agitation and Seizures

Agitation may result in significant increases in intracranial pressure, but it can be controlled through judicious use of sedatives and paralyzing agents.[106] Seizure activity results in local loss of autoregulation with concomitant increases in cerebral blood flow and tissue lactic acidosis, which also increase intracranial pressure. Electrolyte imbalance and fever also may raise intracranial pressure and should be avoided.[116]

Some neurosurgeons feel that all patients with moderate-severe head injuries should receive prophylactic diphenylhydantoin at a loading dose of 18 mg/kg intravenously in normal saline over 30 minutes while blood pressure and the electrocardiogram (ECG) are monitored.[7] Other neurosurgeons feel that one should not give dilantin until at least one or two seizures have occurred. For control of ongoing seizures (with or without prophylactic diphenylhydantoin), 5-10 mg of diazepam can be given intravenously. This may be repeated as needed at 10- to 15-minute intervals to a maximum dose of 30 mg.

Immunization and Antibiotic Prophylaxis

Patients with open wounds who cannot give an up-to-date tetanus immunization status should receive tetanus toxoid.[9] If the wound is grossly contaminated, tetanus immune globulin and antibiotics should also be given and the wound cleaned in the OR.

Patients with open depressed skull fractures and penetrating injuries should be given an antistaphylococcal penicillin or first-generation cephalosporin in full dosage. These drugs cover the most likely pathogens and can achieve adequate levels across the blood-brain barrier. For gunshot wounds, gram negative aerobes and anaerobes should also be covered.

OPERATIVE MANAGEMENT OF HEAD INJURIES

Indications for Operation

> **AXIOM** An intracranial hematoma causing increasing neurological dysfunction or more than 5 mm midline displacement should be evacuated as soon as possible.

CLINICAL STATUS

An operative intracranial decompression is required in about 12% of patients with an acute head injury causing unconsciousness.[7] Such decompression should be performed before the patient shows clinical evidence of tentorial herniation.[83] Progressively diminishing responsiveness, development of unilateral pupillary dilatation, abnormal flexor or extensor posturing, and increasing arterial hypertension and bradycardia associated with periodic breathing are signs that third nerve and brain stem compression have already occurred from tentorial herniation.[83]

Head-injured patients with a GCS of 9-15 who are found to have an intracranial mass lesion causing a midventricular shift of more than 5 mm should have the lesion evacuated immediately.[7] If the shift is less than 5 mm, the patient should be observed closely in the intensive care unit with intracranial pressure monitoring. If the ICP is greater than 25 mm Hg or there is neurological deterioration, the mass should be evacuated. If the clinical status is stable and ICP is controllable, one should continue to observe the patient carefully and repeat a CT scan in 24 hours. Mass lesions should be evacuated quickly in patients with a GCS of 8 or less if further brain damage is to be prevented.

If no mass lesion is seen in a patient with a GCS of 13 or less, the most likely explanation is brain swelling, which does not benefit from operative decompression.[5,7] Since a small extra-axial or intra-axial dense lesion seen on CT scan is usually much larger than expected, if the ICP is persistently greater than 25 mm Hg despite attempts to control it, or if there is further neurological deterioration, the patient should have a repeat CT scan and operative decompression as indicated. Large bilateral lesions, especially if they are clearly causing brain compression with midventricular impingement, should be evacuated promptly.

As a general rule, extra-axial lesions should be removed first and then, depending on the situation, ipsilateral or contralateral intra-axial lesions can be removed. Patients with temporal or temporoparietal hematomas with a volume of more than 30 ml are at significant risk of developing brain stem compression and should be considered for early, aggressive surgery.[19]

Operative Procedure

The patient is placed in whatever position is needed to allow access to known hematomas or other lesions requiring removal. The surgery usually starts with a temporal burr hole.[7] If clot is present, the burr hole is enlarged by craniectomy and the dura opened. This can afford rapid relief of an elevated ICP by evacuation of extra-axial clot or by herniation of contused temporal lobe through the defect. Formal craniotomy is then carried out.

Management of Brain Swelling

Occasionally, sudden massive brain swelling will develop during the operation.[7] This is usually due to hyperemia from defective cerebrovascular autoregulation. Another possible cause is hypoventilation. Consequently, the endotracheal tube position should be promptly checked. Additional mannitol and increased hyperventilation will often reverse such acute swelling, but this therapy may need to be repeated several times. Swelling unrelieved by such means may respond to 500 mg boluses of thiopental, up to a total dose of 1 to 2 grams. If all of these measures fail, internal decompression via frontal or temporal lobectomy has been occasionally performed.

Definitive Treatment of Injuries

SCALP LACERATIONS
Scalp lacerations should be carefully explored for possible fractures or skull penetration. Debridement, irrigation, and closure of the outer scalp in a single layer is usually adequate. If the galea is lacerated or if the scalp injury is extensive or complex, it should be explored and closed in the operating room.[7] Lacerations of the galea should be closed as a separate layer.

AXIOM   Scalp lacerations involving the galea should generally be explored, cleaned, and closed in the OR.

SKULL FRACTURES

Linear Fractures
Undisplaced linear fractures of the cranial vault without associated scalp lacerations do not require specific treatment.[7] Open linear fractures, however, have a small but definite risk of osteomyelitis. The overlying laceration must be carefully cleaned, debrided, and closed, preferably in the O.R. One dose of an antistaphylococcal antibiotic may be of benefit, but longer courses of prophylactic antibiotics are not usually recommended.[9]

Depressed Fractures
A closed, depressed skull fracture does not usually have any effect on neurological deficits that may be present.[7] However, some neurosurgeons feel that a depressed skull fracture, particularly over the motor strip of the cerebral cortex, increases the tendency to post-traumatic epilepsy.

Open depressed fractures require surgery because of the risk of infection. Thorough debridement of the wound, copious irrigation, meticulous hemostasis, and a watertight dural closure are essential.

Basilar Skull Fractures
The treatment of basilar skull fractures is largely concerned with the recognition and care of any associated cranial nerve or vascular injuries and prevention of CSF fistulas. Surgical decompression has been advocated in injuries to the optic and facial nerves if there is evidence of deteriorating function.[130]

The advent of endovascular techniques employing balloon catheters with angiographic guidance has revolutionized the treatment of carotid-cavernous sinus fistulas. In many cases, these intravascular catheter techniques permit occlusion of the fistula with preservation of the carotid lumen.[131]

Because most traumatic CSF rhinorrhea and almost all CSF otorrhea resolve spontaneously, a trial of conservative therapy with bed rest and head positioning to minimize CSF drainage is warranted. If the CSF leakage does not slow after 3 to 4 days, one should begin CSF drainage by repeat lumbar punctures or a lumbar drain. Prophylactic antibiotics are usually not recommended because they do not reduce the incidence of infection, and if infection does occur, it is more likely to be caused by antibiotic-resistant organisms.[7] If the fistula persists for more than 7 to 10 days, repair via an intradural approach is indicated. More immediate closure may be undertaken for a widely diastatic fracture, bone fragments displaced into brain, extremely copious CSF flow, or increasing pneumocephalus.

INTRACRANIAL HEMATOMAS

AXIOM   In areas where neurosurgical help is not readily available, general surgeons should have the ability to make cranial trephine openings (burr holes) to evacuate intracranial hematomas.

Without Preoperative Localization
Even at modern trauma hospitals, there can be an occasional important delay in removal of a rapidly expanding or herniating lesion if one always insists that CT scanning be done first.[17] Although this delay can be life-threatening at times, most neurosurgeons are reluctant to attempt operative decompression without some radiologic guidance. If a neurosurgeon is unavailable to certain remote areas, the neurosurgeons in that area should develop a training program for any surgeon who might have to perform an emergency trephination.

If intracranial hematomas have not been localized by preoperative CT scans or angiography, the trephine openings should be made bilaterally. The use of bilateral frontal, temporal, and parietal burr holes, particularly when supplemented by ultrasound evaluation during surgery, can accurately identify extradural and intracerebral hematomas in more than 90% of cases.[132]

Suggested locations for the initial trephine openings for non-localized hematomas are[1] (Fig. 10-10):

1. Frontocoronal: 3 cm lateral to the midline at the coronal suture (on a line about 2 cm anterior to the ear).
2. Temporal: 2 cm anterior to the ear and 2 cm superior to the zygoma.
3. Parietal: 2 cm above and 2 cm posterior to the top of the ear.

AXIOM   Although the intracranial space can be decompressed to some extent through burr holes, adequate evacuation of the majority of intracranial hematomas requires a bone flap.

Epidural Hematomas
With epidural hematomas, it is important to expose the margins of the clot up to normal dura.[7] After evacuation of the hematoma, a bleeding meningeal vessel will often be seen, and it should be clipped or ligated if possible. Occasionally, control of bleeding from the

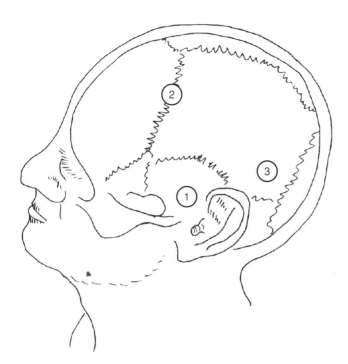

FIGURE 10-10 Suggested sites for emergency trephine openings if the intracranial hematoma has not been localized preoperatively: (a) Temporal: 2 cm anterior to the ear and 2 cm superior to the zygoma, (b) Frontocoronal: 3 cm lateral to the midline at the coronal suture, (c) Parietal: 2 cm above and 2 cm posterior to the ear.

middle meningeal artery can only be accomplished by packing the foramen spinosum.

Subdural Hematomas

After proper exposure, subdural hematomas can usually be removed by irrigation, suction, and gentle traction with forceps.[7] Bleeding from surface vessels is controlled with bipolar coagulation. Avulsed bridging veins are controlled by either coagulation or tamponade with Gelfoam or muscle.

Brain Contusions

Irreparably damaged areas of brain contusion can act as a nidus for edema or hemorrhage, and may be resected by suction if larger than 1 to 2 cm.[7] Over the frontal or temporal areas, one may be relatively aggressive with such debridement. Indeed, Nussbaum et al[132] have recommended early temporal lobectomy for patients with unilateral hemispheric swelling and midline shift. This technique has decreased mortality rates in selected patients without hematomas. In more functionally vital areas, any resection must be done judiciously to avoid adding to the neurologic deficit.

Intracerebral Hematomas

Intracerebral hematomas larger than 3-4 cm diameter (30 ml volume) near the surface may be evacuated.[7] More deeply placed clots require evacuation if they are large enough to produce significant shift, but such aggressiveness should be tempered by the risk of increasing the neurologic deficit.

PENETRATING STAB INJURIES

The management of penetrating stab wounds of the head is analogous to that of compound depressed fractures.[7] In cases where the penetrating object is still in place, no attempt should be made to extract it until the patient is in the operating room with a craniotomy flap turned to expose the wound tract. If it is likely that a major vessel is involved, the preliminary evaluation should include angiography.

GUNSHOT WOUNDS

Patients with penetrating brain injuries resulting from gunshot wounds and any reasonable chance for survival should be given mannitol and broad-spectrum antibiotics as soon as they are seen.[11] The scalp, cranial, and dural entrance wounds are thoroughly debrided. Irreparably damaged cerebral cortex is removed, and the debridement is extended as far as is safely possible along the wound tract to remove all devitalized tissues, bone, missile fragments, hematoma, and foreign bodies. Intraoperative ultrasound may be a useful adjacent for removing foreign bodies safely.

A watertight dural closure at the end of the case is critical, and the wound should be covered by full-thickness scalp which is closed without tension. This may require extensive undermining of the scalp or even rotation flaps.

Continued ICP Monitoring

ICP is monitored until it stabilizes, hopefully at a normal level, for at least 24 hours.[7] This usually means that the ICP catheter and transducer will be in place for 3 to 8 days. If an intraventricular catheter is used, it should probably be removed after 8 days because the incidence of complications, especially infection, increases with time.[107] However, a study in pediatric brain-injured patients suggests that the infection risk declines after 6 days, and a single ICP monitoring device may be used as long as necessary, provided surveillance cultures are obtained daily and the patient observed closely.

CONTINUING POSTOPERATIVE CARE

General Measures

A number of simple measures can help control the ICP. They may include: (a) elevation of the head 20 to 30°, (b) avoidance of fluid overload and high levels of PEEP, and (c) sedation or neuromuscular blockade.[7] If a ventricular catheter is in place, an elevated ICP may also be treated by CSF drainage. Hyperventilation to levels of moderate hypocarbia, between 25 and 30 mm Hg, reduces ICP through reflex constriction of cerebral resistance vessels, causing a decrease in cerebral blood flow and cerebral blood volume.[27]

Drugs

DIURETICS

Mannitol is generally used preoperatively to reduce the ICP; however, sudden discontinuance of osmotic therapy may be associated with a significant ICP "rebound," probably because, when the serum osmolarity falls below that of the tissues, water is shifted from the vasculature into brain tissue. This effect is more pronounced if the serum osmolarity is more than 320 mOsm/kg.[93] The rebound can probably be moderated by limitation of fluid intake, or concomitant furosemide therapy, but this is difficult to recommend in a situation in which hypotension is generally more devastating than a brief elevation of ICP.

AXIOM Abrupt cessation of mannitol therapy can cause a rebound rise in ICP.

BARBITURATES

Barbiturates have been extensively used in patients with severe head injuries. Studies by Marshall et al,[133] Shapiro et al,[134] and Nordby et al[135] have demonstrated that barbiturates can be extremely effective in reducing ICP in patients unresponsive to standard therapy. Sichez et al[136] have also reported favorable results from a regimen of barbiturates and ventricular drainage.

These therapeutic effects of barbiturates may result from any of several different actions.[5] These include: (a) reduction of ICP by cerebral vasoconstriction (probably the major effect), (b) reduction of cerebral metabolism and oxygen requirements,[137] (c) prevention of intravascular coagulation, and (d) reduction of free-radical damage to brain cells.[138]

Although good results have been reported with barbiturates, serious questions remain about their influence on survival and long-term morbidity.[96,138] In a prospective, randomized comparison of mannitol versus pentobarbital in patients with a GCS of 7 or less, Schwartz et al[139] in 1984 noted that pentobarbital was less effective than mannitol in lowering intracranial pressure.

Ward et al[140] in 1985 showed that barbiturate coma increased the incidence of complications when used in the absence of intractable intracranial hypertension. However, more selective studies indicate that high-dose barbiturates were effective in a subset of patients refractory to aggressive therapy that included cerebrospinal fluid drainage, hyperventilation, and mannitol.[121,133]

> **AXIOM** Barbiturates are probably of greatest value in reducing brain damage in patients who have persistently high ICPs in spite of all other therapy.

In a multicenter, prospective study reported in 1988, Eisenberg et al[121] noted that one-third of patients who failed to respond to maximal medical therapy had their intracranial pressure controlled after the addition of high-dose pentobarbital; however, barbiturates do not appear to be effective when given as initial therapy to patients with severe head injury.[140] If high-dose barbiturates are to be used for a prolonged period, they can depress cardiac function, and a pulmonary artery catheter should be used.[140]

Before starting barbiturate therapy, mass lesions should be treated surgically, and the patient should be normotensive (MAP above 70) and normovolemic (pulmonary artery wedge pressure of about 8-12).[5] Thus, a pulmonary artery (PA) catheter, arterial line, and ICP monitor are needed to accurately assess both the cardiovascular and cerebral effects of the barbiturates. The rectal temperature should also be monitored closely and not allowed to fall below 32° C because the combination of barbiturates and hypothermia can cause severe cardiac arrhythmias, particularly in younger patients, and cause problems of gas exchange with resultant hypoxia.[106,141]

The barbiturates are usually administered as intravenous pentobarbital in an initial dose of 5 to 10 mg/kg and continued as a 1.5 mg/kg/hr drip until the ICP falls below 15-20 mm Hg or until serum barbiturate levels are 3 to 5 mg/dl.[106] Levels above 5 mg/dl do not seem to increase the therapeutic effects of barbiturates but can cause the EEG to become isoelectric.[137] Deep tendon reflexes also may disappear at these higher levels, and the patient usually becomes apneic and hypercarbic unless ventilatory assistance is provided.

> **AXIOM** The only way to reliably monitor the neurologic status of a patient in barbiturate coma is with evoked potentials and, if these deteriorate, one should promptly obtain a repeat CT scan.[184]

Barbiturate levels are maintained at 3 to 5 mg/dl by continuous intravenous infusion until the ICP remains normal for at least 24 to 48 hours.[5] The dosage is then tapered gradually over 4 days to avoid the sudden deterioration that may follow abrupt withdrawal.[106] If the ICP increases during the tapering, the barbiturate therapy should be resumed.

ANTICONVULSANTS

Seizure activity in the brain can severely increase cerebral metabolic rate, vasodilation, and ICP.[6] If CBF does not increase adequately during a seizure, there is also danger of severe cerebral hypoxia and acidosis.

> **AXIOM** The deleterious effects of seizures occur even when motor responses are blocked by muscle relaxants or paraplegia.

Although it is controversial, some neurosurgeons feel that any patient whose brain injury is severe enough to require intensive care

should be treated with prophylactic phenytoin loading.[7] The phenytoin should be discontinued within 7 days.[79,142] Delayed surgery may indicate long-term anticonvulsant therapy. Breakthrough seizures are treated initially with intravenous Valium (5-10 mg) repeated × 2 at 5-10 minute intervals if needed. Supplemental doses of phenytoin should also be given if serum levels are subtherapeutic, and/or phenobarbital should be added. Phenobarbital should be used as the primary anticonvulsant in patients who are sensitive to phenytoin or have side effects. The usual dose is 32 mg every 8 hours.[7]

CORTICOSTEROIDS

Although it is well known that corticosteroids can act as antiflammatory agents by reducing cyclooxygenase actively and by acting as free-radical scavengers,[143] most physicians treating head trauma do not believe they are of benefit.

In 1976 reports, Faupel et al[143] and Gobiet et al[144] noted significant reductions in mortality following high dosage schedules of dexamethasone. Faupel et al[143] used 100 mg initially and again after 6 hours, followed by 4 mg every 6 hours. Gobiet et al[144] used 48 mg initially followed by 8 mg every 2 hours during the first and third days and 4 mg every 2 hours on the second and fourth. Miller and Leech in 1975[145] also demonstrated a sustained, beneficial increase in cerebral compliance using betamethasone in head-injured patients.

In spite of these studies, most other authors have not been able to show any benefit with steroids in experimental or clinical head injury. For example, Tornheim and McLaurin[146] could not demonstrate any significant decrease in cerebral edema following dexamethasone in head-injured cats, and Gudeman et al[147] found that high dose methylprednisolone caused no improvement in ICP, cerebral compliance, or survival over low-dose steroids in a clinical study. Similar results were obtained in a group of brain-injured patients who had an increased ICP and were given high-dose dexamethasone.[148] The lack of effect on death rate has also been confirmed in prospective studies by Braakman et al.[149]

It is possible that the doses used in these studies may have been too small. Giannotta et al[150] in 1984 showed significant improvement in mortality and recovery of speech in patients under 40 years of age receiving very high doses of methylprednisolone (30 mg/kg, 2 doses 6 hours apart, then 250 mg every 6 hours for 6 doses, then tapering over 8 days) over those receiving the lower doses used in other studies or placebo. The timing of the first dose appeared to be particularly important because circulatory disturbances in the damaged region may prevent the drug from reaching the involved area after 2 to 4 hours.

> **AXIOM** Steroids should not be routinely used in the management of severe head injury.

Although many centers have used high-dose steroid therapy, questions about its value in brain injury remain unanswered. Currently, most centers do not give steroids to patients with severe head injuries because of the general evidence of its lack of benefit and because its use increases the risk of infection, especially pneumonia and gastrointestinal complications.[79,151]

> **AXIOM** If the ICP remains high in spite of surgery and barbiturate therapy, a fatal outcome is virtually certain.[133]

Ventilatory Support

Mechanical ventilation should be continued until the patient becomes alert enough to follow two-stage commands or until the ICP remains normal for several days.[5] This usually takes a week or less, but in some cases, more than 2 to 3 weeks of ventilatory support may be necessary. Maintenance of hypocarbia for this length of time, however, has not been demonstrated to be beneficial.[152]

In normal subjects, the cerebrovascular response to hypocarbia may begin to wane after only 5 hours.[152] This has raised some questions about the value of long-term hyperventilation in the treatment of cerebral edema. However, the decrease in CBF with prolonged hypocarbia seems to be sustained in many brain-injured children and adults.[61,153] Even after cerebral blood volume (CBV) returns to normal, hypocapnia in some patients produces a continuing increase in CSF absorption, which may help maintain ICP control.[154]

AXIOM In adults, continuous ventilatory support may not only help to control the ICP, but it may also prevent the hypoxic brain damage that might be caused by unexpected apnea, respiratory obstruction, or respiratory insufficiency.[5]

Sedation and/or neuromuscular blockade may be helpful in getting the patient to breathe synchronously with the ventilator. Chlorpromazine (25 mg intramuscularly every 6 hours) or repeated small doses (1 to 3 mg) of intravenous morphine will usually allow proper ventilatory assistance or control without unduly masking the neurologic status.[106] However, these agents may not be sufficient in the presence of severe central hyperventilation, and intermittent doses of intravenous muscle relaxants may be needed. Pancuronium is the agent usually recommended, but vecuronium and atracurium can also be used.[5]

In many patients, inability to monitor neurologic signs is a relatively small price to pay for the benefits obtained from adequate ventilatory control.[5] However, paralysis or sedation alone with nothing for pain should be avoided because even apparently comatose patients may have an elevated ICP because of noxious stimuli.

AXIOM Ventilation in patients with moderate-severe head injuries should be monitored by both arterial blood gases and the ICP.

Hypercarbia, struggling, or coughing during pulmonary physiotherapy, tracheal suctioning, and therapeutic bronchoscopy, even in the presence of coma, can cause severe increases in ICP.[5] The use of sedatives, lidocaine, muscle relaxants, and adequate preoxygenation can help limit the patient's reaction to tracheal stimulation.[155] Occasionally, general anesthesia may be required to perform such procedures safely.[93,106]

Hemodynamic Control

Postoperative patients or patients with moderate-severe brain injuries not requiring surgery should be monitored closely in an ICU to: (a) maintain a normal or slightly higher BP, (b) keep the CVP as low as possible, and (c) attempt to optimize cerebral blood flow.

BP CONTROL

Correcting Hypotension
Obviously, CPP should be kept at 80-100 mm Hg if possible. If the BP tends to fall, one must look carefully for other injuries or problems that may be causing hypovolemia. Although increasing preload is usually the best way to raise the BP in trauma patients, the CVP should be kept as low as possible in patients with an increased ICP.

Preventing and Correcting Hypertension
If a head-injury patient becomes severely hypertensive but the ICP is unchanged and no brain shift has occurred, the logical treatment would seem to be beta-adrenergic blockade.[5] Indeed, propranolol has been shown in a small group of hypertensive head-injury patients to bring cardiovascular indices back toward normal quickly and safely.[156] No ICP changes were noted after administration of propranolol, even in high doses. The drug is usually administered at a rate of 1.0 mg/min intravenously until the systolic pressure falls below 160 mm Hg, the pulse rate decreases to 55, or the pulmonary artery wedge pressure (PAWP) increases above 18 mm Hg. Labetalol, intravenously, in 10-20 mg doses every 5-10 minutes to a total dose of

60-100 mg, is also effective in reducing blood pressure.[157] The drug can also be administered as an infusion (1 to 2 mg/min after the initial bolus dose) under close monitoring.

AXIOM An abrupt decline in BP is usually much more damaging to an injured brain than moderate hypertension.

Nitroglycerine and nitroprusside are rapid, potent, and easily controllable vasodilators, but they are relatively contraindicated in head-injury patients because they can cause significant cerebral vasodilatation and increases in ICP.[158]

Since an expanded intravascular volume in the absence of an abnormality in serum sodium does not usually predispose to brain swelling, fluid restriction is not indicated in head injury.[7] In fact, inadequate fluid replacement may have serious deleterious effects on cerebral perfusion if it causes hypotension or a fall in cardiac output.

KEEPING THE ICP LOW
From a hemodynamic standpoint, the tendency for the ICP to rise can be partially prevented by keeping the CVP as low as possible while maintaining a normal or slightly increased BP and an increased DO_2. Thus, inotropes should be used primarily to achieve these goals if the ICP is 15 mm Hg or more.

OPTIMIZING OXYGEN DELIVERY

AXIOM In severe head-injury patients (GCS below 8), a pulmonary artery catheter should be inserted and efforts made to optimize oxygen delivery to the brain.

Monitoring of DO_2 and VO_2
If possible, one should attempt to optimize DO_2 to the brain by ensuring that the total DO_2 is at least 600 ml/min/m² and that it is increased until the VO_2 will no longer rise or it is a least 150 ml/min/m². This is best done by achieving a cardiac index of at least 4.0 L/min/m² with a hemoglobin level of 12.0-14.0 gm/dl and an SaO_2 of 92-98%.

Jugular Bulb Catheterization
Catheterization of the jugular bulb with a cannula passed retrograde up the internal jugular vein has been used increasingly in some centers in attempts to optimize cerebral blood flow.[159] This permits sampling of venous drainage from the brain. One can then use a modified Fick equation to estimate the adequacy of the cerebral oxygen consumption ($CMRO_2$).

$$CBF = \frac{CMRO_2}{C(a\text{-}jb)O_2}$$

CBF is cerebral blood flow and $C(a\text{-}jb)O_2$ represents the arterial-jugular bulb venous oxygen content difference. This relationship can also be expressed as:

$$C(a\text{-}jb)O_2 = \frac{CMRO_2}{CBF}$$

$C(a\text{-}jb)O_2$ greater than 8.0 vol% generally indicates definite cerebral ischemia, and $C(a\text{-}jb)O_2$ greater than 6.0 vol% in a head-injured patient with an increased ICP is borderline and implies that any further reduction in CBF, such as by decreasing $PaCO_2$, with more hyperventilation may lead to severe cerebral ischemia.[159] In such circumstances, the indicated therapy might be an agent, such as mannitol, which lowers ICP while increasing CBF. Conversely, a patient with cerebral hyperemia tends to have decreased $C(a\text{-}jb)O_2$ and will probably benefit from hyperventilation since the decrease in $PaCO_2$ will bring the CBF into a more normal relation with the $CMRO_2$.[5] The $C(a\text{-}jb)O_2$ may also be helpful in evaluating the effects of antihypertensive medications or barbiturates on the cerebral oxygen supply-demand ratio.

AXIOM If a jugular bulb catheter is in place, one should try to keep the C(a-jb)O$_2$ differences less than 6 vol% and the S$_{jb}$O$_2$ above 50%.

There are at least two limitations to the use of jugular bulb catheterization in the treatment of head-injured patients.[6] First, this technique should be restricted to patients who have a diffuse cerebral injury, have not suffered a stroke, and do not have a large midline shift or other major focal abnormalities on CT scan. Second, the leftward shift in the hemoglobin dissociation curve caused by alkalosis tends to reduce the C(a-jb)O$_2$ and decrease the reliability of this measurement in aggressively hyperventilated patients.[160]

Further experience is needed to determine how often and in which patients knowledge of the C(a-jb)O$_2$ will allow one to optimize therapy. Questions also remain as to whether there are risks associated with inserting a jugular bulb catheter into an already unstable cerebral circulation.

Fluid and Electrolyte Problems

Diabetes insipidus (DI) and the syndrome of inappropriate antidiuretic hormone (SIADH) secretion are both complications of head trauma that can quickly lead to severe fluid and electrolyte imbalance.

AXIOM Urine output and serum electrolytes should be monitored carefully in all severely head-injured patients.

DIABETES INSIPIDUS
Diabetes insipidus (DI) is particularly common after basilar skull fractures[161] producing injury to the pituitary stalk or hypothalamus. The decreased antidiuretic hormone (ADH) secretion results in polyuria and progressive dehydration. In the absence of excess fluid or hyperglycemia, DI should be suspected if the urine output exceeds 200-300 ml/hr. Onset of DI may be abrupt or delayed, is often associated with a "paradoxial" early SIADH phase, and is often self-limited.

The increased free water loss of DI should be replaced with hypotonic saline and appropriate potassium at a rate that includes the previous hour's urine output. Serum sodium and potassium levels should be checked frequently until the DI is controlled. Aqueous vasopressin can be given intermittently, at a dosage adjusted to the urinary output. Prolonged DI may be treated with longer-lasting vasopressin tannate in oil. Desmopressin acetate (DDAVP), a synthetic analogue of 8-arginine vasopressin, has decreased vasopressor activity and can be administered intravenously or intranasally.

SYNDROME OF INAPPROPRIATE ANTIDIURETIC HORMONE
The syndrome of inappropriate ADH secretion (SIADH) occurs frequently in head trauma and should be suspected if hyponatremia is associated with high urine osmolarity and sodium concentrations.[5,7] Clinically significant SIADH is usually the result of overadministration of free water in intravenous fluids to patients who cannot excrete free water because of excess ADH. Excess release of atrial natriuretic peptide (ANP) by the atria in response to stress may mimic SIADH as it can cause increased urinary sodium loss and hyponatremia even in the absence of hypervolemia. This cerebral salt wasting syndrome must be differentiated from SIADH.

SIADH is best treated by dehydration, but isotonic solutions (0.9% normal saline) may be necessary to prevent hypovolemia and hyponatremia early after injury. Hypertonic saline solutions may be required if the patient has central nervous system irritability and/or the serum sodium is less than 120 mEq/L. Rapid correction (faster than 0.5 mEq/L per hour) of chronic hyponatremia with a S$_{Na}$ less than 120 mEq/L may cause central pontine myelinolysis.

Nutrition

Patients with severe cerebral trauma (particularly those with midbrain syndrome) tend to develop a severe hypermetabolic state that peaks around the third day and lasts about a week.[162] In some patients with isolated head injury, the negative nitrogen balance may exceed 30 gm/day. Such patients require a high caloric and protein intake to avoid nitrogen wasting with its attendant possibilities of impaired host defenses, decubitus ulcers, and infections.[163]

At least one study has suggested that early total parenteral nutrition (TPN) is associated with better outcome than enteral feeding, possibly because greater amounts of both protein and calories can be administered earlier by this route.[163] However, a controlled prospective study by Young et al[164] showed no significant long-term advantage with either route.

AXIOM Patients with severe head injury should be started on nutritional support as soon as possible.

Early TPN in head injury may improve survival. The TPN should be supplemented or replaced after 3 or 4 days by oral or tube feeding if there are no gastrointestinal problems to preclude its use. Because patients with severe head injuries have increased gastroesophageal reflux,[165] there appear to be advantages to providing early jejunostomy feedings and gastric decompression with a gastrostomy tube. Use of gastrostomy and jejunostomy tubes inserted at laparotomy plus an early tracheostomy should also reduce the incidence and severity of sinus infections resulting from indwelling nasal catheters.

Blood glucose levels, nitrogen balance, and respiratory quotient should be monitored carefully. The hyperglycemia frequently seen after severe head injury may result from both the nonspecific response to stress as well as from abnormalities of cerebral metabolism.[166] Experimental evidence indicates that hyperglycemia above 200 mg/dl tends to cause harmful lactic acidosis in the injured brain.[55,167] Although high blood glucose levels in adults seem to correlate with poorer survival,[167] it is not known whether these results can be altered by treatment.

General Management
PATIENT POSITION
Patients with head injury should generally be kept in semi-Fowler's position, with 20 to 30° of head elevation, in order to decrease jugular venous pressure and cerebral vascular volume.[168] Even if the cervical spine is uninjured, the head should be maintained in a neutral position, by padding if necessary, since rotation, flexion, or extension of the neck may partially block the jugular veins and increase ICP.[5]

CORE TEMPERATURE
Body temperature should be kept within normal limits. Hyperpyrexia unrelated to infection is seen in about 15% of brain injuries as a result of blood in the ventricles or damage to the hypothalamus or brain stem.[5] If fever develops, therapy, including ice packs, cold blankets, and/or alcohol sponging, should be instituted promptly. Decreasing body temperature might, theoretically, offer the advantage of reducing cerebral oxygen requirements; however, a significant therapeutic benefit from induced hypothermia has not been demonstrated in cerebral trauma.[5]

Monitoring Evoked Potentials

The technique of monitoring evoked potentials (EPs) involves enhancement of the weak signals produced in the brain by sensory stimulation, and elimination of the "noise" from the brain's random electric activity and from outside electrical interference.[5] Three types of EPs may be tested: somatosensory (SSEP), using the median and/or sural nerves; auditory (AEP), using a series of clicks; or visual (VEP), using a flashing light. EPs can be important indicators of functional capacity over a wide area of the brain, in contrast to CT scans which show only anatomic derangements. They may provide the only means of neurologic evaluation of patients receiving muscle relaxants or barbiturates, and they can demonstrate functional improvement or deterioration in the course of these therapies. They can also indicate the degree and localization of cortical or brain stem impairment in the presence of coma and show which sensory areas are preserved. Most important, EPs can be extremely helpful in determining prognosis. A good recovery is likely if there is only a moderately altered EP pattern. In contrast, the patient with marked, diffuse EP abnormalities will almost certainly have a poor result.[169]

Newer Therapy

DIMETHYL SULFOXIDE
Dimethyl sulfoxide (DMSO) has shown beneficial effects in experimental brain injury and early clinical trials.[170] It is quite effective in reducing ICP and increasing CBF, without producing alteration of consciousness or hypotension.[171] However, DMSO is a potent diuretic, and it can cause significant electrolyte disturbances. At high concentrations, DMSO can also cause intravascular hemolysis and some decrease in platelet function.

PROPOFOL
Propofol is a short-acting, rapidly metabolized intravenous anesthetic agent recently introduced in the United States.[5] It does not cause cardiovascular instability, it has no cumulative effect, even after prolonged administration, and it does not inhibit steroidogenesis. It has been administered to a small number of head-injured patients, both for surgical anesthesia and for sedation in the intensive care unit.[172] Arterial blood pressure, ICP, and CPP were well maintained in the ICU throughout a 24-hour infusion at an average dose of 2.9 mg/kg/h.

ADRENOCORTICOTROPHIC HORMONE ANALOGS
Data suggests that certain neuroendocrine mechanisms are involved in the regulation of blood-brain barrier integrity in normal animals.[172] Fragments and analogs of adrenocorticotrophic and alpha-melanocyte-stimulating hormones have been found to reduce blood-brain barrier permeability. Because blood-brain barrier leakiness is an early event after head trauma, Goldman et al[173] used an analog of an adrenocortico-trophic hormone-related neuropeptide 15-30 minutes, 6 hours, and 24 hours post-traumatically and found that it successfully reversed and/or minimized trauma-induced abnormalities of the blood-brain barrier and the subsequent pathologically elevated intracranial pressure. It also reversed the early hypoperfusion that tends to follow head trauma.

21-AMINOSTEROIDS

> **AXIOM** By limiting lipid peroxidation in damaged brain, early administration of 21-aminosteroids (lazaroids) may be beneficial in head-injured patients.

Because of the high-dose nonglucocorticoid antioxidant action of methylprednisolone, various nonglucocorticoid steroid analogs of methylprednisolone have been synthesized in an attempt to find an agent that might be helpful in head trauma.[174] One such compound (U-74006F) is a potent and effective inhibitor of lipid peroxidation in experimental models of CNS trauma and ischemia.[175] It also inhibits lipid peroxidation in systems that do not contain membranes and are free of iron.[176] Other effects include: (a) decreased degradation of vitamin E, another antioxidant, (b) scavenging of hydroxyl and lipid peroxyl radicals, (c) hydroxyl radicals generated during in vitro Fenton reactions (i.e., $Fe^{2+} + H_2O_2 \rightarrow Fe^{3+} + OH^- + \cdot OH$), (d) stabilizing effects on cell membranes, and (e) decreased release of free arachidonic acid from injured cell membranes by inhibition of phospholipase A_2.

In other studies, U-74006F has been shown to localize within the hydrophobic core of cell membranes and to cause decreased fluidity of the phospholipid bilayer.[177] This may help to inhibit the propagation of lipid peroxidation by restricting the movement of lipid peroxyl and alkoxyl radicals within the membrane. Data obtained from a mouse head injury model shows that U-74006F can reduce mortality rates and post-traumatic brain hydroxyl radical concentrations.[178] This agent is now being tested in a multicenter clinical trial for the treatment of closed-head injuries.

TRIS HYDROXYMETHYL AMINOMETHANE
Tris hydroxymethyl aminomethane (THAM), a systemic and intracellular alkalinizing agent that crosses the blood-brain barrier, has been shown to reduce cerebrospinal fluid lactate levels after traumatic brain injury.[179] Thus, THAM can act as a buffering agent to raise cellular pH, thereby countering the adverse effects of excessive lactate production and acidosis, and increasing survival. Other studies, however, have not been so encouraging.[180]

CALCIUM ANTAGONISTS
Calcium antagonists may help inhibit cellular calcium influx, and thereby inhibit phospholipase activity and lipid peroxidation.[8] The activity of some "calcium antagonists" may be produced by interference with calcium activation of calmodulin, which mediates the phospholipase-stimulating action of calcium.[181] For example, flunarizine acts not only as a calcium channel blocker, but also as a calmodulin antagonist in the brain.[182]

IRON CHELATORS
Iron chelators may be useful in closed-head injury because iron is essential for the generation and activity of some of the toxic free radicals causing lipid peroxidation in head trauma.[8] Deferoxamine has also been shown to inhibit the initial hyperperfusion and the delayed hypoperfusion seen during postischemic brain reperfusion. A hetastarch-deferoxamine complex (with a much longer half-life) also improves both survival and neurologic outcome in animals during postischemic reperfusion.[183]

SUPEROXIDE DISMUTASE
Because of data suggesting that superoxide dismutase (SOD) was an effective superoxide scavenger, Zimmerman et al[184] studied the effects of topical SOD and catalase on a model of cryogenic brain injury and found that it reduced the tendency to intracranial hypertension. In that same year (1989), Levasseur et al[185] noted improved survival in rats subjected to fluid percussion brain injury treated with intravenous SOD.

In a randomized, double-blind, controlled phase II trial to evaluate head-injured humans with a GCS of 8 or less, 104 patients were randomized to receive a placebo or 2,000 units/kg, 5,000 units/kg, or 10,000 units/kg intravenous polyethylene glycol-superoxide dismutase as a bolus an average of 4 hours after injury.[23] At 3 months, 43% of patients in the placebo group were vegetative or had died, whereas only 20% of patients who had received SOD in doses of 10,000 units/kg were in those poor outcome categories. However, a larger multicenter phase III trial using a higher dose (20,000 units/kg) compared with placebo and 10,000 units/kg failed to demonstrate a statistically significant beneficial effect.

COMPLICATIONS OF SEVERE BRAIN INJURY

Pulmonary Complications

NEUROGENIC PULMONARY EDEMA

Definition
Neurogenic pulmonary edema (NPE) can be defined as a state of increased interstitial or alveolar lung water occurring in acute diseases of the nervous system, in the absence of cardiac or pulmonary disorders or hypervolemia.[186] It is characterized by a fulminant onset of pulmonary vascular congestion, alveolar hemorrhage, and exudation of protein-rich edema fluid.[5] It is most commonly associated with

subarachnoid hemorrhage (SAH), intracerebral hemorrhage, and head trauma.

Mechanisms

The most popular theory concerning the mechanism of NPE is that a massive sympathetic discharge produces a dramatic increase in peripheral vascular resistance, causing a shift of blood into the pulmonary vasculature.[187] This shift is accompanied by increased arterial and venous pressures in both the systemic and pulmonary circuits. The resultant abrupt dilation of pulmonary capillaries and venules can produce structural damage and altered capillary permeability.

Systemic hypertension causing cardiogenic pulmonary edema is not the major factor causing NPE as this problem can be produced without systemic hypertension, and the edema fluid is much higher in protein content than that seen with cardiogenic pulmonary edema.[188] Experimental models of NPE involving brain stem lesions reveal that lesions in the nucleus tractus solitarius or the adjacent noradrenergic A1 cell group will most reliably produce the condition.[189] Higher brain stem lesions, formerly thought to produce central neurogenic hyperventilation, and hypothalamic lesions in the lateral preoptic nuclei can also produce NPE.

Management

AXIOM   Fluid overload greatly increases the tendency to neurogenic pulmonary edema.

Since high filtration pressures in experimental models promote fluid leakage through pulmonary capillaries, PAWP should be kept as low as possible while maximizing cerebral blood flow. The PAWP should be kept in the 10-12 mm Hg range or lower. When NPE develops, the major problem is oxygenation.[190] Increasing the FiO_2 is important, but these patients quickly get into the range (FiO_2 more than 0.50) commonly thought to produce oxygen toxicity. Adding PEEP often produces a dramatic improvement in oxygenation, but at the cost of decreasing cardiac output and possibly also increasing the ICP.[186]

ACUTE RESPIRATORY DISTRESS SYNDROME

It can be difficult to distinguish between NPE and acute respiratory distress syndrome (ARDS) in head-injured patients; however, they are treated in the same way except for the increased efforts to keep ICP low in NPE. ARDS is usually the result of pulmonary capillary damage produced by shock, sepsis, severe ischemia, and/or tissue damage.[5] There is increased pulmonary vascular resistance and protein-rich fluid leaks into the interstitial spaces and alveoli, decreasing pulmonary compliance and increasing intrapulmonary shunt and hypoxia.

The use of positive end-expiratory pressure (PEEP) in head-injured patients is somewhat controversial. Both animal and clinical studies have indicated that PEEP can reduce jugular venous return and thereby increase cerebral blood volume and ICP.[191] Frost,[192] however, has shown that ICP is less apt to increase if the patient is maintained in a 30° semi-Fowler's position, even at PEEP levels as high as 40 cm H_2O. Nevertheless, high levels of PEEP tend to reduce cardiac output and O_2 delivery to the tissues, unless adequate hydration is maintained and/or inotropic agents are used as needed to maintain the O_2 delivery.

FAT EMBOLISM

Fat embolism is not usually recognized as a common cause of pulmonary failure in acute head injury, but it can be an important cause of hypoxemia in patients who also have multiple extremity fractures.[193] The pulmonary changes of fat embolism usually become evident 12-36 hours after the trauma, and this problem should be strongly suspected if the platelet count is lower than expected.

Cardiac Complications

The catecholamine release associated with severe brain trauma can increase the tendency to heart failure and arrhythmias. Clinical studies[194] have shown CPK-MB elevations occur in almost all brain-injured patients tested for this enzyme. The most frequent ECG changes are prolonged QT intervals and ST segment depression. In a study by McLeod et al,[195] two of seven patients with arrhythmias after head trauma died. Two other patients also showed evidence of myocardial infarction but survived.

Gastrointestinal Bleeding

AXIOM   Gastric pH must be monitored carefully in all head-injured patients and kept above 5.5 with appropriate medications.

Gastrointestinal (GI) bleeding is common after severe head injury and up to 30% of comatose patients treated in an ICU will show clinical evidence of blood loss from the GI tract.[194] In 1932, Harvey Cushing[194] described ulcers of the stomach, duodenum, and/or esophagus in patients with a variety of cerebral problems.

The probable cause of ulcers associated with head trauma is elevated gastric acidity resulting from hypothalamic stimulation of vagal activity.[198] Significant hemorrhage or perforation of Cushing's ulcers should be considered in any head-injured patient who develops abdominal distension, ileus, hypotension, or anemia.[5,196]

A controlled trial of cimetidine (300 mg every 4 hours intravenously until oral feedings were begun and orally thereafter) did not change the incidence of GI problems; however, the patients receiving cimetidine had a lower incidence of lesions requiring transfusion or surgery.[199] The H_2 blockers are now usually given to head-injured patients as a continuous intravenous drip, which appears to be much more effective than intermittent doses.

Coagulation Problems

AXIOM   Damaged brain tissue is a powerful procoagulant and can cause a severe consumptive coagulopathy.

Clotting disorders, particularly disseminated intravascular coagulation (DIC), are quite common after severe brain trauma and may represent a significant contributing factor in patients dying as a result of hemorrhage and/or intractable cerebral edema.[200] Appropriate therapy involves treating the causes, restoring blood volume, and administering clotting factors (such as cryoprecipitate and fresh frozen plasma) and platelets.

OUTCOME

Although the outcome of patients with severe head injury is often poor, some progress is being made. The Glasgow Outcome Scale[201] provides a basis for comparing the results of treatment in different centers and for evaluating new therapeutic measures as they are introduced. There are five categories of results.

1. Good recovery: complete neurologic recovery or presence of only minor deficits that do not prevent the patient from returning to his or her former level of function
2. Moderately disabled: deficits that prevent normal function but allow self-care
3. Severely disabled: marked deficits which prevent self-care
4. Vegetative: no evidence of higher mental function
5. Dead

In adults, the overall mortality for serious head injuries averages 40%, and another 13% of patients are vegetative or severely disabled.[202] Some factors affecting outcome are independent of medical care. As age increases, the chance of a good recovery decreases significantly.[21,203] Compared with adults, children have fewer severe lesions and intracranial hematomas, and have an improved survival and rate of recovery.[22,23,221] Nevertheless, even in children, a low GCS score and absent pupillary reaction and brain stem reflexes after an adequate resuscitation correlate highly with a poor outcome.

The presence of an intracranial mass lesion worsens prognosis, and in one series it increased mortality from 17 to 40%.[16] Outcome, however, also depends on the type of intracranial hematoma present. For example, in a study of 107 patients, a poor outcome (dead, vegetative, or severely disabled) occurred in 24% of patients with an epidural hematoma, 58% of patients with a subdural hematoma, and 79% of patients with intracerebral hematomas.[203] Temporal lobe lesions and all lesions causing a high degree of midline shift increase the likelihood that the patient will have a poor functional outcome.[18,100] The higher morbidity and mortality of subdural and intracerebral hematomas has been attributed to a higher incidence of more severe concomitant cerebral injuries.

The Glasgow Coma Scale (GCS), although not originally intended as a prognostic index, is a strong indicator of outcome. After 6 hours, a GCS of 3 or 4 is almost always associated with a poor outcome, and a score of 5-7 is associated with a poor outcome in more than 50% of patients. Almost all patients with a GCS of 8 or more at 6 hours have a grade 1 or 2 outcome.[204]

Mortality rates for patients who talk and then deteriorate remain high, confirming that any cause of deterioration is ominous.[17] The patients in the Traumatic Coma Data Bank with an initial GCS score of 9 or more and deterioration to a GCS score of 8 or less did substantially worse than patients with an initial GCS score of 6, 7, or 8.[205]

Interestingly, there are questions as to what extent aggressive treatment of severe head injuries really improves survival. The usual standard for comparison is the large multinational survey of 700 cases of brain injury reported by Jennett et al in 1977.[206] Some, but not all, patients received hyperventilation, mannitol, and/or steroids. The overall results at 6 months were: dead, 51%; vegetative or severely disabled, 11%; moderate or no disability, 38%.

When compared with 158 patients who had similar injuries but were treated aggressively with early intubation and ventilation, early surgery for mass lesions, and continuous monitoring of ICP with prompt therapy for ICP elevation, there was a 40% mortality, 12% severely disabled or vegetative, and 47% with moderate or no disability.[207,208] Thus, a significant reduction in mortality was achieved (51% versus 40%) and the incidence of moderate or no disability increased (38% versus 47%). A sophisticated statistical analysis of the predictive power of clinical and laboratory data obtained from head-injured patients has been reported by Narayan et al.[111] They found that although a combination of clinical data (age, GCS, mass lesions, pupillary responses, ocular motility, and motor posturing) provided the best indications of outcome, the addition of laboratory results could further increase the reliability of predictions based on clinical status. It should be possible, then, to determine with some accuracy which patients are likely to benefit from prolonged intensive care.

⊘ FREQUENT ERRORS

In the Management of Head Injury Patients

1. *Inadequate attention to other severe injuries.*
2. *Delay in restoring an adequate blood volume and correcting hypoxemia.*
3. *Delay in intubating patients with severe head injury.*
4. *Assuming that there is little or no neurological defect in patients with "mild head injuries."*
5. *Making strong efforts to reduce an elevated ICP without enough attention to maintaining a more than adequate CPP.*
6. *Delay in obtaining a CT scan in patients with moderate-severe head injury.*
7. *Delay in measuring ICP in patients who have severe brain injury or require a craniotomy to evacuate an intracranial hematoma.*

8. *Inadequate frequency of careful neurological examinations.*
9. *Failure to act on any change in pupil size or reactivity.*
10. *Failure to act on any deterioration of CNS function.*
11. *Failure to take strong steps to rule out or prevent spinal cord injury.*
12. *Failure to get prompt repeat CT scans of the head in patients who deteriorate neurologically.*
13. *Delaying mannitol therapy in a patient with rapid neurological deterioration.*
14. *Overcorrecting hypertension, particularly before evacuating an intracranial mass lesion.*
15. *Failure to give adequate prophylaxis for stress ulceration.*
16. *Failure to closely monitor urine output and osmolarity.*

▼▼▼▼▼▼▼▼▼▼▼▼▼▼▼▼▼▼▼▼▼▼▼▼▼▼▼▼▼

SUMMARY POINTS

1. Head injury is the leading cause of mortality and morbidity after trauma.

2. Although there is usually no specific treatment for primary brain injury, at least some secondary injury is preventable or treatable.

3. Brain edema of sufficient magnitude to significantly alter intracranial pressure is virtually never observed in patients in the absence of either focal shear-strain injuries or hemorrhage.

4. Hypoxemia and hypotension are the most frequent systemic insults causing secondary brain injury.

5. Unless large intracranial hematomas are removed promptly, intracranial pressure can rise rapidly because of further bleeding or edema formation.

6. If subarachnoid hemorrhage is seen on the CT scan, there is an increased likelihood of the patient developing cerebral vasospasm.

7. Increased intracellular calcium can cause a large number of reactions that can directly or indirectly increase secondary brain damage.

8. Free radical damage of brain tissue may be decreased by making iron unavailable.

9. Excessive release of excitatory amino acids after head trauma can greatly aggravate secondary brain injury.

10. Magnesium deficiencies can contribute to the severity of secondary brain injury.

11. Skull fractures greatly increase the likelihood of underlying brain injury.

12. Although cerebral concussions are generally considered mild head injuries, extensive subclinical damage may be present.

13. The magnitude and distribution of diffuse axonal injury ultimately reflect the morbidity of the head injury, particularly in patients who do not have a mass lesion.

14. Much of the relatively poor prognosis associated with acute subdural hematomas is due to the underlying brain damage.

15. Epidural hematomas are uncommon but usually have a good prognosis with prompt surgical evacuation.

16. A lucid interval should warrant special efforts to rule out an acute epidural hematoma.

17. It is now generally felt that an arteriovenous oxygen difference of 8 ml/dl or more or a jugular bulb oxygen saturation less than 50% is an indication of cerebral ischemia after severe head injury.

18. Even in the absence of increased intracranial pressure, hypercarbia, or hypoxemia, endotracheal intubation of patients with severe head injury is generally indicated for prevention of secondary hypoxic brain damage.

19. Although cerebral blood flow does not correlate with outcome in all head injuries, it appears to be a significant factor in patients with severe injury.

20. In head-injured patients with impaired cerebral autoregulation, cerebral blood flow is directly dependent on the arterial BP.

21. Hyperventilation and hypocapnia are most effectively used for early, temporary control of intracranial pressure.

22. After head injury, the ability of the brain to reduce CSF in response to a rising ICP can be severely limited.

23. A declining PVI may be an early warning of an impending dangerous rise in ICP.

24. Regardless of the cause of an elevated ICP in head trauma, failure to promptly reduce it to less than 20 mm Hg is generally indicative of a poor prognosis.

25. ICP monitoring is indicated in patients who have severe head injuries (i.e., GCS of 8 or less) after adequate resuscitation.

26. Although a moderate rise in arterial pressure may help maintain the CPP, an exaggerated effect may be harmful.

27. The management of blood pressure in patients with head injury must tread the fine line between maintenance of adequate cerebral perfusion and exacerbation of cerebral edema.

28. An arterial $PaCO_2$ less than 25 mm Hg may significantly impair cerebral perfusion.

29. If, after head trauma, a decompressive craniotomy is not performed before cerebral herniation occurs, death or severe disability is almost certain.

30. In general, marked and prolonged retrograde amnesia indicates a more serious and prolonged period of initial unconsciousness.

31. Any tendency to hypoxemia or hypotension should be corrected before performing a complete neurologic examination.

32. All patients with major trauma should be assumed to have a head injury and cervical spine fracture until proven otherwise.

33. The sine qua non of head-injury management is repetitive careful neurological examinations and timely intervention.

34. One cannot rely on neurologic assessments until adequate perfusion and oxygenation have been obtained.

35. Any change in the size, shape, or reactivity of a pupil after head trauma may indicate early herniation.

36. A fixed pupil may be caused by head trauma, cerebral aneurysm, hypoxia, hypotension, seizures, eye trauma, injury to the third cranial nerve, and various drugs.

37. A new focal motor deficit is an important sign that the patient needs immediate, aggressive care.

38. Proper observation of a head-injury patient means repeated careful neurological examination.

39. A significant deterioration in the state of consciousness is almost invariably associated with an alteration of the ventilatory pattern.

40. Central neurogenic hyperventilation is the most frequent type of abnormal breathing in patients with moderate-severe head injuries.

41. Hypotension is extremely dangerous in patients with head injury and must be corrected as soon as possible.

42. Hypotension in a patient with adequate or increased ventilation generally results from associated non-cerebral injuries.

43. The presence of alcohol or illicit drugs should be checked in all patients with a head injury.

44. Although skull fractures do not generally require treatment, they indicate a much greater likelihood of severe underlying brain damage.

45. One should assume that all head-injured patients have associated cervical spine fractures until ruled out by complete clinical and radiologic examinations.

46. CT scanning is the most accurate and expeditious method to localize and quantify intracranial mass lesions.

47. Patients who are admitted with signs of cerebral herniation or who deteriorate during their initial evaluation should receive mannitol (1.0 to 1.5 g/kg) by rapid intravenous infusion while attempting to obtain at least a limited CT scan through the cerebral hemispheres before surgery.

48. Cerebral angiography may be the only readily available means of diagnosing traumatic intracranial mass lesions if CT scanning is unavailable.

49. Although not all patients with head injury require neurosurgical consultation, they all require prompt, frequent, and careful neurological assessment.

50. Assisted or controlled ventilation should be provided to severely head-injured patients to ensure adequate oxygenation and a PCO_2 of 350-40 mm Hg for the first 2-3 days.

51. Although emergency intubation of head-injured patients without appropriate premedication can cause an abrupt rise in ICP, there is not always time for such medications.

52. Even if the ICP is elevated, hypotension in head-injured patients is still usually best treated by administering fluids.

53. Vasopressors should be used cautiously, if at all, in head-injured patients, because their effect on CBF is not well-defined.

54. The treatment of hypertension in a head-injured patient should be directed primarily at reducing ICP and/or evacuating intracranial hematomas.

55. Serum osmolarity should be monitored and kept less than 320 mOsm/L during mannitol therapy.

56. An intracranial hematoma causing increasing neurological dysfunction or more than 5 mm midline displacement should be evacuated as soon as possible.

57. Scalp lacerations involving the galea should generally be explored, cleaned, and closed in the OR.

58. In areas where neurosurgical help is not readily available, general surgeons should have the ability to make cranial trephine openings (burr holes) to evacuate intracranial hematomas.

59. Although the intracranial space can be decompressed to some extent through burr holes, adequate evacuation of the majority of intracranial hematomas requires a bone flap.

60. Abrupt cessation of mannitol therapy can cause a rebound rise in ICP.

61. Barbiturates are probably of greatest value in reducing brain damage in patients who have persistently high ICPs in spite of all other therapy.

62. The only way to reliably monitor the neurologic status of a patient in barbiturate coma is with evoked potentials and, if these deteriorate, one should obtain a repeat CT scan.

63. If the ICP remains high in spite of surgery and barbiturate therapy, a fatal outcome is virtually certain.

64. In adults, continuous ventilatory support may not only help to control the ICP, but it may also prevent hypoxic brain damage that might be caused by unexpected apnea, respiratory obstruction, or respiratory insufficiency.

65. Ventilation in patients with moderate-severe head injuries should be monitored by both arterial blood gases and the ICP.

66. An abrupt decline in BP is usually much more damaging to an injured brain than moderate-severe hypertension.

67. In severe head-injury patients (GCS below 8), a pulmonary artery catheter should be inserted and efforts made to optimize oxygen delivery to the brain.

68. If a jugular bulb catheter is in place, one should try to keep $C(a jb)O_2$ differences less than 6 vol% or $S_{jb}O_2$ above 50%.

69. Urine output and serum electrolytes should be monitored carefully in all severely head-injured patients.

70. The deleterious effects of seizures occur even when motor responses are blocked by muscle relaxants or paraplegia.

71. Steroids should not be used routinely in the management of severe head injury.

72. Patients with severe head injury should be started on nutritional support as soon as possible.

73. By limiting lipid peroxidation in damaged brain, early administration of 21-aminosteroids (lazaroids) may be beneficial in head-injured patients.

74. Fluid overload greatly increases the tendency to neurogenic pulmonary edema.

75. Gastric pH must be monitored carefully in all head-injured patients and kept above 5.5 with appropriate medications.

76. Damaged brain tissue is a powerful procoagulant and can cause a severe consumptive coagulopathy.

▲▲▲▲▲▲▲▲▲▲▲▲▲▲▲▲▲▲▲▲▲▲▲▲▲▲▲▲▲▲▲▲▲▲▲▲▲

REFERENCES

1. Thomas LM, Gurdjian ES. Some considerations in the initial management of injuries to the head and spine. In: Walt AJ, Wilson RF, eds. Management of trauma: pitfalls and practice. Philadelphia: Lee & Febiger, 1975:197.

2. Bennett BR, Jacobs LM, Schwartz RJ. Incidence, cost, and DRG-based reimbursement for traumatic brain injured patients: a 3-year experience. J Trauma 1989;29:556.

3. Shackford SR, Mackersie RC, Davis JW, et al. Epidemiology and pathology of traumatic deaths occurring at a level I trauma center in a regional system: the importance of secondary brain injury. J Trauma 1989;29:1392.

4. Cooper PR. Epidemiology of head injury. In: Cooper PR, ed. Head injury. Baltimore: Williams & Wilkins, 1982:12.

5. Miller SM. Management of central nervous system injuries. In: Capan LM, Miller SM, Turndorf H, eds. Trauma: anesthesia and intensive care. Philadelphia: JB Lippincott Co, 1991:321.

6. Shogan SH, Kindt GW. Injuries of the head and spinal cord. In: Zuidema GD, Rutherford RB, Ballinger WF, eds. The management of trauma. Philadelphia: WB Saunders, 1985:207.

7. Lahaye PA, Gade GF, Becker DP. Injury to the cranium. In: Moore EE, Mattox KL, Feliciano DV, eds. Trauma. 2nd ed. Norwalk, CT: Appleton & Lange, 1991:247.

8. White BC, Krause GS. Brain injury and repair mechanisms: the potential for pharmacologic therapy in closed-head trauma. Ann Emerg Med 1993;22:970.

9. Wilberger JE, Rothfus WE, Tabas J, et al. Acute tissue tear hemorrhages of the brain: computed tomography and clinicopathological correlations. Neurosurgery 1990;27:208.

10. Gentry LR, Godersky JC, Thompson B. MR imaging of head trauma: review of the distribution and radiopathologic features of traumatic lesions. Am J Roentgenol 1988;150:663.

11. Povlishock JT, Kontos HA. Continuing axonal and vascular change after experimental brain trauma. Cent Nerv Syst Trauma 1985;2:285.

12. Rose J, Valtonen S, Bennett B. Avoidable factors contributing to death after head injury. Br Med J 1977;2:615.

13. Miller JD, Becker DB. Secondary insults to the injured brain. J Royal Coll Surg Edinburgh 1982;27:292.

14. Ommaya AK, Gennarelli TA. Cerebral concussion and traumatic unconsciousness. Brain 1974;97:633.

15. Hovda DA, Becker DP, Katayama Y. Secondary injury acidosis. J Neurotrauma 1992;9:S47.

16. Seelig JM, Becker DP, Miller JD, et al. Traumatic acute subdural hematoma: major mortality reduction in comatose patients treated under 4 hours. N Engl J Med 1981;304:1511.

17. Rockswold GL, Pheley PJ. Patients who talk and deteriorate. Ann Emerg Med 1993;22:1004.

18. Lobato RD, Rivas JJ, Gomez PA, et al. Head-injured patients who talk and deteriorate into coma. J Neurosurg 1991;75:256.

19. Andrews BT. Management of delayed posttraumatic intracerebral hemorrhage. Contemp Neurosurg 1988;10:1.

20. Marmarou A, Anderson RL, Ward JD, et al. Impact of ICP instability and hypotension on outcome in patients with severe head trauma. J Neurosurg 1991;75:S59.

21. Snoek JW, Minderhoud JM, Wilmink JT. Delayed deterioration following mild head injury in children. Brain 1984;107:15.

22. Martin NM, Doberstein C, Zane CJ, et al. Post-traumatic cerebral arterial spasm: transcranial Doppler ultrasound, cerebral blood flow, and angiographic findings. J Neurosurg 1992;77:575.

23. Muizelaar JP. Cerebral ischemia-reperfusion injury after severe head injury and its possible treatment with polyethyleneglycol-superoxide dismutase. Ann Emerg Med 1993;22:1014.

24. Katayama Y, Becker DP, Tamura T, et al. Massive increases in extracellular potassium and the indiscriminate release of glutamate following concussive brain injury. J Neurosurg 1990;73:889.

25. McCord JM. Oxygen derived free radicals in postischemic tissue injury. N Engl J Med 1985;312:159.

26. Bouma GJ, Muizelaar JP, Choi SC, et al. Central circulation and metabolism after traumatic brain injury: the elusive role of ischemia. J Neurosurg 1991;75:685.

27. Bouma GJ, Muizelaar JP, Stringer WA, et al. Ultra early evaluation of regional cerebral blood flow in severely head-injured patients using xenon-enhanced computed tomography. J Neurosurg 1992;77:360.

28. Shapira Y, Shohami E, Sidi A, et al. Experimental closed head injury in rats: mechanical, pathophysiologic, and neurologic properties. Crit Care Med 1988;16:258.

29. Kumar K, White BC, Kraus GS, et al. A quantitative morphological assessment of the effect of lidoflazine and deferoxamine therapy for global brain ischemia. Neurol Res 1988;10:136.

30. Krause GS, White BC, Aust SD, et al. Brain cell death after ischemia and reperfusion: a proposed biochemical sequence. Crit Care Med 1988;16:714.

31. Siesjo BK. Basic mechanisms of traumatic brain damage. Ann Emerg Med 1993;22:959.

32. Kontos HA. Oxygen radicals in CNS damage. Chem-biol 1989;72:229.

33. Faden AI, Demediuk P, Panter SS, et al. The role of excitatory amino acids and NMDA receptors in traumatic brain injury. Science 1989;244:798.

34. Povlishock JT. Traumatically induced axonal injury: pathogenesis and pathological implications. Brain Pathol 1992;2:1.

35. Hubschmann OR, Nathanson DC. The role of calcium and cellular membrane dysfunction in experimental trauma and subarachnoid hemorrhage. J Neurosurg 1985;62:698.

36. Wei EP, Lamb RG, Kontos HA. Increased phospholipase C activity after experimental brain injury. J. Neurosurg 1982;56:695.

37. Kontos HA, Wei EP. Superoxide production in experimental brain injury. J Neursci 1985;64:803.

38. Halliwell B, Gutteridge JMC. Oxygen toxicity, oxygen radicals, transition metals, and disease. Biochem J 1984;219:1.

39. Thomas CE, Morehouse LA, Aust SO. Ferritin and superoxide dependent lipid peroxidation. J Biol Chem 1985;260:3275.

40. Kontos HA, Povlishock JT. Oxygen radicals in brain injury. Cent Nerv Syst Trauma 1986;3:257.

41. Gentile NT, McIntosh TK. Antagonists of excitatory amino acids and endogenous opioid peptides in the treatment of experimental central nervous system injury. Ann Emerg Med 1993;22:1028.

42. Olney JW. Inciting excitotoxic cytocide among central neurons. Adv Exp Mel Biol 1986;203:631.

43. Rothman SM, Olney JW. Glutamate and the pathophysiology of hypoxic-ischemic brain damage. Ann Neuron 1986;19:105.

44. Choi DW. Ionic dependence of glutamate neurotoxicity. J Neurosci 1987;7:369.

45. Miller LP, Lyeth BG, Jenkins LW. Excitatory amino acid receptor subtype binding following traumatic brain injury. Brain Res 1990;526:103.

46. Dykens JA, Stern A, Trenkner E. Mechanism of kainate toxicity to cerebellar neurons in vitro is analogous to reperfusion tissue injury. J Neurochem 1987;49:1222.

47. Kemp JA, Foster AC, Wang EHF. Noncompetitive antagonists of excitatory amino acid receptors. Trends Neurosci 1987;10:294.

48. Vink R, McIntosh TK, Demuduk P, et al. Decline in intracellular free Mg^{++} is associated with irreversible tissue injury after brain trauma. J Bill Chem 1968;263:757.

49. Ebel H, Gunterh T. Magnesium metabolism: a review. J Clin Chem Clin Biochem 1980;18:257.

50. McIntosh TK, Faden AI, Yamakami I, et al. Magnesium deficiency exacerbates and pretreatment improves outcome following traumatic brain injury in rats: ^{31}P magnetic resonance spectroscopy and behavioral studies. J Neurotrauma 1988;5:1731.

51. McIntosh TK, Vink R, Yamakami I, et al. Magnesium protects against neurological deficit after brain injury. Brain Res 1989;482:257.

52. Crockard HA, Brown FD, Johns LM, Mullan S. An experimental cerebral missile injury model in primates. J Neurosurg 1977;46:776.

53. Braakman R. Emergency craniotomy in severe head injury and the present state of knowledge regarding prognosis. Injury 1983;14:22.

54. McCormick WF. Pathology of closed head injury. In: Wilkins RH, Rengachary SS, eds. Neurosurgery. New York: McGraw-Hill, 1985:1544.

55. Goldman H, Hodgson V, Morehead M, et al. A rat model of closed head injury. J Neurotrauma 1990;8:129.

56. Povlishock JT. Pathobiology of traumatically induced axonal injury in animals and man. Ann Emerg Med 1993;22:980.

57. Adams JH, Graham DI, Murray LS, et al. Diffuse axonal injury due to nonmissile head injury in humans: an analysis of 45 cases. Ann Neurol 1982;12:557.

58. Maxwell WL, Graham DI, Adams JH, et al. Focal axonal injury: the early axonal response to stretch. J Neurocytol 1991;20:157.

59. Adams JH, Grahan DI, Gennarelli TA, et al. Diffuse axonal injury in non-missile head injury. J Neurol Neurosurg Psychiatry 1991;54:481.

60. Markwalder TM. Chronic subdural hematomas: a review. J Neurosurg 1981;54:637.

61. Bruce DA. Management of severe head injury. In: Cottrell JE, Turndorf H, eds. Anesthesia and neurosurgery. 2nd ed. St. Louis: CV Mosby, 1986:150.

62. Miller JD, Bell BA. Cerebral blood flow variations with perfusion pressure and metabolism. In: Wood JH, ed. Cerebral blood flow physiologic and clinical aspects. New York: McGraw-Hill, 1987:119-130.

63. Rosner MJ, Daughton S. Cerebral perfusion pressure management in head injury. J Trauma 1990;30:933.

64. Robertson CS, Narayan RK, Gokaslan ZL, et al. Cerebral arteriovenous oxygen difference as an estimate of cerebral blood flow in comatose patients. J Neurosurg 1989;70:222.

65. Walls RM. Rapid-sequence intubation in head trauma. Ann Emerg Med 1993;22:1008.

66. Woster PS, LeBlanc KL. Management of elevated intracranial pressure. Clin Pharm 1990;9:762.

67. Radan JA, Livingston DH, Tortella BJ, et al. The value of intubating and paralyzing patients with suspected head injury in the emergency department. J Trauma 1991;31:371.

68. Yoshino E, Yamaki T, Higuchi T, et al. Acute brain edema in fatal head injury. Analysis by dynamic CT scanning. J Neurosurg 1985;63:830.

69. Jaggi JL, Obrist WD, Gennarelli TA, et al. Relationship of early cerebral blood flow and metabolism to outcome in acute head injury. J Neurosurg 1990;72:176.

70. Schrader H, Lofgren J, Swetnow NN. Influence of blood pressure on tolerance to an intracranial expanding mass. Acta Neurol Scand 1985; 71:114.

71. Rosner MJ, Coley I. Cerebral perfusion pressure: a hemodynamic mechanism of mannitol and the postmannitol hemogram. Neurosurg 1987; 21:147.

72. Bouma GJ, Muizelaar JP, Bandoh K, et al. Blood pressure and intracranial pressure-volume dynamics in severe head injury: relationship with cerebral blood flow. J Neurosurg 1992;77:15.

73. Muizelaar JP, Lutz HA III, Becker DP. Effect of mannitol on intracranial pressure and cerebral blood flow and correlation with pressure autoregulation in severely head-injured patients. J Neurosurg 1984;61:700.

74. Burke AM, Quest DO, Chien S, et al. The effects of mannitol on blood viscosity. J Neurosurg 1981;55:550.

75. Karaca M, Bilgin UY, Akar M, et al. Dimethyl sulfoxide lowers ICP after closed head trauma. Eur J Clin Pharmacol 1991;40:113.

76. Schmoker JD, Zhuang J, Shackford SR. Hypertonic fluid resuscitation improves cerebral oxygen delivery and reduces intracranial pressure after hemorrhagic shock. J Trauma 1991;31:1607.

77. Fessler RD, Diaz FG. The management of cerebral perfusion pressure and intracranial pressure after severe head injury. Ann Emerg Med 1993;22:998.

78. Muizelaar JP, van der Poel HG. Cerebral vasoconstriction is not maintained with prolonged hyperventilation. In: Hoff JT, Bertz AL, eds. Intracranial pressure VII. Berlin-Heidelberg: Springer Verlag 1989;899.

79. Bullock R, Chesnut RM, Clifton G, et al. Guidelines for the management of severe head injury. Brain Trauma Foundation, 1995.

80. Monro A. Observations on the structure and function of the nervous system. Edinburgh: Greech and Johnson, 1783.

81. Kellie G. An account of the appearances observed in the dissection of two of the three individuals presumed to have perished in the storm of the 3rd, and whose bodies were discovered in the vicinity of Leith on the morning of the 4th November 1821 with some reflections on the pathology of the brain. Trans Med Chir Sci Edinburgh 1984;1:84-169.

82. Burrows G. Disorders of the cerebral circulation. Philadelphia: Leu & Blanchards, 1984.

83. Gudeman SK, Young HF, Miller JD, Ward JD, Beiker DP. Indications for operative treatment and operative technique in closed head injury. In: Becker DP, Gudeman SK, eds. Textbook of head injury. Philadelphia: WB Saunders, 1989:138-181.

84. Marmarou A, Maset AL, Ward JD, et al: Contribution of CSF and vascular factors to elevation of ICP in severely head-injured patients. J Neurosurg 1987;66:833.

85. Kosteljanetz M. Intracranial pressure: cerebrospinal fluid dynamics and pressure-volume relations. Acta Neurol Scand 1987;75(Suppl 111).

86. Maset AL, Marmarou A, Ward JD. Pressure-volume index in head injury. J Neurosurg 1987;66:832.

87. Yano M, Kobayashi S, Otsuka T, et al. Useful ICP monitoring with subarachnoid catheter method in severe head injuries. J Trauma 1988; 28:476.

88. Guillaume J, Janny P. Manometrie intracranienne continue: interet de la methode aux premiers résultats. Revue Neurologique 1951;84:131-142.

89. Lundberg N. Continuous recording and control of ventricular fluid pressure in neurosurgical practice. Acta Psychiatrica et Neurologica Scandinavica 1960;36 (Suppl 149):1-193.

90. Vries JK, Becker DP, Young HF. A subarachnoid screw for monitoring intracranial pressure: technical note. Journal of Neurosurgery 1979;39: 416-419.

91. Ward JD. Intracranial pressure monitoring. In: Champion HR, Robbs JV, Trunkey DD, eds. Rob and Smiths' operative surgery: trauma surgery, part I. 4th ed. London: Butterworths, 1989:217-223.

92. Durward QJ, Del Maestro RF, Amacher A, et al. The influence of systemic arterial pressure and intracranial pressure on the development of cerebral vasogenic edema. J Neurosurg 1983;59:803.

93. Shapiro HM. Intracranial hypertension: therapeutic and anesthetic considerations. Anesthesiology 1975;43:445.

94. DeSalles AA, Muizelaar JP, Young HF. Hyperglycemia, cerebrospinal fluid lactic acidosis, and cerebral blood flow in severely head-injured patients. Neurosurgery 1987;21:45.

95. Overgaard J. The distribution of regional cerebral blood flow values in traumatic coma. In: Grossman RG, Gildenberg PL, eds. Head injury: basic and clinical aspects. New York: Raven Press, 1982:239.

96. Miller JD. Head injury and brain-ischemia: implications for therapy. Br J Anaesth 1985;57:120.

97. Dresser LP, McKinney WM. Anatomic and pathophysiologic studies of the human internal jugular valve. Am J Surg 1987;154:220.

98. Suwanwela C, Suwanwela N. Intracranial arterial narrowing and spasm in acute head injury. J Neurosurg 1972;36:314.

99. Michael BD, Guyot DR, Darmody WR. Coincidence of head and cervical spine injury. J. Neurotrauma 1989;6:177.

100. Marshall LF, Toole BM, Bowers SA. The National Traumatic Coma Data Bank, part 2: patients who talk and deteriorate. J Neurosurg 1983;59:285.

101. Marshall LF, Barba D, Toold BM, et al. The oval pupil: clinical significance and relationship to intracranial hypertension. J Neurosurg 1983; 58:566.

102. O'Malley KF, Ross SE. The incidence of injury to the cervical spine in patients with craniocerebral injury. J Trauma 1988;28:1476.

103. Tabaddor K. Emergency care: initial evaluation. In: Cooper PR, ed. Head injury. Baltimore: Williams and Wilkins 1982:15.

104. Feuerman T, Wackym PA, Gade GF, et al. Value of skull radiography, head computed tomographic scanning, and admission for observation in cases of minor head injury. Neurosurgery 1988;22:449.

105. Gandy SE, Snot RB, Zimmerman RE, et al. Cranial nuclear magnetic resonance imaging in head trauma. Ann Neurol 1984;16:254.

106. Marshall LF, Bowers SA. Medical management of intracranial pressure. In: Cooper PR, ed. Head injury. 2nd ed. Baltimore: Williams & Wilkins, 1987:177.

107. Narayan RK, Kishore DRS, Becker DP, et al. Intracranial pressure: to monitor or not to monitor? J Neurosurg 1982;56:650.

108. Gelb AW, Manninen PH, Mezon BJ, et al. The anaesthetist and the head-injured patient. Can Anaest Soc J 1984;31:98.

109. Bakay RA, Sweeney KM, Wood JH. Pathophysiology of CSF in head injury, part 2. Neurosurg 1986;18:376.

110. Rabow L, DeSalles AF, Becker DP, et al. Cerebral spinal fluid brain creatine kinase levels and lactic acidosis in severe head injury. J Neurosurg 1986;65:625.

111. Narayan RK, Greenberg RP, Miller JD, et al. Improved confidence of outcome prediction in severe head injury: a comprehensive analysis of clinical examination multimodality evoked potentials, CT scanning, and intracranial pressure. J Neurosurg 1981;54:751.

112. Judson JA, Cant BR, Shaw NA. Early prediction of outcome from cerebral trauma by somatosensory evoked potentials. Crit Care Med 1990;18:363.

113. Doberstein CE, Hovda DA, Becker DP. Clinical considerations in the reduction of secondary brain injury. Ann Emerg Med 1993;22.993.

114. McDowall DG. Artificial ventilation in the management of the head-injured patient. In: Fitch W, Barker J, eds. Head injury and the anaesthetist. Amsterdam: Elsevier, 1985:149.

115. Dronen SC, et al. A comparison of blind nasotracheal and succinylcholine-assisted intubation in the poisoned patient. Ann Emerg Med 1987;16:650.

116. Dohi S, Inomata S, Tanaka M, et al. End-tidal carbon dioxide monitoring during awake blind nasotracheal intubation. J Clin Anesth 1990; 2:415.

117. Helfman SM, Gold MI, DeLisser EA, et al. Which drug prevents tachycardia and hypertension associated with tracheal intubation: lidocaine, fentanyl, or esmolol? Anesth Analg 1991;72:482.

118. Bernstein JS, Ebert TJ, Stowe DF, et al. Partial attenuation of hemodynamic responses to rapid sequence induction and intubation with labetalol. J Clin Anaesth 1989;1:444.

119. Miller DR, Wellwood M, Teasdale SJ, et al. Effects of anaesthetic induction on myocardial function and metabolism: a comparison of fentanyl, sufentanil, and alfentanil. Can J Anaesth 1988;35:219.

120. Nagao S, Murota T, Momma F, et al. The effect of intravenous lidocaine on experimental brain edema and neural activities. J Trauma 1988; 12:1650.

121. Eisenberg HM, Frankowski RF, Constant CF, et al. High-dose barbiturate control of elevated intracranial pressure in patients with severe head injury. J Neurosurg 1988;69:15.

122. Cold GE, Eskesen V, Eriksen H, et al. CBF and $CMRO_2$ during continuous etomidate infusion supplemented with N_2O and fentanyl in patients with supratentorial cerebral tumor: a dose-response study. Acta Anesthesiol Scand 1985;29:490.

123. Minton MD, Grosslight K, Stirt JA, et al. Increases in intracranial pressure from succinylcholine. Prevention by prior nondepolarizing blockade. Anaesthesiology 1986;65:165.

124. Tullock WC, Diana P, Cook DR, et al. Neuromuscular and cardiovascular effects of high-dose vecuronium. Anesth Analg 1990;70:86.

125. Rosner MJ, Becker DP. Origin and evolution of plateau waves. J Neurosurg 1984;60:312.

126. Clifton GL, Robertson CS, Kyper K, et al. Cardiovascular response to severe head injury. J Neurosurg 1984;60:687.

127. Feldman Z, Kanter MJ, Robertson CS, et al. Effect of head elevation on intracranial pressure, cerebral perfusion pressure, and cerebral blood flow in head-injured patients. J Neurosurg 1992;76:207.

128. Marshall LF, Smith RW, Rauscher LA, et al. Mannitol dose requirements in brain-injured patients. J Neurosurg 1978;48:169.

129. Yen JK, Bourke RS, Popp AJ, et al. Use of ethacrynic acid in the treatment of serious head injury. In: Popp AJ, Bourke RS, Nelson LR, Kimelberg HK, eds. Neural trauma. New York: Raven Press, 1979:329.

130. Guyer DR, Miller MR, Long DM, et al. Visual function following optic canal decompression via craniotomy. J Neurosurg 1985;62:631.

131. Mehringer CM, Heishima GB, Grinnel V, et al. Therapeutic embolization for vascular trauma of the head and neck. AJNR 1983;4:137.

132. Nussbaum ES, Wolf AL, Sebring L, et al. Complete temporal lobectomy for surgical swelling. Neurosurgery 1991;29:62.

133. Marshall LF, Smith RW, Shapiro HM. The outcome with aggressive treatment in severe head injuries, part I: acute and chronic barbiturate administration in the management of head injury. J Neurosurg 1979;50:26.

134. Shapiro HM, Wyte SR, Loesser J. Barbiturate augmented hypothermia for reduction of persistent intracranial hypertension. J Neurosurg 1974; 40:90.

135. Nordby HK, Nesbakken R. The effect of high dose barbiturate decompression after severe head injury. Acta Neurochir 1984;72:157.

136. Sichez JP, Melon E, Clergues F, et al. Traumatismes craniocerebraux avec signes precoces de souffrance axiale: traitement par drainage ventriculaire externe et barbituriques. Neurochirurgie 1981;27:205.

137. Kassell NF, Hitchon PW, Gerk MK, et al. Alterations in cerebral blood flow, oxygen metabolism, and electrical activity produced by high dose sodium thiopental. Neurosurgery 1980;7:598.

138. Godin DV, Mitchell MJ, Saunders BA. Studies on the interaction of barbiturates with reactive oxygen radicals: implications regarding barbiturate protection against cerebral ischemia. Can Anaesth Soc J 1982;29:203.

139. Schwartz ML, Tator CH, Rowed DW, et al. The University of Toronto head injury treatment study: a prospective, randomized comparison of pentobarbital and mannitol. Can J Neurol Sci 1984;11:434.

140. Ward JD, Becker DP, Miller JD, et al. Failure of prophylactic barbiturate coma in the treatment of severe head injury. J Neurosurg 1985; 62:383.

141. Piatt JH, Schiff SJ. High dose barbiturate therapy in neurosurgery and intensive care. Neurosurgery 1984;15:427.

142. Temkin NR, Dikmen SS, Wilensky AJ, et al. A randomized double-blind study of phenytoin for the prevention of post-traumatic seizures. NEJM 1990;323:497.

143. Faupel G, Reulen HJ, Muller D, et al. Double-blind study on the effects of steroids on severe closed head injury. In: Pappius HW, Feindel W, eds. Dynamics of brain edema. Berlin: Springer-Verlag, 1976:337.

144. Gobiet W. The influence of various doses of dexamethasone on intracranial pressure in patients with severe head injury. In: Pappius HM, Feindel W, eds. Dynamics of brain edema. Berlin: Springer-Verlag, 1976:231.

145. Miller JD, Leech P. Effects of mannitol and steroid therapy on intracranial volume-pressure relationships in patients. J Neurosurg 1975;42:274.

146. Tornheim PA, McLaurin RL. Effect of dexamethasone on cerebral edema from cranial impact in the cat. J Neurosurg 1978;48:220.

147. Gudeman SK, Miller JD, Becker DP. Failure of high dose steroid therapy to influence intracranial pressure in patients with severe head injury. J Neurosurg 1979;51:301.

148. Dearden NM, Gibson JS, MacDowall DG, et al. Effect of high dose dexamethasone on outcome from severe head injury. J Neurosurg 1986;64:81.

149. Braakman R, Schouten HJA, Blaau-Van Dishoeck M, et al. Megadose steroids in severe head injury. J Neurosurg 1983;58:326.

150. Giannotta SL, Weiss H, Apuzzo MLJ, et al. High dose glucocorticoids in the management of severe head injury. Neurosurgery 1984;15:497.

151. Braun SR, Levin AB, Clark KL. Role of corticosteroids in the development of pneumonia in mechanically ventilated head trauma victims. Crit Care Med 1986;14:198.

152. Turner E, Hilfiker O, Braun U, et al. Metabolic and hemodynamic response to hyperventilation in patients with head injuries. Intensive Care Med 1984;10:127.

153. Havill JH. Prolonged hyperventilation and intracranial pressure. Crit Care Med 1984;12:72.

154. Artru AA. Reduction of cerebrospinal fluid pressure by hypocapnia: changes in cerebral blood volume, cerebrospinal fluid volume, and brain tissue water and electrolytes. J Cereb Blood Flow Metab 1987;7:471.

155. Hamill JF, Bedford RF, Weaver DC, et al. Lidocaine before endotracheal intubation: intravenous or intratracheal? Anesthesiology 1981;55:578.

156. Robertson CS, Clifton GL, Taylor AA, et al. Treatment of hypertension associated with head injury. J Neurosurg 1983;59:455.

157. Wilson DJ, Wallin JD, Vlachakis ND, et al. Intravenous labetalol in the treatment of severe hypertension and hypertensive emergencies. Am J Med 1983;75:95.

158. Ghani GA, Sung YF, Weinstein MS, et al. Effects of intravenous nitroglycerin on the intracranial pressure and volume pressure response. J Neurosurg 1983;58:562.

159. Sari A, Matayoshi Y, Yonei A, et al. Cerebral arteriovenous oxygen content difference during barbiturate therapy in patients with acute brain damage. Anesth Analg 1986;65:1196.

160. Cruz J, Miner ME. Modulating cerebral oxygen delivery and extraction in acute traumatic coma. In: Miner ME, Wagner KA, eds. Neurotrauma: treatment, rehabilitation, and related Issues. Boston: Butterworth, 1986:55.

161. Griffin JM, Hartley JH, Crow RW, et al. Diabetes insipidus caused by craniofacial trauma. J Trauma 1976;16:979.

162. Kaufman HH, Bretaudiere JP, Rowlands BJ, et al. General metabolism in head injury. Neurosurgery 1987;20:254.

163. Rapp RP, Young B, Twyman D, et al. The favorable effect of early parenteral feeding on survival in head-injured patients. J Neurosurg 1983; 58:906.

164. Young B, Ott L, Twyman D. The effect of nutritional support on outcome from severe head injury. J Neurosurg 1987;67:668.

165. Saxe JM, Ledgerwood AM, Lucas CE, et al. Lower esophageal dysfunction precludes safe gastric feeding after head injury. J. Trauma 1993; 35:170.

166. Robertson CS, Clifton GL, Grossman RG, et al. Alterations in cerebral availability of metabolic substrates after severe head injury. J Trauma 1988;28:1523.

167. Prough DS, Coker LH, Lee S, et al. Hyperglycemia and neurologic outcome in patients with closed-head injury. Anesthesiology 1988;69:A584.

168. Durward QJ, Amacher AL, Del Maestro RF, et al. Cerebral and cardiovascular responses to changes in head elevation in patients with intracranial hypertension. J Neurosurg 1983;59, 938.

169. Newlon PG, Greenberg RP. Evoked potentials in severe head injury. J Trauma 1984;24:61.

170. Marshall LF, Camp PE, Bowers SA. Dimethyl sulfoxide for the treatment of intracranial hypertension: a preliminary trial. Neurosurgery 1984;14:659.

171. James HE, Camp PE, Harbaugh RD, et al. Comparison of the effects of DMSO and pentobarbitone on experimental brain edema. Acta Neurochir 1982;60:245.

172. Farling PA, Johnston IR, Coppel DL. Propofol infusion for sedation of patients with head injury in intensive care. Anaesthesia 1989;44:222.

173. Goldman H, Morehead M, Murphy S. Use of adrenocorticotrophic hormone analog to minimize brain injury. Ann Emerg Med 1993;22:1035.

174. Hall ED. Lipid antioxidants in acute central nervous system injury. Ann Emerg Med 1993;22:1022.

175. Braughler JM, Hall ED, Jacobsen EJ, et al. The 21-aminosteroids: potent inhibitors of lipid peroxidation for the treatment of central nervous system trauma and ischemia. Drugs Future 1989;14:143.

176. Molofsky WJ. Steroids and head trauma. Neurosurgery 1984;15:424.

177. Audus KL, Guillot FL, Braughler JM. Evidence for 21-aminosteroid association with hydrophobic domains of brain microvessel endothelial cells. Free Radic Biol Med 1991;11:361.

178. Anderson DK, Hall ED, Braughler JM, et al. Effect of delayed administration of U74006F (tirilazed mesylate) on recovery of locomotor function following experimental spinal cord injury. J Neurotrauma 1991; 8:187.

179. Rosner MJ, Elias KG, Coley I. Prospective, randomized trial of THAM therapy in severe brain injury: preliminary results. In: Hoff JT, Betz AL, eds. Intracranial pressure VII. Berlin: Springer-Verlag, 1989:611.

180. Ward JD, Choi S, Marmarou A. Effect of prophylactic hyperventilation on outcome in patients with severe head injury. In: Hoff JT, Betz AL, eds. Intracranial pressure VII. Berlin: Springer-Verlag, 1989:611.

181. Moskowitz N, School W, Puszkin S. Interaction of brain synaptic vesicles induced by endogenous Ca^{++} dependent phospholipase A_2. Science 1982;216:305.

182. Kubo K, Matsuda Y, Kase H, et al. Inhibition of calmodulin-dependent cyclic nucleotide phosphodiesterase by flunarizine, a calcium-entry blocker. Biochem Biophys Res Commun 1984;124:315.
183. Rosenthal RE, Chanderbhan R, Marshall G, et al. Prevention of post-ischemic brain conjugated diene production and neurological injury by hydroxyethyl starch-conjugated deferoxamine. Free Radic Biol Med 1992;12:29.
184. Zimmerman RS, Muizelaar JP, Wei EP. Reduction of intracranial hypertension with free radical scavengers. In: Hoff JT, Betz AL, eds. Intracranial pressure VII. Berlin: Springer-Verlag, 1989:804.
185. Levasseur JE, Patterson JL, Ghatak NR, et al. Combined effect of respirator-induced ventilation and superoxide dismutase in experimental brain injury. J Neurosurg 1989;71:573.
186. Ledingham I McA, Watt I. Influence of sedation on mortality in critically ill multiple trauma patients. Lancet 1983;1:1270.
187. Rosner MJ, Newsome HH, Becker DP. Mechanical brain injury: the sympathoadrenal response. J Neurosurg 1984;61:76.
188. Theodore J, Robin ED. Pathogenesis of neurogenic pulmonary oedema. Lancet 1975;2:749.
189. Simon RP, Gean-Martin AD, Sander JE. Medullary lesion inducing pulmonary edema: a magnetic resonance imaging study. Ann Neurol 1991;30:727.
190. Bleck TP, Vespa P, Brock DA. Oxygenation abnormalities in acute aneurysmal subarachnoid hemorrhage patients. Neurology 1993;43(Suppl 1)A325:651.
191. Cooper PR, Moody S, Clark WK, et al. Positive end-expiratory pressure (PEEP) and cerebrospinal fluid pressure during normal and elevated intracranial pressure in dogs. Intensive Care Med 1981;7:187.
192. Frost EAM. Effects of positive end-expiratory pressure on intracranial pressure and compliance in brain-injured patients. J Neurosurg 1977;47:195.
193. Shier MR, Wilson RF. Fat embolism syndromes: traumatic coagulopathy with respiratory distress. Surg Ann 1980;12:139.
194. Hackenberry LE, Miner ME, Rea GL, et al. Biochemical evidence of myocardial injury after severe head trauma. Crit Care Med 1982;10:641.
195. McLeod AA, Neil-Dwyer G, Meyer DHA, et al. Cardiac sequelae of acute head injury. Br Heart J 1982;47:221.
196. Kamada T, Fusamato H, Kawano S, et al. Gastrointestinal bleeding following head injury: a clinical study of 433 patients. J Trauma 1977;17:44.
197. Cushing H. Peptic ulcers and the interbrain. Surg Gynecol Obstet 1932;51:1.
198. Larson GM, Koch S, O'Dorisio TM, et al. Gastric response to severe head injury. Am J Surg 1984;147:97.
199. Halloran LG, Zfass AM, Gayle WE, et al. Prevention of acute gastrointestinal complications after severe head injury: a controlled trial of cimetidine prophylaxis. Am J Surg 1980;139:44.
200. Clark JA, Finelli RE, Netsky MG. Disseminated intravascular coagulation following cranial trauma. J Neurosurg 1980;52:266.
201. Jenett B, Bond M. Assessment of outcome after severe brain damage. Lancet 1975;1:480.
202. Eisenberg HM. Outcome after head injury: general considerations and neurobehavioral recovery, part I: general considerations. In: Becker DP, Povlishock JT, eds. Central nervous system trauma status report. Washington, DC: NINCDS, 1985:271.
203. Bruce DA, Alavi A, Bilaniuk L, et al. Diffuse cerebral swelling following head injuries in children: the syndrome of "malignant brain edema." J Neurosurg 1981;54:170.
204. Giannotta SL, Weiner JM, Karnaze D. Prognosis and outcome in severe head injury. In: Cooper PR, ed. Head injury. Baltimore: Williams & Wilkins, 1987:464.
205. Marshall LF, Gautille T, Klauber MR. The outcome of severe closed head injury. J Neurosurg 1991;75:S25.
206. Jennett B, Teasdale G, Galbraith S, et al. Severe head injuries in three countries. J Neurol Neurosurg Psychiatry 1977;40:291.
207. Lauerssen TG, Klauber MR, Marshall LF. Outcome from head injury related to patient's age. J Neurosurg 1988;68:409.
208. Miller JD, Butterworth JF, Gudeman SK, et al. Further experience in the management of severe head injury. J Neurosurg 1981;54:289.

Chapter 11 Spinal Cord Injuries

TOM HIGHLAND, M.D.

GINO SALCICCIOLI, M.D.

ROBERT F. WILSON, M.D.

INTRODUCTION

Incidence

Between 8,000 and 10,000 spinal cord injuries occur in the United States annually. This is equivalent to an incidence of about 3 to 4 per 100,000 persons per year.[1] Although it is infrequent, spinal cord injury often causes catastrophic disability and tends to involve young adults who would otherwise have a long life expectancy. The median age in one series was less than 20 years.[2] In another series, 61% of spinal cord injuries occurred between 16 and 30 years of age and the mean age was 29.7 years.[3] According to the National Spinal Cord Registry, in 1975 about 200,000 patients with spinal cord injuries lived in the United States.

Cost

The physical disability and financial losses associated with spinal cord injury can be precisely determined; however, the emotional and psychological problems, which are often much greater, are extremely difficult to quantify. Many quadriplegic patients develop severe psychiatric problems and some have strong suicidal tendencies.

The financial cost of spinal cord injury is immense. Spinal-cord-injured patients typically require hospital stays that can range from 45 to more than 100 days, resulting in average hospital charges exceeding $50,000-70,000 per patient.[4,5] For quadriplegic patients, the average hospital stay is usually longer and more expensive. The cost of caring for a patient who has a spinal cord injury in early adulthood will probably exceed $1,000,000 during the patient's lifetime. It is estimated that the medical cost of treating spinal cord injuries exceeds 1.5-2.0 billion dollars annually.[5,6] In addition, less than 30% of these patients are employed in any type of job after 5 years.

Causes and Location of Spinal Cord Injuries

The most common causes of spinal cord injuries are motor vehicle accidents (48%), falls (21%), assaults (15%), and sports-related accidents (14%).[4] Most sports-related injuries result from diving into shallow water. Spinal cord injuries most frequently occur on weekends and during the summer months. Unfortunately, almost 50% of these injuries involve the cervical spinal cord, particularly the mid-portion, and lead to tetraplegia in 32-45%.[3,6,7] Of injuries below the cervical spinal cord, 54% result in complete paraplegia. The thoracic spine is particularly vulnerable to injury in motorcycle accidents.[8] Because of the increased force necessary to damage the thoracic spine, injuries in this area are much more likely to be complete (62-80%) than are those involving the cervical spine.[3,6] Thoracolumbar and lumbar spine fractures account for 20-30% of all spine fractures, and the neurologic injury usually involves the conus medullaris or cauda equina.

Causes of Immediate Death

In victims of trauma who die immediately or within minutes of the accident, 16-24% have had a high cervical spine injury.[2,3,6] In patients with spinal cord injury above C-4, apnea is the most frequent cause of death. In cases of child abuse, violent shaking of young infants can cause death by damaging the brain-spinal cord junction and/or the upper spinal cord.[9]

Associated Injuries

Problems commonly associated with spinal cord injury include injury to the head, chest, abdomen, and extremities. In a study of 789 head-injured victims in the San Diego Regional Trauma System, the incidence of cervical spine fractures and/or dislocations among patients with Glasgow Coma scores of 10 or less was 7.5%.[10] In patients with cervical spinal cord injury, 67% had associated limb fractures with approximately equal involvement of the upper and lower extremities, 53% had intrathoracic injuries, and 33% had associated head injury. Approximately 70% of patients with thoracic spinal cord injury had pneumothorax, hemothorax, or other associated intrathoracic injuries.

Associated injuries not only make it more difficult to diagnose a spinal cord injury, but they can also cause hypovolemia, impaired ventilation, and release of a wide variety of vasoactive and cytotoxic substances which can aggravate the pathophysiologic changes in the spinal cord.

NORMAL ANATOMY, BIOMECHANICS, AND PHYSIOLOGY

Biomechanical Considerations

The spinal cord normally is well protected by the vertebrae, which are held in alignment by a series of joints and ligaments. Trauma severe enough to injure the spinal cord almost always disrupts the ligaments or joints that maintain the stability of one vertebra on another. Thus, trauma to the spine not only causes immediate injury to the cord, but it also increases the risk of further spinal cord damage if the vertebral fracture is unstable. The cervical spinal cord is most vulnerable to injury because normally more motion occurs in this region and relatively little mechanical support exists for these vertebrae.[11]

Spinal Column Motion and Injuries

The spinal column can be divided into five segments according to the types of movement and facet-joint relationships between adjacent vertebrae.[12] These segments include: (a) the upper cervical spine from the occiput to C-2; (b) the lower cervical spine from C-3 to C-7; (c) the thoracic spine from T-1 to T-11; (d) the thoracolumbar junction at T-12 to L-1; and (e) the lumbosacral spine from L-2 to the sacrum.

The upper cervical spine is particularly vulnerable to axial loading if force is applied to the top of the skull. This tends to cause burst fractures through the lateral masses of C-1 (Jefferson fractures) (Fig. 11–1). Hyperextension of the neck due to force applied to the forehead can cause fractures through the odontoid, usually at its base (Fig. 11–2). More severe hyperextension can cause bilateral fractures of the ring of C-2 (hangman's fractures) (Fig. 11–3).[11]

In the lower cervical spine (C-3 to C-7), the most common types of fractures and dislocations are hyperflexion injuries, which likely cause unstable fractures involving the C5 or C6 vertebra. The joints may be so disrupted that both facets of the upper vertebra are transposed anterior to those of the lower vertebra, a situation referred to as "jumped" or "locked" facets. This injury tends to be associated with significant neurologic injury. Rotation combined with flexion injuries can cause unilateral disruption of a facet joint with minimal

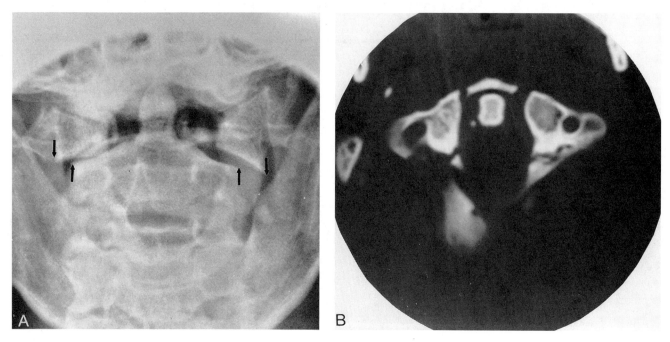

FIGURE 11–1 Jefferson burst fracture. **A.** This odontoid view radiograph shows that the lateral masses of C-1 are displaced laterally from the odontoid, and particularly from the subjacent lateral margins of C-2 (arrows). **B.** This axial CT image demonstrates a classic four-point fracture of the C-1 ring (From: Mirvis SE, Young JWR. Imaging. Trauma and critical care. Baltimore: Williams & Wilkins, 1992; 340).

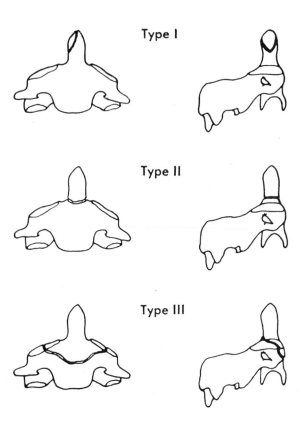

FIGURE 11–2 AP and lateral views of the three types of dens fractures (From: Harris JH Jr, Harris WH, Navelline RA. The radiology of emergency medicine, 3rd ed. Baltimore: Williams & Wilkins, 1993; 221).

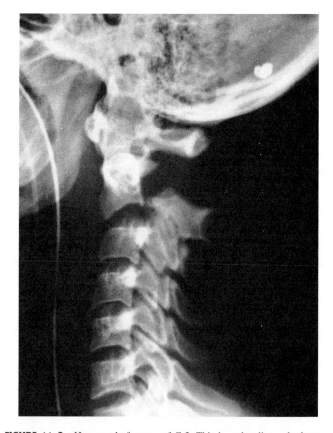

FIGURE 11–3 Hangman's fracture of C-2. This lateral radiograph shows a symmetric fracture through the pars interarticularis of C-2, with moderate fracture displacement. There is anterior tilting of the body of C-2 with respect to C-3 and widening of the intervertebral space (From: Mirvis SE, Young JWR. Imaging. Trauma and critical care. Baltimore: Williams & Wilkins, 1992; 334).

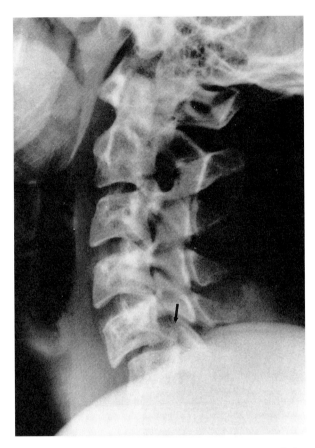

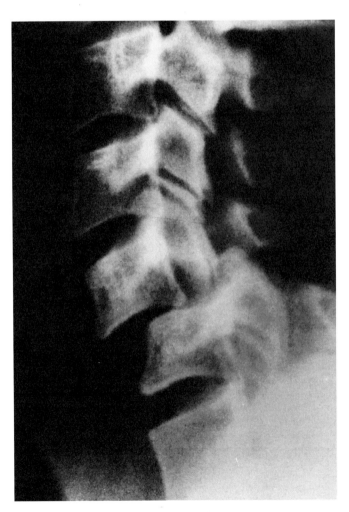

subluxation of the vertebrae.[13] If the force is great enough, it can cause unilateral locked facets with about 25% subluxation of one vertebral body relative to an adjacent vertebral body (Fig. 11–4). This injury is usually stable and not associated with significant ligamentous disruption, abnormal mobility, or neurologic injury.[11] If the injury is more severe, it can cause bilateral facet dislocation with a greater than 50% AP vertebral body length displacement (Figs. 11–5, 11–6).

In the thoracic spine, fractures usually result from direct blows or extreme hyperflexion injuries. Compression or burst fractures from motorcycle or bicycle accidents are generally due to axial loading to the upper thoracic spine, which usually occurs when the cycle is stopped abruptly and the victim is thrown off with his head tucked forward and the thorax hyperflexed.[8]

The thoracolumbar junction is particularly vulnerable to hyperflexion injuries, especially because much of the normal lower back flexion and extension occurs at this level.[14] Extreme hyperflexion with axial loading tends to cause compression fractures of the T-12 or L-1 vertebrae, often with severe ligamentous injury and retropulsion of bone fragments into the spinal canal.

Lumbar spine injuries are most commonly due to hyperflexion, and this tends to cause compression or burst fractures. A burst fracture is a more severe form of a compression fracture. Compression is simply a descriptive term of the fracture caused primarily by axial

FIGURE 11–4 Unilateral facet dislocation. This lateral radiograph demonstrates a C-5 to C-6 unilateral facet lock (arrow) with about 25% of AP vertebral body length anterosubluxation of C-5 with respect to C-6 (From: Mirvis SE, Young JWR. Imaging. Trauma and critical care. Baltimore: Williams & Wilkins, 1992; 318).

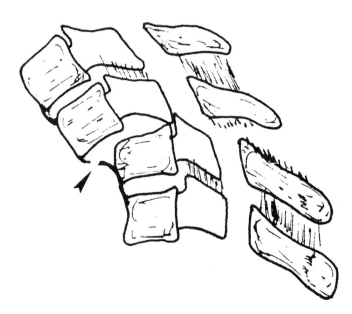

FIGURE 11–5 Bilateral facet dislocation diagram demonstrating complete dislocation of a vertebra in relation to its subjacent neighbor. Disruption of the interspinous, capsular posterior, and anterior longitudinal ligament (arrowhead) is depicted. The inferior facets of the dislocated vertebra are locked between the superior facets and the vertebral body of its subjacent neighbor (From: Mirvis SE, Young JWR. Imaging. Trauma and critical care. Baltimore: Williams & Wilkins, 1992; 307).

FIGURE 11–6 Bilateral locked facets. This lateral radiograph shows a bilateral facet dislocation of C-5 in relation to C-6, with greater than 50% AP vertebral body length displacement of C-4 anteriorly. Note the marked fanning of the spinous processes of the involved vertebral bodies. Minimal corner compression fractures of C-5 and C-6 are observed (From: Eisenberg RL. Diagnostic imaging in surgery. McGraw-Hill Book Company, 1987; 752).

loading. If it is a mild deformity of the vertebra, it is referred to as compression; a more serious deformity from compression is often called a burst fracture.

Spinal Cord Physiology

The blood supply to the spinal cord varies with the region (cervical, thoracic, lumbar) and is critical to its survival and function. The arterial structure of the spinal cord at the T12-L1 level is consistent and lends itself to understanding the blood supply to the cord. One anterior spinal artery supplies the anterior white matter and central gray matter and is discontinuous to the lower thoracic spinal cord in about 30% of patients. Two paired posterior spinal arteries supply the posterior and posterolateral white matter.[15] These arteries are terminal branches of segmental arteries that arise from the aorta. The cervical spinal cord has a more intricate blood supply with more anastomoses, but disrupting its blood flow damages the spinal cord like any other tissue.

AXIOM   If there is any doubt as to the stability of a spinal fracture, the patient should be treated as if the spine were very unstable.

PATHOPHYSIOLOGY OF SPINAL CORD INJURY

Actual mechanical transection of the spinal cord is rare, even in patients with severe neurologic disability. However, functional impairment often is present in such patients because neural action potentials will not cross the injured area. This results in interruption of cerebral interaction with voluntary motor, sensory, and inhibitory areas and activities in the spinal cord distal to the area of damage.

Vascular Changes

Almost immediately following a complete injury to the spinal cord, there is disruption of vascular structures,[16] and a dramatic local decrease in spinal cord blood flow followed by development of punctate areas of hemorrhagic necrosis in the central gray matter of the cord.[17] Within minutes, these small areas of hemorrhagic necrosis tend to coalesce into larger lesions which then extend outward toward the peripheral white matter of the cord. The degree to which the cross-sectional area of the spinal cord is damaged by the hemorrhagic necrosis appears to be related directly to the severity of the initial injury.

The histologic changes within the injured spinal cord reach a maximum approximately 72 hours after trauma and may extend for two segments proximally and distally. If the cord is sectioned at this time, central hemorrhagic softening is usually seen. Later, this softening can progress to central cavitation with surrounding demyelination.

Most of these changes are due to secondary phenomena occurring at a cellular and neurochemical level immediately after injury. These cause a vicious cycle of ischemia, free radical damage to tissue with lipid peroxidation, and then further ischemia. Jansen and Hensebout, using several animal models of spinal cord injury, found that the early biochemical events can be characterized as an uncoupling of oxidative phosphorylation and a shift to anaerobic glycolysis.[18] The resultant depletion of ATP leads to inactivation of calcium-dependent ATPase which helps control levels of intracellular cytoplasmic calcium. As a consequence, a sharp increase occurs in intracellular calcium, which activates calcium-dependent phospholipase A2. This, in turn, acts on membrane phospholipids and liberates arachidonic acid. Ultimately, an accumulation of lipid peroxides and various free radicals develops. These can disrupt the protein and phospholipid bilayer of cell membranes causing an increase in free water, sodium, and lactate and a decrease in potassium in the area of cord injury.[19] Local accumulation of norepinephrine, dopamine, and histamine also occurs.[20]

Although gray matter is usually ischemic after spinal cord injury, blood flow changes in the surrounding white matter vary according to the severity of the injury.[21] White matter hyperemia is often seen after injuries that are incomplete, whereas ischemia tends to be associated with complete spinal cord injuries. Vascular autoregulation is lost in the injured area and, to some extent, spinal cord blood flow varies with systemic arterial blood pressure.

In the areas of the spinal cord immediately surrounding the hemorrhagic necrosis, significant edema forms within a few hours.[22] Axons swell and later rupture, spilling lysosomal enzymes into the extracellular space, forming larger cavities in the medullary substance of the cord and producing gross focal metabolic changes. Histologically, the areas of hemorrhagic necrosis reveal capillary obstruction by fibrin and platelets. Impairment of the microcirculation by these microthrombi is generally seen after a 30-minute delay following injury and may be secondary to the tissue changes rather than a primary effect of the trauma itself.[23]

Using radio-labeled microspheres, it has been demonstrated experimentally that spinal cord compression severe enough to completely block electrical conduction is associated with a significantly reduced local blood flow. The injury to the spinal cord also destroys the autoregulation and carbon dioxide responsiveness of its blood vessels.[24]

Blockage of Electrical Conduction

The precise mechanisms that block electrical conduction in the injured spinal cord are unclear, but several have been suggested: (a) mechanical disruption in axons and other neural elements at cellular and subcellular levels; (b) spinal cord edema; and (c) secondary ischemic damage.[23] Compression applied to a peripheral nerve will halt electrical conduction across that segment, but conduction along the remainder of the axon usually remains intact. This finding suggests that the inability to conduct action potentials after spinal cord injury is a local phenomenon.

Spinal Cord Edema

Swelling of spinal cord tissue in and around the area of injury tends to occur rapidly following local trauma.[22] Initially this appears to be a vasogenic phenomenon, and intravascular fluids rapidly escape into the extravascular space because of increased capillary permeability. The increased capillary permeability is due not only to the trauma but also to the effects of vasoactive substances released from adjacent injured or ischemic neural tissue. These changes, plus the decreased local spinal cord blood flow, result in additional damage to the neural tissue, causing further increases in capillary permeability. During the second 24 hours following trauma, the fluid shifts continue, but they become increasingly cytotoxic in nature.[23] The resultant intracellular swelling can not only deform the neural elements, but can also occlude local capillaries.

Vertebral Artery Injuries

After mid-cervical spine fractures or dislocations, vertebral artery injury is more frequent than commonly believed. In one series of 26 patients with spinal cord trauma reported by Willis et al., 12 (46%) had vertebral artery injury identified radiographically.[25] In nine, the vessel was occluded, and in three, there was an intimal flap, a dissection or a pseudoaneurysm; however, in none of the patients did the vertebral artery injury clearly result in any neurologic dysfunction. However, Miyachi et al. pointed out in two patients with cerebellar infarction after cervical spine trauma, bilateral or dominant vertebral artery occlusion may cause rapid and fatal ischemic damage to the cerebellum and brainstem.[26] Such changes can only be prevented when vertebral artery angiography and treatment are provided early.

EMERGENCY (INITIAL) TREATMENT

Spine Immobilization

DURING EXTRICATION AND TRANSPORT

AXIOM   During the extrication from vehicles, prehospital transport and the initial resuscitation of any patient with a possible spinal cord injury, one should take all necessary precautions for immobilizing the potentially injured spine.

The simplest and perhaps the most effective method of immobilization of the cervical spine is the application of sandbags to both sides of the head and neck with adhesive tape applied across the forehead to a long spinal board (Fig. 11–7). Hard cervical collars, such as the "Philadelphia collar," can provide similar immobilization when adhesive tape is applied across the collar and across the forehead to a long spinal board to secure that portion of the head. However, cervical collars have a disadvantage in that neck structures are hidden from view of the attending medical personnel. The thoracolumbar spine can be effectively immobilized by keeping the patient strapped to a backboard or examining surface, with bedrolls placed on either side of the body to minimize movement.

PRECAUTIONS DURING GENERAL ANESTHESIA

AXIOM   Special precautions with immobilization must be taken during induction and maintenance of general anesthesia in any patient with a known or suspected vertebral fracture.

In patients with unstable fracture dislocations of the spine, there may be further instability imposed on the injured site by relaxation of paraspinal muscles that, while in spasm, splint the injury site.[23] Thus, appropriate precautions with traction, a halo-vest, or a hard collar, must be taken to ensure continued spine stability before, during, and after any anesthetic. If a cervical spine injury is suspected, and endotracheal intubation is required, awake intubation should be considered.

Initial Resuscitation

AXIOM   All severely injured patients should be assumed to have unstable spinal injuries.

Early recognition of spinal column injuries is of utmost importance because up to 10% of spinal cord injuries occur when patients with unstable spine fractures are moved.[27] Although many physicians believe that the nose is the route of choice for endotracheal

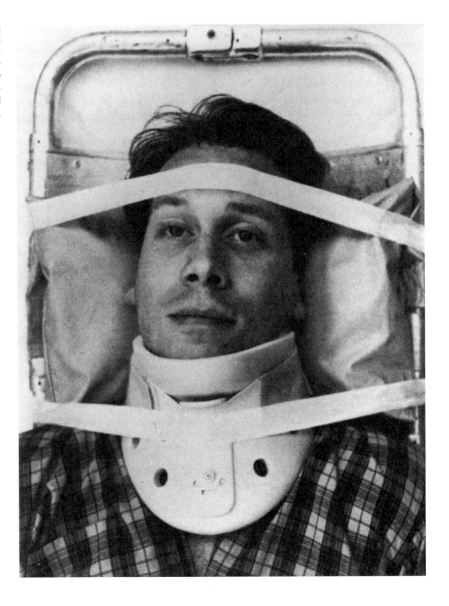

FIGURE 11–7   Good immobilization of the cervical spine is achieved with the patient strapped to a long backboard or scoop stretcher. The head and neck are further immobilized by sandbags placed on both sides of the head and by adhesive tape over the forehead and over the hard collar (From: Kopaniky DR. Pathophysiology of spinal cord disruption and injury. Physiologic basis of modern surgical care. Miller TA, ed. St. Louis: CV Mosby Co., 1988; 791).

intubation of individuals with possible spinal cord injuries, insertion of an orotracheal tube while the head is stabilized by another individual will not cause additional spinal cord injury. In trained hands, use of a flexible laryngoscope or bronchoscope to insert the endotracheal tube when other techniques have been unsuccessful can be effective.

AXIOM	Patients with spinal cord injuries tend to have relative hypovolemia.

Large intravenous lines should be inserted. Even without any blood loss, vascular capacity may be greatly increased by high spinal cord injuries, and fluid may have to be administered rapidly to maintain adequate spinal cord perfusion. In the hypotensive patient who is not responding to fluid resuscitation, the possibility of spinal shock or associated injuries should be considered. When a poor response to fluids occurs, peripheral vasoconstrictors, such as ephedrine or dopamine, can restore adequate blood pressure.

DIAGNOSIS

AXIOM	Early, accurate diagnosis of spinal cord injury is essential to prevent further neurologic damage and to provide optimal therapy.

All victims of trauma who are confused, obtunded, or comatose should be evaluated for possible spinal injuries. These patients should be kept on a rigid back support and their heads stabilized in the midline until it is clear that there is no vertebral fracture or instability.

History

After the patient has respiratory and hemodynamic stabilization, the presence of spinal cord injuries and vertebral fractures or instability must be determined. Special attention should be paid to the mechanism of injury. Hyperflexion injuries or flexion with rotation are more common with motor vehicle accidents. Falls typically cause hyperextension injuries, and axial loading is often due to diving into shallow water.

A head injury with loss of consciousness may be associated with an injury to the cervical spine in 7-15% of patients.[10,28] Falls from a horse or motorcycle with the patient landing on a shoulder frequently result in an unstable injury to the thoracolumbar junction.[11] Injuries sustained in a motor vehicle while wearing a lap belt are often the result of flexion-distraction forces to the thoracolumbar spine, and these fractures are usually unstable.

If the patient is conscious, questions must be asked to determine whether the patient has any pain along the spine or any abnormality of strength or sensation. Radicular pain, numbness, or paraesthesias are important and may indicate at least transient damage to the spinal cord or cauda equina.

AXIOM	Bowel or bladder dysfunction after trauma may be important evidence of a lesion involving the conus medullaris or cauda equina.

Physical Examination

In patients with severe blunt trauma, the entire spine must be palpated very carefully looking for any deformity, tenderness, or hematomas. A high index of suspicion must be maintained whenever tenderness is encountered anywhere along the spine, even in the absence of any neurologic deficit. Such patients should be regarded as having a spine injury until proven otherwise.

AXIOM	All unconscious trauma victims should be assumed to have a spinal cord injury until proven otherwise.

The initial neurologic evaluation must be thorough and should include an accurate description of the level of any sensory and motor dysfunction. Sensory testing should include touch and pain sensation, including sharp-dull discrimination. Joint position sense should be determined carefully because posterior column pathways are apt to remain intact following incomplete cord injuries.

AXIOM	Loss of any motor or sensory function below the level of the neck should be assumed to be the result of a spinal cord injury.

Muscle strength is graded according to the five-point system developed by the Medical Research Council (Table 11–1).[29] Sacral function is tested by evaluating perianal sensation, rectal sphincter tone, and the bulbocavernosus reflex. When this reflex is present, the bulbocavernosus muscle and anal sphincter contract when the glans penis is squeezed or the dorsum of the penis is tapped.

The bladder should be catheterized to detect residual urine as an indication of bladder denervation. The hourly urine output may also be an excellent indicator of the adequacy of fluid resuscitation and blood pressure.

One can diagnose normal cord function and proceed to examine patients for individual spinal nerve roots when the following are present: all muscles in the legs and arms and anal sphincter are normal; all skin sensation is present, including sharp/dull discrimination around the perineum; and all deep tendon reflexes are present. If spotty sensory or motor abnormalities are found, an incomplete cord lesion or peripheral nerve damage is present. If there is no sensory perception or muscle power found distal to the level of injury, a complete cord lesion is present.

To establish the clinical and anatomic functional level of a complete cervical cord lesion (quadriplegic), the lowest nerve root providing good sensation and active muscle control (grade 3 or better) must be established (Table 11–2).[29]

The usual markers for evaluating cervical spinal nerve root function include:

C-4 Sensation over the shoulders and down over the chest, almost to the nipple line; voluntary control of the diaphragm, trapezius, and sternocleidomastoid muscles

C-5 Sensation over the lateral arm; voluntary control of deltoid and biceps muscles (can abduct the arm at the shoulder)

C-6 Sensation over the thumb and index finger; voluntary control of radial wrist extensors (can flex at the elbow and extend at the wrist)

C-7 Sensation over the long and ring fingers; voluntary control of wrist flexors, pronator teres, triceps, and finger extensors (can flex at the wrist and extend at the elbow)

C-8 Sensation over the little finger; voluntary control of finger flexors

T-1 Sensation over the medial arm; voluntary control of intrinsic hand muscles

TABLE 11–1   *The MRC Grading System for Motor Strength*

Grade	Description
0	No contraction
1	Flicker or trace of contraction, but unable to move extremity across a joint
2	Able to move extremity with gravity eliminated
3	Able to move against gravity, but with no resistance
4	Movement against some resistance
5	Normal strength

Rogers LF, Lee C. Cervical spine trauma. In: Dalinka MK, Kaye JJ, eds. Radiology in emergency medicine. New York: Churchill-Livingstone, 1984; 275.[27]

TABLE 11–2 *Functional Levels of Quadriplegia*

Functional Root Level	Sensory Intact	Motor Function Present	Level of Quadriplegia
C-4	Clavicular cape	Diaphragm; trapezius and sternocleidomastoid muscles	High quadriplegia
C-5	Lateral arm	Deltoid, biceps	High quadriplegia
C-6	Thumb, index finger	Extensor carpi radialis brevis; extensor carpi radialis longus	Average quadriplegia
C-7	Long and ring finger	Flexor carpi radialis, pronator teres; extensor digitorum longus and triceps	Low quadriplegia
C-8	Small finger	Finger flexors	Low quadriplegia
T-1	Upper medial arm	Intrinsic muscles	Paraplegia

Stauffer ES. Cervical spine injuries. In: Moore EE, Eiseman B, Vanway CW, eds. Critical decision in trauma. St. Louis: CV Mosby Company, 1984; 92.

The dermatomes for sensory function of the lumbosacral nerve roots include:

L-1 pubis and lower abdomen
L-2 anterior thigh
L-3 knee
L-4 medial lower leg
L-5 lateral lower leg and big toe
S-1 fifth toe and heel
S-2 back of thigh
S-3 buttocks
S-4 perineum
S-5 perianal skin

Although some overlap occurs, the motor functions of the nerve roots to the lower extremities include:

L-2 flexion at the hip
L-3,4 extension at the knee (knee DTR)
L-4 dorsiflexion at the ankle
L-5 dorsiflexion at the toes
S-1 plantar flexion at the toes (ankle DTR)
S-2/3 anal sphincter contraction

Radiologic Examination

BLUNT TRAUMA

The primary goal of the radiologic evaluation is to determine whether an injury to the spinal column is present.

AXIOM The extent of bony deformation seen on radiography after trauma does not represent the full bony excursion and damage occurring at the time of injury.

Plain films are usually the first radiologic studies used to assess spinal trauma (Table 11–3). All severely injured patients must be presumed to have sustained unstable spinal injuries, and the initial assessment of the cervical spine with a cross-table lateral should begin during the initial resuscitation.

In evaluating the cervical spine on lateral radiography, one should see all seven cervical vertebrae plus the top portion of the body of T-1. One should also carefully check: (a) the alignment of the anterior line of the vertebral bodies; (b) the posterior line of the vertebral bodies; (c) the junction of the laminae with the spinous processes; and (d) the tips of the spinous processes (Fig. 11–8A).[30] A number of special measurements may also be helpful (Fig. 11–8B).

It often is not possible to directly determine the integrity of the spinal ligaments and stability of the spine on the basis of radiologic evaluations; however, the presence of ligamentous injury can usually be inferred from certain radiographic characteristics.[11] These include:

1. >5 mm of subluxation.
2. Bilateral jumped facets.
3. Burst fractures with bone fragments in the canal.
4. Widening of the interspinous space.
5. Fractures of the posterior elements associated with a fracture of the vertebral body.

AXIOM Absence of the typical signs of spinal fractures does not guarantee stability.

Spinal stability after traumatic fractures is frequently assessed according to the "three-column theory." The three columns (Fig. 11–9) evaluated by such analysis include: (a) the anterior half of the vertebral body and the anterior longitudinal ligament; (b) the posterior half of the vertebral body, the facets, facet capsules, and posterior longitudinal ligament; and (c) the spinous process, lamina, and interspinous ligament. When two of these columns are damaged, the spine is usually considered to be unstable.

After the patient has been adequately resuscitated, more complete evaluation of the spine can be obtained with additional plain films, tomography, CT scans or MRI. In spinal trauma, CT is a good way to assess the integrity of the spinal canal, to detect its possible compromise by bone fragments, and to investigate the craniovertebral junction. MRI can be especially helpful for evaluating soft tissue changes, such as ligament rupture, herniated disc, and cord trauma.

When the lower cervical and upper thoracic spine cannot be visualized adequately with plain radiography, polytomograms in the sagittal plane or CT scans can be obtained for this region. The degree of stability should be determined on the basis of the severity of bony injury and presence or absence of subluxation. Flexion and extension views to determine stability in patients with known spinal cord injuries are unwise. However, in a patient without spinal cord injury and without spinal fracture, flexion/extension views may be useful to determine stability of the spinal column.

Prevertebral soft-tissue swelling is an important radiologic finding, even though it is usually absent with fractures of the posterior elements. In one study, 50% of patients with cervical spine fractures had no anterior soft-tissue swelling.[31] In addition, significant interobserver variability exists over what constitutes a critical amount of prevertebral soft-tissue swelling. The same study found that 24% of patients whose radiographs were believed to demonstrate soft-tissue swelling subsequently were found to have no spinal cord or vertebral injury.

When trauma victims are alert and have neck, shoulder, or arm pain or neurologic deficits that could be due to spinal cord injury, it is particularly important to conduct an exhaustive radiologic evaluation of the cervical spine. If no abnormalities are seen on lateral and anteroposterior films, one should obtain oblique views or pillar views (to demonstrate facet alignment). If the lower cervical vertebrae cannot be visualized well with conventional studies, including the swimmer's view, sagittal polytomography can be used.

TABLE 11–3 Diagnostic Modalities for Cervical Spine Fractures*

Diagnostic Modality	Indication	Abnormality Diagnosed
Lateral cervical spine radiograph	Any injured patient when cervical fracture is suspected	Alignment; body height; contour; cartilaginous space; soft-tissue signs
Anteroposterior radiograph	Follow-up to lateral cervical spine radiograph	Spinous process; articular masses; vertebral body
Odontoid radiograph	Follow-up to lateral cervical spine radiograph	Atlanto-occipital joint; atlanto-axial joint; odontoid; lateral edge of articular masses of C1 with C2
Horizontal oblique radiograph	Normal trauma series and pain or neurologic deficit	Pedicle; intervertebral foramina; facet alignment; lamina
Pillar radiograph	Same as above; hyperextension injury	Posterior elements: lateral masses; lamina; limitations (visualizes C4–C7)
Flexion/extension radiograph	Same as above	Anterior subluxation; divergence of spinous processes; atlantodens interval (< 3 mm)
Computed tomography	Same as above; neurologic findings not explainable; suspicious radiographic findings; high clinical suspicion	Flexion teardrop; Jefferson; burst; lamina; hyperextension-dislocation
Magnetic resonance imaging	Same as above	Cord transection or contusion; intervertebral disk abnormality; parenchymal hemorrhagic lesions; intrinsic cord abnormality

Rozycki GG, Champion HR. Radiology of the cervical spine. In: Maull KI, ed. Advances in trauma, vol 5. St. Louis: Mosby Year Book, 1990; 37-47.

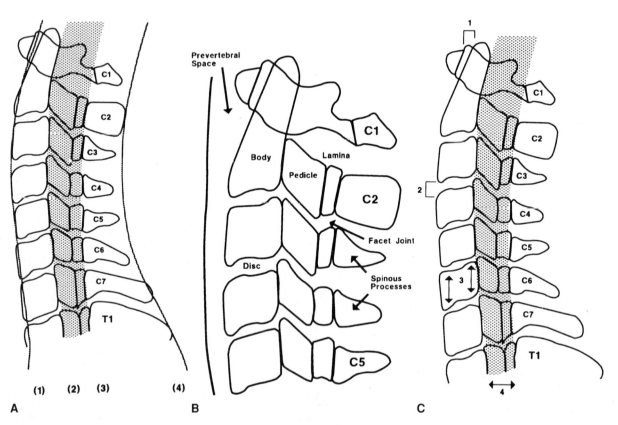

FIGURE 11–8 A. In evaluating the cervical spine on a lateral radiography, one should see all seven cervical vertebrae plus the top portion of the body of T-1. The alignment of the anterior portions of the vertebral bodies, the posterior vertebral bodies, the junction of the laminae with the spinous processes and the tips of the spinous processes should all be checked carefully. **B.** When reviewing radiographs of the cervical spine one should look closely at various components of the prevertebral space, the alignment of the vertebral bodies, the disc spaces, the pedicles, the laminae, the facet joints, and the spinous processes. **C.** Measurements that may be helpful in evaluating a lateral radiography of the cervical spine for injuries include: (a) atlantodental interval (normal: 2.5-3.0 mm), (b) superior vertebral body inferior vertebral alignment (should be < 2.7 mm difference), (c) anterior to posterior bone height in a vertebrae body (should be < 3 mm difference), (d) spinal canal width (should be at least 13 mm), and (e) < 5 mm prevertebral space (From: Rozycki GS, Champion HR: Radiology of the cervical spine. Advances in trauma, vol 5. Maull KI, ed. St. Louis: Mosby Year Book, 1990; 42–44).

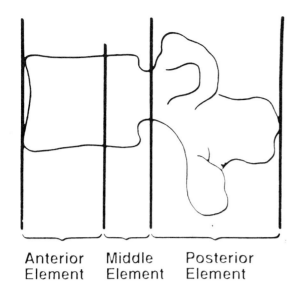

FIGURE 11–9 Three column concept of the spine includes: (a) the anterior half of the vertebral body and the anterior longitudinal ligament, (b) the posterior half of the vertebral body, the facets, facet capsules, and posterior longitudinal ligament, and (c) the spinous process, lamina, and interspinous ligament. If two of these columns are damaged, the spine is usually considered to be unstable. (From: Harris JH Jr, Harris WH, Navelline RA. The radiology of emergency medicine, 3rd ed. Baltimore: Williams & Wilkins, 1993; 152).

In assessing alignment of the vertebrae, polytomography is superior to CT. However, for defining fractures through the posterior elements (spinous processes, laminae, pedicles, and facets), CT windows for bone provide greater detail. CT is also the best way to assess the integrity of the spinal canal, to detect compromise of its lumen by bone fragments, and to investigate the craniovertebral junction.[27,32]

If the radiologic examination is negative or equivocal in patients with suspicious signs or symptoms, one can also obtain either an MRI scan or a myelography followed by a CT scan of suspicious areas. These studies can show a ruptured disk or epidural clots that may be compressing the cord. MRI is increasingly recommended for patients with clinical evidence of spinal cord injury—with or without bony injury—to provide a better understanding of the degree of spinal cord damage and to identify soft-tissue lesions. MRI can be very helpful in defining anatomic spinal cord damage, cord deformity from extrinsic compression (such as herniated disk), cord enlargement, or intramedullary hemorrhage (Fig. 11–10).[33]

AXIOM Cervical spine radiographs are not necessary for victims of blunt head and neck trauma if they are alert, asymptomatic, and have no distracting injuries.

Trauma patients who are alert and oriented at examination, have no signs or symptoms of cervical spine injury, and have no other major injuries that might distract the patient are at extremely low risk for having a cervical spine fracture. Fischer[34] and Bayles and Ray[35] each reported the results of cervical spine radiographs in a combined total of 455 alert and asymptomatic trauma victims; no patient in either series had a significant cervical spine fracture or instability. They emphasized, however, that the patient must not be intoxicated and

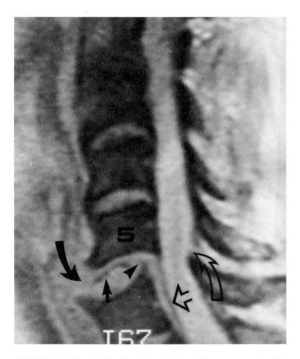

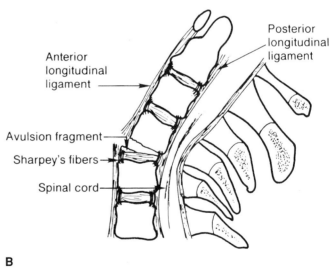

B

FIGURE 11–10 **A.** The Pathophysiology of hyperextension dislocation demonstrated by MRI. C-5 is posteriorly subluxated with respect to C-6. The anterior longitudinal ligament and anterior annulus are disrupted. The intervertebral disk space is abnormally widened and contains a low-intensity signal representing blood within the disk space (solid arrow). The posterior annulus is disrupted (arrowhead), and the posterior longitudinal ligament is stripped from the posterior cortex of the subjacent vertebral body. The spinal cord is compressed between the posterior inferior corner of the involved vertebral body and the subjacent lamina. The ligamentum flavum between C-5 and C-6 is also disrupted (curved open arrow) (From: Harris JH Jr, Harris WH, Navelline RA. The radiology of emergency medicine, 3rd ed. Baltimore: Williams & Wilkins, 1993; 199). **B.** Schematic representation of hyperextension dislocation demonstrating the etiology of the fracture fragment arising from the anterior aspect of the inferior endplate of the involved vertebra avulsed by the intact Sharpey's fibers. (From: Kopaniky DR. Pathophysiology of spinal cord disruption and injury. Physiologic basis of modern surgical care. Miller TA, ed. St. Louis: CV Mosby Co., 1988; 199).

must have no interscapular or shoulder pain through a full range of neck motion. There also should be no pain on palpation over the spinous processes.

PENETRATING TRAUMA

In penetrating wounds of the spine, CT is used to assess the integrity of the spinal canal and cord, to localize foreign bodies and bone fragments, and to study their effect on the spinal cord. These studies are aided significantly by non-ionic, water-soluble, intrathecal contrast media. Multiplanar reconstruction of images allows the radiologist to intensively study these areas without unnecessary manipulation of the patient.

DEFINITION OF SPINAL CORD INJURIES

Injury to the spinal cord is clinically defined by both the completeness of the lesion and its spinal level. When a person with a spinal cord injury is first seen, they may be in spinal shock. Spinal shock is a common manifestation of spinal cord injury and occurs because of disruption of descending autonomic pathways. A patient's precise spinal cord injury may not be known until after spinal shock has cleared, which can take a few hours to a few weeks.

PITFALL ⊘

The prognosis of a spinal cord injury cannot be determined until the patient recovers from spinal shock.

A complete injury is defined as a total loss of neurologic function below the level of cord injury, whereas an incomplete lesion denotes preservation of some neurologic function below the injury site. In the majority of functionally complete spinal cord lesions, anatomic continuity of the spinal cord is maintained.[36] The spinal level of the lesion is designated as the most distal uninvolved segment of the spinal cord. Thus, a patient with a spinal cord lesion causing neurologic dysfunction at C-7 and below would be designated as having a C-6 spinal level injury.

Incomplete Spinal Cord Injuries

Frequently observed syndromes associated with incomplete spinal cord injuries include the central cord syndrome, anterior spinal cord syndrome, Brown-Sequard syndrome, conus medullaris lesions, and injuries to the cauda equina.

CENTRAL CORD SYNDROME

Central cord syndromes tend to occur with cervical spine trauma because of the arrangement of the nerve fibers within the spinal cord. The fibers responsible for lower extremity motor and sensory functions are located in the more lateral portions of the spinal cord, whereas the fibers controlling the upper extremities and voluntary bowel and bladder function are more centrally located (Fig. 11–11). Thus, a central cord syndrome causes more neurologic impairment of the upper extremities than the lower extremities, and greater neurologic loss in the proximal portions of the limbs than distally. Although bowel and bladder control may be lost in the more severe cases, pain perception (sharp/dull) is usually maintained around the anus and in the perineum. These lesions are more likely to occur in traumatized patients who have underlying cervical spondylosis and spinal canal narrowing. Usually some clinical improvement occurs following this injury, but up to 50% of patients will have permanent motor deficits, particularly in their hands.[37]

ANTERIOR SPINAL CORD SYNDROME

Anterior spinal cord syndrome is due to trauma or ischemia to the anterior portion of the spinal cord. It is characterized by complete loss of motor function and pain (including sharp/dull discrimination) and temperature sensation below the injured segment. Because preservation of the dorsal columns occurs, joint position (proprioception) and deep-pressure sensation remain intact. The posterior columns are relatively resistant to ischemia from clamping of the descending thoracic aorta because they are supplied by two fairly uniform posterior spinal arteries. In contrast, the anterior spinal cord receives its blood supply from only a single artery, which is discontinuous to the lower spinal cord in 30% of patients. Anterior spinal cord ischemia is much more apt to cause severe cord damage when aortic clamping is longer

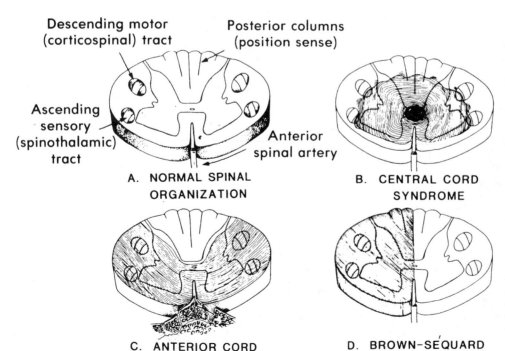

FIGURE 11–11 The neurologic deficits following an incomplete spinal cord injury reflect the neurologic function of the portions of the spinal cord involved in the injury. **A.** Normal spinal cord organization. **B.** Central cord syndrome. The motor deficit affects the upper limbs more than the lower limbs. The extent of the damage in the central spinal cord determines the extent of the neurologic dysfunction. **C.** Anterior cord syndrome. Motor function and pain sensation are lost below the level of spinal cord injury. Position sense, which is carried by the intact posterior columns, is relatively well preserved. **D.** Brown-Sequard syndrome. This syndrome is characterized by loss of motor function on the side ipsilateral to the spinal cord lesion and loss of pain and temperature sensation on the contralateral side (From: Kopaniky DR. Pathophysiology of spinal cord disruption and injury. Physiologic basis of modern surgical care. Miller TA, ed. St. Louis: CV Mosby Co., 1988; 791).

than 30 minutes or when the patient is in shock. The prognosis for recovery from this type of injury is poor, and less than 10% of patients regain functional motor control.[35] Prognosis is especially poor when sharp/dull discrimination does not return quickly.

BROWN-SEQUARD SYNDROME

Brown-Sequard syndrome is the result of injury to half of the spinal cord. Anatomically this should cause interruption of motor function and position and vibratory sensation on the same side as the injury and interruption of pain and temperature on the contralateral side. This rare syndrome most often occurs with penetrating injuries of the spine, such as with knife or gunshot wounds. Clinically, some gross sensory and motor sparing usually is evident, and most patients make a fairly good recovery.[38]

CONUS MEDULLARIS LESIONS

Lesions to the lowest portion of the spinal cord can cause bilateral lower extremity deficits (that are usually symmetric) and disturbances of bowel and bladder function.[23] In contrast to cauda equina lesions, there is little or no radicular pain. Early decompression of a traumatic injury to the conus medullaris is important and may improve the chances of recovery. Although the motor deficit usually resolves completely, there is generally some permanent sensory impairment.

CAUDA EQUINA LESIONS

Lesions of the cauda equina tend to cause asymmetric lower extremity deficits.[23] Radicular pain or dysesthesia in the legs is often a major complaint, but sensation around the anus (S-2,S-3,S-4) and bowel and bladder control are usually retained. Timing of surgery to decompress cauda equina lesions is not as critical in determining outcome as with conus medullaris deficits.

Spinal Cord Concussion (Contusion)

Spinal cord concussion is a rare, temporary injury to the spinal cord that is usually due to deceleration trauma to the neck.[39] Neurologic function below the level of the injury is lost instantaneously and usually entirely, but it usually returns spontaneously within 48 hours. This lesion occurs in 3-4% of all patients with spinal cord injuries and is most common when preexisting degenerative disease has narrowed the spinal canal. Because this lesion may be present, caution is advised in predicting neurologic recovery on the basis of the acute presentation. After a few days, and particularly after several weeks, one can be much more certain of the extent of the spinal cord impairment.

PITFALL ⊘

> *Predicting neurologic outcome within 48 hours of a spinal cord injury.*

SCIWORA Syndrome

Spinal cord injury without radiographic abnormalities (SCIWORA) usually occurs in children and has been called the SCIWORA syndrome.[40] The elasticity of the anterior and posterior longitudinal ligaments in children as well as the immaturity of the osseous elements of the developing vertebrae can allow momentary subluxation of vertebrae in response to deforming forces, without radiographic evidence of injury. This syndrome should be suspected when neurologic signs of a spinal cord injury are demonstrated in a child but no radiographic abnormalities are evident, even on flexion and extension views.[37]

PHARMACOLOGIC TREATMENT OF SPINAL CORD INJURY

Many compounds have been tested in an effort to improve neurologic outcome following spinal cord injury. These include massive doses of adrenocortical-like steroids, gangliosides, opiate analogs

(such as naloxone and thyrotropin-releasing hormone), inhibitors of prostaglandin synthesis (such as indomethacin), and calcium channel blockers. The rationale for using these agents is based on the theory that spinal cord injury is at least partially due to local ischemia and the deleterious effects of toxic free radicals that accumulate as a result of anaerobic metabolism.

Massive Doses of Corticosteroids

The administration of massive doses of corticosteroids prior to spinal cord injury in cats can lessen the severity of posttraumatic demyelination, cavitation, and neuronal loss.[41] Even when given as late as 30 minutes after experimental spinal cord injury, steroids diminish lipid peroxidation and decrease local levels of free radicals and lactate.[41,42] More recently, scientists have developed steroid analogs, known as lazaroids, that lack glucocorticoid or mineralocorticoid activity but maintain the ability to inhibit lipid peroxidation. One such agent, U-74006F, has been found to be very effective in promoting functional recovery after spinal cord injury in cats.[43]

In the first National Acute Spinal Cord Injury Study (NASCIS-1), a 1000 mg infusion of methylprednisolone sodium succinate was given as a bolus and daily thereafter for 10 days and was compared with a 100 mg dose given in a similar manner.[44] No significant difference was manifest in motor or sensory function or overall outcome between these two treatments. However, a control arm was not included in this trial because, at the time, it was considered unethical to omit steroids from the treatment of acute spinal cord injury. Conversely, experimental evidence suggested that the doses of corticosteroids used in the clinical trials were too low.[45] A second national trial (NASCIS 2), therefore, was performed.[46] There were 487 patients recruited into this multicenter, randomized, double-blind, placebo-controlled study. Methylprednisolone was given to 162 patients within 12 hours of sustaining severe spinal cord injuries in initial doses of 30 mg/kg followed by 5.4 mg/kg/hr for 23 hours. The second treatment arm was naloxone, which was given to 154 patients as a bolus of 5.4 mg/kg followed by an infusion for 23 hours at 4 mg/kg; 171 patients received placebos. Motor and sensory functions were assessed on admission and then 6 weeks and 6 months after injury.

Patients who received methylprednisolone within 8 hours of injury showed slight but significant improvement in motor function and sensation at 6 months. These improvements were observed both with initially complete and incomplete lesions. As a result of these data, many believe that one should give massive steroids (30 mg/kg methylprednisolone by IV push, followed by 5.4 mg/kg/hr for 48 hours) to patients as soon as possible after spinal cord injury.

The other mainstays of initial therapy include stabilizing the spine and ensuring an optimal cardiac output and oxygenation of the blood. Interestingly, some recent data by Prendergast et al. questioned the value of steroids in spinal cord injuries, especially when caused by penetrating trauma.[47]

GM-1 Ganglioside

Gangliosides, which are complex acidic glycolipids present in high concentrations in central nervous system cells, form a major component of the cell membrane and are located predominantly in the outer portion of the cell membrane's bilayer.[48] Although the functions of the neuronal gangliosides remain unknown, experimental evidence suggests that they augment neurite outgrowth in vitro, induce regeneration and sprouting of neurons, and restore neuronal function after injury in vivo. In animals, gangliosides stimulate the growth of nerve cells and the regeneration of damaged nervous tissues. These encouraging experimental results have led to clinical trials in stroke and to animal trials for diabetic neuropathy that suggest a positive effect of gangliosides on neurologic recovery.[49]

Recently, the results of a prospective, randomized, placebo-controlled, double-blind trial of GM-1 ganglioside in patients with spinal cord injuries were reported.[50] Of 37 patients studied, 34 (23 with cervical injuries and 11 with thoracic injuries) completed the test-drug protocol. This included 100 mg of GM-1 sodium salt daily or a placebo intravenously for 18-32 doses, with the first dose given within 72 hours of the injury. The follow-up period extended for one year.

The patients treated with GM-1 ganglioside had a significantly greater improvement in neurologic function at one year than patients treated with a placebo. The increased recovery in the GM-1 group was attributable to initially paralyzed muscles that regained useful motor strength rather than to strengthening of weak muscles.

The treatment groups had similar motor recovery over time in the upper extremities, implying that in both groups dysfunctional gray matter at the injury site had similar recovery rates. However, motor recovery over time was significantly more enhanced in the lower extremities in the GM-1 group.

Naloxone

The systemic hypotension seen with experimental cord injury may be caused by the release of endogenous opiates and their inhibition of dopaminergic systems.[51] Because the neurologic deficit following spinal cord trauma is partially the result of spinal cord ischemia, maintaining or increasing spinal cord blood flow could potentially reverse these deficits, particularly if treatment were applied early. By blocking endorphin receptors in the spinal cord, naloxone may help maintain a more physiologic blood flow to the spinal cord after injury.[51] Furthermore, naloxone may also act indirectly through its ability to block the fall in systemic arterial blood pressure seen following spinal cord injury.

Naloxone may also act through nonopiate mechanisms, such as stabilization of lysosomal membranes or inhibition of free-radical reactions.[51] Free-radical particles are presumably formed in the respiratory chain in mitochondria following hypoxic or ischemic episodes. With reperfusion and supplying of oxygen again, the cells can produce these highly reactive substances that can destroy the cell by peroxidizing unsaturated fatty acids in the cellular membranes. Thus, naloxone may prevent or reduce damage to cells by acting as a "free-radical scavenger" inhibiting lipid peroxidation.[52] In experimental spinal cord injury, cats treated with naloxone regained neurologic function substantially faster than those that were untreated. Other opiate antagonists have also been used with success in various models of spinal cord injury.

Dimethyl Sulfoxide

Rapid administration of dimethyl sulfoxide (DMSO) following spinal cord injury results in protection of axons and myelin sheaths, reduced associated tissue swelling, and accelerated return of motor function.[53] DMSO may interact with cyclic AMP, prostaglandins, and thromboxane to inhibit platelet aggregation and reduce vasospasm, thereby maintaining blood flow to the neural tissue. In addition, DMSO appears to have a stabilizing effect on cellular and subcellular membranes.[54]

Growth Factors

Although peripheral nerves have the capacity to regenerate damaged axons, this does not seen to occur with injured neurons in the spinal cord or brain. However, transected spinal cord axons can initiate a "sprouting" process which appears within 10 days after experimental trauma.[23] The failure of the axonal sprouting to continue in an injured spinal cord may indicate a lack of specific nerve growth factors, which are available to peripheral nerves. Because specific nerve growth factors have not been identified, the term "growth factor" may refer to one or more neurotrophic substances or other neurosecretory material.[23] It may also refer to morphologic components that produce a favorable environment for regeneration.

Other Factors

Accumulation of prostaglandins, particularly those causing vasoconstriction, can be toxic to neural tissues following trauma, and indo-

methacin can inhibit their production.[52] Influx of ECF calcium into the cytoplasm can activate phospholipases; calcium channel blockers have been used to prevent this with limited success.[53]

SPINAL CORD COOLING

Experimental local cooling of the spinal cord soon after it has been injured can dramatically improve neurologic function.[23] Although spinal cord cooling can be done through percutaneously placed subarachnoid needles, most investigators prefer an open technique, such as laminectomy. When the spinal cord is cooled to 50°C by constant irrigation within 4 hours of the initial injury, edema can be prevented from forming in the neural tissue and can decrease neuronal metabolism and oxygen requirements.[23] It may also wash out biochemical breakdown products, catecholamines, and histamine-like substances that can have a detrimental effect on injured neural tissue.

MANAGEMENT OF SPINE FRACTURES

Categorizing the Injury

STABLE VERSUS UNSTABLE SPINE INJURIES

A spinal injury is said to be stable when the integrity of the ligamentous and skeletal components of the spine is maintained and further controlled motion has a low risk of producing spinal cord or nerve root damage. Conversely, an unstable spinal injury can allow abnormal excursion of one vertebral segment on another so as to compromise neural elements. The three-column theory of the spine is often used to determine stability of the spine. It is believed that when two of the three columns are damaged, the spine is unstable. Although the degree of stability cannot be predicted in every instance of acute spinal injury, it should be accurately determined as soon as possible to render the most appropriate treatment.

COMPLETE VERSUS INCOMPLETE SPINAL CORD INJURIES

The goals of treatment of spinal cord injuries include: (a) preserve whatever neurologic function is present; (b) prevent further neurologic damage; (c) reduce the time to rehabilitation; and (d) prevent medical complications of spinal cord injury. The decision regarding whether to treat any spine fractures operatively or nonoperatively must consider all these factors as well as the fracture stability.

In patients with incomplete spinal cord injuries, care must be taken to prevent further neurologic injury as well as provide the optimum environment for the spinal cord to recover as much as possible. Thus, when diagnostic studies suggest that compression still exists on the spinal cord, then it must be relieved either operatively or nonoperatively. If a decision has been made to treat the fractures surgically, the use of intraoperative sensory evoked potentials may aid in immediate decision-making concerning the degree of decompression, continued spinal stability during turning or positioning, and surgical manipulation of neural or vascular structures.[54] During spinal surgery, sensory evoked potentials can be recorded from scalp, spinous processes, posterior spinous ligaments, or from the epidural space following stimulation of peripheral nerves below the area of surgery. Although these recordings reflect primarily dorsal column function, motor and other sensory functional changes appear to correspond reasonably well. A steady pharmacologic and physiologic state must be ensured so that the changes in evoked potentials may be correctly attributed to surgical intervention.

Management of Cervical Spine Fractures

GENERAL APPROACH AND INITIAL THERAPY

When no clinical or radiologic evidence of cervical spine fracture is manifest in a patient with neck trauma, one should assess cervical nerve root function.[11] Even if there is no fracture or neurologic deficit, wearing a neck collar for several days can help to reduce local pain and spasm.

When an unstable cervical spine fracture is present, but it is in good position, it can be treated either by tong traction, halo immobilization, or surgical stabilization to maintain proper alignment. If reduction cannot be accomplished with traction, open reduction and internal fixation are performed followed by immobilization as indicated.

Reduction of Fractures and Realignment of Vertebrae

For cervical spine fractures associated with subluxation or angulation, axial traction is generally applied to the skull.[11] Such traction is not only effective in reducing maligned vertebrae, but it also helps to immobilize unstable cervical spine fractures. Attempts at reducing subluxed cervical vertebrae involve the stepwise addition of weight to the skull traction apparatus.

Because the axis of the cervical spine is in line with the mastoid processes, traction applied just above the mastoid processes can produce simple axial distraction.[11] However, most injuries involving locked or perched facets are caused by hyperflexion, and use of slight flexion with the distracting force may facilitate reduction. Consequently, skull traction is usually applied slightly posterior to the external auditory canals to also provide mild extension. Because overdistraction may damage the brainstem or upper cervical spinal cord, it is important to closely monitor the patient's neurologic status and check lateral cervical spine radiographs as each increment of weight is added. Widening of the disk space or interspinous distance is a sign that further distraction may be hazardous.

AXIOM When the patient has an injury to the occipitoatlantal joint, axial traction is often contraindicated.

As a rule, it is suggested that 5 pounds of weight be used per level of injury. Thus, a deformity at C_5-C_6 probably requires an average of about 25 pounds of traction. Weight is added every 30 minutes until reduction is obtained. However, in order to prevent overdistraction, serial radiographs should be obtained after the initial application of traction and after each added weight in order to determine whether more traction is needed or whether it should be reduced.[11] Diazepam and morphine are used liberally as needed to reduce pain and muscle spasm. It is generally recommended that one should not use more than 50 pounds of traction, even for low cervical spine fractures. When reduction cannot be obtained with that amount of weight, intraoperative reduction is recommended.

AXIOM Closed manipulation of the cervical spine to reduce fractures is not recommended.

External Braces

Several different kinds of external cervical spine braces can be used, depending on the degree of neck immobilization desired. The most commonly used brace is the Philadelphia collar. This is a reinforced, synthetic, semirigid foam brace that limits neck flexion only slightly, and it allows significant rotation.[11] The only braces that significantly immobilize the cervical spine enough to allow proper healing of unstable cervical spine fractures are the halo brace (Fig. 11-12) and the Minerva jacket. Stable cervical spine injuries, such as unilateral locked facets, can be treated adequately in a SOMI, four poster, or Yale brace.

FIGURE 11–12 The Halo vest apparatus minimizes movement of the head and neck with respect to the body. The Halo ring is applied to the skull by four-point fixation and is in turn attached to the vest apparatus by sturdy upright bars (From Camp International Inc., Jackson, MI) (From: Kopaniky DR. Pathophysiology of spinal cord disruption and injury. Physiologic basis of modern surgical care. Miller TA, ed. St. Louis: CV Mosby Co., 1988; 794).

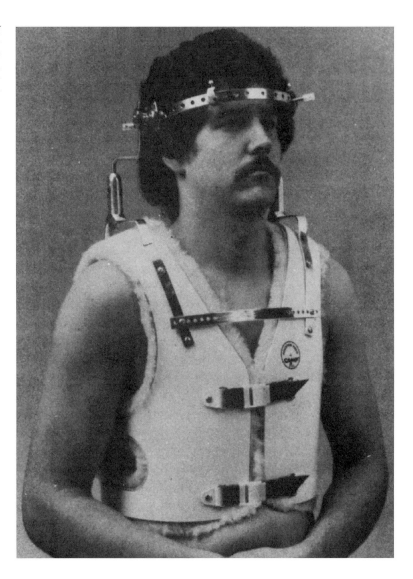

MANAGEMENT OF SPECIFIC UPPER CERVICAL SPINE FRACTURES

Rotatory subluxation of C-1 is rare but it can cause a very painful torticollis. After reduction with traction, continued treatment of this injury is based on the degree of subluxation.[11] Complete subluxation should be treated for three months in a halo brace. Less severe subluxations, commonly seen in children, may be treated for a shorter time with a collar.

Jefferson fractures are usually stable and can be treated with a Philadelphia collar. However, if the fracture is associated with ligamentous injuries, a halo brace is recommended for three months.[11] Spinal cord injury is unusual with this fracture because it tends to widen the spinal canal.

Odontoid fractures are the most common upper cervical spine fractures. Avulsion of the tip of the odontoid (type I fracture) is a stable injury and can usually be treated adequately with a Philadelphia collar for 6 weeks.[11] Type III odontoid fractures extend into the body of the C-2 vertebrae and usually heal well when immobilized with a halo brace for at least three months.

Treatment of type II odontoid fractures, which occur at the base of the odontoid (Fig. 11–2), is somewhat controversial. Young patients with nondisplaced type II odontoid fractures generally heal with only halo brace immobilization. However, internal fixation is often necessary for patients 60 years or older if the odontoid were displaced more than 4 mm.[55] The surgical treatment of type II odontoid fractures usually involves posterior fixation and fusion of the laminae of C-1 to C-2. More recently, anterior screw fixation of the odontoid to the body of C-2 has been used.

Hangman's fractures, (fractures through the pedicles of C-2) result from hyperextension of the cervical spine (Fig. 11–3). This fracture is only rarely associated with neurologic problems in patients admitted to a hospital. They usually are treated with halo brace immobilization for at least three months

MANAGEMENT OF LOWER CERVICAL SPINE FRACTURES

The lower cervical spine is very susceptible to hyperflexion injuries that disrupt the posterior elements. These disruptions of the interspinous ligaments and facet joints are often associated with subluxation of one vertebra on another.[11] Some of these fractures may be difficult to reduce with traction. If reduction were unsuccessful at 50 pounds of traction, operative reduction would be required. Because of severe ligamentous and bony disruption, fracture dislocations of the lower cervical vertebrae usually cannot be treated adequately with external braces alone.[56] After the subluxation is reduced, the involved vertebrae are fused intraoperatively.

Various plate and wire techniques are available for either an anterior or posterior fusion.[11] A posterior approach to fuse the laminae and spinous processes is used most often. A combination of bone and wire is used because wire can provide immediate stability, and by the time the wires fatigue and fail, the bony fusion will have usually matured enough to provide adequate support. Metal clamps, plates, or facet screws are newer devices that may be used in cervical fusion. Patients are usually then kept in a rigid neck support for 6 weeks to 3 months, depending on the stability of the fixation.

For compression or burst fractures (Fig. 11–13), an anterior approach may be necessary to remove retropulsed bone fragments or herniated disk and replace them with a fibular or iliac crest strut-graft. This can be supplemented with internal fixation. Otherwise, external support with a halo brace is recommended.

Thoracic Spine

Simple compression fractures of the thoracic spine without subluxation are usually stable, and surgery is not necessary.[11] However, a rigid external brace for three months may help reduce pain. Severe compression (comminuted or burst) fractures or subluxed vertebrae require internal stabilization. When fragments of bone have been retropulsed into the spinal canal causing neurologic injury, surgical decompression is required; however, the role of surgical treatment in patients with fragments in the canal and no neurologic injury is still debated.

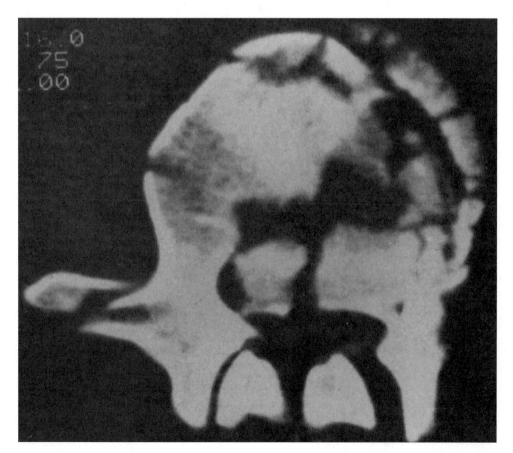

FIGURE 11–13   Axial CT image of burst-compression fracture of L-1 with bone fragments retropulsed into the spinal canal (From Marion D, Clifton G. Injury to the vertebrae and spinal cord. Moore EE, Mattox KL, Feliciano DV, eds. Trauma, 2nd ed. Norwalk: Appelton and Lange, 1991; 269.

Thoracolumbar Spine

Mild compression fractures of the thoracolumbar spine are usually stable and are best managed with a rigid "tortoise shell" thoracolumbar brace to hasten healing and diminish pain.[57] If neurologic deficits were to occur, one would have to search for a herniated disk, epidural hematoma, or bone fragments in the spinal canal. These are best detected with MRI or myelography and CT scan.

If a burst fracture, retropulsed fragments, or subluxation were present with a neurologic deficit, surgical decompression of the spinal cord and stabilization would be required.[57] Rigid external thoracolumbar braces are generally used for at least 3 months after such surgery.

Reid et al. suggested that contact orthosis without surgery may be adequate in selected patients with thoracolumbar burst fractures.[58] In a series of 21 patients treated without surgery, he observed no new neurologic deficits and a change of only 4-6° in the angle of kyphosis after one year. The role of surgery in patients with these fractures and no neurologic injury is still being studied.

Lumbosacral Spine

The principles used in treating fractures of the thoracic and thoracolumbar vertebrae also apply to fractures of the lumbosacral spine. Mild compression fractions can be treated conservatively, but severe fractures and subluxations should be treated surgically.

Penetrating Spine Injuries

AXIOM Because of the risk of meningitis, anyone with a cerebrospinal fluid leak from the spine for more than 24 to 48 hours should have primary closure of the dura.

Patients who sustain gunshot or stab wounds to the spine occasionally require surgery to repair the dura when there is a persistent cerebrospinal fluid (CSF) leak.[11] In patients with gunshot wounds that pierce the small bowel or colon and then penetrate the vertebral column, the need for surgical exploration and debridement of the spine is controversial. Cybulski et al. found that the risk of infection was not diminished by exploration or debridement of the spinal wound, and no improvement in neurologic deficits occurred unless neural elements were compressed by the bullet.[59] Venger et al.[60] and Velmahos and Demetriades[61] also found that removing the bullet did not diminish the incidence of infection or improve neurologic outcome. Thus, removing the bullet from the spinal canal is generally not recommended unless there is incomplete neurologic injury. However, prophylactic antibiotics should be administered to prevent vertebral osteomyelitis.

Timing of Surgical Treatment

The role of early surgery in the management of acute spinal cord injury is controversial. Arguments used to support early surgical intervention in spinal cord injury include: (a) it may provide better restoration of bone alignment; (b) earlier decompression of neural tissue may improve ultimate neural function; (c) early stabilization reduces the risk of secondary spinal cord damage; and (d) early mobilization of the patient reduces the incidence of pulmonary and other complications.[23]

Counterarguments to early surgical intervention in spinal cord injury include: (a) adequate alignment can usually be obtained by skeletal traction and closed manipulation; (b) early removal of bone fragments from the spinal canal usually does not improve neurologic recovery; and (c) the benefits of early mobilization can also be obtained by a program of active physiotherapy.[23] Nevertheless, indications for early surgery may include: (a) a progressively worsening neurologic deficit; (b) persistent leaking spinal cord wounds; and (c) failure to achieve spinal alignment by closed methods.[23]

Patients in whom there is neurologic deterioration during the first few days after injury should be suspected of having increasing compression of the spinal cord.[11] If plain radiographs or CT do not demonstrate bone fragments in the spinal canal, an MRI or myelography is obtained to determine whether there is soft-tissue compression of the cord.

AXIOM When neurologic function deteriorates and objective evidence of epidural compression exists, surgical decompression should be undertaken as soon as possible.

REHABILITATION PROGRAMS

AXIOM An effective rehabilitation program begins at initial admission to the hospital.

Rehabilitation Objectives

The initial objective in spinal cord rehabilitative programs is to maintain a full range of motion in all joints.[23] This requires early attention to proper positioning of all portions of the body and to passive and active range of motion exercises. As soon as practical, self-range techniques should be taught, and the importance of a daily routine to maintain maximal motion should be emphasized. The use of orthotics to maintain joint motion and to assist in stretching contractures is also important for maintaining a functional range of motion. Muscle strengthening should be started simultaneous with the range-of-motion programs to retard atrophy in normal muscle and to assist in regaining strength in neurologically compromised areas. Electrical stimulation may be of some assistance in maintaining strength in marginally functioning muscles until reinnervation occurs.

Choosing Orthotic and Assistance Devices

Once the anticipated range of motion and strength have been achieved, appropriate orthotic and assist devices should be used.[23] The wheelchair is particularly important and should be as light and maneuverable as possible. Patients with high cervical spine lesions require an electrically powered wheelchair, whereas patients with lesions at or below C-6 can often manage manual wheelchairs with appropriate modifications.

For quadriplegic patients with limited hand function, various manually driven or externally powered orthoses may significantly improve upper extremity function. For high quadriplegics, extremely sophisticated control units may be used to manipulate a multitude of electronic devices, enabling patients to open doors, answer telephones, write, and even feed themselves.[23]

Although thoracic level paraplegics usually are nonambulatory, paraplegics with a functional level below L-2 may be able to achieve limited ambulation with lower extremity orthoses and crutches. Individuals with bilateral long leg braces rarely become functionally ambulatory, but patients with a long leg brace on one side and a short leg brace on the other can frequently ambulate satisfactorily with proper training and conditioning.

INTENSIVE CARE AND COMPLICATIONS OF SPINAL CORD INJURIES

Disruption of spinal cord pathways results in changes in multiple body systems. The secondary effects of spinal cord injury on vital organs may have much more of an effect on morbidity and mortality than the spinal cord injury itself.[36]

Cardiovascular Problems

HYPOTENSION

Spinal cord injury above T-1 or T-2 with disruption of the descending sympathetic fibers from the hypothalamus and midbrain results in loss of sympathetic vasomotor tone throughout the body. The resultant vasodilation not only reduces systemic vascular resistance but also increases vascular capacity.[62] There may also be some myocardial dysfunction.[63] The decreases in afterload and preload and contractility can cause significant hypotension, which is often called spinal shock. Consequently, a systolic blood pressure of 80 mm Hg or less is not unusual immediately following spinal cord injury. Although this degree of hypotension may not interfere with tissue perfusion, the ability to compensate for any reduction in venous return because of fluid loss or ventilatory support is greatly decreased, and hypotension may also impair blood flow to the injured spinal cord.[64] Patients with high spinal cord lesions may have a significantly reduced difference between the blood volume that causes hypotension and the blood volume that causes pulmonary edema. Nevertheless, one should probably attempt to keep systolic blood pressure at about 100-110 mm Hg without giving too much fluid.[65]

AXIOM   Fluids must be administered with care to patients with high spinal cord injuries because they have an increased tendency to develop pulmonary edema.

When, in the absence of other injuries, the patient remains hypotensive in spite of rapid infusion of 1.5 - 2.0 L of crystalloid, one should insert a pulmonary artery catheter to monitor the pulmonary artery wedge pressure (PAWP), especially its response to a fluid challenge. If additional fluid were to raise the central venous pressure (CVP) or PAWP rapidly without significant improvement in blood pressure or cardiac output, inotropic and/or vasoconstrictor agents, such as dopamine, should be used. If the hypotension were to persist, the surgeon would have to ascertain that it was not due to associated injuries.

AXIOM   If CVP and blood pressure continue to be low after aggressive fluid resuscitation, one should suspect an associated injury causing continued blood loss.

BRADYCARDIA

Sinus bradycardia following spinal cord injury is caused by loss of sympathetic input to the heart, with unopposed parasympathetic stimulation through intact vagus nerves.[23] Increased parasympathetic stimulation by tracheal suctioning can exacerbate the bradycardia and may even cause asystole. In patients who are extremely sensitive to parasympathetic stimulation, intermittent use of atropine (0.5-1.0 mg) may be necessary. In rare cases, a pacemaker may be required.

AXIOM   Patients with high spinal cord injuries need careful cardiac monitoring during tracheal suctioning.

ANESTHETIC MANAGEMENT

When early surgery is contemplated for a patient with a high spinal cord injury, the preoperative placement of a pulmonary artery catheter to determine optimal filling pressure is increasingly recommended. Optimal cardiac filling pressures are determined by progressively giving fluid until cardiac output stops rising and filling pressures begin to rise rapidly with additional fluid. The optimal PAWP should then be maintained intraoperatively and for at least 24-48 hours postoperatively. If there is intraoperative hypotension in spite of optimal filling pressures, vasoconstrictors, such as phenylephrine, are often preferable to adrenergic agonists.

Denervated muscles tend to have increased sensitivity to acetylcholine, manifested as sustained contractions and a massive release of potassium. Consequently, succinylcholine can precipitate hyperkalemic crises and should be avoided during the first six months after a high spinal cord injury.

AXIOM   Use of succinylcholine is contraindicated for at least 6 months following spinal cord injuries.

ECG CHANGES

Changes in the ECG following cervical spinal cord injury consistent with subendocardial ischemia have been described clinically and experimentally.[63] Other observed ECG changes included: ST segment and T- wave abnormalities, sinus pauses, shifting sinus pacemaker, nodal escape beats, runs of atrial fibrillation, multifocal premature ventricular contractions, and ventricular tachycardia.

CHANGES DUE TO POSITIVE PRESSURE VENTILATION

In patients with marginal cardiovascular function, positive-pressure ventilation, especially with high levels of positive end expiratory pressure (PEEP), can reduce venous return and thereby compromise cardiac output, systemic blood pressure, and tissue perfusion. High inspiratory pressures may also be better tolerated if expiration is at least twice as long as inspiration.[66]

CHANGES DUE TO ACID-BASE AND ELECTROLYTE PROBLEMS

In patients with acute spinal cord injury, acid-base and electrolyte balance may be disturbed by both pathophysiologic respiratory acidosis, iatrogenically-induced respiratory alkalosis (as a result of alveolar hyperventilation), and metabolic alkalosis (from emesis, gastric suction, or hypokalemia).[23] Alterations may also occur from the stress of the trauma and its effects on catabolic hormones and the renin/aldosterone system.

POSTURAL HYPOTENSION

Patients with either complete or nearly complete spinal cord lesions in the cervical or high thoracic regions may experience syncopal episodes when first assuming an upright position.[23] These patients should be brought to an upright position by slowly increasing the elevation of the head with close monitoring of blood pressure. Syncopal episodes in these patients may be minimized by using elastic stockings and an abdominal binder, both of which may aid venous return to the heart.

VENOUS THROMBOEMBOLISM

Patients with spinal cord injury are at great risk for developing deep-vein thrombosis (DVT) of the lower extremities and up to 10% develop significant pulmonary emboli.[67] The use of low-dose heparin to minimize these complications has been advocated by some; however, other clinicians have found more value in instituting a routine of leg elevation (while the patient is confined to bed), thigh high elastic stockings, pneumatic compression stockings, and frequent passive range-of-motion exercises.[23] Use of a rotobed or Keane bed is also helpful in reducing the incidence of DVT in these patients.

AUTONOMIC HYPERREFLEXIA

Immediately following spinal cord injury, there is a period of "spinal shock," which lasts for several days. Some time later, spinal reflexes return to the distal portion of the spinal cord and these can produce chronic or repeated episodes of hypertension, diaphoresis, and diffuse pallor, which are referred to as autonomic hyperreflexia.[68] These episodes usually occur with injuries above T-6 and involve up to 50% of patients with complete cervical spinal cord injuries.

Autonomic hyperreflexia results when a sensory stimulus enters an isolated segment of the spinal cord below the injury level, initiating a "mass reflex" of excessive sympathetic and somatic activity. Common stimuli initiating this response include an overdistended bladder or gut, irritation of cutaneous pressure sores, or sudden decreases in arterial blood pressure, such as during the induction of anesthesia.[69]

AXIOM   After the spinal shock has resolved, an overdistended bladder, pressure sores, or hypotension can initiate a phenomenon known as autonomic hyperreflexia, which can cause severe hypertension, diaphoresis, and diffuse pallor.

The sympathetic mass reflex can produce strong vasoconstriction below the level of the spinal cord lesion, resulting in severe hypertension. This, in turn, can cause seizures or even intracerebral hemorrhage. The hypertension can also trigger a compensatory parasympathetic reaction with vasodilation above the level of the spinal cord lesion and marked bradycardia.

Because autonomic hyperreflexia can be extremely painful and can cause severe damage to the patient, preventive measures should be taken as soon as there is any suggestion that this problem is developing.[23] If a response were not noted soon after removing the apparent stimulus, the use of diazoxide or apresoline would possibly be required to control the blood pressure. In chronic or recurrent cases, dibenzyline has helped to prevent further episodes.

Pulmonary Problems

Atelectasis and pneumonia are common in patients with high spinal cord lesions and are the leading cause of death.[2] In one series, a 40% mortality rate in tetraplegic patients was largely attributed to pulmonary complications,[70] but the percentage who usually die from this cause is closer to 20-25%.[2] Good pulmonary toilet and frequent position changes, with or without rotary beds, can help reduce these problems.

> **AXIOM** Need for chronic ventilatory assistance in tetraplegic patients can frequently be prevented by aggressive, sterile pulmonary toilet.

VENTILATORY MUSCLES

The principal muscles involved in ventilation are the diaphragm and the intercostals. The intercostal muscles are used primarily to increase the anterior-posterior diameter of the middle and upper rib cage during normal breathing. With complete spinal cord injuries above T-1, these muscles are initially flaccid, but eventually become spastic, thereby helping to stabilize the chest wall during efforts at spontaneous ventilation. Adequate spontaneous ventilation may be almost impossible with high cervical spine injuries because the diaphragm, the most important muscle for ventilation, is innervated by the C-3 to C-5 segments. Paradoxic (inward) motion of the abdominal wall during spontaneous efforts at inspiration may be a sign of diaphragm paralysis.[71] In addition, if the diaphragm is weak, the abdominal contents may push cephalad while the patient is supine, thereby restricting pulmonary capacity.[72]

The upper accessory muscles of respiration, such as the trapezius, scalenus, and sternocleidomastoids muscles, are innervated by C-1 to C-3 and usually are spared, but the tidal volume they produce by increasing the anteroposterior diameter of the upper chest is not enough for adequate ventilation.[11]

Because of the impaired respiratory muscle function, the forced vital capacity (FVC) in patients with high spinal cord injuries can decline from a normal of about 65 mL/kg to less than 10-15 mL/kg. The FVC is a good indicator of "ventilatory reserve" in these patients, and a progressive decline in the FVC may be an indication for intubation and ventilatory assistance.[11]

A rigorous program of pulmonary care should be instituted early for quadriplegic patients, particularly when trying to avoid ventilator dependence. Postural drainage on a regular basis can be assisted by devices such as the Roto-rest bed. The "quad" cough or rapid application of upper abdominal pressure every 2-3 hours, can also be helpful in mobilizing secretions.[11]

During the first 7-10 days after high thoracic or low cervical spine injuries, patients who are not ventilator dependent must be watched very closely in an intensive care unit for pulmonary problems. Even in patients with spinal cord trauma below C-5, the level of neurologic dysfunction may ascend in the spinal cord during the first few days after trauma because of hemorrhage and edema in the central portion of the cord.

In many of these patients with excess secretions requiring prolonged ventilatory support, a tracheostomy may greatly increase patient comfort and improve pulmonary toilet. Gastric feedings can greatly increase the risk of aspiration into the lungs, but jejunostomy feedings provide relatively little risk of aspiration unless there is distal obstruction. Nevertheless, gastric decompression should be maintained until it is evident that the stomach is clearing its own secretions adequately. Removal of all catheters, such as nasotracheal and nasogastric tubes, from the pharynx will also help reduce upper airway secretions and will decrease the danger of aspiration of oral contents.

> **AXIOM** Patients with injuries to the low cervical spinal cord must be monitored carefully for delayed decreases in ventilatory ability due to an ascending lesion.

During the first two weeks after injury, in addition to continuous monitoring of pulse-oximetry and FVC, arterial blood gases (ABG) should be measured at least once daily. FVC less than 10 mL/kg or a PCO_2 above 45 mm Hg with an arterial pH < 7.40 is usually an indication for ventilatory assistance.

ONDINE'S CURSE

Injuries to cervical cord segments C-3 through C-5 may be associated with sleep apnea, sometimes referred to as "Ondine's curse."[23] Patients with this problem ventilate adequately while awake, but they lose their central respiratory drive while asleep. This syndrome is more apt to occur if the patient is given CNS depressants.

DIAPHRAGM PHYSICAL THERAPY

Physical therapy for the diaphragm can increase FVC. Weights are placed just below the xiphoid process, and the patient inhales and exhales as deeply as possible 15 times in succession. This therapy should be done three or four times a day. One can usually start with two pounds, increasing the weight by half-pound increments every few days, up to 8-10 pounds.[23]

Gastrointestinal Complications

> **PITFALL** ⊘
>
> *Failure to initiate early gastric suction in patients with spinal cord injury.*

ILEUS

A severe adynamic ileus usually develops promptly following spinal cord injury.[23] In uncomplicated cases, without associated injuries to the abdomen, or retroperitoneum, peristalsis gradually returns over the next 3-5 days. Failure to prevent gastrointestinal dilation prolongs the ileus and greatly increases the risk of aspiration and atelectasis.

STRESS ULCERATION

In patients with high spinal cord injuries, the unopposed parasympathetic stimulation can greatly increase gastric secretions and contribute to the development of stress gastritis or ulcers, particularly when high-dose corticosteroids are given. The incidence of severe ulcer disease causing gross bleeding or perforation is at least 5% in patients with spinal cord injury.[73] Consequently, a combination of intravenous H_2 blockers and frequent instillations of Maalox into the NG tube is often required to keep the gastric pH > 4.5.

> **AXIOM** Continuous intravenous drip of an H2 - blocker and/or frequent instillation of antacids should be given to patients with spinal cord injury to keep gastric pH > 4.5.

PERITONITIS

Because quadriplegic patients cannot feel abdominal pain, progressive bowel distension resulting in necrosis and perforation can go unrecognized.[11] One should be suspicious of peritonitis when there is an unexplained fever, elevation of the white blood cell count or amylase, or increasing abdominal distention or rigidity.

> **AXIOM**   One should obtain abdominal and pelvic CT scans if there is any suspicion of an intra-abdominal problem in a patient with spinal cord injury.

CONSTIPATION

Because most patients with spinal cord injuries lose the urge to defecate and also lose voluntary control of the anal sphincter, the bowel should be trained to empty regularly as soon as the patient receives enteral feedings.[11] A bowel program that is usually effective includes a daily stool softener and a rectal suppository as needed to stimulate peristalsis at appropriate intervals. Daily enemas may also be required.

NUTRITIONAL CONSIDERATIONS

Nutritional problems are frequently encountered in patients with spinal cord injuries.[74] These patients can develop severe negative nitrogen balance (exceeding 20-25 gm/day) after injury as a result of the trauma and the muscle "denervation." The diaphragm may also be weakened if the severe protein catabolism is not balanced by appropriate nutrition.

To deliver adequate calories and protein, intravenous nutrition is usually required initially. If the patient cannot take an adequate oral diet by five days, insertion of a feeding jejunostomy may be beneficial. Feeding via thin nasogastric tube can greatly increase the risk of gastric distention and aspiration of stomach contents. Feeding via nasal tubes advanced into the duodenum can also be helpful, but it can be difficult to keep such tubes from retracting back into the stomach. Recent evidence suggests that early enteral feeding can lower the incidence of many complications, including decubitus ulcers and stress bleeding.[75,76]

Genitourinary Complications

The innervation of the bladder is derived from the autonomic and somatic nervous systems. The sympathetic component is derived from T-11 to L-2, and the parasympathetic innervation from S-2 to S-4. During the period of spinal shock, the contractile ability of the bladder is lost, resulting in an areflexic bladder which tends to distend and develop overflow incontinence.[23] Following resolution of the spinal shock, reflex bladder activity returns because the spinal micturitional reflex arc is usually intact in the spinal cord below the lesion. This results in an "automatic bladder" which has spastic bladder muscles that tend to cause urinary frequency.

The initial management of patients with spinal cord injury usually requires an indwelling bladder catheter to help accurately monitor fluid intake and output. Later, the bladder is only catheterized intermittently to decrease the risk of urinary tract infections, which has a high frequency in both tetraplegic and paraplegic patients.[77] Urinary tract infections are of special concern because of their close association with subsequent renal failure. Both of these problems continue to be major causes of morbidity and mortality in patients with spinal cord injury. In addition, overdistention of the bladder can cause a painful mass reflex. Spinal cord injury patients also have an increased excretion of calcium in the urine and a high incidence of urinary tract calculi.[78] The calculi, plus the presence of bladder catheters for long periods, increase the risk of urinary tract fistulas.

After reflex parasympathetic activity returns, penile erections may occur in response to local stimuli; however, the ability to ejaculate, which is a sympathetic nervous system activity, is lost with a complete cord injury. Because of inability to ejaculate and decreased sperm motility, it is rare for males with spinal cord injury to be fertile.[79] In females, spinal cord injury produces only transient interruption of the menstrual cycle, and these individuals can become pregnant and bear normal children.

Musculoskeletal Problems

HETEROTOPIC OSSIFICATION

Heterotopic ossification (myositis ossificans) is an inflammatory process of unclear etiology involving voluntary muscles below the level of the spinal cord injury, primarily around major joints, such as the hips, knees, and elbows. It is characterized by calcium deposits within the muscle tissue and decreased range of motion. This process, which occurs in approximately 30% of all spinal-cord-injured patients and up to 70% of tetraplegics, results in a significant limitation of motion in at least half of those affected.[80] Although the joints are not affected, the ossification can become massive enough to cause extra-articular ankylosis.

Prophylaxis with salicylates or diphosphonates has been only partially successful and has not eliminated the occurrence of this problem. Therapy includes attempts to reduce the inflammation accompanying the bone formation and to maintain a normal range of motion until maturation of the process is complete. Surgical resection of the main areas of heterotopic ossification may help regain motion in severe cases. Associated extremity fractures should be treated with early internal fixation because immobility increases the risk of hypertrophic ossification and joint contractures.

> **AXIOM**   Gentle passive and active exercises to maintain the range of motion of all joints should be started as soon as possible after spinal cord injury.

JOINT CONTRACTURES

Contractures of joints tend to develop rapidly in patients with spinal cord injuries not only from loss of motion but also from loss of elastic properties and shortening of the ligaments surrounding the bony articulations. This phenomenon can be minimized by appropriate physical and occupational therapeutic interventions as soon as possible after the injury.

> **AXIOM**   Joints that do not move tend to develop contractures.

MUSCLE SPASTICITY

Spasticity, due to increased muscle tone below the level of spinal cord injury, becomes increasingly noticeable a few weeks after the spinal cord injury.[23] Because the cerebral inhibitory influences are lost to the denervated muscles, the local monosynaptic stretch reflex arcs can react in an unrestrained manner. The resulting spasticity can interfere with nursing care and proper positioning of the patient; however, with a program of early muscle stretching, one can often achieve a full range of motion of the joints and decrease muscle tone and spasticity.

> **AXIOM**   Muscle spasticity can often be controlled by early muscle stretching, which helps to maintain a full range of motion and decreased muscle tone.

When noninvasive techniques fail to adequately control muscle spasticity, pharmacologic agents may be of some benefit. Baclofen, beginning at 20 mg/day in divided doses and increasing until maximal benefit is achieved, may be effective. The addition of diazepam in small doses may also help. In cases that are refractory to these medications, clonidine in doses of 0.2-0.4 mg/day has been used with some success.[81]

Skin Complications

> **AXIOM**   Skin breakdown resulting in decubiti is the most common, avoidable complication of spinal cord injury.

Pressure sores developing over bony prominences are the single most frequent cause of prolonged hospitalization and increased medical costs with spinal cord injury. Decubitus ulcers develop in at least 32% of tetraplegic and paraplegic patients, most frequently over the bony prominences of the sacrum (39%), heels (14%), and ischium (9%).[3,11] Loss of sensation to the skin keeps patients from shifting and turning as they normally would. The prolonged pressure causes local ischemia which leads to necrosis and ulcer formation.

> **AXIOM** Prevention of pressure sores begins at admission because decubiti can develop in as short a time as a half hour.

Deep ischial and trochanteric decubiti can cause severe sepsis and death. If the decubiti were to become very large and deep, extensive debridements and reconstruction would frequently be required. These ulcers are best prevented by minimizing the pressure against any body surface and by frequent redistribution of pressure over the body, such as by "log-rolling" the patient side-to-side every two hours.[23]

The presence of traction devices should not interfere with good skin care. A standard hospital bed equipped with appropriate traction devices and a conscientious nursing care team to frequently turn the patient and attend to any unique requirements can be as effective as the wide variety of mechanical beds and special mattress that are presently available. Nevertheless, mechanical beds, such as the Roto-rest or Keane, by providing motorized continuous side-to-side motion, may give better results in selected patients with multiple trauma. This is particularly true in patients with unstable spine fractures associated with severe extremity or pelvic fractures.[23]

> **AXIOM** Decubiti are usually caused either by a lack of attention to details on the part of those caring for the patient or improperly fitting equipment.

Psychiatric Issues

During the past four decades, there has been increased awareness of severe psychiatric complications, such as suicide and alcohol and other drug abuse, in spinal-cord-injured patients. Spinal cord injury almost always causes severe emotional distress, which manifests as overt anger and/or indifferent withdrawal behavior that can last up to 2 years. In addition, at least 5-10% of quadriplegic patients attempt suicide at some point. Overt or covert self neglect is a common sign of this adjustment problem.[82] The divorce rate among patients with spinal cord injury is twice as high as the national average, with most divorces occurring in the second and third years after injury.[3,11]

> **AXIOM** Psychological counseling should begin as soon as possible after injury.

PROGNOSIS

The prognosis for victims of spinal cord injury depends primarily on the severity and location of the injury and the age of the patient; however, early use of comprehensive spinal cord rehabilitation facilities can be the main factor in a successful rehabilitation. Patients with tetraplegia have the highest mortality rate and 15-37% of these patients die during the first year after their injuries.[83] The early mortality rate for all spinal-cord-injured patients is about 11%, but for those 50 years of age or older, it rises to 39%.[84]

The most common causes of death for spinal-cord-injured patients are respiratory problems (21%), cardiovascular problems (15%), accidents, poisonings, or violence (10%), and infections (9%).[2] Up to 20% of those who require ventilator assistance die in the first 3 months.[85]

Recovery of neurologic function is primarily related to the severity of the injury. Those with complete loss of sensory and motor func-

tion below the level of the lesion may regain some sensation to deep pain or vibration, but they usually do not recover any useful motor function. For patients with incomplete lesions, significant improvement in motor strength and sensation can continue for several years after injury.[86]

Unfortunately, up to 7% of patients with spinal cord injuries experience a progressive decrease in neurologic function or develop painful dysesthesias months to years after injury.[86] A common cause of this is posttraumatic spinal cord syrinx that develops when hemorrhagic or necrotic lesions cavitate, leaving a space that can take on fluid and thereby compress surrounding spinal cord tissue. Such patients may have substantial neurologic improvement and pain relief following surgical drainage of the cyst.

Posttraumatic back and radicular pain and extremity contractures of unclear etiology (not caused by a syrinx) are not uncommon following spinal cord injury. These conditions may respond to appropriate physical therapy and intrathecal baclofen injections. Occasionally, cutting of selective dorsal roots may help relieve otherwise intractable pain.[87]

> **AXIOM** Comprehensive spinal cord rehabilitation programs play a vital role in determining the outcome following spinal cord injury.

Tetraplegic and paraplegic patients need long-term care from teams of physicians, nurse practitioners, physical therapists, and other health care professionals, to help prevent the many complications that can occur. The importance of early, skilled, continuous rehabilitation cannot be overemphasized.

SUMMARY

An increasing number of patients with spinal cord injuries survive the initial resuscitation and transportation to a major medical center. The proportion of patients with incomplete neurologic lesions, which carries a much better overall prognosis than does complete injury, has also increased significantly. With proper early management, the life expectancy and quality of life for these patients can be significantly improved. Prevention of the common complications of spinal cord injury and improved, more rapid rehabilitation are important reasons for the development of regional spinal cord injury centers.

⊘ *FREQUENT ERRORS*

In the Management of Spinal Cord Injuries

1. *Not assuming that all unconscious patients and patients with severe blunt injuries have spine injuries until proved otherwise.*
2. *Assuming that the extent of the spine injury seen on plain radiography indicates the amount of deformity that occurred at injury.*
3. *Assuming that absence of the typical signs of spinal fractures guarantees spinal stability.*
4. *Relying on fluids alone to restore BP in patients with high spinal cord injuries.*
5. *Not considering associated injuries as a possible cause of continued hypotension during aggressive fluid therapy.*
6. *Predicting neurologic outcome within 24-48 hours of injury.*
7. *Failing to look for evidence of increasing spinal cord compression as a possible cause of deteriorating neurologic dysfunction.*
8. *Not beginning comprehensive rehabilitation at admission.*
9. *Failure to ensure early gastric decompression with a nasogastric tube.*
10. *Failure to keep the gastric pH > 4.5.*

11. *Delaying passive and active range-of-motion exercises.*
12. *Failure to take special efforts to prevent decubiti.*

▼▼▼▼▼▼▼▼▼▼▼▼▼▼▼▼▼▼▼▼▼▼▼▼▼▼▼▼▼

SUMMARY POINTS

1. If there is any doubt as to the stability of a spinal fracture, the patient should be treated as if the spine were very unstable.

2. During the extrication from vehicles, prehospital transport, and the initial resuscitation of any patient with a possible spinal cord injury, one should take all necessary precautions for immobilizing the potentially injured spine.

3. Special precautions with immobilization must be taken during induction and maintenance of general anesthesia in any patient with known or suspected vertebral fractures.

4. All severely injured patients should be assumed to have unstable spinal injuries.

5. Patients with spinal cord injuries tend to have relative hypovolemia.

6. Early, accurate diagnosis of spinal cord injury is essential to prevent further neurologic damage and to provide optimal therapy.

7. Bowel or bladder dysfunction after trauma may be important evidence for a lesion involving the conus medullaris or cauda equina.

8. All unconscious trauma victims must be assumed to have a spinal cord injury until proved otherwise.

9. Loss of any motor or sensory function below the level of the neck should be assumed to be the result of a spinal cord injury.

10. The extent of bony deformation seen on radiography after trauma does not represent the full bony excursion and damage occurring at time of injury.

11. Absence of the typical signs of spinal fractures does not guarantee stability.

12. Cervical spine radiographs are not necessary for victims of blunt head and neck trauma when they are conscious, alert, and asymptomatic.

13. The prognosis of a spinal cord injury cannot be determined until the patient recovers from spinal shock.

14. If the patient has an injury to the occipitoatlantal joint, axial traction is often contraindicated.

15. Closed manipulation of the cervical spine to reduce fractures generally is not recommended.

16. Because of the risk of meningitis, anyone with a spinal CSF leak for more than 24 to 48 hours should have primary closure of the dura.

17. If there is deteriorating neurologic function and objective evidence of epidural compression, surgical decompression should be undertaken as soon as possible.

18. An effective rehabilitation program begins at initial admission to the hospital.

19. Fluids must be administered with care to patients with high spinal cord injuries because they have an increased tendency to develop pulmonary edema.

20. If the CVP and blood pressure continue to be low after aggressive fluid resuscitation, one should suspect an associated injury causing continued blood loss.

21. Patients with high spinal cord injuries need adequate cardiac monitoring during tracheal suctioning.

22. Use of succinylcholine is contraindicated for at least six months following spinal cord injuries.

23. After spinal shock has resolved, an overdistended bladder, pressure sores or hypotension can initiate a phenomenon known as autonomic hyperreflexia, which can cause severe hypertension, diaphoresis, and diffuse pallor.

24. Need for chronic ventilatory assistance in tetraplegic patients can frequently be prevented by aggressive, sterile pulmonary toilet.

25. Patients with injuries to the low cervical spinal cord must be monitored carefully for delayed decreases in ventilatory ability due to an ascending spinal cord lesion.

26. A continuous intravenous drip of an H_2-blocker and/or frequent instillation of antacids should be used for spinal-cord-injured patients, to keep gastric pH > 4.5.

27. One should obtain abdominal and pelvic CT scans if there is any suspicion of an intra-abdominal problem in a patient with spinal cord injury.

28. Gentle passive and active exercises to maintain the range of motion or all joints should be started as soon as possible after spinal cord injury.

29. Joints that do not move tend to develop contractures.

30. Muscle spasticity can often be controlled by early muscle stretching, which helps to maintain a full range of motion and also decreases muscle tone.

31. Skin breakdown resulting in decubiti is the most common, avoidable, complication of spinal cord injury.

32. Because decubitus ulcers can develop in as short a time as a half hour, prevention of pressure sores begins at admission to the hospital.

33. Decubiti are usually caused by either by lack of attention to details on the part of those caring for the patient or improperly fitting equipment.

34. Psychological counseling should begin as soon as possible after injury.

35. Comprehensive spinal cord rehabilitation programs play a vital role in determining the outcome following spinal cord injury.

▲▲▲▲▲▲▲▲▲▲▲▲▲▲▲▲▲▲▲▲▲▲▲▲▲▲▲▲▲▲▲▲

REFERENCES

1. Woolsey RM. Modern concepts of therapy and management of spinal cord injuries. Crit Rev Neurobiol 1988;4:137.
2. Young JS, et al. Spinal cord injury statistics: experience of the regional spinal cord injury systems, Phoenix: Good Samaritan Medical Center, 1988.
3. Kennedy EJ, ed. Spinal cord injury: the facts and figures. Birmingham: University of Alabama, 1986; 1.
4. Panchal PD. Rehabilitation of the patient with spinal cord injury. Curr Probl Surg 1980;17:254.
5. Young JS, Burns PE, Wilt GA. Medical charges incurred by the spinal cord injured the first six years following injury. Model Systems SCI Digest 1982;4:19.
6. Roye WP Jr, Dunn EL, Moody JA. Cervical spinal cord injury—a public catastrophe. J Trauma 1988;28:1260.
7. Meyer PR. Emergency room assessment: management of spinal cord and associated injuries. Meyer PR, ed. Surgery of spine trauma. New York: Churchill Livingstone, 1989; 23.
8. Kupferschmid JP, Weaver ML, Raves JJ, et al. Thoracic spine injuries in victims of motorcycle accidents. J Trauma 1989;29:593.
9. Hadley MN, Sonntag VK, Rekate HL, et al. The infant whiplash-shake injury syndrome: a clinical and pathological study. Neurosurgery 1989; 4:536.
10. Mackersie RC, Shackford SR, Garfin SR, et al. Major skeletal injuries in the obtunded blunt trauma patient: a case for routine radiologic survey. J Trauma 1988;28:1450.
11. Marian D, Clifton G. Injury to the vertebrae and spinal cord. Moore EE, Mattox KL, Felicians DV, eds. Trauma, 2nd ed. Norwalk: Appleton & Lange, 1991; 261-275.
12. Bunegin L, Hung TK, Chang GL Biomechanics of spinal cord injury. Crit Care Clin 1987;3:453.
13. Allen BL. A mechanistic classification of closed indirect fractures and dislocations of the lower cervical spine. Spine 1982;7:1.
14. Benson DR. Unstable thoracolumbar fractures, with emphasis on the burst fracture. Clin Orthop 1988;May: 14.
15. Domisse GF. The blood supply of the spinal cord. J Bone Joint Surg 1974;56B:225.
16. Sasaki S. Vascular change in the spinal cord after impact injury in the rat. Neurosurgery 1982;10:360.
17. Balentine JD. Pathology of experimental spinal cord trauma. I. The necrotic lesion as a function of vascular injury. Lab Invest 1978;39:236.
18. Janssen L, Hansebout RR. Pathogenesis of spinal cord injury and newer treatments. A review. Spine 1989;14:23.

19. Anderson DK, Prokop LD, Means ED, et al. Cerebrospinal fluid lactate and electrolyte levels following experimental spinal cord injury. J Neurosurg 1976;44:715.

20. Naftchi NE, Demeny M, DeCrescito V. Biogenic amine concentrations in traumatized spinal cords of cats. J Neurosurg 1974;40:52.

21. Fehlings MG, Tator CH, Linden RD. The relationships among the severity of spinal cord injury, motor and somatosensory evoked potentials and spinal cord blood flow. Electroencephalogr Clin Neurophysiol 1989; 74:241.

22. Kao CC, Chang LW, Bloodworth JMB Jr. The mechanism of spinal cord cavitation following spinal cord transection: electron microscopic observation. J Neurosurg 1977;6:745.

23. Kopaniky DR. Pathophysiology of spinal cord disruption and injury. Miller TA, ed. Physiologic basis of modern surgical care. St. Louis, CV Mosby 1988; 789.

24. Smith AJK. Hyperemia, CO_2 responsiveness, and autoregulation in the white matter following experimental spinal cord injury. J Neurosurg 1978;48:239.

25. Willis BK, Greiner F, Orrison WW, et al. The incidence of vertebral artery injury after midcervical spine fracture or subluxation. Neurosurgery 1994;34:435-41.

26. Miyachi S, Okamura K, Watanabe M, et al. Cerebral stroke due to vertebral artery occlusion after cervical spine trauma. Two case reports. Spine 1994;19:83.

27. Rogers LF, Lee C. Cervical spine trauma. Dalinka MK, Kaye JJ, eds. Radiology in emergency medicine. New York: Churchill Livingstone, 1984;275.

28. Micheal DB, Guyot DR, Darmody WR. Coincidence of head and cervical spine injury. J Neurotrauma 1989;6:177.

29. Medical Research Council. Aids to the examination of the peripheral nervous system. Philadelphia: Bailliere Tindall, 1986; 1.

30. Rozycki GS, Champion HR. Radiology of the cervical spine. Maull KI, ed. Advances in trauma, vol 5. St. Louis: Mosby Year Book, 1990;37-47.

31. Miles KA, Finlay D. Is prevertebral soft tissue swelling a useful sign in injury of the cervical spine? Injury 1988;19:177.

32. Handel SF, Lee Y-Y. Computed tomography of spinal fractures. Radiol Clin North Am 1981;19:69.

33. Tracy PT, Wright RM, Hanigan WC. Magnetic resonance imaging of spinal injury. Spine 1989;14:292.

34. Fischer RP. Cervical radiographic evaluation of alert patients following blunt trauma. Ann Emerg Med 1984;13:905.

35. Bayles P, Ray VG. Incidence of cervical spine injuries in association with blunt head trauma. Am J Emerg Med 1989;7:139.

36. Kakulas A. The applied neurobiology of human spinal cord injury: a review. Paraplegia 1988;26:371.

37. Stauffer ES. Rehabilitation of posttraumatic cervical spinal cord quadriplegic and pentaplegia. Sherk HH, et al. eds. The cervical spine. Philadelphia: Lippincott, 1989; 521.

38. Stauffer ES. Diagnosis and prognosis of acute cervical spinal cord injury. Clin Orthop 1975;112:9.

39. Del Bigio MR, Johnson GE. Clinical presentation of spinal cord concussion. Spine 1989;14:37.

40. Pang D, Pollack IF. Spinal cord injury without radiographic abnormality in children. The SCIWORA syndrome. J Trauma 1989;29:654.

41. Braughler JM, Hall ED. Lactate and pyruvate metabolism in the injured cat spinal cord before and after a single large intravenous dose of methylprednisolone. J Neurosurg 1983;59:256.

42. Hall ED, Braughler JM. Effects of intravenous methylprednisolone on spinal cord lipid peroxidation and Na^+–K^+-ATPase activity. J Neurosurg 1982;57:247.

43. Anderson DK, Braughler JM, Hall ED, et al. Effects of treatment with U-74006F on neurological outcome following experimental spinal cord injury. J Neurosurg 1988;69:562.

44. Bracken MB, Collins WF, Freeman DF, et al. Efficacy of methylprednisolone in acute spinal cord injury. JAMA 1994;251:45.

45. Hall ED, Wolf DL, Braughler JM. Effects of a single large dose of methylprednisolone sodium succinate on post-traumatic spinal cord ischemia: dose-response and time-action analysis. J Neurosurg 1984;61:124.

46. Bracken MB, Shepard MJ, Collins WF, et al. A randomized, controlled trial of methylprednisolone of naloxone in the treatment of acute spinal cord Injury. Results of the Second National Acute Spinal Cord Injury Study. N Engl J Med 1990;322:1405.

47. Prendergast MR, Saxe JM, Ledgerwood AM, et al. Massive steroids do not reduce zone of injury after spinal cord injury (SCI) (Abstract). J Trauma 1993;35:168.

48. Ledeen RW. Ganglioside structures and distribution: are they localized in the nerve endings? J Supramol Struct 1978;8:1.

49. Argentino C, Sacchetti M, Toni D, et al. GM1 ganglioside therapy in acute ischemic stroke. Stroke 1989;20:1143-9.

50. Geisler FH, Dorsey FC, Coleman WP. Recovery of motor function after spinal-cord injury—a randomized, placebo-controlled trial with GM-1 ganglioside. N Engl J Med 1991;324:26;1829.

51. Faden AI, Jacobs TP, Mougey E, et al. Endorphins in experimental spinal injury: therapeutic effect of naloxone. Ann Neurol 1981;10:326.

52. Faden AL. Jacobs TP, Smith MT, et al. Comparison of thyrotropin-releasing hormone (TRH), naloxone, and dexamethasone treatments in experimental spinal injury. Neurology 1983;33:673.

53. Kijihara K. Dimethyl sulfoxide in the treatment of experimental acute spinal cord injury. Surg Neurol 1973;1:16.

54. Lim R, Mullan S. Enhancement of resistance of glial cells by dimethyl sulfoxide against sonic disruption. Ann NY Acad Sci 1975;243:358.

55. Sherk HH. Fractures of the atlas and odontoid process. Orthop Clin North Am 1978;9:973.

56. Bucholz RD, Cheung KC. Halo vest versus spinal fusion for cervical injury: evidence from an outcome study. J Neurosurg 1989;70:884.

57. Durward QJ, Schweigel JF, Harrison P. Management of fractures of the thoracolumbar and lumbar spine. Neurosurgery 1981;8:555.

58. Reid DC, Hu R, Davis LA, et al. The nonoperative treatment of burst fractures of the thoracolumbar junction. J Trauma 1988;28:1188.

59. Cybulski GR, Stone JL, Kant R. Outcome of laminectomy for civilian gunshot injuries of the terminal spinal cord and cauda equina: review of 88 cases. Neurosurgery 1989;24:392.

60. Venger BH, Simpson RK, Narayan RK. Neurosurgical intervention in penetrating spinal trauma with associated visceral injury. J Neurosurg 1989;70:514.

61. Velmahos G, Demetriades D. Gunshot wounds of the spine: should retained bullets be removed to prevent infection? Ann R Coll Surg Engl 1994;76:85.

62. Lehmann KG, Lane JG, Piepmeier JM, Batsford WP. Cardiovascular abnormalities accompanying acute spinal injury in humans. J Am Coll Cardiol 10:46, 1987.

63. Greenhoot JH, Shiel FO, Mauck HP Jr. Experimental spinal cord injury: electrocardiographic abnormalities and fuchsinophilic myocardial degeneration. Arch Neurol 1972;26:524.

64. De la Torre JC. Spinal cord injury: review of basic and applied research. Spine 1981;6:315.

65. Silver JR. Immediate management of spinal injury. Br J Hosp Med 1983;29:412.

66. Morgan BC. Hemodynamic effects of intermittent positive pressure respiration. Anesthesiology 1966;27:584.

67. Myllynen P, Kammonen M, Rokkanen P. Deep venous thrombosis and pulmonary embolism in patients with acute spinal cord injury: a comparison with nonparalyzed patients immobilized due to spinal fractures. J Trauma 1985;25:541.

68. Erickson RP. Autonomic hyperreflexia: pathophysiology and medical management. Arch Phys Med Rehabil 1980;61:431.

69. Lambert DH, Deane RS, Mazuzan JE. Anesthesia and the control of blood pressure in patients with spinal cord injury. Anesth Analg 1982;61:344.

70. Ballamy R, Pitts FW, Stauffer ES. Respiratory complication in traumatic quadriplegia. J Neurosurg 1973;39:596.

71. Luce JM, Culver BH. Respiratory muscle function in health and disease. Chest 1982;81:82.

72. Bergofsky EH. Mechanism for respiratory insufficiency after cervical cord injury: a source of alveolar hypoventilation. Ann Intern Med 1964; 61:435.

73. Berly MH, Wilmont CB. Acute abdominal emergencies during the first four weeks after spinal cord injury. Arch Phys Med Rehab 1984; 65:687.

74. Peiffer SC, Blust P, Leyson, JFJ. Nutritional assessment of the spinal cord injured patient. J Am Diet Assoc 1981;78:501.

75. Rodriguez GP, Claus-Walker J. Biochemical changes in skin composition in spinal cord injury: a possible contribution to decubitus ulcers. Paraplegia 1988;26:302.

76. Kuric J, Lucas CE, Ledgerwood AM, et al. Nutritional support: a prophylaxis against stress bleeding after spinal cord injury. Paraplegia 1989; 27:140.

77. Erickson RP, Merritt JL, Opitz JI. Bacteriuria during follow up in patients with spinal cord injury: I. Rate of bacteriuria in various bladder emptying methods. Arch Phys Med Rehabil 1982;63:409.

78. Nikakhtar B, Vaziri ND, Khonsari F. Urolithiasis in patients with spinal cord injury. Paraplegia 1982;20:48.
79. Comarr AE. Sexual function among patients with spinal cord injury. Urol Int 1970;25:134.
80. Finerman GAM, Stover SL. Heterotopic ossification following hip replacement or spinal cord injury. Two clinical studies with EHDP Metab. Bone Dis Relat Res 1981;45:337.
81. Morris JA Jr, Limbird TJ, MacKensie E. Rehabilitation of the trauma patient in trauma, 2nd ed. Moore EE, Mattox KL, Feliciano DV, eds. Norwalk: Appelton & Lange, 1991;820.
82. MacLeod AD. Self-neglect of spinal injured patients. Paraplegia 1988; 26:340.

83. Janssen L, Hansebout RR. Pathogenesis of spinal cord injury and newer treatments. A review. Spine 1989;14:23.
84. Bracken MD, Shepard MJ, Collins WF, et al. Methylprednisolone and neurological function 1 year after spinal cord injury. J Neurosurg 1985; 63:704.
85. Daverat P, Gagnon M, Dartigues JF, et al. Initial factors predicting survival in patients with spinal cord injury. J Neurol Neurosurg Psychiatry 1989;52:403.
86. Piepmeier JM, Jenkins NR. Late neurological changes following traumatic spinal cord injury. J Neurosurg 1988;69:399.
87. Kiwerski J. The natural history of neurological recovery in patients with traumatic tetraplegia. Paraplegia 1989;27:41.

Chapter **12** Ocular Trauma

THOMAS C. SPOOR, M.D.

JOHN M. RAMOCKI, M.D.

GEOFFREY M. KWITKO, M.D.

INTRODUCTION

Incidence of Eye Trauma

Approximately 100,000 work-related and at least 35,000 to 40,000 sports-related eye injuries occur annually.[1] Other major types of trauma account for an additional 300,000 cases; therefore, approximately 500,000 individuals sustain eye injuries every year.[2] Fortunately, only a small percentage of these patients have severe ocular damage. Of the more than 60,000 patients who sustain ocular injuries serious enough to require hospitalization about 20,000 have open wounds of the eyeball or ocular adnexa.[3] Serious eye injuries are more common in men than in women, and the majority occur in patients 10-40 years of age.[4,5] A second peak incidence occurs after 70 years of age.[3]

Prognosis With Eye Trauma

Penetrating ocular injuries generally have the worst prognosis and up to 40% will result in blindness.[6] When the posterior segment of the globe is penetrated, up to 50% of patients will require enucleation.[7] More recent studies, however, indicated that up to 70% of eyes treated with modern microsurgical techniques can regain functional vision.[8-11] Equally important has been the development of techniques that allow the ophthalmologist to enter the vitreous cavity under microscopic control to remove blood, foreign bodies, and inflammatory or proliferative membranes.

Associated Injuries

Many patients presenting to the trauma center with severe ocular injuries have other associated injuries particularly to the head and neck.[2] Facial and skull fractures and associated tissue disruption and hematomas can delay recognition and evaluation of severe associated eye damage.

In one major series, 67% of patients with blunt maxillofacial trauma had associated ocular injuries of which 18% were serious and 3% resulted in blindness.[12] In other series, ocular injuries were present in 10-40% of orbital and periorbital fractures[13] and in up to 8% of head-injured patients.[14]

Consulting an Ophthalmologist

> **AXIOM** The earlier an ophthalmologist sees a badly injured eye, the better the vision is likely to be.

In life-threatening trauma, detailed evaluation of the eyes may have to be delayed; however, early involvement of the ophthalmologist can help to prevent further damage to the globe and can reduce the need for additional surgical procedures.

MECHANISM OF VISION

A common misconception about the eye is that it "sees." In fact, it is the brain that sees, and the eye acts only as a receptor of energy in the form of light.

> **AXIOM** Although the eye is the receptor of light rays, it is the brain that "sees."

Eye Anatomy

GENERAL

From a functional standpoint, the eye itself can be divided into two parts: a smaller anterior chamber with a radius of about 8 mm and containing the cornea and lens, and a posterior chamber with a radius of about 12 mm containing the retina and optic nerve (Fig. 12–1). The eyeball is flattened vertically and has a diameter of about 24 mm in the anterior-posterior axis. The cornea and lens act to refract incident rays of light so that they focus a sharp image on the fovea. The fovea is a special area of the macula which, in turn, is a specialized portion of the retina positioned about 3.5 mm lateral (temporal) to the optic disc. There are more ganglion cells in the macula than in the rest of the retina.

MACULA AND FOVEA

The anatomy of the macula is quite different from the rest of the retina. A progressive decrease occurs in the number of rods and a progressive increase occurs in the number of cones as one moves from the periphery of the macula towards the central fovea. No rods exist in the fovea itself. It has only cones, with each cone being connected to only one ganglion cell instead of many; hence, the impulse at the fovea is much purer and the resultant image received by the brain much sharper than those originating from elsewhere in the retina. Because of this, the fovea is the only part of the retina capable of having 20/20 vision. The resultant visual acuity decreases as the image is focused peripheral to the fovea, dropping to 20/200 at the edge of the macula and over the rest of the retina. When vision cannot be corrected to at least 20/200, the individual is said to be legally blind.

NEURAL ANATOMY

Once the cornea and lens focus a sharp, inverted image of light on the fovea, the light excites the cones in that area; these cones, in turn, convert the light energy into electrical impulses. Each electrical impulse synapses with appropriate ganglion cells, which make up most of the optic nerve. The axons of the ganglion cells then continue, as the intraorbital, intracanalicular, and then intracranial optic nerve without synapsing. Axons arising from ganglion cells nasal to the fovea cross the midline in the optic chiasm and merge with axons nasal to the fovea from the contralateral eye. Axons that arise temporal to the fovea remain uncrossed. These long axons eventually synapse with other neurons at the lateral geniculate body. Fibers arising from the lateral geniculate bodies then form the optic radiations which traverse the temporal and parietal lobes and terminate in the occipital cortex.

> **AXIOM** Because visual pathways cross at the optic chiasm, injury anterior to the chiasm will cause unilateral visual dysfunction, while injury at or posterior to the chiasm will cause bilateral visual dysfunction.

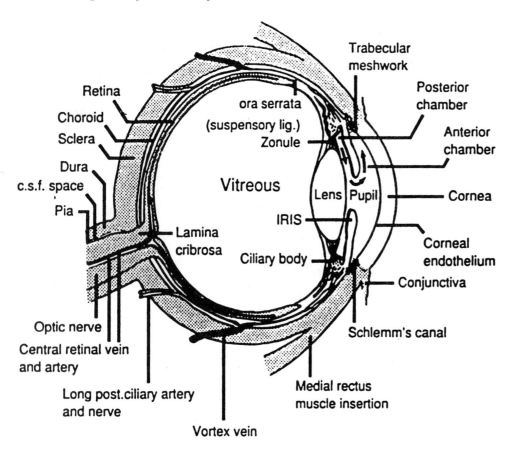

FIGURE 12–1 Anatomical organization of the eye. (From: Capan LM, Mankikar D, Eisenberg WM. Anesthetic Management of ocular injuries. Capan LM, Miller SM, Turndorf H, eds. Trauma: anesthesia and intensive care. Philadelphia: JB Lippincott, 1991; 358.)

MECHANISMS OF VISUAL DYSFUNCTION

Refractive Lesions

If incident light, after being refracted by the cornea and lens, is not focused on the fovea, a refractive error exists. The focal point may be anterior to the fovea because the eye is too long or has a cornea that has too much converging power; this produces myopia (nearsightedness). Conversely, the focal point may be posterior to the fovea because the eye is too short or has a cornea that is too flat; this produces hyperopia (farsightedness).

Myopia may be corrected by optically weakening the eye with a corrective lens so that the incident rays of light diverge before they are perceived by the cornea. This may be accomplished by glasses or by contact lenses. A similar effect can be produced by refractive surgery, which flattens the cornea. Hyperopia may be corrected by adding converging power to the eye, which can also be done with contact lenses or glasses.

Obstructive Lesions

In the normal eye, a clear path exists between the front of the cornea and the fovea. Any opacity that lays between the two may cause visual disturbances. The opacities may take the form of corneal scars, blood in the anterior chamber (hyphema), cataracts, vitreous hemorrhage, or other vitreous opacities. This type of visual dysfunction is not correctable with refractive lenses.

AXIOM Clear vision requires a clear path from the cornea to the fovea and precise focusing of the rays of light on the fovea.

Perceptive Lesions

Once the rays of light traverse a clear ocular media and are precisely focused, a healthy fovea must be present to detect the image being transmitted and subsequently convert the light energy into electrical

energy. Once past the healthy eye, the visual information, now in the form of electrical energy, needs a healthy optic nerve and radiations to transmit the information to the occipital cortex where vision can be perceived. Finally, if the occipital cortex were injured or diseased, the visual image could not be appreciated (cortical blindness), even though the rest of the system would be functioning normally. Functioning eyes, optic nerves, chiasm, tracts, radiations, and occipital cortex are all necessary for normal visual acuity and visual fields. Disease or injury at any point along this path may cause visual dysfunction.

AXIOMS The best screening technique for detecting defective eye function is testing of visual acuity and visual fields.

PATHOPHYSIOLOGY OF EYE TRAUMA

Corneal Abrasions

The cornea is covered with a layer of epithelium overlying a basement membrane (Bowman's membrane).[6] This epithelium protects the corneal stroma against infection and is necessary for the cornea to remain in its normal, relatively dehydrated, clear state. The corneal sensory nerves lay just beneath the corneal epithelium. If the corneal epithelium were removed or damaged, the nerve endings would become exposed, causing severe pain.

Corneal abrasions are most commonly caused by minor mechanical trauma, such as a fingernail or particulate matter striking the eye.[6] Multiple extremely fine linear abrasions of the superior third of the cornea (the "ice rink sign") suggest the presence of a foreign body under the upper lid. Overuse of contact lenses, particularly the hard variety, can also cause corneal abrasions. Another not uncommon cause of corneal injury is exposure to intense ultraviolet light, as from arc welding. The ultraviolet light disrupts nucleoproteins in the corneal epithelium and causes sloughing of the epithelium after about 6-10 hours. Welders with this problem typically come to the trauma center in the evening complaining of eye pain, blurred vision, and the sensation of a foreign body in the eye.

Chemical Injuries

> **AXIOM** Alkali injuries of the eye are generally much more severe than those caused by acid.

The degree of ocular damage caused by a chemical depends primarily on its pH.[6,15] The most severe damage is caused by highly alkaline compounds. Acids do not cause as much ocular damage because they tend to coagulate protein which then acts as a barrier to further penetration. The corneal and conjunctival epithelium also act as barriers to the penetration of toxic chemicals. Although concentrated acids may render the corneal epithelium white and opaque, with time the opaque epithelium sloughs, and it is usually replaced by normal epithelium so that permanent damage to vision is rare.

Alkali, conversely, can quickly penetrate the corneal epithelium and cause direct liquefaction necrosis of the cornea and sclera. Some indirect damage is also caused by the release of proteases and collagenases[6] (Fig. 12–2). Strong alkali can cause complete melting of the cornea and severe intraocular inflammation resulting in dense, permanent corneal scarring, cataracts, glaucoma, ocular ischemia, and necrosis of intraocular contents.

Blunt Ocular Trauma

Severe concussive injury to the eye can produce damage to almost every ocular tissue (Fig. 12–3).[6] A fist or steering wheel striking the eye, pushes the globe back into the orbit. When the eye is deeply set in the orbit, the orbital rim may absorb much of the impact. Generally, however, the globe is compressed to some degree, producing some damage to the soft tissues of the globe, including the choroid, iris, ciliary body, and/or retina.[16]

Blunt trauma to the orbit may also result in an orbital hematoma.[6] Although a mild orbital hematoma may cause only minimal damage, a severe orbital hematoma can cause marked proptosis and raise the intraorbital pressure sufficiently to occlude the central retinal artery, producing pain and an abrupt loss of vision.

> **AXIOM** Posttraumatic posterior intraocular hypertension can rapidly occlude the retinal artery and cause blindness.

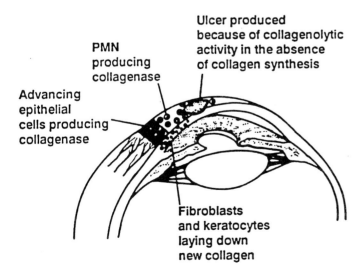

FIGURE 12–2 Pathogenesis of ulceration in the alkali-burned cornea. Ulceration occurs when collagenase production manifests in areas devoid of adequate collagen synthesis. (From: Belin MW, Catalano RA, Scott JL. Burns of the eye. In Catalano RA, ed. Ocular emergencies. Philadelphia: WB Saunders, 1992; 179.)

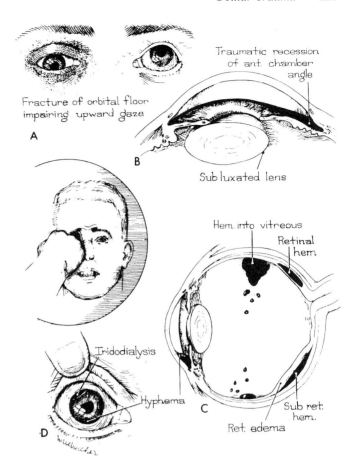

FIGURE 12–3 Some common contusion injuries. (From: Paton and Goldberg's management of ocular injuries. Deutsch TA, Feller DB, eds. Philadelphia: WB Saunders, 1985; 184.)

Fracture of the floor of the orbit may be accompanied by herniation of orbital tissue into the maxillary antrum, producing enophthalmos and double vision (Fig. 12–4). There will also be limitation of upward gaze if the inferior rectus muscle becomes entrapped (Fig. 12–5).[6] Fracture of the roof or medial wall of the orbit can cause orbital emphysema (air in the orbit), which may be followed by orbital cellulitis. Bony fractures at the apex of the orbit may cause damage to the optic nerve by direct contusion, pressure from adjacent hematomas, or lacerations by bony fragments.

Penetrating Ocular Trauma

Penetrating injury to the eye is much less common than blunt trauma or corneal abrasions; however, it generally has a poor prognosis for vision and requires admission to a hospital. The annual hospitalization costs in the United States for patients with penetrating ocular injuries may exceed $120 million.[6]

The prognosis of penetrating eye trauma is related primarily to its location and the extent of damage. In general, the more posterior and larger the laceration is the worse the prognosis. Through-and-through injuries have a particularly dismal prognosis.

> **AXIOM** Posterior penetrations of the eye tend to have much poorer prognoses than anterior injuries.

Penetrations or lacerations of the cornea, anterior chamber and/or lens can generally be repaired by meticulous microsurgical closure, contact lens, intraocular lens, optical corrections, or even corneal transplantation with a high rate of visual rehabilitation.[6]

> **AXIOM** Early microsurgery to correct penetrating eye injuries can save much vision that would otherwise be lost.

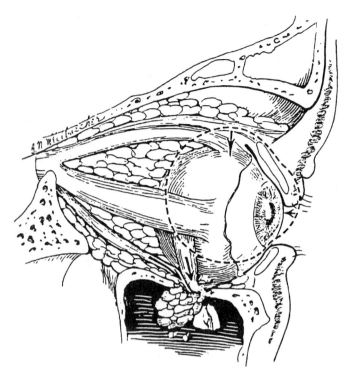

FIGURE 12–4   Blow-out fracture of the orbital floor. The dotted line indicates the normal position of the globe. The inferior oblique and inferior rectus muscles are restrained by the incarcerated orbital tissues. (From: Paton and Goldberg's management of ocular injuries. Deutsch TA, Feller DB, eds. Philadelphia: WB Saunders, 1985; 40.)

Posterior injuries involving the retina are generally severe.[6] In addition to direct damage to the retina, foreign material in the vitreous creates a perfect medium for growth of scar tissue throughout the vitreous cavity.[17] This tissue, derived in part from metaplastic fibroblasts and retinal pigment epithelial cells, also contains contractile proteins which have the potential to contract and induce retinal tears. Despite successful initial reattachment of the retina, the process of cellular proliferation and contracture may cause recurrent retinal detachment.

Although microbial endophthalmitis occurs in < 3% of penetrating eye injuries, > 50% of such cases result in blindness.[6] The risk of blindness is increased further by the presence of intraocular foreign bodies and delayed repair.

AXIOM   Parenterally administered antibiotics penetrate the eye poorly, making it particularly important to reduce the risk of endophthalmitis by prompt surgical repair of open-eye injuries whenever possible.

Sympathetic ophthalmia is a bilateral inflammation of the uveal tract (iris, ciliary body, and choroid) associated with penetrating injury to one eye.[6] Untreated, this inflammation may result in loss of the noninjured eye. Evidence suggests that the risk of sympathetic ophthalmia may be reduced when the injury eye is enucleated within two weeks of the injury. This has prompted some physicians to recommend prompt removal of an injured eye when it has very poor visual potential.

AXIOM   Any patient with a penetrating injury to one eye is potentially at risk for the development of sympathetic ophthalmia, which can cause blindness in the other eye.[18]

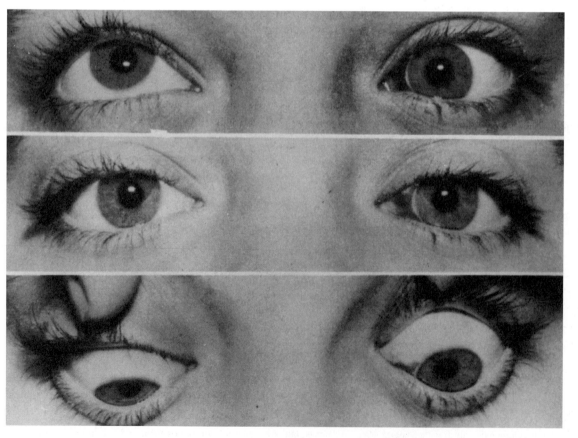

FIGURE 12–5   Fresh blow-out fracture of left orbit with limitation of upward and downward movement of the left eye. (From: Paton and Goldberg's management of ocular injuries. Deutsch TA, Feller DB, eds. Philadelphia: WB Saunders, 1985; 41.)

Although it would be a great misfortune to lose the remaining good eye because a severely injured nonfunctioning eye is left in too long, the risk of sympathetic ophthalmia is exceedingly low; only about 20 new patients are diagnosed in the United States each year. Furthermore, enucleation does not guarantee protection for the other eye against later development of sympathetic ophthalmia. Additionally, early use of corticosteriods or cytotoxic agents can allow retention of good vision in the majority of patients who develop sympathetic ophthalmia. Furthermore, vitreous microsurgery is constantly improving so that even severely injured eyes may recover some useful vision.

AXIOM The risk of sympathetic ophthalmia does not justify the primary removal of a severely traumatized eye unless the vision of that eye is completely lost.

DIAGNOSIS

Patient History

The nature of an ocular injury can obviously have profound effects on the eventual visual outcome, and an accurate history can provide valuable clues for early diagnosis and optimal treatment (Table 12–1). Several items that are particularly important when evaluating the histories of patients with ocular trauma include:[6]

1. How well can the patient see now?
2. Is one eye or both eyes affected?
3. Are there any other symptoms besides decreased vision?
4. What was the vision in the affected eye(s) prior to injury? Was that with or without corrective lenses?
5. Does a history of prior eye disease, injury, or surgery exist?

With chemical injuries, it must be immediately ascertained whether the agent is an alkali, such as ammonium hydroxide (as in ammonia gas plus water vapor or fertilizers), sodium hydroxide (in drain cleaners, lye), potassium hydroxide (potash), calcium hydroxide (in lime, quicklime, mortar, cement, whitewash), or magnesium hydroxide (in sparklers, fireworks, flares).[6] If the causative agent may have been alkaline, treatment with copious irrigation should be begun immediately.

With foreign body or pellet injuries, the probable size, velocity, and chemical constituency of the pellet should be obtained. The toxicity and management of intraocular pellets vary significantly depending upon whether they are lead, steel, or copper.

TABLE 12–1 *Items That Should Be Part of the Ophthalmic Evaluation When Ocular Injury Is Suspected*

History
   Details of the traumatic event
   Any complicating conditions
      Diabetes
      Sickle cell
      Bleeding dyscrasias
   Drug allergies
   Medications, especially anticoagulants
Examination
   Visual acuity
   External inspection of lids and adnexa
   Pupillary light reflexes
   Ocular motility
   Visual fields by confrontation
   Penlight evaluation of the lids, globe, and anterior segment
   Tactile pressure (omit if ruptured globe is suspected)
   Fundus examination with direct ophthalmoscope

Hamil MB. Ophthalmologic complications. In: Mattox KL, ed. Complications of trauma. 1994; 601.

Physical Examination

VISUAL ACUITY TESTING

PITFALL ⊘

If visual acuity and visual fields are not checked during the initial physical examination, the diagnosis of important eye injuries may be delayed.

A check of visual acuity can usually determine how well the eyes and visual pathways are functioning and alert the examiner to the possible existence of less obvious injuries. When the patient has poor vision, even in otherwise normal-appearing eyes, one should suspect a significant injury and make sure that an emergency complete ophthalmic examination is performed.

Visual acuity should be tested in each eye independently, with the examiner making sure that the other eye is properly covered. With a Rosenbaum near-vision card, one can easily check visual acuity at the bedside or in the emergency department. A standard eye chart or near-vision card is preferable so that one can assign a numerical value to the patient's visual acuity; however, when not available, a newspaper, magazine, or even package label may be used.

AXIOM In checking near visual acuity in patients over 40 years of age, it is imperative that the patients wear their reading glasses if they normally use them.

As we age, the ability to accommodate (focus on close objects) is progressively lost and must be replaced by adding plus lenses (reading glasses). If a near-vision card is not available, some other notation of baseline visual acuity should be obtained (newsprint at 12 inches or a standard eye chart at 20 feet).

If the patient cannot even read large print, it is important to determine whether the patient can at least count fingers, see gross movements of the examiner's hands, or perceive light.[6] As long as the patient has any vision, there is some potential for successful repair of the eye, no matter how severely damaged it appears. Conversely, the patient with no light perception has little chance for recovery of vision, and enucleation may be justified as a primary procedure.

AXIOM Pain from a corneal abrasion or chemical injury may result in the vision being assessed as poorer than it really is.

Topical anesthesia (0.5% proparacaine) can relieve much of the pain and tearing than can occur with mild eye injuries and allow patients to keep their eyes open; however, use of any medication that may affect pupil size and reactions in patients with head injury should first be discussed with the physicians evaluating the patient's CNS status.

VISUAL FIELDS

In an alert, cooperative patient, visual fields can be easily determined. As with visual acuity testing, each eye is evaluated individually after covering one eye. The eye being tested fixates on the examiner's nose, and the patient is asked what part of the face is missing. Visual field defects and central scotomas may be detected in this manner. To detect hemianopsias and quadrantanopsias, the patient again is asked to stare at the examiner's nose while fingers are presented in the periphery. The patient is asked how many fingers are being presented while fixating on the examiner's nose.

AXIOM When the patient has normal visual acuity and visual fields, the chance of serious injury to the eye or visual pathways is unlikely. However, when subnormal results are obtained, a vigorous investigation is needed.

GLOBE, LID, AND ORBIT EXAMINATION

AXIOM It is extremely important to make an early diagnosis of ruptures or penetrating wounds of the eye.

During external examination of the globe, lids, and orbit, the primary question to be answered is, "Is the globe ruptured?" Clues to rupture of the globe include: (a) the presence of brown tissue (the iris or ciliary body) protruding through a laceration; (b) an obviously soft, shrunken eye; (c) a teardrop-shaped or eccentric pupil, or (d) sticky, clear material (vitreous) on the surface of the globe. Other evidence suggesting a ruptured or perforated globe include a large hyphema (blood in the anterior chamber) or a history of a high-velocity foreign body injury.

AXIOM Once it is discovered that an eye globe is ruptured, further examination is unnecessary, and the eye should be covered with a protective shield until it can be examined by an ophthalmologist in an appropriate environment.

If the eye is not obviously ruptured, further examination is necessary. Subconjunctival hemorrhages can be very dramatic, but by themselves are usually innocuous and of no functional concern.[6] The cornea should be clear and smooth in contour. Any irregularity of the corneal light reflex suggests the presence of an abrasion or corneal laceration.

When a lid laceration is present, one should determine whether the margin or the nasal aspect of the lid has been violated. With medial lacerations, involvement of the lacrimal drainage system is likely.

Although simple lid lacerations may be repaired by nonophthalmologists, those involving the lid margin or lacrimal system are best repaired by an ophthalmologist who is prepared to cannulate the lacrimal drainage system and deal with the problem of sutures passing through the posterior aspects of the lid and lid margin.

AXIOM Many orbital floor fractures can be diagnosed on the initial physical examination.

Orbital floor fractures can often be diagnosed by palpation of a step-off in the orbital margin. Orbital fractures should also be suspected when the patient has hypesthesia involving the cheek, upper lip, or forehead as a result of injury to the infraorbital or supraorbital nerves.[6]

OPHTHALMOSCOPY

Inability to visualize the fundus with ophthalmoscopy after trauma often denotes the presence of blood in the anterior chamber or vitreous.

PUPILS

The Marcus-Gunn pupil indicates an abnormality in afferent pupillary function and should be considered when unexplained vision loss

TABLE 12–2 *Cardinal Positions of Gaze Used to Test Extraocular Muscle Actions (Right Eye)*

Extraocular Muscle	Movement
Superior rectus	Up and laterally
Lateral rectus	Straight lateral
Inferior rectus	Down and laterally
Superior oblique	Down and medially
Medial rectus	Straight medial
Inferior oblique	Up and medially

occurs in one eye. To perform this test, the reaction of each pupil to light is observed. A bright light shining into the normal eye will cause both pupils to constrict; however, the same light shining into the abnormal eye will cause the pupils to dilate for a short period of time. Situations when this may be encountered following trauma include contusion of the optic nerve, retinal detachment, or vitreous hemorrhage.

OCULAR MOBILITY

Examination of ocular motility is useful for detecting cranial nerve palsies, particularly of the sixth nerve (Fig. 12–6) (Table 12–2). Difficulty in gazing upward may be noted in some patients with orbital floor fractures.

LID EVERSION

Eversion of the upper lid is often necessary to detect and remove conjunctival foreign bodies (Fig. 12–7).[6] Foreign bodies have a tendency to embed themselves in the conjunctiva on the inner surface of the upper lid. Then, as the eye blinks, these foreign bodies rub against the cornea causing areas of corneal abrasion. The eyelids may be everted using Desmarres' retractors, paper clips, or cotton applicator sticks.

FLUORESCEIN STAINING

AXIOM Superficial corneal injuries are diagnosed most readily by fluorescein staining.

Corneal abrasions may be invisible to the observer without the use of fluorescein which stains areas of the cornea that have been denuded of epithelium because of abrasions, chemical injury, or foreign body.[6] The tip of a fluorescein strip should be wet, preferably with a commercial irrigating solution, and then touched to the conjunctiva. By blinking, the patient disperses the fluorescein in the preocular tear film. Then, using a penlight with a blue filter or a Wood's light, the area of fluorescence corresponding to an abrasion can generally be seen quite easily.

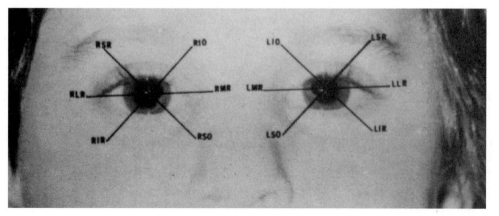

FIGURE 12–6 Cardinal positions of gaze: RSR, right superior rectus; RLR, right lateral rectus; RIR, right inferior rectus; RSO, right superior oblique; RMR, right medial rectus. RIO, right inferior oblique; LIO, left inferior oblique; LMR, left medial rectus ; LSO, left superior oblique; LIR left inferior rectus; LLR, left lateral rectus; LSR, left superior rectus. (From: Catalano RA. Ocular emergencies. Philadelphia: WB Saunders, 1992; 135.)

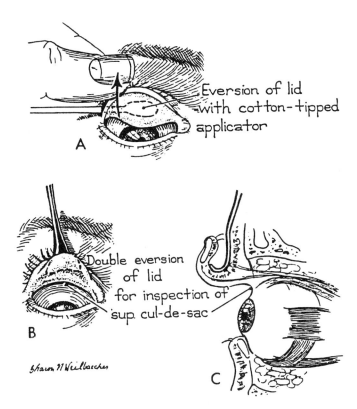

A Eversion of lid with cotton-tipped applicator

B Double eversion of lid for inspection of sup. cul-de-sac

Sharon M Weilbaecher

FIGURE 12–7 Techniques of single and double eversion of the upper lid. (From: Paton and Goldberg's management of ocular injuries. Deutsch TA, Feller DB, eds. Philadelphia: WB Saunders, 1985; 65.

RADIOGRAPHY

Any patient with severe blunt trauma to the mid face or a suspected penetrating eye injury should have a complete set of orbital radiographs, including a Water's view. These radiographs are useful for detection of orbital fractures and radiopaque intraorbital or intraocular foreign bodies. Orbital floor fractures are most easily visualized by using a Water's view. Sometimes the fracture itself cannot be visualized but can be strongly suspected because there is clouding of the maxillary sinus due to herniation of blood or tissue into it through the orbital floor defect. Metallic fragments and foreign bodies made of leaded glass can often be detected on plain anteroposterior (AP) and lateral orbital films.[6]

Precise localization of intraocular foreign bodies requires the use of CT and/or echographic (ultrasonographic) techniques. CT scans may also occasionally be used to diagnose a suspected orbital floor fracture not visualized on plain films. CT scans, however, are unreliable in detecting optic nerve injuries, posterior rupture of the globe, intraocular hemorrhage, or retinal detachment.[6]

One of the newest noninvasive diagnostic studies is MRI. Unfortunately, such testing requires the use of very high magnetic fields which is contraindicated in the patient who may have a metallic intraocular foreign body.[6] These strong magnetic fields, acting on the metallic foreign body could cause significant additional trauma if the foreign body were magnetically pulled through delicate intraocular tissues.

AXIOM MRI should not be used in any patient who may have a metallic foreign body in the eye.

ECHOGRAPHY

Echographic examination of the globe and orbit can be useful for detecting and localizing foreign bodies and for determining the gross anatomy of the eye. When the fundus cannot be visualized because of hemorrhage or cataract, B-scan echography is the only nonsurgical technique for determining whether vitreous or choroidal hemorrhage is present and whether the retina is detached.[6]

INITIAL MANAGEMENT

AXIOM Only three true ocular emergencies exist: chemical burns, orbital hypertension, and central retinal artery occlusions. In all three circumstances, appropriate therapy must be started within minutes.

The eyes or the adnexa may be injured in many ways; however, three conditions that truly require immediate care are chemical burns of the eye, orbital hypertension, and central retinal artery occlusion.

Chemical Burns

Chemical injuries to the eyes range from mild superficial irritation to severe, painful ocular destruction. The severity of the chemical injury depends on the nature of the agent (acid or alkali), its pH, the volume instilled, and the exposure time. Acid generally causes less damage than alkali, but both can rapidly cause blindness. As acid contacts the corneal epithelium, it coagulates the local protein, forming a barrier to further penetration. Additionally, the corneal stroma can buffer solutions with a pH < 4.0.

AXIOM Chemical burns of the eyes are best treated by early, copious irrigation.

The treatment of acid injuries must be immediate and on-site. Copious irrigation with any solution that is nontoxic to the eye must be started as soon as possible. If chemical particulate matter may be involved, the fornices must be inspected and cleaned out as necessary. Once the pH normalizes, topical antibiotics and cycloplegia may be started.

Alkali burns of the eyes are usually quite severe. Alkali rapidly penetrates through the entire cornea into the anterior chamber causing liquefaction necrosis of the cornea and sclera, eventually resulting in an opacified, scarred cornea. If the alkali were to penetrate into the anterior chamber, the pH would rise rapidly and cause coagulation of the aqueous humor and lens, resulting in glaucoma and cataract formation.

Ammonia, which is soluble in both lipids and water, can cause severe eye injuries. Sodium hydroxide (lye) is readily available in many household products (such as Drano® or Liquid Plummer®) and, therefore, is the most common cause of alkali injuries. Calcium hydroxide, which is found in plaster, cement, mortar, and whitewash, is usually less damaging.

AXIOM Treatment of alkali injuries is the same as for acid injuries and primarily involves immediate, copious irrigation with any solution that is nontoxic to the eye.

There is often severe pain with alkali eye injuries and topical anesthesia will facilitate irrigation. During the irrigation, the lids should be held open and the stream of irrigating fluid should be directed into the superior and inferior fornices so as to wash away any particulate matter that may be lodged there.[6] The lids may be held open with fingers, but better exposure can often be obtained with bent paperclips. Even when prolonged irrigation of the eyes occurred at the scene of the accident, additional irrigation should be performed in the emergency department. The fornices should also be cleaned with moistened swabs in order to remove any possible retained particulate matter. If after 30 minutes of irrigation, the pH in the cul-de-sac normalizes, it is safe to discontinue irrigation.

Topical antibiotics and cycloplegia are started once the pH normalizes. Elevated intraocular pressures are reduced with topical beta-blockers or carbonic anhydrase inhibitors as needed. Most patients who have had severe alkali eye injuries eventually require surgery.

The goal is a clear cornea with an intact epithelium, but this outcome is not possible for most of these patients.

With a chemical injury to the eyes, an ophthalmologist should be called immediately, unless the injury is clearly the result of a nonalkali innocuous compound and the damage sustained is no worse than a mild corneal abrasion. When the injury is minor, about 2,000 ml of irrigant will suffice, and the injury can then be managed as a corneal abrasion.[6]

> **AXIOM** The key to treatment of caustic eye injuries is prevention. This is best done with public education about the dangers of commercially available alkalies and the need to wear safety glasses when dealing with such agents.

Orbital Hypertension

Bleeding within the orbit or swelling of retrobulbar tissues can occasionally raise the pressure within the orbit to over 20-30 mm Hg. At such pressure, blood flow to the optic nerve and/or posterior eye may be so impaired that blindness can result. When orbital hypertension is suspected because of evidence of local trauma, severe proptosis, eye pain, and/or decreasing vision, a lateral canthotomy may be required on an emergency basis (Fig. 12–8).

Central Retinal Artery Occlusion

Central retinal artery occlusion (CRAO), although not generally traumatic in origin, is a condition that should be dealt with on an emergent basis.[6] It can result from a severe orbital hematoma, inflammatory eye disease, or emboli from a calcified aortic valve or ulcerated carotid artery. Sudden interruption of blood flow to the inner retina can cause an immediate, severe, unilateral loss of vision so that often only light perception remains. On funduscopic examination, sluggish blood flow may be noted in thready, retinal arterioles as well as a peculiar pale waxy color to the retina with a "cherry-red spot" in the area of the macula. The goal of therapy is to restore blood flow to the retina as soon as possible so as to minimize the extent of retinal necrosis.

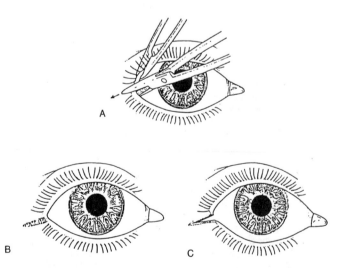

FIGURE 12–8 The technique of lateral canthotomy. The lateral canthus, after being anesthetized with lidocaine, is grasped with toothed forceps and a hemostat is angled laterally and slight inferiorly, with the lateral lower eyelid margin contained within the jaws. **A&B.** The hemostat is advanced with open jaws into the fornix, and then closed, crushing the tissue. **C.** Scissors are then introduced along the same path and the lateral canthal tendon is divided. If additonal relaxation is required, the inferior crus to the lateral canthan tendon can be completely separated. (From: Hamil MB. Ophthalmologic complications. Mattox KL, ed. Complications of trauma. 1994; 606.

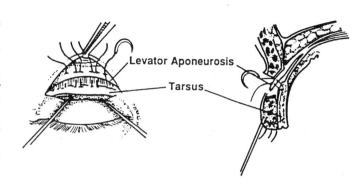

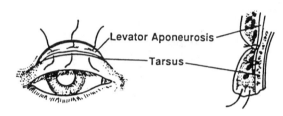

FIGURE 12–9 Technique to repair a disrupted levator aponeurosis. (From: Catalano RA. Ocular emergencies pg 126.)

> **AXIOM** Any patient with a history of painless, sudden loss of vision should be presumed to have CRAO and should be transported immediately to an emergency center for definitive therapy.

Initial management of CRAO includes control of intraocular pressure and attempts to vasodilate the retinal vessels with: (a) osmotic diuretics, such as mannitol, 1 g/kg, (b) acetazolamide, 500 mg IV or IM, (c) 5% CO_2 inhalation or rebreathing into a paper bag, (d) massage of the eye (30 seconds of moderate pressure, 15 seconds off, and repeat cycle four times) and (e) paracentesis of the anterior chamber by an ophthalmologist.

Eyelid Lacerations

DIAGNOSIS

> **AXIOM** Any trauma that has injured an eyelid is also likely to have injured the eye.

Subtle injuries to the eye may be overlooked in patients with eyelid lacerations when the eye is not systematically and completely examined. Complete knowledge of the anatomy of the eyelids is mandatory for proper diagnosis and repair. In complicated upper eyelid lacerations, a thorough search for detachment or laceration of the levator muscle should be conducted in the pretreatment evaluation (Fig. 12–9). When the levator muscle is lacerated but not repaired, the patient is generally left with profound ptosis.

ANESTHESIA

> **AXIOM** All but the simplest eyelid lacerations should be repaired in the operating room in a well-illuminated, controlled, pain-free environment.

Local or regional anesthesia is an alternative to general anesthesia during surgical management of closed-eye injuries and injuries to the ocular adnexae.[2] However, children and uncooperative adults rarely tolerate surgery while conscious, and local or regional anesthesia may not provide optimal operative conditions in all patients. The three important requirements for successful eye surgery under local or regional anesthesia include: adequate sedation; complete anesthesia; and an immobile eye.

The eyelids are supplied by the supraorbital, infraorbital, supratrochlear, infratrochlear, and lacrimal branches of the trigeminal nerve (Fig. 12–10).[19] Although blocking these nerves individually can produce satisfactory analgesia, infiltration of local anesthetic agents through the lacerated wound edges can be equally effective. When this approach is used, the anesthetic should be injected into the neurovascular plane of the eyelid which lays between the tarsal plate and the orbicularis oculi muscle (Fig. 12–11).[2] Topical anesthesia or a retrobulbar block is usually needed to manipulate the conjunctiva during repair of lid lacerations. Local anesthesia for the lids can be provided by injection of a few milliliters of lidocaine (1-1.5%) or bupivacaine (0.5%) with or without epinephrine (1/200,000). Topical anesthesia of the cornea and conjunctiva can be provided by two to three drops of tetracaine (1%). This treatment also allows for the measurement of the IOP and removal of foreign bodies lodged on the eye surface.

REPAIR

A crucial part of eyelid repair is the meticulous reapproximation of lacerated eyelid margins and tarsal plates. Failure to reapproximate the lacerated borders accurately may result in lid notching, which can lead to severe eye damage over time. Eyelid margins can be repaired with 6-0 sutures reapproximating first the Meibomian gland orifices, then the anterior lash line, and finally the gray line (Fig. 12–12). Several 5-0 absorbable sutures can be used to repair the torn tarsus, taking care not to enter the posterior boundary of the lid. If the suture were to enter the posterior boundary of the lid, one might accidentally include the conjunctiva in the repair; this could cause corneal irritation and abrasion. Improper placement of sutures can also cause a malignment of eyelid structures and impair their function.

AXIOM   Any time a lid laceration involves the eyelid margin or the medial canthal area, a canalicular laceration should be suspected (Fig. 12–13).

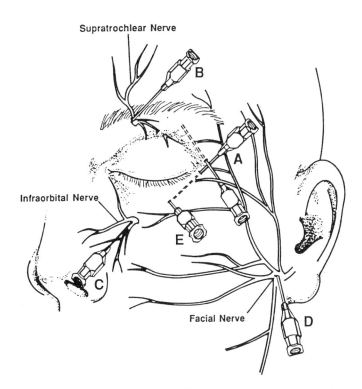

FIGURE 12–10   Regional anesthetic blocks **A.** van Lint, **B.** supraorbital, **C.** infraorbital, **D.** O'Brien, **E.** retrobulbar. (From: Catalano RA. Ocular emergencies Philadelphia: WB Saunders, 1992; pg 116.)

Supratrochlear Nerve

B

A

Infraorbital Nerve

E

C

Facial Nerve

D

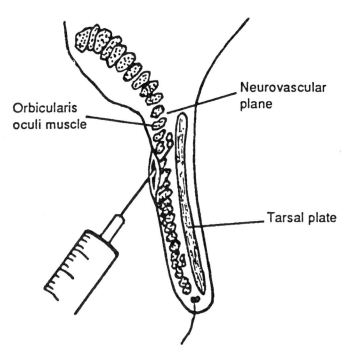

Orbicularis oculi muscle

Neurovascular plane

Tarsal plate

FIGURE 12–11   Sagittal section of the eyelid showing orbicularis oculi muscle anteriorly, tarsal plate posteriorly, and neurovascular plane in the middle. Satisfactory analgesia can be obtained by injection of local anesthetic agent within the neurovascular plane. (From: Capan LM, Mankikar D, Eisenberg WM. Anesthetic management of ocular injuries. In Trauma: anesthesia and intensive care. Capan LM, Miller SM, Turndorf H, eds. Philadelphia: JB Lippincott, 1991; 372.

When either an upper or lower eyelid has been lacerated, thorough examination of the extent of the laceration should be performed to determine the integrity of the lacrimal drainage system. A canaliculus should be probed and irrigated with a fluorescein solution when there is any possiblity that it has been injured.

AXIOM   If a laceration involving a canaliculus of the eye is not repaired properly, persistent tearing can result.

Upper and lower canalicular lacerations must be repaired because both play such important roles in the drainage of tears (Fig. 12–14). Repair consists of identification and isolation of the severed proximal and distal canalicular ends, intubation with silastic tubing, and microsurgical anastomosis of the severed ends, followed by accurate repair of the lid.

AXIOM   A delay of 12-24 hours, until optimum patient and operative conditions can be obtained, will not compromise the outcome of most eyelid lacerations.[20]

Repair of eyelid lacerations can be postponed for up to 12-24 hours until appropriate anesthesia, suitable operating room conditions, and experienced staff are available. Complicated lid lacerations are best referred to an oculoplastic surgeon for primary repair. Proper initial repair can save a patient from multiple secondary or tertiary procedures which seldom are as successful.

Corneal Abrasions

Probably the most frequent ocular problem seen in the emergency room is corneal abrasion. When the corneal epithelium is injured and the corneal nerves are exposed, the resultant pain can be quite severe. Patients with corneal abrasions often present with a red eye, severe pain, tearing, and photophobia. If the corneal abrasion is not obvious, the instillation of a topical anesthetic will bring immediate relief of pain. After the symptoms are relieved, a drop of sterile fluorescein should be instilled in the eye. With fluorescein staining,

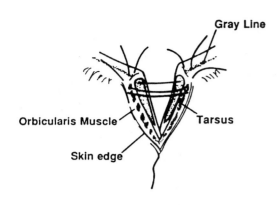

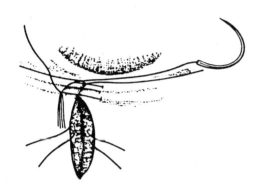

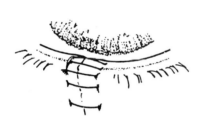

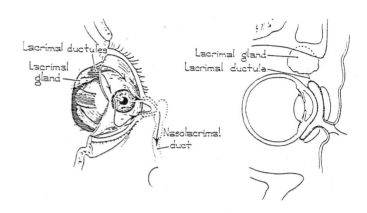

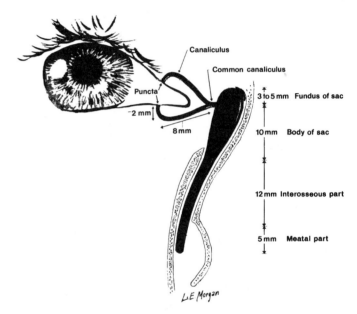

FIGURE 12–12 Three-suture technique to repair eyelid margin laceration with minimal loss of tissue. (From: Catalano RA. Ocular emergencies. Philadelphia: WB Saunders, 1992; 118.)

FIGURE 12–13 Lacrimal apparatus. (From: Putterman AM. Basic oculoplastic surgery. Peyman GA, Sanders D, Goldberg MF, eds. Principles and practice of ophthalmology. Philadelphia: WB Saunders Co, 1980; 2273).

denuded corneal epithelium appears green under white light and fluoresces as bright green under cobalt-blue light. Normal cornea with intact epithelium does not stain.

When the pattern of the defect in the corneal epithelium is multiple vertical streaks, one should search for an upper lid foreign body by everting the upper lid. This is best accomplished by having the patient look down. The examiner then grasps the margin of the upper lid, and pulls it down. A cotton swab is then placed above the tarsus (the firm portion of the upper lid), and the lid is folded up over it.

Corneal abrasions caused by vegetable matter may require intensive treatment to prevent or treat fungal keratitis, but corneal abrasions caused by clean objects, such as a sheet of paper, may require only an eye patch and observation. Thus, obtaining a careful history can be very important because it can often help the examiner obtain an early diagnosis and provide prompt, appropriate treatment.

Treatment of corneal abrasions is best achieved by instilling an antibiotic ointment (e.g., gentamicin) in the eye and applying a pressure patch to prevent the patient from opening the eye. This relieves pain and helps to prevent infection. In addition, the patch immobilizes the eyelids, thereby allowing uninterrupted ingrowth of corneal epithelium.

To place a pressure patch on the eye, two eye pads are placed across the patient's closed lids.[6] The patches are then taped in place

firmly with multiple strips of adhesive paper or plastic tape. Prior to the patching, the examiner should instill a topical cycloplegic agent, either ¼% scopolamine or 1% cyclopentolate, in the affected eye. This will partially relieve patient discomfort.

AXIOM Under no circumstances should a patient with a corneal abrasion be given a bottle of topical anesthetic.

When patients feel no pain, they will not rest their eyes properly so that the cornea can heal. Uncomplicated corneal epithelial defects often heal within 24-48 hours, depending on the size of the defect. The eye should be examined daily by a physician until the abrasion has resolved.

PITFALL ⊘

Steroids should never be used in the presence of a corneal epithelial defect because they can rapidly make undetected herpes simplex or bacterial keratitis much worse.

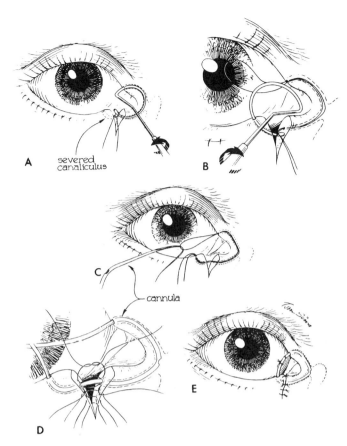

FIGURE 12–14 Worst's method of identifying and repairing a severed canaliculus. (From: Paton and Goldberg's management of ocular injuries. Deutsch TA, Feller DB, eds. Philadelphia: WB Saunders, 1985; 35.)

Corneal Ulcers

If, during the course of treatment of a corneal abrasion, the underlying or surrounding cornea were to develop an infiltrate (which makes it hazy), an early corneal ulcer would have to be assumed. An immediate ophthalmic consult must be obtained and the patient admitted to the hospital. Treatment of corneal ulcers includes scraping the ulcer for Gram stain and culture, cycloplegia, and appropriate topical antibiotic drops hourly around the clock. Occasionally, subconjunctival injection of antibiotics will also be necessary.

Corneal Foreign Bodies

The majority of corneal foreign bodies are superficially embedded, and although they can cause severe pain, they are, in themselves, usually not serious injuries.[6] Following careful examination of the eye to eliminate a penetrating injury, the examiner may attempt removal of the foreign body. A moistened cotton swab can be gently rolled across the cornea in an attempt to loosen and remove the foreign body. If this attempt were unsuccessful, ophthalmologic consultation should be obtained. Some foreign bodies must be removed using a slit lamp and a needle, spud, or high-speed burr. Following removal of the foreign body, the eye should be treated as if a corneal abrasion were present.

Corneal Lacerations

Corneal lacerations may range from small, subtle, self-sealing lacerations to large gashes with prolapse of intraocular contents. Because the cornea contains 70% of the eye's refractive power, an injury to the cornea may have profound effects on vision; however, with small, self-sealing corneal lacerations, normal vision and appearance are usually retained.

AXIOM The optimal treatment of full-thickness corneal lacerations is expeditious surgical repair to restore the eye's integrity and to prevent intraocular infection and complications.

Because corneal lacerations heal with scar formation, vision may be compromised, even after rapid repair of a minimal corneal laceration. If the scar is centered in the visual axis, vision will suffer to some degree. Visually significant corneal scarring is minimized by meticulous microsurgical repair of corneal lacerations with careful attention given to the placement of the sutures.

Penetrating Ocular Injury or Ruptured Globe

GENERAL MANAGEMENT

Prolapse of intraocular contents may occur in any ruptured globe, and for this reason, any eye suspected of having a laceration or perforation should be shielded during transportation. If an instrument, such as a knife or wire is still impaled in the eye or orbit, it should not be removed.

PITFALL ⊘

As soon as it is discovered, a ruptured globe should be protected from further damage by a metal shield until it is formally repaired.

As soon as the diagnosis of an open eye wound is made, broad spectrum intravenous antibiotics are begun. High-dose intravenous Ancef and gentamicin can be started with adjustments made later as needed according to the clinical progress and culture results. The antibiotics are initially given intravenously to achieve high bacteriocidal levels in the eyes. These are continued for only 48-72 hours if no growth is evident on intraoperative culture of the wound. Oral antibiotics will not generally achieve high enough blood levels. When there is concern regarding vegetable-matter contamination of the eye, antibiotics, such as clindamycin, which are active against Bacillus species, are added to provide broad-spectrum coverage.

Tetanus prophylaxis is administered to all patients with an open eye wound or eyelid lacerations. A preoperative CT scan of the orbits aids in eliminating retained intraocular foreign bodies and in delineating any unsuspected concomitant intracranial injuries (Fig. 12–15). The metallic eye shield does not interfere with high-resolution CT.

A culture of the wound is always obtained at the time of the repair. Prior to the repair, magnetic intraocular foreign bodies, if present, may be removed with a giant magnet. Some magnetic fragments and all nonmagnetic fragments are removed from the posterior segment of the eye utilizing vitrectomy and vitreous microsurgery. Primary enucleation should be avoided in the present medicolegal environment.

Surgical repair of an eye that is ruptured or has a full-thickness penetration is performed under general anesthesia. Closure of the sclera is usually accomplished with 8-0 nonabsorbable material, such as silk, and corneal lacerations are generally closed with 10-0 nylon sutures.

TIMING OF EYE SURGERY

Although an open eye should be considered an emergency and should generally be repaired within the first 24 hours, there is little difference in the eventual visual outcome in eyes immediately repaired versus those whose repair is delayed by 24-36 hours. Untrained operating room personnel, inadequate anesthesia, a tired surgeon, and unavailable surgical equipment all serve to make a repair suboptimal. Delaying the repair until appropriate conditions become available is usually advisable.

PITFALL ⊘

A ruptured globe should not be repaired immediately when the circumstances for repair are unfavorable.

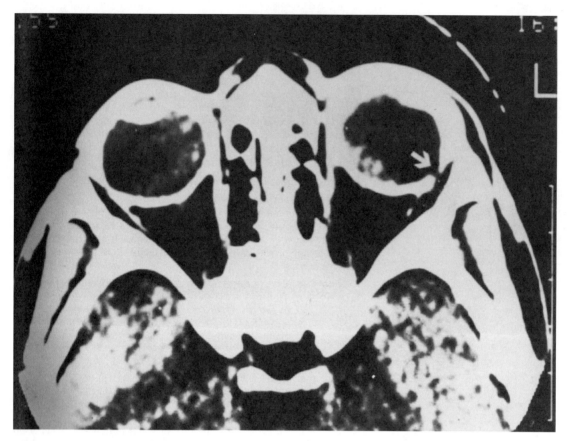

FIGURE 12–15 CT of a patient with posterior segment perforation of the eye (arrow) (From: Capan LM, Mankikar D, Eisenberg WM. Anesthetic management of ocular injuries. In Trauma: anesthesia and intensive care. Capan LM, Miller SM, Turndorf H, eds. Philadelphia: JB Lippincott, 1991; 372.)

Most penetrating ocular injuries are complicated by some degree of intraocular injury, such as lens damage, vitreous hemorrhage, vitreous loss, retinal incarceration in the wound, retinal detachment, or significant choroidal hemorrhage.[5] Many ocular trauma surgeons believe that these cases are managed more effectively by primary wound closure and delayed definitive management rather than by a single, comprehensive surgical procedure.

Delaying definitive intraocular repairs for 5-10 days allows for a decrease in orbital congestion and periocular tissue swelling, partial if not complete resolution of choroidal hemorrhage, and spontaneous separation of the vitreous from the underlying retina. This also allows a more complete preoperative evaluation, including echography. The delayed second operation generally includes removal of the vitreous and its hemorrhage and may also involve removal of the lens and inflammatory membranes, scleral buckling, cryotherapy, and/or laser photocoagulation. Following closure of the globe, the intraocular fluid may be replaced with an expansible gas to tamponade the retina.

Delayed surgical intervention on the eye should be coordinated with other facial procedures, such as repair of fractures that will require placement of external hardware.[6] Such hardware may render introduction of microinstruments into the eye physically impossible. Additionally, when the eye is filled with gas, it may be necessary to keep the patient in a prone position for several days.

Hyphema

Hyphemas (Fig. 12–16) (blood in the anterior chamber) usually result from contusive injuries to the eye that traumatize the vasculature of the iris.[32] Because normal vision depends on a clear path from the cornea to the macula, a large hyphema can interfere with vision. Conversely, small hyphemas may go unnoticed by both the patient and the examiner.

The initial collection of blood in the anterior chamber usually resolves spontaneously without complications; however, in 9-32% rebleeding will occur, usually between the second and fifth day.[21-24] When permanent visual loss is secondary to hyphema, it is almost always due to rebleeding which causes corneal staining or hemorrhagic glaucoma with subsequent optic atrophy. Because of this, the

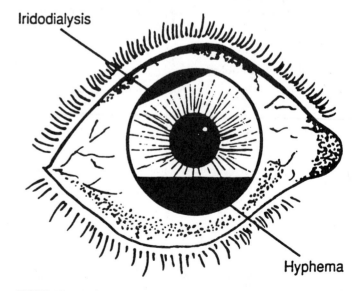

FIGURE 12–16 Blood in the anterior chamber (hyphema) obscures the distal part of the iris. The lesion seen on the upper portion of the iris is caused by iridodialysis. (From: Capan LM, Mankikar D, Eisenberg WM. Anesthetic management of ocular injuries. In Trauma: anesthesia and intensive care. Capan LM, Miller SM, Turndorf H, eds. Philadelphia: JB Lippincott, 1991; 372.)

treatment of traumatic hyphema, although extremely controversial, has two basic principles: prevent rebleeds and control intraocular pressure.

> **AXIOM** All patients with hyphemas, regardless of how small, are admitted and placed on strict bed rest with sedation to prevent anterior chamber hypertension and rebleeding.

Daily ophthalmic evaluations are performed on patients with traumatic hyphema with specific attention to intraocular pressure and the condition of the corneal endothelium. It is important to control intraocular pressure in these patients using osmotic agents, carbonic anhydrase inhibitors, and/or topical beta blockers.[5] Carbonic anhydrase inhibitors, however, should not be used in patients with sickle cell anemia because this agent slows the clearance of sickled red cells from the anterior chamber.

> **AXIOM** All black patients with hyphemas should be checked for the presence of sickle hemoglobin.

Blood staining of the cornea may occur in patients with hyphema, especially those with elevation of intraocular pressure.[5] This is a particularly disastrous complication in small children. Blood staining may render the cornea opaque for many months, leading to a sensory-deprivation amblyopia.

> **AXIOM** When early corneal blood staining or persistently elevated intraocular pressure occurs due to hyphema, blood should be removed surgically from the anterior chamber.

Other frequently employed regimens for the initial management of hyphemas include bilateral patching, prolonged cycloplegia (to reduce the possibility of synechia formation), bed rest, topical steroids, and systemic antifibrinolytic agents, such as epsilon aminocaproic acid (Amicar). Such therapy is continued until the hyphema has totally resorbed and the risk of rebleeding has passed.

> **PITFALL** ⊘
>
> *Aspirin and nonsteroidal antiinflammatory drugs are avoided in patients with hyphema because they increase the risk of rebleeding.*

Rebleeding recurs in approximately 10-30% of hyphema patients, generally within the first five days.[25] Many medical regimens have been advocated to minimize the risk of rebleeding,[21-27] but only Amicar (epsilon aminocaproic acid), an antifibroinolytic agent, has proved effective in randomized, double-blind trials;[23,26,28] however, the systemic side effects of epsilon aminacaproic acid, such as hypotension, dizziness, nausea, and vomiting have limited its widespread use.

> **AXIOM** When hyphema is present, it is important to eliminate injury to other portions of the eye and to the optic nerve.

Common injuries associated with hyphema include traumatic cataract, subluxed lens, choroidal tears, retinal detachment, and macular holes.

Intraocular Injuries

LENS

Severe contusive or penetrating trauma to the eye can cause the lens to opacify, forming a traumatic cataract. Violation of the lens capsule causes the lens fibers to imbibe aqueous humor, lose their clarity, and opacify. A traumatic cataract that is visually significant obscures the fundus and is usually easy to detect with a penlight examination or with an ophthalmoscope. Definitive treatment involves the removal of the cataract and subsequent visual rehabilitation with an intraocular or contact lens.

> **AXIOM** A traumatic cataract in a child with a vague or inconsistent history of trauma should alert the examiner to the possibility of child abuse, and the appropriate agencies should be notified.

VITREOUS

Vitreous hemorrhages are commonly seen in penetrating or severe contusive eye injuries. Normally, the vitreous is a clear hydrogel that permits the uninterrupted passage of light from the posterior aspect of the lens to the macula. Any collection of blood in the vitreous will decrease visual acuity and limit retinal evaluation.

Because retinal detachments and holes frequently are associated with vitreous hemorrhages, nonvisual means of detection are needed. Ocular ultrasonography is a valuable adjunct and allows for "visualization" of the posterior segment through opaque media. The treatment of unresorbing blood from the vitreous cavity is the surgical removal of the blood and the associated vitreous. If a retinal detachment were also present, it could be repaired at the same time.

RETINA

Retinal detachments may be caused by penetrating or contusive eye injuries and need to be detected and repaired surgically as soon as possible. These patients will usually complain of flashing lights and "floaters" or loss of visual field as the retina detaches, but they may remain asymptomatic until the macula detaches, at which time visual acuity is severely diminished.

> **PITFALL** ⊘
>
> *All patients with ocular or periocular trauma need complete fundus examinations, including visualization of the retinal periphery with indirect ophthalmoscopy to detect retinal holes, tears, or detachments.*

Macular edema and hemorrhage are common after contusive injuries. The main symptom is decreased vision, and the cause is usually readily evident on funduscopy. Fortunately, visual acuity usually improves with resolution of macular edema and hemorrhage. Macular holes, which may also be associated with contusive eye injuries, cause a permanent visual deficit and are easily detected on fundus examination.

Optic Nerve Damage

Damage to the optic nerve may occur anywhere along its course from the back of the eye to the optic chiasm; however, the optic canal where the nerve is tightly enclosed by bone and dura is where injury most commonly occurs. Visual loss may occur after blunt trauma because of optic nerve avulsion or infarction, or by compression by a nerve sheath hematoma, edema, or bone fragments.

The history is vital in diagnosing the nature of the optic nerve injury and subsequent treatment. If the patient noticed immediate total loss of vision at injury, it is likely that the patient has optic nerve avulsion or infarction for which there is no successful therapy. Conversely, a history of slowly progressive visual loss after blunt craniofacial trauma suggests the presence of increasing compression of the optic nerve, and prompt neuroradiologic evaluation is mandatory to eliminate optic canal fracture.

> **AXIOM** Gradual loss of vision following blunt eye or face trauma requires emergency evaluation and treatment to save as much vision as possible.

When neuroradiologic evaluation with CT scans demonstrates fractures in the optic canal, visual loss may be due to compression of the optic nerve, and transcranial or transethmoidal decompression of the optic canal may provide dramatic restoration of vision.

Traumatic optic neuropathy may also occur after blunt orbital trauma. This entity may be detected and quantified by serial examinations of the pupils for the presence of an afferent pupillary defect. When a bright light is shined into the normal eye, both pupils constrict, the ipsilateral pupil directly and the contralateral pupil consensually. When the light is directed at the eye with the optic nerve injury, the midbrain detects less light because the optic nerve (afferent fibers) is damaged, and consequently both pupils dilate.

When blunt orbital or cranial trauma causes vision loss in the presence of an afferent pupillary defect, traumatic optic neuropathy exists. Treatment includes megadoses of intravenous corticosteroids given as a 30 mg/kg loading dose of methylprednisolone sodium succinate (Solu-medrol) followed two hours later by 15 mg/kg and then 15 mg/kg every six hours.[31] If visual acuity improves, the steroids should be continued as long as vision is improving for up to 72 hours. In the unconscious patient, grading of the afferent pupillary defect is the only indicator of progression. Although the prognosis for regaining useful vision is guarded, excellent results have been reported.[29-30,32]

ORBITAL FRACTURES

The orbital contents are protected by a thick, bony ring consisting of the supraorbital ridge, the glabella, and the infraorbital and lateral orbital rims (Fig. 12–17). The bones of the medial wall, floor, and roof are almost eggshell thin. Orbital fractures are often associated with other facial fractures. Zygomatic fractures with orbital floor components outnumber isolated orbital floor fractures nearly 10 to 1.[33] In addition, associated injuries to the orbital contents are common, and an ophthalmology consult should be obtained.

AXIOM   Over 60 percent of patients suffering mid-face fractures have injuries to the eyes that should be evaluated by an ophthalmologist.[27]

The initial evaluation of anyone with a possible eye or orbital injury should include visual acuity and any field defects, the presence or absence of an afferent pupillary defect, associated ocular

or adnexal injuries, and any extraocular muscle motility disturbances. Restriction of gaze can usually be explained by the location of the fracture. A patient with a posterior orbital floor fracture may be hypertropic with restricted downward gaze. A patient with an anterior floor fracture may be hypotropic with an upward gaze restriction.

AXIOM   CT is the best method for evaluating the extent of orbital fractures (Fig. 12–18).

Any question of orbital fracture on plain facial radiography requires complete evaluation by CT. The evaluation of orbital floor and medial wall fractures is incomplete without high-resolution CT scanning of the orbits. Orbital fractures can usually be localized well by axial views, but additional helpful information can often be obtained with the aid of oblique and coronal reconstructions. These can help to evaluate the size and extent of any orbital fractures and any involvement of the inferior rectus muscle or the optic nerve. The anterior versus posterior location of the fracture can also be determined by coronal reconstructive views. In patients with decreased visual acuity and the presence of an afferent pupillary defect which may indicate a traumatic optic neuropathy, CT may show extension of the orbital fracture to the orbital apex or optic canal.

With mid-facial fractures, extensive orbital involvement may occur, sometimes with concomitant intracranial and intraocular injuries. Nasolacrimal duct obstruction is not uncommon after midface injuries. If silastic tube stenting of the nasolacrimal drainage system were not performed during the primary repair of these fractures, dacryocystorhinostomy often would be necessary at a later date. Extension of facial fractures to the orbital apex and optic canal should be sought and their presence or absence documented.

PITFALL ⊘

With fractures extending into the orbital apex or orbital canal, orbital surgery may cause traumatic optic neuropathy with marked loss of vision; the patient and family should be notified of this risk preoperatively.

BLOW-OUT FRACTURES

The treatment of blow-out fractures of the orbit is controversial.[29] Many different specialists treat this type of injury, and each has a different set of criteria for its repair. Nevertheless, because the incidence of associated eye injuries is so high, all patients with facial fractures should have thorough eye examinations. When any question of ocular or orbital eye involvement exists, an ophthalmologist should be consulted.

Most authorities believe that significant residual diplopia, entrapment of orbital contents, or large fractures with significant enophthalmos are indications for surgical repair of orbital fractures. Repair of orbital floor fractures is often delayed 7-14 days, so that orbital swelling and hemorrhage can subside. Surgical repair of the orbit should also be delayed until hyphema or other ocular injuries (e.g., ruptured globe) have resolved or have been repaired. Prior to repair of the orbit, visual acuity should again be documented and concomitant medial wall fracture with extension into the medial orbital apex should be evaluated.

PITFALL ⊘

The presence of a medial wall orbital fracture extending to the orbital apex greatly increases the risk of optic nerve injury and blindness with any surgical manipulation of other portions of the orbit.

Impairment of eye motion is generally an indication for surgical correction of a blow-out orbital fracture. If the vision of the other

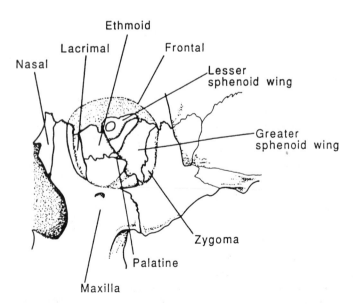

FIGURE 12–17   The roof of the orbit includes the orbital plate of the frontal bone anteriorly and the lesser wing of the sphenoid bone posteriorly. The medial bones of the orbit include the frontal process of the maxillary bone and lacrimal bone anteriorly and the orbital plate of the ethmoid bone. The inferior bones of the orbit include the orbital place of the maxillary bone anteriorly, the palatine bone posteriorly and the zygoma laterally. The bones of the lateral orbit include the zygoma and zygomatic process of the frontal bone anteriorly and the greater wing of the sphenoid bone posteriorly. (From: Catalano RA. Ocular emergencies. Philadelphia: WB Saunders, 1992; 132.)

FIGURE 12–18 Orbital floor fracture with entrapment of orbital contents (fat, inferior rectus muscle, and inferior oblique muscle) in the maxillary sinus (arrow). The patient had diplopia due to limitation of ocular movement. (From: Capan LM, Mankikar D, Eisenberg WM. Anesthetic management of ocular injuries. In Trauma: anesthesia and intensive care. Capan LM, Miller SM, Turndorf H, eds. Philadelphia: JB Lippincott, 1991; 360.

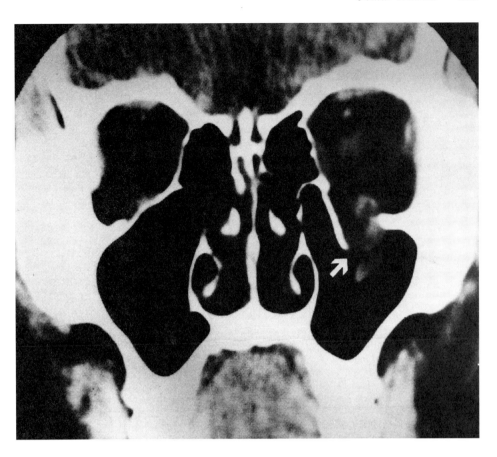

eye has been lost, however, indications for surgery on the orbit of remaining sighted eye must be considered very carefully.

PITFALL ⊘

> *Surgical repair of a blow-out fracture may be contraindicated if it is on the side of the only eye with vision.*

MEDIAL WALL FRACTURES

Blunt trauma can cause a fracture of the medial orbital wall while leaving the rims intact.[35-36] The medial wall (lamina papyracea) is the thinnest portion of the orbit and is easily fractured. These fractures are easily missed, and CT scans may show only a subtle step-off of medial wall bone or blood in the ethmoid sinus. These fractures are particularly easy to miss when the patient is asymptomatic, which is not unusual. The presence of orbital emphysema on radiography or CT should make one suspicious of a medial wall fracture.

Surgical repair of medial wall orbital fractures is needed only rarely and then only when medial rectus entrapment or damage to the nasolacrimal duct or lacrimal sac occurs. If primary placement of silastic tubes were not accomplished and/or repair of the lacrimal system were unsuccessful, dacryocysto-rhinostomy often would be necessary at a later date to relieve symptomatic epiphora (tearing).

ASSOCIATED ZYGOMATIC FRACTURES

Simple fractures of the zygoma are easily missed by the triage physician. A slight flattening of the malar eminence on the involved side may be the only indication; however, the patient may complain of difficulty opening the mouth or chewing. Trimalar (tripod) fractures involve the lateral and inferior orbital rim, the zygomatico-maxillary junction, and the arch of the zygoma. Associated orbital rim fractures

can usually be detected by palpating a step-off at the site of injury. Medial orbital floor fractures often accompany tripod fractures but may only be detected on CT.

ORBITAL ROOF FRACTURES

Orbital roof fractures can involve the frontal sinus and anterior cranial fossa and can be associated with significant intracranial injury. Cerebrospinal fluid leaks and carotid cavernous fistulas can occur when the fracture extends along the base of the skull. Ptosis with upward gaze palsy can occur secondary to injuries to the superior division of the oculomotor nerve.

PITFALL ⊘

> *When critically ill or injured patients cannot completely close their eyes, exposure problems of the eyes are common.*

When patients cannot close their eyes, exposure damage to the cornea can occur despite intensive medical and nursing care. An exposed cornea can dry out quickly, breaking down the corneal epithelial barrier and leaving it susceptible to infection, severe scarring, and loss of vision.

AXIOM Taping the eyelids shut, placing plastic wrap over the orbital areas in unconscious patients, and instilling eye ointment (lacri-lube) can help to prevent the eyes from drying and developing corneal ulcers.

Organisms colonizing the upper airway or local wound sites are the most common causes of corneal infections. Because these are most commonly Gram-negative bacilli that are often resistant to conventional antibiotics, the corneal ulcers they produce can be difficult to treat.

OUTCOME

Visual outcome following ocular trauma is difficult to predict because of the noncomparability of various published series, differences in case recruitment, and differing modes of therapy. Nevertheless, visual loss is exceedingly rare in corneal abrasions and is uncommon with nonalkali chemical burns. With severe alkali burns of the eyes, only approximately 50% will have any visual improvement with treatment.[15] Of the patients with facial fractures and associated eye injuries, 18% will sustain significant visual loss.[33] Less than 50% of eyes with severe contusion injuries will regain reading vision better than or equal to 20/40.[37,38] With hyphemas, 8% of patients have lost vision to a level of legal blindness, and only 60% have retained vision of 20/30 or better.[25] With penetrating ocular injuries, 50-75% of eyes will only achieve vision of 5/200 or better.[10,11] In fact, nearly all eyes with BB or pellet injuries lose a significant amount of functional vision.[39]

⊘ FREQUENT ERRORS

In the Management of Eye Tramua

1. *Failing to promptly check visual activity and visual fields in patients with possible eye trauma.*
2. *Failing to check visual acuity with the patient wearing glasses.*
3. *Failure to promptly and adequately irrigate the eyes after possible chemical injury.*
4. *Failure to promptly consult an ophthalmologist when the patient has a potentially serious eye injury.*
5. *Missing corneal lesions because of failure to use fluorescein staining.*
6. *Failure to completely examine the globe in patients with penetrating eyelid injuries.*
7. *Failure to completely examine the lacrimal apparatus after medial eyelid injury.*
8. *Improper closure of lacerations involving the free margin of the eyelids.*
9. *Using corticosteroids on a corneal lesion that may be due to a viral or bacterial infection.*
10. *Failing to promptly and adequately protect a ruptured or lacerated eye globe.*
11. *Failure to admit and aggressively treat patients with a "minor" hyphema.*
12. *Using agents, such as ASA or other NSAID, that impair bleeding and/or clotting in patients with intraocular injuries.*
13. *Failure to carefully evaluate the eyes in patients with midface fractures, especially when a "tripod" fracture is present.*
14. *Failure to promptly use CT to further evaluate the orbit in patients with suspected but unproved fractures on plain radiography.*
15. *Failure to adequately protect the corneas when the eyelids cannot cover them properly.*

▼▼▼▼▼▼▼▼▼▼▼▼▼▼▼▼▼▼▼▼▼▼▼▼▼▼▼▼▼

SUMMARY POINTS

1. The earlier an ophthalmologist sees a badly injured eye, the better the vision is likely to be.
2. Although the eye is the receptor of light rays, it is the brain that "sees."
3. Because visual pathways cross at the optic chiasm, injury anterior to the chiasm causes unilateral visual dysfunction, while injury at or posterior to the chiasm causes bilateral visual dysfunction.
4. Clear vision requires a clear path from the cornea to the fovea and precise focusing of light rays on the fovea.
5. The best screening technique for detecting defective eye function is testing of visual acuity and visual fields.
6. Alkali injuries of the eye are generally much more severe than those caused by acid.

7. Posttraumatic posterior intraocular hypertension can rapidly occlude the retinal artery and cause blindness.
8. Posterior penetrations of the eye tend to have a much poorer prognosis than anterior injuries.
9. Early microsurgery on penetrating eye injuries can save much vision that would otherwise be lost.
10. Parenterally administered antibiotics penetrate the eye poorly, making it particularly important to reduce the risk of endophthalmitis by prompt surgical repair of open eye injuries whenever possible.
11. Any patient with a penetrating injury to one eye is potentially at risk for the development of sympathetic ophthalmia, which can cause blindness in the other eye.
12. The risk of sympathetic ophthalmia does not justify the primary removal of a severely traumatized eye unless the vision of that eye is completely lost.
13. When visual acuity and visual fields are not checked during the initial physical examination, the diagnosis of important eye injuries may be delayed.
14. In checking visual acuity in patients over 40 years of age, it is imperative that patients wear their reading glasses if they normally use them.
15. Pain from a corneal abrasion or chemical injury may result in the vision being assessed as poorer than it really is.
16. If the patient has normal visual acuity and visual fields, the chances of a serious injury to the eye or the visual pathways is unlikely. However, subnormal results require vigorous investigation.
17. It is extremely important to make an early diagnosis of ruptures or penetrating wounds of the eye.
18. Once it is discovered that an eye globe is ruptured, further examination is unnecessary, and the eye should be covered with a protective shield until it can be examined by an ophthalmologist in an appropriate environment.
19. Many orbital floor fractures can be diagnosed on the initial physical examination.
20. Superficial corneal injuries are diagnosed most readily by fluorescein staining.
21. MRI should not be used in any patient who may have a metallic foreign body in the eye.
22. Only three true ocular emergencies exist: chemical burns, orbital hypertension, and central retinal artery occlusions. In all three circumstances, appropriate therapy must be started within minutes.
23. Chemical burns of the eye are best treated by early, copious irrigation.
24. Treatment of alkali injuries is the same as for acid injuries and primarily involves immediate, copious irrigation with any solution that is nontoxic to the eye.
25. The key to treatment of caustic eye injuries is prevention; this is best done with public education about the dangers of commercially available alkalies and the need to wear safety glasses when dealing with such agents.
26. Any patient with a history of painless, sudden loss of vision should be presumed to have a central artery occlusion and should be transported immediately to an emergency center for definitive therapy.
27. Any trauma that injured an eyelid also likely injured the eye.
28. All but the simplest eyelid lacerations should be repaired in the operating room in a well-illuminated, controlled, pain-free environment.
29. Any time a lid laceration involves the eyelid margin or the medial canthal area, a canalicular laceration should be suspected.
30. If a laceration involving the canaliculus of the eye is not repaired, persistent tearing can result.
31. A delay of 12-24 hours, until optimum patient and operative conditions can be obtained, will not compromise the outcome of most eyelid lacerations.
32. Under no circumstances should a patient with a corneal abrasion be given a bottle of topical anesthetic.
33. Steroids should not be used in the presence of a corneal epithelial defect because they can rapidly make an undetected Herpes simplex or bacterial keratitis much worse.

34. The optimal treatment of full-thickness corneal lacerations is expeditious surgical repair to restore the eye's integrity and to prevent intraocular infection and complications.

35. As soon as it is discovered, a ruptured globe should be protected from further damage by a metal shield until it is formally repaired.

36. A ruptured globe should not be repaired immediately when the circumstances for repair are unfavorable.

37. All patients with hyphemas, regardless how small, are admitted and placed on strict bedrest with sedation to prevent anterior chamber hypertension and rebleeding.

38. All black patients with hyphemas should be checked for the presence of sickle hemoglobin.

39. Early corneal blood staining or persistently elevated intraocular pressure due to hyphema requires the surgical removal of blood from the anterior chamber.

40. Aspirin and nonsteroidal antiinflammatory drugs should not be given to patients with hyphema because these drugs increase the risk of rebleeding.

41. When hyphema is present, it is important to eliminate injury to other portions of the eye and optic nerve.

42. A traumatic cataract in a child with a vague or inconsistent history of trauma should alert the examiner to the possibility of child abuse, and the appropriate agencies should be notified.

43. All patients with ocular or periocular trauma need complete fundus examinations, including visualization of the retinal periphery with indirect ophthalmoscopy, to detect retinal holes, tears, or detachments.

44. Gradual loss of vision following blunt eye or face trauma requires emergency evaluation and treatment to save as much vision as possible.

45. Over 60% of patients suffering mid-face fractures have injuries to the eyes that should be evaluated by an ophthalmologist.

46. CT is the best method for evaluating the extent of orbital fractures.

47. With fractures extending into the orbital apex or orbital canal, surgery may cause traumatic optic neuropathy with marked loss of vision; the patient should be notified of this risk preoperatively.

48. The presence of a medial wall orbital fracture extending to the orbital apex greatly increases the risk of optic nerve injury with resultant blindness after any surgical manipulation of other portions of the orbit.

49. Surgical repair of a blow-out fracture may be contraindicated when it is on the side of the only eye with vision.

50. When critically ill or injured patients cannot completely close their eyes, exposure problems of the eyes are common.

51. Taping the eyelids shut, placing plastic wrap over the orbital areas in unconscious patients, and instilling eye ointment (Lacri-lube) can help to prevent the eyes from drying and developing corneal ulcers.

▲▲▲▲▲▲▲▲▲▲▲▲▲▲▲▲▲▲▲▲▲▲▲▲▲▲▲▲▲▲▲▲▲▲▲

REFERENCES

1. Vinger PF. The incidence of eye injuries in sports. Int Ophthalmol Clin 1981;21:21.
2. Capan LM, Mankikar D, Eisenberg WM. Anesthetic management of ocular injuries. Trauma: anesthesia and intensive care. Philadelphia: JB Lippincott Co., 1991; 357-384.
3. Tielsch JM, Parver L, Shanker B. Time trends in hospitalized ocular trauma. Arch Ophthalmol 1989;107:519.
4. Niiranen M. Perforated eye injuries, treated at Helsinki University Eye Hospital from 1970 to 1977. Ann Ophthalmol 1981;13:957.
5. Blomdahl S, Norell S. Perforating eye injury in the Stockholm population: an epidemiological study. Acta Ophthalmol 1984;62:378.
6. Bracker G, Parke DWII, Hamill MB. Injury to the eye. Moore EE, Mattox KL, Feliciano DV (eds). In Trauma, 3rd ed. Norwalk: Appelton and Lange, 1995; 279-290.
7. Roper-Hall MJ. Treatment of ocular injuries. Trans Ophthalmol Soc UK 1959;79l:57.
8. Brinton GS, Aaberg TM, Reeser FH, et al. Surgical results in ocular trauma involving the posterior segment. Am J Ophthalmol 1982;93:271.
9. Steinberg P, de Juan E, Michels RG. Penetrating ocular injuries in young patients. Initial injuries and visual results. Retina 1984;4:5.
10. Barr CC. Progressive factors in corneoscleral lacerations. Arch Ophthalmol 1983;101:919.
11. de Juan E, Sternberg P, Michels RG. Penetrating ocular injuries. Types of injuries and visual results. Ophthalmology 1983;90:1246.
12. Holt JE, Hot GR, Blodgett JM. Ocular injuries sustained during blunt facial trauma. Ophthalmology 1983;90:14.
13. Petro J, Tooze FM, Bales CR, et al. Ocular injuries associated with periorbital fractures. J Trauma 1979;19:730.
14. Cantore GP, Delfini R, Gambacorta D, et al. Cranio-orbito-facial injuries: technical suggestions. J Trauma 1979;19:370.
15. Pfister RR. Chemical injuries of the eye. Ophthalmology 1983;90:1318.
16. Delori F, Pomerantzeff O, Cox MS. Deformation of the globe under high-speed impact: its relation to contusion injuries. Invest Ophthalmol 1969; 8:290.
17. Cleary PE, Ryan SJ. Method of production and natural history of experimental posterior penetrating eye injury in the Rhesus monkey. Am J Ophthalmol 1979;88:212.
18. Marak GE. Recent advances in sympathetic ophthalmia. Surv Ophthalmol 1979;24:141.
19. Allen ED, Elkington AR. Local anaesthesia and the eye. Br J Anaesth 1980;52:689.
20. Deutsch TA, Feller DB. Paton and Goldberg's management of ocular injuries, 2nd ed. Philadelphia: WB Saunders Co., 1985; 26.
21. Spoor TC, Hammer M, Belloso H. Traumatic hyphema: failure of steroids to alter its course. A double-blind prospective study. Arch Ophthalmol 1980;98:116.
22. Crouch ER, Frenkel M. Aminocaproic acid in the treatment of traumatic hyphema. Am J Ophthalmol 1976;81:355.
23. Rakusin W. Traumatic hyphema. Am J Ophthalmol 1972;74:284.
24. Yasuna E. Management of traumatic hyphema. Arch Ophthalmol 1974; 91:190.
25. Thomas Ma, Parrish RK II, Fener WJ. Rebleeding after traumatic hyphema. Arch Ophthalmol 1986;104:206.
26. Goldberg MF. Antifibrinolytic agents in the management of traumatic hyphema. Arch Ophthalmol 1983;101:1029.
27. Rynne MV, Romano P. Systemic corticosteroids in the treatment of traumatic hyphema. J Pediatr Ophthalmol Strabismus 1980;17:141.
28. Palmer DJ, Goldberg MF, Frenkel M, et al. A comparison of two dose regimens of epsilon aminocaproic acid in the prevention and management of secondary traumatic hyphemas. Ophthalmology 1986;3:102.
29. Fukado Y. Results of 350 cases of surgical decompression of the optic nerve. Trans Fourth Asia-Pac Congr Ophthalmol 1972;4:96.
30. Kennderdell JW, Amsbaugh GA, Myers EM. A transantralethmoidal decompression of optic canal fracture. Arch Ophthalmol 1976;94:1040.
31. Anderson RI, Panse WP, Gross CE. Optic nerve blindness following blunt forehead trauma. Ophthalmology 1982;89:445.
32. Sofferman RA. Spenoethmoidal approach to the optic nerve. Laryngoscope 1982;41:184.
33. Holt JE, Holt GR, Blodgett JM. Ocular injuries sustained during blunt facial trauma. Ophthalmology 1983;90:14.
34. Putterman AM, Stevens T, Urist MJ. Non-surgical management of blow-out fractures of the orbital floor. Am J Ophthalmol 1974;77:232.
35. Converse JM, Smith B, Obear MF, Wood-Smith D. Orbital blow-out fractures: a ten-year survery. Plast Reconstr Surg 1967;39:20.
36. Smith B, Regan WR. Blow-out fracture of the orbit. Mechanism and correction of internal orbital fracture. Am J Ophthalmol 1957;44:733.
37. Canavan YM, Archer DB. The traumatized eye. Trans Ophthalmol Soc UK 1982;102:79.
38. Hutton WL, Fuller DG. Factors influencing final visual results in severely injured eyes. Am J Ophthalmol 1984;97:715.
39. Sternberg P, de Juan E, Green W, et al. Ocular BB injuries. Ophthalmology 1984;91:1269.

Chapter 13 Trauma to the Face

WALTER G. SULLIVAN, M.D.

HISTORIC DEVELOPMENTS

Maxillofacial injury has been described in the medical literature since at least 2500 BC.[1,2] Treating jaw injuries by wiring them together was first described by Hippocrates around 400 BC.[3] This treatment was apparently forgotten until Guglielmo Salicetti of Italy reintroduced Hippocrates' technique in 1275 AD.

Little was written on maxillofacial injuries during the subsequent several centuries. A case report by von Graefe in 1823 described the introduction of an elastic tube through the nose to prevent suffocation of a coachman who was kicked in the face by a horse;[3] this report suggested that the danger of airway obstruction from maxillofacial injury was recognized by this time. In the beginning of the twentieth century Sir Harold Gillies, father of plastic surgery in England, attempted to alert army personnel to the increased tendency and danger of upper airway obstruction in patients with facial injuries when placed in the supine position.[3]

A major advance in the understanding of maxillary fractures was achieved by Rene LeFort's famous work on cadavers in France in 1901.[1,4] During World War I, endotracheal anesthesia was developed, and the introduction of radiologic diagnoses resulted in a quantum leap in maxillofacial trauma management.[3]

After World War II, efforts were made to establish maxillofacial units utilizing the close cooperation of plastic surgery, oral and maxillofacial surgery, otorhinolaryngology, ophthalmology, and neurosurgery departments.[3] Concerns about fragmented care were raised, and the benefits of an interdisciplinary system were emphasized.[5]

> **AXIOM** Severe maxillofacial injuries are probably best treated by an interdisciplinary approach.

Progress in maxillofacial injury care during the past two decades has mainly been a result of: (a) improved diagnoses with CT; (b) improvements in the care of the multiply-injured patient; (c) new surgical techniques, such as open-jaw reduction and bone grafting; and (d) modern anesthetic, airway management, and monitoring techniques.

> **PITFALL** ⊘
>
> *Treating severe maxillofacial trauma before actual or potentially life- or limb-threatening problems are controlled.*

The gruesome appearance of facial injuries can easily distract clinicians from less obvious but more critical injuries;[1] however, one should focus attention on the most life- or limb-threatening-associated injuries until they are adequately controlled. Except for airway problems, massive bleeding, or aspiration of blood into the lungs, patients seldom die of facial injuries; however, for anesthesiologists, severe facial fractures in patients requiring emergency surgery can present a formidable challenge.

INCIDENCE AND ETIOLOGY

It is estimated that about three million facial injuries requiring emergency department or in-hospital care occur in the United States every year; however, more than 90% of these injuries are relatively minor soft-tissue lacerations requiring only local infiltration anesthesia in the emergency department for repair.[6] Although large population-based studies are not available, data from Dane County, Wisconsin (population 324,000) suggested that the national incidence of major

maxillofacial fractures and lacerations is 0.04 to 0.09%,[6] which is roughly comparable to results of population surveys from other countries.[7,8]

The etiology of maxillofacial injuries differs from one locality to the next, depending on socioeconomic characteristics, cultural background, degree of industrialization and urbanization, existing traffic regulations, compliance of motor vehicle drivers with the laws, and the extent of alcohol and drug consumption.[1] Before 1970, motor vehicle accidents were the single most frequent cause of maxillofacial fractures and accounted for almost 50% of all maxillofacial injuries.[6,9-11] Motor vehicle accidents probably remain the predominant cause of this injury for patients treated in private hospitals and in centers located in rural areas near busy highways and in developing countries;[6,12,13] however, in municipal hospitals and in regions where a mandatory seat belt law is enforced, the most common cause of maxillofacial injury is interpersonal violence.[7,9,13-15]

Among motor vehicles, automobiles are responsible for the majority of maxillofacial injuries, followed by motorcycles, trucks, and other vehicles.[10] In regions where bicycling is popular, 5-10% of maxillofacial fractures are caused by bicycle accidents.[16] Sports- and game-related maxillofacial trauma comprises 2.5-28.5% of all facial injuries in published series,[13,17] with contact sports, such as football, soccer, and rugby resulting in the highest incidence. Penetrating trauma is generally responsible for only a small percentage of maxillofacial injuries.

Acute alcohol intoxication is particularly common when the injury is secondary to assault, a motor vehicle accident, or a fall.[1,18] Illicit drugs contribute to trauma in general, but the extent of their involvement in maxillofacial injury is unknown. Fortunately, the victims of maxillofacial injury are usually 15-30 years of age and, therefore, usually have no significant underlying cardiovascular disease.

PATHOPHYSIOLOGY OF MAXILLOFACIAL INJURIES

Mechanism of Injury

In general, the causes of maxillofacial injuries can be divided into four different types of physical insults: blunt trauma, penetrating trauma, thermal trauma, and explosions.[1] In blunt trauma, the facial skeleton is usually more damaged than the soft tissue. When the injury is caused by an automobile accident, concomitant lacerations of soft tissue are likely. Altercation and sports-related blunt trauma are only occasionally associated with severe soft-tissue lacerations, but edema and hematomas almost invariably occur.

Impact interface geometry, which is the shape and texture of the surfaces by which the face is struck, has an important effect on the ultimate type and severity of injury. Car accident victims who strike their faces on soft surfaces in the vehicle are less likely to develop severe injuries than those contacting hard surfaces. Likewise, cushioned boxing gloves reduce the likelihood of jaw fractures in boxers, whereas severe injury occurs commonly in altercation victims.

The type and severity of injuries from penetrating trauma depend on the weapon used.[1] Knives usually only injure soft tissue, but intracranial and orbital penetration can also occur.[19] The severity of low-velocity gunshot wounds ranges from mild soft-tissue damage without bony involvement to severe facial bone fractures. The tongue and the floor of the mouth are frequently injured, and the severity of injury is difficult to predict.[19-20]

242

Close-range shotguns, rifles, and high-velocity military missiles can produce massive facial destruction and loss of tissue.[21,22] Injuries to the face and jaw from bombs may result in massive soft-tissue and skeletal destruction, and the resultant edema often rapidly produces upper airway obstruction.

Amount of Force

Swearingen[23] and Nahum[24] identified the degree of force needed to fracture different parts of the facial skeleton.[25] Using their findings from a series of 1020 patients, Luce et al.[26] subdivided facial fractures into: (a) high-impact injuries involving the supraorbital ridge, anterior mandible, and high maxilla; and (b) low impact injuries involving the condyle, nasoethymoid, and zygomatic regions (Fig. 13–1). They found that high-impact injuries had concomitant major injuries in 50% of patients resulting in a mortality rate of 12%. In contrast, the low-impact injuries were associated with other severe trauma in only 21% of patients. It has also been shown that the longer the duration of the impact, the more likely a fracture is to occur.[27]

AXIOM One should always consider the possibility of brain or cervical spine injuries in patients with severe maxillofacial trauma.

Bucholz et al. found that 25% of fatal automobile accidents were the result of cervical spine fracture dislocations.[28] In surviving patients examined in a trauma center, 2-4% of those with facial fractures have cervical spine injuries as well.

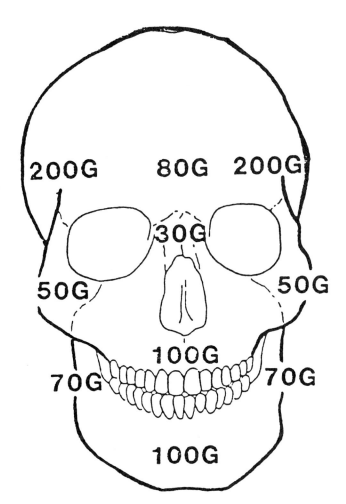

FIGURE 13–1 The forces necessary to fracture individual facial bones. (From: Luce EA, Tubb TD, Moore AM. Review of 1,000 major facial fractures and associated injuries. Plast Reconstr Surg 1979;63:26.)

Tolerance of Facial Bones to Impact

Women tend to have a lower impact tolerance than do men, and individual facial bones also differ in fragility.[26] The nasal bones, the zygoma, the mandibular ramus, and the frontal sinus are less tolerant to impact forces than other facial bones. For instance, a 30-mph collision can easily result in 80-g forces and is sufficient to cause fractures in the more fragile facial bones, while sparing others.[29] This fact explains, at least partially, the common occurrence of nasal, zygomatic, and mandibular fractures.

Direction of the Force

The direction of the force vector usually determines the fracture location.[1] For instance, a force applied to the point of the chin is likely to produce symphyseal and/or bilateral condylar fractures.[13] A lateral blow to the mandibular body tends to cause a direct fracture on the side of the impact and a contralateral fracture of the mandibular angle.

Resilience of the Facial Bones and the Cushioning Effects of Muscles

Even minor impacts in elderly people with osteoporotic facial bones may produce complicated fractures, whereas young persons may have major trauma without fractures.[1] Muscles play a significant role in the genesis of jaw fractures, especially of the mandible. They reduce the likelihood of fractures by cushioning the bones when they are relaxed; however, they may increase the chances of a fracture occurring if they are strongly contracted at the time of the trauma.[13]

Force Dispersion by Facial Bony Buttresses

The middle third of the face is composed of laminar, paper-thin bones reinforced by thick, bony buttresses[2] (Fig. 13–2), which are capable of dispersing physiologic or traumatic forces applied at any point. This distribution of forces helps to prevent, to some extent, fractures of low-resistance facial bones, and also tends to reduce transmission of the impact forces from the face to the skull. The bony reinforcement of the midfacial skeleton is provided by: (a) the palate and the floor of the nose, (b) the alveolar process, (c) the lateral and superior rims of the pyriform aperture, (d) the zygomatic complex with its connections to the inferior and lateral orbital margins and the zygomatic arch, (e) the orbital rims, and (f) posteriorly, the pterygoid plates.[2]

A similar mechanism, although architecturally in a different form, exists in the mandible.[1] The strength of this bone, as with all tubular bones, is located in its dense cortical plates. These comprise the buttresses, surrounding the central cancellous bone. The cortex is particularly thick in the anteroinferior aspect of the mandible, but it becomes thinner posteriorly at the angle and the condyles.[2]

TYPES OF INJURY

Soft-tissue Injuries

Soft-tissue lacerations by themselves rarely result in management difficulties; most can be repaired in the emergency department under local-infiltration anesthesia.[30] Because of the rich vascularity of the face, primary closure, after proper irrigation and debridement, is possible even with wounds in which treatment has been delayed for as long as 36 hours. Surgical management, however, is much more complicated when important structures, such as the facial nerve, the parotid duct, or the lacrimal apparatus, are injured. Repair of these injuries often requires general anesthesia.

Hematomas of the nasal septum or auricular cartilages require urgent surgery. When hematomas in these structures are not drained promptly, they can cause pressure necrosis of the cartilage and secondary, severe septal or external ear deformities.

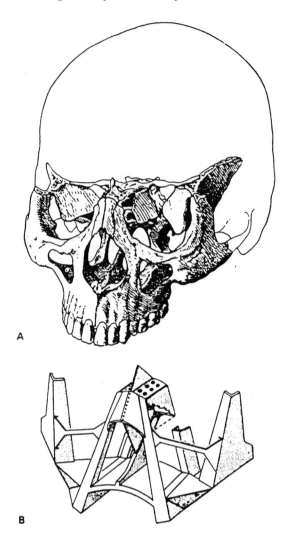

FIGURE 13–2 **A.** Osseous buttresses of the midfacial skeleton. The thin laminar bones are removed. **B.** An architectural concept of the bony buttressing of the face. (From: Bradley JC, et al. Applied surgical anatomy. Rowe NL, Killey HC, eds. Maxillofacial injuries. London: Churchill Livingstone, 1985; 19.)

Mandibular Fractures

TYPICAL LOCATIONS

After the nose and the zygoma, the mandible is the third most frequently fractured facial bone.[1,14] The severity of fracture varies from a simple, nondisplaced or greenstick type to one in which the bone is shattered. Olson et al. noted that mandibular fractures tend to occur in weaker areas of the bone, such as the condyles, the subcondylar area, the angle, or the body in the area of the second bicuspid or the mental foramen.[31] Fractures in the region of the alveolar and coronoid processes occur less frequently[32] (Fig. 13–3A). In elderly edentulous persons with thin cortical bone, the mandible is often broken in the symphyseal and parasymphyseal areas.

CORRELATION WITH TYPES OF TRAUMA

There seems to be a relationship between the etiology of the injury and the site of mandibular fracture.[1,10,14] After automobile accidents, the condylar and symphyseal regions are the most common areas injured[10] (Fig. 13–3B). Motorcycle accidents in which the victim's face strikes the pavement result in a larger percentage of alveolar fractures and fewer symphysis fractures, although angle, condylar, and body fractures occur with similar frequencies (Fig.

13–3C). The pattern of fracture is also different after altercations which most frequently involve the angle, the body, and the condyles[10,14] (Fig. 13–3D).

MULTIPLICITY OF FRACTURE LINES

> **AXIOM** If a mandible has one fracture line, one must look very carefully for other fractures that may not be readily apparent on standard radiography.

The U-shape of the mandible permits transmission of impact forces to the contralateral side; thus, more than 50% of mandibular fractures occur in more than one site.[1,25] Common fracture combinations include the body and opposite angle, the body and opposite subcondylar region, the symphysis and angle, and the symphysis and both condyles. Thus, a careful search for two or more fracture sites is necessary.[33]

ASSOCIATED NEUROVASCULAR INJURIES

The inferior neurovascular dental bundle, which comprises the inferior alveolar nerve, artery, and veins, enters the mandibular canal via the mandibular foramen on the inner surface of the ramus. It emerges from the mental foramen on the lateral surface of the bone midway between the inferior border and the alveolar crest at the level of the second bicuspid[1] (Fig. 13–4). This neurovascular bundle is at risk in fractures occurring between the mental foramen and the mandibular foramen; however, the fibrous sheath surrounding the bundle provides considerable support and explains the low incidence of permanent nerve damage.[34] Lower lip numbness caused by damage to the inferior alveolar nerve or its branches is generally transient, and hemorrhage from a transected inferior alveolar artery often ceases spontaneously because of retraction of the transected vessels and the tamponading effect of the surrounding bone.

FRACTURE FRAGMENT DISPLACEMENT

Muscle Effects

Many strong muscles are attached to the mandible, and they have a tendency to displace fracture fragments.[35] The resulting lack of anterior support for the tongue plus displacement of the fracture fragments and the surrounding swollen soft tissue can rapidly endanger the airway, especially in individuals who are not fully conscious.

Mandibular muscles are divided into four functional categories that include: (a) elevators, (b) depressor-retractors, (c) retractors, and (d) protrusors (Fig. 13–5).

MANDIBLE ELEVATOR MUSCLES

> **AXIOM** The muscles closing the mouth (i.e., elevating the mandible) include the masseter, temporalis, and medial pterygoid.

Of the three elevator muscles, the masseter is the strongest, and it extends from the medial and lateral surfaces and lower border of the zygomatic arch to the anterior and lateral surfaces and angle of the mandibular ramus (Fig. 13–6).[1] The fan-shaped temporalis muscle arises in the temporal fossa, descends medial to the zygomatic arch, and inserts on the coronoid process, the mandibular notch, and the inner surface of the ramus of the mandible. It retracts the mandible in addition to functioning as an elevator. The medial pterygoid muscle originates from the pterygoid fossa of the sphenoid bone and the pyramidal process of the palatine bone and inserts on the inner surface of the ramus and angle of the mandible.

MANDIBLE DEPRESSOR AND RETRACTOR MUSCLES

> **AXIOM** The muscles opening the mouth (i.e., Depressing the mandible) include the anterior belly of the digastric, the geniohyoid, and the mylohyoid.

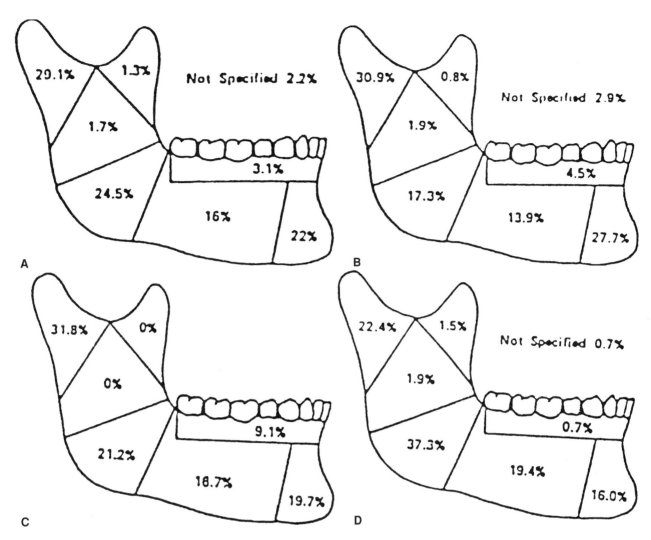

FIGURE 13–3 **A.** Overall anatomical distribution of mandibular fractures. **B.** Anatomical distribution of fractures caused by automobile accidents, **C.** motorcycle accidents, and **D.** altercations. (From: Olson RA, Fonseca RJ, Zeitter DL, et al. Fractures of the mandible: a review of 580 cases. J Oral Maxillofac Surg 1982;40:23.)

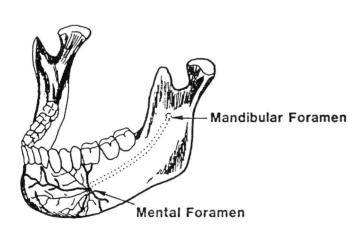

FIGURE 13–4 Mandibular foramen, mandibular canal, and mental foramen. The neurovascular bundle extends through the mandibular canal and is prone to injury in body and ramus fractures. (From: Capan LM, Miller S, Glickman R. Management of facial injuries. Capan LM, Miller SM, Turndorf H, eds. Trauma: anesthesia and intensive care. Philadelphia: JB Lippincott, 1991; 389.)

The depressor-retractors of the mandible are the suprahyoid muscles, and they all originate from the hyoid bone.[1] The digastric and geniohyoid muscles attach to the inferior border of the mentum. The mylohyoid has little effect on movement of the intact mandible because most of its fibers join in the midline at the mylohyoid raphe. Its principal function is to elevate the tongue during swallowing; however, it can exert considerable force on fractured mandibular fragments.

In bilateral parasymphyseal fractures, the fractured segment of the mandible is pulled downward and backward by the digastric, mylohyoid, and geniohyoid muscles.[1] Such a pull may retract the tongue and intraoral soft tissues into the airway, causing obstruction.[13,36] Fragments of the anterior portion of the mandible can also be displaced medially by the mylohyoid muscles, elevating the tongue and sometimes obstructing the oral airway[14] (Fig. 13–7).

MANDIBLE PROTRUSOR MUSCLES. The lateral pterygoid muscle is the protrusor muscle of the chin. After originating in two heads from the infratemporal surface of the great wing of the sphenoid bone and the outer surface of the lateral plate of the pterygoid process, it enters the articular disc of the temporomandibular joint and the anterior surface of the neck of the mandible (Fig. 13–6).

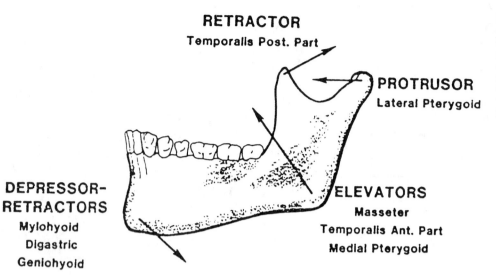

FIGURE 13–5 The elevator, depressor-retractor, retractor, and protrusor muscles of the mandible and the direction of fragment displacement produced by them (arrows). (From: Capan LM, Miller S, Glickman R. Management of facial injuries. Capan LM, Miller SM, Turndorf H, eds. Trauma: anesthesia and intensive care. Philadelphia: JB Lippincott, 1991; 390.)

COMBINED MUSCLE EFFECTS. With fractures of the mandible anterior to the elevator muscles, the posterior fragment is usually displaced upward by the masseter and medially by the medial pterygoid muscle, whereas the anterior fragment is pulled downward by the suprahyoid muscles.[1] In condylar and subcondylar fractures, the lateral pterygoid muscle displaces the condyle anteriorly and medially. If the fracture is unilateral, the mouth deviates toward the side of injury when opened.[37] In bilateral condylar fractures, the victims often present with an open bite deformity because they are unable to occlude the teeth of the anterior lower jaw against the maxillary teeth.

Effects of the Direction of the Fracture Line

The direction of the fracture line can be extremely important in determining the position of fracture fragments.[1] In a fracture of the angle or body of the mandible the posterior fragment is pulled upward only when the fracture line is directed from posteroinferior to anterosuperior[13,34,37] (Fig. 13–8A). A fracture line in the opposite direction does not permit vertical displacement of the posterior fragment by the elevator muscles because of the locking effect of the anterior fragment and its attached muscles (Fig. 13–8B). Medial displacement of the posterior fragment by the medial pterygoid muscle is also affected by the direction of the fracture line. If the fracture line extends from posterolateral to anteromedial, there will be no obstacle to movement of the posterior fragment (Fig. 13–8C). In contrast, a large buccal cortical fragment in fractures extending in a posteromedial to anterolateral direction prevents medial displacement.

Temporomandibular Joint Injuries

Apart from condylar fractures, the two most important injuries occurring at the temporomandibular joint (TMJ) include: TMJ dislocation and condylar impaction into the middle cranial fossa.[1,13,25] TMJ is formed by the condyle, the articulating bony socket, the capsule of the joint, the fibrocartilaginous disc, and two synovial pockets above and below the disc. The mouth cannot open unless an initial rotation of the condyle occurs within the capsule and then the condyle slides forward (also called translation). Anterior translation is limited by the bony articular eminence (or tubercle). The mouth becomes locked in an open position when the condylar head is dislocated anteriorly beyond the articular eminence. If the dislocation were unilateral, the open mouth, in contrast to condylar fractures, would deviate away from the involved side.[37]

TMJ DISLOCATION

Considerable pain and muscle spasm are present in almost all patients with TMJ dislocations; however, injection of a few milliliters of local anesthetic into the connective tissue of the TMJ capsule can relieve the pain and muscle spasm and sometimes results in spontaneous reduction of the dislocation.[37,38] If this measure is ineffective, one can often reduce the dislocation by depressing the mandible with the thumbs pushing down on the back teeth and simultaneously providing gentle elevation with the fingers from outside the mouth. Intravenous narcotics may be necessary to reduce the pain and spasm and thereby facilitate the reduction.

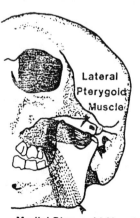
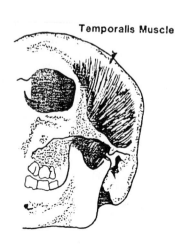
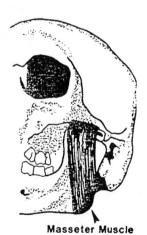

FIGURE 13–6 The bony attachments of lower jaw muscles. (From: Capan LM, Miller S, Glickman R. Management of facial injuries. Capan LM, Miller SM, Turndorf H, eds. Trauma: anesthesia and intensive care. Philadelphia: JB Lippincott, 1991; 390.)

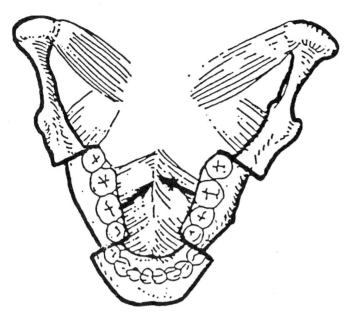

FIGURE 13–7 Bilateral double fractures of the mandibular body. The fragments are pulled medially by the mylohyoid muscle. This displacement may push the tongue upward and backward and cause airway obstruction. (Capan LM, Miller S, Glickman R. Management of facial injuries. Capan LM, Miller SM, Turndorf H, eds. Trauma: anesthesia and intensive care. Philadelphia: JB Lippincott, 1991; 391.)

INTRACRANIAL CONDYLAR IMPACTION

The condyle may become impacted into the cranium through the thin roof of the glenoid fossa when the mandible receives a blow in the mental region with the mouth open.[39] This is, however, a rare phenomenon because the elevated margins of the glenoid fossa prevent upward movement of the medial and lateral poles of the condyle.[40] Another reason for the rarity of this type of injury is that the neck of the condyle breaks readily and absorbs most of the

impact energy. Thus, the force applied to the cranial base is limited.[34]

A potential complication of impaction of the condyle into the cranium is severe intracranial hemorrhage because of damage to the middle meningeal artery, which is close to the glenoid fossa.[39] Rarely, the condylar head may be pushed posteriorly into the thin tympanic plate, which constitutes part of the posterior nonarticular portion of the glenoid cavity.

Central Midface Fractures

Unlike mandibular fractures, the fragments from fractures of membranous midfacial bones are seldom displaced by muscle pull.[1,37] These fractures also occur less frequently than mandibular fractures.[13] Because midface fractures frequently involve important adjacent structures, morbidity is high. Both the initial trauma and secondary infection may involve the nasal cavity, maxillary antrum, orbit, and brain, resulting in major complications. In addition, injuries of adjacent cranial nerves, major blood vessels, and richly vascularized soft tissues are not uncommon.

LEFORT FRACTURES

In an attempt to determine the value of external facial signs and symptoms in predicting the severity of maxillary fractures, Rene LeFort applied various forces to the facial skeletons of cadavers.[1,4] He found little relationship between severity of skeletal injury and external findings, but he did notice surprisingly constant fracture lines in the facial skeleton. Based on these observations, in 1901 he divided midfacial fractures into three categories, which are now designated LeFort I, LeFort II, and LeFort III (Fig. 13–9).

LeFort I Fractures

In LeFort I or Guerin's fractures, a horizontal fracture line separates the maxillary alveolar process from the rest of the maxilla. The fracture line passes above the nasal floor medially and extends laterally at the same level, involving the maxillary sinuses and the lower third of the septum. Consequently, the bony palate and the maxillary alveolar process are separated from the adjacent bones and can be

FIGURE 13–8 LeFort's classification of midfacial fractures. **A.** LeFort I, horizontal fracture of the maxilla, also known as Guerin's fracture. **B.** LeFort II, pyramidal fracture of the maxilla. **C.** LeFort III, craniofacial disjunction. (From: Converse JM. Kazanjian and Converse's surgical treatment of facial injuries. Baltimore: Williams and Wilkins, 1974.)

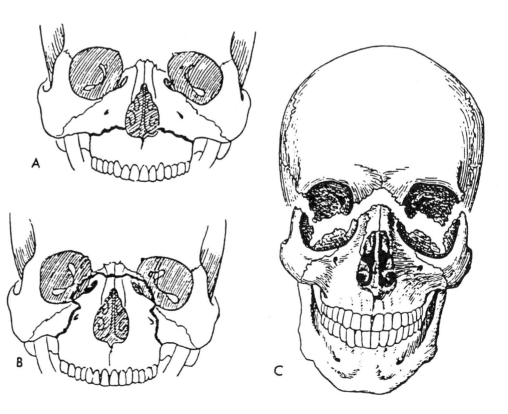

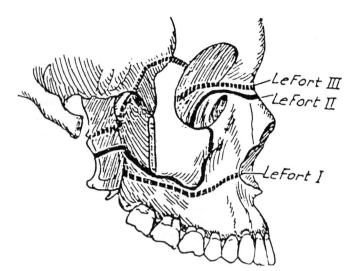

FIGURE 13–9 LeFort's lines of fracture on lateral view. (From: Converse JM. Kazanjian and Converse's surgical treatment of facial injuries. Baltimore: Williams and Wilkins, 1974; 697.)

moved back and forth by the examiner quite freely. Posteriorly the fracture line extends to the palatine bones and the lower third of the-pterygoid plates (Fig. 13–9). An associated fracture of the hard palate is common and clinically manifests as a line of submucosal ecchymosis. The LeFort I fracture differs from isolated alveolar fractures which do not extend to the midline of the palate.

LeFort II Fractures

The LeFort II fracture is pyramidal-shaped and begins in the midline at the thick portion of the nasal bone, extends laterally through the lacrimal bones and inferior rim of the orbit, and then continues downward near the zygomaticomaxillary sutures. The fracture line then crosses the lateral wall of the antrum and extends beneath the malar bone (zygoma) toward the pterygomaxillary fossa. Posteriorly, the LeFort II fracture involves the upper parts of the pterygoid plates (Fig. 13–9). Significant widening of the inner canthus of the eyes, epicanthal deformity of the bridge of the nose, and damage to ethmoidal cells may be present.

> **AXIOM**   Associated basal skull fractures are not uncommon in LeFort II fractures and should be ruled out before embarking on airway manipulation via the nasal route.

LeFort III Fractures

In the most severe LeFort III injuries, a combination of frontal and maxillary fractures may result in complete separation of the midface and the anterior base of the skull from the main body of the cranium resulting in dysjunction of parts of the frontal bone, orbital roof, and/or sphenoid bone.[41,42] Medially, the fracture line originates at the nasofrontal suture and involves the ethmoid bone posteriorly. Laterally, it extends through the orbit below the level of the optic foramen to the pterygomaxillary suture and the sphenopalatine fossa. The fracture then extends laterally and upward, separating the greater wing of the sphenoid and the zygoma up to the frontozygomatic suture. Posteriorly, it extends to the sphenopalatine fossa and the uppermost part of the pterygoid plate. The zygomatic arch is usually fractured at its weakest point which is adjacent to the zygomaticotemporal suture.

When a LeFort III fracture occurs, the entire midface tends to move backward and downward, parallel to the base of the cranium, causing the face to be elongated and flattened.[1] The posteriorly displaced midface can impinge upon the oropharynx and nasopharynx, potentially causing airway obstruction. The cranial base may be fractured at multiple sites. Because the cribriform plate is broken in the majority of patients, rhinorrhea is a frequent complication.

> **AXIOM**   One should look carefully for CSF rhinorrhea and/or airway obstruction in patients with LeForte III fractures.

In practice, LeFort fractures are rarely bilaterally symmetric.[1] Usually one side of the face has one type of LeFort fracture and the other side has another. Various combinations of LeFort fractures and nasal, nasomaxillary, nasoethmoidal, or zygomatic fractures are also observed.

NASAL FRACTURES

The projection of the nose beyond the rest of the face and the delicate structure of its bones make nasal fractures the most commonly encountered bony injury of the face.[1,33] Nasal fractures are usually isolated injuries but they may also be combined with maxillary, ethmoidal, and orbital injuries. This fracture is not difficult to recognize, and a history of trauma to the nose combined with severe external swelling and severe epistaxis strongly suggest the presence of this injury.[42] Radiographic studies add little to the clinical diagnosis. CT may be required, however, to differentiate simple nasal fractures from complex nasoethmoid fractures that require early surgical intervention to prevent infection.

NASOETHMOID FRACTURES

Nasoethmoid fractures should be suspected when severe trauma to the central face causes epistaxis, depression of the nasal dorsum, severe pain and tenderness over the upper nose, bilateral "black eyes" (spectacle hematomas), and/or inferomedial orbital rim fractures[1] (Fig. 13–10). Definitive diagnosis is established by CT. Nasoethmoid fractures differ from nasal fractures in that the cribriform plate of the ethmoid is also broken, potentially resulting in laceration of the dura and CSF rhinorrhea with pneumocephalus and potential CNS infection.[1] The cribriform plate is the most common site of bony injury causing a CSF leak, but damage to other structures in the base of the skull may also cause this complication. Microorganisms can gain access to the brain via the CSF fistula and may cause meningitis, brain abscess, or encephalitis. The bony injuries are easily missed because of the severe soft-tissue swelling, and the clinical findings are often attributed to simple nasal fracture.

> **AXIOM**   A nasoethmoid fracture should be suspected with severe nasal fractures and/or bilateral periorbital ecchymosis (spectacle hematoma or raccoon eyes).

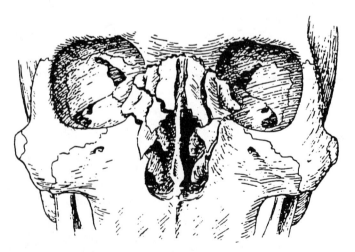

FIGURE 13–10 Comminuted fracture of the nasal bones involving the frontal processes of the maxilla. (From: Converse JM. Kazanjian and Converse's surgical treatment of facial injuries. Baltimore: Williams and Wilkins, 1974; 724).

Bilateral "black eyes" suggest the possibility of fractures in the base of the skull anteriorly. Nasoethmoid fractures may be associated with orbital, maxillary, frontal, and LeFort fractures. In some of these patients, the midface may be separated from the anterior cranial fossa.[41]

Severe ocular injury with initial or subsequent loss of sight may be present in up to 30% of patients with nasoethmoid fractures.[1,41] Telecanthus, which is an increased distance between the medial canthal ligaments, may be observed either immediately after injury or a few days later as the swelling disappears. The canthal ligaments are attached to the inferomedial orbital rim, which is frequently fractured in conjunction with nasoethmoid injuries.[43] Telecanthus suggests the presence of an unstable, complex, maxillofacial injury that often requires aggressive management using a combined craniofacial approach.[42] Nasolacrimal duct lacerations occur in about 20% of these patients.[41] Carotid-cavernous sinus fistula may develop within a few days to months after injury, resulting in a characteristic pulsating eye.[1]

Lateral Midface Fractures

Lateral midface fractures primarily involve the zygomatic arch, but they may also involve the malar bone and the orbit.[1] The zygoma is the second most common facial bone fractured after the nose.[33] The masseter muscle is attached to its anteroinferior aspect, and the temporalis fascia is attached along the junction of the facial and temporal surfaces of its frontal process and the superior aspect of its temporal process. Thus, significant displacement may occur after fractures of the zygomatic arch or the zygomatico-maxillary complex. The displaced zygomatic fragment may impinge on the mandibular coronoid process and produce limited mouth opening, which must be differentiated from trismus secondary to pain and temporalis muscle spasm.[1] The displaced zygomatic fragment may also intrude upon the lateral wall of the maxilla and produce infraorbital nerve damage.

Orbital fractures can affect eye movement when the external ocular muscles are entrapped by fractured segments or when the globe prolapses into the maxillary sinus.[1] Direct eye injury, including optic nerve laceration, may also occur; consequently, a careful eye examination is essential.

Upper Facial Fractures

Upper facial fractures are also called "frontobasilar fractures" and tend to involve the frontal bone, frontal sinus, and anterior cranial fossa.[1] Concomitant nasoethmoid, supraorbital, zygomatic, and cranial base fractures are common associated injuries. Frequent complications of these fractures include frontal lobe contusions or lacerations, CSF rhinorrhea, pneumocephalus, and periorbital emphysema.[42]

Significant brain injuries associated with upper facial fractures may be easily overlooked because of the silent nature of injuries to the frontal lobe and the absence of increased intracranial pressure due to the decompression of the cranial contents by mobile anterior fracture fragments.

In frontal sinus fractures, the nasofrontal ducts may also be damaged, resulting in an accumulation of secretions within the sinus and subsequent abscess formation.[1]

INITIAL MANAGEMENT

General

The rich blood supply and expandable soft tissues of the face allow for rapid edema formation following facial fractures, and the patient's swollen face covered with blood can be dramatic. Because the clinical examination frequently begins with the face, attention may be diverted from life- or limb-threatening injuries.

AXIOM   Facial fractures generally do not pose an immediate threat to life unless they compromise the airway or are associated with extensive bleeding; however, associated injuries of the cervical spine and brain must be suspected when attempting airway management techniques.[1]

The initial examination and management of patients with severe facial injuries should be directed to the airway and cervical spine. Exsanguination from facial injuries is rare, and digital pressure usually controls most external bleeding.

If an associated head injury were present, appropriate measures should be taken to limit secondary brain injury from hypoxia or hypotension. Such therapy includes prompt restoration of blood volume and provision of adequate oxygenation and ventilation. Once the initial resuscitative efforts have been accomplished and a secondary survey of the entire body performed, attention can be directed to the facial injuries.[1]

PITFALL ⊘

Letting dramatic facial trauma divert attention from less obvious but much more critical life or limb-threatening injuries.

Airway Problems

ETIOLOGY

Two to 6% of patients who present to the emergency department with serious maxillofacial injuries require emergency tracheal intubation to relieve airway obstruction, improve oxygenation, and/or initiate hyperventilation for associated head injury.[1,14,44] Respiratory distress in a patient with acute maxillofacial injury is most commonly caused by an upper airway obstruction, but other problems, such as a pneumothorax, pulmonary contusion, pulmonary aspiration, or combination of these factors, must also be considered.

Prompt diagnosis of the respiratory distress mechanism is mandatory. Parasymphyseal mandibular fractures allow the floor of the mouth and the tongue to fall backward, occluding the upper airway.[1,36] In bilateral double fractures of the mandible body, the free mandibular segment may be pulled medially after the mylohyoid muscle pushes the tongue up towards the palate, thus obstructing the oral airway. Similar airway compromise may develop from swelling of the tongue due to edema and/or hematoma.[45] Edema and hematomas may also develop in the pharynx, palate, and floor of the mouth after facial fractures, burns, and penetrating wounds, limiting tongue movement and producing rapid, progressive airway occlusion.[46]

The pterygoid plate is the only buttress preventing posterior shift of midface fractures. When it is broken, the entire midface may move posteriorly, thereby encroaching upon the nasopharynx. In the conscious patient, this shift may not result in airway obstruction because mouth breathing is maintained; however, if consciousness is impaired because of associated craniocerebral trauma or hemorrhagic shock, the tongue could fall back against the posterior wall of the pharynx and occlude the airway.[47]

AXIOM   Even without facial fracture, impaired consciousness can cause upper airway obstruction by allowing the tongue to fall back into the pharynx.

Blood, tooth fragments, dentures, and foreign bodies in the pharynx may occlude the upper airway or may be aspirated into the tracheobronchial tree.[48] Inhaled, loose, oral-tissue fragments or displaced dental prostheses occasionally lodge in the larynx sometimes without causing voice impairment or any signs of respiratory obstruction;[49] however, when the airway is subsequently manipulated, severe signs of airway obstruction may suddenly develop because of displacement of the foreign body or because of increasing traumatic edema.

DIAGNOSIS

Prompt diagnosis of the respiratory distress mechanism is mandatory because treatment of each cause is different.[1] In conscious patients with marginal breathing difficulty, a fairly reliable way to establish the need for immediate airway management is to ask them if they are getting enough air. If these patients cannot answer, stick out their tongues fairly easily or hyperventilate, they should probably be intubated. In unconscious patients, it is probably best to intubate the trachea, even when evaluation of the airway and auscultation and radiographic evaluation of the chest reveal no problems.

AXIOM   Because cyanosis occurs late in the process of respiratory distress and may not develop in anemic patients, lack of cyanosis does not rule out airway or ventilatory compromise.

Breathing is characteristically noisy in a patient with partial airway obstruction, although the respiratory efforts of a totally obstructed patient are silent.[1] When inspiratory stridor occurs, we assume that the upper airway is at least 70% occluded. Intercostal retraction, paradoxical movement of the lower neck and chest, flaring of alae nasi, and stridor are also important signs of upper airway obstruction. When any doubt exists about the airway, the safest course is to intubate the patient.

Meticulous examination of cervical radiographs for foreign objects is important before attempting intubation.[50] Occasionally, hemoptysis or persistent atelectasis may occur if these foreign bodies are inhaled or pushed into lobar or segmental bronchi during endotracheal intubation and mechanical ventilation.[51] Bronchoscopy and sometimes even bronchotomy may be necessary to diagnose and/or remove these objects.

Concomitant neck injury, especially to the larynx, may occasionally be the cause of airway occlusion. Cervical hematomas, voice change, laryngeal deviation, absence of laryngeal protuberance, and subcutaneous emphysema are signs of injury to this region. Flail chest, sucking chest wounds, pneumothorax, and hemothorax are also common causes of respiratory distress and should be promptly corrected.

TREATMENT OF THE PATIENT

Positioning

Many conscious patients with maxillofacial injury breathe more comfortably leaning forward in a sitting position.[1] In this position, the intraoral soft tissues tend to move forward, and may relieve some upper airway obstruction. If the patient tries to assume this position and is hemodynamically stable, he or she should be allowed to do so.[52]

AXIOM   Patients with severe facial injuries who are hemodynamically stable should be allowed to sit up if they can breathe more effectively and comfortably in that position and the cervical spine has been cleared or immobilized.

Oral or Nasal Airway

If airway occlusion following a maxillofacial injury is caused by simple loss of soft-tissue tone, anterior traction on the jaw or tongue or proper placement of an oral or nasal airway usually relieves the problem.[1] A nasal airway is less likely to cause gagging when airway reflexes are still present, but it should not be used when a fracture of the nasoethmoid complex or anterior base of the skull is suspected.

If airway obstruction is caused by a displaced mandibular fracture, anterior traction on the lower jaw using a towel clip or wire passed through the mandible can be very helpful. A chin lift or jaw thrust may also be effective, but the rest of the head must be stabilized if cervical spine injury has not been ruled out.

Removal of Debris or Blood in the Airway

The mouth should be carefully examined for blood clots, foreign bodies, vomitus, and loose teeth or dentures. Any blood, secretions, or vomitus should be removed by suction. It may be necessary to insert fingers in the oral cavity and pharynx to remove blood clots or solid material. When this is done, a blocker should be used to prevent the patient from biting the fingers of the examiner.

Pulling the Palate Forward

Airway obstruction is occasionally caused by posterior displacement of the entire midface after fracture of the pterygoid plates.[1] Insertion of the fingers into the mouth and palpation of the pterygoid plates immediately posterior and medial to the last upper molar tooth can confirm this diagnosis. A characteristic crepitation in this area is also highly suggestive of a pterygoid plate fracture. In these instances, the palate can usually be pulled anteriorly with the fingers. This maneuver can reposition the entire maxilla and relieve any airway obstruction it is causing.[41] Oxygen should be administered by face mask or cannula once the airway is cleared.

Endotracheal Intubation

RISK OF VOMITING.   If emergency laryngoscopy and endotracheal intubation are required urgently, this must be done carefully and expeditiously because attempting this procedure can cause a number of problems. Deeply unconscious patients usually do not gag or vomit during endotracheal intubation; however, conscious patients may be restless, irritable, and uncooperative because of underlying hypoxemia, alcohol intoxication, or respiratory distress. These patients, including those who otherwise seem relatively unresponsive, may vomit during attempted intubation with resultant loss of airway control and aspiration of gastric contents. Struggling by the patient may also increase muscle activity enough to make arterial hypoxemia worse.

SEDATION.   Moderate sedation to facilitate endotracheal intubation of restless or uncooperative patients may be accomplished with diazepam (5-10 mg) or midazolam (1-3 mg) with or without small doses of fentanyl (0.05-0.1 mg). These drugs may also improve the ability to open the mouth in patients who cannot do so because of severe pain and jaw muscle spasm. Irretrievable steps, such as the use of muscle relaxants or large doses of narcotics, should be avoided before placement of the endotracheal tube, unless the likelihood of easy intubation is high. Apnea may lead to death when the establishment of an artificial airway is time-consuming or not possible.

AXIOM   Paralyzing a patient to insert an endotracheal tube may be rapidly fatal if intubation or provision of a surgical airway is not accomplished promptly.

CONTRAINDICATIONS TO NASAL INTUBATION.   Although it is tempting to try nasal intubation in an awake patient, valuable time should not be wasted with this technique.[1] Nasal intubation also carries some risk in patients with fractures of the anterior base of the skull because it is possible to pass the endotracheal tube into the cranium[53] or to cause severe infection of the CNS. Thus, in LeFort II and especially LeFort III fractures, nasal intubation is generally strongly discouraged or contraindicated. Nasally introduced gastric tubes carry similar risks.[54]

AXIOM   Nasal tubes are generally contraindicated in patients with fractures that may involve the anterior base of the skull.

BRONCHOSCOPIC PLACEMENT.   The fiberoptic bronchoscope, although often recommended for airway control in maxillofacial injuries,[55] may be ineffective during the acute stage of trauma because of poor visualization resulting from excessive blood in the pharynx.[1]

INTUBATION OVER A RETROGRADE WIRE.   When it cannot be inserted by the standard techniques, an endotracheal tube can sometimes be inserted by passing a translaryngeal wire or catheter retrograde into the pharynx or mouth; however, one must be able to open the patient's mouth to allow recovery of the wire or catheter.[1,56] This technique, may be difficult if blood in the pharynx obscures a catheter or wire. This problem can be circumvented to a certain extent by continuous pharyngeal suctioning and injection of air through a retrograde catheter.[1] Another difficulty with retrograde intubation may be the tube or wire getting caught on the anterior commissure of the larynx. Once the wire is located, a flexible fiberoptic bronchoscope within an endotracheal tube or an endotracheal tube by itself can be passed over the wire into the proper position.[57]

Cricothyroidotomy

INDICATIONS

AXIOM	One should always be prepared to perform an emergency cricothyroidotomy in adults with severe facial injuries because attempts at endotracheal intubation may fail or cause complete airway obstruction.[1]

A cricothyroidotomy is generally preferred over a tracheostomy for emergency airway control because it is easier and faster to perform and does not require extension of the neck. This procedure, however, is contraindicated when laryngeal injury is suspected, particularly cricotracheal separation. Cricothyroidotomy is usually a temporary measure, and it generally should be converted to a tracheostomy soon after the acute hypoxia is relieved. One of the major problems with cricothyroidotomy is the ease with which the relatively small tube (usually 6 mm or less) can be occluded by blood or secretions.

TECHNIQUE. The technique for performing a cricothyroidotomy (coniotomy) is relatively simple and can often be completed in 15-30 seconds. The cricothyroid membrane is usually incised 1.0-2.0 cm transversely with a pointed scalpel blade, and the opening widened with a medium or large hemostat. A 6 or mm ID cannula is inserted. Alternatively, in children a 14-gauge intravenous catheter may be inserted percutaneously through the cricothyroid membrane in the midline and directed caudally. Ventilation through the intravenous catheter is accomplished by connecting it to a high-pressure (50 psi) oxygen source or a jet ventilator[58] by means of adapters that allow intermittent insufflation of the lung. One potential problem with this technique is that excessive airway pressure may be inadvertently applied to the lung when obstruction to the outflow of air occurs.

Tracheostomy

An emergency tracheostomy is only rarely required during management of maxillofacial injuries, but it is the procedure of choice when evidence of a serious laryngeal injury exists and/or no other type of airway can be rapidly obtained. Whenever possible, however, the airway should be controlled initially by endotracheal intubation, allowing the tracheostomy, if needed, to be performed under much safer conditions. Tracheostomy may also be necessary after intermaxillary fixation if replacement of the orotracheal tube with a nasotracheal tube cannot be accomplished safely.

Cervical Spine Injuries

INCIDENCE AND TYPES OF INJURIES

AXIOM	All patients with maxillofacial trauma—especially those with neck pain, tenderness, or spasm—or neurologic deficits should be assumed to have cervical spine injury until proven otherwise.

Cervical spine injury is reported in 0.2-6% of maxillofacial trauma victims.[1,10,11,14,26] Cervical spine injuries associated with mandibu-

lar fractures typically involve the first or second cervical vertebra, whereas middle or upper facial trauma is typically associated with injuries of the lower cervical spine.[59] These differences are probably due to the direction of the force vectors that accompany trauma to different regions of the facial skeleton.

Because the spinal canal of the upper cervical vertebrae is wide in relation to the spinal cord, neurologic injury is less likely to occur with injuries in those areas.[1] Thus, patients with fractures of the lower face may have an associated cervical spine injury without any initial neurologic deficit.

MANAGEMENT

AXIOM	Airway management without concern for cervical spine protection in patients with maxillofacial fractures may result in unnecessary spinal cord damage.

The head and neck of patients with severe facial injuries should be held rigidly in a firm cervical collar which is taped to a back board and sandbags alongside the head until C-spine films indicate that no cervical spine injury exists. An open mouth view when possible is invaluable for the diagnosis of fractures or dislocations of the first and/or second cervical vertebrae.[1] In hemodynamically unstable patients, an immediate cross-table lateral radiograph of the C-spine is usually done without moving the patient to the radiology suite. When patients need to be intubated emergently, before these films can be obtained, the head must be held in a neutral position by an assistant during the procedure. If an orotracheal tube cannot be inserted rapidly and easily in these circumstances and nasotracheal intubation is contraindicated, a coniotomy may be necessary to control the airway and provide adequate ventilation.

Hemorrhage

ETIOLOGY

Bleeding from soft-tissue lacerations in the mouth and the nose is a common feature of facial injuries.[1] Severe external hemorrhage may result from large lacerations of the scalp. Bleeding from deep lacerations involving major branches of the external carotid artery can also be dangerous; however, bleeding from skin, muscle, or bone injuries associated with facial fractures is usually not excessive and can usually be controlled with local pressure.

AXIOM	In hypotensive patients with facial injuries, other sources of hemorrhage and acute spinal cord injury should be suspected.

Major hemorrhage from the nose and mouth in closed maxillofacial injuries is unusual; however, when it is severe and/or persistent, hemorrhage is often due to lacerations of arteries within the walls of fractured sinuses.[1] Such bleeding is usually from the anterior and posterior ethmoidal, the internal maxillary, the lingual, or the greater palatine arteries.

Persistent bleeding from the nose may also be due to fractures involving the nasoethmoid sinuses, frontal sinus, or anterior cranial fossa. Lacerations of the inferior alveolar artery may be the cause of some bleeding in fractures of the mandible body. Massive bleeding into the nose, sinuses, or pharynx from maxillofacial fractures may sometimes be undetected, particularly in patients with impaired consciousness when the blood is promptly swallowed.[60]

TREATMENT

Severe bleeding from facial lacerations can usually be controlled with digital pressure until the lacerated vessel is identified. Blind probing of facial wounds with surgical clamps should be discouraged because of the potential for damage to important nerves or ducts.

Bleeding into the walls of fractured sinuses may often be stopped by simple manual repositioning of the bone fragments or by intermaxillary fixation. Anterior packing of the nose with half-inch wide adaptic gauze moistened with a petroleum-jelly-based ointment often stops mild-to-moderate bleeding from the nose or sinuses. Combined anterior and posterior nasal packing is occasionally necessary to control more severe and/or persistent posterior epistaxis.

Posterior packing can be performed by inserting a 16F or 18F Foley catheter with a 30-mL balloon via the nostril until its tip is seen in the pharynx. The balloon then is filled with air or water and pulled up gently against the choana. The balloon should be inflated only after the tip is seen in the pharynx because if it entered the cranial vault via a fracture of the cranial base and the balloon was then inflated, it could cause severe damage. Alternatively a 4x4 antibiotic-impregnated gauze pad may be tied into a roll with heavy sutures; this pad is then tied to the tip of a nasally-inserted Foley catheter that is withdrawn until the gauze is snugly secured against the posterior nasal opening into the pharynx. Anterior gauze is then packed up against the posterior pack.

Although packing will control nasal bleeding in most patients, a small percentage may not benefit from this technique.[1] In such patients, angiography can often identify the bleeding site and then occlude it with material injected through the angiography catheter.

In many centers, superselective angiography and embolization with gelfoam or other substances is the treatment of choice for persistent nasal bleeding. Furthermore, this procedure does not produce a surgical scar or peripheral nerve damage. At Bellevue Hospital, this procedure is performed under local anesthesia with sedation and careful monitoring of hemodynamics and cerebral function. In some of their earlier patients, spillage of the embolizing material into the internal carotid artery resulted in neurologic damage; however, this complication has not occurred during the past five years.[1]

When bleeding from an identified vessel is profuse, and radiologic intervention is not available or is not successful, surgical ligation of the feeding vessel is the treatment of choice. External carotid artery ligation alone is seldom effective because of the rich collateral circulation between the facial, maxillary, and lingual arteries.[60] Ligation of the external carotid artery plus clipping of the anterior and posterior ethmoid arteries along the medial orbital wall is a more successful method of dealing with posterior epistaxis.[61] Ligation of the internal maxillary artery within the maxillary sinus can also be effective.[60] Although such procedures can be performed under local anesthesia, general anesthesia is preferred in most instances.

In patients with massive or continued bleeding from facial fractures, observation of the injured sites for the quality of clot formation plus frequent monitoring of coagulation studies are important because such bleeding may be secondary to dilutional coagulopathy or disseminated intravascular coagulation (DIC) caused by release of thromboplastin from concomitantly injured brain or other organs.[62]

Associated Injuries

Concomitant injury to other regions of the body is a common feature of severe maxillofacial trauma.[1] These associated injuries are often more life-threatening than the facial injury itself. Overall, associated trauma is present in approximately 50-70% of motor-vehicle-accident victims and 30-35% of altercation victims.[14,26,44]

As described earlier, a close correlation often occurs between the facial bone(s) fractured and the incidence and severity of the associated injuries.[26] When the fracture is limited to facial bones with low-impact resistance (nasal bones, zygoma, mandible), both the incidence and severity of associated injuries are low. In contrast, the incidence and severity of associated injuries are much higher when facial bones with high-impact resistance, such as the supraorbital rim and mandibular symphysis, are fractured.

BRAIN INJURY
Fractures of facial bones are common with head injuries; brain injuries frequently occur with maxillofacial trauma, especially after automobile accidents.[63,64] The incidence of brain injury, according to published reports, varies from 15-48%.[10,11,14,26] The risk of serious brain injury is particularly high in upper facial injuries.[29]

EYE INJURIES
The incidence of associated eye injuries in patients with maxillofacial fractures is extremely varied and ranges from 3-67% in large series.[10,26,44,65] Fortunately, most of these eye injuries are minor and do not require specialized management.[1] In a series of 727 patients with blunt maxillofacial trauma reported by Holt et al.,[65] 67% of the patients sustained ocular injuries but only 18% of these injuries were serious and 3% caused blindness. The most frequent severe eye injuries included hyphema, lens dislocation, intraocular hemorrhage, retinal detachment, optic nerve damage, and rupture of the globe. In rare instances, retrobulbar hemorrhage, resulting in severe proptosis, may necessitate emergency decompression of the orbit.[66] Sometimes even trivial injuries may cause sudden blindness, probably because of disruption of the optic nerve.[67] In patients with severe facial fractures, recognition of eye injuries may be difficult. Palpebral hematomas and edema often prevent an adequate examination. Consultation should be obtained from an ophthalmologist for such patients before administration of general anesthesia. During induction of general anesthesia, the patient may have a severe Valsalva maneuver that causes the contents of the eye to extrude through a full-thickness laceration of the sclera.

AXIOM When general anesthesia is required and the patient has an eye injury that could not be examined closely, the patient should be considered to have an open globe until proved otherwise.[1]

NECK INJURIES
A wide variety of neck structures may also be damaged in patients who have facial injuries from blunt or penetrating trauma.[1] Associated neck injury is particularly frequent in gunshot injuries of the lower jaw because the bullet, after shattering the mandible, often continues into the neck.[19,68]

In automobile accidents, unrestrained front-seat occupants often strike their faces and necks on the steering wheel, dashboard, or windshield. In addition to the facial injuries, these patients can have a variety of other problems, including shock, airway obstruction, CNS injuries, cervical hematomas, hemoptysis, or absent pulses in the head and neck or upper extremities because of carotid or subclavian artery thrombosis.

THORACOABDOMINAL INJURIES
Thoracoabdominal injuries occur in 5-15% of patients presenting to the emergency department with maxillofacial injuries.[1,10,11,14,26,44] Almost any intrathoracic or intraabdominal organ can be injured along with the face, but one should look carefully for pneumothorax, hemothorax, partial aortic tears, and myocardial contusions. Although they occur often, the recognition of these conditions is often delayed and can result in disastrous intraoperative complications.

EXTREMITY INJURIES
Upper and lower extremity injuries occur in about 10-20% of patients with facial injuries after automobile, motorcycle, and bicycle accidents.[44] Hemorrhage from these extremity lacerations or fractures may be substantial. Extremity vessel and nerve injuries are easily missed, but can usually be detected by careful systematic examination.

DIAGNOSIS OF MAXILLOFACIAL INJURIES

History

The time and mechanism of the injury should be sought from the patient, EMS, police, or any witness. Although the cause of the injury is usually obvious (for example, automobile accident), the exact mechanisms for the injuries, such as striking the face on the steering wheel or dashboard, may require some questioning; the type and direction of the injuring force frequently determines the pattern of facial bone injury. When injury by a high-velocity missile is suspected, one can expect a great deal of surrounding tissue injury.

Symptoms, such as localized pain, tenderness, or crepitation, should make one suspect an underlying fracture even when no palpable deformity exists. Numbness or paralysis in the distribution of a specific nerve, facial asymmetry or deformity, or visual disturbance, should also suggest fracture.[1] Malocclusion, which is an abnormal relation of the upper and lower dentition, is a very important clinical sign of maxillofacial fracture. Any time a conscious patient states that his or her bite is abnormal and/or the teeth of the upper and lower jaw are not meeting in their usual fashion, one should assume that a mandibular and/or maxillary fracture is present.

AXIOM Malocclusion indicates a fracture of the jaws or teeth until ruled out by careful, complete examination radiologic studies.

Any history of drug use, excess alcohol ingestion, or loss of consciousness, should be noted with respect to the diagnosis of occult CNS injury. The patient's dental history and any prior radiographs are important not only to document missing teeth and dentures, but also to use as a guide for later reconstruction. Dentures may be the only record of the patient's occlusal alignment, and similarly, records from prior orthodontic treatment may also be extremely helpful in planning reconstructive surgery.

Physical Examination

SOFT TISSUES

Lacerations

AXIOM Prior to physical examination, the patient should be positioned so that the examination light is centered on the midline to avoid visual distortion of facial asymmetry.

Examination of the face during the secondary survey begins by checking all lacerations for foreign bodies and for their proximity to major nerves or vessels. The scalp must also be closely examined for lacerations because they can bleed excessively but the exact sources are easily obscured by matted hair. All lacerations of the scalp and face should be carefully palpated and examined for any evidence of underlying fractures.

Full thickness lacerations of the eyelids, cheek, or lips should be diagnosed and promptly repaired surgically. All lacerations near an eye should also be carefully screened for associated penetrating trauma to the globe. The nature and extent of the lacerations, abrasions, and contusions should be carefully documented. When readily available, multiple photographs from various angles may also be helpful, especially if later malpractice litigation were to occur.

Parotid Duct

The approximate position of Stensen's duct from the parotid gland is on a line drawn from the tragus to the mid upper lip. Where this line crosses the anterior border of the masseter is the position of its entrance into the oral cavity and also marks the location of the buccal branches of the facial nerve (Fig. 13–11). Any lacerations in this area should lead to suspicion of a parotid duct laceration. Frequently the cut ends of the duct can be seen in the wound; however, when the diagnosis is in doubt, a catheter can be placed into the duct from inside the mouth and passed proximally. A sialogram can then be used to rule out injury.

AXIOM Any injury along the posterior half of a line drawn from the tragus to the mid upper lip should be suspected of involving the parotid duct and/or buccal branches of the facial nerve.

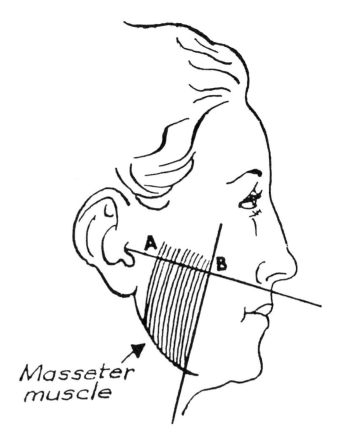

FIGURE 13–11 The course of Stensen's duct is deep to the middle third of a line drawn from the tragus of the ear to the mid-portion of the upper lip. This corresponds roughly to the anterior-posterior limits of the masseter muscle. The hilus of the gland is near point A, and the opening of the duct into the mouth is opposite the second maxillary molar tooth deep to point B. The buccal branch of the facial nerve crosses Stensen's duct near point B. Lacerations involving Stensen's duct usually result in severance of the buccal branch of the seventh nerve. (From: Converse JM. Kazanjian and Converse's surgical treatment of facial injuries. Baltimore: Williams and Wilkins, 1974; 635.)

NEUROLOGIC EXAMINATION

Motor Nerve Function

The major motor nerves of the face are the facial nerve, which supplies the facial muscles, and the motor branch of the trigeminal nerve which supplies many of the muscles of mastication (masseter, temporalis, and the medial and lateral pterygoids). Injury to the motor branch of the trigeminal is rare, but facial nerve injuries are not uncommon and are easily missed.

The patient is inspected for facial asymmetry. Does the oral commissure droop on one side, indicating injury to the buccal branch of the facial nerve? Are the forehead wrinkles absent on one side, indicating injury to the temporal branch of the facial nerve?

Patients are then asked to smile, show their teeth, wrinkle their forehead, and close their eyes. Inability or asymmetry is strongly suspicious of facial nerve injury. Careful examination is necessary, particularly with facial edema which can minimize or hide movement.

Deep lacerations of the central portion of the face may cause facial muscle lacerations which can also result in asymmetry. This is most frequently seen in the nasolabial and lip areas. These muscles, such as the zygomaticus or orbicularis, must be repaired as a separate layer below the skin and subcutaneous tissue.

PITFALL ⊘

Facial edema may limit facial movement and a facial nerve injury can easily be missed under such circumstances.

Sensory Nerve Function

AXIOM Because most of the major sensory nerves of the face traverse facial bones, any area of hypesthesia or anesthesia should make one suspect an underlying facial fracture.

The inferior alveolar nerve enters the mandible medially at the midpoint of the ramus, supplies the lower teeth and gingiva. The branch that exits the mandible through the mental foramen is known as the mental nerve, and it supplies sensation to the lower lip. Although the mental nerve may be injured by deep chin lacerations, numbness of the lip or gum should make one suspect a mandibular fracture until proved otherwise by radiography. Similarly, the infraorbital nerve exits the maxilla after traversing the orbital floor and supplies the side of the nose, cheek, and upper lip. Numbness in those areas, though occasionally due to a direct blow to the cheek, is frequently evidence of an orbital floor or maxillary fracture.

FACIAL BONE EXAMINATION

AXIOM The most accurate method for determining the presence of facial fractures (except for CT) is careful palpation of bony landmarks looking for step-offs, irregularities, or asymmetry.

The bones of the face should be examined very carefully for any bony step-offs, irregularities, or asymmetry. Facial edema can develop so rapidly that a severely depressed zygoma fracture may be quickly obscured visually by overlying swelling and hematoma; however, careful palpation generally reveals the asymmetry. Although radiographic examination is frequently necessary to detect deeper injuries and to determine the extent of injury, virtually all facial bone fractures can be diagnosed by careful palpation. Questionable fractures on radiography are frequently obvious on physical examination.

PITFALL ⊘

Reliance on radiographic evidence alone to diagnose facial fractures will lead to missed fractures that would have been easily detectable by physical examination.

Examination of the facial bones should be performed in a systematic fashion from forehead to mandible.[1] The forehead and supraorbital ridges should be inspected and palpated for depressed fractures first. Loss of supraorbital nerve sensation suggests a fracture involving the supraorbital ridge.

By standing above the patient and looking down the facial axis, the examiner's index finger can be stabilized on the supraorbital margin and then the middle finger used to assess zygomatic depression.[1] Particularly noticeable are "step-offs" at fracture sites. With "tripod" fractures at the zygomaticofrontal, zygomaticomaxillary, and zygomaticotemporal sutures, step-offs usually are palpable at the upper lateral and lower orbital margins, and the zygomatic arch is depressed. The supraorbital margin and glabellar regions are palpated for frontal bone fractures. Step-offs along the mandibular margin usually indicate mandibular fractures. Point tenderness is usually present at fracture sites, but it is not always diagnostic. The nose is examined for asymmetry, and the nasal bones are palpated for depression.

Displacement of the nasal pyramid is also best seen from above.[1] In this position the examiner can also assess the degree of enophthalmos that may be caused by orbital floor fracture. An index finger is placed in the auditory meatus, and the patient is asked to open and close the mouth. Normal TMJ movement is felt symmetrically by the examiner's fingers. Lack of TMJ movement may indicate a condylar fracture or dislocation.

AXIOM One of the most important diagnostic methods for detecting a mandible or maxillary (LeFort) fracture is inspection of occlusion.

While checking for maxillary and/or mandibular fractures, one should ask patients if their teeth fit together the same as they did before the trauma. Even a small degree of misalignment will be obvious to most patients. The dental occlusion should then be directly inspected (Fig. 13–12). Although Class I occlusion is most common (first mesiobuccal cusp of the maxillary first molar is aligned axially with the first mesiobuccal groove of the mandibular first molar), some patients normally have Class II (distoclusion) or Class III (mesioclusion). It is the change from the pretraumatic status that is most important. If most of the teeth are still present, malocclusion caused by maxillary or mandibular fractures is usually very obvious to the patient.

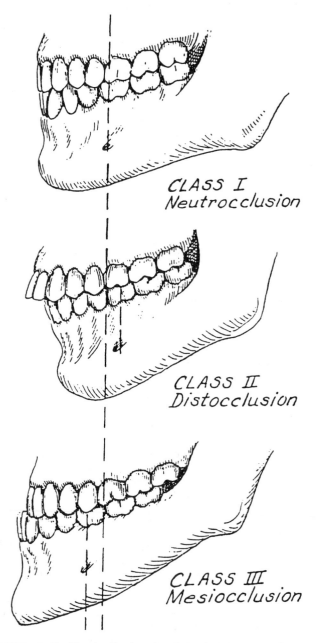

FIGURE 13–12 The classification of occlusion includes three main types. The classification is based upon the position of the mesiobuccal cusp of the maxillary first molar in relationship to the mesiobuccal groove of the mandibular first molar tooth. Subdivisions of the three main classes are identified by differences in mesial or lateral positioning of the teeth in the dental arches. (From: Converse JM. Kazanjian and Converse's surgical treatment of facial injuries. Baltimore: Williams and Wilkins, 1974; 647.)

Failure to ask and look for dental malocclusion can easily lead to a missed maxillary or mandible fracture.

Additional testing involves grasping and pulling on the maxillary alveolus (Fig. 13–13) and then the mandibular alveolus in several areas to determine whether the underlying bone moves. If an isolated segment of the maxilla can be moved from its position with the other bones, an alveolar or sagittal fracture is present. When the upper central teeth and the attached bone can be moved in and out, a LeFort I fracture is probably present. When the maxilla moves only at the nasofrontal area, a LeFort II fracture is present. When the entire midface and the zygoma move, a LeFort III fracture (craniofacial dysjunction) is present. Facial fractures, however, rarely fit one of the LeFort patterns exactly.

Nasoethmoid or nasoorbital fractures are serious injuries requiring special surgical care. These injuries usually present as a depressed nasal dorsum, and if mistaken for a simple nasal fracture, the consequences could be disastrous. With nasoethmoid or nasoorbital fractures, the lacrimal bones are usually also fractured and the medial canthi are displaced laterally causing telecanthus, which is an increased distance between the medial corners of the eye. This is generally associated with significant periorbital ecchymosis and edema ("raccoon eyes"). Nasoethmoid fracture also causes loss of nasal support which is usually telescoped back into the face causing nasal shortening and loss of dorsal projection.

Nasoethmoid fractures, which often require special craniofacial techniques for repair, may easily be mistaken for simple depressed nasal fractures if one does not perform a careful examination.

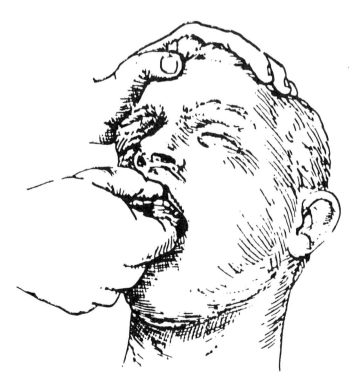

FIGURE 13–13 Examination for fractures of the maxilla. When the patient has a mobile scalp, the stabilizing hand should be repositioned lower on the forehead. (From: Zuidema GD, Rutherford RB, Ballinger WF. The management of trauma, 5th ed. Philadelphia: WB Saunders, 1985; 284.)

EXAMINATION OF THE EYE

One should look carefully for any evidence of an eye injury in patients with facial trauma. Initially, one can compare the level of the globes. Frequently, globe level is lowered with the orbital floor or roof fractures.

Extraocular movement is also tested. Inability to look up (supraduction) or diplopia on supraduction implies an orbital floor fracture or, more rarely, an orbital roof fracture.

AXIOM Diplopia alone is nonspecific, but should alert one to possible occult facial fracture which requires investigation radiographically.

Ptosis of the eyelid may be caused by a direct lid laceration, but it may also signify an underlying fracture of the supraorbital rim or orbital roof. Enophthalmos is best evaluated by looking at the globe from below and noting the projection. A sinking-in of one globe implies an orbital floor or medial wall fracture. Proptosis of the globe should alert one to the possibility of an orbital roof fracture, particularly when the globe is pulsatile.

Failure to look for and appreciate orbital asymmetry may lead to missed orbital fractures.

Following observation, one should palpate the rims of the orbits to determine their symmetry.[1] Widening of the intercanthal distance (telecanthus) occurs with nasoethmoid fractures, and the whole orbit may be shifted (orbital dystopia) in complex midface or zygomatic fractures.

Total loss of lid function may indicate CNS injury or intraorbital injury (superior orbital fissure syndrome).[69] Whether lid function is lost because of tissue destruction or because of a neural defect, the eye must be protected. In emergency situations, standard ophthalmologic ointments and polyethylene film or Op-site protects an exposed cornea from desiccation[25] but one should also look for definitive eye protection.

Visual acuity should be documented carefully before subsequent facial edema makes this impossible.[1] At least, patients must be asked if they are able to discern light shone through their lids.

AXIOM Decreased visual acuity without global injury may indicate a periorbital hematoma that requires urgent decompression.

The corneas are carefully examined for any abrasions. When any question exists, fluorescein strips and the Wood's lamp are used. The iris is examined for pupillary size, symmetry, and degree of responsiveness; the anterior chamber is inspected for the presence of blood (hyphema). Any irregularity of the pupil suggests a globe laceration. Funduscopic examination is also done. When an eye injury is suspected or when the patient reports a change in vision, a visual acuity test should be done, and an ophthalmologist should be consulted.

EXAMINATION OF THE EARS

The ears are inspected for hematomas which may need to be drained before causing damage to cartilage, which can result in a "cauliflower ear." A careful examination of the external ear, the external ear canal, and the tympanic membrane should be performed with an otoscope. Blood in the middle ear cavity often indicates a basal skull fracture;[1] however, bleeding may also occur from small wounds in the external auditory canal. Such wounds may be seen occasionally in condylar fractures and dislocations. One must also look carefully for CSF leak (otorrhea).

AXIOM Bleeding from an ear after trauma should be considered due to a basilar skull fracture until proved otherwise.

EXAMINATION OF THE NOSE

The nasal bones are carefully palpated to assess for deformities and for shifting of the nasal pyramid. An endonasal examination should also be conducted to assess septal deviation and to detect the presence of a septal hematoma. If a septal hematoma is found, it should be drained promptly to prevent necrosis of underlying cartilage.

With severe nasoethmoid fractures, a CSF leak is detected in approximately one-third of patients within the first 24 hours of the injury. By 48 hours, a CSF leak is evident in more than half of patients.[70] CSF rhinorrhea may develop in some of the remaining patients, up to three months after injury.

It is often difficult to recognize rhinorrhea or otorrhea during the initial stages of maxillofacial trauma when the CSF is mixed with blood and mucus.[1] Glucose levels in nasal secretions are generally very low so that a commercial paper reagent test designed to identify glucose in normal CSF can help to determine what type of fluid is draining from the nose; however, when much blood is evident in the nasal fluid, the test can be falsely positive. When the rhinorrhea is clear, this test can fairly accurately differentiate CSF rhinorrhea from common types of nasal secretions.

AXIOM When bloody CSF is placed on filter paper, there will be an outer clear ring caused by the CSF and an inner ring of blood with or without nasal fluid.

A simpler test to differentiate CSF rhinorrhea from nasal discharge involves placing a handkerchief under the nose for a short period and then allowing the material to dry; CSF will dry without starching, whereas nasal discharge will stiffen the cloth.[46] A CSF leak may also be confused with discharge of tears into the wound after injury to the lacrimal apparatus. Tears can be distinguished by depositing fluorescein dye into the lumbar subarachnoid space and examining pledgets inserted into the nose with a Wood's lamp after 30 minutes. Fluorescence of the pledgets suggests CSF leakage.[37]

EXAMINATION OF THE MOUTH

Limitation and/or pain in mouth opening can be important keys to the recognition of facial injury. Condylar movement can be detected by introduction of the little finger in the ear canal; absence of condylar movement with opening and closing of the jaw suggests fracture of this part of the mandible.[1]

In the oral cavity, the locations of loose or missing teeth are documented.[1] Lacerations of the tongue and floor of the mouth that have stopped bleeding can be easily overlooked and are often best palpated. Mandibular fractures are often compound into the mouth either directly or via a tooth socket where a small amount of bleeding may herald the presence of the fracture.

With cheek retractors in place, patients are asked to bring their teeth together so that the actual occlusion can be documented.[1] Loss of dental proprioception; as in a zygomatic fracture, can give a subjective feeling of malocclusion that may be confirmed or ruled out by observing the actual occlusion. Externally, anesthesia over the chin may be due to injury to the mental nerve in fractures of the mandibular body.[1]

Radiographic Examinations

After the airway and ventilation are secured, the blood volume has been adequately restored, and other more serious injuries have been controlled, patients with maxillofacial injury can be transported to radiology for further evaluation of their injuries.[1] Equipment for airway management and other types of resuscitation should also be provided during transport to radiology. Frequent monitoring of the level of consciousness and vital signs should be continued. If available, a pulse oximeter should be attached to a finger to continuously monitor arterial oxygen saturation.

PLAIN VIEWS AND SPECIAL VIEWS

AXIOM As a diagnostic tool, radiographic studies of the face are generally inferior to a careful physical examination.

Except in simple nasal fractures, radiographic studies can help to investigate suggestive physical findings (e.g., limitation of upward gaze), confirm clinical diagnoses, and plan operative treatment. A facial series includes views of the maxilla, zygoma, orbits, and frontal bone. The Waters view is usually included and is particularly useful for evaluating the zygoma, maxilla, and orbits (Fig. 13–14). The symmetry of the zygomatic arches can often be best provided by a submentovertex view. For the mandible and the teeth, Panorex radiography is most useful and shows the lower maxilla and mandible from condyle to condyle on one film. Although it is readily available in

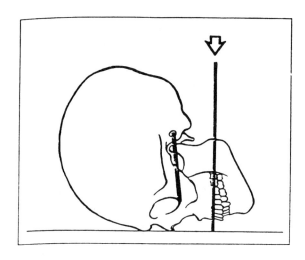

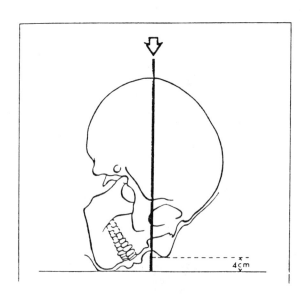

FIGURE 13–14 A. PA view of the mandible (Towne's view of the mandible) gives the best view of ascending rami and subcondylar regions (From: Early care of the injured patient, 4th ed. Moore EE, ed. Philadelphia: BC Decker, 1990; 142). **B.** Positioning of a patient for the Water's view which provides the best view for screening of midface fractures. (From: Early care of the injured patient, 4th ed. Moore EE, ed. Philadelphia: BC Decker, 1990; 140.)

many dental departments, the Panorex may not be available in the emergency department. In such circumstances, a mandibular series is necessary. Particular effort should be expended in visualizing the condyles well. A missed condyle fracture may cause considerable functional disability and deformity.

AXIOM Condyle fractures are missed easily and can cause considerable functional disability and deformity.

Many special radiographic views are available to demonstrate specific fracture sites; however, it must be emphasized that some of these techniques require special positioning and thus cannot be obtained in multiply-injured patients, particularly when there is concern about the integrity of the cervical spine. For instance, the Panorex view of the mandible that demonstrates the angle, rami, and condyles requires that the patient be upright; thus, it cannot be obtained in hemodynamically compromised trauma victims. Likewise, the standard Water's view is obtained with the patient in a prone position. Therefore, a cervical spine injury must be eliminated before obtaining this view.

Subcutaneous emphysema and pneumomediastinum are uncommon complications of facial injury,[1] but rarely, air from fractured maxillary or ethmoid sinuses can communicate via the fascial planes of the neck into the mediastinum. Nevertheless, the presence of a pneumomediastinum should stimulate a careful search for injury to the larynx, tracheobronchial tree, lungs, pharynx, or esophagus.

AXIOM Appropriate radiographic and endoscopic evaluation of the aerodigestive tracts should be performed before one decides that a pneumomediastinum is a harmless consequence of facial injury.[87]

COMPUTED AXIAL TOMOGRAPHY

The problems of positioning patients for special radiographic views have largely been resolved with the availability of CT scans. In fact, CT has replaced plain radiography for evaluating facial fractures in many centers, not only because it eliminates the problems of positioning, but also because of its ability to provide more detailed information.

AXIOM CT is now the radiographic method of choice for the diagnosis and operative planning of facial fractures.

Although they are not required for the treatment of complex facial fractures, the clarity and easy availability of CT scans make them a useful and important tool, particularly when plain radiography is not definitive. When a trauma patient with possible facial injuries is being taken for a CT scan of the brain and his condition permits, the face should be included in the examination. This may substitute for roentgenographic studies of the midface, orbits, and zygoma.

During CT examination of the face for fractures, axial cuts are routinely obtained. For the orbital floor and roof, the coronal cuts are superb and can help quantitate the severity of the fracture; however, for coronal cuts, the patient must extend the neck; consequently the cervical spine must be cleared first. If this is not possible, computer reconstructions of the facial bones can be done from axial views. These will, however, be somewhat inferior in resolution.

With sophisticated computer software, 2-D CT data can be reformatted to create three-dimensional CT images (3-D CT). Some surgeons have found 3-D CT images of the unpredictably shaped facial skeleton in congenital craniofacial abnormalities to be valuable in treatment planning.[71] Several reports have also advocated 3-D CT as an important adjunct in the preoperative evaluation of facial trauma patients.[72,73] Broumand et al.,[74] however, believed that 3-D CT added little to the preoperative assessment.

TOMOGRAPHY

Although it can be very useful for showing certain fractures with relative clarity, tomography has been largely supplemented by CT, which also provides less radiation exposure to the patient.

ARTERIOGRAPHY

In the rare patient with facial fractures and uncontrolled bleeding, arteriography with selective embolization can be extremely useful and can obviate the need for emergency operative intervention.

TREATMENT OF SOFT-TISSUE FACIAL INJURIES

General Directions

Using judicious surgical principles and sound technique, most soft-tissue injuries of the face can be handled well in the emergency department by most physicians. In general, with adequate surgical facilities, most soft-tissue repairs that can be completed in an hour or less can be performed in the emergency department.[1] Special injuries, such as those involving the parotid duct, facial nerve, or eyelids, should be repaired in the operating room.

Contusions and Hematomas

With proper use of ice-cold compresses, most contusions resolve within 24-72 hours.[25] Small hematomas may be treated expectantly; however, large clots should be evacuated through well-placed incisions made along lines of relaxed skin tension.[75] For instance, when a hematoma of the cheek is evacuated, an incision through the lower eyelid in one of the skin crease lines will be well camouflaged. The clot is then milked upward and evacuated. The cavity is irrigated and then allowed to heal spontaneously.[76]

If a large hematoma is neglected, the periphery can organize while the center liquifies. Once this occurs, collection may require repeated aspirations, resulting in an unsightly depressed scar.

Timing of Repairs

It is generally best to repair facial lacerations as soon as they are seen; however, the patient's condition may not allow this. When repair is delayed, an effort should be made to irrigate and cleanse the wound and cover it with a sterile dressing as soon as possible. Fortunately, the luxurious blood flow to most facial tissues makes them remarkably resistant to infection.[25] Because of this long "grace period," most such wounds, with the possible exception of human bites, may be safely closed up to 24 hours after injury.

Anesthesia

For injuries involving the skin and subcutaneous tissues, local anesthesia is the method of choice. Even very young children can be immobilized in a "papoose" device to allow accurate suturing under local anesthesia; however, general anesthesia in an operating room is preferred for very extensive injuries, uncooperative patients, or possible injuries of special structures, such as the facial nerve or parotid duct.

For local anesthesia on the face 0.5% Xylocaine with 1:200,000 epinephrine is generally used. It has been suggested that epinephrine not be used in the ear or the tip of the nose because of possible detrimental effects from the excessive vasoconstriction that it can cause. In most cases, infiltration with a small caliber needle through the cut edge of the laceration is done. Alternatively, if anatomically convenient, a local nerve block can be done which will cause less distortion of the soft tissue. For example, injection of local anesthesia at the mental foramen can often be used to repair lacerations of the lower lip.

Wound Debridement

The skin around any open wound should be thoroughly cleaned and then the wound irrigated with sterile saline. In some cases, the wound must be anesthetized before it can be cleaned adequately. Particularly dirty wounds should be irrigated with several liters of saline and scrubbed with moistened gauze. Pulsatile jet lavage can be very effective for removing hair, dirt, clothing, and other foreign matter from wounds. A mild cleaning agent, such as Hibaclens® or Phisohex®, is recommended for especially dirty wounds.

With severe soft-tissue facial injuries, some tissue may look marginally viable; however, the blood supply to the face is so good, that it will usually survive. When excess tissue is debrided, however, good cosmetic repair may be extremely difficult.

AXIOM   In all facial soft-tissue injuries, wound debridement should be conservative.

Most dog bites of the face can be closed after they are thoroughly cleaned and debrided. Human bites are never closed primarily. These should be cleansed, debrided, and dressed, and after proper wound care and antibiotics for several days, they can usually be closed.

With deep abrasions or partial-thickness loss of skin, the bleeding dermis is usually readily apparent. These areas need to be cleansed and then covered with an antibiotic ointment or an oil-based dressing. Many patients with roadside injuries will have "road burns" with traumatic tattooing secondary to asphalt, tar, or dirt becoming imbedded in the abrasions. Unless this foreign material is removed within 24-48 hours, it can cause permanent pigmentation of the skin; if the debris were allowed to become trapped in the resultant scar, a formal dermabrasion would be needed later. Removing debris embedded in the skin requires adequate local or general anesthesia. A sterile scrub brush can be very helpful for removing these particles. If the particles are deeply imbedded, they may be picked out with a No. 11 blade. Ether or benzene can be used to remove embedded grease. Prompt reepithelialization of these deeply abraded areas usually occurs within 10 days.

Repair of Lacerations

SCALP

The dense fascia surrounding scalp vessels retards proper contraction of cut arteries and veins, and copious bleeding from such wounds is common.[25] When hemostasis is a problem in hair-bearing areas of the scalp, a continuous nylon suture encompassing all layers will usually control the bleeding readily. In general, much less blood will be lost when a continuous suture is inserted immediately than if attempts were made to clamp and tie bleeding vessels. Where debridement is required, incisions should be bevelled parallel to the hair follicles to avoid secondary alopecia.[76]

FACE

AXIOM   Open facial lacerations tend to appear larger than they really are.

Edema and bleeding can cause the edges of facial lacerations to gape far apart, and make it appear as if tissue is missing; however, this is rarely the case. By finding the proper matching points to bring together, such wounds can usually be closed adequately. Although it is true that the rich blood supply of the face will usually allow partially devascularized torn edges of facial wounds to survive, the cosmetic appearance will often be suboptimal secondary to excessive scarring. Ideally, the edges should be debrided of injured tissue until the wound edge is perpendicular to the skin surface. In most cases, this means an elliptical excision of the wound. Although this technique is not possible in some areas of the face where there is limited tissue, it is particularly applicable to the cheek and forehead.

Frequently, the direction of the laceration will determine the direction of the excision; however, in irregular or circular wounds, there is some leeway in the direction of the final scar. It is critically important to visualize the relaxed skin tension lines of the face and to make the wounds parallel to them if possible (Fig. 13–15). In this way, the scar will blend in better with natural skin creases, there will

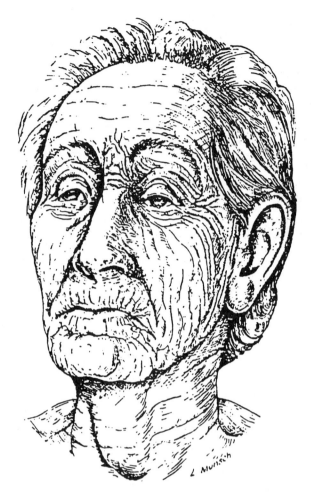

FIGURE 13–15   The lines of minimal tension of the face and neck. (From: Converse JM. Kazanjian and Converse's surgical treatment of facial injuries. Baltimore: Williams and Wilkins, 1974; 42.)

be less tension on the scar, and it is less likely to become hypertrophic.

Absorbable subcutaneous and dermal sutures are initially placed to line up the edges and to relieve tension on the skin closure. These sutures should be placed in a buried, simple fashion so that the knots will not be close to the epidermis. The skin is then closed with a fine, nonabsorbable, nonreactive suture.

AXIOM   Using small sutures is not the essence of a plastic repair; proper technique is.

If small sutures are taken too close to the edge, they will cut through and leave an indented, irregular edge. There is no role for mattress sutures on the face. Simple skin sutures placed properly by taking more tissue in the deeper portion of the wound than superficially will give the slight amount of eversion that is necessary for an optimal result. Eversion is necessary because a perfectly flat repair will become depressed when the inevitable scar contraction occurs. Depressed scars look worse because the irregularity causes harsh shadows to appear; consequently, the scar is more noticeable. When the wound is slightly everted initially, it will usually flatten out somewhat as the scar contracts and result in a much more cosmetically pleasing scar.

PITFALL ⊘

Repairing skin wounds without slight eversion. A repair that is initially flat will become depressed with time, and the scar will be more obvious.

Complex Wounds

Stellate lacerations, traumatic flaps, lacerations made at sharp angles, and actual tissue loss may appear to pose special problems, but the same techniques used on simple lacerations apply here as well. Wound edges and tips of flaps are debrided until healthy perpendicular skin edges remain. Except in areas close to the lips, eyelid, and nasal tip, such debridement usually leaves enough tissue for closure without tension. Occasionally, the skin must be freed up from the deep subcutaneous tissue to allow the skin edges to be brought together without tension.

Where there is extensive tissue loss from an avulsion injury and primary closure is not possible, adequate cleansing and debridement is done, the wound is dressed and the patient is referred to a plastic surgeon for special treatment. Such wounds may require skin grafts or flap repairs; however, this circumstance is the exception.

For the so-called "windshield wounds" which usually involve the forehead, multiple wounds cut at sharp angles may be present. These wounds should be carefully examined for foreign matter because small pieces of glass are often present. These wounds should also be excised to give clean, perpendicular wound edges which can then be closed primarily.

Complete or partial scalp loss may occur when the hair and scalp are avulsed by spinning machinery.[25] Any sizeable avulsed segment of scalp that is retrieved should be considered for microsurgical replantation. When this is not possible, rotation flaps can be used to close small defects. If the periosteum is intact, a split skin graft can be used to cover any residual defects.[77] The alopecia resulting from such skin grafting can be corrected by a secondary procedure using tissue expansion techniques on the remaining scalp.

Special Areas

Lacerations of certain areas of the face must be repaired meticulously, preferably in the operating room where the lighting, equipment, and assistance are the best.

LIPS

Lacerations through the cutaneous vermilion border of the lips require special consideration. The first suture should be placed at this boundary to precisely line up the skin and vermilion so that there is a smooth, continuous line throughout the border (Fig. 13–16). Being off by even a fraction of a millimeter can make the defect very noticeable, and such defects often require secondary repair. After this key suture is placed, the deeper sutures can be placed. It is especially important that the orbicularis oris muscle continuity be restored with deep sutures.

NASAL RIM

For nasal rim lacerations, a key suture is placed at the lower border of the alar rim to ensure a continuous, smooth line without notching. Without perfect approximation, an annoying and unsightly notch results.

HELICAL RIM

The key suture for repair of the helix of the external ear is placed at the outer rim to prevent notching. The underlying cartilage must also be carefully approximated for optimal results.

EYELID

A full-thickness laceration through an eyelid requires meticulous technique. Although relatively complicated repairs have been recommended, the simplest is usually the best. The key suture is placed through the ciliary margin at the "gray line" which is the border of the tarsus and orbicularis. Two additional sutures are then placed, first through the tarsus and then through the orbicularis muscle at the ciliary margin. Once the lid margin is repaired, the orbicularis muscle and skin are closed in layers. No conjunctival repair is necessary. Lacerations at the medial lid margin must be inspected for canalicular

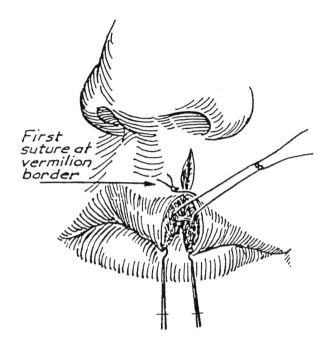

FIGURE 13–16 Repair of vertical lacerations of the vermilion-cutaneous margin. The first suture should be used to approximate the vermilion-cutaneous border. This will avoid conspicuous irregularity of this portion of the lip following healing. (From: Converse JM. Kazanjian and Converse's surgical treatment of facial Iijuries. Baltimore: Williams and Wilkins, 1974; 641.)

injury. The canaliculus is probed; if it is lacerated, it is repaired over a stent utilizing an operating microscope.

PAROTID DUCT

A transected parotid duct should be repaired in the operating room. The buccal branches of the facial nerve are also often involved and should be explored and repaired as necessary. The duct is repaired over a stent brought out through its buccal opening. Utilizing the operating microscope or loupe magnification, 8-0 monofilament suture is usually adequate.

FACIAL NERVE

It is easiest to repair facial nerve lacerations at the time of injury in the operating room using a microscope and microsurgical monofilament suture; however, if microsurgical expertise were not available, the wound should be closed and the patient referred to a plastic surgeon.

Facial nerve repairs done within 2-3 weeks of injury generally provide the same results as early repair. If a facial nerve laceration is missed for a longer period of time, the nerve ends will contract and make later apposition impossible. With this occurrence, later repairs usually require a nerve graft and produce results that are much inferior to those of primary repairs.

The temporal and zygomatic branches are most likely to be injured by lacerations at the lateral eyebrow and zygoma. The buccal branch is usually cut in the mid-cheek, and the marginal mandibular branch is generally injured at the mandibular margin. Because the marginal mandibular branch normally depresses the corner of the mouth, the side with the injured mandibular branch remains elevated after the rest of the face has relaxed.

TREATMENT OF FACIAL FRACTURES

General

There has been a virtual revolution in the treatment of facial fractures following the introduction and application of craniofacial surgery begun by Paul Tessier over 20 years ago. Within the past decade, techniques utilizing wide, direct exposure of fracture sites combined with rigid miniplate fixation and immediate cranial bone grafting have made the most complex facial fractures amenable to primary repair. This obviates the need for extremely difficult secondary reconstruction with its usual inferior results.

Contemporary facial fracture repair is characterized by: (a) precise preoperative imaging of fractures;[13] (b) precise preoperative plans of bony reconstruction; (c) early one-stage repair whenever possible; (d) adequate exposure of all fractures, using "degloving" of the entire facial skeleton as necessary;[14] (e) precise reduction of all fractures in three dimensions using immediate bone grafts as needed; and (f) rigid interosseous fixation, particularly with self-tapping miniplates.

These advances, however, have not supplanted two basic principles of facial bone repair.[25] First, the teeth must be returned to their normal occlusal relationship. Second, the repair proceeds from an unbroken or a stabilized segment to an adjacent fracture fragment which is reduced and then rigidly fixed to the adjacent stable bone. In this way, multiple fractures are repaired in a stepwise fashion, each fixed segment being used to align and stabilize the next.

AXIOM   If a plastic surgeon with craniofacial capabilities is not present, one has 7-10 days to transfer the patient for proper primary treatment.

Contrary to previous beliefs, new experience in craniofacial surgery has shown that facial fractures heal by osseous rather than fibrous union. Secondary procedures requiring involved formal osteotomies are best avoided by prompt recognition and treatment of the fractures. Facial fractures can generally be treated easily within 10 days of injury; however, after two weeks, enough healing may occur so that osteotomies may be necessary to loosen or refracture and then realign the fracture fragments. In children, the healing rate is more rapid, and primary repairs should be performed within the first week.

In some centers, maxillofacial injuries are treated immediately after CT evaluation of the face when no associated injuries exist or when the associated injuries do not interfere with hemodynamic stability.[43] Although definitive facial reconstructions can be performed during emergent repair of associated injuries, most maxillofacial injuries can wait at least 6-10 days without deleterious effects on the outcome of the repair, provided that the soft-tissue injuries are treated and intermaxillary fixation is applied.

Intermaxillary fixation involves closed reduction of the mandibular and maxillary fractures and fixation of the jaws with wires passing through arch bars attached to the upper and lower teeth. In edentulous persons, a prosthesis is placed over the gums to provide fixation. These procedures can usually be done under local anesthesia or regional nerve block in the emergency department without subjecting the patient to the risks of general anesthesia.

Mandible

CLASSIFICATION

Mandible fractures are classified according to the region involved into parasymphyseal, body, angle, ramus, condyle, and coronoid process fractures. Bilateral fractures are common and should always be suspected. Obvious fractures of the mandible body should not distract the physician from a careful examination of the condyles because contralateral condyle fractures are frequently seen.

FRACTURE DISPLACEMENTS

The directional displacement of mandibular fracture fragments will be determined by the line of the fracture and the pull of the attached muscles. The posterior mandible fragment, which is acted on by the powerful "muscles of mastication" (masseter, temporalis, and the medial and lateral pterygoids) will be displaced upward and forward. The anterior mandible fragment, which is acted on by the depressor muscles (geniohyoid, genioglossus, mylohyoid, and anterior digastric), will be moved inferiorly and posteriorly. In bilateral fractures,

particularly in the subcondylar area, the mandible will override and shorten, and the posterior teeth will meet prematurely, creating an open bite anteriorly. Failure to reduce the mandible and bring the teeth into proper occlusion can lead to malocclusion, deformity, and possible TMJ dysfunction. This may necessitate formal mandibular osteotomies and orthodontic surgery.

PITFALL ⊘

Failure to reduce a mandible to a proper occlusal relationship can lead to severe anatomical and functional problems with the jaws.

STABLE FRACTURES

One of the first decisions to make with mandibular fractures is whether they are stable or unstable. A stable fracture may be managed in a closed fashion by bringing the teeth into centric occlusion and then holding the mandible in place with arch bars or interdental wiring. Thus, the maxilla is used as a physiologic splint for four to six weeks.

REGIONAL ANESTHESIA

In cooperative patients, arch bars or interdental wiring can be applied under regional anesthesia with some sedation.[1] Regional anesthesia for intermaxillary fixation includes blocks of the inferior alveolar and greater palatine nerves. Supraorbital, nasal, infraorbital, maxillary, and mandibular blocks may also be employed to repair concomitant facial lacerations. These blocks are often supplemented by topical or local anesthesia. Infiltration of the mucosa with local anesthesia helps to ensure complete analgesia during intraoral procedures. When epinephrine is added, hemostasis is also improved.

UNSTABLE FRACTURES

Unstable fractures cannot be treated simply with arch bars or interdental wiring as there will be movement at the fracture site despite the presence of the interdental fixation. The deciding factor is the obliquity of the fracture line and the pull of muscles attaching to the segments. For example, a fracture of the mandible body, which occurs forward and upward, is displaced by the attached muscles. Occasionally, the presence of a molar tooth keeps a potentially unstable fracture from moving, and a stable reduction may be achieved with simple intermaxillary fixation alone.

Mandible fractures that must be opened are approached through lower labial buccal sulcus incisions for fractures of the symphysis and body and either oral or cutaneous incisions for fractures of the angle and ramus. If an external approach were used, care should be taken to avoid injuring the marginal mandibular branch of the facial nerve. An intraoral approach avoids this risk, but reducing the fragments with this approach can be very difficult without special maxillofacial instruments. Fixation of these fractures classically consists of simple wiring of the fragments together combined with intermaxillary fixation.

Mandible fractures can also be treated by another approach, which is now preferred, using fixation with special miniplates and screws.[78-79] This can provide rigid, stable fixation, and intermaxillary fixation can be avoided. It is critically important, however, that the patient's pretraumatic dental occlusion be reestablished first with interdental fixation. This is followed by rigid fixation of the other fragments with plates. When plates are used and normal centric occlusion can be maintained with the plates alone, the interdental fixation can be removed in the operating room. An intact tooth present in the fracture site should be left in place; however, a fractured tooth should be removed.

PITFALL ⊘

Failure to obtain centric occlusion with intermaxillary fixation before fracture fixation of the remaining fragments can result in severe malocclusion.

SPECIAL AREAS

Condyle Fractures

Although considerable controversy exists, the vast majority of condyle fractures can be managed by the reestablishment of centric occlusion and intermaxillary fixation. Unusual condyle fractures with dislocation into the middle cranial fossa or severe displacement, often require an open approach.

Parasymphyseal Fractures

The depressor group of muscles tends to cause lingual displacement of parasymphyseal fracture fragments, even in the presence of intermaxillary fixation. To obviate this problem, interdental fixation can be combined with a fabricated lingual splint and wire fixation. A simpler approach is rigid-plate fixation through a lower labial-buccal sulcus incision. Following proper plate fixation, the arch bars can be removed in the operating room.

Coronoid Fractures

A simple coronoid fracture will be displaced by the temporalis muscle but will not affect occlusion. The only treatment usually required is a soft diet.

THE EDENTULOUS MANDIBLE

Proper occlusion of a fractured edentulous mandible is reestablished by using intermaxillary fixation to maintain the position of the patient's dentures, when they are available. When dentures are not available, appropriate splints are fabricated and secured to the maxilla and mandible using wires. Centric occlusion is then established and intermaxillary fixation is achieved. Another approach places the maxilla and mandible into approximate occlusion, reduces the fracture fragments, and then fixates them with rigid miniplates. Discrepancies in occlusion may be repaired later when the patient is fitted for new dentures.

EXTERNAL FIXATION

Before the advent of plate fixation, severely comminuted mandibular fractures occasionally necessitated the use of an external fixation device (e.g., Morris biphasic fixation appliance). Even now, if plate fixation were contraindicated, the use of an external fixation device could be extremely helpful in instances of gunshot or shotgun wounds with severe soft-tissue damage or deficiencies, where infection is much more likely.

Centric occlusion is reestablished first and then soft-tissue and oral-lining deficiencies can be addressed with appropriate flaps. Once this is accomplished and the external fixator is applied, mandibular bone grafting and rigid fixation can be undertaken later as needed.

Maxillary Fractures

CLASSIFICATION

The classification system used for maxillary fractures generally follows the work of Rene LeFort (Figs. 13–8, 13–9). Although this system refers primarily to the maxilla, LeFort I fractures also involve the sphenoid bone, LeFort II fractures also involve the sphenoid, nasal, ethmoid, and lacrimal bones. In LeFort III fractures, all of these bones and the zygoma are involved. Sagittal fractures of the maxilla are much less common than LeFort fractures because they occur parallel to the nasomaxillary, zygomaticomaxillary, and pterygomaxillary buttresses rather than through them. They may involve just the maxilla, passing into the pyriform aperture and through the palate. Sagittal fractures may, however, occur more laterally and extend into the orbit.

DISTORTIONS PRESENT

Fractures of the maxilla are usually associated with edema, ecchymosis, and malocclusion; however, malocclusion may be slight. Because no strong muscle attachments exist, maxillary fragments generally displace in the direction of the causative force. Although classically a LeFort III fracture is displaced downward and backward, causing a "dishface" and malocclusion, occasionally the maxilla is impacted superiorly or rotated in such a way as to cause significant displacement superiorly but with minimal malocclusion.

SUSPENSION WIRES OR NONOPERATIVE TREATMENT

AXIOM Treatment of maxillary fractures attempts to reestablish centric occlusion and reconstruct associated injuries.

Because a maxillary fracture may be associated with significant comminution, simple reduction with intermaxillary fixation and craniofacial suspension wires can lead to midfacial shortening and an anterior open bite, particularly if the suspension wires were placed too anteriorly. If such maxillary shortening were allowed to persist, it would be particularly difficult to correct secondarily. If nasal and orbital fractures associated with LeFort II and III fractures were not adequately reduced and fixated, severe secondary deformities could occur from untreated or inadequately treated nasoethmoid and orbital floor fractures.

AXIOM All LeFort fractures should be explored and accurately reduced under direct vision.

OPERATIVE REDUCTION

Maxillary fractures are usually inspected initially through an upper labial-buccal sulcus incision. For LeFort I fractures, the teeth are placed into intermaxillary fixation and the fracture fixed with miniplates across the buttresses. In some cases, the comminution is so severe that bone grafts are used to reconstruct the buttresses and anterior maxilla in order to prevent maxillary shortening. After adequate fixation is secured, the intermaxillary fixation is released. Miniplate fixation is generally so stable that interdental fixation is not required postoperatively.

For LeFort II and III fractures, incisions are made in the lower lids to explore the zygomatic-maxillary sutures, orbital floor, and medial orbital wall. Additionally, a coronal incision is made in the anterior scalp and the upper face is degloved to expose the nasofrontal region and also the zygomatic arch in LeFort III fractures. In this way, the displaced segments can be reduced into anatomic position and secured with miniplates.

When the maxillary fracture is associated with a nasoethmoid fracture, bone grafts from the outer table of the skull may be necessary to restore proper nasal projection. In addition, lateral displacement of the medial canthi in the nasoethmoid component causes a telecanthus. In this circumstance, the medial canthi are found through the coronal incision and secured medially with wire sutures.

PITFALL ⊘

Failure to recognize and properly treat a comminuted maxillary fracture may lead to a shortened face which is difficult to correct secondarily.

SAGITTAL FRACTURES

Sagittal fractures of the maxilla are explored through upper labial buccal sulcus incisions. An arch bar is placed on the maxilla and then cut where the sagittal fracture has occurred. Intermaxillary fixation (IMF) is then established with the mandible. When satisfactory occlusion is established, the reduction is secured with a miniplate across the sagittal fracture line. In addition, a palatal splint may be required to prevent lingual rotation of the lateral segments. Associated orbital fractures are also explored, reduced, and fixated as needed. If wires rather than plates were used to fixate the fracture fragments, IMF would need to be maintained for four to six weeks.

ALVEOLAR FRACTURES

With alveolar fractures, the maxilla is placed into intermaxillary fixation. After proper centric occlusion has been established, only the maxillary arch bar is needed to keep the segment in position, and a soft diet is prescribed for four weeks. With very unstable alveolar segments or with noncompliant patients, complete intermaxillary fixation is maintained for four weeks.

Zygomatic Fractures

Zygomatic fractures can be divided into simple arch fractures and those involving the entire zygoma, so-called "tripod fractures" (Fig. 13–17). Fractures of the zygomatic arch are usually caused by a direct blow. The arch usually fractures in at least two locations and becomes depressed. The depressed zygomatic arch impinges against the coronoid process of the mandible and will limit mandibular motion.

Although the overlying swelling and hematoma may obscure the bony depression, it is readily palpable. Unlike most facial fractures, the arch can simply be elevated into position and generally does not need internal fixation.

The zygomatic arch is approached through a Gillies's incision at the temporal scalp, and an elevator is passed underneath the deep temporal fascia. Staying on top of the temporalis muscle leads to the undersurface of the arch. Arch fragments are elevated into position and when the reduced fragments appear to be stable, the wound is closed.

Occasionally the arch cannot maintain its reduction without some form of fixation. Under such circumstances, the arch is explored directly through a coronal scalp incision. The upper face is degloved exposing the deep temporal fascia, and the arch fragments are then wired directly after being accurately reduced under direct vision.

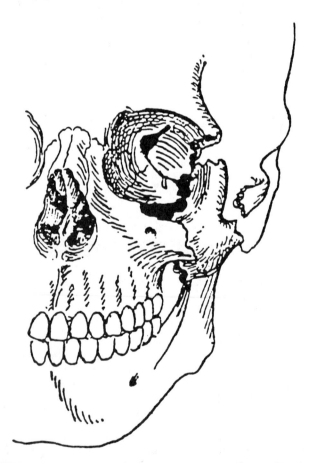

FIGURE 13–17 Fractures involving the entire zygoma are often called tripod fractures because of the presence of three fracture lines: zygomaticomaxillary, zygomaticofrontal, and zygomatic arch. (From: Converse JM. Kazanjian and Converse's surgical treatment of facial injuries. Baltimore: Williams and Wilkins, 1974; 714.)

After reduction, displaced zygoma "tripod" fractures generally cannot predictably maintain their position without fixation. Therefore, the zygomaticomaxillary suture is exposed through a lower eyelid incision and the zygomaticofrontal suture is exposed through an upper eyelid or brow incision. The zygoma is then reduced and fixed with miniplates. When wire is used for fixation, an additional third point of fixation is chosen at the zygomaticomaxillary buttress through an upper labial-buccal sulcus incision. Because "tripod" fractures also include an orbital floor fracture, the floor of the orbit is routinely explored through the lower lid incision at the time of zygoma reduction.

PITFALL ⊘

Simple reduction of zygoma "tripod" fractures without adequate fixation will often lead to displacement and significant deformity.

Orbital Floor Fractures

ETIOLOGY

When blunt force is suddenly transmitted to the eye, both the thin floor and medial wall may "blow out" to relieve the pressure on the globe. Although these are classically described as blow out fractures, many orbital floor fractures actually result from buckling of the floor through a transmitted force applied to the inferior rim.

DIAGNOSIS

The orbital asymmetry with orbital floor fractures may be apparent, and the globe may be inferiorly displaced as compared with the normal side. This will limit upward gaze, but limitation of upward gaze may occur even when true entrapment of the inferior rectus muscle is absent. Enophthalmos may also occur because of the movement of orbital contents into the maxillary or ethmoid sinuses. Less specific signs and symptoms of orbital fractures include diplopia and hypesthesia or anesthesia in the distribution of the infraorbital nerve over the cheek and nasolabial fold.

Plain radiography often does not show orbital floor fractures well, but the maxillary sinus may be opacified. Coronal CT, however, shows the orbital floor very well.

TREATMENT

Enophthalmos or impaired eye motion are clear indications for operative reduction of orbital fractures. Even in the absence of these indications for exploration, a significant floor fracture with herniation of orbital contents should be explored because of the strong likelihood of resultant late enophthalmos. Small floor fractures without limitation of upward gaze, enophthalmos, or inferior displacement of the globe or herniation on CT can be treated without surgery; however, the patient should be followed closely to detect any delayed diplopia or enophthalmos.

Explorations of the orbital floor are performed through a lower lid incision. The full extent of the defect is outlined by reflection of the periosteum of the orbital floor. The orbital contents are returned to the orbit. The optic foramen is located superiorly and medially and is, on average, 45 millimeters from the orbital rim. Dissection is safe when kept within 30 mm of the anterior orbital rim.

Much variation occurs in the techniques used to reconstruct the orbital floor. There is an increasing tendency to use of autogenous material in all facial fracture reconstructions and outer table cranial bone grafts to graft the orbital floor. Although alloplastic material (e.g., silastic sheath), can be used, bone grafts are preferred, particularly when orbital volume must be augmented. The medial wall should be explored because concomitant fractures are common.

PITFALL ⊘

Failure to identify and treat the full extent of an orbital floor fracture will probably result in late enophthalmos.

Nasal Fractures

Of all the facial bones, the nasal bones are fractured most frequently. Nasal fractures are generally the result of direct trauma and are frequently associated with fractures of other bones within the nasal pyramid. The dorsum of the nose may be impacted in a posterior direction and/or displaced to either side. There is usually an obvious deformity, but it may be obscured by developing edema.

The nasal septum should be inspected in all nasal fractures for a septal hematoma which is evacuated, if present, preferably through a small incision rather than aspiration with a needle and syringe.

Reduction of displaced nasal bones is done using Ashe forceps under local anesthesia but the edema that is usually present can make judging the adequacy of the reduction extremely difficult, and a secondary open reduction is not infrequently necessary for residual deformity. A plaster or preformed splint is then applied for one week.

When the patient is examined after a significant amount of edema has already developed, primary reduction may not be possible. In such patients, after the edema has subsided, the nasal bones are refractured and reduced through intranasal incisions.

Despite the frequency of nasal fractures, diagnosis and treatment are not always satisfactory.[25] A review by Barrs and Darn[80] of patients treated for nasal trauma revealed that only about 20% had nasoscopic examination in the emergency department.

Even with correct diagnosis, the results of closed reduction of nasal fractures are not uniformly good. On late evaluation about a third of patients have persistent deformities on late evaluation. In addition, about half of the patients who had a closed reduction performed acutely will have airway problems secondary to nasal septal deviation.[77]

AXIOM Careful follow-up of patients with closed reductions of nasal fractures is important to detect significant residual bony or septal deformities.

Frontonasoethmoid Fractures

Cruse et al.[41] reported the incidence of frontonasoethmoid fractures to be surprisingly high. In addition, patients with these fractures rarely had isolated injuries. Nearly 100% had associated infraorbital rim or orbital floor fractures, and 70% had maxillary complex fractures. Luce[26] reported that 30% of these patients also had severe ocular injuries.

Significant sequelae of these injuries include: (a) traumatic telecanthus, (b) ocular injuries, (c) CSF rhinorrhea, (d) injury to the nasolacrimal apparatus, and (e) depressed nasal dorsum with inward telescoping of the nose.[77] Fracture of the nasal and ethmoid bones with posterior and lateral displacement tends to increase the distance between the medial canthi. Direct trauma or displacement of the medial orbital walls may also cause ocular injury. Disruption of the nasolacrimal apparatus may occur from direct injury or from impingement by bony fracture fragments.[81] A "saddle nose" may result from comminution of the nasal dorsum or the loss of dorsal support plus elevation of the nasal tip. CSF rhinorrhea may result from fractures extending into the base of the skull at the cribriform plate.

AXIOM Nasoethmoid fractures should be accurately reduced under direct vision, preferably through a coronal degloving scalp and face incision.

Simple reduction of the nasoethmoid complex, which is frequently severely comminuted, will not result in stability and the canthi will remain displaced. Consequently, these fractures should be explored through a coronal degloving incision so that the nasoethmoid segment can be reduced to its proper anterior position. Frequently, comminution makes this type of reduction impractical, and the nasal dorsum is then bone grafted to restore dorsal projection and nasal length. Following this, bilateral medial canthoplasties are performed and the medial walls of the orbit are bone grafted as needed.

A CSF leak associated with these fractures is usually initially managed by elevation of the head until the fractures are repaired. Eighty percent of these CSF leaks cease in two weeks and 90% in three weeks. Although it is controversial, most patients are placed on intravenous antibiotics. Edgerton and Kenney reported that use of broad-spectrum antibiotics during CSF leakage appeared to decrease the danger of meningitis.[37]

AXIOM A CSF leak is no reason to postpone treatment of facial fractures. In fact, reduction of facial fractures may stop the leak.

According to some clinicians, reduction of facial fractures during CSF rhinorrhea promotes meningitis.[1] Others believe that positive-pressure ventilation by mask facilitates the development of meningeal infection but no clear evidence for these suppositions exists.

Accurate reduction of frontonasoethmoid fractures is essential when a CSF leak is present; however, when the CSF leak persists for more than three weeks neurosurgical intervention with dural repair should be strongly considered. The incidence of meningitis in patients with CSF rhinorrhea varies from 9-36%.[70] The mortality from this complication is also variable, ranging in published reports from 1-20%.

Persistent CSF leakage is often treated conservatively unless the following conditions exist: (a) large amounts of CSF are draining, (b) drainage is from the cribriform plate and/or posterior ethmoid/sphenoid region, (c) the site of fistula is uncertain or multiple, or (d) the leak is associated with pneumocephalus.[70] Evaluation of the involved craniofacial region with CT is invaluable in assessing these conditions and deciding among therapeutic choices.

Surgery for persistent CSF leaks involves patching the fistulous tract with a fascia lata graft and covering any bony defects with hammered muscle.[70] This procedure is performed by either craniotomy or a transethmoid/sphenoid approach. Accompanying frontal sinus fractures are also treated.

Occasionally the orbital floor is also fractured, and better exposure of this injury is obtained through lower eyelid incisions. Although frequently injured, nasolacrimal duct obstruction is uncommon; when it occurs late, it is treated with a secondary dacryocystorhinostomy.

Frontal Sinus Fractures

Frontal sinus fractures are usually noted on plain radiographic examination and are clearly delineated by CT. Fractures involving only the anterior table are treated if they are displaced. The segments are reduced through a coronal incision or accompanying facial lacerations and wired in place. Unless the mucosa is extensively damaged, no treatment is necessary.

Fractures involving the anterior and posterior tables of the frontal sinus are explored. Significant posterior table fractures may lead to CSF rhinorrhea because of dural injury, and neurosurgical support should be readily available. When the mucosa is severely injured, it is completely stripped from the sinus cavity and the sinus is obliterated. Classically, fat and muscle have been used to obliterate the cavity with good results, but the author prefers outer table cranial grafts.

In severe frontal sinus fractures with comminution, the sinus is cranialized by stripping the mucosa, removing the remains of the posterior table and then the anterior table and the frontal sinus duct outlet are bone grafted. The dura and frontal lobes are then allowed to fill the cavity.

Panfacial Fractures

The treatment of isolated facial fractures is facilitated by adjacent normal anatomy. When multiple adjacent facial fractures are present, the problems are greatly compounded (Fig. 13–18). A well-ordered plan combined with craniofacial techniques, including direct exposure, liberal bone grafting, and miniplate fixation is the only satisfactory approach for these difficult fractures.

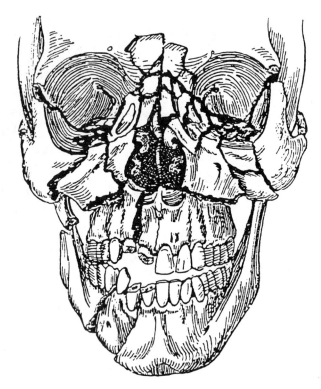

FIGURE 13–18 Panfacial fractures. This drawing shows multiple fractures involving all of the facial bones. (From: Converse JM. Kazanjian and Converse's surgical treatment of facial injuries. Baltimore: Williams and Wilkins, 1974; 733.)

AXIOM   Rigid fixation and liberal use of bone grafts to preserve facial volume and height are particularly important in panfacial fractures.

A systematic approach to reducing and fixing panfacial fractures is essential. First, the mandibular fractures are reduced and fixed. Next, the maxilla is related to the mandible with intermaxillary fixation. The maxilla is then bone grafted and fixated as necessary. The zygoma is then repaired to the maxilla, paying particular attention to the preservation of facial volume at the zygomatic arches. The orbital floor and walls are then bone grafted, and the nasoethmoid and frontal sinuses are repaired.

If the mandible were badly comminuted, facial reconstruction would begin at the zygomatic arch. Remaining nondisplaced zygomatic processes of the temporal bone are good starting points from which to rebuild a zygoma. The maxilla is then related to the zygoma and fixed, and then the frontal bone fractures are repaired. The mandible is then reduced by bringing it into intermaxillary fixation with the reduced and fixated maxilla and then the fracture sites of the mandible are fixed.

PITFALL ⊘

Failure to preserve facial volume with bone grafts and rigid fixation results in secondary deformities which can be extremely difficult to reconstruct.

Without aggressive primary treatment utilizing craniofacial exposure and use of rigid fixation and bone grafts, secondary deformities are common in serious facial fractures; however, even "simple" facial fractures may result in severe deformities if appropriate techniques are not used. With the inevitable soft-tissue contracture that occurs in severe facial injuries, failure to maintain bony volume initially can lead to deformities which can

be extremely difficult to reconstruct even with craniofacial techniques.

AXIOM   The best chance of providing an excellent result with facial fractures is during the initial reduction and fixation.

Facial Fractures in Children

Facial fractures are infrequent in children and comprise only 1-5% of all maxillofacial injuries in most major series;[1,44,82] however, in a recent retrospective study, 14.5% of maxillofacial injuries occurred in children less than 17 years of age.[83] The frequency of this injury decreases to 1% in children less than five years of age.

The highly resilient facial bones of children are often able to withstand significant trauma without fracture or, in many instances, with only greenstick fractures. The three-to-one male-to-female predominance characteristic of adult maxillofacial trauma[52] is not evident in young children; in this age group, male predominance is only slight (60% to 40%).[83]

In the pediatric population, the etiology of maxillofacial injury is similar to that of adults except that in children, motor-vehicle-pedestrian accidents replace altercations as the greatest cause.[83] The pediatric maxillofacial injury victim is also more prone than adults to have other injuries, especially of the head, extremities, and soft tissues.[1]

Children tend to sustain mandibular rather than maxillary injuries.[1] Midface fractures occur in pediatric patients, but they are seen mostly in older children and at a significantly lower rate than mandibular fractures.[83] This is largely due to the relatively small size of the pediatric maxilla and the lack of pneumatization of the maxillary sinuses.

As compared to adults, mandibular fractures in children are more likely to occur at a single site. Unlike adults, pediatric mandibular fractures are generally not displaced by muscle pull because of elasticity of the bone, the developing tooth buds, and the high incidence of greenstick fractures.[84]

The mandibular condyle is a common site of fracture in children,[85] probably because it contains a higher proportion of medullary bone to cortex.[86] These fractures can easily be overlooked because of physician inexperience and diversion of attention to more obvious injuries, such as lacerations and abrasions.[85]

AXIOM   Condylar fractures should be suspected in children presenting with laceration of the chin and fractures of the symphysis or body of the mandible.[85]

In children, facial fractures, especially those close to suture lines, may result in arrest of bone growth.[1] The rapid bone growth of the contralateral side of the face can result in severe facial deformity. This complication may also arise from rapid healing and malunion when treatment of the fracture is delayed or absent.[37]

AXIOM   In pediatric patients, the impact of severe trauma on subsequent facial growth must be carefully monitored and the patient and family advised accordingly.[84]

Diagnosis of maxillofacial injuries in children can be difficult.[1] The apprehension of the child and the anxiety of the parents can make a good physical examination extremely difficult. Complaints, such as pain and malocclusion, can also be difficult for children to express, especially when they are young. Obtaining the patient's cooperation for radiographic studies may also be a problem in this age group. Even with cooperation, the complex anatomy of the small pediatric mandible—which contains multiple tooth buds, a relatively small amount of cortical bone, and a probable greenstick fracture—makes interpretation difficult. Thus, CT evaluation is invaluable for both mandibular and maxillary fractures in this age group. In adults, CT evaluations are usually necessary only for middle and upper facial fractures.[1] Sometimes, the physical examination may need to be performed under general anesthesia to diagnose these injuries properly in children.[37]

AXIOM Generally, the simplest fixation will be the best for most facial bone fractures in children.

The treatment principles of maxillofacial injury in pediatric patients differs somewhat from those of adults.[1] Intermaxillary fixation is maintained for a shorter time than in adults. Early mobilization of the jaw is the mainstay of treatment because long periods of immobilization can result in ankylosis, especially with condylar or subcondylar fractures.[86] The dentition of many pediatric patients is not appropriate for application of arch bars and interdental wire fixation. Deciduous teeth, mixed dentition, and small permanent teeth make such treatment difficult. Therefore, open reduction and internal fixation under general anesthesia shortly after injury are considered the treatment of choice by many surgeons.

IMMEDIATE POSTOPERATIVE CARE

The airway is rarely a serious problem following reduction and fixation of facial fractures, particularly with the use of rigid plate fixation which makes intermaxillary fixation unnecessary. Nevertheless, the endotracheal tube should be left in place at the conclusion of surgery while soft-tissue swelling is evaluated, airway reflexes return, and the patient recovers fully from the anesthetic.[1] Dexamethasone, 4-8 mg intravenously, may help to diminish soft-tissue edema.

AXIOM If intermaxillary fixation is used, a wire cutter should be taped to the patient's chest until full recovery from the anesthetic and surgery.

If intermaxillary fixation were used, a wire cutter should be taped to the patient's chest for immediate release of the wires in case of airway obstruction with blood clot or vomitus, laryngeal spasm, or soft-tissue intrusion on the airway. If one of these problems were to occur, however, only two to four of the wires in the patient's mouth would need to be cut to provide an adequate airway. Identification of these wires, however, can be difficult for individuals who are not involved in surgical management.[87] Covering these key wires to be cut in an emergency with colored rubber or plastic or leaving them long facilitates emergency jaw release.[88]

Postoperatively, attention also is directed to prevention of infection with appropriate antibiotics, adequate nutrition with liquid formulas in patients with intermaxillary fixation, follow-up radiographic studies to ensure optimal fragment alignment, and jaw exercises to prevent ankylosis of TMJ.[1]

OUTCOME

Mortality

Maxillofacial injuries seldom are life-threatening; death is usually due to associated injuries. In a study from Europe only 84 (2.4%) of 3564 motor-vehicle-accident victims who died shortly after trauma had maxillofacial injuries.[89] In only 20 (24%) of these patients was maxillofacial injury believed to contribute to the fatality.[89] Hypoxia, the principal cause of death after maxillofacial trauma, is usually caused by a combination of head injury and massive blood aspiration rather than merely airway obstruction from displaced jaw fractures.[89]

Complications

INFECTION

Infection is an uncommon but important problem in patients with maxillofacial injury.[1] In addition to contamination of the CNS by oral microorganisms, infection in the vicinity of fracture sites can extend into the fascial planes of the face and neck and may even spread to distant sites, such as fractures in the extremities. Although rigid internal fixation (RIF) requires more extensive soft-tissue manipulation and bone exposure for plate application as well as increased operative time, RIF does not appear to contribute to increased postoperative infection rates in midfacial trauma.[90]

Fractures of the mandibular angle, body, or parasymphyseal region appear to have a higher infection rate than zygomatic and maxillary fractures, especially when they are open fractures and involve the teeth.[1,91] Surprisingly, delay of definitive surgical treatment does not appear to increase the infection rate. Prophylactic use of cefazolin, 1 gm intravenously, 1 hour before surgery, and a similar dose 8 hours later, has been shown to diminish the incidence of postoperative infections in facial fractures during electively performed definitive surgery.[91]

Wound infections with collections of pus are drained as needed. Osteomyelitis is uncommon, but when present, usually involves mandibular fractures. This may require debridement of a sequestrum, removal of hardware, and the application of an external fixation device. Late bone grafting may be necessary after the infection has been eradicated. In some instances, simultaneous debridement, reduction, and rigid internal fixation may also be a satisfactory method for treating mandibular fractures complicated by osteomyelitis.[92]

Extension of infection into the fascial planes of the head and neck a few days after a facial fracture may jeopardize the airway.[1] Such infections are characteristically caused by combinations of aerobic and anaerobic mouth organisms.[93] These infections can usually be adequately treated with 400,000 units of aqueous penicillin G every four hours for several days, drainage of the abscess, and further antibiotic therapy depending on the sensitivity of the specific organisms involved.

Tracheal intubation to secure the airway for abscess drainage is performed under direct vision using a fiberoptic bronchoscope with the patient sedated and awake.[1] Preoperative CT scans of the face and neck can help to determine the degree of airway encroachment.

AXIOM A coniotomy or tracheostomy under local anesthesia without attempts at endotracheal intubation is indicated when the patient's clinical condition or CT reveals severe airway compromise.

Concern about the possibility of infective endocarditis after elective dental procedures in patients at risk, such as those with valvular heart disease or prosthetic cardiac valves, has led to the development of an antibiotic prophylaxis protocol by the Committee on Rheumatic Fever and Infective Endocarditis of the American Heart Association.[1,94] These guidelines are largely aimed at preventing infective endocarditis in electively operated patients and may not necessarily prevent this complication in patients with acute maxillofacial injury because the dentition is damaged before antibiotics can be administered. Nevertheless, patients at risk should receive antibiotic prophylaxis as soon after the injury as possible.

For the last decade, an increasing number of injured patients have had concurrent surgery for repair of both facial and orthopedic injuries. The question has been raised whether these patients are at increased risk of orthopedic sepsis due to mouth organisms. Preliminary data suggest that preoperative use of a first-generation cephalosporin eradicates both mouth organisms and Staphylococcus aureus. In these patients, orthopedic sepsis is not likely when only one orthopedic and one oral surgical procedure are performed after injury;[95] however, in multiply-injured patients requiring more than one procedure, the initial cephalosporin may not be adequate. In these circumstances, throat cultures obtained 24 hours before subsequent surgery should reveal the organisms likely to be involved and permit selection of appropriate antibiotics.

NERVE INJURIES OR DYSFUNCTION

Nerve injury is usually due to the initial injury and is only rarely iatrogenic. The temporal branch of the facial nerve is occasionally stretched during the facial degloving incision and results in impaired frontalis function, but this is usually only a temporary problem.

SECONDARY DEFORMITIES

AXIOM Probably the most frequent complication of treatment of severe facial fractures is secondary deformities.

Although secondary facial deformities usually occur because of an inadequate initial operation, secondary reconstruction should be expected with very severe facial trauma. Furthermore, if modern techniques are used, such deformities usually tend to be less severe and more easily corrected.

SUMMARY

Facial injuries are frequent and errors in diagnoses and/or treatments producing poor cosmetic results can have tragic effects on patients and their relationships with others. One must not, however, be side-tracked by these often obvious injuries and thereby delay proper treatment of more life-threatening disorders. Even though a great reliance is placed on radiologic studies—especially CT scans—for diagnosis, a careful history and physical examination are still important for making some diagnoses and for obtaining optimal radiologic studies. Surgical techniques now allow adequate exposure and very accurate direct miniplate fixation of almost all facial fractures. It is apparent that the initial proper management of facial injuries by specially-trained surgeons provides the best assurance of an optimal result.

⊘ FREQUENT ERRORS

In the Treatment of Facial Trauma

1. *Being distracted from life- or limb-threatening injuries by concentrating on facial injuries.*
2. *Blind clamping of bleeding vessels deep in facial lacerations.*
3. *Missing facial fractures by relying primarily on radiographic examinations.*
4. *Missing a facial nerve injury because facial edema limits movement on the unaffected side.*
5. *Not looking carefully for a parotid duct or facial nerve injury in a cheek laceration.*
6. *Missing fractures of the maxilla or mandible because of failure to check the occlusion of the teeth.*
7. *Mistaking a nasoethmoid fracture for a nasal fracture.*
8. *Missing an orbital fracture because of failure to look for orbital asymmetry.*
9. *Missing a condyle fracture of the mandible by relying only on a cursory physical examination or inadequate radiographs.*
10. *Failing to slightly evert skin edges during repair of facial lacerations.*
11. *Failing to obtain centric occlusion when treating fractures of the maxilla and mandible.*
12. *Reducing but not using adequate fixation in "tripod fractures."*
13. *Failing to identify and treat the full extent of orbital floor fractures.*
14. *Failing to treat complex facial fractures with adequate exposure, primary bone grafts, and rigid fixation.*

▼▼▼▼▼▼▼▼▼▼▼▼▼▼▼▼▼▼▼▼▼▼▼▼▼▼▼▼▼▼▼▼

SUMMARY POINTS

1. Severe maxillofacial injuries are probably best treated by an interdisciplinary approach.

2. One should not treat severe maxillofacial trauma until actual or potentially life- or limb-threatening problems are controlled.

3. One should always consider the possibility of brain or cervical spine injuries in patients with severe maxillofacial trauma.

4. When a mandible has one fracture line, one must look carefully for other fractures that may not be readily apparent on standard radiography.

5. The muscles closing the mouth (i.e., elevating the mandible) include the masseter, temporalis, and medial pterygoid.

6. The muscles opening the mouth (i.e., depressing the mandible) include the anterior belly of the digastric, the geniohyoid, and the mylohyoid muscles.

7. Associated basal skull fractures are not uncommon in LeFort II fractures and should be ruled out before embarking on airway manipulation via the nasal route.

8. One should look carefully for CSF rhinorrhea and/or airway obstruction in patients with LeFort III fractures.

9. A nasoethmoid fracture should be suspected with severe nasal fractures and/or bilateral periorbital ecchymosis (spectacle hematoma or raccoon eyes).

10. Facial fractures generally do not pose an immediate threat to life unless they compromise the airway or are associated with extensive bleeding; however, associated injuries of the cervical spine and brain must be suspected when attempting airway management techniques.

11. Letting dramatic facial trauma divert attention from less obvious but much more critical life- or limb-threatening injuries.

12. Even without facial fractures, impaired consciousness can cause upper airway obstruction by allowing the tongue to fall back into the pharynx.

13. Because cyanosis occurs late in the process of respiratory distress and may not develop at all in anemic patients, lack of cyanosis does not rule out airway or ventilatory compromise.

14. Patients with severe facial injuries who are hemodynamically stable should be allowed to sit up when they can breathe more effectively and comfortably in that position and the cervical spine has been cleared or immobilized.

15. Paralyzing a patient to insert an endotracheal tube may be rapidly fatal if intubation or provision of a surgical airway cannot be accomplished promptly.

16. Nasal tubes are generally contraindicated in patients with fractures that may involve the anterior base of the skull.

17. One should always be prepared to perform an emergency cricothyroidotomy in adults with severe facial injuries because attempts at endotracheal intubation may fail or may cause complete airway obstruction.

18. All patients with maxillofacial trauma, especially those with neck pain, tenderness, or spasm, or neurologic deficits, should be assumed to have cervical spine injury until proven otherwise.

19. Airway management without concern for cervical spine protection in patients with maxillofacial fractures may result in unnecessary spinal cord damage.

20. In hypotensive patients with facial injuries, other sources of hemorrhage and acute spinal cord injury should be suspected.

21. When general anesthesia is required and the patient has an eye injury that cannot be examined closely, the patient should be considered to have an open globe until proved otherwise.

22. Malocclusion indicates a fracture of the jaws or teeth until ruled out careful, complete examination and radiologic studies.

23. Prior to the physical examination, the patient should be positioned so that the examination light is centered on the midline to avoid visual distortion of facial asymmetry.

24. Any injury along the posterior half of a line extending from the tragus to the mid-upper lip should be suspected of involving the parotid duct and/or buccal branches of the facial nerve.

25. Facial edema may limit facial movement and a facial nerve injury can easily be missed under such circumstances.

26. Because most of the major sensory nerves of the face traverse facial bones, any area of hypesthesia or anesthesia should make one suspect an underlying facial fracture.

27. The most accurate method for determining the presence of facial fractures (except for CT) is careful palpation of bony landmarks looking for step-offs, irregularities, or asymmetry.

28. Reliance on radiographic evidence alone to diagnose facial fractures leads to missed fractures that would have been easily detected by physical examination.

29. One of the most important diagnostic methods for detecting a mandible or maxillary (LeFort) fracture is inspection of occlusion.

30. Failure to eliminate dental malocclusion can easily lead to a missed maxillary or mandible fracture.

31. Nasoethmoid fractures, which often require special craniofacial techniques for repair, may easily be mistaken for simple, depressed nasal fractures when one does not perform a careful examination.

32. Diplopia alone is nonspecific, but should alert one to a possible occult facial fracture to be investigated radiographically.

33. Failure to look for and appreciate orbital asymmetry may lead to missed orbital fractures.

34. Decreased visual acuity without global injury may indicate a periorbital hematoma that requires urgent decompression.

35. Bleeding from an ear after trauma should be considered due to a basilar skull fracture until proved otherwise.

36. When bloody CSF is placed on filter paper, an outer clear ring is caused by the CSF and an inner ring is caused by blood with or without nasal fluid.

37. As a diagnostic tool, radiographic studies of the face are generally inferior to a careful physical examination.

38. Condyle fractures are missed easily and can cause considerable functional disability and deformity.

39. Appropriate radiographic and endoscopic evaluation of the aerodigestive tracks should be performed before one decides that pneumomediastinum is a harmless consequence of facial injury.

40. CT is now the radiographic method of choice for the diagnosis and operative planning of facial fractures.

41. In all facial soft-tissue injuries, wound debridement should be conservative.

42. Open facial lacerations tend to appear larger than they really are.

43. Using small sutures is not the essence of a plastic repair; proper technique is.

44. Skin wounds should be slightly everted by the repair sutures. A repair that is initially flat will become depressed with time and the scar will be more obvious.

45. If a plastic surgeon with craniofacial capabilities is not present, one has 7-10 days to transfer the patient for proper primary treatment.

46. Failure to reduce a mandible to a proper occlusal relationship can lead to severe anatomical and functional problems with the jaws.

47. Failure to obtain centric occlusion with intermaxillary fixation before fracture fixation of the remaining fracture fragments can result in severe malocclusion.

48. Treatment of maxillary fractures attempts to reestablish centric occlusion and reconstruct associated injuries.

49. All LeFort fractures should be explored and accurately reduced under direct vision.

50. Failure to recognize and properly treat a comminuted maxillary fracture may lead to a shortened face which is very difficult to correct secondarily.

51. Simple reduction of zygoma ("tripod") fractures without adequate fixation often leads to displacement and significant deformity.

52. Failure to identify and treat the full extent of orbital floor fractures probably results in late enophthalmos.

53. Careful follow-up of patients with closed reductions of nasal fractures is important to detect significant residual bony or septal deformities.

54. Nasoethmoid fractures should be accurately reduced under direct vision, preferably through a coronal degloving scalp and face incision.

55. A CSF leak is no reason to postpone treatment of facial fractures. In fact, reduction of facial fractures may stop the leak.

56. Rigid fixation and liberal use of bone grafts to preserve facial volume and height are particularly important in panfacial fractures.

57. Failure to preserve facial volume with bone grafts and rigid fixation results in secondary deformities which can be extremely difficult to reconstruct.

58. The best chance of providing an excellent result with facial fractures is during the initial reduction and fixation.

59. Condylar fractures should be suspected in children presenting with laceration of the chin and fractures of the symphysis or body of the mandible.

60. In pediatric patients the impact of severe trauma on subsequent facial growth must be carefully monitored and the patient and family advised accordingly.

61. Generally, the simplest fixation will be the best for most facial bone fractures in children.

62. If intermaxillary fixation is used, a wire cutter should be taped to the patient's chest until full recovery from the anesthetic.

63. A coniotomy tracheostomy under local anesthesia without any attempts at endotracheal intubation is indicated when the patient's clinical condition or CT reveals severe airway compromise.

64. Probably the most frequent complication of treatment of severe facial fractures is secondary deformity.

▲▲▲▲▲▲▲▲▲▲▲▲▲▲▲▲▲▲▲▲▲▲▲▲▲▲▲▲▲▲▲▲

REFERENCES

1. Capan LM, Miller SM, Olickman R. Management of facial injuries. Capan LM, Miller SM, Turndorf H, eds. Trauma: anesthesia and intensive care. New York: JB Lippincott, 1991; 385-408.
2. Breasted JH. Edwin Smith surgical papyrus. Chicago: University of Chicago Press, 1930.
3. Rowe NL. The history of the treatment of maxillofacial trauma. Ann R Coll Surg Engl 1971;49:329.
4. LeFort R. Etude experimentale sur les fractures de la machoire superieure. Rev Chir 1901;23:208-227,360-379,479-507.
5. Chuong R, Mulliken JB, Strome M. Fragmented care of facial fractures. J Trauma 1987;27:477.
6. Karlson TA. The incidence of hospital-treated facial injuries from vehicles. J Trauma 1982;22:303.
7. Andersson L, Hultin M, Nordenram A, Ramstrom G. Jaw fractures in the county of Stockholm (1978-1980). (I) General survey. Int J Oral Surg 1984;13:194.
8. Nair KB, Paul G. Incidence and aetiology of fractures of the faciomaxillary skeleton in Trivandrum: a retrospective study. Br J Oral Maxillofac Surg 1986;24:40.
9. Eriksson L, Willmar K. Jaw fractures in Malmo 1952-62 and 1975-85. Swed Dent J 1987;11:31.
10. Olson RA, Fonseca RJ, Zeitter DL, et al. Fractures of the mandible: a review of 580 cases. J Oral Maxillofac Surg 1982;40:23.
11. van Hoof RF, Merkx CA, Stekelenburg EC. The different patterns of fractures of the facial skeleton in four European countries. Int J Oral Surg 1977;6:3.
12. Abiose BO. Maxillofacial skeleton injuries in the Western States of Nigeria. Br J Oral Maxillofac Surg 1986;24:31.
13. Kruger GO. Fractures of the jaws. Kruger GO, ed. Textbook of maxillofacial and oral surgery. St. Louis: CV Mosby, 1984; 364.
14. Busuito MJ, Smith DJ, Robson MC. Mandibular fractures in an urban trauma center. J Trauma 1986;26:826.
15. Scherer M, Sullivan WG, Smith DJ, et al. An analysis of 1,423 facial fractures in 788 patients at an urban trauma center. J Trauma 1989; 29:388.
16. Lindqvist C, Sorsa S, Hyrkas T, Santavirta S. Maxillofacial fractures sustained in bicycle accidents. Int J Oral Maxillofac Surg 1986;15:12.
17. Linn EW, Vrijhoef MMA, de Wijn JR, et al. Facial injuries sustained during sports and games. J Maxillofac Surg 1986;14:83.
18. McDade AM, McNicol RD, Ward-Booth P, et al. The aetiology of maxillofacial injuries, with special reference to the abuse of alcohol. Int J Oral Surg 1982;11:52.

19. Gussack GS, Jurkovich GJ. Penetrating facial trauma: a management plan. South Med J 1988;81:297.
20. Calhoun KH, Li S, Clark WD, et al. Surgical care of submental gunshot wounds. Arch Otolaryngol Head Neck Surg 1988;114:513.
21. Goodstein WA, Stryker A, Weiner LJ. Primary treatment of shotgun injuries to the face. J Trauma 1979;19:961.
22. Zaytoun GM, Shikhani AH, Salman SD. Head and neck war injuries: 10 years experience at the American University of Beirut Medical Center. Laryngoscope 1986;96:899.
23. Swearingen JJ. Tolerances of the human face to crash impact. Reprint #AM-65-20. Oklahoma City: Federal Aviation Agency, 1965.
24. Nahum AM. The biomechanics of maxillofacial trauma. Clin Plast Surg 1975;2:59.
25. Robson MC, Smith DJ, Hayward PG. Maxillofacial and mandibular injuries. Moore EE, Mattox KL, Feliciano DV, eds. Trauma, 2nd ed. Norwalk: Appleton & Lange, 1991; 277-294.
26. Luce EA, Tubb TD, Moore AM. Review of 1000 major facial fractures and associated injuries. Plast Reconstr Surg 1979;63:26.
27. Hodgson VR. Tolerance of the facial bones to impact. Am J Anat 1967;120:113.
28. Bucholz RW, Burkhead WZ, Graham W, Petty C. Occult cervical spine injuries in fatal traffic accidents. J Trauma 1979;19:768.
29. Lee KF, Wagner LK, Lee YE, et al. The impact-absorbing effects of facial fractures in closed-head injuries. J Neurosurg 1987;66:542.
30. Seaton JR. Soft tissue facial injuries related to vehicular accidents. Clin Plast Surg 1975;2:79.
31. Olson RA, Fonseca RJ, Zeitter DL, et al. Fractures of the mandible: a review of 580 cases. J Oral Maxillofac Surg 1982;40:23.
32. Schrimshaw GC. Malar/orbital/zygomatic fracture causing fracture of underlying coronoid process. J Trauma 1978;18:367.
33. Bowers DG, Lynch JB. Management of facial fractures. South Med J 1977;70:910.
34. Bradley JC, Haskell R, Rowe NL, et al. Applied surgical anatomy. Rowe NL, Killey HC, eds. Maxillofacial injuries. London: Churchill Livingstone, 1985.
35. Dingman RO, Natvig P. Surgery of facial fractures. Philadelphia: WB Saunders, 1964; 133.
36. Gott AW. Maxillofacial trauma: anesthetic considerations. ASA Refresher Courses 1987;15:39.
37. Edgerton MT, Kenney JG. Emergency care of maxillofacial and otological injuries. The management of trauma, 4th ed. Zuidema GD, Rutherford RB, Ballinger WF, eds. Philadelphia: WB Saunders, 1985; 275.
38. Block C, Brechner V. Unusual problems in airway management. Anesth Analg 1971;50:114.
39. Musgrove BT. Dislocation of the mandibular condyle into the middle cranial fossa. Br J Oral Maxillofac Surg 1986;24:22.
40. Fonseca GD. Experimental study on fractures of the mandibular condylar process. Int J Oral Surg 1974;89:101.
41. Cruse CW, Blevins PK, Luce EA. Naso-ethmoid-orbital fractures. J Trauma 1980;20:551.
42. Gruss JS. Fronto-naso-orbital trauma. Clin Plast Surg 1982;9:577.
43. Manson PN. Maxillofacial injuries. Siegel JH, ed. Trauma: emergency and critical care. New York: Churchill Livingstone, 1987; 983.
44. Gwyn PP, Caraway JH, Horton CE, et al. Facial fractures associated injuries and complications. Plast Reconstr Surg 47:225, 1971.
45. Chase CR, Hebert JC, Farnham JE: Post-traumatic upper airway obstruction secondary to a lingual artery hematoma. J Trauma 1987;27:953.
46. Cawood JI, Thind GS. Supraglottic obstruction. Injury 1983;15:277.
47. Boidin MP. Airway patency in the unconscious patient. Br J Anaesth 1985;57:306.
48. Volpe BT, Bradstetter RD. Delayed pneumonia after aspiration of "dashboard" fragment. J Trauma 1985;24:1173.
49. Mehta RM, Pathak PN. A foreign body in the larynx. Br J Anaesth 1973; 45:755.
50. Jackson CL. Endoscopy for foreign body: report of 178 cases of foreign body in the air and food passages. Ann Otol 1936;45:644.
51. Kahn RMA. An easily missed foreign body in the respiratory passages. Br J Anaesth 1975;47:628.
52. Zachariades N, Rapidis AD, Papademetriou J, et al. The significance of tracheostomy in the management of fractures of the facial skeleton. J Maxillofac Surg 1983;11:180.
53. Horellou MF, Mathe D, Feiss P. A hazard of naso-tracheal intubation. Anaesthesia 1978;33:73.
54. Fletcher SA, Henderson LT, Miner ME, Jones JM. The successful surgical removal of intracranial nasogastric tubes. J Trauma 1987;27:948.
55. Mulder DS, Wallace DEH, Woolhouse FM. The use of the fiberoptic bronchoscope to facilitate endotracheal intubation following head and neck trauma. J Trauma 1975;15:638.
56. Barriot P, Riou B. Retrograde technique for tracheal intubation in trauma patients. Crit Care Med 1988;16:712.
57. Lechman MJ, Donahoo JS, MacVaugh H. Endotracheal intubation using percutaneous retrograde guidewire insertion followed by antegrade fiberoptic bronchoscopy. Crit Care Med 1986;14:589.
58. Wagner DJ, Coombs DW, Doyle SC. Percutaneous transtracheal ventilation for emergency dental appliance removal. Anesthesiology 1985; 62:664.
59. Lewis VL, Manson PN, Morgan RF, et al. Facial injuries associated with cervical fractures: recognition patterns and management. J Trauma 1985; 25:90.
60. Murakami WT, Davidson TM, Marshall LF. Fatal epistaxis in craniofacial trauma. J Trauma 1983;23:57.
61. Hassard AD, Kirkpatrick DA, Wong FS. Ligation of the external carotid and anterior ethmoidal arteries for severe or unusual epistaxis resulting from facial fractures. Can J Surg 1986;29:447.
62. Samman N. Disseminated intravascular coagulation and facial injury. Br J Oral Maxillofac Surg 1984;22:295.
63. Gautman V, Leonard EM. Bony injuries in association with minor head injury; lessons for improving the diagnosis of facial fractures. Injury 1994;25:47.
64. Haug RH, Adams JM, Conforti PJ, Likavec MJ. Cranial fractures associated with facial fractures: a review of mechanism, type, and severity of injury. J Oral Maxillofac Surg 1994;52:729.
65. Holt JE, Holt R, Blodgett JM. Ocular injuries sustained during blunt facial trauma. Ophthalmology 1983;90:14.
66. Ord RA, Awty MD, Pour S. Bilateral retrobulbar hemorrhage: a short case report. Br J Oral Maxillofac Surg 1986;24:1.
67. Wood GD. Blindness following fracture of the zygomatic bone. Br J Oral Maxillofac Surg 1986;24:12.
68. Stanley RB, Cannalis RF, Colman MF. Gunshot wounds to the mandible with secondary neck injuries. Arch Otolaryngol 19981;107:565.
69. Zachariades N. The superior orbital fissure syndrome. Oral Surg 1982; 53:237.
70. Westmore GA, Whittman DE. Cerebrospinal fluid rhinorrhoea and its management. Br J Surg 1982;69:489.
71. Marsh JL, Vannier MW, Bresina S, Hemmer KM. Applications of computer graphics in craniofacial surgery. Clin Plast Surg 1986;13: 441.
72. Mayer JS, Wainwright DJ, Yeakley JW, et al. The role of three-dimensional computed tomography in the management of maxillofacial trauma. J Trauma 1988;28:1043.
73. Alder ME, Deahl ST, Matteson SR. Clinical usefulness of 2-dimensional reformatted and 3-dimensional computerized tomographic images. J Oral Maxillofa Surg 1995; 53:375.
74. Broumand SR, Labs JD, Novelline RA, et al. The role of three-dimensional computed tomography in the evaluation of acute craniofacial trauma. Ann Plast Surg 1993;31:488.
75. Kraissl CJ. The selection of appropriate lines for elective surgical incisions. Plast Reconstr Surg 1951;8:1.
76. Marks MW, Smith DJ. Complications of traumatic wounds of the face. Greenfield LJ, ed. Complications in surgery and trauma. Philadelphia: JB Lippincott, 1989.
77. Robson MC, Smith DJ. Injuries to the maxillofacial complex. Evaluation and management of trauma. McSwain NE, Kerstein MD, eds. Norwalk: Appleton-Century-Crofts, 1987.
78. Touvinen V, Norholt SE, Sindet-Pedersen S, Jensen J. A retrospective analysis of 279 patients with isolated mandibular fractures treated with titanium miniplates. J Oral Maxillofac Surg 1994;52:931.
79. Ellis E, Walker L. Treatment of mandibular angle fractures using two non-compression miniplates. J Oral Maxillofac Surg 1994;52:1032.
80. Barrs DN, Darn EB. Acute nasal trauma: Emergency room care of 250 patients. J Fam Pract 1980; 10:225.
81. Gruss JS, Hurwitz JJ, Nik NA, Kassel EE. The pattern and incidence of nasolacrimal injury in naso-orbital ethmoid fractures: the role of delayed assessment and dacryocystorhinostomy. Br J Plast Surg 1985; 38:116.
82. Rowe NL. Fractures of the facial skeleton in children. J Oral Surg 1968;26:505.
83. Gussack GS, Luterman A, Powell RW, et al. Pediatric maxillofacial trauma: unique features in diagnosis and treatment. Laryngoscope 1987; 97:925.

84. Hall RK. Injuries to the face and jaws and in children. Int J Oral Surg 1972;1:65.
85. Myall RWT, Sandor GKB, Gregory CEB. Are you overlooking fractures of the mandibular condyle? Pediatrics 1987;79:639.
86. James D. Maxillofacial injuries in children. Rowe NL, Williams JL, eds. Maxillofacial trauma. Edinburg: Churchill Livingston, 1985; 538.
87. Goss AN, Chau KK, Mayne LH. Intermaxillary fixation: how practicable is emergency jaw release? Anaesth Intensive Care 1979;7:253.
88. Barclay JK. Intermaxillary fixation—a safety measure. Br J Oral Surg 1979;17:77.
89. Arajarvi K, Lindqvist C, Santavirta S, et al. Maxillofacial trauma in fatally injured victims of motor vehicle accidents. Br J Oral Maxillofac Surg 1986;24:251.
90. Macias JD, Haller J, Frodel JL. Comparative postoperative infection rates in midfacial trauma using intermaxillary fixation, wire fixation, and rigid internal fixation implants. Arch Otolaryngol Head Neck Surg 1993;119:308.
91. Chole RA, Yee J. Antibiotic prophylaxis for facial fractures: a prospective, randomized clinical trial. Arch Otolaryngol Head Neck Surg 1987;113:1055.
92. Koury ME. The use of rigid internal fixation in mandibular fractures complicated by osteomyelitis. J Oral Maxillofac Surg 1994;52(Suppl):105.
93. Schroeder DC, Sarha ED, Hendricksson DA, Healey KM. Severe infections of the head and neck resulting from gas forming organisms: report of case. JADA 1987;114:65.
94. Shulman ST, Amren DP, Bisno AL, et al. Prevention of bacterial endocarditis: a statement for health professionals by the Committee on Rheumatic Fever and Infective Endocarditis of the Council on Cardiovascular Disease in the Young. Circulation 1984;70:1123A.
95. Foster RJ, Collins FJV, Back AW. Concurrent oral surgery and orthopaedic treatment in the multiple injured patient. Is there an increased incidence of orthopaedic sepsis? J Trauma 1987;27:626.

Chapter **14** Injuries to the Neck

ROBERT F. WILSON, M.D.

LAWRENCE DIEBEL, M.D.

HISTORY

Penetrating neck injury was first reported 5,000 years ago in the Edwin Smith papyrus, and the resulting esophagocutaneous fistula was treated by packing the wound with lint.[1] The first record of successful management of a penetrating vascular injury in the neck was in 1552 by Ambroise Pare, who according to de Fourmestranx, stopped the bleeding from a lacerated common carotid artery and internal jugular vein in a man who had been wounded in a duel.[2,3] The patient survived; however, he had aphasia and a hemiplegia. In 1803, Fleming successfully ligated the common carotid artery of a sailor who attempted suicide by cutting his neck.[2,4] In 1811, Abernathy ligated the lacerated left common and internal carotid arteries in a patient who had been gored by a bull. This patient developed profound hemiplegia and subsequently succumbed to his injury.[2,4] In 1872, Vernouil was the first to publish a report on two patients with carotid occlusion due to blunt head and neck trauma.[2,5]

Since the late 1800s, mortality rates due to neck injuries steadily decreased because of improved diagnostic facilities, advanced therapeutic modalities, and reduced time from injury to definitive therapy. The mortality rate due to penetrating neck injuries in the Vietnam war was about 15%; now in civilian practice, it has ranged 2-6%.[5-9]

ANATOMY

The neck has many important structures in a relatively small space. Although they are well protected by the spine posteriorly, the face superiorly, and the chest inferiorly, these structures are very vulnerable to anterior and lateral penetrating and blunt trauma.

The superficial fascia of the anterior neck is a thin layer that encloses the platysma muscle. The deep cervical fascia supports the muscles, vessels, and viscera of the neck and is divided into three distinct layers: the investing fascia, the pretracheal fascia, and the prevertebral fascia. The investing fascia encircles the neck and splits to enclose the sternocleidomastoid and trapezius muscles. The pretracheal fascial layer envelopes the larynx, thyroid gland, trachea, and esophagus, and extends into the mediastinum, where it blends with the pericardium. The prevertebral fascia covers the prevertebral muscles, which include the longus capitis, longus cervices, scalenus anterior, scalenus medius, levator scapulae, and splenius capitis. The carotid sheath, which contains the common and internal carotid arteries, the internal jugular vein, and the vagus nerve, blends in front with the pretracheal and investing layers of the deep cervical fascia and behind with the prevertebral fascia.

The sternocleidomastoid (SCM) muscle which extends diagonally from the mastoid process of the skull to the superior sternum and medial portion of the clavicle divides the neck into the anterior and posterior triangles (Fig. 14-1). The anterior triangle of the neck, bounded by the SCM, the midline, and the mandible, contains most of the major vascular and visceral structures, including the airway. The posterior triangle, which is bounded by the SCM, the trapezius, and the clavicle, has relatively few important structures except inferiorly just above the clavicle.

AXIOM In the posterior triangle of the neck, there are several vital structures just above the clavicle.

In discussing the management of penetrating injuries of the neck, Saletta et al. divided the anterior neck into three anatomic areas.[10]

Zone I, often referred to as the thoracic inlet or outlet, was originally described as the area of the neck below the sternal notch, but it is now usually described as the area below the cricoid cartilage (Fig. 14-2). If a major vessel were injured in this area, it could bleed massively, and frequently required a thoracotomy for control.[6] Vascular injuries in this zone are usually associated with higher mortality rates than those in zones II and III.[11]

Zone II is the mid area of the neck, and it extends from the cricoid cartilage to the angle of the mandible. This is the most frequent site of penetrating neck trauma. Injuries in this area are relatively easy to expose and repair, and they generally have a lower mortality rate than injuries in zones I or III.[10]

Zone III is located above the angle of the mandible. Vascular injuries high in zone III involving the upper portions of the internal carotid or vertebral arteries can be difficult to expose and manage.

AXIOM In stable patients with penetrating neck injuries, preoperative arteriography is particularly important for injuries in zones I and III.

Blunt vascular injuries in the neck are rare, and are easily missed. In about two-thirds of patients studied by Wozasek and Balzer, the hypoglossal nerve and the occipital artery branch of the external carotid arch across the internal carotid artery (ICA) about 1.5-3.0 cm above its origin from the common carotid.[13] Consequently, if the head were hyperextended and rotated contralaterally, these structures could act as a tight band across the ICA and injure it. This may explain why this is the most common site for blunt trauma to the ICA.[14,15]

The neural structures of the neck are located primarily in the lower portion of the posterior neck and are much better protected than the major vessels and the aerodigestive tract. The cervical sympathetic ganglia lie posterior to the carotid sheath.

In the mediastinum, the thoracic duct passes along the left margin of the esophagus up to the level of the transverse process of the seventh cervical vertebra. At this point, the duct bends laterally behind the carotid sheath and in front of the left vertebral artery. As the duct approaches the medial border and then anterior surface of the scalenus anticus muscle, it turns inferiorly in front of the phrenic nerve. It may drain into the first portion of the left innominate vein or into the proximal end of the subclavian or internal jugular vein.

TYPES OF INJURY

Penetrating

AXIOM Although the course of a stab wound is relatively limited and direct, the path of a bullet can be completely unpredictable.

Penetrating injuries of the neck are due to knives in about 50%, gunshot wounds in about 45%, and shotgun wounds in about 4-5%.[16] An injury requiring surgical exploration occurs in about 70-80% of gunshot wounds and 50-60% of stab wounds. Exploration of penetrating neck trauma will, on the average, reveal injuries to major veins (15-25%), major arteries (10-15%), pharynx or esophagus (5-15%), larynx or trachea (4-12%), or major nerves in 3-8%.[16,17] Thus, approximately 40% of penetrating neck wounds will not involve an important structure.

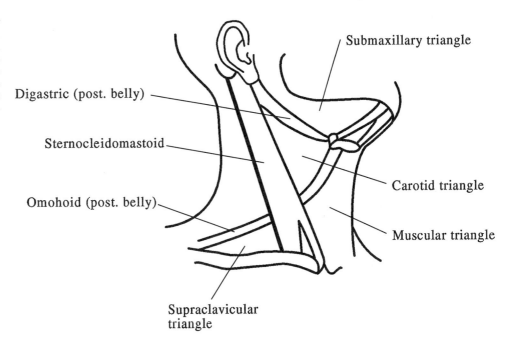

FIGURE 14-1 The anterior triangles of the neck lie between the sternocleidomastoid muscles (SCM) and the mandible. It, in turn, is divided into the carotid triangle formed by the SCM, posterior belly of the digastric muscle and the omohyoid. In the posterior triangle of the neck, most of the important structures lay below the posterior belly of the omohyoid muscle.

AXIOM Penetrating injuries of the neck involve major vessels in 25-40% of patients.

Gunshot wounds, in addition to directly injuring or tearing structures, may produce shock waves that can devitalize tissue, resulting in later necrosis and leakage. This is especially true with high-velocity missiles (>2000-2500 ft/sec) which are characteristic of military weapons or hunting rifles.[18] In Ordog's study, almost 100 percent of patients with high-velocity missile injuries of the neck required surgical repair.[19]

AXIOM All high-velocity gunshot wounds of the neck should be surgically explored.

In civilian centers, stab wounds accounted for 55-70% of patients requiring surgery[20-22] but they usually caused much less morbidity and mortality than gunshot wounds. When the anterior spine is involved by a gunshot wound, frequent associated injuries occur to the aerodigestive tract increasing the risk of osteomyelitis.

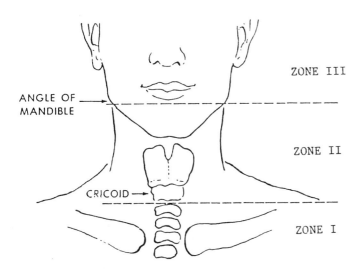

FIGURE 14-2 Regions of the neck. (From: Roon AJ, Christensen N. Evaluation and treatment of penetrating cervical injuries. J Trauma 1979;19:391.)

Blunt Trauma

SPINE INJURIES

Blunt injuries to the neck are usually due to direct blows, sudden deceleration, or strangulation. The cervical spine is the structure most frequently injured by blunt neck trauma. Because of the potential severe neurologic sequelae, cervical spine injury should be suspected in all patients with blunt trauma to the head or neck.

AXIOM Patients with blunt head or neck trauma should have their neck immobilized in the neutral position until radiography and careful examination have eliminated cervical spine fracture or dislocation.

NEUROLOGIC INJURIES

Although neurologic abnormalities seen with cervical spine injuries are usually due to direct trauma to the spinal cord or brachial plexus, associated vascular injuries with hypotension can make the neurologic picture much worse. Blunt trauma itself, however, can indirectly cause severe cerebral damage or dysfunction by causing dissection and subsequent thrombosis of the internal carotid or vertebral arteries.

VASCULAR INJURIES

Injury to the extracranial arteries from blunt trauma is quite rare. Aviv et al. noted that only 96 such patients were reported before 1978, and only an additional 86 patients were reported in the succeeding 10 years.[23] Initial or delayed thrombosis of the internal carotid or vertebral arteries can cause neurologic sequelae which may have mortality rates as high as 40%.[24]

The more frequent causes of nonpenetrating trauma to the carotid artery include: (a) direct blows to the neck, which account for about 50% of these injuries and are usually due to automobile accidents,[25,26] (b) hyperextension and rotation of the neck, which stretches the ICA against the hypoglossal nerve and occipital artery or against the transverse processes of C-2 and C-3, (c) direct blunt intraoral trauma to the ICA in the tonsillar region,[27] (d) basilar skull fracture causing contusion or tearing of the petrous portion of the ICA, and (e) direct compression injuries of the carotid artery by car safety belts.[26,28] Even vertebral artery injury can occur with shoulder straps, hyperextension, and/or manipulation.[28]

AXIOM Neurologic injury after severe blunt neck trauma may occasionally be due to correctable carotid or vertebral arterial damage.[25]

With severe spinal injuries, the carotid and vertebral arteries may be directly compressed by bony structures, or they may be forcefully stretched, resulting in vasospasm or intimal tears with dissection and/or thrombosis.[29,30] It has been shown that when the vertebral arteries are compressed for 15 minutes or less, reversible functional and histologic changes of ischemia can occur in the upper spinal cord; however, ischemia that exceeds 20 minutes can cause arterial thrombosis and severe, permanent spinal cord injury.[28] With such injuries, partial or complete neurologic recovery may sometimes be obtained by immobilizing the head to prevent further injury to the vessels and by specifically treating severe vasospasm or arterial dissection.

LARYNX AND CERVICAL TRACHEA

In a high-speed collision with sudden deceleration, use of a lap belt by itself (without a shoulder harness) can firmly anchor the passenger's pelvis to the back of the seat, while the upper body is propelled forward with the neck in hyperextension. Upon impact of the anterior neck with the dashboard or steering wheel, the larynx may be crushed against the cervical spine, and/or the cricoid cartilage may be torn away from the upper trachea. Although properly worn shoulder straps can prevent many of these injuries, if the passenger were to slip under the shoulder strap, a direct shearing force could damage neck structures.

AXIOM Improperly used seat belts can increase the incidence of serious neck and other injuries.

PHARYNX AND ESOPHAGUS

Mechanisms of blunt injury to the pharynx and upper esophagus include crushing, shearing, and sudden rises in intraluminal pressure. Perforation of the pharynx or esophagus after external blunt neck trauma, however, is extremely rare.[31] Worman and Hurley reviewed the English language literature and found only 30 such patients reported between 1900 and 1962.[32] Blunt trauma causes < 2% of all pharyngoesophageal perforations in the neck.[33]

DIAGNOSIS AND EVALUATION

AXIOM A thorough history and physical examination is important in the diagnosis of neck injuries, but many patients with organ damage in the neck requiring an operation have no clinical evidence of such an injury preoperatively.[20]

Many injuries in the neck are asymptomatic, and diagnosis of an esophageal injury may be particularly difficult. In the series by Weigelt et al., 3 of 10 patients with esophageal trauma had no preoperative signs or symptoms of injury.[22] In addition, of 98 other patients with neck trauma without esophageal injury, 25% had symptoms and 26% had signs suggesting such an injury. Although all patients with gunshot injuries to the esophagus had clinical findings suggesting the diagnosis, these were frequently absent in patients with esophageal stab wounds.

AXIOM Esophageal injuries in the neck are particularly difficult to detect from signs and symptoms.

History

Knowledge of the mechanism of injury, the events observed in the prehospital setting, and the progression of symptoms or physical signs en route to the hospital can facilitate the diagnostic efforts. The patient should be questioned in detail about any pain, including its lo-

cation and character, as well as any difficulty breathing, talking, or swallowing. A careful neurologic history is also important and should include questions about any paresthesias or weakness in the upper and lower extremities.

With blunt injury to the ICA, the time between the injury and appearance of symptoms is extremely variable and may exceed two weeks. In some patients with otherwise occult lesions, extension and/or rotation of the neck can precipitate neurologic symptoms or signs.[13]

Patients with laryngeal trauma frequently complain of neck pain or voice change. Occasionally, they may also have hemoptysis or shortness of breath.

Injury to the food passages is suggested by dysphagia or odynophagia. Hematemesis after neck trauma is usually due to associated nasal or oral injuries, but it may occasionally be due to damage to the pharynx or esophagus.

AXIOM Symptoms are poor predictors of the presence or absence of important neck injuries.

Nine of 46 asymptomatic patients reported by Sclafani et al. had injuries seen arteriographically.[39] Eleven (50%) of 22 injuries of the carotid or vertebral arteries were asymptomatic. One asymptomatic woman had occlusion of both the right internal carotid and the right vertebral arteries and a pseudoaneurysm of the left ICA.

Physical Examination

AXIOM Physical examination of an injured neck is often deceptively negative in spite of severe underlying injuries to major vessels or the aerodigestive system.

In a recent series reported by Walsh, 38% of patients with no clinical signs had significant neck injuries.[35] The author believed that this justified a policy of mandatory exploration. Other recent reports, however, suggested that a well-performed physical examination can be quite accurate. Beitsch et al., for example, found that of 71 patients without signs or symptoms of arterial injury, only one (1.4%) had an arterial injury.[36] Similarly, in a series of 335 patients reviewed by Demetriades et al., 269 had no signs or symptoms of significant injury[37]; of these 269 patients, only two (0.7%) later required surgery.

Patients with possible neck injuries should have systematic and thorough examinations for evidence of injury to: (a) musculoskeletal tissues, (b) blood vessels, (c) aerodigestive tract, and (d) neurologic system.[38]

MUSCULOSKELETAL SYSTEM

When patients are not completely awake and alert, especially following blunt trauma, one should assume that a cervical spine injury is present until it has been eliminated by appropriate clinical examinations and radiologic studies. In particular, the neck should be examined thoroughly for any swelling, tenderness, or deformity.

VASCULAR INJURIES

The presenting signs of a major vascular injury after penetrating trauma may vary from a completely normal neck to varying amounts of hematoma or hemorrhage. The patient must be carefully examined for evidence of pressure on the aerodigestive tract, a bruit or a thrill, or a peripheral pulse deficit. Clinical signs suggesting carotid arterial injury include transient ischemic attacks, a lucid interval, Horner's syndrome,[38] limb paresis or paralysis, or deep coma. These changes, however, may be delayed for up to several days, especially after blunt trauma.

PITFALL ⊘

Failure to consider an occult, blunt carotid artery injury as a cause of neurologic changes, especially when cranial CT is negative and CNS changes are delayed.

Hematomas from major vascular injuries may be quite stable until the neck is manipulated or probed or the patient gags or performs a Valsalva maneuver, especially while a nasogastric or endotracheal tube is being inserted. Occasionally, a hematoma may develop as late as 24-48 hours after the injury and rupture when the patient gags or retches.

PITFALL ⊘

If a penetrating wound of the neck is probed, a clot may be dislodged, allowing massive uncontrollable bleeding to occur.

Patients with neurologic deficits due to direct brain injury or occlusions of the ICA or CCA have much worse prognoses if they have hypotension. In Fabian's series of 31 patients with penetrating neck injuries and evaluable CNS status, 24 had little or no neurologic deficits, and only one of these patients presented in shock; however, of seven patients with severe neurologic deficits, six (86%) were in shock on admission (P < 0.03).[39] Hypotensive patients are much more apt to have neurologic symptoms or signs after neck trauma, but these clinical findings may be due largely to impaired CNS perfusion rather than to direct brain damage.

AXIOM Neurologic signs in patients with penetrating neck injuries may be caused or greatly increased by hypotension.

Following neck trauma, the importance of continued and repeated neurologic evaluations, preferably by the same examiner, cannot be overemphasized. It is important to note that serious vascular injuries in the neck after blunt trauma frequently occur without any overt hematoma formation. Most blunt carotid injuries cause dissection of the wall of the vessel, and a small subadventitial hematoma may be the only indication at the time of exploration of a severe underlying injury. Rarely, a false aneurysm may develop from a small, contained leak.

AXIOM Lack of clinical findings does not eliminate major vascular injury in the neck.

Many surgeons have found a poor correlation between clinical signs and symptoms and the presence of an arterial injury. Moreover, the clinical signs frequently do not differentiate between injury to major and minor vessels. Carducci et al. found that almost a third of patients with major blood vessel trauma had no signs or symptoms of such injury, particularly when only a major vein was involved.[12] Fogelman and Stewart, reporting on 100 consecutive penetrating neck injuries, noted that 43% of patients with vascular injuries were hemodynamically stable, and 70% had no signs of bleeding.[40]

Yoder and Merck described the mandatory exploration of the necks of 48 patients with "innocuous appearing wounds without large hematomas or evidence of tracheal obstruction or massive bleeding".[41] They found arterial injuries in 12 patients, including five with carotid or vertebral arterial injuries. Saletta et al., who were also proponents of mandatory exploration, found that clinical signs were absent in two of 13 patients with major arterial injuries.[10]

INJURIES TO THE AERODIGESTIVE TRACTS
Injuries to the upper aerodigestive tract may be indicated by subcutaneous emphysema, coughing, or hematemesis. In the series by Weigelt et al., however, 30% of patients with esophageal injury had no clinical signs or symptoms of such a problem.[22] Sankaran and Walt emphasized that an important cause of death from penetrating neck wounds is delayed recognition and treatment of esophageal injuries.[43]

AXIOM Suspected airway injuries should be managed emergently in the operating room, especially when evidence exists that blood is being aspirated into the tracheobronchial tree.

Aspiration of blood from a nasogastric tube during or after its insertion may help to identify an injury in the stomach or esophagus; however, blood found in the stomach is frequently swallowed from injuries of the nose or mouth. The tube can also serve to evacuate gastric contents and thereby decrease the chance of later aspiration, particularly in the perianesthetic period.

With a possible vascular injury of the neck, one should defer insertion of the nasogastric tube until the patient is anesthetized in surgery; otherwise, a clot could be dislodged and start massive bleeding if the patient were to gag excessively as the nasogastric tube was being inserted.

NEUROLOGIC INJURIES
A complete neurologic examination should be performed with any neck injury that could damage the spinal cord, brachial plexus, sympathetic ganglia or blood supply to the brain, and it should be repeated frequently. Nerve injury may be manifest by sensory deficits, Horner syndrome, drooping of the corner of the mouth, or deviation of the tongue. Brachial plexus injuries may be detected by motor or sensory deficits in the upper extremities.

AXIOM With injuries in the neck, the neurologic examination should include an evaluation of the patient's mental status, cranial nerves, spinal cord, brachial plexus, and sympathetic nerves.

With carotid injuries, symptoms or signs of dysphagia or changes in affect are considered to be mild deficits. Monoplegia, hemiplegia, or coma are profound deficits.

TRAUMATIC ASPHYXIA
Traumatic asphyxia refers to a rare, but special combination of physical findings, including marked violaceous discoloration of the upper chest, neck, arms, and face following crushing chest trauma.[2,18] This is caused by sudden, severe compression of the chest causing a transient high-grade obstruction of venous return with extravasation of venous and capillary blood into the tissues drained by the superior vena cava. Subconjunctival hemorrhages are often seen with this condition. Any neurologic changes occurring are usually transient, but the sudden, severe venous hypertension can occasionally cause intracerebral hemorrhage with focal neurologic changes ranging from agitation to death.

AXIOM The tissue changes of traumatic asphyxia usually resolve spontaneously, but one must look carefully for associated injuries.

ROUTINE LAB STUDIES
With the exception of a complete blood cell count and type-and-cross match, usually little need exists for other routine laboratory tests in previously healthy individuals; however, in patients with liver disease, severe brain injury, or prolonged shock, a PT, PTT, and platelet count may also be indicated.

FURTHER INVESTIGATION VERSUS IMMEDIATE SURGERY
Once the patient has been resuscitated and stabilized and the history and physical examination are complete, the surgeon must decide whether to operate promptly, perform more diagnostic tests, or just observe. No disagreement exists about the need for immediate surgery on patients who are hemodynamically unstable or who have had severe hemorrhage or expanding hematoma. Patients who are hemodynamically stable, however, may undergo further diagnostic evaluation of the cardiovascular, respiratory, and digestive systems. Such investigations may include radiography, contrast swallows, CT scans, arteriography, laryngoscopy, bronchoscopy, and esophagoscopy.

Radiography

PLAIN

Neck

> **AXIOM** Lateral radiographs of the neck are indicated in all patients who have had penetrating injuries of the neck or severe blunt trauma above the shoulders.

Lateral radiography of the cervical spine should be obtained on all severe blunt trauma, especially when the head or upper chest are involved. Anteroposterior and lateral films of the neck may also reveal subcutaneous emphysema, airway compression, injury to laryngeal structures (especially those that are calcified), tracheal deviation, cervical spine injury, and increased thickness of the anterior paravertebral tissues due to bleeding or edema. The position of missile fragments should also be noted.

Free air in the neck, particularly in the deep perivisceral spaces after any instrumentation, is usually due to an injury to the hypopharynx, but may also be due to an esophageal, laryngeal, or tracheal tear. Following penetrating trauma, free air in the deep tissues may occasionally be due to air passing down the missile tract, but it is much more likely to be due to injury to aerodigestive structures. A lateral view of the neck may be particularly helpful in diagnosing injury to the pharynx or upper esophagus.

> **AXIOM** Increased prevertebral space behind the upper airway is usually due to injuries to the adjacent spine or aerodigestive tract.

Increased space between the posterior margin of the upper airway and the anterior border of the vertebral bodies can be very helpful. Normally, this distance is less than 4-5 mm in front C-3 and C-4 and less than 5-10 mm in front of C-5, C-6, and C-7. Increased space in this area after trauma is usually due to blood from an adjacent injury, and after 48-72 hours, it is often caused by infection.

With suspected airway trauma, the laryngotracheal shadow should be evaluated particularly carefully along its entire length for evidence of disruption. Interstitial emphysema along the fascial planes of the neck or mediastinum following blunt trauma is almost diagnostic of a tear in the aerodigestive tract.

Cervical spine

Cervical spine films are obtained on all patients with penetrating or blunt injuries that may have involved the cervical spine. Any patient with severe blunt trauma to the face or head should also have cervical spine films.

> **AXIOM** If an alert and oriented patient has full range of nonpainful neck motion, no local tenderness, and no distracting injuries, a significant cervical spine injury is effectively ruled out.

Fisher et al., in a report of 333 alert patients admitted for neurologic observation after sustaining blunt head trauma, found no cervical spine injuries in alert and oriented patients who were asymptomatic.[43] They further reported that only 11% of their patients with signs and/or symptoms that were strongly suggestive of cervical spine injuries actually had such damage.

Chest

Posteroanterior and lateral views of the chest may reveal subcutaneous or mediastinal emphysema, tracheal deviation, pneumothorax, hemothorax, fractured ribs, flail segments, pneumo- or hemopericardium, or widening of the mediastinum. With blunt trauma, the first two ribs should be inspected carefully for fracture because such injuries may be associated with an increased incidence of tracheobronchial, myocardial, or vascular injury. Chest radiography is particularly important with zone I injuries because of associated thoracic injuries in at least 27% of patients.[18]

ARTERIOGRAPHY

Fabian et al. summarized the general indications for angiography in patients with neck trauma as: (a) proximity of injury to the carotid artery, with or without hematoma; (b) shotgun blasts in which multiple arterial segments may be injured; (c) precise localization of injury in patients with probable or possible proximal common or high internal carotid injuries to allow planning of appropriate incisions and exposure; (d) blunt trauma with soft-tissue injury to the neck; and (e) blunt trauma with neurologic deficits unexplained by CT.[39]

> **AXIOM** Four-vessel angiography should be performed on all stable patients with suspected penetrating vascular injuries in zones I and III of the neck.

In general, when suspicion of a vascular injury exists, arteriograms of the ipsilateral carotid and vertebral vessels are obtained on all hemodynamically stable patients with penetrating wounds of the neck in zones I and III. With zone I injuries, the arch vessels and subclavian arteries should be visualized. In patients with gunshot wounds that could have transversed the midline, four-vessel studies, including both carotid and both vertebral arteries, are obtained. When vascular injury is obvious in zone II, arteriography is not necessary, but some surgeons believe that it may still provide a helpful road map, especially when zone I or III may also be involved.

> **PITFALL** ⊘
>
> *When the need for surgical exploration of a penetrating injury in zone II is obvious, further diagnostic studies tend to delay surgery and increase the chances of severe bleeding, aspiration, and CNS deterioration.*

Even when the patient is stable and there is no apparent injury in zone II, some authors advocate surgical exploration without routine angiography.[44] In contrast, other authors use angiography fairly routinely to reduce the number of unnecessary surgical explorations.[2,8,43,44] Angiography, however, is not completely without risk,[45] and a selective policy, possibly using duplex scanning, would seem desirable.

Control and repair of injured vessels in zones I and III of the neck may be extremely difficult at times and can carry some risk.[46] Vertebral artery injuries in particular are usually not suspected clinically and are generally only diagnosed by arteriography. In addition, in patients with neurologic deficits, documentation of vessel patency may be important to the intraoperative decision regarding repair or reconstruction of the internal carotid or vertebral arteries. Collateral circulation seen, especially in the circle of Willis, on cerebral angiography may also be helpful in determining whether it may be safer to ligate an injured vessel or perform a bypass procedure.

> **PITFALL** ⊘
>
> *Carotid and vertebral artery injuries may be present in the absence of hematoma, neurologic deficit, or clinically apparent blood loss.*

Several authors have questioned whether angiography is indicated in the patient with a penetrating wound of the neck who has no signs or symptoms[47,48]; however, ample evidence suggests that the physical examination for vascular injuries can be extremely unreliable. Almost three-fourths of patients with carotid artery injuries reviewed by Liekweg and Greenfield had no neurologic deficits.[49] Furthermore, hematomas were present in only two-thirds of carotid artery injuries reported by Thal in 1974. McCormick and Burch reported that 42% of 91 patients clinically suspected of having vascular injuries had normal arteriograms, while in those with no clinical evidence of vascular injury, 20% had angiographic demonstration of vessel trauma.[45] Thal[2] and Thal et al.[50] have noted that, even in the presence of physical signs of vascular injury (such as absent pulses, bruits, hematomas, or alterations of neurologic status), 70% of patients studied had no vascular injuries.

AXIOM In patients with blunt trauma, presence of central neurologic changes in spite of a normal CT of the brain should make one suspect a carotid injury.

The accuracy of angiography in the neck is generally extremely high. A recent, prospective study of 118 patients with penetrating neck trauma by Weigelt et al revealed no false-positive or false-negative arteriograms.[22] All patients in their series had angiography followed by operative exploration. All 11 vascular injuries in the series were properly identified preoperatively, and no missed injuries were found in the 107 patients with normal studies. Similar 100% accuracy with angiography was noted by Cohen et al.[21] and by Noyes et al.[51] Nevertheless, false-negative arteriograms due to clots occluding the injury have been reported.[52]

One of the advantages of preoperative angiography is the establishment of a road map for the approach to the carotid artery. Ideally, carotid angiography with cerebral vessel studies delineates the amount of crossover circulation. This is valuable knowledge to the surgeon who is determining the possibility of ICA ligation. Although it is widely believed that good crossover circulation exists in most patients through the circle of Willis, only 20% of individuals have complete circles. Furthermore, many patients have one or more developmental abnormalities that can restrict the effectiveness of collateral circulation of this vascular ring.[39,42]

AXIOM Whenever a neck is explored for trauma, the vascular and aerodigestive structures should be examined closely, even if preoperative arteriography and other studies do not reveal injuries.

For arteriography in the neck, an arch study using the Seldinger technique via the femoral route is the procedure of choice. The films should be taken in at least two planes. Digital subtraction angiography via the intravenous route can be extremely useful and has the advantages that less contrast medium and time are required and more oblique views can be obtained. However, the detail is not as good as with arterial studies.

Contrast Swallows

A high index of suspicion for pharyngoesophageal injuries must be maintained because they are easily missed clinically, radiologically, and endoscopically, and a delay in diagnosis may be associated with a great increase in morbidity and mortality.[42,53]

PITFALL ⊘

One should not rely on a normal Gastrografin swallow to eliminate pharyngoesophageal leak.

Extravasation of swallowed contrast material is diagnostic of a pharyngeal or esophageal leak; however, a negative contrast swallow is not reliable, particularly in the neck and especially when done with Gastrografin. Up to 50% of esophageal leaks may be missed on Gastrografin swallows. Even with careful barium studies, over 25% of esophageal leaks can be missed.

Some controversy exists as to whether the initial contrast swallow should be done with barium or meglumine diatrizolate (Gastrografin). Gastrografin is used by many physicians because, if a leak were present, the extravasated contrast material would be less likely to increase the severity of the inflammatory response and risk of infection; however, when the patient does not have a good cough and gag reflex and Gastrografin is aspirated into the lungs, severe chemical pneumonitis frequently develops. Barium, conversely, is less irritating to the lungs if it is aspirated, and the incidence of false-negative examinations is usually lower.

AXIOM Barium could cause increased inflammation and infection if it were to enter the mediastinum, but Gastrografin could cause severe pneumonitis if it were to be aspirated into the lungs.

In general, because most patients with a pharyngeal or esophageal leak undergo surgery and adequate drainage soon after demonstration of the perforation, barium is probably the preferred contrast material.

AXIOM When a patient with suspected esophageal injury has a negative Gastrografin swallow, the study should be immediately repeated with barium and/or an esophagoscopy should be performed.

Unless the esophagus is examined very carefully under fluoroscopy as the contrast material is given, the site of leak can be missed or not precisely localized. Weigelt et al. recommended that the initial study be a barium swallow, using anteroposterior and lateral views with cineradiography.[22] With this technique, the sensitivity was 89%, specificity 100%, and accuracy 94%. In reports by Noyes et al.[51] and Ordog et al.[9] the sensitivity was 80% in both, specificity 100% and 94%, and accuracy 95% and 90%, respectively.

AXIOM If a patient were uncooperative during a contrast swallow, if the study were equivocal, or if one were still concerned that esophageal injury may be present, endoscopy should be performed.

CT

Brain

When CT scans of the brain in a patient with a cerebral neurologic defect reveal no abnormality, the patient is usually said to have diffuse axonal injury (DAI). Such patients, however, should also be evaluated for the possibility of blunt carotid injury.

Neck

The ability of CT scans to sharply demonstrate most bony or soft-tissue injuries and to delineate fascial planes with exquisite detail is one of the many advantages of this technique. The extent of soft-tissue injury and hematoma formation can also be convincingly documented with CT. Injuries to the larynx can be examined in any designated plane by use of appropriate windows and level settings using advanced reformatting software.

AXIOM Clinically subtle injuries to laryngeal cartilages can usually be demonstrated clearly on CT.

Vertebrae and Spinal Cord

Neurologic injuries resulting from injury to the spinal cord are usually quite obvious clinically, and CT studies are often used only for confirmation or to document concomitant injuries; however, some patients present with neurologic deficits and no obvious spinal column injuries. In such patients, neurologic impairment may not be attributable to a bony or vascular insult, and the neurologic lesions may be demonstrated only by CT. Such injuries may include occult cervical spine fractures, epidural hematomas, or a partially transected spinal cord. Occasionally, metrizamide myelography may be used to demonstrate an injury. CT may also demonstrate unsuspected concomitant injuries to other vital structures.

VESSEL INJURIES

Aviv et al. recommended CT scans of the neck, followed by carotid angiography where indicated, for the patient with a history of blunt neck injury and ecchymosis of the pharyngeal wall because such findings, may be due to hematoma from an underlying carotid injury.[23]

Angiography with high-resolution dynamic CT can be even more helpful. It can not only identify discrete areas of vascular injury, but it can also detect damage to some vital soft-tissue structures. It should be remembered, however, that CT scanning of the head and neck can sometimes take 60 minutes or longer to perform.

> **AXIOM** Proper CT scanning requires a cooperative or sedated patient and should not be attempted with an acute, unprotected airway injury or unstable vital signs.

MRI

The ability of MRI to display most of the information that can be provided by CT scans with better definition of soft-tissue and vascular injuries may eventually make MRI the preferred diagnostic technique for neck trauma; however, the inability of MRI to reliably identify bone injuries and the constraints of its physical set-up will probably retard extensive use of this technique in recently-injured patients.

DUPLEX SCANS

Duplex (ultrasonographic) scans are used extensively for diagnosing nontraumatic carotid arterial disease, including dissections. This modality should detect most extracranial carotid injuries, but its results are operator dependent.

ENDOSCOPY

LARYNX AND TRACHEA

Endoscopy is the best method for evaluating the airway in the neck. Whenever possible, endoscopy for a possibly injured larynx should be performed in the operating room as soon as possible after injury. Noyes et al. noted that bronchoscopy and laryngoscopy, when done together, are 100% accurate for detecting upper airway injuries[51]; however, when they are done individually, an occasional false-negative result occurs.

Pharynx and esophagus

> **AXIOM** Only a high index of suspicion and a liberal attitude toward operative exploration of penetrating neck injuries can keep the incidence of missed pharyngeal and esophageal perforations to a minimum.

Pharyngoesophageal injuries can be difficult to diagnose and occur in up to 7% of penetrating injuries of the neck.[17] Consequently, surgery is recommended for all patients in whom the course or extent of the penetrating wound makes one suspicious of such damage.

> **AXIOM** Patients with platysma penetration who are suspected of having a vascular or visceral injury should either be promptly explored surgically or have a rapid, complete diagnostic work-up.

The work-up to eliminate visceral injury with penetrating neck trauma includes a contrast swallow, with or without esophagoscopy, plus laryngoscopy and bronchoscopy. Even when studies do not reveal injury, the patient should be closely observed in the hospital without oral intake for at least 24 hours.

If an injury to the pharynx or esophagus is suspected and a contrast swallow is negative or equivocal, one should proceed with esophagoscopy. One must, however, first be sure that the airway is intact or protected with an endotracheal tube or tracheostomy. Flex-

ible esophagoscopy is usually safer and easier to perform than rigid esophagoscopy, but occasionally the latter may be preferable, particularly when a foreign body is present or when a perforation is suspected in spite of a negative contrast swallow.

> **AXIOM** When endoscopy is to be performed under topical anesthesia, it is important that major vascular injuries be eliminated prior to the procedure because gagging or retching could restart bleeding from injured vessels.

Although pharyngeal and esophageal injuries can often be seen fairly readily during endoscopy, in some reports more than half of the perforations have been missed with this procedure,[22] particularly when the lesion is small and in the pharynx or cervical esophagus. Esophageal injuries are particularly apt to be missed when the patient is on a ventilator and the esophagus does not expand well during the examination. Because the conscious, spontaneously breathing patient tends to dilate the esophagus during inspiration, topical anesthesia for endoscopy often provides better visualization than general anesthesia.

A recent prospective study at Parkland Memorial Hospital evaluated the ability of endoscopic and contrast studies to define esophageal injuries after penetrating neck trauma.[22] Barium swallow was performed in 111 patients, flexible endoscopy in 106, and rigid endoscopy in 116. Both the barium swallow and rigid endoscopy had 20% false-negative rates; however, by combining these two studies, no injury was missed. Flexible endoscopy was not reliable, having a 63% (⅝) false-negative rate.

Noyes et al. also found that rigid endoscopy was more accurate than examination with a flexible scope.[51] In that series, three patients had esophageal injuries; endoscopy was positive in two and negative in one. In two other patients, esophagoscopy was considered positive, but no injury was found at surgery.

> **AXIOM** If an ecchymosis of the posterior or lateral pharyngeal wall is seen on endoscopy, one should be concerned about a possible underlying vascular injury.[23]

Summary of Diagnostic Efforts

The selection and value of angiography and panendoscopy in stable patients depend, to some extent, on the zone in which the injury is located. Nonsurgical diagnostic investigations are most helpful in zone III trauma where surgical exposure of injuries can be much more difficult than in zone II. Arteriography may also demonstrate vascular injuries that are: (a) high in the neck, (b) involve the vertebral arteries, and/or (c) are better managed by an interventional radiologist. In addition, when surgical evaluation of a high zone III injury is indicated, the incision may need to be extended and dislocation of the mandible may need to be performed to provide adequate exposure of the distal ICA.

In zone II, adequate surgical exposure of all injuries can usually be readily accomplished through an anterior sternocleidomastoid neck incision. Consequently, the precise site of injury, as defined by preoperative tests, is not as critical as with injuries in zones I and III. Many surgeons now believe that routine exploration of penetrating injuries in zone II without special studies is safer (less pharyngeal and esophageal injuries missed) and less expensive, especially when the patient can go home the next day. Nevertheless, many authors believe that preoperative angiography is indicated in stable patients with zone II injuries to reduce the incidence of false-negative explorations.[10,51,56] In special settings, identification of vascular damage preoperatively may allow for early angiographic vascular control prior to exposing the injury surgically with its attendant risks of bleeding. This may be particularly important with transcervical gunshot wounds in which 83% of explorations may be positive and more than 40% of patients may have bilateral injuries requiring surgical correction.[55]

TREATMENT—GENERAL

Emergent

AXIOM Early death after neck injury is usually due to airway compromise, exsanguination, or CNS injury.

When any suspicion of an inadequate airway after trauma to the neck exists, the problem should be resolved immediately. Despite extensive literature on penetrating neck trauma, little attention has been devoted to this problem.[57] Securing an airway under adverse conditions associated with penetrating neck injuries can be extremely difficult. Of 114 patients with penetration beyond the platysma muscle reviewed by Eggen and Jorden, 26 (23%) were intubated urgently in the emergency department for acute respiratory distress, airway compromise from blood or secretions, extensive subcutaneous emphysema, tracheal shift, or severe alterations in mental status.[57] The maneuvers used to provide an airway included orotracheal intubation (9), nasotracheal intubation (4), surgical airway (9), and passage of the endotracheal tube through the neck wound (4). Eight (31%) of the 26 urgent intubations were initially unsuccessful. Of 6 initially unsuccessful orotracheal attempts, 3 were accomplished via open neck wounds, 2 by repeated attempts at orotracheal intubation, and 1 by emergency tracheostomy. Two unsuccessful nasotracheal attempts were resolved by tracheostomy.

In patients with blunt trauma, the neck should be stabilized in a neutral position until injury to the cervical spine can be eliminated. Patients with evidence of major vessel damage, such as shock, large expanding hematomas, or uncontrollable bleeding are taken directly to the operating room.

Most neurologic injuries are caused by the initial neck injury and are not preventable; however, some patients with no direct brain injury are comatose because of hypovolemic shock or illicit drugs. With blunt trauma, occasional associated injury to the vertebral or internal carotid arteries occurs, and the neck should be immobilized to prevent further injury to these vessels or to the spinal cord and brachial plexus. Care must also be taken to prevent ischemia or hypoxia which could cause secondary damage to the CNS.

Nonemergent Management

AXIOM The management of stable patients with penetrating zone II neck injuries and no evidence of vascular or aerodigestive tract injury remains controversial.[58-60]

The debate centers primarily on whether patients with zone II injuries should have routine surgical neck exploration, or whether there should only be surgical intervention when the diagnostic evaluation reveals significant correctable injury.

MANDATORY EXPLORATION

Mandatory surgical neck exploration was the accepted management for penetrating wounds to the neck during World War II. During this time, the mortality of penetrating neck wounds declined from more than 11% to approximately 5% with adoption of a policy of surgical neck exploration in all patients with deep, penetrating neck wounds.[12] Cohen et al.[21] and Fogelman and Stewart[40] championed mandatory exploration and noted significant injuries in up to 95% of patients with penetrating neck injuries.

AXIOM When thorough diagnostic studies cannot be performed promptly in patients with penetrating neck injuries, early surgical exploration is generally safer than continued clinical evaluation.

The primary advantage to performing routine surgical neck exploration has been believed to be a decreased incidence of missed injuries. Up to 25% of patients undergoing mandatory neck exploration have visceral injuries that were not suspected during the preoperative clinical evaluation.[20,44] In addition, negative neck exploration is usually associated with a morbidity rate of < 5% and no mortality. Roon and Christenson,[6] for example, had only one wound complication and no deaths in 82 negative neck explorations. Conversely, missed or delayed recognition of esophageal injuries can be associated with considerable morbidity and mortality.[61,62] Early operation and repair of an esophageal injury within 12 hours of trauma is usually associated with a mortality rate of less than 10%; in contrast, delay beyond that time may be associated with a mortality rate exceeding 40%. Fogelman and Stewart reported a four-fold increase in mortality rate when surgical repair of an esophageal injury was delayed more than six hours.[40]

In spite of its proved efficacy, mandatory exploration does have some disadvantages. The negative exploration rate has been reported to be as high as 67%.[10] Furthermore, the morbidity of a negative exploration is not negligible.[44] Such concerns have led to a reevaluation of the indications for surgical intervention.

SELECTIVE CONSERVATISM

An alternate method of management that has been gaining increasing acceptance in stable patients with penetrating neck wounds is selective conservatism. This technique requires that patients with penetrating neck wounds be studied promptly with angiography, contrast, or other radiologic studies, and endoscopy as needed. Surgical neck exploration is undertaken when these techniques reveal an injury requiring surgical repair.[54]

AXIOM A policy of selective conservatism for neck injuries will not be successful unless the needed diagnostic tests can be done promptly and accurately.[34]

Using a selective surgical approach, the incidence of negative neck exploration is reduced to approximately 20% and the incidence of missed injuries in many series is negligible.[2,56] No statistically significant difference usually occurs in morbidity, mortality, or financial cost of management.[2,51]

AXIOM Although a policy of selective conservatism reduces the morbidity and mortality rates associated with a negative exploration of the neck, diagnostic studies done to eliminate significant injuries have some costs and risks that should be considered.[37]

Maddison noted a 14% incidence of complications with arteriography in patients with penetrating wounds of the neck.[63] These may include arterial dissection, occlusion, reactions to intravenous contrast, renal failure, false aneurysms, or hemorrhage. Endoscopy can cause iatrogenic perforation, and contrast swallows may result in aspiration of contrast or gastrointestinal secretions into the lungs.

In 1981, Merion et al. reviewed 27 series reported in the literature and documented the clinical courses of 4369 patients (Table 14-1).[64] From this study, it appeared that little or no difference in outcome occurred between mandatory exploration and selective conservatism. If the outcome for mandatory and selective management is similar, cost-effectiveness becomes a major concern.[64,65]

AXIOM With zone II injuries, it is often quicker, safer, and less expensive to explore the neck surgically than it is to get all the studies needed to eliminate vascular or aerodigestive tract injuries.

Weigelt et al. estimated the cost of arteriography, esophagography, and a one-day hospitalization to be $2,670 in 1986 dollars.[22] Rigid esophagoscopy increased the cost to $3,350. If a neck exploration were still required, the charge would increase to $4,790. The hospital cost for mandatory exploration with no diagnostic tests was

TABLE 14-1 *Neck Trauma: Selective versus Routine Exploration*

	2660 Selective (13 series)	*1708 Mandatory (14 series)*
Immediate operation	1394 (52.4%)	1516 (88.7%)
Injury requiring repair	934 (67.0%)	928 (61.2%)
Observed	1266 (46.6%)	193 (11.3%)
Delayed operation for an overlooked injury	30 (2.4%)	15 (7.7%)
Mortality—when significant injury found at immediate operation	86 (9.2%)	77 (8.3%)
Mortality—no operation	21 (1.7%)	8 (4.1%)
Mortality—delayed operation	5 (16.7%)	2 (13.3%)
Total Mortality	112 (4.2%)	87 (5.1%)

From: Merion RM, Haness JK, Rousbergh SR, et al. Selective management of penetrating neck trauma. Ann Surg 1981;116:691.

$2,840 for a negative cervical exploration. Thus, Weigelt et al. found that an aggressive, selective approach is often more expensive than mandatory exploration; however, this comparison ignores the cost of operative complications which could greatly alter the final financial considerations.[22]

In most analyses, the cost of mandatory exploration (including the fees for operating room time, anesthesia, surgeons and recovery room) balances those for all of the diagnostic studies. When the patient with a negative exploration is discharged in a day or two, there is a cost advantage to the mandatory exploration; however, Elerding et al. reported that the duration of hospitalization after a negative exploration actually averaged three days.[66] In three other reports, hospitalization ranged 3-8 days[64,67,68]; however, in more recent years, the length of hospital stays for all procedures tends to be much lower.

Callaham[59] noted that "For the time being, each surgeon will have to resolve this issue (mandatory exploration vs selective conservatism) personally, based on his experience, the hospital resources, and local cost. Evolving and improving diagnostic tests will no doubt make observation more reliable, but may also make it more expensive."[53] A large, controlled, prospective study of patients with penetrating midneck trauma and no obvious clinical signs of injury to aerodigestive or neurovascular structures could help resolve this controversy.

AXIOM Generally, in patients with penetrating neck wounds in zone II, it may be safest to practice mandatory exploration on GSWs and selective conservatism on stab wounds.

SPECIAL SITUATIONS

Evidence of Chest Injury

AXIOM Penetrating neck trauma with associated chest involvement is not an absolute indication for exploration of the neck or chest.

Although many patients with penetrating neck wounds can be treated selectively, some investigators have believed that evidence of skin injury on one side of the neck with evidence of a chest injury on the other side (i.e., a transmediastinal injury) is an indication for exploration of the neck and/or chest.[69] Goldberg et al. from Capetown, South Africa, however, successfully observed 75 of 94 patients who had penetrating neck wounds and evidence of chest penetration by the presence of hemothorax or pneumothorax.[66] The other 19 patients were explored because of shock, hematomas, or other signs of vascular or visceral injury.

AXIOM Most patients with neck injuries that also involve the chest do not require chest exploration; of those who do, obvious clinical evidence of severe bleeding or an aerodigestive tract injury usually exists.

Technical Considerations

ANESTHESIA

AXIOM When a possibility of vascular injury in the neck exists, a nasogastric tube should not be inserted until the patient is anesthetized because gagging or retching during insertion of the tube could restart bleeding.

Insertion of a nasogastric tube, which may cause retching or gagging, should be withheld until there is little risk of such a response. The nasogastric tube can be inserted just after the induction of anesthesia, when rapid exploration and treatment can be initiated if bleeding were to occur.

Whenever possible, neck exploration should be performed under general anesthesia in the operating room; however, one must be very careful with endotracheal intubation in anyone with a possible laryngeal or tracheal injury.

PITFALL ⊘

When an endotracheal tube is too large or is inserted roughly, it can cause severe damage to a normal larynx or trachea or cause complete disruption or occlusion if they were injured.

A wide variety of laryngeal and tracheal injuries may occur at intubation. A tube that is too large is particularly apt to damage the anterior commissure. If the tube were inserted too vigorously, it could cause arytenoid dislocation or postcricoid ulceration and scarring; the resultant scars, webs, or strictures could then cause aphonia and/or airway compromise.

With any neck injury, one must be prepared to immediately provide a surgical airway during endoscopic examination or endotracheal intubation. If the airway suddenly occludes and an endotracheal tube cannot be inserted promptly, the surgeon only has about 2-3 minutes to provide adequate oxygenation via a needle or surgical cricothyroidotomy or tracheostomy.

AXIOM If the airway occludes suddenly and suspicion exists of laryngeal injury, a large needle or surgical tracheostomy should be rapidly provided.

POSITIONING AND SKIN PREPARATION

Once the airway is assured, appropriate preparations for surgery can be made at a less urgent pace. The patient should be placed supine with a roll between the scapulas, with the neck in extension, and the head rotated away from the side to be explored. When cervical spine injury is a possibility, the neck should not be turned to the side; but this makes the surgical dissection and exposure more difficult. Preparation and draping should extend from the chin to the umbilicus and should include all of the anterior and lateral neck and chest so that a median sternotomy or anterolateral thoracotomy can be performed if necessary. The arms should be free-draped. Instruments for vascular repairs and thoracotomy should be immediately available.

Care must be taken during preoperative preparation not to rub the neck vigorously because dislodging a tamponading clot could cause sudden, severe bleeding or embolization. Consequently, it is better to cleanse the skin gently by painting on an antiseptic rather than by scrubbing with soap.

In addition to preparing the surgical area, if time permits, a vascular donor site in one of the thighs should be cleaned and draped when the patient has a known or potential injury that may require an interposition venous graft or patch.

INCISIONS

> **AXIOM** No limited miniexplorations or probing of neck injuries should be conducted in the emergency department.

Limited miniexploration of neck injuries in the emergency department or operating room is generally inappropriate. It provides little information and can cause sudden severe bleeding and/or airway compromise.

Midneck

A low, standard "collar" incision 1-2 cm above the heads of the clavicles is used in patients whose preoperative evaluation suggests bilateral neck injuries or damage to the larynx or trachea. A horizontal incision placed over the midportion of the thyroid cartilage is generally used only when it is certain that the injuries are limited to the larynx.

Unilateral Neck

> **AXIOM** Unilateral neck explorations are usually best done through an incision along the anterior border of the sternocleidomastoid muscle.

An anterior sternocleidomastoid incision usually provides ready access to the trachea, thyroid gland, larynx, and carotid artery in a plane anteromedial to the internal jugular vein. The common carotid artery is exposed by division of the branches of the internal jugular vein as they cross the artery. The esophagus can be exposed by posterolateral or anteromedial retraction of the internal jugular vein, carotid artery, and vagus nerve (which extends posteriorly within the carotid sheath). Care must be taken to avoid damaging the sympathetic chain which lies posterior to the carotid sheath on the prevertebral muscles. When it is difficult to identify the esophagus, a nasogastric tube can be passed to help determine its position.

If a contralateral injury is suspected intraoperatively, exposure of the other side of the neck may be obtained by extending the lower end of this incision transversely as a "collar" incision or by making a separate oblique incision.

> **AXIOM** Any vessel that is in the path of a knife or near the presumed tract of a bullet must be explored to definitely rule out a vascular lesion.

Vessels that have any possibility of injury should be thoroughly explored during surgery, even after obtaining a negative preoperative arteriogram. False-negative arteriograms have been reported in up to 10% of patients.[52]

Lower Neck

The right subclavian artery, both subclavian veins, and the distal two-thirds of the left subclavian artery can usually be exposed through a supraclavicular incision. Exposure of these structures can generally be improved when one performs a subperiosteal resection of the medial third of the clavicle. If one needs to get to the origins of the innominate, left common carotid or left subclavian arteries, a median

sternotomy incision should be performed. If the clavicular head of the sternocleidomastoid is divided and the supraclavicular fat pad is cleared away by blunt dissection, one can examine most of the brachial plexus, the scalenus anticus muscle, and the phrenic nerve crossing it from the lateral side. Division of the scalenus anticus muscle with careful preservation of the phrenic nerve exposes the second part of the subclavian artery.

Access to the distal subclavian artery and vein can be improved by division of the clavicle at its midpoint or by performing a subperiosteal resection of the middle and medial thirds of the clavicle. Although resection of the head of the clavicle can provide more exposure in many cases, simple division of the clavicle tends to cause less pain and less impairment of shoulder girdle motion postoperatively.

Upper Neck

Access to the vessels and structures close to the base of the skull can be improved by: (a) dividing the sternocleidomastoid muscle near its insertion into the mastoid process and/or (b) dislocating the temporomandibular joint and pulling the mandible forward. Care must be taken to avoid injury to the hypoglossal nerve (which usually crosses the internal and external carotid artery about 1.5-3.0 cm above their origin) and the spinal accessory nerve (which enters the deep part of the sternocleidomastoid muscle about 3-4 cm below the mastoid process). The ICA lays posteromedial to the internal jugular vein and the two vessels are separated by the lower four cranial nerves which should carefully be preserved. The wall of the pharynx is the most medial structure.

MANAGEMENT OF SPECIFIC INJURIES

Vascular

PENETRATING INJURIES

ICA and CCA Injuries

The carotid arteries are injured in about 10-15% of all penetrating injuries of the neck.[17] This includes the CCA in 4-8%, ICA in 1-4%, and external carotid (ECA) in 1-5%.

TYPES OF INJURIES

High ICA Injuries. When a high ICA lesion is found, adequate exposure of the vessel can be very difficult. Additional exposure can be obtained by anterior subluxation of the mandible to a more anterior and inferior position. Fry and Fry found that mandibular joint dislocation and maintenance of that position with arch bars allows exposure of another 1-2 cm of ICA.[70] Fisher et al. described another method of mandibular subluxation using a circummandibular-transnasal wiring technique which is said to be quick, easy to perform, and not associated with any TMJ dysfunction.[43] Transection of the omohyoid muscle usually also improves exposure.[17] Other procedures that have been described for improving exposure of the distal ICA include: (a) detachment of the sternocleidomastoid muscle from the mastoid process,[71] (b) division of the digastric muscle and occipital artery,[50] (c) lateral mandibulotomy,[72] and (d) a posterolateral approach.[73]

Bleeding from the distal ICA immediately adjacent to the skull can be extremely difficult to manage. Under such circumstances, the injury may be controlled best by inserting a Fogarty balloon-tipped catheter into the distal segment and then inflating the balloon. If necessary, the catheter can be left in place for several weeks until the vessel has solidly thrombosed.[2]

When it is anticipated that the ICA will be clamped for more than 10-15 minutes, the patient should be systemically heparinized 2-3 minutes prior to clamping the artery, providing no associated injuries are manifest that would preclude its use. Anticoagulation is rarely indicated for patients requiring only a simple rapid repair of the ICA.

Internal Carotid Injuries with Neurologic Deficits. Controversy continues as to whether an injured ICA should be repaired when the patient has a major neurologic deficit. In 1964, Wylie et al. showed that ischemic brain tissue caused by an acute stroke can be converted into a hemorrhagic infarct when the responsible occluded vessel is opened and perfusion is reestablished soon after the infarct.[74] Bradley confirmed that observation in a review of 24 patients with penetrating carotid injuries.[71] Ten of these patients had neurologic deficits, five of whom died following revascularization; two of the five patients who died had hemorrhagic infarcts at autopsy. They concluded that ligation should be considered for patients with severe preoperative neurologic symptoms. Cohen et al. also suggested that there was a high risk of hemorrhage into the infarcted area after carotid artery injury if the area were revascularized[75]; however, they reported no autopsy data to support this belief.

The idea that early repair of internal carotid injuries increases the risk of hemorrhagic infarct has been contested by many authors. In 1980, Ledgerwood et al. recommended that primary arterial repair be performed in all patients who were not comatose.[76] They provided direct evidence of its safety in five patients who presented in coma or with stroke, all of whom underwent primary repair of the injured vessel. Postmortem examination in the patients who died revealed that the deaths were caused by diffuse cerebral edema and not hemorrhagic infarction. Brown et al. reported similar findings in 1982.[77]

Liekweg and Greenfield reviewed 233 patients with carotid artery injury collected from the literature, and concluded that, in patients with any neurologic deficit short of coma, less morbidity and mortality occurred after repair than after ligation.[49] Unger et al., in an extensive review of the English-language literature from 1952 through 1979, analyzed 722 patients.[78] Of the 186 patients presenting with severe neurologic deficits, 34% improved following primary arterial repair. This was much better than the 14% improvement rate in patients who had the injured carotid artery ligated or who did not have surgery. Shock or coma were independent, ominous findings, but no evidence indicated that coma was a contraindication to restoring arterial continuity; however, the authors pointed out that satisfactory follow-up data existed on only 40 patients in the entire literature.

Brown et al. also recommended that all patients who present with central neurologic deficits short of coma after carotid artery injury, undergo revascularization, particularly when there had been minimal ischemic time.[77] In their study, nine patients presenting in coma underwent revascularization, with significant clinical improvement in six. The authors believed that the three patients who died probably would have done so without the procedure.

In 1988, Richardson et al. confirmed good outcomes for primary repair of carotid arterial injuries.[79] In their study, 13 patients whose neurologic conditions were difficult to determine because of the presence of shock or confusion had arterial repair of their injuries, with good neurologic outcomes in 12. The one death resulted from exsanguination not related to the carotid arterial injury. Those authors recommended prompt preoperative angiography to alert the surgeon to occult injuries to the vertebral or subclavian arteries, followed by early repair.[79] They presented five patients with clinically unsuspected findings including one patient with bilateral carotid artery injury, to support their recommendation for preoperative arteriography.

> **AXIOM** Regardless of the absence or extent of neurologic defects, the ICA should be repaired when prograde flow still is manifest. When no prograde flow exists, the vessel should be ligated.

Although controversy still exists concerning repair or ligation of an injured ICA in patients with deep coma, these patients tend to do very poorly regardless what is done. It increasingly appears that there is minimal additional risk to repair, and there may be something to gain. As Fabian et al. reported, some of these comas, or at least part of the coma, may be due to shock, alcohol, or other substances[39]; consequently, one should consider ligation of an injured ICA only in patients who do not have internal carotid flow, particularly when they

have a high intraluminal thrombus that cannot be safely removed surgically and may embolize.

Subadventitial Hematomas. If a subadventitial hematoma is noted at operation, a vertical arteriotomy is made over the area, and the inside of the vessel inspected for injury. If a portion of the ICA must be resected, a saphenous vein graft or the proximal 2-3 cm of the external carotid artery can be used as an in-continuity interposition graft.

Minimal Intimal Defects. Anticoagulation as therapy for small intimal defects in carotid arteries was successful in all six patients in whom this was attempted in a report by Fabian et al.[39] They believed that these lesions are probably similar to the injuries caused by needles during carotid angiography.

TECHNICAL CONSIDERATIONS

Internal Carotid Shunts. Once bleeding from an internal carotid artery injury has been controlled, systemic heparinization is usually recommended (in order to prevent embolic complications) unless concurrent injuries to the eyes, brain, or spinal cord occur. Following this, it may be advisable to insert a temporary intravascular shunt for added protection to the brain when: (a) the backflow from the distal ICA is scant, (b) the stump pressure is < 40-50 mm Hg, or (c) the repair will take more than 5-10 minutes or one must wait while a vein graft or vein patch is obtained. Shunts were used in none of the 31 patients studied by Ledgerwood et al.[76] or the 37 studied by Richardson et al.,[79] but were used in 10 (56%) of the 18 vessels repaired by Liekweg and Greenfield.[49] These data, however, show no advantage or disadvantage to using a shunt.

Shunts are rarely indicated during repair of common carotid injuries, especially when the distal clamp is applied proximal to its bifurcation into the ECA and ICA. It is generally believed that collateral retrograde flow from the ECA is usually quite adequate to supply the ICA.

Bypass Grafts

> **AXIOM** Prosthetic bypass grafts to restore flow to an injured carotid artery should be avoided if possible because of the high rate of later occlusion.

Fabian et al. believed that prosthetic bypass grafts for ICA or CCA injuries should be avoided when possible.[39] Of six patients with normal preoperative CNS examinations who had bypass grafts for carotid injuries, two developed major strokes 3 and 7 days postoperatively, presumably from thrombosis of PTFE grafts. Others have also reported adverse outcomes with the use of prosthetic grafts. Richardson et al. reported a stroke resulting from a clotted PTFE graft[79] and Meyer et al. reported a blowout of a saphenous vein graft from sepsis 10 days postoperatively in a patient with an associated esophageal injury.[80] In some series the need for bypass grafts has been very low. The incidence was 3% for Brown et al.[77] and 7% for Ledgerwood et al.[76]

When a bypass graft must be used, a prosthetic graft is more likely to thrombose and also is more likely to become infected than a saphenous vein graft; however, when a satisfactory vein graft is not available in the arms or legs, the surgeon may be forced to use a prosthesis. Furthermore, Feliciano et al. reported that if a prosthetic graft were to become infected, it would likely occlude or form a pseudoaneurysm at the suture line, while an infected vein graft would be more likely to lyse and bleed massively.[81]

EC-IC Shunts. When an injury to the ICA is extensive or it is necessary to ligate the distal segment, one option available to maintain cerebral blood flow is an extracranial-intracranial (EC-IC) bypass. This is typically accomplished by anastomosing the middle meningeal artery to the middle cerebral artery. This may be indicated in special centers where such surgery is available when the cerebral collateral circulation, proved by arteriography, is inadequate and a neurologic deficit has been present for less than 2-4 hours. Unfortunately, the long-term results with EC-IC bypasses have not been encouraging.

Postrepair Angiography. Intraoperative angiography following restoration of blood flow in injured critical vessels is advisable because of the serious consequences of inadequate reconstruction. When a graft is inserted, postrepair angiography can be particularly important.[39] Approximately 6% of such repairs will be shown on postrepair arteriography to require revision.

> **AXIOM** If any question exists about the adequacy of a vascular repair or its run-off, intraoperative postrepair angiography should be performed.

Vertebral Artery

The vertebral artery is injured in only about 1-2% of penetrating neck injuries. However, Willis et al. found angiographic evidence of vertebral artery injury in 12 (46%) of 26 patients with blunt trauma to the cervical spine.[82]

Patients with vertebral artery injuries have a mortality rate averaging about 11%, primarily from associated injuries.[17] Similarly, Yee et al. reported on 16 patients, eight of whom had neurologic complaints on admission.[83] The treatment for vertebral artery injuries included surgical ligation (2), transcatheter embolization (4), and simple observation (10). Although eight patients had neurologic signs or symptoms on admission, there were no deaths, no late bleeding, and no neurologic complications following treatment. In contrast, Miyachi et al. recently reported two patients with cerebellar infarction due to bilateral or dominant vertebral artery occlusion.[84]

Injuries to a vertebral artery near its origin from the subclavian artery can be managed by ligation of the proximal segment. If any question exists about the blood supply to the brain, an anastomosis of the distal end of the vertebral artery to the side of the CCA can be performed. Higher vertebral artery injuries can usually be controlled by performing proximal and distal ligation. Such ligations should be safe if angiography were to reveal a normal contralateral vertebral artery and if no demonstrable extracranial branches were to extend from the ligated portion of the vertebral artery to the spinal cord.

The proximal part of the vertebral artery may be relatively easy to expose at its take-off from the subclavian vessel; however, exposing the distal end can be much more difficult and may require unroofing the bony canal at the C-1, C-2 interspace. The vertebral vessels can also be ligated, when needed, between C-2 and C-6 by removing the portion of the transverse processes covering the artery.

> **AXIOM** Interventional radiology should be considered in patients with bleeding or A-V fistulas from high vertebral or very high ICA injuries.

When the vertebral artery injury is above the sixth cervical vertebra, one can often use interventional radiology to occlude it with autologous clot or other material.[34] Vertebral arteriovenous fistulas, which occur in up to 10-15% of vertebral arterial injuries, should probably also be treated angiographically whenever possible. Nevertheless, exploration of the neck may still be required to manage any associated injuries. This may include other vascular injuries in 10-25%, pharyngoesophageal injuries in 5-25%, and neurologic or spinal cord injuries in 15-25%.[17]

Arterial Injuries in Zone I

Adequate exposure for zone I arterial injuries can often be obtained with an oblique cervical incision just above the clavicle.[22] Resection of the medial portion of the clavicle can often provide even better exposure. In some instances, the incision will have to be extended into a median sternotomy to obtain adequate proximal control of the injured vessels. In some instance of uncontrolled intrathoracic hem-

orrhage from what is believed to be the proximal left subclavian artery, an anterior third or fourth intercostal space incision on the left will allow one to clamp the artery just above its origin from the arch of the aorta. Injuries to a subclavian artery distal to the vertebral artery origin can generally be ligated rather than repaired because of excellent collateral circulation in this area.

Venous Injuries

> **AXIOM** Asymptomatic venous injuries in the neck are only rarely diagnosed preoperatively, and surgical exploration with ligation or repair is seldom required for an isolated injury.

The jugular vein is the most frequently injured vessel in the neck, but in many cases, no preoperative evidence of such an injury is manifest. Unless the patient is actively bleeding, isolated jugular vein injuries are seldom important and only rarely require surgical treatment. Occasionally, however, a hematoma from such an injury can cause some airway compression. Simple lacerations of the larger veins of the neck encountered during surgical exploration are repaired unless the patient's condition is so unstable that ligation is essential for rapid control of blood loss to conclude the operation. When the contralateral internal jugular vein is patent, moderate-to-severe lacerations of the internal jugular vein can be ligated with relative impunity.

Some surgeons are concerned that repair of a long or irregular laceration of an internal jugular vein may form thrombi which could later embolize to the lungs; however, Asensio et al. noted that such complications appear to be rare.[17] In their extensive review of the literature, they found no patients with these complications. Care must also be taken to prevent air embolism when the venous injury is exposed and manipulated.

Results with Extracranial Vascular Injuries

The mortality rate with carotid injuries averages about 15-20%.[17] The factors thought to influence the outcome of major extracranial vascular injuries, especially those involving the carotids, include shock, ischemia time, location (ICA vs CCA), the adequacy of the collateral circulation, and the presence or absence of prograde flow.[39]

Although about 90% of cranial blood flow comes from the carotid arteries,[85] only about 20% of individuals have a complete circle of Willis.[86] It is the patient with poor collateral cerebral blood flow who is most apt to develop a severe neurologic defect when an ICA is acutely occluded.[49]

> **AXIOM** Shock in patients with neurologic defects should be corrected as rapidly as possible to reduce the amount of cerebral damage.

BLUNT VASCULAR INJURIES

Cogbill et al. noted that although blunt trauma to the carotid artery is rare, it can cause death in up to 40% of patients and permanent neurologic impairment in up to 80% of the survivors.[87]

Etiology and Pathophysiology

> **AXIOM** Blunt carotid artery injuries that cause symptoms usually have a delayed dissection in the media with subsequent thrombotic occlusion.

Okuhn reported that the two main types of carotid dissections are traumatic or spontaneous in origin.[88] Traumatic carotid dissection is usually caused by a severe deceleration or hyperextension injury. In a prospective experience derived from 11 institutions over a six-year period, 60 blunt carotid injuries were found in 49 patients.[87] The most common etiology was motor vehicle accidents and the ICA was involved much more frequently than the CCA.

Spontaneous dissections may involve any part of the ICA, but traumatic dissection usually involves the distal artery, often right up to the skull. A spontaneous dissection may result in a "jelly-roll" appearance of the artery in cross-section due to curling of the dissected intima and inner media with the jelly-like thrombus in the false lumen.

Diagnosis

Spontaneous carotid dissection usually causes transient ischemic attacks (56%) or a completed stroke (30%).[87] An associated sudden onset of ipsilateral headache and neck pain may be helpful in making the diagnosis. Traumatic dissections apparently act similarly, but a delay of 2-7 days often occurs after the trauma before localizing neurologic findings develop. In the series by Cogbill et al. significant neurologic deficits developed more than 12 hours after normal neurologic examinations were obtained in 14 (29%) of their patients.[87]

AXIOM Blunt carotid injury should be suspected in patients who have severe head trauma and localized neurologic changes but have no lesions on CT of the brain to explain the clinical findings.

The diagnosis of carotid dissection is usually made with arteriography which typically shows extensive narrowing of the internal carotid lumen, often extending up to the skull. This "carotid string sign" represents elevation and folding of the intima in the dissected segment. In some instances, carotid arteriography shows a tapered area of narrowing (referred to as a "dunce's cap" deformity) with distal occlusion.

Of 18 patients with blunt carotid injuries who had angiography in the series by Fabian et al., 11 had unilateral ICA dissections and 7 had bilateral dissections.[39] The initial neurologic examinations were normal in 8 of these 18 patients, but later all 18 patients had focal deficits or altered mental status. In the series by Cogbill et al., the diagnosis was confirmed by angiography in 42 (86%).[87] Duplex ultrasonography accurately demonstrated arterial injury in 12 (86%) of 14 patients. The arterial lesions included thrombosis in 20 arteries, arterial dissection alone in 19, dissection with pseudoaneurysm in six, pseudoaneurysm alone in five, frank arterial disruption in seven, and carotid-cavernous fistula in three.

Lebos and Saadia reported on three patients who had penetrating neck trauma with unsuspected blunt carotid injury.[89] They emphasized the need for a high index of suspicion and early angiography to prevent what may be severe neurologic sequelae.

Treatment

If a vascular injury were found in conjunction with damage to any cervical vertebrae, the head and neck should be immobilized to prevent any additional injury to the spinal cord or arteries in the neck. Stabilization of the neck with a Halo vest may be safer than skeletal traction because an injured spinal cord or neck vessels may be further damaged by traction.[28] In the series by Cogbill et al., arterial dissection was managed nonsurgically in 15 (79%) patients, the majority with systemic anticoagulation.[87] Arterial thrombosis was managed with supportive therapy alone in 16 (80%) patients. Six (55%) of the 11 pseudoaneurysms were repaired. Three carotid-cavernous fistulas were successfully treated with balloon occlusion. Cogbill et al. concluded that with blunt carotid trauma: (a) neurologic symptoms may be delayed, (b) arterial dissection without complete occlusion may be managed by anticoagulation, (c) pseudoaneurysms in accessible anatomical locations can be repaired, and (d) injuries with complete arterial thrombosis and severe initial neurologic impairment are associated with high mortality rates and poor neurologic outcomes.[87]

AXIOM When angiography demonstrates blunt carotid injury with dissection of the wall, full anticoagulant therapy should be instituted to prevent thrombus formation.

Anticoagulation for carotid or vertebral artery dissections may help prevent infarction of the spinal cord and may aid in the recovery of neurologic function. Vasospasm has also been shown to be a potentially reversible cause of neurologic deficits in survivors of cervical spine injuries. The full extent of vascular injury is best evaluated by angiography, and the endpoint of therapy for either dissection or vasospasm can be monitored by angiography.

Anticoagulation for carotid dissection can start with full-dose heparin for 7-14 days and then continue with coumadin or antiplatelet agents for 3-6 months[87-90]; however, the artery should be explored and repaired under the following circumstances: (a) anticoagulation is contraindicated because of associated injuries, (b) the carotid artery is not totally occluded, and (c) the dissection does not extend too high. When the vessel is explored and the carotid stump pressure is > 70 mm Hg, the ICA can be ligated with almost no potential of stroke. With lower stump pressures, occlusion of a patent ICA may result in stroke in up to 20-30% of patients.

AXIOM If a carotid artery has an injury that would be very difficult or hazardous to repair and the distal stump pressure exceeds 70 mm Hg, the safest treatment is generally ligation of the damaged vessel.

Li et al. recently presented 7 patients with blunt carotid injury and reviewed 100 patients from the recent literature.[90] One of two patients treated surgically died and all five treated nonsurgically survived with permanent deficits directly related to their pretreatment neurologic status.

The overall mortality rate in the 100 patients reviewed from the literature was 12%. In the series reported by Cogbill et al., the mortality rate was 43%[87]; however, most (71%) of their patients had neurologic deficits before or within 12 hours of admission. Good neurologic outcomes were achieved in only 22 patients, and these results were largely related to the neurologic status of patients on admission.

POSTTRAUMATIC ANEURYSMS

Extracranial carotid artery aneurysms may occur after blunt or penetrating trauma, but are extremely rare. Sharma et al., however, successfully treated eight such lesions over a course of 10 years.[91] These lesions often produce nonspecific symptoms and may mimic neoplastic or inflammatory masses. Intravenous digital subtraction angiography appears to be ideal for preoperative assessment of these lesions.

Pharynx and Esophagus

AXIOM One of the most important reasons for mandatory exploration of penetrating neck injuries is to ensure that injury to the pharynx or esophagus is not missed.

When repair or drainage is required, pharyngeal or cervical esophageal injuries are approached most readily through an incision along the anterior border of the sternocleidomastoid muscle on the side of the injury. The omohyoid muscle can be cut, and the carotid sheath and sternocleidomastoid muscle are retracted laterally and posteriorly to improve exposure. The middle thyroid vein and inferior thyroid artery can also be divided when more exposure is required.

When an injury is found, the tear is debrided, as needed, and then closed with two layers of inverting interrupted slowly absorbable sutures. If it were to become difficult to see the mucosa to close the defect properly, a Foley catheter could be inserted through the injury into the pharynx and the inflated balloon could then be pulled back to bring the mucosa up into the operative field. After the sutures incorporating mucosa are placed, the balloon is deflated, the catheter is withdrawn, and the first layer of sutures is tied. A second layer of sutures is then used to close the muscle layer. Whenever possible, a flap of local muscle, such as the omohyoid, should be used to reinforce or buttress the closure. This is particularly important when the patient has sustained an associated arterial or tracheal injury. A closed drainage tube, such as a Jackson-Pratt catheter, is placed near, but not on, the repair.

One must also look carefully for associated injuries, the more common of which include injury to the trachea (36-50%), major vessels (15-25%), thyroid gland (10-15%), spinal cord (7-15%), thyroid cartilage (6-12%), jugular vein (5-10%) or recurrent laryngeal nerve (4-8%).[92,93]

AXIOM With any soft-tissue infection developing in the neck, one should look for missed injuries of the aerodigestive tract.

Neck infections due to missed injuries of the aerodigestive tract are often indolent and may be hidden for several days or weeks by the fascial planes. Unexplained pain, fever, and leukocytosis should alert the physician to the possibility of a missed injury causing an infection in the neck and/or superior mediastinum. Occasionally, cervical osteomyelitis may develop following gunshot wounds that have traversed the pharynx or esophagus in the neck before entering bone. CT scans with contrast are probably the best method for detecting these deep abscesses or collections, but even these studies may be falsely negative in 10-15% of patients.

In a patient with a delayed diagnosis of esophageal injury, one can still attempt a two-layer closure after thorough debridement if no necrosis or gross suppuration are present. The closure should be reinforced with a good, viable local muscle flap. With such injuries, closed drainage of the area is extremely important to prevent infection from spreading throughout the neck and down into the mediastinum.

AXIOM If a missed pharyngeal or esophageal injury in the neck causes severe infection, extensive irrigation, debridement, and drainage plus intravenous antibiotics, and in some patients, also a cervical esophagostomy, are indicated.

The overall mortality rate for patients with esophageal injuries is about 10%[17]; however, the mortality and morbidity rates are greatly increased when a significant injury is missed for more than 12-24 hours.[42]

AXIOM Repairs of pharyngeal and esophageal injuries have a tendency to leak and form fistulas, especially if these are associated injuries.

In the review by Asensio et al., 15 of 118 patients with penetrating esophageal injuries developed fistulas.[17] Remarkably, all 15 patients recovered fully after wide drainage and intravenous hyperalimentation were provided. Winter and Weigelt reported 4 patients with cervical esophageal fistulas that developed from a total of 46 patients with penetrating trauma to the esophagus.[92] Risk factors significantly increasing the incidence of fistula formation included shock and the performance of an emergency tracheostomy outside the operating rooms.

The question of whether single-layer closures are adequate for esophageal wounds remains unanswered. From their data, Winter and Weigelt could not show a disadvantage to such closures[92]; however, they recommended that all patients who have repairs of cervical esophageal wounds undergo postoperative esophagography prior to eating. Fifty percent of esophageal fistulas in the Winter and Weigelt study were asymptomatic and discovered only on routine postoperative contrast studies.

AXIOM Following repair of penetrating esophageal trauma, the patient should not be allowed to eat until or unless a contrast swallow confirms the clinical impression that no leak is present.

Recently, Ngakune et al. reported success in treating selected penetrating injuries to the pharynx and cervical esophagus nonoperatively.[94] In their study to determine the type of treatment required, all patients with gunshot wounds of the neck and all patients with stab wounds who had severe pain on swallowing a mouthful of wa-

ter underwent a contrast swallow with Dianosil®. Patients with stab wounds who had no pain when swallowing water had no further investigation. Surgery was performed only when the contrast swallow showed gross extravasation. The patients treated nonoperatively were kept NPO, and those with discomfort were given a full course of intravenous antibiotics (cloxacillin 4 gm/24 hrs and metronidazole 1.5 gm/24 hrs). Repeat contrast swallows on day five on the patients treated nonoperatively showed no leak. The 25 patients with negative contrast swallows and 80 other patients with no pain on swallowing had uneventful recoveries.

AXIOM Small perforations of the pharynx or cervical esophagus may be treated nonoperatively as long as sepsis does not supervene.

Complex Combined Injuries

Combined tracheoesophageal injuries can be extremely difficult to manage. Feliciano et al. described the management of 23 patients with combined tracheoesophageal injuries from penetrating trauma.[93] Physical examination, endoscopy, barium swallow, or a combination of these techniques confirmed the diagnoses preoperatively in 19 (83%) patients. A variety of operative techniques were used, with 20 of the 23 patients having primary repairs of the trachea and esophagus with or without tracheostomy. Almost three-quarters (74%) of the patients had significant complications, which included eight with pneumonia, eight esophageal leaks, six tracheoesophageal fistulas, five mediastinal abscesses, four wound infections, and two carotid artery blowouts.

AXIOM Patients with combined tracheoesophageal injuries should be observed carefully postoperatively for the development of anastomotic leaks, infections, and fistulas.

As a result of this experience, Feliciano et al. described various techniques used to decrease the incidence of these complications.[93] For example, they recommended debridement and primary repair of all injuries with an interposed sternocleidomastoid or strap muscle flap between the suture lines. They also recommended avoiding tracheostomy whenever possible. When an extensive esophageal injury is present, they recommended that a cutaneous esophagostomy be created. The authors also recommended that drainage be instituted with closed systems and directed anteriorly, so that the drains do not cross the carotid artery. When a concomitant ipsilateral carotid artery injury has been repaired, the drainage of the neck should be established through the side of the neck opposite the injury.

For transcervical missile injuries or very large neck lacerations, bilateral neck explorations are indicated.[22] The standard anterior sternocleidomastoid incisions on each side may be connected by a transverse incision approximately 2-3 cm above the suprasternal notch. Because patients with bilateral injuries usually undergo extensive dissections and may have severe edema postoperatively, one should consider performing a tracheostomy to prevent the disastrous consequences of inadvertent extubation.

AXIOM Transcervical neck injuries requiring bilateral neck explorations can cause so much neck edema that one should consider a tracheostomy in case of inadvertent endotracheal extubation postoperatively.

A strong association of transpharyngeal gunshot wounds with later cervical spine osteomyelitis has been described by Schafer et al.[94] They noted that contamination with pharyngeal flora, inappropriate antibiotic therapy, inadequate debridement of the bone and soft tissue, and inadequate spinal immobilization as possible contributing factors. The authors described five patients and outlined a management protocol consisting of triple endoscopy to identify the pharyngeal injury, anteroposterior and lateral radiography of the cervical spine to localize the injury, administration of full-dose penicillin and gentamicin intravenously, exploration of the neck with repair of the pharyngeal wounds, thorough debridement of the cervical spine, and external immobilization of the spine for 6 weeks in order to prevent this complication.

AXIOM	Injury to the cervical spine by a transpharyngeal GSW, even with the best therapy, increases risk of severe bone infections.[94]

Neurologic Injuries

CNS and peripheral nerve injuries are not infrequent in patients with neck injuries; however, such injuries are difficult to assess in patients who are comatose, intoxicated, or in shock. CNS deficits secondary to vascular injury are particularly important to diagnose prior to surgical intervention.

Cleanly incised peripheral nerves in stable patients should be repaired primarily using magnification lenses as needed to obtain as exact a nerve bundle to nerve bundle repair as possible. With contaminated injuries or with injuries in unstable patients, the ends of the nerve are tagged with nonabsorbable sutures and repaired 1-2 weeks later, after skin healing appears to be satisfactory. Even with very careful repairs, however, eventual return of function is very unlikely, especially in older individuals.

Thoracic Duct

Thoracic duct injuries with penetrating cervical trauma are rare. In a collected review of six studies, Pollack et al. found only 15 thoracic duct injuries in 1,088 patients with penetrating neck injuries.[95] The injury occasionally occurs in zone II, where the duct may rise as high as 4 cm above the clavicle, but it is more likely to occur in zone I where it enters the venous system. Clinical evidence of ductal injury mandates exploration.

AXIOM	When the thoracic duct is injured, the jugular and subclavian venous systems must be inspected with care.

The presence of a thoracic duct fistula may be confirmed by staining the drainage fluid with Sudan III dye and confirming the presence of fat globules. Recognition of thoracic duct injuries is often delayed. Although they rarely produce large amounts of lymph at surgery, later such injuries may produce more than 1000-1500 ml of drainage per day, especially after an enteral diet is resumed. These injuries may first be noticed as either a persistent cervical fistula, localized swelling (chyloma), or as chylothorax if drainage were to occur into a pleural cavity.

AXIOM	Chylous fistulas should be treated carefully because they can cause severe metabolic and nutritional deficiencies.[96]

A collection of chyle ("chyloma")[97] may form in the neck and persist despite repeated drainage procedures until the source is recognized and definitive therapy undertaken. Chylous leakage into the pleural space (chylothorax) may also occur after a low neck injury, but it is much more apt to occur following intrathoracic trauma to the duct.[98]

AXIOM	With a cervical chyloma or cervical chylous fistula, early ligation of the thoracic duct is often indicated to avoid potential complications.

Ligation of the cervical portion of the thoracic duct causes no known morbidity. If a traumatic chylothorax were to develop after ligation of an injured thoracic duct, it usually would be due to inadvertent operative injury. If a chylothorax is noted, it should be managed with chest tube drainage and TPN and/or a modified diet which

has increased levels or medium-chain triglycerides and little or no long-chain fatty acids. If there is still much chylous drainage after 2-3 weeks, surgical ligation of the thoracic duct is indicated.

⊘ FREQUENT ERRORS

In the Management of Neck Injuries

1. *Delaying needed surgery for a penetrating neck wound to perform various diagnostic tests when significant bleeding exists and/or the aerodigestive tract is obviously injured.*
2. *Failing to obtain preoperative arteriography in stable patients with suspected vascular injuries in zone I or III.*
3. *Failing to adequately stabilize the neck in patients with blunt neck injury until cervical spine injury has been eliminated.*
4. *Failing to consider a carotid injury in someone with CNS changes but a normal CT scan of the brain after blunt trauma.*
5. *Relying on a negative Gastrografin swallow to eliminate esophageal injury.*
6. *Attempting to follow a policy of selective conservatism on penetrating neck wounds when the needed tests are not readily available.*
7. *Failing to bring patients with suspected airway injuries to surgery promptly.*
8. *Failing to repair an internal carotid injury because a neurologic deficit is present.*
9. *Taking time to repair a complex internal jugular vein injury rather than just ligating it, especially when other severe injuries are present.*
10. *Failing to adequately explore all vital structures that may have been injured by a gunshot wound of the neck.*
11. *Failing to look carefully for associated injuries when one finds injury to major vessels or the aerodigestive tract.*
12. *Failing to adequately buttress and separate repairs of the esophagus and blood vessels or the tracheobronchial tree.*
13. *Failing to consider that a neck infection after a penetrating neck wound may be due to a missed aerodigestive tract injury.*

▼▼▼▼▼▼▼▼▼▼▼▼▼▼▼▼▼▼▼▼▼▼▼▼▼▼▼▼▼▼

SUMMARY POINTS

1. In the posterior triangle of the neck, several vital structures lie just above the clavicle.
2. In stable patients with penetrating neck injuries, preoperative arteriography is particularly important for injuries in zones I and III.
3. Although the course of a stab wound is relatively limited and direct, the path of a bullet can be completely unpredictable.
4. Penetrating injuries of the neck involve major vessels in up to 25-40% of patients.
5. All high-velocity gunshot wounds of the neck should be surgically explored.
6. Patients with blunt head or neck trauma should have their necks immobilized in the neutral position until radiography and careful examination have eliminated cervical spine fracture or dislocation.
7. Neurologic injury after severe blunt neck trauma may occasionally be due to correctable carotid or vertebral arterial damage.
8. Improperly used seat belts can increase the incidence of serious neck and other injuries.
9. A thorough history and physical examination is important in the diagnosis of neck injuries, but some patients with organ damage in the neck requiring surgery have no clinical evidence of such injuries preoperatively.
10. Esophageal injuries in the neck are particularly difficult to detect from signs and symptoms.
11. Symptoms are poor predictors of the presence or absence of important neck injuries.

12. Failure to consider an occult blunt carotid artery injury as a cause of neurologic changes, especially when cranial CT is negative and CNS changes are delayed.

13. If a penetrating wound of the neck were probed, a clot could be dislodged, allowing massive, uncontrollable bleeding to occur.

14. Neurologic signs in patients with penetrating neck injuries may be caused or greatly increased by hypotension.

15. Lack of clinical findings does not eliminate major vascular injury in the neck.

16. Suspected airway injuries should be managed emergently in the operating room, especially when evidence exists that blood is being aspirated into the tracheobronchial tree.

17. With injuries in the neck, the neurologic examination should include an evaluation of the patient's mental status, cranial nerves, spinal cord, brachial plexus, and sympathetic nerves.

18. The tissue changes of traumatic asphyxia usually resolve spontaneously, but one must look carefully for associated injuries.

19. Lateral radiographs of the neck are indicated in all patients with penetrating injuries of the neck or severe blunt trauma above the shoulders.

20. Increased prevertebral space behind the upper airway is usually due to injuries to the adjacent spine or aerodigestive tract.

21. If an alert and oriented patient has a full range of nonpainful neck motion, no local tenderness, and no distracting injuries, a significant cervical spine injury is effectively ruled out.

22. Four-vessel angiography should be performed on all stable patients with suspected penetrating vascular injury in zones I and III of the neck.

23. When the need for surgical exploration of a penetrating injury in zone II is obvious, further diagnostic studies tend to delay the operation and increase the chances of severe bleeding, aspiration, and CNS deterioration.

24. Carotid and vertebral artery injuries may be present in the absence of hematoma, neurologic deficit, or clinically apparent blood loss.

25. In patients with blunt trauma, the presence of central neurologic changes in spite of a normal CT of the brain should make one suspect a carotid injury.

26. Whenever a neck is explored for trauma, the vascular and aerodigestive structures should be examined closely even if preoperative arteriograms and other studies did not reveal any injuries.

27. One should not rely on a normal Gastrografin swallow to eliminate pharyngoesophageal leak.

28. Barium could cause increased inflammation and infection if it were to enter the mediastinum, but Gastrografin could cause severe pneumonitis if it were aspirated into the lungs.

29. When a patient with a suspected esophageal injury has a negative gastrografin swallow, the study should be immediately repeated with barium and/or an esophagoscopy should be performed.

30. Endoscopy should be performed for the following: an uncooperative patient during a contrast swallow, equivocal contrast swallow study results, or possible pharyngoesophageal injury.

31. Clinically subtle injuries to laryngeal cartilages can usually be demonstrated clearly on CT.

32. Proper CT scanning requires a cooperative or sedated patient and should not be attempted when there is an acute, unprotected airway injury or unstable vital signs.

33. Only a high index of suspicion and a liberal attitude toward operative exploration of penetrating neck injuries can keep the incidence of missed pharyngeal and esophageal perforations to a minimum.

34. Patients with platysma penetration who are suspected of having vascular or visceral injuries should either be promptly explored surgically or have rapid, complete diagnostic evaluations.

35. When endoscopy is to be performed under topical anesthesia, it is important that major vascular injuries be eliminated prior to the procedure because gagging could restart bleeding from injured vessels.

36. If an ecchymosis of the posterior or lateral pharyngeal wall were seen on endoscopy, one should be concerned about possible underlying vascular injury.

37. Early death after neck injury is usually due to airway compromise, exsanguination, or CNS injury.

38. The management of stable patients with penetrating zone II neck injuries and no evidence of vascular or aerodigestive tract injury remains controversial.

39. When thorough diagnostic studies cannot be performed promptly in patients with penetrating neck injuries, early surgical exploration is generally safer than continued clinical evaluation.

40. A policy of selective conservatism for neck injuries will not be successful unless the needed diagnostic tests can be done promptly and accurately.

41. Although a policy of selective conservatism reduces the morbidity and mortality rates associated with a negative exploration of the neck, the diagnostic studies done to eliminate significant injuries also have some costs and risks which should be considered.

42. With zone II injuries, it is often quicker, safer, and less expensive to explore the neck surgically than it is to get all the studies needed to eliminate vascular or aerodigestive tract injuries.

43. Generally, in patients with penetrating neck wounds in zone II, it may be safest to practice mandatory exploration on GSWs and selective conservatism on stab wounds.

44. Penetrating neck trauma with associated chest involvement is not an absolute indication for exploration of the neck or chest.

45. Most patients with neck injuries that also involve the chest do not require chest exploration; of those who do require it, usually obvious clinical evidence of severe bleeding or an aerodigestive tract injury exists.

46. When a possibility of vascular injury in the neck exists, a nasogastric tube should not be inserted until the patient is anesthetized because gagging during insertion of the tube could restart bleeding.

47. If an endotracheal tube were too large or were inserted roughly, it could cause severe damage to a normal larynx or trachea or cause complete disruption or occlusion if they were injured.

48. If the airway occludes suddenly and there is a suspicion of laryngeal injury, a large needle or surgical tracheostomy should be rapidly provided.

49. No limited miniexplorations or probing of neck injuries should be conducted in the emergency department.

50. Unilateral neck explorations are usually best done through an incision along the anterior border of the sternocleidomastoid muscle.

51. Any vessel that is in the path of a knife or near the presumed tract of a bullet should be explored to definitely rule out a vascular lesion.

52. Regardless of the absence or extent of neurologic defects, the ICA should be repaired if prograde flow is still present. If no prograde flow exists, the vessel should probably be ligated.

53. Prosthetic bypass grafts to restore flow to an injured carotid artery should be avoided if possible because of the high rate of later occlusion.

54. When any question about the adequacy of vascular repair or its run-off exists, an intraoperative postrepair angiography should be performed.

55. Interventional radiology should be considered in patients with bleeding or A-V fistulas from high vertebral or very high ICA injuries.

56. Asymptomatic venous injuries in the neck only rarely are diagnosed preoperatively, and surgical exploration with ligation or repair is seldom required for an isolated injury.

57. Shock in patients with neurologic defects should be corrected as rapidly as possible to reduce the amount of cerebral damage.

58. Blunt carotid artery injuries that cause symptoms usually have a delayed dissection in the media with subsequent thrombotic occlusion.

59. Blunt carotid injury should be suspected in patients with severe head trauma and delayed localized neurologic changes, but no lesion on CT scan of the brain to explain the clinical picture.

60. If angiography were to demonstrate blunt carotid injury with dissection of the wall, full anticoagulant therapy should be instituted to prevent thrombus formation.

61. When a carotid artery has an injury that would be difficult or hazardous to repair and the distal stump pressure exceeds 70 mm Hg, the safest treatment is generally ligation of the damaged vessel.

62. One of the most important reasons for mandatory exploration of penetrating neck injuries is to ensure that an injury to the pharynx or esophagus is not missed.

63. With any soft-tissue infection developing in the neck, one should look for missed injuries of the aerodigestive tract.

64. If a missed pharyngeal or esophageal injury in the neck causes severe infection, treatment includes extensive irrigation, debridement, and drainage plus intravenous antibiotics. In some patients, a cervical esophagostomy may also be indicated.

65. Repairs of pharyngeal and esophageal injuries have a tendency to leak and form fistulas, especially with associated injuries (13%).

66. Following repair of penetrating esophageal trauma, the patient should not be allowed to eat until or unless a contrast swallow confirms the clinical impression that no leak is present.

67. Small perforations of the pharynx or cervical esophagus may be treated nonoperatively as long as sepsis does not supervene.

68. Patients with combined tracheoesophageal injuries should be observed carefully postoperatively for the development of anastomotic leaks, infections, and fistulas.

69. Transcervical neck injuries requiring bilateral neck explorations can cause so much neck edema that one should consider a tracheostomy in case of inadvertent endotracheal extubation postoperatively.

70. Injury to the cervical spine by transpharyngeal GSW, even with the best therapy, increases risk of severe bone infections.

71. When the thoracic duct is injured, the jugular and subclavian venous systems must be inspected with care.

72. Chylous fistulas should be treated carefully because they can cause severe metabolic and nutritional deficiencies.

73. With a cervical chyloma or cervical chylous fistula, early ligation of the thoracic duct is often indicated to avoid potential complications.

▲▲▲▲▲▲▲▲▲▲▲▲▲▲▲▲▲▲▲▲▲▲▲▲▲▲▲▲▲▲▲▲▲▲

REFERENCES

1. Payne JM, Kerstein MD. Penetrating neck injuries. Current surgical therapy 3rd Ed.; BC Decker Inc., 1989; 706.
2. Thal ER. Injury to the neck. EE Moore, KL Mattox, DV Feliciano, eds. Trauma, 2nd ed. Norwalk: Appelton & Lange, 1991; 305-317.
3. Watson, WL, Silverstone, SM. Ligation of the common carotid artery in cancer of the head and neck. Ann Surg 1939;109:1.
4. Fleming D. Case of rupture of the carotid artery with wounds of several of its branches, successfully treated by tying the common trunk of the carotid itself. Med Chir J 1817;3:2.
5. Vernouil. Thrombose de L'artere carotide. Bull Acad Med Paris 1872;1:46-56.
6. Roon AJ, Christensen N. Evaluation and treatment of penetrating cervical injuries. J Trauma 1979;19:391.
7. Campbell FC, Robbs JV. Penetrating injuries of the neck: a prospective study of 108 patients. Br J Surg 1980;67:582.
8. Golueke PJ, Goldstein AS, Sclafani SJA, et al. Routine versus selective exploration of penetrating neck injuries: a randomized prospective study. J Trauma 1984;24:1010.
9. Ordog GJ, Albin D, Wasserberger J, et al. 110 bullet wounds to the neck. J Trauma 1985;25:238.
10. Saletta JD, Lowe RJ, Leonardo TL, et al. Penetrating trauma of the neck. J Trauma 1976;16:579.
11. Rao PM, Bhatti FK, Guadino J, et al. Penetrating injuries of the neck: criteria for exploration. J Trauma 1983;23:47.
12. Carducci B, Lowe RA, Dalsey W. Penetrating neck trauma: consensus and controversies. Ann Emerg Med 1985;15:208-215.
13. Wozasek GE, Balzer K. Strangulation of the internal artery by the hypoglossal nerve. J Trauma 1990;30:332.
14. Burrows PE, Tubman DE. Multiple extracranial arterial lesions following closed cranial facial trauma. J Trauma 1981;21:497.
15. Zilkha A. Traumatic occlusion of the internal carotid artery. Radiology 1970;97:543.
16. Miller RH, Duplechain JK. Penetrating wounds of the neck. Otolaryngol Clin North Am 1991;24:15.
17. Asensio JA, Valenziano CP, Falcone RE, et al. Management of penetrating neck injuries. The controversy surrounding zone II injuries. Surg Clin North Am 1991;71:267.
18. West JG, Eastman AB. Patterns of injury. Mattox KL, Moore EE, Feliciano DV, eds. Trauma. Norwalk: Appleton and Lange, 1988; 94-96.
19. Ordog GJ. Penetrating neck trauma. J Trauma 1987;27:543-554.
20. Bishara RA, Pasch AR, Douglas DD, et al. The necessity of mandatory exploration of penetrating zone II neck injuries. Surgery 1986;100:655-60.
21. Cohen ES, Breaux CW, Johnson PN, et al. Penetrating neck injuries: experience with selective exploration. South Med J 1987;80:26-28.
22. Weigelt JA, Thal ER, Snyder WH, et al. Diagnosis of penetrating cervical esophageal injuries. Am J Surg 1987;154:619.
23. Aviv JE, Berkower AS, Urken ML. Carotid artery laceration secondary to thyroid cartilage fracture: an unusual complication of blunt neck trauma. Otolaryngol Head Neck Surg 1991;104:375.
24. Perry MO, Snyder WH, Thal ER. Carotid artery injuries caused by blunt trauma. Ann Surg 1980;192:74.
25. Benito MC, Garcia F, Fernandez-Quero L, et al. Lesion of the internal carotid artery caused by a car safety belt. J Trauma 1990;30:116.
26. Chedid MK, Deeb CL, Rothfus WE, et al. Major cerebral vessels injury caused by a seat belt shoulder strap: case report. J Trauma 1989;29:1601.
27. Woodhurst, WB, Robertson WD, Thompson GB. Carotid injury due to intraoral trauma: case report and review of the literature. Neurosurgery 1980;6:559.
28. Lee C, Woodring JH, Walsh JW. Carotid and vertebral artery injuries in survivors of atlantooccipital dislocation: case reports and literature review. J Trauma 1991;31:401.
29. Dublin AB, Marks WM, Weinstock D, et al. Traumatic dislocation of the atlantooccipital articulation (AOA) with short-term survival. J Neurosurg 1980;52:541.
30. Pang D, Wildberger JE. Traumatic atlantooccipital dislocation with survival: case report and review. Neurosurgery 1980;7:503.
31. Niezgoda JA, McMenamin P, Graeber GM. Pharyngoesophageal perforation after blunt neck trauma. Ann Thorac Surg 1990;50:615.
32. Worman LW, Hurley JD. Rupture of the esophagus from external blunt trauma. Arch Surg 1962;85:173.
33. Berry BE, Ochsner JL. Perforation of the esophagus: a 30 year review. J Thorac Cardiovasc Surg 1973;65:1.
34. Sclafoni SJA, Cavaliere G, Atweh N, et al. The role of angiography in penetrating neck trauma. J Trauma 1991;31:557.
35. Walsh MS. The management of penetrating injuries of the anterior triangle of the neck. Injury 1994;25:393.
36. Beitsch P, Weigelt JA, Flynn E, Easley S. Physical examination and arteriography in patients with penetrating zone II neck wounds. Arch Surg 1994;129:577.
37. Demetriades D, Charalambides D, Lakhoo M. Physical examination and selective conservative management in patients with penetrating injuries of the neck. Br J Surg 1993;80:1534.
38. Brown AS, Wilson GR. Just a minor neck laceration. Injury 1994;25:269.
39. Fabian TC, George SM, Croce MA, et al. Carotid artery trauma: management based on mechanism of injury. J Trauma 1990;30:953.
40. Fogelman MJ, Stewart RD. Penetrating wounds of the neck. Am J Surg 1956;91:581.
41. Yoder RL, Merck DE. Innocuous appearing stab wounds to the neck: Is exploration always indicated? South Med J 1969;62:113.
42. Sankaran S, Walt AJ. Penetrating wounds of the neck: principles and some controversies. Surg Clin North Am 1977;57:139.
43. Fisher DF, Clagett GP, Perker JL, et al. Mandibular subluxation for high carotid exposure. J Vasc Surg 1984;1:727.
44. Obeid FN, Hadad GS, Horst HM, et al. A critical reappraisal of a mandatory exploration policy for penetrating wounds of the neck. Surg Gynecol Obstet 1985;160:157.
45. McCormick TM, Burch BH. Routine angiographic evaluation of neck and extremity injuries. J Trauma 1979;19:384.
46. Reid JDS, Weigelt JA. Forty-three cases of vertebral artery trauma. J Trauma 1988;28:1007.
47. North CM, Ahmadi J, Segall HD, et al. Penetrating vascular injuries of the face and neck: clinical and angiographic correlation. AJNR 1986;7:855.

48. Rose SL, Moore EE. Trauma angiography: the use of clinical findings to improve patient selection and case preparation. J Trauma 1988; 28:240.

49. Leikweg WG Jr, Greenfield LT. Management of penetrating carotid arterial injury. Ann Surg 1978;188:587.

50. Thal ER, Snyder WH, Hays RJ, et al. Management of carotid artery injuries. Surgery 1974;76:955.

51. Noyes LD, McSwain NE, Markowitz IP. Panendoscopy with arteriography versus mandatory exploration of penetrating wounds of the neck. Ann Surg 1986;204:21.

52. Hewitt RL, Smith AD, Becker ML, et al. Penetrating injuries of the thoracic outlet. Surgery 1974;76:715.

53. Pringle MB, Charig MJ. The use of digital subtraction angiography in penetrating neck injury—a very instructive case. J Laryngol Otol 1994; 108:522.

54. Richardson JD, Martin LF, Borzotta AP, et al. Unifying concepts in treatment of esophageal leaks. Am J Surg 1985;149:157.

55. Hirshberg A, Wall MJ, Johnston RH Jr, et al. Transcervical gunshot injuries. Am J Surg 1994;167:309.

56. Jurkovich GJ, Zingarelli W, Wallace J, et al. Penetrating neck trauma: studies in the asymptomatic patient. J Trauma 1985;25:819.

57. Eggen JT, Jorden RC. Airway management, penetrating neck trauma. J Emerg Med 1993;11:381.

58. Garramone RR Jr, Jacobs LM, Sadhev P. Diagnosis and management of penetrating neck trauma. Contemp Surg 1990;36:11.

59. Callaham M, Dailey RH, Callaham M, eds. Controversies in trauma management. New York: Churchill Livingstone, 1985; 174-175.

60. Bivens BA, Procter CD, Bell RM. Arguments against mandatory exploration. Dailey RH, Callaham M, eds. Controversies in trauma management. New York: Churchill Livingstone, 1985; 163-175.

61. Shireley AL, Beall AC, DeBakey ME. Surgical management of penetrating wounds of the neck. Arch Surg 1963;86:955.

62. Stone HH, Callahan GS. Soft tissue injuries of the neck. Surg Gynecol Obstet 1963;117:745.

63. Maddison FE. Patient evaluation and other clinical considerations: basic principles of angiography. Rutherford RB, ed. Vascular surgery. Philadelphia: Sanders Publishing Co, 1977.

64. Merion RM, Haness JK, Rousbergh SR, et al. Selective management of penetrating neck trauma. Ann Surg 1981;116:691.

65. Narrod JA, Moore EE. Selective management of penetrating neck injuries. Arch Surg 1984;119:574.

66. Elerding SC, Manart FD, Moore EE. A reappraisal of penetrating neck wounds? J Trauma 1980;20:695.

67. Pate JW, Gasini M. Penetrating wounds of the neck: explore or not? Am Surg 1980;46:38.

68. Prakaschandra MR, Bhatti MFK, Gaudino J, et al. Penetrating injuries of the neck: criteria for exploration. J Trauma 1983;23:47.

69. Shama DM, Odell J. Penetrating neck trauma with tracheal and oesophageal injuries. Br J Surg 1984;71:534.

70. Fry RE, Fry WJ. Extracranial carotid artery injuries. Surgery 1980;88:581.

71. Bradley EL III. Management of penetrating carotid injuries: an alternative approach. J Trauma 1973;13:248.

72. Dichtel WJ, Miller RH, Feliciano DV, et al. Lateral mandibulotomy: a technique of exposure for penetrating injuries of the internal carotid artery at the base of the skull. Laryngoscope 1984;94:1140.

73. Shah A, Phillips T, Scalea T, et al. Exposure of the internal carotid artery near the skull base: the posterolateral anatomic approach. J Vasc Surg 1988;8:618.

74. Wylie EJ, Hein MF, Adams JE. Intracranial hemorrhage following surgical revascularization for treatment of acute strokes. J Neurosurg 1964;21:212.

75. Cohen A, Brief D, Mathewson C. Carotid artery injury. Am J Surg 1970;120:210.

76. Ledgerwood AM, Mullins RJ, Lucas CE. Primary repair vs ligation for carotid artery injuries. Arch Surg 1980;115:488.

77. Brown MF, Graham JM, Feliciano DV, et al. Carotid injuries. Am J Surg 1982;144:748.

78. Unger SW, Tucker WS Jr, Mrdeza MA, et al. Carotid arterial trauma. Surgery 1980;87:477.

79. Richardson JD, Simpson C, Miller FB. Management of carotid artery trauma. Surgery 1988;104:673.

80. Meyer JP, Walsh J, Barrett J, et al. Analysis of 18 recent cases of penetrating injuries to the common and internal carotid arteries. Am J Surg 1988;2:96.

81. Feliciano DV, Mattox KL, Graham JM, et al. Five years experience with PTFE grafts in vascular wounds. J Trauma 1985;25:71.

82. Willis BK, Greiner F, Orrison WW, et al. The incidence of vertebral artery injury after midcervical spine fracture or subluxation. Neurosurgery 1994;34:435.

83. Yee L, Olcott EW, Knudson MM. Extraluminal, transluminal, and observational treatment for vertebral artery injuries. J Trauma 1994;37:159.

84. Miyachi S, Okamura K, Watanabe M, et al. Cerebellar stroke due to vertebral artery occlusion after cervical spine trauma. Two case reports. Spine 1994;19:83.

85. Hardesty WH, Whitacre WB, Toole JR. Studies on vertebral artery blood flow in man. Surg Gynecol Obstet 1963;116:662.

86. Roberts B, Hardesty WB, Helling HE. Studies on extracranial cerebral blood flow. Surgery 1964;56:826.

87. Cogbill TH, Moore EE, Meissnr M, et al. The spectrum of blunt injury to the carotid artery: a multicenter perspective. J Trauma 1994;37:473.

88. Okuhn SP. Carotid dissection. Bergan JJ, Yao JST, eds. Vascular surgical emergencies. Orlando: Grune & Stratton, 1986; 125-137.

89. Lebos MR, Saadia R. The overlooked blunt component in penetrating neck injuries: three case reports. J Trauma 1994;36:410.

90. Li MS, Smith BM, Espinosa J, et al. Nonpenetrating trauma to the carotid artery: seven cases and a literature review. J Trauma 1994;36:265.

91. Sharma S, Rajani M, Mishra N, et al. Extracranial carotid artery aneurysms following accidental injury: ten years experience. Clin Radiol 1991;43:162.

92. Ngakane H, Muckart DJJ, Luvuno FM. Penetrating visceral injury of the neck: results of a conservative management policy. Br J Surg 1990;77:908.

93. Winter RP, Weigelt JA. Cervical esophageal trauma: incidence and cause of esophageal fistulae. Arch Surg 1990;125:849.

94. Feliciano DV, Bitondo CG, Mattox KL, et al. Combined tracheoesophageal injuries. Am J Surg 1985;150:710.

95. Schafer SD, Bucholz RW, Jones RE, et al. The management of transpharyngeal gunshot wounds to the cervical spine. Surg Gynecol Obstet 1981;152:27.

96. Pollack CV Jr, Kolb JC, Griswold JA. Chylous drainage from a stab wound of the neck. Ann Emerg Med 1990;19:1450.

97. Stubbs WK, Tabb HG. Thoracic duct injuries. South Med J 1977;70:1062.

98. Sinclair D, Woods E, Saibil EA, et al. "Chyloma:" a persistent posttraumatic collection in the left supraclavicular region. J Trauma 1987;27:567.

99. Ramzy AL, Rodriguez A, Cowley RA. Pitfalls in the management of traumatic chylothorax. J Trauma 1982;22:513.

Chapter **15** Laryngotracheal Trauma

ROBERT F. WILSON, M.D.

RICHARD L. ARDEN, M.D.

INCIDENCE OF LARYNGOTRACHEAL INJURY

AXIOM   Blunt laryngotracheal injuries are rare, but can be rapidly fatal.

Blunt injury to the upper airway is quite uncommon due to its protection by the mandible and sternum anteriorly, the spinal column posteriorly, and the mobility and the elasticity of the upper airway itself. The larynx or cervical trachea is injured in < 1% of patients admitted to the hospital for blunt trauma.[1] In a series of 10,113 patients admitted to one trauma center, only 46 (0.45%) had diagnosed injuries to the upper airway.[1] Angood et al. found only 16 patients with laryngeal injury and 4 patients with cervical tracheal injury treated at the Montreal General Hospital over a 10-year period.[2] Cantrell commented that, because of the rarity of laryngotracheal trauma, it is difficult to draw conclusions about protocols for its treatment, especially when the data from many centers spans a 20-year period.[3] However, the incidence of these injuries has been increasing over the past three decades.[4,5]

Improvements in prehospital care since that time have increased the number of patients who survive to reach tertiary care; however, Kelly et al. found that 21% of patients with airway injuries died in the first 2 hours after admission to a hospital.[6] Of 46 patients with upper airway injuries reported by Cicala et al. 11 (24%) died and four (36%) of these deaths were primarily due to airway injury.[7]

Penetrating airway injuries in the neck are also relatively uncommon. Capan et al reviewed 17 reports published between 1965 and 1989 describing acute cervical airway injuries.[8] Approximately 300 patients were found, and this represented an average case load per reporting center of < 3 patients per year. Penetrating injuries of the neck involve the larynx in up to 5-15% of patients,[9,10] but this incidence was at least doubled in patients who had carotid artery or digestive tract injuries. Of the penetrating upper airway injuries seen by Cicala et al. about one-third involved the larynx and two-thirds involved the cervical trachea.[7]

The site of upper airway injury is quite varied from individual reports. Of the blunt injuries of the upper airway, Cicala et al. found seven (35%) involved the larynx above the cricoid, three (15%) involved the cricoid cartilage, nine (45%) involved the cervical trachea, and one (5%) involved multiple sites.[7] Trone et al. found the thyroid cartilage (47%) to be the most commonly fractured site in blunt and penetrating laryngeal injuries.[11] Injuries involving the arytenoid cartilage (24%) and cricoid cartilage (22%) were next in frequency. The incidence of laryngeal injuries due to intubation is unknown but were reported to be about 0.1% in a prospective study by Kambic and Radsel.[12]

ANATOMY AND PHYSIOLOGY

The superficial fascia of the anterior neck is a thin layer that encloses the platysma muscle. The deep cervical fascia supports the muscles, vessels, and viscera of the neck and is divided into three distinct layers; the investing layer, the pretracheal layer, and the prevertebral layer. The investing fascia encircles the neck, splitting to enclose the sternocleidomastoid and trapezius muscles. The pretracheal layer (deep cervical visceral fascia) encloses the larynx (below the oblique line of the thyroid cartilage), thyroid gland, trachea, and esophagus. Behind the esophagus superiorly, it is continuous with the buccopharyngeal fascia. Below, it extends into the mediastinum, where it blends with the pericardium.

The anterior neck between the sternocleidomastoid muscles has been divided into zone I below the top of the clavicles[13] or the cricoid cartilage,[14] zone II from the top of the clavicles or the cricoid cartilage to the angle of the mandible, and zone III above the angle of the mandible. Zone II includes the larynx and zone I includes the cervical trachea. A prominent area in the anterior neck is the one referred to by Stanley et al. as the "laryngeal trapezium" which is bounded superiorly by the hyoid bone, inferiorly by the cricoid cartilage, and laterally by the anterior borders of the sternocleidomastoid muscles.[15]

Larynx

The larynx consists of an articulated cartilaginous skeleton with ligaments, muscles, and soft-tissue attachments combining to form a sphincter at the entrance to the lower airway.

RELATIONSHIPS

The larynx extends from the epiglottis opposite the third cervical vertebra (C-3) to the cricoid which is at the level of C-6 in adults. It is situated in the anterior and upper part of the neck, below the base of tongue and hyoid bone, and between the great vessels of the neck. Posteriorly, it relates to the prevertebral fascia and muscles and the vertebral bodies of C-3 through C-6. It opens into the hypopharynx above and into the cervical trachea below. In the midline it is covered only by skin, subcutaneous fat, platysma muscle (often deficient in the midline), and cervical fascia. Laterally, it is covered by portions of the strap muscles (including the sternohyoid, sternothyroid, and thyrohyoid muscles) and the origin of the inferior pharyngeal constrictors. Under these muscles, the larynx is encircled by the lateral lobes of the thyroid gland below and by the carotid sheath above. Behind the larynx is the hypopharynx, which also extends down to C-6 where it joins the cervical esophagus at its introitus.

CARTILAGES OF THE LARYNX

The skeleton of the larynx has nine cartilages. These include the epiglottis, thyroid, cricoid, two arytenoids, two corniculates, and two cuneiform cartilages. Accessory triticeal cartilage may be situated in the lateral thyrohyoid ligaments; when calcified, it can be mistaken for a foreign body on soft-tissue radiography of the neck.

Calcification of the laryngeal cartilages progresses with age. On CT examination of the larynx in the adolescent, only the posterior portion of the thyroid cartilage is distinctly calcified, the cricoid cartilage is barely visible, and the arytenoid cartilages are not sufficiently calcified to be visible. Ossification typically commences at 20-30 years of age in the thyroid cartilage at its inferior margin and proceeds in a cephalad direction. By contrast, the cricoid cartilage ossifies after the thyroid cartilage, proceeding in a caudal direction from its superior portion. The arytenoid cartilages usually ossify in the third decade so that by the age of 30 years, these three cartilages are sufficiently calcified to be visualized on CT scans of the larynx.[16]

Epiglottis

The epiglottis is a leaf-shaped structure consisting of fibroelastic cartilage that is situated at the superior aperture of the larynx (Figs. 15-1, 15-2). Its pointed lower end (petiole) is attached firmly by the thyroepiglottic ligament to the posterior surface of the fused wings (alae) of the thyroid cartilage in the midline, just below the thyroid notch. Its expanded upper end projects beyond the hyoid bone and defines a

FIGURE 15-1 Sagittal view of right hemilarynx highlighting the superior and inferior epiglottic attachments: the hyoepiglottic and thyroepiglottic ligaments, respectively. (From: Jeffrey RB, Dillon WP. The larynx. Computed tomography of the head and neck. Modern Neuro Radiology Series, 1988; 12.4.)

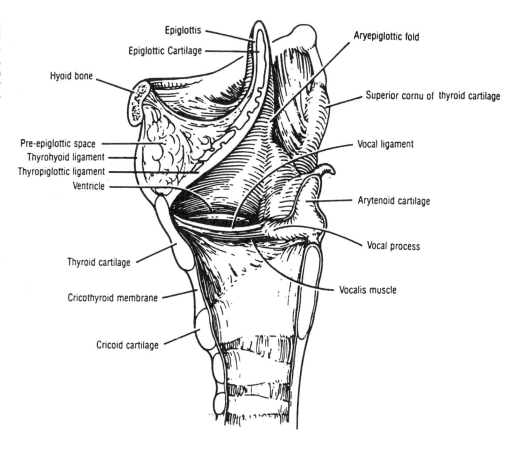

FIGURE 15-2 Posterior view of laryngotracheal skeleton demonstrating cephalad orientation of the epiglottis within the endolarynx and the protected position of the arytenoid cartilages. (From: Jeffrey RB, Dillon WP. The larynx. Computed tomography of the head and neck. Vol 3. Modern Neuro Radiology Series, 1988, pg 12.3.)

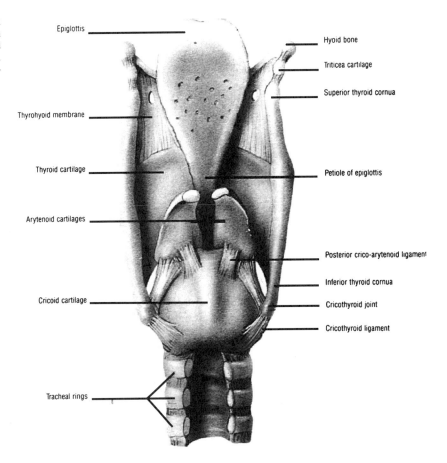

portion of the laryngeal aditus. It is covered by a tightly adherent mucous membrane anteriorly and posteriorly. The anterior (lingual) surface of the epiglottis is attached to the dorsum of the tongue by the median glossoepiglottic fold and the right and left (lateral glossoepiglottic) pharyngoepiglottic folds. The space or depression between these folds is referred to as the vallecula.

Thyroid Cartilage

The thyroid cartilage consists of hyaline cartilage and is the largest of the laryngeal cartilages. Its name is derived from the Greek and means "like a shield." It is formed from two broad quadrilateral laminae or plates that are fused together anteriorly, but are widely divergent posteriorly (Fig. 15-3). At the top of the anterior fusion of the two laminae, the cartilage has a marked prominence which is known as the "Adam's apple." This is more evident in males in whom it has a more acute angle (approximately a right angle) by comparison with a more obtuse anterior vertical thyroid seen in females. The upper halves of the thyroid plates or laminae are separated by a V-shaped thyroid notch. The posterior borders of the thyroid laminae project upwards (approximately 2 cm) as a superior horn on each side and downward as a shorter inferior horn on each side. The superior horn of the thyroid cartilage is attached to the greater cornua of the hyoid bone by the lateral thyrohyoid ligament. The inferior thyroid horn articulates with the cricoid cartilage. The cricothyroid joint is a synovial joint that allows for rotational movement of the thyroid cartilage about a horizontal axis passing through the joints of both sides.

Cricoid Cartilage

The cricoid cartilage consists of hyaline cartilage and is shaped like a signet ring. It is the only completely circumferential structure of the laryngotracheal skeleton. In infants, it represents the narrowest portion of the upper airway. The lamina, which is the larger posterior portion of the cricoid cartilage, is 20-30 mm in height.

The arch, which is the smaller anterior portion, is only 5-7 mm in height (Fig. 15-1). The cricoid is attached below to the cervical trachea via the cricotracheal ligament, and posteriorly it extends upwards inside the inferior horns of the thyroid cartilage. Anteriorly, the space between the lower part of the thyroid cartilage and the top of the cricoid cartilage contains the cricothyroid membrane.

AXIOM   A cricothyroidotomy (coniotomy) may be performed to establish an emergency airway when endotracheal tube insertion is impossible and there is inadequate time to perform a formal tracheotomy.

Arytenoid Cartilages

The two arytenoid cartilages, which are mostly hyaline cartilage, are small, triangular-shaped cartilages situated on the posterosuperior aspect of the cricoid lamina (Fig. 15-2). They are completely shielded anteriorly and laterally by the thyroid cartilage. The anterior angle of the base of each arytenoid cartilage projects forward as a vocal process to which the vocal ligament attaches. The lateral (muscular) process serves as a site of attachment for the thyroarytenoid and the lateral and posterior cricoarytenoid muscles.

Corniculate Cartilages

The two corniculate cartilages (cartilages of Santorini) are small conical structures composed of fibroelastic cartilage that are attached to the apex of each arytenoid cartilage. They cause a posterior prominence in the aryepiglottic fold on each side.

Cuneiform Cartilages

The two cuneiform cartilages (cartilages of Wrisberg) are composed of fibroelastic cartilage and lay in the aryepiglottic folds just anterior to the corniculate cartilages.

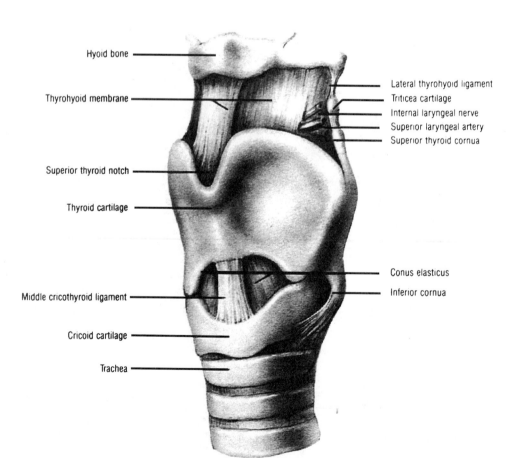

FIGURE 15-3 Anterolateral view of the laryngeal framework. Note the medial and lateral ligamentous attachments and articulatory facets between thyroid and cricoid cartilages. (From: Jeffrey RB, Dillon WP. The larynx. Computed tomography of the head and neck. Modern Neuro Radiology Series, 1988; 12.2.)

Hyoid bone

Thyrohyoid membrane

Superior thyroid notch

Thyroid cartilage

Middle cricothyroid ligament

Cricoid cartilage

Trachea

Lateral thyrohyoid ligament
Triticea cartilage
Internal laryngeal nerve
Superior laryngeal artery
Superior thyroid cornua

Conus elasticus
Inferior cornua

MEMBRANES AND LIGAMENTS OF THE LARYNX

The ligaments of the larynx are either intrinsic or extrinsic. The intrinsic fibrous framework lies beneath the laryngeal mucosa and is divided into an upper and lower part by the laryngeal ventricle (of Morgagni). The upper portion of the elastic membrane is termed the quadrangular membrane and extends from the lateral epiglottic margin to the arytenoid cartilage and false cord inferiorly. The conus elasticus (cricovocal membrane) comprises the lower supportive elastic tissue and extends from the superior border of the cricoid cartilage upward to the vocal ligament. Its thickened anterior portions include the median cricothyroid and thyroepiglottic ligaments.

The extrinsic ligaments include the median and lateral thyrohyoid and cricotracheal ligaments. The thyrohyoid membrane attaches the top of the thyroid cartilage to the hyoid bone and possesses a lateral opening for the superior laryngeal vessels and the internal branch of the superior laryngeal nerve. The cricothyroid membrane connects the cricoid and thyroid cartilages and has a central and two lateral portions. The lateral part of the cricothyroid membrane is attached to the upper border of the cricoid cartilage on each side. Its upper end is free except for an attachment anteriorly between the thyroid laminae and behind to the vocal process of each arytenoid cartilage.

LARYNGEAL CAVITY

The glottis or vocal apparatus of the larynx includes the two true vocal cords (plica vocalis) and the opening between them (rima glottidis). With the glottis as a reference point, the laryngeal cavity can be subdivided into supraglottic, glottic, and subglottic compartments.

Supraglottic Compartment

The supraglottic compartment of the larynx extends from the tip of the epiglottis anterosuperiorly, and the apices of the arytenoids posterosuperiorly, to the base of the laryngeal ventricles inferiorly. Its superior margin is bounded by the aryepiglottic and interarytenoid folds. The vestibule is defined as that portion of the laryngeal cavity extending from its inlet (aditus) to the vestibular folds (false vocal cords). The laryngeal ventricle is a fusiform fossa bounded by the crescentic edge of the false cords superiorly and the straight margin of the true cords inferiorly. The supraglottic compartment is bounded anteriorly by the fat-filled preepiglottic space and the thyroid cartilage (Fig. 15-1). The preepiglottic space, which is the space between the epiglottis and the root of the tongue, is divided in the midline by the median glossoepiglottic fold. The depressions or spaces between the anterior epiglottis and the base of the tongue on either side of the median fold are called the valleculae (Fig. 15-4).

The aryepiglottic folds consist of squamous-mucosa-covered ligaments and muscles which extend from the inferolateral aspect of the epiglottis to the apex of the arytenoid cartilages. These two folds form the border between the lateral pyriform sinuses and the central laryngeal lumen.

In the supraglottic larynx, the laryngeal cavity is symmetric; however, the pyriform sinuses, located lateral to the aryepiglottic folds, may be asymmetrically distended during quiet breathing.

The false vocal cords are two folds of mucous membrane enclosing the vestibular ligament on each side. The vestibular ligament extends posteriorly from the angle of the thyroid cartilage to the anterolateral surface of the arytenoid just superior to the attachment of the true cords on the vocal process of the arytenoid. The lower segment of the ligament forms a free crescentic margin which constitutes the upper boundary of the laryngeal ventricle.

Glottic Compartment

The glottic region includes the vocal cords and the anterior and posterior commissures (Fig. 15-5). The true vocal cords (vocal folds) extend obliquely from the vocal processes of each arytenoid cartilage and join anteriorly in the midline to form the anterior commissure. The anterior commissure is situated at the anterior junction between the true and false vocal cords. The ligamentous attachment (Broyle's ligament) of the vocal cords to the inner aspect of the thyroid cartilage varies in its vertical positioning according to sex. In males, this occurs roughly midway from the thyroid notch to the inferior thyroid cartilage margin. In females, this occurs roughly at the junction of the upper and middle one-third. The posterior commissure consists of the interarytenoid muscles and overlying mucosa, and is located between the arytenoid cartilages above the cricoid lamina.

During quiet respiration, the larynx is in maximum relaxation. The normal arytenoid cartilages are abducted and in close proximity to the inner margin of the posterior portions of the thyroid cartilages. With phonation, the normal arytenoid cartilages move medially and rotate inward, away from the inner margin of the thyroid cartilage (Fig. 15-6). Adduction, or apposition of the vocal cords, is accomplished through the complex interaction of the intrinsic laryngeal mus-

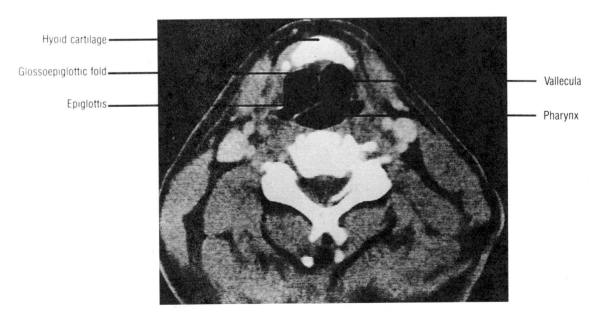

FIGURE 15-4 Axial CT section at the level of the hyoid demonstrating the valleculae bounded by the median and lateral glossoepiglottic folds. (From: Jeffrey RB, Dillon WP. The larynx. Computed tomography of the head and neck. Modern Neuro Radiology Series, 1988; 12.6.)

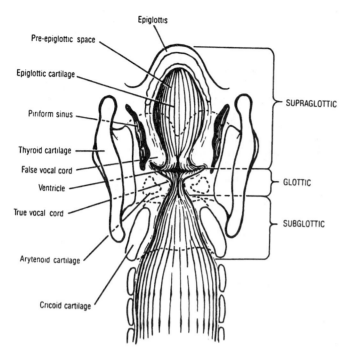

FIGURE 15-5 Schematic coronal view of larynx showing defined limits of the supraglottic, glottic, and subglottic compartments. (From: Jeffrey RB, Dillon WP. The larynx. Computed tomography of the head and neck. Modern Neuro Radiology Series, 1988; 12.5.)

culature, including the thyroarytenoid, the lateral cricoarytenoid, and the interarytenoid muscles. The only muscle that separates (abducts) the vocal cords is the posterior cricoarytenoid muscle on each side.

Subglottic Compartment

The subglottic region of the larynx extends from below the undersurface of the true cords to the inferior margin of the cricoid cartilage (Fig. 15-5). The signet-ring cricoid cartilage forms a complete circle that, together with the cricothyroid membrane, defines the limits of the subglottic region. The conus elasticus is a tentlike condensation of

tissue from the cricothyroid membrane that delineates the lateral borders of the subglottic region (Figs. 15-7, 15-8). On CT, the mucosal surface of the airway is normally applied closely to the inner margin of the cricoid cartilage, below the level of the conus elasticus.

MUSCLES OF THE LARYNX

Extrinsic Muscles

The muscles acting on the outer surfaces of the larynx can be divided into an infrahyoid (depressor) group and a suprahyoid (elevator) group. The former includes the omohyoid, sternohyoid, sternothyroid, and thyrohyoid muscles. The latter includes the mylohyoid, geniohyoid, digastric, and stylohyoid muscles. These muscle groups enable movement and stabilization of the larynx as a whole, and are actively involved in deglutition.

Intrinsic Muscles

The intrinsic muscles of the larynx act to modify the size of the laryngeal aperture (rima glottidis) and to control the degree of tension on the vocal cords. The principal intrinsic laryngeal muscles include the cricothyroid, the transverse and oblique portions of the interarytenoid, the posterior and lateral cricoarytenoids, and the thyroarytenoids. All of these, except the interarytenoid muscle are in pairs, and receive innervation unilaterally. The interarytenoid muscle possesses dual innervation.

CRICOTHYROID MUSCLE. The cricothyroid muscle is the only "intrinsic" laryngeal muscle laying on the exterior of the larynx. Its origin is from the lateral surface of the cricoid arch, and it inserts into the inferior border of the thyroid lamina and anterior border of the inferior horn of the thyroid cartilage. The cricothyroid muscle is the chief tensor of the vocal cords. By pulling the front of the cricoid cartilage upward, or by tilting the thyroid cartilage downward, the vocal cords are lengthened or tensed and mildly adducted.

POSTERIOR CRICOARYTENOIDS. The posterior cricoarytenoid muscle arises from the juxtamedian aspect of the posterior lamina, passes superolaterally, and inserts into the muscular process of the arytenoid. It is the only muscle that separates (abducts) the vocal cords; it does this by rotating the vocal process of the arytenoid laterally. All other muscles of the larynx tend to close the glottis.

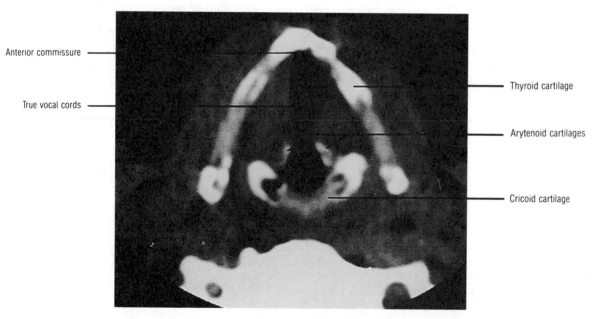

FIGURE 15-6 Axial CT scan at the level of the true vocal folds during adduction. (From: Jeffrey RB, Dillon WP. The larynx. Computed tomography of the head and neck. Modern Neuro Radiology Series, 1988; 12.10.)

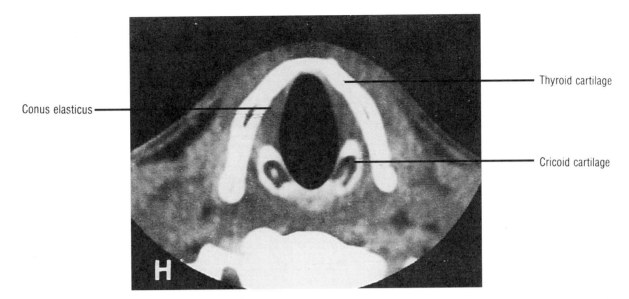

FIGURE 15-7 Axial CT section through the thyroid and cricoid cartilages at the subglottic level. (From: Jeffrey RB, Dillon WP. The larynx. Computed tomography of the head and neck. Modern Neuro Radiology Series, 1988; 12.9.)

LATERAL CRICOARYTENOIDS. Lateral cricoarytenoids are the main adductors of the vocal cords and the principal antagonists to the posterior cricoarytenoids. These muscles extend from the cricoid arch to the muscular process of each arytenoid, and following contraction, rotate the vocal process medially.

THYROARYTENOID MUSCLE. The thyroarytenoid muscle arises from the medial surface of the thyroid cartilage lamina and lateral aspect of the conus elasticus and inserts into the vocal ligament and arytenoid cartilage on each side. Its deepest fibers form the vocalis muscle, which is the principal antagonist to the cricothyroid muscle. The vocalis muscle shortens and thickens the vocal cords to enable fine control of the voice. Following contraction of the thyroarytenoid muscle, the vocal cords relax.

INTERARYTENOID MUSCLE. The interarytenoid muscle has transverse and oblique fibers and subserves an adductor function at two levels; the transverse arytenoid muscle is attached to the medial surfaces of the arytenoid bodies, and during contraction they approximate the posterior commissure. The oblique arytenoid connects the muscular process of one arytenoid to the apex of the contralateral arytenoid and continues superiorly as the aryepiglottic muscle. This muscle assists in closure of the laryngeal aditus.

NERVES OF THE LARYNX. The nerve supply of the larynx is from the vagus nerve via two branches, the superior and inferior (recurrent) laryngeal nerves.

Superior Laryngeal Nerve. The superior laryngeal nerve exits the vagus nerve at the level of the nodose ganglion and passes posteriorly and medially to the internal carotid artery. It subsequently divides into a small, external branch and a thicker, internal one. The external laryngeal nerve passes posterior to the superior thyroid artery that accompanies it and is purely motor to the cricothyroid muscle and some of the inferior pharyngeal constrictor fibers. The internal laryngeal nerve supplies sensation to the larynx above the vocal cords and may contribute some motor or proprioceptive input to the interarytenoid muscle.

Loss of the superior laryngeal nerve makes it difficult for a patient to perceive a foreign body in the larynx, and it also paralyzes the cricothyroid muscle. This reduces the tension of the vocal cord, and initially produces a weak, easily-fatigued, husky voice.

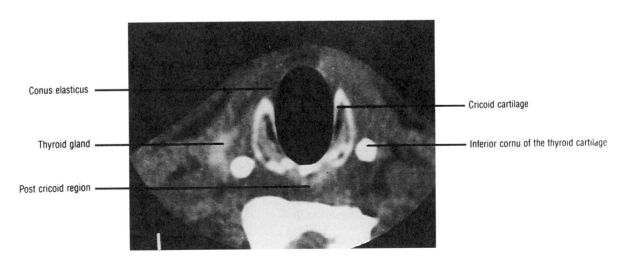

FIGURE 15-8 Axial CT section of the subglottis at the level of the inferior cornu of the thyroid cartilage. (From: Jeffrey RB, Dillon WP. The larynx. Computed tomography of the head and neck. Modern Neuro Radiology Series, 1988; 12.9.)

Inferior (Recurrent) Laryngeal Nerves. The recurrent laryngeal nerves are also branches of the vagus nerves. On the right, the recurrent laryngeal nerve extends upward after crossing the anterior surface of the first part of the subclavian artery to continue medial to the common carotid artery in the tracheoesophageal groove. On the left, the recurrent laryngeal nerve extends from the vagus nerve on the anterior surface of the aortic arch and continues around the descending thoracic aorta just distal to the ligamentum arteriosum. The left recurrent nerve then runs upward in the tracheoesophageal groove. Rarely, a nonrecurrent laryngeal nerve may be encountered, especially on the right side in the patient with an aberrant origin of a subclavian artery, predisposing it to iatrogenic injury.

Both recurrent laryngeal nerves are closely associated with, but variably related to, the branches of the inferior thyroid artery on each side. The nerves enter the larynx under the inferior pharyngeal constrictors, just posterior to the articulation of the inferior horn of the thyroid cartilage with the cricoid cartilage.

The recurrent laryngeal nerves supply sensation to the vocal cords, and to the lower portion of the larynx. It is also the motor nerve to all of the intrinsic muscles except the cricothyroid.

With unilateral, recurrent nerve injury, the airway is typically uncompromised but the initial voice quality is hoarse and breathy, and there is early vocal fatigue. This occurs because of incomplete glottic closure from the paramedian position of the affected vocal cord. Over time, the voice quality typically improves because of compensatory crossing of the midline by the contralateral vocal cord.

With bilateral, recurrent nerve injury, suffocation can occur rapidly because of bilateral vocal cord abductor paralysis. Paralyzed vocal cords become lax and initially tend to be about 3-4 mm apart. At first usually no dyspnea occurs, but immediate loss of voice is manifest. Within 3-5 months, the voice begins to improve, but dyspnea often appears because atrophy and fibrosis of the attached muscles cause the cords to gradually draw toward each other, greatly reducing the size of the rima glottidis. If an upper respiratory infection (or other form of local tissue reaction) were to occur, with its attendant mucosal swelling, an acute complete airway obstruction could be precipitated.

Cervical Trachea

The cervical trachea extends from the cricoid cartilage to the thoracic inlet at the level of the sternal manubrium. The trachea varies from 13-22 mm in width and is supported anteriorly and laterally by 16-20 U-shaped rings of hyaline cartilage which keep its lumen open. The posterior portion of the trachea is closed by a fibrous membrane on which lies the trachealis muscle and mucous membrane. The entire (cervical and thoracic) trachea is about 9-15 cm long, and almost half of it (the cervical trachea) is above the sternum.

The trachea is usually widely open, especially during deep spontaneous inspiration. During forced expiration, especially with coughing, the tracheal lumen may be narrowed to less than 20% of its normal cross-sectional area.

AXIOM Symptoms of airway obstruction are not usually manifest until loss of at least 50-70% of the cross-sectional area of the airway occurs.

ETIOLOGY OF INJURIES

Penetrating

Stab wounds, which make up about half of penetrating neck injuries, cause significant vascular, neural, or aerodigestive injury in 40-60% of patients. Gunshot wounds of the neck are slightly less common, but the significant injuries they cause are more frequent (60-80% of patients) and are usually more severe.[9,10] The most common organs injured by penetrating trauma are major veins in 15-30%, major arteries in 10-20%, digestive tract (pharynx or esophagus) in 5-20%,

TABLE 15-1   Classification of Laryngeal Injuries

Supraglottic tear and fractures
Transglottic injuries
Cricoid fractures
Avulsion of trachea from cricoid
Lacerations or tears of trachea

Harris HH, Ainsworth JZ. Immediate management of laryngeal and tracheal injuries. Laryngoscope 1965;75.

and upper respiratory tract (larynx or cervical trachea) in 5-15%. The incidence of upper airway injury is at least doubled when one of the other systems is also injured.[9,10] Of the airway injuries, the larynx is involved in about a third of patients, and the cervical trachea is damaged in about two-thirds. In 15-20% of gunshot wounds, the airway is injured in two or more locations.[7]

Patients with penetrating trauma of the larynx or cervical trachea are likely to have concurrent vascular, esophageal, and thoracic injuries.[2] Esophageal injuries occur in 25% of patients with penetrating airway trauma,[6] and it is the diagnosis most likely to be missed until late in the patient's hospital course. Death in patients with penetrating airway trauma is usually due to an associated vascular injury and is rarely due to the airway injury itself.[6]

Blunt Injuries

LARYNX

Injuries Related to Mechanism of Trauma

Blunt injuries to the larynx or cervical tracheal can occur in a wide variety of ways, including direct compression (hanging, strangulation, assaults, or shearing injuries). A classification introduced by Harris and Ainsworth divides laryngeal injuries into anatomic sites which tend to be caused by certain types of trauma (Table 15-1).[17] In Schaeffer's classification, (Table 15-2) patient groupings were based on the extent of injury rather than on the anatomic site.[5]

SUPRAGLOTTIC INJURIES

Injuries include fractures, which tend to be oriented vertically, of the hyoid bone and thyroid cartilage. A depression or widening of the thyroid notch with loss of the thyroid prominence is often seen. With disruption of the thyrohyoid membrane and/or thyroepiglottic ligament, posterior and superior displacement of the epiglottis and soft tissues of the larynx can occur. Associated injuries include tears of the false cords, aryepiglottic folds, pharyngeal walls, and ventricles. The injury pattern can be further complicated by avulsion-dislocation of the arytenoid cartilages.

TRANSGLOTTIC INJURIES

Injuries often result from direct right-angle blows to the thyroid cartilage and are usually divided into anterior and posterior types. The anterior type is characterized by midline vertical fractures of the thyroid cartilage with extension of the laceration injury into the true and false cords and the aryepiglottic folds. The resultant foreshortening of the larynx in the anteroposterior dimension causes vocal cord mo-

TABLE 15-2   Classification of Endoscopic Findings

Group I	Minor endolaryngeal hematoma or mucosal disruption
Group II	Moderate mucosal lacerations and edema
Group III	Significant injury requiring exploration
Group IV	Massive injury with exposed cartilage, vocal cord injury, and displaced fractures

Schaeffer SD, Close LG. Acute management of laryngeal trauma. Ann Otol Rhinol Laryngol 1989;98:98.

bility to be impaired. Ipsilateral avulsion-dislocation of the arytenoid may occur when the impact force is concentrated about the lateral thyroid ala. Posterior type injuries typically relate to interarytenoid and thyroarytenoid muscle disruptions with dislocation and/or exposure of the arytenoid cartilages. Recurrent laryngeal nerve injury may occur secondary to compression from cricoarytenoid displacements.

SUBGLOTTIC INJURIES

Subglottic injuries as an isolated entity are rare, and more often occur in conjunction with thyroid cartilage fractures or as part of a laryngotracheal separation pattern. Fractures of the cricoid usually occur in the arch in the midline or paramedian position. Internal displacement with reactive edema and hemorrhage may lead to rapid deterioration of the airway.

LARYNGOTRACHEAL INJURIES

Laryngotracheal injuries typically occur from excessive shearing forces acting on the neck in a hyperextended position. Damage to the strap muscles, recurrent laryngeal nerves, and even the anterior esophageal wall are associated with this injury pattern. With complete transection, the larynx tends to retract upward, while the distal tracheal stump characteristically retracts downward substernally due to the elasticity of the intercartilaginous ligaments. This can result in a gap of 6-10 cm or more between the cricoid superiorly and the torn trachea distally.

Motor Vehicle Accidents

The most frequent cause of blunt laryngeal injuries in most series is high-speed motor vehicle accidents (MVAs). In the unrestrained victim, the usual scenario involves the victim's head striking the windshield and the exposed anterior neck impacting the steering wheel[18] or dashboard ("padded dashboard syndrome").[19] Upon impact of the neck on the dashboard or steering wheel, the larynx can be crushed against the cervical spine. Such trauma may not only produce severe laryngeal fractures but it may also cause separation of the cricoid cartilage from the upper trachea as the larynx is displaced upward. In addition, if the glottis were to close in anticipation of a blow, the trachea would be converted to an air-filled rigid tube. A sudden elevation of intraluminal pressure by a compressive force against the chest can blow out the trachea and increase any other ligamentous or cartilaginous damage. Cervical hyperextension, which pulls the larynx away from the trachea, also facilitates avulsion injury.[20,21]

In the restrained patient, the incidence and extent of laryngeal injury is usually decreased, but this depends on the type of restraint system used.[22] Although a lap belt by itself can prevent a large number of serious injuries, the upper body can still move forward with the neck in hyperextension. Diagonal restraint belts, or shoulder harnesses, can also cause neck injuries. The "seat-belt sign" is a well-known phenomenon, and it may be associated with abrasions or contusions of the neck. This can cause severe underlying laryngeal injury with minimal superficial clinical evidence of damage.

Of 10 patients with laryngeal injury recently reported by Fuhrman et al., six were unrestrained occupants in MVAs, two received direct blows to the neck, one was a pedestrian hit by a car, and one had a "clothesline" type injury while riding a motorcycle.[23]

Blunt trauma from sports, assaults, and hangings can cause a wide variety of injuries.[6,22] Hematoma formation within the vocal cords has been caused by a wide variety of trauma, including prolonged singing and disorders of clotting.

"Clothesline" Injuries

"Clothesline" injuries are described as injuries caused to the neck by high-speed contact with a horizontally suspended cord.[24] These injuries occur with increasing frequency because of the proliferation of snowmobilers who tend to run into fences. Such trauma can cause severe injury to the larynx or cervical trachea and is a frequent cause of cricotracheal disruption in northern states during the winter. In MVAs, cricotracheal membrane rupture often results from the flat-

tening effect of an anterior blow to the U-shaped tracheal rings causing stress on the cricotracheal membrane.[21]

Endotracheal Intubation

> **AXIOM** Laryngeal dysfunction can occur following endotracheal intubation and most often results from laryngeal edema, hemorrhage, or mucosal tears.

Even an apparently uncomplicated endotracheal intubation in a normal upper airway can occasionally cause either arytenoid subluxation by direct trauma or recurrent laryngeal nerve paralysis (RLNP). The mechanism of injury of the latter is believed to be a neuropraxic response of the anterior branch of the RLN, caused by compression of the abducted arytenoid (from endotracheal cuff inflation) against the internal thyroid lamina. Other predisposing factors in endotracheal-tube-associated RLN injury include an overinflated cuff (which may migrate to the cricoid level) and use of high-nitrous-oxide mixtures in an air-inflated cuff (causing expansion of the balloon cuff over time).[25]

Differentiating between arytenoid dislocation and RLNP can be difficult. Both may show an immobile lateralized vocal cord and asymmetrically positioned arytenoid cartilages on examination by indirect laryngoscopy. Usually the arytenoid cartilages are displaced in an anterolateral position with the vocal processes shifted medially. The distinction may be made, however, through videostroboscopy which can demonstrate preserved mucosal wave movements of the vocal cord with arytenoid subluxation. Laryngeal EMG shows absence of fibrillation potentials with acute denervation injury of a vocal cord, but not in arytenoid dislocation. Direct palpation, using a microlaryngeal manipulator, demonstrates a mobile arytenoid cartilage in its joint space when an isolated injury to the RLN occurs.

Arytenoid subluxation refers to abnormal displacement of an arytenoid cartilage which is still partly in contact with the joint space.[26] Arytenoid dislocation describes the complete separation of the arytenoid cartilage from its articulating surface on the cricoid cartilage; this usually results from severe laryngeal injury. Although only eight patients with arytenoid subluxation due to intubation injury have been reported in the English-language literature, the incidence may be much greater. The first patient with isolated arytenoid subluxation resulting from blunt external laryngeal trauma has only recently been reported.[27] Previously, external trauma or surgery in the neck usually was blamed for abnormal laryngeal function.

In one patient with upper airway obstruction, which developed after what seemed to be an uneventful three-hour intubation for surgery, bilateral arytenoid dislocation was noted.[28] Reports suggested that the cricoarytenoid articulation may be particularly prone to subluxation in children, women, and the elderly. Typically these injuries only involve one cartilage, but bilateral dislocation has been described.[29] Up to 30% of injuries occurring after laryngeal instrumentation may be due to arytenoid dislocation.[28]

> **AXIOM** It can be difficult to differentiate between arytenoid dislocation and recurrent nerve injury, particularly after neck surgery.

Several reports indicated that vocal cord paralysis after tracheal intubation[30] was due to damage to the recurrent laryngeal nerves by an overexpanded cuff, toxic neuritis, and various nonspecific causes. Glottic edema is a common finding in these patients. Castella et al. suggested that some of these unexplained vocal cord paralyses with glottic edema at extubation may actually have been caused by arytenoid dislocation.[28]

INJURIES TO THE CERVICAL TRACHEA

Blunt external trauma to the upper cervical trachea is relatively uncommon. Cases have been reported following motor vehicle collisions, and after occupational, sporting, and domestic accidents.[29,30] The most commonly described blunt injury of the cervical trachea is cricotracheal separation. Injuries to the cervical trachea may also be caused or aggravated by endotracheal intubation. In one series, five of seven patients with tracheal rupture were probably made complete by insertion of the endotracheal tube.[30]

LARYNGOTRACHEAL PATHOLOGY

The type of laryngotracheal injury following blunt trauma is determined by multiple factors, including: (a) the magnitude and direction of the force, (b) the position of the cervical spine during impact, (c) the age of the patient, and (d) the consistency of the laryngotracheal cartilages and soft tissue.[8] Depending on these factors, laryngotracheal contusion, edema, hematoma, laceration, avulsion, and/or fracture and dislocation of the thyroid, cricoid, or tracheal cartilages can occur.

The subglottic and supraglottic submucosa allows for rapid accumulation of edema fluid. Because the vertical spread of accumulated edema is limited by the conus elasticus, subglottic endolaryngeal swelling tends to be circumferential, thereby increasing the potential for airway obstruction.[31] Air in the submucosal space further reduces the luminal diameter of the larynx or trachea. Air may also cause epiglottic emphysema and narrow the supraglottic airway.[21,32]

The majority of submucosal edema and hematoma formation developing after trauma presents within several hours.[33] Consequently, airway obstruction due to endolaryngeal swelling is unlikely to occur later than 6 hours after injury unless coughing, straining, or speaking increases the quantity of subcutaneous air or reinitiates intramural bleeding.

Although laryngeal fracture can occur at any age, older persons with calcified cartilages are presumed to be more susceptible to this type of injury. This assumption, however, has never been proved because most patients with laryngeal trauma are younger adults.[34] Fractures are usually vertical, but horizontal or comminuted fractures also occur.

Both the thyroid and cricoid cartilages are composed of hyaline cartilage and, consequently, are especially prone to fracture. The cuneiform, corniculate, arytenoid, and epiglottic cartilages are made of fibroelastic tissue, and consequently they are more likely to avulse or dislocate than fracture.[35] The arytenoid cartilages are especially likely to dislocate, and this greatly interferes with the function of the vocal cords. The hyoid bone, although calcified, is rarely injured because it is protected by the overhanging chin and cushioned by its surrounding muscles.

Frequently, soft-tissue, supraglottic, glottic, and infraglottic injuries are found in varying combinations in the same patient. A system devised by Harris and Ainsworth[17] in 1965, and modified by Potter et al.[36] in 1970, may be used to classify the type, location, and severity of laryngotracheal injury (Table 15-1). CT allows for the noninvasive assessment and classification of these injuries.

The trachea may be lacerated or transected, especially in younger patients in whom intercartilaginous connective membranes are not strong, and thus are susceptible to interruption.[37] A common site of transection is the junction of the cricoid with the trachea because the connective tissue there is relatively weak.[38]

> **AXIOM** Cricotracheal separation is often accompanied by avulsion of the recurrent laryngeal nerves.[39]

ASSOCIATED INJURIES

> **AXIOM** Cervical spine injury is frequently associated with blunt laryngotracheal trauma, and should be considered present until proved otherwise.[40]

The esophagus may be lacerated when it is crushed between the thyroid or cricoid cartilage and the sharp edge of an osteophyte or a fractured fragment of the spine.[41] Tracheoesophageal fistulas usually de-

velop early, but may not become apparent until a few days after corrective surgery. They can sometimes be suspected radiographically because of the presence of an air column in the esophagus. Typically, isolated pharyngoesophageal tears cause limited neck emphysema, in contrast to tears of the laryngotracheal structures which usually lead to massive subcutaneous emphysema.

> **AXIOM** Airway problems in comatose patients with blunt head injury may be due to associated laryngotracheal trauma.

Closed-head injury is frequently seen in patients with blunt laryngotracheal trauma[37] and may give the false impression that the airway obstruction is due to coma which relaxes the tongue and allows it to fall back into the pharynx. Hypoxemia, which is frequently found in laryngotracheal injury, is particularly deleterious in patients with concomitant head injury as it not only deprives the brain of necessary oxygen and results in further neuronal loss, but it also increases cerebral blood flow and intracranial pressure.[42]

Maxillofacial injuries are common in patients with laryngeal trauma, and the airway obstruction may initially be blamed on the facial injuries. This assumption may lead to an emergency cricothyroidotomy that may convert a partial airway obstruction to one that is complete.

> **AXIOM** Associated chest injuries which impair ventilation may divert attention from less obvious laryngotracheal injuries.

DIAGNOSIS

> **AXIOM** Severe laryngeal damage may be associated with minimal initial symptoms or signs. Therefore, a high index of suspicion, partially based on the mechanism of injury, is needed.

Early diagnosis and treatment of laryngeal or tracheal injuries are essential. Concern about the airway is paramount regardless of how minor the trauma or symptoms may seem, which carries great responsibility for the initial examining physician. A high index of suspicion is most apt to lead to early diagnosis and prompt treatment. Often laryngeal injury is not recognized until a sudden, severe airway problem develops. This is particularly apt to occur during endoscopy or anesthetic induction.

> **AXIOM** When an endotracheal tube cannot be passed through the larynx of a trauma victim, one should assume that a laryngotracheal injury is present.[37,43]

Although a thorough physical examination is important, at least 25% of patients with laryngotracheal trauma requiring surgery may have no physical evidence of such injury,[22] and symptoms may not begin until 24-48 hours after trauma.[44] In addition, many of these patients have associated injuries to the head, face, chest, and extremities which can divert the physician's attention.[11,23,45]

Of the 46 patients with upper airway injuries in the series reported by Cicala et al.,[11] 10 (22%) were not diagnosed from the presenting signs and symptoms. Of these 10 patients, five were diagnosed by CT, one by laryngoscopy, one by bronchoscopy, two during the induction of anesthesia, and one at autopsy.

In many patients, the airway problem does not become apparent until an attempt at endotracheal intubation is made during anesthesia. Some laryngeal injuries may remain undetected for weeks or months, until the patient presents later with airway or voice problems. The diagnosis of airway damage is particularly apt to be delayed in patients with relatively minor airway injuries who were intubated on an emergency basis soon after admission.[6]

> **AXIOM** Attempts to intubate a patient with respiratory distress and unsuspected airway injury can easily result in complete obstruction of the airway and death.

Because even major trauma centers may see only a few patients with airway injuries each year, a high degree of suspicion is necessary to recognize and manage patients with upper airway injuries.

History

AXIOM The history and physical examination should make one suspect laryngeal injury, but CT is best for evaluating the cartilages, and laryngoscopy for evaluating the mucosa and cord motion.

LARYNX

The diagnostic process is faciliated by knowledge of the mechanism of injury, events observed in the prehospital setting, and the progression of symptoms or physical signs en route to the hospital, as noted by the ambulance attendants.[46] The patient should be questioned in detail about any pain, including its location and character, as well as any difficulty breathing, talking, or swallowing.

AXIOM Dysphonia is the most common presenting symptom with laryngeal injury.

Voice problems may vary from mild hoarseness to aphonia depending on the structure(s) involved.[18] However, the voice may also be impaired because of cerebral damage causing dysphonia or dysarthria. Hoarseness due to neck trauma is usually caused by injury to the laryngeal nerves, laryngeal edema, or hematoma. Although vocal impairment cannot be taken as a guide to the severity of injury,[31] a progressive change in the voice suggests worsening of the injury and requires prompt surgical intervention in the operating room.[47]

AXIOM Presence of a normal voice on admission does not eliminate significant laryngeal injury.

Although the voice is usually weak with partial tracheal avulsion, or hoarse or even absent when the vocal cords are involved, dysphonia may not be present. In LeMay's series, two-thirds of patients with penetrating laryngotracheal injury had no voice change.[48] Only 13% of the 46 patients in Cicala's series presented with vocal abnormalities, but at least 21 other patients underwent definitive airway management (endotracheal intubation or tracheotomy) before the ability to phonate was assessed.[7] Kelly et al. also noted that voice changes and hemoptysis were uncommon with airway injuries.[6] However, when hoarseness is present, one must also look for recurrent laryngeal nerve paralysis or arytenoid dislocation.[41,49]

Other symptoms seen with laryngeal trauma include dyspnea, neck pain, sore throat, voice change, dysphagia, and odynophagia. Occasionally, these patients may have hemoptysis. A sore throat from endotracheal tube intubation (ETI) usually resolves in 24-48 hours. Increasing or severe discomfort beyond that time should be investigated.[50]

AXIOM A severe sore throat not improving 48 hours after a transient endotracheal intubation should be investigated for laryngeal injury.

Although odynophagia (painful swallowing) or dysphagia (difficulty swallowing) has not been associated with arytenoid subluxation in all patients, it is frequently present for several days and should be considered as a potential etiology in addition to, or exclusive of, recurrent laryngeal nerve paralysis.

Hematemesis following head and neck trauma is usually due to nasal or oral injuries but may occasionally be due to injuries of the aerodigestive tract in the neck.

TRACHEA

The classic symptoms of injury to the cervical trachea include pain, dysphagia, stridor, and hemoptysis; however, none of these may be present at initial assessment. Nevertheless, the patient may have noted some neck swelling due to the subcutaneous emphysema that is usually present when the cervical trachea has been torn.

Physical Examination

PENETRATING INJURIES

Respiratory distress after penetrating neck trauma suggests airway obstruction by various mechanisms including: (a) aspiration of foreign bodies, secretions, or blood, (b) external compression of the airway by hematoma, (c) submucosal edema, or (d) direct injury to the larynx or trachea.[8] Unlike blunt injuries, which often require a high index of suspicion to make an early diagnosis, penetrating injuries to the larynx and trachea are usually obvious and can be dramatic in their presentations.

AXIOM A sucking neck wound and progressive hypoxemia is virtually pathognomonic for a major laryngotracheal laceration.[6,40]

Many patients with stab or GSW injuries to the larynx or cervical trachea will have dyspnea, with an obvious opening into the airway, characterized by air bubbling through the wound and subcutaneous or deep perivisceral emphysema.[6] With lower cervical tracheal wounds, the patient may also have a pneumothorax with decreased breath sounds on one or both sides. Persistent localized neck pain with coughing suggests laryngeal or tracheal injury.[48] Mild-to-moderate hemoptysis immediately after trauma usually stops soon after admission in patients with only laryngeal or tracheal injury.

AXIOM Continued significant hemoptysis suggests a combined airway and major vascular injury.[8]

BLUNT TRAUMA

Unlike penetrating trauma in which the neck wound is a major stimulus to suspect an airway injury, blunt trauma to the neck is often associated with few physical findings even though serious injuries may be present.[2,24,31,37] Associated injuries, most notably to the cervical spine, face, head, and chest are common after blunt neck trauma and frequently complicate diagnosis and treatment.[2,47]

AXIOM A high index of suspicion is needed to diagnose most blunt laryngotracheal injuries.

The most obvious evidence of blunt laryngeal trauma is airway obstruction or voice change. However, the presenting signs of blunt laryngeal injury may be deceptively mild and often correlate poorly with the severity of damage. In some instances, laryngeal edema gradually obstructing the airway may not become evident for 24-48 hours.

AXIOM The most frequent sign of blunt laryngotracheal trauma is subcutaneous emphysema.

Subcutaneous emphysema does not always develop in patients who have deep perivisceral air. In the series by Cicala et al., which included nine patients with GSW's, only four (44%) had clinically apparent subcutaneous air.[7] Of the three patients with blunt laryngeal or cricoid fractures resulting in deep, soft tissue air, only one (33%) was apparent clinically.

AXIOM The extent of subcutaneous emphysema correlates poorly with the extent of injury and should not be used as a guide for inferring injury patterns.

AXIOM Absence of clinically apparent subcutaneous air does not eliminate airway injury.

The neck must be carefully examined for subcutaneous emphysema (swelling with crepitance), palpable laryngeal fractures, loss of the normal external architecture of the larynx, soft-tissue swelling, and ecchymosis. It is noteworthy that even when the larynx is severely fractured, with marked displacement of its component parts, only minimal external evidence of injury may be evident.[17,37,46,47] Even patients with separation and malfunction of the vocal cords may have little or no initial hoarseness.

AXIOM The quality of the voice is often a poor indicator of the severity of the underlying laryngeal damage.

The thyroid notch and the thyroid prominence, which is usually readily felt and identified as the Adam's apple in the male, may not be palpable following neck trauma. This may be due to overlying edema or hematoma formation, or to vertical fracture(s) of the thyroid cartilge with posterolateral splaying of the alar segments. In females, this area of the thyroid cartilage may be difficult to evaluate because the angle of the thyroid prominence is less acute. Loss of the cricoid prominence is a significant finding in either sex.

When a cervical immobilization collar has been applied because of the possibility of concomitant cervical spine injuries, it is important that the anterior component of the collar be removed (while the head is held in a neutral position) so that the neck can be examined for any signs of injury.

AXIOM Difficulty breathing in the supine position may be a sign of upper airway injury.

Intolerance of the supine position is occasionally seen in patients with upper airway injury and was present in 30% of patients reported by Fuhrman et al.[23] Cherry and Hammond noted posttraumatic positional dyspnea (i.e., severe dyspnea on neck extension) in these patients.[29] They believed that this was indicative of severe upper airway obstruction and constituted an absolute indication for immediate exploration.

AXIOM Whenever intubating a patient with blunt trauma to the head or neck, one should be prepared to rapidly provide a surgical airway if needed.

When difficulty occurs in advancing an endotracheal tube or ventilating a patient once the endotracheal tube has supposedly "passed between the vocal cords," one should consider the possibility of a cricoid or tracheal injury. When an airway is still present, one can attempt to intubate the patient using a flexible bronchoscope; however, when the airway is lost, immediate emergency tracheostomy is required. One must also be prepared to manage a laryngotracheal avulsion injury which may necessitate retrieval of the distal tracheal stump from the superior mediastinum.

AXIOM If a nasogastric tube were placed prior to the intubation attempt, the tube may act as a guide to finding an otherwise "lost" dislocated trachea in the mediastinum.

An injury to the trachea should be suspected when evidence of overdistension or abnormal migration of the balloon or tip of an endotracheal tube exists. Tobias et al. noted that the inability to seal a properly placed endotracheal tube with a reasonable amount of air is an ominous sign and is suggestive of airway discontinuity.[51] In one recent series reported by Rollins and Tocino,[52] five of seven cases of tracheal rupture were due to intubation, and it was found that the endotracheal tube balloon plugged the site of rupture and minimized the airleak.

AXIOM If a patient had an emergency intubation soon after arrival in the hospital, one must be alert to the possibility of an airway injury when extubating the patient.

In patients who have had emergency intubation soon after admission, it may be wise to extubate them using a flexible bronchoscope or at least have an anesthesiologist or surgeon standing by. An injury of the upper airway should obviously be suspected when, following extubation, the patient has intermittent noisy inspiration and/or painful swallowing.

ROUTINE LABORATORY STUDIES

With the exception of a complete blood cell count, and a type and cross match, usually little need exists for other routine laboratory tests to be performed in a previously healthy patient.

Radiography

PLAIN RADIOGRAPHY

AXIOM Radiography of the chest, lateral cervical spine, and pelvis should be obtained on all patients with severe blunt trauma.

Angood et al. found that radiography alone was sufficient to diagnose 12 (60%) of 20 patients with cervical airway trauma.[2]

Neck

ABNORMAL AIR OR AIR COLUMNS. Radiography of the neck may reveal deep, soft-tissue (perivisceral) emphysema, airway compression, injury to laryngeal structures (especially in older patients with calcified cartilages), tracheal deviation, cervical spine injury, and increased thickness of paravertebral tissues due to bleeding or edema. A lateral view of the neck can be particularly helpful. Not only may it demonstrate the integrity of the cervical spine in blunt trauma, but it can also demonstrate disruption of the airway in a high percentage of injuries.[53] Posterior displacement of the epiglottis and distortion of the laryngeal air column may be important.[54] With gunshot wounds, the position of missile fragments should also be noted.

AXIOM Free air in the deep (perivisceral) spaces of the neck is usually due to an injury of the aerodigestive tract.

Following penetrating trauma, free air in the deep tissues may occasionally be due to air passing down the missile tract, but it is much more likely to be due to injury to air-containing structures. In most patients with severe, blunt laryngeal or upper tracheal trauma, deep cervical and mediastinal emphysema are manifest.

Radiographic evidence of air in the deep cervical tissue planes may be apparent several hours before there is any clinical evidence of subcutaneous emphysema,[55] and it may be the only indication of tracheobronchial trauma in some patients.[46] Cervical radiographs or CT scans also may demonstrate the location of an interruption of the normal air column.[55]

POSITION OF THE HYOID BONE. Tobias et al. noted that superior displacement of the hyoid bone on a lateral view of the neck can be a valuable sign of tracheal transection.[51] Normally, the body of the hyoid bone is situated entirely below a line drawn along the top of the third cervical vertebral body, and the distance between the cornua of the hyoid bone and the angle of the mandible should be > 2 cm.[56] With tracheal or cricotracheal transection, the hyoid bone is elevated.

Polansky et al. noted that neck flexion and extension do not normally affect hyoid bone position.[56] Even with supine radiographs of the neck, this sign may still be valuable. Ideally, lateral radiographs of the neck should be obtained with the patient's mouth closed and while the patient is not swallowing.

INCREASED RETROPHARYNGEAL SPACE. Increased space between the upper airway and the anterior border of the vertebral bodies of C-3 and C-4 > 4-5 mm often suggests the presence of interstitial edema, blood, or other fluids in that area. From C-5 to C-7, the prevertebral space is usually < 10 mm. Increased space in this area after 48-72 hours may be caused by infection.

CERVICAL SPINE INJURIES. Between 10%[11] and 50%[12] of patients sustaining blunt airway trauma have concurrent cervical spine injuries. Reddin et al. noted that fractures of the bodies of lower cervical vertebrae can cause laceration of the membranous portion of the trachea.[41] Esophageal injury can also occur in conjunction with blunt airway trauma, especially in patients with concurrent cervical spine injuries.[57]

FRACTURED STERNUM. A fractured sternum may also be seen best on lateral chest radiography; this is associated with an increased incidence of myocardial contusion and thoracic tracheal injury.[53]

Chest Radiography

Posteroanterior (PA) and lateral radiographs of the chest may reveal subcutaneous or mediastinal emphysema, tracheal deviation, pneumothorax, hemothorax, fractured ribs, flail segments, pneumo- or hemopericardium, or widening of the mediastinum. Typically, injury to the cervical trachea causes severe pneumomediastinum, often without accompanying pneumothorax.

With blunt trauma, the first two ribs should be inspected carefully for fracture because such injuries are associated with an increased incidence of tracheobronchial, myocardial, or vascular injury.[58]

ARTERIOGRAPHY

AXIOM When vascular injury is suspected in a stable patient with a penetrating wound of the neck, arteriography of the carotid and vertebral vessels should be obtained.

Patients should not be sent for arteriography unless they are hemodynamically stable and have no active bleeding or large hematomas that might rupture and bleed massively. In stable patients with gunshot wounds, especially when the missile has transversed the midline, four-vessel studies including both carotid and both vertebral arteries, should be obtained. When an obvious vascular injury is evident in zone II, arteriography is not necessary.

Vascular injury with blunt trauma is uncommon, but can occur, and delayed diagnosis of blunt carotid thrombosis can be fatal or cause severe neurological changes in up to 85% of patients.[59] When any evidence suggests diminished carotid pulses or neurologic changes, but cranial CT is negative, one should obtain a four-vessel arteriography of the carotid and vertebral vessels.

CONTRAST SWALLOW

AXIOM Injuries to the upper respiratory tract, especially by penetrating trauma, are frequently associated with injuries to the pharynx or esophagus.

A high index of suspicion for pharyngoesophageal injuries must be maintained in the patient with penetrating airway injury because a delay in diagnosis may be associated with a significant increase in morbidity and mortality.[59,60]

PITFALL ⊘

> *Relying on a normal Gastrografin swallow to eliminate a pharyngoesophageal leak.*

Extravasation of swallowed contrast material is diagnostic of a pharyngeal or esophageal leak. However, a negative contrast swallow is not reliable, particularly in the neck, and especially when done with Gastrografin.[61-63] Up to 50 percent of esophageal leaks may be missed on Gastrografin swallows[63]; therefore, because of this and the significant likelihood of aspiration in the face of acute laryngeal

trauma, the diagnosis of pharyngoesophageal injury is often made by esophagoscopy.

CONTRAST LARYNGOGRAPHY

The use of contrast laryngography to diagnose laryngeal trauma is of historic interest only. When initially introduced, extravasation of dye from the larynx served as an important indication for immediate exploration of the neck and larynx. Although some believed that extravasation of dye into the perilaryngeal tissues increased the possibility of infection with delays in wound healing, the series by Ogura and Biller of more than 20 patients demonstrated no evidence of increased infection or delayed healing following laryngography.[64]

CT

AXIOM CT is the examination of choice for the diagnosis and localization of laryngeal cartilage injuries in otherwise stable patients.[31]

Detailed, accurate appraisal of laryngeal damage and airway encroachment can be obtained by CT. CT may be particularly useful in identifying laryngeal cartilage position and structure in patients in whom endoscopic evaluation of the larynx is obscured by edema and hematoma, or when the medical condition of the patient prevents laryngoscopy.[31,65,66]

The ability of CT to sharply demonstrate any bony or soft-tissue injury, to delineate fascial planes, and to detect airway encroachment with exquisite detail is only one of the many advantages of this technique. The extent of soft-tissue injury and hematoma formation can also be convincingly documented by this method. Injuries to the larynx and cervical trachea can be examined in any designated plane by use of appropriate window and level settings with advanced reformatting software.

CT is an important complement to laryngoscopy in patients who demonstrate no evidence of air leak, but who do have suspicious soft-tissue or cartilage injury.[55] CT may also be very helpful for diagnosing arytenoid dislocation due to endotracheal tube injuries.[26,65] However, RLNP may also show an immobile vocal cord and asymmetric positioning of one or both arytenoid cartilages. In general, CT should be employed when the results of the test are likely to influence management decisions. When large cartilage fracture displacements, dislocations, or mucosal disruptions mandate open exploration, CT is unlikely to alter the surgical approach. Similarly, a patient with a history of minimal neck trauma and a normal fiberoptic endoscopic examination is unlikely to benefit from the information gained by CT.[67]

MRI

MRI can display most of the information about soft-tissue injuries that can be provided by CT, and it provides better definition of vascular injuries.

Hoffman et al. found that MRI and CT were equally efficacious in documenting arytenoid subluxation and in demonstrating the degree of laryngeal disruption following intubation injuries.[68] MRI not only offers the advantages of allowing direct sagittal imaging without relying on reformatting of axial images, but also spares the patient exposure to ionizing radiation.

Although MRI is generally superior to CT for imaging the interface between soft tissues, CT may continue to be preferred in situations that require identification of the relationship between adjacent cartilaginous or calcified structures.[68] For these reasons, as well as problems with cost, lack of general availability, and difficulty with motion artifact seen with MRI, CT at present remains the preferred method of imaging arytenoid subluxation.

EMG

Although the use of EMG in the study of the intrinsic laryngeal muscles was first published 50 years ago,[69] it is not used very much except to distinguish recurrent laryngeal nerve paralysis (RLNP) from arytenoid fixation.[26,70] The use of intraoperative EMG in three patients at laryngoplasty helped to distinguish arytenoid subluxation from RLNP.[70]

Endoscopy

LARYNX AND TRACHEA

AXIOM   With penetrating injuries, endoscopy and/or CT are needed to diagnose laryngotracheal injuries in < 15% of patients, but with blunt injury about half of the patients require these tests for diagnosis.[7]

Penetrating injuries of the larynx or cervical trachea are usually obvious, but blunt injuries of the upper airway may be subtle and CT and/or endoscopy are much more likely to be needed for diagnosis.

Types of Endoscopy

INDIRECT LARYNGOSCOPY.   Indirect laryngoscopy can be helpful in alert, cooperative patients who do not have respiratory distress or a threatened airway. It can provide information about vocal cord mobility, mucosal integrity, endolaryngeal hematomas, arytenoid dislocation, and the degree of distortion of the laryngeal lumen. Areas poorly visualized on indirect laryngoscopy include the pyriform apex and postcricoid region. Unfortunately, it is not very useful during the initial evaluation of airway trauma. Associated injuries, hypovolemia, and altered consciousness also preclude its use in most acute trauma patients.

DIRECT LARYNGOSCOPY.   Although some otolaryngologists believe that it is indicated whenever a serious injury of the larynx is suspected but not proved or eliminated by other techniques, direct laryngoscopy should be reserved for physicians who are thoroughly familiar with the procedure and are prepared to handle any complications. The examiner should also be capable of proceeding with immediate, complete surgical reconstruction of the larynx if needed.

AXIOM   Endoscopic examination of a larynx with a suspected injury should be attempted in stable patients before attempting airway intervention.[15,71]

Direct laryngoscopy can provide important information about the type and extent of injury, especially when findings are interpreted in conjunction with those obtained from CT. The conventional laryngoscopic blade (Miller, MacIntosh) is not suitable for this purpose, as it may lead to acute airway obstruction in conscious patients, and it is inadequate for assessment of the cervical trachea. The Holinger anterior commissure laryngoscope provides a bluntly bevelled and narrow tip to adequately expose the pyriform fossae, post-cricoid region, and endolarynx. Consequently, it is the preferred instrument for this purpose.

PITFALL ⊘

When direct laryngoscopy is not performed within 2-4 hours of injury, normal landmarks may be obscured by edema, and the laryngeal injury may be aggravated.

When the patient's condition does not allow for immediate endoscopic examination, a waiting period of three to four days is often advised to allow some of the edema and hematoma to subside.

Although direct laryngoscopy was the definitive procedure for diagnosing laryngeal damage in the past, flexible bronchoscopy is now generally considered to be the single most important technique for the overall diagnosis of airway injury.[7] In the face of significant edema, however, the paralaryngeal and endolaryngeal recesses, as well as the subglottic larynx, are inadequately assessed by this method.

FLEXIBLE BRONCHOSCOPY

AXIOM   Flexible bronchoscopy is probably the best and safest technique for directly examining the luminal structures in the upper and lower airway.

Transnasal, flexible bronchoscopy is generally much more effective than an indirect mirror examination, and it is safer than direct laryngoscopy. Flexible bronchoscopy not only minimizes movement of the cervical spine in patients with blunt trauma, but it can also be very helpful for diagnosis of lesions in the nasopharynx, hypopharynx, larynx, trachea, and bronchi.[1] In addition, it can be used to provide immediate airway control, if needed, with introduction of an endotracheal tube over the instrument.[2,35] It affords the opportunity to evaluate the endolarynx in a more prolonged and deliberate manner without distorting the relationship between tongue base and supraglottic larynx.

Flexible bronchoscopy has been 100% accurate in a few small series[41] and can be used to identify airway pathology at any level, as well as to determine the presence of vocal cord paralysis secondary to recurrent laryngeal nerve injury.[89] Noyes et al. noted that bronchoscopy and laryngoscopy, when done together, are 100% accurate[62]; however, when they are done individually, there is an occasional false negative.

Flexible bronchoscopy performed through an endotracheal tube that is already in place is less accurate, particularly for laryngeal and cricoid injuries.[2] In addition, bleeding from the nose, mouth, or pharynx may make this examination difficult or impossible. Severe edema in the pharynx or epiglottic structures can also reduce the value of the technique.

Specific Features to be Examined

INTERNAL INJURIES.   Specific features that should be visualized during endoscopy include: (a) hemorrhage or hematoma formation, (b) false passages and/or mucosal tears, (c) the position of the arytenoids, (d) the size and shape of the laryngeal and tracheal lumens, (e) the presence of exposed cartilage, and (f) vocal cord mobility. Hematomas are most apt to involve the false cords, true cords, and aryepiglottic folds. False passages in short-necked individuals are more apt to be infraglottic, but in long-necked patients, they tend to be supraglottic. Ogura and Biller reported never encountering a supraglottic injury in a short-necked patient.[64] When the arytenoids are dislocated by blunt trauma, they are usually displaced posteriorly and superiorly. When the larynx is disrupted, the lumen will often seem to end abruptly. Exposed cartilage within the lumen is prima facie evidence of laryngeal fracture.

VOCAL CORD MOBILITY

AXIOM   Laryngeal trauma can cause bilateral vocal cord paralysis without apparent anatomical evidence of external or internal damage.

The mobility of the vocal cords should be noted carefully whenever the larynx is examined. This is one important advantage of performing the examination under topical anesthesia. In the absence of restrictive endolaryngeal edema or hematoma, bilateral cord paresis suggests thyrocricoid disarticulation with either entrapment or avulsion of the recurrent laryngeal nerves.[72] Unilateral cord "paralysis" often indicates a cricoid-arytenoid joint dislocation.

VOCAL CORD POSITION.   Damage to the recurrent laryngeal nerves results in varying and somewhat unpredictable vocal cord positions. The paralyzed vocal cord may be in the midline or partly abducted.[73] A clear explanation of this variability is not available, and the literature on this subject is controversial. Nevertheless, EMG studies conducted by Dedo suggested that the behavior of paralyzed vocal cords is best explained by the Wagner-Grossman theory.[74] According to this concept, complete severance of the recurrent laryngeal nerves results in paralysis of all intrinsic laryngeal muscles except the cricothyroid, which is innervated by the external branch of the superior laryngeal nerve.[8]

Because the cricothyroid muscles act both as an adductor and tensor of the vocal cords, complete transection of a recurrent laryngeal nerve results in the involved cord remaining in the paramedian position. Complete transection of both the superior laryngeal and recurrent laryngeal nerves causes the paralyzed vocal cord to be in the intermediate position. A similar, although very uncommon, situation can result from severance of the vagus nerve high in the neck or at the base of the skull.

When the recurrent laryngeal nerve is not completely transected, the position of the vocal cord depends on the type of nerve fibers damaged. Namiroff and Katz demonstrated that approximately 40% of recurrent laryngeal nerves divide into anterior and posterior branches between 0.6-4 cm from the cricoid cartilage.[75] Gacek et al. using peroxidase tracers, suggested that fibers of the recurrent laryngeal nerve collect into distinct adductor and abductor groups before entering the larynx.[76] Thus, it is possible that damage to an abductor nerve bundle in the presence of an intact external branch of a superior laryngeal nerve, can result in a median or paramedian position of the vocal cord, whereas damage to the adductor nerve bundle can produce an intermediate or abducted position.

ARYTENOID POSITION. When any abnormality of vocal cord function exists, the arytenoids and their location should be assessed carefully. If the arytenoids were not fractured, and were in their normal position, over 95% of patients would have spontaneous return of normal cord mobility.[64] If general anesthesia were used for the examination, the mobility of the cords could be tested somewhat by having the anesthetist lighten the anesthesia to the point of having the patient cough.

Endoscopic findings that suggest acute arytenoid subluxation include reduced vocal cord mobility, arytenoid edema, and anterolateral positioning of the arytenoid body.[49] Long-standing cricoarytenoid subluxation with joint ankylosis may be more difficult to differentiate from RLNP once the edema and pain of the acute injury have resolved. To identify characteristics of arytenoid position that may help differentiate these processes, fiberoptic videolaryngoscopy has been used by Hoffman et al.[68]

Problems in Apprehensive Patients

Laryngoscopy and bronchoscopy can be very difficult to perform in an awake, apprehensive patient. It may be necessary to use general anesthesia to perform the type of direct laryngoscopy and bronchoscopy needed to clearly identify the presence and extent of injury.

AXIOM While examining the larynx for injury, one must be prepared to handle sudden, complete airway obstruction.

Occasionally during endoscopy, fractured or dislocated cartilages may be displaced, causing complete occlusion of the airway. When one is not prepared for this possibility, the airway may not be reestablished in three to five minutes, and the patient may suffer irreparable brain damage.

Esophagoscopy

If esophageal injury is suspected, but esophagraphy is negative or equivocal, one should proceed with esophagoscopy. Many surgeons do not obtain esophagraphy and proceed directly to esophagoscopy. One must, however, first be sure that the airway is intact or protected with an endotracheal tube or tracheotomy. Flexible esophagoscopy is usually much safer and easier to perform, but occasionally rigid esophagoscopy may be preferred. Rigid esophagoscopy is also often preferred when a large foreign body is present, or when a perforation is still suspected in spite of a negative contrast swallow

and flexible esophagoscopy. Although esophageal injury can often be seen fairly readily, in some studies more than half of the esophageal perforations have been missed on flexible esophagoscopy,[65] particularly when the lesion is small and in the cervical esophagus.

Delayed Diagnosis

Delayed diagnosis of laryngotracheal injuries is not unusual, especially when emergency intubation is performed soon after arriving in the emergency department. In the series by Couraud et al., laryngotracheal injury was not diagnosed in 37% (7 of 19) patients until they presented with airway stenosis 8 days to 3 years after the initial trauma.[72] The diagnosis was made in some patients after they had recovered from coma, shock, or respiratory distress, but could not be extubated because of stenosis or complete obstruction of the larynx above a tracheotomy site. These patients were diagnosed with CT and/or laryngoscopy.

AIRWAY MANAGEMENT

Causes of Airway Obstruction

AXIOM Early death after neck injury usually occurs by one of three mechanisms: airway compromise, exsanguination, or CNS injury.

Airway obstruction after trauma may develop from several causes and at various times after admission.[21,47] Dislocated arytenoid cartilages may separate from their attachment to the cricoid and move anteromedially to obstruct the larynx. The larynx or trachea may be distorted enough by fractures to compromise luminal diameter. Submucosal emphysema, hematoma, and edema may further narrow the tracheal lumen.

Partial obstruction of the lumen results in an increase in inspiratory air velocity. According to Poiseuille's Law, the subatmospheric pressure generated in the air column to maintain constant flow causes the tissues to move medially, further increasing the obstruction.[21]

AXIOM The faster a patient with a narrow airway breathes, the greater the airway obstruction produced.

In cricotracheal separations, the soft tissue surrounding the trachea usually remains intact, providing airway continuity even though a gap of as much as 8 cm may be present between the separated ends of the airway.[24,37,47] Paralysis produced by muscle relaxants or weakness from sedatives causes these supporting muscles to lose their tone, and can result in sudden airway occlusion.

AXIOM Muscle relaxants or sedatives in patients with complete cricotracheal separation can rapidly cause complete airway obstruction.

Severe upper airway obstruction may also result from damage to peritracheal tissues caused by the tip of an endotracheal or cricothyroidotomy tube.[37]

Bleeding into the peritracheal tissue may cause a hematoma which can compress the trachea. Damage to both recurrent laryngeal nerves frequently brings the vocal cords close to the midline, resulting in airway narrowing, but this may not occur until several days or weeks after injury.[36] Delayed, recurrent nerve paralysis is often due to entrapment within peritracheal scar tissue.

Subcutaneous emphysema, although rarely a cause of airway obstruction, is capable of making existing respiratory distress much worse. Struggling or coughing increases the rate of air escape into perivisceral tissues by increasing the intratracheal pressure. Air from the neck may also enter the mediastinum or the pleural cavities, resulting in atelectasis or even tension pneumothorax.[8]

Indications for Providing an Emergency Airway

Conservative management can usually be maintained in the patient with laryngotracheal trauma when a clinically stable airway is present, and radiologic and flexible endoscopic examinations fail to show displaced cartilages, mucosal disruptions, or progressing edema or hematoma formation. Such therapy includes bed rest in Semi-Fowlers position, humidification by face mask with supplemental oxygen, intravenous access with hydration, systemic steroids, prophylactic antibiotics, and early vaponephrine mist nebulizer treatments to help curtail reactive edema. Additionally, the use of H_2 blockers in patients with gastroesophageal reflux may prove beneficial in reducing the extent of mucosal irritation and potential for laryngeal stenosis.[77]

Although many patients with injuries to the larynx can be initially managed conservatively, 15-50% of patients with penetrating laryngotracheal injuries have moderate-to-severe respiratory distress requiring immediate airway management.[6,15] Cicala et al. found that three-fourths of their patients (35 of 46) had no apparent airway management problems on admission and were either observed without being intubated (four patients), intubated through an obvious airway defect (six patients), or endotracheally intubated (25 patients).[7] The remaining 11 (24%) patients required emergent tracheotomy.

> **AXIOM** Acute airway problems are most apt to occur with blunt trauma to the cricoid or cervical trachea.

In the series by Cicala et al., the incidence of acute airway problems was 0% (0 of 8) for stabs, 24% (4 of 17) for gunshot wounds, and 40% (8 of 20) for blunt trauma.[7] The incidence of acute airway problems with 21 blunt injuries to various parts of the upper airway was 14% (1 of 7) with the larynx above the cricoid, 60% (3 of 5) with the cricoid, and 44% (4 of 9) with the cervical trachea. Indications for immediate tracheotomy and surgical exploration include: (a) impending or existent airway obstruction, (b) displaced or large fractures of the laryngeal skeleton, (c) increasing surgical emphysema, (d) evidence of internal airway derangement, and (e) continuing airway hemorrhage.[78]

> **AXIOM** Patients with airway injuries and inability to tolerate the supine position need to have their airways secured as soon as possible.

The importance of a patient's inability to tolerate the supine position cannot be overemphasized. Fuhrman et al. believed that this was an indication for immediate tracheotomy without indirect or flexible laryngoscopic evaluation.[23] Patients with evidence of major vessel damage, such as shock, large and expanding hematomas, or uncontrollable bleeding, should also be taken directly to the operating room.

Techniques for Providing an Emergency Airway

IN THE EMERGENCY DEPARTMENT

> **AXIOM** Acute airway problems that may be due to trauma to the larynx or trachea should be handled in the operating room as soon as possible.

Endotracheal Intubation

If the patient has acute, severe respiratory distress and is about to have a cardiac arrest, it is too dangerous to move the patient to the operating room. Such patients should have orotracheal intubation (with stabilization of the head for possible cervical spine injuries). However, this can be potentially hazardous. It may: (a) increase the amount of damage in the airway,[24,51,79] (b) convert a partial airway obstruction into one that is complete, and/or (c) hide a laryngeal or proximal tracheal injury that may not become apparent until an attempt is made to extubate the patient. Entry into a false passage (e.g., cricotracheal separation) is suggested when the attempt at orotracheal

intubation seems successful initially, but difficulty is experienced in advancing the endotracheal tube, and/or a bulging mass appears on the anterior surface of the neck.[80]

> **AXIOM** Nasotracheal intubation should not be attempted in patients with suspected laryngeal or tracheal trauma.

Blind intubation of the larynx can cause severe, additional laryngeal injury and can convert a partial laryngeal or upper tracheal obstruction into one that is complete and life-threatening.

Many surgeons contend that the airway of patients with blunt laryngotracheal trauma, including those with cricotracheal separation, can be intubated safely when the procedure is performed under direct vision of the glottis and trachea, such as with a flexible bronchoscope.[1,2,6,40,81] Occasionally, it may be helpful to use a conventional laryngoscope to visualize the supraglottic structures, and then a fiberoptic bronchoscope passed through the laryngoscope to visualize the glottis and infraglottic structures.[37] Alternatively, in order to expedite airway control, the larynx can be visualized with a laryngoscope blade, and once the tip of the endotracheal tube is introduced, it can be advanced with the aid of a fiberoptic bronchoscope that is inside it.

Tracheotomy

Many surgeons believe that immediate tracheotomy, rather than endotracheal intubation, should be performed in acutely asphyxiating patients whenever possible.[10,36,38] In addition to rapidly relieving any airway obstruction, tracheotomy reduces intrabronchial pressure and decreases the movement of air into the subcutaneous tissue, mediastinum, and pericardium.[6] Unfortunately, the emergency department is not the ideal place to perform a tracheotomy.

> **PITFALL** ⊘
>
> ***Attempting to perform an emergency tracheotomy in the emergency department on an uncooperative patient.***

Tracheotomy may be extremely difficult to perform in uncooperative individuals, such as children or hypoxic adults, and in those with distorted cervical anatomy. In patients with cricotracheal separation, the distal portion of the trachea can retract into the mediastinum and may be difficult to find.[47] Delay in identification of the distal trachea may aggravate hypoxemia, with resulting catastrophic consequence.

Cricothyroidotomy (Coniotomy)

> **AXIOM** Coniotomy can be dangerous in patients with possible laryngeal injury.

Cricothyroidotomy can provide an adequate airway when the injury is limited to the upper larynx. However, it can greatly aggravate the damage already caused by the original trauma, particularly when cricoid cartilage injuries are present.[8] In addition, obliteration of landmarks by edema, blood, or subcutaneous emphysema can result in technical difficulties. The most important disadvantage of this procedure, however, is the possibility of acute airway obstruction by insertion of the cannula into a false passage. This is particularly apt to happen when a cricotracheal separation is present. Even if the cricothyroidotomy tube were to remain within the airway, air could escape through a lacerated tracheal wall, preventing adequate ventilation. Thus, this procedure is generally contraindicated when blunt laryngotracheal trauma is suspected.[1,47,79]

Tracheal Oxygen via a Needle Catheter

If the patient were in severe respiratory distress in the emergency department and could not be intubated, one could consider inserting a large needle into the trachea and maintaining oxygenation of the patient with wall O_2 until a proper tracheotomy could be performed in the operating room. A hole in the tubing can be occluded as needed to provide the patient with enriched wall oxygen on an intermittent basis.

MANAGEMENT IN THE OPERATING ROOM

> **AXIOM** Acute airway problems are best handled in the operating room with the most experienced anesthesiologist and surgeon present.

The anesthesiologist relies on the surgeon to secure the airway when attempts at intubation fail, and the surgeon relies on the anesthesiologist to provide optimum conditions for the performance of a tracheotomy. Except in the gravest emergencies, both should be present and fully prepared before any definitive procedure to secure the airway is undertaken.[78]

Endotracheal Intubation

The anesthetic management of patients can be extremely complicated if the site and extent of possible laryngeal or tracheal injury are unknown. Endotracheal intubation can be extremely hazardous under these circumstances because it can easily cause complete airway obstruction or create false passages.[30]

> **AXIOM** "Rapid sequence" intubation can be extremely hazardous and is usually contraindicated in patients with a possible laryngotracheal injury.[83]

A wide variety of laryngeal and tracheal injuries may occur during endotracheal intubation. A tube that is too large is particularly apt to damage the anterior commissure. If the tube were inserted too vigorously, it could cause arytenoid dislocation and postcricoid ulceration and scarring. The resultant scars, webs, or strictures could then cause dysphonia and progressive respiratory embarrassment.

> **PITFALL** ⊘
>
> *If an endotracheal tube is too large or is inserted roughly, it can cause severe damage, even to a normal larynx or trachea.*

Attempts at intubation in patients with unsuspected cricoid injuries following blunt trauma can be particularly dangerous. When the cricoid cartilage is fractured, manual pressure on the cricoid cartilage (Sellick maneuver)[84] to reduce the risk of regurgitation of gastric contents into the upper airway may completely disrupt the cricotracheal junction.

> **AXIOM** The anesthesiologist and surgeon should have an extremely high index of suspicion for cricoid injury in patients with blunt neck trauma.

Ideally, endotracheal intubation is performed under direct vision over a flexible bronchoscope or with a standard laryngoscope to visualize the upper larynx, and a flexible bronchoscope with an endotracheal tube over it to visualize the infraglottic lumen and structures.[8]

Blood in the tracheobronchial tree can greatly impair the efficacy of flexible bronchoscopes because the suction port of the fiberoptic scope is not large enough to remove massive amounts of blood or formed clots from the airway. In this situation, a small, rigid pediatric bronchoscope can be substituted. The endotracheal tube is placed over the small, rigid bronchoscope and both can then be advanced into the distal trachea. The cuff of the endotracheal tube can then be inflated once the injured segment is passed.

> **AXIOM** Cervical spine injury should be eliminated before rigid endoscopy is performed.

Rigid endoscopic visualization of the larynx and trachea usually requires the neck to be extended. However, when the injury is severe and the risk of airway obstruction is high, the patient can often be ventilated through an adult-sized rigid bronchoscope without an endotracheal tube until the trachea is exposed surgically. Controversy exists, however, over the safety of oral intubation in the presence of cervical spine injury. A recent review suggested that this may be done safely if the head is properly stabilized by another individual.[85]

Tracheotomy

The operating room is the ideal place to perform a tracheotomy. For many surgeons, this provides the optimal initial and definitive airway for management of laryngeal and upper tracheal injuries. However, if the airway were lost during an attempted endotracheal intubation in the emergency department, immediate tracheotomy would be the only appropriate choice.[83] This should be performed via a vertical midline incision which will facilitate superior or inferior access depending on the site of injury.

> **AXIOM** All airway manipulations with a suspected laryngotracheal injury should be performed while the patient is conscious and breathing spontaneously.

The use of muscle relaxants and anesthetics should be avoided in a patient with a suspected airway injury until the integrity of the airway is secured. Because the severed larynx or trachea may be held together by the tone of the surrounding muscle, muscle relaxation can result in airway displacement and obstruction. The risk of aspiration is also much greater in a sedated patient. However, when the patient is extremely uncooperative or apprehensive, a general anesthetic may be necessary.

> **AXIOM** The importance of oxygen administration during a procedure to establish an airway cannot be overemphasized.

In patients with partial airway obstruction but adequate arterial oxygenation, a mixture of helium (50%) and oxygen (50%) may be helpful because the low density of the helium facilitates inspiratory gas flow. Helium reduces the work of breathing by decreasing airway resistance.[8]

> **PITFALL** ⊘
>
> *A tracheotomy, although often lifesaving, is not a simple, harmless procedure. If done poorly, it may cause death or severe respiratory problems.*

Tracheotomy should be performed without extending the neck, and spine protection measures should be used when the possibility of cervical spine injury has not yet been eliminated. These constraints give rise to technical difficulties and may be associated with some risks of airway obstruction if prior airway control is not established by endotracheal intubation.[77,85]

Elective or semielective tracheotomies are usually performed through a 3-4 cm horizontal incision placed midway between the cricoid cartilage and the suprasternal notch of the sternum. In patients whose superficial cervical landmarks are indistinct, or when an emergency tracheotomy is required, a vertical skin incision is preferable. After incising the skin, subcutaneous tissue, and platysma, the investing (deep cervical) fascia is identified and cut vertically between the medial margins of the sternohyoid and sternothyroid muscles.

Not infrequently, the thyroid isthmus will overlie the intended tracheotomy site. In most cases this can be mobilized superiorly or inferiorly by developing the pretracheal plane with a right-angle clamp. This is both time-saving and advantageous with regard to minimizing potential bleeding problems. Maintaining airway stability is essential for rapid intubation of the trachea. If the cricoid ring is intact, this would be facilitated by utilizing a cricoid hook (to pull the trachea anteriorly and superiorly. A vein retractor can also be used to stabilize and distract the thyroid isthmus.

The opening in the trachea should be below the area of injury, and ideally above rings four or five, to reduce tension on the repair (by fixation of trachea with tube), to lessen the likelihood of tracheoinnominate erosion, and to decrease the risk of bacterial contamination of the injured region after repair.[39]

Some of the more frequent, immediate complications of tracheotomy include hemorrhage, pneumothorax, and inadequate ventilation during the procedure. Careful attention to hemostasis and restriction of the dissection to the immediate area of the proposed opening into the trachea help to reduce the incidence of complications. In addition, the smallest tracheotomy tube compatible with adequate ventilation should be utilized.

AXIOM   After completion of the tracheotomy, it is important to auscultate the lungs and obtain chest radiography because it is not unusual for a pneumothorax to develop during or after this procedure.

Nonemergency Airway Management

In patients without respiratory distress, attention is directed first to more life-threatening, associated injuries.[8] However, one should avoid manipulation that may endanger the airway until the integrity of the spine is assured. Maneuvers, such as forceful neck examination, hypopharyngeal suctioning, changing the patient's position from sitting to supine, and nasogastric tube insertion, should not be performed during the initial stages of trauma because they may precipitate airway obstruction.[37]

AXIOM   All laryngeal injuries are dangerous and can suddenly occlude the upper airway.

While awaiting surgery, these patients should be treated with the conservative measures previously outlined. The use of corticosteroids to reduce inflammatory edema in the acute setting is of little value because the onset of clinical action is typically delayed 2-4 hours.

During this preanesthetic period, CT can be obtained and evaluated in patients with stable airways. Findings should be evaluated while airway patency, hemodynamic status, and associated injuries continue to be monitored and compared with previous examinations. With little or no respiratory compromise, initial airway management is somewhat controversial. Many authors advocated immediate tracheotomy without prior endotracheal intubation.[5,11,24,45,86] This avoids acute complications induced by attempts at intubation, such as entry into a false passage, damage to injured laryngeal structures, and complete obstruction of a marginally patent airway.

When endotracheal intubation is elected, irreversible steps, such as administration of intravenous anesthetics or muscle relaxants, should not be taken before the airway is secured.[8] These agents may result in severe and uncontrollable airway obstruction by producing a loss of tone in the peritracheal supportive structures or by displacing of the distal segment of the airway in cricotracheal separation injuries. Such complications can occur even with small sedative doses of hypnotic and opioid agents. Such drugs should be administered only in small doses and repeated only after an adequate time interval and careful assessment of the effect of previous doses.

AXIOM   Adequate topical anesthesia of the upper airway is essential before any airway manipulation is attempted.

Agitation, straining, and coughing during these maneuvers may precipitate hemorrhage, result in increased intratracheal pressure, spread subcutaneous emphysema, and cause complete airway obstruction.[47]

Children may not tolerate endotracheal intubation under sedation and topical anesthesia. Induction of general anesthesia by mask using inhalational agents and maintenance of spontaneous breathing has been recommended by some clinicians for fasted children or adults.[21,43] However, this technique is dangerous, especially in individuals who have evidence of partial airway obstruction. Complete airway obstruction can rapidly occur secondary to laryngeal

spasm and other mechanisms described above.[80] Therefore, tracheotomy under local anesthesia is preferred despite its inherent difficulties.

When no evidence of airway obstruction exists and anesthetic induction with inhalational agents is chosen to facilitate endotracheal intubation, the position that allows the most comfortable breathing while awake should be determined, and anesthetic induction performed in this position.

Atropine (0.02 mg/kg) or glycopyrrolate (0.01-0.02 mg/kg) should be administered intravenously to prevent laryngeal spasm and bradycardia.[8] Muscle relaxants should be avoided. When an adequate level of anesthesia is achieved, an orotracheal tube is placed under direct vision using a pediatric fiberoptic bronchoscope with an external diameter of 2.8 or 3.4 mm.[8] As in adults, the procedure should be attempted only in the presence of complete facilities for performing an emergency tracheotomy.

Timing of Laryngotracheal Repair

Controversy exists regarding the optimal timing for laryngeal repair. Some older reports recommended a delay of 3-5 days plus administration of steroids.[51] This approach provides some time for the traumatic edema to subside, making surgery technically easier.

Most surgeons[31,87,88] now tend to favor a more immediate operative approach (within 24 hours) and have found no advantage in delaying definitive management. Early exploration and repair facilitates healing by reducing the potential for granulation tissue development and allows for the identification of mucosal, muscular, and cartilaginous injuries which may be approximated primarily in most patients. Generally, delayed intervention has been shown to result in poorer voice and airway results.[23,88]

PITFALL ⊘

When displaced laryngeal fractures are not reduced and stabilized within 7-10 days, the resultant scarring may make later correction extremely difficult, and return of normal function is unlikely.

Early diagnosis and prompt treatment of laryngeal fractures can prevent many of the potential crippling sequelae that may otherwise occur. It will usually also provide a satisfactory voice, patent airway, and good protection of the lower respiratory system. However, in the recently fractured larynx, the landmarks may be so distorted that even an experienced laryngeal surgeon using a binocular microscope may have difficulty identifying residual normal laryngeal structures. In such instances, delay for five to six days usually makes the surgery safer and more successful.

Anesthesia

Inhalational induction of general anesthesia is generally the safest technique for patients with possible airway injuries[43,78]; however, for confused and/or uncooperative patients, intravenous induction may be more practical. Relaxants should be avoided if possible, but when they are indicated, the patient should be test-ventilated with a bag and mask prior to administration.

Positioning and Surgical Preparation

Once the airway is secured, appropriate preparations for diagnosis and management can proceed at a less urgent pace. The patient should be placed supine with a roll between the scapulae, with the neck in slight extension. Skin preparation and draping should include all of the anterior neck and extend from the chin to umbilicus so that a sternotomy could be performed if necessary. Care is taken during the preoperative preparation not to dislodge a tamponading clot and thereby cause massive bleeding or embolization. Consequently, it is better to cleanse the skin by painting than by scrubbing. The arms should be free-draped. Instruments for vascular repairs and thoracotomy must be readily available.

AXIOM   With neck injuries one can never be certain when proximal control of a vessel in the chest may be required.

Incisions

MIDNECK EXPLORATIONS

A low standard "collar" incision 1-2 cm above the heads of the clavicles is used in patients whose preoperative evaluations suggest bilateral or anterior neck injuries, especially damage to the larynx or trachea. Improved access to more lateral and superior structures can be provided by designing a superiorly based "apron flap" either unilaterally or bilaterally. A higher horizontal incision (along a relaxed skin tension line), placed over the midportion of the thyroid cartilage, is used only when it is confirmed that the injuries are limited to the larynx.

UNILATERAL NECK EXPLORATIONS

The best incision for most unilateral neck explorations extends along the anterior border of the sternocleidomastoid muscle. With this incision, ready access can be obtained to the trachea, thyroid, larynx, and carotid artery on a plane anteromedial to the internal jugular vein. The carotid artery is exposed by division of the branches of the internal jugular as they cross the artery.

The esophagus is exposed by anteromedial retraction of the internal jugular vein, carotid artery, and vagus nerve (which lays posteriorly within the carotid sheath). Care must be taken to avoid damaging the sympathetic chain on the prevertebral muscles. When difficulty occurs in identifying the esophagus, a nasogastric tube can be passed as an aid to finding it by palpation. When a contralateral injury becomes suspected intraoperatively, exposure of the other side of the neck may be obtained by extending the lower end of this incision transversely into a "collar" incision, or by making a separate oblique incision.

AXIOM   Any vessel in the path of a knife, or near the path of a bullet, should be explored to definitely rule out a vascular lesion because false negative arteriograms have been reported.

Laryngeal Injuries

HEMATOMAS

Hematomas of the aryepiglottic folds, false cords, or true cords may occur with or without associated fractures. The hallmarks of this injury are pain and tenderness in the area of the larynx, often with some airway obstruction. Usually no hemoptysis or crepitation occurs over the laryngeal cartilages, and vocal cord mobility is usually normal unless associated fracture or dislocation of laryngeal cartilages is manifest.

In general, patients with laryngeal hematomas should receive broad-spectrum antibiotics. The role of steroids is controversial, but if they are given, the dose for an average-sized adult male should be the equivalent of 200 mg of hydrocortisone daily.[89] In patients with pure hematoma with no fracture, good return of laryngeal function can be anticipated.

LARYNGEAL FRACTURES AND DISLOCATIONS

Thyroid Cartilage

TYPES OF FRACTURES

Midline Thyroid Cartilage Fractures.   Midline fractures of the thyroid cartilage are generally due to a direct frontal blow to the larynx. These are the most common laryngeal fractures, occurring in more than 80% of patients explored for laryngeal trauma in some series.[90] In about 50% of these patients, the epiglottis is displaced posteriorly with herniation of the periepiglottic contents into the larynx.[89] The cords are separated in about 25% of patients. Unfortunately, associated mucosal tears, which should alert the surgeon to this injury, are recognized in only about half of the patients at the initial endoscopic examination.

Lateral Thyroid Cartilage Fractures.   Fractures of the lateral portions of the thyroid cartilage (Fig. 15-9) result from lateral forces applied against the thyroid cartilage.[89] These are usually associated with ipsilateral arytenoid dislocation with displacement of its attached vocal cord. This injury can usually be readily appreciated on indirect laryngoscopy. On occasion, because of the resilience of the thyroid cartilage, the fragments of thyroid cartilage may snap back to their normal position after the force of the trauma is expended without any evident fracture; however, the arytenoid cartilage and vocal cord may still be dislocated. Without careful endoscopy or CT, this injury may not be detected.

REPAIR.   Fine stainless-steel sutures (28 or 30G) can be used to maintain position of the large cartilage fragments following reduction.[89] If comminution of the fracture were present, placement of a soft conforming endolaryngeal stent, for at least four to six weeks, usually would be recommended.

When moderate-to-severe mucosal tears are present, and/or cartilage is exposed, a laryngofissure should be performed to expose and accurately reapproximate the injured respiratory epithelium, usually with 4-0 or 5-0 chromic suture. Any area in which mucosal continuity is not provided can be a site of excess granulation tissue formation and subsequent scar contracture. Cartilage exposure may also lead to chondritis with secondary resorption and laryngeal stenosis. When primary mucosal closure cannot be accomplished, local advancement-rotation flaps of mucosa may be utilized to form the laryngeal surface of the epiglottis, aryepiglottic folds, or pyriform fossa, depending on the location of injury.

Epiglottic Displacement

If the epiglottis is displaced posteriorly and cannot be returned to its normal position, it should be sutured anteriorly to the remnant of stable thyroid cartilage. In severe epiglottic injuries with associated thyroid cartilage fractures, Ogura and Biller found that a supraglottic laryngectomy often results in good return of voice and protective function of the larynx over time.[64] Laryngeal suspension with cricopharyngeal myotomy may be employed adjunctively to facilitate swallowing rehabilitation in these patients.

Arytenoid Dislocation

Unilateral (Fig. 15-10) or bilateral arytenoid dislocation can occur from a variety of trauma, including intubation. Diagnosis can sometimes be difficult to make except by CT or careful endoscopy while the patient is phonating. In some instances, arytenoid dislocation can be mistakenly diagnosed as recurrent laryngeal nerve paralysis.

Treatment of arytenoid subluxation or dislocation usually consists of surgical reduction by applying gentle pressure with a laryngeal spatula to reposition the arytenoid on the cricoid facet. Early reduction (within 24 hours) must be performed to be of benefit because the cricoarytenoid joint can become fibrosed and the vocal cord fixed in an unfavorable position quickly.[49] In patients with severe disruptive injuries or in those who cannot attain proper repositioning, submucosal resection of the arytenoid should be performed with meticulous mucosal reapproximation. In addition, the vocal process of the arytenoid should be preserved and fixed posteriorly to the midline of the cricoid lamina. When the mobility of the contralateral cord is intact, the protective and phonatory capabilities of the larynx should be adequate.

A more conservative therapy is prolonged tracheal intubation, following arytenoid reduction, in which the tube acts as an internal

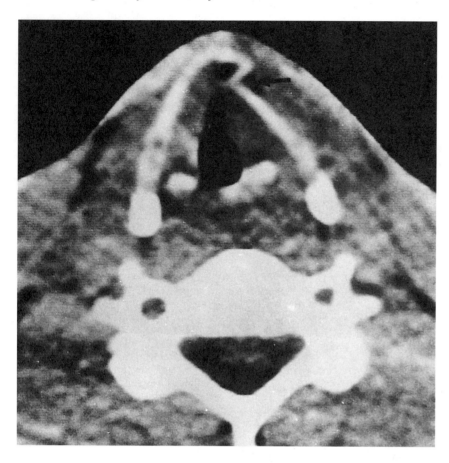

FIGURE 15-9 Axial CT scan demonstrating medial fracture displacement of the thyroid lamina with perilaryngeal soft-tissue swelling. (From: Jeffrey RB, Dillon WP. The larynx. Computed tomography of the head and neck. Modern Neuro Radiology Series, 1988; 12.17.)

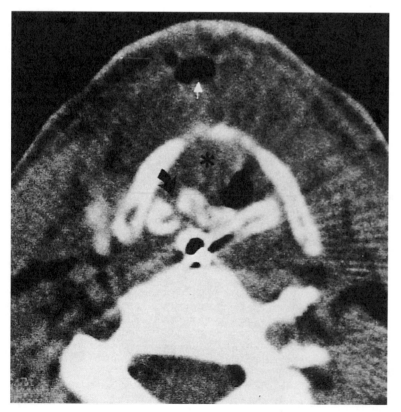

FIGURE 15-10 Axial CT scan demonstrating fracture dislocation of the right arytenoid (black arrow) with compromise of the endolaryngeal lumen secondary to hemorrhage and/or edema (asterisk) and displacement of the true vocal cord. (From Jeffrey RB, Dillon WP: The Larynx. Chap 12. IN Computed Tomography of the Head and Neck. Vol 3. Modern Neuro Radiology Series, 1988, pg 12.18.)

stent.[91] In this way, arytenoid movement is blocked, and healing of the dislocated joint is possible. However, the consequences of prolonged laryngeal intubation outweigh its possible benefits. Tracheotomy, by diverting air flow from the glottis, and allowing the laryngeal muscles to relax, is a more effective treatment for arytenoid dislocation. Even though a certain degree of arytenoid dislocation may persist, symptoms often improve sufficiently to permit later decannulation.[28]

Cricoid Cartilage Fractures

Some authors, such as Cicala et al., consider cricoid cartilage fractures in a category separate from other laryngeal injuries.[7] These injuries are especially treacherous because they may not be recognized until a sudden loss of the airway occurs at intubation.

Two of the three patients with blunt cricoid injuries in the series by Cicala et al. presented with no physical or radiographic findings and were undiagnosed prior to the induction of anesthesia for laparotomy.[7] The distal portion of the trachea was dislodged in two patients, one during attempted nasotracheal intubation, and the other during rapid sequence induction of anesthesia. Complete airway obstruction requiring emergent tracheotomy occurred. In one of these patients, tracheotomy was unsuccessful because of retraction of the distal trachea into the thorax and the patient died. Thus, cricoid cartilage injuries are likely to be associated with serious airway management problems, (Fig. 15-11) particularly laryngotracheal separation.[40]

Treatment of unstable or displaced cricoid cartilage fractures involves open exploration and repair following tracheotomy. Limited anterior arch fractures should be reduced and stabilized with fine stainless steel wires placed extraluminally. When the arch is too comminuted to lend itself to interfragmentary repair, but it still retains perichondrial attachments, manual reduction through the injury site or tracheotomy incision should be accomplished with internal stenting (finger cot or Montgomery T-tube) for 2-4 weeks. In patients with missing or divitalized fragments and loss of anterior subglottic support, a pedicled sternohyoid (with or without omohyoid muscle) interposition graft can be transferred to effect repair. With more extensive comminuted injuries involving anterior and lateral walls, local resection with direct thyrotracheal anastomosis is recommended.

Avulsion of the Larynx from the Trachea

Avulsion of the larynx from the trachea (cricotracheal separation) has been found in up to 18% of patients explored for laryngeal trauma.[90] It is usually due to high-speed MVAs but also occurs with "clothesline" injuries. In a series of 19 patients reported by Couraud in 1989, 11 injuries were caused by direct impact with a steering wheel, dashboard, or handle bar.[72] Eight injuries were due to strangulation with a seat belt (6 patients) or a rope (2 patients).

The anatomical lesions found by Couraud et al. in 19 patients with laryngotracheal disruption included[72]: (a) complete disruption in 14 patients, (b) recurrent laryngeal nerve paralysis in 18 patients (bilateral in 14 and unilateral in 4), (c) cricoid fracture in nine patients, and (d) mucosal retraction exposing the cricoid cartilage in all 19 patients. The mucosal injury, especially when not properly repaired, can contribute to airway insufficiency and will increase the incidence of infection and subsequent stenosis.

Because patients with cricotracheal separation are usually in severe respiratory distress on arrival, emergency attempts at endotracheal intubation are often made in the emergency department. However, such manipulation may convert a partial cricotracheal separation into one that is complete, and the distal trachea can be displaced deep into the mediastinum causing rapid asphyxia.

When a cricotracheal separation is suspected, and the patient can tolerate the trip to the operating room, intubation over a flexible bronchoscope has been advocated.[59,92] Conversely, many authors would argue that major tracheal lesions should be managed by immediate neck exploration with a tracheotomy performed through a vertical midline incision. When intubation over a bronchoscope is chosen, preparations must be made for potential emergency tracheotomy if rapid deterioration of the airway were to occur.[59,92] A coniotomy is

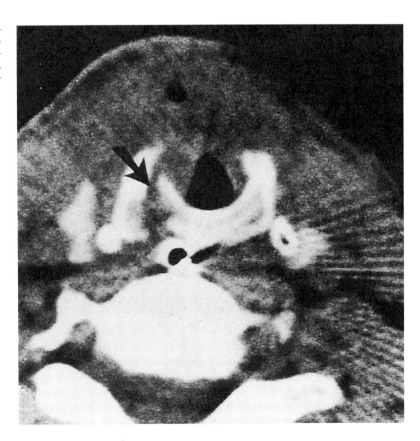

FIGURE 15-11 Axial CT scan showing a cricoid cartilage fracture with intrusion of the subglottic lumen by anterolateral displacement of the cricoid body. Extensive subcutaneous emphysema is also seen. (From: Jeffrey RB, Dillon WP. The larynx. Computed tomography of the head and neck. Modern Neuro Radiology Series, 1988; 12.18.)

contraindicated and typically inadequate to restore the airway because of the proximity of the injury, and it can make the damage much more severe.

After the airway is secured, one can then examine the cricoid and tracheal cartilages through the injury site to determine how best to handle the injury. In many patients with blunt laryngotracheal separation, the injured cricoid and uppermost tracheal cartilage must be partially or totally resected.[89] When the cricoid is severely damaged and must be removed, the trachea can be anastomosed directly to the thyroid cartilage. The disparity in size of the trachea and thyroid cartilage can make such a thyrotracheal anastomosis a delicate procedure. With such injuries, Couraud et al. preferred to perform a horizontal resection of the damaged lower portion of the cricoid cartilage so that an intact mucosal covering over the remaining cricoid segment could be retained.[72] In Alonso's experience many patients with laryngotracheal disruption have associated telescoping of the posterior cricoid mucosa into the trachea leaving exposed cartilage. Failure to recognize this injury can result in delayed subglottic stenosis. With these repairs, it is recommended that a stent be left in place for approximately six weeks to prevent stenosis at the anastomotic site.

Partial cricotracheal disruptions can usually be repaired directly, and smaller lesions may be sealed with laser photocoagulation.[105] If a primary repair cannot be performed, the distal trachea should be sutured to the skin as a low tracheostomy to provide an airway.[45]

Complete cricotracheal separations have a high incidence of recurrent laryngeal nerve injury with vocal cord paralysis, as well as associated esophageal injuries, particularly in the postcricoid region. Therefore, esophagoscopy is essential with these types of injuries. Failure to identify and effectively repair an esophageal disruption can result in mediastinitis, tracheoesophageal fistula, and dehiscence of the thyrotracheal repair. When esophageal injury is recognized, a meticulous inverting myomucosal closure is required. This should be followed by interposition of strap muscle, between the tracheal and esophageal repairs.

RECURRENT LARYNGEAL NERVE PARALYSIS

Owing to the position of the recurrent laryngeal nerves, entering the larynx close to the cricothyroid articulation posteriorly, vocal cord paralysis can occur either with the initial laryngotracheal trauma or during surgical attempts to treat the injuries.

The function of the vocal cords and, hence, the recurrent laryngeal nerves should be closely examined both pre- and postoperatively. With injuries to the cricoid cartilage or cervical trachea, direct neural trauma is more apt to occur (particularly with cricotracheal separation) and a high index of suspicion for this injury must exist.

When the nerves are transected, proper epineural repair should be attempted employing microsurgical technique. In most patients, however, restitution of muscle tone and some degree of bulk to the vocal fold is the best outcome possible. If the neural injury occurred proximal to the point of selective distribution into adductor and abductor muscle fibers, synkinetic function following laryngeal renervation would be the anticipated result. Consequently, the long-term functional results have been poor.[39] Most surgeons prefer not to search for recurrent nerves during the initial procedure because they are difficult to identify and there is a danger of damaging adjacent structures.[82]

PEDIATRIC LARYNGEAL INJURIES

PITFALL ⊘

If reconstruction of laryngeal injuries in children is delayed, the resultant excessive scarring is apt to prevent normal growth of the larynx.

It is particularly important in children to recognize and treat laryngeal injuries promptly and accurately.[89] Delayed or inadequate repairs can result in excess scarring which can prevent normal growth of the larynx and cause severe distortion of the vocal cords and airway.

When it is impossible to perform an immediate laryngeal repair in a child, it is the recommendation of Holinger and Schild that any stenotic areas that develop later be treated by dilatation and conservative treatment.[93] Definitive repair should be delayed, if possible, until the conclusion of puberty. This gives the larynx an opportunity to achieve maximal adult growth and maturity. Beyond puberty the treatment is the same as in adults.

Tracheal Injuries

Open tracheal injuries caused by penetrating trauma can often be managed by direct intubation through the wound to establish an airway. However, the dissection is greatly facilitated by the placement of an endotracheal tube guided by flexible bronchoscopy prior to exploration.

Most cervical tracheal injuries can be adequately treated through a neck incision. In a review of 17 patients with penetrating injuries of the trachea by Sulek et al. only one patient required thoracotomy.[94] If the tracheal injury is small, it can be repaired without a tracheotomy. If the injury is larger and involves the first portion of the trachea, a tracheotomy should be placed through the site of the injury.

Tracheal fracture sites from blunt trauma should generally be debrided and an end-to-end primary anastomosis performed. Because the blood supply enters laterally, dissection and mobilization of the trachea should be restricted to the anterior and posterior walls.[95]

When more than 3 cm of trachea needs to be resected, the tension on the suture line often exceeds 1000g and is associated with an unacceptable incidence of short- and long-term sequelae. In these patients, several options can minimize closing tension and permit an end-to-end anastomosis.

Mobilization of the cervical trachea typically provides 1-2 cm of added length. A laryngeal release, performed by sectioning the suprahyoid or infrahyoid muscle attachments, can provide 2.5-5 cm of length.[96,97] The suprahyoid release is generally preferred because this causes fewer problems with dysphagia.[96] Incising the annular ligaments between the tracheal rings may add an additional 1.5 cm.[98] A right thoracotomy can also be performed to divide the inferior pulmonary ligament and mobilize the thoracic trachea and the hilum of the right lung. This may provide another 5.0 cm of tracheal length[99,100]; however, 7 cm of tracheal loss (about half the tracheal length) is the upper limit of resection that is still compatible with primary closure utilizing release procedures.

During repair, the mucosa and tracheal walls are approximated with absorbable synthetic (Dexon or Vicryl) or minimally reactive (Prolene) suture. The ideal submucosal (extraluminal) placement of these sutures is technically difficult, if not impossible, secondary to the tightly adherent relationship of the thin mucosal layer to the tracheal rings. This layer of sutures is usually sufficient to allow healing, but placing extraluminal, stainless steel or prolene sutures above and below the anastomosis to relieve tension on the suture line is usually recommended. Tension on the suture line is also reduced by keeping the neck in flexion for 5-10 days by means of a heavy silk suture between the skin over the sternum and the chin. Alternatively, a similar flexed positioning of the head can be maintained by utilizing a high back, internally padded, modified rigid cervical collar which has been cut low anteriorly.

A tracheotomy is usually not necessary following tracheal repairs unless the patient requires prolonged intubation for concomitant injuries.[75] Laryngeal fractures, recurrent nerve injuries, high spinal cord lesions, severe chest trauma, and closed-head injury are some of the other indications for tracheotomy. Drainage of the neck incision is usually not necessary unless heavy contamination has occurred, such as with delayed repair of esophageal injury.

Patients with cervical tracheal injuries often have severe postoperative morbidity. Many patients develop some subglottic or tracheal stenosis due to excess granulation tissue or scar contracture. These patients should be followed closely for months or years to diagnose and treat such stenoses before critical narrowing (> 50% of cross-sectional area) occurs.

Because the recurrent laryngeal nerves may also be damaged, subsequent voice and airway problems can also result. This is an additional reason for frequent bronchoscopic and CT scan follow-ups for years.

PROBLEMS DUE TO PROLONGED INTUBATION

Endotracheal Tubes

> **AXIOM** Although endotracheal tubes may be lifesaving, their prolonged use may damage the larynx and trachea, especially if a high-pressure balloon cuff is used.

Even if the initial intubation were completely atraumatic, prolonged endotracheal intubation, especially with an over-inflated, high-pressure (low compliance) balloon, could cause severe mucosal and cartilaginous changes with eventual stricture formation in the larynx and trachea. This is especially apt to occur in the trachea when the tube has a high-pressure balloon cuff or is inflated excessively in attempts to completely seal the airway for more effective ventilation of noncompliant lungs with a respirator.

The newer endotracheal tubes, with "soft" compliant balloon cuffs, are much less likely to damage the trachea, especially when they are not completely inflated and a small amount of air is allowed to escape during expiration. However, the balloon pressure should be monitored and kept below 20-25 cm H_2O.

In his classic study, Bryce showed that mucosal changes may develop in the trachea within three hours after insertion of an endotracheal tube and inflation of the balloon to excessive pressure.[100] With more prolonged intubation, superficial ulcerations extend into the underlying cartilage producing perichondritis and subsequent chondromalacia. After removal of the endotracheal tube, the fibrosis and scar formation can cause progressive narrowing of the trachea with eventual stricture formation or tracheomalacia. Many surgeons perform a tracheotomy when endotracheal intubation is required for more than 7-10 days. The advantages of an early tracheotomy over prolonged endotracheal intubation are being increasingly recognized.[102]

TRACHEOTOMY TUBES

Prolonged use of a tracheotomy tube can produce many of the same tracheal problems as prolonged endotracheal intubation. Perhaps the most frequent and serious complication is tracheal stricture. The most frequent site of stricture formation in the trachea following a tracheotomy is the tracheotomy stoma itself. The next most frequent site is the junction of the superior and middle third of the trachea where the inflated cuff can cause pressure necrosis of the tracheal cartilages. The combined incidence of stenosis at these two sites in patients requiring ventilator support for more than two weeks had been reported in the past, with less compliant endotracheal balloons, to be as high as 20%.[103] With more compliant balloons, the incidence of tracheal stricture has been greatly reduced.

Strictures at the tracheotomy stoma can often be treated adequately by dilations or relatively simple plastic surgical procedures. Strictures at the cuff site, however, are often circumferential. They usually respond poorly to dilations and frequently require segmental resection of the involved area and reanastomosis. As an alternative, prolonged intraluminal stenting (Montgomery T-tube) following open exploration and resection of the stenotic tissue may be utilized.

Associated Injuries

Vascular and digestive tract injuries are frequently associated with penetrating laryngotracheal trauma. Vascular injuries, especially to the larger arteries, are usually obvious, but may occasionally not be found unless sought for carefully.

Although endoscopy and/or contrast swallows have been recommended for diagnosis of pharyngeal or esophageal injuries after neck trauma, there is no substitute for a thorough examination of the neck at the time of surgery. False-negative flexible endoscopy and/or

esophagraphy may occur in 25-50% of patients with pharyngeal or esophageal trauma.

When both the airway and esophagus or pharynx require repair, it has been recommended that a viable muscle patch be used to buttress the esophageal and/or tracheal repair to help prevent fistula formation.

OUTCOME

Mortality

Mortality rates after airway injury in the neck have been reported as high as 15%[6] and 30%.[4] Death is usually caused by massive aspiration of blood, associated cervicothoracic vascular injuries, irreversible shock, and injuries to distant organs. Unsuccessful intubation attempts during emergency management may also result in airway obstruction and death.[15]

Up to one-third of all patients who survive an airway injury and reach a hospital alive suffer delays in treatment before the diagnosis is made.[3,6] Preventable deaths occur in up to 10% of patients with airway trauma, and these are most likely to occur in patients whose airway injuries are undiagnosed.

The recent report by Cicala et al. on deaths due to laryngotracheal trauma had more detail than many other series.[7] They reported a mortality rate of 24% (11 of 46) for patients admitted with upper airway injuries. When one excluded the patients arriving in cardiac arrest, the mortality rate was 17% (7 of 42). The mortality rate was 22% (2 of 9) for stab wounds, 25% (5 of 20) for blunt trauma victims, and 35% (6 of 17) for gunshot wounds. When looking at the location of the injuries, the mortality rate was 8% (1 of 13) for laryngeal injuries, 25% (6 of 24) for tracheal injuries, and 44% (4 of 9) for combined or cricoid injuries. The causes of death were exsanguination in five (45%), airway problems in four (36%), brain injury in one (9%), and sepsis in one (9%).

Morbidity

> **AXIOM** Most surviving patients with severe laryngotracheal injuries will have some permanent voice and airway impairment, and/or pulmonary aspiration.

These complications are largely due to scar contracture and/or excess granulation tissue formation.[45,47,88] Granulation tissue, subsequent scar formation, and voice and airway problems are more frequent after blunt than penetrating neck trauma, probably because the injury is usually more extensive.[48,88] Results of surgical repair from many series are inconsistent and often disappointing. Although severity of injury is an important determinant of long-term sequelae,[86] delay of treatment for more than 24 hours appears to be the main contributor to the development of late complications.[18,35,40,45,47,86,88] Leopold,[88] Reece and Shatney,[104] and Bent and Porvbsky[105] noted that the quality of the voice and airway are directly related to the timing of the repair. Delay in airway repair is particularly apt to be associated with an increased frequency of late airway stenosis.[104] It has been reported that all patients who have undiagnosed airway injuries for more than 24-48 hours will eventually develop strictures.[106]

> **AXIOM** Early diagnosis and treatment of laryngotracheal injuries, based largely on a high index of suspicion, offers the best chance of survival and reduced complications.

Additional factors contributing to poor results include multisystem injuries, prolonged systemic hypotension, and laryngeal rather than tracheal injury.[2,8,36,86] Although vocal cord mobility after injury suggests that the airway and the voice will be preserved,[88] the airway can often eventually be restored with a functional voice even when the cords are paralyzed.[45] However, this is a potentially dangerous situation because even a mild upper respiratory tract infection may cause acute airway embarrassment.

Infection at the surgical site is an important cause of long-term morbidity. Early drainage, interposition of muscle flaps between the trachea and an injured esophagus, and broad-spectrum antibiotics may reduce the frequency of this complication.[45,86]

Many patients suffering from blunt laryngotracheal trauma require multiple operative procedures for complications of the injury or surgery itself.[8] In this setting, anesthesia is administered most frequently for bronchoscopy, laryngoscopy for assessment of repair and stent removal, endoscopic laser procedures to remove adhesions or a nonfunctioning arytenoid cartilage, repositioning of arytenoids, Teflon or Gelfoam paste injection of the vocal cords, nerve-muscle pedicle grafts to improve vocal cord function, thyroplasty, or laryngeal renervation procedures.[1,8,36,45,106-109]

UNRESOLVED QUESTIONS

Alfille and Hurford outlined many of the continuing questions concerning laryngotracheal injury, including[83]: (a) Should all patients with even minimal evidence of neck trauma undergo CT and/or bronchoscopy to exclude occult laryngotracheal injuries? (b) Which associated injuries or signs should make one suspect an occult airway injury? (c) How frequently do late complications occur with unrecognized laryngotracheal injuries? and (d) Should all patients with severe laryngotracheal injuries receive an immediate tracheotomy, or are bronchoscopic intubations preferable for some or all of these patients?[83]

SUMMARY

Laryngotracheal injuries are uncommon but must be suspected in all patients who have even minimal evidence of neck trauma. Such injuries can rapidly cause death either at the scene of the accident or in the hospital, especially when intubation or endoscopic examination of the digestive tract is attempted by an unsuspecting emergency physician, anesthesiologist, or surgeon.

With the more severe injuries, the airway should be secured with intubation over a flexible endoscope, or a tracheotomy preferably performed under local anesthesia and in the operating room. Early definitive diagnosis and management can reduce the incidence of complications, but some residual voice and/or airway problems can be expected in most patients with severe injuries.

Prolonged follow-up with endoscopy and/or CT is recommended to detect late stenoses before they become critical.

⊘ FREQUENT ERRORS

In the Management of Laryngotracheal Trauma

1. *Not suspecting blunt laryngotracheal injury in a patient with severe trauma to the head, posterior neck, or upper chest.*
2. *Not suspecting a laryngeal injury because the voice seems normal.*
3. *Not realizing that a little inspiratory stridor actually means a subtotal upper airway obstruction.*
4. *Assuming that an airway problem in an unconscious patient is only due to prolapse of the tongue.*
5. *Inserting an endotracheal tube with a little more force than usual if it is through the cords but does not seem to want to advance.*
6. *Failure to immediately protect the lower airway when bleeding occurs in the upper airway.*
7. *Not pursuing the cause of deep air in the neck after trauma.*
8. *Relying on a negative Gastrografin swallow and/or flexible endoscopy to definitely rule out an esophageal or laryngotracheal injury.*
9. *Using muscle relaxants in a patient with possible cricotracheal separation.*

10. *Attempting to perform an emergency tracheotomy on an uncooperative patient in the emergency department.*
11. *Failing to provide viable mucosal coverage over exposed portions of laryngeal cartilage.*
12. *Failing to separate tracheal and esophageal suture lines following transection injury.*
13. *Attempting blind endotracheal intubation in a patient with suspected laryngeal lacerations or fractures.*
14. *Not performing early surgical exploration of a badly injured larynx when medically feasible.*
15. *Attempting to reposition a completely avulsed or displaced arytenoid.*
16. *Failing to employ stenting when the laryngeal injury involves traumatic disruption of the anterior commissure.*
17. *Inadequately assessing the esophagus for associated injuries in patients with blunt or penetrating laryngotracheal trauma.*
18. *Assuming that vocal cord dysfunction following blunt laryngeal trauma is only the result of reactive edema or hematoma formation.*
19. *Adopting a false sense of security when a patient, who sustained blunt laryngeal trauma, has an adequate airway at initial examination.*

▼▼▼▼▼▼▼▼▼▼▼▼▼▼▼▼▼▼▼▼▼▼▼▼▼▼▼▼▼▼

SUMMARY POINTS

1. Blunt laryngotracheal injuries are rare, but they can be rapidly fatal.
2. A cricothyroidotomy (coniotomy) may be performed through the cricothyroid membrane to establish an emergency airway when endotracheal tube insertion is impossible and there is no suspicion of laryngeal or distal tracheal injury.
3. Laryngeal dysfunction can occur following endotracheal intubation and most often results from laryngeal edema, hemorrhage, or mucosal tears.
4. It can be difficult to differentiate between arytenoid dislocation and recurrent nerve injury, particularly after neck surgery.
5. Cricotracheal separation is often accompanied by avulsion of recurrent laryngeal nerves and esophageal injury.
6. Cervical spine injury is frequently associated with blunt laryngotracheal trauma and should be considered present until proved otherwise.
7. Airway problems in comatose patients with blunt head injury may be due to associated laryngotracheal trauma.
8. Associated chest injuries that impair ventilation may divert attention from less obvious laryngotracheal injuries.
9. Severe laryngeal damage may be associated with minimal initial symptoms or signs. Therefore, a high index of suspicion, partially based on the mechanism of injury, is needed.
10. When an endotracheal tube cannot be passed through the larynx of a trauma victim, one should assume that a laryngotracheal injury is present.
11. Attempts to intubate a patient with respiratory distress and unsuspected airway injury can easily result in complete obstruction of the airway and death.
12. The history and physical examination should make one suspect laryngeal injury, but CT is best for evaluating the cartilages, and laryngoscopy for evaluating the mucosa and cord motion.
13. Dysphonia is the most common presenting symptom of laryngeal injury.
14. Presence of a normal voice on admission does not eliminate significant laryngeal injury.
15. A severe sore throat not improving 48 hours after transient endotracheal intubation should be investigated for laryngeal injury.
16. A sucking neck wound and progressive hypoxemia is virtually pathognomonic for a major laryngotracheal laceration.
17. Continued significant hemoptysis suggests a combined airway and major vascular injury.

18. A high index of suspicion is needed to diagnose most blunt laryngotracheal injuries.
19. The most frequent sign of blunt laryngotracheal trauma is subcutaneous emphysema.
20. The quality of the voice is often a poor indicator of the severity of the underlying laryngeal damage.
21. Absence of clinically apparent subcutaneous air does not eliminate an airway injury.
22. Difficulty breathing in the supine position may be a sign of upper airway injury.
23. Whenever intubating any patient with blunt trauma to the head or neck, one should be prepared to rapidly provide a surgical airway if needed.
24. When a nasogastric tube has been placed prior to the intubation attempt, this tube may act as a guide to finding an otherwise "lost" tracheal stump in the mediastinum during emergency exploration of the neck.
25. When a patient had an emergency intubation soon after arrival in the hospital, one must be alert to the possibility of an airway injury when extubating the patient.
26. Radiography of the chest, lateral cervical spine, and pelvis should be obtained on all patients with severe blunt trauma.
27. Free air in the deep (perivisceral) spaces of the neck is usually due to an injury to the aerodigestive tract.
28. When suspicious of a vascular injury in a stable patient with a penetrating wound of the neck, arteriography of the carotid and vertebral vessels should be obtained.
29. Injuries to the upper respiratory tract, especially by penetrating trauma, are frequently associated with injuries to the pharynx or esophagus.
30. A normal Gastrografin swallow cannot eliminate the possibility of a pharyngoesophageal leak.
31. CT is the examination of choice for the diagnosis and localization of laryngeal cartilage injuries in otherwise stable patients.
32. With penetrating injuries, endoscopy and/or CT are needed to diagnose laryngotracheal injuries in $< 15\%$ of patients, but with blunt injury about half of the patients require these tests for diagnosis.
33. Endoscopic examination of a larynx with a suspected injury should be attempted in stable patients before attempting airway intervention.
34. If direct laryngoscopy is not performed within 2-4 hours of injury, the normal landmarks may be obscured by edema, and the laryngeal injury may be aggravated.
35. Flexible bronchoscopy is probably the best and safest technique for directly examining the luminal structures in the upper and lower airway.
36. Laryngeal trauma can cause bilateral vocal cord paralysis without any apparent anatomical evidence of external or internal damage.
37. While examining a larynx that may be injured, one must be prepared to handle sudden complete airway obstruction.
38. Early death after neck injury usually occurs by one of three mechanisms: airway compromise, exsanguination, or CNS injury.
39. The faster a patient with a narrow airway breathes, the greater the airway obstruction that is produced.
40. Muscle relaxants or sedatives in patients with complete cricotracheal separation can rapidly cause complete airway obstruction.
41. Patients with airway injuries and inability to tolerate the supine position need to have their airways secured as soon as possible.
42. Acute airway problems that may be due to trauma to the larynx or trachea should be handled in the operating room if possible.
43. Nasotracheal intubation should not be attempted in patients with suspected laryngeal or tracheal trauma.
44. Attempting to perform an emergency tracheotomy in the emergency department on an uncooperative patient is potentially disastrous.
45. Cricothyroidotomy can be dangerous in patients with possible laryngeal injuries.
46. Acute airway problems are best handled in the operating room with the most experienced anesthesiologist and surgeon present.

47. If an endotracheal tube is too large or is inserted too roughly, severe damage can occur, even in a normal larynx or trachea.
48. The anesthesiologist and surgeon should have an extremely high index of suspicion for cricoid injury in patients with blunt neck trauma.
49. Cervical spine injury should be eliminated before rigid endoscopy is performed.
50. All airway manipulations with a suspected laryngotracheal injury should be performed while the patient is conscious and breathing spontaneously.
51. The importance of oxygen administration during procedures to establish an airway cannot be overemphasized.
52. A tracheotomy, although often lifesaving, is not a simple, harmless procedure. If done poorly, it may cause death or severe respiratory problems.
53. After completion of the tracheotomy, it is important to auscultate the lungs and obtain a chest radiography because it is not unusual for a pneumothorax to develop during or after this procedure.
54. All laryngeal injuries are potentially dangerous and can suddenly occlude the upper airway.
55. Adequate topical anesthesia of the upper airway is essential before any airway manipulation is attempted.
56. If displaced laryngeal fractures are not reduced and stabilized within 7-10 days, the resultant scarring may make later correction extremely difficult and return of normal function unlikely.
57. With penetrating neck injuries, one can never be certain when proximal control of a vessel in the chest may be required.
58. Any vessel in the path of a knife or near the path of a bullet should be explored to definitely eliminate a vascular lesion because false-negative arteriograms have been reported.
59. When reconstruction of laryngeal injuries in children is delayed, the resultant excessive scarring is apt to prevent normal growth of the larynx.
60. Although endotracheal tubes may be lifesaving, their prolonged use may damage the larynx and trachea, especially when a high-pressure balloon cuff is used.
61. Most surviving patients with severe laryngotracheal injuries will have some permanent voice and airway impairment and/or recurrent pulmonary aspiration.
62. Early diagnosis and treatment of laryngotracheal injuries based largely on a high index of suspicion offers the best chance of survival and reduced complications.

▲▲▲▲▲▲▲▲▲▲▲▲▲▲▲▲▲▲▲▲▲▲▲▲▲▲▲▲▲▲▲▲▲

REFERENCES

1. Gussack GS, Jurkovich GJ, Luterman F, et al. Laryngotracheal trauma: a protocol approach to a rare injury. Laryngoscope 1986;96:660-665.
2. Angood PB, Attia EL, Brown RA, et al. Extrinsic civilian trauma to the larynx and the cervical trachea—important predictors of long-term morbidity. J Trauma 1986;26:869-873.
3. Cantrell RW. Laryngeal trauma reviewed (Commentary). Arch Otolaryngol 1983;109:112.
4. Mulder DS. Blunt neck injury. Hurst JM, ed. Common problems in trauma. Chicago: Year Book Medical Publishers, 1987; 135.
5. Schaefer SD, Close LG. Acute management of laryngeal trauma. Ann Otol Rhinol Laryngol 1989;98:98.
6. Kelly K, Webb WR, Moulder PV, et al. Management of airway trauma. I. Tracheobronchial injuries. Ann Thorac Surg 1985;40:551-555.
7. Cicala RS, Kudsk KA, Butta A, et al. Initial evaluation and management of upper airway injuries in trauma patients. J Clin Anesth 1991; 3:91.
8. Capan LM, Muller S, Turndorf H. Management of neck injuries. Capan LM, Miller S, Turndorf H, eds. Trauma: anesthesia and intensive care. Philadelphia: JB Lippincott, 1991; 409-446.
9. Asensio JA, Valenziano CP, Falcone RE, et al. Management of penetrating neck injuries—the controversy surrounding zone II injuries. Surg Clin North Am 1991;71:267-296.
10. Miller RH, Duplechain JK. Penetrating wounds of the neck. Otolaryngol Clin North Am 1991;24:25.

11. Trone TH, Schaefer SD, Carder HM. Blunt and penetrating laryngeal trauma: a 13 year review. Otolaryngol Head Neck Surg 1980;88: 257-261.

12. Kambic V, Radsel Z. Intubation lesions of the larynx. Br J Anaesth 1978;50:587-590.

13. Saletta JD, Lowe RJ, Lim LT, et al. Penetrating trauma of the neck. J Trauma 1976;16:579.

14. Roon AJ, Christensen N. Evaluation and treatment of penetrating cervical injuries. J Trauma 1979;19:391.

15. Stanley RB, Crockett DM, Persky M. Knife wounds into the airspaces of the laryngeal trapezium. J Trauma 1988;28:101.

16. Jeffrey RB, Dillon WP. The larynx. Newton TH, Hasso AN, Dillon WP, eds. Modern neuroradiology: computed tomography of the head and neck. New York: Raven Press, 1988; 12.1-12.19.

17. Harris HH, Ainsworth JZ. Immediate management of laryngeal and tracheal injuries. Laryngoscope 1965;75:1103-1115.

18. Black RJ. External laryngeal trauma. Med J Aust 1981;1:644.

19. Butler RM, Moser FH. The padded dash syndrome: blunt trauma to the larynx and trachea. Laryngoscope 1968;78:1172-1182.

20. Rogers LF. Injuries peculiar to traffic accidents: seat belt syndrome, laryngeal fracture, hangman's fracture. Texas Med 1974;70:77.

21. Seed RF. Traumatic injury to the larynx and trachea. Anaesthesia 1971; 26:55-65.

22. Guertler AT. Blunt laryngeal trauma associated with shoulder harness use. Ann Emerg Med 1988;17:838-839.

23. Fuhrman GM, Stieg FH III, Buerk CA. Blunt laryngeal trauma: classification and management protocol. J Trauma 1990;30:87-92.

24. Sofferman RA. Management of laryngotracheal trauma. Am J Surg 1981;141:412-417.

25. Peppard SB, Dickens JH. Laryngeal injury following short-term intubation. Ann Otol Rhinol Laryngol 1983;92:327-330.

26. Close LG, Merkel M, Watson B, Schaefer SD. Cricoarytenoid subluxation, computed tomography, and electromyography findings. Head Neck Surg 1987;9:341-348.

27. Stack BC, Ridley MB. Arytenoid subluxation from blunt laryngeal trauma. Am J Otolaryngol 1994;15:68-73.

28. Castella X, Gilabert J, Perez C. Arytenoid dislocation after tracheal intubation: an unusual cause of acute respiratory failure. Anesthesiology 1991;74:613.

29. Chatterji S, Gupta N, Mishra T. Valvular glottic obstruction following extubation. Anaesthesia 1984;39:246-247.

30. Dash HH, Gode GR. Blunt trauma to the cervical portion of the trachea. Br J Anaesth 1983;55:1271-1272.

31. Stanley RB. Value of computed tomography in management of laryngeal injury. J Trauma 1984;24:359-362.

32. Sacco JJ, Halliday DW. Submucosal epiglottic emphysema complicating bronchial rupture. Anesthesiology 1987;66:555.

33. Miles WK, Olson NR, Rodriguez A. Acute treatment of experimental laryngeal fractures. Ann Otol 1971;80:710-720.

34. Schaefer SD. The treatment of acute external laryngeal injuries: state of the art. Arch Otolaryngol Head Neck Surg 1991;117:35-39.

35. Cavo J, Leonard G, Tzadik A. Laryngeal trauma. Maull KI, Cleveland HC, Stauch GO, Wolfert CC, eds. Advances in trauma. Chicago: Year Book Medical Publishers, 1986; 157.

36. Potter CR, Sessions DG, Ogura JH. Blunt laryngotracheal trauma. Otolaryngology 1978;86:909-923.

37. Hermon A, Segal K, Har-El G, et al. Complete cricotracheal separation following blunt trauma to the neck. J Trauma 1987;27:1365.

38. Alonso WA, Pratt LL, Zollinger WK, Ogura JH. Complications of laryngotracheal disruption. Laryngoscope 1974;84:1276-1290.

39. Snow JB. Diagnosis and therapy for acute laryngeal and tracheal trauma. Otolaryngol Clin North Am 1984;17:101-106.

40. Lambert GE, McMurry GT. Laryngotracheal trauma: recognition and management. JACEP 1976;5:883-887.

41. Reddin A, Stuart ME, Diaconis JN. Rupture of the cervical esophagus and trachea associated with cervical spine fracture. J Trauma 1987; 27:564-566.

42. Allen SJ. Management of intracranial pressure after head injury. ASA Refresher Course Lectures 1987;15:1.

43. Flood LM, Astley B. Anaesthetic management of acute laryngeal injury. Br J Anaesth 1982;54:1339-1342.

44. Hartman PK, Mintz G, Verne D, et al. Diagnosis and primary management of laryngeal trauma. Oral Surg Oral Med Oral Pathol 1985;60:252-257.

45. Mathisen DJ, Grillo H. Laryngotracheal trauma. Ann Thorac Surg 1987;43:254-262.

46. Kirsh MM, Orringer MB, Behrendt DM, et al. Management of tracheobronchial disruption secondary to nonpenetrating trauma. Ann Thorac Surg 1976;22:93-101.

47. Camnitaz PS, Shepherd SM, Henderson RA. Acute blunt laryngeal and tracheal trauma. Am J Emerg Med 1987;5:157.

48. Le May SR. Penetrating wounds of the larynx and cervical trachea. Arch Otolaryngol 1971;94:558-565.

49. Quick CA, Merwin GE. Arytenoid dislocation. Arch Otolaryngol 1978;104:267-270.

50. Blanc VG, Tramblay NAG. The complications of endotracheal intubation with a review of the literature. Anesth Analg 1974;53:202-213.

51. Tobias ME, Sack AD, Carter G, et al. Cricotracheal separation in blunt neck injury—the sign of hyoid bone elevation. S Afr J Surg 1991;27:189.

52. Rollins RJ, Tocino I. Early radiographic signs of tracheal rupture. Am J Roentgenol 1987;148:695-698.

53. Spencer JA, Rogers CE, Westaby S. Clinico-radiological correlates in rupture of the major airways. Clin Radiol 1991;43:371.

54. Greene R, Stark P. Trauma of the larynx and trachea. Radiol Clin North Am 1978;16:309.

55. Mancuso AA, Hanafee WN. Computed tomography of the injured larynx. Radiology 1979;133:139-144.

56. Polansky A, Resnick D, Sofferman RA, et al. Hyoid bone elevation: a sign of tracheal transection. Radiology 1984;150:117.

57. Jones WS, Mavroudis C, Richardson JD, et al. Management of tracheobronchial disruption resulting from blunt trauma. Surgery 1984;5:319-322.

58. West JG, Eastman AB. Patterns of injury. Mattox KL, Moore EE, Feliciano DV, eds. Trauma. Norwalk: Appleton and Lange, 1988; 94-96.

59. Sankaran S, Walt AJ. Penetrating wounds of the neck: principles and some controversies. Surg Clin North Am 1977;57:139.

60. Richardson JD, Martin LF, Borzotta AP, et al. Unifying concepts in treatment of esophageal leaks. Am J Surg 1985;149:157-162.

61. Kelly JP, Webb WR, Moulder PV, et al. Management of airway trauma II: combined injuries of the trachea and esophagus. Ann Thorac Surg 1987;43:160.

62. Noyes LD, McSwain NE, Markowitz IP. Panendoscopy with arteriography versus mandatory exploration of penetrating wounds of the neck. Ann Surg 1986;204:21-31.

63. Weigelt JA, Thal ER, Snyder WH, et al. Diagnosis of penetrating cervical esophageal injuries. Am J Surg 1987;154:619.

64. Ogura JH, Biller HF. Reconstruction of the larynx following blunt trauma. Ann Otol 1971;80:492-506.

65. Dudley J, Mancuso A, Fonkalsrud E. Arytenoid dislocation and computed tomography. Arch Otolaryngol 1984;110:483-484.

66. Maceri DR, Mancuso AA, Rinaldo RC. Value of computed axial tomography in severe laryngeal injury. Arch Otolaryngol 1982;108:449-451.

67. Schaefer SD, Brown OE. Selective application of CT in the management of laryngeal trauma. Laryngoscope 1983;93:1473-1475.

68. Hoffman HT, Brunberg JA, Winter P, et al. Arytenoid subluxation: diagnosis and treatment. Ann Otol Rhinol Laryngol 1991;100:1.

69. Weddel G, Feinstein B, Pattle RE. The electrical activity of voluntary muscle in man under normal and pathological conditions. Brain 1944; 67:178-257.

70. Miller RH, Rosenfield DB. The role of electromyography in clinical laryngology. Otolaryngol Head Neck Surg 1984;92:287-291.

71. Symbas PN, Hatcher CR, Vlasis SE. Bullet wounds of the trachea. J Cardiovasc Surg 1982;83:235.

72. Couraud L, Velly JF, Martignel N'Daiye M. Post-traumatic disruption of the laryngotracheal junction. Eur J Cardio-thor Surg 1989;3:441.

73. Stevens MH, Stevens CN. Vocal cord paralysis. Ear Nose Throat J 1983; 62:519.

74. Dedo HH. The paralyzed larynx: an electromyographic study in dogs and humans. Laryngoscope 1970;80:1455-1517.

75. Namiroff PM, Katz AD. Extralaryngeal divisions of the recurrent laryngeal nerve. Surgical and clinical significance. Am J Surg 1982;144:466.

76. Gacek RR, Malmgren LT, Lyon MJ. Localization of adductor and abductor motor nerve fibers to the larynx. Ann Otol 1977;86:770-776.

77. Koufman JA. The otolaryngologic manifestations of gastroesophageal reflux disease (GERD): a clinical investigation. Laryngoscope 1991;101:1-78.

78. Goodie D, Paton P. Anesthetic management of blunt airway trauma. Anesth Intens Care 1991;19:271.

79. Mace SE. Blunt laryngotracheal trauma. Ann Emerg Med 1986;15:836.

80. Dash HH, Rode GR. Blunt trauma to the cervical portion of the trachea. A case report. Br J Anaesth 1983;55:1271.

81. Grewel H, Rao PM, Mukerji S, et al. Management of civilian penetrating laryngotracheal injury (Abstract). J Trauma 1994;36:153.
82. Soothill EF. Closed traumatic rupture of the cervical trachea. Thorax 1960;15:89.
83. Alfille PH, Hurford WE. Upper airway injuries (editorial). J Clin Anesth 1991;3:88.
84. Sellick BA. Cricoid pressure to control regurgitation of stomach contents during induction of anesthesia. Lancet 1961;2:404.
85. Walls RM. Airway management. Emerg Med Clin North Am 1993;11:53-60.
86. Schaefer SP. Primary management of laryngeal trauma. Ann Otol Rhinol Laryngol 1982;91:399.
87. Gussack AS, Jurkovich GJ. Treatment dilemmas in laryngotracheal trauma. J Trauma 1988;28:1439.
88. Leopold DA. Laryngeal trauma. Arch Otolaryngol 1983;109:106.
89. McKenna J, Jacob HJ. Trauma to the larynx. Walt AJ, Wilson RF, eds. Management of trauma: pitfalls and practice. Philadelphia: Lea & Febiger, 1975; 294.
90. Middleton P. Traumatic laryngeal stenosis. Ann Otol 1975;84:139.
91. Roberts D, McQuinn T, Beckerman RC. Neonatal arytenoid dislocation. Pediatrics 1988;81:580.
92. Minard G. Laryngotracheal transection. J Tenn Med Assoc 1990;83:402.
93. Holinger PH, Schild JA. Pharyngeal, laryngeal, and tracheal injuries in the pediatric age group. Ann Otol 1972;81:538.
94. Sulek M, Miller RH, Mattox KL. The management of gunshot and stab injuries of the trachea. Arch Otolaryngol 1983;109:56.
95. Gregor RT, Davidge-Pitts KJ. The management of laryngotracheal injury. S Afr J Surg 1984;22:79.
96. Montgomery WW. Suprahyoid release for tracheal anastomosis. Arch Otolaryngol 1974;99:255.
97. Dedo MM, Fishman NH. Laryngeal release and sleeve resection for tracheal stenosis. Ann Otol Rhinol Laryngol 1969;78:285.
98. Som ML. Reconstruction of the larynx and the trachea: report of a case of extensive cicatricial stenosis. J Mt Sinai Hosp 1951;17:1117.
99. Grillo HC. Circumferential resection and reconstruction of the mediastinal and cervical trachea. Ann Surg 1965;162:374.
100. Barclay RS, McSwan N, Welsh TM. Tracheal reconstruction without the use of grafts. Thorax 1957;12:177.
101. Bryce DP. The surgical management of laryngotracheal injury. J Laryngol Otol 1972;86:547-587.
102. Rodriguez JL, Steinberg SM, Luchetti FA, et al. Early tracheostomy for primary airway management in the surgical critical care setting. Surgery 1990;108:655-659.
103. Montgomery WW. The surgical management of supraglottic and subglottic stenosis. Ann Otol 1968;77:534.
104. Reece GP, Shatney CH. Blunt injuries of the cervical trachea: review of 51 patients. South Med J 1988;81:1542.
105. Bent JP, Porubsky ES. The management of blunt fractures of the thyroid cartilage. Otolaryngol Head Neck Surg 1994;110:195.
106. Dedo HH, Rowe LD. Laryngeal reconstruction in acute and chronic injuries. Otolaryngol Clin North Am 1983;16:373.
107. Sessions DG, Ogura JH, Heeneman H. Surgical management of bilateral vocal cord paralysis. Laryngoscope 1976;86:559.
108. Isshiki N, Morita H, Okamura H, Hiramota M. Thyroplasty as a new phonosurgical technique. Acta Otolaryngol (Stockh) 1974;78:451.
109. Crumley RL. Selective reinnervation of vocal cord abductors in unilateral vocal cord paralysis. Ann Otol 1984;93:351.

Chapter 16 Thoracic Trauma: Chest Wall and Lung

ROBERT F. WILSON, M.D.

ZWI STEIGER, M.D.

INCIDENCE

> **AXIOM** Chest injuries cause or contribute to 25-50% of the deaths due to trauma in the United States annually.

Chest injuries are directly responsible for over 25% of the trauma deaths that occur annually, and they contribute significantly to at least another 25% of these fatalities.[1] At Detroit Receiving Hospital from 1988 through 1994, 20% of deaths occurring in patients who arrived at the hospital alive were due to chest injuries; chest injuries also contributed to the deaths in another 15% (Table 16-1). Not only are thoracic injuries increasing in number, but more rapid transportation by trained ambulance personnel is bringing increasing numbers of critically injured patients who previously would have died before arriving at the hospital.

When treatment under such circumstances is to be successful, it must be applied vigorously and accurately according to procedures formulated and practiced prior to their actual need. Many patients with chest trauma can be saved by rapidly ensuring the adequacy of ventilation with an endotracheal tube, chest tubes, and/or rapid infusion of fluids. Only 5-15% of patients admitted with chest trauma require thoracotomy.[4]

INITIAL RESUSCITATION

Ventilatory Problems

As with all trauma victims, the initial step in resuscitation is to ensure the patency of the airway and adequacy of ventilation. The minute ventilation (V_E) should be at least 1.5-2.0 times normal and "normal" for average-sized adult males is about 6.0 L/min. If the V_E were < 9-12 L/min, one should rapidly and systematically examine the patient for the possible cause(s) and begin therapy immediately (Table 16-2).

INCIDENCE

Patients with chest trauma who develop acute, severe respiratory distress have high mortality rates. In one series, 11% of 1132 patients admitted with chest trauma were in acute respiratory distress and required endotracheal intubation almost immediately upon entrance to the emergency department.[2] Of these patients, 58% died.

> **AXIOM** The combination of shock and acute respiratory distress is often lethal.

In this same series, the mortality rate was 7% for those with an admission systolic BP < 80 mm Hg.[2] When shock was accompanied by acute respiratory distress, the mortality rate rose to 73%. No one past the age of 43 years survived with both shock and acute respiratory distress on admission. Acute respiratory distress or inadequate ventilation on arrival in the emergency department was more frequent in patients with blunt trauma (17%) than in those with penetrating injuries (8%). The most frequent injuries associated with respiratory distress were rib fractures (Table 16-3).

ETIOLOGY

In patients with blunt chest trauma, the most frequent factors associated with acute respiratory distress included shock, coma, multiple rib fractures, and hemopneumothorax. The severity of lung injuries has been quantified by the Organ Injury Scaling Committee of the American Association for the Surgery of Trauma[3] (Table 16-4).

DIAGNOSIS

Depending upon the amount of air or blood that leaks into the pleural space and the magnitude of the parenchymal injury, the patient with a penetrating lung wound may be relatively asymptomatic or suffer various degrees of respiratory or circulatory embarrassment. The main clinical manifestations of this type of wound are commonly pneumothorax or hemopneumothorax,[2] but occasionally hypoxia may be the primary manifestation. Hemoptysis usually accompanies missile wounds; when severe, it may be an indication for emergency thoracotomy to prevent continued flooding of dependent alveoli and possible air embolism.

Diagnosis of the cause of respiratory distress must be made promptly. If the patient were to make little or no effort to breathe, CNS dysfunction due to head trauma or drugs would be the most likely problem. If the patient were attempting to breathe but was moving little or no air, upper airway obstruction should be suspected.

If the patient were attempting to breathe and the upper airway appeared to be intact but the breath sounds were poor, thoracic problems, such as flail chest, hemopneumothorax, diaphragmatic injury, or parenchymal lung damage, should be considered. If an endotracheal tube were inserted and the breath sounds were poor on one side, one should check the positioning of the tip of the endotracheal tube.

TREATMENT

Airway Control

DISPLACING THE MANDIBLE FORWARD. When upper airway obstruction occurs, the mandible should be pulled or pushed forward while the neck is stabilized in the midline by another individual. The mouth and pharynx should then be aspirated with a suction catheter and examined digitally or endoscopically. An oral airway can then be inserted if the patient will tolerate it without gagging or vomiting.

ENDOTRACHEAL INTUBATION

Indications. With any airway or ventilatory problem in a severely injured patient, endotracheal intubation is usually preferable to mask ventilation or nasal oxygen administration because it: (a) allows better control of ventilation, (b) helps to protect against aspiration of gastric contents, and (c) provides a means for removal of tracheal secretions.

Technique. In someone without midfacial injury who is breathing spontaneously, the safest, most comfortable airway is a nasotracheal tube. When it is not possible to rapidly insert such a tube, an orotracheal tube should be inserted carefully while someone stabilizes the head in the midline. In some instances, a fiberoptic laryngoscope or bronchoscope can be used to visualize the glottis and then the endotracheal tube can then be threaded down over the scope.

TABLE 16-1 Etiology and Primary Organs Involved in 1000 Deaths at Detroit Receiving Hospital (1-1-88 → 8-15-94)

Body Region Injured	Type of Trauma				
	Blunt	GSW	Stab	Other	Total
Head	275	168	4	0	447
Neck	21	22	2	0	45
Chest	41	137	36	0	214
Abdomen	24	111	11	0	146
Extremities	36	8	2	0	46
Other (burns etc.)	-	-	-	102	102
Total	397	446	55	102	1000

Although many physicians prefer nasotracheal intubation when any suspicion of a cervical spine injury exists, some problems do occur with nasotracheal tubes. The nasotracheal tube usually has an inner diameter that is 1.0-1.5 mm smaller, and it is also at least 5 cm longer than an orotracheal tube; consequently, it is more difficult to aspirate pulmonary secretions and blood through it. It also occasionally causes significant nasal hemorrhage as it is inserted. Because the nasal mucosa is very sensitive, the nostril of a conscious patient should be anesthetized with a topical anesthetic spray. When time is available, packing the nose with gauze soaked in 4% cocaine provides even better anesthesia and also helps shrink the turbinates. Phenylephrine nasal drops can also be used to shrink the turbinates.

AXIOM Cardiac arrests in the emergency department frequently occur during or just after endotracheal intubation.

Complications

Although early intubation and positive-pressure ventilation of critically-injured patients with severe respiratory distress can be life-saving, the most frequent time for cardiac arrest of trauma patients in the ED is just after or during such intubations. Possible causes for cardiac arrest at that time include:

1. Inadequate preintubation oxygenation and ventilation
2. Unrecognized esophageal intubation
3. Intubation of the right (or left) mainstem bronchus
4. Excess ventilatory pressures, further reducing venous return
5. Development of a tension pneumothorax
6. Systemic air embolism

TABLE 16-2 Causes of Inadequate Ventilation After Chest Trauma

CNS dysfunction	Pleural collections
Due to trauma	Hemothorax
Due to drugs	Pneumothorax
Airway obstruction	Simple
Pharynx	Tension
Vomitus, foreign bodies	Diaphragmatic injuris
Relaxed tongue	Parenchymal dysfunction
Larynx and Trachea	Contusion
Foreign bodies	Aspiration
Direct trauma	Intrabronchial hemorrhage
Chest wall injury	Previous pulmonary disease
Pain from fracture	
Flail Chest	
Open (sucking) wounds	

TABLE 16-3 Injuries Associated with Acute Respiratory Distress After Chest Trauma

Trauma	Incidence (%)
Blunt	
Thoracic	95
Rib fracture	75
Hemothorax, pneumothorax	55
Lung contusion	39
Intracranial injury	39
Diaphragmatic injury	9
Spinal cord injury	4
Penetrating	
Intrathoracic	
Pulmonary damage with hemopneumothorax	55
Cardiac injury	29
Diaphragmatic injury	17
Chest wall defects	7

7. Vasovagal response (rare)
8. Development of severe alkalosis

Whenever possible, prior to attempts at endotracheal intubation, one should ventilate the patient for at least 6-8 breaths with a bag and mask and 100% oxygen. This will wash out at least 90% of the nitrogen present and can allow at least 2-3 minutes of apnea without great danger. Ideally, an attached pulse oximeter should also show 100% saturation for several breaths.

With emergency endotracheal intubations, it is easy to insert the tube into the esophagus without knowing it. Some ways to ensure that the endotracheal tube is in the trachea include: (a) visualizing the tube going between the vocal cords, (b) noting the compliance of the pilot balloon; the pressure in the pilot balloon is less while the cuff is being inflated if the tube is in the esophagus, (c) looking for breath condensation in the tube; this is not 100% reliable, but it is helpful, (d) looking and feeling for chest wall motion as the Ambu bag is squeezed, (e) noting the compliance of the ventilating bag; it is easier to ventilate the stomach than the chest, and (f) auscultating the lateral sides of the chest and epigastrium. When capnography is

TABLE 16-4 Lung Organ Injury Scale

Grade*	Injury Type	Injury Description†	AIS-90
I	Contusion	Unilateral, <1 lobe	3
II	Contusion	Unilateral, single lobe	3
	Laceration	Simple pneumothorax	3
III	Contusion	Unilateral, >1 lobe	3
	Laceration	Persistent (>72 hrs), airleak/distal airway	4
	Hematoma	Nonexpanding intraparenchymal	
IV	Laceration	Major (segmental or lobar) airway leak	4-5
	Hematoma	Expanding intraparenchymal	
	Vascular	Primary branch intrapulm. vessel destruction	3-5
V	Vascular	Hilar vessel disruption	4
VI	Vascular	Total, uncontained transsection of pulmonary hilum	4

*Advance one grade for bilateral injuries; hemothorax is graded according to the thoracic vascular OIS.
†Based on most accurate assessment at autopsy, operation, or radiologic study.
From: Moore EE, Malangoni MA, Cogbill TH, et al. Organ injury scaling IV: Thoracic vascular, lung, cardiac, and diaphragm. J Trauma 1994;36:299.

available, an exhaled $PCO_2 > 10\text{-}20$ mm Hg indicates that exhaled gases are coming back through the endotracheal tube.[4]

PITFALL ⊘

> *Assuming that the endotracheal tube is properly situated because some breath sounds can be heard bilaterally in the chest.*

If breath sounds are heard better in the epigastrium, you should assume that the endotracheal tube is in the esophagus, no matter how certain you are that the tube is in the trachea. When any question exists about the location of the endotracheal tube, it should be replaced after ensuring adequate tissue oxygenation using bag-mask ventilation with 100% oxygen. Many anesthesiologists will leave the misplaced tube in the esophagus as an anatomical guide while attempting to insert a new endotracheal tube.

Even if the endotracheal tube were correctly placed initially, it would be easy for it to move down into the right mainstem bronchus later, especially if the patient were small and uncooperative. Dronen et al. noted that up to 28% of patients who received cardiopulmonary resuscitation (CPR) had their endotracheal tubes in the right mainstem bronchus at the end of resuscitation.[5]

AXIOM When breath sounds are poor over the left hemithorax, one should check the position of the endotracheal tube before treating for a hemopneumothorax.

When the patient has poor venous return because of hypovolemia, excessive ventilatory pressures can further reduce venous return and cause cardiac arrest. Hypovolemic patients should probably be ventilated with only 8-10 ml/kg tidal volumes at 10-14 times a minute until venous return and BP are adequate. If a lung injury or subpleural blebs are present, bagging the patient vigorously could cause a tension pneumothorax to develop rapidly, further reducing venous return.

PITFALL ⊘

> *Excessive ventilator pressures after intubation can be rapidly fatal.*

Any patient with a lung injury, especially with hemoptysis, should be considered at risk for developing systemic air emboli.[6,7] During general anesthesia or assisted ventilation, the airway pressure should be maintained as low as possible to avoid this complication. Patients with intrabronchial bleeding are also at risk for flooding normal alveoli with blood and rapidly causing severe hypoxemia.

Vasovagal responses are rare in injured patients, but they can occur during insertion of endotracheal, nasogastric, or chest tubes. One should be alert for this problem developing during any invasive procedure when the patient has an inappropriately slow pulse rate.

Patients who have emergency intubation are usually hyperventilated aggressively, often driving the PCO_2 down to 20-30 mm Hg or lower. When plasma bicarbonate levels are normal (24 mEq/L), arterial PCO_2 of 20 mm Hg will increase the pH to 7.70. When the plasma bicarbonate level is 30 mEq/L or higher, as it can be in some patients with chronic obstructive pulmonary disease, the pH will increase even further to 7.80. A pH rise of 0.10 decreases ionized calcium levels about 4-8%. Thus, a sudden, severe alkalosis can reduce ionized calcium levels abruptly, and this, in turn, can produce serious arrhythmias.

SURGICAL AIRWAY

AXIOM One must be prepared to supply a surgical airway any time difficulty occurs in intubating a patient with acute respiratory distress.

If the patient were in severe respiratory distress and an endotracheal tube could not be inserted promptly, an emergency cricothyroidotomy (coniotomy) should be performed immediately. A cricothyroidotomy is performed much more rapidly than a tracheostomy, but will not correct a cricotracheal separation, which fortunately is extremely rare. Cricothyroidotomy is generally recognized as the airway of choice in adults in emergency situations when endotracheal intubation cannot be accomplished promptly.

In many adults, the largest tube that can be inserted via the cricothyroid membrane safely is only 6 mm in diameter. When the tube inserted is < 8 mm in diameter, it can easily be occluded by blood or secretions and should be changed to a tracheostomy in the operating room as soon as possible.

In children, the cricothyroid space is usually too small for an endotracheal tube; a 12-14 gauge "catheter-over a needle" through the cricothyroid membrane and attached to wall oxygen may be preferable as the initial effort to prevent severe hypoxemia. The tubing attached to the cricothyroid catheter should have a hole near the attachment, which can be occluded briefly 10-30 times a minute, to insufflate the lungs with oxygen. This will usually provide oxygenation for up to 20-30 minutes, but CO_2 retention can be a problem until the airway is properly intubated.

Relief of Hemopneumothorax

PITFALL ⊘

> *Waiting for chest radiography to confirm the presence of a tension pneumothorax before treating it.*

If a hemothorax or pneumothorax were suspected in a patient with acute severe respiratory distress, a "blind" chest tube (i.e., a chest tube inserted without waiting for a chest roentgenogram) should be inserted through the fourth or fifth intercostal space in the anterior axillary line on the affected side. Digital examination of the pleural cavity before the chest tube is inserted reduces the chances of inserting the chest tube either into lung parenchyma (if the lung were stuck to that area by adhesions) or through a high diaphragm. Even with these precautions, however, it is easy to inadvertently place the chest tube into lung parenchyma when any pleural adhesions are present.

AXIOM Blind chest tubes should be inserted high and only after finger exploration indicates that it is safe to insert the tube.

Once a properly functioning chest tube is in place, it should be connected to 20-30 cm H_2O suction. When a tension pneumothorax is present, a large needle can be inserted into the pleural cavity through the second intercostal space in the midclavicular line to produce temporary decompression while a chest tube is being inserted.

Ventilatory Support

AXIOM In patients with chest trauma, persistent impaired ventilation or persistent hypoxemia in spite of other efforts (i.e., an open airway, relief of chest wall pain, and drainage of any hemopneumothorax) is an indication for ventilatory support.

Severe respiratory distress associated with a flail chest is best treated by prompt endotracheal intubation and ventilatory support, particularly if the patient has associated injuries. Ventilatory assistance should also be strongly considered in the patient with a flail chest and marginal ventilation if the patient is in shock, has other multiple injuries, is comatose, requires multiple transfusions, is elderly, or has underlying pulmonary disease. Respiratory rate $> 30\text{-}35$/min, vital capacity $< 10\text{-}15$ ml/kg, negative inspiratory force $< 25\text{-}30$ cm H_2O, and increased ventilatory efforts should also be considered indications for early ventilatory support.

Pulse oximeter should be attached to all severely injured patients. Blood gases should also be obtained because pulse oximeter can overestimate arterial oxygen saturation by 3-5%. Arterial and central or mixed and venous samples should be drawn soon after admission and at frequent intervals thereafter. If the cardiac output is very low, arterial PCO_2 may be normal but the mixed venous PCO_2 can be quite high. Metabolic acidosis with an arterial $PCO_2 > 40$-45 mm Hg is evidence of a significant reduction in pulmonary function and indicates the need for ventilatory support.

AXIOM Serial arterial and mixed venous blood gas values are more informative than isolated levels.

When the arterial PO_2 is < 55 mm Hg while the patient is breathing room air, or < 80 mm Hg while breathing supplemental oxygen (equivalent to an FiO_2 of 0.4 or more), the patient should generally be given ventilatory support.

AXIOM Continuous pulse oximetry should be part of the initial evaluation in anyone with severe chest trauma.

Pulse oximetry allows one to rapidly determine the effect of ventilator or drug changes and can reduce the need for multiple blood gas determinations. In many instances, significant trends in the arterial PO_2 may not be apparent clinically until the process is so far advanced that treatment may be difficult. Consequently, more objective parameters, such as pulse oximetry and/or frequent blood gases, can be very helpful.

Shock

ETIOLOGY

Once adequate ventilation has been attained, efforts should be directed toward rapidly restoring tissue perfusion, particularly for respiratory distress. In the study by Wilson et al, the most frequent causes of shock in patients with blunt chest trauma have been pelvic or extremity fractures (59%), intraabdominal injuries (41%), and intrathoracic bleeding (26%)[2] (Table 16-5). In addition, 15% had myocardial contusion and 7% had spinal cord injuries.

In patients with penetrating chest trauma, the cause of shock was an intrathoracic injury in 74%[2] (Table 16-6). The most frequent intrathoracic injuries causing massive bleeding included: lung (36%), heart (25%), great vessels (14%), and intercostal

TABLE 16-5 Injuries Present in 27 Patients with Shock with Blunt Chest Trauma

Injury	Incidence	Mortality Rate
Flail Chest/Multiple Rib Fx.	77.8%	66.7%
Extremity Fx.	59.3%	50.0%
Cranial	48.1%	84.6%
Intra-abdominal	40.7%	54.5%
Hemothorax	29.6%	37.5%
Lung Contusion	25.9%	71.4%
Myocardial Contusion	14.8%	75.0%
Diaphragm	7.4%	50.0%
Paraplegia	7.4%	100.0%
Other	18.5%	80.0%
Totals	3.3/pt	59.3%

Wilson RF, Gibson DEB, Antonenko D. Shock and acute respiratory failure after chest trauma. J Trauma 1977;17:697.

TABLE 16-6 Injuries in 147 Patients with Shock after Penetrating Trauma

Injury	Incidence	Mortality Rate
Lung	35.6%	51.9%
Intra-abdominal	33.6%	51.0%
Heart	24.7%	36.1%
Hemothorax	14.4%	19.0%
Diaphragm	13.7%	40.0%
Chest Wall	10.3%	20.0%
Superficial Extensive Lacerations	6.8%	10.0%
Extremity Vessels	6.1%	11.1%
Paraplegia	4.8%	14.3%
Subclavian/Innominate	4.1%	33.3%
Pulmonary A or V	3.4%	80.0%
Aorta	3.4%	80.0%
SVC/IVC	2.7%	50.0%
Totals	1.3/pt.	32.8%

Wilson RF, Gibson DEB, Antonenko D. Shock and acute respiratory failure after chest trauma. J Trauma 1997;17:697.

or internal mammary arteries (10%). In addition, 40% of patients with penetrating chest trauma had extrathoracic injuries contributing to shock. These included intraabdominal bleeding (14%), bleeding from extremity injuries (12%), and spinal cord injuries (5%).[2]

TREATMENT

Fluid

AXIOM Failure to correct hypotension within 15-30 minutes greatly increases mortality rate.

In previously healthy patients who require massive blood transfusions (10 or more units in 24 hours) but have hypotension for < 30 minutes, the mortality rate averages 9-10%.[8,9] If hypotension were more prolonged in young, healthy individuals, the mortality rate rises to about 50%. If massively transfused patients were to have preexisting disease, were over 65 years of age, or were to have shock for > 30 minutes, the mortality rate exceeds 90%. About two-thirds to three-fourths of these deaths occur within 48 hours and are due primarily to hemorrhagic shock. Most of the remaining later deaths are due to sepsis or its complications.

When intravenous lines are inserted, a peripheral site is preferred. When peripheral sites are unavailable and/or monitoring of the CVP or PAWP is required a central line should be inserted, usually via a subclavian vein. The catheter is inserted on the side of the injury so that there is no opportunity for both lungs to be injured. If one lung were injured and the other lung collapsed by insertion of a central line on the other side, the impaired function of both lungs could be rapidly fatal. Some believe that one should use internal jugular veins for central lines because attempts at insertion of internal jugular veins are less apt to cause pneumothorax.

Rarely, the pleural cavity is so full of blood that a misplaced needle enters the pleural cavity and then blood is aspirated from the hemothorax making one believe that the needle, and subsequently the catheter, is in a vein. Obviously, fluid administered through such a line only makes the hemothorax worse and does not improve the patient's vital signs.

PITFALL ⊘

One should not attempt to insert a catheter into a subclavian vein on the side opposite an injured lung because injuring both lungs can be rapidly fatal.

Emergency Thoracotomy

A large hemothorax or pneumothorax can seriously interfere with ventilation and venous return, and, consequently, it should generally be evacuated as rapidly as possible. However, if blood is pouring out rapidly through the chest tube, vital signs should be followed closely. If vital signs are improving, as the hemothorax is drained and more intravenous fluids are given, blood should continue to be evacuated. However, when vital signs deteriorate, the patient may be exsanguinating into the chest as the tamponading effect of the hemothorax is removed. In these unusual circumstances, the chest tube should be clamped and the patient taken directly to the operating room for emergency thoracotomy.

DIAGNOSIS

Symptoms of Lung and/or Chest Wall Injury

The most frequent symptoms of thoracic trauma are chest pain and shortness of breath. The pain is usually well localized to the involved area of the chest wall, but not infrequently it is referred to the abdomen, neck, shoulders, or arms. Dyspnea and tachypnea are important symptoms of lung and chest-wall damage, but they are nonspecific and can also be caused by anxiety or pain from other injuries.

Physical Examination

PITFALL ⊘

Excessive reliance on chest radiography may lead to delay in performing lifesaving procedures.

Careful physical examination of patients with chest trauma can be extremely important and may provide valuable information to help confirm or eliminate equivocal findings on radiography. Tension pneumothorax should be diagnosed and treated before chest radiography is performed.

INSPECTION

Chest Wall

In some patients, a chest wall contusion may be the only external evidence of severe thoracic trauma. The paradoxical motion of a flail chest may be minimal when the patient is first examined, especially when it involves the lateral or posterior thorax.

PITFALL ⊘

Without careful inspection of the chest wall, one can easily overlook contusions, flail chest, and open or "sucking" chest wounds.

Although external bleeding is easily recognized, it may be difficult to determine if the actual source were intrathoracic or the chest wall itself. Most chest wounds that communicate with the pleural cavity are readily apparent because of the noise made as air passes through the tissue of the chest wall; some of these wounds, however, are open only intermittently and may be discovered only in retrospect.

Neck

Distended neck veins, especially when the patient is sitting upright, may indicate the presence of pericardial tamponade, tension pneumothorax, or cardiac failure. The distended neck veins, how-

ever, may not appear until hypovolemia has been at least partially corrected. When the face and neck are cyanotic and swollen, injury to the superior mediastinum with occlusion or compression of the superior vena cava should be suspected. Severe subcutaneous emphysema from a torn bronchus or laceration of the lung may cause much swelling of the neck and face, quickly obliterating landmarks and, in some instances, shutting the eyelids.

Abdomen

A scaphoid abdomen may indicate a diaphragmatic injury with herniation of abdominal contents into the chest. Excessive abdominal movement with breathing may indicate chest-wall damage that may not otherwise be apparent. A rocking-horse type of ventilation may indicate a high spinal cord injury with paralysis of intercostal muscles.

PALPATION

Palpation should begin with determining whether the trachea is in its normal position, which is in the midline or slightly to the right. Palpation of the chest wall may reveal areas of severe, localized tenderness or crepitation from fractured ribs or subcutaneous emphysema. If radiography were not to reveal any fractures, the areas of severe pain and localized tenderness over ribs would be referred to as "clinical" rib fractures.

AXIOM Well-localized and consistent tenderness over ribs after chest trauma should be considered due to rib fractures, even when initial chest radiography or rib detail films appear to be normal.

Many rib fractures (up to 50%) may not show on initial chest radiography.[10-12] These fractures, however, can often be seen 2-4 weeks later when callus or a lytic line at the fracture site develops. Motion of a portion of the sternum or severe localized tenderness may be the only objective evidence of a fractured sternum. When a patient is coughing or straining, the physician can sometimes palpate abnormal motion of an unstable portion of the chest wall better than can be seen. Sternal fractures can easily be missed on routine chest radiography, and a special lateral view is often required.

PERCUSSION

Percussion of the chest wall sometimes can be of great help in differentiating between hemothorax and pneumothorax. Dullness to percussion over one side of the chest following trauma may be the first evidence of hemothorax; hyperresonance, conversely, often indicates the presence of pneumothorax.

AXIOM Moderate hemothorax can easily be missed on chest radiographys taken while the patient is lying flat.

When the pericardial cavity is greatly distended by an effusion or tamponade, the area of cardiac dullness may extend beyond the midclavicular line on the left or the sternal border on the right. Pericardial dullness extending more than an inch past the point of maximal cardiac impulse may indicate the presence of pericardial tamponade or a large effusion.

AUSCULTATION

Whenever possible, the chest should be auscultated systematically and thoroughly, anteriorly, laterally, and posteriorly at both the bases and apices. When breath sounds are equal bilaterally at the bases and apices, the major bronchi are probably intact. Decreased breath sounds on one side usually indicate the presence of hemothorax or pneumothorax, but this may also occur when the endotracheal tube is in too far and is only ventilating one lung.

AXIOM Before inserting a chest tube into a patient with acute respiratory distress and decreased breath sounds on one side, one should check the position of the endotracheal tube.

Occasionally decreased breath sounds on one side are due to a foreign body or ruptured bronchus. The presence of bowel sounds high in the chest may be the first indication of a diaphragmatic injury.

INJURY TO THE CHEST WALL

Soft-tissue Injuries

BLEEDING

AXIOM Probing of chest wounds can be dangerous.

Probing of penetrating chest wounds to determine their depth or direction can be dangerous because it can damage underlying structures and/or cause severe, recurrent bleeding, pneumothorax, or a sucking chest wound. Bleeding from larger muscles can be profuse and is best controlled initially by local pressure. Later, one can explore the wound in the operating room and use ligatures to control bleeding from the bottom of the wound up, and carefully close the wound.

OPEN (SUCKING) CHEST WOUNDS

AXIOM Occluding a sucking chest wound without almost simultaneously inserting a chest tube can rapidly cause a tension pneumothorax.

Small open chest wounds can act as one-way valves, allowing air to enter during inspiration, but none to leave during expiration, thereby causing increasing pneumothorax. This not only reduces tidal volume but can also interfere with venous return to the heart. With larger chest wall wounds, air may come into the pleural cavity through the wound rather than through the tracheobronchial tree.

AXIOM If an open chest wound were to exceed two-thirds of the cross-sectional area of the trachea, effective ventilation may cease.

Sucking wounds of the chest should be covered immediately by a sterile, airtight dressing, such as a petrolatum gauze, and a chest tube inserted at a separate site to relieve pneumothorax.

AXIOM Chest tubes should not be inserted through penetrating wounds because they are apt to follow the missile tract into the lung or diaphragm and damage those organs or restart massive bleeding.

TISSUE LOSS

Injuries caused by close-range shotgun blasts or high-powered rifles may destroy such large quantities of tissue that it may be impossible to close the chest wall in the usual manner. Occasionally, severe congestion or edema in an injured lung may preclude closure of the rib cage at the conclusion of thoracotomy[13]; however, it is important to provide some type of coverage for the lungs and heart, even with just a skin closure, and to close the diaphragm.

Large chest wall defects, after thorough debridement, can be closed with various types of muscle flaps.[14] When such flaps cannot be utilized, the defect may be temporarily closed with prosthetic material. The prosthetic material can then be covered with a skin or composite pedicle graft. With large, low chest wounds, the diaphragm may

be detached and reimplanted to the chest wall above the wound. The open subdiaphragmatic wound can then be packed with gauze. Thoracostomy tubes are inserted into the involved pleural cavities through separate incisions for pleural drainage.

SUBCUTANEOUS EMPHYSEMA

Subcutaneous emphysema usually develops because air from lung parenchyma or the tracheobronchial tree has gained access to the chest wall through an opening in the parietal pleura. The air may also reach the chest wall by dissecting back along the bronchi into the hilum and mediastinum and then into the extrapleural spaces. Subcutaneous emphysema may also be caused by injury to the pharynx, larynx, or esophagus.

Swelling from subcutaneous emphysema may occasionally reach massive proportions, causing the eyelids to swell shut and/or distending the scrotum to several times normal. Although the patient's appearance may be greatly distorted and severe discomfort may be experienced, subcutaneous emphysema by itself does not cause any significant ventilatory or hemodynamic problem unless there is an associated pneumothorax.

AXIOM Patients with subcutaneous emphysema after chest trauma should have a chest tube inserted before being placed on a ventilator.

It should be assumed that patients with subcutaneous emphysema have underlying pneumothorax, even when it is not visible on chest radiography. If the patient were to require general anesthetic or were to be placed on a ventilator, a chest tube should be inserted on the involved side(s), being careful not to damage lung which may be stuck to the chest wall. If subcutaneous emphysema were severe, major bronchial injury should be suspected and sought for by bronchoscopy.

When any respiratory difficulty appears to be due to mediastinal emphysema, tracheostomy—around which the skin and fascia are closed only loosely—may serve to maintain adequate ventilation and also allow a route for air to escape from the mediastinum and subcutaneous tissue. Rarely, a large pneumomediastinum may retard venous return to the heart, and a small (2-3 cm), transverse incision just above the suprasternal notch and then down along the anterior trachea can help relieve the mediastinal tension. Once the initiating cause is controlled, subcutaneous emphysema usually disappears gradually over a period of several days.

Bony Injuries

CLAVICULAR FRACTURES

Isolated clavicular fractures due to blunt trauma are usually relatively harmless. Occasionally, however, direct trauma produces sharp bone fragments that may injure the subclavian vein and produce a moderately large hematoma or venous thrombosis. Rarely, excess callus forming at the site of clavicular fracture may press against the subclavian artery or brachial plexus, producing a thoracic outlet syndrome.

SCAPULA FRACTURES

The scapula is usually strong and relatively well protected by thick muscles so that it generally takes great force to cause it to fracture. Consequently, when a fracture of the scapula occurs, one should look for underlying damage to ribs, lungs, and great vessels. However, it is easy to miss scapula fractures on chest radiography.

Harris and Harris reported that scapular fractures were missed on initial chest radiographs in 43% of 100 patients with major blunt thoracic trauma.[15] When examined in retrospect, 72% of the missed scapular fractures were visible on initial supine chest radiographs. The fracture lines were often obscured by rib or clavicular fractures, pulmonary contusion, pleural effusion, subcutaneous emphysema, film identification labels, or monitoring leads.

RIB FRACTURES

Simple Fractures

DIAGNOSIS

AXIOM Many clinically significant rib fractures cannot be visualized on initial radiography.

In some series, rib fractures are the most frequently "missed" fractures after trauma.[10] In a classic study by Nahum et al.,[11] embalmed and unembalmed cadavers were impacted by a 42.5-pound device at the midsternum at the level of the fourth-fifth interspace.[11] PA and right and left oblique radiographs were taken before and after impact. The ribs were then dissected to determine the number of fractures present. Of 98 rib fractures dissected from eight cadavers, radiographs were positive in only 47 (48%) and questionable fractures were seen on radiographs in 4 (4%) others. Hunt and Schwab also noted that 10-50% of incomplete or nondisplaced rib fractures may not be identified on initial chest radiographs.[12] Missing rib fractures radiologically is particularly apt to occur during the first few days after injury. Later, many of these fractures may be noted much more easily because of a lytic line or callus developing at the fracture site. Furthermore, injuries to the cartilaginous portions of the ribs may never be seen on radiography. Unfortunately, there is some reluctance for third-party payers to accept hospital admission for "clinical" rib fractures, even if there is point tenderness over specific ribs after trauma, and the patient cannot cough or take deep enough breaths to maintain adequate pulmonary toilet.

AXIOM The main purpose of chest radiography in patients with possible fractured ribs is to eliminate associated hemothorax, pneumothorax, lung contusion, and other organ injury.

The principal diagnostic goal in patients with possible rib fractures is the detection of significant complications, especially hemopneumothorax, pulmonary contusion, or major vascular injury. Of the readily available tests, a simple upright PA chest radiograph is most likely to detect associated injuries and/or complications. Expiratory, oblique, "coned-down" views, and tomography should probably not be done except for specific indications, such as trauma to ribs 1 or 2, or 9-12, or suspicion of multiple rib fractures, especially in the elderly.

When suspicion of pneumothorax exists and it is not seen on initial chest radiography, the patient should have inspiratory and expiratory PA radiography. Generally, pneumothorax is seen better on expiratory chest films because the pneumothorax space takes up a larger percentage of the involved hemithorax after the patient has exhaled. When the patient has experienced severe trauma, when rib fractures have sharp fragments, or when the patient has other injuries, serial chest roentgenography (every 6-12 hours for 24-48 hours) should be obtained. Delayed pneumothorax or hemothorax (due to trauma to the lung parenchyma or intercostal vessels by rib fragments) may occasionally develop more than 12-24 hours after initial injury.

TREATMENT

AXIOM Rib belts and taping of the chest wall to relieve pain from fractured ribs should be avoided except in young, previously healthy individuals.

The pain of rib fractures can greatly interfere with ventilation. Strapping the chest with adhesive tape or a rib belt to relieve the pain may be effective in young, athletic individuals with only a few rib fractures; however, in less vigorous patients, strapping may further reduce ventilation and cause progressive atel-

ectasis. If one were to use external support, rib belts would be more pleasant to use than adhesive tape. They also do not blister the skin and can be adjusted by the patient to provide optimal pain relief.

Probably the best analgesics for mild-to-moderate chest wall pain are Tylenol #3® every 4-6 hours or ibuprofen 600-800 mg every 6-8 hours as needed. Demerol® or morphine is apt to suppress the cough reflex too much.

Intercostal Nerve Blocks. The administration of an intercostal nerve block is a relatively good way to control severe chest wall pain because it can be accomplished without suppression of the patient's cough and without oversedation. This can usually be accomplished readily by the injection of 2-4 ml of a local long-acting anesthetic, such as 0.5-1% bupivacaine (Marcaine) mixed 2:1 with 1% lidocaine with epinephrine at each rib to be blocked. Because of the crossover of nerve fibers, it is necessary to not only infiltrate the intercostal nerves of the involved ribs but also two above and two below the fracture site(s).

The technique used to anesthetize each intercostal nerve is standard. After the skin is cleansed and the overlying skin is infiltrated over each rib where the nerves are to be blocked with a 26-gauge needle and 1% lidocaine, a 20- to 22-gauge needle is inserted through the skin wheal. The needle is inserted down to the underlying rib and gradually "walked" down the rib until the tip of the needle makes contact with the lower edge of the rib (Fig. 16-1). The needle is advanced under the lower rib edge for 3-4 mm. Its tip should now be located in the area of the neurovascular bundle. One then aspirates with the syringe to make certain that the tip of the needle is not in the pleural space or in a blood vessel, and 2-4 ml of the bupivacaine-lidocaine-epinephrine mixture is injected. This process is repeated for each rib to be blocked. Any portions of the chest wall that are still tender 5-10 minutes later should be directly infiltrated. Unless a functioning chest tube is already in place, chest roentgenography should be obtained after this procedure to ensure that a pneumothorax has not developed.

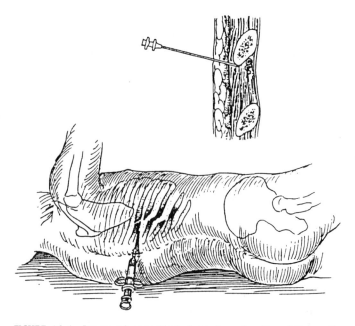

FIGURE 16-1 Intercostal nerve block. Inset shows insertion of the needle tip beneath a rib. Ideally, the needle should be angled up a little to get nearer to the intercostal nerve. (From: Kirsh MM, Sloan H. Blunt chest trauma general principles of management. Boston: Little, Brown and Company, 1977; 101.)

Epidural Analgesia

AXIOM Epidural analgesia is frequently the ideal method for controlling chest wall pain so that a patient can cough and breathe deeply.

When time is available, periodic injection of morphine-like agents into a spinal epidural catheter can relieve pain more effectively than intercostal blocks.[16] The catheter, however, must usually be inserted by an anesthesiologist, and the patient should have apnea monitoring in an ICU or stepdown-ICU environment because apnea or severe hypoventilation may develop up to 12-16 hours after the last dose. Another drawback with epidural analgesia is that it may cause some hypotension.

Intrapleural Analgesia. In 1986, Reiestad and Stromskag reported their results with injecting local anesthetics through an intrapleural catheter into the chest to control postoperative pain after mastectomy and various types of abdominal surgery.[17] In 1987, Rocco et al. from the same group reported significant pain relief and improved minute ventilation with this technique in patients with multiple rib fractures.[18]

The technique recently reported by Luchette et al. involves insertion of a 17-gauge Touhy needle in the eighth intercostal space 10 cm lateral to the posterior midline while the patient is in the lateral decubitus position.[19] Entry into the pleural space is noted by loss of 3 ml of air in a syringe attached to the Touhy needle. An epidural catheter is passed into the pleural cavity about 5 cm beyond the tip of the Touhy needle. Chest radiography is obtained to ascertain the position of the catheter, prior to infusing 20 ml of 0.5% bupivocaine. The patient is maintained in a 45° lateral position, with the injured side up, to facilitate a uniform spread of the local anesthetic into the paravertebral gutter. If the patient has a chest tube, it is removed from negative suction during positioning of the patient to avoid draining the local anesthetic. The dose of local anesthetic is repeated every 8 hours for 72 hours. When Luchette et al. compared the effectiveness of the intrapleural and epidural catheter techniques, epidural analgesic was significantly better.[19] It caused less pain at rest, reduced the use of parenteral narcotics, and provided better negative inspiratory pressure and tidal volumes.

Special Rib Fractures

FIRST AND SECOND RIB FRACTURES

AXIOM First rib fractures usually have a higher incidence of associated injuries and death than other rib fractures.

Except with direct trauma, such as with a hammer, it usually takes great force to fracture the first and second ribs. In a series reported by Wilson et al., 40% of patients with fractures of the first and second ribs had severe associated injuries, including myocardial contusion, bronchial tear, or major vascular injury.[20] Apparently, some first rib fractures may also be caused by sudden contraction of neck muscles or by stress because of repeated muscle pull.[21] With stress fractures, brachial plexus palsy may also occur.

First rib fractures are usually associated with higher mortality rates (15-36%) than any other rib fractures because of frequently severe associated injuries.[22] (Table 16-7). However, in the series by Richardson et al., 49 patients with second rib fractures had a higher mortality (27%) than did 71 patients with first rib fractures (15%).[23] Two-thirds of the deaths were due to head injury or rupture of major vessels.

LOWER RIB FRACTURES. When a patient with fractured ribs, especially ribs 9-11, becomes hypotensive and does not have a large hemothorax, tension pneumothorax or extremity fractures, intraabdominal bleeding must be suspected. In one series of 783 patients with rib

TABLE 16-7 Mortality with Fractures of Individual Ribs Detroit Receiving Hospital

Position of Rib Fracture	Number of Times Fractured	Number of Deaths	Mortality Rate (%)
1st	36	6	16.7%
2nd	116	13	11.2%
3rd	168	15	8.9%
4th	232	24	10.3%
5th	283	26	9.2%
6th	338	26	7.7%
7th	339	24	7.1%
8th	341	24	7.0%
9th	294	19	6.5%
10th	229	15	6.6%
11th	109	5	4.6%
12th	38	1	2.6%
Total # Fractures	2523	—	
Total # Patients	783	56	7.2%

Bassett JS, Gibson RD, Wilson RF. Blunt injuries to the chest. J Trauma 1968;8:418.

fractures from blunt chest trauma, 71% of patients admitted in shock had a ruptured intraabdominal viscus.[22]

In general, it is wise to hospitalize patients with chest trauma (with or without radiologic evidence of fractured ribs) for at least 24-48 hours when they cannot cough and clear their secretions adequately, especially the elderly or those with preexisting pulmonary disease. Admitting such patients also provides time to observe them for associated injuries that may not be apparent initially. Aspiration pneumonitis or fat embolism often does not become apparent clinically for 24-48 hours or longer. Some authors[24] feel that patients with fractures of three or more ribs should be transferred to a level I trauma center. In a Pennsylvania trauma study, 58% of the patients with chest trauma had rib fractures.[25] Of these, 91% had associated extrathoracic injuries and 14.7% died.

FLAIL CHEST

The term "flail chest" was probably derived from the instrument called a flail, which was used to thresh grain. As it was moved up and down or from side to side, use, the distal portion with grain stalks moved in the opposite direction from handle, just as the unstable chest wall segment moves in the opposite direction from the rest of the chest wall during inspiration and expiration.

Pathophysiology

Segmental fractures (i.e., fractures in two or more locations on the same rib) of three or more adjacent ribs anteriorly or laterally often result in an unstable chest wall (Fig. 16-2). This injury is characterized by a paradoxical inward movement of the involved portion of the chest wall during spontaneous inspiration and outward movement during expiration.

AXIOM Although the paradoxical motion of the chest wall in traumatic flail chest injuries can greatly increase the work of breathing, the main cause of hypoxemia is the underlying lung contusion.

In the past, it was believed that, with the paradoxical movement of the involved chest wall segment, a to-and-fro movement of air from one lung to the other (referred to as pendelluft by Brauer[26] in 1907) occurred without adequate movement of air through the tracheobronchial tree; however "pendelluft" does not generally occur with flail chest unless there is some airway obstruction. It is also now clear that the underlying pulmonary contusion is the main cause of the hypoxemia.[27]

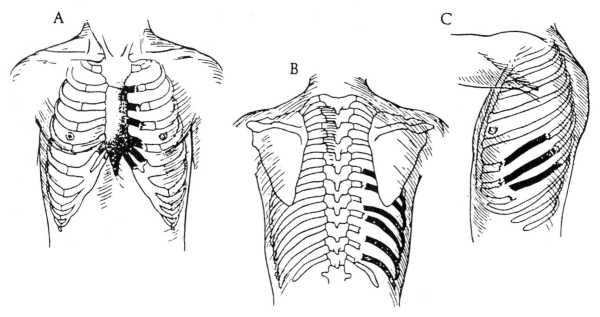

FIGURE 16-2 Flail chest may be caused by **(A).** anterior rib fractures, **(B).** posterior rib fractures, or **(C).** lateral rib fractures. (From: Kirsh MM, Sloan H. Blunt chest trauma general principles of management. Boston: Little, Brown and Company, 1977; 99.)

In the patient with an unstable chest wall segment, ventilatory impairment is associated with decreased vital capacity, functional residual capacity, total lung volume, and lung compliance; it also is associated with increased airway resistance and work of breathing. Patients with a flail chest are also unable to cough effectively, resulting in a tendency toward accumulation of tracheobronchial secretions, atelectasis, and pneumonitis. It is the associated contusion of the lung, however, that is the main cause of the alteration of the alveolar ventilation/perfusion ratio, shunting, and hypoxemia.[28]

Immediately after injury, little or no flail may be apparent. Later, as fluid moves into the injured lung and pulmonary compliance decreases, more transpleural pressure change is needed to inflate the lungs. The increasing pressure differential inside and outside the chest wall may then overcome the resistance of the muscles attached to the fractured ribs, thereby allowing the involved chest wall to develop increasing paradoxical motion. This may result in the diagnosis of flail chest being delayed for 24-48 hours or longer.[29]

In addition to increasing evidence of a flail chest with time, the patient may fatigue rapidly because of the decreased efficiency of ventilation and increasing muscle effort. Thus, a vicious cycle of decreasing efficiency of ventilation, increasing fatigue, and hypoxemia may develop. In many instances, the increasing fatigue with breathing results in a relatively sudden cessation of ventilatory efforts and respiratory arrest.[30]

AXIOM Prolonged increased work of breathing without relief is apt to result in respiratory arrest.

Treatment

INITIAL THERAPY. For many years, the treatment of flail chest had consisted of external stabilization with sandbagging, strapping, or application of towel clips. Subsequently, internal stabilization by mechanical ventilation was introduced and was considered the treatment of choice.[31] Later, selective management of flail chest without mechanical ventilation was advocated.[32]

Because the magnitude of the flail chest, the underlying pulmonary contusion, and the associated injuries varies from patient to patient, the treatment should be individualized but provided in an ICU or step-down ICU where the patient can be easily monitored. The treatment is directed toward the relief of pain and prevention of respiratory complications. As in the treatment of simple rib fractures, the pain of flail chest may be controlled with the administration of analgesics, intercostal blocks or epidural analgesia. Analgesics, however, particularly narcotics, should be administered judiciously to control the pain so as not to suppress the patient's cough. Other supportive measures, including deep breathing and incentive spirometry, should be administered to prevent atelectasis and pneumonia.

The forces that cause multiple rib fractures seldom spare the underlying lung from injury. Various degrees of lung contusion are present in virtually all patients with flail chest, even when it is not apparent on plain chest radiographs. Therefore, the treatment for patients with flail chest or pulmonary contusion should be primarily directed toward preventing pulmonary complications.

AXIOM Fluid overloading should be prevented or rapidly corrected in patients with pulmonary contusion or ARDS.

Fluid overload can rapidly result in worsening of the pathophysiologic changes of lung contusion.[32,33] Consequently, close attention to fluid balance is extremely important in patients with flail chest. Although large volumes of colloid and crystalloids may be required during resuscitation and during the period of obligatory third-spacing of fluid, restriction of fluids thereafter should reduce the movement of water into the contused lung.

NONVENTILATORY THERAPY. One of the major advances in the definitive management of patients with severe flail chest injuries has been the use of early ventilatory assistance. Nevertheless, patients with mild-to-moderate flail chest, little or no underlying pulmonary contusion and no major associated injuries can often be managed without a ventilator.[30,32]

AXIOM Patients with isolated flail chest injuries can often be managed without ventilatory support, especially if the chest pain can be adequately relieved.

Trinkle et al. reported that mechanical ventilation is not necessary in many patients with flail chest and may even be deleterious.[32] Important aspects of their nonventilatory therapy included: (a) relief of pain by analgesics or intercostal nerve block, (b) frequent coughing and chest physiotherapy, and (c) restriction of intravenous fluids to prevent fluid overload. They also advised the use of steroids and albumin, but the value of such agents is extremely controversial now. Aggressive respiratory therapy kept many of their patients off the ventilator; however, ventilatory support was provided when, in spite of this regimen, the arterial PO_2 remained < 80 mm Hg on supplemental oxygen.

When during the course of treatment of flail chest the patient develops atelectasis or excessive pulmonary secretions that cannot be ameliorated with pulmonary physiotherapy and orotracheal or nasotracheal suctioning, bronchoscopy is performed.

VENTILATORY SUPPORT

The usual indications for early ventilatory support of patients with flail chest include shock, three or more associated injuries, severe head injury, previous severe pulmonary disease, fracture of eight or more ribs, or age greater than 65 years.[30] Although the mortality rate of flail chest injuries is largely related to the numbers and types of associated injuries,[34] early (prophylactic) ventilatory assistance in patients with flail chest and only one or two significant associated injuries has been associated with a mortality rate of only 7%.[30] This is in sharp contrast to a mortality rate of 69% that occurred in similar patients in whom ventilatory assistance was delayed until there was clinical evidence of respiratory failure.

AXIOM When a patient will require ventilatory support, it is much safer to apply it "prophylactically" before actual ventilatory failure develops.

Our ventilated patients with flail chest seem to do better when intermittent mandatory ventilation (IMV) is used rather than controlled mandatory ventilation (CMV). In the series by Cullen et al., the mean ventilator time of patients treated with IMV and positive end-expiratory pressure (PEEP) (5.1 ± 4.7 days) was significantly less than that of patients treated with standard CMV (11.2 ± 6.2 days).[34]

OPERATIVE STABILIZATION (FIG. 16-3)

Recently there has been increased interest in operative stabilization of the chest wall if the flail is severe. In patients with a large, unstable chest wall segment who require thoracotomy for other injuries, the flail segment should also be fixed at that time with appropriate devices, e.g., intramedullary nails, struts, or wires.[35,36] Nevertheless, even after all rib fractures are healed, a significant number of these patients continue to have some disability consisting of chest pain, dyspnea, and impaired pulmonary function regardless what form of treatment was used.[37]

STERNAL FRACTURES

Before the advent of the automobile, fractures of the sternum were extremely rare and were usually due to direct blows or falling on the sternum. With the increase of vehicular travel and the increased incidence of motor vehicle accidents, the incidence of sternal fracture has increased pari passu.[38] Vehicular accidents are the most common cause of this injury, which usually occurs when the victim's anterior chest strikes the steering wheel. With increased use of collapsible steering wheels, the incidence of this injury appears to be decreasing; however, seat belt use may cause sternal fractures.[39,40] A specific pattern of injuries, including multiple rib fractures, sternal fractures, and myocardial and pulmonary contusions, has been referred to as the "seat belt syndrome" by Hamilton et al.[38] Fracture of the sternum usually occurs in adults. Such injuries seldom occur in children because of the elasticity of the anterior chest. Sternal fractures may be difficult to detect and may not be diagnosed until weeks later when excess callus on the sternum indicates that a fracture was present (Fig. 16-4).

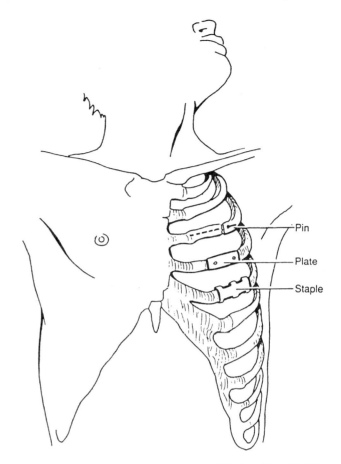

FIGURE 16-3 Technique of internal fixation of flail chest. (From: Rodriguez A. Injuries of the chest wall, the lungs and the pleura. Turney SZ, Rodriguez A, Cowley RA, eds. Management of cardiothoracic trauma. Baltimore: Williams & Wilkins, 1990; 162.)

AXIOM Sternal fractures should make one look carefully for an associated myocardial contusion.

In some series, up to 70% of patients with fractured sternums have myocardial contusions as well.[38,41,42] Consequently, in patients with fractured sternums from severe trauma, serial ECGs and creatine phosphokinase (CPK-MB) studies should be done every 8-12 hours for the first 24 hours and an echocardiography should be performed. Unstable sternal fractures with multiple costochondral disruptions may produce a significant flail chest without any fractured ribs visualized on chest radiography. In some patients with fractured sternums, external fixation may permit earlier extubation and mobilization.[43]

INJURIES TO THE LUNGS

Pulmonary Contusions

ETIOLOGY

Pulmonary contusion may result from penetrating, explosive, compressive, or decelerating trauma to the chest. The precise mechanism for the development of contusion of the lung from both penetrating or blunt trauma is not known, but a variety of forces has been considered as being responsible for this injury.

During blunt or explosive traumatic impact, the force delivered to the chest wall results in a decrease of the chest cavity size and compression of the lung. At the termination of the impact, the distorted chest wall returns to its normal position and the lung is rapidly decompressed.[44] The three physical effects generated by this trauma are referred to as spalling, inertial, and implosion.

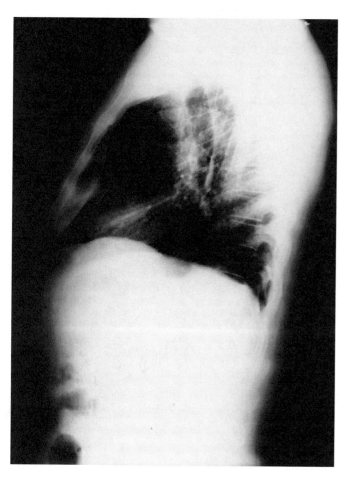

FIGURE 16-4 Delayed diagnosis of a sternal fracture. A 44-year-old truck driver had hit his chest against the steering wheel in a motor vehicle accident six weeks earlier. Initial radiographs were considered normal. He continued to have localized pain over his midlower sternum and this lateral chest radiography taken six weeks later showed excessive callus formation related to the missed fracture.

The spalling effect occurs when the compressive wave generated from the impact meets the liquid/air interface at the alveolus.[44] This results in disruption of the alveoli as energy is released by the transmission and partial reflection of the shock wave into the gas. The inertial effect appears to result from different rates of acceleration of the pulmonary tissues causing stripping of low-density alveoli from the high-density bronchi. The implosion effect is generated by the rebound effect of overexpansion of lung tissue following its compression from the impact. This causes rapid stretching and tearing of the alveoli.

PATHOPHYSIOLOGY

AXIOM The major cause of hypoxemia after blunt thoracic trauma is pulmonary contusion.

The pathologic changes seen with pulmonary contusion include capillary damage resulting in interstitial and intra-alveolar edema. The increasing interstitial edema plus some peribronchial extravasation of red blood cells can cause a progressive decrease in compliance and an increasing physiologic shunt. Hypoxemia usually gets progressively worse over the next 24-72 hours as a result of increasing physiologic shunt and a progressively greater oxygen diffusion barrier.[45,46] The $PaCO_2$ and pH changes are less consistent, but typically, increasing respiratory alkalosis occurs. In addition, pulmonary vascular resistance and usually increases, and pulmonary blood flow tends to

decrease. When atelectasis and pneumonia can be prevented, the lungs usually improve rapidly after 48-72 hours. These pulmonary changes seem to be worst in patients with severe associated injuries who also have the highest mortality rates.[47] Hoff et al. found that poor outcomes in patients with pulmonary contusion occurred when: (a) the contusion was seen on the admission chest radiography, (b) three or more rib fractures were manifest, (c) a chest tube was required, or (d) the PaO_2/FiO_2 ratio on admission was < 250.[48]

DIAGNOSIS

In the majority of the patients, chest radiographic changes of lung contusion appear during the first 4-6 hours after injury, and in the remaining patients, within the next 24 hours.[39] In the series by Hoff et al., radiographic changes were not present on the admission chest radiography in 36% of patients eventually diagnosed as having pulmonary contusions.[48] These changes are usually a patchy infiltration or consolidation of the lung at the site of injury. The roentgenographic changes frequently progress during the first 24-48 hours after injury (Figs. 16-5,16-6). Because the pathophysiologic changes tend to be progressive, repeat chest radiographs and blood gas determination should be performed at 6-12-hour intervals to help guide patient management.

Aspiration pneumonia and fat embolism are not usually seen on chest radiography during the initial six hours after injury. At thoracotomy or autopsy, the severity of lung contusions is usually much greater than suspected from the original chest radiographs. CT tends to give a much better impression of the extent of lung damage than does chest radiography (Fig. 16-7). Generally, chest radiographic changes tend to lag at least 24 hours behind blood gas changes.

AXIOM Pulmonary contusions are generally much larger than one would suspect from initial chest radiographs.

TREATMENT

Treatment of pulmonary contusions primarily involves maintenance of adequate ventilation of the lungs and prevention of pneumonia. Chest physiotherapy, nasotracheal suction, intercostal nerve blocks, and epidural analgesia are used as needed. When ventilatory assistance is required, use of IMV and PEEP usually provides much better ventilation-perfusion matching, better venous return, and quicker weaning than standard assisted or controlled ventilation. The initial use of positive end-expiratory pressure in patients with penetrating injury should be avoided or applied judiciously to minimize the risk of systemic arterial air embolization.[9,10]

Although the type and amount of fluids to be administered to patients with pulmonary contusion are somewhat controversial, blood loss should be replaced with blood or blood components, and the amount of crystalloid solutions given should probably be kept to a minimum. Administration of excessive amounts of crystalloids has been shown to accentuate pathophysiologic changes.[48] Sufficient crystalloids are given to keep the hourly urine output at about 0.5 ml/kg body weight. In severely injured patients continuous monitoring of the PAWP and/or right ventricular end-diastolic volume index (RVEDVI) should be considered.[49]

Patients who have severe unilateral lung injuries and are responding poorly to conventional mechanical ventilation may benefit from synchronous independent lung ventilation (SILV) provided through a double-lumen endobronchial catheter.[50] This technique helps prevent overinflation of the normal lung and underinflation of the damaged lung.

Pulmonary Hematomas

Pulmonary hematomas are large parenchymal tears filled with blood. Hematomas generally resolve spontaneously over a few weeks; however, when they become infected, hematomas can form lung abscesses that may be very difficult to manage. Hematomas are more likely to be-

FIGURE 16-5 AP chest radiograph revealing mild bilateral infiltrates characteristic of early pulmonary contusions. (From: Kirsh MM, Sloan H. Blunt chest trauma general principles of management. Boston: Little, Brown and Company, 1977; 25.)

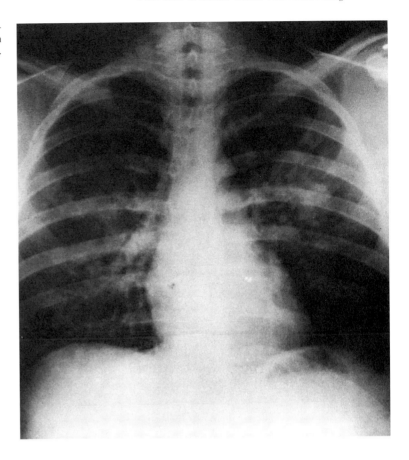

FIGURE 16-6 Later AP chest radiograph revealing severe, advanced pulmonary contusion with a tracheostomy present. (From: Kirsh MM, Sloan H. Blunt chest trauma general principles of management. Boston: Little, Brown and Company, 1977; 26.)

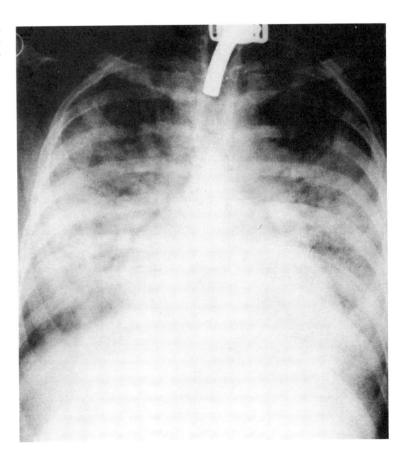

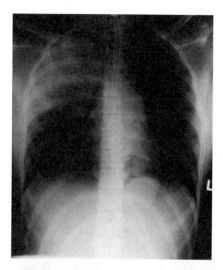

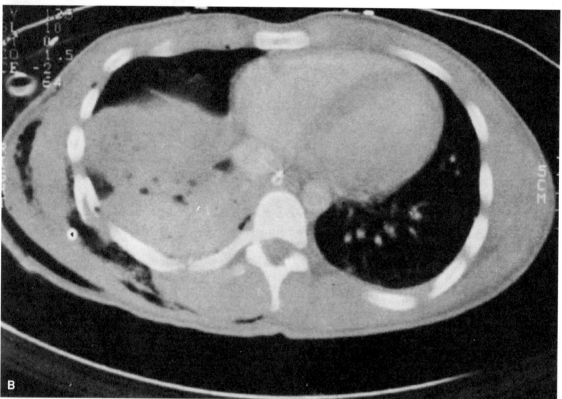

FIGURE 16-7 CT scans usually allow a more accurate assessment of the extent of lung contusions. (From: Rodriguez A. Injuries of the chest wall, the lungs and the pleura Turney SZ, Rodriguez A, Cowley RA, eds. Management of cardiothoracic trauma. Baltimore: Williams & Wilkins, 1990; 163,164.)

come infected after thoracotomy or with prolonged chest tube drainage, especially if the lung is not completely expanded or if there is a persistent air leak.

Pulmonary Lacerations with Hemopneumothorax

Major hemorrhages from lacerations of the lung following blunt trauma are usually caused by the sharp ends of fractured ribs. Occasionally they may be caused by tearing of the lung at previous pleural adhesions as the lungs move away from the chest wall during rapid deceleration. In some instances, the adhesions themselves are vascular, and a torn adhesion may occasionally bleed enough to cause shock.

Antibiotics, aggressive physiotherapy, and drainage of the hemo-

pneumothorax usually result in progressive resolution and obliteration of the cavity. If the cavity, fever, and purulent sputum persist, a foreign body should be sought on chest radiography and by bronchoscopy. If no improvement occurs after 4-6 weeks of vigorous therapy, resection of the cavity as a segmentectomy or lobectomy should be considered.[51]

Systemic Air Embolism

AXIOM In patients with penetrating chest wounds and particularly those with hemoptysis, aggressive positive-pressure ventilation increases the risk of systemic air emboli.

High-ventilatory pressures may force air from an injured bronchus into an adjacent, injured pulmonary vein producing systemic air emboli. This probably accounts for many of the severe arrhythmias or CNS changes that occur when patients with penetrating chest wounds are intubated and ventilated.[9,10] Campbell and Kerridge recently emphasized the high risk of traumatic air embolism in patients with penetrating wounds of the chest requiring positive-pressure ventilation.[52]

If systemic air embolism causes cardiac arrest, the head should be lowered and immediate thoracotomy performed to clamp the injured area of lung and then aspirate air from the left heart and aorta. Open cardiac massage with clamping of the ascending aorta may help push air through the coronary arteries. Cardiopulmonary bypass should be instituted promptly when available.

Traumatic Asphyxia

Sudden, severe crushing of the chest, especially by heavy weights, may result in a typical clinical picture referred to as traumatic asphyxia. Patients with this injury typically have subconjunctival hemorrhage or petechiae together with vascular engorgement, edema, and cyanosis of the head, neck, and upper extremities. Rusato et al. reported that Ollivier provided the first autopsy description of a syndrome of cranial cyanosis, subconjunctival hemorrhage, and vascular engorgement of the head, in a person crushed to death by a panicked crowd in Paris.[53] He referred to the skin changes on the face as "masque ecchymotique." Subsequently, various other terms were given to this syndrome, including traumatic cyanosis, Perth's symptom complex, cervicocutaneous asphyxia, and cervicofacial static cyanosis.[53]

By 1979, only 202 patients with traumatic asphyxia were reported.[54] This clinical picture appears to be due to an abrupt, sustained rise in superior vena caval pressure. The preferential passage of blood from the right atrium into the superior caval venous system is due to the lack of valves in these vessels. The sudden venous hypertension causes massive capillary engorgement of the head, neck, shoulders, and upper chest with stagnation of blood. Subsequent desaturation of the relatively stagnant blood gives the characteristic bluish discoloration to the skin. Periorbital ecchymosis, subjunctival hemorrhages, retinal hemorrhages, and slight exophthalmos are typically also present, with or without visual disturbances.[54]

Patients with only traumatic asphyxia are usually asymptomatic and require no special treatment. If CNS signs or symptoms are present, the head of the patient's bed should be elevated about 30° and supplemental oxygen administered. The prognosis of this syndrome is good; the skin ocular and neurologic manifestations usually disappear within 3-4 weeks.[55,56]

Intrabronchial Bleeding

AXIOM Intrabronchial bleeding can rapidly cause flooding of dependent alveoli and severe hypoxemia.

Intrabronchial bleeding is poorly tolerated and can rapidly cause death from severe hypoxemia by flooding of dependent alveoli.[57] Patients with intrabronchial bleeding tend to die from "drowning" rather than from hypovolemic shock. Relatively small amounts of blood infused into a dog trachea over 30-60 minutes can cause severe hypoxemia with minimal changes in $PaCO_2$ or airway resistance. The combination of shock and intrabronchial bleeding is highly lethal and can rapidly reduce oxygen transport to less than 25% of normal.[57]

In patients with hemoptysis due to trauma, the noninvolved lung must be kept as free of blood as possible, and nasotracheal suction and bronchoscopy should be used as often as necessary to keep the tracheobronchial tree clear. When thoracotomy is necessary, it should be performed with the patient supine (through a midsternot-

omy or anterior thoracotomy) to prevent the noninvolved lung from being flooded with blood. If the bleeding were severe, a double-lumen endotracheal (Carlens) tube could be used to confine the bleeding to one lung. When a Carlens or similar tube is not available or cannot be inserted, one may insert a smaller (5-6 mm diameter) endotracheal tube over a flexible bronchoscope into the left mainstem bronchus. The balloon on the endotracheal tube can then be inflated as needed. If the bleeding were from the left lung, the endotracheal tube would prevent blood from passing into the right lung, and ventilation of the right lung could then be maintained either spontaneously, via a mask, or through another small endotracheal tube.

In some instances, bleeding can only be controlled by occluding the involved bronchus with a Fogarty balloon catheter or by packing it with gauze. Obviously, these are temporary measures until the bleeding site can be controlled surgically.

Arteriovenous Fistulas

Pulmonary arteriovenous fistulas after penetrating chest trauma are uncommon because of the small-pressure differential between the pulmonary arteries and veins. However, a high degree of shunting in the lung or unexplained hypoxemia with residual pulmonary density should make one suspect this problem.

Aspiration

Aspiration of gastric contents is common after severe trauma, especially when the patient is unconscious. After removing as much material as possible from the tracheobronchial tree by standard suction, the patient should have bronchoscopy to remove whatever fluid or food particles remain. When the tracheobronchial tree is irrigated immediately with buffered saline, it may reduce the severity of the chemical pneumonitis.

AXIOM With suspected aspiration, intubation and bronchoscopy should be performed as soon as possible.

The radiologic changes characteristic of aspiration pneumonitis tend to be delayed for at least 12-24 hours. Suctioning of food particles, bile-stained fluid, or coffee-groundlike material from the trachea right after vomiting should be an indication for urgent bronchoscopy. Although gastric acid will probably already have caused most of its damage within 5-15 minutes, any remaining food particles should be removed.

When the patient is lying flat, aspiration pneumonitis tends to involve the posterior portions of the lung, especially the superior segment of the right lower lobe, the posterior segment of the right upper lobe, and the superior segment of the left lower lobe. These pneumonias are often necrotizing and frequently progress to form lung abscesses.

The early use of intravenous corticosteroids in doses equivalent to 100-200 mg hydrocortisone every 4-6 hours for 3-4 doses following aspiration is controversial. Corticosteroids may help to reduce inflammatory changes in the lungs, but they probably only help when begun within 1-2 hours of aspiration.

If an opaque foreign body is aspirated into the tracheo-bronchial tree, it usually is readily diagnosed. Radiolucent foreign bodies, however, can be extremely difficult to detect. They can remain lodged in a bronchus, causing repeated pulmonary infections or hemoptysis for years before being discovered. Persistent or recurrent cough, hemoptysis, atelectasis, or pneumonia after trauma should be an indication for bronchoscopy. If the bronchoscopic findings are unclear bronchography can be performed. Inspiratory and expiratory chest films may help to diagnose a foreign body in a main bronchus. If the foreign body causes a one-way-valve effect in a major bronchus, the involved lung will fail to empty properly during expiration and the mediastinum will tend to be pushed away from the side containing the foreign body.

HEMOTHORAX

Etiology

Hemothorax is most frequently caused by bleeding from lung injuries[58]; however, the compressing effect of the shed blood, the large concentration of thromboplastin in the lungs, and low pulmonary arterial pressures combine to help reduce bleeding from torn lung parenchyma. Consequently, when persistent, severe intrathoracic bleeding occurs, it usually arises from central lung injuries or from damage to major vessels. Bleeding from intercostal or internal mammary arteries may also be brisk and persistent.

Pathophysiology

AXIOM   Blood in the pleural cavity should be removed as completely and rapidly as possible.

Large clots release fibrinolysins and fibrinogenolysins that can act as local anticoagulants. Thus, a large hemothorax may not only restrict ventilation and venous return, but it also releases substances that can act as anticoagulants and contribute to continued intrathoracic bleeding. Bleeding from smaller intrathoracic vessels often stops if the hemothorax is completely removed at thoracotomy.

Diagnosis

Hemothorax should be suspected following trauma when breath sounds are reduced and the chest is dull to percussion on the involved side. Fluid collections > 200-300 ml can usually be seen on good upright or decubitus radiographs of the chest. If the patient is supine, however, up to 1000 ml of blood may not be readily apparent. Occasionally, hemothorax will be subpulmonic so that it only gives the impression that the diaphragm is elevated (Fig. 16-8); however, on decubitus films, blood layers out against the dependent chest wall.

Treatment

EMERGENCY THORACOTOMY

Most patients with intrathoracic bleeding can be treated adequately by intravenous administration of fluids and evacuation of the hemothorax with a chest tube. In a study by Washington et al., only 9% of patients with penetrating chest wounds have required thoracotomy to treat hemorrhage.[58] Thoracotomy for intrathoracic bleeding is generally indicated when: (a) patient's vital signs remain or become unstable, (b) > 1500-2000 ml of blood is lost from the chest tube in the first 12-24 hours, (c) drainage of blood from chest tubes exceeds 300 ml/hour for 3-4 hours or longer, or (d) the chest remains more than half full of blood on radiography. With these last three criteria, emergency thoracotomy is not always necessary when evidence suggests that the bleeding has stopped or has become < 100-200 ml/hr.

PITFALL ⊘

Delaying thoracotomy in patients with severe intrathoracic bleeding or unstable vital signs can result in sudden cardiac arrest.

If possible, emergency thoracotomies should be performed in the operating room; however, when the patient's condition is so precarious that transfer to the operating room could cause cardiac arrest, thoracotomy should be performed in the emergency department. It is becoming increasingly evident that emergency department thoracotomies can be lifesaving in selected patients. In a study by Washington et al., the survival rate for patients with emergency department thoracotomies for cardiac arrest due to penetrating trauma to the chest, neck, or extremities was 30%.[58] In contrast, no patients survived with no vital signs at the scene or with abdominal or head injuries. Patients requiring CPR for blunt trauma have also done poorly in all reported series. In general, thoracotomy should be performed in the emergency department when the patient remains unstable to move to the operating room safely, has a cardiac arrest in the emergency de-

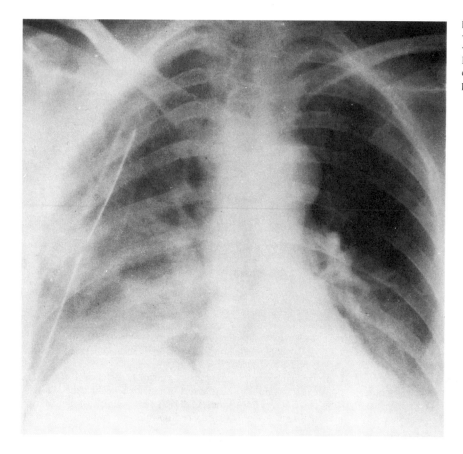

FIGURE 16-8 PA chest radiograph demonstrating what appears to be a very high right diaphragm, but what is actually a right subpulmonic effusion. (From: Kirsh MM, Sloan H. Blunt chest trauma general principles of management. Boston: Little, Brown and Company, 1977; 72.)

partment, or has a cardiac arrest within five minutes of arriving to the department because of a chest wound.[58,60]

THORACENTESIS

A small, stable hemothorax does not always need to be removed, but it should be carefully observed. When the hemothorax seems large enough to drain, one should avoid needle aspiration and rely on chest tubes. Needle aspiration of a hemothorax is usually incomplete and may cause a pneumothorax or an infected hemothorax.

PITFALL ⊘

> *Attempts to drain a traumatic hemothorax with needle thoracenteses are seldom completely successful and can cause air leaks, infections, or other complications.*

CHEST TUBE (THORACOSTOMY) DRAINAGE

Indications

Blood in the pleural cavity should be removed as completely and rapidly as possible. Blood entering the pleural cavity slowly does not usually clot because its fibrinogen quickly layers out on the pleural surface. However, if hemorrhage were rapid, much of the blood would clot before it could defibrinate.

Technique

Chest tubes for the treatment of traumatic pneumothorax or hemothorax should be inserted in the anterior axillary line just behind the lateral edge of the pectoralis major muscle. For pneumothorax, place the tube as high and anteriorly as possible. For hemothorax, the tube is inserted at the level of the nipple and directed posteriorly and laterally.

Once the insertion site is selected, the area around it is painted liberally with an iodophor preparation, and then widely draped with a fenestrated sheet. A 22-gauge needle infiltrates the skin, subcutaneous tissue, intercostal muscles, and parietal pleura with 1% lidocaine (Xylocaine) with adrenalin, keeping the total dose < 0.5 ml/kg (5 mg/kg).

A transverse skin incision, 2-3 cm in length, is then made. The skin incision for the chest tube should be at least one inch below the interspace through which the tube will be placed (Fig. 16-9). A large (Mayo) clamp is then inserted through the muscles in the next higher intercostal space, taking care to prevent the tip of the clamp from penetrating the lung. The resulting oblique tunnel

through the subcutaneous tissue and muscle usually closes promptly after the tube is removed, thereby reducing the chances of recurrent pneumothorax.

Once it is through the internal intercostal fascia, the clamp is opened to enlarge the hole to at least 1.5 cm in diameter. The clamp is then withdrawn and a finger is inserted through the hole as needed to verify the position of the hole within the thorax and to make sure the lung is not stuck to the chest wall.

AXIOM Insertion of an exploratory finger before placing a chest tube is important when chest radiography has not been taken or when radiography does not clearly show that the lung is away from the chest wall.

For a simple pneumothorax, a 24 or 28 F chest tube can be inserted. For a hemothorax, a 32-40 F chest tube is preferred. The chest tube is grasped at its tip with the clamp and directed through the hole into the pleural space and advanced in the appropriate direction. The tube is advanced until the last side hole is at least 1.0-2.0 cm inside the pleural cavity. The tube is secured in place with a long, heavy nonabsorbable skin suture (2-0 or 1-0) placed in a "U" fashion around the tube. The suture is tied so as to pull the soft tissues firmly around the tube and provide an airtight seal without necrosing the tissue. The tails of the suture can be wrapped around the tube in opposite directions approximately half a dozen times and then tied so as to secure the tube firmly to the chest wall. The open end of the tube is attached to a combination collection-water-seal suction device, such as the Pleur-evac with 20-30 cm H_2O suction.

After it appears that the chest tube is properly placed and is functioning satisfactorily, sterile occlusive dressing is placed on the chest around the tube and additional layers of tape are used to secure the tube to the chest wall so that it will not accidentally be pulled out when the patient is moved.

PITFALL ⊘

> *Failure to carefully note the location of the last hole of a chest tube on postinsertion chest radiography can result in air leaks and/or chest wall infections.*

The intrathoracic position of the chest tube and its last hole and the amount of air or fluid remaining in the pleural cavity should be checked with an upright chest film as soon as possible after the tube is inserted. When significant air leak occurs, chest films are best done

FIGURE 16-9 Placement of chest tube. The skin incision is below the site of penetration of the tube through the intercostal muscle. The oblique placement of the chest tube through chest wall also tends to cause the tube to spiral upward and apically. (From: Millikan JS, Moore EE, Steiner E, et al. Complications of tube thoracostomy for acute trauma. Am J Surg 1980;140:738.)

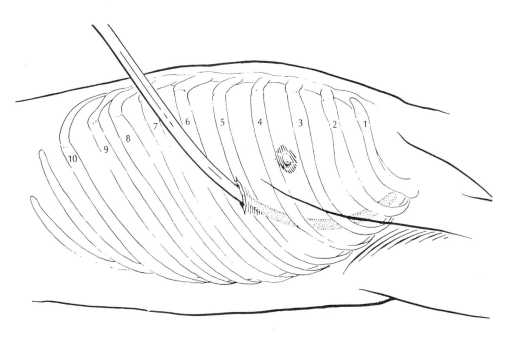

as portables at the patient's bedside so as not to risk the development of pulmonary collapse or tension pneumothorax while the patient is without suction en route to radiology.

AXIOM   When the patient has an air leak, the chest tube should not be clamped, even when the patient is being transported.

When the patient is sent to the radiology department for radiography, the chest tube should not be clamped because any continuing air leak can collapse the lung or cause a tension pneumothorax. While the tube is unclamped, the water-seal bottle should be kept 1-2 feet lower than the patient's chest.

Serial chest auscultation plus daily chest radiography and careful recording of the drainage volume and the severity of any air leak are important guides to the functioning of the chest tubes. When a chest tube becomes blocked and a significant pneumothorax or hemothorax is still present, the tube should be replaced. This can often be done easily through the same incision that the previous chest tube occupied. Irrigating an occluded chest tube or passing a Fogarty catheter through an occluded chest tube increases the risk of infection.

When the chest tube is functional and well-placed, but a decubitus film shows a fluid shift, the hemothorax then is partly clotted or loculated and another chest tube—placed as directed by ultrasound—may be helpful. If a tube were inserted because of a pneumothorax, it would be left in place on suction until at least 24 hours after all air leaks have stopped. If a tube were inserted for bleeding, it would be left in place until the drainage was serous and < 100 ml/24 hours. However, while the patient is on a ventilator, many physicians prefer to keep the chest tubes in place to act as a safety valve in case a new pneumothorax suddenly develops.

When a chest tube is to be removed, sutures securing the chest tube are cut and the patient is trained to take deep breaths and bear down with a Valsalva maneuver on command. While the intrathoracic pressure and lung volume are at their maximum, the tube is quickly pulled out and vaseline gauze immediately placed over the chest tube site as an airtight dressing. Some surgeons put only one knot in the securing suture so that the ends can be unwound from the chest tube and then tied down to provide the airtight seal at the chest tube site.

The patient should be in full inspiration when the tube is pulled. Patients have a tendency to gasp with a quick inspiratory effort because of the pleural pain caused as the tube is removed. This sudden gasp can rapidly pull in large quantities of air into the pleural cavity just as the tube is being removed.

Following removal of a chest tube, chest radiographs should be obtained to rule out any residual or recurrent pneumothorax. Another chest radiograph should be obtained 12-24 hours later to confirm continued, complete expansion of the lungs. If chest radiography after chest tube removal were to show a small, stable pneumothorax, it should be observed for 24-48 hours; another chest tube should be inserted when a moderately large pneumothorax is present, causes symptoms, or increases in size.

Antibiotics

Much controversy exists concerning the value of prophylactic antibiotics in patients with chest tubes for traumatic hemothorax or pneumothorax. Grover et al., in a prospective, randomized double-blind study, showed that 300 mg of intravenous clindamycin every six hours while the chest tubes were in place reduced the total intrathoracic infection rate from 35.1% (13 of 37) in controls to 10.5% (4 of 38) in the patients receiving antibiotics.[61] Three other prospective double-blind studies have also shown a significant reduction in infections with the use of antibiotics.[62-64] Mandal et al. found no infections in 40 patients receiving intravenous doxycycline (200 mg initially and then 100 mg every 12 hours), but this was not significantly better than the infection rate of 2.5 (1 of 40) in those receiving placebos.[65] LeBlanc and Tucker also found no significant reduction in infections with antibiotics (3.9% vs 8.7%).[66]

Unfortunately, great variation occurred in the incidence of infection in patients not receiving antibiotics (0-3.5% for pneumonia and

2.5-16.2% for empyema). Nevertheless, when the data from the first six prospective studies on the use of prophylactic antibiotics for chest tubes after trauma are pooled, antibiotics reduced the empyema rate from 9.4% (22 of 234) to 0.8% (2 of 230) and the infection rate from 11.1% to 2.5% (p < 0.001). Total intrathoracic infections were reduced from 17.5% (41 of 234) with placebos to 2.9% (7 of 238) with antibiotics. The validity of those data were confirmed in a metanalysis by Fallon and Wears.[67]

AXIOM   Although antibiotics can reduce the incidence of empyema and pneumonia in the patient requiring a chest tube for traumatic hemopneumothorax, the ideal duration of such treatment is not clear.

In the six studies described above, antibiotics were given as long as the chest tube was in place. However, studies by Cant et al. suggested that antibiotics given for 24 hours are adequate[68]; a study by Demetriades et al. suggested that only one dose of antibiotic needed to be given.[69]

Autotransfusion

In the patient with massive bleeding into a body cavity, autotransfusion may reduce the need for donor blood and its associated risks. Intrathoracic bleeding is generally ideal for this technique because there is usually no contamination of the blood by bile or intestinal contents.[70] To use the blood for autotransfusion, one needs to add citrate or heparin to the blood as it is removed to keep it from clotting and collect it in a special sterile container. In emergency situations with continued shock, however, attempts at autotransfusion may seem excessively difficult, particularly when adequate type-specific blood is readily available. Autotransfused blood may contribute to the development of coagulopathy.

Thomas found that more than 1,000 ml of blood that is directly autotransfused can lead to coagulopathy and irreplaceable blood loss.[71] When red blood cells are washed in a cell saver, more autotransfusions can be given, but one should still be concerned about coagulopathy. At Detroit Receiving Hospital, it is generally easier and faster to use donor blood unless: (a) the bleeding is massive and not rapidly controllable by surgery, or (b) the blood bank is running short of that type of blood.

TREATMENT OF RETAINED BLOOD

If the chest were to remain more than one-third to one-half full of blood after 3-4 weeks, the retained blood should be removed to prevent delayed empyema or fibrothorax. If the blood were allowed to remain in place for more than 4 weeks, increasing capillary growth could develop into the clotted blood via visceral and parietal pleural capillaries. This makes later removal of the blood much more difficult.

TREATMENT OF EMPYEMA

When evidence of infection exists in a retained hemothorax as reflected by spiking fevers and/or radiologic studies, the empyema should be drained promptly. If the empyema were loculated or if it were inadequately controlled with chest tube drainage and antibiotics, thoracotomy and decortication are usually required. Recently, however, thoracoscopy has been used successfully to drain and decorticate these empyema.[72]

PNEUMOTHORAX

Pathophysiology

Collections of air or blood within the pleural cavity reduce vital capacity and increase intrathoracic pressure, thereby decreasing minute ventilation and venous return to the heart. During spontaneous inspiration, negative intrapleural pressure increases the tendency for air or blood to leak into the pleural cavity through any wound in the lung or chest wall. When any obstruction to the upper airway occurs or chronic obstructive lung disease is present, additional air may be forced into the pleural cavity during expiration causing tension pneumothorax with intrapleural pressures exceeding atmospheric pressure.

Diagnosis

PITFALL ⊘

Failure to obtain chest radiography soon after admission and again six hours later may result in significant intrathoracic injuries being overlooked.

The presence of a chest injury is usually readily apparent from the history and physical examination; however, accurate assessment of the damage, especially to the intrathoracic organs, often requires serial chest radiographs. Pneumothorax is not apt to cause severe symptoms unless it: (a) is a tension pneumothorax, (b) occupies more than 20-40% of one hemithorax, or (c) occurs in a patient with shock or preexisting cardiopulmonary disease.

When suspicion of a pneumothorax exists, but is not clearly seen on the first chest radiograph, repeat films during expiration may be helpful (Fig. 16-10, 16-11). Apical-lordotic films may allow better visualization of an apical pneumothorax. Pneumothorax after a stab wound is only rarely delayed for more than six hours. A deep lateral sulcus on chest radiography is also evidence of pneumothorax (Fig. 16-12).

In a study of 4106 patients with initially asymptomatic stabs of the chest by Ordog et al,[73] only 12% required tube thoracostomy for delayed pneumothorax or hemothorax in spite of two normal chest radiographs within six hours of admission. The authors also found that patients with nonprogressive, small (< 20%) pneumothoraces not requiring chest tubes could be discharged after 48 hours of observation; however, 32% of patients with "small" pneumothoraces experienced progression and required tube thoracotomy. Consequently, when a repeated chest radiograph at six hours is normal, it is un-

likely that additional radiographs are needed except in selected patients. Occasionally, a small pneumothorax is not apparent on chest radiography, but is seen on CT of the chest or abdomen. This is referred to as an occult pneumothorax.[74] An occult pneumothorax should be drained with a chest tube or catheter if the patient is to be placed on a ventilator in the operating room or in the ICU.

One should assume that a tension pneumothorax is present and begin treatment without waiting for chest radiography when the patient has: (a) severe respiratory distress, (b) decreased breath sounds and hyperresonance on one side of the chest, (c) distended neck veins (not caused by hypervolemia), and/or (d) deviation of the trachea away from the involved side (Fig. 16-13). Insertion of a large needle into the involved side through the second intercostal space in the midclavicular line may help to confirm the diagnosis and to provide temporary relief while a chest tube is being inserted.

Treatment

TENSION PNEUMOTHORAX

AXIOM When a tension pneumothorax is suspected in an unstable patient, it must be relieved as rapidly as possible.

When a chest tube cannot be inserted almost instantly, the pleural cavity should be immediately aspirated anteriorly in the second intercostal space with a needle and syringe. One or more chest tubes should then be inserted as rapidly as possible and connected to a water-seal/collection/suction device.

OBSERVATION OF SMALL, STABLE PNEUMOTHORAX

A small pneumothorax (< 1.0 cm wide and confined to the upper one-third of the chest) that is unchanged on two chest roentgenograms taken 4-6 hours apart in an otherwise healthy individual can usually be treated by observation alone. However, in most instances after

FIGURE 16-10 Inspiratory PA supine chest radiograph showing what appears to be a small, right-sided pneumothorax (arrows). (The pleural line is also retouched for clarity.) (From: Kirsh MM, Sloan H. Blunt chest trauma general principles of management. Boston: Little, Brown and Company, 1977; 51.)

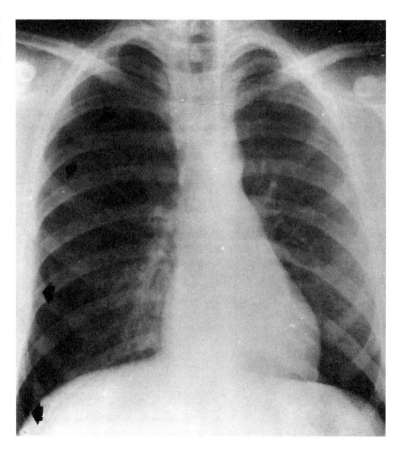

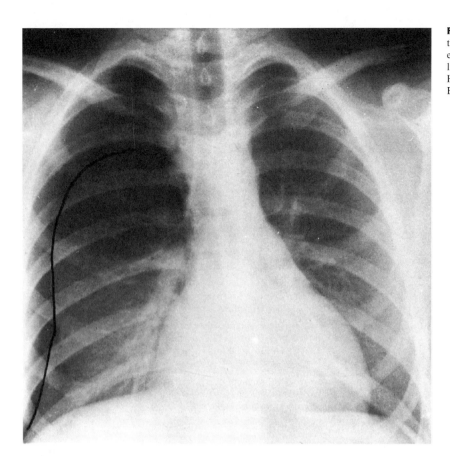

FIGURE 16-11 Expiratory PA supine chest radiograph of the same patient showing the pneumothorax more readily, especially in the upper portion of the chest. (The pleural line was retouched for clarity). (From: Kirsh MM, Sloan H. Blunt chest trauma general principles of management. Boston: Little, Brown and Company, 1977; 55.)

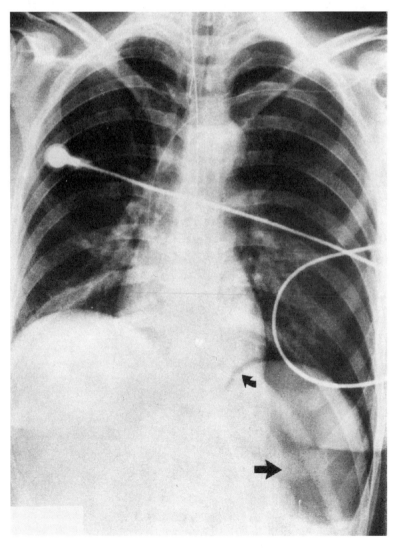

FIGURE 16-12 The "deep sulcus" sign of a pneumothorax. In the supine position, air may collect anteriorly, outlining the diaphragm and cardiac apex. The lateral sulcus is deepened (straight arrow). Subpulmonary air is also frequently seen posteromedially outlining the lung base (curved arrow). (From: Shulman HS, Samuels TH. The radiology of blunt chest trauma. J Can Assoc Radiol 1983;34:204.)

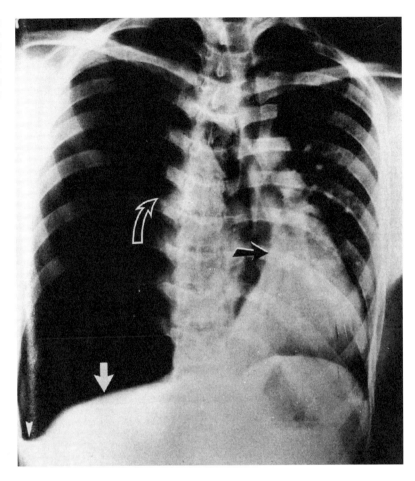

FIGURE 16-13 Tension pneumothorax. Signs indicating that the right hemithorax is under tension include depression of the hemidiaphragm (straight white arrow), herniation of lung across the midline (black arrow), and flattening of the right lung against the mediastinum (curved open arrow). Note the small, right hemothorax (arrowhead). (From: Shulman HS, Samuels TH. The radiology of blunt chest trauma. J Can Assoc Radiol 1983; 34:204.)

trauma, a chest tube or small catheter should be inserted as a precautionary measure, especially when the patient cannot be observed closely. An occult pneumothorax seen only CT scan can be just observed in most cases.

CHEST TUBE DRAINAGE

When only a pneumothorax is present, a small-to-moderate-sized (24-28 French) chest tube may be inserted anteriorly in the second intercostal space in the midclavicular line; however, a high midaxillary tube is generally preferable. Although some physicians insert chest tubes over trocars because it is less painful, especially if the lung were well away from the chest wall, we believe it is safer to avoid the trocar and insert chest tubes using a large hemostat.

CATHETER ASPIRATION OF SIMPLE PNEUMOTHORAX

Obeid et al. treated simple, uncomplicated traumatic pneumothorax with catheter aspiration.[75] This technique of catheter aspiration of a simple pneumothorax (CASP) using a 16-gauge catheter, three-way stopcock, and 50 ml syringe successfully reexpanded the lung in 16 of 17 patients without admission to the hospital. However, the CASP technique was suitable in only 6% of all traumatic pneumothoraces seen; the major complication was a continued air leak.

Complications of Pneumothoraces

CONTINUED AIR LEAK

AXIOM The combination of a pneumothorax space plus a continued air leak almost invariably results in a pleural infection unless the pneumothorax can be corrected within 24-48 hours.

In general, a small- or moderate-sized pneumothorax does not cause complications unless it occurs with a continuing air leak. Also, a continuing air leak does not usually cause problems when the lung is completely expanded; however, if the combination of a pneumothorax and continued air leak were allowed to exist for more than 24-48 hours, the incidence of empyema and bronchopleural fistula would be greatly increased. If the pneumothorax space cannot be eradicated with another chest tube, bronchoscopy, and ventilatory support, one should perform a thoracotomy. Autologous fibrin gel administered by means of a chest tube has successfully controled traumatic bronchopleural fistulas in some patients.[76]

CONTINUED PNEUMOTHORAX

The most frequent reasons for the failure of a chest tube attached to suction to completely expand the lungs include: (a) improper connections in the external tubing or to the water-seal-collection device, (b) improper position of the chest tubes(s), (c) occlusion of bronchi by secretions or a foreign body, (d) a tear of one of the larger bronchi, or (e) a large tear of the lung parenchyma. When the lung is not expanded and a large air leak occurs, emergency bronchoscopy should be performed to clear the bronchi and identify any damage to the tracheobronchial tree that may need repair. Continued large air leak and failure of the lung to expand adequately within 24-48 hours in spite of the above measures are often indications for early thoracotomy. Occasionally, as pointed out by Rankin et al., a massive traumatic air leak can be treated successfully with prolonged double-lumen intubation and high-frequency ventilation on the side of injury.[77]

POSTTRAUMATIC PULMONARY PSEUDOCYST

Occasionally following trauma, an air space without a bronchial or pleural connection develops within the injured lung parenchyma. This may cause cough, chest pain, leukocytosis, and/or low-grade fever.

Most pulmonary pseudocysts resolve spontaneously over a few weeks or months. If they enlarge or become infected, resection or drainage may be required.[78]

PNEUMOMEDIASTINUM

Pneumomediastinum is an important finding in patients with chest trauma. The diagnosis is usually made on chest radiography. It should also be suspected with subcutaneous emphysema in the neck, but this finding can easily be missed. The diagnosis of pneumomediastinum should also be suspected from the presence of a crunching sound (Hamman's sign) over the heart during systole. This finding is present in about 50% of patients with pneumomediastinum, and it is usually accentuated when the patient is in the left lateral decubitus position. Bruit de Moulin, a loud precordial murmur caused by turbulence of air and fluid in the pericardial cavity, may also be heard.[79]

> **AXIOM** Most posttraumatic pneumomediastinums are idiopathic, but if their source were not sought aggressively, rapidly lethal injuries may go untreated until too late.

Usually little or no disability occurs from a pneumomediastinum except perhaps in the newborn; rarely, tension pericardium may develop in older individuals.[79] Nevertheless, one should look closely for an injury to the airway or the digestive tract. In the great majority of patients, no obvious injury or source can be found. Most "spontaneous" pneumomediastinums are seen in patients with asthma or emphysema. Even in these patients, however, with histories of trauma, one must look carefully for injury to the larynx, trachea, major bronchi, pharynx, or esophagus. One must also look carefully for associated pneumothorax, which may develop later, especially when the patient requires mechanical ventilation.

TRACHEOBRONCHIAL INJURIES

The trachea in adults is a 10-12 cm long tube that extends from the larynx, which is at the level of the sixth cervical vertebra, to the lower border of the fifth thoracic vertebra. At that level, the trachea divides into right and left main bronchi. The anterolateral wall, making up 60-70% of the circumference of the trachea is cartilaginous and the posterior one-third is membranous. The trachea is situated next to the great vessels, and its membranous portion is loosely attached to the anterior wall of the esophagus. The first portion of the trachea, from the level of the sixth cervical to the second thoracic vertebra, is surrounded anterolaterally by soft-tissue structures and posteriorly by the cervical spine. The remainder of the trachea is situated behind the sternum and is enclosed by the bony structures of the thorax.

Blunt Trauma

INCIDENCE AND ETIOLOGY

Blunt tracheobronchial injuries are rare and most patients with such trauma die before they reach the hospital, primarily from severe associated injuries. Ecker et al. reviewed tracheobronchial injuries over a 10-year period in Dallas County.[80] Of 27 patients with blunt tracheobronchial injuries (14 vehicular, 11 air crash, and 2 crush- or fall-related), only 9 (33%) reached the hospital alive. Bertelsen and Howitz, reviewing 1178 postmortem reports of persons dying of trauma, reported that only 33 (0.03%) had tracheobronchial disruptions, and 27 (82%) of these patients died almost immediately.[81] Iwasaki et al. documented that five (2.1%) of their patients admitted with blunt chest trauma had tracheobronchial injuries.[82]

> **AXIOM** Blunt tracheobronchial injuries are rare, but when they occur, they are frequently fatal.

PATHOGENESIS

Three mechanisms are believed to be involved in the pathogenesis of blunt tracheobronchial rupture.[83] First, a sudden decrease in the an-

teroposterior diameter of the thorax causes abrupt widening of transverse diameter. This tends to pull the lungs apart, causing vertical tears at the carina or transverse tears of the mainstem bronchi.[84] Second, if the trachea and major bronchi were crushed between the sternum and vertebral column while the glottis was closed, the sudden increase in intrabronchial pressure may cause a "blow-out" rupture of the bronchi and/or a longitudinal tear of the membranous trachea.[85] Third, rapid deceleration may result in shearing forces at the areas of fixation at the carina and cricoid cartilage.[84] These forces may act alone or in concert.

As expected from these mechanisms of action, blunt tracheobronchial rupture is usually reported to be in the main bronchi within 2.5 cm of the carina.[86] Taskinen et al. had similar findings in 7 of 9 patients[87]; however, only 5 (42%) of the 12 patients reported by Shimazu et al. were near the carina,[88] and of the 18 patients reported by Limet et al., 7 (39%) were below the bronchus intermedius.[89]

Because high-energy trauma is required to bluntly tear the trachea or bronchi, one would expect a high incidence of associated injuries. Although one series in the older literature had associated injuries in only 50% of patients with tracheobronchial disruption from blunt trauma,[84] a recent series reported 48 associated injuries in 13 patients.[86] Baumgartner et al[83] found blunt tracheobronchial disruption as an isolated injury in only 2 (22%) of their 9 patients.

Review of the older literature seems to indicate that blunt tracheobronchial injuries are equally divided between the right and left sides; however, Baumgartner et al. found right bronchial injuries in 5 of 9 patients and left bronchial injuries in only 2 of 9 patients.[83] This right-sided preponderance supports the finding of another recent series in which 7 of 13 tracheobronchial injuries involved right bronchi and none involved the left.[86]

DIAGNOSIS

Symptoms and Signs

The most common presenting symptoms of tracheobronchial disruption include dyspnea, cough, and hemoptysis.[86] The most frequent signs include subcutaneous emphysema, diminished breath sounds, mediastinal crunch, and persistent air leaks after chest tube placement. Most of these findings are nonspecific, but they should increase suspicion of a tracheobronchial injury.[83,87,90]

Traditionally, subcutaneous emphysema and dyspnea have been the most frequent initial signs and symptoms of blunt tracheobronchial rupture. In one recent series of 13 patients sustaining blunt tracheobronchial disruptions, 85% had subcutaneous emphysema and 77% had dyspnea.[86] All 9 of the patients reported by Baumgartner et al. had subcutaneous emphysema, although it was delayed up to 4 hours in two patients.[83] Dyspnea was an initial or early symptom in 6 of their 9 patients. Other signs included sternal tenderness in 6 of 9, hemoptysis in 4 of 9, and Hamman's sign in 3 of 9.[83] Occasionally, subcutaneous emphysema in the neck may be due to a pharyngeal injury occurring during an attempt at endotracheal intubation (Fig. 16-14).

> **AXIOM** A large air leak, mediastinal air, and persistent pneumothorax are due to tracheobronchial tear until proved otherwise.

Early diagnosis of tracheobronchial rupture is aided by the presence of a persistent, large air leak after a chest tube is inserted for treatment of pneumothorax.[91] The majority of patients with tracheobronchial injury have this finding.[92] The lack of a pneumothorax or air leak makes early diagnosis of tracheobronchial injury much more difficult.

Blood Gases

> **AXIOM** Elevated PCO_2 in patients with hypoxemia and/or metabolic acidosis can be highly lethal unless corrected rapidly.

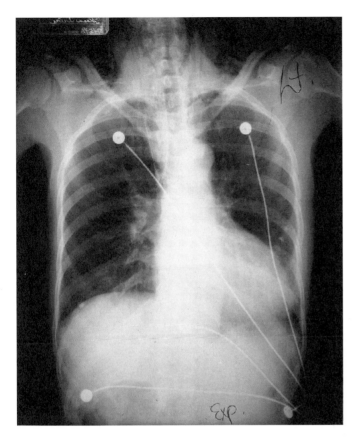

FIGURE 16-14 Pharyngeal injury causing subcutaneous emphysema in the neck. A 54-year-old comatose female had an unsuccessful attempt at endotracheal intubation. Subcutaneous emphysema from a torn pharynx was noted immediately on palpation of the neck and on the subsequent chest radiographs.

The average ($\pm$ SD) values found on admission blood gas analyses in 12 patients with tracheobronchial injuries reported by Shimazu et al. included a mean PaO_2 of 49 ± 12 mm Hg, $PaCO_2$ of 43 ± 12 mm Hg, and base excess of -4.1 ± 5.1 mEq/L.[88] The mortality rate correlated well with the $PaCO_2$ in that 4 of 7 (57%) of the hypercapnic patients died, but all patients with $PaCO_2 < 40$ mm Hg survived (P = 0.012).

Radiologic Studies

CHEST RADIOGRAPHY. Rupture of major bronchi is frequently accompanied by pneumothorax and a partially or completely atelectatic lung, pneumomediastinum, and subcutaneous emphysema. Some of these patients present with a tension pneumothorax. In patients with complete transection of the bronchus, progressive atelectasis leading to complete collapse of the involved lung occurs immediately or develops over the next 2-3 weeks. Roentgenographic evidence of persistent lobar atelectasis or atelectasis of one lung may be the only manifestation of a bronchial rupture. Failure of the lung to expand after a chest tube is inserted should make one even more suspicious.

AXIOM A "dropped lung" on an upright chest radiograph is virtually pathognomonic of a complete tear of a major bronchus.

A very pathognomonic radiographic sign of a main bronchus rupture is a drop of the superior margin of the collapsed lung below the level of the transected bronchus.[92] However, this "dropped lung" sign is uncommon. For example, only one of seven patients with a bronchial rupture reported by Taskinen et al. demonstrated this sign, but

it is not clear how many of the other mainstem bronchial tears were complete.[87] Barnhart et al. reported that occasionally pneumoperitoneum may be the first sign of tracheobronchial disruption.[91] Bronchoscopy should be performed in patients with the combination of pneumoperitoneum and pneumomediastinum, even if pneumothorax were not present.[91]

RIB FILMS

AXIOM Fractures of the first two ribs may be associated with an increased incidence of cardiovascular and tracheobronchial injuries.

In the review of 200 reported patients with tracheobronchial rupture described by Chesterman and Stasangi's, chest wall fractures were found in only 33% of patients.[93] However, Burke mentioned in a review of 167 reported patients that fractures of the upper three ribs were common in patients with tracheobronchial injuries.[94] No patients were over 30 years of age with a bronchial rupture who did not also have rib fractures.

Of the 12 patients in the series by Shimazu et al., seven had broken ribs (58%) and six had fractures of the first three rib(s).[88] Of these six, five (83%) were associated with one or more ruptured segmental bronchi, suggesting that chest wall fractures are associated with an increased incidence of rupture of more distal bronchi.

BRONCHOGRAPHY. The value of bronchography in acute blunt tracheobronchial injury is questionable. It was done twice in the series reported by Baumgartner et al. and did not assist the diagnosis in either patient.[83]

Bronchoscopy

AXIOM Bronchoscopy should be performed in any patient with a suspected airway injury.[83,87]

Although identifying the site and nature of a tracheobronchial injury is critical for planning anesthetic and surgical strategy, in emergency situations, one may have no time for bronchoscopy or other investigations. Nevertheless, when it was done in the study by Taskinen et al., bronchoscopy revealed the diagnosis in all patients.[87]

AXIOM The accuracy of bronchoscopy in diagnosing tracheobronchial injuries depends largely on the expertise of endoscopists and the timing of endoscopy.

Although only 3 of 9 of the initial fiberoptic bronchoscopies in the series by Baumgartner et al. had correct diagnoses, 5 of the 6 incorrect endoscopies were performed by physicians who were not cardiothoracic surgeons.[86] Conversely, six (86%) of the seven correct endoscopies in these patients were performed by cardiothoracic surgeons and the seventh was performed by a pulmonologist. The one lesion missed by a cardiothoracic surgeon was later identified by the same surgeon, suggesting that it had changed to a more easily identifiable form. Although the high accuracy of the bronchoscopies performed by the cardiothoracic surgeons was impressive, they tended to perform the later bronchoscopies when the lesion is often much easier to recognize.

Rigid bronchoscopy was performed in 5 of the 9 patients reported by Baumgartner et al. and showed a lesion requiring operation in 4 (80%) of these patients.[83] The one endoscopy that missed the lesion was performed by a surgical resident. Thus, in at least one study, rigid endoscopy in the hands of a trained cardiothoracic surgeon provides 100% sensitivity, specificity, and accuracy. Thus, if the patient's clinical condition were to suggest tracheobronchial disruption, bronchoscopy should be performed by an experienced physician.

AXIOM Negative bronchoscopy by a relatively inexperienced endoscopist does not eliminate tracheobronchial injury.

Tracheobronchial injury in burn patients is usually diagnosed by bronchoscopy revealing tracheobronchial inflammation and carbonaceous sputum. Mausarines et al. performed bronchial biopsies in addition to bronchoscopy to confirm the bronchoscopist's findings.[95] Complete agreement between the bronchoscopist and the histologic findings occurred in 107 of 130 patients (81 with negative and 26 with positive findings). In nine other patients in whom bronchoscopy was considered negative, histology was considered indeterminate in six and positive in three. In 14 patients, bronchoscopy was considered positive for inhalation injuries but on histology, the biopsy was considered indeterminate in 9 and normal in 5. If the indeterminate histologic readings were considered to be negative, the sensitivity of bronchoscopy for detecting definite tracheobronchial inflammation from inhalation of toxic gases would be 89% and specificity 87%.

ASSOCIATED INJURIES

All nine patients with tracheobronchial trauma in the series reported by Taskinen et al. had some concomitant injuries with an average of two injuries per patient.[87] Six patients had other life-threatening injuries, including: severe pulmonary contusion, splenic or pancreatic rupture, or dislocation of the heart because of rupture of the pericardium. Minor concomitant injuries included rib, clavicle, and radius fractures.

With blunt linear tears of the membranous portion of the trachea, one should look carefully for associated injuries to the esophagus. Stothert et al., in a review of blunt tracheobronchial injuries, found 17 patients in the world literature with associated esophageal injuries and added a patient of their own.[96] All were relatively young patients (18-38 years of age) and associated rib fractures were unusual. All of the tracheal tears were longitudinal and above the pulmonary hilum, ranging in length from 3-8 cm.

Only three (17%) of the 18 associated esophageal injuries were discovered and treated within 48 hours of injury, and 13 (83%) were repaired after 30 days.[96] Only three (17%) of these 18 patients died. Obviously, the leaks must have been fairly well contained and did not cause severe suppurative mediastinitis.

DELAYED DIAGNOSIS

> **AXIOM** Many blunt tracheobronchial injuries are not diagnosed until after they cause stenosis and/or severe distal pulmonary infections.

Because of a lack of specific findings, the diagnosis of blunt tracheobronchial injury is delayed in 25-69% of patients.[92,94,97] In the series by Taskinen et al., the diagnosis was overlooked initially in five (55%) of their nine patients.[87] One reason for the delay is that peribronchial tissue may remain sufficiently intact to permit ventilation in the involved lung. Within 2-6 weeks, however, bronchial obstruction can develop due to increased granulation tissue at the site of injury. Distal to the obstruction, the lung tends to become atelectatic and infected.[86,97]

> **AXIOM** Physicians treating MVA victims must maintain a high index of suspicion for tracheobronchial disruptions in order to detect these rare lesions promptly.

TREATMENT

Ventilation

The two major problems that can occur in patients with tracheobronchial rupture include early ventilatory insufficiency and the development of stricture at the site of rupture causing atelectasis and/or infection.[81] Although strictures can usually be prevented by early repair, a massive air leak can cause death before a repair can be performed. Ventilatory management to maintain an adequate gas exchange and control air leakage before and during operation is essential to reduce the early mortality of tracheobronchial rupture.[88]

Intubation

Shimazu et al. found that endobronchial intubation (two patients) or a double-lumen endobronchial tube (two patients) greatly improved ventilation in patients with torn major bronchi.[88] Similar benefits were noted by Iwasaki et al. who used a Univent tube, which has a movable blocker capable of excluding the injured lung to prevent aspiration of blood into the uninjured lung.[82] The double-lumen endobronchial tube has several advantages over single-lumen tubes. Most importantly, it permits independent ventilation of each lung with selective PEEP, while preventing aspiration of blood or secretions into the contralateral lung.

> **AXIOM** Double-lumen (split-function) endotracheal tubes can be helpful in managing torn bronchi, but they can be difficult to insert promptly and properly.

Previous results with endobronchial tubes were often poor because the tubes were composed of material which elicited inflammatory changes in the airway mucosa and had high-pressure cuffs that would cause mucosal necrosis. The newer polyvinyl chloride, double-lumen endobronchial tubes have low-tissue reactivity and are equipped with high-volume, low-pressure cuffs.[98] Although a narrow fiberoptic bronchoscope can often be passed through these tubes, endobronchial suction may be difficult, even when using the special suction catheters that are included in the tube package. Other disadvantages of the endobronchial tube include difficulty in placement and fixation of the tube as compared to a single-lumen endotracheal tube and the necessity for oral intubation because the tube cannot be passed transnasally. Although intraoperative bronchial rupture has been reported in one patient in whom such a tube was used,[98] such complications can probably be prevented by carefully checking the position of the tube and the pressure in the tube cuffs.

The use of the double-lumen endobronchial tube should not be limited to patients with tracheobronchial injuries because independent ventilation of the lungs is advantageous in patients with severe pulmonary parenchymal injuries as well.[94] Although selective mainstem bronchial intubation of the uninjured lung with a standard endotracheal tube may occasionally be necessary in an emergency, the double-lumen endobronchial tube should be considered for use in any patient with symptoms suggestive of major tracheobronchial injury.

> **AXIOM** Flexible bronchoscopy can be of great help in diagnosing and intubating injured bronchi.

Occasionally, a rigid bronchoscope can be used to secure the airway or to bridge the gap between ends of a transected trachea or mainstem bronchus.[100] However, one may also elect not to attempt intubation of the distal segment before thoracotomy for fear of further compromising the airway. When intubation from the operative field is planned, a sterile anode tube and sterile extension ventilator tubing should be ready for use when the chest is opened.

To facilitate the ventilatory management of patients with tracheobronchial injury, high-frequency jet ventilation has been recommended by a number of authors.[101,102] Dreyfuss et al. reported two patients with tracheobronchial rupture successfully managed intraoperatively and postoperatively by high-frequency ventilation[101]; in one of these patients, a double-lumen endobronchial tube was also used.[93] However, the efficacy of high-frequency ventilation during the acute phase of tracheobronchial rupture with progressive hypercapnia remains to be determined. Kaiser et al. compared high-frequency ventilation and conventional mechanical ventilation in dogs under methacholine inhalational challenges and reported significantly higher mean airway pressure and arterial PCO_2 values during high-frequency ventilation.[103] These results suggest that high-frequency ventilation may not always be a solution to ventilatory problems caused by tracheobronchial disruptions.

Surgical Repair

HISTORY. The first successful primary repair of a bronchial rupture caused by blunt trauma was reported in 1947 by Kinsella and Johnsrud.[104] In 1959, Hood and Sloan reported significantly improved results with prompt primary repair of these injuries.[105] Since then, several series demonstrated that early diagnosis and primary repair of these injuries lead to the fewest complications and best long-term results.[80,84,86,94]

INCISIONS. In deciding on which side to perform a thoracotomy for exploration and repair, one should be aware that the side of the largest pneumothorax or air leak may not be the side of the injury. Taskinen et al. noted that the mainstem bronchial ruptures that 2 of 3 patients had were left-sided injuries with massive air leakages to the right side and only 1 to the left.[88] The adventitial tissue surrounding the left main bronchus is so tight that it can often prevent air leakage to the left.

AXIOM Posterolateral right thoracotomy is generally the best incision for exploring tracheal and proximal right and left mainstem bronchial injuries.

Isolated distal tracheal injuries are best exposed through right-sided thoracotomy. However, when an associated vascular injury requires the use of a median sternotomy, division of the innominate vein and extensive mobilization of the aorta, superior vena cava, and arch vessels allows complete exposure of the trachea to the level of the carina.

TRACHEAL DISSECTION. Extensive dissection of the intrathoracic trachea prior to repair should be avoided. In most patients with tracheal transection, the two segments can easily be brought together without tension, and only rarely should additional length be needed because of loss of tracheal tissue.[100] However, up to 5 or even 6 cm of the trachea can be excised, if necessary, and a primary tracheal anastomosis can still be performed.[106]

AXIOM Tracheal dissection must be performed carefully to avoid disrupting the tracheal blood supply which comes in laterally or posterolaterally.

Tracheal dissection should be limited to the anterior and posterior surfaces of the trachea.[98,99] The tracheal blood supply, which comes in laterally, should be disturbed as little as possible. Martinez et al., however, found from cadaver dissections that the tracheal vessels join the distal trachea posterolaterally rather than directly lateral,[100] as previously described by Salassa et al.[107] Martinez et al. also observed that a substantial number of vessels from the esophagus join the trachea at its left posterolateral angle.[92] In addition, the anterior branch of the superior bronchial artery often enters the carina anteriorly and is an important source of collateral blood flow to the distal trachea.[107]

INTRAOPERATIVE AIRWAY MANAGEMENT. Airway management of a completely transected trachea requires close cooperation between surgeon and anesthesiologist. Direct cannulation of the distal trachea with a small (7.0 mm), sterile, cuffed tube can provide uninterrupted ventilation while the transected ends of the trachea are mobilized.[90]

TECHNIQUE OF REPAIR. Most reported repairs of a ruptured bronchus have been done with nonabsorbable sutures with good success.[66,92,97] However, most surgeons now use slowly absorbable materials because of the danger of suture granulomas.[108] The only patient who developed a scar obstruction in the series by Taskinen et al. was in a patient in whom Prolene suture was used.[87]

PROTECTING ANASTOMOSES

AXIOM Tracheal or bronchial repairs should be buttressed with viable tissue.

Use of a pedicled flap of pericardium, pleura, or intercostal muscle to wrap a tracheal or bronchial anastomosis reduces the risk of air leak and may promote healing.[90] When the tracheal repair is directly adjacent to the repair of a vascular injury, a pedicle flap should be used to separate the suture lines.

ASSOCIATED INJURIES. Goldfaden et al. believe that, with both tracheobronchial disruption and mediastinal contamination, associated major vascular injuries should be managed without using a prosthetic graft.[90] When the bronchial tear cannot be covered well, one should consider treating the vascular injury with a vein patch, vein interposition, or extraanatomical bypass through a separate sterile field.

DELAYED BRONCHIAL SURGERY

AXIOM Chronically atelectatic lung distal to traumatic bronchial strictures is usually worth preserving.

Delay in repair of injured bronchi increases the risk of infection and later stenosis. When bronchial stenosis develops, the stenotic segment can be excised and the bronchus reconstructed after the distal bronchus is thoroughly cleaned.[87] Reconstruction of the bronchus should be attempted regardless of the age of the injury when the lung tissue distal to the bronchial tear is functional. Successful reconstruction has been reported up to 26 years later.[109] However, if bronchial injury were extensive, if severe infection were present, or if the rupture were situated in a small bronchus, resection would be preferable to reconstruction.[66,84,92]

Postoperative Care

AXIOM Bronchial hygiene is especially important and can be difficult after bronchial repairs.

Postoperative management of the patient with tracheal or bronchial anastomosis requires careful attention to keeping the bronchi clear of secretions which tend to build up distal to suture lines. Careful endotracheal suctioning is needed so as not to disturb the suture line. Bronchoscopy may be required daily or more frequently when secretions are excessive or any atelectasis is present.[83] When the patient is alert and cooperative and has satisfactory ventilatory reserve, early extubation and restoration of the normal coughing mechanism are probably the best method for keeping the airway clear of secretions and preventing atelectasis.

OUTCOME

Mortality
In 1966, Chesterman and Satsangi reported an in-hospital mortality rate of 30% with major tracheobronchial injuries, and half of these victims died within the first hour.[93] Ecker et al. noted that the two major factors influencing survival in patients with tracheobronchial trauma were the associated injuries and the site of the tear.[80] Of 24 patients alive on arrival, only nine (38%) had major associated injuries; however, of 70 patients who were dead on arrival, an average of two associated injuries were present. In the patients alive on arrival, the cervical trachea was the predominate site of injury, whereas in those dead on arrival, the intrathoracic trachea was most frequently involved.

Complications
Delayed recognition of tracheobronchial injuries leads to chronic atelectasis and to the possibility of distal bronchopulmonary suppuration.[84,91,92] Of the 5 patients diagnosed promptly in the series by Baumgartner et al., 4 had excellent surgical outcomes.[83] The only complication was that of unilateral vocal cord paralysis, which may have been present before surgery. The fifth patient died as a direct result of the severity of the injury, which required a pneumonectomy, a procedure associated with high mortality.[83,110]

AXIOM Prompt diagnosis and treatment appear to be the best way to ensure a reduced incidence of complications after tracheobronchial trauma.

Delay in diagnosis was also detrimental in all 4 patients in the series by Baumgartner et al.[83] Two of the patients developed postoperative empyema or hilar abscess. The third patient developed hypertrophic granulation tissue which obstructed the repaired bronchus, and the fourth patient developed pneumonia, mediastinitis, and multiple-system organ failure.

Pulmonary Function

Normal pulmonary function cannot generally be expected when bronchial repair is delayed for more than six months; however, successful results have been reported after delays of nine and 11 years.[111,112] Taskinen et al. could not demonstrate functional differences in the distal lungs in patients with early or delayed bronchial repairs.[87]

Endotracheal Flame Burns

Many patients requiring prolonged ventilatory support have tracheostomy performed, usually some time between day 5-14. Because many of these patients require an $FiO_2 > 0.30$ during the procedure, the endotracheal tube may become ignited if electrocautery were used to control tracheal bleeding.[113] The resulting tracheobronchial burn is usually fatal.

Penetrating Trauma

AXIOM Penetrating injuries of the intrathoracic trachea or mainstem bronchi are unusual in patients who reach the hospital alive.

Kelly et al. reported on 106 patients with penetrating tracheobronchial injuries treated over 20 years at the Tulane Medical Center Hospital or the Charity Hospital of New Orleans; (Table 16-8) 78 of these injuries involved the cervical trachea.[114] Thus, the incidence of intrathoracic penetrating tracheobronchial injuries in this large trauma center was only about one per year. Of the patients with penetrating injuries in this area, most die before arrival at the hospital from associated cardiovascular injuries. Most of the injuries of the intrathoracic trachea or mainstem bronchi are caused by gunshot wounds. Most knives will not reach beyond the upper thoracic trachea.[115]

In the earlier series by Kelley et al., 55% of the penetrating tracheobronchial injuries were through-and-through and 45% were tangential.[115] The most significant associated injuries involved the esophagus or adjacent major vessels. Of 12 patients with penetrating thoracic tracheal injuries, associated injuries included adjacent major vessels in seven (58%) and esophagus in four (33%). Of ten patients with mainstem bronchial injuries, none had associated esophageal injury and only one (10%) had associated vascular injury.

The diagnosis of penetrating tracheobronchial injuries is made in a manner very similar to that used to diagnose blunt injuries; however, more emergency operations for severe bleeding from associated injuries are required for penetrating trauma.

AXIOM Penetrating tracheal trauma often has associated major vascular and/or esophageal injuries.

Associated vascular and esophageal injuries should be ruled out in any patient who has penetrating tracheal injury.[115] If the patient were hemodynamically stable, one could begin to rule out an injury with water-soluble contrast given by mouth. Because the incidence of false-negative examinations with gastrographin may exceed 25-50%, barium should be given when no leak is evident. Because

TABLE 16-8 Injuries Associated with Tracheobronchial Trauma

Associated Injury or Condition	Site of Primary Injury		
	Cervical Trachea (n=80)	Thoracic Trachea (n=13)	Bronchi (n=13)
Esophagus	20	4	0
Hemopneumothorax	17	12	13
Major vessel	9	7	1
Cardiac	1	2	1
Paraplegia	0	3	0
Pulmonary	0	2	14
Recurrent laryngeal nerve	6	1	0
Spinal cord	2	0	0
Horner's syndrome	1	0	0
Intraabdominal	4	7	3
Total	60	38	31

Kelly JP, Webb WR, Moulder PV, et al. Management of airway trauma I: tracheobronchial injuries. Ann Thorac Surg 1985;30:551.

barium esophagograms can have a false-negative rate of 10-25%, esophagoscopy should also be performed if the study is negative and one is still suspicious of esophageal injury. Winter and Weigelt believed that rigid esophagoscopy is more accurate than flexible endoscopy.[116] Nevertheless, even if all these studies are negative, the esophagus should be examined closely at surgery.

Treatment of penetrating tracheobronchial injuries is similar to that used for blunt trauma, and the outcome is largely dependent on the type and severity of the associated injuries. When the patient is not in shock on admission and has not aspirated large quantities of blood into the lungs, the mortality rate should be quite low.

⊘ FREQUENT ERRORS

In the Management of Trauma to the Chest Wall and Lungs

1. *Delaying intubation of patients with chest trauma and severe or persistent shock.*
2. *Aggressive hyperventilation following emergency endotracheal intubation.*
3. *Assuming an endotracheal tube is properly positioned because breath sounds can be heard over both sides of the upper chest anteriorly.*
4. *Promptly inserting a chest tube (without checking the position of the endotracheal tube) when the breath sounds are reduced on one side after endotracheal intubation.*
5. *Insisting on chest radiography prior to insertion of a decompressing needle or a chest tube in a patient with severe respiratory distress and/or shock that may be due to tension pneumothorax.*
6. *Failing to provide early monitoring with pulse oximetry or frequent arterial blood gases in patients with severe chest wall or lung trauma.*
7. *Assuming that a hemothorax or a pneumothorax is not present because they were not seen on a supine chest radiograph.*
8. *Closing or covering a sucking chest wound without prior or prompt insertion of a chest tube on that side.*
9. *Delay in inserting a chest tube in trauma patients with only subcutaneous emphysema when the patient will require ventilatory assistance.*
10. *Delayed or inadequate local pain relief in patients with multiple fractured ribs.*

11. *Delay in providing ventilatory assistance to a patient who has a flail chest and other significant injuries or severe preexisting pulmonary disease.*
12. *Failure to look carefully for possible associated injuries to the heart or great vessels in patients with fractures of the sternum or the first two ribs.*
13. *Delay in operating on patients with moderate-to-severe hemoptysis and/or air embolism after chest trauma.*
14. *Inadequate or delayed protection of the uninvolved lung in patients with intrabronchial bleeding.*
15. *Delayed or inadequate evacuation of a hemothorax after chest trauma.*
16. *Delayed thoracotomy in patients with thoracic trauma and continued unstable vital signs or persistent significant bleeding (> 200-300 mL/hr).*
17. *Failure to promptly perform bronchoscopy in a patient with a persistent pneumothorax and large air leak after insertion of a chest tube.*
18. *Failure to look for tracheobronchial or esophageal injury in patients with traumatic pneumomediastinum.*
19. *Failure to carefully look for vascular or esophageal injury in patients with penetrating thoracic tracheal trauma.*

▼▼▼▼▼▼▼▼▼▼▼▼▼▼▼▼▼▼▼▼▼▼▼▼▼▼▼▼▼▼

SUMMARY POINTS

1. Chest injuries frequently cause or contribute to 25-50% of deaths due to trauma in the United States annually.
2. The combination of shock and acute respiratory distress is highly lethal.
3. Cardiac arrests in the emergency department frequently occur during or just after endotracheal intubation.
4. One should not assume that the endotracheal tube is properly situated because breath sounds can be heard bilaterally in the upper chest.
5. When breath sounds are poor over the left hemithorax, one should check the position of the endotracheal tube before treating a hemopneumothorax.
6. Excessive ventilator pressures after endotracheal intubation in patients with severe trauma can be rapidly fatal.
7. One must be prepared to provide a surgical airway when any difficulty occurs in intubating a patient with acute respiratory distress.
8. Waiting for chest radiography to confirm the presence of a tension pneumothorax before treating it.
9. "Blind" chest tubes (without prior chest radiography) should be inserted high and only after finger exploration indicates that it is safe to insert the tube.
10. In patients with chest trauma, persistent impaired ventilation or hypoxemia in spite of other efforts (i.e., open airway, relief of chest wall pain, and drainage of hemopneumothorax) is an indication for ventilatory support.
11. Serial arterial and mixed venous blood gas values are more informative than isolated levels.
12. Continuous pulse oximetry should be part of the initial evaluation in anyone with severe chest trauma.
13. Failure to correct hypotension within 15-30 minutes greatly increases mortality rate.
14. One should not attempt to insert a catheter into a subclavian vein on the side opposite an injured lung because injuring both lungs can be rapidly fatal.
15. Excessive reliance on chest radiography may lead to delay in performing lifesaving procedures.
16. Without careful inspection of the chest wall, one can easily overlook contusions, flail chest, and open or "sucking" chest wounds.
17. Well-localized and consistent tenderness over ribs after chest trauma should be considered due to rib fractures even when initial chest radiographs or rib detail films appear to be normal.

18. Moderate hemothorax can easily be missed on chest radiographs taken while the patient is lying flat.
19. Before inserting a chest tube into a patient with acute respiratory distress and decreased breath sounds on one side, one should check the position of the endotracheal tube.
20. Probing of chest wounds can be dangerous.
21. Occluding a sucking chest wound without inserting a chest tube almost simultaneously can rapidly cause tension pneumothorax.
22. When an open chest wound exceeds two-thirds of the cross-sectional area of the trachea, effective ventilation may cease.
23. A chest tube should not be inserted through a penetrating chest wound because it is apt to follow the missile tract into the lung or diaphragm and damage those organs or restart massive bleeding.
24. Patients with subcutaneous emphysema after chest trauma should have a chest tube inserted before being placed on a ventilator.
25. Many clinically significant rib fractures cannot be visualized on initial radiography.
26. The main purpose of chest radiography in patients with possible fractured ribs is to eliminate associated hemothorax, pneumothorax, lung contusion, and other organ injury.
27. Rib belts and taping of the chest wall to relieve pain from fractured ribs should generally be avoided except in young, previously healthy individuals.
28. Epidural analgesia is frequently the ideal method for controlling chest wall pain so that a patient can cough and breathe deeply.
29. First-rib fractures usually have a higher incidence of associated injuries and death than other rib fractures.
30. Although the paradoxical motion of the chest wall in traumatic flail chest injuries can greatly increase the work of breathing, the main cause of hypoxemia is underlying lung contusion.
31. Prolonged, increased work of breathing without relief is apt to result in a respiratory arrest.
32. Fluid overloading should be prevented or rapidly corrected in patients with pulmonary contusion or ARDS.
33. Patients with isolated flail chest injuries can often be managed without ventilatory support, especially if the chest pain can be adequately relieved.
34. When a patient will require ventilatory support, it is much safer to apply it "prophylactically" before ventilatory failure develops.
35. Sternal fractures should make one look carefully for associated myocardial contusion.
36. The major cause of hypoxemia after blunt thoracic trauma is a pulmonary contusion.
37. Pulmonary contusions are generally much larger than one would suspect from initial chest radiography.
38. In patients with penetrating chest wounds, and particularly in those with hemoptysis, aggressive positive-pressure ventilation increases the risk of systemic air emboli.
39. Intrabronchial bleeding can rapidly cause flooding of dependent alveoli and severe hypoxemia.
40. With suspected aspiration, intubation and bronchoscopy should be performed as soon as possible.
41. Blood in the pleural cavity should be removed as completely and rapidly as possible.
42. Delaying thoracotomy in patients with severe intrathoracic bleeding or unstable vital signs can result in sudden cardiac arrest.
43. When one attempts to drain a traumatic hemothorax with needle thoracenteses, it is seldom completely successful and can cause air leaks, infections, or other complications.
44. Insertion of an exploratory finger before a chest tube is important if a chest radiograph has not been taken or when radiographs do not clearly show that the lung is away from the chest wall.
45. Failure to carefully note the location of the last hole of a chest tube on postinsertion chest radiography can result in air leaks and/or chest wall infections.
46. When the patient has an air leak, the chest tube should not be clamped, even when the patient is being transported.

47.   Although antibiotics can reduce the incidence of empyema and pneumonia in patients requiring a chest tube for a traumatic hemopneumothorax, the ideal duration of such treatment is not clear.

48.   One should obtain chest radiographs soon after admission and again in six hours or significant intrathoracic injuries may be overlooked

49.   When a tension pneumothorax is suspected in an unstable patient, it must be relieved as rapidly as possible.

50.   The combination of a pneumothorax space and continued air leak almost invariably results in pleural infection unless the pneumothorax can be corrected within 24-48 hours.

51.   Most posttraumatic pneumomediastinums are idiopathic, but when their source is not sought aggressively, rapidly lethal injuries may go untreated until too late.

52.   Blunt tracheobronchial injuries are rare, but frequently are rapidly fatal.

53.   A large air leak, mediastinal air, and persistent pneumothorax are due to tracheobronchial tear until proved otherwise.

54.   Elevated PCO_2 in patients with hypoxemia and/or metabolic acidosis can be highly lethal unless corrected rapidly.

55.   A "dropped lung" on an upright chest radiograph is virtually pathognomonic of a complete tear of a major bronchus.

56.   Fractures of the first two ribs may be associated with an increased incidence of cardiovascular and tracheobronchial injuries.

57.   Bronchoscopy should be performed in any patient with suspected airway injury.

58.   The accuracy of bronchoscopy in diagnosing tracheobronchial injuries depends to a large extent on the expertise of the endoscopist and the timing of endoscopy.

59.   Negative bronchoscopy by a relatively inexperienced endoscopist does not eliminate tracheobronchial injury.

60.   Many blunt tracheobronchial injuries are not diagnosed until after they cause stenosis and/or severe pulmonary infections.

61.   Physicians treating MVA victims must maintain a high index of suspicion for tracheobronchial disruptions in order to detect these rare lesions promptly.

62.   Double-lumen (split-function) endotracheal tubes can be very helpful in managing torn bronchi, but they can be difficult to insert promptly and properly.

63.   Flexible bronchoscopy can be of great help in diagnosing and intubating injured bronchi.

64.   Posterolateral right thoracotomy is generally the best incision for exploring tracheal and proximal right and left mainstem bronchial injuries.

65.   Tracheal dissection must be performed carefully to avoid disrupting the tracheal blood supply which enters laterally or posterolaterally.

66.   Tracheal or bronchial repairs should be buttressed with viable tissue.

67.   Chronically atelectatic lung distal to traumatic bronchial strictures is usually worth preserving.

68.   Bronchial hygiene is especially important but can be difficult after bronchial repairs.

69.   Prompt diagnosis and treatment appear to be the best way to ensure a reduced incidence of complications after tracheobronchial trauma.

70.   Penetrating injuries of the intrathoracic trachea or mainstem bronchi are unusual in patients who reach the hospital alive.

71.   Penetrating tracheal trauma often causes major associated vascular and/or esophageal injuries.

▲▲▲▲▲▲▲▲▲▲▲▲▲▲▲▲▲▲▲▲▲▲▲▲▲▲▲▲▲▲▲▲▲

REFERENCES

1. LoCicero J, Mattox KL. Epidemiology of chest trauma. Surg Clin North Am 1989;59:15.
2. Wilson RF, Gibson DEB, Antonenko D. Shock and acute respiratory failure after chest trauma. J Trauma 1977;17:697.
3. Moore EE, Malangoni MA, Cogbill TH, et al. Organ injury scaling IV: thoracic vascular, lung, cardiac, and diaphragm. J Trauma 1994; 36:299.
4. O'Flaherty D, Adams AP. The end-tidal carbon dioxide detector. Assessment of a new method to distinguish esophageal from tracheal intubation. Anesthesia 1990;45:653.
5. Dronen S, Chadwick O, Nowak R. Endotracheal tip position in the arrested patient. Ann Emerg Med 1982;11:116.
6. Yee ES, Verrier ED, Thomas AN. Management of air embolism in blunt and penetrating chest trauma. J Thorac Cardiovasc Surg 1983;85:661.
7. Estrera AS, Pass LJ, Platt MR. Systemic arterial air embolism in penetrating lung injury. Ann Thorac Surg 1900;50:257.
8. Wilson RF, Mammen E, Walt AJ. Eight years of experience with massive blood transfusions. J Trauma 1971;11:275.
9. Wilson RF. Complications of massive transfusions. Surgical Rounds 1981;4:47.
10. Freed HA, Shields NN. Most frequently overlooked radiographically apparent fractures in a teaching hospital emergency department. Ann Emerg Med 1984;13:900.
11. Nahum AM, Gadd CW, Schneider DC, et al. The biomechanical basis for chest impact protection: I. force-deflection characteristics of the thorax. J Trauma 1971;11:874.
12. Hunt DM, FJ Schwab. Chest Trauma. Rosen P, ed. Diagnostic radiology in emergency medicine. St. Louis: Mosby Yearbooks, 1992; 77.
13. Rosenblatt MS, Aldridge SC, Millham FH, et al. Temporary thoracotomy wound closure following penetrating thoracic aorta injury. Milit Med 1993;158:58.
14. Chaikhouni A, Dyaas CL Jr, Robinson JH, et al. Latissimus dorsi free myocutaneous flaps. J Trauma 1981;21:398.
15. Harris RD, Harris JH Jr. The prevalence and significance of missed scapular fractures in blunt chest trauma. AJR 1988;151:747.
16. Luchette FA, Radfshar MR, Kaiser R, et al. Prospective evaluation of epidural versus intrapleural catheters for analgesia in chest wall trauma. J Trauma 1993;35:165.
17. Reiestad F, Stromskag KE. Intrapleural catheter in the management of postoperative pain: a preliminary report. Reg Anaesth 1986;11:89.
18. Rocco A, Reiestad F, Gudman J, et al. Intrapleural administration of local anesthetics for pain relief in patients with multiple rib fractures: preliminary report. Reg Anaesth 1987;12:10.
19. Luchette FA, Radafshar SM, Kaiser R, et al. Prospective evaluation of epidural versus intrapleural catheter for analgesia in chest wall trauma. J Trauma 1994;36:865.
20. Wilson JM, Thomas AN, Goodman PC, et al. Severe chest trauma: morbidity implications of first and second rib fractures in 120 patients. Arch Surg 1978;113:846.
21. Ochi M, Sasashige Y, Murakami T, et al. Brachial plexus palsy secondary to stress fracture of the first rib: case report. J Trauma 1994; 38:128.
22. Bassett JS, Gibson RD, Wilson RF. Blunt injuries to the chest. J Trauma 1968;8:418.
23. Richardson JD, McElvein RB, Trinkle JK. First rib fracture—a hallmark of severe trauma. Ann Surg 1975;181:251.
24. Lee RB, Bass SM, Morris JA, MacKenzie EJ. Three or more rib fractures as an indicator for transfer to a level I trauma center: a population-based study. J Trauma 1990;30:689.
25. DB Campbell. Trauma to the chest wall, lung, and major airways. Semin Thorac Cardiovasc Surg 1992;4:234.
26. Brauer L. Erfahrungen and Uberlegungen zur Lungenkollapstherapie. Beitr Klin Tuberk 1909;12:49.
27. Maloney JV Jr, Schnutzer KJ, Raschke F. Paradoxical respiration and "pendelluft." J Thorac Cardiovasc Surg 1961;41:291.
28. Parham AM, Yarbrough DR III, Redding JS. Flail chest syndrome and pulmonary contusion. Arch Surg 1978;113:900.
29. Landercasper J, Cogbill TH, Strutt PJ. Delayed diagnosis of flail chest. Crit Care Med 1990;18:611.
30. Sankaran S, Wilson RF. Factors affecting prognosis in patients with flail chest. J Thorac Cardiovasc Surg 1970;60:402.
31. Avery FF, Morch ET, Benson WD. Critically crushed chests. A new method of treatment with continuous mechanical hyperventilation to produce alkalotic apnea and internal pneumatic stabilization. J Thorac Surg 1956;32:291.
32. Trinkle JK, Richardson JD, Franz JL, et al. Management of flail chest without mechanical ventilation. Ann Thorac Surg 1975;19:355.
33. Richardson JD, Franz JL, Grover FL, et al. Pulmonary contusion and hemorrhage: crystalloid versus colloid replacement. J Surg Res 1974; 16:330.

34. Cullen P, Modell JH, Kirby RR, et al. Treatment of flail chest: use of intermittent mandatory ventilation and positive end-expiratory pressure. Arch Surg 1975;110:1099.

35. Landreneau RJ, Hinson JM Jr, Hazelrigg SR, et al. Strut fixation of an extensive flail chest. Ann Thorac Surg 1991;51:473.

36. Borioni R, Ciani R, Guglielmo M, et al. Surgical stabilization of the chest wall. Ann Thorac Surg 1992;54:394.

37. Landercasper J, Cogbill TH, Lindesmith LA. Long-term disability after flail chest injury. J Trauma 1984;24:410.

38. Hamilton JR, Dearden C, Rutherford WH. Myocardial contusion associated with fracture of the sternum: important features of the seat belt syndrome. Injury 1984;16:155.

39. Restifo KM, Kelen GD. Case report: sternal fracture from a seatbelt. J Emerg Med 1994;12:321.

40. Shapira AR, Levi I, Khoda J. Sternal fractures: a red flag or red herring? J Trauma 1994;37:59.

41. Harley DP, Mena I. Cardiac and vascular sequelae of sternal fractures. J Trauma 1986;26:553.

42. Wojcik JB, Morgan AS. Sternal fractures—their natural history. Ann Emerg Med 1988;17:912.

43. Henley MB, Peter RE, Benirschke SK, et al. External fixation of sternum for thoracic trauma. J Ortho Trauma 1991;5:493.

44. Eijgelaar A, Homan van der Heide JN. A reliable early symptom of bronchial or tracheal rupture. Thorax 1970;25:120.

45. Fulton RL, Peter ET. The progressive nature of pulmonary contusion. Surgery 1970;67:499.

46. Trinkle JK, Furman RW, Hinshaw MA, et al. Pulmonary contusion. Ann Thorac Surg 1973;16:568.

47. Stellin G. Survival in trauma victims with pulmonary contusion. Am Surg 1981;57:780.

48. Hoff ST, Shotts SD, Eddy VA, et al. Outcome of isolated pulmonary contusion in blunt trauma patients. Am Surg 1994;60:138.

49. Diebel L, Wilson RF, Tagett MG, et al. End-diastolic volume: a better indicator of preload in the critically Ill. Arch Surg 1992;127:817.

50. Adoumie R, Shennib H, Brown R, et al. Differential lung ventilation. Applications beyond the operating room. J Thorac Cardiovasc Surg 1993;105:229.

51. Ganske JG, Dennis PL, Vanderveer JB. Traumatic lung cyst: case report and literature review. J Trauma 1981;21:493.

52. Campbell PR, Kerridge R. Fatal traumatic air embolism following a stab wound to the chest. Aust NZ J Surg 1993;63:307.

53. Rosato RM, Shapiro MJ, Keegan MJ, et al. Cardiac injury complicating traumatic asphyxia. J Trauma 1991;31:1387.

54. Ectors P, Bosschaert T, Vincent G, et al. Traumatic asphyxia: an unusual cause of traumatic coma and paraplegia. J Neurosurg 1979;51:375.

55. Landercasper J, Cogbill TH. Long-term follow-up after traumatic asphyxia. J Trauma 1985;25:838.

56. Jongewaard WR, Cogbill TH, Landercasper J. Neurologic consequences of traumatic asphyxia. J Trauma 1992;32:28.

57. Wilson RF, Soullier GW, Wiencek RG. Hemoptysis in trauma. J Trauma 1987;27:1123.

58. Washington B, Wilson RF, Steiger Z, Bassett JS. Emergency thoracotomy: a four-year review. Ann Thorac Surg 1985;40:188.

59. Esposita TJ, Jurkovich GJ, Rice C, et al. Reappraisal of emergency room thoracotomy in a changing environment. J Trauma 1991;31:881.

60. Ivatury RR, Kazigo J, Rohman M, et al. "Directed" emergency room thoracotomy: a prognostic prerequisite for survival. J Trauma 1991;31:1076.

61. Grover FL, Richardson JD, Fewel JG, et al. Prophylactic antibiotics in the treatment of penetrating chest wounds. J Thorac Cardiovasc Surg 1977;74:528.

62. Stone HH, Panagiotis NS, Hooper CA. Cefamandole for prophylaxis against infection in closed tube thoracostomy. J Trauma 1981;21:975.

63. LoCurto JJ Jr, Tischler CD, Swan KG, et al. Tube thoracostomy and trauma—antibiotics or not? J Trauma 1986;26:1067.

64. Brunner RG, Vinsant GO, Alexander RH, et al. The role of antibiotic therapy in the prevention of empyema in patients with an isolated chest injury (ISS 9-10): a prospective study. J Trauma 1990;30:1148.

65. Mandal AK, Montano J, Thadepalli H. Prophylactic antibiotics and no antibiotics compared in penetrating chest trauma. J Trauma 1985;25:639.

66. LeBlanc KA, Tucker WY. Prophylactic antibiotics and closed tube thoracostomy. Surg Gynecol Obstet 1985;160:259.

67. Fallon WF, Wears RL. Prophylactic antibiotics for the prevention of infectious complications including empyema following tube thoracostomy for trauma: results of meta-analysis. J Trauma 1992;33:110.

68. Cant PJ, Smyth S, Smart DO. Antibiotic prophylaxis is indicated for chest stab wounds requiring closed tube thoracostomy. Br J Surg 1993;80:464.

69. Demetriades D, Breckon V, Breckon C, et al. Antibiotic prophylaxis in penetrating injuries of the chest. Ann R Coll Surg Engl 1991;73:348.

70. Symbas PN. Autotransfusion from hemothorax: experimental and clinical studies. J Trauma 1972;12:689.

71. Thomas AN. Discussion of Graham et al. Innominate vascular injury. J Trauma 1982;22:655.

72. O'Brien J, Cohen M, Solit R, et al. Thoracoscopic drainage and decortication as definitive treatment for empyema thoracis following penetrating chest injury. J Trauma 1994;36:536.

73. Ordog GJ, Wasserberger J, Balasubramanian S, et al. Asymptomatic stab wounds of the chest. J Trauma 1994;36:680.

74. Collins JC, Levine G, Waxman K. Occult traumatic pneumothorax: immediate tube thoracostomy versus expectant management. Am Surg 1992;58:743.

75. Obeid FN, Shapiro MJ, Richardson HH, et al. Catheter aspiration for simple pneumothorax (CASP) in the outpatient management of simple traumatic pneumothorax. J Trauma 1985;25:882.

76. Nicholas JM, Dulchavsky SA. Successful use of autologous fibrin gel in traumatic bronchopleural fistula: case report. J Trauma 1992;32:87.

77. Rankin N, Day AC, Crone PD. Traumatic massive air leak treated with prolonged double lumen intubation and high frequency ventilation: case report. J Trauma 1994;36:428.

78. Carroll K, Cheeseman SH, Fink MP, et al. Secondary infection of posttraumatic pulmonary cavity lesions in adolescents and young adults: role of computed tomography and operative debridement and drainage. J Trauma 1989;29:109.

79. Hudgens S, McGraw J, Craun M. Two cases of tension pneumopericardium following blunt chest injury. J Trauma 1991;31:1408.

80. Ecker RR, Libertini RV, Rea WJ, et al. Injuries of the trachea and bronchi. Ann Thorac Surg 1971;11:289.

81. Bertelsen S, Howitz P. Injuries of the trachea and bronchi. Thorax 1972;27:188.

82. Iwasaki M, Kaga K, Ogawa J, et al. Bronchoscopy findings and early treatment of patients with blunt tracheo-bronchial trauma. J Cardiovasc Surg (Torino) 1994;35:269.

83. Baumgartner F, Sheppard B, de Virgilo C, et al. Tracheal and main bronchial disruptions after blunt chest trauma: presentation and management. Ann Thorac Surg 1990;50:569.

84. Kirsh MM, Orringer MB, Behrendt DM, et al. Management of tracheobronchial disruption secondary to nonpenetrating trauma. Ann Thorac Surg 1976;22:93.

85. McGrath JP. Burst trachea. Br J Surg 1968;55:77.

86. Jones WS, Mavroudis C, Richardson JD, et al. Management of tracheobronchial disruption resulting from blunt trauma. Surgery 1984;95:319.

87. Taskinen SO, Salo JA, Halttunen PEA, Sovijarvi ARA. Tracheobronchial rupture due to blunt chest trauma: a follow-up study. Ann Thorac Surg 1989;48:846.

88. Shimazu T, Sugimoto H, Nishide K, et al. Tracheobronchial rupture caused by blunt chest trauma: acute respiratory management. Am J Emerg Med 1988;6:427.

89. Limet R, Kerzman R, Janvier C, et al. Traumatic tracheobronchial ruptures. Acta Chir Belg 1981;80:41.

90. Goldfaden D, Seifert P, Milloy F, et al. Combined tracheal transection and innominate artery disruption from blunt chest trauma. Ann Thorac Surg 1986;41:213.

91. Barnhart GR, Brooks JW, Kellum JM. Pneumoperitoneum resulting from tracheal rupture following chest trauma. J Trauma 1986;26:486.

92. Deslauriers J, Beaulieu M, Archambault G, et al. Diagnosis and long-term follow-up of major bronchial disruptions due to nonpenetrating trauma. Ann Thorac Surg 1982;33:32.

93. Chesaterman JT, Stasangi PN. Rupture of the trachea and bronchi by closed injury. Thorax 1966;21:21.

94. Burke JF. Early diagnosis of traumatic rupture of the bronchus. JAMA 1962;181:682.

95. Masanes MJ, Legendre C, Lioret N, et al. Fiberoptic bronchoscopy for the early diagnosis of subglottal inhalation injury: comparative value in the assessment of prognosis. J Trauma 1994;36:59.

96. Stothert JC, Buttorff J, Kaminski DL. Thoracic esophageal and tracheal injury following blunt trauma. J Trauma 1980;20:992.

97. Roxburgh JC. Rupture of the tracheobronchial tree. Thorax 1987;42:681.

98. Burton NA, Watson DC, Brodsky JB, et al. Advantages of a new polyvinyl chloride double-lumen tube in thoracic surgery. Ann Thorac Surg 1983;36:78.

99. Burton NA, Fall SM, Lyons T, et al. Rupture of the left main stem bronchus and a polyvinyl chloride double-lumen tube. Chest 1983; 83:928.

100. Martinez MJ, Hotzman RS, Salcedo VM, Garcia-Rinaldi R. Successful repair of a transected intrathoracic trachea after chest trauma—brief communication. J Thorac Cardiovasc Surg 1986;91:307.

101. Dreyfuss D, Jackson RS, Coffin LH, et al. High-frequency ventilation in the management of tracheal trauma. J Trauma 1986;26: 287.

102. Hanzawa T, Yoshioka O, Fujiwara S, et al. The effects of high-frequency jet oscillation on severe respiratory failure accompanied by injuries of the major bronchus. J Intensive Care Med 1982;6:961.

103. Kaiser KG, Davies NJH, Rodriguez-Roisin R, et al. Efficacy of high-frequency ventilation in presence of extensive ventilation-perfusion mismatch. J Appl Physiol 1985;58:996.

104. Kinsella TJ, Johnsrud LW. Traumatic rupture of the bronchus. J Thorac Surg 1947;16:571.

105. Hood RM, Sloan HE. Injuries of the trachea and major bronchi. J Thorac Cardiovasc Surg 1959;38:458.

106. Grillo HC. Surgical treatment of postintubation tracheal injuries. J Thorac Cardiovasc Surg 1979;78:860.

107. Salassa JR, Pearson BW, Payne WS. Gross and microscopical blood supply of the trachea. Ann Thorac Surg 1977;24:100.

108. Juttner FM, Pinter H, Popper H, et al. Reconstructive surgery for tracheobronchial injuries including complete disruption of the right main bronchus. Thorac Cardiovasc Surg 1984;32:174.

109. Webb WR. Diagnosis and long-term follow-up of major bronchial disruptions due to nonpenetrating trauma. Ann Thorac Surg 1992;33:38.

110. Bowling R, Mavroudis C, Richardson JD, et al. Emergency pneumonectomy for penetrating and blunt trauma. Am Surg 1985;51:136.

111. Mahaffey DE, Greech O, Boren HG, DeBakey ME. Traumatic rupture of the left main bronchus successfully repaired eleven years after injury. J Thorac Surg 1956;32:312.

112. Nonoyama A, Masuda A, Kasahara K, et al. Total rupture of the left main bronchus successfully repaired nine years after injury. Ann Thorac Surg 1976;21:445.

113. Lew EO, Mittleman RE, Murray D. Endotracheal tube ignition by electrocautery during tracheostomy: case report with autopsy findings. J Forensic Sci 1991;36:1586.

114. Kelly JP, Webb WR, Moulder PV, et al. Management of airway trauma II: combined injuries of the trachea and esophagus. Ann Thorac Surg 1987;43:260.

115. Kelly JP, Webb WR, Moulder PV, et al. Management of airway trauma I: tracheobronchial injuries. Ann Thorac Surg 1985;40:551.

116. Winter RP, Weigelt JA. Cervical esophageal trauma, incidence and cause of esophageal fistulas. Arch Surg 1990;125:849.

Chapter 17 Thoracic Trauma: Heart

ROBERT F. WILSON, M.D.

LARRY W. STEPHENSON, M.D.

The insulting victor withdrew the weapon from his panting heart. From the wide wound gush'd out a stream of blood. And the soul issued in the purple flood. —The Iliad, Homer

PENETRATING INJURY TO THE HEART

Introduction

HISTORY

Hippocrates realized the fatal nature of cardiac wounds.[1] In 1679, Roilanus suggested pericardiocentesis as a treatment for cardiac wounds, and in 1829 Larrey successfully drained a hemopericardium due to a stab wound.[2]

In spite of the usual fatal consequences of untreated cardiac injury, Theodore Billroth (1829-1894), is often quoted as having said "anyone who attempts to surgically correct an injury to the heart will lose the respect of his colleagues."[1] There are scholars, however, who claim that he never made that statement.[3] Nevertheless, surgeons were becoming more interested in the heart. In 1882, Block first successfully sutured a heart (in rabbit), and in 1895 deVecchio sutured stab wounds of the heart in dog and demonstrated successful healing. The first successful repair of a stab wound of the heart was performed by Ludwig Rehn in Frankfurt-am-Main, in Germany in 1896.[4] Daniel Halo Williams in 1893 closed a tear in the pericardium in a patient with a stab wound that apparently also injured the right ventricle. The ventricle was not sutured, however, because it was not bleeding. He reported this case four years later.[5] In 1902, Luther Hill of Montgomery, Alabama, repaired a stab of the heart in a 13-year-old boy by the light of kerosene lamps on a kitchen table.[6] In 1926, Claude Beck gave the first English description of the steps to be used in repair of heart wounds.[4] He reviewed the history of this type of surgery, translated Sauerbruch's earlier work on the subject, and presented his own experimental observations on the techniques to be employed.

PROGNOSIS

In various studies, it has been shown that 50-81% of patients with cardiac wounds succumb shortly after the injury, either from cardiac tamponade or bleeding.[7,8] Bullet wounds are particularly likely to cause death quickly.[1] Of patients lucky enough to reach medical attention, the most important factors for survival are early diagnosis and immediate treatment. One recent attempt to quantitate anatomical and physiologic cardiac injuries correlated quite well with survival rates.[9] All patients admitted with penetrating chest injuries anywhere near the heart plus shock should be considered to have cardiac injuries until proved otherwise.[10,11] Even when no evidence of cardiac involvement exists and the patient is asymptomatic and hemodynamically stable, sudden deterioration can occur later, as did four patients of Ordog et al.[12] resulting in two deaths.

AXIOM Patients with penetrating wounds of the chest, especially from stab wounds, can often be successfully resuscitated from a recent (<5 min) cardiac arrest by emergency resuscitative thoracotomy.

With early, aggressive resuscitation and surgery, up to one-third of patients arriving at a trauma center "in extremis" with cardiac injuries can be saved.[13] For patients who can be brought to the operating room with signs of life and a recordable blood pressure, the survival rate should exceed 70% for gunshot wounds of the heart and 85% for stab wounds of the heart.[12] In one series, 23 consecutive patients with isolated penetrating injuries of the heart reaching the operating room alive survived.[11]

Pathophysiology

Penetrating wounds of the heart are usually rapidly fatal, generally because of massive hemorrhage. Patients surviving more than 15-30 minutes usually have relatively small cardiac wounds or some component of pericardial tamponade.[14] In a sense, pericardial tamponade is a two-edged sword; although it may prolong life by reducing the severity of the initial blood loss, it can also be fatal by interfering with venous return and diastolic filling of the heart. Thus, its effects on survival are not clear.[15]

AXIOM Pericardial tamponade increases the likelihood of emergency resuscitative thoracotomy for penetrating heart wound being successful.

The parietal pericardium sac normally contains tough, inelastic tissue that cannot easily accommodate rapid accumulation of more than 80-100 ml of fluid without greatly affecting the intrapericardial pressure and cardiac output. At that point, an additional 20-40 ml of pericardial fluid can almost double the intrapericardial pressure, thereby greatly restricting cardiac filling and cardiac output.[16]

The increased intrapericardial pressure during tamponade causes an increased diastolic pressure in all chambers.[17] The decreased diastolic filling of the heart reduces stroke volume, cardiac output, and arterial blood pressure. The decreased blood pressure initially causes a decrease in subendocardial perfusion and with further increase in pericardial pressure, a decrease in both subendocardial and subepicardial myocardial perfusion occurs.[18]

To compensate for the decreasing arterial pressure and cardiac output caused by the tamponade, sympathetic stimulation causes an increased heart rate and arterial, venous, and splenic constriction.[2,15-17] This raises BP and causes an increased venous return. If the tamponade is not too severe, these can help restore cardiac output and tissue perfusion back to normal.

Diagnosis

CLINICAL FEATURES

AXIOM All patients in shock with penetrating chest wounds between the midclavicular line on the right and anterior axillary line on the left should be considered to have cardiac injuries until proved otherwise.

If the only problem with a penetrating heart wound is tamponade and the patient is not hypovolemic, the Beck I triad may be present. This includes distended neck veins, hypotension, and muffled heart tones. The Beck I triad can be very deceptive, and many false-positive and false-negative findings do occur.[10] Although patients with penetrating heart wounds are usually hypotensive, the neck veins will generally not be distended until the blood volume is at least partly restored.

AXIOM The neck veins in patients with shock from pericardial tamponade will not usually become distended until coexistent hypovolemia is at least partly corrected.

When fluids are given rapidly to a patient with a cardiac wound who has stopped bleeding and now has only pericardial tamponade, the vital signs often improve rapidly after the filling pressures are increased by rapid administration of crystalloids and other blood volume expanders.[19]

AXIOM Distended neck veins after chest trauma are not always due to pericardial tamponade.

Chest injuries can cause patients to breathe abnormally or strain, thereby raising the CVP and distending the neck veins in the absence of tamponade. A tension pneumothorax, mediastinal hematoma, or heart failure can also cause the CVP to rise and BP to fall.

AXIOM Muffled heart tones are a very insensitive and nonspecific sign of pericardial tamponade.

Even with a large, acute pericardial tamponade, which seldom is more than 150-200 ml, the heart tones are usually fairly clear, and muffled heart sounds are the least reliable sign in Beck's triad. Although the experience of Wilson and Basset suggested that the Beck I triad is falsely positive or negative at least one-third of the time,[10] Demetriades found it positive in 77% of patients with proved tamponade.[7]

Tamponade may also cause two Kussmaul signs. One is increased distension of neck veins during inspiration and the other is pulsus paradoxus. Paradoxical pulse is characterized by a decrease in systolic blood pressure of >10-15 mm Hg during normal inspiration. The "paradoxical" pressure decrease is best determined by listening carefully while taking multiple cuff blood pressures. One notes the highest systolic blood pressure at which only one Korotkoff's sound is heard during a ventilatory cycle and then subtracts the highest systolic blood pressure at which all of the Korotkoff's sounds are heard. The difference between these two pressures is the amount of paradox present. The amount of paradox may be increased by hypovolemia; bronchospasm is the most frequent cause of pulsus paradoxus in hospitalized patients.

INVASIVE MONITORING

An increasing volume of blood in the pericardial cavity causes a rise in diastolic pressures in all cardiac chambers; so an equalization of diastolic pressures in all chambers should make one suspicious of pericardial tamponade. At the same time, stroke volume tends to fall. The rise in filling pressure and fall in stroke volume and blood pressure may be difficult to differentiate from heart failure of other causes. The circumstances of the injury and the equalization of diastolic pressures on both the right and the left sides of the heart, however, should increase the suspicion of tamponade.

AXIOM Equalization of cardiac diastolic filling pressures following chest trauma should make one suspicious of pericardial tamponade.

An abrupt decrease in atrial pressures at the beginning of diastole followed by a high, flat-pressure wave may produce a wave form that has been referred to as the "square-root sign" (Fig. 17-1). Acute right ventricular infarction can cause similar changes; it tends to flatten the atrial waves somewhat and reduce the amount of the X descent.[20] With constrictive pericarditis, the X descent may almost disappear and the wave pattern is even flatter. Although central venous pressure (CVP) measurements can also help make these diagnoses, a CVP catheter that is inserted too far can perforate the heart. Aldridge and Jay studied 61 such patients who had a mortality rate exceeding 50%.[21]

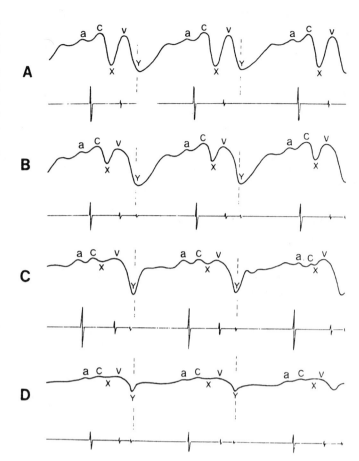

FIGURE 17-1 **A.** Normal right atrial or central venous pressure waves. **B.** A right ventricular infarction or acute right ventricular failure can flatten the atrial waves somewhat and reduce the amount of the X descent. **C.** With constrictive pericarditis, the X descent may almost disappear. **D.** With tamponade, there may be no X descent and the Y descent may become much smaller; the atrial waves also tend to be very flat. With right ventricular infarction, constrictive pericarditis, and pericardial tamponade, the right and left heart diastolic pressures tend to be equal. (From: Wilson RF. Injury to the heart and great vessel. Henning RJ, Grenvik A, eds. Critical care cardiology. New York: Churchill Livingstone, 1989; 414.)

RADIOGRAPHY

If at all possible, a chest radiograph should be obtained on all trauma victims before they are brought to the operating room. Chest films are of little help, however, in diagnosing acute cardiac injury except in unusual cases with intrapericardial air. Because the average acute tamponade has only 150-200 ml of blood and clots, significant early enlargement of the cardiac shadow is unusual.[10] For example, if the heart were considered a sphere with a radius of 5.0 cm, its volume would be 524 cm^3; if the radius were increased by only 0.5 cm, the volume would increase by 176 cm^3 to 700 cm^3. Chest radiography may, however, reveal hemopneumothorax or other mediastinal pathology that may make one more suspicious of cardiac injury.

ECG

ECG changes following cardiac injury are usually nonspecific. ST-T-wave changes may indicate pericardial irritation, ischemia, or myocardial damage. New Q waves generally indicate a full thickness myocardial infarction.

ECHOCARDIOGRAPHY

Two-dimensional echocardiography is a fairly reliable method of detecting the presence of increased quantities of intrapericardial fluid and can be used to diagnosis tamponade rather reliably.[22] It may also help localize missile fragments in the pericardium;[16] however, it is often not immediately available, and occasional false-positive and -negative results occur. In some instances, the intrapericardial blood moves to the most dependent portions of the pericardial cavity and can be missed with this technique. Hemothorax may also interfere with the accuracy of the ECHO diagnosis of pericardial effusion.[23]

PERICARDIOCENTESIS

AXIOM   If blood is obtained on pericardiocentesis and the patient's vital signs improve promptly, a tamponade was almost certainly present.

Accuracy

The use of pericardiocentesis as a diagnostic procedure is increasingly avoided in acutely injured patients with possible tamponade. In at least one series, the incidence of false-negative pericardiocentesis was 80%, and the incidence of false-positives was 33%.[7] In addition to its inaccuracy, pericardiocentesis may injure the heart and/or cause dangerous delays in needed surgery.

Technique

Almost all pericardiocenteses are now done via the paraxiphoid approach (Fig. 17–2). An 18-gauge, 10 cm spinal needle attached to a stopcock and then a 20 ml syringe can be used. Pericardiocentesis should be done with continuous ECG monitoring if possible. The needle is passed upward and backward at an angle of 45° for 4-5 cm and advanced slowly until the tip seems to enter a cavity. Most authors direct the needle toward the left scapula tip; however, directing the needle toward the right scapula is more likely to parallel the right border of the heart and less likely to penetrate the right ventricle.

One should aspirate frequently as the needle is advanced; when no blood is obtained, one can insert a stylet or inject 0.2-0.5 ml of saline at intervals to be certain that the needle is not plugged. The

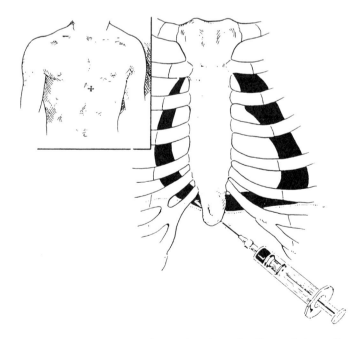

FIGURE 17–2   The paraxiphoid technique for pericardiocentesis is usually performed with the needle directed toward the left scapula tip. However, when one aims toward the tip of the right scapula, the needle tends to go parallel to the lateral border of the right heart and is less apt to penetrate the myocardium. (From: Wilson RF. Injury to the heart and great vessel. Henning RJ, Grenvik A, eds. Critical care cardiology New York: Churchill Livingstone, 1989; 415.)

needle is then carefully pushed farther, about 1-2 mm at a time, until blood is obtained, cardiac pulsations are felt, or ECG shows an abrupt change, usually PVCs or abrupt ST-T-wave changes.

AXIOM   When a large amount (>20 ml) of blood can be aspirated rapidly and easily during attempted pericardiocentesis, it is likely that one is aspirating blood from the right ventricle rather than the pericardial cavity.

Generally, with penetrating trauma, one-half to two-thirds of the blood in the pericardial cavity is clotted. Consequently, one can usually remove only 4-5 ml of blood without manipulating the end of the needle. When 20 ml of blood can be drawn out easily and rapidly, it usually indicates that the blood is being aspirated from the right ventricular cavity.

When immediate thoracotomy is not possible in a patient with positive pericardiocentesis, a plastic catheter inserted over a needle or Seldinger wire can be left in place for continuous or intermittent drainage of intrapericardial blood until the cardiac wound can be repaired.

Complications

Pericardiocentesis is not without danger. Holes in the right ventricle are frequently found at thoracotomy after attempts at pericardiocentesis. The needle occasionally can cause a fairly large hole or laceration in the right ventricle or a coronary artery and produce a tamponade. This is most apt to happen if the procedure were performed on a restless, uncooperative patient. Other complications, such as arrhythmias, may also occur. A negative pericardiocentesis may also give a false feeling of security that cardiac injury is not present.

SUBXIPHOID PERICARDIAL WINDOW

Another alternative for diagnosis of pericardial tamponade is a subxiphoid pericardial window.[24,25] (Fig. 17–3). This can be done under local anesthesia in cooperative individuals, but is generally performed more safely under general anesthesia. When blood is found and the patient is under general anesthesia, the incision can be extended up as a mid sternotomy to repair the cardiac wound. Unfortunately, if the pericardial window were done under local anesthetic on a restless patient, it could be extremely difficult to perform. Furthermore, if a cardiac wound were found, massive exsanguination may occur by the time the surgeon would be able to perform a thoracotomy and control the bleeding.

An ideal situation for this procedure is an individual who has a penetrating wound near the heart, but has always been hemodynamically stable. In such patients, a subxiphoid pericardial window may reveal a pericardial injury with or without myocardial injury in up to 18% of patients.[26,27] However, it is not known whether any of those patients would have had a problem if the cardiac wound had not been discovered. It is estimated that only a small percentage of such patients would have difficulty without surgery.

A subcostal or subxiphoid window is also an excellent technique for draining pericardial fluid and/or biopsying the pericardium in less emergent situations.[28] If bowel obstruction and signs of tamponade were to develop following blunt trauma, one should suspect a pericardial diaphragmatic hernia.[29]

Treatment

FLUID REPLACEMENT

In patients who are hypotensive and have low cardiac output or poor tissue perfusion, the intravascular volume should be expanded by rapid intravenous infusion of normal (0.9%) saline or Ringer's lactate to increase right atrial and ventricular filling.[26] If the patient's blood volume status is not clear, one should watch the response of the CVP to the fluid challenges. When the CVP does not rise as fluid is given rapidly, one can continue to give fluid until the BP and tissue perfusion are adequate. When the CVP rises abruptly with no

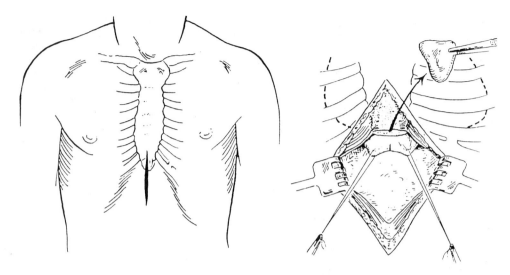

FIGURE 17–3 A subxiphoid pericardial window can be performed under local anesthesia in stable patients with suspected paricardial tamponade. The xiphoid process may be removed or split. The diaphragmatic pericardium is pulled inferiorly with traction sutures to facilitate incision of the pericardium. When blood is present in the pericardium, general anesthesia is immediately administered and the incision is extended superiorly into a median sternotomy. (From: Wilson RF. Injury to the heart and great vessel. Henning RJ, Grenvik A, eds. Critical care cardiology. New York: Churchill Livingstone, 1989; 416.)

improvement in tissue perfusion, the patient probably needs inotropic agents to improve tissue perfusion.

Although the quickest way to correct hypotension due to pericardial tamponade is to increase preload by rapid infusion of intravenous fluids, the patient's condition can deteriorate rapidly if the increased preload and intracardiac pressures restart bleeding from the cardiac wound prior to thoracotomy.[30]

> **AXIOM** One of the quickest and most effective ways to restore adequate tissue perfusion in a hemodynamically unstable patient is aggressive fluid resuscitation.

PERICARDIOCENTESIS

If it is not possible to perform emergency thoracotomy almost immediately in a patient with cardiac injury and hypotension, a pericardiocentesis should be performed promptly to relieve suspected tamponade. Ideally, this is done with a catheter over a needle to continue to aspirate pericardial fluid as necessary.

Pericardiocentesis is primarily a diagnostic procedure, but removal of as little as 5-10 ml of blood from the pericardial sac in a hypotensive patient may increase stroke volume by 25-50% with dramatic improvement in cardiac output and blood pressure. In selected patients who have small puncture wounds of the heart, pericardiocentesis may be curative, and the patient may not require thoracotomy as long as the vital signs remain stable.[31]

NONOPERATIVE MANAGEMENT

An occasional, highly selected, stable patient with a small, penetrating cardiac injury may be successfully treated without surgery;[32] however, virtually all patients with shock and suspected injuries to the heart should have emergency thoracotomy to completely relieve the tamponade and to repair any injuries found. An almost immediate thoracotomy is particularly important when the patient's condition deteriorates and/or the patient has a cardiac arrest.

EMERGENCY DEPARTMENT THORACOTOMY

> **AXIOM** Penetrating wounds of the heart are best treated with emergency thoracotomy and cardiorrhaphy.

In hospitals where adequate facilities, equipment, and trained personnel are present, an emergency department (ED) thoracotomy may be lifesaving.[33] In one study, it was believed that ED thoracotomy for penetrating cardiac injuries is essential for patients who are: (a) clinically dead on arrival in the ED but had some signs of life in transit

(survival: 32%), or (b) deteriorating and have no obtainable blood pressure (survival: 33%). However, ED thoracotomies for patients with no signs of life at the scene or within five minutes of arrival in the ED are almost invariably futile. Cardiac arrest from blunt trauma or from penetrating brain or abdominal injuries is also almost uniformly fatal.[11,33-40]

Cardiac arrest in the hospital from penetrating heart trauma is most apt to occur as the patient enters the ED. The second most frequent time for an injured patient to have cardiac arrest in the ED is during or just after endotracheal intubation (Table 17–1). Such cardiac arrests are usually due to: (a) inadequate preintubation oxygenation, (b) intubation of the esophagus or right mainstem bronchus, or (c) excessive ventilatory pressures reducing venous return or causing tension pneumothorax or air embolism.

ED thoracotomy for penetrating cardiac injury may be lifesaving for patients deteriorating so rapidly that it is not likely that they will survive movement from the ED to the operating room;[11] however, implementation of ED thoracotomy should be selective. Indiscriminate use of this technique is wasteful of time and supplies, and it may increase mortality and morbidity.[4] Furthermore, one must have the appropriate backup from the operating room and surgeons.

> **AXIOM** Resuscitative thoracotomy for trauma should not be performed unless rapid, appropriate backup by the operating room and surgeons is available to properly manage intrathoracic injuries that are likely to be found.

The goal of ED thoracotomy is not merely resuscitation of cardiovascular activity, but also salvage of central neurologic function. Factors that correlate with survival following ED thoracotomy include the site of injury,[31-43] mechanism of injury,[11,44] signs of life at the scene and on admission to the ED,[32,43] cardiac activity at thoracotomy,[43] EKG activity,[33,44] systolic blood pressure response to thoracic aortic occlusion,[42] and the depth of shock on admission.[44] Patients

TABLE 17–1 Causes of Cardiac Arrest During or Just After Endotracheal Intubation

1. Inadequate oxygenation of the patient before intubation
2. Esophageal intubation
3. Mainstem bronchial intubation
4. Excessive ventilatory pressures retarding venous return
5. Excessive ventilatory pressures causing a tension pneumothorax
6. Air embolism
7. Vasovagal response
8. Excessive respiratory alkalosis

with isolated stab wounds of the heart and obtainable BPs on admission have survival rates often exceeding 90%.[45]

Prior to ED thoracotomy, prediction of the amount of neurologic recovery to be expected is extremely difficult. Cogbill et al. noted a correlation between spontaneous respirations at the time of ambulance pickup and ultimate neurologic recovery,[41] while Baker et al. suggested that a response to verbal and noxious stimuli prior to ED thoracotomy is an important prognosticator of neurologic recovery.[46] Postoperatively, early return to consciousness within 12 hours usually indicates an excellent ultimate neurologic recovery.[42]

ANESTHESIA

Whenever the patient can be moved to the operating room with reasonable safety, emergency thoracotomy should be performed there. Thoracotomy is performed with the patient under light general anesthesia administered through an orotracheal tube. If the patient is deeply comatose or in extremis, the operation may be begun without general anesthesia.

General anesthesia with drugs such as ketamine that have little or no cardiodepressant action, cause the least hemodynamic impairment. In both animals and humans, ketamine has been shown to increase blood pressure, heart rate, and cardiac output, and it has antiarrhythmic properties.

INCISION FOR ED THORACOTOMY

Once the patient is intubated, anterolateral thoracotomy is performed in the left fifth intercostal space, one interspace below the male nipple (Fig. 17–4). The incision should be as long as possible, extending

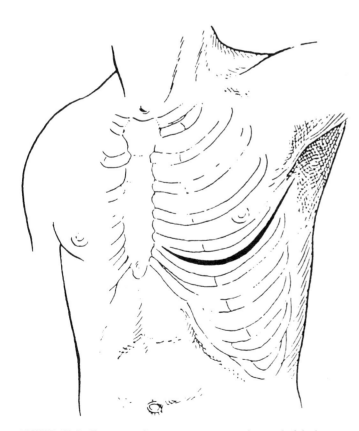

FIGURE 17–4   Emergency thoracotomy to treat a stab wound of the heart or to perform open cardiac massage is usually done through an anterolateral thoracotomy incision. The incision extends along the fifth intercostal space with the skin incision placed in the inframammary crease. It extends from just lateral to the sternum to the midaxillary line. (From: Wilson RF. Injury to the heart and great vessel. Henning RJ, Grenvik A, eds. Critical care cardiology. New York: Churchill Livingstone, 1989; 418.)

from about 1.5 cm lateral to the sternum, to the midaxillary line in the axilla. In females, the breast is displaced upward, and the skin incision is made through the breast crease. The incision extends through the intercostal muscles just above the sixth rib into the pleural cavity, being careful not to injure the underlying lung or heart. A rib-spreader is then inserted and opened widely until two hands can fit inside the chest. Cutting the intercostal cartilages above and below the incision may help increase exposure. Not infrequently the internal mammary vessels, which lay about 0.5-1.0 cm lateral to the sternum, are cut with the medial extension of this incision; when this occurs, the vessels must be securely clamped and tied or suture-ligated. Unfortunately, one could waste 5-10 minutes gaining control of the internal mammary vessels if they were accidently cut. Therefore, one should make an effort to avoid this problem.

> **AXIOM**   Injuries to the mid or left chest in unstable patients are best explored through the left chest and lesions on the right are explored through the right chest.

When the injury is to the right of the sternum, right thoracotomy is initially performed to control any bleeding sites, but strong consideration should be given to extending the incision across the sternum as bilateral thoracotomy so as to be able to also compress or clamp the descending aorta and to massage the heart, if needed, more effectively. The right and left anterolateral incisions are connected by transverse division of the sternum using a rib cutter. This allows wide exposure to both sides of the heart and to the proximal great vessels, but requires control of both internal mammary arteries.

In the patient with cardiac arrest, usually minimal bleeding occurs from the thoracotomy incision until circulation is restored; however, when spontaneous cardiac activity is restored, incisional bleeding may become severe, especially from the internal mammary vessels.

> **AXIOM**   If the patient were relatively stable and the cardiac injury were likely to be anterior (as with anterior stab wounds), median sternotomy could be used to explore the chest.

Although anterolateral incision may be preferred in the ED for patients who have arrested and/or are profoundly hypotensive and may need to have the descending aorta clamped, a median sternotomy has many advantages in the operating room. A median sternotomy can provide exceptional exposure of the anterior heart. This incision is preferred by most surgeons who routinely perform cardiac surgery.

PERICARDIOTOMY

Even when the pericardial sac is not distended with blood at thoracotomy, it can be difficult to grasp the pericardium with a pickup or forceps. It may be necessary, at times, to "hook" the pericardium with one blade of a scissors and then grab it with a forceps or clamp. Another technique is to carefully incise the pericardium near the apex of the heart with a knife to produce a hole just big enough to allow the tip of one blade of a scissors. However, if a scalpel were used to open the pericardial sac, inadvertent injury to the underlying myocardium or left anterior descending coronary artery could easily occur.

The pericardial sac should be opened with a scissors in a longitudinal direction 1-2 cm anterior to the left (or right) phrenic nerve. The pericardial incision should extend from the diaphragm below up to the pericardial reflection anteriorly on the ascending aorta. When the pericardial sac is still tight around the heart, a transverse cut of the pericardium inferiorly along the diaphragm may greatly help with exposure. After the pericardium is open, the surgeon should evacuate any liquid blood and clots and begin open cardiac massage if it is needed. If a cardiac wound is seen, it should quickly be sutured, in between episodes of cardiac massage. If it is not convenient to suture the myocardial wound at that time, finger pressure can usually control the bleeding. A Foley catheter balloon can also be used to occlude the hole while it is being repaired.

CLAMPING THE DESCENDING AORTA

The second maneuver in the patient with severe hypotension or cardiac arrest is compression or clamping of the descending thoracic aorta to help improve coronary and cerebral arterial flow. Because >60% of cardiac output goes through the descending thoracic aorta, cross-clamping it can increase blood flow to the coronary and cerebral arteries by two- to three-fold.

> **AXIOM** Compressing the descending aorta in a severely hypotensive patient can greatly increase coronary and cerebral blood flow.

To expose the descending aorta, an assistant on the right side of the patient pulls the left lung anteromedially as far as safely possible. The surgeon then dissects the lower descending thoracic aorta under direct vision. The tissue can usually be in front of the aorta opened bluntly, but the tougher posterior tissue between the aorta and the vertebral bodies often has to be incised sharply. When the aorta has been adequately exposed and freed from its investing tissue, the surgeon can pass a finger or a vascular clamp around the aorta. In this way, the aortic clamping is performed under direct vision, and the chances of intercostal arterial or esophageal injuries are reduced. After the clamp is applied, the time is noted, and the left lung is allowed to drop back into the thorax. To be sure that the clamp is applied properly, one should feel pulsations above the clamp, but none below. If a nasogastric tube were not in place and little or no blood pressure were evident, one could easily mistake the esophagus for the aorta.

CLAMPING INJURED LUNG

> **AXIOM** The first step to control bleeding from injured lung and to reduce the risk of air emboli and aspiration of blood into dependent, uninjured lung tissue is to clamp the hilum.

If the lung injury were peripheral, it should be controlled promptly with a vascular or lung clamp to prevent systemic air embolism and to stop the bleeding and air leak until more definitive control could be accomplished. When a large, central lung injury occurs with bleeding, one should apply a vascular clamp across the hilum proximal to the injury. If the hilar clamp does not control the bleeding because the injury is too close to the heart, one may have to clamp the pulmonary vessels inside the pericardium.

EXPOSING THE HEART

Once the heart is in view, the surgeon should rapidly inspect the chambers that are most likely to be injured. When the stab wound is on the right side of the sternum, the cardiac injury almost always involves the right ventricle (RV) or right atrium (RA). When the entrance wound is on the left side of the sternum, the right and left ventricles are almost equally involved. If a cardiac injury cannot be seen, the heart can be swung out laterally and anteriorly into the left hemithorax to allow better examination. If it were necessary to lift the tip of the heart up, the surgeon should be cautious because this would increase the possibility of air entry into left-sided or posterior cardiac wounds. This could result in sudden, fatal coronary or cerebral air embolism.

CONTROLLING CARDIAC WOUNDS

Most atrial wounds can be temporarily controlled by the application of a Satinsky vascular clamp and then sewn with a running 3-0 or 4-0 polypropylene suture. One can also frequently control bleeding with finger compression or an inflated Foley catheter. Wounds of the ventricles can generally be tamponaded by the surgeon's finger while pledgetted horizontal mattress sutures of 2-0 silk or prolene are passed under the finger and tied by an assistant. When a wound

is situated next to a major coronary artery, a pledgetted horizontal mattress suture is placed beneath the artery so as to avoid ligation or compression of the vessel[47] (Fig. 17–5). When the left anterior descending coronary artery is involved, use of unnecessarily wide or multiple sutures can cause increased damage to the septal perforating branches.

> **AXIOM** Many open cardiac wounds can be controlled well by inserting a Foley catheter, blowing up its balloon, and then pulling the catheter back until the balloon occludes the hole.

For handling larger or complex cardiac wounds, several techniques are available. The insertion of a 5-ml- or 30-ml-balloon Foley catheter into a large or inaccessible (posterior) defect may allow for control of hemorrhage until a relatively deep purse string suture can be applied around the hole. Such a catheter can also be used to infuse fluids rapidly into the right heart. Infusion of fluid directly into the left heart has the risk of also infusing air or clots which, in even small amounts, can cause disastrous occlusion of a coronary or cerebral vessel.

Wide, horizontal mattress sutures placed on either side of a large defect and pulled together may control most of the hemorrhage until cardiopulmonary bypass can be instituted. When cardiopulmonary bypass is not readily available, occlusion of the superior vena cava and

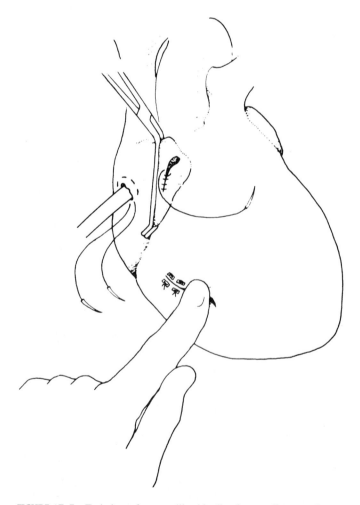

FIGURE 17–5 Techniques for controlling bleeding from cardiac wounds may include an inflated Foley catheter pulled against the hole, a Satinsky clamp across the base of an auricle torn at its top, and direct finger compression. (From: Williams JB, Silver DG, Laws HL. Successful management of heart rupture from blunt trauma. J Trauma 1981;21:534.)

inferior vena cava by vascular tapes or clamps slows the heart and finally stops it, allowing for quick repair of larger defects without causing exsanguinating hemorrhage. When this latter technique is used, all air is evacuated from the heart by allowing bleeding through the hole prior to tying the final suture.

CARDIAC MASSAGE

AXIOM Compressing the heart with two hands or with one hand against the sternum reduces the risk of inadvertently entering the heart with a fingertip.

Once the cardiorrhaphy has been completed, internal cardiac massage can be performed as needed by compressing the heart between the palms of two hands or between one palm and the sternum. Warm (preferably 104° F) saline poured over the heart may help prevent ventricular fibrillation, which is often associated with the hypothermia of shock and resuscitation. If ventricular fibrillation were to occur, defibrillation with internal paddles, starting at 20-40 watt-seconds and increasing the energy as needed should be performed. Lidocaine, magnesium, and correction of severe acidosis or alkalosis may also be of some benefit for recurrent ventricular fibrillation.[48]

Demetriades and Vanderveen performed a two-year, prospective study analyzing penetrating heart injuries in Johannesburg, South Africa.[48] This series included 125 hospital patients and 407 who died before arrival. Twenty-three of the victims had sustained bullet wounds, and 384 stab wounds. Aortic lacerations generally caused rapid death (93% were dead before admission). The next highest mortality rate was seen with injuries to the left ventricle. Cardiac tamponade was more than twice as common in patients who reached the hospital alive versus the dead-before-admission group. The mortality rate for those who reached the operating room alive was 14.4%. For those who had thoracotomy in the ED, the mortality rate was 88%. The prognosis among the hospitalized patients was poorest for aortic injuries (60% mortality rate) and best for right ventricular injuries (8% mortality rate).

AIR EMBOLISM

AXIOM The sudden onset of arrhythmia or hypotension in a patient with open veins or lung injury, especially with hemoptysis, should be considered due to air emboli until proved otherwise.

If severe arrhythmias or cardiac arrest were to develop during endotracheal intubation or while the chest were being opened, systemic air embolism should be suspected. The head should be lowered and cardiac chambers aspirated for air immediately. Systemic air embolism is most frequently diagnosed by seeing small air bubbles in the coronary arteries. This serious complication is seldom mentioned; however, in one series, needle aspiration of cardiac chambers was performed on 25 patients with cardiac arrest after trauma and a significant amount of air was aspirated in seven (28%).[7] Four of these air embolism patients survived with no significant neurologic defect.

CONTINUED CARE

When the patient develops a satisfactory rhythm, the descending thoracic aorta can be gradually declamped as infusions of fluid and blood are administered, being careful to keep the systolic blood pressure >90-100 mm Hg. One should avoid systolic blood pressures >160–180 mm Hg when the aorta is clamped because it may tear open cardiac repairs, excessively dilate the left ventricle (causing irreversible LV failure), or cause intracerebral bleeding. The use of powerful inotropes, such as intravenous adrenalin, should be avoided at this point, as they may cause sudden, severe hypertension and also increase the risk of recurrent ventricular fibrillation.

AXIOM Hypertension and/or severe tachycardia can greatly increase the work load and oxygen requirements of an injured heart and can cause infarction and/or overt heart failure.

After the cardiac wounds and all bleeding vessels are controlled and an adequate cardiac output has been obtained, all residual blood and clots are washed out of the pericardial and pleural cavities. One must look closely to make sure that the internal mammary arteries are intact or carefully suture-ligated. If the heart were edematous or dilated, the pericardium could be left open. Occasionally, the sternum or chest wall incision cannot be completely closed because of edema or congestion of the lungs, but in such instances, the skin can usually be sutured. The sternum or chest wall muscles can then usually be closed after several days when cardiac dilatation and pulmonary congestion have resolved.

CORONARY ARTERY INJURIES

The incidence of traumatic coronary artery injury is not accurately known because not all victims are examined. Even when autopsy is performed, it is likely that this injury is often overlooked, particularly when concomitant massive heart injury occurs. In a review of 500 patients with penetrating wounds of the heart, coronary artery injury was found in only 4.4%.[49]

A penetrating wound of the coronary artery may result in immediate cardiac tamponade, intrathoracic bleeding, or myocardial infarction. Later, the patient may develop coronary arteriocameral or arteriovenous fistulas or a coronary artery aneurysm.[50] Although the left anterior descending coronary artery is the most commonly injured vessel,[47] the most frequent coronary arteriocameral fistulas in decreasing order of frequency include: the right coronary artery to the right atrium or ventricle, and the left anterior descending coronary artery to the right or left ventricle.[50,51] An isolated, traumatic coronary artery aneurysm without a coronary arteriovenous or arteriocameral fistula is rare.

Ligation of the cut ends is the treatment of choice for lacerations of small coronary vessels. Torn proximal coronary arteries may also be ligated when no evidence of cardiovascular dysfunction exists. Such patients, however, must be observed closely. When a large, proximal coronary artery is lacerated and results in arrhythmias, myocardial ischemia, and/or impaired hemodynamic function, the vessel should be repaired primarily or, if not feasible, it should be bypassed with an internal mammary artery or reversed saphenous vein graft.[52]

VENTRICULAR SEPTAL DEFECTS

The development of an interventricular defect following a penetrating cardiac wound is relatively rare.[53,54] Among 177 patients with penetrating cardiac injury, a ventricular septal deficit was diagnosed in only 1.1%,[55] and in another study of 102 patients treated over a 10-year period, four had ventricular septal defects (3.9%).[56] During a 10-year period at Grady Memorial Hospital, five patients were treated for ventricular septal defects, four from bullet wounds of the heart and one from blunt trauma.[57,58] When the patient is in intractable heart failure, emergency cardiac catheterization and surgery are generally required. In most instances, however, the patient is only mildly-to-moderately symptomatic, and one can usually wait 2-3 months to repair the defect.

VALVE INJURIES

A penetrating wound of the heart or its attached great vessels may involve valve cusps, leaflets, chordae tendineae, or papillary muscles.[59] Most valvular injuries detected postoperatively can be corrected 3-6 months later on an elective basis after cardiac catheterization. Occasionally, however, severe cardiac failure or dysfunction at the initial procedure necessitates an emergency valve repair or replacement.[60,61] During a 10-year period at Grady Memorial

Hospital, Symbas et al. treated five patients with cardiac valve injury from penetrating trauma.[59] One patient had a stab wound of a pulmonic valve cusp with an aorticopulmonary fistula, and four had injuries to the mitral valve (2 gunshot wounds and 2 stabs).

ANEURYSMS

Traumatic aneurysms of the heart are rare, and most reported cases have been the result of nonpenetrating injuries to the heart.[62] During a 10-year period at Grady Memorial Hospital, Symbas et al. treated five patients with traumatic ventricular aneurysms, all of which resulted from penetrating trauma. One patient had a true aneurysm, two had a pseudoaneurysm, and one patient had two pseudoaneurysms and a ventricular septal defect. The left ventricle is the most common cardiac chamber to develop a traumatic aneurysm, but it may also occur in the right ventricle or in the atria.[62] Traumatic aneurysms of the heart may be either true aneurysms or pseudoaneurysms.

AXIOM Pseudoaneurysms of the heart caused by penetrating trauma should be treated surgically because they are basically a contained rupture of the heart.

True aneurysms of the heart are treated surgically when they cause heart failure, arrhythmias, or emboli. In most instances, an aneurysm is either plicated or resected back to its fibrotic edges, and the defect is closed directly or with a prosthetic patch.

BLUNT INJURIES TO THE HEART

Introduction

INCIDENCE

AXIOM Cardiac injury is frequently found in individuals dying immediately after blunt chest trauma.

It has been estimated that at least 200,000 patients suffer blunt cardiac trauma annually in the United States.[63] It has been said that cardiac injury is the most frequent, unsuspected visceral injury responsible for death in fatally-injured accident victims and accounts for about 25% of such deaths.[64] The reported incidence of cardiac injury after blunt chest trauma in patients who reach the hospital alive probably averages about 15-25%, but reports vary from 16% in an autopsy series[65] to 76% in clinical studies.[66]

ETIOLOGY AND MECHANISMS OF INJURY

The most common cause of blunt cardiac trauma is high-speed motor vehicle accidents. However, myocardial injury has also been documented in accidents involving vehicles going less than 20 mph.[67] Other causes include direct blows to the chest, industrial crush injuries, falls from heights, blast injuries, and athletic trauma. One study suggested that use of seat belts may increase the incidence of myocardial contusion in motor vehicle accidents.[68]

AXIOM Myocardial contusion should be suspected in anyone with severe trauma to the anterior chest.

The heart seems to be relatively well protected within a bony case formed by ribs, sternum, and vertebrae. However, it is suspended relatively freely within the chest cavity from the great vessels, and this mobility plus its location between the sternum and the thoracic vertebrae make it susceptible to injury as a result of several mechanisms: (a) sudden horizontal acceleration and/or deceleration causing the heart to impact against the sternum or vertebrae, (b) compression between the sternum and vertebrae following a direct, forceful blow to the chest, (c) sudden increase in intrathoracic and intracardiac pressures causing disruption of myocardium or cardiac valves, (d) "hydraulic ram effect" with compression of the abdomen forcibly displacing abdominal viscera against the heart with sudden, great force,[68] and (e) strenuous or prolonged cardiac massage, particularly when performed through the intact chest wall.

TYPES OF INJURIES

Blunt trauma to the heart can cause a wide spectrum of injuries, including: (a) pericardial tears (b) rupture of an outer chamber wall with resulting death from tamponade or bleeding, (c) septal rupture, (d) valvular injuries of which the aortic valve is the most frequent, (e) direct myocardial injury (contusion), and (f) laceration or thrombosis of coronary arteries.[69]

Some authors stressed the differences between myocardial concussion and myocardial contusion.[70] With myocardial concussion, no anatomical cellular injury occurs, but some functional damage is demonstrated on 2-D echocardiography or other wall-motion studies. With contusion, anatomical injury is demonstrated either by elevated CPK-MB enzymes or by direct visualization at surgery or autopsy.

DIAGNOSTIC PROBLEMS

Blunt cardiac trauma can be difficult to detect. The victim may have experienced severe, multiple-system trauma, and the presence of cardiac injury may be overshadowed by other more obvious injuries. In addition, the forces that produce blunt cardiac trauma may cause little or no external evidence of injury. Therefore, a history of moderate-to-severe chest or upper abdominal injury, even without abnormalities on physical examination, should make one suspect cardiac injury.

Types of Injuries

PERICARDIAL TEARS

Of the 59 patients with blunt cardiac injuries reported by Fulda et al., 22 (37%) had pericardial tears.[71] Left pleuropericardial tears were most common, occurring in 14 (24%) of these patients. Other sites included four diaphragmatic pericardial tears, two right pleuropericardial tears, and two superior mediastinal tears. All of the pleuropericardial tears were linear and located on the lateral aspect of the pericardium, either just anterior or just posterior to the phrenic nerve and coursing in the same direction as the nerve. Tears ranged in length from 2 cm to the entire length of the pericardium. The three diaphragmatic tears were transverse and ranged from 3-10 cm in length. No patients had herniation of abdominal contents into the pericardial sac.

CARDIAC RUPTURE

The most severe form of cardiac injury is rupture of the myocardium. This is usually due to a motor vehicle accident, but it may also result from other forms of severe blunt trauma. Blunt cardiac rupture was first reported by Berard in 1862[71] and was first successfully repaired by Desforges et al. in 1955.[72]

Cardiac rupture due to blunt chest trauma is the heart lesion most frequently found at autopsy in patients dying at the scene of an accident[73] (Table 17–2). Most patients with such damage succumb at the time of trauma or shortly thereafter, and only a few (7-20%) live more than 30 minutes.[71] Although some believe that the anterior

TABLE 17–2 Predominant Injury in 546 Patients with Fatal Nonpenetrating Cardiac Trauma

Predominant Injury	Number
Myocardial rupture, including septum	353
Myocardial contusion or surface laceration	129
Pericardial laceration	36
Hemopericardium	25
Papillary muscle rupture or lacerations	1 (23)[a]
Coronary artery injury	1 (9)
Laceration of valve	1 (6)
Coronary artery thrombosis	0
Total	546

[a] ( ) = number combined with other more serious cardiac injury.
(Modified from Parmley et al.,[37] with permission.)
Wilson RF. Injury to the heart and great vessel. In: Henning RJ, Grenvik, A, eds. Critical care cardiology. New York: Churchill Livingstone, 1989; 422.

right ventricle is the most frequent location for blunt cardiac rupture, our own experience suggests that tears of the right atrium at its junction with the superior or inferior vena cava are much more common in patients reaching the hospital alive.

Santavirta and Arajarvi analyzed the records of 4169 victims of traffic collisions in Finland who were fatally injured from 1972 to 1985.[74] Chest injuries were the main cause of death in 1121 (27%), 207 of whom had worn seatbelts. Cardiac rupture was found at autopsy in 75 (36%) of the seatbelt wearers. Precise information on the location and size of the heart rupture was available in 47 patients. For a control group, the authors analyzed 47 randomly chosen unbelted victims who sustained fatal heart ruptures in comparable collisions. Analysis of the data suggested that the mechanism leading to heart rupture in frontal impact collisions was usually crushing of the chest against the steering wheel, even in seatbelt wearers (Table 17–3).

> **AXIOM** Occasionally, patients with blunt rupture of the right atrium reach the hospital alive, but they usually die rapidly in the ED unless their injuries are recognized and corrected promptly.

About 80% of patients with cardiac rupture die almost immediately at the scene of the accident.[73] With today's rapid transport systems, however, some patients, especially those with only small tears of the right atrium, may arrive in the emergency department with little or no evidence of hemorrhagic shock or tamponade. Calhoon et al. reported on 30 patients, including 7 who had undergone surgery for blunt cardiac rupture during the past decade.[25] Unfortunately, most of these patients suddenly deteriorated a short time later and died before appropriate surgery could be performed. Cardiac rupture may also occur 7–14 days after trauma when a softened area of severely contused myocardium may give way.[71]

Four factors in determining whether cardiac rupture will occur include: the direction of the chest compression, the phase of the cardiac cycle in which the compression occurs, the velocity with which the force is applied, and the rise of intracardiac pressure produced.[65]

Trauma of the anterior chest wall can result in compression of the heart between the sternum and vertebral column. Violent compression of the legs and abdomen has also produced rupture of the heart supposedly by a sudden increase of venous return causing sudden severe distension of the heart.

Cardiac rupture should be suspected when shock exists out of proportion to the degree of recognized injury or when shock persists despite rapid fluid resuscitation and control of all other possible sources of hemorrhage. An immediate median sternotomy, preferably with cardiopulmonary bypass, is usually necessary to repair these devastating injuries successfully. Blunt right atrial and right ventricular injuries are frequently not accessible through a left thoracotomy incision. Therefore, when a left anterior thoracotomy incision has been

made and the right heart is injured, the incision generally needs to be extended across the midline into the right chest.

In spite of the poor results in most reports, in a recent series of 10 patients with blunt heart rupture seen in a single trauma center during an 11-year period, seven (70%) survived.[75] These excellent results were attributed to prompt performance of a pericardial window with subsequent immediate thoracotomy. Similar results were presented in another report of four survivors of five patients presenting with tamponade after right atrial rupture.[76] Kato et al., who reported on 63 patients with blunt cardiac rupture seen over a period of 18 years, noted a 54% survival rate in patients who arrived with an obtainable blood pressure.[77]

SEPTAL DEFECTS

Fragmentation and laceration of muscle fibers of the interventricular septum may be seen following blunt cardiac injury, but rupture of the septum is an uncommon complication.[71] In a postmortem examination of 546 victims of blunt trauma, rupture of the ventricular septum was found in only 30 (5%) and in another study of 152 victims, septal rupture was found in 11 (7%).

> **AXIOM** Septal defects after blunt chest trauma should be evaluated carefully to determine whether a new murmur plus evidence of myocardial damage exist.

Patients with an interventricular septal defect (VSD) from blunt trauma are generally critically ill as a result of the cardiac defect and the associated myocardial and pulmonary contusion.[71] The symptoms and signs of traumatic VSD are similar to those following acute myocardial infarction. The muscular interventricular septum near the apex is particularly susceptible to perforation after blunt trauma. VSD is characterized by a systolic thrill and a harsh, holosystolic murmur that is usually loudest along the left sternal border in the third and fourth intercostal spaces and is transmitted to the right.

The appearance of the characteristic murmur and thrill may be delayed for several hours or days.[71] This may result from low cardiac output or from contused, hemorrhagic septal muscle fibers that may not rupture until days or weeks later. Occasionally, patients with VSD may also have A-V conduction abnormalities or complete heart block.

> **AXIOM** ECG evidence of cardiac damage plus a new murmur after trauma suggest a valve lesion or VSD.

One should suspect a septal injury in patients with chest trauma who immediately develop severe hypoxemia.[78] Any right-to-left shunt increases hypoxemia, and high ventilatory pressures tend to increase the amount of right-to-left shunting. If severe heart failure were to occur, prompt cardiac catheterization and rapid surgical repair may be required to restore adequate oxygen delivery to the tissues. Although small, traumatic VSDs in the muscular septum may close

TABLE 17–3 *Anatomical Location of Heart Ruptures in Drivers and Right-Front Passengers, Including Those With and Without Seatbelts*

Location of Heart Rupture	Drivers				Passengers				Totals	
	Belted		Unbelted		Belted		Unbelted			
	Number	%	Number	%	Number	%	Number	%	Number	%
Left ventricle	22	56.4	14	36.8	5	62.5	0	0.0	41	43.6
Right ventricle	10	25.6	13	34.2	1	12.5	6	66.7	30	31.9
Left atrium	0	0.0	1	2.6	0	0.0	0	0.0	1	1.1
Right atrium	4	10.3	2	5.3	1	12.5	2	22.2	9	9.6
Atrial appendage	3	7.7	6	15.8	0	0.0	0	0.0	9	9.6
Other	0	0.0	2	5.3	1	12.5	1	11.1	4	4.3
Totals	39	100.0	38	100.0	8	100.0	9	100.0	94	100.0

From: Santavirta S, Arajarvi E. Ruptures of the heart in seatbelt wearers. J Trauma 1992;32:275.

spontaneously,[79] surgical repair, preferably six to eight weeks after trauma, is the treatment of choice.

Isolated atrial septal defects (ASD) due to blunt trauma are extremely rare, and most patients with traumatic ASD die within minutes of injury.[80] Furthermore, because ASD is the congenital cardiac lesion most apt to be first diagnosed in adulthood, ASD found after trauma is not always a new lesion. Nevertheless, if ASD were suspected, cardiac catheterization should be performed as soon as the patient's condition stabilized. The defect can then be repaired when appropriate. The associated murmur may be difficult to hear and such defects may not become apparent unless pulmonary problems cause right heart pressures to rise high enough to cause a right-to-left shunt resulting in increased hypoxemia.

VALVE INJURY

Aortic Valve

AXIOM The valve injury most apt to be caused by blunt trauma is aortic insufficiency.[59]

Valvular injury from nonpenetrating trauma, although uncommon, has been reported with increasing frequency.[59] Patients with bioprosthetic heart valves are particularly likely to have traumatic valve injury.[81] During a 10-year period at Grady Memorial Hospital, Symbas et al. treated four patients for valve injury from blunt trauma;[59] the aortic valve was injured in three patients and the mitral valve in one.

Aortic valve injury is usually in the form of rupture of the cusp itself, at its free border, at its base, or at one of its commissural attachments. Similar lesions of the aortic valve have been produced in human cadavers by a sudden increase in intraaortic pressure by 116-484 mm Hg.[59] Symptoms of traumatic aortic valve rupture immediately after the injury are usually those of acute, severe heart failure; however, with mild tears, symptoms such as chest pain, easy fatigability, faintness, or syncope, may be present or delayed for months or years.

Mitral Valve

Trauma to the mitral valve may include rupture or avulsion of a papillary muscle or chordae tendineae or, rarely, a tear of the valve leaflets.[82,83] Mitral valve rupture is believed to occur when sudden, severe force is applied during the short interval of isovolemic contraction between the closure of the mitral valve and the opening of the aortic valve. Rarely, mitral insufficiency may develop when the valve and adjacent myocardium are sufficiently contused to cause scar formation with later contraction and distortion of the valve apparatus.

A review of autopsy findings in 546 patients with nonpenetrating trauma to the chest revealed no isolated mitral valve injuries.[84] Consequently, the initial clinical manifestations are variable and dependent upon associated cardiac damage. Rupture of a papillary muscle or leaflet may cause death from severe heart failure developing within a few days after injury.[85]

Tricuspid Valve

The mechanism for tricuspid valve injury is believed to involve violent compression of the heart and sudden pulmonary outflow obstruction.[59,86] Isolated tricuspid valve injury has been only rarely reported, and it is generally of less serious hemodynamic consequence than isolated injury of the mitral valve. The endocarditis study by Arbulu et al. indicated that a patient can do well without a tricuspid valve for prolonged periods when pulmonary vascular resistance is normal.[87] The most frequent indication for late tricuspid valve insertion is the development of hepatic dysfunction from chronic, excessive congestion.

MYOCARDIAL CONTUSION

History

Myocardial contusion following blunt chest trauma has intrigued physicians since its initial description by Burch in 1676 in an eight-year-

old boy.[88] In 1859, Schnabel described a 49-year-old workman who died several hours after severe blunt injury to the chest and who, at autopsy, had a mediastinal hematoma, widespread hemorrhage on the anterior wall of the right atrium, a number of hemorrhages in the wall of the left ventricle, and a tear of the aorta.[88] In 1954, Burchell wrote[89]

> "And always with a heart contusion
> Arise both doubt and much confusion."

Incidence

AXIOM Cardiac contusion has been reported to be the most common visceral injury responsible for death immediately after trauma.

Over 90% of cardiac injuries found in patients admitted to a hospital after blunt trauma are myocardial contusions.[88] The reported incidence of myocardial contusion varies from 16% in an autopsy series of motor vehicle accidents[65] to 76% with clinical diagnoses;[66] the reported average is about 15-25% in patients admitted with severe blunt chest trauma. It has been suggested that approximately one quarter of patients will be found to have cardiac contusion if serial ECGs are obtained in all patients with suspected chest injuries.[90] In unstable patients admitted to an ICU, the incidence, as determined by radionuclide angiography, may approach 75%.[91]

PATHOLOGIC CHANGES

The typical pathologic changes seen at autopsy with myocardial contusion include subendocardial and interstitial hemorrhage, large surrounding areas of focal myocardial edema, myofibrillar degeneration, and myocytolysis and infiltration of polymorphonuclear leukocytes.[64] This injury may resemble an acute myocardial infarction, but contusions tend to be more patchy. The anterior right ventricular wall is the area most frequently involved, with the anterior interventricular septum and anterior-apical left ventricle next in frequency. Additional myocardial injury may occur when concomitant coronary arterial problems occur, such as spasm, intimal tears, or compression from adjacent hemorrhage and edema.[92]

PHYSIOLOGIC CHANGES

Physiologic changes seen with myocardial contusions are extremely variable. In an attempt to help investigators in this area, the Organ Injury Scaling Committee of the American Association of the Surgery of Trauma has devised a scaling system for various types of cardiac injuries (Table 17–4).[93]

Myocardial contusion can cause rhythm and/or conduction disturbances, and can significantly impair myocardial contractility in 10-20% of patients studied.[94] In otherwise normal individuals without severe, associated injuries, hemodynamic impairment may not even be noticed; however, in patients who have preexisting cardiac disease, multiple other injuries, or require prolonged general anesthetic, this impairment can greatly reduce myocardial function and prognosis.[88]

AXIOM Myocardial contusions are usually clinically insignificant unless patients have preexisting cardiac disease, other severe injuries, or need general anesthesia.

A significant reduction in cardiac output has been found in 65% of patients tested and this is directly related to the amount of contused myocardium. This has been confirmed in experimental animal studies, and such impairment may persist for two to three weeks or longer.[95]

In an attempt to evaluate hemodynamic changes due to myocardial contusion, Torres-Mirabal et al. inserted a PA catheter into a series of myocardial contusion patients and noted the response to a fluid challenge.[96] Of seven patients who developed either major complications or died, biventricular failure was demonstrated in three, cardio-

TABLE 17–4 Cardiac Injury Organ Scale

Grade	Injury Description	AIS-90
I	Blunt cardiac injury with minor ECG abnormality (nonspecific ST- or T-wave changes, premature atrial, ventricular contraction or persistent sinus tachycardia)	3
	Blunt or penetrating pericardial wound without cardiac injury, cardiac tamponade or cardiac herniation	
II	Blunt cardiac injury with heart block (right or left bundle branch, left anterior fascicular, or atrioventricular) or ischemic changes (ST depression or T-wave inversion) without cardiac failure	3
	Penetrating tangential myocardial wound up to, but not extending through endocardium, without tamponade	3
III	Blunt cardiac injury with sustained ($\geq$ 5 beats/min) or multifocal ventricular contractions	3-4
	Blunt or penetrating cardiac injury with septal rupture, pulmonary or tricuspid valvular incompetence, papillary muscle dysfunction, or distal coronary arterial occlusion without cardiac failure	
	Blunt pericardial laceration with cardiac herniation	
	Blunt cardiac injury with cardiac failure	3-4
	Penetrating tangential myocardial wound up to, but not extending through endocardium, with tamponade	3
IV	Blunt or penetrating cardiac injury with septal rupture, pulmonary or tricuspid valvular incompetence, papillary muscle dysfunction or distal coronary arterial occlusion producing cardiac failure	3
	Blunt or penetrating cardiac injury with aortic or mitral valve incompetence	
	Blunt or penetrating cardiac injury of the right ventricle, right atrium, or left atrium	5
V	Blunt or penetrating cardiac injury with proximal coronary arterial occlusion	
	Blunt or penetrating left ventricular perforation	5
	Stellate injuries causing < 50% tissue loss of the right ventricle, right atrium or left atrium	5
VI	Blunt avulsion of the heart; penetrating wound producing > 50% tissue loss of a chamber	6

*Advance one grade for multiple penetrating wounds to a single chamber or multiple chamber involvement.
Moore EE, Malangowi MA, Cogbill TH, et al. Organ injury scaling IV: Thoracic vascular, lung, cardiac, and diaphragm. J Trauma 1994;36;299.

genic shock in two, and left ventricular dysfunction in one. It was also found that the cardiac index was only slightly reduced, and PAWP only slightly increased in most of these patients. However, when a fluid challenge was administered, the PAWP rose rapidly and little or no rise in cardiac output occurred. These authors concluded that although screening tests, such as the ECG, CPK-MB and MUGA scan can be relatively sensitive for diagnosing myocardial contusion, they do not indicate the severity of the injury and are not predictive of major morbidity or mortality.[96]

> **AXIOM** The reduced ejection fraction of a contused heart can be compensated for by increased preload and is not usually a problem unless the patient has multiple other injuries and/or requires general anesthesia.

In another study of blunt chest injury and focal ventricular wall-motion defects as defined by gated cardiac scintigraphy, Sutherland et al. found that the reduced right ventricular (RV) ejection fraction (29 $\pm$ 5% vs 47 $\pm$ 7% in those without wall-motion defects) was compensated for quite well by an increased RV end diastolic volume (143 $\pm$ 63 vs 93 $\pm$ 26 ml/m^2).[97]

In spite of these abnormalities most patients with myocardial contusions have relatively few problems unless: (a) an arrhythmia, especially PVCs, atrial fibrillation, or a conduction defect is present, (b) clinical evidence of heart failure exists, (c) multiple other injuries occur, (d) preexisting cardiac disease is present, or (e) general anesthesia is required, especially when surgery will be prolonged or associated with clamping of the aorta or significant blood loss.

> **AXIOM** General anesthesia within a month of a diagnosed myocardial contusion can be a significant risk for the development of arrhythmias or hypotension.

In a group of patients studied at the Mayo Clinic by Frazee et al., the incidence of hypotension during general anesthesia was significantly higher in chest trauma patients who had abnormal cardiac wall motion on 2-D echocardiogram than those with normal myocardial motion (23% vs 11%).[70] Furthermore, the incidence of an increased CVP during hypotension was 50% if the 2-D echocardiogram were abnormal. None of the patients with normal heart motion who developed hypotension had an elevated CVP.

DIAGNOSIS

Much debate continues over how to diagnose myocardial contusion. The value of various diagnostic tests varies greatly in the large number of reports written on this subject.

> **AXIOM** The diagnosis of a myocardial contusion can be made on the basis of new ECG findings, arrhythmias, heart failure, impaired cardial function ($\downarrow$ EF etc.), or increased CPK-MB levels, but evidence of anterior heart wall-motion abnormalities is probably most definitive.

Clinical Features

Many forces producing blunt cardiac injury are of such a nature that the external evidence of injury may not be detectable in up to one-third of injured individuals.[98] Frequently internal thoracic damage occurs with nonpenetrating trauma even when no rib or other skeletal fractures are present. Nevertheless, the majority of patients with myocardial contusion have severe extracardiac injuries and up to 60% have other thoracic injuries.[97]

> **AXIOM** Any patient involved in a head-on motor vehicle accident at speeds exceeding 35 mph and having any chest symptoms or signs should be suspected of having myocardial contusion.

Rarely, a patient with myocardial contusion will have angina-like pain which is not relieved by nitroglycerin. Differentiation from an acute myocardial infarction may be difficult under such circumstances.

Tachycardia that is out of proportion to the degree of trauma or blood loss may be the first sign of myocardial contusion. Aside from evidence of significant chest wall injury, the only other helpful physical signs may include a friction rub or abnormality in heart sounds. Occasionally, an irregular rhythm due to atrial fibrillation or premature atrial or ventricular contractions may be noted.

Radiologic Examination

Chiu et al. demonstrated radiographically that acute dilation of the heart often follows experimental cardiac injury,[100] but this is seldom seen clinically. Chest radiography has its greatest value in the recognition of associated injuries.

> **AXIOM**   Plain chest radiography is unlikely to help with the diagnosis of myocardial contusion unless evidence of otherwise unexplained pulmonary edema and/or cardiomegaly exists.

The closest radiographic correlates of myocardial contusion are pulmonary contusion or fractures of the first two ribs, clavicles, or sternum. Sternal fractures are particularly important. In many series, the presence of a fractured sternum is the clinical finding most significantly associated with myocardial contusion. In a series of 11 patients with sternal fractures studied with radionuclide angiography, ten (91%) had functional defects involving the anterior heart.[101] Only four of these patients had ECG abnormalities and none had elevated CPK-MB isoenzymes. Another series, however, suggested that sternal fractures are relatively benign and do not require a special work-up unless evidence of heart failure or an arrhythmia is present.[102]

ECG

ECG should be obtained initially and at 12 and 24 hours postinjury in anyone suspected of having a myocardial injury. If no ECG changes were noted by 24 hours, it would be unlikely that any would develop later; however, in a series reported by Soliman and Waxman, 24 (23%) of the patients had initially normal ECGs, but then developed 12-lead ECG abnormalities on the second or third hospital day.[98] Although 64% of the patients studied developed abnormalities on 12-lead ECG, few required therapy. Only six patients needed antiarrhythmic therapy, and only 15% of the study patients with abnormal ECGs experienced any episodes of hypotension or oliguria during hospitalization.[103] This is one of the few reports showing a significant incidence of arrhythmias after 24 hours, unless there was new added stress, such as a general anesthetic. New atrial fibrillation, multiple PVCs, or conduction disturbances are much more important than ST-T-wave changes and are virtually diagnostic of direct or indirect (ischemic or hypoxic) myocardial injury.[103]

> **AXIOM**   Myocardial contusion seldom causes new arrhythmias more than 24 hours after admission unless significant stress, such as general anesthesia, is added.

ECG changes have been noted in 33-88% of patients with contusions.[66,91,99] In one series of 108 clinically diagnosed myocardial contusions, 12% had normal ECGs, 22% had ventricular rhythm disorders, 32% had other arrhythmias or disturbances of conduction, 61% had disturbances of repolarization, and 3% had ECG evidence of myocardial infarction.[104]

The ECG abnormalities that are usually attributed to myocardial contusion are generally nonspecific, and may be due to hypotension, hypoxia, stress, electrolyte abnormalities (especially hyperkalemia), head trauma, or associated injuries.[82] Furthermore, in some cases of myocardial contusion found at autopsy, no ECG abnormalities were demonstrated before the patient's death.[105]

> **AXIOM**   Holter monitoring reveals many more arrhythmias than the usual ECG monitoring systems, but it is unlikely that they are significant.

Fabian et al. reported that Holter monitoring revealed far more cardiac problems than routine or continuous ECG monitoring.[106] Of 90 patients monitored for 4-5 days for severe anterior chest trauma, 24 had significant arrhythmias (SARR) demonstrated by Holter monitoring. These included episodes of ventricular tachycardia (18), supraventricular tachycardia (3), bigeminy (2), and atrial fibrillation (1). Of these arrhythmias, only 6% were documented by other techniques. The average CPK-MB level in the 24 patients with SARR was 8.3% (vs. 2.6% in patients without SARR). The patients with SARR also had lower cardiac indices (2.4 vs 3.2 L/min/m^2). It is not clear, however, how many SARR required treatment.

Enzymes

SGOT, LDH, and CPK levels are often elevated in patients with severe blunt chest trauma because of associated injuries to the liver, lung, bone, brain, or skeletal muscle. Consequently, they are of relatively little value in diagnosing cardiac injuries. Myocardial (CPK-MB) isoenzyme levels, however, are believed to be more accurate.[107] These should be drawn initially when the patient is first seen in the emergency department and at 8, 16, 24, and 48 hours postinjury. With acute myocardial contusions, the CPK-MB peaks at about 18-24 hours.

> **AXIOM**   CPK-MB levels are of little or no value in predicting the outcome of patients with myocardial contusions.

Most authors consider a ratio of CPK-MB to total CPK of 5% or more to be indicative of myocardial damage;[67,99] however, at least one other author considers 6% as only suspicious and 8% as highly suggestive of a diagnosis of myocardial contusion.[103] Because CPK-MB isoenzyme can also be found in skeletal muscle, pancreas, lung, colon, liver, stomach, and small bowel, CPK-MB fraction may be elevated from a variety of injuries, particularly if the total CPK were very high. Although one series found that no patient whose EKG and CPK-MB results were both negative had a clinical course compatible with important cardiac injury,[108] no correlation appeared to exist between the severity of injury and the level of CPK-MB isoenzyme. Likewise, normal CPK-MB levels do not entirely eliminate blunt myocardial injury. In one study, up to two-thirds of patients with impaired ventricular motion on gated radionuclide angiography had normal CPK-MB levels.[91]

Technetium Pyrophosphate Scan (99m-Tc PYP)

Myocardial cell death is accompanied by an influx of calcium ions that bind to the crystalline lattice of hydroxyapatite within the mitochondria.[102] Technetium pyrophosphate (99m-Tc PYP) is normally used as a bone scanning agent, but it also labelled the hydroxyapatite in infarcted myocardium.[109] Although experimentally inflicted cardiac contusion in dogs could be accurately detected with 99m-Tc PYP,[57] Go et al. successfully diagnosed myocardial contusion in only two of eight patients using PYP, and both had greatly elevated total CPK levels.[110]

> **AXIOM**   Technetium pyrophosphate scans are of no diagnostic value for myocardial contusion except with full-thickness, left ventricular injuries.

Although one investigator believed that technetium pyrophosphate scans may be more sensitive than ECG or CPK-MB studies for diagnosing myocardial contusion,[111] most authors do not agree. For example, Brantigan et al. studied 29 patients suspected of having myocardial contusions.[112] Of 13 patients with ECG abnormalities, only two (6.8%) had positive PYP scans.

Several reasons can explain why 99m-Tc PYP scans lack sensitivity in most patients with myocardial contusions.[113] In order for a technetium pyrophosphate scan to be positive, a transmural injury is necessary to bind enough scintigraphic tracer to distinguish the lesion from background noise. The sensitivity of the scan is further hampered because it cannot differentiate a contusion of the right ventricle from an overlying sternal fracture or chest-wall contusion.

Radionuclide Angiography

First-pass biventricular radionuclide angiography (RNA), including left ventricular segmental wall-motion analysis (LVSWM), can now be performed at bedside, as well as in the radiology department.[91,101] The study can be performed with the patient in any position, although the 30° RAO is preferable. An intravenous injection of 15 mg of stannous pyrophosphate is followed by a 15-mCi bolus injection of sodium pertechnetate Tc 99m about 10-20 minutes later. Raw data are transferred from a single-crystal camera to magnetic tape, and the acquisitions are analyzed with a digital computer in an event-to-event mode for 30 seconds. These are processed for both right- and left-ventricular ejection fractions (RVEF and LVEF) and for right- and left-ventricular segmental wall-motion analysis.

The normal LVEF is 62 ± 5% (mean ± SD) and the normal RVEF is 50 ± 4%.[100] A LVEF < 50% (< 2.5 SD below the mean) and a RVEF < 40% have been interpreted as abnormal. Using this technique, Harley and Mena found that 11 of 12 patients with sternal fractures had abnormalities of ventricular contraction and motion;[101] however, only four had ECG changes and none had abnormal CPK-MB. Sutherland et al. had similar findings with less than one-third of the patients with abnormal radionuclide angiography having ECG or CPK-MB abnormalities.[91]

AXIOM   Gated RNA appears to be a sensitive technique to assess cardiac function, including left- and right-ventricular ejection fractions, and wall-motion abnormalities.[110]

As a result of these studies of ED patients with first-pass RNA, some authors[113,114] recommended the use of RNA on all trauma patients with no other problems except suspected cardiac injury. They believed that patients with normal RNA can be observed in the ED for four to six hours and then safely discharged and followed as outpatients.

Single-Photon Emission Computed Tomography

Another technique, utilizing thallus chloride, has been described for imaging the heart.[115] Following intravenous injection of this radioactive potassium analogue, thallium is extracted from the blood into normally functioning myocardial cells. This technique has been used effectively for some time to detect myocardial ischemia or infarction; however, it appears that conventional thallus chloride T1 201 imaging is unreliable for detecting small, partial-thickness lesions, especially in the right ventricle.[115]

To offset these problems, a process has been developed so that the thallium images of the heart can be processed, reconstructed, and displayed by computer in the form of tomographic slices in different planes of the heart. This process, referred to as single-photon-emission computed tomography (SPECT), has been shown to add significantly to the accuracy of thallus chloride T1 201 myocardial imaging.[115] In a recent series of 48 patients with blunt chest trauma, 23 had normal SPECT studies and none of these 23 developed any serious arrhythmias; however, five of 25 with abnormal or ambiguous studies did develop arrhythmias requiring treatment.[116]

Echocardiography

Two-dimensional echocardiography (2-D ECHO) has many advantages in attempting to make a diagnosis of acute myocardial contusion. Although the initial results of echocardiography in experimental studies in dogs were inconsistent, subsequent reports using improved techniques suggested that it is a valuable diagnostic tool.[112,113,117]

Quantitative and qualitative information can be obtained noninvasively on the status of the cardiac chambers, wall-motion abnormalities, the functional integrity of the valves, cardiac tamponade, and intracardiac thrombus or shunts. Additionally, 2-D ECHO can differentiate right- from left-ventricular contusions, as well as right-ventricular contusions from pericardial tamponade.

Pandian et al. found that contused myocardium could be identified on 2-D ECHO by: (a) increased ECHO brightness, (b) increased end-diastolic wall thickness, and (c) impaired regional systolic function.[118] The most common abnormality seen with myocardial contusion on 2D-ECHO is right-ventricular free-wall dyskinesia, often with some dilation.[117] In addition, some of the patients studied have had mural thrombi attached to the contused myocardium.[102]

Some authors[70] advocated obtaining 2-D ECHO on all patients with suspected cardiac injuries and particularly when they have abnormal ECGs or elevated cardiac isoenzymes.[99] This can be done safely and rapidly in the ICU or ED without transporting the patient to another area. Others, however, believed that echocardiography is really only indicated when the patient develops complications, such as arrhythmia or heart failure.[119]

Transesophageal Echocardiography

Recently, Shapiro et al. reported that transesophageal echocardiography (TEE) can be of great help in the cardiovascular evaluation of patients with blunt thoracic trauma.[120] They observed regional wall-motion abnormalities consistent with cardiac contusion in 26% of their patients. In their study, performance of the TEE enabled them to make a rapid diagnosis of myocardial contusion and to exclude other causes of circulatory failure, particularly hypovolemia and cardiac tamponade. Orliquet et al. performed TEE on a patient receiving mechanical ventilation with PEEP.[121] They noted that this procedure can be very helpful diagnostically, is noninvasive, and can be performed at the bedside. Unlike transthoracic echocardiography, it is unaffected by recent cardiac or abdominal procedures, mechanical ventilation hemodynamic monitoring lines, chest tubes, or dressings.

AXIOM   A patient with a normal 2-D ECHO after blunt trauma is unlikely to have a physiologically significant myocardial contusion.

Monitoring of PAWP and Cardiac Output

AXIOM   Patients with myocardial contusions tend to have relatively flat cardiac function curves in response to fluid-loading, indicating impaired responses to stress.

A pulmonary artery catheter should be inserted to monitor pulmonary artery pressures and cardiac output in anyone with a suspected myocardial contusion and (a) any hemodynamic impairment or (b) need for a major operative procedure under general anesthesia. Although the baseline cardiac output may be relatively normal, a poor response to fluid-loading often occurs. Torres-Mirabel et al. also found that patients with biventricular dysfunction had a 40% incidence of major morbidity or mortality, but usually only in the presence of other significant injuries.[96]

Summary of Diagnostic Approach

It has generally been suggested that all trauma patients with suspected cardiac injury or with any other factors that increase the risk of arrhythmias or heart failure should be admitted to an ICU for continuous ECG and other monitoring. However, a panel of trauma experts recently suggested that asymptomatic patients with blunt cardiac injuries with minor ECG or enzyme abnormalities not be admitted to an ICU for extensive monitoring.[122]

When the CPK-MB and ECGs are all negative for 48 hours, it is unlikely that a significant cardiac injury exists; however, 2-D ECHO or RNA provides more clinically significant information and should be performed in individuals who have other cardiac risk factors or other injuries that may require general anesthesia. Determination of ejection fractions and/or studying the response to a fluid challenge with a PAWP catheter can provide important information on the degree of myocardial dysfunction. Cardiac catheterization and coronary angiography should be performed when cardiac symptoms or signs persist for more than a few days.

TREATMENT

AXIOM   Patients with myocardial contusions and wall-motion abnormalities should, when possible, not receive general anesthesia for at least 30 days.

The distinction between myocardial concussion and contusion has allowed some authors to develop what they believe is a rational acute management protocol.[70] They believe that patients without identifiable CPK-MB changes or wall-motion abnormalities on 2-D ECHO or RNA do not require continuous cardioscopic monitoring and cardiac precautions, unless indicated by other severe injuries.

Supplemental oxygen should be administered, as needed, to keep the PO_2 > 80 mm Hg, and analgesics should be given, as needed, to reduce any tachycardia or increased BP that may be caused by pain. Coronary vasodilators should not be used unless patients have suspected, preexisting coronary artery disease. Cardiac dysrhythmias should be diagnosed early and treated with appropriate medication; prophylactic treatment is generally not indicated.

Low-cardiac output or hypotension should be treated with fluids and/or inotropic agents, guided by the response of the PAWP and cardiac output. In patients with possibly impaired right ventricular function, monitoring of the right ventricular end-diastolic volume index (RVEDVI) with a special PA catheter may be important.[123]

Because patients with cardiac contusion tend to have decreased myocardial compliance and cardiac output, preload should be adjusted carefully. In one series, no operative deaths were recorded in 27 patients with myocardial contusions who were carefully monitored.[99] However, in another series of 19 patients with myocardial contusions proved by RNA, 11 patients requiring surgery for associated injuries required perioperative inotropic support and one needed intraaortic balloon pumping (IABP).[124]

AXIOM   Intraaortic balloon pumping may be lifesaving in patients with acute myocardial contusions who have persistent severe hypotension in spite of inotropes and adequate preload.

If a patient remains in a low-cardiac output state despite adequate volume, inotropic support, and correction of any mechanical problems (e.g., tamponade), IABP should be begun. Beneficial hemodynamic effects of IABP include; (a) arterial diastolic augmentation with increased coronary perfusion; (b) left ventricular unloading and (c) blood pumping action by the balloon pump. Diastolic augmentation of intraaortic pressure with IABP was shown by Saunders and Doty to improve cardiac output in a group of dogs with experimentally inflicted cardiac contusions.[125] The intervention was most successful in the group whose cardiac output was reduced 26-50% below that of controls. These authors also found that IABP was most effective when applied as early as possible. Snow et al. used this device in several patients with low-cardiac output resulting from cardiac contusion and obtained a significant improvement in circulatory dynamics in all of them.[99]

When intramural thrombus is found on 2-D ECHO in patients with myocardial contusions, it is not clear whether they should have prophylactic anticoagulation.[126] Although five of seven patients with chest trauma in one series had echocardiographically-proved, right ventricular thrombi, none of these patients had subsequent systemic or pulmonary embolization.[127] Furthermore, anticoagulation is contraindicated in many patients with multiple trauma because of the risk of severe hemorrhage. Nevertheless, in patients with proven intramural thrombosis and no contraindication to anticoagulation, one may consider using "mild" to "moderate" heparinization (i.e., 500-800 units/hr).[67]

Coronary Arterial Injury

Direct injury to the coronary arteries from blunt chest trauma occurs rarely, but if it caused pericardial tamponade or intrathoracic bleeding, immediate operation would be required. Coronary artery thrombosis due to chest trauma is also rare but has been reported. In a large autopsy series, Parmley at el. found coronary lacerations in only 10 (1.8%) of 546 patients with fatal blunt chest trauma.[73]

Several investigators studied postmortem angiograms of experimental myocardial trauma in dogs and after trauma in humans.[92,95,100] In dogs, transmural redistribution of small-vessel perfusion to the myocardium distal to the site of injury could be demonstrated almost immediately following impact.[92,100] They found no associated coronary artery spasm; in fact, a significant decrease in distal small-vessel resistance was noted. However, when dogs were killed immediately after experimental contusion and postmortem angiographic studies were performed, large collections of contrast material were found accumulated in the terminal branches of small vessels in the area of the

damaged muscle. These collections appeared to be dilated vascular channels or "giant capillary sinusoids" which are probably a type of arteriovenous communication. They concluded that these channels with their associated local A-V shunting, and not coronary artery problems, lead to regional myocardial ischemia.

AXIOM   Myocardial contusion may precipitate severe coronary insufficiency in patients with preexisting coronary artery disease.

A more common clinical problem is the role of myocardial contusion causing myocardial ischemia in patients with preexisting coronary artery disease. In patients who already have decreased cardiac reserves, the added loss of myocardial contractility from contusions may severely compromise cardiac output. Thus, cardiac catheterization plus coronary arteriography may be important in evaluating such patients.

Pericardial Injury and Effusion

Hemopericardium or pericardial effusion can occur without evidence of blunt cardiac injury. This may develop acutely or be delayed a week or longer.[67,128] As with other causes of pericardial effusion, the rate of fluid accumulation is the important determinant of hemodynamic consequences.

AXIOM   Although rarely documented, blunt pericardial injury can cause pericardial tamponade without concomitant myocardial injury.

Pericardial injury from blunt trauma should be suspected when no ECG or other evidence of myocardial damage exists; however, a normal ECG does not eliminate traumatic pericarditis. In some instances, only echocardiography or autopsy may provide the diagnosis.[121] If blood were found on pericardiocentesis following blunt trauma, thoracotomy should be performed, preferably with cardiopulmonary bypass available.

Small pericardial effusions are usually of no consequence. They generally remain asymptomatic and resolve without therapy. Nevertheless, a rare patient with an effusion develops late, constrictive pericarditis, occasionally with extensive calcification of the pericardium.[129] Like chronic hemopericardium, this condition may eventually necessitate pericardiectomy.

Occasionally, severe blunt chest trauma may tear the parietal pericardium.[129] If the hole is large enough and near the apex, the heart will, rarely, herniate through the defect causing sudden, severe shock or cardiac arrest. This problem should be suspected in patients with abnormal cardiac silhouettes and/or traumatic diaphragmatic hernias.

Follow-Up

Most patients discharged after blunt cardiac injury will do well. When RNA has been repeated after myocardial contusion, significant improvement is almost uniformly documented by three to four weeks.[130] By one year, follow-up studies indicate that right- and left-ejection fractions during maximal workload are essentially the same as other patients with chest injuries who have not had evidence of cardiac trauma.[131]

It is important that patients with proved or suspected cardiac injury be closely observed not only throughout their hospital stay, but also later for initially undiagnosed injuries or complications. One should evaluate the patient for posttraumatic pericarditis, ventricular septal defect, valvular defects, and ventricular aneurysms. When such problems are found early, and it appears that the defect endangers the patient's life, cardiac catheterization and surgical repair should be performed as soon as possible; however, when the patient tolerates the lesion well, cardiac catheterization can be performed electively six to eight weeks later.

Posttraumatic Pericarditis

A variable number of patients develop pericarditis following either penetrating[132] or nonpenetrating trauma[128,129] to the heart and pericardium. This syndrome is usually similar to that seen in patients who have had elective heart surgery or suffered acute myocardial infarction.[132,133]

ETIOLOGY/PATHOGENESIS

The cause of the this syndrome is still largely unknown, but it may be a delayed hypersensitivity reaction to the presence of damaged blood, pericardium, or myocardium in the pericardial cavity similar to that of postpericardiotomy syndrome.[132-134] This damaged tissue can act as a foreign protein, inducing the production of autoantibodies against similar tissues. Antiheart antibodies can be measured in these patients, and the serum concentration of these antibodies correlates to some extent with the severity of symptoms.[135] Autogenous blood and lipids in the pericardium can also cause an intense inflammatory response which may also be a contributing factor.[136]

AXIOM Blunt cardiac damage can produce delayed immune responses similar to those caused by acute myocardial infarction or cardiac surgery.

DIAGNOSIS

Post traumatic pericarditis should be suspected in individuals who develop chest pain, fever, and pleural or pericardial effusions two to four weeks after trauma. These patients may also have friction rubs, arthralgia, and even pulmonary infiltrates. The blood count often reveals lymphocytosis, and the ECG frequently shows ST-T-wave changes consistent with pericarditis.

TREATMENT

Treatment is primarily symptomatic. Salicylates and rest can often reduce symptoms dramatically within 12-24 hours. When no improvement occurs, corticosteroids may be required; these also usually reduce symptoms within 48-72 hours. Occasionally, drainage of pleural or pericardial fluid may be necessary to relieve symptoms or to rule out other more serious problems.[127]

Traumatic Aneurysms

True aneurysms of the heart usually result from blunt trauma to the heart or to a major coronary artery branch.[62] The injured muscle, either as a result of contusion or as a result of ischemia from injury and occlusion of a coronary artery, undergoes necrosis, stretching, and thinning, and eventual dilatation and fibrosis.

No symptoms are characteristic of traumatic cardiac aneurysms. The patient may be asymptomatic and able to perform ordinary activity without discomfort, but an abnormal cardiac silhouette may be discovered during routine chest roentgenography.[62] The most common symptom of aneurysm of the heart is congestive heart failure. Occasionally, symptoms of systemic embolization from mural thrombi or dysrhythmias are the main manifestations. The excellent prognosis following surgical repair suggests that these larger aneurysms should be treated by resection, even in asymptomatic patients.[62]

⊘ FREQUENT ERRORS

In the Management of Injuries to the Heart

1. *Rejecting a diagnosis of pericardial tamponade because the neck veins are not distended.*
2. *Assuming a pericardial tamponade is not present because an attempted pericardiocentesis was negative.*
3. *Delaying thoracotomy to perform pericardiocentesis in a patient in severe shock when thoracotomy can be started almost as quickly.*
4. *Failure to provide adequate fluid resuscitation in an unstable patient with pericardial tamponade because the neck veins are distended.*
5. *Performing resuscitative thoracotomy on a patient with chest trauma when there is inadequate OR and/or surgical backup.*
6. *Performing a resuscitative thoracotomy when the patient has had no signs of life at the scene or for more than five minutes prior to reaching the hospital.*
7. *Turning a patient who is hemodynamically unstable or has intrabronchial bleeding onto one side to perform posterolateral thoracotomy.*
8. *Inadequate or delayed compression of the aorta during thoracotomy or laparotomy in severely hypotensive patients.*
9. *Allowing the proximal systolic BP to exceed 160 mm Hg during clamping of the descending thoracic aorta.*
10. *Admitting patients with uncomplicated, but suspected myocardial contusion to an ICU for prolonged monitoring.*
11. *Inadequate pursuit of a diagnosis of valve injury or septal defect in the patient with a murmur after severe chest trauma.*
12. *Assuming that normal ECG and CPK-MB levels eliminate acute myocardial contusion.*
13. *Inadequate cardiovascular monitoring of a patient with suspected myocardial contusion before and during general anesthesia.*

▼▼▼▼▼▼▼▼▼▼▼▼▼▼▼▼▼▼▼▼▼▼▼▼▼▼▼▼▼▼

SUMMARY POINTS

1. Patients with penetrating wounds of the chest, especially from stab wounds, can often be successfully resuscitated from a recent (< 5 minutes) cardiac arrest by emergency resuscitative thoracotomy.
2. Pericardial tamponade increases the likelihood of survival after an emergency resuscitative thoracotomy for penetrating cardiac trauma
3. All patients in shock with penetrating wounds of the chest between the midclavicular line on the right and anterior axillary line on the left should be considered to have a cardiac injury until proved otherwise.
4. The neck veins in patients with shock from pericardial tamponade usually do not become distended until coexistent hypovolemia is at least partly corrected.
5. Distended neck veins after chest trauma are not always due to pericardial tamponade.
6. Muffled heart tones are an insensitive and nonspecific sign of pericardial tamponade.
7. Equalization of cardiac diastolic filling pressures following chest trauma should make one suspicious of pericardial tamponade.
8. If blood is obtained on pericardiocentesis and the patient's vital signs improve promptly, a tamponade was almost certainly present.
9. When a large amount (> 20 ml) of blood can be aspirated rapidly and easily during an attempted pericardiocentesis, it is likely that one is aspirating blood from the right ventricle rather than the pericardial cavity.
10. One of the quickest and most effective ways to restore adequate tissue perfusion in a hemodynamically unstable patient is aggressive fluid resuscitation.
11. Resuscitative thoracotomy for trauma should not be performed unless rapid, appropriate backup by the operating room and surgeons is available to properly manage the likely intrathoracic injuries.
12. Injuries to the mid or left chest in unstable patients are best explored through the left chest, and lesions on the right are best explored through the right chest.

13. When the injury is likely to be confined to the heart, a median sternotomy is perferred because all areas of the heart can be treated and cardiopulmonary bypass initiated easily through this incision.

14. Penetrating wounds of the left heart in an arrested or severely hypotensive patient are usually best treated with a left anterior thoracotomy because compression or clamping of the descending aorta may also be required.

15. Compressing the descending aorta in a severely hypotensive patient can greatly increase coronary and cerebral blood flow.

16. Clamping the hilum of a severely injured lung has three benefits: (a) control of blood loss from the injured lung, (b) reduced risk of air emboli and (c) reduced aspiration of blood into dependent, uninjured lung tissue.

17. Many open cardiac wounds can be controlled surprisingly well by inserting a Foley catheter, blowing up the balloon, and then pulling the catheter back until the balloon occludes the hole.

18. Compressing the heart with two hands or with one hand against the sternum reduces the risk of inadvertently entering the heart with a finger-tip.

19. A sudden onset of an arrhythmia or hypotension in a patient with open veins or a lung injury, especially in patients with hemoptysis, should be considered due to air emboli until proved otherwise.

20. Hypertension and/or severe tachycardia can greatly increase the workload and oxygen requirements of an injured heart and can cause infarction and/or overt heart failure.

21. Cardiac injury is frequently found in individuals dying immediately after blunt chest trauma.

22. Myocardial contusion should be suspected in anyone with severe trauma to the anterior chest.

23. Occasionally, patients with blunt rupture of the right atrium reach the hospital alive, but they usually die rapidly in the ED unless their injuries are recognized and corrected promptly.

24. One should look carefully for septal defects after blunt chest trauma if the patient has a new murmur plus evidence of myocardial damage.

25. ECG evidence of cardiac damage plus a new murmur after trauma suggest a valve lesion or VSD.

26. The valve injury most apt to be caused by blunt trauma is aortic insufficiency.

27. Cardiac contusion has been reported to be the most common visceral injury responsible for death immediately after trauma.

28. Myocardial contusions are usually clinically insignificant unless preexisting cardiac disease, other severe injuries, or a need for general anesthesia are present.

29. The reduced ejection fraction of a contused heart can be compensated for by increased preload and is not usually a problem unless the patient has multiple other injuries and/or requires general anesthesia.

30. General anesthesia within a month of a diagnosed myocardial contusion can be a significant risk for the development of arrhythmias or hypotension.

31. The diagnosis of a myocardial contusion can be made on the basis of new ECG findings, arrhythmias, heart failure, impaired cardiac function (↓ EF etc.), or increased CPK-MB levels, but evidence of anterior heart wall-motion abnormalities is probably most definitive.

32. Any patient involved in a head-on motor vehicle accident at speeds exceeding 35 MPH and having any chest symptoms or signs should be suspected of having myocardial contusion and injuries to the great vessels.

33. Plain chest radiography is unlikely to help with the diagnosis of myocardial contusion unless evidence of otherwise unexplained pulmonary edema and/or cardiomegaly exists.

34. Myocardial contusion seldom causes new arrhythmias more than 24 hours after admission, unless a significant stress, such as general anesthesia is added.

35. Holter monitoring reveals many more arrhythmias than the usual ECG monitoring systems, but it is unlikely that they are significant.

36. CPK-MB levels are of little or no value in predicting the outcome of patients with myocardial contusion.

37. Technetium pyrophosphate scans are of no diagnostic value for myocardial contusion except with full-thickness left ventricular injuries.

38. Gated RNA appears to be a sensitive technique to assess cardiac function, including left- and right-ventricular ejection fractions, and wall-motion abnormalities.

39. A patient with a normal 2-D ECHO after blunt trauma is unlikely to have a physiologically significant myocardial contusion.

40. Patients with myocardial contusions tend to have relatively flat cardiac function curves in response to fluid-loading, indicating impaired responses to stress.

41. Patients with myocardial contusions and wall-motion abnormalities should, when possible, not be given general anesthesia for at least 30 days.

42. Intraaortic balloon pumping may be lifesaving in patients with acute myocardial contusions and persistent, severe hypotension in spite of inotropes and adequate preloads.

43. Myocardial contusion may precipitate severe coronary insufficiency in patients with preexisting coronary artery disease.

44. Although rarely documented, blunt pericardial injury can cause pericardial tamponade without concomitant myocardial injury.

45. Blunt cardiac damage can produce delayed immune responses similar to those sometimes caused by acute myocardial infarction or cardiac surgery.

▲▲▲▲▲▲▲▲▲▲▲▲▲▲▲▲▲▲▲▲▲▲▲▲▲▲▲▲▲▲▲▲▲▲▲▲

REFERENCES

1. Symbas PN. Penetrating wounds of the heart. Symbas PN, ed. Cardiothoracic trauma. Philadelphia: W.B. Sanders Co., 1989; 27-54.
2. Symbas PN. Cardiac tamponade. Symbas PN, ed. Cardiothoracic trauma. Philadelphia: W.B. Sanders Co., 1989; 18-26.
3. Absolon KB. Theodore Billroth and cardiac surgery. J Thorac Cardiovasc Surg 1983;86:451.
4. Meade RH. A history of thoracic surgery. Thomas CC, ed. Springfield, 1961.
5. Henderson VJ, Smith RS, Fry WR, et al. Cardiac injuries: analysis of an unselected series of 251 cases. J Trauma 1994;36:341.
6. Bordley J, Harvey AM. Two centuries of American medicine. Philadelphia: WB Saunders, 1976; 502.
7. Demetriades D. Cardiac wounds. Ann Surg 1985;203:315.
8. Moreno C, Moore EE, Majure JA, Hopeman AR. Pericardial tamponade. A critical determinant for survival following penetrating cardiac wounds. J Trauma 1986;26:821.
9. Ivatury RR, Nallathambi MN, Stahl WM, Rohman M. Penetrating cardiac trauma. Ann Surg 1987;205:61.
10. Wilson RF, Basset JS. Penetrating wounds of the pericardium or its contents. JAMA 1966;195:513.
11. Washington B, Wilson RF, Steiger Z, Bassett JS. Emergency thoracotomy: a four year review. Ann Thorac Surg 1985;40:188.
12. Ordog GJ, Wasserberger J, Balasubramanian S, et al. Asymptomatic stab wounds of the chest. J Trauma 1994;36:680.
13. Martin LF, Mavroundis C, Dyess DL, et al. The first 70 years experience managing cardiac disruption due to penetrating and blunt injuries at the University of Louisville. Am Surg 1986;52:14.
14. Buckman RF, Badellino MM, Mauro LH, et al. Penetrating cardiac wounds: prospective study of factors influencing initial resuscitation. J Trauma 1993;34:717.
15. Aaland MO, Sherman RT. Delayed pericardial tamponade in penetrating chest trauma: case report. J Trauma 1991;31:1563.
16. Pories W, Gaudiani V. Cardiac tamponade. Surg Clin North Am 1975; 55:573.
17. Reddy PS, Curtiss EI, O'Toole JD, et al. Cardiac tamponade: hemodynamic observations in man. Circulation 1978;58:265.
18. Wechsler AS, Auerbach BJ, Graham TC, et al. Distribution of intramyocardial blood flow during pericardial tamponade. J Thorac Cardiovasc Surg 1974;68:847.
19. Cooley DA, Dunn JR, Brockman HL, et al. Treatment of penetrating wounds of the heart: experimental and clinical observations. Surgery 1955;37:882.

20. Lorell B, Leinbach RC, Pohost GM, et al. Right ventricular infarction: clinical diagnosis and differentiation from cardiac tamponade and pericardial constriction. Am J Cardiol 1979;43:465.
21. Aldridge HE, Jay AWL. Central venous catheters and heart perforation. Can Med Assoc J 1985;135:1082.
22. Aaland MO, Bryan FC 3rd, Sherman R. Two-dimensional echocardiogram in hemodynamically stable victims of penetrating precordial trauma. Am Surg 1994;60:412.
23. Meyer DM, Grayburn PA, Jessen ME, et al. The use of echocardiography to detect cardiac injury after penetrating thoracic trauma—a prospective study. J Trauma 1994;37:150.
24. Arom KV, Richardson JD, Webb G, et al. Subxiphoid pericardial window in patients with suspected traumatic pericardial tamponade. Ann Thorac Surg 1977;23:545.
25. Calhoon JH, Hoffmann TH, Trinkle JK, et al. Management of blunt rupture of the heart. J Trauma 1986;26:495.
26. Duncan AO, Scalea TM, Sclafani SJ, et al. Evaluation of occult cardiac injuries using subxiphoid pericardial window. J Trauma 1989;29:955.
27. Mayor-Davies JA, Britz RS. Subxiphoid pericardial windows—helpful in selected cases. J Trauma 1990;30:1399.
28. Steiger Z, McAlpin G, Wilson RF. Left subcostal approach to the pericardium. SGO 1985;160:414.
29. Nelson RM, Wilson RF, Huang CL, et al. Cardiac tamponade due to an iatrogenic pericardial-diaphragmatic hernia. Crit Care Med 1985;13:607.
30. Gyhra A, Pierart J, Torres P, Pieto L. Experimental cardiac tamponade with a myocardial wound: the effect of rapid intravenous infusion of saline. J Trauma 1992;33:25.
31. Ravitch MM, Blalock A. Aspiration of blood from the pericardium in treatment of acute cardiac tamponade after injury. Arch Surg 1949; 58:463.
32. Michelow BJ, Bremner CG. Penetrating cardiac injuries: selective conservatism—favorable or foolish? J Trauma 1987;27:398.
33. Baxter BT, Moore EE, Moore JB, et al. Emergency department thoracotomy following injury: critical determinants for patient salvage. World J Surg 1988;12:671-675.
34. Esposito TJ, Jurkovich GJ, Rice CL, et al. Reappraisal of emergency room thoracotomy in a changing environment. J Trauma 1991;31:881.
35. Boyd M, Vanek VW, Bourguet CC. Emergency room resuscitative thoracotomy: when is it indicated? J Trauma 1992;33:714.
36. Jurkovich GJ, Esposito TJ, Maier RV. Resuscitative thoracotomy performed in the operating room. Am J Surg 1992;165:463.
37. Millham FH, Grindlinger GA. Survival determinants in patients undergoing emergency room thoracotomy for penetrating chest trauma. J Trauma 1993;34:332.
38. Rohman M, Ivatury RR, Steichen FM, et al. Emergency room thoracotomy for penetrating cardiac injuries. J Trauma 1983;23:570.
39. Lorenz HP, Steinmetz B, Lieberman, et al. Emergency thoracotomy: survival correlates with physiologic status. J Trauma 1992;32:780.
40. Mazzorana V, Smith RS, Morabito DJ, et al. Limited utility of emergency department thoracotomy. Am Surg 1994;60:516.
41. Carrasquilla MD, Wilson RF, Walt AJ, et al. Gunshot wounds of the heart. Ann Thorac Surg 1972;13:2089.
42. Cogbill MH, Moore EE, Millikan JS, et al. Rationale for selective application of emergency department thoracotomy in trauma. J Trauma 1983;23:453.
43. Shimazu S, Clayton HS. Outcomes of trauma patients with no vital signs on hospital admission. J Trauma 1983;23:213.
44. Baker CC, Thomas ANM, Trunkey DD. The role of emergency room thoracotomy in trauma. J Trauma 1980;20:848.
45. Velmahos GC, Degiannis E, Souter I, et al. Penetrating trauma to the heart: a relatively innocent injury. Surgery 1994;115:694.
46. Baker CC, Caronna JJ, Trunkey DD. Neurologic outcome after emergency room thoracotomy for trauma. Am J Surg 1980;19:677.
47. Williams JB, Silver DG, Laws HL. Successful management of heart rupture from blunt trauma. J Trauma 1981;21:534.
48. Demetriades D, Van Der Veen BW. Penetrating injuries of the heart: experience over two years in South Africa. J Trauma 1983;23:1034.
49. Rea WJ, Sugg WL, Wilson LC, et at. Coronary artery laceration: an analysis of 22 patients. Ann Thorac Surg 1969;7:518.
50. Symbas PN. Coronary artery injuries. Cardiothoracic trauma Philadelphia: W.B. Saunders Co., 1989; 127-135.
51. Lowe, JE, Adams DH, Cummings RG, et al. The natural history and recommended management of patients with traumatic coronary artery fistulas. Ann Thorac Surg 1983;36:295.
52. Espada R, Whisennand HH, Maddox KL, et al. Surgical management of penetrating injuries to the coronary arteries. Surgery 1975;78:755.
53. Symbas PN. Traumatic ventricular septal defect. Symbas PN, ed. Philadelphia: W.B. Saunders Co., 1989; 95-107.
54. Von Berg VJ, Moggi L, Jacobson LF, et al. Ten year's experience with penetrating injuries of the heart. J Trauma 1961;1:186.
55. Beall AC Jr, Hamit HF, Cooley DA, et al. Surgical management of traumatic intracardiac lesions. J Trauma 1965;5:133.
56. Symbas PN, Harlaftis N, Waldo WJ. Penetrating cardiac wounds: a comparison of different therapeutic methods. Ann Surg 1976;183:377.
57. Symbas PN, Ware RE, Belenkiel I, et al. Traumatic biventricular pseudoaneurysm of the heart with ventricular septal defect. J Thorac Cardiovasc Surg 1972;64:4.
58. Symbas PN. Residual or delayed lesions from penetrating cardiac wounds. Chest 1974;66:408.
59. Symbas PN. Traumatic cardiac valve injury. ed. Cardiothoracic trauma. Philadelphia: W.B. Saunders Co., 1989; 108-120.
60. Rustad DG, Hopeman AR, Murr PC, Van Way CW. Aortocardia fistula with aortic valve injury from penetrating trauma. J Trauma 1986;26:266.
61. Borkon AM, Schneider R, Sarr M, Reitz B. Immediate mitral valve replacement following gunshot wound to the heart. J Trauma 1987;27:96.
62. Symbas PN. Traumatic aneurysms of the heart. (ed) Cardiothoracic trauma. Philadelphia: W.B. Saunders Co., 1989; 121-126.
63. Jackson DH, Murphy GW. Nonpenetrating cardiac injuries. Med Concepts Cardiovasc Dis 1976;45:123.
64. Leidtke AJ, DeMuth WE. Nonpenetrating cardiac injuries: a collective review. Am Heart J 1973;86:687.
65. Leinoff HD. Direct nonpenetrating injuries of the heart. AMA Ann Intern Med 1940;14:653.
66. Sigler LH. Traumatic injury of the heart—incidence of its occurrence in forty-two cases of severe accidental bodily injury. Am Heart J 1945; 30:459.
67. Tenzer ML. The spectrum of myocardial contusion: a review. J Trauma 1985;25:620.
68. Muwanga CL, Cole RP, Sloan JP, et al. Cardiac contusion in patients wearing seat belts. J Accid Surg 1986;17:37.
69. Van Loehout RMM, Schiphorst TJMJ, Wittens CHA, Pinkaers JA. Traumatic intrapericardial diaphragmatic hernia. J Trauma 1986;26:271.
70. Frazee RC, Mucha P, Farnell MB, Miller FA. Objective evaluation of blunt cardiac trauma. J Trauma 1986;26:510.
71. Fulda G, Brathwaite CEM, Rodriguez A, et al. Blunt traumatic rupture of the heart and pericardium: a ten-year experience (1979-1989).
72. Desforges O, Ridder WP, Lenoci RJ. Successful suture of ruptured myocardium after nonpenetrating injury. N Engl J Med 1955;252:567.
73. Parmley LF, Manion WC, Mattingly TW. Nonpenetrating traumatic injury to the heart. Circulation 1958;18:371.
74. Santavirta S, Arajarvi E. Ruptures of the heart in seatbelt wearers. J Trauma 1992;32:276.
75. Calhoon JH, Hoffmann TH, Trinkle JK, Harman PK, Grover FL. Management of blunt rupture of the heart. J Trauma 1986;26:495.
76. Getz BS, Davies E, Steinberg SM, et al. Blunt cardiac trauma resulting in right atrial rupture. JAMA 1986;255:761.
77. Kato K, Kushimoto S, Mashiko K, et al. Blunt traumatic rupture of the heart: an experience in Tokyo. J Trauma 1994;36:859.
78. Jenson BP, Hoffman I, Follis FM, et al. Surgical repair of atrial septal rupture due to blunt trauma. Ann Thorac Surg 1993;56:1172.
79. Krajcer Z, Cooley DA, Leachman RD. Ventricular septal defect following blunt trauma: spontaneous closure of residual defect after surgical repair. Cathet Cardiovasc Diagn 1977;3:409.
80. Rao G, Garvey J, Gupta M. Atrial septal defect due to blunt thoracic trauma. J Trauma 1977;17:405.
81. Rumisek JD, Robinowitz MM, Virmani R, et al. Bioprosthetic heart valve rupture associated with trauma. J Trauma 1986;26:276.
82. Bailey CP, Vara CA, Hirose T. Regurgitation from rupture of chordae tendineae due to a "steering wheel" compression. Geriatrics 1969;24:90.
83. Allen DB, Wilson RF. Clinical management of mitral valve injury: in current concepts in cardiac dynamics. Cardiac Chronicle 1992;6:1-7.
84. Bright EF, Beck CS. Nonpenetrating wounds of the heart: a clinical and experimental study. Ann Heart J 1935;10:293.
85. Munin A, Chodoff P. Traumatic acute mitral regurgitation secondary to blunt chest trauma. Crit Care Med 1983;11:311.
86. Kessler RM, Foianin JE, Davis JE, et al. Tricuspid insufficiency due to nonpenetrating trauma. Am J Cardiol 1976;37:442.
87. Arbulu A, Thoms NW, Wilson RF. Valvulectomy with prosthetic replacement: a life-saving operation for tricuspid pseudomonas endocarditis. J Thorac Cardiovasc Surg 1972;64:103-7.
88. Symbas PN. Contusion of the heart. Symbas PN, ed. Cardiothoracic trauma. Philadelphia: W. B. Saunders Co., 1989; 55-76.

89. Burchell HB. Unusual forms of heart disease. Circulation 1954;10:574.

90. Jones JW, Hewitt RL, Drapanas T. Cardiac contusion: a capricious syndrome. Ann Surg 1975;181:567.

91. Sutherland GR, Driedger AA, Holliday RL, et al. Frequency of myocardial injury after blunt chest trauma as evaluated by radionuclide angiography. AM J Cardiol 1983;52:1099.

92. Leidtke AJ, Allen RP, Nellis SH. Effects of blunt cardiac trauma on coronary vasomotion, perfusion, myocardial mechanics and metabolism. J Trauma 1980;20:777.

93. Moore EE, Malangoni MA, Cogbill TH, et al. Organ injury scaling IV: thoracic vascular, lung, cardiac and diaphragm. J Trauma 1994; 36:299.

94. McLean RF, Devitt JH, Dubbin J, et al. Incidence of abnormal RNA studies and dysrhythmias in patients with blunt chest trauma. J Trauma 1991;31:968.

95. Doty DB, Anderson AE, Rose EF, et al. Clinical and experimental correlations of myocardial contusion. Ann Surg 1974;180:452.

96. Torres-Mirabal P, Gruenberg JC, Talbert JG, et al. Ventricular function in myocardial contusion—a preliminary study. Crit Care Med 1982; 10:19.

97. Sutherland GR, Cheung HW, Holliday RL, et al. Hemodynamic adaptation to acute myocardial contusion complicating blunt chest injury. Am J Cardiol 1986;57:291.

98. DeMuth WE Jr, Lerner EH, Liedtke AJ. Nonpenetrating injury of the heart: an experimental model in dogs. J Trauma 1973;13:639.

99. Snow N, Richardson JD, Flint LM Jr. Myocardial contusion: implication for patients with multiple traumatic injuries. Surgery 1982; 92:744.

100. Chiu CL, Roelofs JD, Go RT, et al. Coronary angiographic and scintigraphic findings in experimental cardiac contusion. Radiology 1975; 116:679.

101. Harley DP, Mena I. Cardiac and vascular sequelae of sternal fractures. J Trauma 1986;26:553.

102. Shapira-Roy A, Levi I, Khoda J. Sternal fractures: a red flag or a red herring. J Trauma 1994;37:59.

103. Soliman MH, Waxman K. Value of a conventional approach to the diagnosis of traumatic cardiac contusion after chest injury. Crit Care Med 1987;15:218.

104. Glinz W. Problems caused by the unstable thoracic wall and by cardiac injury due to blunt injury. Injury 1986;17:322.

105. Blair E, Topuzlu C, Davis JH. Delayed or missed diagnosis of cardiac damage in blunt chest trauma. J Trauma 1971;11:129.

106. Fabian TC, Cicala RS, Croce MA, et al. A prospective evaluation of myocardial contusion: correlation of significant arrhythmias and cardiac output with CPK-MB measurements. J Trauma 1991;31:653.

107. Reynolds M, Jones JM. CPK-MB isoenzyme determinations in blunt chest trauma. JACEP 1979;8:304.

108. Miller FB, Richardson JD. Blunt cardiac injury. Common problems in trauma. Ann Emerg Med 1982;11:319.

109. Coleman RE, Klein MS, Ahmad SA, et al. Mechanisms contributing to myocardial accumulation of technetium-99m stannous pyrophosphate after coronary arterial occlusion. Am J Cardiol 1977;39:55.

110. Go RT, Doty DB, Chiu CL, et al. A new method of diagnosing myocardial contusion in man by radionuclide imaging. Radiology 1975;116:107.

111. Kumar SA, Puri VK, Mittal VK, et al. Myocardial contusion following nonfatal blunt chest trauma. J Trauma 1983;23:327.

112. Brantigan CO, Burdick D, Hoperman AR, et al. Evaluation of technetium scanning for myocardial contusion. J Trauma 1978;18:460.

113. Rodriguez A, Shatney C. The value of technetium (99-m pyrophosphate scanning in the diagnosis of myocardial contusion. Am Surg 1982; 48:472.

114. Rothstein RJ, French RE, Mena I, et al. Myocardial contusion diagnosed by first-pass radionuclide angiography. Am J Emerg Med 1986;4:210.

115. Jaszczak RJ, Whitehead FR, Lim CB, et al. Lesiondetection with single photon emission computerized tomography (SPECT) compared with conventional imaging. J Nucl Med 1982;23:97.

116. Waxman K, Soliman MH, Braunstein P, et al. Diagnosis of traumatic cardiac contusion. Arch Surg 1986;121:689.

117. King RM, Mucha P, Seward JB, et al. Cardiac contusion: a new diagnostic approach utilizing two-dimensional echocardiography. J Trauma 1983;23:610.

118. Pandian NG, Skorton DJ, Dothy DB, et al. Immediate diagnosis of acute myocardial contusion by two-dimensional echocardiography—studies in a canine model of blunt chest trauma. JACC 1983;2:448.

119. Karalis DG, Victor MF, Davis GA, et al. The role of echocardiography in blunt chest trauma: a transthoracic and transesophageal echocardiographic study. J Trauma 1994;36:53.

120. Shapiro MJ, Yanofsky SD, Trapp J, et al. Cardiovascular evaluation in blunt thoracic trauma using transesophageal echocardiography (TEE). J Trauma 1991;31:835.

121. Orliaguet G, Jacquens Y, Riou B, et al. Combined severe myocardial and pulmonary contusion: early diagnosis with transesophageal echocardiography and management with high-frequency jet ventilation: case report. J Trauma 1993;34:455.

122. Mattox KL, Flint LM, Carrico CJ. (Editorial) Blunt cardiac injury (Formerly termed "Myocardial Contusion"). J Trauma 1992;33:649.

123. Diebel LN, Wilson RF, Tagett MG, et al. End-diastolic volume: a better indicator of preload in the critically ill. Arch Surg 1992;127:817-21.

124. Flancbaum L, Wright J, Siegel JH. Emergency surgery in patients with post-traumatic myocardial contusion. J Trauma 1986;26:795.

125. Saunders CT, Doty DB. Myocardial contusion—effect of intra-aortic balloon counterpulsation on cardiac output. J Trauma 1978;18:706.

126. Timberlake GA, McSwain NE. Thromboembolism as a complication of myocardial contusion: a new capricious syndrome. J Trauma 1988; 28:535.

127. Miller FA, Seward JB, Gersh BJ, et al. Two-dimensional echocardiographic findings in cardiac trauma. Am J Cardiol 1982;50:1022.

128. Solomon D. Delayed cardiac tamponade after blunt chest trauma: case report. J Trauma 1991;31:1322.

129. Symbas PN. Traumatic injury of the pericardium. Cardiothoracic trauma. Philadelphia: W.B. Saunders Co., 1989; 77-78.

130. Rosenbaum RC, Johnston GS. Post-traumatic cardiac dysfunction: assessment with radionuclide ventriculography. Radiology 1986;160:91.

131. Sturaitis M, McCallum D, Sutherland G, et al. Lack of significant long-term sequelae following traumatic myocardial contusion. Arch Intern Med 1986;146:1765.

132. Tabatznik B, Issacs JP. Postpericardiotomy syndrome following traumatic hemopericardium. Am J Cardiol 1961;7:83.

133. Dressler W. Management of pericarditis secondary to myocardial infarction. Prog Cardiovasc Dis 1960;3:134.

134. Kirsh MM, McIntosh K, Kahn DR, et al. Postpericardiotomy syndromes. Ann Thorac Surg 1970;9:158.

135. Engle MA, McCabe JC, Ebert PA, et al. The post pericardiotomy syndrome and antiheart antibodies. Circulation 1974;49:401.

136. Ehrenhaft JL, Taber RE. Hemopericardium and constrictive pericarditis. J Thorac Surg 1952;24:355.

Chapter 18 Trauma to Intrathoracic Great Vessels

ROBERT F. WILSON, M.D.

LARRY W. STEPHENSON, M.D.

PENETRATING WOUNDS OF THE GREAT VESSELS OF THE CHEST

Introduction

Although thoracic trauma may directly or indirectly account for 30-50% of the 150,000 deaths from trauma occurring annually in the United States,[1-4] injury to thoracic great vessels is uncommon and occurs in < 5% of patients reaching a trauma center alive.[2-4] Over a period of 10 years (1980 to 1990), during which approximately 30,000 trauma patients were admitted to Detroit Receiving Hospital, only 108 patients were documented to have great-vessel injuries in the chest. Although in-hospital mortality rates have been reported to be 8-30%,[1,3,5] prehospital mortality rates resulting from such injuries have been estimated at 48%,[5] emphasizing the importance of early, aggressive management.

AXIOM Patients with injured thoracic great vessels may suddenly begin to bleed massively again when their BPs are restored or when they gag or wretch as an esophageal or tracheal tube is inserted.

Patients with penetrating injuries of major intrathoracic vessels who survive long enough to reach a hospital generally have their bleeding sites temporarily occluded with blood clot and/or vessel adventitia. Subsequently, with a Valsalva maneuver or restoration of a normal BP, the blood clot or seal may become dislodged, causing recurrent, massive bleeding. Occasionally, vascular injury results in the formation of a traumatic aneurysm or arteriovenous fistula, and patients with thoracic vascular trauma are more likely to survive when the injury is within the pericardial cavity where the bleeding may become tamponaded.[3]

AXIOM Penetrating extrapericardial injuries to thoracic great vessels are usually rapidly fatal.

History

The first successful repair of a penetrating injury of the thoracic aorta was reported by Dshanelidge in 1923.[4] Although a number of penetrating aortic injuries within the pericardial cavity were successfully repaired in the 1940s and 1950s, it was not until 1958 that Perkins and Elchos were able to report the first successful repair of a penetrating injury of the thoracic aorta outside the pericardium.[6]

Injuries involving great vessels at the thoracic inlet tend to have a much better prognosis than injuries more centrally located within the chest. In 1977, Richardson et al. noted that patients with injuries of the subclavian or innominate artery at the thoracic inlet had a survival rate of 70%.[7] Nevertheless, in 1978, Rich and Spencer indicated that "probably less than 20 successful repairs of acute injuries to the intrathoracic great vessels have been reported in the English literature.[8]"

In 1987, Demetriades et al.[9] reported on 228 patients with penetrating wounds of subclavian vessels. Most (61%) of the 138 patients were certified dead on arrival at the hospital. In the remaining 90 patients, six died in the operating room and eight died within hours or days of surgery; the in-hospital mortality rate was 16%.

In a 1993 review of 23 years experience in Memphis, Pate et al. reported 93 patients with penetrating injuries of the aortic arch and its branches which included 31 common carotid, 29 subclavian, 27 aortic arch, and 6 innominate artery injuries.[10] Twelve of 93 patients could not be resuscitated. Of those having surgery, the mortality rates for the various vessel injuries were aortic arch 39%, innominate 17%, subclavian 14%, and common carotid 11%.

Recently, the organ injury scaling committee of the American Association for the Surgery of Trauma has developed a thoracic vascular organ injury scale to facilitate clinical research and to allow more valid comparison of results with various types of treatment (Table 18–1).

Anatomy

ARCH OF THE AORTA

The aortic arch begins at the upper border of the second chondrosternal articulation on the right side, and passes upward and backward and then across and down to the left side of the lower border of the fourth dorsal vertebra.[14] The upper border of the arch is usually about an inch below the sternal notch.

Relationships

The anterior surface of the aortic arch is covered by the lungs and the remains of the thymus gland. It is crossed on the left side by the left vagus and phrenic nerves. Its posterior surface is situated on the lower third of the trachea, the esophagus, thoracic duct, and left recurrent laryngeal nerve. The upper border is adjacent to the left innominate vein, and the lower border is adjacent to the bifurcation of the pulmonary artery and the remains of the ductus arteriosus.

Aortic Arch Anomalies

AXIOM When the aortic arch or one of its branches is injured, one must be prepared to handle an anatomical variant of aortic arch branching in one-third to one-fourth of the patients.

A great deal of variation in the number of vessels coming off the aortic arch has been noted.[11] The incidence of three branches (innominate, left common carotid, and left subclavian arteries) extending from the aortic arch is about 65-75%.[15,16] A common origin for the right subclavian and right and left common carotid arteries from the innominate artery is seen in 10-27% of individuals. In 0.5-2.5% of patients, both carotids and both subclavians extend from the aortic arch. In 0.5-1.2% of patients, the left vertebral artery arises from the arch just proximal to the origin of the left subclavian artery. In 0.5-2.5% of patients, there are two innominate arteries, and in about 0.5% of persons with a left aortic arch, the right subclavian artery arises as a fourth branch posterior and to the left of the origin of the left subclavian. This vessel extends behind the esophagus to reach the right upper extremity. A right aortic arch is present in 0.1-0.14% of the population.

TABLE 18–1   Thoracic Vascular Organ Injury Scale

Grade*	Injury Description†	AIS-90
I	Intercostal artery/vein	2-3
	Internal mammary artery/vein	2-3
	Bronchial artery/vein	2-3
	Esophageal artery/vein	2-3
	Hemiazygous vein	2-3
	Unnamed artery/vein	2-3
II	Azygous vein	2-3
	Internal jugular vein	2-3
	Subclavian vein	3-4
	Innominate vein	3-4
III	Carotid artery	3-5
	Innominate artery	3-4
	Subclavian artery	3-4
IV	Thoracic aorta, descending (intrathoracic)	4-5
	Inferior vena cava	3-4
	Pulmonary artery, primary intra-parenchymal branch	3
	Pulmonary vein, primary intra-parenchymal branch	3
V	Thoracic aorta, ascending and arch	5
	Superior vena cava	3-4
	Pulmonary artery, main trunk	4
	Pulmonary vein, main trunk	4
VI	Uncontained total transection of thoracic aorta or pulmonary hilum	5
		4

*Increase one grade for multiple grade III or IV injuries if >50% circumference; decrease one grade for IV and V injuries if <25% circumference.
†Based on most accurate assessment at autopsy, operation, or radiologic study.

INNOMINATE ARTERY

The innominate (brachiocephalic) artery is the largest branch off the arch of the aorta. It arises at the level of the border of the second right costal cartilage and ascends obliquely for 1½-2 inches to the upper border of the right sternoclavicular joint where it divides into the right common carotid and right subclavian arteries.

Relations

The innominate artery is separated from the upper sternum by the sternohyoid and sternothyroid muscles, the thymus gland, and the left innominate and right inferior thyroid veins. It lays on the trachea, which it crosses obliquely.

Branches

The innominate artery typically divides into the right subclavian and common carotid arteries. It usually has no branches, but in about 10% of patients, a branch, the thyroidea ima, ascends in front of the trachea up to the thyroid isthmus. The thyroid ima varies greatly in size to compensate for any deficiency or absence of one of the other thyroid vessels.

SUBCLAVIAN ARTERIES

The right subclavian artery arises from the innominate artery opposite the right sternoclavicular joint, and passes upward and outward behind the scalenus anticus muscle where it ascends slightly above the clavicle. It is covered, in front, by the clavicular origin of the sternomastoid and the sternohyoid and sternothyroid muscles. It is crossed by the internal jugular and vertebral veins and by the right vagus nerve. Below and behind the artery is the pleura and apex of the lung. The right recurrent laryngeal nerve winds around the lower and back part of the vessel.

The left subclavian artery typically arises from the end of the arch of the aorta, opposite the fourth dorsal vertebra. From there it ascends nearly vertically to the inner margin of the scalenus anticus muscle. The vagus and phrenic nerves lay anterior and parallel the left subclavian artery. Posteriorly, it is adjacent to the esophagus, thoracic duct, and inferior cervical ganglion. More distally, the esophagus and

thoracic duct lay on its right, with the thoracic duct arching over the vessel to enter the venous system between the subclavian and internal jugular veins.

The second portion of the subclavian artery is covered anteriorly by the scalenus anticus muscle. On the right side the phrenic nerve is separated from the second part of the artery by the anterior scalene muscle, while on the left side the nerve crosses the first part of the artery at the inner edge of the scalenus anticus muscle. The artery is in relation to the pleura and middle scalene posteriorly and the brachial plexus superiorly. The subclavian vein lays below and in front of the artery, and is separated from it by the scalenus anticus muscle.

The third portion of the subclavian arteries passes downward and outward from the outer margin of the scalenus anticus to the outer border of the first rib, where it becomes the axillary artery.

The branches from the subclavian artery are the vertebral, internal mammary, thyrocervical trunk, and superior intercostal arteries. On the left side, all four branches generally arise from the first portion of the vessel, but on the right side, the superior intercostal usually arises behind the scalenus anticus muscle.

Etiology

KNIVES

The survival rate of patients with great-vessel injuries caused by stab wounds is generally much higher than with those caused by gunshot wounds.[3] Small stab wounds are often sealed rapidly by the vascular adventitia. This limits the amount of blood loss, particularly after blood pressure decreases to hypotensive levels. Furthermore, an occasional stabbing victim comes in with the knife still in place, and the retained foreign body may seal the opening in the involved vessel, at least temporarily.

GUNSHOT WOUNDS

AXIOM   One cannot assume that bullets travel in straight lines.

Bullets sometimes take unexpected paths as they travel through tissue. The amount of tissue destruction caused by a bullet is determined partially by the kinetic energy (KE) lost after the missile enters the tissue and partially by the orientation or tumbling of the bullet as it passes through the tissues. The KE imparted to the tissues can be calculated as $KE = 1/2m(V_1^2 - V_2^2)$. Thus, the tissue destruction is proportional to the mass (m) of the missile and the entering velocity squared (V_1^2) minus the exiting velocity squared (V_2^2) as the bullet leaves the tissue. When the bullet remains in the patient, V_2^2 is zero. Thus, a rifle bullet with a velocity of 3000 ft/s can impart 25 times as much damage to tissue as a similar weight pistol bullet going at 600 ft/s. A shotgun blast from close range (< 20 feet), particularly by 12-gauge shotgun pellets, can be even more destructive.

Types of Vascular Injuries

SIMPLE LACERATIONS

Simple lacerations of the great arteries of the chest can cause exsanguination, tamponade, and/or hemothorax. Other vascular injuries, which may present as delayed problems, include arteriovenous fistulas and false aneurysms.

ARTERIOVENOUS FISTULAS

AXIOM   Major thoracic arterial injuries can easily be missed until an arteriovenous fistula or false aneurysm is detected.

Systemic

Injuries to a systemic artery and vein situated side by side within a contained hematoma can lead to formation of an arteriovenous (AV) fistula. As time passes, the fistula tends to enlarge and have increasing flow. When more than 25% of the cardiac output goes through the AV fistula, high-output cardiac failure is likely to develop.

Pulmonary

Pulmonary AV fistulas after penetrating chest trauma are said to be extremely rare because of the small-pressure differential that usually exists between the pulmonary arteries and veins.[12] Nevertheless, injuries to adjacent major pulmonary arteries and veins can lead to this problem, especially when pulmonary arterial pressures are high or rise as they often do following severe trauma.

AXIOM Severe arterial hypoxemia in spite of what appears to be normally functioning lungs should make one search for a pulmonary AV fistula.

FALSE ANEURYSMS

A small injury to an artery associated with a contained hematoma will often stop bleeding, and the hematoma will gradually resolve. In some instances, however, the opening into the hematoma remains patent, and the hematoma may develop into a false aneurysm with a pseudoendothelial lining. These false aneurysms often enlarge and rupture within a few days, but they occasionally remain for many years.

Diagnosis

HISTORY

Most penetrating wounds of the chest are quite obvious, and little or no additional information is required to make a diagnosis; however, certain historic facts can be helpful in planning the diagnostic steps and treatment. For example, the amount of time the patient spent at the scene and in transit may be extremely important in considering whether to perform an emergency department (ED) thoracotomy on a patient who arrives in cardiac arrest. Cardiac arrest for more than five minutes rarely, if ever, allows one to perform a successful resuscitation so that the patient leaves the hospital alive with an intact CNS.

AXIOM Cardiac arrest for more than five minutes before resuscitative thoracotomy is performed rarely results in a patient leaving the hospital alive with a normally functioning brain.

The size of a knife and its depth and angle of penetration may indicate the vessels or organs most likely to be injured. When two skin wounds are present, it may be helpful to know whether they represent two entrance wounds or single exit and entrance wounds. In some instances, a bullet that entered the chest without exiting is missed on chest or abdominal radiography because it is in subcutaneous tissues or has entered a major vessel and embolized. It is also extremely important to know, if possible, the caliber of the bullet and whether it was a high-velocity missile (2000 ft/sec), which tends to cause far more tissue destruction than knives or low-velocity (< 1000ft/sec) bullets. High-velocity missile injuries are much more likely to require thoracotomy, even when the bullet does not enter the chest cavity.

PHYSICAL EXAMINATION

AXIOM Although most penetrating injuries of the chest are obvious, small wounds (especially in the axilla, skin folds, or areas covered with thick hair) may easily be missed.

Presence or absence of pulses in the upper extremities is not a reliable sign of the presence or absence of innominate or subclavian artery injury. The excellent collateral circulation about the shoulder may result in a normal pulse when injury occurs; however, vascular spasm occasionally occurs secondary to adjacent soft-tissue or boney injury when no demonstrable vessel injury is present at surgery. In a recent study by Calhoon et al., 14 (64%) of 22 patients with proxi-

mal thoracic vascular injuries had normal peripheral pulses.[13] Nevertheless, if pulse loss were accompanied by another sign of vascular injury, such as bruit or expanding hematoma (present in 68% of patients reported by Calhoon et al.), arterial injury would be present at least 80% of patients. Loss of a peripheral pulse caused by embolization of a bullet is also occasionally seen.

AXIOM Generally, one should not probe chest wounds because it may restart bleeding or an air leak or may cause pneumothorax.

Although probing of penetrating thoracic injuries is not recommended, careful superficial instrumentation may provide useful information on the direction of the tract. One should auscultate the entire chest and back for bruits after penetrating injury. A systolic bruit, particularly when heard over the back or upper chest, should make one suspect a false aneurysm involving one of the great vessels. A continuous bruit should make one suspect an AV fistula.[12] Bruits were present in all three of the patients with AV fistulas reported by Calhoon et al.[13]

A millwheel murmur, believed to be due to air being churned in the heart, may be diagnostic of air embolism. Hamman's sign, which is a crunching sound heard over the precordium during systole, indicates the presence of a pneumomediastinum or pneumopericardium. Loss of a peripheral pulse caused by embolization of a bullet from an injured thoracic vessel is occasionally seen.

Severe, blunt intrathoracic injuries can occur with little or no external evidence of injury. Occasionally, a large upper mediastinal hematoma can cause an acute superior vena caval syndrome, tracheal compression, and/or respiratory distress.[5]

AXIOM Distended neck veins plus hypotension are usually due to pericardial tamponade, tension pneumothorax, or excessive straining in a hypovolemic patient.

Distended neck veins may indicate pericardial tamponade, tension pneumothorax, heart failure, systemic air embolism, or damage to or compression of the superior vena cava; however, these conditions usually do not cause neck vein distention while the patient is severely hypovolemic. Neck vein distention often does not become apparent until the hypovolemia is at least partly corrected.

AXIOM Pericardial tamponade or tension pneumothorax usually does not cause distended neck veins while the patient is severely hypovolemic.

Some patients with major intrathoracic vascular injuries exhibit few or no signs of injury initially. Flint et al. found that 45 (32%) of 146 patients with 206 injuries of major vessels at the thoracic inlet had none of the usual diagnostic signs of significant vascular injury.[14] Early diagnosis of such injuries usually requires a high index of suspicion and careful evaluation of the patient.

A careful neurologic examination is also indicated with injuries near the thoracic inlet. In the study by Calhoon et al., upper extremity neurologic deficits were present in 31% of patients, and bruits were audible as evidence of arteriovenous fistulas in 14%.[13]

RADIOGRAPHY

AXIOM Virtually all patients with major trauma should have chest radiography soon after admission.

Plain Radiography

Virtually all patients with major trauma should have chest radiography soon after admission. With penetrating injuries of great vessels, a hemothorax is generally apparent on routine radiography of the chest, particularly when an associated pneumothorax provides an air-fluid level. When the patient is lying flat, however, up to 500-1000 mL of blood may cause only a slightly increased haziness over the lung on the involved side. Occasionally, even on an upright chest film, several hundred milliliters of blood may be difficult to identify if it were to settle under the lung as a subpulmonic hematoma where it could be mistaken for an elevated diaphragm. Decubitus chest radiography, however, usually demonstrates layering of the blood, unless it is loculated or clotted.

Evidence of cervical or supraclavicular swelling and/or widening of the upper mediastinal silhouette on chest radiography is often present in patients with injury to the aortic arch or its branches. With innominate artery injuries, the widening is usually more superior and to the right than that seen after aortic injury.

In the study by Calhoon et al., initial chest radiographs were interpreted as normal in four of 22 patients and revealed only hemopneumothorax or pneumothorax in seven of 22.[13] In eight (36%) of the patients, either an apical density or mediastinal widening occurred. Aortography was used in only seven stable patients who had equivocal signs and symptoms of vascular injury.

AXIOM A "fuzzy" bullet should be considered a radiologic sign of a major vascular injury until proven otherwise.

One should not assume that a "fuzzy" foreign body (bullet) on a radiograph is due to poor radiologic technique.[15] When a foreign body pulsates because it lays next to a major vessel, its margins tend to be indistinct on chest films. Therefore, a fuzzy foreign body contiguous with mediastinal structures can be an important radiographic clue to vascular injury. Fluoroscopy showing pulsation of the foreign body may lend additional support to the suspicion of vascular involvement. Even when angiography is performed and is normal, McFadden et al. believed that a fuzzy foreign body should still be considered an indication for surgery because of the strong likelihood that vascular injury is present.[15] Although magnetic resonance imaging (MRI) can be as valuable as an arteriogram in most situations, it should not be attempted in patients with bullets in or adjacent to great vessels because the metal object may blur the image, and more importantly, the MRI could cause the bullet to move, with resultant further tissue damage and bleeding.

In hemodynamically stable patients presenting with no clinical signs of great-vessel injury and with normal chest radiographs, it may be important to also obtain repeat chest radiographs at 6 hours and again at 24 hours.

CT Scans

AXIOM CT scans of the chest should not be performed while a patient is hemodynamically unstable.

In stable patients, CT scans can identify localized hematomas or other collections of blood that may not be apparent on routine radiography. When a persistent extravascular "mass" is adjacent to a great vessel and does not move with position changes by the patient, one should assume a contained hematoma is present. Intravenous contrast is essential for reliably demonstrating a mediastinal hematoma or false aneurysm on CT. One should also look for an irregular aortic contour, divided aortic lumen, or intimal flap.

Arteriography

Arteriography may be particularly helpful for identifying major intrathoracic vascular injuries within contained hematomas, especially those resulting from penetrating wounds of the lower neck; however, even with no clinical evidence of vascular injury, proximity of the missile trajectory is often considered to be an indication for arteriography.[16]

The type of arteriography performed depends on the location of the hematoma and the experience of the radiologist. Graham et al. described percutaneous retrograde upper-extremity arteriography or venography performed in the ED by surgeons to visualize the entire subclavian, carotid, and innominate arteries and their associated

veins.[17] More frequently, however, the angiographic evaluation of the thoracic aorta and its major branches is performed by percutaneous retrograde studies via the femoral artery in a radiology suite.

Although valuable information concerning the choice of incision can be derived from arteriography, the penetration site may be temporarily "sealed off" or the radiologic projection may not be appropriate for demonstrating a vascular abnormality. Although Buscaglia et al. noted that subclavian artery injuries could always be identified by angiography, their experience was unique.[18] Furthermore, in those patients with arteriovenous communication, the extent of arterial injury was difficult to assess because of associated venous blush.

Perry et al. reported three false-negative arteriograms for subclavian injuries in three patients who had widened mediastinums on chest radiography and were hemodynamically stable.[19] In a study by Fisher and Ben-Menachem, 3 (17%) of 18 patients with surgically-proved, penetrating injuries to the thoracic aorta or brachiocephalic arteries had false-negative preoperative angiograms.[20] Allen et al.[21] and Hewitt et al.[22] each reported one false-negative thoracic aortogram in patients with a gunshot and stab wound, respectively.

AXIOM A "negative" aortogram may convey a false sense of security in a patient with significant injury.[20]

Venograms
Venograms are seldom performed to identify major venous injuries in the chest. A patient who is actively bleeding from a major venous injury is usually explored emergently because of unstable vital signs and/or continued blood loss via the chest tubes. After a venous injury stops bleeding, however, the hemorrhage often does not recur, and the damaged vessel usually does not require thoracotomy. Nevertheless, we have had at least two isolated innominate vein injuries which bled massively after the patient was hemodynamically stable for more than 24 hours.

Contrast Swallows
A contrast swallow should be performed when the patient is hemodynamically stable and when concern exists about the possibility of an associated esophageal injury. The patient should be awake and have a good swallowing and cough reflex before attempting a contrast swallow, otherwise there can be severe aspiration of the contrast material into the lungs. One usually uses Gastrographin first because, if a leak were to occur, it is believed to be less of an adjuvant to infection than barium; however, if the patient were to aspirate Gastrographin into the lungs, it would be extremely irritating and could cause severe chemical pneumonitis.

One should not, however, completely rely on a negative Gastrographin swallow to eliminate esophageal injury. Contrast swallows with Gastrographin may miss 25-50% of esophageal leaks. Barium swallows are less likely to result in false negatives, but they may aggravate the mediastinitis if a perforation were present.

ENDOSCOPY
With penetrating wounds of the chest or lower neck in hemodynamically stable patients, it is prudent to perform bronchoscopy and esophagoscopy to eliminate injury to the aerodigestive tract. In some patients with "hemoptysis" after trauma, the source may not be clear, but such bleeding may result from a wide variety of injuries, including injury to the nose, mouth, pharynx, larynx, lung parenchyma, trachea, or a major bronchus.[20] Mediastinal air can also be a problem because it can also be caused by a wide variety of trauma, including esophageal, pulmonary, or tracheobronchial.

Treatment

INITIAL RESUSCITATION
The standard ABCs of initial resuscitation should be followed aggressively when the patient is in shock. These steps include (a) rapid clearing and maintenance of the airway, (b) establishment of adequate ven-

tilation using a ventilator, oxygen, and/or chest tubes as necessary, and (c) establishment of adequate circulation using intravenous fluids and control of bleeding. With some injuries to the great vessels in the thoracic outlet, mediastinal hematoma may cause severe tracheal compression. Consequently, early endotracheal intubation should be performed when such an injury is suspected. Tracheostomy should be avoided initially in patients with injuries at the thoracic inlet because of the possibility of precipitating massive bleeding from an otherwise controlled hematoma.

> **AXIOM** Shock plus inadequate ventilation are a rapidly fatal combination.

When the patient is in shock, two or three veins are cannulated with large gauge needles or catheters. At least one, and preferably two, of the intravenous lines should be started in the lower extremities. In patients with severe shock (systolic BP < 50 mm Hg), immediate surgery is required. With mild-to-moderate shock (systolic BP 50-89 mm Hg), 2000-3000 mL of balanced electrolyte solution is infused in 10-15 minutes. When shock is persistent or recurs in spite of this fluid, immediate surgery is required.

FINGER CONTROL OF HEMORRHAGE
Occasionally, external hemorrhage from either the suprasternal notch or supraclavicular fossa may be the sole manifestation of major intrathoracic vascular injury.[5] If no pleural connection is present, insertion of a finger or pack into the stab or gunshot wound site can often control much of the hemorrhage until the patient is transferred to the operating room. Sometimes, one can control the intrathoracic hemorrhage by digital pressure on the injured vessel itself.

TRANSCUTANEOUS BALLOON CATHETER TAMPONADE
DiGiacomo et al. recently reported on their success in treating two patients; 18 F Foley catheters were placed directly into the depths of actively bleeding infraclavicular stab and gunshot wounds. Inflating the balloon with 10 mL of sterile saline in each case immediately controlled the hemorrhage from what were later proven to be injuries to axillary veins.[23]

CHEST TUBE (THORACOSTOMY) DRAINAGE

Indications
Blood in the pleural cavity should usually be removed as completely and rapidly as possible. Blood entering a mesothelial-lined cavity slowly often does not clot because its fibrinogen quickly adheres to the pleural surfaces. When hemorrhage is rapid, however, much of the blood will clot before it can defibrinate. If the hemothorax were not removed, it not only would restrict ventilation and venous return, but the clots present would release fibrinolytic and fibrinogenolytic substances that could act as local anticoagulants and contribute to continued intrathoracic bleeding.

> **AXIOM** Moderate or large hemothorax should be promptly evacuated with a chest tube unless the patient requires emergency thoracotomy.

When a patient needs emergency thoracotomy because of massive intrathoracic bleeding, one should not insert a chest tube first because it will delay the surgery and may greatly increase the blood loss prior to surgical control of the bleeding site.

Autotransfusion
In patients with massive bleeding into a body cavity, the addition of citrate or heparin to the blood in the suction container prevents it from clotting. This may allow the blood to be given back to the patient as an autotransfusion, preferably after washing the red blood cells to remove anticoagulants and any contaminants. Unfortunately, in emergency situations with continued shock, attempts at autotransfusion

may seem troublesome and time-consuming, particularly when adequate type-specific blood is available. Large amounts of autotransfused blood may also contribute to development of coagulopathy.[24] Thomas found that more than 1000 mL of blood that is directly autotransfused may lead to coagulopathy and increased blood loss.[25] When cells are washed in a cell-saver, however, 5-6 units of packed autotransfused red blood cells can usually be given relatively safely.[26]

ED (Resuscitative) Thoracotomy

> **AXIOM** ED resuscitative thoracotomy is seldom successful if cardiac arrest is present for more than five minutes before arrival or when due to blunt trauma.

Although ED thoracotomies can be lifesaving, especially in patients with penetrating wounds of the chest, the results seem to be about twice as good for equivalent injuries when the patient has the emergency thoracotomy in the operating room. In an earlier series of 314 patients requiring emergency thoracotomies for intrathoracic injuries, 127 (40%) required ED thoracotomies because of cardiac arrest or rapidly deteriorating vital signs.[2] The survival rate for individuals with ED thoracotomies for cardiac arrest in the ambulance or ED resulting from penetrating trauma to the chest, neck, or extremities was 30% (8 of 27).

Antibiotics

Large doses of an antibiotic, such as Cefazolin, primarily to cover staphylococcal and/or streptococcal contamination, should be given as soon as the chest tube is inserted. Another dose can be given immediately preoperatively when there is more than a 3- or 4-hour delay in performing the surgery. When much blood is lost, antibiotics should be repeated after the major blood loss has been controlled.

OPERATING ROOM THORACOTOMY

Indications

Although most patients with intrathoracic bleeding can be treated adequately with intravenous fluids and evacuation of the hemothorax with a chest tube, 9% of our patients with penetrating chest wounds required thoracotomy for continuing hemorrhage.

SEVERE OR PERSISTENT SHOCK

> **AXIOM** If it is obvious that the patient has exsanguinating intrathoracic bleeding, thoracotomy should be performed as quickly as possible and with little or no resuscitation until the bleeding is controlled.

As mentioned previously, when the patient is in severe shock (systolic BP < 50 mm Hg), ED thoracotomy should be performed or the patient should be rapidly moved to the operating room for the thoracotomy to control bleeding. If shock were persistent or recurred in spite of 2,000 to 3,000 mL of balanced electrolyte solution given rapidly, the patient should be rushed to the operating room while type-specific blood and further fluid are administered rapidly.

CONTINUED BLEEDING
Even when the patient's vital signs are stable, one should perform thoracotomy for severe, continued bleeding as demonstrated by: (a) more than 1500-2000 mL of blood loss from the chest within the first 4-8 hours, (b) blood loss from the chest tubes exceeding 300 mL/hr for four or more hours, or (c) the chest staying more than half full of blood on radiography in spite of properly inserted and functioning chest tubes.

HYPOTENSION DEVELOPING WITH CHEST TUBE DRAINAGE

AXIOM Hypotension that develops or gets worse while a chest tube is draining blood from the chest is an indication for emergency thoracotomy.

When the chest tube is initially inserted, blood may come out at an alarmingly rapid rate. If the patient's condition were to improve as blood was removed and additional intravenous fluids were given, continued chest tube drainage of the hemothorax and observation of the patient would be appropriate. However, if the patient's vital signs were to deteriorate as blood was removed, it would be assumed that drainage of the hemothorax has removed a tamponading effect on the bleeding site(s). In such cases, the chest tube should be clamped and the patient taken immediately to the operating room.

Skin Preparation

Most patients with possible major vascular injuries in the upper chest or thoracic inlet should have anterior incisions, and skin preparation should include: (a) the anterior and lateral neck, chest, and abdomen, (b) the entire upper extremity on the side of the potential subclavian arterial or venous injury, and (c) one lower extremity from thigh to toe to allow harvesting of an appropriately-sized saphenous vein, if necessary. If a posterolateral thoracotomy incision is to be used, that area should also be prepared.

Incision

The six basic incisions used for managing vascular injuries in the upper chest and/or thoracic inlet include: posterolateral thoracotomy, anterolateral thoracotomy, bilateral anterior thoracotomy, midsternotomy, anterior flap (trapdoor) thoracotomy, and a high (third intercostal space) anterior thoracotomy.

POSTEROLATERAL THORACOTOMY

Standard posterolateral thoracotomy (Fig. 18–1) provides excellent exposure to almost all parts of the hemithorax; however, the lateral position of the patient tends to reduce venous return and can cause a precipitous drop in blood pressure if the patient were hypovolemic. When the patient has blood in the tracheobronchial tube, the dependent lung could be flooded, even with a split function endotracheal tube in place. Consequently, the patient should not be turned onto one side for a posterolateral thoracotomy when significant intrabronchial bleeding occurs or when the patient is hypotensive.

MEDIAN STERNOTOMY

For penetrating wounds of the thoracic inlet or injuries involving the innominate artery or proximal portions of the carotid or subclavian arteries, a median sternotomy incision is usually ideal (Fig. 18–2). Extension of the median sternotomy into the neck along the anterior border of the sternocleidomastoid muscle (Fig. 18–3) also provides excellent exposure to the proximal right subclavian and midleft subclavian arteries, as well as the more distal portions of the right common carotid artery. The more distal portions of the right subclavian arteries can generally be readily approached via a supraclavicular extension with resection of the medial third of the clavicle. As the distal subclavian artery is approached and one cuts the sternocleidomastoid and scalenus anticus muscles, care should be taken to avoid damaging the phrenic nerve that is situated on the anterior surface of the latter muscle.

Occasionally, it can be difficult to approach the proximal left subclavian artery via a median sternotomy; however, the exposure can be improved by having a vertical sheet roll placed between the shoulder blades so that the shoulders can be pulled back.

When the stab or GSW has damaged posterior structures, such as the esophagus or azygous or hemizygous veins, it may be difficult to get adequate exposure without an additional incision along one of the intercostal spaces. Another problem with a median sternotomy is the

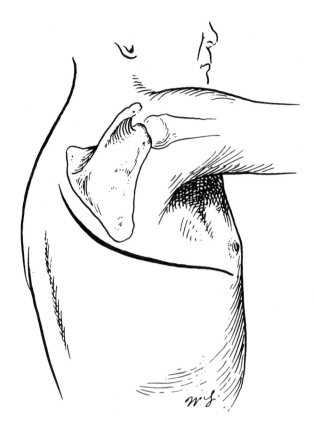

FIGURE 18–1 Standard posterolateral thoracotomy incision. This incision is made with the patient lying on one side. It extends from behind the scapula down below its tip and out to the anterior axillary line. One can then enter the chest through the fourth, fifth, sixth, or seventh interspace or through the bed of one of these ribs. It provides very good exposure to the hilum of the lung and, on the left, it provides excellent exposure to the descending thoracic aorta. It should not be used in patients who are hypotensive or who have hemoptysis because the lateral position of the patient interferes with venous return and can allow flooding of the dependent lung with intrabronchial blood. (From: Wilson RF. Injury to the heart and great vessels. Henning RJ, Grenvik A, eds. Critical care cardiology, New York: Churchill Livingstone, 1989; 441.)

increased time it can take to perform when a sternal saw is not readily available and/or the surgeon does not have a great deal of experience with this approach.

ANTEROLATERAL THORACOTOMY

When the patient is in severe shock, has moderate-to-severe hemoptysis, or requires internal cardiac massage, the patient is kept supine and a left anterolateral thoracotomy is performed in the fourth or fifth intercostal space. The incision should start about 2.0 cm lateral to the sternum (to miss the internal mammary artery, which is subpleural and about 1.0 cm lateral to the sternum) and continued into the axilla. The ribs are widely separated with a rib-spreader. Cutting the costal cartilages of one or two ribs above and below the incision can also help with the exposure.

BILATERAL THORACOTOMY

A left anterolateral thoracotomy can be extended into a bilateral anterolateral thoracotomy (clamshell incision) rapidly by cutting the sternum transversely with rib shears. Exposure of both pleura cavities and the mediastinum can thus be quickly attained without the need for a sternal saw. If the incision were extended into both axillas, one would have excellent exposure to virtually all organs in the chest. An upper median sternotomy and cervical extension can be added if additional exposure in the neck is needed. One must be sure to obtain secure control of the internal mammary vessels, preferably with suture ligatures, which are cut when this incision is used.

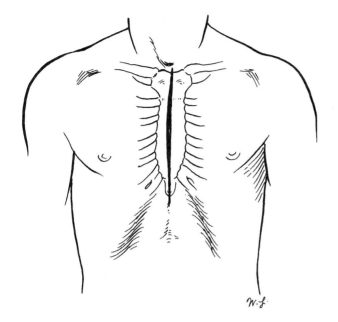

FIGURE 18–2 Median sternotomy. This incision is made from the top of the manubrium down past the xiphoid. The sternum is usually cut with a special electric saw after the soft tissue has been cleared from behind the superior and inferior borders of the sternum. This incision provides excellent exposure to the heart (especially anteriorly), to the ascending aorta, and to most of the aortic arch and its branches. The origin of the left subclavian artery may not be accessible through this incision in some patients. (From: Wilson RF. Injury to the heart and great vessels. Henning RJ, Grenvik A, eds. Critical care cardiology. New York: Churchill Livingstone, 1989; 442.)

TRAPDOOR INCISIONS

Steenburg and Ravitch described a trapdoor (cervicothoracic) approach to expose the proximal and midsubclavian vessels[27] (Fig. 18–4). They used a transverse supraclavicular incision connected to a median sternotomy that, in turn, was connected to an anterior thoracotomy in the third intercostal space. The medial portion of the clavicle was resected, and the flap of the sternum and ribs was reflected laterally "like the pages of a book."

Some of the problems with this incision include difficulty in folding back the chest wall, excessive time to get vascular exposure, increased bleeding, iatrogenic injury to subclavian or innominate veins, iatrogenic rib fractures, suboptimal exposure, and difficulty in wound closure.[25] These incisions can also cause significant paradoxical respiration so that the patient may require mechanical ventilation for at least several days. A high incidence of postoperative "causalgia-type" neurologic symptoms also occurs.

HIGH ANTERIOR THORACOTOMY

When penetrating wounds of the subclavian vessels communicate with the corresponding pleural cavity, rapid exsanguination can occur. In such patients a high right or left anterolateral thoracotomy (Fig. 18–5) at the level of the third intercostal space above the nipple can be performed to obtain proximal innominate or subclavian control.[28] The second and third portion of the subclavian arteries can then be controlled through a supraclavicular incision.[29]

Buscaglia et al. positioned the patient with a pillow under the shoulder to effect a 15-20° anterior rotation.[18] The arm can be extended or placed to the side. When a supraclavicular incision is also required, try to avoid connecting it to the anterolateral thoracotomy to create an "open book" approach.

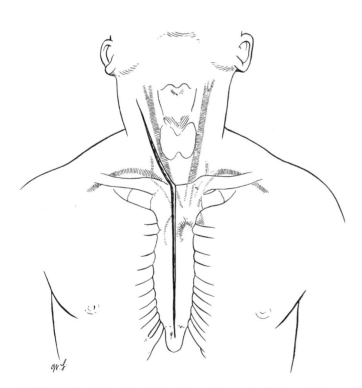

FIGURE 18–3 Incision for right brachiocephalic vessels. The innominate artery and the origins of the right common carotid and right subclavian arteries can usually be readily approached through a sternal splitting incision which is extended either into the right neck or along and just above the right clavicle. Resecting the medial portion of the clavicle subperiosteally can further improve exposure to the mid portion of the right subclavian artery. (From: Wilson RF. Injury to the heart and great vessels. Henning RJ, Grenvik A, eds. Critical care cardiology. New York: Churchill Livingstone, 1989; 443.)

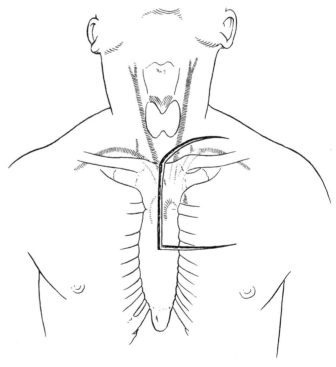

FIGURE 18–4 Approach to the left subclavian artery. One of the techniques used to approach the entire left subclavian artery is the "trapdoor" incision popularized by Steenburg and Ravitch. A midsternotomy is performed down to and into the third intercostal space. This is connected with a supraclavicular incision. The resultant block of sternum, ribs, and clavicle is then swung out laterally to get adequate exposure. In most instances this requires that the clavicle and first three ribs be broken causing much postoperative pain and some disability. (From: Wilson RF. Injury to the heart and great vessels. Henning RJ, Grenvik A, eds. Critical care cardiology. New York: Churchill Livingstone, 1989; 444.)

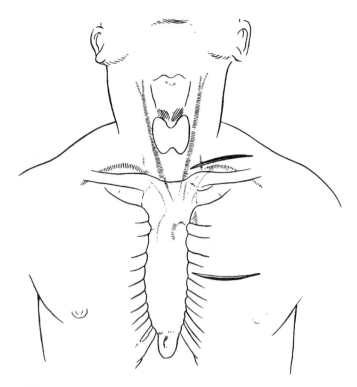

FIGURE 18–5 Approach to massive bleeding from the left subclavian artery. Some surgeons prefer to approach a rapidly bleeding left subclavian artery by clamping it at its origin via a relatively small anterior third intercostal space incision. A separate left supraclavicular incision can then be performed to expose the more distal portions of the vessel. (From: Wilson RF. Injury to the heart and great vessels. Henning RJ, Grenvik A, eds. Critical care cardiology. New York: Churchill Livingstone, 1989; 445.)

CLAVICULAR INCISIONS

If subperiosteal or complete removal of the medial portion of the clavicle were combined with division of the scalenus anticus muscle, all three portions of the right subclavian artery and the entire right subclavian vein would be easily visualized. Injuries to the second or third portion of the right (or left) subclavian artery can often be exposed adequately through a supraclavicular incision without the addition of a median sternotomy, especially when the clavicle is resected or divided.

Although there should be little reluctance to perform claviculectomy to properly expose subclavian injuries, Elkin and Cooper reported that it is easy to injure the underlying subclavian vein or transverse scapular artery.[36] This can, however, be avoided by performing an anterior subperiosteal resection of the entire convex portion of the clavicle between the medial portion of the sternocleidomastoid muscle and the border of the trapezius muscle.

When one tries to remove the clavicle with its attached periosteum, great care must be taken not to injure the subclavian vein.[30] When further exposure of the first and second portions of the right subclavian artery is desired, the scalenus anticus muscle can be cut (avoiding the phrenic nerve which lays on or near the scalenus anticus). The right internal jugular vein can also be ligated and divided at its junction with the right subclavian vein. If the injury is near the junction of the right common carotid and subclavian arteries, great care must be taken to preserve the right recurrent laryngeal nerve as it loops around the subclavian artery in this area.

When distal vascular control is still difficult to obtain, it may be necessary to extend the incision infraclavicularly and laterally. Transverse division of the fibers of the pectoralis major and minor muscleson the coracoid process then allows control of the first portion of the axillary artery.

Once the vascular repair is completed, Feliciano et al. occasionally reattached the resected clavicular fragment to the stump(s) of the remaining clavicle using either dynamic compression plates and screws or sternal wires passed around Steinmann pins in the ends of the fragment and stump.[31] Buscaglia et al., however, reported that replacement of the clavicular fragment tends to cause more complications than it prevents.[18] Furthermore, claviculectomy proximal to the coracoid process is not associated with shoulder instability or disability. With subperiosteal excision of a portion of the clavicle, complete regeneration takes place in 6-8 weeks.[30]

Control of Bleeding Sites at Surgery

RIGHT SUBCLAVIAN VESSELS

For right-sided injuries causing severe intrathoracic bleeding, finger or pack control in the right pleural cavity through a high right thoracotomy, coupled with manual pressure on the right supraclavicular fossa, will tamponade most major subclavian hemorrhage until vascular control can be obtained in the operating room.[31]

LEFT SUBCLAVIAN VESSELS

Because the proximal left subclavian artery is an intrapleural structure (in contrast to the mediastinal course of the proximal right subclavian artery), it can often be visualized and directly clamped via a high thoracotomy incision.[31] If back-bleeding from the distal artery or concomitant hemorrhage from the left subclavian vein were to continue, finger or pack pressure through the thoracotomy incision should be combined with supraclavicular pressure, as described for the right side.

Intraoperative Resuscitation

Once the bleeding sites are controlled, further dissection or other surgery should be delayed until the anesthesiologist can administer enough fluid and blood to restore adequate BP, urine output (at least 1.0 mL/kg/hr), core temperature ($\geq$ 35°C), and acid-base balance.

AXIOM   When systolic BP does not rise to 90 mm Hg within 5 minutes of clamping the descending thoracic aorta, controlling bleeding, and providing aggressive fluid resuscitation, the patient will almost certainly die intraoperatively.

When control of the bleeding sites and aggressive fluid therapy does not raise the systolic BP to at least 90 mm Hg, one can consider temporarily compressing or clamping the descending thoracic aorta. When cross-clamping of the descending thoracic aorta or distal arch (plus control of the bleeding sites and aggressive blood and fluid administration) does not raise the systolic BP to at least 90 mm Hg within 5-10 minutes, terminal cardiovascular failure is present and the patient will almost invariably die intraoperatively.[32] When large doses of epinephrine or dopamine are also used in such circumstances, a transient rise in BP can usually be obtained while the aorta is cross-clamped, but death is still almost invariably the outcome.

Surgical Exploration

AXIOM   All hematomas on major vessels should be explored surgically.

It is extremely important to explore all hematomas over major arteries and possibly also the larger veins. We are aware of at least three patients with aortic injuries that were missed at various hospitals and bled later because the obvious great vessel injuries that were bleeding were controlled and other smaller nonbleeding hematomas were not carefully explored. When possible, one should have proximal and distal control of vessels before an overlying hematoma is explored.

Clamping the Thoracic Aorta

INDICATIONS

In some instances, one may have to temporarily clamp the aorta above and below the injured area to obtain control. This should not be done in the ascending aorta or proximal arch without the patient being on cardiopulmonary bypass, but it is usually possible to clamp the distal arch proximal to the left subclavian artery or the descending aorta safely for at least a few minutes. However, this could be dangerous if one were to allow proximal aortic pressure to rise over 180 mm Hg because it could cause acute LV failure or intracerebral bleeding or edema. Temporarily occluding the venous return to the heart may help to prevent such a pressure rise, but this can cause cardiac arrest, especially in older or hypovolemic patients.

TECHNIQUES OF THORACIC AORTIC CLAMPING

When adequate repair of the aorta, especially the ascending aorta or the arch, cannot be performed with direct suturing or side-clamping, the aorta must be completely clamped. Four techniques are used currently: (a) simple cross-clamping of the aorta ("cut and sew") without shunt or bypass, (b) external heparin-bonded shunts without systemic heparinization, (c) partial or complete cardiopulmonary bypass using an oxygenator and systemic heparinization, and (d) left atrial or left ventricular bypass via a centrifugal pump to the distal aorta or femoral artery without an oxygenator.

"Clamp and Sew" Technique

AXIOM Clamping the upper descending thoracic aorta for more than 30 minutes without providing some blood flow to the distal aorta will result in a high incidence of paraplegia.

Although great controversy exists over this point, it is believed that the clamp-and-sew technique should be avoided by surgeons who do not have experience and special expertise in this type of such surgery. Clamping of the thoracic aorta in the distal arch or isthmus for more than 30 minutes is associated with a high risk of paraplegia.[33] Monitoring of somatosensory evoked potentials and distal aortic pressure appears to be useful for preventing ischemic spinal cord damage, although their exact role is still unclear.[34,35]

Cardiopulmonary Bypass

Although it may take more than 30-60 minutes to setup cardiopulmonary bypass, especially at night and on weekends, the bleeding site(s) can generally be controlled by direct pressure during that time. Nevertheless, because patients who sustain intrathoracic vascular injury frequently have associated injuries, the use of cardiopulmonary bypass with systemic heparinization can be hazardous.

External Shunts

Because of the risk of systemic heparinization, techniques other than full or partial cardiopulmonary bypass have been developed. Symbas and Sehdeva, in 1970, reported the use of a temporary external shunt from the ascending aorta to the innominate artery for repair of a stab wound of the arch.[36] In 1973, DeMeester et al. used a heparinized shunt from the ascending aorta to the femoral artery to maintain distal circulation and to decompress the heart during repair of an arch injury.[37] In 1982, Graham et al. introduced the use of a permanent prosthetic bypass graft from the ascending aorta to the distal carotid or innominate artery for injuries of the arch or innominate artery.[37] In 1984, Pate described the use of Y grafts to both carotid arteries before disturbing the hematoma on such injuries.[13]

Partial Bypass Without an Oxygenator

AXIOM Probably the safest bypass to the distal aorta is via a centrifugal pump from the left atrium to the distal aorta or femoral artery with little or no systemic heparinization.

Another technique utilizes heparin-bonded cannulas and a centrifugal (Biomedicus) to pump blood from the left atrium or the apex of the left ventricle into the descending aorta or femoral artery. When no oxygenator is used with this type of pump, little or no heparin is required, and improved results have been obtained.[16,39]

Aortic Repairs

EXPOSURE OF INJURED AREA

With a contained hematoma, limited dissection is performed to obtain proximal and distal control without disturbing the hematoma. Care must be taken not to injure the left vagus nerve where it crosses over the left subclavian artery and distal aortic arch. If the distal aortic arch were involved, proximal control generally would be obtained within the pericardium by cross-clamping the aortic arch between the left common carotid and left subclavian arteries and by clamping the left subclavian artery distal to the hematoma and proximal to its branches. The distal aorta is cross-clamped below the hematoma. The hematoma can then be opened. Obviously, any blood lost should be recovered for autotransfusion.

If exposure of the concavity and/or posterior surface of the aorta is necessary, the pulmonary artery and aorta should be separated by sharp incision, followed by division of the attached pericardial and fascial tissue from within the pericardium. Dissection of the concave and posterior surfaces of the arch from outside the pericardium is hazardous because the fibrous layer of the pericardium blends into the aortic adventitia, and extrapericardial dissection can easily develop an apparent cleavage plane, within the aortic wall.[40]

VESSEL REPAIR

In most instances, the hole in the aorta is rather small (or the patient would have rapidly exsanguinated), and lateral aortorrhaphy is often easily accomplished. Mattox noted that the survival rate exceeds 90% for patients who are normotensive on arrival and have an ascending aortic injury repaired in the operating room.[1]

When inspection of the superior mediastinum reveals pulsatile hemorrhage from the transverse aortic arch, a finger (or vascular clamp) can be placed over the hole as the operating surgeon sews under it with a 4/0 polypropylene or polyester suture. An assistant can tie the knots as the surgeon withdraws finger pressure. Closure of a posterior hole usually requires much more extensive dissection.

AXIOM Whenever possible, aortic sutures should be pledgetted and tied while the blood pressure in that area is as low as possible.

Whenever possible, aortic sutures should be pledgetted. Larger diameter sutures are also less apt to tear through the vessel. When a 2-3-inch long aortic tear must be repaired, the best technique known to this author is to use a horizontal mattress suture, which everts about 2-3 mm of vessel wall on each side, followed by a simple suture over the everted wound edges. This should be done with the injury isolated by side-clamping or total clamping of the involved aorta.

Unfortunately, sometimes the aorta does not take sutures well. Because the tension in a vessel wall is proportional to its radius and the internal pressure (law of LaPlace), whenever possible sutures in the aorta and large arteries should be tied while the intraluminal pressure is low. If the anesthesiologist cannot decrease the systemic pressure while the aortic sutures are tied, one can sometimes temporarily apply a side-clamp around the involved aorta.

The use of inflow occlusion by digital compression of both vena cavae combined with pharmacologic reduction of blood pressure has been used to suture a penetrating aortic arch injury to allow enough time to place the sutures while the systolic pressure was low (± 30 mm Hg).[41] The safe time for inflow occlusion is believed to be about 1.5 minutes, and it can be repeated after a recovery period of 3 minutes. No additional equipment is necessary.

In a recent patient with through-and-through injury of the lower aspect of the transverse arch, Robicsek and Matos-Cruz induced temporary ventricular fibrillation to prevent exsanguination when their efforts by conventional means failed to bring the hemorrhage under control.[42]

With all repairs on an opened aorta, the proximal and distal aorta should be flushed before the first knot is tied at the completion of the final suture line. As the first knot is being tied, the distal clamp and then the proximal clamp is partly released to evacuate air from the graft. After the sutures have been tied securely, the distal clamp is removed again, to check for any obvious suture line leaks. The proximal clamp is then gradually released so that no abrupt decrease in the patient's blood pressure occurs.

If the repair of a small portion of the aorta is not as good as one would like, one can apply fibrin glue and/or place a 2-inch wide prosthetic graft completely around the aorta in that area and tighten it so as to indent the lumen. This can often successfully control any tendency for the vessel to tear at the site of injury.

Innominate Artery Repairs

Exposure of the innominate artery is best obtained through a median sternotomy and complete mobilization of the overlying left innominate vein, which is often also injured. With some injuries to the innominate artery, it is prudent to bypass the injury before entering the surrounding hematoma.[3,4,38] The proximal ascending aorta is exposed, and an 8 mm knitted Dacron bypass graft can be sewn onto it using a partial occlusion clamp and a 4/0 polypropylene or polyester suture. The hematoma around the proximal innominate artery is not entered until the aortic arch at the origin of the artery and the innominate bifurcation have been dissected free. At this point a partial occlusion clamp is placed on the arch around the origin of the innominate artery. A vascular clamp is then placed on the distal innominate artery or the origins of the right subclavian and common carotid arteries are clamped separately.

After vascular isolation is achieved, the hematoma is entered, and the distal innominate artery is transected. The previously inserted Dacron bypass graft, which has been cut longer than necessary, can then be sewn end-to-end to the distal innominate artery using a 4/0 polypropylene or polyester suture. If the distal innominate artery and the origins of both the right common carotid artery and right subclavian artery must be replaced, a 12 mm x 6 mm Dacron bifurcation graft can be used.[3]

AXIOM When a common carotid artery must be clamped for more than 2-5 minutes in a hypotensive patient, one should try to shunt some blood flow to the distal vessel.

Although repairs of the right (or left) proximal common carotid artery in young patients often do not require internal or external shunting, with complete clamping for more than 2-5 minutes, one should have some concern about maintaining adequate blood flow to the brain. If the "stump pressure" of the right carotid artery distal to the cross-clamp on the innominate artery is 50 mm Hg or greater, the repair can generally be performed safely without a shunt. If the stump pressure is < 50 mm Hg or cannot be measured, it would be prudent to insert a temporary external or internal shunt to ensure adequate blood flow to the brain.[43] The proximal end of the graft shunt can be placed into the intrapericardial aorta and the other end is usually placed in the carotid artery distally, before the hematoma is entered. Use of systemic heparinization is not advised by Feliciano and Graham[44] in trauma patients, especially those who have suffered blunt injuries.

The external shunt may consist of heparin-bonded plastic tubing or a 0.25-inch vascular tubing connected to two arterial cannulas that are 7.5 or preferably 9.0 mm in diameter. While the bleeding is controlled with local pressure, two 3-0 arterial pulse-string sutures are placed to secure the bypass cannulas proximal and distal to the selected point of the aortic cross-clamping. The shunt is primed with heparinized 0.9% sterile saline solution. Stab wounds are then made in the centers of the purse-string stitches and dilated slightly. The ar-

terial cannulas on the ends of the heparin-bonded plastic tubes are inserted into the aorta. The two purse-string sutures around each cannula are then tied to make the openings water-tight and to secure the tubes. The ends of the tubes are then connected with a T-piece, and the aorta is cross-clamped above and below the injury. The clamps are then removed from the external shunt. The wounds of the aorta are repaired while the distal aorta is perfused via the temporary shunt.

CAROTID ARTERIES

Common carotid injuries are treated much the same as innominate artery injuries, but with particular concern for the neurologic status of the patient and preservation of an adequate cerebral blood flow while the vessel is occluded, particularly when the patient is hypotensive. The collateral flow to the internal carotid artery via the external carotid system generally is adequate when: (a) the blood pressure and cardiac output are good, (b) the distal clamp is below the carotid bifurcation, and (c) the other common carotid artery is open.

If, at the time of exploration, the injured vessel were completely transected and no neurologic deficit were manifest, the collateral circulation to brain would be adequate and a shunt would not be necessary; otherwise, the decision of whether to use a shunt should be made according to "stump pressure." When a shunt is required, an internal type is preferred.

Management Decisions in Patients With Neurologic Deficits

Much controversy exists among trauma surgeons as to whether repairing or ligating a common or internal carotid artery should be done after a penetrating injury in a patient who presents with deep coma or other major neurologic findings. It can be difficult to distinguish severe cerebral ischemia from cerebral infarction immediately after a carotid injury, and some surgeons attempt to repair all acute carotid injuries.[45]

Liekweg and Greenfield reported a collective review of 233 injuries of the common and internal carotid arteries and categorized the patients according to presenting neurologic status and method of surgical treatment.[46] This review indicated that carotid reconstruction was beneficial in all patients except those in severe coma. Of 34 patients with neurologic deficits—other than coma—who had carotid repair, 29 (85%) improved or remained stable, 2 (6%) had progressive deficits, and 3 (9%) died. In six similar patients in whom the carotid artery was ligated, three (50%) improved or remained stable, one (17%) deteriorated neurologically, and 2 (33%) died. Twenty-three other patients who presented in deep coma did poorly with ligation or repair. Contrary to general belief, autopsy examination of the patients with major neurologic defects who had repair of carotid injuries revealed ischemic rather than hemorrhagic infarcts.

AXIOM Penetrating carotid injuries should probably be repaired if the vessel is not already occluded even if a severe neurologic defect is present.

Based on the available data, carotid arterial injuries should be repaired in the vast majority of patients. Ligation should probably be reserved for patients who are in deep coma preoperatively or who have an occluded internal carotid artery. When the patient has no neurologic defect and the injured internal carotid artery is occluded, one can ligate the artery or attempt to extract the clot and repair the vessel. If the clot cannot be extracted easily and safely, the vessel should be ligated.

A continuing point of controversy is the patient who presents in deep coma but has some flow demonstrated by arteriography. In this situation, repair should probably be performed to prevent propagation of thrombus and potential irreversible ischemia.[28]

Whenever possible, the head should be lowered during any procedure involving a vessel that may allow air emboli to reach the brain. When a graft is inserted, care must be taken to allow the distal vessel to flush backwards before and after establishing shunt flow to remove all air, clots, and other debris.

Maintaining Cerebral Blood Flow

Of major concern in the repair of injuries to the innominate or common carotid arteries in the chest is the maintenance of adequate cerebral blood flow during occlusion of the artery. Since Binet et al. reported the first successful repair of an innominate artery avulsion using deep hypothermia, a variety of techniques has been used.[47] Cardiopulmonary bypass, moderate or profound hypothermia, separate distal carotid artery catheters, internal and external shunts, and surface hypothermia have all been employed to help protect against cerebral ischemia.[3] Although successful repair without the aid of these adjuncts has been reported, it is probably safer to try to protect against cerebral ischemia in some way.

AXIOM Unless a carotid or innominate artery repair will be extremely rapid, one should evaluate distal carotid blood flow and pressure clinically or with stump pressure measurements to determine the need for a temporary shunt.

Despite limited experience with injury to the innominate or proximal common carotid arteries, some authors recommend the use of cardiopulmonary bypass with temporary internal carotid shunts for repairs of these vessels.[46] The threat of uncontrollable hemorrhage, possible extension of the injury into the aortic arch, tracheal compression, enlarging hematoma, intimal retraction into the aorta, and the presence of a large pseudoaneurysm have all been cited as indications to use cardiopulmonary bypass in the repair of innominate artery injuries.[14] The experience at Ben Taub Hospital in Houston, however, has demonstrated that cardiopulmonary bypass and temporary carotid shunts are not necessary in most patients.[17] Furthermore, experience with elective carotid revascularization has documented the safety of temporary carotid occlusion, particularly when the distal common carotid is unclamped and collateral flow can occur from the external carotid into the internal carotid artery.[48] Graham et al. believed that use of intraarterial shunts should be confined to patients in whom simultaneous occlusion of both the innominate and left common carotid arteries is required or intraoperative hypotension occurs.[17]

Subclavian Artery Repairs

APPROACH

AXIOM The proximal left subclavian artery is one of the more difficult sites to expose in vascular surgery, especially during an emergency.

Many authors recommend a high, standard, left posterolateral thoracotomy for injuries involving the proximal left subclavian artery, but some prefer an initial small left anterior thoracotomy in the second or third intercostal space to insert a long clamp to control the proximal portion of the artery.[49,50] For all proximal injuries of aortic arch branches, irrespective of side, Demetriades et al. used a supraclavicular incision combined with a median sternotomy.[9]

The more common distal injuries are exposed through a supraclavicular incision with or without resection or division of the clavicle. When associated mediastinal or cardiac injuries occur, anterolateral thoracotomy and supraclavicular incisions may be connected by adding a partial median sternotomy.

REPAIRS

Isolated injuries of the right subclavian artery or the origin of the right common carotid artery are repaired by lateral arteriorrhaphy, resection with end-to-end anastomosis, or resection with interposition grafting. Autogenous saphenous vein, Dacron and polytetrafluoroethylene have all been used successfully, with 5/0 polypropylene or polyester sutures. However, the subclavian artery can be thin and fragile, and can be easily torn by vascular clamps or forceps.[12,25] One should also use extreme caution to avoid any tension on the sutures, especially with end-to-end anastomoses. Tension on end-to-end anasto-

moses can usually be avoided by sacrificing subclavian artery branches, such as the vertebral, internal mammary, and/or thyrocervical trunk.

Schimpf et al. showed in autopsy studies that a primary end-to-end subclavian artery anastomosis can almost always be achieved by mobilizing the axillary artery and passing it through the first intercostal space.[51] With this technique, up to 7.5 cm of the subclavian artery can be resected and primary anastomosis still achieved.

Although distal gangrene of the upper extremity is unusual with ligation of the subclavian artery,[52] the injured vessel should be repaired whenever possible. Claudication of the arm may occur, and if the ligation is proximal to the vertebral artery, subclavian steal syndrome may develop. It is also preferable to repair subclavian vein injuries, but when any technical problems occur, ligation can be performed without serious consequences. Any associated brachial plexus injuries should be primarily repaired if possible.

Superior Vena Cava

In a review of 93 patients with penetrating injuries of the aortic arch and its branches, Pate et al. noted frequent, associated injuries, including: major veins 23%, trachea 9%, esophagus 8%, lung 8%, spinal cord 7%, brachial plexus 5%, heart 4%, and abdomen 4%.[10]

Few patients with superior vena cava injury live long enough to receive treatment. Ochsner et al., in 1961, noted that of 27 patients with superior vena cava injuries, only two reached the hospital alive, and one died almost immediately after admission.[53] Mattox estimated the mortality rate for the few patients who reach the operating room alive with these injuries at about 50%.[1]

AXIOM When possible, the superior or inferior vena cava should not be cross-clamped while a patient is hypovolemic. When a proximal cava must be clamped, the descending thoracic or proximal abdominal aorta should usually also be clamped.

In most instances, holes in the superior vena cava can be repaired with a lateral venorrhaphy; however, when the inferior or superior vena cava must be completely clamped in the chest, the sudden, severe reduction in venous return can cause cardiac arrest, particularly with hypovolemic patients. If the descending thoracic or proximal abdominal aorta is clamped, not as much preload is required, and clamping of an intrathoracic cava is generally tolerated much better.

When possible, the bleeding sites should be controlled with local pressure until adequate fluid and blood can be given to the patient. One can also insert a Foley catheter through the holes in the vessel and blow up the balloon just enough to occlude the injured area with external traction. In rare instances, it may be necessary to clamp both vena cavas to produce inflow occlusion to the heart to be able to effect a repair. Cardiac arrest is almost certainly apt to occur, but this can often be tolerated well when it is not allowed to persist for more than 2-3 minutes.

If the superior vena cava is irreparably damaged, a portion of the internal jugular or left innominate vein is probably the ideal graft; however, one internal jugular vein should be left intact. If an internal jugular vein is not readily available, a PTFE or Dacron prosthesis may be used, but such prostheses would likely occlude within 2-4 days.

Innominate or Subclavian Veins

In the report by Graham et al. on innominate artery injuries, penetrating injuries to the overlying left innominate vein occurred three times more frequently than to the short right innominate vein.[38] Ligation of the vein was the most common treatment, being performed in 21 of 25 injuries. However, if possible, one innominate vein should be left intact to reduce the likelihood of a superior vena caval syndrome developing postoperatively.

With penetrating subclavian artery trauma, the incidence of associated venous injuries is extremely varied. Agarwal et al. found no associated subclavian venous injuries,[54] but the incidence of Buscaglia et al. was 20%,[18] and the incidence of Lim et al. was 44%.[55]

In the series by Demetriades et al., the subclavian arterial and venous injury groups were similar with regard to associated injuries and operative mortality rates (21% and 18%, respectively); the overall mortality was 82% and 60%, respectively (P < 0.01).[9]

Injuries of the subclavian vein can be extremely difficult to repair, even with excellent exposure. Numerous small venous branches are easily avulsed during rapid dissection. This can cause further hemorrhage which may require proximal and distal ligation of the vein, rather than repair.

Azygous and Hemizygous Veins

The azygous and hemizygous veins run posteriorly in the chest alongside the vertebral bodies and return blood from the posterior chest wall to the superior vena cava. When the patient is cirrhotic, the azygous vein may also return much of the splanchnic blood flow to the heart.

Injuries to the azygous or hemizygous system can be extremely difficult to control at times, and not infrequently they can cause exsanguination in spite of the surgeon's best efforts to control them with multiple suture ligatures. One must also remember that opening the chest and using the rib spreader to provide better exposure can cause preexisting holes in these veins to enlarge markedly. Under such circumstances, it may be better to cut or remove ribs to improve exposure.

Associated Injuries

NERVE INJURIES

Penetrating wounds of the thoracic inlet and/or upper chest can injure a variety of nerves. Injuries to the brachial plexus are particularly common if the second or third portion of a subclavian artery is involved. In a recent report of 28 patients with arterial injuries of the thoracic inlet, Abouljoud et al. noted eight (29%) brachial plexus injuries, but repair was performed in only one patient who had moderate improvement in motor function on long-term follow-up.[56] The remaining patients had contusions with variable motor and sensory deficits which recovered slowly. Four patients had direct bullet injury to the spinal cord. Two patients had perioperative stroke after repair of common carotid injuries, and two patients had Horner syndrome.

Donohue and McGuire reported that delayed neurologic changes after penetrating injury may be due to expanding pseudoaneurysms.[57] Rarely, a phrenic or recurrent laryngeal nerve is injured either by the initial trauma or iatrogenically during surgery. Consequently, documentation of the preoperative neurologic status of the patient should be as complete as possible.

TRACHEOBRONCHIAL INJURIES

Penetrating injuries of the thoracic inlet or upper central chest may also involve the trachea or major bronchi. Such injuries should be considered a source of contamination so that a prosthetic graft should be avoided if possible. Bronchial and vascular repairs should be separated and buttressed with normal tissue as much as possible.

ESOPHAGUS

With any injury involving the thoracic inlet or upper central chest, one should also look carefully for esophageal injury, which can be missed easily on endoscopy and contrast studies. When the esophagus is injured, one should assume that the area is contaminated and avoid the use of prosthetic vascular grafts if possible. One should also attempt to separate and buttress the vascular and esophageal repairs with viable tissue, such as muscle or pleura.

POSTOPERATIVE CARE

In patients with major thoracic vascular injury who present with exsanguinating hemorrhage requiring ED thoracotomy for temporary control, the intraoperative and postoperative courses are often characterized by severe hypothermia, coagulopathies, and profound metabolic acidosis. Chest tubes should be connected to an autotransfusion collection device so that shed blood can be returned to the patient if necessary. Hypothermia is reversed with heating blankets, warmed fluids, and heated ventilator gases. Coagulopathies are corrected by making the patient normothermic and giving fresh frozen plasma or cryoprecipitate and platelets, as necessary. However, one should remember that excess bleeding following surgery for trauma is usually due to inadequate hemostasis by the surgeons.

Optimal resuscitation is best obtained with rapid crystalloid and blood administration, guided by oxygen delivery (DO_2I) and oxygen consumption (VO_2I) studies. One should attempt to obtain a $DO_2I \geq 600$ ml/min/m^2 and VO_2I of ≥ 170 ml/min/m^2 as soon as possible.[58] If hypotension or inadequate DO2I persists despite adequate cardiac filling, various inotropes, such as dopamine and dobutamine, should be infused.

Complications of Penetrating Thoracic Vascular Trauma

EXSANGUINATION

AXIOM The vast majority of deaths in thoracic vascular trauma are due to exsanguination.

Many patients with penetrating thoracic vascular injuries arrive with no obtainable BP and, in spite of aggressive resuscitation, arrest in the ED or arrive in the operating room with continued, severe shock. According to a report by Wiencek and Wilson, when rapid control of bleeding sites and cross-clamping of the descending thoracic aortic arch did not raise systolic BP to at least 90 mm Hg within five minutes, terminal cardiovascular failure was present and all patients died in the operating room.[32] If it required large doses of epinephrine or dopamine combined with aortic cross-clamping to raise the systolic BP over 90 mm Hg, the cardiovascular system generally became less and less responsive to these agents, and the patients would still die in the operating room.

PULMONARY

The most frequent complications following chest trauma and/or thoracotomies are atelectasis and pneumonia. This is best prevented and/or treated with good pulmonary toilet, encouraging deep breaths and coughing after extubation, and nasotracheal suction and/or bronchoscopy as needed. Epidural analgesia can also be helpful.

Adult respiratory distress syndrome (ARDS) is apt to develop in patients with severe, prolonged shock and multiple transfusions. These patients should be treated with a volume-cycled ventilator with positive end-expiratory pressure added to decrease the FiO_2 to 0.5 or less as soon as possible. If severe pulmonary hypertension were to develop, an infusion of amrinone plus dobutamine could be helpful. When the ARDS does not respond to good standard therapy, one should look closely for uncontrolled sepsis.

RETAINED HEMOTHORAX

During the past 10 years, increasing enthusiasm has developed for early decortication of moderate- or large-sized persistent hemothoraces to prevent later empyema and fibrothorax. Most thoracic surgeons, however, still manage small, residual hemothoraces in an expectant manner because they will usually almost completely resorb spontaneously within three to four weeks. If a relatively large hemothorax were to persist for more than four weeks, capillaries would begin to grow from the lungs and chest wall into the fibrous tissue which developed around these hematomas. This can make the decortication much more difficult and may result in multiple air leaks and large blood loss.

AXIOM Hemothorax should be evacuated via a formal thoracotomy when it remains large in spite of well-placed, functioning chest tubes and/or when it is infected.

A retained hemothorax should probably be removed when it: (a) continues to occupy more than one-third of a hemithorax for more than 3 weeks, (b) causes atelectasis of two or more lung segments, or (c) is associated with continuing fever exceeding 101.4°F. Delay in performing decortication may result in empyema or atelectasis with pneumonitis.

INFECTION

AXIOM	Retained hemothorax without infection can cause some leukocytosis (up to 12,000-15,000/mm^3) and fever (up to 101.4°F); higher fever or white cell counts or systemic evidence of sepsis is an indication for prompt removal of a retained hemothorax.

When intrathoracic fluid collection is believed to be infected, it should be rapidly removed before the resultant sepsis can cause multiple organ failure or disruption of any adjacent vascular, bronchial, or esophageal repairs. This is particularly important if a prosthetic graft is inserted. When suspicion exists that a prosthetic graft is infected, it should be removed early, if possible, and an extraanatomical bypass should be inserted well away from the infected area.

AV FISTULAS

Although few individuals survive penetrating injury of the thoracic aorta, those who do frequently have cardiac or venous fistulas that are not diagnosed initially. Symbas and Sehdeva, in a review of 48 patients with successful repairs of penetrating thoracic aortic injuries, noted that 14 had a fistulous communication with a cardiac chamber, nine had a fistulous communication with an innominate vein, and eight had aortopulmonary artery fistulas.[36] Only 17 of 48 patients surviving thoracic aortic wounds did not have fistulas. Most of the 17 patients without fistulas had injuries to the intrapericardial portion of the ascending aorta or a small wound to the lower descending thoracic aorta.

NEUROLOGIC COMPLICATIONS

The major morbidity in many series of thoracic outlet vascular injuries is related to permanent neurologic loss from associated brachial plexus injuries.[59] When the aorta is cross-clamped, paraplegia may also occur. Severe pain syndromes may result from incisions or trauma, but these can usually be helped by anesthetic blocks.

BULLET EMBOLI

Bullet emboli via large intrathoracic arteries or veins are relatively uncommon, but they can be extremely important. Bullets entering large systemic veins or the right heart can embolize to the lungs, whereas bullets entering the pulmonary veins, left heart, or major systemic arteries can embolize to carotid, iliac, femoral, or even popliteal arteries. Many of these emboli apparently cause no symptoms or signs.

When a bullet embolus is diagnosed, the entrance wound into the vascular system should be controlled first, even when bleeding has stopped, and then the bullet removed from its new position. Fluoroscopy in the operating room can be important in tracing these bullets, especially in the central veins or heart, because they can change position rapidly.

Follow-up

AXIOM	Some intrathoracic great vessel injuries may not be detected until or unless follow-up examinations reveal pseudoaneurysm or arteriovenous fistula.

Follow-up of patients with intrathoracic vascular injuries is important.

Late complications of thoracic vascular repairs may occur in up to 5-10% of patients. These include distal ischemia, pseudoaneurysms, and edema. As noted previously, the most frequent late manifestation of missed vascular injuries in the chest are arteriovenous fistulas and pseudoaneurysms. Another concern is late infections of vascular grafts, and these may not be apparent until several weeks or months later. With venous injuries, reports of chronic edema and/or recurrent thrombophlebitis are uncommon, even if major veins are ligated or if they thrombose after a repair. Neurologic deficits, usu-

ally due to cerebral or spinal cord ischemia, account for many of the late continuing morbidities in patients having emergency thoracic great vessel surgery. In addition, up to 40% may have excess pain of other neurologic problems, including causalgia, that may not be diagnosed until late, but may persist for several months after injury. Patients with upper extremity causalgia often respond to repeat stellate ganglion blocks or upper thoracic sympathectomy.

BLUNT TRAUMA TO THE GREAT VESSELS IN THE CHEST

Introduction

INCIDENCE

Approximately 80-90% of patients with blunt trauma to thoracic great vessels, particularly the aorta, die at the scene of the accident or assault, and up to 50% of the remaining patients die within 48 hours if not properly treated.[60-62] Strassman reviewed 7000 autopsy reports from New York City from 1936 through 1942 and found 51 cases of traumatic rupture of the aorta (TRA) secondary to motor vehicle accidents.[60] In 1958, Parmley et al. reviewed 1174 autopsy reports of trauma to the heart and aorta and found 296 cases of TRA.[61] In 1966, Greendyke reported 41 cases of blunt trauma to the aorta in 1259 medicolegal autopsy reports.[62] He also noted that 16% of the victims of immediately fatal motor vehicle accidents had rupture of the aorta. Thus, it can be estimated that each year about 8,000 individuals in the United States suffer traumatic rupture of the thoracic aorta or of one of the other great arteries in the chest.

MECHANISMS OF INJURY

For the descending aorta at the level of the isthmus, which is the most frequent site of injury in patients reaching the hospital alive with thoracic aortic damage, the three mechanical factors believed to contribute to injury include shearing stress, bending stress, and torsion stress.[63] The difference in deceleration between the mobile aortic arch and the relatively immobile descending aorta puts the aortic isthmus under tension, and the resultant shearing stress can theoretically lead to rupture opposite the site of fixation.

Bending stress is another factor and is produced as the heart exerts downward traction on the aortic arch, resulting in hyperflexion of the blood-filled aortic arch on a transverse mechanical bar and fulcrum created by the hilar structures of the left lung.[63] Torsion stress occurs when anteroposterior compression of the chest causes displacement of the heart to the left and a pressure wave of blood is transmitted to the aorta. The combination of smearing, bending, and torsion stress can combine to produce maximum stress on the inner surface of the aorta just above its point of greatest fixation, the ligamentum arteriosum.

AXIOM	Patients reaching the hospital alive with blunt aortic trauma generally have injury to the isthmus of the aorta.

A sudden increase in intraluminal pressure also may be a factor in rupture of the aorta. In one study, the bursting pressures of a healthy adult human aorta ranged 580-2500 mm Hg.[63] The fact that multiple aortic ruptures occasionally occur supports the hypothesis that these bursting pressures can be reached or exceeded.

AXIOM	Aortography to look for TRA should include the entire thoracic aorta and its major branches, including the distal subclavian arteries.

Rupture of the innominate or left subclavian artery at their origins probably results from the interaction of two forces.[63] One is a compression force that displaces the heart into the left chest and places the brachycephalic vessels under tension at their attachments to the aortic arch. The other force involves hyperextension of the neck with rotation of the head to one side placing the contralateral subclavian vessels under additional stretch. The resulting tension leads to maximum shearing stresses at the origins of these vessels. Injuries to the subclavian arteries can also occur just over the first rib due to direct trauma and/or stretching over that structure.

AXIOM	Blunt injuries to aortic arch branches tend to occur at their origins or where they cross the first rib.

PATHOLOGIC CHANGES

Blunt aortic tears tend to extend obliquely up the isthmus from just above the ligamentum arteriosum.[63] Preexisting disease, such as atherosclerosis or medial necrosis, does not appear to predispose one to traumatic rupture. When the aortic tear involves all layers of the aortic wall, death by exsanguination is almost instantaneous. When the tear does not involve the adventitia, and the parietal pleura and the surrounding mediastinal tissues remain intact, a false aneurysm may be formed. The false aneurysm tends to expand with time, and when BP is not adequately controlled, about 50% rupture within 24 hours.[39] Some false aneurysms, however, may remain intact and may not be detected for 20 years or longer. Although lacerations of the subclavian artery occasionally form a false aneurysm, an occluded vessel seldom causes distal ischemia. Occasionally, aortic injury causes a dissection that may occlude distal vessels.[64]

It should be emphasized that the small hemothorax that is often present with blunt trauma to the aorta does not result from the aortic injury itself, but rather from tears to adjacent, small mediastinal veins. Although it may be partly due to aortic pseudoaneurysm, much of the widened mediastinum is actually caused by bleeding from adjacent structures.

NATURAL HISTORY

Parmley et al. found that, of the patients with traumatic rupture of the thoracic aorta who reach a hospital and survive for 1 hour, without appropriate therapy, 20-30% die within 6 hours, 40-50% die within 24 hours, 60-80% die within 7 days, 80-90% die within 4 weeks, and 90-95% die within 3 months.[61]

AXIOM	When aortic injury is suspected because of the mechanism of injury, associated injuries, or chest radiography or CT findings, systolic BP should be kept below 110-120.

Many early deaths are caused by associated injuries, but even when aortic injury is an isolated problem, the diagnosis should be made promptly and therapy started immediately. Although the emphasis has generally been to get the patient to the operating room as soon as possible, it is probably much more important to keep the systolic BP < 110-120 mm Hg and to prevent powerful Valsalva maneuvers. These lesions should be treated somewhat like a dissection of the descending thoracic aorta, in which surgery is only performed when BP cannot be controlled properly or when the conditions for surgical repair are optimal.

LOCATION

In patients with traumatic rupture of the thoracic aorta who die rapidly without a cardiac injury, 50-60% occur at the aortic isthmus and only 10-20% in the ascending aorta.[61-63] However, in patients dying rapidly with associated cardiac injuries, 52% of ruptures occurred in the ascending aorta, with only 32% in the isthmus.[61] Ascending aortic tears are particularly apt to occur in plane crashes and falls from great heights.

At least 90% of blunt thoracic aortic injuries in patients who reach the hospital alive occur in the isthmus of the aorta between the left subclavian artery and the ligamentum arteriosum. The next most common thoracic great artery injury from blunt trauma in patients reaching a hospital alive is the innominate artery, usually at its origin. Tears in the lower aorta below the ligamentum arteriosum are uncommon, but tend to occur adjacent to comminuted fractures of vertebral bodies.

Diagnosis

CLINICAL FINDINGS

History

AXIOM	The single most important factor in diagnosing acute traumatic aortic rupture is a high index of suspicion because of the mechanism of injury (Table 18–2).

Even when no external evidence of chest injury exists, one should still be acutely aware of the possibility of this injury in anyone who has sustained an accident characterized by sudden, severe deceleration. This is particularly true of a motor vehicle striking an immovable object. "T-bone" motor vehicle accidents in which a car runs into the victim's side of the car at high speed is becoming an increasingly frequent cause of this injury.[65,66]

Patients with traumatic aortic rupture usually complain primarily of severe, associated injuries and generally have few or no symptoms related to the aortic injury itself. The most common symptom that may be due to aortic injury is retrosternal or interscapular pain from "stretching" or dissection of the adventitia of the aorta. Recurrence or exacerbation of the pain, particularly when associated with an increase in BP (which may be due to increased pain, excess fluid administration, or a Valsalva maneuver), may herald an impending rupture of the pseudoaneurysm. Less frequent symptoms, due primarily to pressure from the associated hematoma on adjacent structures, include dysphagia, stridor, dyspnea, voice change, or hoarseness.

Physical Examination

AXIOM	Up to one-third of patients with blunt trauma to the thoracic aorta or its major branches have little or no external evidence of thoracic injury.[63]

Only 15 (27%) of 55 patients with traumatic rupture of the aorta in one series sustained identifiable chest-wall contusion or rib fractures.[65] However, almost all of our patients at DRH with TRA since our initial report[63] have had some clinical evidence of chest trauma.

Physical findings that suggest aortic injury include: (a) upper extremity hypertension, (b) decreased pulsations or blood pressure in the lower extremities, and (c) the presence of a harsh systolic murmur over the precordium or posterior interscapular area. This systolic murmur is believed to be caused by turbulent blood flow across the area of transection and is found in about 25% of patients with acute aortic rupture.[67,68]

Upper extremity hypertension has been noted in 31-43% of patients reported in the literature and has been attributed to compression of the aortic lumen by periaortic hematoma.[63] Nevertheless, hypertension may also be due to stretching or stimulation of special receptors located in the vicinity of the aortic isthmus.[69] This mechanism could account for the upper extremity hypertension that occurs without aortic narrowing and for the slowly resolving postoperative hypertension that is seen in up to one-third of patients successively repaired.

TABLE 18–2   Clinical Features Suggesting Possible Traumatic Rupture of the Aorta

1. History of high-speed deceleration injury
2. Multiple rib fractures or flail chest
3. Fractured first or second rib
4. Fractured sternum
5. Pulse deficits
6. Hypertension, especially in the upper extremities
7. Systolic murmur, especially interscapular
8. Hoarseness or voice change without laryngeal injury
9. Superior vena cava syndrome

If the torn intima and media form a flap that acts as a "ball valve," partial or complete aortic obstruction can occur. With partial obstruction, an "acute pseudocoarctation syndrome" can develop, with upper extremity hypertension and increased pulse amplitude.[69] This "acute pseudocoarctation syndrome" was reported in 37% of 204 patients reviewed by Symbas et al.[67] We have also had two patients with a negative aortogram who developed severe upper extremity hypertension and a pseudocoarctation syndrome during laparotomy for associated abdominal injuries.

When complete obstruction of the descending thoracic aorta occurs, anuria and paraplegia can develop almost immediately, particularly when the patient is hypotensive.[70] Compression of the second through the fifth intercostal arteries by mural and mediastinal hematomas with subsequent ischemia of the spinal cord from T-3 to T-7 has also been described as a mechanism for causing paraplegia.[71]

Other less frequently encountered physical findings include superior vena cava syndrome and swelling at the base of the neck, with an increase in collar size. Because the aorta is covered with a periadventitial sheath that extends up to the neck, a partial aortic tear may allow blood to extravasate along the branches of the aorta. MacKenzie was able to demonstrate the presence of blood in the carotid sheath in 16 (44%) of 17 accident victims who died from aortic rupture.[72]

RADIOGRAPHY

Plain Chest Radiography

Although the circumstances of the accident and the physical examination may be helpful, the diagnosis of TRA is usually suspected from findings on routine chest radiography (Table 18–3). The most frequent radiologic finding noted is widening of the superior mediastinum, usually to more than 8.0-8.5 cm, caused primarily by an associated mediastinal hematoma (Figs. 18–6, 18–7).

AXIOM One of the main reasons that many unnecessary aortograms are performed for possible TRA is a technically poor radiograph.

The upper mediastinum tends to appear wider than it really is when chest radiography is taken: (a) anteroposteriorly (AP) rather than posteroanteriorly (PA), (b) with the patient < 100 cm from the origin of the x-ray beam, (c) with the patient lying flat, and (d) with poor inspiration. The optimal chest radiography is taken with the patient in the so-called Ayella position: an upright PA chest radiography taken at a distance of 6 ft (150 cm) with the patient leaning forward about 15°.[73]

The most accurate chest radiographic sign of TRA is usually deviation of the esophagus or trachea > 1-2 cm to the right of the spinous process of T-4 (Fig. 18–8). In the series by Ayella et al., none of the patients with the esophagus < 1.0 cm from the midline had TRA.[73] In a series of 45 patients, Gerlock noted that none of the patients with a nasogastric tube in its normal position had TRA.[74]

TABLE 18–3 Some Chest Radiographic Findings Associated with Traumatic Rupture of the Aorta

1. Deviation of esophagus to the right at T4 more than 1.0-2.0 cm
2. Superior mediastinal widening
3. Obscuration of the aortic knob
4. Obliteration of the outline of descending aorta
5. Tracheal deviation to the right
6. Apical cap
7. Depression of left main stem bronchus more than 40°
8. Obliteration of the aortopulmonary window
9. Obscuration of medial aspect of left upper lobe
10. Widened paravertebral stripe
11. Thickened and/or deviated paratracheal stripe
12. Fracture of first or second ribs
13. Fractured sternum, especially in younger individuals

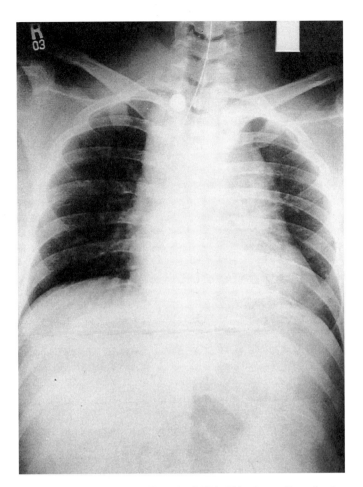

FIGURE 18–6 Plain chest radiograph of TRA. This chest radiograph of a patient with a traumatic rupture of the aorta shows widening of the superior mediastinum, obscuration of the aortic knob, loss of the usual clear space between the aorta and left pulmonary artery, and deviation of the trachea to the right. (From: Wilson RF. Injury to the heart and great vessels. Henning RJ, Grenvik A, eds. Critical care cardiology. New York: Churchill Livingstone, 1989; 451.)

AXIOM A deviation of the esophagus or trachea > 2.0 cm to the right after severe blunt trauma is frequently due to TRA.

Blurring or obscuration of the aortic knob or descending aorta is almost as accurate an indication of TRA as esophageal or tracheal deviation. In one study of 86 patients with blunt chest trauma, of whom 13 patients had TRA, Marnocha et al. noted that none of the patients with a normal aortic contour and no deviation of the trachea or nasogastric tube to the right on chest radiography had TRA.[75]

Other chest radiographic signs of TRA include a left apical cap, displacement of the left main stem bronchus more than 40° below the horizontal, widening of the right paratracheal stripe, and displacement of the right paraspinous interface.[75,76] In 1975, Simeone et al. stressed the value of the extrapleural left apical cap as a sign of an aortic isthmus tear.[77] However, in 1981, they observed that if no other signs of TRA were present, aortography was not indicated.[78]

The paratracheal stripe is a linear density on the right side of the tracheal air column[79] (Fig. 18–9). It extends from the thoracic inlet to the proximal right bronchus and normally measures < 5 mm in thickness at a level 2 cm above the azygous vein. When the paratracheal stripe is > 5 mm wide and/or is deviated to the right, this may be another sign of mediastinal hemorrhage.[79]

The right paraspinal line is usually not visible on routine chest radiography, but if it is seen and is displaced to the right in the

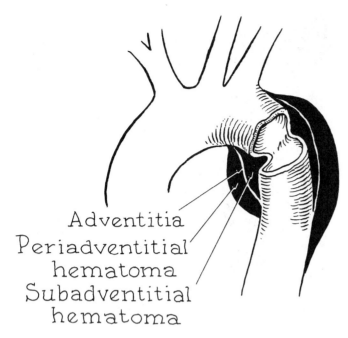

Adventitia
Periadventitial
    hematoma
Subadventitial
    hematoma

FIGURE 18–7 The widening of the mediastinum around a traumatic rupture of the aorta usually results from hematoma in the subadventitial and periadventitial spaces. The periadventitial hematoma may be very large and is due primarily to bleeding from small mediastinal vessels. (From: Wilson RF. Injury to the heart and great vessels. Henning RJ, Grenvik A, eds. Critical care cardiology. New York: Churchill Livingstone, 1989; 452.)

absence of spinal or sternal fractures, it may be of some diagnostic value. Peters and Gamsu found this sign in 8 of 14 patients with TRA and in none without this injury.[76] The paraspinal lines lay between the pleura and the lung, projected away from the lateral margin of the thoracic spine. The left paraspinal line may be distinguished from the image of the descending aorta by the fact that it is not continuous with the aortic knob. When displaced more than one-half the distance from the spine to the left margin of the descending aorta without spine or sternal fractures, it was 83% specific.[80]

AXIOM Fracture of the first or second ribs should make one suspect the presence of severe intrathoracic injuries.

It often takes great force to fracture the first or second ribs or the sternum, especially in young patients. Consequently, such fractures tend to be associated with an increased incidence of major intrathoracic injuries. Although fractures of the first or second ribs have been believed to be associated with an increased incidence of traumatic aortic rupture,[81] this association has not been noted in other reports.[82] In a report by Sadow et al., one patient with TRA had a fracture of the sternum; because of the individual's young age, the fracture led to a request for aortography which showed the aortic injury.[83]

AXIOM An initially normal chest radiograph does not eliminate TRA.

One should not assume that a TRA has been eliminated when initial chest radiography is normal. Unfortunately, in up to one-third of patients, widening of the mediastinum and other radiographic changes may not be apparent on initial chest radiography.[84] Consequently, serial chest films should be taken in any patient with severe chest trauma at 6-8 hour intervals during the first day and then daily for at least the next 2-3 days. Up to two-thirds of patients older than 65 years with traumatic aortic rupture may not show mediastinal widening.[85] In such individuals, the circumstances of the accident should be the main indication for ordering aortography.

CT Scans

Early diagnosis of traumatic rupture of the aorta is essential to improve a patient's chance of survival. Aortography, as indicated by high clinical suspicion of injury and/or chest radiographic findings, has been the gold standard for evaluation of the aorta in such cases.

The potential value of CT in screening for traumatic rupture of the aorta is controversial. Fenner et al., in 1990, reported that CT and arteriography had comparable specificity (CT 96%, arteriography 92%) and false-positive rates (CT 3.8%, arteriography 7.7%) when CT was used as a screening tool for aortic rupture.[86] Madayag et al. used dynamic CT to screen for aortic injury in patients with blunt chest trauma who had normal initial chest radiographic findings.[87] They concluded that emergent aortography should be performed only when abnormal chest radiography or CT findings occur.

AXIOM Mediastinal hematoma seen on CT of the chest after blunt chest trauma is an indication for complete thoracic aortography.

Miller et al., in a series of 104 patients who had CT scans of the chest and aortography, had five patients with TRA.[88] Two were apparently interpreted as not having mediastinal hematoma seen on CT scan, but one was apparently performed without intravenous contrast and one was misread by a radiology resident at night. Three major aortic branch injuries were also missed. In a more recent discussion

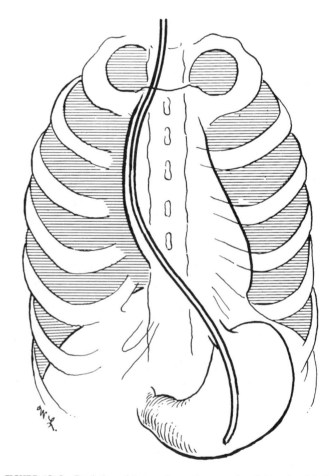

FIGURE 18–8 Deviation of the esophagus (nasogastric tube) to the right is generally an accurate sign of traumatic rupture of the aorta. When the distance from the nasogastric tube to the spinous process of the fourth thoracic vertebra is > 2.0 cm, it is strongly indicative of a torn descending thoracic aorta. (From: Wilson RF. Injury to the heart and great vessels. Henning RJ, Grenvik A, eds. Critical care cardiology. New York: Churchill Livingstone, 1989; 452.)

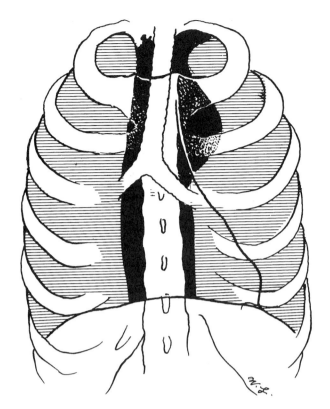

FIGURE 18–9 Mediastinal hematomas, indicated by the blackened areas, may thicken and displace the paratracheal stripe laterally by more than 5 mm. Mediastinal hematomas may also displace the right and left paraspinal lines in the lower thorax rather widely from the edge of the thoracic spine. (From: Wilson RF. Injury to the heart and great vessels. Henning RJ, Grenvik A, eds. Critical care cardiology. New York: Churchill Livingstone, 1989; 453.)

of another report, Miller noted that an additional two aortic injuries have been missed with CT scans.[89]

In another study comparing CT scans of the chest with aortography in 144 stable patients with suspected blunt aortic injury, Durham et al. reported that six aortic injuries were detected by aortography, but only 4 had positive CT scans for a sensitivity rate of only 67%;[90] however, some interreader variation occurred and the quality of CT scans was not known.

In a review and commentary, Raptopoulos indicated that normal findings on chest CT scan exclude aortic injury quite well.[91] Fisher et al. found that CT was at least as good as chest radiography for excluding aortic injury.[92] Of 679 patients who had normal results on CT in eight recent studies, only five (0.7%) had abnormalities on aortography. One or two additional case reports described similar findings. These results were similar to those for chest radiography: of 352 patients with normal radiographic findings in the same eight studies, findings on aortography were abnormal in three (0.9%).

In a report, Agee et al. had no TRA missed on CT scans.[93] Fisher et al. agreed that chest CT scans with normal findings excluded aortic/brachiocephalic injury, but only 25% of their patients had unequivocally normal CT findings and three of four patients with aortic injuries had only suggestive (1), or subtly positive (2) CT findings.[92]

It is clear that patients who are hemodynamically unstable or whose mechanism of injury or clinical examination strongly suggests aortic injury should have immediate aortography or surgery. In the absence of either of these criteria, Raptopoulos believed that overwhelming evidence suggests that CT can be used in the workup and screening of patients with suspected aortic transection, especially those who are hemodynamically stable and are undergoing CT for other injuries.[91] This additional examination, which may increase the workup time by no more than 10 minutes, requires one technologist

and one resident, all in-house. Usually one physician, one technologist, and one nurse are required for aortography. This may necessitate up to a 45-minute delay, during which time several CT scans could be done.

Tomiak et al, however, were not convinced that normal CT scan excludes the possibility of significant vascular injury in the chest.[94] This is primarily due to the possibility of missing transversely oriented injuries inherent in the axial scanning technique. In stable patients with equivocal chest radiographs, but with low clinical suspicion of vascular injury, CT can differentiate mediastinal hematoma from other causes of mediastinal widening.[95] CT often shows additional unsuspected findings, such as sternal or vertebral fractures, which could implicate a greater severity of injury than initially believed and provide an indication for arteriography. Finally, in cases where aortography is unclear, as in ductus diverticulum, acute dissection, or atherosclerotic aneurysm, CT may help elucidate confusing arteriographic findings.

We have yet to see a TRA without a mediastinal hematoma in our own practice. One of us (RFW), however has personally had two patients with a false negative aortogram and knows personally of two others. Nevertheless, when a reasonable suspicion of TRA exists because of the mechanism of injury, physical findings, or chest radiography, aortography or transesophageal echocardiography (TEE) should be performed promptly. When only mild-to-moderate suspicion of TRA exists, CT of the chest can be performed. When no evidence of mediastinal hematoma is present, there is no need for further study. It is important while ordering these tests in patients with severe blunt chest trauma, to keep the systolic BP < 120 mm Hg to greatly reduce the chances of an injured aorta completely rupturing.

AXIOM When the mechanism of injury, clinical findings, or chest radiogram make one suspicious of aortic injury, one should obtain a complete thoracic aortogram. When relatively little suspicion of thoracic injury exists, CT of the chest can be an excellent screening technique.

MRI

The newer generations of MRI seem to be particularly good for diagnosing dissecting aneurysms and, therefore, should be ideal for posttraumatic studies of the thoracic vessels when the patient: (a) is hemodynamically stable, (b) does not require a ventilator, (c) can lie still long enough for a proper study, and (d) does not have a pacemaker or other metallic objects that will be affected by the powerful magnetic field.

Transesophageal Echocardiography For Chest Injuries

Because of the difficulty in obtaining aortography, particularly at night and on weekends in some hospitals and occasional false-negative results with CT scans of the chest, there has been increasing interest in the use of TEE to examine the great arteries of the chest after severe blunt chest trauma.

Shapiro et al., in one of their first reports on the use of TEE to evaluate the thoracic aorta for injury, studied 19 patients who had blunt chest trauma with widened mediastinum and TEE detected aortic injuries in two patients; both injuries were confirmed by aortography.[96] In one patient in their study, TEE failed to detect an intimal tear that was visualized by aortography.

Soon thereafter, Brooks et al. reported 450 trauma patients who had TEE.[97] Of 21 patients with wide mediastinum, TEE identified 3 aortic disruptions, and these were confirmed by aortography. Two patients, however, showed intimal aortic irregularities on TEE just distal to the left subclavian artery which was missed on aortography.

In a similar study, Kearney et al. studied 39 patients for possible thoracic aortic injury after blunt trauma using both aortography and TEE.[98] TEE correctly identified 5 aortic injuries which were confirmed by aortography (4) or thoracotomy (1) for a sensitivity and specificity of 100%.

In a more recent study, Buckmaster et al. evaluated 145 patients with TEE and/or aortography.[99] Of 110 patients having TEE, 11 had aortic injuries. Five of these were confirmed with aortography, 4 were identified at thoracotomy, and two were identified at autopsy. TEE was suspicious in two patients who had negative aortograms; however, one of these two patients had an injury involving the aortic arch. There was one false-positive aortogram and three false-negative aortograms.

In an another study of the value of TEE in 105 patients with severe blunt chest trauma, Karalis et al. found that biplane TEE correctly diagnosed aortic transection in one patient and correctly excluded the diagnosis in another seven patients with suspected aortic injury.[100] TEE was also more sensitive than aortography in detecting small, intimal tears in the descending thoracic aorta not requiring surgery in four other patients.

Thus, TEE is safe and effective,[6] it is generally more accurate than aortography for diagnosing TRA, and it can be much quicker (30 min vs 75 min; P < 0.001).[99] Aortography, however, should be used when TEE is equivocal, not tolerated, or contraindicated (as with cervical spine injuries) or when arteriography is needed for other suspected vascular injuries. In addition, a negative TEE obviates the need for aortography, and a definite positive TEE probably does not need aortography.

Aortography

AXIOM	If an aortic rupture is suspected because of the mechanism of injury, physical findings, or chest radiographic changes, aortography should be performed.

While waiting for aortography or surgery, it is important to ensure that the systolic BP does not rise above 110-120 mm Hg, as may easily occur in patients who have severe pain and are given large quantities of intravenous fluids. It is also important to prevent the patient from forcefully gagging or retching, as may occur during insertion of a nasogastric or endotracheal tube.

In the 1950s and 1960s, almost 50% of the aortograms that Wilson et al. performed for suspected TRA were positive.[84] Now, because of our greatly increased sensitivity to this problem, we tend to perform aortograms when a TRA is even minimally suspected, partly because of the fear of malpractice litigation. In a recent personal survey, 95-98% of the aortograms performed at trauma hospitals in Detroit to look for TRA were negative.

AXIOM	Thoracic aortography is still considered the "gold standard" for diagnosing TRA, and most trauma surgeons believe that it should be done on all patients who possibly have TRA.

The most common finding on aortography of a TRA is a pseudoaneurysm of the isthmus of the aorta between the origin of the left subclavian artery and the ligamentum arteriosum (Fig. 18–10). A slight pouching out of the inferior or inner border of isthmus, sometimes referred to as a "ductus bump" is normal, but it can easily be confused with a traumatic pseudoaneurysm. Bulging of the aorta laterally or a linear filling defect caused by torn intima and media is strong evidence that a TRA is present.

AXIOM	Aortography obtained to eliminate TRA should visualize the entire thoracic aorta and its major branches to the thoracic inlet.

The left anterior oblique (LAO) radiography appears to be optimal for examining the aortic arch and proximal descending aorta. In addition, the entire aorta and its branches, particularly those extending from the arch, should be visualized to eliminate the less common great artery injuries or multiple injuries that may otherwise be missed.[72] However, a patient who is in shock from a suspected traumatic aortic rupture or has a rapidly expanding mediastinal hematoma should be taken directly to the operating room without undergoing aortography.

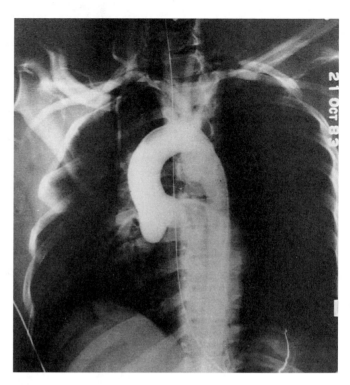

FIGURE 18–10 This aortogram shows a tear of the isthmus of the aorta distal to the left subclavian artery. Not only is a pseudoaneurysm present, but one can also see a faint filling defect representing the torn intima and media. (From: Wilson RF. Injury to the heart and great vessels. Henning RJ, Grenvik A, eds. Critical care cardiology. New York: Churchill Livingstone, 1989; 454.)

AXIOM	Aortography is the "gold standard" for diagnosing TRAs, but it is not infallible.

We have personally seen two injuries of the thoracic aorta in the isthmus missed on aortograms. We also know of an injury at the take-off of the left subclavian artery, that was missed on two aortograms.

Although it is generally believed that aortography should be performed on anyone with even a slight chance of having an injury to the aorta or other great vessel in the chest, the test requires movement of the patient to the radiology suite and places the patient in a suboptimal area for monitoring and treatment.

Angiographic complications may result from puncturing the vessel, passing the catheter through diseased or injured vessels, and the injection of contrast material under pressure. In a report by Waugh and Sacharias, it was noted that local complications with conventional angiography may occur in 4.1-23.2% of patients and systemic complications may occur in 2.2-9.4%.[101] Although the rates of amputation (0.1%) or death (0.3%) resulting from transfemoral studies are relatively low,[102] one is apt to be much more selective in future aortography requests if such a complication occurs in an individual with a negative study. Death has also occurred in at least two instances when the angiographic catheter was manipulated thorough the aorta at the level of a tear.[103] In addition, the incidence of renal dysfunction may exceed 7%,[104] especially if the patient is hypotensive, with about 20% of these patients requiring dialysis. If the angiography is done in a hospital where only a few aortograms are done each year, the incidence of fatal and/or neurologic complications may be up to 32 times greater than at busier institutions.[102]

Digital Subtraction Angiography

In an effort to improve the speed and accuracy of angiography and to reduce the dose of contrast material, Mirvis et al. studied 61 consecutive patients who had blunt thoracic trauma and obscuration of the aortic knob or mediastinal widening on chest radiography, using intraarterial digital subtraction angiography (IA-DSA) of the thoracic aorta.[105] Ten of these patients had aortic ruptures diagnosed by IA-DSA. Digital subtraction aortography proved 100% accurate, as indicated by results of surgery, conventional arteriography, serial chest x-rays, and clinical follow-up. The method was 50% faster than conventional aortography and significantly reduced radiographic film costs. The use of smaller caliber catheters for the intraaortic injection and a decrease in radiographic contrast media requirements also make this method safer than conventional arteriography.

Treatment

PREVENTION OF COMPLETION OF RUPTURE

Although it is essential to rapidly correct hypotension and hypoxemia following severe injuries, patients with possible TRA should be treated as if an aortic dissection were present and should not be allowed to develop a systolic BP exceeding 110-120 mm Hg or to retch or perform a Valsalva maneuver. Fluid administration should be watched carefully, and administration of analgesics and/or vasodilators may be required to keep the patient's systolic BP from getting too high. Walker and Pate reviewed the literature and showed that medical management of traumatic rupture of the aorta can be successful.[106] Pharmacologic therapy to keep the systolic BP and rate of pressure rise (dp/dt) low may be particularly useful in individuals would be at high-risk for any major emergency operation.

AXIOM When one suspects TRA because of the mechanism of injury or chest radiographic findings, the patient should be treated as if a dissecting aneurysm of the descending thoracic aorta were present and the systolic BP should be kept < 110-120 mm Hg.

Although it is generally important to insert a nasogastric tube in patients with multiple injuries, it is essential that the patient with a suspected TRA not perform vigorous Valsalva maneuvers. Sudden, severe gagging or bearing-down can cause intraaortic pressure to rise abruptly to well over 200 mm Hg and complete the rupture of a partially torn aorta. Similar precautions must be undertaken when inserting an endotracheal tube.

ELECTIVE DELAYS IN SURGICAL INTERVENTION

Since the initial report of a successful repair of an acute traumatic thoracic aortic disruption by Passaro and Pace[107] in 1959, emergency operation has become the accepted standard for treatment. However, in selected patients, medical management with a delay in surgical intervention may be warranted and safe.[106] In a report by Akins et al. in 1981, 14 of 44 patients with TRA had operative therapy delayed for 2-79 days with only 2 (14%) deaths, and 5 did not have operative repairs (i.e., surgery was delayed indefinitely with no deaths).[108] Of 21 patients having operative repair within 48 hours, 5 (24%) died. The 14 patients with elective delays of surgery included 12 patients with severe head injuries, 9 patients with extensive pelvic or extremity fractures, 3 with severe burns, 2 with large pulmonary contusions, and 1 with a ruptured colon.

AXIOM When the BP of a patient with proven TRA can be controlled properly, surgery for TRA should be delayed until the best possible circumstances for operative success are available.

A similar experience was reported by Stiles et al. in 1985.[109] They had 24 patients with thoracic and abdominal aortic injuries who became stable after initial fluid replacement. BPs were carefully controlled with vasodilators and beta-blockers while awaiting elective repair of the torn aorta. Only one patient died and no stabilized patient bled during the elective delay. The mortality rate was much higher in patients who were rushed to surgery at night in spite of being hemodynamically stable.

Delaying aortic surgery so that it can be performed under optimal conditions has also worked well for acute, nontraumatic dissecting

aneurysms of the descending thoracic aorta. Such delay should be considered for TRA when: (a) the patient is hemodynamically stable, (b) the systolic BP can be maintained at ideal levels (<110-120 mm Hg systolic), (c) the conditions for surgery are not ideal, or (d) the patient represents an extremely high operative risk because of associated injuries or preexisting medical conditions.[108-111] Kipfer et al. recently reported on 10 consecutive patients in whom TRA was initially treated medically to reduce aortic shear forces until the patient could safely tolerate cardiopulmonary bypass.[112] It recently was pointed out by Lamp et al. that because they had a higher mortality rate (83 versus 125%) than younger individuals with TRA, patients over 55 years of age may also be candidates for nonsurgical management.[113]

MANAGEMENT PRIORITIES WITH ASSOCIATED INJURIES

Priority of therapy is an important consideration in patients with a TRA and other severe injuries. Patients who sustain aortic rupture in association with an injury to an extremity or another thoracic organ usually pose little problem. In such instances, it is usually obvious that the aortic injury takes precedence. However, when intraabdominal injuries also require emergency surgery, determination of priorities can be difficult.

AXIOM Unless one is exsanguinating from associated abdominal injuries, TRA should generally be treated prior to laparotomy for abdominal injuries.

In an early experience at the University of Michigan,[68] six patients with TRA and intraabdominal bleeding had laparotomy before thoracotomy. Five died because of rupture of the aorta. Six others with similar injuries had repair of the TRA before laparotomy, and all six survived. This experience has influenced many surgeons to perform the thoracotomy first in most patients. Nevertheless, one should first correct whatever seems to be the most life-threatening injury. If the TRA appeared to be stable and the patient were bleeding rapidly inside the abdomen, laparotomy would take precedence. However, when patients' injuries require both thoracotomy for TRA and laparotomy for intraabdominal bleeding, the survival rate may be less than 40%.[112]

SURGICAL TECHNIQUES

Descending Thoracic Aorta

Great controversy exists concerning the best techniques for controlling the torn thoracic aorta during repair. Some believe that the surgeon should simply clamp the aorta above and below the tear and repair the aorta (clamp/repair technique) with no provision for blood flow to the distal aorta. Others believe that an external shunt or partial cardiopulmonary bypass should be used to decompress the proximal aorta and perfuse distally during aortic clamping and repair.

"CLAMP/REPAIR" TECHNIQUE

AXIOM The clamp/repair technique should not be used if the surgeon is unaccustomed to thoracic aortic surgery or if the repair is likely to require more than 30 minutes of aortic clamp time.

Most centers reporting success with the "clamp/repair" technique have had extensive experience with various types of aortic surgery.[113,114] Such authors believe that this technique may not only be much faster but also safer; however, the greatest successes quoted for the clamp/repair technique have been seen in patients with chronic TRA or arteriosclerotic aneurysms of the descending thoracic aorta.[115,116]

With the clamp/repair technique, the proximal clamps are usually on the arch between the left common carotid and left subclavian arteries. A clamp is also placed on the left subclavian artery. The distal clamp is as close to the hematoma as possible so as not to interfere with the upper intercostal arteries (Fig. 18–11). By avoiding cardiopulmonary bypass (CPB) and its attendant heparinization, the risk of

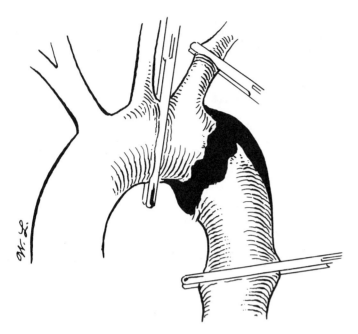

FIGURE 18–11 The usual technique for obtaining vascular control above and below the aortic injury involves clamping (1) the aortic arch between the left subclavian and left common carotid arteries, (2) the left subclavian artery, and (3) the descending thoracic aorta as close to the injury as possible without disturbing the contained hematoma. With the clamp-repair technique, interruption of the flow to the distal aorta for more than 30 minutes greatly increases the risk of postoperative paraplegia. (From: Wilson RF. Injury to the heart and great vessels. Henning RJ, Grenvik A, eds. Critical care cardiology. New York: Churchill Livingstone, 1989; 456.)

excessive bleeding is reduced. This may be particularly important in patients with injuries to the brain, eyes, or retroperitoneum.

Clamp/repair enthusiasts also note that the ascending aorta or the apex of the left ventricle can be damaged during insertion of the proximal end of the shunt. Use of the clamp/repair technique also avoids damage to the descending aorta and/or the femoral artery during insertion of the distal end of the shunt. Nevertheless, aortic cross-clamping without distal perfusion because of sudden complete aortic rupture or by relatively inexperienced surgeons may result in high mortality and morbidity rates, especially when the aorta is clamped for more than 30 minutes. In addition, significant hemodynamic and metabolic changes can occur in patients without a shunt or bypass to the distal aorta.[117] Forbes and Ashbaugh recently noted that simple aortic cross-clamping to repair TRA resulted in a 44% incidence of new neurologic deficits, longer hospitalization, and higher incidence of pulmonary, gastrointestinal, and septic complications than mechanical circulatory support.[118]

In one of the largest experiences with TRA (80 patients in 15 years), Schmidt et al. noted that the most important factor determining the incidence of paraplegia was the duration of the cross-clamp time.[119] The majority of patients (54%) were treated with the clamp/repair technique with only two postoperative paraplegias. However, they stressed the importance of primary aortic repair, rather than graft interposition, which they were able to accomplish in 61 patients, including the last 32 consecutive patients.

EXTERNAL SHUNTS. A frequently used alternative technique for maintaining blood flow to the distal aorta without systemic heparinization is the use of heparin-bonded tubing as a shunt to divert blood around the involved aorta. The shunts usually extend from the ascending aorta to the apex of the left ventricle to the descending aorta or to a femoral artery (Fig. 18–12). These shunts can reduce the danger of distal ischemia to the spinal cord and abdominal viscera and can prevent proximal hypertension damage to the heart

and brain. When heparin-coated polyvinyl tubing is used, the patient does not require systemic heparinization.

The safety of the shunt technique has been demonstrated well by Verdant et al. who reported operating on 114 consecutive shunted patients with descending thoracic aortic disease and no postoperative paralysis.[120] In that same report, the use of a Gott shunt between the ascending and descending aorta in 20 patients with acute traumatic aortic rupture and in 20 patients with chronic traumatic aortic aneurysms resulted in only two deaths (both in the acute group) and no renal dysfunction or paraplegia in the survivors. A more recent report further confirmed the safety of this technique.[121]

CARDIOPULMONARY BYPASS. Repair of traumatic rupture of the thoracic aorta is often performed under partial CPB because it allows increased time for a meticulous repair. When the patient with TRA is stable, transfer to a hospital where CPB is available seems prudent.

A number of CPB techniques can be used for TRA. Complete CPB is seldom used now except when repairing tears of the ascending aorta or arch. For lesions involving the aortic isthmus, partial bypass is usually adequate. Probably the most frequent type of partial CPB used in the past for TRA was a femoral vein to femoral artery bypass. This involves use of an oxygenator and requires heparinization of the patient.

AXIOM A vortex pump with a left atrial-femoral artery bypass requires little or no heparin and is probably the safest technique for preserving distal aortic flow in patients with TRA.

When a left atrial to femoral artery partial CPB is used, an oxygenator is not needed, further reducing the need for heparin. When a special vortex (Biomedicus) pump is used with a left atrial-femoral artery bypass, an oxygenator is not needed and little or no hepariniza-

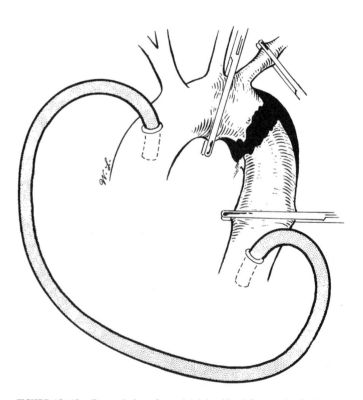

FIGURE 18–12 One technique for maintaining blood flow to the distal aorta while clamps are placed above and below the aortic injury is to use a heparin-bonded tube to shunt blood from the ascending aorta to the descending thoracic aorta. The cannula is filled with heparinized saline before insertion and secured in place with double purse-string sutures. (From: Wilson RF. Injury to the heart and great vessels. Henning RJ, Grenvik A, eds. Critical care cardiology. New York: Churchill Livingstone, 1989; 460.)

tion of the blood is required (Fig. 18–13). Olivier et al. reported two groups of patients in whom either a heparinized (Gott) shunt or the Biomedicus pump was used.[122] In the control group of 10 patients treated with heparinized shunts, 4 died and 2 had paraplegia postoperatively. In contrast, when the Biomedicus pump was used without heparin on 9 patients, only one died and none experienced paraplegia postoperatively. In four published series in which this technique was used, only two deaths (7%) and no paraplegia were reported.[16,122-124] This is increasingly becoming the preferred technique for treating this injury; however, it is important to maintain distal aortic flow at > 1.0 L/min to prevent clotting and to maintain adequate distal BP. Kim et al. from Denver General Hospital recently noted a survival rate of 89% (16 of 18) of their patients without paraplegia using this technique.[39]

Blunt Injuries to the Ascending Aorta

Few patients with blunt ascending aortic injury survive long enough for the diagnosis to be established and the repair to be effected. These injuries are frequently associated with cardiac rupture or severe myocardial contusion, and aortic tears are multiple in up to 15-20% of these patients. Most victims have been hit by or thrown from moving vehicles or have fallen from great heights, and multiple, severe associated injuries are usually present.

Most ascending aortic tears occur within the pericardium so that if the tear is complete, there is generally evidence of both shock and pericardial tamponade. Chest radiographic findings often show a widened superior mediastinum with or without obscuration of the aortic knob. Aortography must usually be performed for the diagnosis to be established preoperatively. Aortography usually shows a pseudoaneurysm with an intimal tear seen as an irregular filling defect within the lumen. When an associated aortic valvular injury occurs, aortic insufficiency of varying magnitude may also be seen.

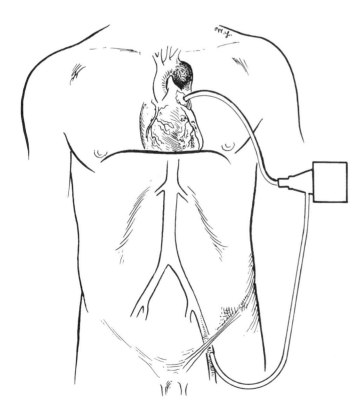

FIGURE 18–13 Partial cardiopulmonary bypass with a centrifugal pump. Using this pump to move oxygenated blood from the left atrium directly into the femoral artery allows one to use little or no heparin because an oxygenator is not in the circuit. (From: Wilson RF. Injury to the heart and great vessels. Henning RJ, Grenvik A, eds. Critical care cardiology. New York: Churchill Livingstone, 1989; 463.)

In most instances, complete cardiopulmonary bypass will be required to repair or replace the injured ascending aorta. If the tear is long and spiral, a graft from just above the coronary arteries to just below the innominate artery would probably be safest.

Injury to Lower Thoracic Aorta

Thoracic aortic injuries distal to the isthmus should be suspected with severe chest trauma in which a lower thoracic vertebra is crushed. Aortography is the diagnostic test of choice and should visualize the entire aorta and all of the arch branches up to and including the thoracic inlet. Repair techniques should be similar to those used with injuries to the aortic isthmus, but a little less difficulty should be encountered with clamp/repair technique in this area compared with more proximal aortic injuries.

Other Great Vessel Injuries

INNOMINATE ARTERY

Incidence. In patients reaching the hospital alive, blunt injuries of the innominate artery are second in frequency only to rupture of the aorta at the isthmus. However, Kirsh and Sloan were able to find fewer than 40 patients treated for this condition in the literature.[41] Associated injuries, such as rib fractures, flail chest, hemopneumothorax, fractured extremities, head injuries, facial fractures, and/or abdominal injuries, were found in more than 75% of these patients.

Diagnosis. The diagnosis of blunt injury to the innominate artery may be difficult because no characteristic physical findings are manifest except for some diminution of the right radial or brachial pulse, which occurs in about 50% of patients.[3,33] Signs and symptoms of distal ischemia are uncommon. Occasionally, a localized systolic murmur may draw attention to a possible lesion in this area.

Chest radiographic findings are similar to those seen with TRA (i.e., widened superior mediastinum); however, the outline of the descending aorta may be preserved. In this instance, the trachea and esophagus may be deviated to the left.

Aortography must generally be performed for the diagnosis to be established preoperatively. The right posterior oblique position is best for visualization of the proximal aorta and the origin of the innominate artery. It may be the only projection that demonstrates a partial innominate artery tear.

Tears of the innominate artery typically show bulbous dilation of the vessel just distal to its origin, associated with a crescentic line across its base representing retraction of the torn intima into the lumen of the vessel. Associated injuries in other brachycephalic vessels or the aorta are found in about 10% of patients. This emphasizes the need for visualization of the entire thoracic aorta and its major branches during aortography.[36]

Management. Because of the ever-present danger of sudden rupture of the pseudoaneurysm, the ideal treatment is generally immediate surgical repair; however, one can postpone this surgery to provide optimal conditions for repair as long as one can keep the systolic BP < 110-120 mm Hg and prevent excessive Valsalva maneuvers.

The best approach to the innominate artery is through a median sternotomy incision extended into the right side of the neck or above the right clavicle. Maintenance of cerebral perfusion should be attempted during the period of innominate arterial occlusion because the incidence of paralysis after occlusion of the common carotid artery may be as high as 25%.[36] This is best avoided by placing an external or internal bypass shunt from the ascending aorta to the distal common carotid artery. Cardiopulmonary bypass or an external bypass shunt should be available for all patients with aortic or innominate artery injury in the event that the tear extends into the aortic arch.

Reconstruction of the innominate artery is usually carried out with a prosthetic graft, using a direct end-to-end anastomosis whenever possible. The in-hospital survival of patients reaching the operating room alive with this injury is about 75%.[36]

In the patient with an associated injury of the aortic arch, which requires graft reconstruction, cardiopulmonary bypass with selective cerebral perfusion and moderate hypothermia (20-28°C) may be used.[36] The femoral artery is used for arterial perfusion, and both common carotid arteries are cannulated and perfused separately. The total flow rates through the carotid vessels should be about 400-800 mL/min, but the pressure in the perfusion lines should not exceed 120 mm Hg. Myocardial preservation is maintained with topical cooling and intermittent intracoronary cardioplegic infusions. Deliberate, severe hypothermia (15-20°C) with complete cessation of all blood flow and close monitoring with EEG is another technique that can be used to protect the brain during aortic arch surgery, particularly when any problem cannulating or perfusing the distal common carotid arteries occurs.

SUBCLAVIAN ARTERY INJURY

Etiology. Although an occasional subclavian artery is avulsed at its origin because of sudden deceleration, direct trauma to the distal artery with occlusion associated with fractures of the first rib or clavicle are much more likely.[3,17]

Diagnosis. The most important sign of a subclavian artery injury is absence of a radial pulse; however, the collateral is so good across the shoulder and upper arm that 15-25% of the patients with occlusion of the subclavian, axillary or high brachial artery have a palpable radial pulse.[36] Other physical findings that are highly suggestive of subclavian artery injury are a pulsatile mass or hematoma or a bruit in the root of the neck. An occasional patient may develop a subclavian steal syndrome when the subclavian artery occludes proximally to the origin of the vertebral artery.

Up to 60% of patients with blunt injury to the subclavian artery, especially from motor vehicle accidents, also have damage to the brachial plexus.[36] Consequently, a complete neurologic examination preoperatively is important in these patients. When evidence of brachial plexus injury exists, one should strongly consider obtaining arteriography. Horner's syndrome with a penetrating wound at the thoracic inlet often also indicates avulsion of nerve roots from the spinal cord.

In patients with subclavian artery injuries, chest radiography may show a widened superior mediastinum without blurring or obscuration of the aortic knob shadow. Angiography usually shows occlusion, but a pseudoaneurysm is occasionally found. One should also remember that blunt subclavian artery injuries are associated with other major vascular injuries in about 10% of patients.[36]

Treatment. The treatment of acute subclavian artery injury is usually immediate repair; however, in certain high-risk patients who are doing poorly, ligation or angiographic occlusion may be the treatment of choice. When the artery is already occluded, nonoperative care with close observation may be all that is required. The survival rate of patients treated for isolated, acute subclavian artery injuries should exceed 90%.

AXIOM When a subclavian artery is occluded by trauma and no AV fistula, false aneurysm, or distal ischemia is present, no critical need exists for exploring the artery, particularly if the patient has severe associated injuries.

The collateral circulation for the distal portions of the subclavian arteries is usually very good, but many of the collateral vessels may be damaged by severe blunt trauma to the shoulder girdle. In one series, 53% (8 of 15) patients with blunt subclavian artery injuries had critical ischemia of the hand.[125] In addition, during World War II, ligation of subclavian arteries resulted in upper extremity gangrene in 29% of patients.[8] When reconstruction of a blunt injury to the distal subclavian artery is required, a graft is usually necessary because the involved vessel may be quite fragile and may not mobilize well. Gore-Tex (PTFE) grafts usually work well in this circumstance.

AXIOM Blunt subclavian artery injuries usually require a graft to provide successful repair.

The optimal incisions to approach the subclavian arteries are somewhat controversial. If the injury involves the proximal right subclavian artery, exposure is best provided by a median sternotomy with extension along or above the right clavicle. Removal of the medial portion of the right clavicle can greatly improve exposure of almost all of the right subclavian artery.

The ideal exposure of the proximal left subclavian artery is provided by a fourth interspace posterolateral thoracotomy, but the patient should not be turned onto one side when hypovolemic. For injuries of the mid or distal left subclavian artery, an anterolateral fourth intercostal incision can be made for proximal control of the artery. This can be extended over to the sternum and then joined to a total or upper midsternotomy incision. For the more distal subclavian artery, a supraclavicular incision with excision of the medial clavicle may be needed.

Complications of Blunt Thoracic Great Artery Injuries

PARAPLEGIA

Flaccid paraplegia with varying degrees of sensory loss below T-6 to T-10 is characteristic of the ischemic myelopathy that occurs after prolonged thoracic aortic cross-clamping.[95] Most patients preserve partial function of the posterior column and have at least some pain and temperature sensation below the level of the spinal injury.

AXIOM The best way to prevent paraplegia with thoracic aortic clamping is to maintain an adequate blood flow to the mid and lower intercostal arteries.

Ischemic damage to the spinal cord with thoracic aortic clamping is believed to be due to inadequate anterior spinal artery flow. Collaterals to the anterior spinal artery (ASA) in the lower chest are inadequate in many patients. Ligation and division of mid and lower thoracic intercostal arteries, particularly the arteria radicularis magna (ARM) of Adamkiewicz which is believed to be the major blood supply to the lower spinal cord, can lead to paraplegia, even without prolonged aortic cross-clamping.[126] Although this occasionally occurs in other aortic operations, particularly those for arteriosclerotic aneurysms of the descending aorta, the number of intercostal arteries divided (and their location) have not been clearly related to the development of paraplegia after trauma.[127]

In the study by Svennson et al., the ARM originated from T-9 to T-12 intercostal arteries in 7 of 8 humans.[128] One arose from T-7. In most baboons the ARM arises from the T-9 to L-1 segment. Studies with larger sample sizes showed that the ARM in humans arises from the T-5 to T-8 segment in 15%, T-9 to T-12 in 75%, L-1 to L-2 in 10%, and L-3 to L-5 in 1.6%.

Of particular interest in the studies by Svensson et al. was the discrepancy between the diameter of the ASA above and below its junction with the ARM in both nonhuman and human primates.[128] This is of interest because the blood supply to the distal (lumbar) aspect of the spinal cord by distal aortic perfusion reaches the spinal cord predominantly via the ARM. The mean diameter of the distended human ASA is 0.231 mm above the ARM junction and 0.941 mm below (P = .0057).[128] The difference in size has profound implications for spinal cord protection during thoracic aortic cross-clamping. Because resistance to blood flow is inversely proportional to the fourth power of the radius (Poiseuille's equation), the resistance to flow up the ASA past the ARM in humans is about 250 times greater than downward. Thus, if a shunt were used to bypass an occluded segment of the descending aorta, blood would preferentially flow via the ARM and then down the ASA to perfuse the lumbar spinal cord rather than the lower thoracic spinal cord.

From communications with thoracic surgeons, Pate noted that many instances of paraplegia are not reported in the medical literature but frequently result in extremely expensive malpractice cases.[129] In one rehabilitation center, five young people were admitted with paraplegia within a 2-year period following repair of a traumatic rupture of the thoracic aorta.[126] Paraplegia, therefore, may be more common than the 5-10% that the surgical literature generally indicates. Some surgeons believe that draining cerebrospinal fluid via a lumbar tap during surgery will improve blood flow to the lower spinal cord. Some experimental evidence suggests that this technique can be helpful, and several centers are using it.

A study evaluated somatosensory evoked potentials (SEPs) in patients undergoing descending thoracic or thoracoabdominal aortic surgery.[127] They found a 71%-incidence of paraplegia in patients who had SEP losses of > 30 minutes duration. No paraplegia occurred in patients in whom SEP loss was prevented or limited in duration to < 30 minutes.

The reasons for the low incidence of neurologic deficit observed by Crawford and Rubio[115] and DeBakey et al.[116] using the clamp/repair technique are not completely known. However, in patients with chronic aneurysms or atherosclerotic disease, collateral vessels are likely to have developed to intercostal arteries distal to the aortic lesion. This collateral flow may then provide protection to the spinal cord during aortic cross-clamping.[67] Furthermore, these surgeons have an almost unparalleled experience with thoracic aortic surgery of all types.

AXIOM Thoracic aortic cross-clamp times should not exceed 30 minutes unless a bypass or shunt maintains an adequate flow to the mid and lower thoracic aorta.

If aortic cross-clamp time were < 30 minutes, the incidence of paraplegia would be rather low. A number of investigators reported no patients developing paraplegia under such circumstances;[107,114,126,127,129-136] however, if the aortic cross-clamp time exceeds 30 minutes in patients without functioning distal shunts or bypasses, up to 73% have become paraplegic. When shock is present during surgery or when intercostal arteries have to be ligated and divided, the incidence of paraplegia increases.

In a review of the literature, it appears that the paraplegia rate with the clamp/repair technique from 1970 to 1990 (Table 18–4) and 1985 to 1990 (Table 18–5) is over twice as high as with the other techniques that provide some blood flow to the distal portions of the aorta. Thus, it appears that repair of acute aortic transections without a shunting procedure should be limited to those patients in whom the surgeon believes, with reasonable certainty, that the operation can be completed with < 30 minutes of aortic cross-clamp time. Pate paraphrased this requirement, stating that "repair of acute aortic rupture without distal circulation should be recognized as a serious gamble."[129] Surgeons without much thoracic aortic surgical experience should probably avoid this technique.

Reports have documented paraplegia/paraparesis following other types of thoracic trauma, including ED thoracotomy for a stab of the heart with aortic cross-clamping.[137] Three other patients developed permanent neurologic injury after oxidized regenerated cellulose

TABLE 18–4 Techniques for Repairing Traumatic Rupture of the Aorta 1970-1990

Technique	Number of Papers	Mortality Rate	Paraplegia Rate*
Clamp/Repair	27	46/184 (25%)	23/167 (13.8%)
Shunt	31	44/298 (14.8%)	20/285 (7.0%)
Bypass	33	49/251 (19.5%)	8/238 (3.4%)
Biomedicus	2	2/ 23 (8.7%)	0/ 23 (0%)
Total	49	141/756 (18.7%)	51/713 (7.2%)

*Excluding intra-operative deaths.

TABLE 18–5 Techniques for Repairing Traumatic Rupture of the Aorta 1985-1990

Technique	Number of Papers	Mortality Rate	Paraplegia Rate*
Clamp/Repair	12	35/112 (31.3%)	16/ 98 (16.3%)
Shunt	10	13/115 (11.3%)	10/110 (9.1%)
Bypass	8	10/ 91 (11.0%)	5/ 87 (5.8%)
Biomedicus	1	1/ 14 (7.1%)	0/ 14 (0%)
Total	14	59/332 (17.8%)	31/309 (10.0%)

*Excluding intra-operative deaths.

which was used to achieve hemostasis in the posterior angle of the thoracotomy incision migrated into the spinal canal.[138]

LEFT HEART FAILURE

AXIOM Maintaining a systolic BP above 160-180 mm Hg can cause acute left heart failure in patients with recent severe blunt chest trauma.

Increasing data are available to demonstrate the potentially deleterious effects of thoracic aortic cross-clamping on the heart and lungs. Pulmonary artery wedge pressure (PAWP) can double after two minutes of thoracic aortic clamping distal to the left subclavian artery.[139] Verdant et al. observed that substantial elevations of left atrial pressure occur when the proximal aortic systolic pressure is maintained above 160 mm Hg, suggesting that any pressure above 160 mm Hg can result in left ventricular overload.[120] In a related clinical study by Ross and Braunwald,[140] it was noted that virtually all patients in whom the systolic BP was raised above 160 mm Hg by angiotension doubled their left ventricular end diastolic pressures.

CEREBRAL HYPERTENSION

It is generally believed that raising arterial blood pressure in the head to levels much greater than normal increases the likelihood of aggravating associated brain injury. Although a high systolic blood pressure may increase intracranial pressure in patients with head injury, there does not seem to be any clinical data demonstrating that there is increased brain damage in patients when the clamp/repair technique is used to repair TRA.

RENAL ISCHEMIA

Although overt renal insufficiency is only rarely described in retrospective studies of patients having the clamp/repair technique,[134] Carlson et al. found some renal dysfunction in all patients studied after that procedure.[141]

ATELECTASIS AND PNEUMONIA

Pulmonary problems, particularly atelectasis and pneumonia, are the most frequent postoperative complications after almost all thoracic operations. However, careful attention to pulmonary management postoperatively and use of a double-lumen endotracheal tube intraoperatively have decreased the incidence and severity of these problems.[63]

POSTOPERATIVE HYPERTENSION

Hypertension in both the upper and lower extremities may persist for several days after repair of TRA, possibly because of stretching or stimulation of baroreceptors located in tissues near the aortic isthmus.[69] If hypertension is severe, it should be treated with antihypertensive agents.

HOARSENESS

Hoarseness caused by damage to the left recurrent laryngeal nerve as it passes around the aorta just beyond the ligamentum arteriosum is common after TRA. This may be due to the initial trauma, pressure from an expanding pseudoaneurysm, or iatrogenic damage in spite of the surgeon's efforts to avoid this structure. In most instances, hoarseness is only temporary.

ESOPHAGEAL INJURY

Necrosis or tearing of the esophagus is an infrequent but dreaded complication of repair of a ruptured thoracic aorta. Such damage may be caused by initial trauma, direct compression by mediastinal hematoma, damage to esophageal blood supply, or surgical dissection or clamps. Iatrogenic injury, particularly by vascular clamps intended only for the aorta, may also occur easily. When the esophagus has a full thickness injury, the prognosis is very poor because, even if the patient were to survive the surgery, the suture line or prosthetic graft would have an increased chance of becoming infected.

Mortality Rates

In most reports, the mortality for patients reaching the hospital alive is 10-25%. In those who reach the operating room conscious and with stable vital signs, the mortality rate should be < 10%.

In a review of the literature from 1985 to 1990 (Table 18–5), the mortality rates with the clamp/repair technique (31.3%) were significantly higher than with techniques that maintain some distal aortic blood flow (7.1-11.3%). Thus, although the mortality rates seen with traumatic rupture of the aorta are due primarily to the multiple, severe associated injuries that frequently accompany this problem, the technique of repair may also be an important factor.

⊘ FREQUENT ERRORS

IN THE MANAGEMENT OF INJURIES TO INTRATHORACIC GREAT VESSELS

1. *Failure to promptly obtain arteriography on stable patients with penetrating chest wounds anywhere near a great vessel or across the mediastinum.*
2. *Delaying needed surgery to obtain arteriography on patients who are even marginally unstable from penetrating chest wounds.*
3. *Discounting the possible importance of a penetrating wound that may have injured a great vein of the chest.*
4. *Turning a patient with hypotension or significant hemoptysis onto one side to perform a posterolateral thoracotomy.*
5. *Taking time to repair a badly injured subclavian artery rather than just ligating it in patients who are hemodynamically unstable because of other injuries.*
6. *Failing to repair a lacerated carotid artery because a mild-to-moderate neurologic defect is present.*
7. *Failing to evaluate the adequacy of collateral blood flow to the brain or to maintain cerebral blood flow when a carotid or innominate artery must be clamped.*
8. *Completely clamping or occluding the superior or inferior vena cava while the patient is still hypovolemic.*
9. *Allowing the systolic BP to exceed 120 mm Hg when one suspects a TRA.*
10. *Assuming that TRA is not present in spite of a suspicious mechanism of trauma because the initial chest radiograph appears to be normal.*
11. *Failing to obtain a CT of the chest when one is already obtaining a CT of the brain after a severe deceleration injury.*
12. *Assuming that aortography is harmless and is needed on everyone who has even a slight chance of TRA.*
13. *Assuming radiographically-proved TRA must be repaired immediately regardless of the associated injuries, available surgical support, and surgical risk.*
14. *Using a clamp-repair technique when the surgeon does not have extensive aortic surgery experience and/or the repair is apt to require more than 30 minutes of aortic cross-clamp time.*

15. *Repairing other less critical injuries before attempting to repair TRA.*
16. *Inadequate warning of the patient and family of the risk of paraplegia when repairing TRA.*

▼▼▼▼▼▼▼▼▼▼▼▼▼▼▼▼▼▼▼▼▼▼▼▼▼▼▼▼▼▼

SUMMARY POINTS

1. Penetrating extrapericardial injuries to thoracic great vessels are usually rapidly fatal.
2. Major thoracic arterial injuries can easily be missed until an AV fistula or false aneurysm is detected.
3. Severe arterial hypoxemia in spite of what appear to be normal lung function should make one search for pulmonary AV fistula.
4. Cardiac arrest for more than five minutes before resuscitative thoracotomy is preformed rarely results in a patient leaving the hospital alive with a normally functioning brain.
5. Generally, one should not probe chest wounds because it may restart bleeding or an air leak or may cause a pneumothorax.
6. Distended neck veins plus hypotension are usually due to pericardial tamponade, tension pneumothorax, or excessive straining in a hypovolemic patient.
7. Pericardial tamponade or tension pneumothorax will usually not cause distended neck veins while the patient is severely hypovolemic.
8. Virtually all patients with major trauma should have chest radiography soon after admission.
9. A "fuzzy" bullet should be considered a radiologic sign of a major vascular injury until proven otherwise.
10. CT scans of the chest should not be performed while a patient is hemodynamically unstable.
11. When a mediastinal hematoma is not seen on a properly performed CT scan of the chest with intravenous contrast, it is unlikely that the patient has a major systemic thoracic vascular injury.
12. Shock plus inadequate ventilation are a rapidly fatal combination.
13. A moderate or large hemothorax should be promptly evacuated with a chest tube unless the patient requires emergency thoracotomy.
14. Penetrating carotid injuries should probably be repaired if the vessel is not already occluded even if a severe neurologic defect is present.
15. Unless a carotid or innominate artery repair is extremely rapid, one should evaluate distal carotid blood flow and pressure clinically or with stump pressure measurements to determine the need for a temporary shunt.
16. When possible, the superior or inferior vena cava should not be cross-clamped while a patient is hypovolemic. If a proximal cava must be clamped, the descending thoracic or proximal abdominal aorta should also be clamped.
17. The vast majority of deaths in thoracic vascular trauma are due to exsanguination.
18. A hemothorax should be evacuated via formal thoracotomy when it remains large in spite of well-placed, functioning chest tubes and/or when it is infected.
19. A retained hemothorax without infection can cause some leukocytosis (up to 12,000-15,000/mm^3) and fever (to 101.4°F). Higher fever or white cell counts or systemic evidence of sepsis are indications for prompt removal of a retained hemothorax.
20. Some intrathoracic great vessel injuries may not be detected until or unless follow-up examinations reveal a pseudoaneurysm or arteriovenous fistula.
21. Patients reaching the hospital alive with blunt aortic trauma generally have injury to the isthmus of the aorta.
22. Aortography to eliminate TRA should include the entire thoracic aorta and its major branches, including the distal subclavian arteries.
23. Blunt injuries to the aortic arch branches tend to occur at their origins or where they cross the first rib.
24. If an aortic injury is suspected because of the mechanism of injury, associated injuries, or chest radiography or CT scan findings, the systolic BP should be kept below 110-120 systolic.

25. The single most important factor in diagnosing acute traumatic aortic rupture is a high index of suspicion because of the mechanism of injury.

26. Up to one-third of patients with blunt trauma to the thoracic aorta or its major branches have little or no external evidence of thoracic injury.

27. One of the main reasons that many unnecessary aortograms are performed for possible TRA is a technically poor chest radiograph.

28. A deviation of the esophagus or trachea > 2.0 cm to the right after severe blunt trauma is frequently due to TRA.

29. Fracture of the first or second ribs should make one suspect the presence of severe intrathoracic injuries.

30. An initially normal chest radiograph does not eliminate TRA.

31. A mediastinal hematoma seen on CT scan of the chest after blunt chest trauma is an indication for complete thoracic aortography.

32. When the mechanism of injury, clinical findings, or chest radiography make one suspicious of aortic injury, one should obtain a complete thoracic aortogram. When relatively little suspicion of thoracic injury exists, CT scan of the chest can be an excellent screening technique.

33. If an aortic rupture is suspected because of the mechanism of injury, physical findings, or chest radiographic changes, aortography should be performed.

34. Thoracic aortography is still considered the "gold standard" for diagnosing TRA, and most trauma surgeons believe it should be done on all patients with possible TRA.

35. Aortography obtained to eliminate TRA should visualize the entire thoracic aorta and its major branches out to the thoracic inlet.

36. Aortography is the "gold standard" for diagnosing TRAs, but it is not infallible.

37. When one suspects TRA because of the mechanism of injury or chest radiographic findings, the patient should be treated as if a dissecting aneurysm of the descending thoracic aorta were present and the systolic BP kept < 110-120 mm Hg.

38. When the BP of a patient with proved TRA can be controlled properly, surgery for TRA should be delayed until the best possible circumstances for operative success are available.

39. Unless one is exsanguinating from associated abdominal injuries, TRA should generally be treated prior to laparotomy for abdominal injuries.

40. The clamp/repair technique should not be used if the surgeon is unaccustomed to thoracic aortic surgery or if the repair is likely to require more than 30 minutes of aortic clamp time.

41. A vortex pump with a left atrial-femoral artery bypass requires little or no heparin and is probably the safest technique for preserving distal aortic flow in patients with TRA.

42. When a subclavian artery is occluded by trauma and no AV fistula, false aneurysm, or distal ischemia is present, no critical need exists for exploring the artery, particularly if the patient has severe associated injuries.

43. Blunt subclavian artery injuries usually require a graft to provide a successful repair.

44. The best way to prevent paraplegia with thoracic aortic clamping is to maintain an adequate blood flow to the mid and lower intercostal arteries.

45. Thoracic aortic cross-clamp times should not exceed 30 minutes unless a bypass or shunt maintains an adequate flow to the mid and lower thoracic aorta.

46. Maintaining a systolic BP > 160-180 mm Hg can cause acute left heart failure in patients with recent, severe blunt chest trauma.

▲▲▲▲▲▲▲▲▲▲▲▲▲▲▲▲▲▲▲▲▲▲▲▲▲▲▲▲▲▲▲▲▲▲▲▲▲▲

REFERENCES

1. Mattox KL. Symposium: new approaches in vascular trauma. J Vasc Surg 1988;7:725.
2. Wilson RF, Gibson DEB, Antonenko D. Shock and acute respiratory failure after chest trauma. J Trauma 1977;17:697.
3. Symbas PN. Trauma to the great vessels. Cardiothoracic trauma. Philadelphia: WB Saunders, 1989; 160-231.
4. Clarks CP, Brandt PWT, Cole DS, et al. Traumatic rupture of the thoracic aorta: diagnosis and treatment. Br J Surg 1967;54-353.
5. Robbs JV, Baker LW, Human RR, et al. Cervicomediastinal arterial injuries. Arch Surg 1981;116:663.
6. Perkins R, Elchos T. Stab wound of the aortic arch. Ann Surg 1958;147:83.
7. Richardson JD, Smith JM, Grover FL, et al. Management of subclavian and innominate artery injuries. Am J Surg 1977;134:780.
8. Rich NM, Spencer FC. Injuries of the intrathoracic branches of the aortic arch. eds. Vascular trauma. Philadelphia: WB Saunders Co., 1978; 287.
9. Demetriades D, Rabinowitz B, Pezikis A, et al. Subclavian vascular injuries. Br J Surg 1987;74:1001.
10. Pate JW, Cole FH Jr, Walker WA, Fabian TC. Penetrating injuries of the aortic arch and its branches. Ann Thorac Surg 1993;55:586.
11. Nugent EW, Plauth WH, Edwards JE, et al. The pathology, abnormal physiology, clinical recognition, and medical surgical treatment of congenital heart disease. Hurst JW, Schlant RC, Rackley CE, et al. eds. The heart, arteries and veins. New York: McGraw-Hill, 1990; 655-794.
12. Symbas PN, Goldman M, Erbesfeld MH, Vlasis SE. Pulmonary arteriovenous fistula, pulmonary artery aneurysm, and other vascular changes of the lung from penetrating trauma. Ann Surg 1980;191:336.
13. Calhoon JH, Grover FL, Trinkle JT. Chest trauma—approach and management. Clin Chest Med 1992;13:55.
14. Flint LM, Snyder WH, Perry MD, et al. Management of major vascular injuries in the base of the neck. Arch Surg 1973;106:407.
15. McFadden PM, Jones JW, Ochsner JL. The fuzzy foreign body fragment: a subtle roentgenographic clue to mediastinal vascular injury. Am J Surg 1985;149:809.
16. Hess PJ, Howe HR, Robicsek F, et al. Traumatic tears of the thoracic aorta: improved results using the Bio-Medicus pump. Ann Thor Surg 1989;48:6.
17. Graham JM, Feliciano DV, Mattox KL, et al. Management of subclavian vascular injuries. J Trauma 1980;20:537.
18. Buscaglia LC, Walsh JC, Wilson JD, Matolo NM. Surgical management of subclavian artery injury. Am J Surg 1987;154:88.
19. Perry M, Thal E, Shires E. Management of arterial injuries. Ann Surg 1971;173:403.
20. Fisher RG, Ben-Menachem Y. Penetrating injuries of the thoracic aorta and brachiocephalic arteries: angiographic findings in 18 cases. ARJ 1987;149:607.
21. Allen TW, Reul GJ Jr, Morton JR, Beall AC Jr. Surgical management of aortic trauma. J Trauma 1972;12:862.
22. Hewitt RL, Smith AD, Becker ML. Penetrating vascular injuries of the thoracic outlet. Surgery 1974;76:715.
23. DiGiacoma JC, Rotondo MF, Schwab CW. Transcutaneous balloon catheter tamponade for definitive control of subclavian venous injuries: case reports. J Trauma 1994;37:111.
24. Silva R, Moore EE, Bar-Or D, et al. The risk: benefit of autotransfusion—comparison to banked blood in a canine model. J Trauma 1984;24:557.
25. Thomas AN. Discussion of Graham et al: Innominate vascular injury. J Trauma 1982;22:655.
26. Jacob LM, Hsieh JW. A clinical review of autotransfusion and its role in trauma. JAMA 1984;251:3283.
27. Steenburg R, Ravitch M. Cervico-thoracic approach for subclavian vessel injury from compound fracture of the clavicle. Ann Surg 1963;157:839.
28. Buttil RW, Acker B. Management of injuries to the bracheocephalic vessels. Surg Gynecol Obstet 1982;154:737.
29. Schaff HV, Brawley RK. Operative management of penetrating vascular injuries of the thoracic outlet. Surgery 1977;82:182.
30. Elkin DC, Cooper FW. Resection of the clavicle in vascular surgery. J Bone Joint Surg 1946;28:117.
31. Feliciano DV, Bitondo CG, Mattox KL, et al. Civilian trauma in the 1980s: a one-year experience with 456 vascular and cardiac injuries. Ann Surg 1984;199:717.
32. Wiencek RG, Wilson RF. Injuries to the abdominal vascular system: how much does aggressive resuscitation and pre laparotomy thoracotomy really help? Surgery 1987;102:731.
33. Wilson RF. Injury to the heart and great vessels. Henning RJ, Grenvik A, eds. Critical care cardiology. New York: Churchill Livingstone, 1989; 411-172.
34. Crawford ES, Mizrahi EM, Hess KR, et al. The impact of distal aortic perfusion and somatosensory evoked potential monitoring on prevention

of paraplegia after aortic aneurysm operation. J Thorac Cardiovasc Surg 1988;95:357.

35. Williams GM. Thoracoabdominal aneurysm. Cameron JL, ed. Current surgery - 3. Philadelphia: BC Decker, 1989; 531.

36. Symbas PN, Sehdeva JS. Penetrating wounds of the thoracic aorta. Ann Surg 1970;171:441.

37. DeMeester TR, Cameron JL, Gott VL. Repair of a through-and-through gunshot wound of the aortic arch using a heparinized shunt. Ann Thorac Surg 1973;16:1931973.

38. Graham JM, Feliciano DV, Mattox KL, Bealle AC Jr. Innominate vascular injury. J Trauma 1982;22:647.

39. Kim FJ, Moore EE, Moore FA, et al. Trauma surgeons can render operative care for major thoracic injuries. J Trauma 1994;36:871.

40. Raseretnam R, Tissera W. Penetrating wound of the arch of the aorta. Injury 1980;12:145.

41. Vosloo SM, Reichart BA. Inflow occlusion in the surgical management of a penetrating aortic arch injury: case report. J Trauma 1990;30:514-515.

42. Robicsek F, Matos-Cruz M. Artificially induced ventricular fibrillation in the management of through-and-through penetrating wounds of the aortic arch. A case report. Surgery 1991;110:544.

43. Marvasti MA, Parker FB Jr, Bredenberg CE. Injuries to arterial branches of the aortic arch. J Thorac Cardiovasc Surg 1984;32:293.

44. Feliciano DV, Graham JM. Major thoracic vascular injury. Champion HR, Robbs JV, Trunkey DO, eds. Rob & Smith's operative surgery—trauma surgery part 1, 4th ed. London: Butterworths, 1989; 283-293.

45. Phillips CV, Jacobsen DC, Brayton DF, Bloch JH. Central vessel trauma. Am Surgeon 1979;45:517.

46. Liekweg WG Jr, Greenfield LJ. Management of penetrating carotid arterial injury. Ann Surg 1978;188:587.

47. Binet JP, Langlois J, Cormier JM, et al. A case of recent traumatic avulsion of the innominate artery at its origin from the aortic arch. J Thorac Cardiovasc Surg 1962;43:670.

48. Crawford ES. Surgical treatment of occlusion of the innominate, common carotid, and subclavian arteries: a 10-year experience. Surgery 1969;65:17.

49. Zelenock G, Kazmers A, Graham L, et al. Non-penetrating subclavian artery injuries. Arch Surg 1985;120:685.

50. Sturn J, Dorsey J, Olson F, Perry J. The management of subclavian artery injuries following blunt thoracic. Ann Thorac Surg 1984;38:188.

51. Schimpf P, Burt D, Wagner R. Left subclavian artery trauma: in situ vs rib interspace mobilization for primary anastomosis. J Trauma 1985;25:1069.

52. Rich NM, Hobson RW, Jarstfer BS, et al. Subclavian artery trauma. J Trauma 1973;13:485.

53. Ochsner, JL, Crawford, ES, DeBakey, ME. Injuries of the vena cava caused by external trauma. Surgery 1961;49:397.

54. Agarwal N, Shah PM, Clauss RH, et al. Experience with 115 civilian venous injuries. J Trauma 1982;22:827.

55. Lim LT, Saletta JD, Flanigan DP. Subclavian and innominate artery trauma: 5 year experience with 17 patients. Surgery 1979;86:890.

56. Abouljoud MS, Obeid FN, Horst HM, et al. Arterial injuries to the thoracic outlet: a ten-year experience. Am Surg 1993;59:590.

57. Donohoe CD, McGuire TJ. Delayed weakness following a gunshot wound. Postgrad Med 1991;90:219.

58. Shoemaker WC, Kram GB, Lee TS. Prospective trial of supranormal values of survivors as therapeutic goals in high-risk surgical patients. Chest 1988;94:1176.

59. Johnson SF, Johnson SB, Strodel WE, et al. Brachial plexus injury: association with subclavian and axillary vascular trauma. J Trauma 1991; 31:1546.

60. Strassman G. Traumatic rupture of the aorta. Am Heart J 1947;33:508.

61. Parmley LF, Mattingly TW, Manion WC. Nonpenetrating traumatic injury of the aorta. Circulation 1958;17:1086.

62. Greendyke RM. Traumatic rupture of the aorta: with special reference to automobile accidents. JAMA 1966;195:527.

63. Kirsh MM, Sloan H. Blunt chest trauma. Boston: Little, Brown & Co, 1977.

64. Gates JD, Clair DG, Hechtman DH. Thoracic aortic dissection with renal artery involvement following blunt thoracic trauma: case report. J Trauma 1994;36:430.

65. Ben-Menachem Y. Rupture of the thoracic aorta by broadside impacts in road traffic and other collisions: further angiographic observations and preliminary autopsy findings. J Trauma 1993;35:363.

66. Feczko JD, Lynch L, Pless JE, et al. An autopsy case review of 142 nonpenetrating (Blunt) injuries of the aorta. J Trauma 1992;33:846.

67. Symbas PN, Tyras DH, Ware RE, et al. Traumatic rupture of the aorta. Ann Surg 1973;178:6.

68. Kirsh MM, Behrendt DM, Orringer MB, et al. The treatment of acute traumatic rupture of the aorta: a 10 year experience. Ann Surg 1976; 184:308.

69. Laforet EG. Acute hypertension as a diagnostic clue in traumatic rupture of the thoracic aorta. Am J Surg 1965;110:948.

70. Herendeen TL, King H. Transient anuria and paraplegia following traumatic rupture of the thoracic aorta. J Thorac Cardiovasc Surg 1968; 56:599.

71. Hughes JT. Spinal cord infarction due to aortic trauma. Br Med J 1964;2:356.

72. MacKenzie JR. Discussion of acute treatment of traumatic aortic rupture. J Trauma 1970;11:12.

73. Ayella RJ, Hankins JR, Turney SZ, et al. Ruptured thoracic aorta due to blunt trauma. J Trauma 1977;17:119.

74. Gerlock AJ, Muhletaler CA, Coulam CM, et al. Traumatic aortic aneurysm: validity of esophageal tube displacement sign. AJR 1980;135:713-718.

75. Marnocha KE, Maglinte DDT, Woods J, et al. Blunt chest trauma and suspected aortic rupture: reliability of chest radiograph findings. Ann Emerg Med 1985;14:644.

76. Peters DR, Gamsu G. Displacement of the right paraspinous interface: a radiographic sign of acute traumatic rupture of the thoracic aorta. Radiology 1980;134:599.

77. Simeone JF, Minagi H, Putman CE. Traumatic disruption of the thoracic aorta: significance of the left apical extrapleural cap. Radiology 1975; 117:265-268.

78. Simeone JF, Deren MM, Cagle F. The value of the left apical cap in the diagnosis of aortic rupture. Radiology 1981;139:35.

79. Woodring JH, Pulmano CM, Stevens RK. The right paratracheal stripe in blunt chest trauma. Radiology 1982;143:605.

80. Barcia TC, Livoni JP. Indications for angiography in blunt thoracic trauma. Radiology 1983;147:15-19.

81. Wilson JM, Thomas AN, Goodman PC, et al. Severe chest trauma: morbidity implication of first and second rib fracture in 120 patients. Arch Surg 1985;113:846.

82. Bassett JS, Gibson RD, Wilson RF. Blunt injuries to the chest. J Trauma 1968;8:418.

83. Sadow SH, Murray CA, Wilson RF, et al. Traumatic rupture of ascending aorta and left main bronchus. Ann Thorac Surg 1988;45:682.

84. Wilson RF, Arbulu A, Basset J, et al. Acute mediastinal widening following blunt chest trauma: critical decisions. Arch Surg 1972; 104:551.

85. Gundry SR, Williams S, Burney RE. Indications for aortography in blunt thoracic trauma: a reassessment. J Trauma 1982;22:664.

86. Fenner MN, Fisher KS, Sergel NL, et al. Evaluation of possible traumatic thoracic aortic injury using aortography and CT. Am Surg 1990;56:497.

87. Madayag MA, Kirsenbaum KJ, Nadimpalli SR, et al. Thoracic aortic trauma: role of dynamic CT. Radiology 1991;179:853.

88. Miller FB, Richardson JD, Thomas HA, et al. Role of CT in diagnosis of major arterial injury after blunt thoracic trauma. Surgery 1989;106: 596.

89. Miller FB. Discussion of "computed tomography in the management of blunt thoracic trauma." J Trauma 1993;35:301.

90. Durham RM, Zuckerman D, Wolverson M, et al. Computed tomography as a screening exam in patients with suspected blunt aortic injury. J Trauma 1993;35:161.

91. Raptopoulos V. Chest CT for aortic injury: maybe not for everyone. Am J Roentgenol 1992;162:1053.

92. Fisher RG, Chasen MH, Lamki N. Diagnosis of injuries of the aorta and brachiocephalic arteries cause by blunt chest trauma: CT vs aortography. Am J Roentgenol 1994;162:1047.

93. Agee CK, Metzler MH, Churchill RJ, et al. Computed tomographic evaluation to exclude traumatic aortic disruption. J Trauma 1992;33: 876.

94. Tomiak MM, Rosenblum JD, Messersmith RN, et al. Use of CT for diagnosis of traumatic rupture of the thoracic aorta. Ann Vasc Surg 1993;7:130.

95. Wilson D, Voystock JF, Sariego, et al. Role of computed tomography scan in evaluating the widened mediastinum. Am Surg 1994;60:421.

96. Shapiro MJ, Yanofsky SD, Trapp J, et al. Cardiovascular evaluation in blunt thoracic trauma using transesophageal echocardiography (TEE). J Trauma 1991;31:835.

97. Brooks WS, Young JC, Cmolik B, et al. The use of transesophageal echocardiography in the evaluation of chest trauma. J Trauma 1991; 31:1024.

98. Kearney PA, Smith DW, Johnson SB, et al. The use of transesophageal echocardiography in the evaluation of traumatic aortic injury. J Trauma 1992;33:155.

99. Buckmaster MJ, Kearney PA, Johnson SB, et al. Further experience with transesophageal echocardiography in the evaluation of traumatic aortic injury. J Trauma 1993;35:983.

100. Karalis DG, Victor MF, Davis GA, et al. The role of echocardiography in blunt chest trauma: a transthoracic and transesophageal echocardiographic study. J Trauma 1994;36:53.

101. Waugh JR, Sacharias N. Arteriographic complications in the DSA era. Radiology 1992;182:243.

102. Hessel SJ, Adams DF, Abrams HL. Complications of angiography. Radiology 1981;138:273.

103. LaBerge JM, Jeffrey RB. Aortic lacerations: fatal complications of thoracic aortography. Radiology 1987;165:367.

104. Gomes AS, Baker JD, Martin-Paredero V, et al. Acute renal dysfunction after major arteriography. AJR 1985;145:1249.

105. Mirvis SE, Pais OS, Gens DR. Thoracic aortic rupture: advantages of intraarterial digital subtraction angiography. Am J Radiol 1986; 146:987.

106. Walker WA, Pate JW. Medical management of acute traumatic rupture of the aorta. Ann Thorac Surg 1990;50:965.

107. Passaro E, Pacc WG. Traumatic rupture of the aorta. Surgery 1959; 46:787.

108. Akins CW, Buckley MV, Daggett W, et al. Acute traumatic disruption of the thoracic aorta: a ten-year experience. Ann Thorac Surg 1981;31:305.

109. Stiles QR, Cohlmia GS, Smith JH, et al. Management of injuries of the thoracic and abdominal Aorta. Am J Surg 1985;150:132.

110. Hilgenberg AD, Logan DL, Akins CW, et al. Blunt injuries of the thoracic aorta. Ann Thorac Surg 1992;53:233.

111. Fisher RG, Oria RA, Mattos KL, et al. Conservative management of aortic lacerations due to blunt trauma. J Trauma 1990;30:1562.

112. Hanschen S, Snow JN, Richardson JD. Thoracic aortic rupture in patients with multisystem injuries. South Med J 1982;75:653.

113. Vasko JS, Raess DH, Williams TE Jr, et al. Non-penetrating trauma to the thoracic aorta. Surgery 1977;82:400.

114. Mattox KL, Holzman M, Pickard LR. Clamp/repair: a safe technique for treatment of blunt injury to the descending thoracic aorta. Ann Thorac Surg 1985;40:456.

115. Crawford ES, Rubio RA. Reappraisal of adjuncts to avoid ischemia in the treatment of aneurysms of the descending thoracic aorta. J Thorac Cardiovasc Surg 1973;66:693.

116. DeBakey ME, McCollum CH, Graham JM. Surgical treatment of aneurysms of the descending thoracic aorta. J Cardiovasc Surg (Torino) 1978;19:571.

117. Van Norman GA, Pavlin EG, Eddy AC, Pavlin DJ. Hemodynamic and metabolic effects of aortic unclamping following emergency surgery for traumatic thoracic aortic tears in shunted and unshunted patients. J Trauma 1991;31:1007.

118. Forbes AD, Ashbaugh DG. Mechanical circulatory support during repair of thoracic aortic injuries improves morbidity and prevents spinal cord injury. Arch Surg 1994;129:494.

119. Schmidt CA, Wood MN, Razzouk AJ, et al. Primary repair of traumatic aortic rupture: a preferred approach. J Trauma 1992;32:588.

120. Verdant A, Cossette R, Dontigny L, et al. Acute and chronic traumatic aneurysms of the descending thoracic aorta: a 10-year experience with a single method of aortic shunting. J Trauma 1985;25:601.

121. Verdant A, Page A, Cossett R, et al. Surgery of the descending thoracic aorta: spinal cord protection with the Gott shunt. Ann Thorac Surg 1988;46:147.

122. Olivier HF, Maher TD, Liebler GA, et al. Use of the Biomedicus centrifugal pump in traumatic tears of the thoracic aorta. Ann Thorac Cardiovasc Surg 1984;38:586.

123. Walls JT, Curtis JJ, Boley T. Sarns centrifugal pump for repair of thoracic aortic injury: case reports. J Trauma 1989;29:1283.

124. McCroskey BL, BL, Moore EE, Moore FA, Abernathy CM. A unified approach to the torn thoracic aorta. Am J Surg 1991;162:473.

125. Costa MC, Robbs JV. Nonpenetrating subclavian artery trauma. J Vasc Surg 1988;8:71.

126. Lynch C, Weingarden SI. Paraplegia following aortic surgery. Paraplegia 1982;20:196.

127. Cunningham JN. Discussion of "clamp/repair": a safe technique for blunt injury to the descending thoracic aorta. Ann Thorac Cardiovasc Surg 1985;40:462.

128. Svensson LG, Klepp P, Hinder RA. Spinal cord anatomy of the baboon: comparison with man and implications on spinal cord blood flow during thoracic aortic cross-clamping. S Afr J Surg 1986;24:32.

129. Pate JW. Traumatic rupture of the aorta: emergency operation. Ann Thorac Surg 1985;39:531.

130. Kieffer E, Richard T, Chivas J, et al. Preoperative spinal cord arteriography in aneurysmal disease of the descending thoracic and thoracoabdominal aorta: preliminary results in 45 patients. Ann Vasc Surg 1989; 3:34.

131. Katz NM, Blackstone EH, Kirklin JW, et al. Incremental risk factors for spinal cord injury following operation for acute traumatic aortic transection. J Thorac Cardiovasc Surg 1981;81:669.

132. Ketonen P, Jarvinen A, Luosto R, et al. Traumatic rupture of the thoracic aorta Scand. J Thorac Cardiovasc Surg 1980;14:233.

133. Najafi H, Javid H, Hunter J, et al. Descending aortic aneurysmectomy without adjuncts to avoid ischemia. Ann Thorac Cardiovasc Surg 1980; 30:326.

134. Grande AM, Eren EE, Hallman GL, Cooley DA. Rupture of the thoracic aorta: emergency treatment and management of chronic aneurysms. Texas Heart Inst J 1984;11:244.

135. Hartford JM, Fayer RL, Shaver TE, et al. Transection of the thoracic aorta: assessment of a trauma system. Am J Surg 1986;151:224.

136. DeMuth WE, Roe H, Hobbie W. Immediate repair of traumatic rupture of thoracic aorta. Arch Surg 1965;91:602.

137. Connery C, Geller E, Dulchavsky S, Kreis DJ Jr. Paraparesis following emergency room thoracotomy: case report. J Trauma 1990;30:362.

138. Short HD. Paraplegia associated with the use of oxidized cellulose in posterolateral thoracotomy incisions. Ann Thorac Surg 1990;50:288.

139. Kouchoukos NT, Lell WA. Hemodynamic effects of aortic clamping and decompression with a temporary shunt for resection of the descending thoracic aorta. Surgery 1979;85:25.

140. Ross J, Braunwald E. The study of left ventricular function in man by increasing resistance to ventricular ejection with angiotensin. Circulation 1964;24:739.

141. Carlson DE, Karp RB, Kouchoukos NT. Surgical treatment of aneurysms of the descending thoracic aorta: an analysis of 85 patients. Ann Thorac Cardiovasc Surg 1983;35:58.

Chapter 19A Esophageal Injuries

ROBERT F. WILSON, M.D.

ZWI STEIGER, M.D.

INTRODUCTION

History

The first description of a penetrating wound of the pharynx or esophagus is found in the Edwin Smith papyrus[1] which notes that ". . . when he drinks water, it will choose to come out of the opening of his wound; . . . and as a result he develops fever . . . this is a man who has a wound of his throat that has perforated all the way to his gullet."

Repair of esophageal wounds was apparently not considered until 1876, when Wiseman suggested that tears in the esophagus should be sutured.[1] Trauma to the esophagus continued to receive little attention until World War II. In a review published in 1939, Jensen could find only 172 published cases of trauma to the esophagus. He added one case of his own and advocated early drainage as a form of therapy. In the early 1940s, Brewer suggested immediate surgery for esophageal wounds, and Barrett[2] and Olsen and Claget[3] in 1947 reported the first two successful repairs of a spontaneous rupture of the esophagus.

Incidence

The incidence of intrathoracic esophageal injury resulting from external trauma is quite low in most centers. Indeed, most busy trauma centers cite only two to four cases per year. These injuries, however, are important because of the high mortality and morbidity rates likely to occur if definitive treatment is not accomplished within 12 to 24 hours. As Sealy[4] has pointed out, injuries of the esophagus, particularly in the chest, are the most rapidly fatal perforation of the gastrointestinal tract.

Mortality Rate

AXIOM The mortality rate for esophageal injuries rises abruptly if treatment is delayed more than 12-24 hours.

In spite of all our technical and nutritional advances in recent years, the mortality rate of esophageal injuries is still about 5 to 25% for those treated definitively within 12 hours, 10 to 44% for those treated at 12 to 24 hours, and 25 to 66% or higher for those treated after 24 hours.[5,6] Mortality rates tend to be low with instrumental perforations of the cervical esophagus, but they are much higher with thoracoabdominal perforations resulting from external trauma. Mortality rates are particularly high with perforations of the thoracic esophagus because of the severe suppurative mediastinitis that can develop within 6-12 hours.[7,8]

Surgical Anatomy

The esophagus is a muscular tube connecting the pharynx and stomach. It is lined by stratified squamous epithelium. In adult males, it is 25 to 30 cm in length and in its collapsed state measures about 1.5 cm in diameter. The esophagus begins at the cricopharyngeus muscle at the level of the cricoid cartilage opposite the sixth cervical vertebrae. In the neck and upper chest, it lies slightly to the left of the midline (Fig. 19A–1). In the mid and lower chest, it is anterior and slightly to the right of the vertebral bodies. It is in immediate contact with the membranous trachea down to the carina at the level of the

fourth thoracic vertebra (T-4). The prevertebral space posterior to the cervical and upper thoracic esophagus permits direct communication between an esophageal perforation in the neck and the upper mediastinum. The lower thoracic esophagus lies behind the left atrium and slightly to the left of the lowest thoracic vertebrae. It then enters the abdomen through the esophageal hiatus of the diaphragm to the left of T-11, anterior to the aorta.

The muscular layers of the esophagus consist of an inner circular layer and an outer longitudinal layer that is striated in its proximal one-third and smooth in the distal two-thirds. The cervical and thoracic esophagus are devoid of serosa, but are surrounded by a filmy adventitia.

AXIOM Lack of a serosal covering for the cervical and thoracic esophagus increases the likelihood of an anastomotic leak in those areas.

The major blood supply of the esophagus is segmental and originates from the inferior thyroid artery, bronchial arteries, esophageal branches of the descending thoracic aorta, and the left gastric artery.

Gastroesophageal competence is maintained by the diaphragmatic crura, an intra-abdominal segment of esophagus, and most importantly, a physiologic internal lower esophageal sphincter (LES), which is about 3-5 cm in length.

TYPES OF INJURIES TO THE ESOPHAGUS

Until recently, most esophageal injuries were iatrogenic. Most of the remainder were spontaneous or due to a foreign body. However, injuries resulting from gunshot and stab wounds are becoming more common in many hospitals.

Penetrating Injuries

INSTRUMENTATION

AXIOM Most injuries to the esophagus are iatrogenic.

Up to two-thirds of esophageal injuries are iatrogenic, and over half of these occur during efforts to dilate a stricture.[1] Most of the remainder occur during diagnostic endoscopy, usually in a diseased esophagus.[2] Occasionally, injury occurs because of an intraoperative misadventure, particularly while performing a truncal vagotomy, hiatal hernia repair, endotracheal intubation, Sengstaken-Blakemore tube inflation, or esophageal obturator airway insertion.

The risk of iatrogenic injury with rigid endoscopy is approximately 0.25 to 0.4%.[9,10,11] With the advent of flexible endoscopy, the risk of perforation during diagnostic studies has been greatly reduced. However, deep biopsies, dilatation of strictures, forceful dilatation for achalasia, laser surgery for obstructions, and removal of sharp foreign bodies still cause some esophageal injuries.

AXIOM Most esophageal perforations occur at natural or acquired areas of narrowing.

The most common sites of iatrogenic perforation are just above areas that are narrowed anatomically or because of disease. Normally the esophageal introitus at the cricopharyngeus is the narrowest por-

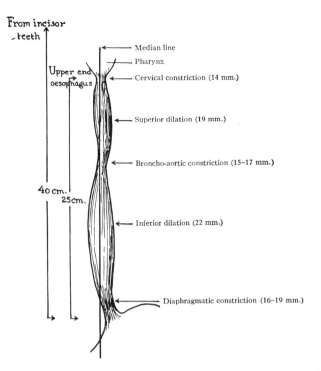

FIGURE 19A–1 The esophagus from the front, showing its constrictions and measurements. The length of the esophagus in the adult is about 25-30 cm, and the distance from the upper incisor teeth to the beginning of the esophagus at the cricoid cartilage is about 15 cm. The esophagus has three distinct narrowings. The narrowest is at its beginning at the level of the cricoid cartilage. The second is at the bifurcation of the trachea (bronchoaortic constriction) at the level of the fourth thoracic vertebra. The third constriction is the point where the esophagus passes through the diaphragm into the abdominal cavity. In the neck and upper chest, the esophagus is a little to the left of the midline; in the mid and lower chest, it lies a little to the right of the midline. (From: Anson BJ, Maddock WG. Callander's surgical anatomy. 4th ed. Philadelphia: WB Saunders Company, 1958.)

tion of the esophagus and is the area most prone to perforation. The other frequent sites of perforation, because of anatomical narrowings, are the diaphragmatic hiatus and the area of slight narrowing produced by the left main stem bronchus.

Complications of endoscopic variceal sclerotherapy are quite common. In a recent review, Edling and Bacon[12] noted mediastinitis in 0-63%, pleural effusions in 0-50%, atelectasis in 16%, bronchitis in 8%, pneumonia in 0-5%, and esophageal fistulas in 0-2%. The pleural effusions were moderate sized (10-50% of a hemithorax) in about 32% and large in about 3%. The effusion is usually a sterile non-bloody exudate and requires no treatment unless there is fever, chest pain, dysphagia, or dyspnea. If deep esophageal ulcers develop from the sclerotherapy, one may see delayed esophagopleural or esophagobronchial fistulas.

Stab and Gunshot Wounds

AXIOM If a penetrating wound involves the tracheobronchial tree, one should look carefully for injury to the adjacent esophagus.

External trauma accounts for only 10 to 20% of all esophageal injuries and 20 to 50% of those that are non-iatrogenic.[13-16] Stab and gunshot wounds may injure the esophagus anywhere along its course, but patients coming to surgery most frequently have involvement of the cervical esophagus.[9,11,14] The majority of injuries to the cervical esophagus are caused by stab wounds, whereas most intrathoracic or intra-abdominal esophageal injuries result from gunshot wounds.[17,18]

Reviews of penetrating wounds of the neck show an incidence of 3.9 to 5.5% for esophageal injury.[19,20]

From August 1964 to August 1979, 48 patients with gunshot wounds of the esophagus were treated at Grady Memorial Hospital.[17] Of these, 24 (50%) involved the cervical esophagus, 17 (35%) involved the thoracic portion, and seven (15%) involved the abdominal esophagus. Because approximately 20-25% of the esophagus is cervical, 5-15% is abdominal, and 60-75% is thoracic, the relative incidence of injury per cm of esophagus is 2.5 to 4.0 times greater for the abdominal and cervical portions than for the thoracic esophagus.

There are several reasons for the relative infrequency of thoracic esophageal injuries. The thoracic esophagus is too deep for most stab wounds, the structures are much more compact or crowded in the neck, and penetrating trauma that injures the midthoracic esophagus is also likely to involve the heart and/or great vessels and be rapidly fatal. In our own experience of 200 emergency thoracotomies for penetrating trauma, only three (1.5%) had an esophageal injury.[21]

Blunt External Forces

Esophageal rupture resulting from blunt trauma is rare. In our own studies, we found no esophageal injuries in 340 patients admitted with blunt chest trauma.[22] Kemmerer et al,[23] in their study of thoracic injuries in 585 fatal traffic accidents, noted only one esophageal injury (0.2%), and this patient died before hospital care. Indeed, most reports cite only one or two cases.[24-26]

Beal et al,[27] in a review of the world experience from 1900 to 1987, found 96 reported cases of blunt esophageal trauma of which 70% involved the cervical esophagus. Motor vehicle accidents were the most frequent cause, followed by falls, pedestrian-motor vehicle collisions, and assaults. Although the mortality rate was not noted, we expect that it would be relatively high, especially with perforation involving the thoracic esophagus. The most recent literature includes two reports with a total of 12 patients with blunt pharyngoesophageal perforation resulting in five (42%) deaths.[28,29]

The rarity of blunt esophageal injury is probably related to the elasticity and mobility of the esophagus, its relatively secluded position, and the protection afforded it by other viscera and the vertebrae. Most instances of blunt rupture are probably a result of much the same mechanism as spontaneous rupture, namely a sudden increase in intraesophageal pressure. Intragastric pressure transmitted to the esophagus may also play a role.

If the cricopharyngeus muscle is contracted during forceful retching or vomiting, a sudden rise of the endoesophageal pressure may cause esophageal rupture.[1] Experimentally, a sudden increase in intraluminal pressure of 5 to 10 pounds per square inch may result in esophageal rupture.[30,31] During injury from blunt trauma, the esophagus also may be compressed against preexisting osteoarthritic prominences (resulting in tearing of the esophageal wall) or be severely contused (which subsequently may result in necrosis and perforation).[24,32] Esophageal injury may also occur during anterior cervical spine fusion or later by dislodged bone grafts, wires, or other hardware.[33]

Barotrauma

Pharyngoesophageal barotrauma with perforation has been reported, following the explosive discharge of compressed carbon dioxide into the mouths from soft-drink containers overpressurized by the addition of dry ice. Accidental insufflation of pressured air may also rupture the esophagus.[34,35]

Spontaneous (Effort or Emetogenic) Injuries

Spontaneous (effort) rupture is the most common of the noniatrogenic esophageal perforations, accounting for 30 to 50% of such injuries.[36,37] Factors that appear to be involved in spontaneous perforation include increased intraluminal pressure, neurogenic deterioration leading to esophagomalacia, and preexisting alcoholic or regurgitation esophagitis.

Emetogenic injuries of the esophagus (i.e., those from vomiting or retching) may be divided (by their depth) into three types: (a) longitudinal tears of the esophageal mucosa near the area of the gastroesophageal junction (Mallory-Weiss syndrome), (b) intramural hematomas (due to tears extending into the muscle layers),[38] and (c) complete rupture of the esophagus (Boerhaave's syndrome). Mallory-Weiss tears are most frequently on the gastric side of the GE junction. The next most frequent site is across the GE junction, and the least common location is on the esophageal side. In contrast, complete ruptures usually occur just above the diaphragm as a 3 to 5 cm tear on the left posterior aspect where there is a reduced amount of smooth muscle and a relative lack of local buttressing structures.

AXIOM   Esophageal ruptures occurring after blunt trauma may resemble those caused by vomiting or retching.

PATHOPHYSIOLOGY

Injuries to the cervical esophagus will initially drain into the neck, and later with continued leakage, the oral-pharyngeal secretions will tend to dissect down into the upper mediastinum. With injuries to the thoracic esophagus, the leak is initially confined within the mediastinum, often producing a small sympathetic pleural effusion. Later, the mediastinal pleura breaks down, and the pleural effusion rapidly increases.

Most of the toxicity of intrathoracic esophageal ruptures results from regurgitated acidic gastric secretions rather than swallowed saliva. The resulting chemical mediastinitis causes increasing loss of fluid into the inflamed tissues, and this is further increased when infection develops. The suppurative mediastinitis that develops can cause severe fever and toxicity and can be rapidly lethal unless treated promptly.

AXIOM   Tears of the thoracic esophagus can rapidly cause severe mediastinal inflammation and damage from regurgitated gastric secretions and/or swallowed oral bacteria.

DIAGNOSIS OF ESOPHAGEAL INJURY

The key to successful treatment of esophageal injuries is early diagnosis. This usually requires a high index of suspicion, which is often absent because the injury is so uncommon. In addition, the clinical changes caused by the esophageal injuries can closely resemble those caused by damage to adjacent organs.[17,39] For this reason, a penetrating wound of the esophagus should be suspected in all patients who have a penetrating wound in the thoracic inlet or mediastinum. One should also look for this injury with any bullet that traverses the mediastinum or any trauma causing a pneumomediastinum or hydropneumothorax.

History

INSTRUMENTATION

AXIOM   Any new cervical, thoracic, or abdominal symptoms, signs, or x-ray changes after esophageal instrumentation are a result of an esophageal leak until proven otherwise.

After operative or endoscopic procedures involving the esophagus, any new symptoms or signs in the neck, chest, or abdomen should be considered a result of an esophageal injury until proven otherwise. The index of suspicion should be particularly high for any symptoms developing after dilatation of an esophageal stricture.

VOMITING

Only a small number of patients who vomit or retch develop esophageal perforation; however, chest pain or dysphagia after such an activity, particularly in a patient who has consumed large amounts of alcohol, should make one suspect an emetogenic injury. Because of

the prominence of chest pain in patients with spontaneous perforations, many are initially admitted to a coronary care unit with a diagnosis of possible acute myocardial infarction.[36] Over half of the patients that we have seen with a spontaneous rupture of the esophagus were initially admitted to a CCU for a possible acute myocardial infarction.

AXIOM   Patients to be admitted to a coronary care unit for a possible myocardial infarction should have a chest x-ray to rule out other intrathoracic processes.

Symptoms

The clinical manifestations of a penetrating wound of the esophagus depend upon the site and size of the wound, the trauma to neighboring organs, and the time elapsed since the injury.[17,18,37] The type of pain is extremely varied and may radiate up or down from the injured area. Thus, cervical perforations may cause upper thoracic pain, while diaphragmatic irritation may cause shoulder pain. When chest pain occurs, it is often of acute onset (30%), and it is usually severe and continuous.[14,40] Back pain tends to develop later, but it tends to be relatively well-localized to the actual area of thoracic or abdominal esophageal injury.

A sore throat and slight pain with swallowing are not uncommon for a day or two after any esophageal instrumentation; however, increasing dysphagia (difficulty swallowing) or odynophagia (painful swallowing) should make one suspect esophageal injury.

Vomiting or spitting up blood after any type of trauma should be viewed with suspicion; however, blood from nose, mouth, or upper airway injuries is often swallowed and may be vomited or coughed up later. Significant bleeding from esophageal injuries, except from Mallory-Weiss tears, is unusual. Traumatic insertion of a nasogastric tube, particularly in an uncooperative patient, is not an infrequent cause of some nasal bleeding. The swallowed blood brought up in the NG tube may then be interpreted as originating from a lower site.

Physical Examination

Although subcutaneous emphysema over the chest usually results from pulmonary injuries, if it is confined to the neck, it is often the first sign of perforation of the esophagus or pharynx. In some instances, subcutaneous emphysema from a digestive tract injury will spread to the chest.

Decreased breath sounds resulting from hydrothorax or pneumothorax after instrumentation or swallowing of a foreign body is virtually diagnostic of an esophageal injury. In many instances, a significant amount of atelectasis may also develop due to restriction of ventilation by chest pain, local inflammation, or associated hydropneumothorax.

AXIOM   Mediastinal air without a pneumothorax is a result of esophageal or tracheobronchial injury until proven otherwise.

Occasionally, Hamman's sign, which is a crunching precordial sound synchronous with cardiac systole, can be heard in patients with mediastinal emphysema. This is often heard better if the patient is in the left lateral decubitus position. The cause of most instances of mediastinal emphysema is unknown. The second most common cause is interstitial emphysema resulting from asthma or a lung injury. Nevertheless, bronchial or esophageal injury should be ruled out if there is any evidence of a pneumomediastinum after trauma.

Fever may occur rapidly with mediastinitis. In older, more critically ill individuals or those with a contained leak, however, little or no fever may be present until quite late in the process.

Upper abdominal tenderness and guarding is expected with perforations of the abdominal esophagus; however, in patients with perforation of the lower thoracic esophagus, abdominal pain and guarding are often the first indications that the chest pain is not cardiac in origin.

AXIOM Abdominal pain and tenderness may be the first signs and symptoms of perforation of the lower thoracic esophagus.

Tachypnea can occur with any type of stress, but it may be an early sign of intrathoracic injury or infection, and its cause should be sought. Cyanosis is usually a late sign of injury or infection. Indeed, cyanosis may not occur at all, regardless of how low the arterial PO_2 or cardiac output are, if the patient has a hemoglobin concentration less than 10 gm/dl.

Nasogastric Tube

When a nasogastric tube is inserted, it will usually bypass the esophageal tear and enter the stomach, as it normally does, unless there is a distal stricture. Occasionally, an esophageal injury will be diagnosed on a chest x-ray showing the end of the NG tube outside the esophagus. If bloody fluid is aspirated after an otherwise atraumatic nasogastric tube insertion, and there has been no bleeding from the head and neck, the blood is probably coming from the esophagus, stomach, or duodenum.

Radiological Studies

PLAIN FILMS

Plain films of the chest and neck, when combined with the history, can be almost diagnostic in 20 to 25% of esophageal injuries.

Neck

AXIOM Mediastinal or deep cervical emphysema is a result of an aerodigestive injury until proven otherwise.

Free air in the neck after trauma or any instrumentation, particularly in the deep perivisceral spaces, is usually from an injury to the hypopharynx, but may also result from a tear of the larynx, trachea, or esophagus. After penetrating external trauma, such as a stab wound, free air in the deep tissues may occasionally result from air passing down the knife tract, but is much more likely from injury to the aerodigestive tract.

A lateral view of the neck while it is extended may be particularly helpful in diagnosing injury to the upper esophagus. An increase in the prevertebral space between the posterior pharynx or larynx and the anterior border of the C2-C4 vertebral bodies greater than 0.5 cm suggests the presence of retro-pharyngeal inflammation or hematoma. Below C5 the prevertebral space may normally be up to 1.5 cm wide.[41]

AXIOM Increased prevertebral "tissue" or space in the neck may result from pharyngoesophageal trauma or a retropharyngeal infection.

Chest

With perforations of the thoracic esophagus, plain films of the chest may reveal mediastinal emphysema. With cervical or upper thoracic perforations, the superior mediastinum may be widened by fluid and/or inflammatory reaction. Air-fluid levels in the mid and upper mediastinum may be a result of abscess formation. Air-fluid levels in the lower mediastinum may be from an abscess, paraesophageal hernia, or retained fluid in the esophagus resulting from achalasia or some other distal esophageal pathology.

AXIOM Pleural effusions with increased amylase levels after trauma are a result of esophageal injury until proven otherwise.

Pleural effusions frequently accompany injuries to the thoracic esophagus. The presence of air with a pleural effusion causing a pneumothorax or hydropneumothorax is less frequent. With perforations of the upper two-thirds of the thoracic esophagus, a right pleural effusion often occurs, but with low thoracic esophageal injuries, the left pleural cavity is more likely to be involved.

When a nasogastric tube is passed, and it enters a pleural cavity, this is diagnostic of an esophageal tear. Occasionally, an upright chest x-ray may show free air under the diaphragm from an abdominal esophageal injury, but this was found in only 7 (29%) of 24 cases of abdominal esophageal injury reported by Glatterer.[15]

CONTRAST STUDIES

As soon as the patient's condition is stable, esophagography should be performed on all patients suspected of pharyngoesophageal injuries. This test may be performed with either absorbable or nonabsorbable radiopaque material, although the visual resolution with barium swallow is usually much better. Both frontal and lateral projections should be obtained before, during, and after the swallowing of the radiopaque material.

Extravasation of the swallowed contrast material is diagnostic of an esophageal leak; however, a negative contrast swallow is not a reliable indicator of the absence of injury, particularly if the study is done with Gastrografin.

There is some controversy as to whether the initial contrast swallow for a suspected esophageal leak should be done with barium or meglumine diatrizoate (Gastrografin). Gastro-grafin is used as the initial contrast by many physicians because, if a leak is present, extravasated Gastrografin is less likely to aggravate the infection and the local inflammatory response in the mediastinum.

AXIOM Aspiration of Gastrografin can cause severe pneumonitis.

If Gastrografin is aspirated, a much more severe chemical pneumonitis is apt to develop than with barium. Consequently, many surgeons will not perform an esophogram if the patient is unconscious or has an absent gag reflex.[42] Under such circumstances, the contrast can be carefully administered through a Foley catheter placed high in the upper esophagus with the balloon inflated to prevent regurgitation of the material.

Gastrografin may fail to demonstrate 42% of proven esophageal leaks.[15,18,36,42] Some of the higher false negative rates reported include those by Glatterer et al[15] (25%), Cheadle and Richardson[45] (33%), and Defore et al[18] (42%). Barium, however, is less irritating to the lungs if aspirated, and the incidence of false-negative examinations is usually less than 25%.

AXIOM Gastrografin swallows will frequently miss an esophageal leak.

All in all, because most of these patients will undergo surgery and adequate drainage soon after demonstration of the perforation, barium is probably the preferred contrast material. If one uses Gastrografin, and the contrast swallow reveals no lesions, the study should be repeated with barium and performed with the patient lying down to reduce the speed of transit of the contrast material. Some investigators have found it useful to administer the contrast under some pressure through an endoesophageal catheter.[46] The esophagus should be examined carefully under fluoroscopy as the contrast material is given, otherwise even if extravasated extraluminal contrast material is seen, the site of the leak can be missed.

Esophagoscopy

If esophageal injury is suspected and the esophogram is negative, one should proceed with esophagoscopy. Flexible esophagoscopy is usually safer and easier to perform, but occasionally rigid esophagoscopy may be preferable, particularly if a foreign body is suspected. Recent studies by Weigelt et al[44] and Winter and Weigelt[47] suggest that rigid endoscopy is more accurate than flexible esophagoscopy.

Esophageal injury can often be seen readily, but more than half the perforations have been missed in some studies, particularly with smaller lesions in the cervical esophagus. In a review of several studies, Symbas[1] noted a false negative rate with endoscopy ranging from 11 to 70%, with an average of 44%. Some typical false negative endoscopy rates reported include those by Glatterer et al[15] (17%),

Defore et al[18] (29%), and Sheely et al[48] (40%). In a recent study of 31 patients with suspected esophageal injury by Flowers et al,[49] however, flexible endoscopy resulted in true positives in four, a false positive in one, and true negatives in 26 (as demonstrated by exploration in five and clinical follow-up in 21).

Esophageal injuries are especially likely to be missed if the esophagus does not expand during endoscopy. Consequently, whenever possible, esophagoscopy should be done without ventilatory assistance so that the spontaneous breaths will dilate the esophagus.

Thoracentesis/Chest Tube

If a patient with blunt chest trauma has a hydropneumothorax and the fluid evacuated resembles swallowed saliva or gastric contents (food or a pH below 6.0), the diagnosis of esophageal injury is virtually certain. If the patient is asked to swallow methylene blue or some other dye while a chest tube is in place, almost instantaneous appearance of the dye is virtually diagnostic. Delayed appearance of the dye may be a result of gastrointestinal absorption and leakage of torn lymphatics in the chest.

Operative Diagnosis

With any penetrating injury of the neck, one should look carefully for an esophageal wound. Although some penetrating esophageal injuries may produce acute symptoms, many may only be detected early if one routinely explores all neck wounds that penetrate the platysma. Although "selective conservatism" is increasingly applied to the management of neck wounds, operative exploration is indicated in all patients with symptoms or signs suggesting vascular or aerodigestive tract injury.

Esophageal injuries in the neck are more likely to be found by surgical exploration of all suspicious neck wounds than by contrast studies or endoscopy. Interestingly, most stab wounds of the cervical esophagus occur on the left side of the neck (because most assailants are right-handed), but if an empyema develops because of a missed cervical esophageal injury, the resulting effusion is usually in the right chest.

> **AXIOM** The esophagus should be examined carefully for injury at surgery if an adjacent organ was damaged by blunt or penetrating trauma.

With esophageal injuries resulting from penetrating trauma, one must also look carefully for associated injuries, the more common of which include injury to the trachea (36 to 60%), major vessels (18 to 45%), thyroid gland (10 to 18%), spinal cord (5 to 13%), thyroid cartilage (9 to 10%), and recurrent laryngeal nerve (5 to 11%).[18,48] If a suspected esophageal injury cannot be found at the time of surgery, a nasogastric tube or Foley catheter can be passed into the cervical esophagus, and air can be injected by the anesthetist while the esophagus is occluded distally by the surgeon. Alternatively, air may be insufflated into the oropharynx using a mask over the nose and mouth. These maneuvers should distend the esophagus with air, and escape of any bubbles can assist in locating transmural injuries. If there is still a question, one may perform esophagoscopy while the esophagus is exposed.

> **AXIOM** If the patient has a tracheobronchial or vascular injury associated with an esophageal tear, the repairs should be separated by a substantial buttress of viable tissue.

When surgery is performed for blunt injury to the trachea, associated injury to the esophagus should be ruled out by careful examination at the time of exploration. In some instances, although the initial esophageal injury is only a contusion, it may later necrose and leak. Consequently, any seriously contused area should probably be buttressed or covered with a well-vascularized flap of adjacent muscle.

As with other penetrating visceral injuries, the surgeon should be reluctant to accept a single defect as a tangential wound, and thorough exploration is mandatory to avoid missing a distant or occult entrance or exit wound.

If a laparotomy has been performed because of severe abdominal pain and tenderness after blunt trauma, but the intra-abdominal examination is negative, one should suspect a thoracic injury. One can then enlarge the esophageal hiatus to examine the distal esophagus. In some instances, a thoracotomy is required to adequately exclude an intrathoracic injury.

> **AXIOM** The longer it takes to diagnose and treat an esophageal injury, the greater the tendency to develop severe sepsis, especially if the mediastinum is involved.

TREATMENT OF ESOPHAGEAL LACERATIONS AND RUPTURES

Treatment of lacerations or rupture of the esophagus should be individualized according to: (a) the amount of delay between injury and diagnosis, (b) the amount of local inflammation, necrosis, or infection present, (c) the location of the injury (neck, chest, or abdomen), and (d) the preexisting pathology.

> **AXIOM** If an esophageal injury is more than 24 hours old, but there is no evidence of tissue necrosis or infection, one can still attempt to close it, but the repair should be well-buttressed with viable adjacent tissue.

Although it is often felt that esophageal perforations more than 24 hours old cannot be repaired successfully, time is not the only important factor when determining treatment. Sometimes an injury less than 6 to 12 hours old is associated with advanced inflammation and necrosis, whereas some older injuries may show relatively minor local changes, even after 48 hours.

Nonoperative Management

INDICATIONS

Although nonoperative management of patients with spontaneous perforation of the esophagus is generally associated with mortality rates approaching 100%, certain other types of esophageal injuries, particularly small contained iatrogenic tears in the neck, can often be managed successfully without surgical intervention. As a general rule, a nonoperative approach to the management of pharyngoesophageal injuries can be considered if: (a) the injury is small, (b) there is no free flow of contrast material into surrounding tissues, (c) there are no other lesions requiring surgical intervention, (d) antibiotic treatment is started promptly after the injury, (e) there continue to be minimal or no symptoms, and (f) there is no evidence of infection.[50-51]

> **AXIOM** Small iatrogenic injuries of the cervical esophagus or pharynx with a contained leak can often be managed nonoperatively.

Within the past 10 to 15 years there have been increasing recommendations for a nonoperative approach to penetrating wounds of the neck when there is no apparent major vascular or aerodigestive tract injury.[52] However, esophageal injuries can easily be missed by such an approach, and there is usually a significant increase in the mortality rate if operative treatment of an esophageal perforation is delayed more than 24 hours.[53] Before electing to not explore a penetrating wound of the neck, one should be fairly certain that the aerodigestive tract is not injured.

Nonoperative treatment of pharyngoesophageal injuries includes: (a) nothing by mouth, (b) nasogastric suction (with lesions in the thoracic or abdominal esophagus) to remove any regurgitated gastric acid, (c) adequate nutrition (preferably via a jejunostomy tube), and

(d) antibiotic therapy. Improved early enteral nutrition, preferably into the small intestine just beyond the ligament of Treitz, may help reduce infection and mortality rates. The antibiotics used should cover organisms apt to be present in the mouth, and these are usually quite sensitive to penicillin. In some instances, particularly in more debilitated patients, one may also wish to cover gram-negative aerobes, such as Escherichia coli, particularly if the patient is receiving antacid or H2 blocker therapy. One should also be looking for Candida species, particularly in older, immunocompromised patients.[54] Postoperative Candida mediastinitis has a mortality rate of nearly 75%, which is almost double that for acute bacterial mediastinitis.

AXIOM Antibiotics for treating esophageal perforations should cover mouth organisms well.

A technique reported for managing full-thickness injuries of the thoracic esophagus without a thoracotomy involves using a combination of continuous peroral transesophageal irrigation of the mediastinum and drainage of the irrigating fluid by one or two accurately positioned chest tubes connected to suction.[55] If the patient cannot swallow, the mediastinal irrigation can be accomplished via a tube positioned in the upper esophagus proximal to the perforation. Most surgeons are reluctant to follow this nonoperative approach unless the patient is too great a risk for almost any type of treatment.

Operative Therapy

EARLY DIAGNOSIS AND MINIMAL LOCAL CHANGES

Cervical Esophagus

Cervical esophageal injuries are approached most readily through an incision along the anterior border of the sternocleidomastoid muscle. Except for penetrating injuries to the right side of the neck, incisions to explore the esophagus are preferably made through the left neck. The omohyoid muscle is cut, and the carotid sheath and sternocleidomastoid muscle are retracted laterally and posteriorly (Fig. 19A–2). The middle thyroid vein and inferior thyroid artery often also have to be ligated and divided to provide adequate exposure.

Once the esophageal wounds are defined, the edges are debrided back to healthy tissue. If a nasogastric tube has not been previously inserted, it is placed now, under the direct control of the surgeon, so that the repair is not jeopardized. Small wounds can be closed with a single layer of interrupted nonabsorbable sutures placed in Lembert fashion.

Larger wounds require an inner layer of interrupted inverted sutures of slowly absorbable material and an outer layer of interrupted sutures. The outer layer is closed with simple Lembert sutures or with horizontal mattress sutures. Some surgeons feel that particular attention should be directed toward incorporating adequate submucosal tissue (which is the strongest layer) in both the inner and outer layer of sutures. Other surgeons feel that a single-layer suture with 3-0 polyglycolic acid is as effective as a two-layer closure.

AXIOM The submucosal layer is the strongest layer of the esophagus.

Routine external drainage of esophageal suture lines is mandatory because of the frequency with which leaks occur, even in the most carefully performed repairs. Drainage of the area should also be performed if the site of the pharyngeal or esophageal injury cannot be found. A Jackson-Pratt drain is positioned about an inch away from the site of injury and brought out via the most direct and dependent tract through an opening separate from the primary incision. The drain tract should traverse behind the sternocleidomastoid muscle and exit laterally. Whenever possible, the drainage system should be of the closed type rather than "open" Penrose drainage.

AXIOM Esophageal repairs should be drained by closed catheter systems placed near, but not on, the area of repair.

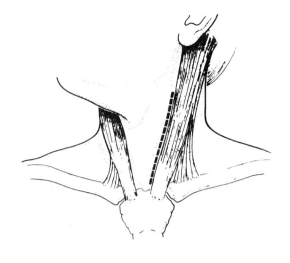

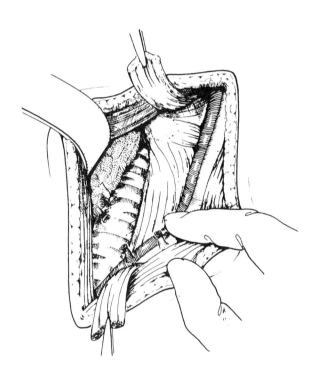

FIGURE 19A–2 Exploring the cervical esophagus. Cervical esophageal injuries are approached most readily through an incision along the anterior border of the left sternocleidomastoid muscle. The omohyoid muscle is cut, and the carotid sheath and sternocleidomastoid muscle are retracted laterally and posteriorly. The middle thyroid vein and inferior thyroid artery usually have to be ligated and divided to provide adequate exposure. (From: Wilson RF, Steiger Z. Oesophageal injuries. In: Champion HR, Robbs JV, Trunkey DD, eds. Rob and Smith's operative surgery: trauma, part 1. 4th ed. London: Butterworths, 1989; 331.)

If the trachea or carotid artery are also injured, their repairs should be kept separate from the repaired esophagus by healthy tissue. The sternohyoid, omohyoid, and/or sternothyroid muscles can be used for this purpose by detaching the muscle from its origin or insertion. This viable muscle flap is carefully sutured in place over the esophageal repair.

Parenteral antibiotics are continued postoperatively for at least 48 hours. The nasogastric tube can be removed as soon as gastrointestinal function returns; however, oral intake is avoided until a contrast esophagogram is obtained 8 to 10 days after surgery. If the repair is intact, clear liquid oral intake can begin. If there is no drainage from the wound after a day or two of oral intake, the drain can be completely removed.

Thoracic Esophagus

INCISIONS

> **AXIOM**   The upper two-thirds of the thoracic esophagus is best approached through a right posterolateral incision; the lowest third is best exposed via a left posterolateral incision.

For perforations of the upper or middle third of the thoracic esophagus, a standard right posterolateral thoracotomy provides the best exposure. The incision begins between the medial border of the scapula and vertebral column and extends down parallel to the scapula and then along the fifth or sixth intercostal space to the anterior axillary line. As the incision is deepened, one incises the trapezius, latissimus dorsi, and serratus anterior muscles. The lower portions of the rhomboid muscles medial to the scapula are also often incised.

To expose the upper thoracic esophagus, the azygos vein is divided near its connection to the superior vena cava and the mediastinal pleura is incised (Fig. 19A–3). The lung is retracted medially and anteriorly. For injuries of the esophagus below the pulmonary hilum, a left posterolateral thoracotomy through the sixth or seventh intercostal space can be used. A celiotomy may be the optimal approach for repair of perforations of the abdominal esophagus and the lowest inch or two of the thoracic esophagus. The most distal thoracic esophagus can be exposed through the abdomen by enlarging the diaphragmatic hiatus. The celiotomy also facilitates applying a gastric fundic patch.

ISOLATING AND REPAIRING THE ESOPHAGUS.   If there is a large mediastinal hematoma, and the esophagus is difficult to delineate from the surrounding tissue, palpating a nasogastric tube in the esophagus can be helpful. The nasogastric tube can also help localize the site of injury if one uses it to instill air or saline, with or without methylene blue.

The mucosal tear in an injured esophagus is often longer than the muscle injury, and it is important to clearly visualize the mucosal injury even if one has to extend the muscle opening at both ends of the perforation. The mucosa and submucosa should be accurately defined, debrided, and closed with interrupted inverting absorbable sutures because most of the strength of the closure will be in that layer. A second layer of nonabsorbable or slowly absorbable sutures incorporating muscle and some of the submucosa should be used to further invert and seal the closure.

BUTTRESSING THE REPAIR

> **AXIOM**   Whenever possible, esophageal repairs, especially in the chest, should be buttressed with adjacent viable tissue.

Esophageal repairs in the chest should be buttressed whenever possible with adjacent viable tissue, such as pleura, intercostal muscle, gastric fundus, or omentum. Pericardial and diaphragmatic flaps have also been recommended for buttressing esophageal repairs, but if an infection develops, such procedures increase the chance that the infection will spread into the pericardial or peritoneal cavities. Consequently, use of parietal pleura or intercostal muscle for the buttresses may be preferable. Such flaps can be wrapped around the entire esophagus or sutured in place as onlay flaps (Fig. 19A–4). Bardaxoglou et al[56] described covering a primary suture repair with absorbable polyglactin mesh and then applying fibrin glue in five patients with success in four (Fig. 19A–5).

> **AXIOM**   With severe injuries in the upper thoracic esophagus, it is safer to reestablish continuity with a gastric bypass and an anastomosis in the neck.

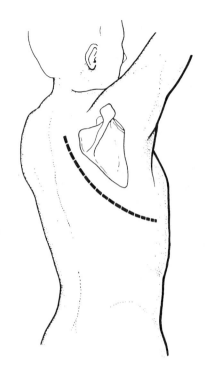

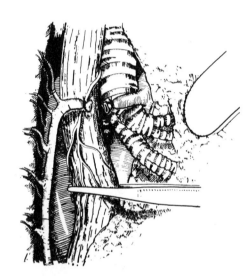

FIGURE 19A–3   Exploring the thoracic esophagus. For perforations of the thoracic esophagus, a standard right posterolateral thoracotomy provides the best exposure. The incision begins between the medial border of the scapula and vertebral column, and extends anteriorly parallel to the medial and lower border of the scapula. It then extends along the fifth or sixth intercostal space to the anterior axillary line. As the incision is deepened, the trapezius, the latissimus dorsi, and serratus anterior muscles are cut. The lower portions of the rhomboid muscles are also incised medial to the scapula. Once inside the pleural cavity, the azygos vein is divided over the esophagus, and the mediastinal pleura is incised. The lung is retracted medially and anteriorly. For injuries of the esophagus below the pulmonary hilum, a left posterolateral thoracotomy can be used. (From: Wilson RF, Steiger Z. Oesophageal injuries. In: Champion HR, Robbs JV, Trunkey DD, eds. Rob and Smith's operative surgery: trauma, part 1. 4th ed. London: Butterworths, 1989; 332.)

If there is destruction or complete transection of the upper thoracic esophagus, it is safer to bring up a gastric or colonic bypass to the cervical esophagus than to construct a major repair in the upper chest. Gouge et al,[57] in a review of 10 reports, found that 99 but-

FIGURE 19A–4 Repair of injuries of the thoracic esophagus. The thoracic esophagus is prone to leak after just a standard two-layer repair of injuries. To buttress the repair, a local flap of parietal pleura sutured or (as depicted here) wrapped around the esophagus provides better protection of the closure. If the opening in the esophagus is large, the pleura itself may be sutured over the hole. (From: Wilson RF, Steiger Z. Oesophageal injuries. In: Champion HR, Robbs JV, Trunkey DD, eds. Rob and Smith's operative surgery: trauma, part 1. 4th ed. London: Butterworths, 1989; 333.)

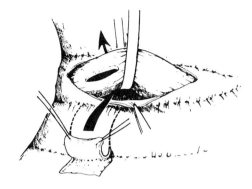

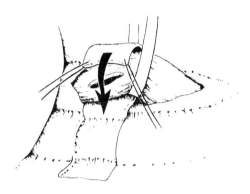

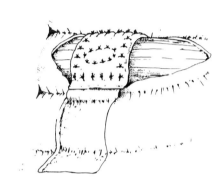

tressed repairs (versus 158 simple repairs) had a lower fistula rate (13% versus 39%) and a lower mortality rate (6% versus 25%).

> **AXIOM** An esophageal leak in the neck tends to be relatively harmless, whereas esophageal leaks in the mediastinum can rapidly cause severe sepsis.

For lower thoracic perforations, a gastric fundic patch is extremely effective for buttressing the closure (Fig. 19A–6). If the repair narrows the esophagus significantly, a flap of intact gastric fundus can be sutured over the hole as a patch as described by Thal and Hatafuku.[58] With such flaps, the inner layer has gastric fundus serosa sutured to the edges of the injury. The second layer should cover the esophagus at least 1.0 to 1.5 cm beyond the injury. Thus, two lines of sutures are used to hold the flap securely in place.

DRAINAGE. Regardless of the type of procedure used to repair the lower thoracic esophagus, the mediastinum and pleural cavity must be drained well. (Fig. 19A-7) The mediastinal pleura is incised from the diaphragm up to the thoracic inlet, and two large-bore (32-36F) chest tubes are inserted to provide ample drainage of the pleural cavity. In addition, a nasal tube can be inserted into the esophagus just proximal to the repair to reduce the amount of swallowed air and oral secretions coming into contact with the repair.

These tubes should be left in place for at least 6 to 7 days. At that time, a contrast swallow can be performed around the nasogastric tube. If the repair is intact, oral fluids can be started cautiously. If the repair does not leak and the pleural drainage remains less than 100 ml per day, the chest tubes can be removed.

GASTROSTOMY TUBE. A sump-type gastrostomy tube should be inserted to decompress the stomach and reduce the chances of gastric acid regurgitating into the esophagus and breaking down the repair. A jejunostomy catheter should also be inserted to begin early enteral feedings.

> **AXIOM** The best method for preventing leakage of gastric acid through an esophageal tear is to keep the stomach decompressed with a gastrostomy tube.

Abdominal Esophagus

REPAIR AND BUTTRESSING. For lacerations of the abdominal esophagus, a repair in two layers followed by coverage with a patch or wrap of

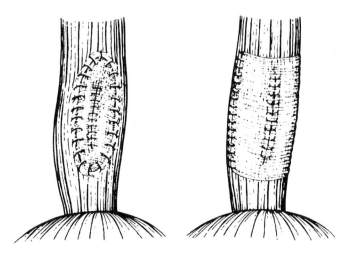

FIGURE 19A–5 Technique of esophageal repair. When using absorbable mesh and fibrin glue to repair esophageal injuries, the mesh can be sutured to the edges of the defect, or the mesh can be wrapped around the repaired injury. (From: Bardaxoglou JP, Champion SL, Manganas D, et al. Oesophageal perforation: primary suture repair reinforced with absorbable mesh and fibrin glue. Brit J Surg 1994;81:399.)

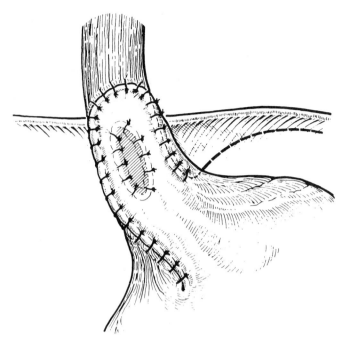

FIGURE 19A–6 Gastric fundic patch. For perforations of the lower thoracic esophagus, a gastric fundic patch can be used to close the defect. If closure of the distal esophageal tear or perforation would narrow the esophagus significantly, no attempt should be made to close the lesion primarily. Instead, a flap of intact gastric fundus should be sutured over the hole as a patch. With such flaps, at least half of the esophageal circumference should be covered at least 2 cm above and below the injury. Two lines of sutures should be used to hold the flap securely in place. One line should be at the edge of the esophageal hole and the other line about 1.0 cm from the hole. Another technique is a complete wrap of the involved lower esophagus with gastric fundus similar to that used for a Nissen fundoplication. (From: Wilson RF, Steiger Z. Oesophageal injuries. In: Champion HR, Robbs JV, Trunkey DD, eds. Rob and Smith's operative surgery: trauma, part 1. 4th ed. London: Butterworths, 1989; 334.)

gastric fundus will usually be satisfactory. If the gastric fundus cannot be mobilized adequately, a wrap of omentum should be used.

DECOMPRESSION.   A large gastrostomy, particularly of the sump type, in addition to the nasogastric tube, may help to protect the esophageal repair by keeping the stomach completely decompressed.

ENTERAL FEEDING.   With injuries to the esophagus, it is prudent to insert a feeding tube into the proximal jejunum about 25 cm distal to the ligament of Treitz whenever possible. Alimentation should be started postoperatively as soon as the patient is hemodynamically stable. In general, enteral feedings are much safer, more effective, and less expensive than intravenous alimentation.

AXIOM   Jejunostomy feedings provide the best and safest nutrition for patients with esophageal lacerations.

DRAINAGE.   Repairs of the abdominal esophagus are not usually drained because the presence of a nearby foreign body may increase the risk of leak and/or infection.

EARLY DIAGNOSIS IN PATIENTS WITH PREEXISTING ESOPHAGEAL DISEASE

If a benign stricture of the distal esophagus can be dilated to 50-60F, repair of a proximal perforation along with a primary antireflux procedure can be performed. If distal esophageal stenosis or stricture cannot be adequately dilated or cannot be corrected with a gastric fundic patch, the perforation and stenotic area should be resected, excluded, or bypassed, depending upon the condition of the patient and the con-

dition and location of the injured esophagus. In the sickest patients, an esophageal exclusion with a cervical esophagostomy and chest tube drainage of one or both pleural cavities. If possible, a gastrostomy and feeding jejunostomy should also be performed.

If the esophagus is perforated proximal to a carcinoma, the perforation and carcinoma should be resected if possible. With favorable conditions, a primary gastroesophagostomy anastomosis can then be performed. If this is not feasible, one can perform an esophagogastrostomy to bypass the injured area and staple off the distal esophageal lumen. The esophagus can also be functionally excluded with just a cervical esophagostomy and gastrostomy. In addition, a jejunostomy feeding tube should be inserted. In patients with far-advanced malignancies who have a perforation during palliative intubation of a neoplastic stricture, an aggressive nonsurgical approach

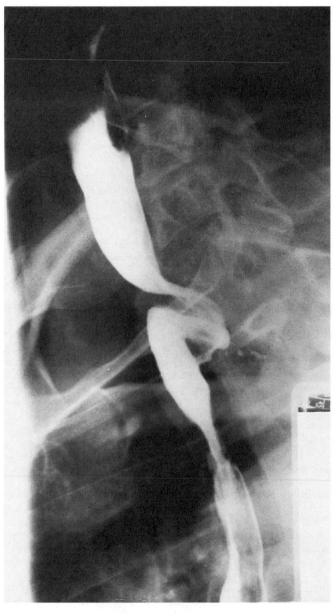

FIGURE 19A–7 Esophagopleurocutaneous fistula. This patient had a gunshot wound to the chest, injuring the trachea and thoracic esophagus. The trachea and esophagus were repaired primarily, but a leak at the site of the esophageal repair resulted in an empyema. This was drained, and the esophagopleurocutaneous fistula eventually closed. The strictured portion of the esophagus at the fistula was later bypassed with stomach brought up substernally to the cervical esophagus.

with continuous mediastinal irrigation and drainage via chest and/or neck tubes can be tried.[59]

DELAYED DIAGNOSIS

If an esophageal injury is not diagnosed until late, the main therapeutic efforts are to reduce the incidence and severity of sepsis.

Cervical Esophagus

If the involved area of the esophagus is necrotic and/or gross suppuration is present, closure of the esophageal tear should not be attempted. After thorough debridement of necrotic and/or infected tissue, the area is carefully drained to prevent the infection from spreading throughout the neck and down into the mediastinum. Exclusion of the esophagus with a cervical esophagostomy is usually indicated if the patient is septic.

AXIOM Severe sepsis resulting from an esophageal leak is best treated by completely defunctionalizing the esophagus.

The type of cervical esophagostomy used may vary depending on the case and surgeon. The advantage of a side cervical esophagostomy is that a later gastric or colonic bypass is usually unnecessary to reestablish esophageal continuity. However, it does exclude oral contents from the distal esophagus as well as an end cervical esophagostomy. In many instances, however, one does not have a choice because the cervical esophagus will not reach the lateral neck unless it is cut off at the thoracic inlet. Under such circumstances the distal esophagus must be closed or drained with a tube, and a gastric or colon bypass is needed later to reestablish continuity of the cervical esophagus of the GI tract.

Thoracic Esophagus

DELAYED REPAIR. The mortality rate with thoracic esophageal perforations treated more than 24 hours after injury often exceeds 50%, primarily because of sepsis. Occasionally, however, a tear of the thoracic esophagus that is more than 24 hours old can be debrided and closed successfully. If one does attempt closure of the esophagus under such circumstances, the area of injury should be generously and securely covered with a flap of viable, adjacent tissue.

ESOPHAGEAL EXCLUSION

AXIOM Whenever possible, severe mediastinitis should be treated via a thoracotomy incision by incising the mediastinal pleura over the entire esophagus and completely debriding and draining the involved tissues.

If the patient is already toxic from mediastinitis, a complete exclusion of the esophagus should be performed. This is usually accomplished with a cervical esophagostomy and gastrostomy.[37]

AXIOM Mediastinitis resulting from an esophageal leak requires exclusion of oral and gastric contents from the area of injury.

A cervical esophagostomy with a distal ligature or band at the gastroesophageal junction was popularized by Urschel[60] as a method for achieving complete exclusion of gastric contents from the area of injury. Originally, an umbilical tape was used to occlude the lower esophagus, but a double strand of catgut is now recommended. Ergin et al[61] have described a temporary tube cervical esophagostomy with a band below it to provide esophageal exclusion. Such a diversion may allow one to reestablish esophageal continuity to the stomach later without using a gastric or colon bypass.

ESOPHAGECTOMY. In spite of all our technical and nutritional advances in recent years, the mortality rate of esophageal injuries is still about 5 to 25% for those treated definitively within 12 hours, and 25 to 66% or higher for those treated after 24 hours.[5,62] As a consequence, there is increased interest in resecting the injured esophagus if there is any delay or if there is significant underlying esophageal disease.[63]

Griffin et al[64] described 11 patients who underwent one- or two-staged esophageal resections following endoscopic perforation of the esophagus, including seven patients with carcinoma. Seven were resected within 24 hours and four between 2 and 10 days after perforation. All four patients with benign disease survived. Four of the seven cancer patients died, but results with perforations in patients with esophageal cancer tend to be poor regardless of what is done.

Orringer and Stirling[65] described their results with esophagectomy in 24 patients with esophageal disruption. They felt that with esophageal disruption accompanying preexisting esophageal disease and/or sepsis or fluid and electrolyte problems, esophageal resection often provides the only chance for patient salvage. Only three of these patients had cancer. The esophagectomy was performed within 12 hours of perforation in 10 patients, in 12-24 hours in three, and in 3-45 days (average of 6.6 days) in 11 patients. GI continuity was established with an immediate cervicogastric anastomosis in 11 patients, and 11 had a cervical or anterior cervical esophagostomy. There were only three hospital deaths (13%), and 19 (90%) of the 21 survivors were able to swallow comfortably. The authors concluded that "conservative" measures (repair, diversion, or drainage) of a perforation with preexisting esophageal disease often inflicts more morbidity than esophageal resection, which eliminates the perforation, the source of sepsis, and the underlying esophageal disease.[65]

T TUBE INTUBATION. In 1970, Abbott et al[66] described the use of T tubes for treating spontaneous ruptures of the esophagus in which the diagnosis was delayed. In a similar manner, Andrade-Alegre[67] described the use of a T tube to treat a gunshot wound of the esophagus not diagnosed until more than 66 hours after injury. At thoracotomy, blood and suppurative material were removed and a 24F biliary T tube was inserted and held in place with a purse-string suture. Gastrostomy and feeding jejunostomy tubes were also inserted. The esophageal T tube was removed by esophagoscopy 2 weeks later. A small catheter was placed in the esophagopleurocutaneous fistula and gradually removed over the next few days.

Abdominal Esophagus

Even with a 24-48 hour delay in diagnosis, some lacerations of the abdominal esophagus can be closed and then buttressed with a gastric fundic patch.

If the area is badly inflamed or there is established infection, it should be managed by an exclusion technique similar to that used with infected thoracic esophageal lesions. Wide drainage of the periesophageal subdiaphragmatic area with a sump tube is important if the distal esophagus is left in place and an abscess was present.

ESOPHAGEAL FOREIGN BODIES

Etiology

Most foreign bodies are ingested by small children or adults with psychiatric disease, alcohol abuse, or mental retardation.[11] Food impaction in the esophagus typically occurs in patients who are elderly or have a preexisting esophageal stricture, ring, or web. Other predisposing factors include false teeth and poor dentition, resulting in poor chewing of food.

Location

About 80 to 90% of ingested foreign bodies pass through the gastrointestinal tract without difficulty, but 10 to 20% lodge at the lower border of the cricopharyngeus muscle, at the level of the aortic arch, or at the LES. Children with a vascular ring or aberrant right subclavian artery have an increased incidence of retained foreign bodies at the site of esophageal compression.[68]

The narrowest part of the gastrointestinal tract is the pharyngoesophageal junction at the cricopharyngeus muscle; however, the constrictors of the pharynx are strong and can propel relatively large and/or irregular objects into the upper esophageal lumen. Once the foreign body has passed the cricopharyngeus, the peristaltic muscular activity of the esophagus is much weaker, and the foreign body may obstruct in an area of the esophagus that is wider than the glottic opening.

Natural History

Objects that lodge within the esophagus may predispose to a number of complications, including: (a) respiratory compromise resulting from aspiration of secretions or pressure on the trachea, (b) perforation and fistula formation, or (c) pressure necrosis leading to mediastinitis or fistulas in adjacent structures.[6,7] Although less than 1% of all swallowed objects perforate the gastrointestinal tract, one may see perforation rates as high as 15 to 35% with sharp foreign bodies, such as toothpicks and pins.[41,69-70] If mediastinitis develops from an ingested foreign body, the mortality rate may be as high as 60%.[14]

Accidentally swallowed sharp foreign bodies may perforate the esophagus at the time they are swallowed or after several hours because of continued local pressure. Foreign bodies may also cause perforation during their removal, particularly if they have sharp hook-like projections.

In a recent series of retropharyngeal abscesses in which 21 of the 23 patients were adults, 13 (57%) resulted from an esophageal foreign body of which 9 were removed at the time of endoscopy.[41] Warner et al[71] reported two children with respiratory distress and stridor associated with a middle mediastinal mass resulting from a retained radiolucent esophageal foreign body.

Diagnosis

An infant who cannot swallow properly or is salivating excessively should be considered to have an esophageal foreign body until proven otherwise. Most older patients with this problem will have additional symptoms, including choking, dysphagia, odynophagia, and/or sialorrhea.[11] The sensation of something sticking in the throat is often also present. With foreign bodies in the esophagus, the sensation of where the object is stuck is usually a few inches above its actual site. Bulky foreign bodies in the cervical esophagus may also produce some upper airway obstruction by extrinsic pressure against the membranous posterior wall of the trachea.

Foreign bodies in the esophagus can generally be identified on plain x-rays if they are radiopaque. Coins, for example, will appear "on face" on a PA film and "on edge" in the lateral film (i.e., opposite to a tracheal foreign body). If the foreign body is radiolucent but holds the esophageal walls apart, air may be seen in that portion of the esophagus. If a swallowed foreign body cannot be located on a lateral neck x-ray, PA and lateral chest x-rays are taken. If the foreign body is not seen on those films, an esophagogram may demonstrate it. If a small pledget of cotton saturated with barium sulfate is swallowed, it may hang on a sharp foreign body that might not otherwise be detected.

If the contrast swallow is negative or only a filling defect is seen, esophagoscopy may be diagnostic and therapeutic. Some authors feel that rigid esophagoscopy for these purposes is superior to flexible endoscopy.[71]

Initial evaluation of unexplained stridor in a child should also include flexible laryngoscopy and bronchoscopy, performed under general anesthesia.[71] However, if the trachea is compromised by an esophageal inflammatory process, bronchoscopic differentiation of anterior and posterior tracheal compression may be difficult.

If a middle mediastinal mass is suggested by the plain x-ray films or if endoscopy of the aerodigestive tract suggests tracheal compression, the patient should be evaluated further by either CT or MRI. Such information is also useful from an anesthetic standpoint because life-threatening airway obstruction, cardiovascular collapse, and death have occurred during the induction of general anesthesia in patients with a compromised airway from a mediastinal mass.[71]

Treatment

AXIOM   Ingestion of a foreign body is an emergency if: (a) it causes an acute obstruction, (b) the foreign body is sharp or irregular, or (c) the foreign body is a disk battery.[11]

Patients with an esophageal foreign body should usually be kept in an upright position. Suctioning of oral secretions should be performed as needed, and airway stability should be guaranteed.[11] In general, objects that cause complete obstruction or that may cause perforation should be removed as soon as possible endoscopically. Some feel that flexible endoscopy is preferred because of its relative safety and ease of performance.[6,7] Others feel that rigid esophagoscopy is more accurate and allows use of larger retrieval forceps.[71] General anesthesia is often needed for rigid endoscopy, particularly for very young or uncooperative patients, as well as in cases of proximal impaction.

AXIOM   Esophageal foreign bodies can cause perforation during their ingestion and even larger tears if forcefully removed.

If the foreign body is seen, it is usually grasped with a forceps appropriate to the object, disengaged from the esophageal wall, and then either removed through a rigid esophagoscope or removed along with the scope as a trailing foreign body. The longer a foreign body remains in the esophagus, the greater the local edema, the greater the difficulty of removal, and the greater the risk of perforation before or during removal.

If the swallowed object is not sharp and is not causing respiratory symptoms, one can try to have the foreign body pass by itself. Although there have been no controlled studies performed to confirm efficacy, smooth muscle relaxants such as sublingual nifedipine or intravenous diazepam, glucagon, or anticholinergics may be helpful in this regard.[11] Glucagon may be particularly helpful because it relaxes smooth muscle and decreases lower esophageal sphincter tone. A dose of 0.5 mg is injected intravenously and may be repeated once or twice at 10 to 20 minute intervals.[11] Aspiration precautions should be used because glucagon may stimulate nausea.

Use of enzymatic digestion of boneless meat with papain, administered orally or by catheter, is controversial. There have been reports of papain causing esophageal perforations, and if it is aspirated, it can induce hemorrhagic pulmonary edema.[67] Consequently, it is no longer recommended, except when endoscopy is not available, and then only when the bolus impaction is of short duration and confirmed by a contrast study.

Effervescent agents to distend the esophagus are generally no longer recommended because of risk of perforation. Nevertheless, Karanja and Rees[72] have reported success using cola in six of six food bolus obstructions.

With varying results, balloon-tipped catheters (e.g., Foley catheters) have been passed with or without fluoroscopic guidance to help in the removal of some blunt foreign bodies in the proximal esophagus. Typically, a small Foley catheter is inserted past the object, the head and neck are lowered, the balloon is inflated, and the catheter is gently pulled back into the hypopharynx. One should take care to prevent aspiration of the foreign body into the larynx or trachea while it is removed from the esophagus.

If a foreign body cannot be removed in any other manner, surgical removal is required. If the foreign body can be moved at all, it can sometimes be removed endoscopically at surgery without an esophageal incision. If an incision into the esophagus is necessary, it should be in a normal area of the esophagus, proximal to the impacted foreign body.

After the foreign body has passed or has been removed, radiographic or endoscopic evaluation of the esophagus should be performed to evaluate the presence of a perforation or underlying esophageal disease.

CHEMICAL INJURIES OF THE ESOPHAGUS

Etiology

An estimated 26,000 caustic ingestions occur in the United States annually.[73] Ingestions in infants and young children are usually accidental and comprise approximately 80% of the reported incidents. In teenagers and adults, the majority of caustic ingestions are suicide attempts.

A wide variety of chemicals may damage the esophagus, but the worst injuries are those caused by strong alkali. The damage is due to dissolution of protein and collagen and to thrombosis of local blood vessels.[74] Rapid penetration of successive tissue layers occurs within seconds of contact. The heat of hydration, generated when the caustic mixes with local secretions, can also contribute to the injury. Ingestants with a pH greater than 12 are responsible for the most serious injuries, whereas household bleaches with a pH less than 11 rarely cause serious problems.[75]

In describing the depth of caustic injuries, first-degree burns involve hyperemia, edema, and/or desquamation of mucosa. Second-degree burns extend through the mucosa into the muscularis as friable lesions with white membranes and deep ulcers. Third-degree burns are transmural. Associated damage to the larynx, skin, eyes, and lungs is not unusual with caustic ingestions.

In second- and third-degree burns, there is increased scar tissue and dysmotility by the second to third week.[74-75] Strictures form in approximately 20 to 30% of cases of third-degree injuries and are evident within 3 to 4 weeks of the ingestion.[75]

Acid causes only about 5% of reported caustic ingestions, and those requiring treatment are usually caused by hydrochloric or sulfuric acid.[76] Acids cause damage by coagulation of protein, and this retards its continued penetration into the tissues. Because of limited contact with the esophagus, the most severe damage from acid ingestion tends to occur in the stomach, predominately along the lesser curvature and in the antrum. This can result in gastric stricture, achlorhydria, dysmotility, and possible later gastric outlet obstruction. Serious esophageal involvement is reported in only 10 to 20% of acid ingestions.[76]

Disk or button batteries used in watches or cameras can cause severe corrosive injury to the gastrointestinal tract when ingested.[78] Injury usually occurs with batteries greater than 21 mm in diameter that lodge within the esophagus and leak sodium or potassium hydroxide and mercuric oxide. Electrical burns may result from contact of the battery with conducting gastrointestinal fluids.

Pill-induced esophageal injury occurs when the caustic contents of a capsule or tablet remain in the esophagus long enough to produce mucosal damage.[79] Since the first reported cases of pill-induced esophageal injury in 1970, at least 679 cases resulting from more than 70 different medications in pill form have been reported.[79-80] Anyone who ingests caustic pills is susceptible to pill-induced esophageal injury because a moderate delay in pill transit through the esophagus is common, even in persons with normal esophageal motility.[81] The agents implicated most frequently are quinidine (198), doxycycline (140), tetracycline (94), emepronium bromide (80), pirmecillinan (32), potassium chloride (28), and aspirin (17).[79]

The mechanism of injury is not clear in all cases. Doxycycline, tetracycline, ascorbic acid, ferrous sulfate, and emepronium bromide produce a pH below 3.0 when dissolved in saliva.[79] Caustic pills such as clindamycin, potassium chloride, and quinidine, however, do not alter the local pH. Esophageal hemorrhage or stricture is unusual with antibiotic or antiviral pills (10/412), but it is quite common with antiinflammatory agents (21/57) and potassium chloride (20/28). Clinitest tablets contain 40 to 50% potassium or sodium hydroxide. After ingestion, they can produce severe burns that are usually circumferential.[82]

AXIOM Alkali tends to cause much deeper and more severe esophageal injuries than acid does.

Diagnosis

HISTORY

With caustic ingestions, the history may provide the only clinical evidence of the injury. With accidental caustic ingestions, a history of dysphagia after drinking an unexpectedly bitter or strange-tasting fluid may be the first indication that caustic material might have been ingested.

AXIOM Anyone who suddenly develops difficult or painful swallowing should be considered to have ingested caustic material or a foreign body until proven otherwise.

Patients with acute caustic ingestions may have a variety of signs and symptoms. Perioral pain may be the predominant symptom, but dysphagia, odynophagia, chest pain, and sialorrhea suggest substantial esophageal damage. Fever and vomiting are not uncommon, and one may occasionally see hematemesis. Hoarseness, dyspnea, and stridor suggest laryngeal or tracheobronchial involvement. Epigastric pain suggests damage to the stomach or gastroesophageal junction. One should also be alert for delayed chest pain and/or dyspnea, which may not develop for up to 48 hours.[83]

In 1984, Crain et al[84] noted a strong correlation between the presence of three specific symptoms (oropharyngeal burns or dysphagia, stridor, and vomiting) and significant esophageal injury. If all three symptoms were present, 50% had significant injuries. If none of these three symptoms was elicited, no grade II or III esophageal injuries were found. In a similar study by Gorman et al,[85] it was found that if the patient refused to swallow and had drooling, dysphagia, vomiting, or abdominal pain, it was very likely (P less than 0.001) that a significant caustic burn was present. Vergauwen et al,[86] in a series of 51 children with accidental caustic ingestion, noted that if vomiting or respiratory distress occurred, the incidence of significant esophageal injury was 84% (16/19) and 75% (6/8), respectively.

AXIOM Although severe symptoms tend to indicate an increased likelihood of severe esophageal damage, absence of symptoms cannot be relied upon to rule out significant injury.[11]

Examination begins with close inspection of the lips, mouth, and hypopharynx which may reveal edema, hyperemia, ulcerations, and friability with white mucosal plaques or brown-to-black ulcerations. With an alkali injury of the esophagus, 50 to 90% of patients will have a pharyngeal burn, and about 25 to 50% of patients with oral or pharyngeal burns will have an esophageal injury.[11] However, even if there are no obvious burns of the mouth or pharynx, it cannot be assumed that the esophagus is uninjured. If subcutaneous emphysema is found, an aerodigestive perforation of some type is usually present. Rebound epigastric tenderness is frequent with gastric involvement, but such a finding is generally not indicative of a perforation.

Radiographs of the neck, chest, and abdomen should be obtained after a suspected caustic ingestion to rule out perforation. After appropriate resuscitation, endoscopy should be performed to guide further therapy and determine prognosis; however, there is probably no need for esophagoscopy if: (a) there are no symptoms of esophageal injury, and (b) one is confident that the ingestant is weak in nature and/or in small volume.[11]

The initial endoscopy should be performed with a flexible instrument. If there is any evidence of airway damage, flexible laryngoscopy should be performed first. Introduction of the esophagoscope should be with direct visualization of the lumen. During the acute phase, the burned area is covered with a grayish slough. The esophageal mucosa is edematous, and the lumen is narrowed. Because the esophagus is friable and easy to perforate, the scope is not passed beyond the first deep circumferential burn, which indicates a need for full antistricture management.

Treatment

Patients with minimal or no gastric or esophageal damage may be discharged with careful medical and psychiatric follow-up, and they may advance their diet as tolerated. If there is respiratory compromise, the patient should be endotracheally intubated via the oral approach with direct visualization.[11]

If there are extensive burns, much fluid may be lost into the involved tissues. Intravenous catheters should be inserted and the patient given crystalloid to promptly restore adequate hydration and perfusion. Nothing should be administered by mouth until the evaluation is complete. In cases of lye ingestion, emetic agents, charcoal, and nasogastric lavage are contraindicated. Immediate surgery is necessary if there is perforation.

In stable patients who have ingested a small amount of mild alkali (bleaches), one may cautiously give milk, dilute vinegar, or citrus juice.[11] In pure acid ingestion, early aspiration of the stomach with a tube, followed by cold fluid lavage, may be of use. Antacids are contraindicated because the heat of neutralization they can produce may cause more damage.

For many years after 1950, when Spain et al[87] documented that corticosteroids can suppress inflammation, glucocorticoids and antibiotics were used extensively to reduce the risk and severity of stricture formation after caustic ingestions. In 1980, however, Hawkins et al[88] published a prospective clinical trial which showed no significant advantage to corticosteroids. They also felt that the risks of the corticosteroids outweighed their potential benefits and were probably contraindicated in these injuries. In another study of patients with corrosive ingestive by Estrera et al,[74] the standard treatment of esophagoscopy, steroids, antibiotics, and dilatation showed disappointing results. Five of nine patients with second-degree esophageal injuries developed strictures, and four with full thickness esophagogastric necrosis died. In contrast, early surgical intervention with use of intraluminal esophageal stents and radical resection of all necrotic tissue greatly reduced the mortality rate and incidence of severe stricture. Oakes et al[89] noted similar poor results when steroids were used to treat severe lye injuries.

Although the current tendency seems to be to avoid corticosteroids, an extensive review by Howell et al[90] of more than 2000 cases published between 1956 and 1991 suggested that corticosteroids are helpful for second- and third-degree esophageal burns. There were 361 cases in which esophageal injury was documented either by esophagoscopy or exploratory surgery, and patient management was either with corticosteroids plus antimicrobials for at least 2 weeks or was without either modality. The steroid treatment group included 283 patients from nine retrospective and two prospective publications. The no-treatment group included 78 patients from three retrospective and three prospective studies. Only one retrospective[91] and two prospective publications[87,92] reported both corticosteroid-treated and untreated patients. Of 72 patients with only first-degree esophageal burns, none developed a stricture; however, of the patients with second- and third-degree esophageal burns, the incidence of stricture was 24% (54/228) in the corticosteroid-treatment group and 52% (13/25) in the no-corticosteroid group.[90] This difference was significant (P less than 0.01). In addition, the steroid-treated patients tended to have a lower mortality rate (9% = 7/76) than those not receiving corticosteroids (19% = 7/37) (P less than 0.15).

If prednisone is used, the usual initial dose is 2 mg/kg/day in children and 80 mg/day in adults. The dose is tapered over 4 to 5 days to maintenance doses of 0.5 mg/kg/day and 20 mg/day, respectively. The steroids are continued for up to 6 to 8 weeks, at which time re-epithelialization is felt to have occurred. Initially the steroids are given intravenously and then orally as tolerated. Antibiotics, such as ampicillin 50 mg/kg/day in 4 divided doses, are usually given initially with the steroids, particularly if there is any evidence of pneumonitis or tissue necrosis with fever. Antacids or H_2 blockers should also be given to reduce the incidence of gastric complications from the steroids.

AXIOM   If corticosteroids are used to prevent esophageal strictures after caustic ingestions, care should be taken to prevent the severe complications that they can cause.

In patients with second- and third-degree burns, barium swallows to assess for stricture formation should be performed at approximately 2, 4, 8, and 12 weeks, even if the patient is swallowing solid food easily.[11] Contrast studies are performed sooner if there are any symptoms suggesting the development of a stricture.

If the patient appears to be developing a stricture clinically or radiologically, he should have a string passed as soon as possible for later dilatations. Many physicians feel that the dilatations should be delayed for at least 2 to 3 weeks after the caustic ingestion to reduce the chances of perforating the esophagus, which is still friable. Others have advocated the use of early, frequent dilation of the esophagus beginning one week after ingestion to retard stricture formation.[88] There is, however, no good evidence that early prophylactic "bougienage" is more effective. Nevertheless, patients with severe cicatricial injury should be treated with early nutrition, either parenteral or preferably via a jejunostomy tube.

If the esophagus cannot be dilated properly, it may be better to excise it early. With severe involvement in children, there is an estimated 1000-fold increase in the incidence of squamous cell carcinoma in the affected areas of the esophagus.[93] Consequently, the development of dysphagia decades after the injury should be anticipated and investigated carefully for a possible malignancy.

In cases of a disk battery lodged within the esophagus, the battery should be removed as soon as possible via endoscopy. If the battery reaches the stomach, daily plain films of the abdomen are obtained to assess its progress. After one week, cathartics may be given if there is retarded evacuation. Surgery should generally be reserved for intestinal perforation or obstruction.

COMPLICATIONS OF PERFORATING ESOPHAGEAL INJURY

Sepsis

The most devastating complication of undetected esophageal perforation is infection, and this is usually a result of delayed diagnosis and treatment. Periesophageal inflammation can rapidly extend to the mediastinum and result in severe generalized sepsis with multiorgan system failure. Mediastinitis usually develops within 12 to 24 hours of an esophageal leak. With neck infections resulting from delayed diagnosis and treatment of cervical esophageal injuries, the mortality rate is usually less than 10%; however, with delayed treatment of suppurative mediastinitis, the mortality rate may exceed 50%.

Diagnosis of sepsis resulting from an esophageal leak may be difficult, especially in older, malnourished patients. These patients may be so immunodepressed that they have little or no fever, and the WBC count may be normal or low. The only evidence of sepsis in such patients may be a "failure to thrive" or a gradual development of multiple organ failure. CT scans can be helpful for detecting mediastinal abscesses in such patients, but they may be falsely negative in 10 to 20% of cases.

AXIOM   A "negative" contrast swallow or esophagoscopy does not rule out a mediastinal infection or abscess in a septic patient who has had esophageal surgery or instrumentation.

The most important aspect of the treatment of mediastinitis is early and complete drainage and debridement of all grossly infected and necrotic tissue. Small to moderately large suppurative collections above the fourth thoracic vertebra resulting from cervical or high thoracic esophageal injuries can often be drained adequately through a neck incision. Abscesses that are large or located in the lower chest require a thoracotomy to obtain complete drainage of the mediastinum and pleural cavity. Posterior intra-abdominal collections can often be drained through the bed of the twelfth rib; however, if the abscess is not obvious and/or not well-positioned, a formal anterior celiotomy is indicated. In patients who develop severe sepsis, esophageal exclusion with a cervical esophagostomy and gastrostomy should be strongly considered.

Although antibiotics are only a second line of defense, they should be given in full dosage for at least 5 to 7 days after esophageal perforation to cover both mouth and gram-negative enteric organisms. Using data from 13 reports, Friedman and Pickul[7] noted that the most frequent organisms in post-traumatic or post-surgical mediastinitis are Staphylococcus aureus and Staphylococcus epidermidis. The next most frequent are gram-negative aerobes, streptococci, and mixed gram-negative and gram-positive organisms. With prolonged delays in therapy, larger numbers of gram-negative organisms, especially pseudomonas, and candida are found. With non-surgical causes of mediastinitis, such as from esophageal carcinoma or adjacent infections, beta-hemolytic streptococcus is the most frequent organism, followed by Staphylococcus aureus, Streptococcus pneumoniae, Bacteroides fragilis, Peptostreptococcus, Klebsiella, and Proteus species.

Fistulas

ESOPHAGOCUTANEOUS FISTULAS

Most esophageal fistulas resulting from trauma in the neck go directly from the cervical esophagus to the skin, and most of these heal spontaneously within 2-3 weeks. Esophagopleurocutaneous fistulas usually result from delayed or inadequate treatment of a thoracic esophageal leak and are much more likely to persist and/or cause the death of the patient.

AXIOM	Esophageal fistulas in the neck often heal spontaneously in 2-3 weeks; however, fistulas in the chest are much more apt to persist and/or cause severe sepsis.

Diagnosis of esophagocutaneous fistula is often made when saliva or swallowed food or liquids come out of a prior thoracotomy incision or a chest tube. In many instances, the material draining is nonspecific, and the presence of a fistula needs to be confirmed by a contrast swallow.

AXIOM	Most enterocutaneous fistulas will eventually heal if there is no distal obstruction or local infection.

Treatment of most enterocutaneous fistulas is conservative and is designed to provide adequate drainage of any suppurative collections. One should also look for factors that tend to keep fistulas open and correct them as soon as possible. These factors include distal obstruction, foreign bodies, malignancy, epithelialization of the tract, and infection. Acute severe malnutrition may also play a role.

With thoracic esophagocutaneous fistulas, cervical esophageal exclusion or bypass of the involved esophagus with stomach or colon is frequently necessary.

TRACHEOESOPHAGEAL FISTULAS

Etiology

Most esophageal fistulas in the adjacent trachea or a bronchus are a result of carcinoma of the esophagus or lung. The next most frequent cause is penetrating trauma, usually in the neck or upper chest. Occasionally, particularly in patients with prolonged sepsis, a tracheostomy tube will erode in the esophagus and cause a high tracheoesophageal fistula (TEF).[94] TEF may also develop in patients with severe esophagitis and prolonged nasogastric tube suction.[11]

Only rarely does blunt trauma result in a tracheoesophageal fistula. The few that do develop tend to result from steering wheel trauma with severe compression and damage to both the trachea and

esophagus. This often results in a small tear in the trachea adjacent to a contusion of the esophagus that becomes necrotic, particularly if local infection is present.

Diagnosis

In the majority of tracheoesophageal fistulas resulting from trauma, subcutaneous emphysema and/or pneumothorax or pneumomediastinum develop almost immediately. After 3 to 5 days, the patient may develop greatly increased bronchial secretions, pneumonia, and/or severe coughing, particularly when taking liquids. Delayed recognition may occur in individuals with head trauma, particularly if an endotracheal tube or tracheostomy tube is in place, but even then, excessive tracheobronchial secretions, especially if they are thin and watery, should make one suspect the diagnosis. If the amylase levels in this fluid are high, this should heighten suspicion of a fistula; however, some individuals aspirate large quantities of oropharyngeal secretions into their lungs without a fistula.

Ideally, the diagnosis should be made by esophagoscopy showing tracheobronchial mucosa or an endotracheal or tracheostomy tube. Occasionally, bronchoscopy will reveal either the fistula or an indwelling nasogastic tube. If possible, contrast agents should not be used to make the diagnosis; however, if the diagnosis cannot be made in any other manner, small amounts of barium can be given and the path of the contrast recorded with cineradiography.

In a collected review of 28 patients with tracheoesophageal fistula after blunt trauma, 16 (57%) of the fistulas were at or just above the carina, and 3 (11%) were in the neck. In 8 cases (29%), the location of the fistula was unknown.[95]

Treatment

Once the diagnosis of traumatic tracheoesophageal fistula has been made, an early attempt should be made to exclude, bypass, or close the fistula to prevent continued aspiration pneumonia. A tracheoesophageal fistula in the cervical area, often resulting from erosion of a tracheostomy tube into the adjacent posterior esophagus, is best corrected through a long collar incision. Tracheoesophageal fistulas in the upper and mid-chest are best approached through a right posterolateral thoracotomy.[14]

As the trachea and esophagus are gently freed from the surrounding tissue, the lateral blood supply of the trachea must be preserved carefully. The area of the tracheal fistula is completely excised. The edges of the underlying esophageal fistula are then debrided and closed in two layers, using a nasogastric tube as a stent. The esophageal closure can be fairly tight around the nasogastric tube, because if stenosis does develop later at the suture line, it is usually relatively easy to dilate.[14]

After the esophagus is repaired, the ends of the remaining trachea are approximated with interrupted sutures. Laryngeal release can provide about 2 to 4 cm of extra tracheal length. If this is not adequate to close the trachea, a midline sternotomy to mobilize both lungs by dividing the inferior pulmonary ligaments and the fascia around hilar structures can provide another 3 to 5 cm of tracheal length. Sternohyoid and sternothyroid strap muscles can be used to buttress both the esophageal and tracheal closures. A pectoral musculocutaneous flap will provide ideal tissue for closure of any remaining esophageal defects and for separating the esophagus from other structures. The chin is sutured down to the chest for about seven days to help take tension off the tracheal anastomosis.[14]

If the tracheal and esophageal tissues are not suitable for closure, one can bypass the involved esophagus with stomach or colon brought up substernally to the proximal normal cervical esophagus. The fistula in the esophagus can then be excluded from the bypassed esophagus with staples or sutures. If the involved tissues are not suitable for closure and the patient is too sick for an esophageal bypass, esophageal exclusion and wide drainage of the involved area should be performed. If the tracheal injury can be bypassed with an endotracheal tube, this should also be done.[14]

ESOPHAGOVASCULAR FISTULAS

Esophageal fistulas into major vessels are rare, and there is only an exceptional survivor.[96] Levine and Alverdy[97] reported one case and found only ten others in the literature. These usually resulted from carcinomas, foreign bodies (usually fish bones), or graft infections. Scher et al[98] reported a fish-bone perforation of the esophagus with resultant mild-moderate bleeding and survival without operation. Nandi and Ong in 1978[99] reported 2394 cases of a foreign body in the esophagus, 86 of which had an aortic injury with no survivors.

Strictures

ETIOLOGY

The most severe benign esophageal strictures usually result from caustic ingestion, which can induce the formation of large amounts of granulation tissue which subsequently cause a scar contracture. Strictures are particularly severe if all layers of the esophagus were damaged by the caustic.

Rarely, a patient will develop an esophageal stricture because of reflux of acid and/or bile around a chronic indwelling nasogastric tube. To help prevent such reflux, only flexible narrow-bore tubes should be placed in the esophagus for long-term enteral feeding.[11] Alternatively, a percutaneous gastrostomy tube may benefit patients requiring prolonged nutritional support. If the possibility of gastroesophageal reflux is a concern, particularly in patients with severe head injuries, a jejunostomy may be performed or an endoscopic technique may be used to pass a percutaneous feeding tube from the stomach into the duodenum or proximal jejunum.

DIAGNOSIS

One should suspect an anatomic or functional obstruction of the esophagus if the patient has a great deal of saliva and is drooling excessively; however, one should not assume that the esophagus is normal if the patient has no dysphagia. A patient may have no dysphagia until more than 70-80% of the normal esophageal lumen is obstructed.

AXIOM	A "little" dysphagia is often a result of rather severe (greater than 70-80%) stenosis.

Strictures can be confirmed by endoscopy, but contrast swallows are generally preferred because they are less hazardous and are more apt to show multiple areas of narrowing if they exist.

TREATMENT

Short, early strictures can usually be dilated relatively easily to at least 40 to 50F. Dilatations are safer if performed over a string or flexible wire which has been passed through the stricture into the small bowel or stomach. If a wire or string cannot be passed in the normal direction (prograde), it is often possible to perform a gastrostomy and pass a small semiflexible probe or Jackson dilator up (retrograde) from the stomach into the esophagus and then into the mouth. A string can then be attached to the probe or dilator and pulled out of a gastrostomy. Linked Tucker dilators of gradually increasing size, drawn retrograde through the esophagus via a string through a gastrostomy, are especially useful and safe for esophageal dilatation in children.

AXIOM	Dilatation of the esophagus is best done over a wire or string to make sure that the dilator does not press excessively against one of the side walls.

Blind dilation without a string or wire to guide the tip of the dilator through the lumen is more apt to result in tears of the esophagus. Mercury-weighted dilators, however, can be used by the patient at home to help maintain the patency of the esophagus once it has been adequately dilated. If the esophagus of an adult can be dilated to 50F, swallowing will usually be relatively normal, and repeat dilatations may not be required for a least several weeks. If the esophagus cannot be dilated to at least 40F in an adult, even after repeated

attempts, swallowing will often be impaired and an esophageal resection or bypass should be considered.

If the esophagus is torn while dilating a chronic stricture, periesophageal fibrosis will often cause the leak to remain localized and cause little or no infection. With perforation of acute strictures, however, surgical drainage plus exclusion or bypass is often needed, especially if sepsis develops.

Occasionally a stricture is so severe that it cannot be dilated. In such instances, bypass of the esophagus with stomach or colon (stomach is preferable in adults and colon in children) may be required. Because of an increased incidence of late carcinoma in chronic lye strictures, it may also be wise to resect the esophagus if it is ruptured during a dilatation. This is particularly important in young patients with severe lye strictures. However, in our institutions we know of only two patients who developed an esophageal carcinoma associated with a long-standing lye stricture.

Mortality Rates

The results of the treatment of traumatic esophageal injury depend on the site of the esophageal injury, the magnitude of the associated injuries, and the degree of contamination and necrosis adjacent to the esophageal wound.[95] The amount of tissue damage and inflammation is usually related to the time elapsed between the injury and the time of the repair.[5,17,39,100] The greater the extent of the infection and/or necrosis of the tissues, the greater the morbidity and mortality are likely to be.[10] In a collected series,[18,36,42,101-103] the overall mortality rate with esophageal injuries was 24% (36/149). The mortality rate with esophageal injuries was lowest in the neck (11%), intermediate in the abdomen (24%), and highest in the chest (40%).

In the past, the mortality rate after spontaneous rupture of the esophagus was 80 to 90%, largely because of delays in diagnosis. Over the past 40 years, the mortality rate has declined to about 20 to 30% with virtually all of the more recent deaths occurring in patients in whom treatment was delayed for more than 24-48 hours or who were severely immunosuppressed.

SUMMARY

The key to preventing esophageal complications is early, definitive management of all injuries. Because many of the diagnostic tests for esophageal injury can be falsely negative, a high index of suspicion is essential. Once severe complications develop, management can be extremely difficult and often involves esophageal exclusion or bypass.

⊘ FREQUENT ERRORS

In the Management of Esophageal Injuries

1. *Delay greater than 6-12 hours in repairing esophageal injuries.*
2. *Failing to understand that an esophageal injury may be present in spite of normal chest x-rays, contrast swallow, and esophagoscopy.*
3. *Failing to aggressively search for an esophageal rupture or leak if the patient has increased chest pain or fever or a chest x-ray abnormality after an esophagoscopic examination or procedure.*
4. *Pulling foreign bodies out of the upper esophagus in spite of a great deal of resistance.*
5. *Failure to appreciate the severity of the sepsis that can result from minor esophageal leaks into the mediastinum.*
6. *Failing to adequately appreciate the potential importance of an increased width of the prevertebral soft tissue space in the neck after esophageal instrumentation or trauma.*
7. *Failing to adequately examine the patient for an esophageal injury intraoperatively if there is an associated vascular or tracheobronchial injury.*
8. *Delay in treating a patient with a "minor" esophageal leak surgically if there is any evidence of infection.*

9. *Failure to appreciate that fluid loss from a drain placed near an esophageal repair is indicative of a leak until proven otherwise.*

10. *Placing an anastomosis in the upper chest when it might have been possible to put it in the neck.*

11. *Failing to buttress an esophageal repair with a flap of viable adjacent tissue.*

12. *Assuming that insertion of a chest tube without a thoracotomy can completely drain an infected mediastinum.*

13. *Failure to provide early jejunal enteral feedings and adequate gastric emptying (preferably with a sump-type gastrostomy tube) in patients with a thoracic esophageal leak.*

14. *Delay in defunctionalizing the esophagus of patients who become septic because of a leaking esophagus.*

15. *Inadequate resuscitation of patients with caustic injuries of the esophagus.*

16. *Passing an esophagoscope beyond the most proximal site of severe circumferential caustic esophageal injury.*

17. *Using corticosteroids to treat a caustic injury of the esophagus without adequate protection from their side effects.*

▼▼▼▼▼▼▼▼▼▼▼▼▼▼▼▼▼▼▼▼▼▼▼▼▼▼▼▼▼▼

SUMMARY POINTS

1. The mortality rate for esophageal injuries rises abruptly if treatment is delayed more than 12-24 hours.

2. Lack of a serosal covering for the cervical and thoracic esophagus increases the likelihood of an anastomotic leak in those areas.

3. Most injuries to the esophagus are iatrogenic.

4. Most esophageal perforations occur at natural or acquired areas of narrowing.

5. If a penetrating wound involves the tracheobronchial tree, one should look carefully for injury to the adjacent esophagus.

6. Esophageal ruptures occurring after blunt trauma may resemble those caused by vomiting or retching.

7. Tears of the thoracic esophagus can rapidly cause severe mediastinal inflammation and damage from regurgitated gastric secretions and/or swallowed oral bacteria.

8. Any new cervical, thoracic, or abdominal symptoms, signs, or x-ray changes after esophageal instrumentation are a result of an esophageal leak until proven otherwise.

9. Patients to be admitted to a coronary care unit for a possible myocardial infarction should have a chest x-ray to rule out other intrathoracic processes.

10. Mediastinal air without a pneumothorax is a result of esophageal or tracheobronchial injury until proven otherwise.

11. Abdominal pain and tenderness may be the first signs and symptoms of perforation of the lower thoracic esophagus.

12. Mediastinal or deep cervical emphysema is a result of an aerodigestive injury until proven otherwise.

13. Increased prevertebral "tissue" or space in the neck may result from pharyngoesophageal trauma or a retropharyngeal infection.

14. Pleural effusions with increased amylase levels after trauma are a result of esophageal injury until proven otherwise.

15. Aspiration of Gastrografin can cause severe pneumonitis.

16. Gastrografin swallows will frequently miss an esophageal leak.

17. The esophagus should be examined carefully for injury at surgery if an adjacent organ was damaged by blunt or penetrating trauma.

18. If the patient has a tracheobronchial or vascular injury associated with an esophageal tear, the repairs should be separated by a substantial buttress of viable tissue.

19. The longer it takes to diagnose and treat an esophageal injury, the greater the tendency to develop severe sepsis, especially if the mediastinum is involved.

20. If an esophageal injury is more than 24 hours old, but there is no evidence of tissue necrosis or infection, one can still attempt to close it, but the repair should be well-buttressed with viable adjacent tissue.

21. Small iatrogenic injuries of the cervical esophagus or pharynx with a contained leak can often be managed nonoperatively.

22. Antibiotics for treating esophageal perforations should cover mouth organisms well.

23. The submucosal layer is the strongest layer of the esophagus.

24. Esophageal repairs should be drained by closed catheter systems placed near, but not on, the area of repair.

25. The upper two-thirds of the thoracic esophagus is best approached through a right posterolateral incision; the lowest third is best explored via a left posterolateral incision.

26. Whenever possible, esophageal repairs, especially in the chest, should be buttressed with adjacent viable tissue.

27. With severe injuries in the upper thoracic esophagus, it is safer to reestablish continuity with a gastric bypass and an anastomosis in the neck.

28. An esophageal leak in the neck tends to be relatively harmless, whereas esophageal leaks in the chest can rapidly cause severe sepsis.

29. The best method for preventing leakage of gastric acid through an esophageal tear is to keep the stomach decompressed with a sump-type gastrostomy tube.

30. Jejunostomy feedings provide the best and safest nutrition for patients with esophageal lacerations.

31. Severe sepsis resulting from an esophageal leak is best treated by completely defunctionalizing the esophagus.

32. Whenever possible, severe mediastinitis should be treated via a thoracotomy incision by incising the mediastinal pleura over the entire length of the esophagus and completely debriding and draining the involved tissues.

33. Mediastinitis resulting from an esophageal leak requires exclusion of oral and gastric contents from the area of injury.

34. Ingestion of a foreign body is an emergency if: (a) it causes an acute obstruction, (b) the foreign body is sharp or irregular, or (c) the foreign body is a disk battery.

35. Esophageal foreign bodies can cause perforation during their ingestion and even larger tears if forcefully removed.

36. Alkali tends to cause much deeper and more severe esophageal injuries than acid does.

37. Anyone who suddenly develops difficult or painful swallowing should be considered to have ingested caustic material or a foreign body until proven otherwise.

38. Although severe symptoms tend to indicate an increased likelihood of severe esophageal damage, absence of symptoms cannot be relied upon to rule out significant injury.

39. If corticosteroids are used to prevent esophageal strictures after caustic ingestions, care should be taken to prevent the severe complications that they can cause.

40. A "negative" contrast swallow or esophagoscopy does not rule out a mediastinal infection or abscess in a septic patient who has had esophageal surgery or instrumentation.

41. Esophageal fistulas in the neck often heal spontaneously in 2-3 weeks; however, fistulas in the chest are much more apt to persist and/or cause severe sepsis.

42. Most enterocutaneous fistulas will eventually heal if there is no distal obstruction or local infection.

43. A "little" dysphagia is often a result of rather severe (greater than 70-80%) stenosis.

44. Dilatation of the esophagus is best done over a wire or string under fluoroscopy to make sure that the dilator does not press excessively against one of the side walls.

▲▲▲▲▲▲▲▲▲▲▲▲▲▲▲▲▲▲▲▲▲▲▲▲▲▲▲▲▲▲

REFERENCES

1. Symbas PN. Esophageal injuries. In: Cardiothoracic trauma. WB Saunders Co., 1989; 285-302.
2. Barrett NR. Report of a case of spontaneous perforation of the oesophagus successfully treated by operation. Br J Surg 1947;35:216.

3. Olsen AM, Clagett OT. Spontaneous rupture of the esophagus: report of a case with immediate diagnosis and successful surgical repair. Postgrad Med J 1947;2:417.

4. Sealy, WC. Rupture of the esophagus. Am J Surg 1963;105:505.

5. Wilson RF, Steiger Z. Oesophageal injuries. In: Champion HR, Robbs JV, Trunkey DD, eds. Trauma surgery. 4th ed. London: Butterworths, 1989; 327-340.

6. Symbas PN, Hatcher CR, Harlaftis N. Spontaneous rupture of the esophagus. Annals of Surg 1978;187:634.

7. Friedman BC, Pickul DC. Acute mediastinitis. Postgrad Med 1990; 87:273.

8. Burnett CM, Rosemurgy AS, Pfeiffer EA. Life-threatening acute posterior mediastinitis due to esophageal perforation. Ann Thorac Surg 1990;49:979.

9. Urschel HC Jr, Razzuk MA. Esophageal injuries. In: Moore EE, Eiseman B, Van Way CW III, eds. Critical decisions in trauma. St. Louis: CV Mosby Co., 1984; 168-171.

10. Jones WG, Ginsberg RJ. Esophageal perforation: a continuing challenge. Ann Thorac Surg 1992;53:534.

11. Shwartz HM, Traube M. Esophageal emergencies. In: Carlson RW, Geheb MA, eds. Principles and practice of medical intensive care. Philadelphia: WB Saunders, 1993; 1432.

12. Edling JE, Bacon BR. Pleuropulmonary complications of endoscopic variceal sclerotherapy. Chest 1991;99:1252.

13. Mulder DS, Barkun JS. Injury to the trachea bronchus and esophagus. In: Mattox KL, Moore EE, Feliciano DV, eds. Trauma II. Norwalk, CT: Appleton & Lange, 1991; 343.

14. Michel L, Grillo HC, Malt RA. Operative and nonoperative management of esophageal perforations. Ann Surg 1981;197:57.

15. Glatterer MS Jr, Toon RS, Ellestad C, et al. Management of blunt and penetrating external esophageal trauma. J Trauma 1985;25:784.

16. Attar S, Hankins JR, Suter CM. Esophageal perforation: a therapeutic challenge. Ann Thorac Surg 1990;50:45.

17. Symbas PN, Hatcher CR Jr, Vlasis SE. Esophageal gunshot injuries. Ann Surg 1980;191:703.

18. Defore WW Jr, Mattox KL, Hansen HA, et al. Surgical management of penetrating injuries of the esophagus. Am J Surg 1977; 134:734.

19. Golueke PJ, Goldstein AS, Sclafani SJ, et al. Routine versus selective exploration of penetrating neck injuries.

20. Weaver AW, Sankaran S, Fromm SH, et al. The management of penetrating wounds of the neck. Surg Gynecol Obstet 1971; 133:49.

21. Washington B, Wilson RF, Steiger Z, Bassett JS. Emergency thoracotomy: a four-year review. Ann of Thor Surg 1985;40:188.

22. Wilson RF, Antonenko D, Gibson DB. Shock and acute respiratory failure after chest trauma. J Trauma 1977;17:697.

23. Kemmerer WT, Eckert WG, Gathright JB, et al. Patterns of thoracic injuries in fatal traffic accidents. J Trauma 1961;1:595.

24. Goudarzi HA, Hall WW, Mason LB. Rupture of the cervical esophagus from blunt trauma. South Med J 1983;76:1563.

25. Stothert JC Jr, Buttorff J, Kaminski DL. Thoracic esophageal and tracheal injury following blunt trauma. J Trauma 1980;20:992.

26. Sharma DM, Whitton ID. Tracheoesophageal fistula from blunt trauma: a case report. S Afr Med J 1982;25:1044.

27. Beal SL, Pottmeyer EW, Spisso JM. Esophageal perforation following external blunt trauma. J Trauma 1988;28:1425.

28. Niezgod JA, McMenamin P, Graeber GM. Pharyngoesophageal perforation after blunt neck trauma. Ann Thorac Surg 1990;50:615.

29. Chen JY, Chen WJ, Huang TJ, et al. Spinal epidural abscess complicating cervical spine fracture with hypopharyngeal perforation: a case report. Spine 1992;17:971.

30. Mackler SA. Spontaneous rupture of the esophagus. Surg Gynecol Obstet 1952;94:345.

31. Derbes VJ, Michell RE. Rupture of the esophagus. Surg 1956;39:688.

32. Morrison A. Hyperextension injury of the cervical spine with rupture of the esophagus. J Bone Joint Surg 1960;42:356.

33. Yee GKH, Terry AF. Esophageal penetration by an anterior cervical fixation device: a case report. Spine 1993;18:522.

34. Gefland ET, Fisk RL, Callighan JC. Accidental pneumatic rupture of the esophagus. J Thoracic Cardiovasc Surg 1977;74:142.

35. Badruddoja M, MacGregor JK. Rupture of the intrathoracic esophagus by compressed air blast. Arch Surg 1971;103:417.

36. Wilson RF, Sarver EJ, Arbula A. Spontaneous perforation of the esophagus. Ann Thorac Surg 1971;12:291.

37. Wilson RF. Discussion of traumatic esophageal perforation. Ann Thor Surg 1972;14:676.

38. Steadman C, Kerlin P, Crimmins F, et al. Spontaneous intramural rupture of the oesophagus. Gut 1990;31:845.

39. Symbas PN, Tyras DH. Penetrating wounds of the esophagus. Ann thorac Surg 1972;13:552.

40. Nevens F, Janssens J, Piessens J, et al. Prospective study on prevalence of esophageal chest pain in patients referred on an elective basis to a cardiac unit for suspected myocardial ischemia. Dig Dis Sci 1991; 36:229.

41. Sethi DS, Chew CT. Retropharyngeal abscess: the foreign body connection. Ann Acad Med 1991;20:581.

42. Mulder DS, Barkun JS. Injury to the trachea, bronchus, and esophagus. In: Mattox KL, Moore EE, Feliciano DV, eds. Trauma. Norwalk, CT: Appleton & Lange, 1988; 335-347.

43. Sawyers JL, Lane CE, Foster JH, Daniel RA. Esophageal perfusion: an increasing challenge. Ann Thorac Surg 1975;19:233.

44. Weigelt JA, Thal ER, Snyder WH. Diagnosis of penetrating cervical esophageal injuries, 1987; 154:619.

45. Cheadle W, Richardson JD. Options in management of trauma to the esophagus. Surg Gynecol Obstet 1982;155:380.

46. Parker EF. Esophageal gunshot injuries. Ann Surg 1980;191:707.

47. Winter RP, Weigelt JA. Cervical esophageal trauma: incidence and cause of esophageal fistulas. Arch Surg 1990;125:849.

48. Sheely CH II, Mattox KL, Beall AC, DeBakey ME. Penetrating wounds of the cervical esophagus. Am J Surg 1975;130:707.

49. Flowers JL, Graham SM, Ligarte MD, et al. Flexible endoscopy for the diagnosis of esophageal trauma. J Trauma 1994;37:160.

50. Mandal AK, Bui HD, Oparah SS. Surgical and nonsurgical treatment of penetrating injuries to the cervical esophagus. Laryngoscope 1984; 93:801.

51. Haffner JF, Fausa O, Royne T. Nonoperative treatment of subcervical esophageal perforations after forced dilation for nonmalignant disease. Acta Chirurgica Scandinavica 1984;150:389.

52. Narrod JA, Moore EE. Selective management of penetrating neck injuries: a prospective study. Arch Surg 1984;119:574.

53. Sankaran S, Walt AJ. Penetrating wounds of the neck: principles and some controversies. Surg Clin N Am 1977;57:139.

54. Weil RJ. Candidal mediastinitis after surgical repair of esophageal perforation. S Med J 1991;84:1052.

55. Santos GH, Frater RW. Transesophageal irrigation for the treatment of mediastinitis produced by esophageal rupture. J Thorac & Cardiovasc Surg 1986;91:57.

56. Bardaxoglou JP, Campion SL, Manganas D, et al. Oesophageal perforation: primary suture repair reinforced with absorbable mesh and fibrin glue. Brit J Surg 1994;81:399.

57. Gouge TH, Depan HJ, Spencer FC. Experience with the Grillo pleural wrap procedure in 18 patients with perforation of the thoracic esophagus. Ann Surg 1989;209:612.

58. Thal AP, Harafuku T. Improved operation for esophageal rupture. JAMA 1964;188:826.

59. Hine KR, Atkinson M. The diagnosis and management of perforations of the esophagus and pharynx sustained during intubation of neoplastic esophageal strictures. Dig Dis Sc 1986;31:571.

60. Urschel HC Jr, Razzuk MA, Wood RE, et al. Improved management of esophageal perforation: exclusion and diversion in continuity. Annals of Surg 1974;179:587.

61. Ergin MA, Wetstein L, Griepp RB. Temporary diverting cervical esophagostomy. Surg Gynecol Obstet 1980;151:97-98.

62. Richardson JD, Martin LF, Borzotta AP, et al. Unifying concepts in treatment of esophageal leaks. Am J Surg 1985;149:157.

63. Tilanus HW, Bossuyt P, Schattenkerk ME, Obertop H. Treatment of oesophageal perforation: a multivariate analysis. Br J Surg 1991; 78:582.

64. Griffin SC, Desai J, Townsend ER, Fountain SW. Oesophageal resection after instrumental perforation. Eur J Cardiothorac Surg 1990;4:211.

65. Orringer MB, Stirling MC. Esophagectomy for esophageal disruption. Ann Thorac Surg 1990;49:35.

66. Abbott O, Mansour K, Logan W, et al. A traumatic so-called "spontaneous" rupture of the esophagus. J Thor Cardiovasc Surg 1970;59:67.

67. Andrade-Alegre, R. T tube intubation in the management of late traumatic esophageal perforations: case report. J Trauma 1994;37:131.

68. Carrarino G, Nikaidoh H. Esophageal foreign bodies in children with vascular ring or aberrant right subclavian artery: coincidence or causation? Pediatr Radiol 1991;21:406.

69. Johnson JA, Landreneau RJ. Esophageal obstruction and mediastinitis: a hard pill to swallow for drug smugglers. Am Surg 1991;57:723.

70. Wu MH, Lai WW. Aortoesophageal fistula induced by foreign bodies. Ann Thorac Surg 1992;54:155.

71. Warner BW, Plecha FM, Torres AM, et al. Chronic respiratory distress caused by radiolucent esophageal foreign body. Am J Otolaryn 1992.

72. Karanjia ND, Rees M. The use of Coca-Cola in the management of bolus obstruction in benign esophageal stricture. Ann Royal Coll Surg Engl 1993;75:94.

73. Lovejoy FH. Corrosive injury of the esophagus in children: failure of corticosteriod treatment emphasizes prevention. N Engl J Med 1990; 323:668.

74. Estrera A, Taylor W, Mills LJ, et al. Corrosive burns of the esophagus and stomach: a recommendation for an aggressive surgical approach. Ann Thorac Surg 1986;41:276.

75. Howell JM. Alkaline ingestions. Ann Emerg Med 1986;15:820.

76. Zagar SA, Kochhar R, Nagi B, et al. Ingestion of corrosive acids: spectrum of injury to upper gastrointestinal tract and natural history. Gastroenterology 1989;97:702.

77. Penner GE. Acid ingestion: toxicology and treatment. Ann Emerg Med 1980;9:374.

78. Litovitz TL. Button battery ingestions: a review of 56 cases. JAMA 1983;249:2495.

79. Kikendall JW. Pill-induced esophageal injury. Gastroenterology. Clin N Am 1991;10:835.

80. Carlberg B, Densert O. Esophageal lesions caused by orally administered drugs. Eur Surg Res 1980;12:270.

81. Hey H, Jorgensen F, Sorensen K, et al. Oesophageal transit of six commonly used tablets and capsules. Br Med J 1982; 285:1717.

82. Lacouture PG, Gaudreault P, Lovejoy FH Jr. Clinitest tablet ingestion: an in vitro investigation concerned with initial emergency management. Ann Emerg Med 1986;15:143.

83. Postlethwait RW. Chemical burns of the esophagus. Surg Clin North Am 1983;63:915.

84. Crain EF, Gershel JC, Mezey AP. Caustic ingestions: symptoms as predictors of esophageal injury. Am J Dis Child 1984;138: 863.

85. Gorman RL, Khin-Maung-Gyi MT, Slein-Schwartz W, et al. Initial symptoms as predictors of esophageal injury in alkaline corrosive ingestions. Am J Emerg Med 1992;10:189.

86. Vergauwen P, Moulin D, Buts JP, et al. Caustic burns of the upper digestive and respiratory tracts. Eur J Pediatr 1991;150:700.

87. Spain DM, Molomut N, Haber A. The effect of cortisone on the formation of granulation tissue in mice. Am J Pathol 1950;26:710.

88. Hawkins DB, Demeter JM, Barnett TE. Caustic ingestion: controversies in management. A review of 214 cases. Laryngoscope 1980;90:98.

89. Oakes DD, Sherck JP, Mark JBD. Lye ingestion: clinical patterns and therapeutic implications. J Thorac & Cardiovasc Surg 1982;83:194.

90. Howell JM, Dalsey WC, Hartsell FW, et al. Steroids for the treatment of corrosive esophageal injury: a statistical analysis of past studies. Am J Emerg Med 1992;10:421.

91. Bikhazi HB, Thompson ER, Shumrick DA. Caustic ingestion. Current status. Arch Otolaryngo 1969;89:112.

92. Anderson KD, Rouse TM, Randolph JG. A controlled trial of corticosteriods in children with corrosive injury of the esophagus. N Engl J Med 1990;323:637.

93. Appleqvist P. Lye corrosion carcinoma of the esophagus: a review of 63 cases. Cancer 1980;45:2655.

94. Payne DK, Anderson WM, Romero MD, et al. Tracheoesophageal fistula formation in intubated patients: risk factors and treatment with high frequency jet ventilation. Chest 1990;98:161.

95. Symbas PN, Logan WD, Hatcher CR Jr, et al. Factors in the successful recognition and management of esophageal perforation. South Med J 1966;59:1090.

96. Ctercteko G, Mok CK. Aortoesophageal fistula induced by a foreign body: the first recorded survival. J thorac Cardiovasc Surg 1980;80:233.

97. Levine EA, Alverdy JC. Carotid-esophageal fistula following a penetrating neck injury: case report. J Trauma 1990;30:1588.

98. Scher RL, Tegtmeyer CJ, McLean WC. Vascular injury following foreign body perforation of the esophagus. Ann Otol Rhinol Laryngol 1990;99:698.

99. Nandi P, Ong GB. Foreign body in oesophagus: review of 2394 cases. Br J Surg 1978;65:5.

100. Popovsky J, Lee YC, Berk JL. Gunshot wounds of the esophagus. 1976;72:609.

101. Braun RA, Goldward RR, Flores LM. Cervical tracheal transection with esophageal fistula. Arch of Otolaryngology 1972;96:67.

102. Rea WJ, Gallivan GJ, Ecker RR, Sugg WL. Traumatic esophageal perforation. Ann Thorac Surg 1972;14:671.

103. Sharma DM, Odell J. Penetrating neck trauma with tracheal and oesophageal injuries. Br J Surg 1984;71:534-535.

Chapter 19B Thoracic Duct Injuries

ROBERT F. WILSON, M.D.

INTRODUCTION

Dulchavsky et al[1] in their review of chylothorax after blunt chest trauma noted that "although chylothorax was described in the seventeenth century, Quincke in 1875 made the first authoritative report on the etiology and treatment". They also noted that DeForest in 1907 suggested that "the wounded thoracic duct should be treated like a bleeding vessel and ligated." In 1943, Peet and Campbell[2] described a massive chylorothorax after splanchnicectomy that they treated by ligation. Unfortunately, the patient died postoperatively from an allergic reaction to an intravenous chyle infusion, which was used not infrequently at that time. In 1948, Lampson[3] performed the first successful thoracic duct ligation for a chylothorax.

ANATOMY

Although there is great anatomic variability in the course of the thoracic duct (Fig. 19B–1), it generally starts in the abdominal cavity just anterior to the first or second lumbar vertebra. At that point, the paired lymphatic trunks from the lower extremities and one or more lymphatic trunks from abdominal viscera converge and form a dilated structure called the cisterna chyli.[4,5] The thoracic duct continues superiorly, anterior to the vertebral column and the right intercostal vessels, between the azygos vein on the right and the descending aorta on the left. It is posterior to the esophagus until it reaches the inferior aspect of the superior mediastinum at the level of the fourth to seventh thoracic vertebra. It then curves slightly to the left and occupies a position to the left of the esophagus and just anterior to the vertebral column. It continues into the neck along the left margin of the esophagus up to the level of the transverse process of the seventh cervical vertebra. At this point, it bends laterally behind the carotid sheath and in front of the left vertebral artery (Fig. 19B–2). As the duct approaches the medial border of the scalenus anticus muscle, it turns inferiorly in front of the phrenic nerve and the first part of the subclavian artery. It then typically enters the venous system at the point where the left internal jugular and left subclavian veins meet to form the left innominate vein. However, it may also enter any one of these three veins near that point.

The thoracic duct is usually a single structure between T12 and T8, but the course of the thoracic duct is quite unpredictable. It also has many collaterals with the azygous and intercostal veins, making it quite susceptible to all types of thoracic trauma.[4,5]

PHYSIOLOGY

The lymphatic system performs three major functions: drainage of interstitial and edema fluid back into the venous circulation, immunologic responses to infection and tumors, and transport of lipids absorbed by the intestines.[6,7]

Ingested triglycerides and cholesterol are first emulsified by bile acids and lecithin into droplets approximately 1 μm in diameter. Digestion by pancreatic enzymes leads to formation of micelles (5nm) that are aggregates of bile acids, monoglycerides, fatty acids, phospholipids, and cholesterol. These are then absorbed by small intestinal epithelial cells, and are resynthesized and ejected via exocytosis. They then form chylomicrons (1 nm), which are transported by intestinal lymphatics to the cisterna chyli and the thoracic duct. The high chylomicron content of lymph after a fatty meal gives chyle and the thoracic duct their milky-white appearance.

Chyle is alkaline and has a specific gravity greater than 1.012.[8] After a meal, chyle will usually separate into three layers upon standing: a creamy uppermost layer containing chylomicrons, a milky intermediate layer, and a dependent layer containing cellular elements, mostly small lymphocytes.[9] During fasting, however, chyle may appear to be only slightly turbid because of its reduced lipid content. Because of its high fatty acid content, chyle is bacteriostatic.[10] The presence of chyle in the pleural space is nonirritating and usually does not induce the formation of a pleural peel or fibroelastic membrane.[9]

> **AXIOM** Because chyle is nonirritating to the pleura and is bacteriostatic, there is generally minimal inflammation and no fibrin peel around a chylothorax.

Chyle has a variable protein content (2.2 to 6.0 gm/dl) and a variable fat content (0.4 to 6.0 gm/dl) that includes fat-soluble vitamins.[8] Its electrolyte composition is similar to that of serum. Of the cellular elements, lymphocytes of the T-cell type predominate.[10,11] A few erythrocytes (50 to 60/mm^3) are also present.

Between 1500 and 2500 ml of chyle empty into the venous system daily.[8,10] Both the volume and the flow rate of chyle vary considerably, depending on the amount of food and its fat content. The ingestion of fat can increase the flow of lymph in the thoracic duct to two to ten times the resting level of 10-15 ml/hr for several hours. Ingestion of water also increases the flow of chyle; however, the ingestion of proteins or carbohydrates has little effect.[6] Severe, prolonged fasting can reduce the amount of chyle greatly.[10] The movement or flow of chyle in the thoracic duct depends on the contraction of its walls, adjacent arterial pulsations, and intrathoracic and intraabdominal pressure changes.[10,12]

> **AXIOM** Prolonged external loss of chyle can result in severe malnutrition, water and electrolyte loss, and lymphopenia with T-cell suppression.[10,13]

ETIOLOGY OF CHYLOTHORAX

Injuries to the thoracic duct or one of its major tributaries can cause a fistula, a localized collection of chyle (a chyloma), or an intrapleural collection referred to as a chylothorax.

Light[14] has divided the etiology of chylothorax into four major categories: tumors, trauma, idiopathic, and miscellaneous. Tumors are responsible for over 50% of chylothoraces in some series and occur primarily in adults.[14] The responsible tumor is a lymphoma in 75%.[15] Hence, a nontraumatic chylothorax in an adult demands a careful search for malignancy, especially lymphomas. A chyloperitoneum is also frequently present in lymphomas.[16,17] The occurrence of chylothorax with a carcinoma suggests mediastinal involvement.[10] Chylothorax can develop as a result of the tumor extrinsically compressing or directly invading the thoracic duct or from obliteration of the lymphatics following radiation therapy.[18]

Although Sasson and Light[8] consider trauma to be the second leading cause of chylothorax and the cause of approximately 25% of chylothoraces, Teba et al,[19] in a special review, indicated that trauma, of either accidental or iatrogenic origin, is the most frequent type of chylothorax. More chylothoraces result from surgical (iatrogenic) trauma than accidental (nonsurgical) trauma. Chylothorax has been reported after a wide variety of surgery of the heart, diaphragm, esophagus, and neck, and the incidence is about 0.20 to 0.56%.[20,21] Superior vena cava and subclavian vein obstruction related to central parenteral hyperalimentation has also resulted in chylothorax.[22]

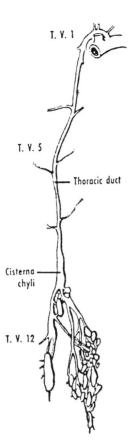

FIGURE 19B–1 The thoracic duct begins in the abdomen at the junction of the intestinal, lumbar, and descending intercostal lymphatic trunks. The junction usually consists of a dilatation called the cisterna chyli. The thoracic duct usually passes through or near the aortic opening of the diaphragm and ascends in the posterior mediastinum on the right side of the aorta, and between the aorta and the azygos vein. At about the level of the fifth or sixth thoracic vertebra, it crosses obliquely to the left behind the esophagus. It then ascends on the left side of the esophagus, passes behind the left subclavian artery, and enters the neck, where it forms an arch that may reach as high as the seventh cervical vertebra. It then turns forward and downward, uniting with multiple other lymphatic channels into a common trunk that usually ends in the left subclavian vein near its junction with the internal jugular vein. (From: Anatomy. 4th ed. In: Gardner E, Gray DJ, O'Rahilly R, eds. Philadelphia: WB Saunders, 1975; 330.)

Nonsurgical ("accidental") trauma leading to chylothorax includes penetrating injuries to the thoracic duct resulting from gunshot or stab wounds and a variety of nonpenetrating injuries. The acute angle between the right crus of the diaphragm and the thoracic duct may promote a shearing injury to the duct when the back is hyperextended, especially after a heavy meal when the duct is dilated and more prone to injury.[1,23]

AXIOM A chylothorax should be suspected if the patient has a pleural effusion after severe blunt chest or back trauma, especially if the patient has no rib or spine fractures.

Thoracic duct injuries have been described with all sorts of blast and crush injuries causing fractures of vertebrae or ribs. However, activities such as weight lifting, straining, severe coughing or vomiting, and vigorous stretching while yawning can induce chylothorax by producing sudden severe changes in the hydrostatic pressure within the thoracic duct.[1,8,19] Chylothorax also has been seen after traumatic amputation of the left upper arm in a young man who later developed subclavian vein thrombosis.[24] Cadaver studies, however, have shown that the thoracic duct may be rapidly and forcefully dilated four or fivefold without rupture.[25]

The third etiologic category of chylothorax, idiopathic, accounts for about 15% of cases including neonatal chylothorax.[8] Spontaneous neonatal chylothorax is the most common cause of pleural effusion in the first few days of life.[26] The pathogenesis is unknown, but it is probably a result of increased fetal venous pressure during delivery. In adults, most cases of idiopathic chylothorax are probably a result of minor, forgotten trauma.

The fourth or miscellaneous etiologic category accounts for less than 10% of chylothoraces and includes such entities as filariasis, tuberculosis, sarcoidosis, cirrhosis, heart failure, aneurysm of the thoracic aorta, and pulmonary lymphangiomyxomatosis.[14]

CLINICAL MANIFESTATIONS

The symptoms, physical findings, and roentgenologic features of chylothorax are usually those seen with any pleural effusion.[8] The actual presence of chyle, however, is usually suspected only after a thoracentesis is performed. Pleuritic chest pain and high fever are rare because chyle is nonirritating to the pleural surface and it is bacteriostatic.

The degree of disturbance caused by a chylothorax is directly related to the rate with which it forms. In slowly developing chylothorax, the clinical picture is usually one of fatigue, dyspnea on exertion, heaviness, and discomfort in the affected side. After trauma, however, a chylothorax may form at rates exceeding 200 ml/hr, and

FIGURE 19B–2 A. The termination of the thoracic duct. **B.** A horizontal section in which the arch formed by the thoracic duct is seen between the scalenus anterior muscle behind, and the internal jugular vein and the common carotid artery in front. (From: Anatomy. 4th ed. In: Gardner E, Gray DJ, O'Rahilly R, eds. Philadelphia: WB Saunders, 1975; 709.)

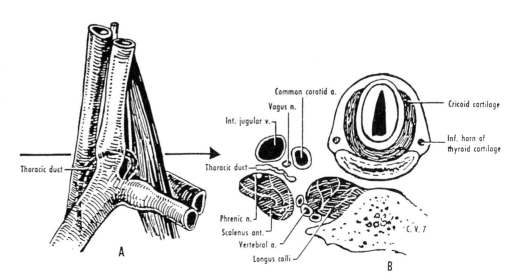

even without any accompanying blood, this can produce serious respiratory distress within hours.[12]

In traumatic chylothorax, there is usually a latent period of 2 to 10 days between the time of the trauma and the onset of the chylothorax, but sometimes symptoms do not develop until weeks or months later.[8] This latent period occurs because the chyle from the ruptured thoracic duct is initially confined to the posterior mediastinum to form a chyloma. The chyloma may expand quite slowly initially, because of the pressure within it, and because the patient may not eat a regular diet for several days or more.[27] Eventually, however, the chyloma ruptures through the mediastinal pleura to produce the chylothorax.[10]

AXIOM   Chylothoraxes are often delayed in their appearance, therefore, the causal relationship with trauma may be forgotten by the patient.

The metabolic effects of chylothorax can be a serious threat to life and are proportional to the duration and volume of the lymph drainage.[8] The loss of proteins, fats, electrolytes, bicarbonate, fat-soluble vitamins, and lymphocytes can be substantial and can lead to malnutrition, compromised immunologic status, and metabolic acidosis.[28] Indeed, before the introduction of thoracic duct ligation, chylothoraces caused mortality rates of up to 45%.[8,28]

DIAGNOSIS

At the Initial Surgery

Any time there is trauma involving structures adjacent to the thoracic duct anywhere along its course, one should look for a major lymphatic injury; however, at the time of surgery, the lymphatic leak may be of small volume and difficult to recognize. Consequently, any injured tissues in the presumed path of the thoracic duct should be securely ligated.

Later Signs and Symptoms

Failure to look carefully for a thoracic duct injury may result in a missed injury that may first be noticed as either a persistent fistula, a localized collection of chyle (i.e., a chyloma), or a chylothorax.

As mentioned previously, the accumulation of chyle in the pleural space may not be apparent for several days after injury. However, one may notice that, as the chylothorax is rapidly forming, there will be a decline in the total leukocyte count, and the absolute lymphocyte count may fall to almost zero.[19] Injury to the thoracic duct at lower thoracic levels, below T4-T7, usually presents as a right chylothorax; injury at upper thoracic levels usually presents as a left-sided effusion.[29]

In postoperative chylothorax, the effusion will usually not be milky or chylous until the patient resumes an enteral diet containing fat. Staats et al[15] reported that about half of their adult patients with chylothorax had yellow, green, serous or serosanguineous effusions.

LABORATORY ANALYSIS

Acute Pleural Effusions

In a fasting patient, chyle will resemble extracellular fluid (ECF) with a slightly higher protein content. If a thoracentesis in a trauma patient reveals an exudate, the differential diagnosis should include a hemothorax and a pseudomeningocele (containing blood and CSF). If almost all of the white blood cells are lymphocytes, one should suspect a chylothorax.

Staats et al[15] have noted that if the triglyceride value of the pleural effusion is greater than 110 mg/dl, the patient probably has a chylous effusion, although at times a pseudochylothorax has a triglyceride level exceeding this value.[30] An effusion with a triglyceride value below 50 mg/dl has a low probability of being chylous.[15] If the triglyceride value is between 50 and 100 mg/dl, or if there is any doubt

about the diagnosis, lipoprotein electrophoresis should be performed. Lipoprotein electrophoresis of chyle will typically demonstrate a chylomicron band with triglyceride levels higher than plasma, cholesterol levels lower than plasma, and a cholesterol/triglyceride ratio of less than 1.0.[15,31]

Chronic Effusions

PITFALL ⊘

Assuming that a milky-white pleural effusion is always a chylothorax.

Determining the etiology of chronic milky-white pleural effusions can be difficult, and the differential diagnosis will include a chronic chylothorax, a pseudochylothorax, and empyema.[8] Pseudochylothorax (referred to as chyliform pleural effusion) is the accumulation of a high concentration of cholesterol and/or lecithin-globulin complexes in a long-standing pleural effusion.[8] The milky appearance of an empyema is due to the presence of white blood cells in suspension.[8] With centrifugation, the supernatant will clear.

In both chylothorax and pseudochylothorax the pleural fluid appears milky or turbid. This characteristic persists after centrifugation and is the result of the high lipid content of the pleural fluid; however, addition of 2 ml of ethyl ether will clear the turbidity in chylothorax, but not in pseudochylothorax.[8]

The incidence of chylothorax is low, and that of pseudochylothorax even lower. Chylothorax is characterized by a relatively acute onset and normal pleural surfaces, while pseudochylothorax is characterized by chronicity and thickened pleural surfaces.[30] Thus, a CT scan of the thorax demonstrating pleural thickening tends to rule out a chylothorax.

Another test used in diagnosing chylothorax involves the ingestion of butter mixed with a lipophilic dye, preferably Drug and Cosmetic Green Number 6. Fluid collected one hour after the patient ingests the green butter should yield green fluid if a chylothorax is present.[12] Alternatively, the patient could ingest radiolabeled triglyceride (^{131}I-triolein). Samples of pleural fluid collected within 48 hours after ^{131}I-triolein administration are counted using a scintillation detector. A high level of radioactivity in the pleural fluid confirms the presence of a chylothorax.[32]

RADIOLOGY

When a patient with severe blunt trauma presents with mediastinal widening, the differential diagnosis includes injury to the aorta, spine, or esophagus.[6] Consequently, the patient may require an extensive radiologic workup, including an aortogram.

In some cases, there may be a long delay between the discovery of a mediastinal mass (chyloma) and the appearance of a chylothorax. Thorne[33] described a case of post-traumatic chylothorax that was preceded by a lower mediastinal mass 3 months before rupture.

If the fluid collection continues to expand without any change in CT attenuation, this tends to rule against a chronic hematoma.[6] The MR characteristics of the fluid may also show evidence of blood degradation products, such as methemoglobin (high T1 intensity) or hemosiderin (low T1 and low T2 intensities). A CSF leak can usually be excluded by premyelogram and postmyelogram CT scan.[6]

A detailed MR examination may diagnose chyle before the effusion is aspirated.[6] Because chyle is nonirritating, the pleura adjacent to a chylothorax should be relatively normal. Also, since the chemical composition of chyle can change from that of a thin proteinaceous liquid to that of a lipid emulsion after eating,[6] one would also expect the MR characteristics to change from those of a proteinaceous liquid to those of a lipid after eating.

AXIOM   A lymphangiogram can be helpful for confirming the diagnosis and source of a chylothorax.

A lymphangiogram can also be a helpful diagnostic test. Teba et al[19] and Janzing et al[28] believe that this test should be considered for every chylothorax that does not respond to nonoperative management and is a candidate for surgery. This test may also demonstrate the exact site of the leak or obstruction.

PRINCIPLES OF MANAGEMENT

The first principle in the management of a patient with chylothorax is to maintain adequate nutrition and to minimize chyle formation.[8] This is necessary to prevent severe nutritional and immunologic derangements from developing because of the removal of large amounts of protein, fat, fat-soluble vitamins, electrolytes, and lymphocytes with repeated thoracenteses or chest tube drainage. Second, when indicated, definitive treatment, such as thoracic duct ligation, should be performed before the patient becomes malnourished or immunodepressed.

TREATMENT

Nonsurgical

An initial trial of conservative treatment has been advocated for traumatic chylothorax because the defect in the thoracic duct frequently closes spontaneously.[1,6,8,9] Conservative treatment includes complete decompression of the pleural space. The chyle is best drained from the pleural space with tube thoracostomy, which allows the lung to fully expand. The placement of a chest tube also allows wide apposition of the parietal and visceral pleura and may result in pleurodesis. The chest tube also allows one to measure the rate of chyle leakage more accurately.

If the enteral fat content is reduced to 1.0 gm/liter, the chest tube drainage may decrease to less than 50 ml/day.[19] Because water ingestion may stimulate chyle formation,[18] one may have to switch to total parenteral nutrition to stop the leak of chyle.[34,35] If the chyle leak can be greatly reduced and the pleural cavity is effectively drained by a chest tube, the leak will stop in at least 50% of patients.[8]

AXIOM Most chylous fistulas will close spontaneously if the bowel is put at rest.

Bozzetti et al[36] reported that the lymphatic fistula occurring postoperatively closed spontaneously in eight of nine patients receiving total parenteral nutrition. Medium-chain triglycerides are absorbed into the portal system rather than into the intestinal and thoracic lymphatics. Therefore, in the management of chylothorax, oral dietary fats should be replaced by medium-chain triglycerides.[37,38] However, many clinicians prefer total parenteral nutrition to oral diet, because the flow of chyle is maximally reduced when the patient is given nothing by mouth.[10,12]

Surgery

INDICATIONS

Patients with high outputs of chyle are not likely not to respond successfully to medical manipulations and should be considered for early surgical intervention. Selle et al[39] described the following criteria for surgical therapy: (a) average daily loss of chyle exceeding 1500 cc per day in an adult (or 100 ml per year of age in a child) for 5 or more days, or (b) persistent flow of chyle for 14 days, or (c) when insurmountable nutritional complications develop. Most authors agree with these recommendations.[1,6,8,19,28,34]

AXIOM Large-volume chylous fistulas that do not close after 2 weeks of nonoperative therapy should be closed surgically.

NONTHORACOTOMY PROCEDURES

If conservative medical therapy has failed, a variety of surgical procedures have been attempted, including pleurodesis with talc,[40] fibrin glue,[41] and tetracycline,[8] as well as insertion of a pleuroperitoneal shunt.[42] Thoracoscopic application of fibrin glue has also been successfully employed.[43]

Successful ligation of a thoracic duct with a thoracoscope was described by Kent and Pinson.[34] The authors assert that this procedure offers the dual advantage of a successful duct ligation and avoidance of a thoracotomy. The obvious advantages of the thoracoscopic approach include the use of limited incisions which minimize postoperative pain and recovery time. In addition, because of the low morbidity of thoracoscopic ligation, early operative intervention should be considered rather than a prolonged conservative trial.

THORACOTOMY

Overall, thoracic duct ligation via a thoracotomy has been the most successful method for treating persistent chylothorax. The surgical exploration is usually performed on the side of the chylothorax. With a bilateral chylothorax, the right side should be explored first.[10]

At thoracotomy, one generally attempts to first identify the thoracic duct just superior to the diaphragm between the aorta and azygos vein, and an earnest effort should be made to locate the site of chyle leakage.[8] There are several aids in finding the site of leakage,[12] but probably the best method is to inject 1% Evans blue at a dose of 0.7 to 0.8 mg per kg body weight into the subcutaneous tissue of the leg.[44] Within 5 minutes, the chyle will be stained dark blue. One can also give 1-2 ounces of cream orally or via an NG tube 30-45 minutes before surgery.[8] If the leak is identified, the duct is ligated on both sides of the leak.[9] Unfortunately, even with dye injections or enteral fat, in most instances, the leak cannot be localized and one will be forced to place mass ligatures incorporating tissue between the aorta, esophagus, and vertebral bodies.

AXIOM If the origin of a chylous leak in the chest cannot be identified at surgery, the tissue between the aorta, esophagus, and vertebra just above the diaphragm should be ligated.

In a series by Patterson et al,[45] mass or "blind" ligation achieved immediate cessation of chyle drainage in four of five patients. It is also suggested that subdiaphragmatic ligation of the duct can be effective when thoracic procedures fail to locate the site of injury.[46] If the duct or the site of leakage cannot be identified at thoracotomy, a parietal pleurectomy to completely obliterate the pleural space should be performed along with the "blind" ligation.[9]

Ligation of the thoracic duct at any point in its course does not produce chylothorax in either humans or experimental animals because of its extensive collateral vessels and anastomoses. Although the lymphocyte count in the peripheral blood may decline dramatically within a few hours of thoracic duct ligation, it usually returns to normal within 7 to 10 days.

⊘ FREQUENT ERRORS

In the Management of Thoracic Duct Injuries

1. *Not looking for thoracic duct injuries in patients with trauma involving the mediastinum or neck near the usual path of the thoracic duct.*
2. *Failure to make strong efforts to look for and ligate injured lymphatic ducts during surgical explorations for trauma.*
3. *Not adequately monitoring and preventing the complications associated with the malnutrition, fluid and electrolyte losses, and lymphopenia that can occur in patients with chylous fistulas.*
4. *Not suspecting thoracic duct injuries in patients who develop pleural effusions or mediastinal fluid collections after neck or chest trauma.*
5. *Failure to pursue a history of possible trauma that may have occurred weeks earlier in patients with pleural effusions.*

6. *Assuming that a nonwhite pleural effusion, even in a patient who is not eating, is not a chylothorax.*
7. *Assuming that a white pleural effusion after chest or neck surgery or trauma is always a chylothorax.*
8. *Not allowing chylous fistulas to close spontaneously by putting the bowel at rest and/or using medium-chain triglycerides for up to 2 weeks.*
9. *Delay of surgery to ligate a thoracic duct injury if it is causing complications.*
10. *Not giving fat or dye that will by picked up by lymphatics at the time of a thoracotomy to identify and/or ligate a thoracic duct injury.*

▼▼▼▼▼▼▼▼▼▼▼▼▼▼▼▼▼▼▼▼▼▼▼▼▼▼▼▼▼▼▼▼

SUMMARY POINTS

1. Because chyle is nonirritating to the pleura and is bacteriostatic, there is generally minimal inflammation and no fibrin peel around a chylothorax.

2. Prolonged external loss of chyle can result in severe malnutrition, water and electrolyte loss, lymphopenia, and T-cell suppression.

3. A chylothorax should be suspected if the patient has a pleural effusion after severe blunt chest or back trauma, particularly if there are no rib or spine fractures.

4. Chylothoraxes are often delayed, therefore, the causal relationship with trauma may be forgotten by the patient.

5. One should not assume that a milky-white pleural effusion is always a chylothorax.

6. A lymphangiogram can be helpful for confirming the diagnosis and source of a chylothorax.

7. Most chylous fistulas will close spontaneously if the bowel is put at rest.

8. Large-volume chylous fistulas that do not close after 2 weeks of nonoperative therapy should be closed surgically.

9. If the origin of a chylous leak cannot be identified at surgery, the tissue between the aorta, esophagus, and vertebral bodies just above the diaphragm should be ligated.

▲▲▲▲▲▲▲▲▲▲▲▲▲▲▲▲▲▲▲▲▲▲▲▲▲▲▲▲▲▲▲▲

REFERENCES

1. Dulchavsky SA, Ledgerwood AM, Lucas CE. Management of chylothorax after blunt chest trauma. J Trauma 1988;28:1400.
2. Peet MM, Campbell KN. Massive chylothorax following splanchnicectomy. Univ Hosp Bull (Ann Arbor) 1943;9:2-3.
3. Lampson RS. Traumatic chylothorax. J Thorac Surg 1948;17:778.
4. Schulman A, Fataar S, Dalrymple R. The lymphographic anatomy of chylothorax. Br J Radiol 1978;51:420.
5. Kausel HW, Reeve TS, Stain AA, et al. Anatomic and pathologic studies of the thoracic duct. J Thorac Surg 1957;34:631.
6. Hom M, Jolles H. Traumatic mediastinal lymphocele mimicking other thoracic injuries: case report. J Thorac Imaging 1992;7:78.
7. Brooks FP. Absorption. In: West JB, ed. Best and Taylor's physiological basis of medical practice. 11th ed. Baltimore: Williams & Wilkins, 1985; 759-762.
8. Sassoon CS, Light RW. Chylothorax and pseudochylothorax. Clin Chest Med 1985;6:163.
9. William KR, Burford THE. The management of chylothorax. Ann Surg 1964;160:131.
10. Ross IK. A review of the surgery of the thoracic duct. Thorax 1961; 16:12.
11. Machleder HI, Paulus H. Clinical and immunological alterations observed in patient undergoing long-term thoracic duct drainage. Surgery 1978; 84:157.

12. Bessone N, Ferguson TB, Burford THE. Chylothorax. Ann Thorac Surg 1971;12:527.
13. McWilliams BC, Fan LL, Murphy SA. Transient T-cell depression in postoperative chylothorax. J Pediatr 1981;99:595.
14. Light RW. Pleural diseases. Philadelphia: Lea & Febiger, 1983; 209.
15. Staats BA, Ellefson RD, Budahn LL, et al. The lipoprotein profile of chylous and nonchylous pleural effusions. May Clin Proc 1980;55:700.
16. Swensson NL, Kurohara SS, George FW. Complete regression following abdominal irradiation alone, or chylothorax complicating lymphosarcoma with ascites. Radiology 1966;87:635.
17. Kostiainen S, Meurala H, Mattila S, et al. Chylothorax: clinical experience in nine cases. Scand J Thor Cardiovasc 1983;Surg 17:79.
18. Strausser JL, Flye MW. Management of nontraumatic chylothorax. Ann Thorac Surg 1981;31:520.
19. Teba L, Dedhia HV, Bowel R, Alexander JC. Chylothorax review. Crit Care Med 1985;13:49.
20. Cevese PG, Vecchioni R, D'Amico DF, et al. Postoperative chylothorax. J Thorac Cardiovasc Surg 1975;69:966.
21. Verunelli F, Giorgini V, Luisi VS, et al. Chylothorax following cardiac surgery in children. J Cardiovasc Surg 1983;24:227.
22. Seibert JJ, Golladay ES, Keller C. Chylothorax secondary to superior vena caval obstruction. Pediatr Radiol 1982;12:252.
23. Birt AB, Connolly NK. Traumatic chylothorax: a report of a case and a survey of the literature. Br J Surg 1951;39:564.
24. Lowman RM, Hoogerhyde J, Waters LL, et al. Traumatic chylothorax: the roentgen aspects of this problem. Am J Roentgenol 1951;65:529.
25. Narasimharao KL, Mitra SK. Chylothorax following traumatic amputation of the upper arm. J Trauma 1988;28:711.
26. Chernick V, Reed MH. Pneumothorax and chylothorax in the neonatal period. J Pediatr 1970;76:624.
27. Janzing H, Tonnard P, Brande FV, Derom F. Chylothorax after blunt chest trauma. Acta Chir Belg 1992;92:26.
28. Siegler RL, Pearce MB. Metabolic acidosis from the loss of thoracic lymph. J Pediatr 1978;93:465.
29. DeHert S, Heytens L, Van Hee R, Adriaensen H. Current management of traumatic chylothorax. Acta Anaesth Belg 1988;39:101.
30. Coe JE, Aikawa JK. Cholesterol pleura effusion. Arch Intern Med 1961;108:163.
31. Seriff NS, Cohen ML, Samuel P, et al. Chylothorax: diagnosis by lipoprotein electrophoresis of serum and pleural fluid. Thorax 1977;32:98.
32. Woolfenden JM, Struse TB. Diagnosis of chylothorax with ^{131}I-triolein: case report. J Nucl Med 1977;18:128.
33. Thorne PS. Traumatic chylothorax. Tubercle 1958;39:29.
34. Kent RB, Pinson TW. Thoracoscopic ligation of the thoracic duct. Surg Endosc 1993;7:52.
35. Spiro JD, Spiro RH, Strong EW, et al. The management of chyle fistula. Laryngoscope 1990;100:771.
36. Bozzetti F, Arullani A, Baticci F, et al. Management of lymphatic fistulas by total parenteral nutrition. JPEN 1982;6:526.
37. Ramzy AI, Rodriguez A, Cowley RA. Pitfalls in the management of traumatic chylothorax. J Trauma 1982;22:513.
38. Hughes RL, Mintzer RA, Hidvegi DF, et al. The management of chylothorax. Chest 1979;76:212.
39. Selle JG, Snyder WH, Schrider JT. Chylothorax: indications for surgery. Ann Surg 1973;177:244.
40. Adler RH, Levinsky L. Persistent chylothorax: treatment by talc pleurodesis. J Thorac Cardiovasc Surg 1970;76:859.
41. Akaogi E, Mitsui K, Shoara Y, et al. Treatment of postoperative chylothorax with intrapleural fibrin glue. Ann Thorac Surg 1989;48:116.
42. Kitchen ND, Hocken DB, Greenhalgh RM, et al. Use of the Denver pleuroperitoneal shunt in the treatment of chylothorax secondary to filariasis. Thorax 1991;46:144.
43. Shirai T, Amano J, Takabe K. Thoracoscopic diagnosis and treatment of chylothorax after pneumonectomy. Ann Thorac Surg 1991;52:306.
44. Merrill K. The use of Evans blue to outline the course of the thoracic duct. J Thorac Surg 1955;29:555.
45. Patterson GA, Todd TRJ, Delarne NC, et al. Supradiaphragmatic ligation of the thoracic duct in intractable chylous fistula. Ann Thorac Surg 1981;32:44.
46. Goorwitch J. Traumatic chylothorax and pseudochylothorax. Clin Chest Med 1985;6:163.

Chapter 20 General Considerations in Abdominal Trauma

ROBERT F. WILSON, M.D.

ALEXANDER J. WALT, M.D.

INCIDENCE

Of the injuries that require surgery after civilian trauma, approximately 20% occur in the abdomen.[1] The causes of abdominal trauma vary in urban and rural areas. In a large series from Houston,[2] the causes of the abdominal injuries were gunshot wounds in 65%, stab wounds in 25%, and blunt abdominal trauma in 10%. In contrast, the causes of abdominal injuries in a series from the entire state of Connecticut were blunt trauma in 69%, stab wounds in 17%, and gunshot wounds in 14%.[3] Of the blunt abdominal injuries, approximately 60% are caused by automobile accidents.[1,4]

In a consecutive group of 307 patients with blunt abdominal trauma treated at Detroit General Hospital, the two most common organs injured were the spleen (30%) and liver (19%).[5] With penetrating trauma the most frequent organs injured were small intestine (38%), liver, (33%), and colon (32%).

Certain distinctive constellations of injuries should also be kept in mind because they frequently occur together, especially in blunt trauma. Falls from heights frequently cause fractures involving the os calcis, lumbar spine, and pelvis with rupture of the bladder. Seat belt injuries are often associated with "chance fractures" (horizontal fractures through the body of the vertebra) of the lumbar spine and tears of the small bowel or mesentery. Steering-wheel injuries frequently damage the liver and spleen in addition to the sternum, ribs, and lungs. The possibility of myocardial contusion must also be considered.

PITFALL ⊘

If individual injuries are viewed in isolation, diagnosis of other problems is apt to be delayed.

Multiple injuries associated with abdominal organ damage are usually due to blunt trauma, and motor vehicle accidents are the most frequent cause of serious blunt trauma. With frontal impacts, it is estimated that seat beats can reduce the number of organ injuries by at least 27%, and a lap belt shoulder harness can reduce the number of organ injuries by at least 42%.[6]

HISTORICAL PERSPECTIVE

One of the first published reports of a successfully treated wound to the abdomen is in Xenophon's "Persian Expedition."[7] In the year 401 BC, Cyrus of Sparta invaded Persia with 10,000 warriors.[1-6] The Persian Tissaphernes induced some of the Greek leaders to come to his camp, where they were treacherously seized and killed except for Nicarchus the Arcadian, who escaped and returned to the Greek camp "with a wound in his stomach and holding his intestines in his hands." Xenophon does not document how he was treated except to note that there were "appointed eight doctors, as there were a number of wounded." Since Nicarchus survived, it seems unlikely that any of the intestines were actually wounded.

Bowden is known to have used celiotomy for treating penetrating abdominal trauma in 1836.[1,8] Possibly Samuel D. Gross[9] knew of Bowden's work, but he does not mention it in his 1843 treatise, "An Experimental and Critical Enquiry in the Nature and Treatment of Wounds of the Intestines." Even though Gross served in the Civil War,

it has never been documented that he practiced his technique on humans, and it was not until 1881 that an exploratory laparotomy was considered for treating penetrating abdominal trauma, and this was during President Garfield's term.[10]

Trunkey et al[1] have noted that surgeons began to report trauma series in 1882. At that time, celiotomy for abdominal trauma was noted to improve survival rates significantly when compared with nonoperative management, which resulted in mortality rates of 67% to 81%.[11] Advances over the next 70-80 years in the management of abdominal trauma, primarily due to the early use of celiotomy, have resulted in mortality rates reported to be as low as 6.4% in 1960[12] and 2.5% in 1978.[13] Nevertheless, it was noted that many of these laparotomies were "negative" or "non-therapeutic." This observation stimulated a change from prompt laparotomy on all patients with suspected abdominal trauma to a more selective approach. This approach has been facilitated greatly by the development of diagnostic peritoneal lavage (DPL) in 1965[14] and computed tomography (CT) scans in 1981.[15]

PATHOPHYSIOLOGY

Injuries to solid organs occur with blunt trauma because the energy of deceleration and compression tends to fracture the capsule and parenchyma of these relatively incompressible structures.[16] Hollow organ injury occurs frequently with penetrating trauma because the intestine takes up the largest portion of the intra-abdominal volume.

With stab wounds, the injury is usually confined to the weapon tract;[1] however, with gunshot wounds, injury can be outside the presumed tract.

AXIOM One should never assume that bullets will travel in a straight line. The bullet, or the secondary missiles it causes, can often injure structures far outside the presumed trajectory.

The wounding potential of gunshot wounds depends on the missile's velocity, caliber, mass, expandability, fragmentation, yaw, pitch, and tumbling. Secondary missiles (bone) and the specific gravity of the target tissue are also important. Transfer of kinetic energy occurs more readily from a missile to a high specific gravity tissue such as bone than to low specific gravity tissue such as fat or lung.[17,18]

AXIOM Because of the unpredictable path and possible blast effect of bullets, all abdominal gunshot wounds require surgical exploration.

As many as 96-98% of gunshot wounds that penetrate the abdomen produce significant intra-abdominal injury.[19] Although all gunshot wounds thought to have entered the abdomen should be explored, an exception can occur in circumstances in which a low velocity bullet has passed tangentially through the wall of the abdomen, with obvious non-involvement of intra-abdominal structures. With high velocity missiles (>2000 ft/sec), however, the abdomen must be explored because the blast effect may extend 2-4 inches beyond the path of the bullet.

INITIAL MANAGEMENT

Immediate Management of Life-threatening Injuries

The primary cause of death in trauma is head injury, and at least 50-55% of the deaths in most trauma centers are due to this problem.[1] Thoracic injuries are the second most common cause of death; they are the direct cause of death in at least 25% of deaths, and they are a contributory cause of death in another 25% of patients. Abdominal injuries account for 13-15% of trauma deaths, primarily due to hemorrhage, but in deaths occurring more than 48 hours after injury, sepsis or its complications are the most frequent causes.

The physician faced with a patient who appears to have suffered abdominal trauma must ask certain critical questions: (a) Are there intra-abdominal injuries? (b) If so, is surgery required? (c) If surgery is required, what is the optimal time for operation? and (d) Are there any extra-abdominal injuries which take precedence?[20]

AIRWAY, VENTILATION, INTRAVENOUS FLUIDS

> **AXIOM**   The initial resuscitation of patients with severe truma must assure an adequate airway and the maintenance of a minute ventilation that is at least 1.5-2.0 times normal.

As with all injuries, the most important initial consideration in resuscitation is maintenance of adequate respiratory and cardiovascular function. An open airway must be assured and minute ventilation in the most severely injured patients must usually be at least 1.5-2.0 times the normal of about 6 L/min.

After adequate ventilation has been assured, two or more large-gauge intravenous catheters should be inserted, ideally in the upper extremities. Blood is simultaneously drawn for type and cross-matching, hematocrit and hemoglobin measurements, and any other tests suggested by the location or extent of the injury or by pre-existing medical problems. If there is any evidence of pre-existing cardiac disease or an associated chest injury, an intravenous catheter should be advanced into the superior vena cava for central venous pressure (CVP) monitoring. If there is evidence of intra-abdominal injury, leg veins should generally be avoided for intravenous catheter sites.

A major determinant of the amount of time spent on fluid resuscitation in the ED depends on the likelihood that the patient has active internal bleeding. If the patient is bleeding actively, giving large quantities of fluid prior to the control of bleeding sites can increase mortality rates significantly. On the other hand, if the bleeding has stopped, aggressive continued fluid resuscitation in the ED is appropriate.

> **AXIOM**   Fluid resuscitation should be kept to a minimum in patients who are bleeding actively, until the bleeding is controlled.

If the patient is in severe shock on admission and this appears to be related to controllable internal bleeding, the patient should be rushed to the OR as soon as possible. On the other hand, if the patient is in relatively mild shock and there is a rapid sustained response to the initial resuscitation fluids, further fluid resuscitation is appropriate. Nevertheless, if the vital signs deteriorate later, indicating that bleeding has recurred, the patient should be rushed to the OR.

The failure of 2000-3000 ml of Ringer's lactate given over 10-15 minutes to restore adequate blood pressure and tissue perfusion strongly suggests that the patient is bleeding rapidly and requires urgent surgical exploration to control the sites of hemorrhage.[20]

MONITORING

> **AXIOM**   The trend of vital signs in relation to treatment is much more important than isolated levels.

Close monitoring of vital signs, particularly in patients who have multiple injuries, is extremely important. If enough fluid and blood to replace estimated losses from fractures or lacerations have been administered, continued or later deterioration of vital signs is an important clue to intra-abdominal bleeding.

In a 70-kg man, the blood volume is normally about 5,000 ml. If the blood volume falls by 25%, the patient will usually have a systolic BP <80 mm Hg plus other signs of shock. If the blood volume is less than 50% of normal, the patient will usually be dead. Thus, the margin between the blood volume deficit that can cause hypotension and that which is generally lethal in a 70-kg man is only about 1250 ml; consequently, failure of the BP to rise if 2-3 liters of fluid are given rapidly, indicates the presence of massive bleeding.[20]

Monitoring must be done frequently and carefully in patients with severe trauma, especially in elderly individuals who have a much smaller blood volume margin between hypotension and death. These patients are also prone to an acute myocardial infarction if hypotension is allowed to develop in the presence of significant coronary artery disease.

GASTRIC DECOMPRESSION

> **PITFALL** ⊘
>
> *Failure to decompress the stomach in patients with severe trauma increases the risk of aspiration, impaired diaphragmatic motion, and prolonged ileus.*

Early gastric decompression, usually with a nasogastric tube, is particularly important where there is a possibility of intra-abdominal visceral damage or when the patient may have eaten or drunk recently.[20] The nasogastric tube also may be of value in diagnosing an injury to the upper gastrointestinal tract. If red blood is found in the stomach, this may indicate damage to that organ, but it can also be swallowed blood from other injuries.

Aspiration of gastric contents, particularly in unconscious trauma victims, occurs much more frequently than is usually recognized.[20] Furthermore, the pulmonary damage following acid aspiration can occur so quickly that even immediate bronchoscopy and lavage may be of relatively little benefit, except for the removal of large solid particles of food. In many instances, aspiration of gastric contents is not suspected until a pneumonic process is noted in the dependent portions of the lungs on the chest roentgenograms taken 24-48 hours later. The mortality rate of aspiration in severely traumatized individuals has been estimated to be as high as 70%.[21]

> **AXIOM**   All trauma patients should be assumed to have full stomachs.

Injured patients, particularly anxious adults and crying children, tend to swallow air, especially if they have any respiratory distress. Patients resuscitated with a face mask can also have large amounts of air forced into their stomachs. The resulting distension of the stomach not only increases the chances of vomiting and aspiration, but also raises the diaphragm, increasing the resistance to ventilation.

Once air has entered the small bowel, it can be extremely difficult to remove, and distended small bowel can make exploration and subsequent closure of the abdomen extremely difficult. In addition, bowel distention interferes with the return of peristalsis in the postoperative period.

> **AXIOM**   One should avoid nasal tubes in patients who may have fractures of the mid-face or anterior base of the skull.

Fractures involving the mid-face or the base of the skull anteriorly may involve the cribriform plate with a resultant cerebrospinal fluid rhinorrhea. Under such circumstances, insertion of a nasal tube can increase the risk of meningeal infection, and there is also a chance that the tube will enter the cranial cavity instead of proceeding down into the pharynx.

FOLEY CATHETER

A urinalysis should be performed on any patient with suspected abdominal or pelvic damage as a guide both to possible injury of the urinary tract and to the detection of diabetes mellitus or concomitant renal parenchymal disease.[20] If the urine on the dipstick is positive for hemoglobin but has few or no red blood cells, one should suspect hemoglobinuria or myoglobinuria. A spontaneously voided specimen is preferable to one obtained with a catheter because the trauma of catheter insertion may in itself cause hematuria.

AXIOM   Prior to inserting a Foley catheter in patients with severe blunt trauma, one should do a rectal exam to check the position of the prostate, look for any rectal blood, and check sphincter tone.

If there is any suspicion of damage to the urethra because of: (a) blood at the urethral meatus, (b) penile or perineal hematomas, (c) a displaced prostate, or (d) a severe anterior pelvic fracture, a retrograde urethrogram should be performed before a Foley catheter is inserted. If the patient has gross hematuria or other evidence of a bladder injury, a cystogram and then a CT scan of the abdomen with intravenous contrast should be performed as soon as the patient's condition is stabilized. If a CT scan cannot be done prior to a laparotomy, an emergency IVP may be achieved by the rapid infusion of 150-200 ml of Renografin-60. A scout film is obtained prior to infusing the contrast, and then films are taken one minute and five minutes after the contrast has been injected.

The urinary output monitored via a Foley catheter can be valuable as a guide to the adequacy of vital organ perfusion, especially if there is evidence of severe hemorrhage or cardiac dysfunction. A sustained urinary output of 0.5-1.0 ml/kg/hr in a patient who is not receiving a diuretic and does not have glycosuria or excess ethanol in the blood is usually reasonable evidence of an adequate tissue perfusion.[20]

ANTIBIOTICS

If there is any suspicion of intra-abdominal contamination, intravenous antibiotics should be started preoperatively so that adequate blood and tissue levels may be achieved during operation, when hypotension and/or further disruption of protective mechanisms against the invasion of bacteria may occur.[20,22-24] If the patient has much blood loss, the antibiotics should be given again as soon as the major hemorrhage has been controlled. If no peritoneal soilage is found at celiotomy, no further antibiotics are required for the abdomen.[24] If much peritoneal contamination with distal small bowel or colon contents is found, the antibiotics can be continued for at least another 24-48 hours.

AXIOM   Intravenous prophylactic antibiotics that cover enteric gram-negative aerobes and anaerobes are given as soon as possible if intra-abdominal contamination is suspected.

A number of different prophylactic antibiotic regimens have been recommended for penetrating abdominal trauma. Most regimens attempt to cover the Enterobacteriaceae (gram-negative aerobic enteric bacteria) and Bacteroides species (gram-negative anaerobes).

A combination of gentamicin and metronidazole should provide adequate coverage for most contamination caused by bowel injuries. Aztreonam can be used instead of an aminoglycoside if there is evidence of renal failure. If one wishes to use a single antibiotic, Timentin, Unasyn, or Cefotetan can be given. Some surgeons also attempt to cover for enterococci, especially in patients who are apt to be immunosuppressed. If ampicillin or vancomycin is also given, the enterococci will usually be well covered. Imipenen by itself can cover all three types of organisms, but this agent it is usually reserved for treating infections by bacteria that are resistant to most other antibiotics.

TETANUS PROPHYLAXIS

Tetanus immunization will depend on the patient's previous immunization status and the nature of the wound. Patients with an uncertain tetanus immunization history and tetanus-prone wounds should receive tetanus-toxoid and tetanus-immune globulin at different sites as well as antibiotics that should be effective against C. tetani.

PREPARING FOR SIMULTANEOUS PROCEDURES

In the patient with multiple injuries, it is useful to make arrangements for other procedures to be done simultaneously with the exploratory celiotomy to keep anesthetic time to a minimum.[1] For example, patients with an intracranial hematoma requiring early decompression may be able to have their surgery at the same time as the celiotomy. If the patient has multiple extremity fractures and requires immediate life-saving surgery on the chest or abdomen, some of these fractures may be debrided, reduced, and/or immobilized simultaneously if the orthopedic surgeon can work in the positions the patient must assume for the laparotomy and/or thoracotomy. In some instances, because of the urgency of abdominal, chest, or neurosurgery, a complete x-ray series will not have been accomplished in the emergency room. After the life-saving surgery has been completed, x-rays can be obtained in the operating room or radiology department as needed, and a decision can then be made as to what types of further treatment may be most beneficial to the patient.

DIAGNOSIS

General Principles

UNSTABLE PATIENTS

In general, the three most common sources of exsanguinating hemorrhage are the abdominal cavity (including the pelvis), the chest, and major vessels in the extremities.[1] If the chest is clear to auscultation and/or on chest x-ray and there are no major wounds, hematomas, bleeding or deformities in the extremities, the abdomen is the most likely source of hemorrhage, and it must be promptly explored. In such patients, the need for immediate laparotomy reduces the time available for a careful physical examination or needed x-rays.

If patients with potentially life-threatening injuries stabilize rapidly in the emergency department during the initial resuscitation, the surgeon has some time to perform a more complete secondary survey.[1] If the patients continue to be stable, the surgeon has the luxury of doing additional diagnostic studies before any operative intervention.

Early diagnosis of intra-abdominal injuries may severely tax the clinical acumen of even the most experienced physician.[20] The multiplicity of organs within the peritoneal cavity and the varied symptoms which may arise from injuries to these structures can provide numerous potential pitfalls. The severity of the impact or the size of the missiles often fail to reflect the degree or extent of internal damage. Blunt trauma is particularly deceptive because clinical manifestations of the injuries may be delayed for 12 to 24 hours or even days.

The organs injured and the extent of the injuries depends on the position of the patient, the tension of the abdominal wall, and the amount of energy applied at the time of impact. It is not unusual for patients with serious abdominal trauma from high-speed automobile accidents to have minimal symptoms and physical findings initially, only to deteriorate rapidly after 6, 12, or even 24 hours. Conversely, patients occasionally develop extensive guarding and rebound tenderness after what is later proven to be minimal internal damage.

AXIOM   It is essential to view the patient with abdominal injury as a whole and not to be distracted from recognizing important concomitant extra-abdominal lesions.

About 75% of patients with nonpenetrating intra-abdominal visceral damage have concomitant injuries of the head, chest, or extremities which alter prognosis and also affect the timing of any projected operations.[20] Injury to a single intra-abdominal organ is unlikely to be fatal, but the mortality rate rises sharply with the number of associated injuries. Extra-abdominal injuries involving the brain, major vessels, or the lungs have a very high priority in treatment and will take precedence over an abdominal injury which is not bleeding.

Diagnostic Procedures

HISTORY

A careful history, when available, may provide valuable clues to the diagnosis of the patient's injuries and also any underlying medical problems. Any such data obtained should be accurately recorded for medical and medicolegal reasons.[20] Changes in symptoms with time or with posture can be extremely important and should be sought by direct questioning. For example, while pain over the shoulder may be due to an injury to that area, it may also be referred there from a diaphragm which is injured or irritated by intra-abdominal blood or bile.

Conscious patients can often give useful information on circumstances surrounding their injuries. The type of accident and the direction of the forces can be of great help in diagnosing certain injuries. The direction of the impact, speeds involved, the location of the patient during the trauma (e.g., driver versus passenger), and whether a seat belt was worn are also important data.

Additional information can often be obtained from EMS personnel, family, friends, or witnesses. Physical evidence at the accident site may also provide clues about possible injuries. For example, knowing about a "bull's eye fracture" of the windshield, a deformed steering column, extrication requirements, and/or the presence of other victims who were injured or dead at the scene can be extremely helpful. The EMTs can also describe the amount of blood seen at the scene or lost en route to the hospital.

A past history, particularly in older individuals, should also be obtained from either the patient or his family. Using the mnemonic "ample" one can inquire about allergies, medications, past illnesses, last meal, and events preceding the injury. Diabetes, coronary artery disease, hypertension, and previous abdominal surgery are particularly important in patients who may need emergency surgery.

Unfortunately, the history is often unobtainable, incomplete, inaccurate, or misleading.[20] The patient may be under the influence of alcohol or drugs, or may have injuries to the head, neck or chest which prevent adequate communication. Severe emotional stress may profoundly influence the interpretation of the event by the patient and bystanders. Occasionally, the history may be deliberately falsified because of anticipated legal action by police or by projected plans for the claiming of future compensation.

PHYSICAL EXAMINATION

AXIOM Careful repeated examination of the patient is frequently the key to the early diagnosis of intra-abdominal injuries.

In many cases of abdominal trauma, the physical examination is the most informative portion of the diagnostic evaluation, and should be as complete as the time available and the condition of the patient permit.[20] A systematic approach is highly desirable, leaving the obviously injured areas until last. The more frequently and carefully these examinations are performed in cases of doubt, the earlier and more accurately the diagnosis can be made and treatment instituted.

AXIOM Narcotics should not be given to patients who are hypovolemic or who are being observed for possible CNS or abdominal injuries.

Even with similar visceral injuries, striking variations in the signs and symptoms may exist in different patients.[20] In addition, hematoma or rupture of the rectus abdominus muscle, fractures

of the ribs or pelvis, extreme obesity, and/or an altered sensorium due to head injury, alcohol, or drugs may make physical examination difficult to interpret and even grossly deceptive at times.

Techniques of Physical Examination

INSPECTION. The initial examination of a patient with suspected abdominal trauma is no time for excessive social niceties.[20] Severely injured patients should be rapidly stripped of all clothing without moving injured areas any more than is absolutely necessary. After the initial visualization of the entire body, inspection of the neck veins, and auscultation of the chest to help rule out tension pneumothorax and pericardial tamponade, areas of ecchymosis and abrasion should be noted and considered as possible clues to internal hemorrhage in the unstable patient. The abdomen is also carefully inspected for distension, contusions, abrasions, or lacerations.

AXIOM Every patient has a back as well as a front.

The back of the patient should be examined as carefully or sometimes even more carefully than the front. Gunshots or stab wounds can easily be missed in creases of the body, especially if the patient has large quantities of body hair.[20] If the patient has a possible cervical spine injury that has yet to be ruled out radiologically, two or three individuals are needed to log-role the patient carefully so that the back and flanks can be examined properly.

Physical examination of the penetrated abdomen is conducted in the same manner as that for blunt trauma, with the following exceptions: (a) contamination of open wounds should be avoided, and (b) the entrance wounds of stabs may be explored to determine visually if there is penetration of the anterior abdominal fascia.

All entrance and exit wounds should be examined and documented. No attempt should be made to label these as exit or entrance wounds in the medical record since this often requires a forensic pathologist.[1] It is prudent to cover each of these wounds with a sterile dressing and a radiopaque marker so that when x-rays are obtained, the location of these wounds can be correlated with the clinical and x-ray findings. Patients with blunt trauma from automobile accidents must be carefully examined for tire marks, abrasions, and bruises. One should also look for skin damage or marking due to seat belts.

Occasionally, intra-abdominal or retroperitoneal blood may cause ecchymosis or purplish discoloration around the umbilicus (Cullen's sign) or in the flanks (Grey-Turner's sign).[20] Such discoloration, however, usually requires a few hours to develop. Watching the abdominal response to a cough can also help one determine if there is peritoneal irritation.

Increasing abdominal distension can be a valuable sign of intra-abdominal damage.[20] If reliance is placed on subjective evaluation, however, increasing distension may not be appreciated until it is rather severe. Consequently, measurement of the abdominal girth at the umbilical level soon after the patient's admission can provide a baseline from which subsequent significant changes can be determined early and accurately. For example, if a patient's girth or circumference (C) increases from 34 inches to 35 inches and if one assumes that an enlarging abdomen assumes a somewhat spherical shape, the volume (V) of the abdomen will have increased from 10,876 cm^3 to 11,865 cm^3 (i.e., an increase of 989 ml).

AXIOM Increases in abdominal girth are best detected with serial tape measurements at the umbilicus.

PALPATION. Palpation is used primarily to determine the presence or absence of peritoneal signs or masses. The palpation must be done carefully and systematically. Sudden deep palpation may cause so much discomfort that the remainder of the exam may be difficult to interpret. Gentle palpation, beginning away from any areas of pain, is followed by examination for rebound tenderness, but only if peritonitis is not diagnosed by more gentle means. A sign that is rarely used involves gentle scratching of the skin in all four quadrants. If this elicits hyperesthesia, peritonitis is apt to be present.

If the patient has pronounced involuntary guarding, no other diagnostic studies are indicated, and the patient requires a prompt celiotomy.[1] If the patient has a "doughy" abdomen, i.e., there is some resistance but not rigidity to palpation, this may indicate a retroperitoneal process, and this finding should lead to further assessment of the pancreas, duodenum, and kidneys.

Many of the symptoms and signs seen with injury to intra-abdominal organs (pain, tenderness, guarding, and rigidity) may also be produced by a hematoma of the abdominal wall.[20] The hematoma usually results from hemorrhage into a torn rectus muscle with or without accompanying tears of the inferior or superior epigastric vessels. If the abdomen is tender when the abdominal muscles are relaxed but not when the muscles are tensed, this tends to indicate an intra-abdominal process. Diagnosis of an abdominal wall hematoma may also be aided by the demonstration of a mass which is palpable when the patient sits up or raises his legs, thereby tensing his rectus muscle, and which cannot be moved from side to side.

Although abdominal rigidity and tenderness can be important signs of peritoneal irritation by blood or intestinal contents, such signs may also be caused by fractures or contusions involving the lower ribs, iliac wings, or spine.[20] While abdominal muscle rigidity is a variable sign and sometimes difficult to assess, it is a dangerous sign to ignore. In cases of doubt, infiltration of a local anesthetic at the sites of severe rib tenderness may relieve the pain from the fractures, but it will not abolish abdominal guarding or rigidity which is due to an intra-abdominal injury.

AXIOM When doubt exists as to whether abdominal rigidity and/or severe tenderness is due to intra-abdominal trauma or an injury to the abdominal wall, one should assume that an intra-abdominal injury is present.

An abdominal mass following blunt trauma is uncommon, but it is an extremely important finding. Such masses generally represent hematomas of the liver, spleen, mesentery, or omentum.[20] Subcutaneous emphysema is an uncommon finding after abdominal trauma, but it can be very important. Crepitation in the abdominal wall is usually due to intrathoracic injury with downward dissection of air, but it may also occasionally result from injury to the retroperitoneal duodenum or distal colon.[20]

Pelvic fractures can be assessed by manual compression on both iliac wings and the pubic symphysis and hip motion. Absence of discomfort on performing these three maneuvers usually rules out a significant pelvic fracture.[25] Genital examination should include noting the presence or absence of blood at the urethral meatus or hematomas involving the penis or vagina and perineum.

On rectal examination, sphincter tone, the integrity of the rectal wall, the presence or absence of blood, and the position of the prostate should be noted. If a nonpalpable, dislocated, or high riding prostate is found, a prostato-membranous disruption of the urethra should be suspected. Vaginal lacerations or disruptions may also be caused by pelvic fractures and should be assessed by digital and speculum examination. Both flanks should also be carefully examined and palpated.

PERCUSSION. Gentle percussion of the abdomen can sometimes localize the area of maximal tenderness better than palpitation. Percussion can also be used sometimes to determine the location of the top of the liver in the chest to detect hepatomegaly even if the liver is not palpable in the abdomen. Percussion over the spleen may also reveal an enlarged area of dullness which does not move when the patient is turned (Ballance's sign). This suggests the presence of a hematoma around an injured spleen. Free blood or fluid in the peritoneal cavity will generally not cause dullness to percussion over the spleen while the patient is lying on his right side.

AUSCULTATION

AXIOM The presence of bowel sounds is a reassuring indicator of peristalsis, but it is not reliable for ruling out visceral injuries.[20]

Active bowel sounds have been thought to rule out significant intraperitoneal injuries, but up to 30% of patients will have active bowel sounds in the presence of intraperitoneal bleeding or rupture of hollow viscera.[1] Conversely, about 30% of patients who have absolutely no bowel sounds after careful listening for at least 5 minutes have no visceral damage.

Although only rarely present, a bruit, often heard better over the back than over the anterior abdomen, may be a valuable sign of an intra-abdominal arterial injury.[20]

Accuracy of Physical Examination

A careful physical examination is important, but its unreliability in the evaluation of blunt abdominal trauma has been frequently noted. A classic study from Los Angeles County Hospital in 1972 by Rosoff et al[26] pointed out that 40% of patients with significant hemoperitoneum had no clinical abdominal signs of this problem. In another study, 45% of liver injuries were discovered only at the time of autopsy and were not suspected clinically prior to death.[27] Similarly, up to 20% of splenic injuries may present as "delayed rupture," which is more accurately defined as "delayed diagnosis." It has also been found that up to 9% of patients suddenly dying after trauma may do so because of unrecognized hemorrhage from an isolated splenic injury.[28]

Olsen and Hildreth,[29] in a series of 70 trauma patients without any sensory impairment, noted that only 48% of their patients with positive findings for intra-abdominal injury on physical examination had significant injuries at the time of surgery. Conversely, 46% of their patients with negative physical findings were found to have important intra-abdominal injuries. In another study of 58 patients who sustained blunt abdominal trauma, Bivens et al[30] reported a 56% false-positive rate and a 34% false-negative rate for physical examination.

AXIOM Using physical findings as the only guide for performing a laparotomy can lead to unacceptable delays in treatment with resultant increased mortality and morbidity rates.

Physical examination for penetrating wounds of the anterior abdomen is more reliable than it is for blunt abdominal trauma.[1] Nevertheless, Bull and Mathewson[31] reported a false-positive rate of 18% and a false-negative rate of 23% for physical signs for their patients with penetrating trauma. Thal et al[32] reported a 16% false-positive rate and a 20% false-negative rate for physical examination of abdominal gunshot wounds. Thompson et al[33] reported similar results.

LABORATORY STUDIES

Complete Blood Count

The initial hemoglobin and hematocrit levels do not usually reflect the amount of recent hemorrhage that has occurred and tend to be deceptively high.[20] At least several hours are usually required for hemodilution due to transcapillary refill or exogenous fluid to be accurately reflected in the hematocrit. Nevertheless, these values can serve as a baseline and are important if a general anesthetic is necessary. A progressive fall in hemoglobin and hematocrit levels in the absence of hypotension can also serve as a warning of continuing bleeding, but this tends to be a relatively late finding.

AXIOM A hemoglobin level less than 10.0 g/dl may not provide adequate oxygen transport during anesthesia if the patient is elderly or has a relatively low cardiac output.

Trauma usually causes some leukocytosis, but injury to the spleen should be suspected in the well-hydrated patient in whom the leukocyte and platelet counts rise rapidly to above 20,000/mm^3 and 600,000/mm^3 respectively.[20]

Serum Amylase

Serum amylase levels must be interpreted with caution following abdominal trauma. A rising level of serum amylase and/or a persistent hyperamylasemia is suggestive, but not pathognomonic, of pancreatic injury.[20,34] In a series of 179 patients with blunt abdominal trauma, only three of 36 patients with hyperamylasemia had pancreatic injuries proven at operation.[35] Equally important, many patients with pancreatic injury have no rise in serum amylase.

AXIOM   Many false-positive and false-negative results occur when using serum amylase levels to diagnosis pancreatic injury.

An elevated serum amylase must be placed in proper perspective following abdominal trauma, recognizing that many patients with hyperamylasemia do not have pancreatic injuries and may in fact have no demonstrable visceral damage. Presumably, in this latter group, injury to organs making non-pancreatic amylase has occurred. In some cases, the hyperamylasemia may have been due to spasm of the sphincter of Oddi, possibly because certain narcotic drugs, such as morphine, had been given.[20]

RADIOLOGIC STUDIES

When the condition of the patient permits, important information can sometimes be derived from radiologic examinations, particularly in patients with gunshot wounds and patients with multiple injuries.[20] In patients with abdominal trauma, flat and upright films of the abdomen and an upright film of the chest are desirable. Not infrequently, however, upright films may not be possible because of the poor clinical condition of the patient. In such circumstances, a lateral decubitus film of the abdomen may be substituted. In the presence of severe hemorrhage and shock, it is necessary to exercise judgment in the use of x-rays. Volume replacement and laparotomy obviously have priority if the patient is hemodynamically unstable.

PITFALL ⊘

The delay and extra movement caused by an insistence on "routine" radiologic examinations can be extremely dangerous in patients with abdominal trauma.

X-rays of the Chest

One of the most important initial diagnostic studies in patients with multiple severe trauma is the chest x-ray. This can rapidly indicate whether or not the pleural cavities are a source of major blood loss or may have damage or disease that can interfere with adequate ventilation and oxygenation.

It is also important to examine the lower lung fields and the outlines of the diaphragms very carefully to rule out a possible diaphragmatic injury.[20] Even minimal abnormalities, especially in the dyspneic patient, may provide significant clues. The presence of stomach or intestines in the left chest may be clearly evident with the patient supine but may be difficult to determine when the patient is upright. The organs may also be pushed back into the abdominal cavity if the patient is on a ventilator.

X-rays of the Abdomen

Flat films of the abdomen can be of great help in detecting: (a) radiopaque foreign bodies such as bullets, (b) separation of loops of intestine by fluid, (c) loss of the psoas shadow, or (d) air around the right kidney or along the right psoas margins.[20] The entrance and exit wounds of any penetrating wound should be covered with a sterile dressing with a radiopaque marker so that the presumed trajectory of the missile or weapon can be determined on the x-rays.

Plain films can diagnose intraperitoneal blood and disruption of a hollow viscous in up to a third of patients.[1] A general haziness or ground glass appearance of the abdomen on x-ray may be caused by the accumulation of fluid or blood in the peritoneal cavity; however, this generally requires a considerable quantity of fluid, and it is a late sign of intraperitoneal hemorrhage.

Intraperitoneal blood should be suspected on x-ray if one sees: (a) a prominent flank stripe due to fluid separating the ascending or descending colon from the peritoneal wall; (the flank stripe often results from blood accumulation in the lateral pericolic gutters with medial displacement of the colon); (b) the "hepatic angle sign" which is loss of definition of the usually distinct inferior and right lateral borders of the liver due to blood accumulation between the hepatic angle and the right lateral peritoneal wall; and (c) the "dog ear sign" which consists of bilateral zones of increased density lying superior to the bladder due to blood accumulating in the space between the pelvic viscera and its side walls.[1] The presence of one or more of these signs indicates the presence of at least 800 ml of intraperitoneal blood. False-positive results are not uncommon, but these can generally be ruled out with diagnostic peritoneal lavage.[30]

Free air on a right or left lateral decubitus abdominal x-ray generally indicates a torn viscus. An abnormal gas pattern or air bubbles in or around the right kidney or along the psoas should make one suspect retroperitoneal rupture of the duodenum or right colon. Occasionally, mediastinal air will accumulate because of an external chest injury or from interstitial emphysema caused by mechanical ventilatory support, and this air can then dissect down into the abdomen.

Free air is most reliably seen if the patient is able to remain upright or on his side for at least 10 minutes prior to the radiologic examination. This allows time for air to accumulate under the diaphragm or along the flank.[20] Absence of free air does not, however, rule out intraperitoneal rupture of a hollow viscus.

Fractures of lower ribs, spine, or pelvis should direct attention to possible injuries of adjacent organs such as the liver, spleen, or bladder.[20] Changes in the outline or position of these organs or the gastric air bubble should be noted.

Pelvic X-rays

X-rays of the pelvis should be obtained on all patients with severe blunt trauma to the abdomen, especially if the patient is hypotensive without any obvious source of bleeding or if physical examination reveals any localized tenderness in that area. If a plain x-ray of the pelvis is negative, it is unlikely that the pelvis is a source of major blood loss, even if further x-rays or a CT scan reveal some fractures. If a severe pelvic fracture is seen on plain x-rays, it could be a source of major hemorrhage, and an orthopedic surgeon should be consulted for possible emergency external fixation.

Contrast GI Studies

A gastrographin swallow and upper GI series may be helpful for diagnosing injury to the stomach, duodenum, proximal jejunum or diaphragm. More distal small intestinal studies require a barium follow-through. A gastrographin or barium enema may be helpful for diagnosing rectal or colonic injury.

Retrograde Urethrograms or Cystograms

If injury to the bladder or male urethra is suspected, a retrograde urethrogram and cystogram should be performed. Urethral injuries should be suspected if there is blood at the urethral meatus, perineal or penile hematomas, displacement of the prostate, or severe anterior pelvic fractures. Injuries to the bladder should also be suspected with anterior pelvic fractures, especially if the patient has gross hematuria and/or cannot urinate.[36]

Intravenous Pyelography (IVP)

The role of the IVP for diagnosis of renal injury is increasingly questioned because CT scans of the abdomen with intravenous contrast will usually provide much clearer delineation of renal anatomy and injuries. If the mechanism of injury, its location, physical examination, or urinalysis suggest a renal injury and the patient is unstable or CT scanning is not rapidly available, one can attempt to get an emergency one-shot IVP in the ED or OR by rapidly infusing 150-200 ml of 60% Renografin and getting flat films of the abdomen prior to the infusion and 1 and 5 minutes later.

If there is only minor microscopic hematuria (<50 red cells per high power field), a repeat urinalysis may be indicated before determining the need for contrast urography. It should be remembered, however, that up to 25% of patients with renal injuries requiring a nephrectomy have no hematuria because the renal pedicle or ureter is torn and, in such patients, the mechanism and/or location of the injury is the main indication for urography.

Abdominal Angiography

Angiography is used infrequently now for evaluating abdominal injuries, but it can be extremely helpful in selected patients with trauma to solid organs or various vessels that are actively bleeding.[20,37,38] Interventional radiology can be particularly helpful for managing continued severe bleeding in the pelvis.[39]

If a kidney is not visualized on an IVP or CT scan with intravenous contrast, renal arteriography has generally been considered to be mandatory.[40] Arteriography is also indicated if physical examination reveals an abdominal thrill or bruit.

RADIOISOTOPE SCANNING

Although radioisotope scanning is a relatively simple noninvasive technique for outlining the liver, spleen, and kidneys, it has only a limited role to play in the management of blunt abdominal trauma.[41] Liver-spleen and renal scans can display a distorted organ contour in cases of subcapsular hematoma, or areas of absent or poor uptake representing major organ disruption. Unfortunately, fine anatomic detail is not obtainable, and small areas of parenchymal injury can easily be missed.[1] In addition, false-positive images can be caused by congenital defects or other lesions not related to trauma (e.g., cysts or hemangiomas). Although this technique has revealed a number of clinically occult lesions in solid organs after trauma, many of these otherwise inapparent defects return to normal without operation.

LOCAL WOUND EXPLORATION

During the past 25 years, three different approaches have been used on stable patients with stab wounds of the abdomen: (a) mandatory celiotomy for all penetrating trauma to the abdomen; (b) selective celiotomy based on physical examination and laboratory findings; and (c) local wound exploration, with or without diagnostic peritoneal lavage, followed by celiotomy as needed.[1] Because more than 25% of stab wounds of the anterior abdominal wall do not penetrate the peritoneal cavity,[42] a policy of mandatory exploration can be a costly and inefficient method for evaluation.

Selective celiotomy based on physical examination and laboratory findings has been practiced to some degree in many institutions (Fig. 20-1). Patients who are hemodynamically stable and without evidence of visceral penetration may be observed, regardless of whether or not peritoneal penetration has been demonstrated. In a 10-year retrospective study in which 219 stab wound patients were managed selectively, the negative celiotomy rate was 7.8%, the false-negative examination rate was 5.5%, and the overall mortality was 2.3%.[43]

Another approach to stable patients who have anterior abdominal stab wounds is to perform local wound exploration to determine whether peritoneal penetration has occurred. Local wound exploration consists of extending the stab wound entrance site under local anesthesia so that one can examine the tract and the anterior abdominal fascia visually for penetration.[44] If it is clear that the stab wound does not penetrate the anterior fascia, the patient can be discharged home. If the stab wound does penetrate the fascia, one can elect to explore the patient, perform a DPL, or just observe the patient.[45] The incidence of a negative or non-therapeutic celiotomy

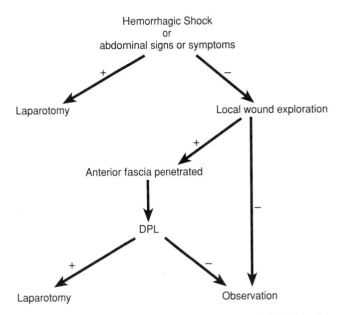

FIGURE 20-1 Management of abdominal stab wounds. (Modified from Keating JP, Yeaton NS. Diagnostic peritoneal lavage: indications, results, and complications. Resident and Staff Physician 1991;37:31.)

in patients with evidence of anterior fascial penetration on local wound exploration is about 22-26%.[46,47] Many surgeons consider this negative exploration rate to be acceptable because the morbidity associated with a negative celiotomy in stab wound victims is only 1.5-3.0%.[31,46]

Although many surgeons would automatically explore the abdomen if exploration of the tract revealed that the stab wound penetrated the anterior fascia, others would like more proof that a laparotomy is really needed. For example, if a DPL is performed and is negative, a laparotomy is not indicated. If the DPL results are positive only because of increased RBCs, one can elect either to observe the patient carefully or explore the abdomen. If the DPL reveals an elevated WBC count or bile, amylase, or food particles are present, the abdomen should be explored.

Digital or probe exploration of a stab wound alone provides very little information unless the finger or probe goes directly into the abdomen and, under such circumstances, the probe could damage bowel or restart bleeding that had previously ceased. In general, one should not probe abdominal stab wounds.

AXIOM The safest policy with stab wounds is to explore the abdomen if any question of visceral injury exists.

Stabograms

As long as the accepted practice was to perform a laparotomy for all stab wounds which penetrated into the peritoneal cavity, knowledge of the depth of penetrating wounds was extremely important.[20] To facilitate this determination Cornell et al[48] developed the technique of introducing 60-80 ml of contrast material via a Foley catheter sutured tightly into the anesthetized stab wound. Anterior, posterior, and lateral roentgenograms were taken to reveal whether or not the contrast material entered the peritoneal cavity. This technique, however, has generally been abandoned because of an unacceptable number of false-negative results.[49]

ABDOMINAL PARACENTESIS

In the 1950s, the technique of four-quadrant needle taps to attempt aspiration of fluid from the peritoneal cavity was frequently used as a diagnostic tool in cases of suspected intra-abdominal injury.[20] The recovery of nonclotting blood, bile, intestinal fluid, or fluid with a high amylase content was highly suggestive of intra-abdominal bleeding or organ damage. This approach was thought to be particularly useful in comatose patients and in those in whom an unnecessary laparotomy might be extremely deleterious. Unfortunately, false-negative results are so common with this technique that a negative tap has no diagnostic significance.

> **AXIOM** Although a positive abdominal tap in an injured patient is of great diagnostic value, a negative tap should never be regarded as definitive.

As an improvement on this technique, tube paracentesis (without lavage) using a polyethylene catheter through a 15-gauge short-bevel needle was advocated, and a false-negative result of only 1% was claimed;[50] however, this procedure was never very popular.

DIAGNOSTIC PERITONEAL LAVAGE

Indications

Diagnostic peritoneal lavage (DPL) was introduced in 1965 by Root et al to find a more accurate method than simple abdominal taps (paracenteses) for determining if significant abdominal injuries are present after trauma.[14] It is generally accepted that an exploratory celiotomy is indicated in patients with blunt trauma if they have: (a) hemodynamic instability, (b) severe tenderness and guarding, (c) progressive abdominal distension, (d) bleeding into the gastrointestinal tract, or (e) free intraperitoneal air. In the absence of these rather obvious indications for celiotomy on trauma patients, DPL can be of great help in deciding if exploratory surgery is indicated.

Some general indications for DPL after blunt abdominal trauma include: (a) patients in whom the physical examination is apt to be falsely negative (such as patients with head or spinal cord injuries, severe intoxication, or general anesthesia for another injury), (b) patients in whom the physical examination is apt to be falsely positive (e.g., lower rib fractures, fractures of lumbar vertebrae, abdominal wall hematomas etc), or (c) patients who will not be available for continuous examination (e.g., during angiography or multiple x-rays, etc) (Table 20-1).

In patients with head injury who require an immediate craniotomy, the DPL should be performed in the operating room. If the lavage is positive, the craniotomy and celiotomy should be performed simultaneously if at all possible. Positioning of the patient for craniotomies in certain areas of the skull, however, can make a simultaneous celiotomy extremely difficult.

Previous abdominal surgery is a relative contraindication to DPL (Table 20-2), because adhesions can compartmentalize the peritoneal cavity and also predispose the patient to iatrogenic bowel injury. One can, however, make an incision in the midline as far away from the previous incisions as possible and do an open DPL.

TABLE 20-1   Indications for DPL in Blunt Trauma

1. Unexplained hypotension, tachycardia, or anemia
2. Suspicion of false-positive abdominal findings because of:
   a. fractured lower ribs, lumbar vertebrae, or pelvis
   b. abdominal wall contusions or hematomas
3. Suspicion of false-negative abdominal findings because of:
   a. head or spinal cord injury or disease,
   b. alcohol or drug intoxication,
   c. major orthopedic or chest injuries, or
   d. psychological withdrawal or denial
4. Slight to moderate suspicion of abdominal injury when the patient will be unavailable for continued observation
   a. because of mechanism of injury, clinical findings, or other factors
   b. during diagnostic studies or major operations on other systems

TABLE 20-2   Contraindications to Diagnostic Tests

DPL
  obvious need for celiotomy
  uncooperative patient
  severe obesity ($\pm$)
  prior abdominal incisions ($\pm$)
  pregnancy ($\pm$)
CT Scan
  obvious need for celiotomy
  hemodynamic instability
  uncooperative patient
  allergy to contrast agents
  renal dysfunction $\pm$
  pregnancy $\pm$
Ultrasound
  obvious need for celiotomy
  severe obesity[a]
  subcutaneous emphysema[a]

($\pm$) = relative contraindication
[a] = main problem is poor visualization

Techniques

> **AXIOM** A diagnostic peritoneal lavage can be performed with relative safety if it is done as an open technique and avoids scars, hematomas, or a pregnant uterus.

There are basically three techniques for performing diagnostic peritoneal lavage: (a) the open technique, (b) the semi-open technique, and (c) the closed technique. The open technique is generally very safe, but it usually takes more time, and the semi-open technique is almost as safe.[51] The closed technique, which consists of blind insertion of the catheter with a sharp stylet through the skin, midline fascia, and peritoneum just inferior to the umbilicus has been associated with an unacceptably high rate of morbidity (6-8%) in some series.[52]

The open and semi-open techniques are performed with a local anesthetic, such as lidocaine with epinephrine. The stomach should first be emptied with a nasogastric tube and the bladder should be emptied with a urinary catheter.

The open technique usually begins with a 1-2 cm vertical midline infraumbilical incision (Fig. 20-2). In pregnant women and patients with pelvic fractures or previous lower abdominal incisions, the incision is made supraumbilically. The incision is extended down to the fascia and then a purse-string suture is placed in the peritoneum. The peritoneum is opened and the lavage catheter is passed through the incision into the peritoneal cavity under direct vision. The purse-string suture is then tied around the catheter.

The semi-open technique involves exposure of the midline fascia by sharp dissection followed by a transfascial and transperitoneal puncture using an 18-gauge needle with a stylet.[52] If desired, the fascia can be lifted up on either side of the proposed immature site with stay sutures of clamps to decrease the chances of injury to retroperitoneal vessels. A guide wire is then threaded through the needle, and the lavage catheter is advanced over the guide wire into the abdomen toward the pelvic cavity. The semi-open technique is generally safer than the open technique if a non-surgeon is called upon to perform the peritoneal lavage.[1]

Once the lavage catheter is in place, an attempt is made to aspirate any free intraperitoneal fluid that may be present. If 10 to 20 ml of gross blood is obtained on the initial aspiration, the DPL is considered "positive," and an exploratory celiotomy is usually mandatory. If the initial aspiration recovers no blood, then 15 ml/kg or 1000 ml (whichever is less) of 0.9% saline solution is allowed to drain by gravity rapidly into the peritoneal cavity. After the fluid has infused, the patient is turned from side to side for about 30 seconds (except in patients with suspected spinal injury) to assure good mixing of the infusate fluid with any intraperitoneal fluid. The lavage fluid is then

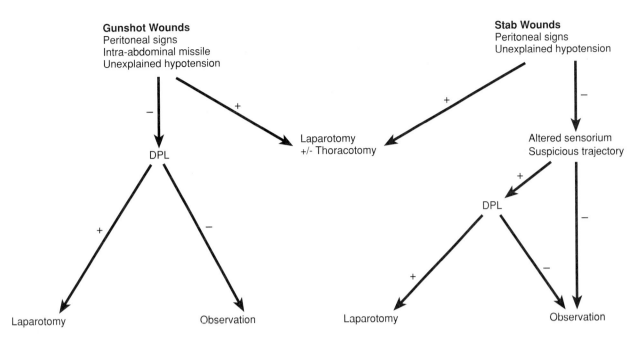

FIGURE 20-2 The open technique of diagnostic peritoneal lavage (DPL) consists of an incision into the peritoneum under direct visualization. The DPL catheter is inserted without the trocar, and directed toward the pelvis (From: Danto LA. In Blaisdell WF, Trunkey DD, eds. Trauma management 1: abdominal trauma. New York, Thieme-Stratton 1982:55.)

allowed to drain out the same tubing, using gravity, by placing the now empty bottle or container on the floor. At least 200 ml of solution should be recovered, 75 ml of which should be sent to the laboratory for analysis.[1]

Interpretation

Several parameters for interpretating the content of the lavage fluid have evolved.[53,54] Inability to read newsprint through the return fluid in the lavage tubing is interpreted as "positive." If the fluid is pink but one can read newsprint through the tubing, the result is interpreted as "indeterminate." Drainage of lavage fluid from a previously placed chest tube signifies a lacerated or ruptured diaphragm. A red blood cell (RBC) count of 100,000/mm³ or more or a white blood cell (WBC) count of 500/mm³ or more is also considered positive (Table 20-3).

TABLE 20-3 *Criteria for Interpretation of Lavage Results in Blunt Abdominal Trauma*

Positive
  Aspiration >10 ml nonclotting blood
  Lavage fluid comes out Foley catheter or chest tube
  Grossly bloody lavage return
  RBC >100,000/mm³
  WBC >500/mm³
  Amylase >175 K.U./dl
  Presence of bile, bacteria, and/or particulate matter
Indeterminate
  Aspiration <10 ml of nonclotting blood
  RBC 50,000 to 100,000/mm³
  WBC 100 to 500 mm³
  Amylase 75 to 175 K.U./dl
Negative
  No blood aspirated
  RBC <50,000/mm³
  WBC <100/mm³
  Amylase <75 K.U./dl

(From Keating KP, Yeston NS. Diagnostic peritoneal lavage: Indications, results, and complications. Resident and Staff Physician 1991;37:31.)

In penetrating trauma, the RBC criterion for a positive averages about 10,000/mm³ but varies from 1,000 to 100,000/mm³ in various centers[55,56] (Fig. 20-3). A retrospective study[57] of 235 patients with penetrating abdominal wounds showed that when 100,000 red blood cells/mm³ was used as a criteria for celiotomy, no false-positives resulted, but there was an 11.4% false-negative rate. When 10,000 red blood cells/mm³ was used as a criterion for celiotomy, there were 13.6% false-positives and a more acceptable 1.0% false-negative rate.

> **AXIOM** The decision to perform an exploratory celiotomy in patients with stab wounds should not be based on set criteria or a single test, but should be individualized and based on all the information available.

The presence of feces, bile, or bacteria in the lavage fluid is also considered positive and is an indication for surgery. The WBC count is relatively reliable if the DPL is performed more than 3 hours after injury.[55,58] If the DPL is "indeterminate" or the number of WBC/mm³ is suspicious, the DPL can be repeated 3-6 hours later. The amylase level of lavage fluid has not been shown to increase the diagnostic yield,[56] but it is still frequently checked.

Results

> **AXIOM** Diagnostic peritoneal lavage is currently considered to be one of the best methods for diagnosing intraperitoneal injury after blunt trauma.

In many surgeons' hands, DPL has been extremely sensitive (98-99%) and accurate (97-98%), and missed injuries are seldom a problem.[59,60] One of main problems with DPL is that as many as 20-40% of the laparotomies done because of a positive test reveal only minor injuries that could have been treated non-operatively. Based on the report of Rosoff et al,[26] one can assume that physical examination missed about 40% of the abdominal injuries, but about half of these patients had injuries, such as a small non-bleeding laceration of the liver, that did not need surgery. Thus, DPL does not discriminate between the patients needing and those not needing a therapeutic laparotomy.

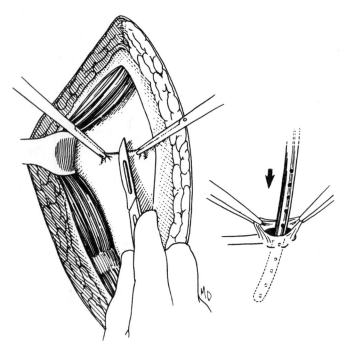

FIGURE 20-3 Management of penetrating lower chest wounds. (Modified from: Keating JP, Yeaton NS. Diagnostic peritoneal lavage: indications, results, and complications. Resident and Staff Physician 1991;37:31.)

One of the techniques suggested for increasing the sensitivity of DPL for bowel injury is measurement of the alkaline phosphatase (ALP) in the effluent. In a study of 545 DPL fluids analyzed for AP by Jaffin et al,[61] 528 had ALP levels <10. Of the 17 patients with increased ALP in the DPL fluid, 11 had small bowel injuries, three had colon injuries, and two had ruptured ovarian cysts. The only bowel injury missed was one involving the colon. Thus, the specificity was 99.4% and sensitivity 93.3%.

It has also been pointed out that, with bowel injuries, at least 3 hours usually must elapse before the WBC on a DPL rises to ≥500/mm^3. As a consequence, McAnena et al[62] evaluated the accuracy of DPL amylase (AMY) and DPL alkaline phosphatase (ALP) in 51 patients with injuries limited to one or more hollow viscera. In the 23 patients with a negative DPL based on RBC or WBC counts, all 11 with isolated SB injury had an AMY of 20 IU/L or higher and six had an ALP of 3 IU/L or higher. All six patients with colon injury and two with gallbladder injury had negative AMY and ALP studies. A patient with a stomach injury had an increased ALP but negative AMY.

In another effort to improve the accuracy of DPL, Mackart et al[63] checked DPL effluent with a urine dipstick for a protein concentration ≥1.0 gm/L and a WBC ≥500 mm^3 in 46 patients with abdominal stab wounds and equivocal physical examination. The lavage effluent was a true-positive for significant injury in 23, and false-positive in three. The 18 patients with a negative DPL dipstick did not have injuries requiring laparotomy. Thus, the sensitivity of the dipstick on DPL fluid was 100% and the specificity was 86%. The negative predictive value was 100%.

The value of DPL in the presence of a pelvic fracture is not clear. There is a fairly high incidence of red blood cells passing from the retroperitoneal pelvic hematoma into the peritoneal cavity so that up to 40% of patients with pelvic fractures may have a false-positive result by red blood cell criteria. Indeed, some investigators have found that unless more than 10-20 ml of gross blood is aspirated at the beginning of the procedure or the red cell count in the lavage fluid is 200,000/mm^3 or more, it is unlikely that a laparotomy is required. Mendez et al,[64] however, in a study of pthe accuracy of DPL in 278 patients with pelvic fractures found 80 true-positives, 194 true-

negatives, two false-positives and two false-negatives. It is not clear, however, how many of the laparotomies performed for positive DPLs were therapeutic.

The relative roles of diagnostic peritoneal lavage (DPL) and CT scans of the abdomen and pelvis in patients with abdominal trauma are still not completely clear to many surgeons. Perhaps the clearest indication for DPL is continued hemodynamic instability in a patient with multiple injuries, especially if physical examination of the abdomen cannot be performed reliably.

In evaluating the usefulness of DPL versus CT scan in blunt abdominal trauma in 301 hemodynamically stable patients, Meyer et al[65] noted a sensitivity of 96% for DPL and 74% for CT scans. Both had a specificity of 99%. The resulting accuracy was 98.2% for DPL and 92.6% for CT scans. The intra-abdominal injuries most apt to be missed on DPL are those involving bowel, diaphragm, and retroperitoneal structures.

DPL can be unreliable for evaluating patients with gunshot wounds to the abdomen,[1] and an immediate exploratory celiotomy should be performed if it is suspected that the bullet entered the peritoneal cavity or could have damaged any retroperitoneal structures. When DPL has been used in patients with gunshot wounds, false-negative rates have been reported to exceed 25%, mainly due to small bowel and colon injuries.[66]

Regarding pediatric patients, there seems to be increasing agreement that if CT scans are not available, peritoneal lavage is only indicated if the child: (a) has a neurologic injury, (b) is obtunded, (c) has multiple injuries requiring a general anesthetic, or (d) has hypotension of unknown etiology.

Computed Tomography

The concept of using CT as a diagnostic adjunct for abdominal trauma was introduced in 1981.[15] CT scans can be very helpful for diagnosing many types of intra-abdominal injury (Table 20-4). Intraperitoneal and retroperitoneal blood and most solid organ injuries can be detected in a highly reliable manner with CT scans. Whereas peritoneal lavage often cannot evaluate retroperitoneal injuries accurately, CT scans done with intravenous and oral contrast can provide rather clear images of the duodenum, liver, spleen, and kidneys.[15,66] CT scans can be very helpful for grading liver or spleen injuries and can thereby help the surgeon to make decisions regarding operative or nonoperative management. CT scans can also be extremely helpful for assessing pelvic and spinal fractures. CT scans, however, are of little help for detecting mid- or distalsmall bowel injuries. They are also not very reliable for diagnosing pancreatic or diaphragmatic injuries. The sensitivity of CT scanning for pancreatic injuries is only 85%.[1] This is partly due to the time that it takes for the pancreas to manifest injury, particularly periglandular edema. This is not too dissimilar to the brain, where approximately 12-15% of the injuries take 6-12 hours to manifest CT evidence of injury.[1]

At the present time, CT scans are generally not done in hemodynamically unstable patients. Newer generation CT scanners which can perform these examinations very rapidly, however, may obviate this

TABLE 20-4   Changes in Pulmonary Function Occurring with Pneumoperitoneum

Pulmonary Function	Change
Peak inspiratory pressure (PIP)	↑
Pulmonary compliance (dV/dT)	↓
Vital capacity (V$_c$)	↓
Functional residual capacity (FRC)	↓
Intrathoracic pressure*	↑

* The intrathoracic pressure may be further increased if the Trendelenburg position is used.
(From: Safran DB, Rocco O III. Physiologic effects of pneumoperitoneum. Am J Surg 1994;167:281.)

problem to some degree, particularly if the CT scanner is in the emergency eepartment or immediately adjacent to it.

Patients who have blunt torso trauma and are hemodynamically stable can be evaluated using contrast-enhanced CT imaging of the chest and abdomen.[1] If this test is normal, these patients should continue to be observed closely with serial abdominal examinations, hematocrits, white blood cell counts, and amylase determinations. Any deterioration in the patient's clinical condition mandates a celiotomy or repeat CT scan. Repeat CT scans can also be useful in patients who are suspected of having a pancreatic injury. If the initial CT scan is positive, appropriate operative management should be carried out as soon as possible.

One of the problems with using CT scans to diagnose intra-abdominal injuries is the need for a qualified radiologist to interpret the study. In some reports, lack of readily-available, well-trained radiologists to perform the studies and interpret the results has led to misdiagnoses and inadequate studies.[38]

> **AXIOM** The accuracy of abdominal ultrasonography and CT scans is largely determined by the expertise of the radiologists performing and interpreting them.

Although DPL can be extremely useful for directing therapy in adult abdominal trauma, it has lost its popularity in the pediatric setting, primarily because the presence of blood in the peritoneal cavity is not in itself an absolute indication for surgery in children.[3,8] Increasingly, CT has become the diagnostic study of choice in the management of pediatric abdominal trauma.[2,5,8,9]

Abdominopelvic CT scanning has been recommended as the preferred initial method for evaluation of hemodynamically stable blunt trauma patients. Unlike diagnostic peritoneal lavage (DPL), CT scanning is organ-specific and can detect injuries of retroperitoneal structures.

In a study of abdominal injuries discovered by CT scans performed 8-72 hours after admission, Freshman et al[68] noted that the delayed positive CT scans were done for a falling hematocrit (67%), associated injuries (28%), or abdominal tenderness (5%). They concluded that a significant number of occult injuries, some of which are life-threatening, can be detected by delayed CT scans; however, a hematocrit drop under observation is not a good predictor of occult abdominal injury.

One of the more important criticisms of CT scanning of the abdomen after trauma has been the delay caused by insisting on administration of oral contrast. In a recent study, Kinnunen et al[69] found that the upper GI contrast was not really necessary. Of 32 patients not given peroral contrast, 18 had an emergency laparotomy after the initial CT examination. The CT revealed all but one of the severe parenchymal organ injuries found at surgery, and in that one patient, a hemoperitoneum was seen. Bowel and mesenteric lesions also caused a hemoperitoneum which was seen on CT. Fourteen other patients also had some findings on the abdominal CT but did not have a laparotomy. Ten of these 14 patients had a repeat CT within three days, but none of the repeat CT scans revealed a lesion requiring surgery. There were no problems related to the nonoperative management of these patients. Thus, in this study, omission of the oral contrast did not jeopardize making the essential diagnoses, and it did save time.

Contrast-enhanced CT Enema

Contrast-enhanced CT enemas (CECTE) using double contrast (intravenous and colonic) or triple contrast (intravenous, oral, and colonic) CT scans are an important advance in the selective management of penetrating injuries to the flank and back. This technique can also be very useful in evaluating suspected renal and renal vascular injuries. In one series of patients with penetrating injuries of the flank or back, an injury requiring a celiotomy was successfully ruled out in 92% of the patients on the basis of a CECTE.[67]

In a recent study by McAllister et al[70] on 53 patients with stab wounds of the back, 51 (96%) either had negative findings on CECTE (n = 31) or injuries not requiring exploration (n = 20). In the two patients in which CECTE revealed injuries requiring surgery, other clinical indications for surgery were also present.

THE ROLE OF LAPAROSCOPY IN ABDOMINAL TRAUMA

Laparoscopy is being performed increasingly in many areas of surgery. In trauma patients, it may be particularly helpful for determining if a laparotomy is required, and for certain mild or moderate injuries, it can be therapeutic.

Salvino et al[71] compared the sensitivity and specificity of diagnostic laparoscopy (DL) and diagnostic peritoneal lavage (DPL) in 59 patients with blunt trauma and 16 with stab wounds. Of the 75 DPLs, 70 (93%) were performed in the ED. Forty-two patients had a negative DPL and DL. Of 25 who had a negative DPL and abnormal DL, 4 had diaphragmatic injuries requiring surgery. Three patients had a positive DPL but insignificant DL findings which were confirmed at laparotomy.

In a study of 28 hemodynamically stable patients with no overt signs of peritoneal penetration by Sosa et al,[72] laparoscopy showed that there was no peritoneal violation in 22 (79%), and all of these patients successfully avoided laparotomy. Townsend et al[73] performed diagnostic laparoscopy in 15 patients with CT evidence of solid organ injury. Seven patients had a laparotomy based on laparoscopic findings which included hollow viscus injury in two, ongoing bleeding in four, and poor visualization of the solid organ injury in one. The remaining eight patients did well with non-operative management.

In a similar study by Brandt et al[74] on 21 trauma patients with clinical criteria for laparotomy, laparoscopy was found to be 100% accurate for preventing non-therapeutic laparotomies. Although it missed some specific injuries, this did not contribute to any complications.

Ivatury et al[75] evaluated laparoscopy in 100 patients with penetrating abdominal trauma. The laparoscopy was very accurate for hemoperitoneum, solid organ and diaphragmatic injuries and retroperitoneal hematomas. Gastrointestinal damage, however, was detected in only two of the nine patients with such injuries. The authors concluded that the major role of laparoscopy in penetrating abdominal trauma is in avoiding unnecessary laparotomy in tangential injuries. Dalton et al[76] also found that laparoscopy significantly reduced the incidence of non-therapeutic celiotomies for abdominal stab wounds from 54% (7/13) to 19% (5/26).

In a report by Sosa et al[77] on 100 patients with abdominal gunshot wounds, diagnostic laparoscopy was positive for peritoneal violation or intraperitoneal blood in 36%. Of these, a therapeutic laparotomy was performed in 28 (78%). There were no delayed laparotomies and no false-negative laparoscopies. In the patients with isolated abdominal injury and a negative laparoscopy, the mean hospital stay was 1.4 days.

Although diagnostic laparoscopy can be very helpful in evaluating patients with penetrating abdominal injuries, there is some concern that bowel injuries could be missed. In addition, there is some concern that the increased intra-abdominal pressure might have some adverse ventilatory effects (Table 20-4). Indeed, if an abdominal vein is injured and venous pressures are very low, in theory one could quickly cause large amounts of CO_2 to enter the vascular system with resulting CO_2 emboli to the heart and lungs, and even portions of the systemic circulation.

Another concern is possible creation of a tension pneumothorax in patients with penetrating injuries involving the diaphragm. However, Rudston-Brown et al[78] have found that the risk of producing a tension pneumothorax during laparoscopy under such circumstances using intra-abdominal pressures up to 20 mm Hg appears to be very low.

In patients with marginal cardiovascular function requiring positive end-expiratory pressures (PEEP), there might be adverse cardiovascular effects (Table 20-5). Indeed, in a study of the hemodynamic effects of laparoscopy on swine that were mechanically ventilated and had varying amounts of positive end-expiratory pressure (PEEP),

TABLE 20-5 *Hemodynamic Reponse to Hypercarbia and Pneumoperitoneum*

Hemodynamic Measurement	Change with Hypercarbia*	Change with Increased IP[+]*
Mean arterial pressure (MAP)	↑	↑
Systemic vascular resistance (SVR)	↓	↑
Cardiac output (CO)	↑	↑↓+§
Central venous pressure (CVP)	↑	↑↓+
Inferior vena caval resistance		↑
Heart rate (HR)	↑	↑
Stroke volume (SV)	↑	↑↓

* The pCO_2 ranged from 55 to 75 mm Hg
** The intraperitoneal pressure was 15 mm Hg
+ Changes correlated with intravascular volume status
§ Changes may be dependent upon the baseline myocardial reserve

(From: Safran DB, Rocco O III. Physiologic effects of pneumoperitoneum. Am J Surg 1994;167:281.)

Moffa et al[79] found a 15 mm Hg pneumoperitoneum increased systemic and pulmonary vascular resistance. This increased ventricular afterload may not be tolerated in individuals with marginal cardiac function and could exacerbate the adverse effects of any PEEP that is being used.

Diagnostic laparoscopy might also interfere with intra-abdominal blood flow, especially in the presence of hypovolemia. Diebel et al[80] showed that at just 10 mm Hg intra-abdominal passive in pigs, hepatic artery flow was reduced by 39%, portal venous blood flow was reduced by 27% and hepatic microvascular blood flow (HMVBF) was reduced by 19%. As IAP was increased, all of these flow parameters decreased even more.

Josephs et al[81] recently showed that diagnostic laparoscopy with a pneumoperitoneum of 15 mm Hg might be injurious in patients with severe head injuries. In normovolemic ventilated pigs, a pneumoperitoneum of 15 mm Hg increased ICP about 5.3 mm Hg ($13.5 \pm 0.7 \rightarrow 18.7 \pm 1.5$ mm Hg) ($P < 0.001$). If an epidural balloon was inflated to raise the ICP to 22.6 ± 1.9 mm Hg, the pneumoperitoneum increased the ICP to 27.4 ± 0.9 mm Hg ($P < 0.001$). These changes occurred in spite of maintaining the P_aCO_2 at about 35 mm Hg. Thus, diagnostic laparoscopy must be used cautiously in the 30% of patients with blunt abdominal trauma who also have an intracranial injury.

THORACOSCOPY

If a diaphragmatic injury is possible, if appropriate laparoscopic or thoracoscopic skills are available, and if the patient can be intubated with a split function endotracheal tube, one can examine the diaphragm through the chest with a thoracoscope.[82,83] One must, however, be concerned about the pneumothorax produced during the procedure, particularly if the patient has any pulmonary insufficiency.

ULTRASOUND

There has been increasing interest in the use of ultrasound, particularly in emergency departments, to diagnose intrathoracic and abdominal injuries. It can be used to detect collections of fluid in the pericardial, pleural, or peritoneal spaces quite accurately and easily. It can also be helpful for detecting abnormalities of the gallbladder and bile ducts. Evaluation of the pancreas largely depends on how obese the patient is and whether gas-filled loops of bowel are interposed between the pancreas and the anterior abdominal wall. Ultrasound can also be used in the pelvis to detect fluid collections or abnormal masses.

In a retrospective study of 1151 patients in a nonrandomized control trial by Glaser et al[84] at the University Hospital of Innsbruck (Austria), all patients with blunt abdominal or thoracic trauma were divided into three groups based on US findings: immediate operation

for US finding, primary conservative treatment in spite of positive US findings, and non-operative treatment for normal ultrasonographic findings. US was repeated when clinical findings or laboratory tests showed the development of intra-abdominal hemorrhage or signs of hollow organ laceration. US showed a sensitivity of 99%, a specificity of 98%, a positive predictive value of 0.97, and a negative predictive value of 0.99; however, they found that US was not reliable in patients with intestinal perforation or large retroperitoneal hematomas.

Lin et al[85] in a prospective study reported in 1993 compared the accuracy of US with DPL and CT in 55 hemodynamically stable patients with blunt trauma and equivocal findings on physical examination. Surgery was performed in 39 patients and 36 of these patients had abdominal injuries. The results of the three tests were as follows:

	DPL	CT	US
Sensitivity	100%	97%	92%
Specificity	89%	95%	95%
Accuracy	95%	96%	93%

With bowel perforation DPL detected 7/7, CT detected intra-abdominal fluid in 6/7, and US detected intra-abdominal fluid in 4/7. In general, DPL had a slightly greater sensitivity than CT (100% versus 97%), but CT had a higher specificity (95% versus 84%). The authors emphasized that these examinations should be considered complementary to each other.

In a somewhat similar study, McKenney et al[86] compared US with CT and DPL in 200 patients with blunt abdominal trauma. For US, the sensitivity was 83%, specificity 100%, and accuracy 97%. Six injuries were missed, but only one was seen to be significant. Consequently, the authors felt that US would have resulted in appropriate care in 199 of the 200 patients.

In a similar study by Goletti et al[87] US was performed on 250 patients with blunt abdominal trauma. The sensitivity was 98% for detecting free intra-abdominal fluid. The overall sensitivity and specificity for solid organ injuries were: spleen 93% and 99%, liver 80% and 100%, and kidney 100% and 100%. Three stable patients also had a therapeutic laparotomy on the basis of US-guided paracentesis.

In the largest US study from the United States, Rozycki et al[88] reported on its use in 250 patients with blunt trauma and 55 with penetrating injuries. The time for each US exam averaged 2.5 minutes. There were 41 (13.4%) true-positive examinations and only two (5%) of these had non-therapeutic laparotomies. There were no false-positive US studies. There were 253 (83%) true-negative and 11 (3.6%) false-negative exams. The 11 patients with false-negative exams had a laparotomy because of mechanism of injury (seven penetrating) or change in clinical exam (four blunt). The costs for the CT exams ($650/patient) and DPLs ($150/patient) that were not done resulted in an $80,000 savings.

It has been found that US can be used to quantify the amount of intra-abdominal fluid rather accurately. To quantify further the amount of intra-abdominal fluid seen on US, Huang et al[89] performed abdominal US before and after infusion of 1000 ml of fluid used for a DPL study in 10 patients. Following the peritoneal infusion, all 10 patients had a score of 3 or more on the scoring system the authors developed. This system of US scoring of hemoperitoneum was then used in 49 patients with blunt trauma. Of 15 patients with an US score ≥3, 24 (96%) required a therapeutic laparotomy. In contrast, of 24 patients with an US score of only 1 or 2, only nine (38%) required a therapeutic laparotomy.

In a prospective clinical study by Akgur et al[90] on 68 children with blunt abdominal trauma, all patients with "pathologic" US findings underwent CT examination before DPL to confirm the pathology. US revealed free-intraperitoneal fluid (FIF) in 11 patients and intraperitoneal solid organ injuries in 11 patients, but DPL was positive in only 10 of these. While US detected renal injuries in six patients and intrapleural fluid in two patients, DPL was positive in only two of these patients as a result of the concomitant FIF. Thus, US detected FIF with a high rate of accuracy. In addition, US had advantages over DPL in the detection of intraperitoneal, retroperitoneal and intrathoracic injuries. The authors recommended US as the routine first-choice screening tool in the initial evaluation of children sustaining blunt abdominal trauma.

ENDOSCOPY

Injuries that may involve the stomach or duodenum can be investigated with esophagogastroduodenoscopy (EGD). In most circumstances this can allow fairly good visualization down to the second and sometimes even the third part of the duodenum. If there is a perforation, however, the air insufflated into the bowel can cause a fairly severe pneumoperitoneum. If there is also a diaphragmatic injury, a rather severe pneumothorax can result.

With injuries that may involve the rectum or colon, flexible sigmoidoscopy and/or colonoscopy may be extremely helpful; however, the bowel will usually be unprepared. A Fleet's enema may allow exam of the rectum and distal sigmoid colon, but to be able to examine more of the large intestine, a more prolonged cleansing of the colon is required.

ERCP

Endoscopic retrograde cholangiopancreatography (ERCP) may be indicated in a stable patient if an injury to the pancreatic duct or the extrahepatic biliary tract is suspected and a celiotomy is not planned.[91] ERCP may also be helpful in patients with severe pancreaticoduodenal trauma when one is debating whether to perform a Whipple procedure (pancreatico-duodenectomy), some type of duodenal diverticulization procedure, or just local repairs with drainage.

NON-OPERATIVE MANAGEMENT

Children

With known intra-abdominal solid organ injuries in children, there is an increasing tendency for non-operative management. In a prospective study by Haller et al,[92] all severely injured children with evidence of intra-abdominal solid organ injury who remained hemodynamically stable after 40 ml/kg fluid replacement were placed in a prospective non-operative management protocol. The organs injured included 28 spleens, 25 livers, 18 kidneys, and seven pancreases. The incidence of eventual operation for each of these organs was 11%, 8%, 6%, and 43%, respectively. Three (33%) of the nine patients requiring a laparotomy died but their deaths were primarily related to head injuries in two and chest injuries in one. There were no deaths or complications in the children treated non-operatively.

Adults

In hemodynamically stable adults with injuries involving the spleen, liver, or kidney, there is an increasing tendency to treat them nonoperatively but with careful observation for several days. However, if the patient requires more than two units of blood to maintain stable vital signs or if there is clinical evidence of peritonitis, an exploratory celiotomy is indicated.

INDICATIONS FOR LAPAROTOMY (Table 20-1)

> **AXIOM** Of the patients with intra-abdominal trauma who reach a hospital alive, 20-30% of those who die do so because of delayed, inadequate, or inappropriate treatment.

Blunt Trauma

CONTINUED HYPOTENSION

With Isolated Abdominal Trauma

Significant intra-abdominal bleeding and/or visceral damage are the main indications for laparotomy following trauma. Intra-abdominal bleeding should be strongly suspected if the patient comes to the hospital in severe shock or if mild-moderate shock is persistent or recurs despite what should be adequate replacement of blood and fluid.[20]

In a Patient Who Also Has a Widened Mediastinum

If a blunt trauma victim is hemodynamically unstable on arrival and does not respond to resuscitation but is also noted to have a widened mediastinum, the surgeon must assume that the widened mediastinum is *not* the cause of shock, and an immediate celiotomy should be performed.[1] Once a traumatic tear of the aorta begins to bleed into the pleural cavity, death from exsanguination generally occurs very rapidly. If a patient is suspected of having a traumatic rupture of the aorta, the systolic BP should not be allowed to rise above 110-120 mm Hg. Adequate pain relief with analgesics or local blocks and alpha and/or beta-adrenergic blockers may be required to accomplish this.

> **AXIOM** Diagnosis and treatment of a suspected traumatic rupture of the aorta has precedence over all but the most life-threatening other injuries.

As soon as the intra-abdominal hemorrhage has been controlled and the laparotomy rapidly completed, a thoracotomy should be performed or the patient should be taken to the arteriogram suite to determine if a contained rupture of the thoracic aorta is present. If a contained thoracic aortic rupture is present, the patient should be returned to the operating room for repair; however, if the patient is an extremely high operative risk because of severe associated injuries, one can treat the patient medically as for a dissecting aneurysm of the descending thoracic aorta until the risk of surgery is reasonable.

If the patient arrives in or is rapidly converted to a hemodynamically stable condition with evidence of abdominal trauma and is found to have a widened mediastinum, an aortogram should be performed. If the patient remains hemodynamically stable, and a contained aortic tear is found, it can be repaired according to the guidelines mentioned above.

Abdominal Bleeding and Pelvic Fractures

If the patient has an unstable pelvic fracture and is hemodynamically unstable in spite of aggressive fluid and blood resuscitation, an immediate celiotomy should be performed. If no intra-abdominal injury is found or if the major bleeding can be controlled but the patient remains hypotensive and there is a large pelvic hematoma, the abdomen should be closed, and an external fixator should be applied. In the experience of Trunkey et al,[1] 85% of the severe bleeding seen with pelvic fractures is venous in origin and only 15% is arterial. The venous bleeding will usually tamponade if the peritoneum is intact and an external fixator is applied to the anterior pelvis. If the bleeding continues in spite of pelvic fixation, the patient should be taken to the arteriogram suite immediately for localization and embolization of any arterial bleeders.

> **AXIOM** Massive bleeding from an unstable pelvic fracture should have prompt external fixation and therapeutic angiography.

If the patient has an open pelvic fracture and is exsanguinating, the perineal wound should be packed, and a pneumatic anti-shock garment can be applied. With large perineal wounds associated with a pelvic fracture, a diverting sigmoid colostomy should be performed after the major bleeding is controlled and the patient is no longer hypotensive.

If the patient has an emergency urethrogram or cystogram and it reveals a tear in the urethra or bladder, no further diagnostic studies are indicated because suprapubic drainage of the bladder should be carried out in the operating room, and a thorough exploration of the abdomen can be carried out at the same time.

BLOOD TRANSFUSIONS

An important factor in the equation for determining operative versus nonoperative management is whether or not the patient can be managed without administering blood. Although this is controversial, some surgeons feel that the risks inherent in receiving more than two units of blood outweigh the risks of a negative or non-therapeutic laparotomy.[93,94]

> **AXIOM** The risks of receiving more than two units of blood generally outweigh the risks of a negatve or non-therapeutic laparatomy.

BOWEL PERFORATION/PERITONITIS

If there is any clinical or radiologic evidence of bowel perforation or peritonitis, the patient should be explored promptly. Unfortunately, if a duodenal perforation is missed for more than 24 to 48 hours, the mortality rate may exceed 50%.[95] Diagnosis of perforations of the stomach or duodenum is facilitated by the oral contrast on the CT scan. Distal colon injuries may be detected by a contrast CT enema. With the remaining bowel, the first evidence of injury may be an elevated WBC on DPL. One should also suspect bowel or mesentery injury if the DPL after blunt trauma shows more than 25,000 RBC/mm^3 and there is no solid organ injury on the CT scan.

CLINICAL FACTORS

Cushing and Morris,[96] in an analysis of 9462 blunt trauma victims, recently reported a number of clinical, laboratory, and radiologic findings that were associated with an increased incidence of abdominal organ injuries. The incidence of abdominal injury with some of the more important indicators included: an admission systolic P <90 mm Hg (39% = 176/449), hemopneumothorax (34% = 232/691), pulmonary contusion or laceration (32% = 140/442) and lower rib (7-12) fractures (30% = 169/572).

Stab Wounds

SELECTIVE OBSERVATION

Anterior Stab Wounds

The management of abdominal stab wounds in patients who are hemodynamically stable and have no peritoneal irritation or radiologic evidence of penetration is controversial. One approach increasingly being advocated is continued observation unless there is clear evidence that a laparotomy is needed. Advocates of this approach point out that a negative laparotomy causes needless expense and may be associated with significant morbidity and mortality rates[20] Nance et al,[97] following a policy of selective observation of 393 patients with stab wounds, reduced the percentage of patients explored for abdominal stab wounds from 95% to 45% with a clear improvement in overall results.

Although condemned by many surgeons, a similar policy was used by Nance for patients with abdominal gunshot wounds, with no complications occurring in 52 patients who were observed and did not have surgery.[97] Considering the likelihood of significant injuries following a gunshot wound of the abdomen, however, it is unlikely that many surgeons would be comfortable with such a strongly selective approach.[70,71]

Stab Wounds of the Back or Flank

Lateral or posterior abdominal stab wounds in hemodynamically stable patients cause visceral injury in about 12% and 7% of patients, respectively.[1] In such patients, a CT scan done with triple contrast

(intravenous, gastric, and colonic) can generally rule out a retroperitoneal colon or duodenal injury quite well.[1] If this study is negative, the patient can be carefully observed for 24 to 48 hours. If the clinical condition deteriorates or signs of peritonitis develop, the patient is promptly explored. Although such a policy can work well with experienced trauma teams, for the surgeon who treats trauma patients only occasionally, routine celiotomy is probably the safest approach.[1]

INDICATIONS FOR SURGERY

The most frequent indications for surgery in patients with a stab wound of the abdomen include unstable vital signs, need for more than two units of blood, evidence of peritonitis or bowel injury, and evidence of diaphragmatic injury. Some surgeons believe that any evidence that the stab wound extends through the anterior abdominal fascia is an indication for surgery; however, such a regimen will result in non-therapeutic laparotomies in at least 40% of those patients.

Whether or not to explore the abdomen of patients in whom omental or intestinal evisceration occurs through a stab wound is somewhat controversial.[1] Most surgeons think such eviscerations are obvious evidence of peritoneal penetration and are an indication for immediate exploratory celiotomy. In one series of 75 patients with eviscerations through abdominal stab wounds, major intra-abdominal injuries were found in 83%. Furthermore, a negative celiotomy in these patients did not contribute to significant morbidity. Thompson et al,[33] however, reported a 29% rate of unnecessary celiotomies and a 35% morbidity using omental evisceration as an indication for abdominal exploration.

Gunshot Wounds

It is generally thought that all patients with gunshot wounds that may have entered the peritoneal cavity should have an exploratory laparotomy. There are, however, a certain number of gunshot wounds in hemodynamically stable patients which appear to be tangential, and it is questionable whether any of the abdominal organs have been injured. In individuals with flank gunshot wounds, abdominal and pelvic CT examinations with rectal and intravenous contrast can be extremely helpful. In tangential abdominal or flank gunshot wounds, laparoscopy may be very helpful for determining if the peritoneal cavity was entered.

It can also be difficult to determine which hemodynamically stable patients with pelvic and/or gluteal gunshot wounds require exploration. With gluteal gunshot wounds, only 22-32% have major injuries. In a recent report by DiGiacomo et al,[98] the hospital records of 52 patients with gunshot injuries to the gluteal region were reviewed. Of the 52 patients, 18 were operated acutely and 15 had therapeutic laparotomies; 33 patients were managed non-operatively, but one of the patients required a laparotomy for a retroperitoneal colon injury on his second hospital day. The only mortality occurred in a patient with a concomitant gunshot wound to the head.

The presence or absence of gross blood in the urine or on rectal exam was 100% accurate in identifying GU and rectosigmoid injuries respectively.[98] Rigid proctosigmoidoscopy was falsely negative in one of four cases, but 100% accurate when positive. The abdominal exam and the location of the wound above or below the intertrochanteric line was not predictive of the presence or absence of major intra-abdominal injury. X-rays which demonstrated a transpelvic trajectory or a bullet within the pelvis correlated with major injury in 14 of 16 patients. No patients whose pelvic x-rays lacked bony injury or trajectory across the ring of the pelvis had major abdominal injuries.

EXPLORATORY LAPAROTOMY

Preoperative Preparation

Once the decision to perform an exploratory laparotomy has been made, the surgery should not be delayed.[20] Concomitant medical problems, such as electrolyte or acid-base imbalance or hyperglycemia, however, should be corrected prior to surgery, if at all possible. On the other hand, rapid correction of chronic defects or excessive operative delays can cause deterioration of the clinical situation and can greatly increase the operative risk.

Although patients respond better to anesthesia and surgery if adequate blood and fluid replacement can be accomplished preoperatively, delaying surgery in an attempt to restore the blood volume while severe hemorrhage continues can greatly increase morbidity and mortality rates.[20]

Changes During General Anesthesia

AXIOM General anesthesia can cause a severe drop in BP and cardiac output if the patient is hypovolemic during induction.

Most general anesthetics reduce cardiac contractility, cause systemic vasodilation, and increase vascular capacitance, thereby increasing the tendency to hypotension, especially if the patient is hypovolemic.[20] Consequently, these patients must be closely monitored as the general anesthetic is induced. Rapid replacement of blood and other fluids may be required before, during, and after induction of the anesthetic to reduce the chances of the patient developing severe hypotension.

The initiation of general anesthesia can be an extremely dangerous period for the patient, and the anesthetic team should be prepared to deal with a number of emergencies, including sudden hypotension, cardiac arrhythmias, and aspiration.[20] In patients who are in shock, minimal anesthesia may be supplemented by oxygen and muscle relaxants. In some instances, it may be advantageous to begin the procedure under local anesthesia. This is especially true in poor-risk patients in whom there is some doubt as to whether or not the wounding agent has entered the peritoneal cavity.

Preparation and Draping of the Patient

Prior to exploring the abdomen for trauma, especially gunshot wounds, the skin should be prepped and draped widely from the chin to the knees and laterally as far as possible, so that the surgeon can gain access to any body cavity or the groin expeditiously and can properly place drains and chest tubes as needed. The prepping should not take more than a few minutes and, if the patient is severely hypotensive, it can be carried out before the anesthetic induction so that, should deterioration occur, an immediate celiotomy or thoracotomy can be performed.

If it is known before the operation that it is likely that a thoracotomy will also be needed, it is sometimes helpful to elevate the patient's hip and shoulder on the involved side on sand bags. This allows a more lateral extensive of an anterior thoracotomy incision if it is needed. Such positioning, however, must be done very cautiously, if at all, if the patient has a possible spine injury.

Abdominal Incisions

Stabs in the flanks or lateral abdomen with well-localized signs or symptoms can sometimes be approached satisfactorily through a transverse or oblique incision.[20] In general, however, a midline incision is preferred because it is relatively bloodless, can be performed rapidly, and allows good exposure to virtually all parts of the abdomen. For gunshot wounds, the midline incision is particularly desirable because the bullet may ricochet unpredictably and cause widely separated injuries. Occasionally the incision may have to be extended into the left or right side of the chest to obtain adequate exposure to structures immediately under the diaphragm or to treat concomitant thoracic injuries. In severe hepatic trauma involving the hepatic veins or retrohepatic vena cava, extension of the midline incision into the chest by splitting the sternum is a quick and effective approach to these structures, especially if an atriocaval shunt may need to be inserted.

AXIOM A midline laparotomy incision is preferred for most types of abdominal trauma, and one should not hesitate to extend it to obtain better exposure of potentially life-threatening injuries.

If the patient has a very distended abdomen and is in profound shock in spite of rapid infusions of large quantities of fluid and blood, the incision into the abdominal cavity may be followed by torrential bleeding.[20] Release of the abdominal tamponade can also result in a sudden severe reduction in the venous return to the heart because previously compressed intra-abdominal veins are permitted to distend. This can result in a rapid cardiac arrest.

In such seriously injured patients, placement of an adequate number of intravenous cannulas, ready availability of sufficient blood and fluid and suitable vascular instruments, including an aortic compressor, must be assured preoperatively. Only the top part of the incision is opened initially so that the surgeon can reach in and compress the abdominal aorta at the diaphragm. The aortic compressor should then be positioned and held in place while the rest of the incision is opened and the abdomen is explored.

Prelaparotomy Thoracotomy

AXIOM Patients with massive hemoperitoneum and continued severe hypotension may benefit from a prelaparotomy thoracotomy and aortic cross-clamping.

Although the results of an ED thoracotomy for cardiac arrest from intra-abdominal bleeding are poor,[99] there is a definite role for prelaparotomy thoracotomy in the OR to obtain proximal aortic control in patients with massive hemoperitoneum and continued severe hypotension (systolic BP <70 mm Hg).[100-104] Prelaparotomy thoracotomy with thoracic aortic cross-clamping can help to: (a) maintain blood flow to the heart and brain, (b) reduce the amount of intra-abdominal blood loss, (c) keep the duration of central hypotension to less than 30 minutes, and (d) reduce the number of blood transfusions. It may greatly reduce mortality and morbidity rates in these patients. In patients with high-risk abdominal vascular injuries, (admission systolic BP <70 mm Hg and four or more associated injuries) if the shock duration was kept to <30 minutes and the number of blood transfusions was kept to less than 10 units, the mortality rate was reduced from 92% (24/26) to 0% (0/12).[102-104]

AXIOM For patients arriving in the OR with massive intra-abdominal bleeding and a systolic BP <70 mm Hg, a prepaparotomy cross-clampiing of the thoracic aorta should be considered.[104]

If, following thoracic aortic cross-clamping, the systolic BP does not rise to at least 90 mm Hg within 5 minutes, the patient has terminal cardiovascular failure and will almost certainly die in the OR. Prolonged surgical efforts for many hours using multiple units of blood have been uniformly futile. Infusions of epinephrine and/or norepinephrine may raise the blood pressure to adequate levels for some time, but these patients still virtually always die in the OR.

Following laparotomy, the thoracic aortic clamp should be moved to the abdominal aorta as soon as possible. Care must be taken not to let the systolic BP in the proximal aorta exceed 160-180 mm Hg. If proximal hypertension develops, the resultant left ventricular dilation can cause acute cardiac failure to develop within a few minutes.

AXIOM If the aorta is cross-clamped, the proximal aortic pressure in previously normal individuals should not be allowed to exceed 160-180 mm Hg.

If the abdominal injury involves a major artery in the upper abdomen, there may not be room to apply an aortic compressor in the abdomen and definitively repair the bleeding site. If the aortic hiatus is free of hematoma, the gastrohepatic ligament should be divided, and the aorta should be encircled as it emerges through the crura of the diaphragm.

Combined Thoracic and Abdominal Injuries

In penetrating trauma causing significant bleeding in both the chest and abdomen, it may be difficult to determine which cavity to explore first. The causes and patterns of difficulties and errors in making these operative decisions in 82 consecutive patients were recently reported by Hirshberg et al.[105] The mean ISS and RTS were 42 and 8.6, respectively. There was a 41% mortality rate. Continuing chest tube output, need for resuscitation, and cardiac tamponade led to 49 formal thoracotomies, 24 resuscitative thoracotomies and nine pericardiotomies. In 16 (20%) of the thoracotomies, no significant injury was found, with the major misleading factor being intra-abdominal bleeding draining into the chest. Of 74 laparotomies, 16 (22%) were negative but were performed because of tangential or misleading bullet trajectories (six patients), abdominal tenderness (four patients), or to "rule out" an injury (four patients).

Forty-seven operations began with laparotomy, and one half were interrupted to explore the chest or pericardium.[105] Appropriate sequencing apparently occurred in only 19 patients (23%). The two main causes of the incorrect sequence of operations were misleading chest tube output (eight patients) and a decision to perform laparotomy first despite high chest tube output (seven patients). Twelve patients (15%) required early reoperation.

Initial Control of Bleeding

When a major intra-abdominal injury is expected because of continued severe hypotension, the abdominal incision should be extended from the xiphoid to below the umbilicus to gain adequate exposure. Free blood and clot is removed rapidly, and the small bowel is eviscerated as needed so that each quadrant of the abdomen can be inspected rapidly for bleeding. Packs can be placed temporarily to absorb excess free blood and apply pressure to any suspected bleeding areas.

If the patient is severely hypotensive, the aorta should be compressed at the diaphragm and packs should be used to help control the bleeding until the anesthesiologist can resuscitate the patient adequately. Further exploration should wait until the systolic BP rises to 100 mm Hg or more, the urine output is at least 0.5 ml/kg/hr, and the core (esophageal) temperature is at least 34-35° C.

> **AXIOM**   Repeated bouts of hypotension while attempting definitive control of bleeding sites frequently results in death.

Technique of Exploration

Once all significant bleeding has been controlled and the patient has been adequately resuscitated, an orderly exploration of the abdomen should be performed. As intestinal injuries are encountered, they can be controlled temporarily with Babcock clamps or a rapid running absorbable suture.

> **AXIOM**   The number one priority during a celiotomy for trauma is to control bleeding. A second consideration is keeping intestinal contamination to a minimum.

If one has a fairly good idea of the main source of the patient's blood loss and it is controlled by packs, the other areas of the abdomen can be explored first. If the packs are not controlling the bleeding, the suspected source should be explored first. If one does not really know the site of the major blood loss, one can start in the left upper quadrant. The retractors are placed to provide optimal exposure and the packs are removed one by one, looking carefully for bleeding sites, especially the spleen. If the spleen is bleeding, a de-

cision must be made immediately as to whether to remove the spleen promptly or control the bleeding temporarily with local pressure. If this appears to be the major site of bleeding, one can mobilize the spleen carefully while controlling the bleeding to see if a repair or partial splenectomy will be possible. If there are other sources of major blood loss in the abdomen, the spleen should be removed rapidly.

If there is obvious injury to the liver with gross hemorrhage, proper application of packs can often control the bleeding. If this does not stop the hemorrhage, compression of the liver between two hands will often suffice. If this is also unsuccessful, a Pringle maneuver (clamping of the hepato-duodenal ligament which encloses the hepatic artery and portal vein at the foramen of Winslow) may help. If there is still continued bleeding from the depths of a liver laceration, one should suspect a major injury to a hepatic vein. If the bleeding appears to be coming from the back of the liver, injury to the retrohepatic inferior vena cava or attached hepatic veins should be strongly suspected. This area should be compressed manually and/or repacked while consideration is given to possible use of an atriocaval shunt, a venous bypass of the inferior cava, packing as definitive treatment, or clamping the infra-diaphragmatic aorta, portal triad and suprahepatic and intrahepatic inferior vena cava to gain control of the bleeding.[81,82]

After the major hemorrhage has been controlled and obvious intestinal leaks contained, a thorough exploration of the abdominal cavity should be performed. One can begin at the esophageal hiatus, examining all organs in the left upper quadrant, the left lower quadrant, right lower quadrant, right upper quadrant, and then running the bowel and its mesentery.

A Kocher maneuver is done to facilitate exploration of hematomas or bile staining of the upper central retroperitoneum. A perirenal hematoma is usually not explored unless it is expanding or radiologic studies have identified a problem that needs to be addressed. Pelvic hematomas should not be explored if they are due to blunt trauma.

Access to central retroperitoneal hematomas above the pelvic brim is best achieved by taking down the attachments of the right colon (as part of an extended Kocher maneuver to examine the duodenum and head of the pancreas) or left colon with mobilization of the corresponding viscera to the midline (to examine the aorta and the origins of its major branches).

The bowel must be inspected systematically and meticulously. If a penetrating injury is present, one should demonstrate an even number of holes or attempt to prove that the injury to the small intestine was tangential.[20] This concept is extremely important because small perforations on the mesenteric side of the small intestine can easily be overlooked.

> **PITFALL** ⊘
>
> *If an odd number of holes in the intestine is attributed to a tangential injury, small wounds on the mesenteric aspect can easily be overlooked.*

Once an intestinal injury is recognized, it should be closed temporarily by a nontraumatic clamp or rapid suturing until the initial inspection of the abdomen is completed.[20] Allowing continuing escape of intestinal contents into the peritoneal cavity can result in later severe peritonitis or abscess formation.

If there is any suspicion of injury in the lesser sac, this area should be examined by making an opening in the gastrocolic omentum.[20] The transverse colon, posterior wall of the stomach, and pancreatic region can then be thoroughly inspected. Single holes in blood vessels should always be viewed with skepticism. Obviously, if a second hole is missed, subsequent hemorrhage, a false aneurysm, or an arteriovenous fistula can be anticipated.[20] A search must also be made to ensure that the missile has not migrated down an injured vessel.

> **AXIOM**   At the conclusion of the operation, it is advisable to re-explore the abdomen again carefully, to ensure that no area of injury has been overlooked.[20]

Peritoneal Irrigation

Once the bleeding and all intestinal leaks are controlled, one should lavage the peritoneal cavity carefully with saline to reduce the bacterial load from any contamination and to remove any residual free blood or blood clots. Excessive irrigation, however, may adversely affect resident macrophages. The addition of antibiotics to the last liter of irrigant is often recommended, but its usefulness remains to be proven. Furthermore, if neomycin or another aminoglycoside is added to the irrigating solutions, some respiratory depression may result. This can be a severe problem at the end of the operation if the anesthesiologist wants to extubate the patient promptly.[20]

Drains

The indications, numbers, and types of drains used for any particular intra-abdominal injury vary greatly from surgeon to surgeon. Drains can be extremely beneficial by removing any bile or pancreatic secretions that may continue to leak from an injured liver, biliary tract, or pancreas. They can, however, cause problems by: (a) serving as a conduit for bacteria to enter the peritoneal cavity, or (b) eroding into adjacent vessels or organs.

Drains should be of the closed type (i.e., not directly open to the air) whenever possible. They should be soft, accurately placed, and brought out through stab wounds of adequate size in the abdominal wall away from the surgical incision. They should also be carefully dressed and intermittently moved ("tweaked"). Drains should not be used routinely and should not be left in situ once they cease to function. With pancreatic or liver injuries, however, drains should not be removed until there is no drainage after the patient has resumed a regular diet. Open drains of the Penrose type tend to increase the risk of intra-abdominal infection, whereas closed drainage systems generally do not.[83]

> **AXIOM** Drains placed near pancreatic or hepatic injuries should not be removed until the patient is eating and there is no drainage.

Planned Reoperations

Planned reoperations are being used increasingly in the management of critically injured patients. At the first operation, measures are taken to control bleeding rapidly, prevent further spillage of intestinal contents or urine, and to close the abdomen and chest.[106] The patient is then warmed and resuscitated in the intensive care unit. The patient is usually returned to the OR within 24-72 hours, when the patient appears to be sufficiently stable to tolerate definitive repair of all injuries. Occasionally, however, more bleeding is encountered at the second operation, necessitating repeat packing and another reoperation.

An aggressive approach to reoperation seems to stem from the growing realization that many critically injured patients are unlikely to survive major definitive procedures at the initial operation. Prolonged operations and massive blood replacement in such patients often leads to a triad of hypothermia, acidosis, and coagulopathy, which is frequently self-propagating and lethal. In other patients, definitive direct control of bleeding or abdominal closure is not technically feasible at the first operation.

In a recent review of 124 patients treated over two years by Hirshberg et al,[106] an abbreviated initial procedure was performed when direct hemostasis was impossible (102 patients), abrupt termination was required because of the patient's condition (56 patients), or the abdomen or chest could not be closed (20 patients). The techniques employed included packing, rapid skin closure, gastrointestinal interruption, rapid vascular control, temporary urinary diversion, stapled lung resections, and/or plastic bag closure. Seventy-three patients survived to undergo 101 reoperations. The first reoperation was planned in 52 patients, and unplanned but performed for bleeding or for abdominal compartment syndrome in 21 patients. Missed injuries were found at reoperation in 14 patients. The overall mortality rate was 58%. Survival was better when the decision to terminate the initial procedure abruptly was made early.

Abdominal Wall Injuries

BLUNT INJURY

Disruptions of abdominal wall muscles, which are increasingly encountered among wearers of seat belts, should be repaired. If there has been a large hematoma or much tissue damage, the area should be left open or drained for a day or two, particularly if any potential dead space is present after the repair or if continued oozing occurs. In patients with persistent abdominal pain after blunt trauma, damage to the abdominal muscles is not infrequent. If the pain and/or tenderness is worse when the abdominal wall muscles are tensed, the diagnosis of an abdominal wall problem is relatively clear. If no hematoma is present and the pain is well localized, it can often be controlled with one to three injections of a combination of 1.0 ml of 1% lidocaine with 1:100,000 epinephrine, 1.0 ml of 0.5% bupivacaine (Marcaine) and 1.0 ml of triamcinolone (Kenolog).

PENETRATING INJURIES

Penetrating injuries of the abdominal wall which are superficial to the peritoneum are relatively easy to treat. After thorough debridement and cleansing under local anesthesia, they can be sutured or left open and drained, depending upon the contamination and age of the wound.

Large defects of the abdominal wall, such as those caused by shotgun blasts at close range, are met increasingly in civilian life and present some unique problems. In some patients the abdominal wall defect may be too large to close with the patient's own tissues. As a further complication, underlying organs, particularly the colon, can be so severely damaged that sepsis is almost inevitable. Wounds likely to become infected should be thoroughly debrided after the intraperitoneal injuries have been treated. If the abdominal wall cannot or should not be closed, the bowel should be covered with silk or rayon cloth and then covered with a pack. This can be held in place by fascial retention type sutures or by abdominal binders.

There is sometimes a temptation to ask a plastic surgeon to rotate a muscle or muscle-skin flap into the defect so as to be able to close the abdomen; however, formation of such flaps at the initial operation is not recommended because they tend to become infected and/or necrotic because of underlying contamination and/or an inadequate blood supply.

> **PITFALL** ⊘
>
> *Muscle flaps to cover large areas of tissue loss immediately following trauma, especially in contaminated areas, often become infected or necrose and should be avoided.*

Another technique for closing large open wounds is the suturing of omentum to the edges of the defect. The omentum is then covered with Owen's cloth or a similar material. After a healthy base of granulation tissue forms on the omentum, split-thickness skin grafts can be applied. The ultimate objective is skin closure, which may be speeded by the use of pigskin as a biologic dressing which is changed every 24 to 48 hours. Used in this manner, pigskin may speed up the development of granulations which will accept skin grafts rapidly.

> **AXIOM** Survival is the primary goal for patients with large abdominal wall defects; hernias may be repaired later.

Closure of Abdominal Incisions

The method of final closure of abdominal fascia is usually a matter of personal preference. Special precautions, however, should be taken in patients who have had extensive trauma and are apt to develop peritonitis, severe ileus, and/or respiratory failure.

Although closures of the linea alba with wire are stronger and less likely to become infected, the use of wire tends to be associated with an increased risk of injury to the surgeon's gloves and hands as well as contamination of the wound.[20] Consequently, most surgeons use nonabsorbable or slowly-absorbable sutures.

Large full-thickness retention sutures tied over dental rolls or rubber tubing may add considerable strength to the abdominal wall closure.[20] If the abdomen cannot be closed except under some tension, but it is important to make the closure water-tight, the skin can be closed and the fascia left open temporarily.

If the abdomen is closed and there is concern about continued intra-abdominal bleeding, the intra-abdominal pressure (IAP) should be monitored closely. This is usually done via a Foley catheter in the bladder. To measure the IAP, the drainage portion of the Foley catheter is clamped a few inches from the penis and a CVP manometer is hooked up to the proximal portion of the Foley catheter via a needle in its side. After instilling 25-50 ml of sterile saline into the bladder, the pressure inside the bladder, which reflects intra-abdominal pressure, can then be measured with the CVP manometer with the zero point at the level of the midaxillary line. If the IAP exceeds 20-30 mm Hg (26-39 cm H_2O) and/or the abdomen feels taut and there is severe oliguria in spite of more than adequate BP and cardiac output, one should suspect the development of an abdominal compartment syndrome, and the abdomen should be opened promptly.[107] Ideally, any coagulopathy that was present should have been corrected by that time by warming the patient and infusing platelets and FFP or cryoprecipitate, as needed. For severe coagulopathies, more than 8-12 units of FFP may have to be infused fairly rapidly.

Leaving the Abdomen Open

In patients with severe abdominal trauma, infusions of large quantities of intravenous fluid may result in excessive swelling of bowel, the mesentery and the retroperitoneal tissues. In addition, increased edema can make the abdominal wall less compliant. Under such circumstances, closing the abdominal fascia may result in increased intraperitoneal pressure with a resultant decrease in hepatic, renal, and intestinal mucosal blood flow.[107] Other problems with excessively tight abdominal closures include respiratory compromise, because of the elevated diaphragms, and fascial necrosis with resulting infection or dehiscence.

A variety of techniques have been used to manage an abdomen that is too tight to close with safety. Bender et al[108] recently described a technique developed at Detroit Receiving Hospital by Anna Ledgerwood and Charles E. Lucas. At the completion of the laparotomy, the swollen intestines are covered with a large piece of sterile rayon, nylon, or silk cloth which is placed under the fascial edges. Four or five widely spaced retention sutures are then placed. Generous gauze packs are inserted between the sutures and the rayon cloth. The sutures are then tied to make certain the intestines are kept within the peritoneal cavity below the plane of the abdominal fascia. The patient is returned to the OR every 24-72 hours to change the dressings and tighten the retention sutures. This process is repeated until the fascia comes together without too much tension. Ostomies are usually not opened until the fascia can be closed properly.

An open abdominal technique can also be used to treat diffuse peritonitis. Sleeman et al[109] recently reported on the use of a zipper technique with daily irrigations of the abdomen in the Surgical Intensive Care Unit (SICU). Once the abdominal problem has resolved, the mesh and zipper are removed. The wound is then allowed to contract and a skin graft is placed. Surgeons, however, are usually reluctant to reoperate on such patients later due to the anticipation of a hostile abdomen with severe adhesions.

Of 12 patients admitted to their trauma service and treated by their open abdomen technique, reoperations were performed for closure of enteric fistula in four, closure of jejunostomy/ileostomy in three and closure of a colostomy in five.[108] Reconstruction of the abdominal

wall was undertaken in nine patients and Prolene Mesh was used in five patients. In the other three patients, a lateral incision was used to enter the abdomen and reanastomose the bowel.

All of the patients survived. There were five complications. Four patients had ischemic skin grafts that responded to hyperbaric oxygen (HBO) therapy. One patient developed a low-output enteric fistula that closed after two weeks of total parenteral nutrition.

Leaving the Skin and Subcutaneous Tissue Open

Where there has been gross contamination of the peritoneal cavity and subcutaneous tissue, as with massive colonic wounds, the skin and subcutaneous tissue should be left open for at least several days.[20]

AXIOM   One of the best ways to prevent wound infections after abdominal trauma with contaminations is to leave the skin and subcutaneous tissue open.

⊘ FREQUENT ERRORS

In the Management of Abdominal Trauma

1. *Failure to recognize the need for emergency abdominal surgery at an early stage.*
2. *Failure to examine the patient with possible intra-abdominal injuries carefully and repeatedly.*
3. *Performance of a laparotomy on all patients with penetrating abdominal wounds with little or no attention to types of injury, signs, symptoms, or the age of the injury.*
4. *Concentrating on an abdominal injury to the extent that serious or life-threatening extra-abdominal injuries are overlooked.*
5. *Insistence on "routine" preoperative radiologic studies in hemodynamically unstable patients.*
6. *Failure to insert a gastric decompression tube in patients who have an injury that may cause vomiting or a severe ileus.*
7. *Failure to resuscitate the patient's blood volume and core temperature adequately once the major bleeding is controlled.*
8. *Unsystematic examination of the abdomen during laparotomy, thereby increasing the likelihood of missing lesions.*
9. *Insistence on performing a one-stage operation, including skin closure, when a staged procedure might be much safer.*
10. *Delayed, inappropriate, or prolonged use of antibiotics.*
11. *Failure to repeat antibiotic therapy after massive bleeding has been controlled.*
12. *Early discontinuation of nasogastric suction in patients recovering from severe abdominal trauma.*
13. *Removing "non-functioning" drains from around hepatic or pancreatic injuries before the patient is eating.*

▼▼▼▼▼▼▼▼▼▼▼▼▼▼▼▼▼▼▼▼▼▼▼▼▼▼▼▼▼▼▼▼

SUMMARY POINTS

1.   If individual injuries are viewed in isolation, diagnosis of other problems is apt to be delayed.

2.   One should never assume that bullets will travel in a straight line. The bullet or secondary missiles can often injure structures far outside the presumed trajectory.

3.   Because of the unpredictable path and possible blast effect of bullets, all abdominal gunshot wounds require surgical exploration.

4.   The initial resuscitation of patients with severe trauma must assure an adequate airway and the maintenance of a minute ventilation that is at least 1.5-2.0 times normal.

5.   Fluid resuscitation in patients who are actively bleeding should be kept to minimum until the bleeding is controlled.

6.   The trend of vital signs in relation to treatment is much more important than isolated levels.

7. Failure to decompress the stomach in trauma patients with severe trauma increases the risk of aspiration, impaired diaphragmatic motion, and prolonged ileus.

8. All trauma patients should be assumed to have full stomachs.

9. One should avoid nasal tubes in patients who may have fractures of the mid-face or anterior base of the skull.

10. Prior to inserting a Foley catheter in patients with severe blunt trauma, one should do a rectal exam to check the position of the prostate, look for any rectal blood, and check sphincter tone.

11. Intravenous prophylactic antibiotics that cover enteric gram-negative aerobes and anaerobes are given as soon as possible if intra-abdominal contamination is suspected.

12. It is essential to view the patient with abdominal injury as a whole and not to be distracted from recognizing important concomitant extra-abdominal lesions.

13. Careful repeated examination of the patient is frequently the key to the early diagnosis of intra-abdominal injuries.

14. Narcotics should not be given to patients who are hypovolemic or who are being observed for possible CNS or abdominal injuries.

15. Every patient has a back as well as a front.

16. Increases in abdominal girth are best detected with serial tape measurements at the umbilicus.

17. Where doubt exists as to whether abdominal rigidity and/or tenderness is due to intra-abdominal trauma or an injury to the abdominal wall, one should assume that an intra-abdominal injury is present.

18. The presence of bowel sounds is a reassuring indicator of peristalsis, but it is not reliable for ruling out visceral injuries.

19. Using physical findings as the only guide for performing a laparotomy can lead to unacceptable delays in treatment with resultant increased mortality and morbidity rates.

20. A hemoglobin level less than 10.0 gm/dl may not provide adequate oxygen transport during anesthesia if the patient is elderly or has a relatively low cardiac output.

21. Many false-positive and false-negative results occur when using serum amylase levels to diagnosis pancreatic injury.

22. The delay and extra movement caused by an insistence on "routine" radiologic examinations can be extremely dangerous in patients with severe abdominal trauma.

23. The accuracy of abdominal ultrasonography and CT scans is largely determined by the expertise of the radiologist performing and interpreting the studies.

24. Although a positive abdominal tap is of great diagnostic value, a negative tap should never be regarded as definitive.

25. A diagnostic peritoneal lavage can be performed with relative safety if it is an open technique and avoids scars, hematomas, or a pregnant uterus.

26. The decision for performing an exploratory celiotomy in patients with stab wounds should not be determined by set criteria or a single test, but should be individualized and based on all the information available.

27. Diagnostic peritoneal lavage is currently considered to be one of the best methods for diagnosing intraperitoneal injury after blunt trauma.

28. The safest policy with stab wounds is to explore the abdomen if any question of visceral injury exists.

29. Of the patients with intra-abdominal trauma who reach a hospital alive, 20-30% of those who die do so because of delayed, inadequate, or inappropriate treatment.

30. Diagnosis and treatment of a suspected traumatic rupture of the aorta has precedence over all but the most life-threatening other injuries.

31. Patients with massive bleeding from an unstable pelvic fracture should have prompt external fixation of the pelvis and therapeutic pelvic angiography.

32. The risk of receiving more than two units of blood generally outweigh the risks of a negative or non-therapeutic laparotomy.

33. General anesthesia can cause a severe drop in BP and cardiac output if the patient is hypovolemic during induction.

34. A midline laparotomy incision is preferred for most types of abdominal trauma, and one should not hesitate to extend it to obtain better exposure of potentially life-threatening injuries.

35. Patients with massive hemoperitoneum and continued severe hypotension often benefit from a prelaparotomy thoracotomy and aortic cross-clamping.

36. For patients presenting to the OR with massive intra-abdominal bleeding and a systolic BP <70 mm Hg, a prelaparotomy cross-clamping of the thoracic aorta should be considered.

37. If the aorta is cross-clamped, the proximal aortic pressure in previously normal individuals should not be allowed to exceed 160-180 mm Hg.

38. The number one priority during a celiotomy for trauma is to control bleeding. The second consideration is keeping contamination to a minimum.

39. If an odd number of holes in the intestine is attributed to a tangential injury, small wounds on the mesentery aspect may be easily overlooked.

40. At the conclusion of the operation, it is advisable to explore the abdomen again carefully, to ensure that no area of injury has been overlooked.

41. Drains should be avoided whenever possible.

42. Drains placed near pancreatic or hepatic injuries should not be removed until the patient is eating and there is no drainage.

43. Muscle flaps to cover large areas of tissue loss immediately following trauma, especially in contaminated areas, should be avoided.

44. Survival is the primary goal for patients with large abdominal wall defects; hernias may be repaired later.

45. One of the best ways to prevent wound infections after abdominal trauma is to leave the skin and subcutaneous tissue open.

▲▲▲▲▲▲▲▲▲▲▲▲▲▲▲▲▲▲▲▲▲▲▲▲▲▲▲▲▲▲▲▲▲▲

REFERENCES

1. Trunkey DD, Hill AC, Schecter WP. Abdominal trauma and indications for celiotomy (Ch 27). In: Moore EE, Mattox KL, Feliciano DV, eds. Trauma. 2nd ed. Norwalk: Appleton & Lange, 1991; 409–426.

2. Jordan GL Jr. Hepatic trauma. Contemp Surg 1985;27:19.

3. Strauch GO. Major abdominal trauma in 1971: a study of Connecticut by the Connecticut Society of American Board of Surgeons and the Yale Trauma Program. Am J Surg 1973;125:413.

4. Nahum AM, Siegel AW. The changing panorama of collision injury. Surg Gynecol Obstet 1971;133:783.

5. Walt AJ, Grifka T. Blunt abdominal trauma: a review of 301 cases. In: Gurdjian ES, Lange WA, Patrick WM, Thomas LM, eds. Impact injury and crash protection. Springfield: Charles C. Thomas, 1970.

6. Evaluating the 1974 and 1975 Restraint Systems. Ann Arbor, Michigan Highway Safety Research Institute, 1976; 1.

7. Xenonophon. The Persian Expedition. Rex Warner, tr. New York: Penguin Books, 1949; 128.

8. Loria FL. Historical aspects of abdominal injuries. Springfield: Chas. C. Thomas, 1968: 10.

9. Mullins R, Trunkey DD. Samuel D. Gross. J Trauma 1990;30:528.

10. Coley WB. The treatment of penetrating wounds of the abdomen. Am J Med Sci 1891;101:243.

11. Wilson H, Sherman R. Civilian penetrating wounds of the abdomen: factors in mortality and differences from military wounds in 494 cases. Ann Surg 1961;153:639.

12. Shaftan GW. Indications for operation in abdominal trauma. Am J Surg 1960;99:657.

13. McAlvanah MJ, Shaftan GW. Selective conservatism in penetrating abdominal wounds: a continuing appraisal. J Trauma 1978;18:296.

14. Root HD, Houser CW, McKinley CR, et al. Diagnostic peritoneal lavage. Surgery 1968;57:633.

15. Federle MP, Goldberg HI, Kaiser JA, et al. Evaluation of abdominal trauma by computed tomography. Radiology 1981;138:647.

16. Blaisdell WF. General assessment, resuscitation and exploration of penetrating and blunt abdominal trauma. In: Blaisdell WF, Trunkey DD, eds, Trauma Management 1: Abdominal Trauma. New York: Thieme-Stratton, 1981;1.

17. Charters AC III, Charters AC. Wounding mechanisms of very high velocity projectiles. J Trauma 1976;16:464.

18. Fackler ML, Malinowski JA. The wound profile: a visual method for quantifying gunshot wound components. J Trauma 1985;25:522.

19. Moore EE, Moore JB, Van Duzer-Moore S, et al. Mandatory laparotomy for gunshot wounds penetrating the abdomen. Am J Surg 1980;140:847.

20. Walt AJ, Wilson RF. General considerations in abdominal trauma. In: Walt AJ, Wilson RF, eds. Management of trauma: pitfalls and practice. Philadelphia: Lea & Febiger, 1975;22:336–347.

21. Cameron JL. Aspiration pneumonia: a clinical and experimental review. J Surg Res 1967;7:44.

22. Fullen WD, et al. Prophylactic antibiotics in penetrating wounds of the abdomen. J Trauma 1972;12:287.

23. Jones RC, Thal ER, Johnson RC, et al. Evaluation of antibiotic treatment following penetrating abdominal trauma. Ann Surg 1985;201:576.

24. Wilson RF, ed. Antibiotic therapy for surgery related infections. 2nd ed. Philadelphia: Scientific Therapeutics Inc, 1994: 20.

25. Trunkey DD, Chapman MW, Lim RC, et al. Management of pelvic fractures in blunt trauma injury. J Trauma 1974;14:912.

26. Rosoff L, Cohen JL, Telfer N, et al. Injuries of the spleen. Surg Clin North Am 1972;52:667.

27. Engav LH, Benjamin CI, Strake RG, et al. Diagnostic peritoneal lavage in blunt abdominal patients. J Trauma 1975;15:854.

28. Ayala LA, Williams LF, Widrich WC. Occult rupture of the spleen: the chronic form of splenic rupture. Ann Surg 1974;179:472.

29. Olsen WR, Hildreth DH. Abdominal paracentesis and peritoneal lavage in blunt abdominal trauma. J Trauma 1971;11:824.

30. Bivens BA, Sachatello CR, Daugherty ME, et al. Diagnostic peritoneal lavage is superior to clinical evaluation in blunt abdominal trauma. Am Surg 1978;44:637.

31. Bull JC Mathewson C. Exploratory laparotomy in patients with penetrating wounds of the abdomen. Am J Surg 1968;116:223.

32. Thal ER, May RA, Beesinger D. Peritoneal lavage. Its unreliability in gunshot wounds of the lower chest and abdomen. Arch Surg 1980;115:430.

33. Thompson JS, Moore EE, Van Duzer-Moore S, et al. The evolution of abdominal stab wound management. J Trauma 1980;20:478.

34. White PH, Benfield JR. Amylase in the management of pancreatic trauma. Arch Surg 1972;105:158.

35. Olsen WR. The serum amylase in blunt abdominal trauma. J Trauma 1973;13:200.

36. Gibson GR. Urologic management and complications of fractured pelvis and ruptured urethra. J Urol 1974;111:353.

37. Freeark RJ. Role of angiography in the management of multiple injuries. Surg Gynec Obstet 1969;128:761.

38. Lim RC, et al. Angiography in patients with blunt trauma to the chest and abdomen. Surg Clin N Am 1972;52:551.

39. Margolies MN, Ring EJ, Waltman AC, et al. Arteriography in the management of hemorrhage from pelvic fractures. N Engl J Med 1972;287:317.

40. Lang EK. Arteriography in assessment of renal trauma. J Trauma 1975;15:553.

41. Little JM et al. Radioisotope scanning of liver and spleen in upper abdominal trauma. Surg Gynec Obstet 1967;125:725.

42. Thal ER. Evaluation of peritoneal lavage and local wound exploration in lower chest and abdominal stab wounds. J Trauma 1977;17:642.

43. Lee WC, Uddo JF Jr, Nance FC. Surgical judgement in the management of abdominal stab wounds. Utilizing clinical criteria from a 10-year experience. Ann Surg 1984;199:549.

44. Markovchick VJ, Moore ED, Moore JB, et al. Local wound exploration of anterior abdominal stab wounds. J Emerg Med 1984;2:287.

45. Moore EE, Marx JA. Penetrating abdominal wounds. The rationale for exploratory laparotomy. JAMA 1985;10:253.

46. Petersen FR, Sheldon GF. Morbidity of a negative finding at laparotomy in abdominal trauma. Surg Gynecol Obstet 1979;148:23.

47. Moss LK, Schmidt FE, Creech O. Analysis of 550 stab wounds of the abdomen. Am Surg 1962;28:483.

48. Cornell WP, et al. A new nonoperative technique for the diagnosis of penetrating injuries to the abdomen. J Trauma 1967;7:307.

49. Aragon GE, Eiseman B. Abdominal stab wounds: evaluation of sinography. J Trauma 1976;16:792.

50. Montegut FJ. Tube paracentesis without lavage. J Trauma 1973;13:142.

51. Bivins BA, Sachatello CR. Diagnostic exploratory celiotomy: an outdated concept in blunt abdominal trauma. South Med J 1979;72:969.

52. Moore JB, Moore EE, Markovchick VJ, et al. Diagnostic peritoneal lavage for trauma: superiority of the open technique at the infraumbilical ring. J Trauma 1981;21:570.

53. Pachter HL, Hofstetter SR. Open and percutaneous paracentesis and lavage for abdominal trauma. Arch Surg 1981;116:318.

54. Lazarus HM, Nelson JA. A technique for peritoneal lavage without risk or complication. Surg Gynecol Obstet 1979;149:889.

55. Feliciano DV, Bitondo PA, Steed G, et al. Five hundred open taps or lavages in patients with abdominal stab wounds. Am J Surg 1984;148:772.

56. Alyono D, Perry JF Jr. Value of quantitative cell count and amylase activity of peritoneal lavage fluid. J Trauma 1981;21:345.

57. Merlotti GJ, Marcet E, Sheaff CM, et al. Use of peritoneal lavage to evaluate abdominal penetration. J Trauma 1985;25:228.

58. Root HD, Keizer PJ, Perry JF. The clinical and experimental aspects of the peritoneal response to injury. Arch Surg 1967;95:531.

59. Fisher RP, Beverlin BC, Engrave LH, et al. Diagnostic peritoneal lavage. Fourteen years and 2586 patients later. Am J Surg 1979;136:701.

60. DuPriest RW Jr, Rodriguez A, Khenja SC, et al. Open diagnostic peritoneal lavage in blunt trauma victims. Surg Gynecol Obstet 1979;148:890.

61. Jaffin JH, Ochsner MG, Cole FJ, et al. Alkaline phosphatase levels in diagnostic peritoneal lavage as a predictor of hollow visceral injury. J Trauma 1992;33:155.

62. McAnena OJ, Marx JA, Moore EE. Contributions of peritoneal lavage enzyme determinations to the management of isolated hollow visceral abdominal injuries. Ann Emerg Med 1991;20:834.

63. Mackart DJJ, McDonald MA. Evaluation of diagnostic peritoneal lavage in suspected penetrating abdominal stab wounds using a dipstick technique. Br J Surg 1991;78:698.

64. Mendez C, Gubler KD, Maier RV. Diagnostic accuracy of peritoneal lavage in patients with pelvic fractures. Arch Surg 1994;129:477.

65. Meyer DM, Thal ER, Weigelt JA, et al. Evaluation of computed tomography and diagnostic peritoneal lavage in blunt abdominal trauma. J Trauma 1989;29:1168.

66. Thal ER, May RA, Beesinger D. Peritoneal lavage. Its unreliability in gunshot wounds of the lower chest and abdomen. Arch Surg 1980;115:430.

67. Trunkey DD, Federle MP. Computed tomography in perspective. Editorial. J Trauma 1986;26:660.

68. Freshman S, Wisner DH, Weber J. After the emergency department: delayed detection of occult abdominal injuries in patients under observation. J Trauma 1991;31:1029.

69. Kinnunen J, Kivioja A, Poussa K, Laasonen EM. Emergency CT in blunt abdominal trauma of multiple injury patients. Acta Radiol 1994;35:319.

70. McAllister E, Perez M, Albrink MH, et al. Is triple contrast computed tomographic scanning useful in the selective management of stab wounds to the back? J Trauma 1994;37:401.

71. Salvino CK, Esposito TK, Marshall W, et al. The role of diagnostic laparoscopy in trauma patients: a preliminary assessment. J Trauma 1992;33:162.

72. Sosa JL, Markley M, Sleeman D, et al. Laparoscopy to avoid nontherapeutic laparotomy. J Trauma 1993;35:178.

73. Townsend MC, Flancbaum L, Choban PS, Cloutier CT. Diagnostic laparoscopy as an adjunct to selective conservative management of solid organ injuries after blunt abdominal trauma. J Trauma 1993;36:647.

74. Brandt CP, Priebe PP, Jacobs DG. Potential of laparoscopy to reduce nontherapeutic trauma laparotomies. Am Surg 1994;60:416.

75. Ivatury RR, Simon RJ, Stahl WM. A critical evaluation of laparoscopy in penetrating abdominal trauma. J Trauma 1993;34:822.

76. Dalton JM, DeMarie EJ, Gore DC, et al. Prospective evaluation of laparoscopy in abdominal stab wounds (abstract). J Trauma 1994;36:149.

77. Sosa JL, Puente I, Arrillaga A, et al. Laparoscopy in 100 consecutive patients with abdominal gunshot wounds (abstract). J Trauma 1994;37:159.

78. Rudston-Brown B, Phang BT, Studer W, et al. Laparoscopic diagnosis of penetrating wounds of the diaphragm (abstract). J Trauma 1993;35:178.

79. Moffa S, Quinn JV, Slotman GJ, et al. The hemodynamic effects of carbon dioxide pneumoperitoneum, during mechanical ventilation and positive end-expiratory pressure (PEEP). J Trauma 1992;32:953.

80. Diebel LN, Saxe JM, Dulchavsky SA, et al. Hepatic perfusion responses to increased intra-abdominal pressure. J Trauma 1991;31:1714.

81. Josephs LG, Este-McDonald JR, Birkett DH, Hirsh EF. Diagnostic laparoscopy increases intracranial pressure. J Trauma 1994;36:815.

82. Uribe RA, Pachon CE, Frame SB, et al. A prospective evaluation of thoracoscopy for the diagnosis of penetrating thoracoabdominal trauma (abstract). J Trauma 1993;35:985.

83. Koehler RH, Smith RS. Thoracoscopic repair of missed diaphragmatic injury in penetrating trauma: case report. J Trauma 1994;36:424.
84. Glaser K, Tschmelitsch J, Klinger P, et al. Ultrasonography in the management of blunt abdominal and thoracic trauma. Arch Surg 1994;129:743.
85. Lin M, Lee C, Pleg F. Prospective comparison of diagnostic peritoneal lavage, computed tomographic scanning, and ultrasonography for the diagnosis of blunt abdominal trauma. J Trauma 1993;35:267.
86. McKenney M, Lentz K, Nunez D, et al. Can ultrasound replace diagnostic peritoneal lavage in the assessment of blunt trauma? J Trauma 1994;37:439.
87. Goletti O, Ghiselli G, Vincenzo P, et al. The role of ultrasonography in blunt abdominal trauma: results in 250 consecutive cases. J Trauma 1994;36:178.
88. Rozycki GS, Ochsner MG, Frankel HL, et al. A prospective study of surgeon-performed ultrasound as the initial diagnostic modality for injured patient assessment (abstract). J Trauma 1994;37:160.
89. Huang MS, Liu M, Wu JK, et al. Ultrasonography for the evaluation of hemoperitoneum during resuscitation: a simple scoring system. J Trauma 1994;36:173.
90. Akgur FM, Aktug T, Kovanhkaya A, et al. Initial evaluation of children sustaining blunt abdominal trauma: ultrasonography versus diagnostic peritoneal lavage. Eur J Ped Surg 1993;3:278.
91. Taxier M, Sivak MV Jr, Cooperman AM, et al. ERCP in the evaluation of trauma to the pancreas. Surg Gynecol Obstet 1980;150:65.
92. Haller JA Jr, Papa P, Drugas G, Colombani P. Nonoperative management of solid organ injuries in children. Is it safe? Ann Surg 1994;219:615.
93. Luna GK, Dellinger EP. Non-operative observation therapy for splenic injuries: a safe therapeutic option? Am J Surg 1994;153:462.
94. Cogbill TH, Moore EE, Jurkovich GJ, et al. Nonoperative management of blunt and splenic trauma: a multicenter experience. J Trauma 1989;29:1312.
95. Lucas CE. Diagnosis and treatment of pancreatic and duodenal injury. Surg Clin North Am 1977;57:49.
96. Cushing BM, Morris JA. Practice guidelines for evaluation of the abdomen in blunt trauma victims; step one, identifying clinical risk factors (abstract). J Trauma 1994;36:152.
97. Nance FC, Wenner NH, Johnson LW, et al. Surgical judgement in the management of penetrating wounds of the abdomen: experience with 2212 patients. Ann Surg 1974;179:639.
98. DiGiacomo JC, Schwab CW, Rotonds MFR, et al. Who warrants exploration for a gluteal gunshot wound (abstract). J Trauma 1994;36:149.
99. Washington B, Wilson RF, Steiger Z, Bassett JS. Emergency thoracotomy: a four-year review. Ann Thor Surg 1985;40:188.
100. Ledgerwood AM, Kazmers M, Lucas CE. The role of thoracic aortic occlusion for massive hemoperitoneum. J Trauma 1976;16:610.
101. Sankaran S, Lucas C, Walt AJ. Thoracic aortic clamping for prophylaxis against sudden cardiac arrest during laparotomy for acute massive hemoperitoneum. J Trauma 1975;15:290.
102. Wiencek RG, Wilson RF. Abdominal venous injuries. J Trauma 1986;26:771.
103. Wiencek RG, Wilson RF. Injuries to the abdominal vascular system: how much does aggressive resuscitation and prelaparotomy thoracotomy really help? Surgery 1987;102:731.
104. Wilson RF, Wiencek RG Jr, Balog M. Factors affecting mortality rate with iliac vein injuries. J Trauma 1990;30:320.
105. Hirshberg A, Mattox KL, Wall MJ Jr. Double jeopardy: thoracoabdominal injuries requiring surgery in both cavities (abstract). J Trauma 1994;37:151.
106. Hirshberg A, Wall MJ, Mattox KL. Planned reoperation for trauma: a two year experience with 124 consecutive patients. J Trauma 1994;37:365.
107. Diebel, L.N., Kozol, R., Wilson, R.F., et al. Gastric intramucosal acidosis in patients with chronic kidney failure. Surgery 1993;113:520.
108. Bender JS, Bailey CE, Saxe JM, et al. The technique of visceral packing: recommended management of difficult fascial closure in trauma patients. J Trauma 1994;36:182.
109. Sleeman D, Gonzales A, Sosa J, et al. Closure of the open abdomen (abstract). J Trauma 1994;36:150.

Chapter 21 Diaphragmatic Injuries

ROBERT F. WILSON, M.D.

JEFFREY BENDER, M.D.

INTRODUCTION

Diaphragmatic injury in and of itself is seldom acutely fatal, but it can be associated with severe life-threatening abdominal or thoracic injuries. This can result in initial mortality rates as high as 27-40% for blunt trauma[1,2] and 10-15% for penetrating trauma.[1-7] In addition, if the injury is not recognized initially and bowel herniates into the chest and later strangulates, the resultant sepsis is frequently fatal.

A diaphragmatic injury should serve as an important marker in alerting the surgeon to search for associated injuries.[3-7] In addition, the anatomical defect may be associated with a host of late complications if the diagnosis is delayed or missed completely. These delayed complications usually first appear as acute respiratory embarrassment or bowel obstruction. Rarely, they present initially as sepsis when a herniated viscus strangulates or perforates. Occasionally, the hernia is discovered only incidentally in an asymptomatic patient.

HISTORY

The earliest record of a diaphragmatic injury is attributed to Sennertus.[8] In 1541 he described the autopsy finding of a post-traumatic herniation of the stomach through the diaphragm of a man who had been stabbed in the chest seven months previously. In 1578 Ambroise Paré recorded in an autopsy that the cause of death in an artillery captain shot eight months earlier was strangulation of transverse colon that had herniated into the chest through a "finger-tip-size" diaphragmatic defect. Paré later described another autopsy case of post-traumatic diaphragmatic herniation following severe blunt abdominal trauma.[9-11] In 1853, Bowditch was the first American to report the antemortem diagnosis of a post-traumatic diaphragmatic hernia and added a review of 83 autopsy reports from the literature.[12]

The first successful surgical correction of a diaphragmatic injury was performed in 1886 by Riolfi, who repaired a knife wound of that structure after reducing the prolapsed omentum.[13] Excellent discussions of traumatic diaphragmatic hernias include recent reviews by Root[14] and Orringer.[15]

Incidence

> **AXIOM** One should suspect diaphragmatic injuries with all penetrating wounds of the lower chest and with severe blunt abdominal trauma.

Although penetrating trauma accounts for more than 90%[7,16-18] of diaphragmatic injuries in many large trauma centers in the U.S., blunt trauma causes the diaphragmatic injuries in 40% of the cases in Rumania and 75% of the cases in Switzerland.[5,7,14,18-21] Over the 12-year period 1980-1992, 420 patients at Detroit Receiving Hospital were noted to have diaphragmatic injuries, and only 28 (6.7%) were due to blunt trauma. Of 573 patients with blunt trauma to intra-abdominal organs, only 4.9% involved the diaphragm.

The diaphragm is lacerated in at least 10%-15% of penetrating wounds to the chest in most series.[18] If the chest wound is anterior and below the nipple line, the diaphragm is injured up to 50% of the time.[19,20] Moore et al[23] noted that abdominal injuries were found in 15% of stab wounds and 46% of gunshot wounds of the lower chest. Although anterior stab wounds of the chest are more likely to cause diaphragmatic injury, Borlase et al[24] found a 27% incidence of diaphragmatic perforation by posterior stab wounds. In the 1980-1992 series at Detroit Receiving Hospital, the incidence of diaphragmatic injuries was 20% (273/1358) with GSW of the abdomen, and 14.7% (119/810) with stab wounds.

It is estimated that 2-3% of all patients with blunt chest trauma have a diaphragmatic injury.[20,26] In those hospitalized for multiple injuries following motor vehicle accidents, the incidence doubles to about 4-8%.[20,21,27-30]

> **AXIOM** If the mechanism of injury does not cause diaphragmatic trauma to be suspected, there is a good chance it will be missed.

ANATOMY AND FUNCTION OF THE DIAPHRAGM

Composition

The word diaphragm comes from the Greek and means a partition or wall. The thoracoabdominal diaphragm is a large fan or dome-shaped sheet of skeletal muscle and fascia separating the chest and abdominal cavities (Fig. 21-l). The diaphragm is attached anteriorly by fleshy fibers to the xiphoid cartilage and to the inner surface of the cartilages and bony portions of the six lowest ribs where it interdigitates with the transversalis muscle. Posteriorly it is attached to two aponeurotic arches (the internal and external arcuate ligaments) and to the lumbar vertebrae by its crura.

The peripheral portion of the diaphragm is composed of three groups of muscle fibers on each side: a sternal portion, a costal portion, and a lumbar portion, arising from the medial and lateral arcuate ligaments and lumbar vertebral bodies. The central tendon is a thin aponeurosis at the convergence point of the muscular portions.[31] Physiologically, the diaphragm acts as if it were composed of two muscles, the costal portion and the crural portion. The costal portion, attached to the lower ribs, lifts those ribs and displaces the abdominal viscera outward.[32,33]

On fluoroscopy, the diaphragm moves down with inspiration and up with expiration, with an average excursion of 3.5 cm for the left hemidiaphragm and 3.2 cm for the right hemidiaphragm.[32,33] Seventy-five percent of patients have 3-6 cm of excursion. Two percent have more than 6 cm, and 23% have less than 3 cm. In addition to having a slightly greater excursion, the left hemidiaphragm also moves more rapidly.

Between its attachments to the xiphoid cartilage and the cartilages of the adjoining ribs, the fibers of the diaphragm are somewhat deficient. The resultant weak spot on either side of the sternum is referred to as the space of Larrey. It is filled by areolar tissue and is the site for Morgagni hernias (Fig. 21-2).

CRURA

The diaphragm is connected to the lumbar spine by two crura or pillars, which lie on the bodies of the lumbar vertebra, on either side of the aorta. The right crus is larger and longer than the left and arises from the anterior surface of the upper three of four lumbar vertebrae. The left crus arises from the first two lumbar vertebrae. The tendinous portions of the crura converge slightly to the left of the midline to form an arch, beneath which pass the aorta, azygous vein and thoracic duct. The muscular fibers decussate in front of the aorta, and then diverge again so as to surround the esophagus before ending in the central tendon.

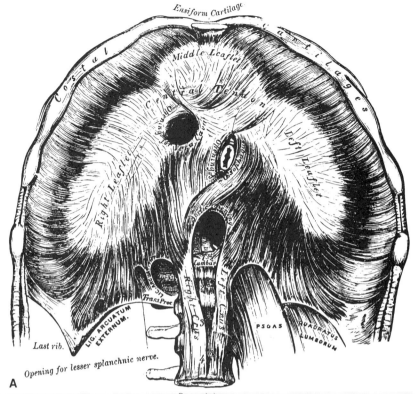

A

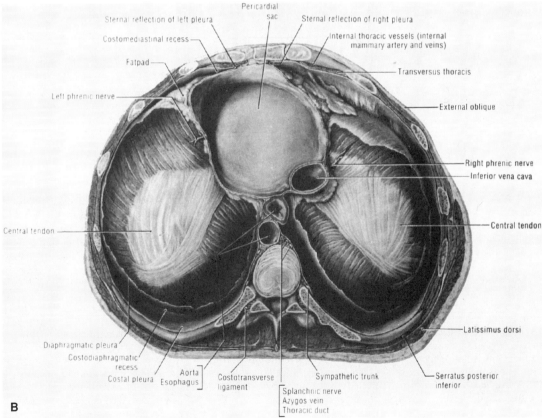

B

FIGURE 21-1 **A.** Inferior (abdominal) surface of the diaphragm (From: Gray H. Anatomy, descriptive and surgical. Pickering T, Howden R, eds. New York: Bounty Books, 1977; 353.) **B.** Superior (thoracic) surface of the diaphragm (From: Agur AMR, Lee MJ, eds. Grant's atlas of anatomy, 9th ed. Baltimore: Williams & Wilkins, 1991; 42.)

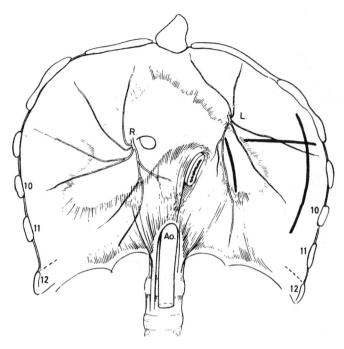

FIGURE 21-2 Inferior aspect of the diaphragm, showing its origins, the course of the phrenic nerves, and the relation of three common incisions to the phrenic nerve branches (From: Gibbon JH, ed. Surgery of the chest. Philadelphia: WB Saunders Co, 1962; 526.)

CENTRAL TENDON

The central tendon is a thin but strong tendinous aponeurosis, situated at the center of the diaphragm immediately below the pericardium, with which it is partly blended. It is shaped somewhat like a trefoil leaf with three divisions or leaflets.

DIAPHRAGMATIC OPENINGS

There are three large and several smaller openings in the diaphragm. The three larger openings are for the aorta, the esophagus and inferior vena cava. The aortic opening, at the level of the eleventh thoracic vertebra, is the lowest and most posterior of the three large openings. It is slightly to the left of the midline and is immediately in front of the body of the first lumbar vertebra. The aortic opening also contains the azygous vein and thoracic duct.

The esophageal opening at the level of the tenth thoracic vertebra contains the esophagus, vagus nerves and some small esophageal arteries. The opening for the inferior vena cava is at a level between the eighth and ninth thoracic vertebra at the junction of the right and middle leaflets of the central tendon.

INNERVATION

The left and right halves of the diaphragm are innervated primarily by the ipsilateral phrenic nerves. The phrenic nerves arise from the third, fourth, and fifth anterior cervical nerve roots and course along the posterolateral mediastinum on the pericardial surface. Each phrenic nerve inserts into the diaphragm at the junction of the pericardium and central tendon, at which point a crow's foot configuration of four to five branches splays laterally (Fig. 21-2). Some diaphragmatic innervation also comes from the lower intercostal nerves and the phrenic plexus of the sympathetic nervous system.

BLOOD SUPPLY

The arterial supply to the diaphragm arises inferiorly from the phrenic arteries which are direct branches off the aorta. Superiorly it is supplied by pericardiacophrenic vessels traveling with the phrenic nerves. The most peripheral portions of the diaphragm are supplied by intercostal vessels.

FUNCTION

The diaphragm is the primary muscle of inspiration, and it can also participate in expiration. The diaphragm is a vital pump for the respiratory system, just as the heart is for the circulatory system. Inspiration is an active process resulting from an increase in intrathoracic volume. On quiet inspiration, the diaphragm provides 75% of the tidal volume.[30] When larger intrathoracic volumes are needed, the accessory muscles (the scalenes, sternocleidomastoid, and external oblique muscles) provide progressively more help with inspiration. The expiratory muscles of the chest wall include the internal intercostal muscles which are used only for forced expiration. During passive exhalation, the right leaflet rises anteriorly to the fourth intercostal space and the left leaflet rises anteriorly to the fifth intercostal space. With forced inspiration and expiration, the total excursion of the top of the diaphragm may exceed 10 cm.

ETIOLOGY AND PATTERNS OF DIAPHRAGMATIC INJURY

Penetrating Injuries

The most common penetrating diaphragmatic injuries are downwardly directed stab wounds to the left lower anterior chest wall. Because the diaphragm normally rises to the level of the fourth and fifth ribs, it is frequently perforated by stab wounds to the anterior chest below the nipple line. Gunshot wounds can traverse the diaphragm in virtually any direction from almost any entrance site in the chest or abdomen. Wounds from knives and bullets usually produce small (1-2 cm) holes in the diaphragm. In the series of Wise et al, 84% of the penetrating injuries measured less than 2.0 cm in length.[25] However, because of the continuous movement of the diaphragm and the gradient between the negative pressure in the thorax and positive pressure in the abdomen, many holes in the diaphragm will not heal spontaneously, and abdominal viscera can gradually herniate into the chest. Marchand[34] has pointed out that the pressure gradient between the pleural and peritoneal cavities varies between 7 and 20 cm H_2O normally, and with maximum inspiration, it may exceed 100 cm H_2O.

AXIOM No injury to the diaphragm is so small that it can be considered safe from future sequelae.

BLUNT TRAUMA

Etiology

Blunt trauma in which the intra-abdominal pressure rises abruptly can create burst injuries of the left and/or right diaphragm which typically radiate posterolaterally out from the central tendinous portion of the diaphragm.[14] During blunt abdominal trauma, intraperitoneal pressure may rise from a normal of +2 to +10 cm H_2O to over 1000 cm H_2O.[35] Although the fusion lines of the individual leaflets during the development of the diaphragm have been considered weak spots that are predisposed to rupture,[36-37] blunt disruptions of all areas of the diaphragm have been described.[38-39] The lesion is usually at least five cm long, and one or more intra-abdominal organs have usually herniated through this defect into the chest.

A properly placed lap belt can be life-saving, but if the belt is placed improperly across the waist instead of the lap, it can cause a diaphragmatic tear in motor vehicle accidents with rapid deceleration. While unusual, such injuries may also be caused by displaced rib fragments that penetrate the diaphragm and produce jagged, irregular peripheral lacerations. These lacerations are frequently associated with severe pulmonary contusions.

Side of Injury

With blunt trauma, the rupture is in the left diaphragm in 65-85%, in the right diaphragm in 15-35%, and bilateral in 1% of the injuries.[4,40-42] However, at the Montreal General Hospital, Angood and Muller noted a 12% incidence of bilateral diaphragmatic rupture.[43] Sharma[44] reported an incidence of 74% of left hemidiaphragm injuries in his collective review covering the 1980s. Ilgenfritz and Stewart[45] found a nearly identical distribution in a study of rural injuries.

The left diaphragm is more often torn because the liver protects the right side. Kearney et al[46] have noted that diaphragmatic injuries due to motor vehicle accidents seem to result more from lateral impact than from frontal collisions and that right lateral impact accounts for the majority of right-sided diaphragmatic injuries.

Recent literature reports indicate that right-sided injuries are more common than previously thought.[47-49] In one recent autopsy series, the incidence of diaphragmatic rupture was 5%, and the tears were equally distributed between the right and left-sides.[29] This may be partly due to increased use of shoulder harness types of restraints.[14]

Organs Herniating into the Chest

Abdominal viscera are more likely to herniate into the chest immediately following blunt injury than after penetrating injury because the defect resulting from non-penetrating trauma is usually considerably larger.[7,30] In addition, the transient but greatly increased intra-abdominal pressure during the blunt trauma helps promote prompt herniation.

In Van Loeuhout et al's review of 58 cases, approximately equal numbers of patients presented in the acute and delayed phases, with the delay averaging 2.3 years.[35] In most series, only one organ is herniated into the chest,[43] and the stomach is involved more than half the time. The other organs that tend to herniate into the left chest are, in decreasing order of frequency, the colon, omentum, spleen, and small bowel.[4,5,7]

> **AXIOM** Blunt disruptions of the right diaphragm are usually associated with herniation of all or part of the liver into the chest.

Traumatic diaphragmatic herniations on the right diaphragm usually involve the liver.[50] With some of the larger and more anterior injuries, the colon may also herniate into the chest.[51] Unusual hernias may also present at the sites of previous surgery.[52-54]

UNUSUAL INJURIES

Hernias Through Pre-existing Hiatuses or Weaknesses

The diaphragm has three major openings, referred to as the esophageal, aortic, and caval hiatuses. In addition, pre-existing congenital diaphragmatic defects or weaknesses may be present posterolaterally (Bochdalek's Hernia) and anteromedially (Morgagni's Hernia). These orifices may be forcefully dilated or torn as a result of the extreme forces developed during blunt trauma, allowing herniation of abdominal structures through them.[55,56]

Posterior Disruption

> **AXIOM** Ruptures of the most posterior portions of the diaphragm may involve displacement of retroperitoneal structures into the chest.

Rarely, following severe blunt trauma, the posterior diaphragm will separate from the ribs, producing a large retroperitoneal extrapleural tunnel. Although intraperitoneal organs generally are not damaged and usually do not herniate through these posterior retroperitoneal defects, the ipsilateral kidney may be displaced into the chest.[14] This defect is most likely to be found during thoracotomy for concurrent chest injuries. In such instances, renal function should be monitored very carefully, and attention must be given to the possibility of a renal vascular injury.

PHRENIC NERVE INJURY

> **AXIOM** The phrenic nerve is more likely to be injured during the repair of a diaphragmatic tear than by the original trauma.

It is rare that more than one of the three to five peripheral branches of a phrenic nerve are injured by blunt trauma.[14] There is, however, an increased possibility of injuring one of the phrenic nerve branches while suturing the tear in the diaphragm. The location of the phrenic nerve branches is difficult to assess from the abdominal approach. It is very easy to catch one of them with the diaphragmatic repair sutures, especially where the medial end of the laceration approaches the point where the main phrenic nerve divides, immediately lateral to the junction of the pericardium and diaphragm. The more peripheral the diaphragmatic tear, the less likely that a significant iatrogenic phrenic nerve injury will occur. If it is necessary to widen a diaphragmatic defect to facilitate reduction of herniated organs into the abdomen, the incision in the diaphragm should be extended laterally toward the periphery of the diaphragm away from the phrenic nerve branches.

CONSEQUENCES OF DIAPHRAGMATIC INJURY

The pathophysiology of diaphragmatic disruption may include immediate hemodynamic and respiratory dysfunction; gastrointestinal (GI) sequelae tend to develop later and insidiously, particularly with penetrating injuries.

Cardiopulmonary

> **AXIOM** Shock in patients with acute diaphragmatic injury is generally due to associated injuries.

The hemodynamic instability so often seen with blunt diaphragmatic injury is usually due to associated injuries; however, herniation of bowel into the chest can closely mimic a hemothorax or pneumothorax.[57,58] The herniated viscera can decrease vital capacity and cause a further reduction in an already impaired venous return. Any concomitant pulmonary contusion further reduces pulmonary function. In addition, in the rare instances in which the diaphragmatic pericardium is torn, displacement of visceral organs into the pericardial cavity can interfere with ventricular filling and produce severe hypotension by a mechanism similar to pericardial tamponade.[35,59,60] The abdominal organs in the pericardium may also push the heart out through any defect in the lateral pericardium that may have been caused by the trauma.[61]

> **AXIOM** A clinical picture of pericardial tamponade and bowel obstruction after blunt abdominal trauma should suggest the presence of an intrapericardial rupture of the diaphragm.

At the Montreal General Hospital, roughly one-third of the patients with diaphragmatic injury were hypotensive while in the emergency department.[43] All of the hypotensive patients were hypoxic to varying degrees, and almost a third required emergency department endotracheal intubation and ventilatory support as part of their initial management. Leppaniemi et al[62] found that about half of their patients with diaphragmatic injury required prolonged postoperative ventilatory support.

> **AXIOM** In older individuals with a delayed diaphragmatic hernia, symptoms of dyspnea, chest pain, and fatigue may be presumed erroneously to be myocardial in origin.[63]

Gastrointestinal

Bowel sounds high in the chest are rarely found in the acute phase, but they should make one highly suspicious of gastrointestinal herniation.[52] Hollow viscera in the chest eventually become incarcerated and obstructed. The diaphragmatic opening often acts as a one-way valve, causing the bowel to distend progressively, enough to rupture. Leaking gastrointestinal contents can cause a severe chemical pleuritis which will usually become infected within 22-24 hours. Spillage of colon contents into the chest almost invariably causes a rapidly progressive and severe sepsis.

ASSOCIATED INJURIES

AXIOM   Most diaphragmatic trauma has associated injuries.

Penetrating Trauma

Penetrating trauma of the diaphragm will have associated injuries in at least 80% of cases.[14] The liver is usually injured in more than half of these patients and the spleen and stomach each are involved in approximately 25%[28] (Table 21-1). In the 1980-1992 Detroit Receiving Hospital series, the incidence of associated liver injuries was 48% (57/119) with stab wounds involving abdominal organs, and 69% (128/273) with gunshot wounds (Table 21-1). The next most common associated injuries with penetrating diaphragmatic trauma were the stomach (30%, 116/392) and spleen (26%, 102/392).

In a series of 154 patients collected by Wiencek et al,[1] there were an average of 2.9 other injuries caused by gunshot wounds and 1.8 by stab wounds. These included: liver 51%, stomach 26%, and spleen and colon 16% each. The pulmonary injuries associated with penetrating wounds of the diaphragm are often placed peripherally and usually require no treatment except a chest tube. However, in Wiencek's series, 18% required a thoracotomy for repair of a lung injury.

Blunt Trauma

GENERAL

The majority of patients with blunt diaphragmatic injuries have associated orthopedic injuries (especially pelvic fractures) and neurological and solid viscus injuries. Wiencek's series had an average of 3.2 associated injuries per patient.[1] Hood, in a collective review of 261 patients with blunt traumatic diaphragmatic hernias, found that 78% had associated rib or skeletal fractures and 18% had major intracranial injuries.[5]

The lung is the most common organ injured after either blunt or penetrating diaphragmatic trauma. A hemothorax or pneumothorax is found in about 60% of the patients after blunt and penetrating trauma.[1,4,18] In Wiencek's series, the incidences of various associated intra-abdominal organ injuries were liver 64%, spleen 45%, and co-

lon 36%.[1] Fractured ribs and pulmonary contusion were also common concurrent injuries.

An increased incidence of blunt diaphragmatic rupture has been reported in patients with pelvic fractures. In one series, more than 50% of the patients with blunt diaphragmatic injury also had a pelvic fracture.[64]

Right versus Left Diaphragm Injuries

Boulanger et al[69] recently reported on 80 patients with blunt diaphragmatic rupture seen over a period of about 5 ⅓ years. There were 59 (74%) on the left, 16 (20%) on the right, and five (6%) bilaterally. Although the mortality rates and complications were similar for the right- and left-sided ruptures, there were some differences. The patients with diaphragmatic injuries on the right were more likely to: (a) have a lower GCS (8 vs 11), (b) be hypotensive with a systolic BP <90 mm Hg (56% vs 22%), (c) have a positive DPL (100% vs 84%), (d) have more liver injuries (93% vs 34%), (e) have more intra-abdominal injuries (100% vs 77%), and (f) less frequently diagnosed from chest films (0% vs 37%).

Diagnosis

GENERAL

In 1951, Carter et al[66] divided the initial presentation of traumatic diaphragmatic hernias into three phases: acute, interval, and obstructive. The latter two groups have been termed the delayed phase of presentation.[66-69] Price et al[70] suggested adding a fourth phase: perforation of the herniated bowel.

It has been estimated that a correct diagnosis of acute diaphragmatic injury is made in 40-60% of patients with blunt trauma within 24-48 hours of injury.[4-5,7,18,68,69] Furthermore, Beeson and Popovici[20] have noted that up to 75% of patients with blunt diaphragmatic rupture have herniation of abdominal structures into the chest, and this should be apparent on the chest radiographs.

If the injury is not diagnosed during the acute phase, the latent phase begins. The patient may either be completely asymptomatic during this phase or have only vague, nonspecific complaints, which are often attributed to problems with other organ systems (e.g., biliary or coronary artery disease).

The obstructive phase may begin from weeks to years after the original injury and starts when an abdominal organ becomes incarcerated or strangulated in the diaphragmatic defect.

History

PENETRATING INJURY

AXIOM   One should suspect injury to the diaphragm with any penetrating trauma to the lower chest or upper abdomen.

Any stab wound of the chest below the nipple, especially anterior, but also lateral and posterior, should be suspected of injuring the diaphragm.[19] Even "trivial" knife wounds can result eventually in destruction or strangulation of herniated bowel.[71]

BLUNT TRAUMA

PITFALL ⊘

Failure to consider the possibility of diaphragmatic rupture in patients sustaining major thoracoabdominal trauma greatly increases the likelihood that the injury will be missed.

A history of sudden severe deceleration or crushing should make one suspect a diaphragmatic injury.[52] Information on the severity of a motor vehicular accident, the condition of the automobile, and the location of the patient in the automobile may be useful. Any patient

TABLE 21-1   Penetrating Trauma to the Diaphragm—Detroit Receiving Hospital (1980-1992)

Organ Injured	Type of Trauma			
	Stab	GSW	SGW	Total
Liver	(57) 35%	(183) 22%	(5) 40%	(245) 20%
Stomach	(25) 12%	(86) 20%	(5) 60%	(116) 20%
Spleen	(21) 5%	(73) 19%	(8) 50%	(102) 19%
Colon	(9) 11%	(66) 12%	(6) 33%	(81) 14%
Kidney	(6) 17%	(49) 18%	(7) 43%	(62) 21%
Abd. Vessels	(5) 40%	(42) 62%	(1) 100%	(48) 60%
Pancreas	(5) 20%	(39) 26%	(3) 67%	(47) 28%
Small Bowel	(6) 0%	(37) 22%	(3) 67%	(46) 22%
Duodenum	(2) 0%	(18) 22%	—	(20) 20%
Total	(119) 8%	(261) 21%	(12) 42%	(392) 18%

with sternal or multiple displaced rib fractures has clearly sustained severe chest trauma and should be watched closely for the possibility of a diaphragmatic injury. This is particularly important in young patients, who tend to have a resilient chest wall.

Symptoms

In most instances, the symptoms in a patient with an acute diaphragmatic tear are very non-specific (nausea, shortness of breath or vague abdominal or chest pain)[4,72,73] or are related to obvious associated injuries. Occasionally, a patient will have shoulder top pain (Kehr's sign) with an injury to the diaphragm.[25,74] If the herniation is large, it may shift the mediastinum toward the opposite side and may even cause cardiac insufficiency from obstruction of venous return.[75-78]

PHYSICAL EXAMINATION

There are no external signs that are pathognomonic for diaphragmatic injury. Moreover, many victims of motor vehicle accidents who have sustained a diaphragmatic rupture will have little more than an abdominal abrasion from the seatbelt. However, if there are decreased breath sounds in the left chest, if the abdomen is scaphoid and if bowel sounds are heard high in the chest, one should suspect a diaphragmatic injury. Patients with a large diaphragmatic injury who require urgent surgery are usually tachycardic, hypotensive, and dyspneic to a greater degree than the magnitude of the external or apparent injuries would suggest. Absent or diminished breath sounds over one hemithorax is most likely to be due to a pneumothorax or hemothorax, but in a small percentage of patients this finding is due to herniation of abdominal contents into the chest.

Pneumatic Antishock Garment (PASG)

AXIOM   Shock or severe dyspnea developing when the abdominal portion of a PASG is inflated should make one very suspicious of a diaphragmatic injury.

Use of a pneumatic antishock garment (PASG) for the treatment of severe hypotension may be very deleterious in patients with diaphragmatic trauma. If sudden severe respiratory distress develops when the abdominal portion of a PASG is inflated, the abdominal portion should be immediately deflated and the possibility of a diaphragmatic injury investigated. Maull et al demonstrated severe respiratory impairment in swine on whom PASG was applied following diaphragmatic laceration.[76] Inflation of the extremity portions of the PASG in severely hypotensive individuals for brief periods can be helpful and benign. However, if ventilatory function appears to be diminished or respiratory effort is increased, the abdominal portion of the PASG should not be inflated.

RADIOLOGICAL STUDIES

Chest Radiograph

AXIOM   The single most frequent and useful non-invasive technique for diagnosing diaphragmatic injury is a chest radiograph.

Following penetrating injuries, the chest radiograph is interpreted as normal in about 40% of patients with penetrating injuries.[1,13,34,78] In the remaining patients, the radiographic findings are usually limited to a small to moderate sized pneumothorax or hemothorax. In Wiencek's series, 56% of the patients with penetrating trauma had a hemothorax and/or a pneumothorax.[1] In patients with entrance wounds in the chest, this is a nonspecific finding. However, in the 65 patients with abdominal entrance wounds, x-ray evidence of a hemopneumothorax in 22 (34%) was considered diagnostic. Wilkinson[77] has noted that metal markers on the sites of entrance and exit wounds can assist in the radiographic diagnosis of diaphragmatic injury since the paths of bullets can then be traced.

Although the chest radiograph is almost always abnormal with blunt diaphragmatic injury, the radiological findings are diagnostic in only about 16-30% of the cases.[1,78,79] Radiograph findings strongly suggestive of a diaphragmatic injury include a very high diaphragmatic shadow (Fig. 21-3), the presence of herniated bowel in the chest (Fig. 21-4), or the nasogastric tube passing from the abdomen high up into the left hemithorax (Fig. 21-5, Table 21-2).[80]

AXIOM   Any abnormal shadows in the left lower lung fields after trauma should make one suspect a diaphragmatic injury.

Payne and Yellin[73] described the radiologic characteristics on routine chest radiographs that should make one suspect a diaphragmatic injury. These include:

1. an arch-like shadow suggesting an abnormally high diaphragm;
2. extraneous shadows such as gas bubbles or densities above the usual level of the diaphragm suggesting bowel in the chest;
3. shift of heart and mediastinal shadows to the side opposite the defect;
4. plate-like atelectasis adjacent to the archlike shadow of the diaphragm.

Intrapleural and intrapulmonary lesions, however, may lead to false interpretation of the chest radiographs.[81] Ventilatory assistance, especially with PEEP, can push herniated bowel back into the abdomen. End-expiratory films with the patient in the Trendelenburg position, off ventilator assistance, is most apt to show herniated bowel.

Multiple displaced fractures of the lower ribs on either side suggest the possibility of a diaphragmatic rupture or puncture.

AXIOM   Patients with penetrating injury to the lower chest and a hemothorax should have an over-penetrated radiograph taken prior to placing a chest tube because it may reveal herniated viscera above the diaphragm.

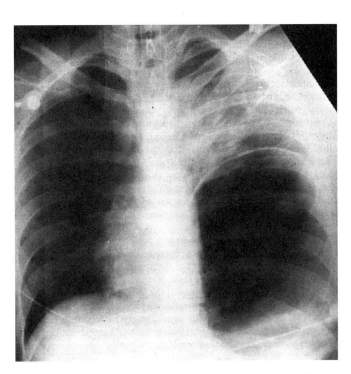

FIGURE 21-3 Traumatic rupture of the diaphragm. Plain chest radiograph showing displacement of air-filled viscera, especially the stomach, into the left lower chest (From: Orringer MB, Kirsh MM. Traumatic rupture of the diaphragm. In Kirsh MM, Sloan H, eds. Blunt chest trauma—general principles of management. Boston: Little, Brown & Company, 1977;6:134.)

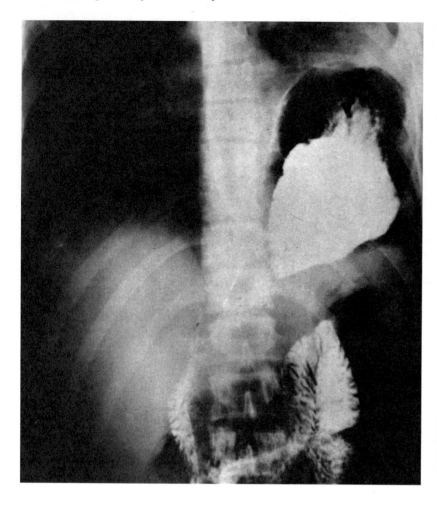

FIGURE 21-4   Displacement of the stomach into the chest, shown by barium meal examination (From: Orringer MB, Kirsh MM. Traumatic rupture of the diaphragm. In Kirsh MM, Sloan H, eds. Blunt chest trauma—general principles of management. Boston: Little, Brown & Company, 1977;6:138.)

With opacification of the lower hemithorax and slight shifting of the mediastinal structures to the opposite side, it is easy to assume that a hemothorax is present. However, caution must be taken when inserting a chest tube until diaphragmatic rupture has been ruled out.[65,81] This can be done relatively simply by obtaining overpenetrated radiographs, which may reveal a typical bowel gas pattern in the chest. If the diagnosis is still not clear, additional studies should be considered.

With an injured diaphragm on the right, all that is usually seen on chest radiograph is an apparently elevated diaphragm because of the herniated dome of the liver. However, separate inspiratory and expiratory chest radiographs may demonstrate a stationary lateral diaphragmatic leaflet with movement of the herniated liver. Fluoroscopy may also be diagnostic, but this is not practical with severely injured patients.

TABLE 21-2   *Radiographic Findings on Chest Radiograph Patients (102)—San Antonio Series*

	Blunt	*Penetrating*	*Totals*
Hemo- and/or pneumothorax	6	51	57
Normal chest radiograph	0	40	40
Herniated abdominal contents	3	1	4
Pneumoperitoneum	0	1	1
Total	9	93	102

From Miller OL, Grover F. Abdominal trauma—injuries of the diaphragm. In Kreis DJ, Jr, Gomez GA, eds. Trauma management. Boston: Little, Brown & Company, 1989; 244.

If suspicion of a diaphragmatic injury is raised in the emergency room, a nasogastric tube should be carefully inserted and connected to low continuous suction.[70,82] If the nasogastric tube enters the abdomen normally and then curls up into the left chest above the diaphragm, this is virtually diagnostic of a ruptured diaphragm. However, distortion of the esophagogastric junction may occur from acute gastric herniation into the chest, and there may be difficulty passing the nasogastric tube into the stomach. Under such circumstances, the tube should be left in the distal esophagus where it can evacuate swallowed air and saliva. Vigorous efforts to pass the esophagogastric junction are dangerous.

AXIOM   Aggressive bag-mask ventilation can greatly increase herniation of bowel through a diaphragmatic defect.

Bag-mask ventilation may be a problem because it can result in rapid insufflation of air or oxygen into the stomach and intestines, increasing the amount of diaphragmatic herniation. A diaphragmatic hernia that enlarges rapidly may cause severe impairment of pulmonary and/or cardiac function.

Positive pressure ventilation may prevent herniation of abdominal viscera into the chest through a diaphragmatic defect. The injury may become apparent only when the patient begins to breathe spontaneously and the intra-thoracic pressure falls below that of the abdominal cavity. It is important, therefore, to repeat the chest radiograph whenever a patient with thoraco-abdominal trauma is taken off the ventilator.[21]

AXIOM   A nasogastric tube can often help detect herniation of stomach into the chest.

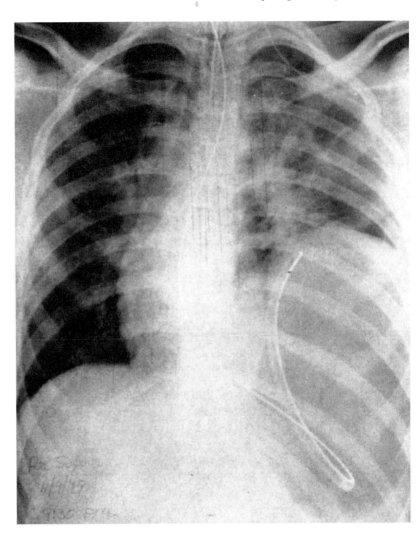

FIGURE 21-5 Ruptured left hemidiaphragm with gastric herniation. AP chest radiograph demonstrates the gastric fundus in the left hemithorax, the nasogastric tube going back up into the chest, left perihilar lung contusion, and a mediastinal shift to the right (From: Mirvis SE, Rodriguez A. Diagnostic imaging of thoracic trauma. In Mirvis SE, Young JWR, eds. Imaging in trauma and critical care. Baltimore: Williams & Wilkins, 1992;3:127.)

If the nasogastric tube goes through a normally positioned gastroesophageal junction and then up into the chest, the presence of a diaphragmatic tear is quite clear. However, sometimes the portion of the tube in the herniated stomach is behind the cardiac silhouette and not easy to see. The diagnosis may also be suspected if air injected through a nasogastric tube which extends into the abdomen is heard gurgling high in the chest.[38,83]

Abdominal Radiographs

Radiographs of the abdomen can sometimes be of help in diagnosing a diaphragmatic injury. Upward displacement of the silhouette of the transverse colon suggests herniation of colon or omentum into the chest.[30]

Contrast Studies

AXIOM A contrast study of the GI tract is the most accurate radiological test for diaphragmatic rupture.

The stomach, small bowel, spleen, liver, and colon are the organs most apt to herniate into the chest. Contrast material delivered through an indwelling nasogastric tube can clearly demonstrate displacement of the stomach into the chest (Fig. 21-2). Follow-through films may also show small bowel which has herniated through the diaphragm. However, if the barium is instilled under pressure, it could distend the herniated viscus, causing GI or cardiorespiratory distress.[84] A barium enema may be helpful if colon has herniated into the chest.

If the traumatic diaphragmatic tear is posterior, accurate localization of a herniated hollow viscus using intraluminal contrast may require lateral views of the torso as well as the standard anteroposterior radiographs.

Ultrasound

Ultrasound evaluation of the integrity of the diaphragm can be valuable, especially for ruptures of the right diaphragm,[85,86] and it is easily performed in most individuals. In skilled hands, it can be used to obtain coronal and sagittal planes through the diaphragm.[86,87] A properly performed ultrasound study can sometimes detect diaphragmatic injuries even if no organs are herniated through the defect. Ultrasonography can also help localize peridiaphragmatic fluid collections, and may be especially helpful in patients whose condition is too poor to permit safe transportation to the radiology department.[88,89] However, the value of ultrasonography is largely dependent on the skills of the individuals performing and interpreting the study.

CT Scans

On CT scans, the diaphragm may be visible as a circular or oval soft-tissue density with fat below and aerated lung above.[90-94] The diaphragm is not visible where it is tangential to the scanning plane or where there is no fat or air separating it from soft-tissue structures such as the liver, spleen, stomach, or colon.[95,96] The integrity of the diaphragm is largely inferred by examining the relationship of the organs above and below it. Thus, a diaphragmatic hernia can be diagnosed positively with CT only if there is protrusion of abdominal viscera above the remaining visualized portions of the diaphragm. This sign is especially helpful if superior displacement of the viscera is noted at the peripheral, more inferior portions of the diaphragm. A more central superior herniation of bowel and omental fat may be indistinguishable on CT from diaphragmatic eventration or paresis, particularly since the torn edges of the central portion of the diaphragm are thinner and more difficult to detect with CT.

Computerized tomography may be particularly useful if obstruction is suspected;[90,91] however, although CT scanning can usually demonstrate herniated viscera very clearly,[93] it seldom shows the actual structure of the diaphragm.[94]

Small focal herniations, particularly of the liver, may be difficult to differentiate.[37] Reformation of CT images in the sagittal and coronal planes may help to make this differentiation at times. Current CT scanners, with their faster scanning times and reduced motion artifact, also facilitate direct visualization of the diaphragm.

Shapiro et al[79] noted that of 10 patients who had a blunt diaphragmatic rupture and CT scan preoperatively, only three were diagnostic because of a nasogastric tube or stomach bubble in the chest; however, these findings were also seen on the chest radiograph.

Magnetic Resonance Imaging

Magnetic resonance imaging (MRI) of soft tissue may be able to differentiate the involved organs associated with diaphragmatic injury more clearly than CT scans.[95] On MRI scans, the diaphragm appears similar to its configuration on CT if the cuts are axial. However, the unique ability of MRI to visualize the body in all planes allows easier coronal and sagittal depiction of the diaphragm.[24]

Unfortunately, patients having MRI must be remarkably stable, and this is difficult to ensure immediately after severe trauma. Another problem is the motion of the diaphragm during the scanning times; however, respiratory gating programs eliminate many of the problems associated with imaging the moving diaphragm.[96]

Radionuclide Studies

Although liver and liver-spleen radionuclide scans are used only rarely to diagnose acute diaphragmatic injuries, they can be helpful, especially in patients with an unexplained elevation of the right hemidiaphragm following severe blunt trauma.[97-99] The radionuclide study may show a characteristic distortion of the hepatic image with superior and posterior displacement of the right lobe.[68,100] Some authors also believe that these scans can show colonic and splenic herniation.[68]

Peritoneoscintigraphy using technetium-99M diethylene-triamene pentacetic acid has also been suggested by Ramirez et al.[101]

Pneumoperitoneum

AXIOM Pneumoperitoneum can help delineate diaphragmatic tears.

If an acute diaphragmatic injury is suspected but not confirmed in a patient who would not otherwise be explored, pneumoperitoneography[5,6,83,102,103] and pleurography[104] have been described as useful, but are seldom employed. The technique requires a chest radiograph before and 15-30 minutes after inducing a pneumoperitoneum with 500 cc of air in a patient sitting erect. However, these methods can be time-consuming and inaccurate, and there is a risk of inducing air embolism.[28] This maneuver is safer if the pneumoperitoneum is limited to less than 500 ml and CO_2 is used instead of air.

False-negative results can occur when an acute diaphragmatic tear is plugged by omentum, liver, or a partial circumference of bowel wall, as is often the case.

Echocardiogram

An echocardiogram can be particularly helpful in diagnosis if the pericardium is injured or there is intrapericardial herniation.[105] An echocardiogram may also detect bowel in the chest.

Thoracoscopy

The most direct method, short of formal surgery, for diagnosing diaphragmatic injury is laparoscopy or thoracoscopy, and this may play a significant role in the management of urgent cases.[106-107] Indeed,

Jackson and Ferreia[107] have suggested that all patients with penetrating injuries below the fourth intercostal space on the left side should undergo routine thoracoscopy to help identify patients with diaphragmatic injuries as early as possible.

Ochsner et al[108] recently described the use of thoracoscopy to rule out diaphragmatic injury in 14 patients with penetrating injuries of the lower chest. A rigid thoracoscope was used in the first five patients, but videothoracoscopy was used on the remaining nine. The diaphragmatic injuries found in nine of the patients were repaired at laparotomy. Two major complications occurring with the thoracoscopy included a subphrenic abscess and empyema in one patient and bleeding from a laceration of the lung in another.

Ivatory et al[109] recently reported on their use of diagnostic laparoscopy to reduce the number of negative abdominal explorations and to assess the diaphragm for occult injury. Diagnostic laparoscopy was performed in 23 patients with a total of 17 stab wounds and six gunshot wounds of the lower chest or upper abdomen. Laparoscopy provided excellent visualization of the upper abdominal viscera as well as both diaphragms. Thirteen patients (59%) had a negative laparoscopy with no peritoneal penetration and, consequently, laparotomy was avoided. Laparoscopy demonstrated organ injury in eight patients, including liver and spleen lacerations, and a perinephric hematoma. Unsuspected diaphragmatic injury was found in five of these eight patients.

In a recent study of the role of diagnostic laparoscopy in the management of trauma patients, Salvino et al[110] found that three of 15 patients with stab wounds had injuries to the diaphragm. All three had less than 10,000 RBC/mm³ on DPL but the injury was easily seen on diagnostic laparoscopy (DL).

In a study of six pigs given a 2.0 cm laceration of the diaphragm, Rudston-Brown et al[111] found that laparoscopy diagnosed the injury in all six pigs. They also noted no tendency to tension pneumothorax in any animal using insufflation pressures as high as 20 mm Hg. Methylene blue instilled into the abdomen did not come out chest tubes often enough for this to be a sensitive test.

Diagnostic Peritoneal Lavage (DPL)

AXIOM A negative DPL does not rule out diaphragmatic injury.

Diagnostic peritoneal lavage (DPL) is an established diagnostic method for assessing abdominal trauma, but false-negative DPL has been noted in 14-36% of blunt diaphragmatic disruptions[14,112,113] and in 12-40% of penetrating diaphragmatic injuries.[14,113,114]

At least two reports have shown that the most common abdominal injury associated with a negative DPL is isolated diaphragmatic trauma.[113,115] Sealing of the perforation by an abdominal viscus, negative intrathoracic pressure sucking the peritoneal blood into the chest, and hemorrhage into the lesser sac have all been blamed for these disappointing results.

The number of red cells that constitutes a positive DPL, for a diaphragmatic injury varies considerably from author to author. A red blood cell (RBC) count of 100,000/mm³ is often defined as a positive lavage even in penetrating injuries, even though Thal et al found it unreliable in gunshot wounds of the lower chest and abdomen.[116] As a consequence, lower RBC counts have been suggested.

Oreskovich and Carrico[117] considered a DPL with an RBC count of 1000/mm³ as positive. Moore and Marx[118] have shown an increased sensitivity for DPL after lower chest wounds if the RBC criteria for celiotomy were lowered to 5,000/mm³. Merlotti et al[119] advocated using an RBC count of 10,000/mm³ as indicating a positive DPL. Hornyak and Shaftan[120] recommended a red blood cell count of 20,000 cells/mm³. However, even with these greatly reduced RBC criteria, diaphragmatic perforations can still be missed by DPL. Interestingly, even though the RBC count on the DPL may be negative, a diaphragmatic injury will occasionally cause the DPL WBC count to exceed 500/mm³.[121]

Other evidence suggesting a diaphragm injury during diagnostic peritoneal lavage is increasing dyspnea, and/or reduced return of the lavage fluid.

TABLE 21-3   Indications for Operations*—San Antonio Series

	Blunt	*Penetrating*	*Totals*
Penetrating wounds to lower chest and upper abdomen	0	91	91
Positive diagnostic peritoneal lavage	6	3	9
Herniated abdominal viscera	3	1	4
Pericardial tamponade	1	1	2
Intrathoracic hemorrhage	0	10	10

From Miller OL, Grover F. Abdominal trauma—injuries of the diaphragm. In Kreis DJ, Jr, Gomez GA, eds. Trauma management. Boston: Little, Brown & Company, 1989; 244.

AXIOM A diagnostic peritoneal lavage for suspected diaphragmatic injury is more apt to be positive if a chest tube is already in place.

If a chest tube is in place, drainage of lavage fluid out of it is diagnostic of a diaphragmatic injury.[88,122,123] However, this seldom occurs.

FINGER THORACOTOMY
It has been suggested by Feliciano et al[124] that one should try to palpate the diaphragm for defects with penetrating wounds of the lower chest, especially if one is going to insert a chest tube.

Diagnosis at Surgery

AXIOM Most penetrating injuries of the diaphragm are initially silent and are discovered incidentally during exploratory surgery.[7]

Victims of penetrating lower chest and upper abdominal trauma often require an aggressive approach to make the definitive diagnosis of diaphragmatic injury.[18,125] In an effort to reduce the incidence of missed diaphragmatic injury, Madden et al[125] reported on 95 patients who had a laparotomy for penetrating injury to the lower chest or abdomen. Eighteen (19%) had diaphragmatic injury but only one had any evidence of herniation on radiograph. Thirty (31%) of the 95 patients had otherwise negative laparotomies. On the basis of their findings, the authors proposed that stab wounds of the epigastrium or of the left chest in the "D-zone" (below the fourth intercostal space anteriorly, the sixth intercostal space laterally, and the eighth interspace posteriorly), require celiotomy until a reliable non-operative method is described. Stylianos and King[20] agree with this approach. Stab wounds of the right chest in the absence of peritoneal sepsis, free air, unexplained hypotension, evisceration, or bilious effusion, can be treated expectantly.[125]

AXIOM The most common reason for missing diaphragmatic trauma during laparotomy is failure to thoroughly inspect the leaflets, especially posteriorly.

Two patients in the series of Ebert et al[126] and Miller et al[18] had diaphragmatic injuries missed at laparotomy. Proper inspection involves pulling the spleen and the fundus of the stomach down on the left and the liver down on the right. Blind palpation of the diaphragm is not adequate. In addition, if the diaphragmatic rupture is extraperitoneal, it can easily be missed at the time of surgery.[100]

Treatment of Acute Injuries (Figs. 21-6, 21-7)
PREOPERATIVE RESUSCITATION

AXIOM With diaphragmatic injury, one should assume that associated injuries are present.

Patients with diaphragmatic injuries frequently have multiple associated intra-abdominal or thoracic injuries. The abdominal injuries may result in significant blood loss, and the associated thoracic injuries, including myocardial contusion and pulmonary contusion, may

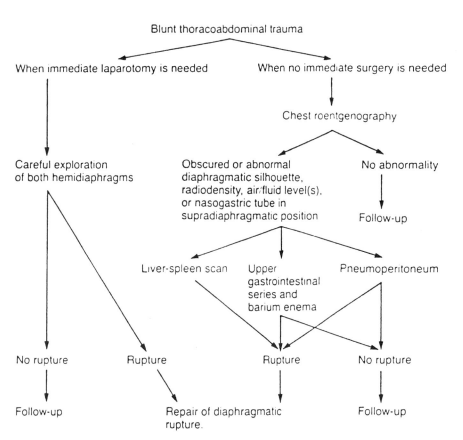

FIGURE 21-6 Algorithm for the diagnosis and management of blunt injury to the diaphragm (From: Symbas PN. Cardiothoracic trauma. Philadelphia: WB Saunders Company, 1989; 348.)

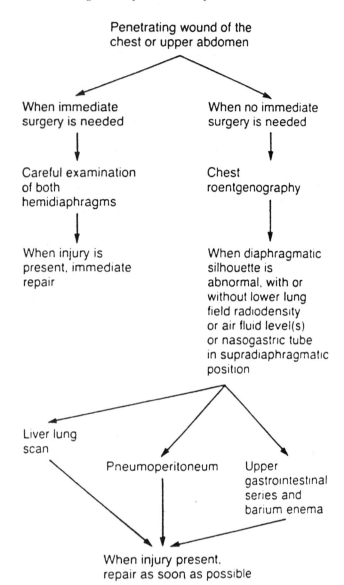

FIGURE 21-7   Algorithm for the diagnosis and management of penetrating injury of the diaphragm (From: Symbas PN. Cardiothoracic trauma. Philadelphia: WB Saunders Company, 1989; 355.)

add to the cardiorespiratory dysfunction. These patients require aggressive resuscitation in the emergency room followed by an urgent laparotomy.

If the patient is in respiratory distress in spite of an open airway and careful correction of any obvious hemothorax or pneumothorax, early endotracheal intubation should be considered. Bagging with a mask can increase the amount of bowel distension and herniation into the chest. This combination of shock and acute respiratory distress is particularly lethal and may have a mortality rate of 70% or more.[127]

AXIOM   Preoxygenation with a bag-mask prior to induction of anesthesia should be done very cautiously in patients with a possible diaphragmatic injury.

INDICATIONS FOR SURGERY

If an obvious diaphragmatic injury is present, surgical exploration should be undertaken as soon as optimal preoperative resuscitation has been achieved. However, even if there is no obvious diaphragmatic injury, early laparotomy is recommended for all patients with

penetrating injuries, particularly gunshot wounds, that reasonably could have injured the diaphragm (Table 21-4). Operation is justified because of the tendency for abdominal organs to herniate eventually through even very small diaphragmatic defects. Since the path of a bullet can be totally unpredictable, the chest and abdomen should be prepped widely prior to exploring a patient for a GSW of the chest or abdomen (Table 21-3).

ANESTHETIC CHOICES

PITFALL ⊘

Nitrous oxide should be avoided in patients with a possible diaphragmatic hernia, as it can greatly increase the volume of gas within an entrapped viscus.

Virtually any type of general anesthetic can be used; however, N_2O should be avoided because it tends to enter the lumen of the bowel and cause it to become increasingly distended if it is obstructed. This could cause the herniated bowel to distend enough to become strangulated.

CHOICE OF INCISIONS

A laparotomy is generally the incision of choice for exploring a patient with a suspected acute diaphragmatic injury.[52] Virtually all acute diaphragmatic injuries can be repaired from within the abdomen through a midline vertical incision. This approach also affords exposure for the repair of the associated intra-abdominal injuries which are frequently present.

Although most acute injuries to the diaphragm can be repaired from the abdominal approach, occasional defects occur in locations, such as posterior to the bare area of the liver, which are very difficult to repair through a laparotomy incision. In these instances, a separate anterolateral or posterolateral thoracotomy incision can be made. Many surgeons believe one should not connect thoracic and abdominal incisions because of the increased incidence of postoperative complications. Although we tend to agree with this axiom, we will not go to great lengths to avoid a thoracoabdominal incision if it is difficult to repair the injuries without it.

If the entrance wound is in the chest and it appears that the main injuries are intrathoracic and not in the abdomen, the optimal initial incision is thoracic. A thoracotomy certainly offers a better approach to associated lung or cardiac injuries. Furthermore, a limited exploration of the upper abdomen can be done through the diaphragmatic tear or through a separate diaphragmatic incision. If there is still difficulty assessing the abdomen for injuries, a separate laparotomy incision should be performed.

If a thoracotomy incision is to be used, a double-lumen endotracheal tube and one-lung anesthesia can assist in providing optimal conditions for exposing the diaphragmatic injury.

TABLE 21-4   Operative Approach

	Blunt	Penetrating	Total
Laparotomy	8	81	89
Thoracotomy	0	4	4
Sternotomy	0	1	1
Laparotomy and thoracotomy	0	6	6
Laparotomy and sternotomy	1	1	2
Total	9	93	102

From Miller OL, Grover F. Abdominal trauma—Injuries of the diaphragm. In Kreis DJ, Jr, Gomez GA, eds. Trauma management. Boston: Little, Brown & Company, 1989; 244.

REPAIR TECHNIQUES

Simple Lacerations

Diaphragmatic wounds less than two cm in length can be securely repaired by interrupted horizontal mattress sutures of 1-0 or 2-0 slowly absorbable or nonabsorbable material. The sutures at the medial end of the tear can inadvertently include branches of the phrenic nerve and should be placed carefully. With defects larger than 2 cm, a two-layer closure should be considered because of the ease with which diaphragm muscle can tear. An initial layer of horizontal mattress sutures can be used to evert the torn edges of the diaphragm toward the abdomen, and this can be reinforced with a running suture. The relatively watertight seal provided by a second (running) suture layer reduces the likelihood that later subphrenic abscess will extend into the pleural space. This may be especially important if the patient also has had an injury to the colon with moderate or severe contamination.

With very large diaphragmatic injuries, it may be difficult to expose the most posterior portion of the tear. Under such circumstances, one can start the repair anteriorly. Placing traction on previously placed anterior sutures can help expose the more posterior portions of the wound.

Recently, Koehler and Smith[128] have described repair of two penetrating diaphragmatic injuries that were repaired via a thoracoscope. One injury was stapled and the other was sutured.

Detachment from the Chest Wall

If the diaphragm has been torn from its attachments to the posterior chest wall, it can often be reattached best through a thoracic incision. The repair itself can often be accomplished by placing a series of figure-of-eight sutures through the leaf of the diaphragm and then around the corresponding rib.

Injuries Through Normal Diaphragmatic Openings

If there has been a forceful dilatation or disruption of the esophageal hiatus, the herniated organs are reduced into the abdomen and the crural fibers are reapproximated posterior to the esophagus. Diaphragmatic tears extending radially from the esophageal hiatus are closed primarily. One can prevent making the closure too tight by inserting a 50 F Maloney dilator in the esophagus prior to placing the repair sutures. A Nissen fundoplication should be added if there has been injury to the distal esophagus.

Injuries involving the aortic hiatus are often fatal because of associated damage to the aorta. However, if such an injury is found, the diaphragmatic repair is achieved by simple reapproximation of the deep posterior crural fibers.

Injuries involving the hiatus of the inferior vena cava (IVC) often have associated vascular injuries either at the junction of the IVC and the right atrium or at the junction of the hepatic veins with the IVC. A sternotomy incision connected to the midline laparotomy incision is often required to properly expose and repair such vascular injuries. An atriocaval shunt, with or without aortic cross-clamping, may reduce blood loss and maintain a reasonable venous return and cardiac output during the repair.

Pericardial Injuries

Pericardial avulsions from blunt trauma are uncommon, but their repair can be extremely difficult. Extension of the laparotomy incision as a median sternotomy may be required to improve the exposure of such an injury. Priority should be given to placing the heart back in its anatomic position and minimizing hemodynamic instability. The pericardium in the chest can be left open, but the diaphragmatic pericardium should be closed, even if a prosthetic patch is required.

PHRENIC NERVE INJURY

Direct phrenic nerve injury is quite rare. The phrenic nerves are more likely to be damaged iatrogenically during the repair of the diaphragm. In the very rare circumstances that one of the phrenic nerves is transected, it can usually be sutured primarily using magnifying loops to provide a more exact repair.

CHEST TUBES

Even if a hemopneumothorax is not already present, exposure and repair of a tear in the diaphragm almost always allows entry of significant amounts of air into the chest. The resultant pneumothorax should be evacuated following the repair. This can be accomplished by placing a tube through the tear and then removing it after the repair is completed; however, we prefer to leave a chest tube in place for at least 24-48 hours in case there is any unrecognized injury causing continued bleeding or an air leak. The chest tube also will evacuate more completely any residual pleural effusion that might become infected later. If an empyema does develop, it must be drained promptly before it can disrupt the diaphragmatic repair.

OUTCOME

AXIOM The morbidity and mortality of patients with diaphragmatic injury is primarily related to the associated injuries.

Post-operative complications are frequent and most commonly include atelectasis and pneumonia. These patients may require prolonged postoperative ventilator support because of the diaphragmatic injury as well as the high incidence of associated injuries to the lung and chest wall. Another major complication related to delayed treatment is bowel strangulation in the chest. Blunt injuries which disrupt considerable portions of the left and/or right diaphragm can cause significant impairment of pulmonary function even after an early adequate repair.

The injured diaphragm tends to remain elevated and portions of it may move paradoxically (i.e., move up during inspiration) for several weeks after the repair. Compression and stretch injuries to the phrenic nerve will usually resolve within 3-4 weeks. However, if the nerve is transected, even if it is repaired primarily, eventration of the ipsilateral diaphragm invariably ensues while the nerve is regenerating. If the eventration is severe and interferes with pulmonary function, plication of the involved leaflet may result in a significant return of function.

The mortality rate for blunt diaphragmatic rupture ranges from 16-41%.[6,14,39,41,50,129,130] In the 12 year Detroit Receiving Hospital series, it was 15% (3/20) for the 20 patients with no, one, or two associated injuries; for those with three or more associated injuries, it was 50% (4/8). Although a diaphragm organ injury scale has been developed by the Organ Injury Scaling Committee of the American Association for the Surgery of Trauma (Table 21-5),[131] deaths in patients with these injuries are almost entirely due to associated injuries. The mortality rate for penetrating diaphragmatic injuries is usually lower, and averages 1-5% for stab wounds and 10-20% for gunshot wounds.[2,7,34,50] In the 1980-1992 Detroit Receiving Hospital series, it was 8% for stab wounds, 21% for GSW, and 42% for SGW. Stab wounds cause a much lower mortality and morbidity than gunshot wounds because they tend to cause fewer and less severe associated injuries.

TABLE 21-5 Diaphragm Organ Injury Scale

Grade	Injury Description	AIS-90
I	Contusion	1
II	Laceration ≤2 cm	2
III	Laceration 2-10 cm	3
IV	Laceration >10 cm with tissue loss ≤25 cm^2	4
V	Laceration with tissue loss >25 cm^2	5

From Moore EE, Malangoni MA, Cogbill TH, et al. Organ injury scaling IV. Thoracic vascular, lung, cardiac, and diaphragm. J Trauma 1994;36:299.

DELAYED RECOGNITION

Diagnosis (Fig. 21-8)

Diaphragmatic injury can easily be overlooked in the acute phase. The frequency of missed diagnosis and subsequent late presentation is difficult to estimate, but de la Rocha et al[132] have estimated that about 30% of diaphragmatic injuries are diagnosed late.

The percentage of patients with diaphragmatic rents who will eventually require surgery because of obstruction and/or strangulation of herniated viscera is unknown. If strangulation of herniated bowel does develop, it occurs within three years of the initial injury in about 85% of cases.[133]

Most cases of delayed presentation can be suspected from a plain chest radiograph. In the less obvious cases, a high degree of suspicion is important, and a history of previous trauma should be sought. In some cases, the incident has been forgotten by the patient.

AXIOM Absence of a history of trauma from the patient does not rule out a delayed traumatic diaphragmatic hernia.

HISTORY

Stab wounds are the most common cause of delayed traumatic hernia, and the risk of strangulations is high because the defects are generally quite small.[73] Victims of penetrating or blunt trauma who have survived the acute phase of injury without repair of their diaphragmatic injury usually have minimal or no symptoms until a significant amount of intra-abdominal viscera herniates into the chest or bowel strangulates. The interval phase can last for days to years before symptoms develop due to compression of the lung or heart or obstruction or strangulation of herniated bowel. Over 85% of patients will develop symptoms of intestinal obstruction because of incarceration of bowel in the diaphragmatic hernia.[31] Without prompt therapy, this can rapidly progress to strangulation and necrosis.

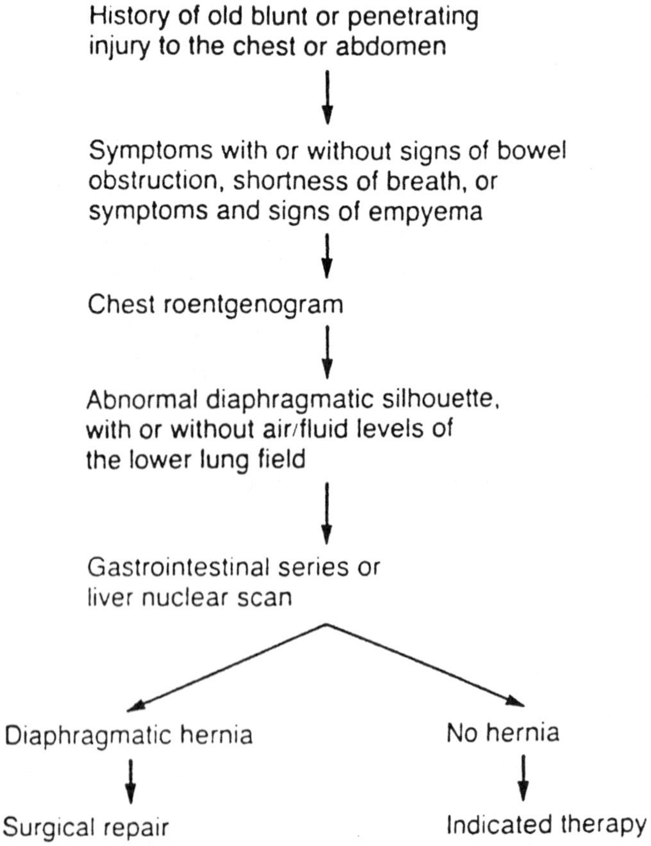

AXIOM Signs and symptoms of a bowel obstruction after remote trauma are usually due to adhesions, but one should be looking for hernias, especially in the diaphragm.

As abdominal viscera increasingly herniate into the chest, the patient may develop vague symptoms of abdominal cramping and nausea, suggesting the presence of an incomplete bowel obstruction.[73,134] In some instances the patient may develop chest pain and/or shortness of breath,[50,81,134] suggesting pulmonary or cardiac disease. Repeated pulmonary infections or empyema may also occur, especially in children.[135]

AXIOM Rapid dilatation of bowel herniated into the chest can cause severe shortness of breath and will occasionally resemble a loculated pneumothorax.

Occasionally, massive dilatation of the stomach or intestine in the chest can produce severe dyspnea with what we have referred to as a "tension enterothorax." Perforation of bowel can produce a similar picture with pneumothorax and a large pleural effusion. If the herniated bowel becomes strangulated, up to 30% of patients will die of severe sepsis, particularly if the colon is involved.[134] Rarely, abdominal contents will herniate into the pericardial cavity and cause a clinical picture of acute pericardial tamponade.[61]

AXIOM If a diaphragmatic hernia is not diagnosed until the herniated bowel becomes strangulated and perforated, the mortality rate is very high.

RADIOLOGIC STUDIES

The chest radiograph usually remains normal in the presence of old penetrating injuries of the diaphragm until significant abdominal contents have herniated into the chest. With blunt injuries, the herniated viscera above the diaphragm are often obvious on the initial chest radiograph. However, interval chest radiographs may only reveal a slightly to moderately elevated diaphragm or an indistinct abnormality in the lower lung fields.

Upper and lower intestinal contrast studies are the most sensitive diagnostic tests if bowel has herniated into the chest.[87] Liver scans can be useful for the evaluation of a stationary or elevated right hemidiaphragm.[97,112] CT scanning, particularly with contrast, has also been helpful occasionally.[87] However, Tocino and Miller,[136] as well as many others, have found CT to be quite insensitive.[137] Right-sided diaphragmatic injuries can be particularly difficult to visualize on CT scan since the torn portion of the diaphragm blends into the liver contour. As a consequence, contrast studies to outline the bowel or liver are usually much more accurate.

AXIOM Once a delayed presentation of a traumatic diaphragmatic hernia is suspected, barium studies of the gastrointestinal tract are the most reliable means of confirming the diagnosis.[87]

It can be extremely difficult to differentiate a traumatic diaphragmatic hernia from an eventration of the diaphragm. Three of four patients with eventrations of diaphragm seen recently at DRH had relatively urgent surgery for what was interpreted initially as a posttraumatic diaphragmatic hernia. A pneumoperitoneum should be helpful in making this differentiation; however, this test may be negative in delayed diaphragmatic hernias if adhesions have sealed the tear.[87]

Graivier and Freeark[103] stated that the possibility of a traumatic diaphragmatic hernia should be considered in any patient with bowel obstruction if there is/are:

History of old blunt or penetrating injury to the chest or abdomen

↓

Symptoms with or without signs of bowel obstruction, shortness of breath, or symptoms and signs of empyema

↓

Chest roentgenogram

↓

Abnormal diaphragmatic silhouette, with or without air/fluid levels of the lower lung field

↓

Gastrointestinal series or liver nuclear scan

⟋   ⟍

Diaphragmatic hernia   No hernia

↓   ↓

Surgical repair   Indicated therapy

FIGURE 21-8 Algorithm for the diagnosis and management of chronic traumatic diaphragmatic hernia. (From: Symbas PN. Cardiothoracic trauma. Philadelphia: WB Saunders Company, 1989; 359.)

1. a history of prior chest or abdominal trauma;
2. a left pleural density;
3. abdominal scars or hernias; or
4. a large bowel obstruction in a young individual.[28]

Bowel Preparation

Patients undergoing surgery after the acute phase of injury should undergo a full cathartic and antibiotic bowel preparation if obstruction is not present. This can help reduce the incidence and severity of sepsis if an enterotomy is inadvertently performed during the release of bowel which has become adhesed to the lung and other structures.

AXIOM Distended ischemic bowel in a diaphragmatic hernia is often extremely friable. As a consequence inadvertent bowel injury is not infrequent during corrective surgery.

Incision and Technique

AXIOM Surgery for a diaphragmatic hernia due to old trauma is usually best done through a posterolateral thoracotomy incision.

Diaphragmatic injuries away from the pericardium that are repaired more than a week following trauma are often approached best through a thoracotomy incision, particularly if there is a significant amount of herniated bowel in the chest.[12] Intrapericardial diaphragmatic hernias have been missed at thoracotomy,[35] and they are best approached through the abdomen.[138] Herniated bowel quickly adheres to the lung because there is no peritoneal hernia sac, and release of these adhesions through a laparotomy incision can be extremely difficult. Tedious dissection is often required to remove the bowel from the lung without inadvertent enterotomies or lung injuries.

Incarcerated organs may be ischemic or even infarcted and consequently more friable and prone to injury or rupture during the operation. Caution must also be taken when manipulating the abdominal organs back into the peritoneal cavity. Unrecognized injury to the herniated organs may lead to severe complications and morbidity. In some instances, a separate abdominal incision may be required in addition to the initial thoracotomy incision. This can facilitate return of the organs to the abdomen or even resection if the organs are damaged too badly. After the bowel and any other herniated abdominal viscera are returned to the peritoneal cavity, a standard two-layer diaphragm closure is performed.

In spite of these concerns, some surgeons prefer using an abdominal approach for the repair of chronic diaphragmatic injuries. Taylor et al,[28] for example, believe that the adhesions in the chest are rarely significant enough to prevent a successful reduction of the herniated viscera and repair transabdominally. Nevertheless, use of prosthetic material or muscle flaps to repair very large defects is best done through the chest.[10]

Prosthetic Material and Muscle Flaps

Occasionally, long-standing large diaphragmatic hernias will require closure of the defect with prosthetic material, such as Marlex, Dacron, or Prolene mesh. This is most common following chronic rents in which large portions of the liver or bowel have herniated into the chest for several months, leaving a defect which may exceed 10-15 cm in diameter. Experience with latissimus dorsi or external oblique muscle flaps and omentum for reconstruction has been relatively good.[139,140] In these circumstances, successful repair from below is difficult, if not impossible, and the preferred approach is a posterolateral thoracotomy.

OUTCOME FOR CHRONIC DEFECTS

Correction of a chronic diaphragmatic hernia in the absence of strangulation or a bowel leak is usually tolerated very well. However, the mortality rate may be as high as 20% for late incarceration and range from 25-66% if the bowel becomes strangulated.[14,15,67,72] Indeed,

Hegarty et al[36] noted mortality rates as high as 80% when strangulation progressed to gangrene. This emphasizes the importance of early diagnosis and treatment.

There are few data concerning the long-term function of ruptured diaphragms. Taylor et al[36] did a two-year follow-up on 13 patients. All but one patient (with a serious head injury) were enjoying good health. One patient had an asymptomatic tear of the right hemidiaphragm which had been observed for 5 years. The remaining 12 patients with repair of the left hemidiaphragm underwent chest radiography and fluoroscopy. All 12 had elevated diaphragms on plain chest radiograph. Fluoroscopy demonstrated partial or total paradoxical motion in eight patients. Only three patients had normal descent of the diaphragm. These preliminary data suggest that there is sub-clinical loss of function of the diaphragm on long-term follow-up.

⊘ FREQUENT ERRORS

1. *Failing to suspect a diaphragmatic injury with penetrating trauma to the lower chest or upper abdomen or with severe blunt thoracoabdominal trauma.*
2. *Failing to suspect a pericardiacophrenic herniation if a patient develops signs of pericardial tamponade and bowel obstruction following blunt trauma.*
3. *Failing to suspect a diaphragmatic injury of the chest if a chest radiograph shows abnormal shadows in the lower lung fields or does not show the diaphragms well.*
4. *Failing to look carefully for associated injuries in patients with diaphragmatic trauma.*
5. *Failing to suspect a diaphragmatic injury when inflation of the abdominal portion of a PASG causes increasing dyspnea.*
6. *Failure to rule out herniated viscera in patients who appear to have a loculated lower lung field pneumothorax after thoracoabdominal trauma.*
7. *Ruling out a diaphragmatic injury because a diagnostic peritoneal lavage is negative.*
8. *Use of nitrous oxide for anesthesia in a patient with a diaphragmatic hernia.*
9. *Attempting to reduce distended, friable bowel in an old diaphragmatic hernia back into the abdomen through a laparotomy incision.*
10. *Failure to be aware of the possibility of catching phrenic nerve branches with the sutures used to repair the medial portion of a diaphragmatic tear.*

▼▼▼▼▼▼▼▼▼▼▼▼▼▼▼▼▼▼▼▼▼▼▼▼▼▼▼▼▼▼

SUMMARY POINTS

1. One should suspect diaphragmatic injuries with all penetrating wounds of the lower chest and with severe blunt abdominal trauma.

2. If the mechanism of injury does not cause diaphragmatic trauma to be suspected, there is a good chance it will be missed.

3. No injury to the diaphragm is so small that it can be considered safe from future sequelae.

4. Traumatic disruptions of the right diaphragm are usually associated with herniation of all or part of the liver into the chest.

5. Ruptures of the most posterior portions of the diaphragm may cause displacement of retroperitoneal structures into the chest.

6. The phrenic nerves are more likely to be injured during the repair of a diaphragmatic tear than by the original trauma.

7. Shock in patients with acute diaphragmatic injury is generally due to associated injuries.

8. A clinical picture of pericardial tamponade and bowel obstruction after blunt abdominal trauma should suggest the presence of an intrapericardial rupture of the diaphragm.

9. In older individuals with a delayed diaphragmatic hernia, symptoms of dyspnea, chest pain, and fatigue may be presumed erroneously to be myocardial in origin.[62,63]

10. Most diaphragmatic trauma has associated injuries.

11. One should suspect injury to the diaphragm with penetrating trauma to the lower chest or upper abdomen.

12. If one doesn't consider the possibility of diaphragmatic rupture in patients sustaining major thoracoabdominal trauma, it greatly increases the likelihood that the injury will be missed.

13. Shock or severe dyspnea developing when the abdominal portion of a PASG is inflated should make one very suspicious of a diaphragmatic injury.

14. The single most frequently abnormal non-invasive method for diagnosing diaphragmatic injury is a chest radiograph.

15. Any abnormal shadows in the left lower lung field after trauma should make one suspect a diaphragmatic injury.

16. Patients with penetrating injuries to the lower chest and a hemothorax should have an overpenetrated radiograph taken prior to placing a chest tube because it may reveal herniated viscera above the diaphragm.

17. Aggressive bag-mask ventilation can greatly increase herniation of bowel through a diaphragmatic defect.

18. A nasogastric tube can often help detect herniation of the stomach into the chest.

19. A contrast study of the gastrointestinal tract is the most accurate radiological test for diaphragmatic rupture.

20. Pneumoperitoneum can help delineate diaphragmatic tears.

21. A negative DPL does not rule out diaphragmatic injury.

22. A diagnostic peritoneal lavage for suspected diaphragmatic injury is more apt to be positive if a chest tube is already in place.

23. Most penetrating injuries of the diaphragm are initially silent and are discovered incidentally during exploratory surgery.

24. The most common reason for missing diaphragmatic trauma during laparotomy is failure to inspect the leaflets thoroughly, especially posteriorly.

25. With diaphragmatic injury, one should assume that associated injuries are present.

26. Preoxygenation with a bag-mask prior to induction of anesthesia can be dangerous in patients with a possible diaphragmatic injury.

27. Nitrous oxide should be avoided in patients with a possible diaphragmatic hernia as it can greatly increase the volume of gas within a herniated viscus.

28. Absence of a history of trauma from the patient does not rule out a delayed traumatic diaphragmatic hernia.

29. Signs and symptoms of a bowel obstruction after prior trauma are usually due to adhesions, but one should also be looking for hernias, especially in the diaphragm.

30. Rapid dilatation of bowel herniated into the chest can cause severe shortness of breath, and the radiographic appearance will occasionally resemble a pneumothorax.

31. If a diaphragmatic hernia is not diagnosed until herniated bowel becomes strangulated and perforated, the mortality rate is very high.

32. Surgery for old diaphragmatic hernias is usually best done through a thoracotomy incision.

▲▲▲▲▲▲▲▲▲▲▲▲▲▲▲▲▲▲▲▲▲▲▲▲▲▲▲▲▲▲▲▲▲▲▲

REFERENCES

1. Wiencek RG, Wilson, RF, Steiger Z. Acute injuries of the diaphragm. An analysis of 165 cases. J Thorac Cardiovasc Surg 1986;92:989.
2. Arendup HC, Jensen BS. Traumatic rupture of the diaphragm. Surg Gynecol Obstet 1982;154:527-530.
3. Carter JW. Diaphragmatic trauma in southern Saskatchewan—an 11 year review. J Trauma 1987;27:987.
4. Brown G, Richardson JD. Traumatic diaphragmatic hernia: a continuing challenge. Ann Thor Surg 1985;29:170.
5. Hood RM. Traumatic diaphragmatic hernia. Ann Thor Surg 1971;12:311.
6. McElwee TB, Myers RT, Pennell TC. Diaphragmatic rupture from blunt trauma. Am J Surg 1984;50:143.
7. Symbas PN, Vlasis SE, Hatcher CR Jr. Blunt and penetrating diaphragmatic injuries with or without herniation of organs into the chest. Ann Thorac Surg 1986;42:158.
8. Schneider CF. Traumatic diaphragmatic hernia. Am J Surg 1956;91:290.
9. Hamby WB. The case reports and autopsy records of Ambroise Paré. Springfield, IL: Thomas CC, 1960; 50.
10. Johnson T. The works of that famous chirageon Ambroise Paré. London: M. Clark, 1678.
11. Schwindt WD, Gale JW. Late recognition and treatment of traumatic diaphragmatic hernias. Arch Surg 1967;94:330-334.
12. Bowditch HI. Diaphragmatic hernia. Buffalo Med J 1853;9:1.
13. Pomerantz M, Rogers BM, Sabiston DC Jr. Traumatic diaphragmatic hernia. Surgery 1968;64:529-534.
14. Root HD. Injury to the diaphragm. In Moore EE, Mattox KL, Feliciano DV, eds. Trauma, 2nd ed. Norwalk, Connecticut: Appleton-Lange, 1991; 28:427-439.
15. Orringer MB, Kirsch MM, Sloan H. Congenital and traumatic diaphragmatic hernias exclusive of the hiatus. Curr Probl Surg 1975;3:3.
16. Reid J. Case of diaphragmatic hernia produced by a penetrating wound. Edinb Med Surg J 1840;53:104.
17. Miller L, Bennett EV, Root HD, et al. Management of penetrating and blunt diaphragmatic injury. J Trauma 1984;24:403.
18. Stylianos S, King TC. Occult diaphragmatic injuries at celiotomy for left chest stab wounds. Ann Surg 1992;58:364.
19. Madden MR, Paull DE, Finkelstein JL, et al. Occult diaphragmatic injury from stab wounds to the lower chest and abdomen. J Trauma 1989;29:292.
20. Beeson A, Popovici Z. Diaphragmatic injuries. Invited comment in thoracic surgery: surgical management of chest injuries. In Webb WR, Beeson A, eds. St. Louis: Mosby Year Book, 1991; 317-322.
21. Johnson CD. Blunt injuries of the diaphragm. Br J Surg 1988;75:226.
22. Robison PD, Harman PK, Grover, FL, et al. The management of penetrating lung injuries in civilian practice. J Thorac Cardiovasc Surg 1988;95:184.
23. Moore JB, Moore EE, Thompson JS. Abdominal injuries associated with penetrating trauma in the lower chest. Am J Surg 1980;140:724.
24. Borlase BC, Moore EE, Moore FA, et al. Penetrating wounds to the posterior chest: analysis of exigent thoracotomy and laparotomy. J Emerg Med 1989;7:455.
25. Wise L, Connors J, Hwang YH, et al. Traumatic injuries to the diaphragm. J Trauma 1973;13:946.
26. Rodkey GV. The management of abdominal injuries. Surg Clin North Am 1966;46:627.
27. Alonyo D, Perry J. Impact of speed limit: chest injuries, review of 966 cases. J Thorac Cardiovasc Surg 1982;83:519-522.
28. Taylor GA. Traumatic rupture of the diaphragm. In McMurtry RY, McLellan BA, eds. Management of blunt chest trauma. Baltimore: Williams & Wilkins, 1990;16:199-205.
29. Estrera AS, Platt MR, Mills LJ. Traumatic injuries of the diaphragm. Chest 1979;75:306.
30. Symbas PN. Diaphragmatic injuries. (Ch 29). In Symbas, PN, ed. Cardiothoracic trauma. Philadelphia: WB Saunders, 1989; 344-363.
31. Tarver RD, Conces DJ, Cory DA, et al. Imaging the diaphragm and its disorders. J Thorac Imag 1989;4:1-18.
32. Roussas C, Mackleon PT. The respiratory muscles. N Engl J Med 1982; 307:786-797.
33. De Troyer A, Sampson M, Sigrist S, et al. The diaphragm: two muscles. Science 1981;213:237-238.
34. Marchand P. A study of the forces productive of gastro-oesophageal regurgitation and herniation through the diaphragmatic hiatus. Thorax 1957;12:189.
35. Van Loenhout RM, Schiphurst TJ, Wittens CH, et al. Traumatic intrapericardial diaphragmatic hernia. J Trauma 1986;26:271.
36. Hegarty MM, Bryer JV, Angorn IB, et al. Delayed presentation of traumatic diaphragmatic hernia. Ann Surg 1978;188:229-233.
37. Heiberg E, Wolverson MK, Hurd RN, et al. CT recognition of traumatic rupture of the diaphragm. AJR 1980;135:369.
38. Lucido JL, Wall CA. Rupture of the diaphragm due to blunt trauma. Arch Surg 1963;86:989.
39. Melzig EP, Swank M, Salzberg AM. Acute blunt traumatic rupture of the diaphragm in children. Arch Surg 1976;111:1009.
40. Humphreys TR, Abbuhl S. Massive bilateral diaphragmatic rupture after an apparently minor automobile accident. Am J Emerg Med 1991;9:246-249.
41. Ginz W. Injuries of the diaphragm. Chest trauma. New York: Springer-Verlag, 1981; 246-257.
42. Wyffels PL, Kenny JN. Primary repair of bilateral diaphragmatic rupture with crural involvement. Am J Surg 1984;147:414.
43. Angood PB, Mulder DS. Rupture of the diaphragm. In JL Cameron, ed. Current surgical therapy. Philadelphia: BC Decker, Inc, 1989; 657-661.

44. Sharma OP. Traumatic diaphragmatic rupture: not an uncommon entity—personal experience with collective review of the 1980s. J Trauma 1989;29:678.

45. Ilgenfritz FM, Stewart DE. Blunt trauma of the diaphragm. A 15 county private hospital experience. Am Surg 1992;58:334.

46. Kearney PA, Rouhana SW, Burney RE. Blunt rupture of the diaphragm mechanism; diagnosis and treatment. Ann Emerg Med 1990;18:105.

47. Epstein LI, Lempke RE. Rupture of right diaphragm due to blunt trauma. J Trauma 1968;8:19.

48. Mansour KA, Clements JL, Hatcher CR Jr, et al. Diaphragmatic hernia caused by trauma: experience with 35 cases. Am Surg 1975;41:97.

49. Meads CE, Carroll SE, Pitt DF. Traumatic rupture of the right hemidiaphragm. J Trauma 1977;17:797.

50. Olin C. Traumatic rupture of the diaphragm. Report of eleven cases. Acta Chir Scand 1975;141:282.

51. Peck WA Jr. Right-sided diaphragmatic liver hernia following blunt trauma. Am J Roentgenol Radium Ther Nucl Med 1957;78:99.

52. Wilson RF, Murray C, Antonenko D. Nonpenetrating thoracic injuries. Surg Clin N Am 1977;57:17.

53. Steiger Z, Wilson RF, Nelson RM, et al. Iatrogenic hiatal and diaphragmatic hernias. Am Surg 1984;50:217.

54. Wilson RF. Controversies and problems in the management of penetrating wounds of the chest. In Najarian JS, Delaney JP, eds. Trauma and critical care surgery. Chicago Yearbook Medical Publishers, Inc, 1987;93.

55. Friedman AI. Hiatus hernia and peptic esophagitus following trauma. Am J Gastroenterol 1960;34:269.

56. Johnson CD. Acquired hernia of the diaphragm. Postgrad Med J 1988; 64:317.

57. Bryant LR, Schechter FG, Rees R, et al. Bilateral diaphragmatic rupture due to blunt trauma—a rare injury. J Trauma 1978;18:280.

58. Kanowitz A, Marx JA. Delayed traumatic diaphragmatic hernia simulating acute tension pneumothorax. J Emerg Med 1989;7:619.

59. Beless DJ, Organ BC. Delayed presentation of intrapericardial diaphragmatic hernia, an unusual cause of colon obstruction. Ann Emerg Med 1991;20:415.

60. Nelson RM, Wilson RF, Huang CL, et al. Cardiac tamponade due to an iatrogenic pericardial-diaphragmatic hernia. Crit Care Med 1985; 13:607.

61. deRooji PD, Haarman MJT. Herniation of the stomach into the pericardiac sac combined with cardiac luxation caused by blunt trauma: a case report. J Trauma 1993;34:453.

62. Leppaniemi A, Pohjankyro A, Haapiainen R. Acute diaphragmatic rupture after blunt trauma. Ann Chir Gynaecol 1994;83:17.

63. Moore TC. Traumatic pericardial diaphragmatic hernia. Arch Surg 1959; 79:827.

64. Rodriquez-Morales G, Rodriquez A, Shatney CH. Acute rupture of the diaphragm in blunt trauma. J Trauma 1986;26:438.

65. Boulanger BR, Milzman DP, Rosati C, et al. A comparison of right and left blunt traumatic diaphragmatic rupture. J Trauma 1986;35:255.

66. Carter BM, Giuseffi J, Felson F. Traumatic diaphragmatic hernia. Am J Roentgenol 1951;65:56.

67. Strug B, Noon GP, Beall AC. Traumatic diaphragmatic hernia. Ann Thor Surg 1974;17:444.

68. Ball T, McCrory R, Smith JO, et al. Traumatic diaphragmatic hernias; errors in diagnosis. AFJA 1982;138:633.

69. Morgan AS, Flancbaum L, Esposito T, et al. Blunt injury to the diaphragm: an analysis of 44 cases. J Trauma 1986;26:565.

70. Price BA, Elliott MJ, Featherstone G, et al. Perforation of intrathoracic colon causing acute pneumothorax. Thorax 1983;38:959.

71. Bush CA, Margulies R. Traumatic diaphragmatic hernia and intestinal obstruction due to penetrating trunk wounds. S Med J 1990;83:1347.

72. Saber WL, Moore EE, Hopeman AR et al. Delayed presentation of traumatic diaphragmatic hernia. J Emerg Med 1986;4:1.

73. Payne JH Jr, Yellin AE. Traumatic diaphragmatic hernia. Arch Surg 1980;111:18.

74. Christophi C. Diagnosis of traumatic diaphragmatic hernia: analysis of 63 cases. World J Surg 1983;7:277.

75. Jones KW: Thoracic trauma. Surg Clin North Am 1980;60:957.

76. Maull KI, Krahwinted DJ, Rozycki GS, et al. Cardio-pulmonary effects of the pneumatic antishock garment on swine with diaphragmatic hernia. Surg Gynecol Obstet 1986;162:17.

77. Wilkinson AE. Traumatic rupture of the diaphragm. An analysis of 121 cases. S Afr J Surg 1989;27:56.

78. Miller OL, Grover FL. Abdominal trauma. Injuries of the Diaphragm. In. Kreis DJ Jr, Gomez GA, eds. Trauma management. Boston: Little Brown & Co, 1989; 238-245.

79. Shapiro MJ, Heilberg E, Durham RM, et al. The unreliability of initial chest radiographs and CT scans in evaluating diaphragmatic rupture (abstract). J Trauma 1994;36:155.

80. Voeller GR, Reisser JR, Fabian TC, et al. Blunt diaphragm injuries. Am Surg 1990;56:28.

81. Lernau U, Bar-Mar JA, Nissan S. Traumatic diaphragmatic hernia simulating acute tension pneumothorax. J Trauma 1974;14:880.

82. Perlman SJ, Rogers LF, Mintzer RA, et al. Abnormal course of nasogastric tube in traumatic rupture of the left hemidiaphragm. AJR 1984; 142:85.

83. Brooks JW. Blunt traumatic rupture of the diaphragm. Ann Thor Surg 1978;26:199.

84. Adamthwaite DN, Snijders DC, Mirwis J. Traumatic pericardiophrenic hernias: a report of 3 cases. Br J Surg 1983;70:117.

85. Rao KG, Woodlief RM. Grey scale ultrasonic demonstration of ruptured right hemidiaphragm. Br J Radiol 1980;53:812.

86. Ammann AM, Brewer WH, Maull KI. Traumatic rupture of the diaphragm: real time sonographic diagnosis. AJR 1983;140:915.

87. McHugh K, Ogilvie BC, Brunton FJ. Delayed presentation of traumatic diaphragmatic hernia. Clin. Rad 1991;43:246.

88. Troop B, Myers RM, Agarwal NN. Early recognition of diaphragmatic injuries from blunt trauma. Ann Emerg Med 1991;14:97.

89. Sukul DM, Kats E, Johannes EJ. Sixty-three cases of traumatic injury of the diaphragm. Injury 1991;22:303.

90. Sperber RG. Diaphragmatic hernia mimicking pyopneumothorax and colonic mass. NY State J Med 1987;87:122.

91. Fagan CJ, Schreiber MH, Amparo EG, et al. Traumatic diaphragmatic hernia into pericardium: verification of diagnosis by tomography. J Comput Assist Tomogr 1979;3:405.

92. Flancbaum L, Dauber M, Demas C, et al. Early diagnosis and treatment of blunt diaphragmatic injury. Am Surg 1988;54:195.

93. Goldstein AS, Sclafani SJA, Kupferstein N, et al. The diagnostic superiority of computerized tomography. J Trauma 1985;25:938-943.

94. Chen JC, Wilson SE. Diaphragmatic injuries: recognition and management in sixty-two patients. Ann Surg 1991;57:810.

95. Mirvis SE, Keramati B, Buckman R, et al. MR imaging of traumatic diaphragmatic rupture. J Comput Assist Tomogr 1988;12:147.

96. Boulanger BR, Mirvis SE, Rodriguez A. Magnetic resonance imaging in traumatic diaphragmatic rupture. Case Report. J Trauma 1992; 32:89.

97. Pecoravo JB, et al. Radioisotope-assisted diagnosis of traumatic rupture of the diaphragm. Am Surg 1985;51:687.

98. Blumenthal DH, Raghu G, Rudd T, et al. Diagnosis of right hemidiaphragmatic rupture by liver scintigraphy. J Trauma 1984;24:536.

99. Kim EE, McConnell BJ, McConnell RW, et al. Radionuclide diagnosis of diaphragmatic rupture with hepatic herniation. Surgery 1983; 94:36.

100. Lorimer JW, Reid KR, Raymond F. Blunt extraperitoneal rupture of the right hemidiaphragm: case report. J Trauma 1994;36:414.

101. Ramirez JS, Moreno AJ, Otero C, et al. Detection of diaphragmatic disruptions by peritoneoscintigraphy using technetium-99M diethylene triamine pentacetic acid. J Trauma 1988;28:818.

102. Clay RC, Hanlon CR. Pneumoperitoneum in the differential diagnosis of diaphragmatic hernia. J Thor Surg 1951;21:57.

103. Gravier L, Freeark RJ. Traumatic diaphragmatic hernia. Arch Surg 1963; 86:363.

104. Nelson JW. Traumatic rupture of the diaphragm: a method of diagnosis. J Can Assoc Radiol 1980;31:99.

105. Larrieu AJ, Wiener I, Alexander R, et al. Pericardio-diaphragmatic hernia. Am J Surg 1980;139:436.

106. Adamthwaite DN. Diaphragmatic hernia presenting itself as a surgical emergency. Injury 1984;15:367-369.

107. Jackson AM, Ferreira AA. Thoracoscopy as an aid to the diagnosis of diaphragmatic injury in penetrating wounds of the left lower chest: a preliminary report. Injury 1976;7:213.

108. Ochsner MG, Rozycki GS, Lucente F, et al. Prospective evaluation of thoracoscopy for diagnosing diaphragmatic injury in thoracoabdominal trauma: a preliminary report. J Trauma 1993;34:704.

109. Ivatury RR, Simon RJ, Weksler B, et al. Laparoscopy in the evaluation of the intrathoracic abdomen after penetrating injury. J Trauma 1992; 33:101.

110. Salvino CK, Esposito TJ, Marshall WJ, et al. The role of diagnostic laparoscopy in the management of trauma patients: a preliminary assessment. J Trauma 1993;34:507.

111. Rudston-Brown B, Phang PT, Studer W, et al. Laparoscopic diagnosis of penetrating injuries to the diaphragm (abstract). J Trauma 1993; 35:178.

112. Freeman T, Fisher RP. The inadequacy of peritoneal lavage in diagnosing acute diaphragmatic rupture. J Trauma 1976;16:538.
113. Aronoff RJ, Reynolds, J, Thal ER. Evaluation of diaphragmatic injuries. Am J Surg 1982;144:671.
114. Thal ER. Evaluation of peritoneal lavage and local exploration in lower chest and abdominal stab wounds. J Trauma 1977;17:642.
115. Flancbaum L, Morgan AS, Esposito T. Non-left sided diaphragmatic rupture due to blunt trauma. Surg Gynecol Obstet 1985;161:266.
116. Thal ER, May RA, Beesinger D. Peritoneal lavage: its unreliability in gunshot wounds of the lower chest and abdomen. Arch Surg 1980; 115:430.
117. Oreskovich MR, Carrico CJ. Stab wound of the abdomen—analysis of a management plan using local wound exploration and quantitative peritoneal lavage. Ann Surg 1983;198:411.
118. Moore EE, Marx JA. Penetrating abdominal wounds. Rationale for exploratory laparotomy. JAMA 1985;253:2705.
119. Merlotti GJ, Marcet E, Sheaff CM, et al. Use of peritoneal lavage to evaluate abdominal penetration. J Trauma 1985;25:228.
120. Hornyak SW, Shaftan GW. Value of inconclusive lavage in abdominal trauma management. J Trauma 1979;19:329.
121. Soyka JM, Martin M, Sloan EP, et al. Diagnostic peritoneal lavage: is an isolated WBC count > 500/mm^3 predictive of intra-abdominal injury requiring celiotomy in blunt trauma patients? J Trauma 1990;30:874.
122. Fallazadeh H, Mays ET. Disruption of the diaphragm by blunt trauma; new dimensions of diagnosis. Am Surg 1975;41:337.
123. Shea LS, Graham AD, Fletcher JC, et al. Diaphragmatic injury: a method of early diagnosis. J Trauma 1982;22:539.
124. Feliciano DV, Cruse PA, Mattox KL, et al. Delayed diagnosis of injuries to the diaphragm after penetrating wounds. J Trauma 1988;28:1135.
125. Madden M, Paull D, Shires GT, et al. Occult diaphragmatic injury from stab wounds to the lower chest and abdomen. J Trauma 1989;29:292.
126. Ebert PA, Baertner RA, Zuidema JD. Traumatic diaphragmatic hernia. Surg Gynecol Obstet 1967;125:59.
127. Wilson RF, Antonenko D, Gibson DB. Shock and acute respiratory failure after chest trauma. J Trauma 1977;17:697.
128. Koehler RH, Smith RS. Thoracoscopic repair of missed diaphragmatic injury in penetrating trauma: case report. J Trauma 1994;36:424.
129. Beal SL, McKennan M. Blunt diaphragmatic rupture. Arch Surg 1988; 123:828.
130. Van Vugt AB, Schoots FJ. Acute diaphragmatic rupture due to blunt trauma. J Trauma 1989;29:683.
131. Moore EE, Malangoni MA, Cogbill TH, et al. Organ injury scaling IV. Thoracic vascular, lung, cardiac, and diaphragm. J Trauma 1994;36:299.
132. de la Rocha AG, Creel RJ, Mulligan GW, et al. Diaphragmatic rupture due to blunt abdominal trauma. Surg Gynecol Obstet 1982;154:175.
133. Carter BN, Giuseffi J. Strangulated diaphragmatic hernia. Ann Surg 1948;128:210.
134. Dajee A, Schepps D, Hurley EJ. Diaphragmatic injuries. Surg Gynecol Obstet 1981;153:31.
135. Adeyemi SD, Stephens CA. Traumatic diaphragmatic hernia in children. Can J Surg 1981;24:355.
136. Tocino I, Miller MH. Computed tomography in blunt chest trauma. J Thor Imaging 1987;2:45.
137. Brandt ML, Luks FL, Spigland NA, et al. Diaphragmatic injury in children. J Trauma 1992;32:298.
138. Meng RL, Straus A, Milloy A, et al. Intrapericardial diaphragmatic hernia in adults. Ann Surg 1979;189:359.
139. Shimoninura YL, Gienven PA, Ishii MS, et al. Repair of diaphragm with external oblique muscle flap. Surg Gynecol Obstet 1989;169:159.
140. Edington HD, Evans SL, Sindelar WF. Reconstruction of functional hemidiaphragm with omentum and latissimus dorsi flaps. Surgery 1989;105:442.

Chapter **22** Injuries to the Liver and Biliary Tract

ROBERT F. WILSON, M.D.

ALEXANDER J. WALT, MB, CHB

INTRODUCTION

Injury to the liver remains a major challenge to surgeons caring for injured patients. Despite extensive military and civilian experience, overall mortality rates range between 6% and 15%, and morbidity rates continue to exceed 25%.[1] In a series of 891 patients with liver injuries treated at Detroit General Hospital between 1961 and 1971, the mortality rate among patients was 2% with stab wounds, 17% with gunshot wounds and 30% with blunt injuries.[2] In most series, penetrating injuries result in mortality rates of less than 5%, but with blunt hepatic injuries mortality rates approach 25%.[3-5] In our most recent series of 910 patients from 1980 to 1992 (12 years), the mortality rates for stab wounds, gunshot wounds and blunt trauma were 8%, 22%, and 35%, respectively (Table 22-1). If concomitant injuries to the retrohepatic cava or main hepatic veins are included, mortality rates often exceed 80%. In addition, morbidity rates in patients surviving severe liver injuries usually exceed 50%.

AXIOM Major liver injuries, particularly with blunt trauma, continue to have extremely high mortality and morbidity rates.

The continuing high morbidity and mortality rates with major liver trauma have prompted re-evaluation of the techniques utilized to manage these injuries. In general, the surgical decisions on most patients with liver trauma are straightforward, and the postoperative course is uncomplicated in about 80-90%.[1] In the remaining 10-20%, however, management decisions may be difficult and can have a great influence on morbidity and mortality. Consequently, surgeons caring for liver trauma should possess a broad knowledge of the techniques available for treatment as well as the wisdom with which to apply them and recognize complications if they develop.

HISTORICAL PERSPECTIVE

Descriptions of injuries to the liver date back to Greek and Roman mythology, particularly to the myth of the titan, Prometheus.[3,6] Prometheus was chained to a mountain in the Caucasus by Zeus because he had stolen fire from the heavens for mankind to use. Every day a portion of his liver was "plucked out" by a giant bird, but it would "regenerate" overnight. In his epic poems "The Iliad" and "The Odyssey," Homer vividly describes sword and piercing arrow injuries to the liver.

While various treatment modalities have been advocated for hepatic injuries since ancient times, surgical control of bleeding from an injured liver was not attempted with any regularity until the latter part of the 19th century.[7] Indeed, the modern management of hepatic injuries did not really begin until the work of Madding and Kennedy.[8] Based on their experience during World War II,[8] they emphasized the need for early laparotomy and establishment of adequate drainage.[3] Using these principles, along with improvements in anesthesia, blood transfusions, antibiotics, and early evacuation from the battlefield, the mortality from hepatic injuries decreased from an average of about 30% to 17%. Although gauze packing of severe liver wounds was discouraged during World War II, this technique can be very helpful in selected cases.

Refinements in pre- and postoperative care were responsible for some additional improvement in the management of hepatic injuries in the Korean conflict and the Vietnam War. Complex hepatic injuries continue, however, to challenge trauma surgeons, and juxtahepatic venous injuries, despite all these advances, continue to have a very high mortality rate.[3]

SURGICAL ANATOMY

Lobar Anatomy

Early anatomists considered the liver to be separated by the falciform ligament into a right and left lobe.[3] Subsequent anatomical studies of the major intrahepatic vessels and bile ducts, however, have demonstrated that the right and left lobes of the liver are actually separated by a plane running from the gallbladder fossa to the inferior vena cava[9,10] (Fig. 22-1). This cleavage plane is devoid of major branches of the portal vein, hepatic artery, and bile ducts, but it frequently contains a portion of the middle hepatic vein.

Ligaments

AXIOM To explore and treat certain types of liver injuries properly, especially posterior wounds, the liver must be completely mobilized.

Complete mobilization of the liver can only be achieved by fully incising the appropriate ligamentous attachments[3] (Fig. 22-2). The coronary ligaments represent the peritoneal attachments of the diaphragm onto the parietal surface of the liver. These consist of anterior and posterior leaflets, but these leaflets do not meet on the posterior surface of the liver where a "bare area" exists. The triangular ligaments are the free lateral margins of the more centrally located coronary ligaments.[3]

AXIOM Extreme caution should be exercised when incising the most medial portions of the coronary ligaments to avoid inadvertent laceration of hepatic veins.

Juxtahepatic Venous Structures (Fig. 22-3)

HEPATIC VEINS

The three main hepatic veins are valveless and thin-walled and have high flow rates. For the most part, these are intra-parenchymal structures, and their extrahepatic length before entering the cava is only about 1-2 cm.[3] The right and left hepatic veins enter the cava directly, but 84% of the time the middle hepatic vein drains into the left hepatic vein near its junction with the inferior vena cava.

RETROHEPATIC INFERIOR VENA CAVA

The retrohepatic inferior vena cava is approximately 8-10 cm in length, and on its anterior surface it receives blood from the main hepatic veins plus about 20 small hepatic veins.[3] The short extrahepatic length of the major hepatic veins, and a relatively inaccessible retrohepatic cava can make exposure and control of these vessels, when they are injured, extremely difficult.

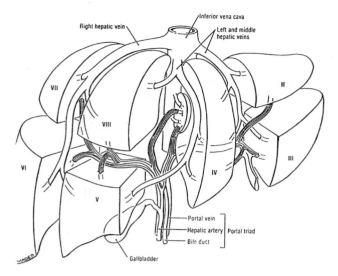

FIGURE 22-1   Segmental and vascular anatomy of the liver: Each segment of the liver is supplied by a branch of the hepatic artery, bile duct, and portal vein. The hepatic veins do not follow the structures of the portal triad and are considered intersegmental in that they drain portions of adjacent segments (From Agur AMR, Lee MJ, eds. Grant's atlas of anatomy. 9th ed. Williams & Wilkins, 1991;115.)

ETIOLOGY

Penetrating Injuries

In major urban trauma centers in the United States, stabs and gunshot wounds are the most frequent injuries of the liver.[1] In the latest series of patients from Detroit Receiving Hospital (1980-1992), penetrating trauma accounted for over 82% of the 910 patients with liver injuries (Table 22-1). Of the 750 patients with penetrating liver injuries, 475 (63%) were caused by gunshot wounds (GSW), 251 (34%) by stabs, and 24 (3%) by shotgun wounds (SGW).

Of 2168 patients with penetrating abdominal trauma, 750 (35%) involved the liver. The only abdominal organ injured more frequently by penetrating trauma was the small bowel (jejunum and ileum) which was injured in 1001 cases (46%). In a series of 686 gunshot wounds of the trunk, 81 (13%) involved the liver or biliary tract.[11] The only injuries that were more frequent were those involving small intestine (15%) or colon and rectum (15%).

TABLE 22-1   *Mortality Rates with Abdominal Injuries Seen in 12 Years at Detroit Receiving Hospital (1980-1992)*

	Type of Trauma			
Organ Injured	*Blunt*	*GSW*	*Stabs*	*Total*
Liver	(160) 35%	(499) 22%	(251) 8%	(910) 20%
Small Bowel	(58) 24%	(551) 14%	(150) 7%	(759) 13%
Colon	(43) 16%	(462) 14%	(122) 6%	(627) 12%
Diaphragm	(28) 25%	(273) 22%	(119) 8%	(420) 18%
Kidney	(145) 7%	(229) 17%	(45) 13%	(420) 13%
Spleen	(172) 15%	(131) 24%	(42) 10%	(345) 18%
Stomach	(6) 50%	(241) 22%	(93) 11%	(340) 19%
Abd. Vessels	(23) 70%	(257) 53%	(53) 32%	(333) 58%
Pancreas	(33) 6%	(140) 24%	(37) 30%	(210) 22%
Duodenum	(10) 30%	(124) 23%	(33) 21%	(167) 23%
Bladder	(44) 18%	(84) 6%	(6) 17%	(134) 10%
Gallbladder	(3) 100%	(59) 24%	(19) 5%	(81) 22%
Total	(573) 16%	(1358) 14%	(810) 5%	(2741) 12%

Stab wounds and the low-velocity gunshot wounds that are typically seen in civilian practice usually result in relatively minor parenchymal injury requiring modest treatment, and the outcome with such injuries is generally good. Of the deaths occurring in hepatic trauma, almost two-thirds are due to associated injuries to other solid organs or to the juxtahepatic vessels. In about one-third, however, death is due primarily to a severe liver parenchymal injury.

AXIOM   Delayed, inadequate, or inappropriate treatment of liver injuries, resulting in hematomas or bile collections, can combine with associated injuries to cause significant morbidity or even death of an otherwise salvageable patient.

Blunt Trauma

The spleen and the liver are generally the two most frequently injured solid organs in patients suffering blunt abdominal trauma.[1] Of 573 patients seen at DRH from 1980 to 1992 with blunt abdominal injuries, 160 (28%) had liver trauma, making the liver second only to the spleen, which was injured in 30%.

Blunt abdominal trauma can cause extensive destruction of hepatic parenchyma, often in the form of stellate lacerations or major fractures extending across anatomic planes. These may be so severe as to be fatal, even without major associated injuries. Such liver damage can be a severe challenge to the surgeon's ability to combine techniques of adequate hemostasis with those of liver repair, management of torn bile ducts, and debridement of any devitalized tissue. Concomitant injuries, the need for massive transfusions, and shock can increase the morbidity and mortality rates exponentially in these patients.

Iatrogenic Injuries

Surgeons are periodically asked to treat patients with significant iatrogenic liver injuries due to percutaneous liver biopsies, CT-guided placement of drainage catheters, or the insertion of biliary stents. Such patients occasionally suffer major injury causing hemorrhage or bile leaks. These complications are more apt to occur when the invasive procedures above are performed in patients with pre-existing liver disease, especially cirrhosis and obstructive jaundice.

AXIOM   One should anticipate complications whenever a percutaneous procedure is performed on the liver, particularly in patients with portal hypertension.

Spontaneous Rupture

Certain medical problems, such as sickle cell disease, pregnancy, coagulopathies, and various neoplasms may lead to "spontaneous" massive hemorrhage from the liver, requiring operation.[12]

Associated Injuries

In most series, more than 90% of blunt hepatic injuries are accompanied by damage to other intra-abdominal organs, especially the spleen, kidney, and intestine.[1] With penetrating injuries of the liver, the diaphragm is usually injured in more than 50% of the patients, and pulmonary complications should be anticipated.

In the 910 patients with liver injuries seen at Detroit Receiving Hospital from 1980 to 1992, the most frequently associated injuries were to the diaphragm (29%), lungs (23%), abdominal vessels (23%), stomach (20%), and colon (19%) (Table 22-2). For the 160 patients with blunt liver trauma, the most frequent associated abdominal injuries were to the spleen (24%), abdominal vessels (14%), and kidney (13%). For the 750 patients with penetrating wounds, the most

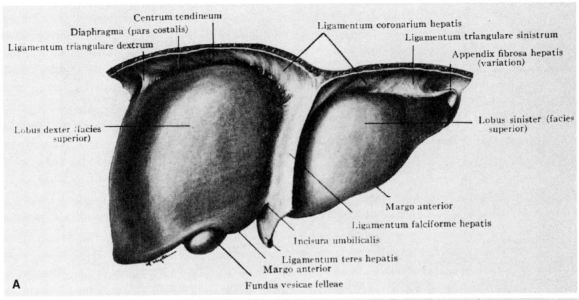

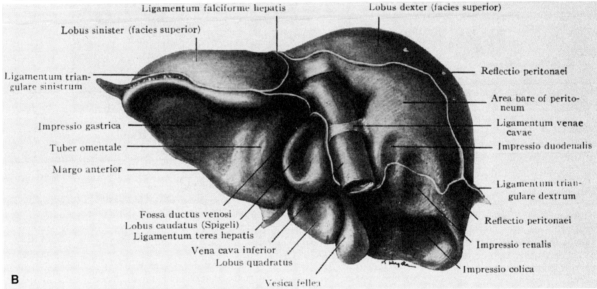

FIGURE 22-2 Hepatic ligaments: **A.** Anterosuperior surface of the liver and its connection with the diaphragm **B.** Posterior view of the liver (From McVay CB, ed. Anson & McVay surgical anatomy. 6th ed. WB Saunders Co., 1984, 616-617.)

frequent associated abdominal injuries were the diaphragm (32%), abdominal vessels (24%), stomach (23%), colon (19%), and jejunum and ileum (15%). Only 162 (18%) of the patients had isolated liver injuries (Table 22-3). The incidence of isolated liver injuries with blunt trauma, stabs, and gunshot wounds was 13%, 43%, and 6%, respectively.

INITIAL MANAGEMENT

When severely injured patients arrive in the emergency department (ED), the initial management should be uniformly directed toward the immediate restoration of adequate ventilation and oxygenation and toward prompt diagnosis and control of any ongoing blood loss.

AXIOM The single greatest danger following liver injury is severe hemorrhage.[1]

Patients presenting with severe hypotension following liver trauma require the rapid placement of two or three large-bore intravenous cannulas. Rapid access to the central venous circulation may be gained through the percutaneous placement of subclavian or internal jugular venous catheters, but the potential hazard of an iatrogenic pneumothorax in the shocked patient must be recognized. Alternatively, large volumes of resuscitative solutions may be administered rapidly through sterile intravenous tubing introduced directly into the basilic or saphenous veins by means of cutdowns.

AXIOM As a general rule, intravenous access in the arms is preferred over lower extremity sites if the patient is in shock from abdominal trauma.

Patients responding promptly to less than 2-3 liters of crystalloid fusion may be carefully monitored while the infusion rate is

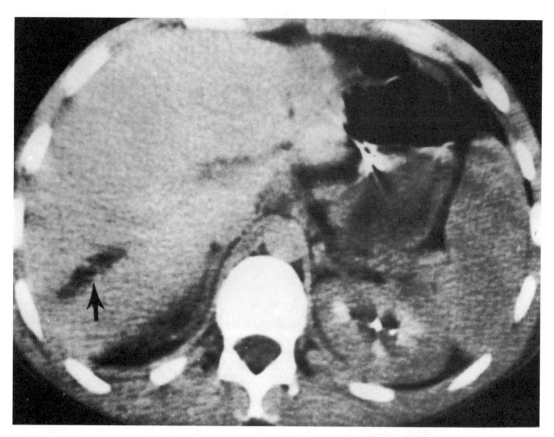

FIGURE 22-3 Simple hepatic laceration. This CT image shows a lucent defect in the posterior aspect of the right lobe that represents a simple laceration (arrow). (From Mirvis SE, Whitley NO. CT in hepatobiliary trauma. In: Ferrucci JT, Mathieu DG, eds. Advances in hepatobiliary radiology. St. Louis: CV Mosby, 1989.)

decreased and evaluation continues. Prompt initiation of blood transfusions and operative intervention is recommended in: (a) patients who have no obtainable BP on admission, (b) patients remaining hypotensive after 2-3 liters of rapid crystalloid infusion, or (c) patients who again become hypotensive after initial normalization of blood pressure.

TABLE 22-2 Mortality Rate and Associated Injuries Seen with Liver Trauma (Detroit Receiving Hospital 1980-1992)

| Associated Injuries | Types of Trauma | | | | |
	Blunt	Stabs	GSW	SGW	Total
Diaphragm	56%[13]	11%[57]	22%[184]	40%[5]	21%[259]
Lung	50%[48]	8%[37]	27%[123]	40%[5]	29%[213]
Abd. Vessels	68%[22]	30%[37]	53%[141]	60%[5]	50%[205]
Stomach	50%[2]	18%[28]	24%[141]	10%[10]	23%[181]
Colon	33%[15]	0%[19]	21%[126]	17%[12]	19%[173]
Jej. & ileum	56%[20]	15%[13]	26%[100]	22%[9]	28%[139]
Kidney	35%[20]	29%[7]	23%[97]	33%[9]	26%[133]
Spleen	45%[38]	17%[6]	25%[55]	100%[2]	34%[101]
Pancreas	8%[12]	36%[11]	27%[69]	33%[6]	25%[99]
Duodenum	100%[3]	25%[12]	25%[67]	17%[6]	27%[88]
Gallbladder	100%[3]	7%[14]	20%[45]	25%[4]	21%[66]
Total	35%[160]	8%[251]	22%[475]	25%[24]	20%[910]

( ) = number of patients in each category.
% = mortality rate.

An absolute prerequisite to the successful outcome of any operative intervention for major traumatic injuries is a well-supplied blood bank.[3] In the emergency situation, type-specific uncrossmatched blood should be available within 10 minutes. In addition, ample amounts of fresh frozen plasma, cryoprecipitate, and platelets may also be needed promptly. In patients with continuing or recurrent hypotension, transfusion with type-specific blood should be begun as the patient is transported rapidly to the operating suite.

TABLE 22-3 Mortality Rate Associated with Liver Trauma (Detroit Receiving Hospital 1980-1992)

| Number of Associated Injuries | Types of Trauma | | | | |
	Blunt	Stabs	GSW	SGW	Total
0	19%[21]	2%[109]	0%[31]	0%[1]	4%[162]
1	23%[40]	3%[66]	13%[93]	50%[4]	13%[203]
2	35%[31]	14%[42]	22%[110]	0%[4]	22%[187]
3	32%[31]	26%[23]	29%[93]	0%[2]	29%[149]
4+	60%[37]	27%[12]	28%[148]	31%[13]	33%[210]

( ) = number of patients in each category.
% = mortality rate.

AXIOM Hypothermia in trauma patients should be rapidly corrected as soon as the major bleeding is controlled.

An extremely important component of the initial management of patients with complex hepatic injuries is the prevention of systemic hypothermia. This potentially fatal complication results from a number of factors including administration of cold intravenous solutions and blood, prolonged shock, and a prolonged surgical operation. Steps to prevent and to correct hypothermia rapidly from the time of admission to the ED are essential if fatal intraoperative coagulopathies and arrhythmias are to be prevented.[13,14]

As part of the initial resuscitation, nasogastric and Foley catheters are inserted, and tetanus and antibiotic prophylaxis is initiated. A second-generation cephalosporin or any drug combination effective against gram-negative aerobes and colonic anaerobes should be begun in anticipation of possible concomitant gastrointestinal injuries.[2]

INJURY CLASSIFICATION

In order to compare the efficacy of management techniques in patients suffering a variety of hepatic injuries, a uniform classification system is mandatory.[3] A number of classifications of hepatic injuries have been published;[15-18] however, until very recently, no one classification has been accepted as definitive. Consequently, the Organ Injury Scaling Committee of the American Association for the Surgery of Trauma has set forth a comprehensive new classification system for hepatic injuries[18] (Table 22-4).

DIAGNOSIS

Gunshot wounds to the abdomen cause intraperitoneal vascular or visceral injury in 96-98% of cases. Consequently, patients with this type of trauma are explored routinely at most institutions and do not generally present any diagnostic problem as regards liver injury. Blunt abdominal trauma, however, may be a diagnostic challenge in even the most experienced hands, particularly in patients who are inebriated or have concomitant head or high spinal cord injury.

The variability in presentation of patients suffering liver trauma reflects the broad range of the underlying injuries. Relatively minor injuries are often asymptomatic, and many such injuries are detected only incidentally at laparotomy performed for other injuries. Individuals suffering more extensive hepatic injuries tend to present with a clinical picture of hypotension or increasing abdominal tenderness and distension. Such a presentation generally leads to an early laparotomy and treatment. Between these extremes, however, is a group of patients with injuries to the liver that may be subtle in presentation but nonetheless significant and requiring prompt operation. It is this group that demands a high degree of suspicion and which can challenge the expertise of even the most experienced trauma surgeon.

History

Any recent history of trauma to the right upper quadrant of the abdomen or right lower chest should signal the presence of a possible hepatic injury. In stable patients, significant hepatic injuries can also be suspected from the mechanism of injury, such as a high-speed motor vehicle accident.

Physical Examination

Right-sided rib fractures, a right pleural effusion, and penetrating injury at or below the right fourth intercostal space are frequent indirect indications of liver trauma. Similarly, injury to the diaphragm and the underlying liver may be reflected in bilious drainage from a tube thoracostomy. Pain referred to the right shoulder may also be caused by a liver injury.

AXIOM As in all aspects of medicine, a careful history and thorough physical examination are of paramount importance in the diagnosis of liver injuries.

The ability to accurately assess the presence or absence of significant intra-abdominal injuries in blunt trauma patients by physical examination alone is notoriously poor.[17-21] Olsen et al[21] found that 21% of the patients thought to have an intra-abdominal injury based on physical examination alone were found to have trivial or insignificant injuries not requiring a therapeutic laparotomy. More importantly, 43% of Olsen's patients thought to have a "benign abdomen" on physical examination were found to have significant intra-abdominal injuries at celiotomy.

Laboratory

Laboratory examinations, with the possible exception of serial hematocrit determinations, are rarely helpful. These studies are not sensitive indicators of acute liver damage and should not be relied on to rule out significant injury.

Adjunctive Diagnostic Tests

LOCAL EXPLORATION OF STAB WOUNDS

Any patient sustaining a stab wound to the abdomen presenting with hypotension, abdominal distention, or tenderness requires immediate operative intervention without any diagnostic tests.[3] If there are no definite signs of intraperitoneal bleeding or irritation, however, one can explore the entrance wound under local anesthesia. If the end of the wound tract can be seen clearly as non-penetrating, no further studies need to be performed. If the wound is seen to penetrate the anterior abdominal fascia or if the end of the wound cannot be defined, the abdomen can either be explored or a diagnostic peritoneal lavage can be performed.

TABLE 22-4 *Liver Injury Scale*

	Grade*	Injury Description+	AIS 90
I.	Hematoma:	Subcapsular, nonexpanding, <10% surface area	1
	Laceration:	Capsular tear, nonbleeding, <1 cm parenchymal depth	
II.	Hematoma:	Subcapsular, nonexpanding, 10-50% surface area	2
		Intraparenchymal, nonexpanding, <2 cm in diameter	
	Laceration:	Capsular tear, active bleeding, 1-3 cm parenchymal depth, <10 cm	
III.	Hematoma:	Subcapsular, >50% surface area or expanding	3
		Ruptured subcapsular hematoma with active bleeding	
		Intraparenchymal hematoma >2 cm or expanding	
	Laceration:	>3 cm parenchymal depth	3
IV.	Hematoma:	Ruptured intraparenchymal hematoma with active bleeding	4
	Laceration:	Parenchymal disruption involving 25-50% of hepatic lobe	4
V.	Laceration:	Parenchymal disruption involving >58% of hepatic lobe	5
	Vascular:	Juxtahepatic venous injuries; i.e., retrohepatic vena cava/major hepatic veins	5
VI.	Vascular:	Hepatic avulsion	6

*Advance one grade for multiple injuries to the same organ.
+Based on most accurate assessment at autopsy, laparotomy, or radiologic study.
From: Moore EE, Shackford SR, Pachter HL, et al. Organ injury scaling: spleen, liver, kidney. J Trauma 1989;29:1664.

DIAGNOSTIC PERITONEAL LAVAGE

The techniques of abdominal paracentesis and diagnostic peritoneal lavage (DPL) have been extensively studied, and these procedures can be extremely helpful for evaluating patients with suspected intra-abdominal injuries when: (a) suspicion is high and clinical signs are lacking and/or (b) patients have an altered sensorium as a result of drugs, alcohol, or head trauma.[3,19] The accuracy of detecting blood in the peritoneal cavity when diagnostic peritoneal lavage is used is approximately 90-98%.[18,20,21] If a tractotomy reveals the abdominal fascia has been penetrated, diagnostic peritoneal lavage can be performed with an accuracy rate of 90-95% for determining the presence of intra-abdominal injury.[20] Few, if any, contraindications exist to the use of the "open" or "semi-open" methods of DPL.[22]

AXIOM A hemodynamically stable patient with a positive DPL because of increased red cells from what is probably an isolated solid organ injury usually can be treated nonoperatively.

In spite of its accuracy, there are two basic drawbacks to diagnostic peritoneal lavage.[3] First, it lacks specificity as to which organ is injured. Second, and more important, it is oversensitive in detecting blood, and therefore, fails to distinguish between significant injuries requiring surgical correction and insignificant injuries. In addition, injuries to retroperitoneal structures, such as the pancreas and kidney, may be missed on DPL. It is for this reason that computed tomography (CT) scanning has gained popularity and has been advocated by some as being superior to diagnostic peritoneal lavage.

CT SCANNING

Much of the support for CT scanning being the optimal procedure for evaluating patients with possible intra-abdominal injuries after blunt trauma stems from the work of Federele and the San Francisco group.[23-26] Federele et al reported a high degree of sensitivity and specificity with this diagnostic modality in evaluating patients with hepatic injuries after blunt abdominal trauma. It has been pointed out, however, that Federele's results cannot be duplicated by all hospitals.[3] The members of the San Francisco group were very selective with this modality and performed CT scans on only 14% of their patients with abdominal trauma. Additionally, each of the scans was read by experienced radiologists with a dedicated interest in trauma.[27]

AXIOM The value of most diagnostic modalities is directly proportional to the experience and interest of the individual performing the test and interpreting the results.

It is becoming more evident that many patients who are stable but have minor hepatic injuries, especially those classified as grade I and grade II injuries (Figs. 22-3, 22-4), would have undergone an unnecessary celiotomy based on a positive diagnostic peritoneal lavage.[3] Consequently, it seems reasonable that when a hepatic injury is strongly suspected in a stable patient, CT scanning might supersede diagnostic peritoneal lavage. If, after the diagnosis has been confirmed by CT scan and other intra-abdominal injuries requiring surgery have been excluded, a nonoperative approach may be undertaken in hemodynamically stable and alert patients.

Unfortunately, CT scans are not accurate in excluding injuries to the small bowel, especially past the proximal jejunum. In addition, some diaphragmatic and pancreatic injuries can be missed. Consequently, careful observation and repeat physical examinations are mandatory in patients whose liver injuries are to be treated nonoperatively. An equivocal abdominal examination or inability to closely monitor the patient, such as during prolonged nonabdominal operations, is an indication for diagnostic peritoneal lavage.

AXIOM DPL and abdominal CT scanning should be considered complementary, rather than competing, diagnostic tests in patients with abdominal trauma.

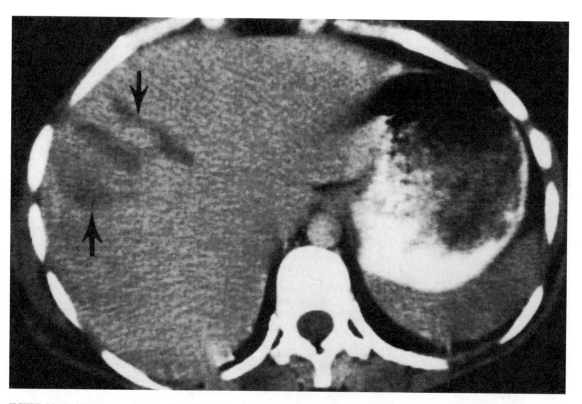

FIGURE 22-4 Multiple lacerations of the liver. This CT image demonstrates three jagged, radially oriented linear lacerations in the anterolateral right lobe (arrow). (From Mirvis SE, Whitley NO, Vainwright JR, Gens DR. Blunt hepatic trauma in adults: CT-based classification and correlation with prognosis and treatment. Radiology 1989;171:27.)

Diagnostic peritoneal lavage (DPL) and CT scanning in patients with possible hepatic injuries should be used selectively.[3] Although both procedures have their advocates, neither is perfect. In specific clinical situations, one may supersede the other, or they may in fact be complementary in many clinical situations.[28-32]

At present, the exact role of CT scanning to evaluate the presence or absence of intra-abdominal injuries in patients with stab wounds of the abdomen is unclear.[3] Marx et al[28] had an 87.5% false negative rate when a CT scan was used as the initial diagnostic modality in 35 patients with stab wounds to the abdomen. Thus, it becomes difficult to endorse CT scanning as superior to diagnostic peritoneal lavage in such circumstances.

> **AXIOM** In patients with stab wounds that may have entered the abdomen, DPL appears to be more accurate than CT scans for determining such penetration.

NONOPERATIVE MANAGEMENT OF BLUNT HEPATIC INJURIES

Hemodynamically Stable Patients

In patients with blunt abdominal trauma who have evidence of liver injury by CT scan, but who do not demonstrate clinical signs of significant continuing hemorrhage or peritoneal irritation, nonoperative management with close observation and serial CT, ultrasonographic, or scintigraphic scanning has been shown to be safe in selected cases, particularly in children.[33,34] These data suggest that if there are no other intraperitoneal injuries requiring operative intervention, a subset of patients can be selected and treated nonoperatively. Strict criteria, however, must be met. Patients with grade I, II or III hepatic injuries but without active bleeding or an expanding hematoma, may be considered for nonoperative management. Essential to the management of these patients is in-hospital serial radiological scanning examinations to document healing or resorption of intrahepatic or perihepatic fluid collections.[3]

> **AXIOM** Need for more than 2 units of blood in adults or replacement of more than half of the estimated blood volume in children to maintain stable vital signs is generally an indication for surgery in patients with isolated splenic or hepatic injuries.

If more than 2 units of blood are required to maintain stable vital signs in an adult, the risk of transmitting a blood-borne disease is probably greater than the risk of surgery.[3] Meyer[40] reported a 100% success rate in 24 patients with hepatic injuries who were treated nonoperatively.

Meredith et al[35] recently reported on 72 hemodynamically stable patients with blunt hepatic trauma who initially were thought to be candidates for nonoperative treatment. Of the 70 injuries successfully treated nonoperatively, 11 (15%) were Grade I, 28 (39%) were Grade II, 16 (22%) were Grade III, 10 (14%) were Grade IV, and 5 (7%) were Grade V. The average blood transfusion requirement in the patients treated nonoperatively was 1.2 ± 1.7 units. Two of the 72 patients picked for nonoperative management eventually came to surgery because of falling hematocrits. There were no hepatic or biliary complications in the patients treated nonoperatively. Fifty-five other patients with blunt liver injuries were treated with early operation primarily because of bleeding or associated injuries.

In a more recent report, Sherman et al[36] noted that 30 (50%) of 60 patients with blunt hepatic injury were initially designated for nonoperative therapy because they were hemodynamically stable, had no other injuries requiring laparotomy and were available for controlled monitoring. The grades of liver injury in the nonoperative group were I-3, II-7, III-14, IV-6, and V-0. There were no deaths, delayed laparotomies, or missed intra-abdominal injuries in the nonoperative group. One patient, however, required angiographic embolization of her hepatic injury eight hours after admission because of continued bleeding from the liver. Continued CT scanning of the liver to resolution of the hepatic injury was performed in 19 patients. The time for resolution ranged from 18-88 days with a mean of 57 days. Occasionally, resolution of the injury on CT scan may take 3-4 months[5] (Fig. 22-5).

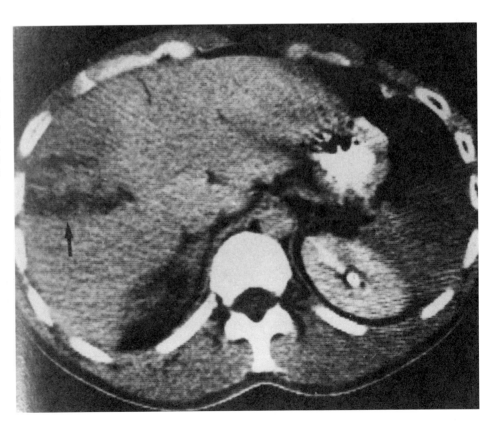

FIGURE 22-5 A. This admitting CT scan shows a large hepatic laceration with a significant parenchymal hematoma which was managed nonoperatively. **B.** A CT scan 1 mo. later showed significant improvement of the hepatic laceration and the parenchymal hematoma. A CT scan 3.5 mo. after the injury showed complete resolution of the laceration and minimal residua of the hepatic hematoma. (From Pachter HL, Spencer FC, Hofstetter SR, et al. Experience with finger-fracture technique to achieve intrahepatic hemostasis in 75 patients with severe injuries to the liver. Ann Surg 1983;197:771.)

Of 106 patients with blunt liver trauma reported by Sugimoto et al,[37] 64 (60%) were treated nonoperatively. Of these 64 patients, 28 had endoscopic retrograde cholangiography (ERC). Bile duct injury was found in six (21%), and five of these patients developed a biloma. Consequently, the authors thought that patients with severe liver injuries treated nonoperatively should be considered for ERC to exclude major bile duct injuries.

Both Foley[38] and Farnell[39] reported a 10% failure rate with nonoperative therapy of blunt liver trauma. This figure, which is probably more realistic, may have been prompted by their decision to operate whenever the hemoperitoneum extended outside Morrison's pouch or if a hemoperitoneum greater than 250 ml existed. While these were considered failures of nonoperative treatment by Farnell et al,[39] other authors might not have operated under similar circumstances.

Aside from signs of hemorrhage, more conventional criteria for operative intervention are evidence of sepsis or biliary obstruction. Either of these two findings is an indication for an immediate CT scan or ERCP. If a collection of fluid is seen, one should attempt percutaneous drainage under ultrasound or CT guidance. Patients in whom percutaneous drainage is not possible or who do not respond to this maneuver should be operated on expeditiously to establish better drainage and to debride nonviable tissue.

In patients in whom a nonoperative approach to blunt liver trauma is pursued, close in-hospital observation for at least a week is recommended. If serial CT scans and hematocrit determinations (after fluid resuscitation) show no evidence of hematoma expansion, the patient is discharged on limited activity to be followed with serial scanning. As resolution of the hematoma is demonstrated, activity is slowly increased over the next 6-8 weeks. The development of peritoneal signs or evidence of serious hematoma expansion usually mandates prompt surgical exploration.

> **AXIOM**   Nonoperative management of liver injuries is not advisable in uncooperative patients.

Nonoperative management should not be viewed as "conservative management," for it is not.[3] Indeed, it is usually much more difficult to manage a patient nonoperatively than operatively. In addition, nonoperative management should not lead to use of more than two blood transfusions in adults nor should it involve any delay in operative intervention if surgery becomes necessary.

Nonoperative management of hemodynamically stable patients with blunt hepatic injuries appears to be an acceptable form of treatment; however, extensive experience in adult patients is lacking.[3] It is likely, moreover, that a certain number of patients will have delayed hemorrhage at some time following the injury.[40]

Subcapsular and Intrahepatic Hematomas (Fig. 22-6)

The management of subcapsular or intrahepatic hematomas due to blunt trauma remains controversial.[3] If the diagnosis is made preoperatively, Richie and Fonkalsrud[41] favor nonoperative management. Geis et al,[42] on the other hand, advocate operative decompression and drainage based on failure in six (40%) of 15 observed patients. Only two of the six "failures" reported by Geis et al, however, required their operation for continued hemorrhage. The other four patients were operated on for hepatic abscesses. It is possible that use of percutaneous drainage guided by CT scanning or ultrasound might have obviated the need for surgery in those four patients.

Pachter et al[3] reported ten patients with subcapsular or intrahepatic hematomas who were treated nonoperatively with uniform success. Serial CT scans demonstrated resolution of the injury in all 10 patients. Criteria for switching to operative intervention during

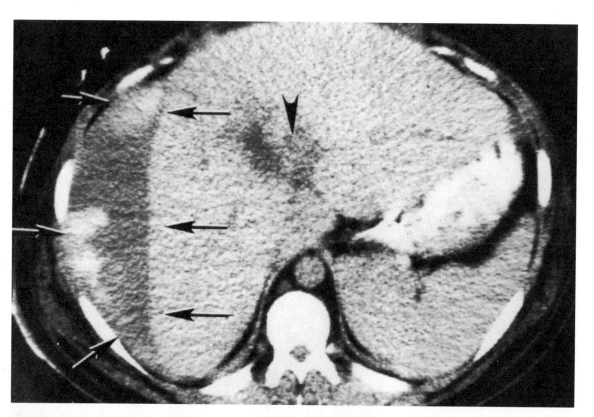

FIGURE 22-6   Subcapsular liver hematoma. This CT image reveals a large subcapsular hematoma indenting the liver parenchyma (arrows). A complex laceration involving the medial segment of the left lobe and extending into the porta hepatis (arrowhead) is also present. (From Mirvis SE, Whitley NO. CT in hepatobiliary trauma. In: Ferrucci JT, Mathieu DG, eds. Advances in hepatobilary radiology. St. Louis: CV Mosby, 1989.)

the observation period were: (a) evidence of ongoing hemorrhage; (b) progressive expansion of the hematoma; (c) signs of sepsis; or (d) deterioration in liver function tests.

A more difficult question is the approach the surgeon should take in patients in whom a nonexpanding subcapsular or intrahepatic hematoma is found at operation.[3] Geis et al[42] favor opening the hematoma, evacuating the clot, obtaining hemostasis, and providing external drainage. Operative intervention, however, without a clear demonstrable need may result in an unnecessary morbidity and mortality. Once Glisson's capsule is opened, the raw surface of liver may ooze, and precise control of multiple bleeding points over a large surface may be difficult. Hepatic resection, which carries an inordinate mortality under these circumstances, may be required occasionally to arrest the intrahepatic hemorrhage which has restarted. The management of these injuries should, therefore, be individualized.

AXIOM Nonexpanding intrahepatic hematomas are best managed conservatively if at all possible.

OPERATIVE MANAGEMENT

Incision

On the operating room table, any patient requiring a laparotomy for trauma should be prepped from chin to knees and draped widely in case the surgeon inserts drains or performs ostomies.[1] An upper midline incision provides rapid and adequate exposure of most injuries, and it is easily extended up into the chest as a median sternotomy or as a right or left anterolateral thoracotomy if this should prove necessary.

Initial Exploration

Once the abdomen is entered, any free blood and clots present are rapidly evacuated. Packs are placed in any abdominal quadrants that may be bleeding. As each quadrant is subsequently explored, injuries are evaluated and hemorrhage and bowel perforations controlled. With the possible exception of injuries to the inferior vena cava or juxtahepatic veins, perihepatic packing is usually effective for obtaining adequate hemostasis for liver injuries while attending to more active bleeding or torn bowel in other quadrants.[1]

After adequate hemostasis has been obtained in the other quadrants and any intestinal disruption has been controlled, the packs are serially removed from each quadrant, usually beginning with the quadrants most apt to have easily controlled problems. Often, much of the bleeding has ceased by this time.

The overwhelming majority (80-90%) of hepatic injuries are minor (grades I and II) and require nothing more than simple sutures, electrocautery, or topical hemostatic agents.[3] Complex hepatic injuries, on the other hand, often are still bleeding when the abdomen is opened and/or the liver is mobilized, and can be a challenge to any trauma surgeon. The actions of the operating surgeon during the first 15-30 minutes of the operation on such injuries will often determine the outcome.[3]

PITFALL ⊘

One should avoid attempts at definitive surgical control of bleeding sites within the liver without prior adequate resuscitation.

Regardless of the severity of the injury, bleeding from the majority of hepatic injuries can be controlled initially by manual compression directly on the liver over lap pads.[3] The importance of this simple maneuver cannot be overemphasized, as it gives the anesthesiologist some time to correct what might otherwise be lethal hypovolemia and hypothermia.

AXIOM It is extremely important to adequately compress the liver manually or control the bleeding in some way so that the patient can be properly resuscitated before further surgery is performed.[47]

Mobilization of the Liver

AXIOM Knowledge of liver anatomy is essential for proper mobilization of the liver.

When the hepatic wound is not directly visible, complete mobilization of the liver may be needed to expose it clearly.[1] Such mobilization is usually begun by division of the round ligament anteriorly and inferiorly and then the falciform ligament over the anterior and superior aspect of the liver. Those maneuvers should be performed early and routinely for almost all liver injuries that require sutures or any other efforts at hemostasis.

Further mobilization of the individual hepatic lobes may be provided by division of the right or left triangular ligaments, leading to exposure of the anterior and superior surfaces of the respective lobes. The left triangular ligament can usually be divided under direct vision. The right triangular ligament, however, often must be divided blindly, and at times ongoing hemorrhage will also obscure the area. Care must be taken to palpate the tips of the scissors with the opposite and retracting hand to protect the inferior vena cava and right hepatic vein from injury, especially as the dissection is continued posteriorly. One must also be careful to avoid injury to the inferior phrenic vessels coursing along the underside of the diaphragm. Division of the triangular ligaments allows mobilization of the liver toward the midline where hemostasis and debridement of the parenchymal injury may be more easily performed.

Controlling Bleeding

Most hepatic injuries will have stopped bleeding by the time the abdomen is opened. Injuries that are still bleeding can usually be controlled by compression with packs for the period necessary to complete the abdominal survey and deal with any associated major injuries. In those instances where bleeding continues in spite of the packs or resumes when the pack is removed later, other measures, such as the Pringle maneuver, may be necessary (Fig. 22-4).

PRINGLE MANEUVER

Technical Considerations

AXIOM The next step to control continued liver bleeding which continues in spite of packs and/or manual compression is the Pringle maneuver.

The Pringle maneuver refers to occlusion of the portal triad at the foramen of Winslow, usually by application of a "soft" vascular clamp to the margin of the hepatoduodenal ligament.[43] Failure of such inflow occlusion to adequately control hemorrhage suggests either an anomalous blood supply to the liver or the possibility of retrohepatic caval or juxtahepatic venous injury. In 10-25% of patients, the hepatic arteries have an anomalous origin. The main or right hepatic artery comes off the superior mesenteric artery (SMA) in about 10-20% of cases, an accessory right hepatic artery comes off the SMA in about 5% of cases, and an anomalous left hepatic artery comes off the left gastric artery in about 5% of cases. These anomalies may be responsible for continued arterial bleeding after the portal triad is occluded.[1] When the Pringle maneuver provides adequate hemostasis, the vascular clamp is left in place until adequate exposure and local hemostasis at the wound site are accomplished.

Traditionally, the clamp on the portal triad was released every 15-20 minutes to allow intermittent hepatic perfusion. More recently, periods of inflow occlusion have been extended to more than an hour without evidence of ischemic damage to the liver. Currently, it is common practice to provide continuous inflow occlusion to the liver until local hemostasis is obtained.[44]

Based on experimental studies in dogs by Raffucci in 1953,[45] the limit of warm ischemia time for the liver was thought to be no more than 15-20 minutes. It is now clear that differences in splanchnic circulation between species render experimental studies in dogs inapplicable to humans.[3] Unfortunately, this misconception was adopted as surgical dogma and undoubtedly has restricted the use of prolonged portal triad occlusion for complex hepatic injuries.

The upper limit of normothermic occlusion of the liver in humans is presently unknown. Reports from France,[46,47] however, have documented occlusion times up to 1 hour during elective hepatic cancer surgery without untoward effects. Indeed, a study by Delva et al[48] reported normothermic liver ischemia times up to 90 minutes without subsequent complications. In addition, Delva et al compared two groups of patients, one cross-clamped for less than 45 minutes (119 patients) and another cross-clamped for more than 45 minutes (23 patients). There were no differences among the two groups with regard to mortality or rate or severity of liver failure.

The ability of the liver to tolerate normothermic ischemia when resected for carcinoma cannot, however, be extrapolated to the severely injured patients.[3] Two major theoretical differences are: (a) the ability of the liver to tolerate normothermic ischemia when resected for carcinoma may in large part be due to spontaneous collateral blood vessels that often accompany large hepatic tumors, and (b) severely injured hypotensive patients may already have experienced significant hypoperfusion and ischemic damage to the hepatic parenchyma. Under these circumstances, normothermic portal triad occlusion may result in permanent dysfunction of already damaged hepatocytes.

Methods for Prolonging Normothermic Hepatic Ischemia

TOPICAL HEPATIC HYPOTHERMIA. Experimental work by both Bernhard et al[49] and Goodall et al[50] demonstrated that dogs subjected to normothermic portal triad occlusion for greater than 40 minutes always died.[3] When the dogs were made hypothermic (28-32° C), however, portal triad occlusion for up to one hour was tolerated by all the dogs. Based on this work and the clinical experience of Fortner et al,[57] the value of hypothermia in increasing the liver's tolerance to ischemia is well documented. The methods described by Fortner et al,[51] however, are too complex to be used effectively in trauma patients. Nevertheless, topical hypothermia can be achieved, preferably prior to portal triad occlusion, by applying cold saline "slush" directly onto the liver surface.

Ideally, an intrahepatic temperative probe should be used to ensure that the liver is cooled to 27-32° C. When central liver temperature readings exceed 32° C, additional "slush" should be applied to the liver to lower the temperature back to the desired range. Previously, iced Ringer's lactate was used, but this method often required application of 500 ml of the solution every 15 minutes.[5] The advantage of the cold "slush" is that the reapplication is usually required only one or two times during surgery.

STEROIDS. The rationale for using large doses of corticosteroids to prolong the safe hepatic ischemia time is based on the reports of Delpin and Figueroa.[52,53] By pretreating experimental animals with methylprednisolone sodium succinate (Solu-medrol), they were able to decrease the mortality from 100%-10% when the portal triad was occluded for 30 minutes and to only a 50% mortality rate if the portal triad was occluded for 60 minutes. Objections to the use of steroids have been voiced by DeMaria et al,[54] whose work suggests that patients with central nervous system trauma who are given steroids are more prone to develop septic complications.

COMBINATIONS. The benefits of topical hypothermia and large doses of steroids (30 mg/kg of Solu-medrol) have not been verified by ran-domized prospective trials.[3] Pachter et al[5] reported on 44 patients with complex hepatic injuries in whom a combination of topical hypothermia and intravenous corticosteroids was used to prevent hepatic ischemic damage when their portal triad was occluded. Seventy percent of these patients had their portal triad cross-clamped for more than 20 minutes, 40% for longer than 30 minutes, and 7% for more than 1 hour. Serial measurements of liver function tests revealed a rise in hepatic enzymes corresponding to the length of ischemia time; however, all of the laboratory values returned to virtually normal levels before hospital discharge, and no patient experienced clinical hepatic dysfunction.[5]

AXIOM If it appears that the portal triad may be occluded for more than 20– 30 minutes, one should consider the use of massive intravenous corticosteroids and topical hypothermia prior to performing the Pringle maneuver.

It seems clear that the 15–20-minute upper limit of portal triad occlusion is a myth for most patients. Whether the combination of hypothermia and corticosteroids or their individual use is actually beneficial is still unknown; however, Pachter et al have apparently had success with these methods.[4,5,55]

CALCIUM BLOCKERS. It has been noted that diltiazem, a calcium channel blocker, can be beneficial in the treatment of hemorrhagic shock,[56] possibly because of its effects on gluconeogenesis, which involves several calcium-sensitive steps.[57,58] In a recent study on rats bled into hemorrhagic shock by Geller et al,[59] resuscitation was performed with Ringers' lactate, with or without diltiazem. In the animals in which the hemorrhagic shock was limited to 30 minutes, the diltiazem significantly improved hepatic gluconeogenesis.

LIVER SUTURING

Many techniques have evolved to achieve hepatic hemostasis from severe liver wounds. The placement of hepatic sutures is the most frequently employed hemostatic method.[1] The careful placement of sutures, usually 2-0 chromic on a long blunt-tipped liver needle in a mattress fashion across the site of injury, will frequently provide hemostasis.[1] Care must be taken to avoid undue tension when tying the sutures because they can easily tear through the enclosed hepatic tissue or cause it to necrose.

AXIOM If sutures incorporating a great deal of liver tissue are used to control bleeding, the incidence of later liver necrosis and abscesses will be increased.

Cogbill et al[60] have also noted that liver sutures can control hemorrhage, but they can also cause liver necrosis and increase the risk of subsequent hepatic abscess formation.[64] Deep liver sutures were employed in 25% of the grade III injuries in their multicenter study.[60] Of the 23 patients who had this type of treatment, a 30% morbidity followed. Two patients developed abscesses, one patient hemorrhaged and four patients developed bile leaks. Stain et al[61] at UCLA have been using the technique of deep liver suturing with success for many years. They recommend it as frequently life-saving when dealing with injuries in inaccessible portions of the liver. In the 66 instances in which "liver sutures" were employed by Stain et al,[61] abscesses developed in 12%; however, they say this incidence of infection is relatively low in comparison to the lives that were saved.

While many of the objections to deep sutures placed into the liver to control hemorrhage may be valid, the trade-off of a postoperative abscess or other nonlethal complications in exchange for controlling exsanguinating hemorrhage in a critically injured patient cannot be ignored.[3] Thus, a role does exist for this method of treatment, but caution should be exercised in applying the technique routinely when more direct methods of controlling hemorrhage are possible.

HEPATORRHAPHY BY THE FINGER-FRACTURE TECHNIQUE

AXIOM Persistent bleeding from deep hepatic wounds is usually best managed with hepatorrhaphy to control the bleeding vessels under direct vision. If this is not practical or successful, stuffing the wound with a viable omental pack should be considered.

When the depth of the liver wound precludes safe use of direct vessel ligation or simple hepatic sutures, the wound should be opened further to permit direct ligation of the injured vessels and biliary radicles.[1,5] With portal triad occlusion achieved by an atraumatic vascular clamp, the injuries can be approached by incising Glisson's capsule with electrocautery and then finger fracturing the hepatic parenchyma in the direction of the injury[3,62] (Fig. 22-5). The blood vessels and bile ducts encountered are ligated or clipped under direct vision. When employing the finger-fracture technique, the position of the main right and left hepatic ducts should be kept in mind, so that they are not injured inadvertently.[3]

After hemostasis has been achieved, the vascular clamp occluding the portal triad is slowly released. Any additional points of hemorrhage are then ligated or clipped. Once adequate hemostasis is obtained, the margins of the wound may then be reapproximated with liver sutures. The liver closure should begin at the bottom of the wound so that no dead space is left. If the hepatic wound cannot be closed without leaving dead space, the wound should be left open and packed with omentum.

Although extensive experience with the finger-fracture technique exists,[62,63] some surgeons feel that incision of normal hepatic parenchyma along nonanatomic planes can cause prohibitive bleeding;[64] however, the published data on using the finger-fracture technique to handle complex liver injuries seem to indicate that the dangers of in-

cising normal hepatic parenchyma along nonanatomical planes are probably exaggerated.[3-5,55]

Feliciano et al[44] reported using this technique in 48% of their patients with complex hepatic injuries. Additionally, in a multicenter experience with over 1000 hepatic injuries, Cogbill et al[60] used the finger-fracture technique in 41% of the patients with grade III injuries. This method was found to be especially useful for exposing bleeding deep in wounds caused by penetrating trauma.

VIABLE OMENTAL PACK

While some surgeons think all deep hepatic wounds that are actively bleeding should be treated by means of hepatotomy to allow accurate ligation of the bleeding points under direct vision,[3] there are times when this is not practical. One such example is an actively bleeding penetrating injury tract that traverses the depths of the right hepatic lobe (Figs. 22-7, 22-8). While superficial tracts should be opened and direct vascular control obtained, the large volume of normal hepatic tissue that may have to be divided to expose a deep injury tract precludes ready application of this technique to all patients. However, the temptation to close both ends of a through-and-through bullet tract to control deep bleeding should generally be resisted because of the risk of forming a large intrahepatic hematoma.[65]

Packing with pedicled omentum can be extremely useful in obtaining hemostasis in deep hepatic wounds when the surgeon is reluctant to use a hepatotomy. It is important that the omentum be freed up enough and the opening to the liver be made large enough for the omentum to be packed down to the bottom of the wound in the liver.[1] This will control most deep hepatic bleeding quite well. Some of the advantages of using a viable omental pedicle to fill hepatic dead space include: (a) the omentum's ability to tamponade major bleeding and minor oozing;[66,67] (b) decreased chances of developing an abscess;

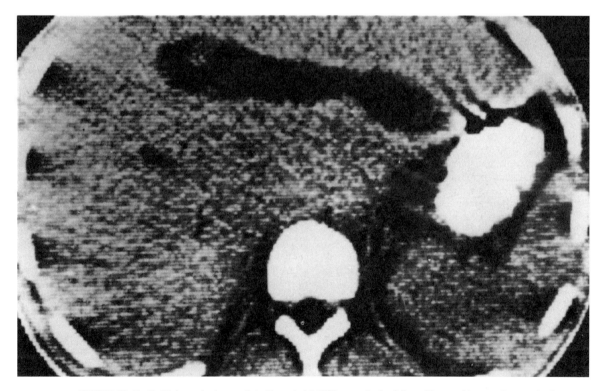

FIGURE 22-7 Ballistic cavitation track in liver. Axial CT image obtained from 23-year-old man who sustained a transabdominal bullet wound. Note the track of the bullet is visualized by the cavitation wound extending across the anterior liver. The hepatic injury became infected and required transhepatic percutaneous catheter drainage later. (From Mirvis SE, Whitley NO. Computed tomography in hepatobiliary trauma. In: Ferrucci JT, Mathieu DG, eds. Advances in hepatobiliary radiology, 1990; 239.)

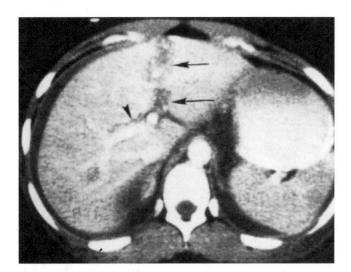

FIGURE 22-8 Liver laceration and segmental devascularization. This CT image reveals a major hepatic laceration extending across the right lobe to the hilus (arrows). An anterior splenic contusion may also be observed. (From Mirvis SE, Whitley NO, Vainwright JR, Gens DR. Blunt hepatic trauma in adults: CT-based classification and correlation with prognosis and treatment. Radiology 1989;171:27.)

(c) supplying a rich source of macrophages, which can also reduce the incidence of infection.[71]

Although the viable omental pack can control venous bleeding,[66,67] it may not be as effective with severe arterial hemorrhage. If the finger-fracture technique is used to achieve hemostasis and then debridement of nonviable parenchyma, this can result in a rather large dead space in the depths of the liver. Pachter et al[3] prefer to fill this dead space with a viable pedicle of omentum (Fig. 22-6). The liver edges are then coapted loosely around the omentum pack with 0-chromic liver sutures.

SELECTIVE HEPATIC ARTERY LIGATION

AXIOM Hepatic artery ligation should only be considered if arterial bleeding from a deep hepatic wound cannot be controlled by any other means.

When bleeding from a hepatic wound is not amenable to other techniques or when active arterial bleeding recurs from a deep liver laceration upon unclamping the portal triad, selective hepatic artery ligation may provide hemostasis.[83,84] Ideally, hepatic artery ligation is reserved for those instances where intrahepatic arterial bleeding can be controlled only by clamping a right and/or left hepatic artery.[1] The ligation should be performed close to the liver to preserve as much collateral flow as possible. Ideally, the right or left hepatic artery should be ligated but, where necessary, the common hepatic artery may be ligated with relative impunity. While usually safe, this technique does entail some risk of hepatic necrosis, particularly if used in combination with placement of perihepatic packs.

Hepatic artery ligation has been performed frequently in humans without significant impairment of liver function or development of subsequent hepatic necrosis.[84,85] The high oxygen saturation in the portal vein of humans, with the absence of intra-hepatic bacteria, and an extensive collateral hepatic arterial flow, has allowed hepatic artery ligation to be performed safely in most patients. The work of Aaron et al[86] and Mays et al[87] was met with enthusiasm initially because the technique could easily be performed and, contrary to previous surgical dogma, it produced only temporary hepatic dysfunction. Collateral vessels to the ischemic hepatic segment apparently often developed within 10-12 hours.[87]

Following hepatic artery ligation, subsequent hyperbilirubinemia and enzymatic derangements were generally only moderate and seldom persisted for more than a week.[87] In conjunction with hepatic artery ligation, however, strenuous efforts must be made to maintain a normal or increased blood pressure, cardiac output, and oxygen delivery. Madding[88] has also advocated the use of glucagon as an intravenous bolus of 2 mg followed by an infusion of 2 mg/hr as a method of increasing the liver blood flow during the first critical 72 hours.

Widespread adoption of hepatic artery ligation has never occurred. In 1986, Feliciano et al[44] reported that selective hepatic artery ligation was employed in only six (0.6%) of 1000 consecutive patients with hepatic injuries treated at the Ben Taub General Hospital. Corroborating these observations, Cogbill et al[60] cited use of selective hepatic artery ligation in only 10 (0.74%) of 1333 injuries collected from six major trauma centers.

Although hepatic artery ligation can safely be performed electively, its role in hepatic trauma appears to be very limited because: (a) selective hepatic artery ligation is unnecessary in the vast majority of hepatic injuries, (b) hepatic artery ligation is ineffective in controlling hemorrhage from major branches of the portal or hepatic veins, (c) hepatic artery ligation in a persistently hypotensive patient may cause severe hepatic ischemia which can go on to extensive hepatic necrosis and sepsis,[89] and (d) mortality rates exceed 50% when hepatic artery ligation fails to control the hemorrhage.[83]

HEPATIC RESECTION

Only rarely does bleeding from a hepatic injury require a major liver resection.[90,91] Except for the left lateral segment, a formal hepatic lobar or segmental resection in the presence of continuing hemorrhage and/or hypotension can be extremely difficult, and it is usually much safer to continue to attempt control with perihepatic or intrahepatic packing and other maneuvers.[92] In a review of 5000 hepatic injuries by Pachter and Spencer in 1983,[93] hepatic resection was employed in only 7.5% of the cases and the mortality rate was 52%. More recently, Cogbill et al[60] reported that hepatic resection for trauma was required in only 12 (0.89%) of 1333 patients, and seven (58%) of these 12 patients died.

AXIOM Hepatic resections should be reserved for situations in which the trauma has almost completed the dissection and/or there is no other reasonable way to control the bleeding.

The realization that hemostasis can generally be achieved successfully with a considerably lower mortality by less dramatic techniques has probably been responsible for the less-than-enthusiastic acceptance of hepatic resection by American surgeons. Some surgeons, such as Balasegaram and Joishy[64] and Blumgart et al,[94] however, report mortalities of only 10% and 21% with hepatic resection for trauma.

In a recent report by Menegaux et al,[95] it was noted that the current trend to perform fewer hepatic resections for severe liver trauma (Grades III, IV, and V) has not resulted in fewer deaths in their series [20% (8/41) for 1973-1981 versus 21% (13/62) for 1982-1990]. The excellent results reported in some series of hepatic resections are probably more reflective of the authors' abilities rather than the merits of resection, and they do not reflect the general experience with this approach.[3] The current indications for major hepatic resections for trauma generally include: (a) total destruction of an anatomic hepatic lobe or segment; (b) instances in which the extent of the injury precludes successful "perihepatic packing"; (c) injuries which have performed much of the dissection, and completion can be achieved with minimal additional surgery, and (d) injuries in which resection is the only method of controlling exsanguinating hemorrhage.[3]

In bilateral severe liver trauma with massive bleeding that cannot be controlled in any other way, total hepatic resection with liver transplantation has been attempted.[103]

ADJUNCTIVE HEMOSTATIC AGENTS

Synthetic Topical Agents

Topical agents, such as Surgicil (oxidized regenerated cellulose, Johnson & Johnson, New Brunswick, New Jersey), Avitene (microfibrillary collagen hemostat, Med Chem Products Inc, Woburn, Massachusetts) and Instat (Johnson & Johnson) are useful adjuncts for achieving topical hemostasis once major hemorrhage has been controlled.[3] These agents have most often been placed on oozing raw hepatic surface. These are manually compressed against the bleeding surface with lap pads for a period of 10-15 minutes. After the compression is released, the raw liver surfaces are inspected for further bleeding. Any continuing spots of bleeding can then usually be controlled with additional applications of a hemostatic agent, sutures, or cautery.

> **AXIOM**   If a topical hemostatic agent controls hemorrhage from a large area of denuded liver, the hemostatic agent can often be left in place, especially if bleeding tends to recur after its removal.

Not infrequently, hemorrhage from a large raw liver surface is controlled as long as the hemostatic agent is left in place but resumes if the agent is removed. Under such circumstances, these agents can be left in situ with relatively little fear that they will contribute to a subsequent infection. For less severe liver injuries (grades I and II), topical hemostatic agents often suffice as the sole means of controlling hemorrhage.[3] Under these circumstances, drainage of the liver injury is usually unnecessary.

Fibrin Glue

> **AXIOM**   Localized surface bleeding which persists in spite of surgical efforts and other topical agents can frequently be controlled by applying fibrin glue.

Fibrin glue mimics the last step in the natural coagulation cascade. Factor XII and fibrinogen are activated by thrombin in the presence of calcium ion, converting fibrinogen to fibrin. Activated factor XIII then polymerizes fibrin to form a stable clot. The thrombin which is added to the clotting factors to form fibrin glue is heterologously derived from bovine sources and is available in a variety of strengths. Although anaphylaxis to bovine thrombin protein is a theoretical possibility, it is rarely of clinical importance, especially if care is taken to avoid injecting it directly into large open vessels. Calcium ion is also added to neutralize any citrate that is present. It also serves as a cofactor for the activation of factor XIII to enhance fibrin cross-linking.

The original fibrin glue, described in European trials and in early United States experiences, used pooled cryoprecipitate as the source of fibrinogen and factor XIII. Although there is always some risk of hepatitis and/or AIDS transmission when a non-heated blood product is used, this has not been documented in over 3000 uses.[68-70] Numerous methodologies, including pre-donation of blood, rapid concentration of native plasma, and solvent detergent treatment of donor plasma have been suggested as methods to decrease the potential viral transmission risk with fibrin glue.[68-70]

> **AXIOM**   Fibrin glue and fibrin gel work best when they can be applied to a surface which is at least temporarily dry.

Fibrin glue can be effective in either superficial injuries or deep parenchymal lacerations of the liver.[3] It can also be used in the presence of a severe coagulopathy.[71] Moreover, fibrin glue can either be sprayed onto the injury site or directly injected into involved hepatic parenchyma when deep and/or inaccessible injuries are present. The versatility of fibrin glue makes it superior to other topical hemostatic agents which are usually limited to injuries that are relatively superficial.

To be most effective, fibrin glue should be applied to surfaces which are temporarily rendered dry. Clots forming directly on tissue are much more secure than those forming on a bleeding surface. Fibrin glue may also be used to pre-clot knitted vascular grafts.[72] An intriguing application of fibrin glue or fibrin gel is to incorporate an antibiotic into it when it is placed in a potentially contaminated field.[73] Several animal models have documented the efficacy of this approach for preventing localized sepsis, but its clinical applicability remains to be defined.[73,74]

To date there have been few complications reported with the use of fibrin glue, and postoperative intra-abdominal sepsis or re-bleeding has been rare.[75,76] Berguer et al,[71] however, have described a fatal reaction following fibrin injection into a deep hepatic wound.

Fibrin Gel

Fibrin gel is a physiologic variant of fibrin glue produced by rapid centrifugation of 30-60 ml of autologous plasma to provide the fibrinogen and factor XIII necessary for the preparation.[75] Cryoprecipitate (2-4 units) can also be used as the source of the coagulation factors. The resulting compound can provide an effective hemostatic agent. No cumbersome concentrating steps are necessary for the production of fibrin gel, thereby simplifying preparation and reducing costs. The fibrin gel may also have the added benefit of a localized antibacterial effect secondary to activation of complement; however, the tensile strength and adhesive properties of the gel are less than fibrin glue because the fibrinogen concentration is lower.

PERIHEPATIC MESH

Use of an absorbable mesh to wrap severely injured, bleeding spleens has gained support[77,78] (Fig. 22-9). As a consequence, this technique has also been used in experimental liver trauma[79] and in several clinical cases.[79,80] In a recent report by Brunet et al,[81] 35 liver injuries (Grade II-V) were repaired using a polyglactin perihepatic wrap. There were only two (6%) deaths (one from hepatic coma and one from an inferior vena cava avulsion). No hemobilia and no liver abscesses developed. The authors said that early use of the mesh also resulted in a large saving of blood.

BALLOON TAMPONADE

If a patient has a deep penetrating wound to the liver and it is causing severe, continuing bleeding in spite of all other attempts to control it, one can insert a Foley catheter with a large balloon into the depths of the wound.[82] The balloon is inflated just enough to control the hemorrhage. Hemostatic agents might also be injected into the depths of the wound through the lumen of the Foley catheter.

PERIHEPATIC PACKING

Indications

When other techniques have failed to achieve adequate hemostasis from liver wounds, the surgeon must consider resorting to the placement of perihepatic packs and abdominal closure to prevent death from exsanguination.[1] Perihepatic packing was frequently used early in World War II by surgeons confronted with complex hepatic injuries; however, in the patients who survived, rebleeding frequently followed the removal of the intrahepatic packs and the incidence of perihepatic abscesses was very high.[3] The poor results attained with "packing" of the more complex hepatic injuries resulted in a widespread condemnation of this technique.[8]

The last 10-12 years, however, have witnessed survival of a number of patients with severe bleeding from complex hepatic injuries that could only be controlled by packing.[96-99] As a consequence, perihepatic packing has again become an acceptable means of controlling hemorrhage from the liver, and in certain instances, it may be the treatment of choice. Primary indications for perihepatic packing include: (a) transfusion-induced coagulopathy; (b) presence of extensive bilobar injuries in which bleeding cannot be controlled; (c) large expanding or ruptured subcapsular hematomas; and (d) profound hy-

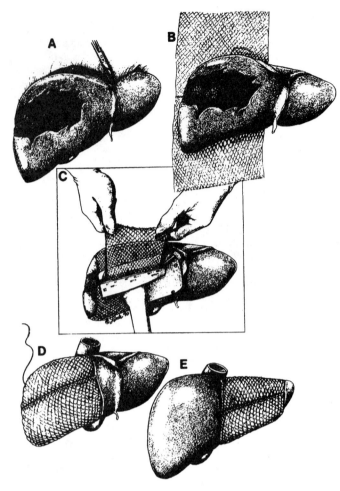

FIGURE 22-9 A. The liver is mobilized by dividing the attachments of the right and left triangular and coronary ligaments and faciform ligament form diaphragm. **B.** Two 7×9 inch pieces of absorbable mesh are stapled end to end and positioned posterior to the injured lobe. **C.** The mesh is wrapped around the right lobe and stapled under tension. The gallbladder is excluded. **D.** Completed wrap with the lateral edges of mesh being sutured. **E.** A similar wrap may be applied to the left lobe. (From Surgery 1992;111:455.)

pothermia and hemodynamic instability.[3] In the presence of exsanguinating bleeding from large intrahepatic vessels, the hepatic veins, or the retrohepatic cava, however, perihepatic packs are not apt to be effective.[3]

> **AXIOM** Perihepatic packing can control most types of parenchymal bleeding from the liver, but whenever possible, standard techniques should be employed to control the hemorrhage from major vessels.[18]

While the technique of perihepatic packing is often reserved as a last-ditch effort to get the patient off the operating table, recent experiences support earlier employment of the technique before massive blood loss has occurred.[1,96,98,100] Perihepatic packing has also been employed successfully in the management of large intraparenchymal hematomas. This technique helps prevent expansion of the hematomas and may avoid the need for a deep hepatotomy, selective hepatic artery ligation, or a large hepatic resection.

Techniques
Perihepatic packing can be accomplished in a variety of ways. A relatively effective technique of perihepatic packing has been described by Pachter et al.[3] A Steri-Drape (3M, St. Paul, Minnesota) with the adhesive bands removed, is folded upon itself and placed directly on

the surface of the involved portion of liver. Lap pads are then applied until there is no space under the ipsilateral hemidiaphragm. The interposition of the plastic drape between the injured liver and the lap pads serves a twofold purpose: (a) it eliminates the bleeding that often ensues when lap pads or gauze rolls are removed later and peeled off raw liver surface, (b) the plastic Steri-Drape helps to keep the packs relatively dry to maintain their effectiveness.[18]

> **AXIOM** Perihepatic packs can cause severe ischemia to portions of the liver which have had their arterial supply ligated.

Compression of liver tissue by packs should be avoided following hepatic artery ligation because this combination greatly increases the tendency to hepatic ischemia and necrosis. After hepatic artery ligation, blood flow to the liver largely depends on portal venous flow, and this low pressure system can be occluded relatively easily by the packs. Posterior compression of the inferior vena cava by the packs should also be avoided, especially in patients who are hypovolemic and have marginal venous return to the heart.

> **AXIOM** Compression of the suprahepatic inferior vena cava by perihepatic packs should be avoided in hypovolemic patients because the abrupt fall in venous return to the heart can cause a cardiac arrest.

Postoperatively, because diaphragmatic movement can be severely impaired by perihepatic packs, the patient's ventilation should be mechanically assisted.[3] Antibiotic coverage is maintained during the period that the packs are in place.

Timing of Packing Removal
The patient may be returned to the operating room for pack removal after 24-48 hours or more, but all hemodynamic, acid-base, core temperature, and coagulation-abnormalities should be corrected first. At the time the packs are removed, one should also debride any nonviable hepatic tissue, control any active bleeding points or lacerated bile ducts, irrigate the abdomen of any clots or bile, and establish new perihepatic drainage.[18]

Results of Perihepatic Packing
A recent collection of 145 patients with complex hepatic injuries treated with perihepatic packing from seven different centers revealed that 105 (72.4%) survived.[3,96-102] Since this maneuver was generally used only in the most desperate circumstances, the salvage rate of 72% would suggest that perihepatic packing should be considered more than just a last ditch effort to control bleeding.[3] Conflicting data exist with regard to the incidence of postoperative sepsis with the use of packing, but reported rates average about 10-25%.

DEBRIDEMENT
Adequate debridement of devitalized tissue is required in the treatment of the traumatized liver to avoid subsequent septic complications.[1] Such debridement should be limited to removal of obviously non-viable tissue and should not stir up excessive bleeding. This may be accomplished with electrocautery or blunt finger-fracture techniques. Precise anatomic resection is seldom indicated except in unusual instances where hepatic artery ligation or the injury leads to obvious severe lobar or segmental necrosis. The only accurate criterion of hepatic viability is arterial bleeding from the parenchyma.[3]

> **AXIOM** After hemostasis is obtained, non-viable tissue should be debrided to reduce the incidence of later septic complications.

Although there may be some reluctance to perform an adequate debridement because of a fear of restarting bleeding; if the debridement is not adequate, there is a greatly increased risk of later abscess formation. During the debridement, hepatic venous drainage of the involved liver should be preserved to the extent possible.[1] Resectional debridement should not, however, be confused with formal hepatic resections, which should be avoided whenever possible.

DRAINS

Indications

Although the quantity of blood and bile leaking from a hepatic injury may be small, the combination of the two, if left undrained, greatly increase the likelihood of subsequent sepsis.[3] For many years after World War II, most hepatic injuries were routinely drained.[3] The most common form of drainage for many years consisted of several large Penrose drains.

AXIOM Even a relatively small collection of bile in contact with a hematoma greatly increases the risk of later sepsis.

In 1954, Sparkman et al,[104] based on their experience with 100 consecutive hepatic trauma patients, questioned the necessity of "routine liver drainage," particularly in patients with relatively minor hepatic injuries. In 1978, Fischer et al[105] also raised the question of whether routine drainage of hepatic injuries was necessary. Indeed, there appeared to be growing evidence that the incidence of perihepatic infections was increased when drains were used for Grade I or II liver injuries.[105,106]

Perihepatic drainage of a liver with a grade I or II injury is unnecessary if the patient is hemodynamically stable, hemostasis has been adequate, and no apparent bile leaks exist.[1] Major complex hepatic injuries, on the other hand, usually result in considerable parenchymal destruction and should be drained to prevent the accumulations of bile and/or blood that would otherwise develop.

Cogbill et al[60] reported an abscess rate of 9% and a biliary fistula rate of 8% in patients with grade III hepatic injuries in whom closed Jackson-Pratt drainage was used. These authors postulated that the incidence of biliary fistula and abscess formation might have even been higher had drainage not been instituted. In addition, they recommended sump drains for grade IV and V injuries where the incidence and severity of necrotic hepatic tissue is likely to be much greater. Pachter et al[5] have reported comparable results in complex hepatic injuries when using closed Jackson-Pratt drains (for bile and blood) in combination with open Penrose drains (for necrotic hepatic tissue).[5]

Type of Perihepatic Drainage

There has been an increasing tendency to use closed (Jackson-Pratt) drainage systems rather than open (Penrose) drainage systems for perihepatic damage. Bender et al[107] showed that patients with Grade I, II, or III hepatic injuries who had open (Penrose) drainage had a 10% incidence of intra-abdominal abscesses while patients with either no drainage or closed drainage had no postoperative abscesses.

AXIOM Closed drainage systems are generally thought to be associated with fewer postoperative abscesses after trauma than open (Penrose) systems.

Additional support for the concept of using closed systems if drainage is required was provided by Noyes et al.[106] Although they believe that liver injuries should generally not be drained, they reported no abscesses when using closed (Jackson-Pratt) drains versus a 2% abscess rate in patients in whom no drains were used. Additionally, they demonstrated that factors independent of the drains themselves influenced the ultimate morbidity rate. In their study, the presence of hypotension resulted in a threefold increase in the incidence of hepatic sepsis;[106] however, increased blood transfusion requirements played an even more significant role because this factor resulted in a tenfold increase in the incidence of subsequent hepatic abscesses.

Gillmore et al[108] have also compared the incidence of infectious complications with open Penrose drainage versus closed suction drainage or no drainage, but they found no differences in comparable groups of patients.

AXIOM Penrose or large sump drains are more effective and less apt to be occluded if necrotic tissue or blood clots need to be drained.

Although closed suction drainage, such as with a large Jackson-Pratt drain, is preferred over open Penrose drainage for removing any blood or bile leakage, large sump drains or Penrose drains may be required if significant amounts of necrotic hepatic tissue remain. It has also been shown that closed suction drains are more prone to be occluded by clots.

If multiple large Penrose drains are left in the perihepatic region but are dressed on the operating table with a sterile wound drainage bag to provide a more closed system, the incidence of infection is reduced, and one can continually monitor the volume and character (bile or blood) of the drainage fluid.

MANAGEMENT OF PERIHEPATIC DRAINS

Perihepatic drains should be kept as sterile as possible and handled only with sterile gloves. If there is any fever, the blood or bile drainage should be smeared and Gram-stained. Culture and sensitivity studies should also be performed to help guide antibiotic therapy.

Drains are left in place after severe liver trauma until the output is negligible, there is no gross evidence of bile in the drainage fluid, and the patient is taking an enteral diet. Drains are often removed on the third or fourth postoperative day after an initial shortening and/or "tweaking" to make sure they are not occluded. Any leakage of bile from the injured liver should be readily apparent by the third postoperative day if the patient is eating and the drains are properly placed. If there is any evidence of a bile leak, the drain(s) should not be removed until there is no further evidence of a bile leak and the patient is eating.

Biliary Tract Drainage

AXIOM Drainage of the common bile duct does not reduce the incidence of hepatic bile leaks or postoperative infections after liver trauma.

In a prospective randomized study of 189 patients with moderate to severe hepatic trauma and no extrahepatic biliary tract injury, Lucas and Walt[109] demonstrated that the presence of a T-tube in the common bile duct was associated with a significant increase in morbidity. In many of these patients, the common bile duct was quite small and insertion of a T-tube was often difficult and hazardous. Furthermore, it did not appear to reduce the tendency for injured intrahepatic ducts to leak.

Antibiotics

Minor isolated liver injuries do not require prophylactic antibiotics; however, severe liver injuries with devitalized liver tissue plus drainage of blood and bile may be benefited by at least 24-48 hours of a broad spectrum antibiotic.

AXIOM The administration of antibiotics does not substitute for adequate debridement and perihepatic drainage after liver trauma.

Continued use of prophylactic antibiotics should generally be discouraged. It is unlikely that continued use of antibiotics will prevent later infection, but they increase the tendency of any organisms causing later infections to be antibiotic-resistant.

RESULTS

Mortality

The overall mortality from hepatic trauma continues to be approximately 10-15%;[3] however, in the DRH series, it was 20%. Over 75% of the deaths in the immediate perioperative period are due to hemorrhage, whereas after 48 hours most of the morbidity and mortality is due to sepsis. In the DRH series, 144 (78%) of the deaths occurred within 48 hours of admission and were due primarily to bleeding from associated injuries. Of the 162 patients with isolated hepatic injuries, only six (4%) died (Table 22-3). In contrast, of the 358 patients with three or more associated injuries, 113 (32%) died. Also, if the 207 patients with abdominal vascular injuries are excluded from this data, the mortality rate was only 11.5%.

Over the last 10-15 years, great strides have been made in the management of complex hepatic injuries (grade IV-V) as reflected by a decrease in the mortality rates from 50% to approximately 30%.[3] It must be noted, however, that this data has been obtained from the institutions dealing with large volumes of hepatic trauma.[110]

Blunt injuries to the liver are generally more lethal and more difficult to manage than penetrating injuries. Nevertheless, advances have also been made with this type of trauma. Cox et al[110] in 1988 reported a mortality rate of only 31% in 323 consecutive patients with blunt hepatic trauma.

Complications

CLOTTING DEFECTS

Most patients with severe liver trauma will have complications, especially if operative therapy is required. Indeed, Knudson et al[111] noted complications in 52% of their patients with Grade IV-V liver injuries due to penetrating trauma.

Most clotting defects after liver trauma are related to platelet deficiencies caused by multiple transfusions of bank blood, which contains few, if any, functional platelets.[2] Following destruction or surgical removal of large amounts of liver tissue, the levels of prothrombin, Factor V, Factor VIII and fibrinogen may also fall, but seldom to levels which could cause excessive bleeding.

AXIOM   Hypothermia and acidosis should be prevented or corrected promptly in patients with liver trauma. Fresh frozen plasma and platelets should be administered rapidly if a coagulopathy develops.

POSTOPERATIVE BLEEDING

After hemostasis has been achieved at the initial operation, all intraperitoneal blood is evacuated, and adequate drains are placed in proximity to the wounds to drain off whatever bile, blood, or other fluid might otherwise accumulate. This allows postoperative assessment of the quantity and character of the drainage fluid as an indication of postoperative hemorrhage. Serial hematocrit determinations on the drainage fluid may also aid in assessing blood loss. Blood clots within the drainage bag are usually evidence of rapid and continuing hemorrhage, suggesting that the bleeding is too rapid for intra-abdominal defibrination of the blood.

Continued postoperative bleeding from severe liver injuries is not uncommon; however, the incidence of significant postoperative hemorrhage should not exceed 3% of all hepatic injuries.[3,4,6] For the most severe liver injuries, however, the postoperative hemorrhage rate may exceed 7%.[60]

AXIOM   The most frequent cause of postoperative bleeding is inadequate technical control of bleeding vessels.

Even if a coagulopathy cannot be excluded, recurrent bleeding in the early postoperative period is usually due to inadequate surgical hemostasis.[1] If the patient's condition is reasonable, reoperation and definitive control of specific bleeding sites is the procedure of choice, preferably after first correcting any hypothermia and/or coagulopathy that may be present.

At reoperation, one may have to cut some previously placed liver sutures or even remove an omental pack from within the liver. Continued arterial bleeding from deep within the hepatic parenchyma, where further hepatotomy is hazardous and may sever major vessels or hepatic bile ducts, may be controlled by selective hepatic artery ligation.[3] If a skilled interventional radiologist is present, the bleeding vessels may be occluded without surgery.[112]

If the patient has surgery and no specific bleeding points are found, but a coagulopathy is encountered, one should not hesitate to use perihepatic packing to control the hemorrhage; however, if hepatic artery ligation was performed, aggressive perihepatic packing should be avoided.

AXIOM   The combination of perihepatic packing and hepatic artery ligation, particularly in hypotensive patients, is likely to cause extensive hepatic necrosis.

Recently, DeToma et al[112] have emphasized the value of selective or superselective hepatic artery embolization for control of continued bleeding after surgery for liver trauma. The authors successfully managed a patient with bleeding from several intrahepatic vessels which included a branch of the right hepatic artery to segment VIII as well as two collateralizing arteries from segments VI and VII.

HYPERPYREXIA

AXIOM   Fever soon after major liver trauma is probably related to localized hematomas or hepatic necrosis; fever after 5-7 days is usually due to an infection.

Fevers ranging from 38°C-39°C have been frequently noted in the first few days following hepatic injuries.[3] Cogbill et al[60] were among the first to document hyperpyrexia as a consistent finding in a fairly large group of patients with complex hepatic trauma. Of 129 patients reported, 53% experienced some fever. Of the patients with persistent postoperative temperatures of 39° C or more, 79% had sustained blunt trauma.

The mechanism of post-liver trauma fever is unclear, but it is probably related to resorption of nonviable hepatic tissue.[3] Interestingly, this phenomenon usually resolves within 3-5 days. Fevers that persist after five days usually reflect the presence of an infection.[60] If pneumonitis can be excluded, intra-abdominal sepsis should be strongly considered, and a prompt CT scan of the abdomen and pelvis should be performed.[3]

INTRA-ABDOMINAL ABSCESSES

Intra-abdominal abscesses are frequent after severe liver trauma, especially if hemostasis and debridement of nonviable liver tissue have been incomplete. The combination of a bile leak with postoperative bleeding frequently results in an infected hematoma. Such hematomas, particularly in association with a concomitant injury to the gastrointestinal tract, greatly increase the likelihood that the patient will develop intra-abdominal sepsis.

AXIOM   For the most part, abscesses around or within the liver can be avoided if early precise hemostasis, meticulous debridement, and adequate drainage have been achieved.

The frequency of intra-abdominal abscesses in the largest series of hepatic trauma varies from 1.9-9%.[44,60] The incidence of such sepsis will vary with several factors, including the extent of the hepatic injury, the presence of shock and associated enteric injuries, the number of transfusions required, and the types of drains used.[18,107,113] The development of a perihepatic abscess is usually manifested seven to 14 days following the trauma, but it may occur earlier in patients who have had prolonged shock or massive transfusions, or later in patients receiving multiple antibiotics.

The presence of a postoperative abscess in septic patients is confirmed by finding a subdiaphragmatic, subhepatic, and/or intrahepatic fluid collection on ultrasonography or CT scan. In the past, management of these abscesses usually consisted of a laparotomy to drain anterior abscesses and a twelfth rib resection for drainage of posterior abscesses.

The need to move patients to the operating room and perform a major operation to drain an established abscess has been reduced by the increasing expertise of interventional radiologists.[3] Success rates with CT or ultrasound guided percutaneous drainage of perihepatic abscesses has been reported to approach 95%;[114-116] however, if the patient's sepsis does not respond promptly to percutaneous drainage, prompt surgical exploration should be considered.

If surgery is necessary to drain a subphrenic abscess, an extraperitoneal approach is generally preferred.[3] Formal reoperation and exploration through the initial midline scar is reserved for instances in which the abscess is anterior and/or percutaneous drainage and extraperitoneal drainage have failed. Although a midline transperitoneal approach is associated with an increased morbidity, it may become necessary if one is to eliminate this source of sepsis and to establish adequate drainage.[3] Appropriate antibiotic coverage is also important, and this is provided by performing Gram stains and cultures and sensitivities on whatever fluid or tissue is drained or debrided.

BILIARY FISTULAS

Biliary fistulas are often defined as the persistence of more than 50 ml of biliary drainage daily for at least two weeks.[3,64] The reported incidence of biliary fistulas following liver trauma varies but should generally not exceed 10%.[3] The patients most prone to develop this complication are those sustaining severe hepatic injuries with major parenchymal destruction. Despite the most diligent search to identify all disrupted biliary tributaries in torn liver parenchyma, some will escape detection. Some torn biliary radicals will retract or be too small to be identified if they are not leaking bile at the time of the exploration. It is essential, therefore, to establish wide dependent drainage and prevent bile peritonitis.

AXIOM   If adequate drainage of the hepatic injury had been accomplished at the initial surgery and the flow of bile into the duodenum is unimpeded, virtually all adequately drained biliary fistulas will close spontaneously.

Persistent drainage of more than 300 ml of bile per day for more than 4-5 days should lead to the performance of a fistulogram to determine its anatomy.[3] If it is found that a major intrahepatic duct has been completely lacerated, spontaneous closure is unlikely. Additional therapy is often necessary, but an immediate reoperation is not usually required. The ability under radiological control to place a catheter percutaneously into a major severed bile duct to control external or internal drainage has obviated the need for urgent surgery. The advantages of an initial percutaneous drainage: (a) it allows for better preparation of the patient if surgery becomes necessary, (b) it can at times be therapeutic, and (c) it can serve as an invaluable "road map" should a Roux-en-Y hepaticoje junostomy be required at a later date.[3]

Recently, Horattas et al[119] have emphasized that traumatic biliary fistulas can frequently be treated nonoperatively if there is an accurate early diagnosis of the exact source of the bile leak, early adequate drainage of any collections, and early adequate decompression of the biliary tract by stents and/or sphincterotomy.

LIVER FAILURE

AXIOM   Jaundice in the first five days after liver trauma may be due to hematomas, hepatic ischemia, or bile duct injuries; jaundice after 7-10 days is usually due to infection.

Enough hepatic regeneration to maintain normal liver function is possible if at least 20% of the normal liver tissue remains following elective resection.[2] In liver trauma, with its associated shock, multiple transfusions, and/or gross bacterial contamination, the results of large liver resections are far less satisfactory. Efforts to prevent failure of a severely damaged liver include maintenance of optimal hepatic perfusion, adequate perihepatic drainage, prompt control of sepsis, intestinal rest, and provision of adequate oxygen and glucose.[2]

Early profound jaundice following hepatic trauma is usually due to an occluded major biliary duct or a biliary-venous fistula, and the work-up should include delineation of the bile ducts by ERCP and/or radionuclide studies. Visner et al[120] recently reported a patient who had early profound jaundice after blunt trauma with bile pooling in the left lobe without antegrade obstruction. A left hepatic lobectomy cured the problem, which was thought initially to be due to a biliary-hepatic vein fistula.

The concept of Merendino et al[117] that drainage of the common bile duct can prevent the formation of biliary fistulas after major hepatic injuries, or can treat established biliary fistulas effectively, is unsubstantiated. Indeed, it has been shown that T-tube drainage of normal common bile ducts does not prevent biliary fistula formation, but tends to cause a higher incidence of intra-abdominal sepsis, cholangitis, and bile duct strictures.[109,118]

HEMOBILIA

Hemobilia, sometimes referred to as hematobilia, is due to a fistula between a biliary duct and a branch of a hepatic artery. It is extremely uncommon and was seen in only 0.3% of patients with liver trauma treated at Detroit Receiving Hospital.[2] This lesion can result from a routine liver biopsy and has been noted with indwelling percutaneous transhepatic catheters, but most reported cases occur after accidental trauma.[121]

AXIOM   Gastrointestinal bleeding after trauma in a patient with a normal EGD and colonoscopy is due to hemobilia until proven otherwise.

Approximately a third of the patients with hemobilia present with the classic triad of hemorrhage, colicky right upper quadrant pain, and jaundice.[122,123] Bleeding may occur as early as the fourth post-injury day or may occur more than a month later.[1] In the majority of patients, it presents as gastrointestinal bleeding without an apparent source. Endoscopy and upper GI contrast studies are usually negative. With a history of recent trauma, hemobilia must be considered in any patient who develops gastrointestinal bleeding within the next 2-8 weeks. The diagnosis is confirmed by angiography.

AXIOM   The diagnosis of hemobilia is best accomplished angiographically, and the best treatment is immediate angiographic embolization of the bleeding vessel.

The efficacy of angiographic embolization to treat hemobilia has clearly been established.[122,124] Surgical intervention is seldom necessary, except in the rare instances when hemobilia is associated with a large intrahepatic cavity. Should this occur, resection of the pseudoaneurysm and drainage of the intrahepatic cavity may be required; however, occlusion of the bleeding vessel angiographically and then percutaneous drainage of the cavity by an interventional radiologist is probably much safer.

Bile Duct Stenosis

Jaundice in the later post-traumatic period may occasionally be due to a late stenosis of a major biliary radical.[125] In such instances, a biliodigestive bypass with a Roux-Y loop of jejunum sutured to a distal radical may be curative.

INJURY TO THE RETROHEPATIC VENA CAVA OR HEPATIC VEINS

Diagnosis

Injury to a hepatic vein or the retrohepatic vena cava remains a formidable challenge and is frequently lethal. The injury may be suspected preoperatively by the trajectory of a penetrating missile. Massive hemorrhage may be delayed for a number of hours or until the abdomen is opened. Not uncommonly, the bleeding is only moderate until the liver is mobilized to provide better exposure of the injury.

> **AXIOM**   Failure of properly placed perihepatic packs to control bleeding from the posterior liver should strongly suggest injury to retrohepatic veins.

When the Pringle maneuver fails to arrest hemorrhage significantly from within or behind the liver, a juxtahepatic venous injury should be suspected.[3] Major venous injury is also suggested by retrohepatic bleeding after the liver is compressed manually or with packs.[1] Indeed, the usual practice of placing packs on the diaphragmatic surface of the liver to achieve compression may greatly exacerbate the bleeding.

Exposure

> **AXIOM**   Attempts to expose the source of bleeding behind an injured liver may result in massive exsanguinating hemorrhage.

An abdominal incision plus mobilization of the liver often will not provide adequate exposure of injuries to the retrohepatic vena cava.[1] Under such circumstances, extension of the abdominal incision into the chest may be necessary. Extension of the incision as a median sternotomy is the preferred approach because this can usually be accomplished quite rapidly. This can provide excellent exposure and can also be used to insert an atrio-caval shunt.[1,3] Following division of the sternum, the diaphragm is divided in the sagittal plane from the xiphoid to the inferior vena cava.

An alternative approach involves extension of the midline abdominal incision obliquely across costal cartilages into the right thorax in the seventh or eighth intercostal space.[1] This thoracoabdominal approach with division of the right hemidiaphragm can provide excellent access to the posterior aspect of the right lobe of the liver and juxtahepatic veins, but it is more painful postoperatively than a median sternotomy, and it has a higher incidence of pulmonary complications. It also does not provide optimal exposure of the heart if an atrio-caval shunt becomes necessary. In patients exhibiting unrelenting shock and a tense hemoperitoneum, a prelaparotomy thoracotomy and aortic clamping has been utilized successfully in an effort to prevent the increased bleeding and hypotension often accompanying the release of the abdominal tamponade.[126-130]

Efforts at encircling the infradiaphragmatic inferior cava often require retraction of the liver, leading to increased hemorrhage. If adequate exposure is obtained, local control of the bleeding point may allow direct repair of the injured cava or hepatic vein, with or without a thoracotomy.

Atriocaval Shunts

The optimal method of managing juxtahepatic venous injuries remains controversial. Although a number of surgeons have had experience with atriocaval shunts (Fig. 22-7),[131,132] mortality rates reported with their use are still extremely high.[3] Data from eight papers on 115 patients in whom an atriocaval shunt was inserted revealed that there were only 32 (28%) survivors.[85,96,122,133-136] Blunt injuries to these vessels are particularly lethal, with very few survivors. Kudsk et al[131] and Cogbill et al[60] both reported no survivors in patients treated with an atriocaval shunt for blunt juxtahepatic venous

injuries. Rovito,[136] on the other hand, reported four survivors out of eight patients with blunt trauma who were managed with an atriocaval shunt for injuries to either the retrohepatic cava or hepatic veins.

> **AXIOM**   For atriocaval shunts to be successful, they must be done early, before the patient has developed prolonged hypotension, hypothermia, acidosis, and a coagulopathy.

Although the severity of the injury and the resultant bleeding are the primary causes of the excessive death rate, Burch et al[135] and Pachter et al[55] have defined other specific causes that may be responsible for the poor success rate with atriocaval shunts. They have pointed out that death in these patients may be related to recognition of the juxtahepatic venous injury only after there has been significant blood loss and prolonged hypotension so that the shunt is inserted only as a last "desperate" maneuver, when all other methods have failed. At this point, hypothermia, acidosis, and a coagulopathy are frequently present.[3] The combination of "nonmechanical bleeding," lactic acidosis, and hypothermia greatly reduce the chance for salvage, even with a successfully inserted and functioning atriocaval shunt.

To provide improved shunting of caval blood around the liver for major juxtahepatic venous injuries, Diebel et al[137] have described a modification of the venovenous bypass used in liver transplantation. Using a porcine model, hemodynamic comparisons were made between active shunting with an interposed Bio-Medicus pumo: (n=6) and passive shunting (n=4) around the liver for 60 minutes. One end of the shunt was placed in the infrahepatic cava and the other end was inserted into the right atrium (Fig. 22-10). Systolic blood pressure (sBP) and cardiac output (CO) were well maintained in the pigs with the active shunt. However, with passive shunting, sBP fell from 134 ± 28 to 83 ± 28 mm Hg (p <0.05) and CO fell from 4.1 ± 0.7 to 1.3 ± 0.5 L/min (p <0.001) after 1 hour. The well-maintained sBP and CO with the active shunt were associated with much better shunt flow rates than with the passive shunt (31 ± 7 versus 11 ± 3 ml/kg/min) (p <0.001).

Balloon Shunts

Poor results and difficulties in rapid and efficient shunt insertion have lead to a search for alternative methods of attaining vascular isolation.[3] Testas et al[138] and Pilcher et al[139] have reported achieving vascular isolation with balloon-tipped shunts inserted through the saphe-

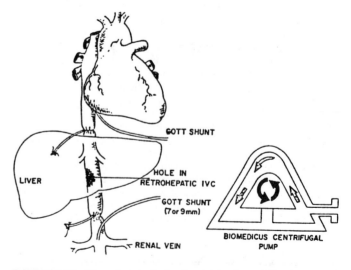

FIGURE 22-10   The active shunt circuit consists of a centrifugal pump and flow probe and a Gott shunt inserted into the infrahepatic vena cava with return to the right atrium via a Gott shunt in the suprahepatic vena cava. The passive shunt circuit consisted of a Gott shunt and flow probe only. (From Diebel LN. J Trauma 1991;31:987.)

nofemoral junction up into the retrohepatic inferior vena cava. The appealing aspect of these shunts is that neither a thoracotomy nor sternotomy with cannulation of the right atrial appendage is necessary.[3] The original balloon shunts were limited by their small internal diameter and thus could not provide adequate preload to the heart. Systemic arterial pressure was usually decreased by 50% while the shunt was in place and functioning. Pilcher et al[139] improved on Testas' design by increasing the internal diameter of the shunt by nearly 50% while increasing the external diameter by only 15%.

In comparison to atriocaval shunts, the number of patients in whom balloon shunts have been inserted through the groin is relatively small.[3] Nevertheless, Cogbill et al[60] were not able to discern any differences in survival between a group of 21 patients treated with an atriocaval shunt and a comparable group of 17 patients managed with the Moore-Pilcher shunt inserted through the groin.

Non-shunt Management of Juxtahepatic Venous Injuries

VASCULAR ISOLATION OF THE LIVER
Sequential vascular clamping of the upper abdominal aorta, the porta hepatis, the suprarenal inferior vena cava, and the suprahepatic inferior vena cava is another technique that has been described to achieve vascular isolation of the liver.[140] Although a few instances of patient salvage have been reported with this technique, it has not been used extensively enough in adults to really comment on its value.[3]

PRINGLE MANEUVER PLUS FINGER-FRACTURE OF THE LIVER
Survival of patients with juxtahepatic venous injuries treated without a shunt has been reported in children by Coln et al.[141] The excellent results achieved by Coln may in part be due to the fact that the hepatic veins and the retrohepatic cava in children are substantially more extrahepatic than in adults. Nevertheless, based on the results achieved by Coln et al,[141] Pachter et al[3] managed five consecutive adult patients with juxtahepatic venous injuries without resorting to the use of a shunt. The technique used in these five patients involved prolonged portal triad occlusion (mean occlusion time 46 minutes) and finger-fracture of the hepatic parenchyma, almost always through normal hepatic tissue, down to the site of the vascular injury for primary repair or ligation. Further clinical trials will be necessary to ascertain the effectiveness of this approach.

INJURIES TO THE PORTA HEPATIS

Injuries to the porta hepatis are best treated by direct repair of the involved structures.[1] This may be facilitated by a Pringle maneuver during the initial dissection. In patients with severe hypotension and a technically difficult repair of the common hepatic artery, it may be preferable to ligate the artery if the portal blood flow is intact and liver viability is not otherwise compromised from prolonged hypotension or cirrhosis. The patient, however, may not tolerate ligation of the proper hepatic artery distal to the gastroduodenal and right gastric artery branches.

Injury to the portal vein can cause massive hemorrhage and is often fatal. Lateral repair or reconstruction with a patch or panel vein graft should be attempted whenever possible.[1] Simple ligation of the injured portal vein may be associated with a high mortality rate and is generally used only as a last resort;[1] however, early ligation with continuing aggressive fluid resuscitation to make up for fluid accumulating in the intestine may be successful.

EXTRAHEPATIC BILIARY TRACT INJURIES

Incidence

Injuries to the extrahepatic biliary tract are uncommon and are noted in less than 5% of all abdominal trauma victims; however, they may be present in up to 10-15% of patients with liver trauma.[1] The vast majority of such injuries are penetrating, with the gallbladder being involved most often[3] (Table 22-3). Blunt injuries to the gallbladder are less common. Kitahama et al[142] found that the gallbladder was injured in only about 2% of blunt trauma. In the DRH series, it was injured in only 3/573 cases (0.5%). Indeed, only 250 cases of blunt gall bladder trauma have been reported in the literature.[3]

The common bile duct is more susceptible to blunt injury than hepatic ducts and is most apt to be injured at its junction with the pancreas. In the porta hepatis, the hepatic artery is tortuous and elastic and the valveless portal vein can rapidly lengthen by emptying the blood it contains. Nevertheless, a sudden, severe deceleration or compression of the right upper quadrant of the abdomen can suddenly move the mobile liver upward, causing a tear in the common bile duct at its junction with the pancreas.[143,144]

Classification

GALLBLADDER INJURIES
Injuries to the gallbladder are usually due to direct trauma whether by gunshot wound, stab wound, motor vehicle accident, or a direct blow. Thin-walled, normal gallbladders that are distended with bile at the time of injury may be more likely to perforate or be torn by a deceleration injury.

Rapid deceleration injuries may cause a shearing force strong enough to tear a fluid-filled gallbladder from its liver bed. If the avulsion is complete, the gallbladder may be left hanging by its attachment to the cystic duct and artery.

Mild contusions will usually resolve spontaneously, but severe contusions may cause ecchymosis of the wall and/or fill the lumen with blood. Furthermore, it has been postulated that an intramural hematoma of the gallbladder wall may be severe enough to interfere with the local blood supply and cause a delayed rupture to occur.[2]

Blood in the gallbladder can cause hematobilia.[142] It can also block the cystic duct and the resulting stasis with secondary bacterial proliferation can result in acute cholecystitis.

BILE DUCT INJURIES

Types of Injuries
Simple injuries of the extrahepatic bile ducts include tangential lacerations involving less than 50% of the ductal wall circumference. These can usually be repaired quite easily, and the incidence of later complications is quite low.

Complex injuries of the bile ducts include lacerations involving more than 50% of the ductal wall circumference, those with segmental loss of a portion of the ductal wall, and those with complete transections. These injuries are much more difficult to repair and are much more likely to develop early leaks and late strictures.

Diagnosis

When an injury to the extrahepatic biliary tract occurs, there are usually significant associated injuries, particularly to the liver or adjacent blood vessels. These associated injuries usually determine the clinical presentation and eventual outcome of the patients.[145-148]

Diagnosis of an extrahepatic biliary tract injury is seldom made preoperatively.[3] Peritoneal lavage may be negative for bile, but even if bile is found in the lavage fluid, it can also come from the injuries to the liver or small bowel.

AXIOM   Free bile anywhere in the abdomen suggests injury to the liver, extrahepatic bile ducts, or duodenum and demands a thorough exploration of these structures.[2]

Failure to identify injuries to the extra-hepatic biliary tract or adjacent structures may result in lethal complications. The acute complications include hemorrhage, cholangitis, and bile peritonitis. The more chronic complications include biliary strictures and hepatic failure.

AXIOM If there is bile staining of tissues in the right upper quadrant of the abdomen without an obvious source after thorough exploration, one should consider performing an intraoperative cholangiogram and duodenoscopy.[2]

In some instance, the bile duct injury is very subtle, and the only clue to its presence may be some bile staining of the adjacent tissues. If such staining is present, the proximal small bowel and the extrahepatic ducts must be examined very carefully. If the source of the bile staining is still not clear, a cholangiogram should be performed. If this is also negative, duodenoscopy should be performed in the OR.

Unconcentrated and uninfected bile from hepatic bile ducts does not initially cause chemical irritation, and thus, there may be no peritoneal signs. Moreover, if there is any abdominal pain because of leakage of bile from an injured gallbladder, it often abates after a few hours.[149] Consequently, the diagnosis of an isolated biliary tract injury may be delayed for days or even weeks after the initial trauma.

If the index of suspicion is not high, patients with isolated extrahepatic bile duct injuries are apt to be discharged from the hospital, only to return later with a clinical picture varying from an "acute abdomen" (due to bile peritonitis with infection) to obstructive jaundice.[143,150-151] When there has been a long time lag between the injury and the presentation of symptoms, abdominal CT, HIDA scan, endoscopic retrograde cholangiopancreatography (ERCP), or percutaneous transhepatic cholangiography (PTC) may be needed to diagnose an isolated extrahepatic bile tract injury.[152,153]

Treatment in General

GENERAL PRINCIPLES

Irrespective of the anatomical location of the injury, the surgical approach to patients with extrahepatic biliary tract damage is initially directed at control of hemorrhage from the associated injuries.[3] Unstable patients, however, are best treated by stenting of the bile duct, external drainage, and staged repair. Hemodynamically stable patients, however, may undergo definitive repair of their biliary tract as a primary procedure.[144]

As with all traumatic injuries, adequate debridement of nonviable tissue is essential to prevent necrosis, fistulization, and stricture.[3] Meticulous dissection and reconstruction without tension are essential. With small injuries, a meticulous mucosa-to-mucosa approximation and T-tube drainage is usually performed. Major or complete lacerations of the common bile duct or hepatic duct are best treated by a stented anastomosis to a Roux-en-Y loop of jejunum. The anatomy of the blood supply to the bile ducts must also be constantly kept in mind.[155] Mobilization of the common bile duct may accidentally injure the longitudinal arteries supplying it along its lateral borders. Ischemia due to excess freeing up of the common bile duct alone may lead to a bile duct stricture.

TREATMENT OF SPECIFIC INJURIES

Gallbladder

AXIOM Cholecystectomy is the preferred treatment for trauma to the gallbladder or cystic duct.[3]

Removing an injured gallbladder eliminates the theoretical risk of future gallstone formation from sutures placed during a cholecystostomy or cholecystorrhaphy. Cholecystectomy removes the risk of bile leakage from a gallbladder suture line, and it should also be performed if there is injury to the cystic or right hepatic artery so that the blood supply to the gallbladder is in question.[1]

Although cholecystectomy is the preferred maneuver for gallbladder injuries, this technique may not be desirable in:(a) patients with a severe coagulopathy because of multiple trauma or cirrhosis, (b) hemodynamically unstable patients with minor damage to the gallbladder, and (c) patients with minimal gallbladder contusions. Minor gallbladder injuries may resolve without any surgical manipulation.[154]

AXIOM The subhepatic space should probably be drained in most patients with a gallbladder injury.[3]

Extrahepatic Bile Ducts

SIMPLE INJURIES. If an injury to the bile duct is a simple laceration involving less than 50% of the ductal wall circumference, treatment usually consists of primary repair T-tube placement, and external drainage.[3] If at all possible, the T-tube should be brought out at least 1-2 cm from the site of the repair. Although no evidence exists that placement of a T-tube is mandatory in bile duct trauma, the tube permits early postoperative decompression of the biliary tree when edema may restrict drainage into the distal common duct. It also permits ready access for postoperative cholangiography. When confronted with an extremely small duct, a ureteral catheter brought out through the duodenum and then the abdominal wall can be used as a substitute for a T-tube.

COMPLEX INJURIES

AXIOM Construction of a biliary-enteric anastomosis and external drainage is the treatment of choice for complex, extrahepatic bile duct injuries.[3]

Injuries to the right or left hepatic ducts from accidental trauma are even rarer than those to the common bile duct and can cause much more difficult problems because of the small size of these structures.[2] In desperate circumstances, in a hemodynamically unstable patient, the severed duct may be drained externally or ligated with the knowledge that the risk of subsequent hepatic sepsis is substantial. Where possible, however, the optimal repair is a biliary-enteric anastomosis performed over a small stent (such as a ureteral catheter) which may be left in place for several months. One must be careful, however, to preserve the tenuous blood supply of the bile duct during the dissection and to keep the anastamosis tension-free.[156]

Cholecystojejunostomy with ligation of the common bile duct is generally inadvisable.[3] Ligation of the common duct may inadvertently result in ligation of a long intramural cystic duct. This would, of course, result in a nonfunctioning anastomosis which would not be recognized at the time of surgery. Postoperative jaundice would then require reoperation in a more complex setting. Consequently, a cholangiogram prior to ligation and after the anastomosis is important.

With damage to the right or left hepatic duct, it may be necessary to use the finger-fracture technique through liver parenchyma to expose and identify the right and left ductal system. The jejunum can then be anastomosed to a common channel formed by suturing the right and left hepatic ducts together.

Complications

Major late morbidity from bile duct trauma is usually in the form of a biliary stricture.[3] Attempts at primary repair or duct-to-duct anastomoses usually result in a stricture rate exceeding 50%. The late stricture rate drops to about 5% when biliary-enteric anastomoses are used for similar injuries.[146,157,158]

Postoperative biliary strictures may not become apparent until months or years later.[3] Reoperation is almost always necessary to prevent recurring cholangitis or biliary cirrhosis. Balloon dilatation of traumatic strictures by an interventional radiologist is a technique that has occasionally proved successful on an acute basis, but the follow-up period is short in most reports, and this technique needs further evaluation.

When reoperation for a bile duct stricture is anticipated, selective angiography can often visualize the biliary ductal blood supply and increases the chances for success, which approaches 85% at the most experienced medical centers. Prolonged stenting, for at least 3-6 months, may also improve the long-term patency rate of the bile duct following reoperation.[159] The overall mortality from extrahepatic biliary tract trauma is primarily from associated injuries, particularly adjacent major vessels.[146,147] The risk of biliary tract complications is particularly high if the injury is not diagnosed during the initial hospitalization.

⊘ FREQUENT ERRORS

1. *Continued resuscitation in the ED rather than prompt surgical control if there is continued severe bleeding.*
2. *Operating on hemodynamically stable patients with an isolated liver injury only because of an increased RBC count in DPL fluid.*
3. *Attempting nonoperative management of moderately-severe liver injuries in uncooperative patients.*
4. *Failure to obtain prompt control of severe hepatic bleeding with packs or manual pressure as soon as the abdomen is opened.*
5. *Prolonged occlusion of the portal vein and hepatic artery in a hypotensive patient when the bleeding could be controlled by more localized means.*
6. *Attempting to control bleeding from deep hepatic wounds with superficial closure of the injury tract.*
7. *Applying perihepatic packs to a portion of liver that has had its arterial supply ligated.*
8. *Failure to anticipate a need for fibrin glue in patients with continuing bleeding from raw hepatic surfaces.*
9. *Performing a major hepatic resection to control bleeding if extensive dissection is required and/or the bleeding might be controlled by simpler techniques.*
10. *Inadequate debridement after successful control of bleeding in a patient who is now hemodynamically stable.*
11. *Prolonged open (Penrose) drainage of minor hepatic wounds.*
12. *Failure to adequately evaluate a patient for sepsis if jaundice develops more than 6-7 days after hepatic trauma.*
13. *Failure to consider hemobilia in patients who develop gastrointestinal bleeding after liver trauma.*
14. *Delaying performance of an atrial-caval shunt until the patient has had prolonged hypotension and is hypothermic.*
15. *Attempts to control gallbladder trauma with a procedure other than a cholecystectomy.*
16. *Direct repair of complex common bile duct injuries in hemodynamically stable patients.*

▼▼▼▼▼▼▼▼▼▼▼▼▼▼▼▼▼▼▼▼▼▼▼▼▼▼▼▼▼▼

SUMMARY POINTS

1. Major liver injuries, particularly with blunt trauma, continue to have extremely high mortality and morbidity rates.
2. To properly explore and treat certain types of liver injuries, especially posterior wounds, the liver must be adequately mobilized.
3. Extreme caution should be exercised when incising the most medial portions of the coronary ligaments to avoid inadvertent laceration of hepatic veins.
4. Delayed, inadequate, or inappropriate treatment of liver injuries, resulting in hematomas or bile collections, can combine with associated injuries to cause significant morbidity or even death of an otherwise salvageable patient.
5. One should anticipate complications whenever a percutaneous procedure is performed on the liver, particularly in patients with portal hypertension.
6. The single greatest danger following liver injury is severe hemorrhage.
7. As a general rule, intravenous access in the arms is preferred over lower extremity sites if the patient is in shock from abdominal trauma.
8. If the patient is moribund on admission or there is evidence of continued major bleeding, prompt surgical control, rather than continued resuscitation, is required.

9. Hypothermia in trauma patients should be rapidly corrected as soon as the major bleeding is controlled.
10. As in all aspects of medicine, a careful history and thorough physical examination are of paramount importance in diagnosis.
11. A hemodynamically stable patient with a positive DPL because of increased red cells from what is probably an isolated solid organ injury usually can be treated nonoperatively.
12. The value of most diagnostic modalities is directly proportional to the experience and interest of the individual performing the test and interpreting the results.
13. DPL and abdominal CT scanning should be considered complimentary, rather than competing, diagnostic tests in patients with abdominal trauma.
14. In patients with stab wounds that may have entered the abdomen, DPL appears to be more accurate than CT scans for determining such penetration.
15. Need for more than two units of blood to maintain stable vital signs is generally an indication to operate on patients with isolated splenic or hepatic injuries.
16. Nonoperative management of liver injuries is not advisable in uncooperative patients.
17. Nonexpanding intrahepatic hematomas are best managed conservatively if at all possible.
18. One should avoid attempts at definitive surgical control of bleeding sites within the liver without prior adequate resuscitation.
19. It is extremely important to compress the liver manually or control the bleeding in some way so that the patient can be properly resuscitated before further surgery is performed.
20. Knowledge of liver anatomy is essential for proper mobilization of the liver.
21. The first step to control continued liver bleeding during exploration of hepatic injuries is the Pringle maneuver.
22. If it appears that the portal triad may be occluded for more than 20-30 minutes, one should consider the use of topical hypothermia with or without massive intravenous corticosteroids prior to clamping.
23. If sutures incorporating a great deal of liver tissue are used to control bleeding, the incidence of later liver necrosis and abscesses will be increased.
24. Persistent bleeding from deep hepatic wounds is usually best managed with hepatorrhaphy to control the bleeding vessels under direct vision. If this is not practical or successful, stuffing the wound with a viable omental pack should be considered.
25. Hepatic artery ligation should only be considered if arterial bleeding from a deep hepatic wound cannot be controlled by any other means.
26. Hepatic resections should be reserved for situations in which the trauma has almost completed the dissection and/or there is no other reasonable way to control the bleeding.
27. If a topical hemostatic agent controls hemorrhage from a large area of denuded liver, the hemostatic agent can often be left in place, especially if bleeding tends to recur after its removal.
28. Localized surface bleeding which persists in spite of surgical efforts and other topical agents can frequently be controlled by applying fibrin glue.
29. Fibrin glue and fibrin gel work best when the blood supply to the area to which they are applied is temporarily occluded.
30. Perihepatic packing can control many types of bleeding from the liver, but whenever possible, standard techniques should be employed to control the hemorrhage from major vessels.
31. Perihepatic packs can cause severe ischemia to portions of the liver which have had their arterial supply ligated.
32. Occlusion of the inferior vena cava by perihepatic packs should be avoided in hypovolemic patients because the abrupt fall in venous return to the heart can rapidly cause a cardiac arrest.
33. After hemostasis is obtained, necrotic tissue should be debrided to reduce the incidence of later septic complications.
34. Even a relatively small collection of bile in contact with a hematoma greatly increases the risk of later sepsis.

35. Closed drainage systems are generally thought to be associated with fewer postoperative abscesses after trauma than open (Penrose drain) systems.

36. Penrose or large sump drains are more effective and less apt to be occluded if necrotic tissue or blood clots need to be drained.

37. Drainage of the common bile duct does not reduce the incidence of hepatic bile leaks or postoperative infections after liver trauma.

38. The administration of antibiotics does not substitute for adequate debridement and perihepatic drainage after liver trauma.

39. Hypothermia and acidosis should be prevented or corrected promptly in patients with liver trauma. Fresh frozen plasma and platelets should be administered promptly if a coagulopathy develops.

40. The most frequent cause of post-operative bleeding is inadequate technical control of bleeding vessels.

41. The combination of perihepatic packing and hepatic artery ligation, particularly in hypotensive patients, is likely to cause extensive hepatic necrosis.

42. Fever soon after major liver trauma is probably related to localized hematomas or hepatic necrosis; fever after 5-7 days is usually due to an infection.

43. For the most part, abscesses around or within the liver can be avoided if early precise hemostasis, meticulous debridement, and adequate drainage have been achieved.

44. If adequate drainage of the hepatic injury had been accomplished at the initial surgery and the flow of bile into the duodenum is unimpeded, virtually all adequately drained biliary fistulas should close spontaneously.

45. Jaundice in the first five days after liver trauma may be due to hematomas, hepatic ischemia, or bile duct injuries; jaundice after 7-10 days is usually due to infection.

46. Gastrointestinal bleeding after trauma in a patient with a normal EGD and colonoscopy is due to hemobilia until proven otherwise.

47. The diagnosis of hemobilia is best accomplished angiographically, and the best treatment is immediate embolization of the offending vessel.

48. Failure of properly placed perihepatic packs to control bleeding from the posterior liver should strongly suggest injury to retrohepatic veins.

49. Attempts to expose the source of bleeding behind an injured liver may result in massive exsanguinating hemorrhage.

50. For atriocaval shunts to be successful, they must be done early, before the patient has developed prolonged hypotension, hypothermia, acidosis, and a coagulopathy.

51. Free bile anywhere in the abdomen suggests injury to the liver, extrahepatic bile ducts, or duodenum and demands a thorough exploration of these structures.

52. If there is bile staining of tissue in the right upper quadrant of the abdomen without an obvious source after thorough exploration, one should consider performing an intraoperative cholangiogram and duodenoscopy.

53. Cholecystectomy is the preferred treatment for trauma to the gallbladder or cystic duct.

54. The subhepatic space should probably be drained in most patients with a gallbladder injury.

55. Construction of a biliary-enteric anastomosis and external drainage is the treatment of choice for complex, extrahepatic bile duct injuries.

▲▲▲▲▲▲▲▲▲▲▲▲▲▲▲▲▲▲▲▲▲▲▲▲▲▲▲▲▲▲▲▲▲

REFERENCES

1. Geller ER, Walt AJ. Liver injuries. In Trauma management. Kreis DJ Jr, Gomez GA, eds. Boston: Little, Brown and Company, 1989; 183-194.
2. Walt AJ, Wilson RF. Specific abdominal injuries. In Management of trauma: pitfalls and practice. Walt AJ, Wilson RF, eds. Philadelphia: Lea & Febiger, 1975;348-374.
3. Pachter HL, Liang HG, Hofstetter SR. Liver and biliary tract trauma. In Trauma. 2nd ed. Moore EE, Mattox KL, Feliciano DV, eds. Norwalk, Connecticut: Appleton & Lange, 1991; 441-463.
4. Pachter HL, Spencer FC. Recent concepts in the treatment of hepatic trauma: facts and fallacies. Ann Surg 1979;190:423.
5. Pachter HL, Spencer FC, Hofstetter SR. Experience with the finger-fracture technique to achieve intrahepatic hemostasis in 75 patients with severe injuries to the liver. Ann Surg 1983;197:771.
6. Hamlyon P: Greek mythology. Fourth impression. London, Paul Hamlin, 1967; 19.
7. Beck C. Surgery of the liver. JAMA 1902;38:1063.
8. Madding GF, Lawrence KB, Kennedy DA. Forward surgery of the severely injured. Second Aux Surg Group 1942;1:307.
9. McIndole AH, Counseller VS. Bilaterality of the liver. Arch Surg 1927;15:589.
10. Healey JE. Clinical anatomic aspects of radical hepatic surgery. J Int Coll Surg 1954;22:542.
11. Payne JE, Berne TV, Kaufman RL et al. Outcome of treatment of 686 gunshot wounds of the trunk at Los Angeles County- USC Medical Center: implication for the community. J Trauma 1993;34:276.
12. Golan A, White RG. Spontaneous rupture of the liver associated with pregnancy: a report of five cases. S Afr Med J 1978;56:133.
13. Luna GK, Maier RV, Pavlin EG, et al. Incidence and effect of hypothermia in seriously injured patients. J Trauma 1987;27:1014.
14. Jurkovich GJ, Greiser WB, Luterman A, et al. Hypothermia in trauma victims: an ominous predictor of survival. J Trauma 1987;17:1019.
15. Flint LM Jr, Polk HC. Selective hepatic artery ligation: limitations and failures. J Trauma 1976;16:442.
16. Lucas CE, Ledgerwood AM. Prospective evaluation of hemostatic techniques for liver injuries. J Trauma 1976;16:442.
17. Moore EE, Eiseman B, Dunn EL. Current management of hepatic trauma. Contemp Surg 1979;15:91.
18. Feliciano DV, Pachter HL. Hepatic trauma revisited. Curr Prog Surg 1989;26:453.
19. Root HD, Hauser CW, McKinley CR, et al. Diagnostic peritoneal lavage. Surgery 1965;57:633.
20. Fischer RP, Beverlin BC, Engrav LH. Diagnostic peritoneal lavage: fourteen years and 2,586 patients later. Am J Surg 1978;136:701.
21. Olsen WR, Redman HC, Hildreth DH. Quantitative peritoneal lavage in blunt abdominal trauma. Arch Surg 1972;104:536.
22. Pachter HL, Hofstetter SR. Open and percutaneous paracentesis and lavage for abdominal trauma. A randomized prospective study. Arch Surg 1981;116:318.
23. Federele MP. Computed tomography of blunt abdominal trauma. Radiol Clin N Am 1983;21:461.
24. Federele MP, Goldberg HI, Kaiser JA, et al. Evaluation of abdominal trauma by computed tomography. Radiology 1981;138:637.
25. Federele MP, Crass RA, Jeffrey BB Jr, et al. Computed tomography in blunt abdominal trauma. Arch Surg 1982;117:645.
26. Moon KL, Federele MP. Computed tomography in hepatic trauma. AJR 1983;141:309.
27. Trunkey D, Federele MP. Computed tomography in perspective. J Trauma 1986;26:660.
28. Marx JA, Moore EE, Jorden RC, et al. Limitations of computed tomography in the evaluation of acute abdominal trauma: a prospective comparison with diagnostic peritoneal lavage. J Trauma 1985;25:933.
29. Goldstein AS, Scaflani SJA, Kupterstein NH, et al. The diagnostic superiority of computerized tomography. J Trauma 1985;25:939.
30. Davis RA, Shayne JP, Max MH, et al. The use of computerized axial tomography versus peritoneal lavage in the evaluation of blunt abdominal trauma. A prospective study. Surgery 1985;98:845.
31. Peitzman AB, Makaroun MS, Slasky BS, et al. Prospective study of computed tomography in initial management of blunt abdominal trauma. J Trauma 1986;26:585.
32. Fabian TC, Mangiante EC, White TJ, et al. A prospective study of 91 patients undergoing both computed tomography and peritoneal lavage following blunt abdominal trauma. J Trauma 1986;26:602.
33. Cywes S, Rode H. Miller AJW. Blunt liver trauma in children: nonoperative management. J Pediatr Surg 1985;20:14.
34. Vock P, Kehrer B, Tschaeppeler H. Blunt liver trauma in children: the role of computed tomography in diagnosis and treatment. J Pediatr Surg 1986;21:413.
35. Meredith JW, Young JS, Bowling J, et al. Nonoperative management of blunt hepatic trauma: the exception or the rule? J Trauma 1994;36:529.
36. Sherman HF, Savage BA, Jones LM et al. Non-operative management of blunt hepatic injuries: safe at any grade? J Trauma 1994;37:616.

37. Sugimoto K, Asari Y, Sakaguchi T, et al. Endoscopic retrograde cholangiography in the non-surgical management of blunt liver injury. J Trauma 1993;35:192.

38. Foley WD, Cates JD, Kellman G, et al. Treatment of blunt hepatic injuries: role of CT. Radiology 1987;164:635.

39. Farnell MB, Spencer MP, Thompson E, et al. Nonoperative management of blunt hepatic trauma in adults. Surgery 1988;104:748.

40. Gates JD. Delayed hemorrhage with free rupture complicating the nonsurgical management of blunt hepatic trauma: a case report and review of the literature. J Trauma 1994;36:572.

41. Richie JP, Fonkalsrud EW. Subcapsular hematoma of the liver—nonoperative management. Arch Surg 1972;104:781.

42. Geis WP, Schulz KA, Giacchino JL, et al. The fate of unruptured intrahepatic hematomas. Surgery 1981;90:689.

43. Pringle JH. Notes on the arrest of hepatic hemorrhage due to trauma. Ann Surg 1908;48:541.

44. Feliciano DV, Jordan GL, Mattox KL, et al. Management of 1000 consecutive cases of hepatic trauma (1979-1984). Ann Surg 1986;204:437.

45. Raffacci FL. The effects of temporary occlusion of the afferent hepatic circulation in dogs. Surgery 1953;33:342.

46. Huguet C, Nordlinger B, Galopin JJ, et al. Normothermic hepatic vascular exclusion for extensive hepatectomy. Surg Gynecol Obstet 1978;147:689.

47. Huguet C, Nordlinger B, Bloch P. Tolerance of the human liver to prolonged normothermic ischemia. Arch Surg 1978;113:1448.

48. Delva E, Camus Y, Nordlinger B, et al. Vascular occlusions for liver resections: operative management of tolerance to hepatic ischemia: 142 cases. Ann Surg 1989;209:211.

49. Bernhard WF, McMurrey JD, Curtis GW. Feasibility of partial hepatic resection under hypothermia. N Engl J Med 1955;253:159.

50. Goodall GW, Hyndman WWB, Gurd FN. Studies on hypothermia in abdominal surgery. Arch Surg 1957;75:1011.

51. Fortner JG, Shiu MH, Kinne OW, et al. Major hepatic resection using vascular isolation and hypothermic perfusion. Ann Surg 1974;180:644.

52. Delpin EA, Figueroa I, Lopez R, Vazquez J. Protective effect of steroids on liver ischemia. Ann Surg 1975;41:683.

53. Figueroa I, Delpin EA. Steroid protection of the liver during experimental ischemia. Surg Gynecol Obstet 1975;140:368.

54. DeMaria EJ, Reichman W, Kenney PR. Septic complications on corticosteroid administration after CNS trauma. Ann Surg 1985;202:248.

55. Pachter HL, Spencer FC, Hofstetter SR. The management of juxtahepatic venous injuries without an atrial-caval shunt: preliminary clinical observations. Surgery 1986;99:569.

56. Maitra SR, Geller ER, Pan W et al. Altered cellular calcium regulation and hepatic glucose production during hemorrhagic shock. Circ Shock 1992;33:121.

57. Kraus-Friedmann N. Hormonal regulation of hepatic gluconeogenesis. Physiol Rev 1984;64:170.

58. Ljungquist O, Khan A, Ware J. Evidence of increased gluconeogenesis during hemorrhage in fed and 24-hour food deprived rats. J Trauma 1987;29:87.

59. Geller ER, Higgins LD, Drourr N, et al. Diltiazem preserves hepatic gluconeogenesis following hemorrhagic shock. J Trauma 1993;35:703.

60. Cogbill TH, Moore EE, Jurkovich GJ, et al. Severe hepatic trauma: a multicenter experience with 1,335 liver injuries. J Trauma 1988;28:1433.

61. Stain SC, Yellin AE, Donovan AJ. Hepatic trauma. Arch Surg 1988;123:1251.

62. Lin TY, Hsu KY, Hsieh CM, Chen CS. Study on lobectomy of the liver. J Formosan Med Assoc 1958;57:750.

63. Ton TT. A new technique for operation on the liver. Lancet 1963;1:192.

64. Balasegaram M, Joishy SK. Hepatic resection: the logical approach to surgical management of major trauma to the liver. Am J Surg 1981;142:580.

65. Mays ET. The hazards of suturing certain wounds of the liver. Surg Gynecol Obstet 1976;143:201.

66. Fabian TC, Stone HH. Arrest of severe liver hemorrhage by an omental pack. South Med J 1980;73:1487.

67. Stone HH, Lamb JM. Use of pedicled omentum as an autogenous pack for control of hemorrhage in major injuries in the liver. Surg Gynecol Obstet 1975;141:92.

68. Siedentop KH, Harris DM. Autologous fibrin tissue adhesive. Laryngoscope 1985;95:1074.

69. Durham LH, Willatt DJ, Yung MW, et al. A method for preparation of fibrin glue. J Laryngol Otol 1987;101:1182.

70. Lerner L, Binuer NS. The current status of surgical adhesives. J Surg Res 1990;48:165.

71. Berguer R, Staerkel RL, Moore EE, et al. Warning: fatal reaction to the use of fibrin glue in deep hepatic wounds. J Trauma 1991;31:408.

72. Jones RA, Schoen FJ, Ziemer G, et al. Biologic sealants and knitted Dacron conduits: comparison of collagen and fibrin glue pretreatments in circulatory models. Ann Thorac Surg 1987;44:283.

73. Ney AL, Kelly PH, Tutu T, et al. Fibrin glue antibiotic suspension in the prevention of prosthetic graft infection. J Trauma 1990;30:1000.

74. Ing RD, Saxe J, Hendrick S, et al. Antibiotic-primed fibrin gel improves outcome in contaminated splenic injury. J Trauma 1992;33:118.

75. Dulchavsky SA, Geller ER, Maurer J, et al. Autologous fibrin gel: bactericidal properties in contaminated hepatic injury. J Trauma 1991;31:991.

76. Kram HB, Nathan RC, Klein SR, et al. Clinical use of nonautologous fibrin glue. Am Surg 1988;54:570.

77. Delany HM, Rudavsky AX, Lan S. Preliminary clinical experience with the use of absorbable mesh splenorrhapy. J Trauma 1985;25:909.

78. Lange DA, Zaret P, Merlotti GJ, et al. The use of absorbable mesh in splenic trauma. J Trauma 1988;28:269.

79. Stevens SL, Maull KI, Enderson BL, et al. Total mesh wrapping for parenchymal liver injuries: a combined experimental and clinical study. J Trauma 1991;31:1103.

80. Jacobson LE, Kirton OC, Gomez GA. The use of an absorbable mesh wrap in the management of liver injuries. Surgery 1992;111:455.

81. Brunet C, Sielezneff I, Thomas P, et al. Treatment of hepatic trauma with perihepatic mesh in 35 cases. J Trauma 1994;37:200.

82. Thomas SV, Dulchavsky SA, Diebel LN. Balloon tamponade for liver injuries. Case Report 1993;34:448.

83. Flint LM, Polk HC. Selective hepatic artery ligation: limitations and failures. J Trauma 1979;19:319.

84. Mays ET, Conti S, Fallahzadeh H, Rosenblatt M. Hepatic artery ligation. Surgery 1979;86:536.

85. Walt AJ: The mythology of hepatic trauma—or Babel revisited. Am J Surg 1978;135:12.

86. Aaron WS, Fulton RL, Mays ET. Selective ligation of the hepatic artery for trauma of the liver. Surg Gynecol Obstet 1975;141:187.

87. Mays ET, Wheeler CS. Hepatic artery ligation. New Engl J Med 1874;290:993.

88. Madding GF, Kennedy PA. Hepatic artery ligation. Surg Clin N Am 1872;52:719.

89. Lucas CE, Ledgerwood AM. Liver necrosis following hepatic artery transection due to trauma. Arch Surg 1978;113:1107.

90. Balasegaram DM. Hepatic resection in trauma. Adv Surg 1984;17:129.

91. Donovan AJ, Michaelian MJ, Yellin AE. Anatomical hepatic lobectomy in trauma to the liver. Surgery 1973;73:833.

92. Moore FA, Moore EE, Seagraves A. Non-resectional management of hepatic trauma: an evolving concept. Am J Surg 1985;50:725.

93. Pachter HL, Spencer FC. The management of complex hepatic trauma. Controv Surg 1983;II:241.

94. Blumgart LH, Drury JK, Wood CB. Hepatic resection for trauma, tumor, and biliary obstruction. Br J Surg 1979;66:762.

95. Menegaux F, Langlois P, Chigot JP, et al. Severe blunt trauma to the liver: study of mortality factors. J Trauma 1993;35:865.

96. Feliciano DV, Mattox KL, Jordan GL Jr. Intra-abdominal packing for control of hepatic hemorrhage: a reappraisal. J Trauma 1981;21:285.

97. Feliciano DV, Mattox KL, Birch JM. Packing for control of hepatic hemorrhage: 58 consecutive patients. J Trauma 1986;26:738.

98. Carmona RH, Peck D, Lim RC. The role of packing and reoperation in severe hepatic trauma. J Trauma 1984;24:779.

99. Svoboda JA, Peter ET, Dang CU, et al. Severe liver trauma in the face of coagulopathy—a case for temporary packing and early re-exploration. Am J Surg 1982;144:717.

100. Calne RY, McMaster P, Pentlow BD. The treatment of major liver trauma by primary packing with transfer of the patients for definitive treatment. B J Surg 1979;66:338.

101. Ivatury RR, Nallathambi M, Gunduz Y, et al. Liver packing for uncontrolled hemorrhage. A reappraisal. J Trauma 1986;26:744.

102. Mullins RJ, Stone HH, Dunlop WE, et al. Hepatic trauma: evaluation of routine drainage. South Med J 1985;78:259.

103. Esquivel CO, Bernardos A, Makowka L, et al. Liver replacement after massive hepatic trauma. J Trauma 1987;27:800.

104. Sparkman RS, Fogelman MJ. Wounds of the liver. Review of 100 cases. Ann Surg 1954;139:690.

105. Fischer RP, O'Farrell KA, Perry JF Jr. The value of peritoneal drains in the treatment of liver injuries. J Trauma 1978;18:393.

106. Noyes LD, Doyle DJ, McSwain NE. Septic complications associated with the use of peritoneal drains in liver trauma. J Trauma 1988; 28:337.

107. Bender JS, Geller ER, Wilson RF. Intra-abdominal sepsis following liver trauma. J Trauma 1989;29:1140.

108. Gillmore D, McSwain NE Jr, Browder IW. Hepatic trauma: To drain or not to drain? J Trauma 1987;27:898.

109. Lucas CE, Walt AJ. Analysis or randomized biliary drainage for liver trauma in 189 patients. J Trauma 1972;12:925.

110. Cox EF, Flancbaum L, Dauterive AH, et al. Blunt trauma to the liver: analysis of management and mortality in 323 consecutive patients. Ann Surg 1988;207:126.

111. Knudson MM, Lim RC, Olcott EW. Morbidity and mortality following major penetrating liver injuries. Arch Surg 1994;129:256.

112. De Toma GD, Mingoli A, Modini G, et al. The value of angiography and selective hepatic artery embolization for continuous bleeding after surgery in liver trauma: case Reports. J Trauma 1994;37:508.

113. Scott CM, Gras Berger RC, Heerdan TF, et al. Intra-abdominal sepsis after hepatic trauma. Am J Surg 1988;155:284.

114. Johnson RD, Mueller PR, Ferrucci JT. Percutaneous drainage of pyogenic liver abscesses. AJR 1985;144:463.

115. Gerzof SG, Johnson WC, Robbin AH. Intrahepatic pyogenic abscesses: treatment by percutaneous drainage. Am J Surg 1985;149:487.

116. Gerzof SG, Coggins AH, Johnson WC, et al. Percutaneous catheter drainage in abdominal abscesses. N Engl J Med 1981;305:653.

117. Merendino KA, Dillard DH, Cammock EE. The concept of surgical biliary decompression in the management of liver trauma. Surg Gynecol Obstet 1963;17:285.

118. Lucas CE, Ledgerwood AM. Controlled biliary drainage for large injuries of the liver. Surg Gynecol Obstet 1973;137:587.

119. Harattas MC, Lewis RD, Fenton AH, et al. Modern concepts in nonsurgical management of traumatic biliary fistulas. J Trauma 1994; 36:186.

120. Visner SL, Helling TS, Watkins M. Early profound jaundice following blunt hepatic trauma: resolution after lobectomy— case report. J Trauma 1994;36:576.

121. Goodnight JE, Blaisdell FW. Hemobilia. Surg Clin North Am 1981;61:973.

122. Cyret P, Baumer R, Roche A. Hepatic hemobilia of traumatic or iatrogenic origin. Recent advances of diagnosis and therapy. Review of the literature from 1976-1981. World J Surg 1984;8:2.

123. Czerniak A, Thompson JN, Hemingway AP, et al. Hemobilia: a disease in evolution. Arch Surg 1988;123:718.

124. Sarr MG, Kaufman SL, Zuidema G. Management of hemobilia associated with transhepatic internal biliary drainage catheters. Surgery 1984; 95:603.

125. Halme L, Orko R, Tierala E, et al. Late biliary stenosis after conservative management of traumatic liver rupture: case report. J Trauma 1994; 36:740.

126. Ledgerwood AM, Kazmers M, Lucas CE. The role of thoracic aortic occlusion for massive hemoperitoneum. J Trauma 1976;16:610.

127. Greig JD, Washington BC, Wilson RF, Whelan TJ Jr. Intra-abdominal venous injuries. Curr Surg 1984;41:10.

128. Wiencek RG, Wilson RF. Abdominal venous injuries. J Trauma 1986; 26:771.

129. Wiencek RG, Wilson RF, Steiger Z. Acute injuries of the diaphragm. J Thor Cardiovas Surg 1986;92:989.

130. Wiencek RG, Wilson RF. Inferior vena cava injuries— the challenge continues. Am Surg 1988;54:423.

131. Kudsk KA, Sheldon GF, Lim RC Jr. Atrial-caval shunting (ACS) after trauma. J Trauma 1982;22:81.

132. Schrock T, Blaisdell W, Mathewson C Jr. Management of blunt trauma to the liver and hepatic veins. Arch Surg 1968;96:698.

133. DeFore WW, Mattox KL, Jordan GL. Management of 1590 consecutive cases of liver trauma. Arch Surg 1976;111:493.

134. Millikan JA, Moore EE, Cogbill TH. Inferior vena cava injuries—a continuing challenge. J Trauma 1983;23:207.

135. Burch JM, Feliciano DV, Mattox KL. The atriocaval shunt. Ann Surg 1988;207:555.

136. Rovito PF. Atrial caval shunting in blunt hepatic vascular injury. Ann Surg 1987;205:318.

137. Diebel LN, Wilson RF, Bender J, et al. A comparison of passive and active shunting for bypass of the retrohepatic IVC. J Trauma 1991; 31:987.

138. Testas P, Benichou J, Benhamou M. Vascular exclusion in surgery of the liver: experimental basis, technic and clinical results. Am J Surg 1977;123:692.

139. Pilcher DB, Harman PK, Moore EE. Retrohepatic vena cava balloon shunt introduced via the sapheno-femoral junction. J Trauma 1977; 17:837.

140. Yellin AE, Chaffee CB, Donovan AJ. Vascular isolation in treatment of juxtahepatic venous injuries. Arch Surg 1971;102:566.

141. Coln D, Crighton J, Schorn L. Successful management of hepatic vein injury from blunt trauma in children. Am J Surg 1980;140:858.

142. Kitahama A, Elliot LF, Overby JL, et al. The extrahepatic biliary tract injury perspective in diagnosis and treatment. Ann Surg 1982;196:536.

143. Gately JF, Thomas EJ. Post-traumatic ischemic necrosis of the common bile duct. Can J Surg 1985;28:32.

144. Thal AP, Wilson RF. A pattern of severe blunt trauma to the pancreas. Surg Gynecol Obstet 1964;119:773.

145. Bade PG, Thomson SR, Hirschberg A, et al. Surgical options in traumatic injury to the extrahepatic biliary tract. Br J Surg 1989;76:256.

146. Ivatury RR, Rohman M, Nallathambi M. The morbidity of injuries of the extrahepatic biliary system. J Trauma 1985;25:967.

147. Kitahama A, Elliot LF, Overby JL. The extrahepatic biliary tract injury. Ann Surg 1982;196:536.

148. Posner MC, Moore EE. Extrahepatic biliary tract injury: operative management plans. J Trauma 1985;25:833.

149. Ackerman NB, Sillin LF, Suresh K. Consequences of intraperitoneal bile: bile ascites versus bile peritonitis. Am J Surg 1985;149:244.

150. Abou-Mourad NN, Rogers LS. Extrahepatic biliary steering-wheel trauma simulating pancreatic carcinoma. J Trauma 1980;20:180.

151. Burt TB, Nelson JA. Extrahepatic biliary duct trauma— a spectrum of injuries. West J Med 1981;134:283.

152. Gottesman L, Marks RA, Khoury PT. Diagnosis of isolated perforation of the gallbladder following blunt trauma using sonography and CT scan. J Trauma 1984;24:280.

153. Spigos DG, Tan WS, Larson G. Diagnosis of traumatic rupture of the gallbladder. Am J Surg 1981;141:731.

154. Soderstrom CA, Maekawa K, DuPriest RW Jr. Gallbladder injuries resulting from blunt abdominal trauma. Ann Surg 1981;193:60.

155. Northover JMA, Terblanche J. A new look at the arterial supply of the bile duct in man and its surgical implications. Br J Surg 1979;66:379.

156. Feliciano DV. Biliary injuries as a result of blunt and penetrating trauma. Surg Clin North Am 1994;74:897.

157. Busuttil RW, Kitahama A, Cerise E. Management of blunt and penetrating injuries to the porta hepatis. Ann Surg 1985;191:539.

158. Sheldon GF, Lim RC, Yee ES. Management of injuries to the porta hepatis. Ann Surg 1985;202:539.

159. Teplick SK, Goldstein RC, Richardson PA. Percutaneous transhepatic choledochoplasty and dilatation of choledochoenterostomy strictures. JAMA 1980;244:1240.

Chapter 23 Injury to the Spleen

ROBERT F. WILSON, M.D.

CHRISTOPHER P. STEFFES, M.D.

JAMES TYBURSKI, M.D.

INTRODUCTION

Historically, the management of splenic injuries has been extremely controversial.[1,2] Most trauma surgeons now agree that an injured spleen should be treated non-operatively or repaired whenever possible; however, the management of the injured spleen has undergone a radical change in the past 15-20 years.[3]

Once regarded as a mysterious organ of unestablished function, the spleen is now recognized for its importance as an immunologic factory and a vital reticuloendothelial filter. Although the risk of overwhelming postsplenectomy sepsis (OPSS) is greatest in children less than 2 years of age, especially those who have their spleens removed for non-traumatic reasons,[4-6] adults who have had a splenectomy may also be vulnerable.[7-13]

> **AXIOM** The spleen is an important immunological organ, especially in children less than 2 years of age.

Recognition of the immunologic consequences of splenectomy has stimulated increasing efforts to save the injured spleen, regardless of the patient's age. This philosophy in conjunction with increased use of computed tomography (CT) scans has provided increased opportunity for nonoperative management of splenic trauma, particularly in younger patients.[14-26]

With increased appreciation of the spleen's segmental anatomy, advances in operative technique, and the development of improved topical hemostatic agents, such as fibrin glue,[27] splenorrhaphy has proved to be both feasible and safe;[28-32] however, immediate total splenectomy is indicated when the spleen is pulverized or when other life-threatening injuries mandate rapid control of bleeding.[33] In this setting, splenic autotransplantation can be a simple, safe alternative;[30,34] however, even though some splenic implants survive with variable degrees of function, the clinical benefit of these implants is unknown.

HISTORICAL PERSPECTIVES

Partial splenectomy for trauma was first recorded in 1650. This was accomplished by Viaird in a soldier with a partial splenic evisceration so that only the extruded portion was resected.[2] Sporadic reports of similar operations appeared in the 17th and 18th centuries. These reports must be viewed with some skepticism because it would be extremely difficult to mobilize a spleen via a stab wound so that it would present on the abdominal wall.[26] One wonders whether these surgeons actually removed eviscerated omentum congested with blood. The first successful total splenectomy, however, was performed in 1893 by Reigner in a 14-year-old-boy sustaining blunt trauma with splenic avulsion.[35]

During the early decades of the 20th century, splenectomy was done frequently for trauma, but mortality rates in most series averaged between 30% and 40%.[36,37] In contrast, the nonoperative approach, reported by Bland-Sutton[38] in 1912, resulted in a 90% mortality. Indeed, Kocher's admonition that "injuries of the spleen demand excision of the gland. No evil effects follow its removal while the damage of hemorrhage is effectively stopped" was virtually unchallenged for the next 60 years.

Since antiquity, the spleen has been regarded as the "mysterii pleni organon," (an organ full of mystery), and its physiologic importance has been appreciated only recently. Early investigations of the spleen's role in host defense against infection were poorly controlled, and conflicting results were often obtained. A classic study by Morris and Bollock in 1919[26,39] conclusively demonstrated the susceptibility of splenectomized rats to overwhelming infection; however, the accuracy and clinical relevance of this observation was thought to have been refuted in subsequent years by several small retrospective clinical reports.

In 1952 a revolutionary change in the concept of managing injured spleens began when King and Schumacker[4] reported a syndrome of overwhelming postsplenectomy infection (OPSI) in five infants who had splenectomies for congenital hemolytic anemia. Similar reports from Huntley[40] and Horan and Colebatch[41] confirmed a 5-8% incidence of life-threatening infection in children under the age of 1 year who had undergone splenectomy for various diseases or for trauma.

In 1972, a multicenter survey was performed by the American Academy of Pediatrics to determine the incidence of postsplenectomy complications. This survey reported that of 342 children who had a splenectomy for trauma, three (0.88%) died of overwhelming sepsis.[42] In 1973, Singer[5] reviewed 2795 patients from the literature and noted a 1.5% incidence of sepsis following splenectomy for trauma and a 2.1% incidence of sepsis for incidental splenectomy. The overall incidence of sepsis was 1.6%, with a mortality rate of 65% in those who become septic. Subsequent reports also estimated the risk of OPSI in adults to be about 1-2% (Table 23-1).[1,9-12]

> **AXIOM** Although the risk of OPSI is only about 1-2%, it is many times higher than in nonsplenectomized individuals, and the risk of death is very high.

At the same time, when the spleen's immunologic significance became increasingly apparent, the anatomic work of Michels[43] and of Nguyen et al[44] delineated the segmental end-arterial system of the spleen. With this work, it became increasingly clear that blunt fractures tend to occur along avascular intersegmental planes which could provide an anatomic basis for operative salvage.[45-47] Development of topical hemostatic agents further aided the performance of splenic repairs and/or partial resections.[48]

Lucas[26] has pointed out that the first splenic salvage was probably performed by Zirkoff in 1897. He also pointed out that Dretzka reported the first successful repair of an injured spleen in a child.

Since the work of Campos in 1961,[46] the principles of anatomic dissection of the human spleen have been promulgated by several authors.[44,47] Favorable results of splenic salvage in children led to increasing enthusiasm for splenorrhaphy in adults.[29,33] Early experience, relying predominantly on hemostasis agents, attested to the feasibility of splenorrhaphy in adults. Ensuing salvage efforts have become more aggressive,[49] and now formal anatomic resections are performed more or less routinely. As an extension of this philosophy, the nonoperative approach of known splenic injuries has been increasingly used in children[15-17] and is also being applied to selected adults.[18-25] Diagnostic laparoscopy may also help to determine which hemodynamically stable patients with splenic injuries can be treated nonoperatively.[50]

TABLE 23-1 *Mortality Rates With Abdominal Injuries Seen in 12 Years at Detroit Receiving Hospital (1980-1992)*

Organ Injured	Type of Trauma			
	Blunt	GSW	Stabs	Total
Liver	56 (160)	110 (499)	19 (251)	185 (910)
	35%	22%	8%	20%
Small Bowel	14 (58)	75 (551)	10 (450)	99 (759)
	24%	14%	7%	13%
Colon	7 (42)	69 (498)	7 (122)	83 (662)
	17%	14%	6%	13%
Diaphragm	7 (28)	59 (273)	10 (199)	76 (420)
	25%	22%	8%	18%
Kidney	10 (145)	40 (229)	6 (45)	56 (419)
	7%	17%	13%	13%
Spleen	26 (172)	31 (131)	4 (42)	61 (345)
	15%	24%	10%	18%
Stomach	3 (6)	53 (241)	10 (93)	66 (340)
	50%	22%	11%	19%
Abd. Vessels	16 (23)	135 (257)	17 (53)	168 (333)
	70%	53%	32%	58%
Pancreas	2 (33)	34 (140)	11 (37)	47 (210)
	6%	24%	30%	22%
Duodenum	3 (10)	29 (124)	7 (33)	39 (167)
	30%	23%	21%	23%
Bladder	8 (44)	5 (84)	1 (6)	14 (134)
	18%	6%	17%	10%
Gallbladder	3 (3)	14 (59)	1 (19)	18 (81)
	100%	24%	5%	22%
Total	92 (573)	192 (1358)	40 (810)	326 (2741)
	16%	14%	5%	12%

ANATOMY

Development

The spleen appears in the 8-10 mm embryo, during the fifth week of fetal development, as a thickening in the dorsal mesogastrium near the tail of the pancreas.[51] The mass increases rapidly in size, and by three months it has acquired its typical shape and has rotated into its normal position in the left upper quadrant. Vascularization occurs early, and from the fourth to the eighth month, the spleen actively forms erythrocytes.

This activity accounts for much of the size of the spleen at this age. Erythrocytogenesis generally ceases entirely by the eighth fetal month, but it may continue in diseases, such as hemolytic disease of the newborn, or it may be revived in the adult in certain other diseases. Lymphoid tissue in small quantities appears in the spleen early, but the characteristic Malpighian corpuscles are not seen until the sixth to the eighth month. Eventually the majority of splenic tissue is lymphoid.

At birth, the spleen is proportionately large, but it remains functionally immature and continues to enlarge until puberty.[52] After puberty, the spleen gradually regresses so that after 60 years of age, its size has decreased by about 30%. The normal spleen in an adult is about 10-14 cm long, 6-10 cm wide, 3-4 cm thick, and weighs 80-300 grams. Accessory spleens have been reported in 14-30% of patients and are much more common in patients operated on for hematologic disorders.[52]

AXIOM Surgeons performing a splenectomy for hypersplenism must look carefully for accessory spleens, which may be present in more than a third of cases.

Position and Ligaments

The spleen is bounded in the deep left upper quadrant by the gastric fundus, left hemidiaphragm, superior pole of the left kidney, and splenic flexure of the colon (Fig. 23-1).[3] It is firmly attached to the retroperitoneum by the lienorenal and phrenicolienal ligaments as well as the tail of the pancreas, and to mobile structures of the abdomen via the gastrolienal and the splenocolic ligaments. The spleen is encapsulated by an external serous coat derived from the peritoneum and an internal fibroelastic coat, which is invaginated at the hilum and carried inward with the splenic artery and its branches. In the child, there is more functional smooth muscle and elastic tissue in the parenchyma, and the capsule is relatively thick compared to the adult.[53,54]

Vascular Segmentation

The arterial blood supply of the spleen, which is about 5% of the cardiac output, arrives via the splenic artery and the short gastric vessels.[3] Gupta et al[47] demonstrated that 84% of adult human spleens had two major lobes (superior and inferior), while the remainder had three (superior, intermediate, and inferior). Each of these is divided into two segments with essentially no vascular communications between these segments.

AXIOM The anatomical division of the spleen's vasculature into 4-6 segments facilitates the performance of partial splenectomy after trauma.

The arterial pedicle at the splenic hilum has a Y shape in 70-80% of patients[55] with the splenic artery dividing into two major vessels

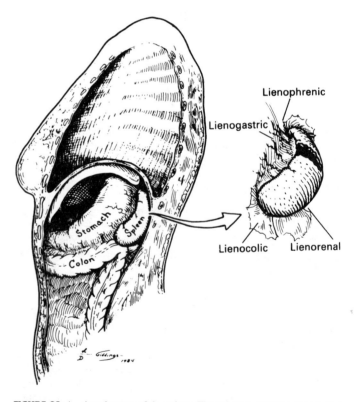

FIGURE 23-1 Attachments of the spleen. The spleen is tethered deep in the left upper abdomen by four connective tissue "ligaments." The splenophrenic and splenorenal ligaments are generally avascular, but the splenocolic ligament may contain sizeable blood vessels, and the splenogastric ligament has the short gastric and left gastroepiploic vessels. (From Moore EE. Splenic injury. In Champion HR, Robbs JV, Trunkey DV, eds. Rob and Smith's operative surgery—trauma surgery, 4th ed. Boston: Butterworths, 1989;1:367.)

2-5 cm away from the hilum; these two branches divide into smaller segmental branches at the edge of the spleen itself. The second most common pattern of the hilar vessels is described as the T type, which occurs in about 20% of patients. In this type, the splenic artery comes straight up to the hilum of the spleen and then divides into a superior and inferior branch, each giving off additional branches. A comparable segmentation of splenic veins has also been demonstrated, but intercommunications are fairly common.

Additional vessels to the superior or inferior pole of the spleen are common and come either from the splenic artery or from branches of the celiac axis.[3] The lobar arteries of the spleen further divide into cephalic and caudad branches thus providing four anatomic segments in the majority of patients.

The splenic artery trifurcates in the remaining 15% of people, and each of these major branches has a cephalic and caudal branch so that a total of six anatomic segments may be defined. Each of the major four or six branches of the splenic artery then runs transversely in the splenic tissue within a trabecular sheath and without anastomosing with adjacent vessels.

Within the splenic parenchyma, the blood passes through a large capillary bed, which gives it intimate contact with resident plasma cells, lymphocytes, and fixed macrophages. The blood then drains into large venous sinusoids. This parenchymal architecture allows for maximal contact between the formed elements of the blood and the reticuloendothelial system. Unlike the arteries,[55] the veins can be highly interconnected and often do not follow a predictable segmental anatomy.

Internal Structure

The spleen's internal architecture or stroma is described as a rich vascular network consisting of: (a) white pulp (which contains lymphocytes and macrophages), (b) red pulp (which is a storage area for red blood cells, granulocytes, and platelets), (c) marginal zones (containing additional macrophages and plasma cells where cellular interactions take place), and (d) ellipsoids (which contain dense periarteriolar concentrations of phagocytes).[1,52] Awareness of this highly organized morphologic arrangement has led some authorities to question the practicality of autotransplanting fragments of splenic tissue.

Unlike the documented successful piecemeal autotransplantation of endocrine tissue (such as parathyroid gland or islet cells), autotransplanting fragments of spleen with the goal of preserving splenic function might be analogous to autotransplanting pieces of kidney or liver. Although immunologic benefits in humans have yet to be absolutely confirmed, precisely reimplanted slices of splenic tissue do demonstrate revascularization and viability for long periods and can correct some of the functional abnormalities seen after splenectomy, including higher levels of pneumococcal antibody production following immunization.[56-59]

AXIOM Although reimplanted slices of spleen can revascularize and develop some splenic function, it is not yet clear how beneficial they are.

PHYSIOLOGY

The total circulation of the spleen is estimated at about 250 ml per minute, representing about 5% of the total cardiac output.[1] Blood passes first through the central arteries of the germinal centers, bringing particulate matter into contact with lymphocytes for antigen processing.[3] More than 90% of the blood is then forced through the cords of Bilroth. During this percolation process the fixed macrophages (Fig. 23-2) actively phagocytose aged blood cells and any bacteria that may be present.[1] This unique anatomy increases the contact time between the fixed macrophages and the blood, thereby decreasing opsonic requirements. If the spleen is absent, the spleen's filtration function must be performed largely by the RES in the liver. As a general rule, encapsulated organisms require much greater opsonization to be removed by hepatic macrophages.

As a consequence, patients with chronic liver disease and impaired hepatic RES function are more prone to develop postsplenectomy infections.

AXIOM Although it is often harder to repair the injured spleen or save part of it in patients with liver disease, it is particularly important in such patients.

The spleen's other major role is that of an immunologic factory, producing immunoglobulins (especially IgM and IgG), properdin, and tuftsin.[3,53,60-65] As the first antibody formed in response to an antigen, the primary role of IgM is initiation of other immune mechanisms. In comparison to IgG, IgM has a shorter half-life and lower serum concentrations.[3] Its large size limits it to the intravascular space but enhances its ability to activate complement and agglutinate bacteria. IgG is produced later, remains longer, and is free to exude into the interstitial space. The body has immunologic memory in respect to IgG production, and on second exposure to an antigen, there is an anamnestic response that more rapidly provides higher antibody titers.

Complement activation is also vital to host defense. It increases vascular permeability and promotes chemotaxis, phagocytosis, and intracellular killing. Complement is activated in the classic sense by antibody-antigen interaction or via the alternative pathway.[66]

Tuftsin is a substance made predominantly by spleen.[62,63] This tetrapeptide binds to leukokinen, which coats circulating neutrophils, inducing a nonspecific enhancement of phagocytosis. Interestingly, Zoli et al[67] have shown that there is a direct relationship between residual splenic function, the percentage of pitted red blood cells in the circulation, and tuftsin activity. In 10 patients who had splenectomies for trauma, the mean tuftsin activity was 4.4% versus 21.6% in control patients with normal spleens. In contrast, 13 patients who had elective splenectomy had no tuftsin activity. The authors said this data confirms that some residual function is often present in patients having splenectomies for trauma.

AXIOM Asplenic patients have low levels of IgM, properdin, and tuftsin, and these deficiencies contribute to an increased susceptibility to OPSI.[3]

The spleen contains 25% of the total lymphoid mass of the body and has been shown to have a direct impact on T and B lymphocytes.[68-71] As a consequence, the asplenic state is characterized by: (a) impaired capacity for clearance of blood-borne particles,[69] (b) decreased phagocytic activity directed against encapsulated bacteria,[72,73] (c) decreased antibody response to specific antigens,[58,62,74,75] (d) decreased opsonization of bacteria,[63,76] (e) an absence of circulating tuftsin,[64,77,78] (f) decreased antibody responses[73,79] and (g) decreased properdin.[66] Additionally, the spleen tends to increase the helper to suppressor T-cell ratio[3,81-83] and modulate distant monocyte function.[84,85] The spleen is also important in immune surveillance and may protect against the induction of cancer.[86]

Beginning with the 1952 report of King and Shumacker,[4] showing increased susceptibility of asplenic infants to infection, there have been numerous additional examples of "overwhelming postsplenectomy infection" (OPSI) in asplenic patients.[3,8-13] The typical clinical course starts with a mild upper-respiratory infection followed by an abrupt onset of fever, chills, nausea, and vomiting. This progresses rapidly to fulminant sepsis, which is frequently associated with disseminated intravascular coagulation and adrenal insufficiency.

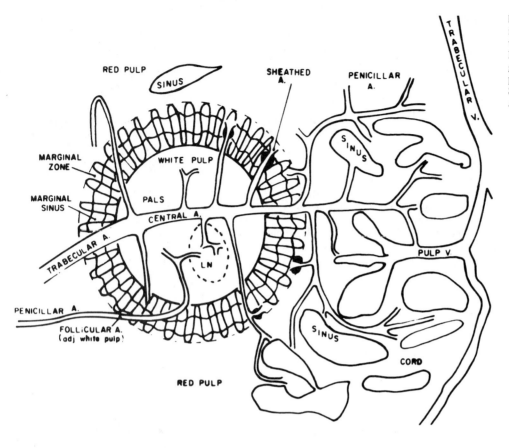

FIGURE 23-2 Diagram illustrating the intrasplenic compartments and associated vessels. A=artery or arteriole; V=vein; LN=lymphatic nodule which may include germinal center; PALS=periarterial lymphatic. (From Barnhart MI, Lusher JM. Structural physiology of the human spleen. Am J Pediatr Hematol Oncol 1979;1:311.)

The large numbers of bacteria found in peripheral blood smears of some of these patients with OPSI have been estimated as at least 1 million per ml.

AXIOM   Patients with lower respiratory infections, particularly by encapsulated organisms, are particularly likely to develop overwhelming postsplenectomy infections (OPSI).

The microorganisms most often found in OPSI are typically encapsulated and include Streptococcus pneumoniae—the pneumococcus (50%), meningococcus (12%); Escherichia coli (11%), Haemophilus influenzae (8%); staphylococci (8%), and other streptococci (7%). The remarkable virulence of the pneumococcus is related to its rapid multiplication and its capsule, which resists opsonization and phagocytosis. The incidence of OPSI in asplenic patients is estimated to be 50-200 times more than in the normal population.[1,5,9,87,88] Mortality rates from OPSI vary from 40-70%. Early recognition and aggressive treatment with antibiotics are mandatory. Although 50% of OPSI occurs within two years of splenectomy, the syndrome has been reported as long as 37 years later.

AXIOM   The incidence of severe sepsis after splenectomy is only about 0.5-2.0%, but this is up to 200 times more frequent than in patients with a normal spleen.

Healthy individuals splenectomized for trauma appear to be at slightly less risk than those who are splenectomized for hematologic disease, and young children, especially those less than 2 years of age, seem to fare worse than older children and adults.[89] Interestingly, however, the severity of sepsis appears to be worse in older patients. The majority of serious infections following splenectomy are said to occur within 24 months,[87,89] but there is no time limit beyond which an asplenic person can be considered safe.

In addition to an increased tendency to overwhelming bacterial sepsis, asplenic patients also seem to have an increased susceptibility to infection by other organisms.[1,8,10,89,90] Of particular concern is the high incidence of viral illnesses in asplenic individuals,[10,87,90] pro-viding evidence that the phenomenon of postsplenectomy sepsis is not confined to encapsulated bacteria.

Long-term follow-up of 740 American servicemen splenectomized for trauma during World War II (1939-1945) revealed a statistically significant increased mortality from pneumonia and ischemic heart disease.[91] The mortality from cirrhosis in this same study was also increased somewhat but not significantly. Thrombocytosis and hypercoagulability have been postulated as reasons for the increased risk of fatal myocardial ischemia after splenectomy, while an increased susceptibility to viral illnesses might account for the increased mortality rate in asplenic cirrhotic patients.[1]

At present, there is considerable evidence supporting a conservative surgical approach to the injured spleen. The main controversy remains as to how best to accomplish splenic preservation following trauma. The enthusiasm of those espousing nonoperative management or splenic repair must be balanced against the threats of a missed associated injury or exsanguination during or after attempted splenic repair.[1] Paramount is the need to confirm that these different techniques do preserve normal or near normal splenic function without jeopardizing the trauma victim's chances for a complete recovery.

INCIDENCE

The spleen is the organ most frequently injured with blunt abdominal trauma in many centers, but the exact incidence is unknown.[1] In addition, the only controlled general population study addressing the issue of sepsis following splenectomy was projected at more than 40,000 splenectomies per year.[9] The age-adjusted incidence of splenectomy per 100,000 person-years in the upper Midwest population studied was 20.5 for men, and 15.3 for women. Only 25% of these splenectomies, however, were performed for trauma. Excluding primary splenic disease or hematologic malignancies, 46% were incidental splenectomies performed because of accidental injury to the spleen at the time of abdominal surgery on other organs.

In a 12 year period at Detroit Receiving Hospital (1980-1992), the spleen was injured in 345 patients who were admitted (Table 23-

1). Of 573 patients admitted with blunt abdominal injuries, the spleen was injured in 172 (30%), making it the abdominal organ most commonly injured by blunt trauma. Of 1358 patients with abdominal injuries from gunshot wounds, the spleen was injured in 131 (9.6%). Of 810 patients with stabs of abdominal organs, it was injured in 42 (5.2%). The mortality rates with each of the main types of trauma were blunt-15%, GSW-24%, and stabs-10%.

Demographically, the peak incidence of splenic injury is usually noted in the second and third decades of life with males predominating. A secondary small peak is observed in women over the age of 70.[1]

AXIOM Most early deaths in patients with splenic trauma are due to associated injuries.[92]

With isolated splenic injury, the mortality rate is only about 1-2%. If all trauma victims with nonpenetrating injuries to the spleen are included (those dead on arrival and those who expired in the emergency room), mortality rates range from 18-25%.[1,2,19,31,93,94] This alarmingly high death rate primarily reflects the magnitude of the multisystem injury and, in particular, associated injuries to the head and chest.

Until the advent of diagnostic peritoneal lavage (DPL) and computed tomography (CT), part of this high mortality could be attributed to difficulties in the diagnosis of abdominal injuries and delays in operative intervention. Spleens which are enlarged due to a variety of conditions (e.g., infectious mononucleosis, hemolytic anemia, leukemia, agnogenic myeloid metaplasia, etc) are felt to be more susceptible to injury. Patients with these problems have an increased incidence of splenic injury occurring spontaneously or after trivial injuries.

AXIOM An enlarged spleen is much more susceptible to accidental trauma than a normal spleen.

MECHANISMS OF INJURY

Blunt Trauma

The type of trauma most often responsible for blunt injury to the spleen continues to be motor vehicle accidents (MVA).[1] The high speeds involved in many of these accidents account for the high incidence of other intraabdominal injuries (30-60%) and extraabdominal injuries (80-85%).[19,22,27,95,96] Traub and Perry[95] found serious associated intraabdominal injuries in 37% of their patients with blunt splenic trauma, and Fisher et al[96] found a 27% incidence of gastrointestinal disruption in adults with blunt splenic injury (versus 7% in children). This high incidence of associated intraabdominal injuries in adults is one of the strongest arguments supporting routine abdominal exploration for blunt splenic injury in that age group.[10,22,95,97]

Although a high incidence of associated intraabdominal injuries would argue against nonoperative management of splenic trauma, less than 12% of blunt splenic trauma victims in some series have sustained other intraabdominal injuries that required operative intervention.[1,22] Buckman et al[97] found that of 142 patients with blunt splenic injuries, only 16 (11.2%) had associated bowel or diaphragmatic injuries that would require laparotomy. This included 12 (8.4%) diaphragmatic ruptures, four (2.8%) bowel perforations, and one (0.7%) bowel ischemia. Of the 45 minor splenic injuries (less than 1 cm deep and not involving the hilum), only 2 (4.4%) had diaphragmatic rupture and none had a full-thickness bowel injury. Of the 97 with more severe splenic injuries, 15.5% had associated major injuries requiring laparotomy. This included 10 diaphragmatic ruptures, four bowel perforations, and one ischemic bowel.

Of 172 patients with blunt splenic injury seen at Detroit Receiving Hospital during a 12-year period, 13 (7.6%) had a major vascular injury, 12 (6.9%) had a diaphragmatic injury, and 12 (6.9%) had a gastrointestinal injury (Table 23-2). Thus, it is important to aggressively look for other organ injuries, using CT scans, DPL, and/or ultrasound techniques.[1]

AXIOM If there is evidence of a splenic injury, one must look carefully for associated intraabdominal injuries, especially in adults, before considering nonoperative treatment in hemodynamically stable adults.

Isolated blunt splenic injury may occur in less than one-fourth of all the cases of splenic trauma and usually involves less destructive force, such as direct blows to the left upper abdomen in minor falls and in contact sports. With access to effective emergency care systems, the mortality of isolated blunt splenic injuries, regardless of the definitive method of management, should be less than 1.0%.[1]

Penetrating Trauma

The incidence of splenic injury in patients having a celiotomy for penetrating abdominal trauma is generally less than 10%.[1,94] The relative infrequency of penetrating splenic injury probably reflects the small volume of intraperitoneal space normally occupied by the spleen as compared to that of other intraabdominal organs.

Mortality rates with penetrating splenic trauma vary with the mechanism of injury and range from 0-1% with stab wounds to 4-10% with gunshot wounds.[31,94,97] The majority of patients with penetrating splenic trauma have associated injuries that require surgical correction, thereby justifying the universal consensus that penetrating splenic trauma demands operative intervention.[1]

AXIOM Virtually all patients with acute penetrating splenic trauma should have a surgical exploration because of the high incidence of associated injuries requiring treatment.

Iatrogenic Injuries

Virtually any surgical maneuver or procedure performed in the left upper quadrant of the abdomen can cause splenic injury. The spleen is particularly vulnerable during surgery on the proximal stomach (especially fundoplication and vagotomy), left kidney, left adrenal gland and splenic flexure of the colon.[1] Other procedures causing iatrogenic splenic injury include external cardiac massage, the Heimlich maneu-

TABLE 23-2 *Most Frequent Associated Injuries With Splenic Trauma Correlated With Mortality Rates*

Associated Injuries	Blunt	Penetrating	Total
Diaphragm	4 (12) 33%	19 (103) 18%	23 (115) 20%
Lung	15 (42) 36%	15 (69) 22%	30 (111) 27%
Liver	17 (38) 45%	17 (63) 27%	34 (101) 34%
Stomach	1 (2) 50%	22 (84) 26%	23 (86) 27%
Pancreas	1 (10) 10%	25 (70) 36%	26 (80) 33%
Kidney	4 (21) 19%	19 (59) 32%	23 (80) 29%
Colon	3 (8) 38%	10 (61) 16%	13 (69) 19%
Major Vessels	7 (13) 54%	24 (42) 57%	31 (55) 56%
Head	11 (35) 31%	1 (2) 50%	12 (37) 32%
Small Bowel	1 (2) 50%	11 (26) 42%	12 (28) 43%
Pelvic Fractures	8 (23) 35%	0 (1) —	8 (24) 33%
Total	26 (172) 15%	35 (173) 20%	16 (345) 18%

ver, pericardiocentesis, and chest tube thoracostomy.[1] Awareness of the consequences of the asplenic state has caused most practicing surgeons to make a strong effort to repair the incidentally injured spleen rather than remove it.

DIAGNOSIS

Prior to the advent of radionuclide imaging and, more recently, DPL and CT, the diagnosis of splenic injury was based largely on clinical findings.[1] Signs and symptoms suggestive of a ruptured spleen are those associated with intraabdominal bleeding from any cause and vary according to the severity of the hemorrhage, associated injuries, and the temporal relationship to the traumatic event.

AXIOM   Delayed recognition of splenic injury is one of the most common causes of preventable death following blunt trauma.

With the modern philosophy of identifying any and all organ injuries aggressively as soon as possible to optimize trauma care, delayed diagnosis of splenic injury should be uncommon.[1] An increasingly aggressive diagnostic approach also explains the marked reduction in the incidence of "delayed rupture" of the spleen, previously reported to occur in up to 40% of splenic injuries, to less than 2% in more recent series.[22,99,100]

Kluger et al[61] noted that Ballance[102] in 1898 suggested that capsular tears occur in the spleen at the time of the initial injury rather than later. In addition, later rupture of a contained perisplenic hematoma is what causes serious secondary bleeding. Baudet[103] in 1907 suggested the term "latent period" (period de latanec) to describe the time elapsed from the original injury to the later splenic rupture. McIndoe,[104] who collected 46 cases of "delayed rupture of the spleen" arbitrarily chose a period exceeding 48 hours to define this delay. He emphasized that the term was a misnomer. The incidence of "delayed rupture" of the spleen has been reported to be as low as 0.6-2.0%.[100,105] Zabinski and Harkins[106] in a collective review, however, found the incidence of delayed rupture to be 14%. The main significance of the delayed rupture lies in its high mortality rates (5-15%)[107-109] compared with mortality rates as low as 1% when acute splenic injury is recognized promptly.[18]

AXIOM   Delayed rupture of the spleen is usually only a delayed diagnosis of a significant splenic injury.

Patient History

Injury mechanisms and preexisting diseases are important risk factors in patients with suspected splenic trauma.[3] Critical details related to the trauma include whether injury was deceleration or compressive, the location of the driver, use of seat belts, and the amount of deformation of the vehicles. With penetrating injuries, it is helpful to know the type of weapon used, the caliber of the bullet, and its muzzle velocity.

Patients with a large abnormal spleen are much more apt to have a severe splenic injury with trivial trauma. Splenomegaly can be produced by a wide variety of hematologic disorders, including bloodborne arterial and viral infections and portal hypertension. Recognition of these diseases is important not only for diagnosing splenic injuries but also for helping to guide preoperative treatment of these patients.

Generalized abdominal pain and nausea are common following splenic injury.[1] Pain localized to the left upper quadrant is reported in about 30% of patients. The reported incidence of pain over the top of the left shoulder when the patient lies down (Kehr's sign) has varied from 15-75%, but averages about 20% and can be enhanced by placing the patient in the Trendelenburg position.[92]

About 75% of delayed splenic bleeding after trauma occurs during the first two weeks after the injury, but some occur only after many months.[110] The hemorrhage with the initial trauma or the delayed rupture may be sudden and sufficiently severe to produce hypovolemic shock rapidly, or it may increase slowly over a period of a few days.

Some patients develop "delayed rupture of the spleen" following minimal and unappreciated trauma, which may not be remembered until or unless the patient or family is questioned very closely. The possibility of a delayed rupture of the spleen must always be explained to patients with unoperated splenic trauma and their families before they are discharged from the hospital. In addition, a note indicating that these warnings and instructions were given to the patient should be documented in the chart.

AXIOM   All patients with an injured spleen that has been observed or repaired should be aware of the possibility of a delayed splenic rupture.

Physical Examination

The clinical manifestations of splenic injury are due to the irritating effect of intraperitoneal blood, acute blood volume loss, or adjacent chest and abdominal wall injury.[3] Fractures of the ninth, tenth, and/or eleventh ribs are frequent in adults with splenic trauma.[92] In children, however, because of the flexibility of the rib cage, the chest wall injury may be minimal.

AXIOM   Children, in contrast to adults, may have a severe splenic injury with little or no evidence of chest or abdominal wall trauma.

Inspection of the chest and abdominal wall in adults with splenic trauma may reveal telltale contusions, abrasions, or penetrating wounds.[3] Posterior penetrating wounds, particularly in obese hirsute adults, may be overlooked if the patient does not have a complete back examination. Systematic palpation of the chest wall may demonstrate point tenderness over associated rib fractures. Intraperitoneal hemorrhage may produce peritoneal signs of tenderness and guarding as well as evidence of diaphragmatic irritation.

On occasion, a large clot in the left upper quadrant or a large subcapsular hematoma may be palpable at the left costal margin. This may also be a positive Ballance's sign, which is an area of "fixed" dullness to percussion over the left lower lateral ribs. In other words, this area is dull to percussion when the patient is in both the right and left lateral decubitus positions. Free fluid in contrast to a large perisplenic hematoma, would not cause the left flank to be dull to percussion when the patient is lying on the right side.[92]

Observation

One should be reluctant to discharge any patient with significant trauma to the left upper abdomen or left lower chest without at least 24 hours of observation.[1] It is far better to observe patients who have had significant trauma over the spleen for 24-48 hours, even if all studies appear to be normal, than to have them return later in profound shock. It should be remembered that mild-to-moderate injuries of the spleen may be diagnosed by physical examination alone in only 42% of cases.[111]

AXIOM   Any patient who has had significant trauma to the abdomen should be observed for at least 24-48 hours, with frequent, careful examinations.

Laboratory Studies

With an appropriate history of trauma, a falling hematocrit and rising WBC and platelet count should make one suspect an injury to the spleen. The white blood cell count usually rises rapidly after severe splenic injury, and a leukocytosis of 12,000-30,000/mm^3 may be present;[92] however, the hemoglobin level may not fall significantly for 6-12 hours, even with fairly substantial blood loss unless large quantities of intravenous fluids are given.

AXIOM Splenic injury should be suspected in patients with abdominal trauma if the patient has a falling hematocrit and/or abruptly rising WBC or platelet count.

Occasionally, a splenic injury will be suspected when the platelet count rises abruptly, to values approaching $10^6/mm^3$. Splenic injury should also be suspected if there is a persistent rise in serum amylase levels.

Diagnostic Peritoneal Lavage

The introduction of diagnostic peritoneal lavage (DPL) by Root et al[112] in 1965 provided a rapid, inexpensive, accurate, and relatively safe diagnostic adjunct which, when properly performed, is very sensitive for detecting hemoperitoneum. However, a high RBC does not necessarily mandate laparotomy, especially in children.

AXIOM An RBC count >100,000/mm³ in the DPL aspirate is positive for intraabdominal bleeding, but it does not necessarily mean that a laparotomy is required, especially in children.

DPL is considered by many surgeons to be the gold standard in the assessment of blunt abdominal trauma. It is about 98% sensitive and, with modification of the diagnostic criteria, has proven to be of increasing value in patients with penetrating wounds to the abdomen, flank, or lower thorax.[1] One of the major limitations of DPL in the assessment of splenic trauma has been its lack of specificity as to exactly what organ might be injured and whether there is continued bleeding. Additional criticisms include its invasive nature and the inability of DPL to consistently identify injuries to the diaphragm and to retroperitoneal structures, such as the duodenum, pancreas, or kidneys. Nevertheless, DPL represents an efficient and economical diagnostic tool in identifying abdominal trauma, particularly when there is any degree of urgency, such as when the cause of hypotension in trauma victims is unknown. With stable patients, many physicians now rely primarily on CT scans of the abdomen to diagnose intraabdominal injuries.

AXIOM DPL and CT scans should be viewed as complementary and not competing examinations in patients with suspected intraabdominal injuries.

Radiologic Evaluation

PLAIN FILMS FOR THE CHEST AND ABDOMEN

Plain chest radiographs may be abnormal in up to half the patients with splenic injury, but none of the changes are specific.[113] Up to 40% of patients with blunt trauma to the spleen have fractures of the ninth, tenth, or eleventh ribs on the left.[92] A left pleural effusion, elevated left hemidiaphragm, and left lower lobe pulmonary contusion are additional evidence of significant left upper abdominal trauma.

Seven radiograph signs considered to be relatively characteristic of a ruptured spleen on plain radiographs of the abdomen include: (a) increased density or a mass in the LUQ of the abdomen, (b) displacement of the gastric bubble to the right, (c) distortion of the left side of the gastric bubble, (d) increased space between the top of the gastric bubble and the diaphragm, (e) an elevated left diaphragm with a pleural effusion (f) loss of definition of the normal outline of the left kidney, and (g) indentation of the splenic flexure of the colon.[3] One or more of these signs are present in about 50% of patients with splenic trauma.[92] Fractures of the left transverse processes of the upper lumbar vertebrae should also suggest possible splenic injury.

Another frequent radiologic finding with splenic injury is free blood within the abdomen; however, at least 500-1000 ml of intra-peritoneal blood is often required to be evident on plain abdominal radiographs. Other radiograph findings supporting the presence of intraabdominal blood or fluid include; (a) the "flank stripe sign" which is a dense line separating the ascending and descending colon from the lateral peritoneal wall, with the colon displaced medially, (b) the "dog ear sign" resulting from accumulations of blood between the pelvic viscera and the side walls of the pelvis on either side of the bladder, and (c) the "hepatic angle sign" which is loss of definition of the usually distinct inferior and right lateral borders of the liver as blood accumulates between the liver and the right side of the abdomen. With extensive hemoperitoneum, the small bowel may float toward the center of the abdomen which may have a general "ground-glass" appearance.

AXIOM Although plain chest and abdominal radiographs may be highly suggestive, they are only occasionally specific for splenic injury.

Computed Tomography

Computed tomography (CT) of the abdomen with intravenous and upper GI contrast can play an important role in the evaluation of blunt abdominal trauma in the appropriate clinical setting.[110,114,117] It should be viewed as complementary to, and not competitive with, diagnostic peritoneal lavage (DPL).[3] DPL should serve as the primary triage tool in unstable patients when the etiology of the hypotension is unclear to determine the need for emergent laparotomy.[16] If the patient is or becomes hemodynamically stable and the lavage is positive or indeterminate, CT scanning has the potential to delineate injuries to specific organs, depending on the resolution of the CT scanning machine, the expertise of the radiologist, and the condition of the patient.

AXIOM A properly performed CT scan with intravenous and upper GI contrast often provides the best anatomic description of a splenic injury.

Abdominal CT scans are routinely performed with 100-150 ml of 60% iodinated intravenous contrast plus 300-1000 ml of oral Gastrografin or barium. A contrast enema can be added to identify colonic wounds in patients with penetrating injury to the back or flank.

Solid organ parenchymal lesions and extravasation of blood can often be detected with great accuracy. Splenic lacerations and transections appear as dense bands across the splenic parenchyma.[3] Recently, Schurr et al[118] have reported on the value of a new sign, a "CT vascular blush", to predict failure of nonoperative management. The vascular blush is defined as a well-circumscribed, intraparenchymal contrast collection which is hyperdense with respect to the rest of the splenic parenchyma. The authors believe that this represents a small false aneurysm that gradually enlarges and ruptures. Of the 17 patients (8.0%) who had this, none were treated nonoperatively with success.

Hiraide et al[119] recently reported a delayed rupture of the spleen caused by an intrasplenic pseudoaneurysm following blunt trauma. The initial CT and US showed a small effusion in the pouch of Douglas and in Morison's pouch. On the fifth day, US revealed a new round (1.5 × 2.0 cm) hypoechoic lesion in the spleen. CT identified the lesion as a slight contrast-enhanced cystic lesion. MRI clearly identified the lesion as an intrasplenic pseudoaneurysm which ruptured two days later. A splenorrhaphy was successfully performed at that time.

Subcapsular hematomas are often seen as low-density peri-splenic masses, and intraparenchymal injuries are frequently seen as intrasplenic accumulations of contrast (Fig. 23-3). Free intraperitoneal blood may be identified in the left pericolic gutter, Morison's pouch, or the pelvis. Some investigators feel that CT evaluation of splenic injuries allows them to identify high-risk patients who require early operation versus those who can be managed nonoperatively.[111]

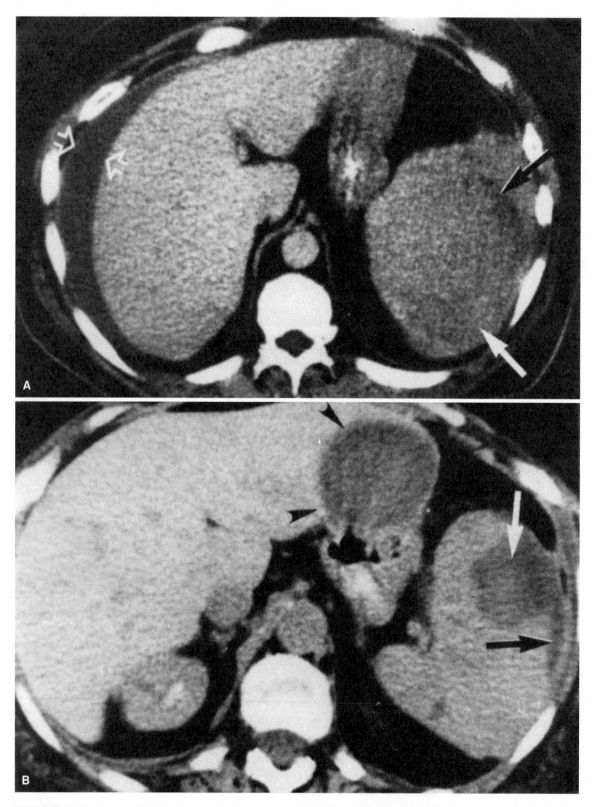

FIGURE 23-3 A. A repeat CT done 3 days after initial scan (because of abdominal pain and hypotension) shows intrasplenic rupture with a large subcapsular hematoma (solid arrows) containing partially clotted and liquefied blood. A large amount of fluid is present around the liver (open arrows). **B.** Repeat abdominal CT scan obtained 3 weeks later to investigate a left hepatic lesion noted by sonography revealed intrasplenic and subcapsular hemorrhage (arrows). A large low-attenuation mass present in the left hepatic lobe was thought to represent a delayed subcapsular hepatic hematoma (arrowheads). (From Pappas D, Mirvis SE. Crepps JT. Case report—splenic trauma: false-negative CT diagnosis in cases of delayed rupture. AJR 1987;149:727-728.)

CT scans can also assess the retroperitoneum and provide valuable information about the extent and configuration of acute pelvic fractures. Many surgeons believe than CT scans can (a) reduce the number of ancillary tests required for evaluation of traumatized patients, (b) provide accurate information regarding the extent and severity of solid-organ injuries, and (c) assist with decisions regarding the need for exploration versus nonoperative management.[115-117,120-122]

AXIOM   CT scans can provide excellent information about most intraabdominal organ injuries, except the pancreas and distal small bowel.

Unfortunately, there have been several reports suggesting that CT scanning of spleen injuries is not very accurate. Sutyak et al,[123] for example, reported that two radiologists disagreed on the grade of splenic injury in 6 (22%) of 27 scans. In addition, the CT injury grade matched the OR grading of the spleen injury in only three of 10 cases. In five cases the CT scan underestimated the injury and in two cases, it overestimated the injury found at surgery.

In a recent report by Kohn et al,[124] two radiologists (blinded to each patient's outcome), reviewed the CT scans of 70 patients with blunt splenic injury and graded them according to three published scoring systems. Interestingly, the higher grades of splenic injury were not associated with an increased risk of nonoperative failure, and three patients with very low splenic injury scores required urgent surgery. The ISS and age were much better guides to the success of nonoperative therapy than the severity of the injury seen on the CT scan. An increased ISS significantly increased the likelihood of failure of nonoperative management, and no failures occurred in patients less than 17 years of age. The authors concluded that properly selected patients can be safely observed regardless of the magnitude of the splenic injury seen on CT scan.

Additional criticisms of CT scans include their cost and their impractical application in patients requiring aggressive resuscitative efforts.[1] In addition, CT scanning often misses blunt pancreatic fractures and is unreliable for detection of small bowel injuries distal to the ligament of Treitz.

Radioisotope Scintiscan

In 1967, Little et al[125] described photoscanning with colloidal gold 190 to detect hepatic and splenic injuries after upper abdominal trauma.[3] Following that report, liver and spleen scanning with technetium-99m sulfur colloid was used increasingly as a reliable, noninvasive technique to delineate splenic parenchymal injury.[126-129] Following intravenous injection, technetium-99m sulfur colloid is phagocytozed by the reticuloendothelial cells of the liver and spleen.

Static images of the spleen are obtained from anterior, posterior, lateral, and oblique positions. Evidence of splenic injury includes focal areas devoid of radioactivity as well as overt splenic fragmentation (Fig. 23-4). The overall sensitivity of technetium splenic scanning for acute injury approaches 98% in some series.[130,131] False negative studies occur when the lesion is small or acutely evolving at the time of the examination.

False-positive scintiscans can occur in 3% of examinations on injured patients due to deep fetal lobulations in the spleen.[3] Direct comparisons of scintigraphy and CT scans for hepatosplenic trauma have found that scintiscans are superior with respect to sensitivity, but are less specific than CT scans in regard to grading splenic injuries, and obviously can not quantitate intraperitoneal hemorrhage. The ability to assess restless or uncooperative children is a major advantage of scintigraphy over CT scans.

Because the scope of radionuclide scans is limited to the liver, spleen, and kidney, it is better suited for the evaluation of suspected isolated solid visceral injury caused by mild-moderate trauma. CT scans, on the other hand, are preferred in patients sustaining severe trauma because it can evaluate both intraperitoneal and retroperitoneal structures.[132,133]

AXIOM   Scintiscanning is probably the most convenient, accurate method for following the process of healing in an injured spleen.

Radioisotope spleen scans are useful during healing and are indirect measures of residual splenic function. They have proved particularly valuable in the follow-up of nonoperatively managed patients and those undergoing partial splenectomy or splenorrhaphy.[134-136] A

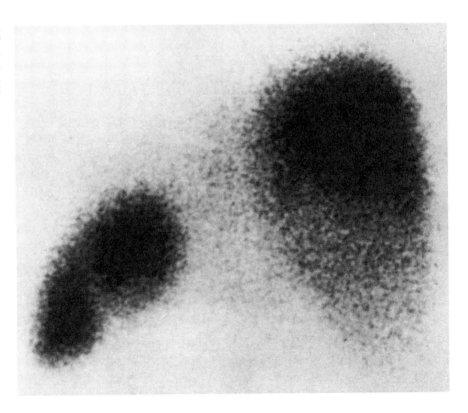

FIGURE 23-4   Posterior liver and spleen scan, demonstrating a small focal defect in the inferior pole of the spleen. This is consistent with either a splenic fracture or a fetal lobulation. (From Moore FA, Moore EE, Abernathy CM. Injury to the spleen. In Moore EE, Mattox KL, Feliciano DV, eds. Trauma, 2nd ed. East Norwalk, CT: Appleton-Lange., 1991; 471.)

major disadvantage in the evaluation of acute abdominal trauma is the time required for nuclear scanning and its qualitative limitation in assessing intraabdominal structures other than the liver and the spleen.[1]

Angiography

Before the introduction of radioisotopic scintiscanning and CT scans, angiography was necessary to localize splenic injury.[3] Angiographic findings in acute splenic trauma include nodular intraparenchymal extravasation, early venous filling, and splenic artery spasm. In some cases of intraparenchymal hemorrhage, there may be no extravasation of contrast, but one can see a mass effect with stretching of vessels or distortion of the normal splenic architecture (Fig. 23-5). With penetrating injuries, the splenic anatomy is less apt to be distorted, and the injury may be detected only by extravasation of contrast or arterial occlusion.

The reported sensitivity and accuracy of angiography for splenic injuries is high.[3] Haertel and Ryder,[113] for example, were able to identify splenic injury correctly in all 48 patients with this problem before surgery. Ward et al,[137] in a series of 123 abdominal angiograms, diagnosed 25 splenic injuries accurately. There was, however, one false-negative study, manifested by delayed rupture of the spleen at 12 days. Fisher and his associates[138] also formulated a classification of splenic injuries based on their arteriographic findings.

Currently, angiography is seldom performed for suspected splenic injury unless the patient already requires angiography for another problem such as a suspected traumatic transection of the aorta, diagnostic and therapeutic embolization of pelvic fracture bleeding, or peripheral vascular trauma. In patients requiring such arteriography, one should also assess the spleen, thereby avoiding unnecessary duplication of diagnostic effort. It has also been suggested that angiography is the best means of identifying CT-diagnosed splenic injuries that are actively bleeding and thus are candidates for operative intervention or therapeutic selective embolization.[111,139]

AXIOM Trauma patients having an arteriogram for possible injuries in the thoracic aorta, pelvis, or extremities should also have a splenic arteriogram if there is any chance that the spleen has been injured.

Ultrasonography

Ultrasonography (US) is an additional noninvasive diagnostic modality that can be useful in the assessment of splenic trauma.[1] It is becoming quite popular in European trauma centers because it can rapidly be brought to the patient's bedside in the E.D. and interpreted. Free intraperitoneal blood and splenic capsular disruption can often be identified, but limitations include a lack of specificity as well as decreased sensitivity when compared to other diagnostic measures, especially CT scans. In one controlled study comparing US to CT for abdominal trauma in children, US had an unacceptable false-negative rate of 50%.[132]

In contrast, in a recent report from Pisa, Italy, on the use of US in 250 consecutive cases of blunt abdominal trauma, using 250 ml of abdominal fluid as an indication for immediate celiotomy, Goletti et al[140] identified 29/31 (94%) of the splenic lesions present.

Diagnostic Laparoscopy

Recently, Townsend et al[50] have reported on the use of diagnostic laparoscopy as an adjunct to the selective conservative management of solid organ injuries after blunt trauma. Of 15 hemodynamically stable patients with solid organ injury documented on CT scan, nine had spleen injuries and eight had liver injuries. At diagnostic laparoscopy, occult hollow viscus injuries (one colon and one small bowel) were found in two patients. The diagnostic laparoscopy also revealed ongoing hemorrhage in four patients and poor visualization in one patient. These problems prompted laparotomy, which resulted in four splenorrhaphies and one hepatorrhaphy. Conservative management was employed in the remaining eight patients, all of whom had adequate hemostasis and no other injuries requiring a laparotomy.

In a recent experimental study in 20 dogs given hepatic and splenic injuries, Salvino et al[141] were able to control the bleeding by laparoscopic injection of fibrin glue into the parenchyma of the injured organs. All the animals did well, and there was no evidence of fibrin glue pulmonary emboli.

CLASSIFICATIONS OF SPLENIC INJURIES

A number of different classification schemes have been suggested for splenic injury.[1] Shackford et al,[142] with slight modifications by Feliciano,[31] developed one of the first detailed classifications of splenic

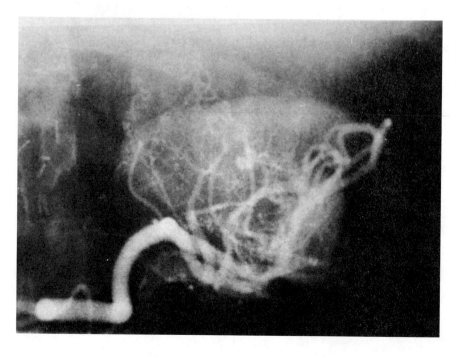

FIGURE 23-5 Selective splenic artery angiogram, demonstrating lack of lower pole vessels and intrasplenic extravasation of contrast. (From Moore FA, Moore EE, Abernathy CM. Injury to the spleen. In Moore EE, Mattox KL, Feliciano DV, eds. Trauma, 2nd ed. East Norwalk, CT: Appleton-Lange., 1991; 472.)

injury and attempted to correlate it with the type of treatment probably needed.

It has been suggested that splenic salvage should be achievable in 90-100% of mild (grade 1 and 2) injuries, 60-65% of moderate (grade 3) injuries, and 5-10% of severe (grade 4) injuries, with the ultimate success rate depending on the surgeon's experience, ingenuity, and persistence.[31]

Barrett and his associates[143] and Buntain and Lynn,[144] independent of one another, outlined remarkably similar classifications of splenic injuries based on CT findings. Each type of injury was also subclassified as an isolated splenic injury or with associated intraabdominal injuries (B1 indicated associated injuries involving a solid viscus, and B2 indicated an associated injury involving a hollow viscus. An E was added if there were associated extraabdominal injuries.

Splenic injuries have most recently been classified anatomically by the Organ Injury Scaling Committee of the American Association for the Surgery of Trauma (Table 23-3)[144] to reflect the impact of a specific injury on management decisions as well as patient outcome. This last classification will probably be the one used by most investigators in the future.

TREATMENT OF SPLENIC TRAUMA

Initial Management

The initial resuscitation and evaluation should be like that for any acutely injured patient.[3] Following spine immobilization in blunt trauma victims, assurance of airway patency, and provision of adequate ventilation and/or oxygen, efforts should be made to restore an adequate intravascular circulating blood volume.

HEMODYNAMICALLY UNSTABLE PATIENTS

Emergent celiotomy is clearly appropriate for acutely injured patients, regardless of age, who are actively bleeding as demonstrated by he-

modynamic instability in spite of resuscitative efforts. In patients with blunt trauma who have multiple potential sites of bleeding, DPL may be extremely helpful for confirming the clinical suspicion of intraabdominal bleeding.

Hemodynamically Stable Patients

Individual management of hemodynamically stable patients is based largely on the injury mechanism and its site (Fig. 23-10). Gunshot wounds to the anterior abdomen are routinely explored, while stab wounds can be selectively managed by local wound exploration and DPL. Penetrating injuries of the lower chest, with the exception of minor stab wounds, should probably also undergo DPL.

In patients sustaining major blunt trauma, DPL should be performed early, and a laparotomy should generally follow if the DPL is positive. However, if a CT scan shows that only the liver or spleen is injured and the DPL was positive only for an increased RBC count, nonoperative treatment may be attempted, especially in young children. If the CT scan shows a grade 4 or grade 5 injury or a vascular blush, Schurr et al[118] feel that the patient should have operative therapy.

Nonoperative Management

For many reasons, including the technical ease of splenectomy and old reports of nonoperative management of blunt splenic trauma resulting in mortality rates greater than 90%,[36] the prevailing attitude toward splenic trauma for many years was one of prompt surgical intervention.[1] In the late 1970s, once the risks of the asplenic state, especially in children, became better known, pediatric surgeons increasingly endorsed the concept of nonoperative management. The pioneering work of Upadhyaya et al[14] from Toronto, as well as other groups,[15,16] has shown that the majority of isolated splenic injuries in children heal without surgical intervention.

AXIOM Criteria for nonoperative management of pediatric splenic injuries documented by imaging techniques include: (a) hemodynamic stability, and (b) absence of serious associated intraabdominal injury.[3]

Although the Toronto group does not advocate laparotomy unless the estimated blood loss exceeds 40 ml/kg, others have adopted much lower blood loss criteria. In addition, anything which precludes a reliable abdominal examination, such as an altered level of consciousness, is an indication for prompt laparotomy. In the acute trauma setting, Rothenberg et al[17] use DPL as an adjunct to their nonoperative management protocol. Lavage indices suggesting other visceral injury, such as an elevated white blood count, amylase, or alkaline phosphatase in the effluent, warrant an immediate laparotomy.[3] CT scans of the abdomen can also be used to assist in the decision for continued nonoperative care.

Well over 1000 nonoperatively managed children with splenic trauma have been reported during the past two decades.[15,16,143,145-152] Although stringent criteria were not always well defined, there appears to be general agreement that less than 40 ml of blood/kg of body weight should be required over 24 hours to maintain hemodynamic stability.[56,87] If more blood is required, the patient should be explored and an attempt made to repair the spleen or salvage as much of it as possible without giving the patient an increased risk of bleeding. Published series now indicate that over two-thirds of children are successfully being managed nonoperatively without apparent significant risk or need for later surgery.[15,16,87,143,148,153]

While nonoperative therapy has become well established in the management of selected children with splenic injuries, application of this practice to adults remains less clear.[3] Initial reports by Morgenstern and Shapiro,[28] and Hebeler et al[19] were encouraging and several investigators[22,54,154] have independently published a cumulative experience with over 100 adult splenic trauma patients managed nonoperatively. This represented 24-38% of all adults with blunt splenic

---

TABLE 23-3 Splenic Injury Scale

	Grade	Injury Description	AIS 90
I.	Hematoma:	Subcapsular, nonexpanding <10% surface area	1
	Laceration:	Capsular tear, nonbleeding, <1 cm parenchymal depth	—
II.	Hematoma:	Subcapsular, nonexpanding, 10-50% surface area	2
		Intraparenchymal, nonexpanding, <2 cm in diameter	—
	Laceration:	Capsular tear, active bleeding; 1-3 cm parenchymal depth which does not involve a trabecular vessel	2
III.	Hematoma:	Subcapsular, >50% surface area or expanding; Ruptured subcapsular hematoma >2 cm or expanding; Intraparenchymal hematoma >2 cm or expanding	3
	Laceration:	>3 cm parenchymal depth or involving trabecular vessels	3
IV.	Hematoma:	Ruptured intraparenchymal hematoma with active bleeding	4
	Laceration:	Laceration involving segmental or hilar vessels producing major devascularization (>25% of spleen)	4
V.	Laceration:	Completely shattered spleen	5
	Vascular:	Hilar vascular injury which devascularizes spleen hematoma >2 cm expanding	5

From: Moore EE, Shackford SR, Pachter HL, et al: Organ injury: scaling: Spleen, liver, kidney. J Trauma 29:1664, 1989.

trauma seen at their respective institutions.[1] To date, standardized selection criteria have not yet been adopted for adults, but Mucha et al[22] noted a failure rate of 29% for nonoperative management early in their experience before specific selection criteria were defined.[22]

Unfortunately, the experience of others[18,20-25] with attempted nonoperative management of blunt splenic injury has been less favorable. Indeed, Malangoni et al[20] noted that nonoperative management of adult splenic trauma has uniformly failed in their hands.

AXIOM   Nonoperative management of adult splenic trauma appears to be most applicable to patients who have remained stable hemodynamically.

Even transient posttraumatic hypotension which responds rapidly to fluid resuscitation may indicate that operative intervention is preferable.[1] Mucha et al[22] noted seven adult patients who were only transiently hypotensive immediately after their injury and were intentionally treated nonoperatively; however, five (71%) of these patients subsequently required splenic surgery. Of the adults in whom nonoperative management was successful, none ever exhibited any hemodynamic instability.[22] In a recent series reported by Sutyak et al,[123] no patient had successful nonoperative management of a splenic injury if: (a) the ED systolic BP was less than 100 mm Hg, (b) the Glasgow coma score was less than 14, or (c) if the trauma score was less than 12.

Although some have accepted transfusion requirements of up to half of the estimated blood volume for nonoperative management of pediatric splenic injury, Mucha et al,[22] Luna and Dellinger[155], and Morgenstern and Shapiro[28], have independently established a maximum transfusion requirement of 2 or 3 units of blood for continued nonoperative management.[1] Patients with isolated mild-to-moderate blunt splenic injury are most apt to fulfill these criteria. Nevertheless, there can be no substitute for experienced surgical judgment and repeated careful examinations for assessing the magnitude of the total body injury, establishing priorities, and noting subtle signs and symptoms of other intraabdominal injuries that, by themselves, might demand operation.

AXIOM   If more than 2 units of blood are needed to maintain hemodynamic stability in an adult, nonoperative management of an isolated splenic injury should be terminated.

One of the most consistently voiced arguments against nonoperative management, in both adults and children, has been the reported high incidence of associated abdominal injuries.[28,56,81,95,96] Traub and Perry[95] noted serious concomitant intraabdominal injuries in 37% of their patients with blunt splenic trauma. Fisher et al[96] documented gastrointestinal disruption after blunt trauma to the spleen in 27% of their adult patients compared to 7% of the children.[27] Buckman et al,[98] however, found associated intraabdominal injuries requiring surgery in only 4.5% (2/45) of those with mild blunt injuries and in 15.5% (15/97) with more severe splenic injuries.

Another criticism promulgated by opponents of nonoperative management has been that splenic salvage is not successful in patients who fail observation.[3] This experience, however, is not uniform. In a multicenter prospective study sponsored by the Western Trauma Association (WTA), where nonoperative management was successful in 60 (83%) of 72 adults, seven (58%) of the 12 nonoperative patients who had surgery eventually were managed effectively with splenic preservation techniques.[18]

AXIOM   Attempted nonoperative management of an injured spleen does not necessarily decrease the chances of splenic repair if surgery is required later.

Another argument voiced against nonoperative management in adults has been the theorized decreased ability of injured splenic vessels in older patients to contract and/or retract sufficiently to stop bleeding.[28] Supporting the presumed difference in vascular integrity

is the fact that nonoperative management is more often successful in the pediatric age group.[1] Nevertheless, nonoperative management in selected adults has been well documented.[22,53,154]

A third argument against nonoperative management has been the need for prolonged hospitalization and restriction of the patient's physical activity.[1] This fact, however, is somewhat misleading because patients who require surgery for splenic injuries tend to have more severe trauma and more associated injuries that may account for much of the longer hospitalization and convalescence. Patients hospitalized and convalescing from long bone fractures or head injuries with minor, nonoperatively managed splenic injuries diagnosed by CT scan also do well and could be home much earlier if it were not for their other problems.[1]

Operative Management

INCISION AND INITIAL INTRAABDOMINAL MANEUVERS

Celiotomies for acute severe trauma are often performed via a midline incision started at the xiphoid process and continued inferiorly below the umbilicus.[3] In patients appearing late after injury with what is almost certainly an isolated splenic injury, a left subcostal incision may be preferred.

At the time of laparotomy, the initial step is a quick evaluation of the abdomen to identify life-threatening injuries.[1] After removing as much free blood as rapidly as possible, the surface of the spleen and then the liver should quickly be palpated for fractures or other defects that could be bleeding. Areas of obvious palpable injury should be packed, and then the remaining intraperitoneal structures should be rapidly examined to detect other major bleeding injuries. One should then palpate the aorta, preferably at the diaphragmatic hiatus, to estimate the adequacy of the systemic blood pressure. This should be compared with the anesthesiologist's ongoing assessment of vital signs.

AXIOM   In injured patients who remain in shock or have other life-threatening injuries, bleeding splenic injury is an indication for splenectomy.

One should not make an effort to save a significantly injured spleen if the patient is hemodynamically unstable after the initial resuscitation and/or has other life-threatening injuries. Attempts to save an injured spleen in such circumstances could result in a greatly increased mortality rate.

Splenic Mobilization

Except for extremely simple avulsions of the anterior capsule of the spleen, effective splenic repair demands a complete atraumatic mobilization to thoroughly assess the extent and severity of the injury.[1,28,87,132] The phrenicolienal and lienorenal ligaments are generally avascular, but the lienocolic ligament may contain sizeable blood vessels and the gastrolienal ligament contains the short gastric vessels (Fig. 23-1).

AXIOM   Gentle, adequate mobilization and exposure are the keys to safe and successful surgery on the spleen.

The stomach should be decompressed well with a nasogastric tube which may need to be adjusted to work more efficiently. Following careful manual extraction of any remaining blood and clot from the left upper quadrant, one should assess the spleen and the extent of any ongoing hemorrhage. The finding of either a totally shattered spleen or one avulsed from the splenic pedicle leaves the surgeon no alternative but to gain immediate control of the bleeding by manual compression of the splenic pedicle.[1]

If the spleen does not have to be removed rapidly, care must be taken to avoid making the already existing injury worse during the mobilization. Whenever possible, the lienocolic ligament, which may contain sizable vessels, is visualized and divided first after displacing the splenic flexure of the colon downward to visualize this area more clearly.

To visualize the phrenicolienal and lienorenal ligaments posteriorly, the left lobe of the liver is retracted to the right by an assistant, while the surgeon applies medial traction on the greater curve of the stomach and gastrocolic ligament. A moist laparotomy pad on the anterior surface of the spleen can help the surgeon move it anteromedially to allow better visualization of the peritoneum behind the spleen. The lienorenal ligament should be incised at least 2 cm from the spleen to prevent tearing of the splenic capsule[3] (Fig. 23-6). Once the incision in this ligament is started, its depth is best controlled by freeing it up for several centimeters at a time with a finger prior to cutting. The incision is continued into the phrenicolienal ligament, which should be divided around to the level of the esophagus.

Following complete division of the lienorenal and phrenicolienal ligaments, a plane can be developed posterior to the pancreas with its attached splenic artery and vein by blunt finger dissection. Care is taken to avoid injury to the underlying left kidney and adrenal gland[3] (Fig. 23-7).

The superior pole of the spleen frequently cannot be mobilized adequately without transection and ligation of the upper short gastric vessels. Extreme care is required to avoid catching the wall of the stomach in clamps while this is done because it can result in local necrosis and a subsequent gastric leak. The spleen should then be rotated medially up into the incision. If there is resistance to this maneuver, the stomach may have to be mobilized and further division of the lienocolic ligament may be required inferiorly.[3]

Once the spleen is adequately mobilized, it is helpful to place several large packs in the splenic bed to help support the elevated spleen. These packs also help to tamponade any oozing from small vessels that were cut while the spleen was being mobilized.

SPLENORRHAPHY

Indications

AXIOM Whenever possible, repair rather than splenectomy should be the goal of surgery to control bleeding from the spleen.

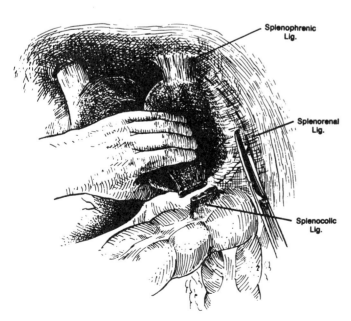

FIGURE 23-6 Techniques for transecting the ligamentous attachments of the spleen. (From Schwartz SI. Spleen. In Schwartz SI, Ellis H, eds. Maingot's abdominal operations, vol. II, 9th ed. East Norwalk, CT: Appleton-Lange, 1990;81:1692.)

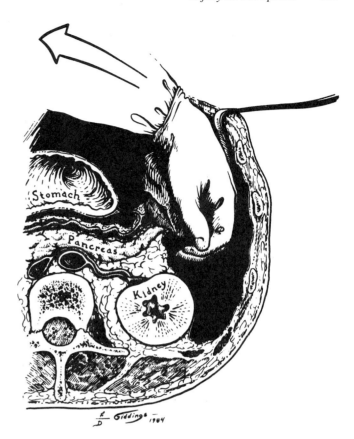

FIGURE 23-7 Mobilizing the spleen. Following complete division of the splenorenal, splenocolic, and splenophrenic ligaments, a plane is developed posterior to the pancreas with blunt finger dissection. Once mobile, the spleen is gradually rotated into the abdominal wound. (From Moore EE. Splenic injury. In Champion HR, Robbs JV, Trunkey DV, eds. Rob and Smith's operative surgery—trauma surgery, 4th ed. Boston: Butterworths, 1989;1:367.)

There is little disagreement today that if operative intervention is indicated for splenic trauma, splenorrhaphy, rather than splenectomy, is preferred;[1] however, this should only be done if the patient is hemodynamically stable, does not have other life-threatening injuries, and the splenic injury is not too severe to repair.

Topical Hemostasis

When a superficial avulsion has stopped bleeding spontaneously, no further treatment is required. If bleeding persists, several materials are available for topical control and include microcrystalline collagen (Avitene), Surgicel, Gelfoam, topical thrombin, and fibrin glue. If the surface bleeding persists after applying one or more of these agents with gentle pressure for 5-10 minutes, the procedure may be repeated. Most superficial injuries will stop bleeding with this technique. Electrocautery can sometimes be effective for one or two spot bleeders, but one must be very careful because it is easy to penetrate the splenic parenchyma with the cautery tip. Moore et al[3] and others have found the Argon Beam Coagulator (Bard Electro Medical Systems, Englewood, Colorado) to be very effective for controlling bleeding from superficial lesions of the spleen, liver and other organs. Others have advocated ultrasonic scalpels[156] or fibrin glue.[153,157-158] Currently, we have been using fibrin glue, which we make by mixing cryoprecipitate with thrombin and calcium just before application to the bleeding site.

Suture Techniques

Actively bleeding vessels in a parenchymal laceration are ligated or controlled with mattress sutures. Loose or devitalized tissue should be gently debrided, but this must be done with great care so as not to start more bleeding. Four basic suture techniques, alone or in combination, will usually manage most bleeding splenic lacerations. These include: (a) direct suture of the splenic parenchyma and capsule, preferably with horizontal mattress sutures using buttressing pledgets of omentum or Surgicel; (b) suture ligation of individual splenic vessels; (c) ligation of segmental vessels in the hilum; or (d) through-and-through absorbable mattress sutures incorporating the entire edge of the cut spleen.

Bleeding from fracture sites in the parenchyma should be controlled with direct suture ligature of the bleeding vessels whenever possible. Diffuse bleeding may require interlocking mattress sutures from one side of the spleen to the other. In children, the relatively thick capsule permits direct suturing, In the adult, pledgets are recommended to reduce the tendency for the horizontal mattress sutures to pull through the tissue. Moore et al[3] use 2-0 polyglycolic acid sutures and Teflon or collagen sheets for bolsters (Fig. 23-8). Absorbable bolsters or pledgets are preferred in patients who have associated gastrointestinal injuries, which may have contaminated the perisplenic area.

Grade III or IV splenic injuries require clear exposure of the hilar vessels to accomplish definitive control.[3] Further blunt dissection may be required medially between the pancreas and Gerota's fascia to obtain such exposure. This dissection must be carried out on the surface of the kidney, since manipulation close to the pancreas may injure the adjacent splenic hilum. If even better exposure is needed, one may have to divide the gastrolienal ligament completely by sequential clamping, cutting, and ligation of the short gastric vessels. To be sure that ties on the short gastric vessels do not come off when the stomach distends, we prefer to use 3-0 suture ligatures incorporating some gastric serosa.

Temporary control of the splenic artery is advisable for complex injuries with active bleeding. The artery usually follows a tortuous course on the superior margin of the pancreas, and it can be con-

trolled safely with a silastic vascular loop. Permanent splenic artery ligation, however, may be associated with a significant loss of immunologic function.[159] If the splenic artery cannot be found and/or dissected out readily, one may have to use a wide vascular clamp on the splenic hilum itself.

Some reluctance has been voiced about suture repair of the spleen because of the potential complications of (a) delayed rupture, (b) development of traumatic splenic cysts, and (c) abdominal splenosis; however, these problems have been virtually nonexistent following splenorrhaphy.[1] Dulchavsky et al[160] have demonstrated a higher wound breaking strength of suture-repaired wounds of the spleen in dogs and pigs as compared to uninjured sites. When measured 3 weeks postinjury, the wound-breaking strength appears to be the same for normal spleen, repaired spleen, and unrepaired but healed splenic injuries.

> **AXIOM**   After several weeks, an area of previous injury in the spleen appears to have more tensile strength than normal splenic tissue.

Partial Splenectomy
Complex splenic fractures with deep parenchymal lacerations often require a partial anatomic resection.[3] It is now clear that the spleen is composed of 4-6 segments, each of which has an autonomous blood supply based on segmental divisions of the splenic artery[46,56,111-161] (Fig. 23-9).

> **AXIOM**   In the absence of other life-threatening problems, an injured spleen that cannot be repaired should be considered for partial splenectomy.

To perform an anatomic partial resection of the spleen, the segmental arteries to the devascularized segments of the spleen are identified and ligated (Fig. 23-10). This should help demarcate the location of the avascular intersegmental plane in the parenchyma.[3] Any segmental veins that were not ligated and cut with the segmental arteries are now clamped, cut, and tied. The ischemic portion of the spleen can then be removed.

Dissection through splenic parenchyma must be done very gently. Some surgeons use a finger-fracture technique, but if the ischemic margin is clear, cautery may also be used. Any vessels identified in the retained cut surface of the spleen should be individually ligated with fine slowly absorbable sutures. Horizontal mattress sutures running from the capsule on one side to the capsule on the other side can help compress bleeding from the raw edges (Fig. 23-11). Such bleeding may also require topical hemostatic agents, especially fibrin glue. Ideally, when contemplating partial resection, one should try to retain at least a third, but preferably half, of the splenic mass along with its blood supply.[1]

> **AXIOM**   During partial splenectomies, one should attempt to save at least half of the spleen.

Splenic Artery Ligation
Splenic artery ligation, either alone or in combination with topical hemostatic agents and/or suture techniques, has been proposed for injuries causing continued bleeding in spite of other attempts at hemostasis and where the only other alternative would be a splenectomy.[162,163] If the short gastric vessels were divided at the time of splenic mobilization, the spleen will be almost completely devascularized and probably of little immunologic value.

Pabst et al[164] demonstrated experimentally in piglets that splenic artery ligation produced no evidence of infarction, and at 6 months the spleen maintained its normal size with enlarged vessels in the gastrolienal ligament. If the splenic remnant was left attached only to a ligated splenic artery, however, no obvious growth of the spleen could be demonstrated. Sherman and Asch[146] have reported similar findings in children.

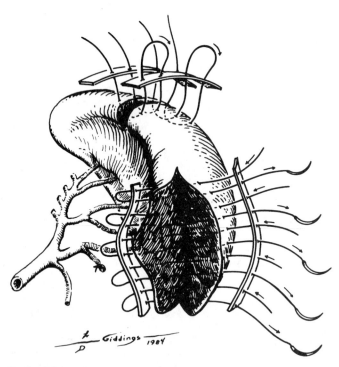

FIGURE 23-8   Splenorrhaphy. Deep parenchymal lacerations may require individual vessel ligation with transfixion sutures. Persistent bleeding from large defects may require interlocking mattress sutures. The thickened capsule in a child permits direct suturing, but in the adult, bolsters are often required. (From Moore EE. Splenic injury. In Champion HR, Robbs JV, Trunkey DV, eds. Rob and Smith's operative surgery—trauma surgery, 4th ed. Boston: Butterworths, 1989;1:370.)

FIGURE 23-9 The spleen has several autonomous vascular segments, based on
secondary divisions of the splenic artery.
In 85% of the patients, the splenic artery
bifurcates into two primary branches, supplying the superior and inferior lobes. The
splenic artery trifurcates in the remaining
15% of individuals. The feasibility of segmentectomy depends on the hilar architecture. This varies from early branching
(magistral type or "Y" configuration-30%)
to that occurring on the surface of the
spleen (distributed type or "T" pattern-
70%). (From Moore EE. Splenic injury. In
Champion HR, Robbs JV, Trunkey DV,
eds. Rob and Smith's operative surgery—
trauma surgery, 4th ed. Boston: Butterworths, 1989;1:371.)

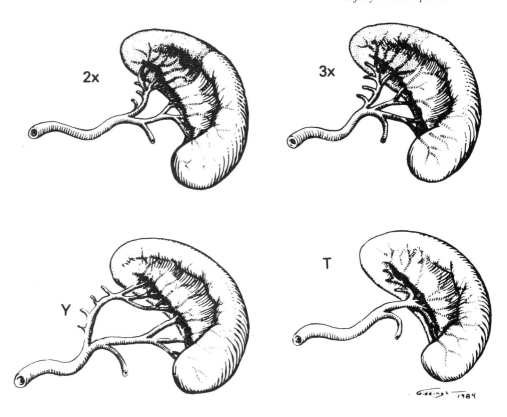

AXIOM   A spleen without a patent splenic artery or intact short gastric vessels is probably of little immunologic use to the patient.

Splenic Wrapping

Performing a splenorrhaphy in patients with delayed splenic hemorrhage can be extremely difficult at times. The spleen in such indi-

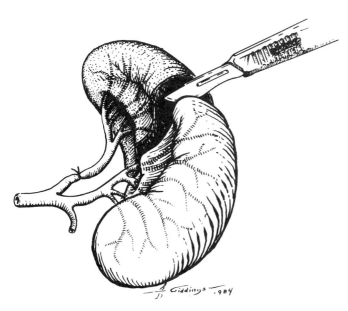

FIGURE 23-10 Hemisplenectomy. Segmental artery ligation will produce demarcation at an avascular intersegmental plane. Hilar disjunction is completed
by interruption of the respective segmental veins. The ischemic portion of the
spleen is then resected. (From Moore EE. Splenic injury. In Champion HR,
Robbs JV, Trunkey DV, eds. Rob and Smith's operative surgery—trauma surgery, 4th ed. Boston: Butterworths, 1989;1:371.)

viduals often has one or more deep parenchymal lacerations and an
expanding subcapsular hematoma that, when evacuated or ruptured,
leaves an extensive area of denuded, bleeding splenic pulp. Moore et
al[3] have successfully managed a number of patients with major de-
capsulating injuries by topical microfibrillar collagen application and
splenic wrapping. Self-made buttressing Vicryl ladders have also been
described as holding the injured spleen together and compressing the
bleeding surfaces.[1] Others have employed omentum or the falciform
ligament of the liver to wrap the spleen.[35] More recently, Delany et
al[149] and Lange et al[165] have employed commercial woven polyglycolic acid (Dexon) mesh like a hair net to hold the pulverized pieces
of spleen together.

To perform a splenic wrap properly, the spleen must be completely
mobilized (Fig. 23-12).[3] A window is fashioned in the mesh to accommodate the splenic artery and vein, and the spleen is enveloped by approximating the free edges of the mesh with absorbable suture. One
may also place hemostatic agents in selected spots to obtain better
control of localized bleeding. If some bleeding continues, localized
pressure on the spleen through the net should be continued. If the
bleeding will not stop, all or part of the spleen will have to be removed.

Complications of Splenorrhaphy

Although a major criticism directed toward splenorrhaphy has been
the additional time required for repair, several studies have revealed
relatively little difference in the time required for splenorrhaphy as
compared to splenectomy.[1,19,22,30,31,87,166] Similarly, there appears to
be no increased risk in regard to mortality and morbidity. In fact, patients who undergo repair often appear to have fewer complications
than those who had a splenectomy.

Nevertheless, one should not hesitate to abandon repair if, in the
surgeon's judgment, splenic hemostasis is inadequate. Finally, if one
cannot salvage at least one-third of the functioning splenic mass along
with its inherent vascular supply, splenorrhaphy should be abandoned.[1]

AXIOM   If bleeding is persistent, one should abandon prolonged efforts to repair or save a substantial part of an injured spleen,
especially in older patients.

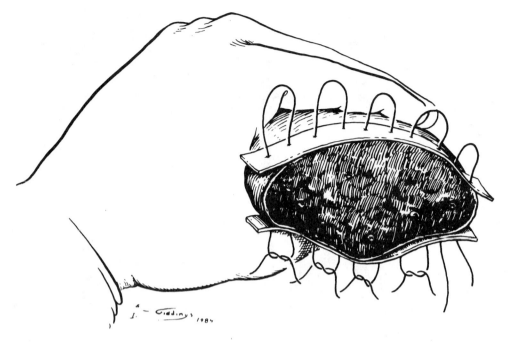

FIGURE 23-11 Closing the cut end of the spleen. The cut end of the spleen is sutured over pledgets while manual compression is maintained by an assistant. An alternative is to place the pledgeted sutures prior to resection of the devascularized segment. (From Moore EE. Splenic injury. In Champion HR, Robbs JV, Trunkey DV, eds. Rob and Smith's operative surgery—trauma surgery, 4th ed. Boston: Butterworths, 1989;1:371.)

SPLENECTOMY

Indications

Total splenectomy should be performed promptly if: (a) the spleen is pulverized, (b) the patient has other life-threatening injuries, or (c) hemostasis cannot be secured after splenorrhaphy or partial splenectomy.[3]

Technique

If the patient is not bleeding significantly or if the bleeding can be controlled by compressing the hilar vessels, the gastrolienal ligament should be taken down first. Division of the short gastric vessels should proceed carefully with sequential clamping, cutting, and ligation with suture ligation of the vessels on the gastric wall under direct vision.

AXIOM   Every effort should be made to avoid damage to the tail of the pancreas while ligating the splenic artery and its major branches in the hilum of the spleen.

Prior to clamping the splenic artery and vein, one should clearly identify the tail of the pancreas and its relationship to the splenic hilum. In 90% of the instances, it lies adjacent to the caudal part of the spleen and, therefore, is easily injured during splenectomy.[3] Theoretically, if conditions permit, the splenic artery should be clamped first and the spleen squeezed in an attempt to autotransfuse any splenic blood back into the circulation.[1] The splenic artery and vein should be ligated separately if possible to prevent later development of an arteriovenous fistula; however, this complication is quite rare, and it is not worthwhile spending much time to accomplish this. Most surgeons either suture ligate or doubly ligate the splenic artery and vein. If possible, one should avoid placing deep sutures to control iatrogenic bleeding from the tail of the pancreas and rely primarily on local pressure and topical hemostatic agents.

After splenectomy, two or three large packs are placed in the splenic bed in the left upper quadrant while the surgeon evaluates the remainder of the peritoneal cavity and performs any needed additional surgery. At the end of the operation, the packs in the splenic bed are removed and the area is inspected carefully. If any clotted blood is present, this is evidence of some ongoing bleeding, and all of the ligatures and all raw surfaces in the splenic fossa should be carefully reinspected.[1]

Autotransplantation

A consideration in any trauma patient requiring splenectomy is whether one should take time to autotransplant thin slices of the spleen.[1] Experimental studies have confirmed the viability of autotransplanted splenic tissue and also its capability of phagocytozing pneumococcal organisms and contributing to a higher level of antibody formation following pneumococcal vaccination.[57,58,167,168] It is doubtful, however, if such implants significantly reduce the incidence or danger of later OPSI.[1]

Several types and sites of autotransplantation[34,57,168-170] have been described. The most popular technique involves cutting the spleen into slices 3-5 mm thick. These are then strategically implanted into a pouch of greater omentum. Moore et al[29] have routinely reimplanted five fragments measuring 40 mm × 40 mm × 3 mm into a pouch of greater omentum. The fragments are secured with silk sutures and marked with radiopaque surgical clips. The omental pouch compartmentalizes the splenic fragment from the small intestine, theoretically preventing splenosis-induced small bowel adhesions.[171,172] Additionally, this site is preferred because of its portal venous drainage.

Several clinical reports corroborate the viability of splenic implants and indicate that the procedure is safe.[30,34,173] The implants regenerate after a period of necrosis[174] and in animal models, growth is progressive over 2 years.[175]

The suggestion that a critical spleen mass of 30-50% of normal is needed to ensure adequate function remains controversial. Cases of overwhelming sepsis reported in patients who have undergone autotransplantation[176] and following the natural phenomenon of splenosis[176] have suggested that preservation of enough splenic function to prevent OPSI appears to require both an inherent blood supply[159] and retention of at least one-third of the splenic mass.[177] In rats, some degree of immunologic protection is afforded with any splenic tissue, and there is an inverse linear relationship between the amount of tissue successfully transplanted and the subsequent susceptibility to infection.[168,170,178]

In the work of Velcek et al[160] on pneumococcal clearance, postimmunization pneumococcal titers for control in dogs who had splenic autotransplants were maintained well, while those in splenectomized animals were significantly depressed. Failure to demonstrate an immunologic advantage to the autotransplanted splenic tissue may be attributed to inappropriate route of bacterial inoculation.[3] Following aerosolized transtracheal *Streptococcus pneumoniae*, survival was

FIGURE 23-12 Wrapping an injured spleen. In patients with an extensive area of denuded splenic pulp, woven polyglycolic acid mesh may be particularly helpful in achieving secure hemostasis. Topical hemostatic agents are applied to the bleeding areas, and the entire spleen is wrapped firmly in the mesh. The spleen is completely mobilized, attached only by its hilar vessels. A window is fashioned in the mesh to accommodate the splenic artery and vein, and the spleen is enveloped by approximating the free edges of the mesh with polyglycolic acid sutures. (From Moore EE. Splenic injury. In Champion HR, Robbs JV, Trunkey DV, eds. Rob and Smith's operative surgery—trauma surgery, 4th ed. Boston: Butterworths, 1989;1:372.)

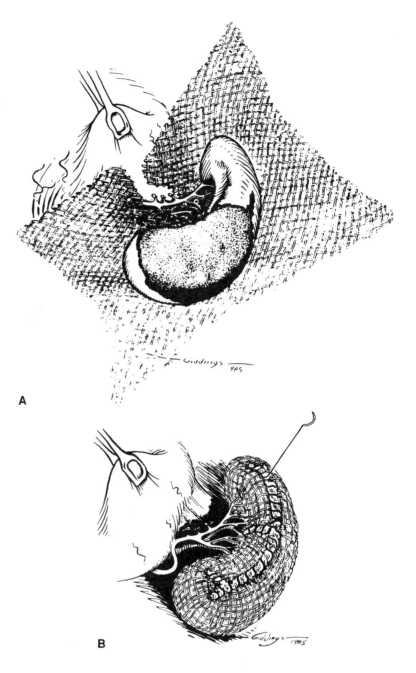

A

B

unquestionably enhanced in animals with splenic autotransplants;[179] however, this benefit was not as clear following an intravenous inoculation.[180]

AXIOM   Although splenic implants may be viable and may grow, it is not completely clear that they are of immunologic benefit to the patient.

While the data from some animal studies seem compelling, supporting clinical data are scant. In 1978, Millikan et al[29] found uniform viability of splenic implants by technetium scanning at 6 months, and this was associated with normalization of IgM levels and platelet counts. Patel et al[34] confirmed these findings, and they also noted the disappearance of target cells and Howell-Jolly bodies which are not usually present if the spleen is working normally. Traub et al[173] found on a 1-year follow-up that seven autotransplanted splenic patients who initially had 25-30 grams of tissue placed in a properitoneal position had at least intermediate reticulo-endothelial function. Moore et al[3] have also reported a case of fivefold growth of intraperitoneal splenic implants at 7 years. This patient survived an episode of pneumococcal sepsis with oral penicillin, suggesting some graft function. Histology also demonstrated normal splenic tissue.

The lack of complete preservation of splenic function has led many surgeons not to consider autotransplantation as a practical clinical alternative at this time. One concern might be a false sense of security.[1] In fact, evidence would suggest that patients who have undergone autotransplantation of splenic fragments should still receive Pneumovax and penicillin prophylaxis.

To date, there appear to be no significant adverse sequelae from autotransplantation as originally theorized, such as a propensity for bowel obstruction or spontaneous rupture of regenerated fragments. Nevertheless, at present, clinical application of splenic autotransplantation in humans must be considered experimental.

DRAINAGE OF THE SPLENIC BED

AXIOM Unless there is damage to the adjacent pancreas, splenic injuries should not be drained.

The question of routine drainage of the splenic bed following repair or removal of the injured spleen has been challenged by Cohn,[181] who demonstrated an 11-fold increase in complications when drainage was employed. If the splenic bed is dry and there is no concern about the pancreas or any other injuries in the left upper quadrant, one should not drain. If there is any concern, however, Pachter et al[182] have demonstrated that there are no apparent increased complications among patients drained with closed systems (Jackson-Pratt or Hemovac). Pachter et al[182] also noted that the type of drains and the length of time that the drains were left in place probably accounted for the high complication rates noted with them in earlier studies.

If drains are employed, they should be of the closed system type and should usually be removed within 72-96 hours, unless there is suspected pancreatic injury. If there is, the drains should not be removed until it is demonstrated that there is no drainage of amylase-rich fluid even after the patient is back on a regular diet. If there is no drainage at all from these drains, they should be moved slightly from time to time to make sure that they are not obstructed.

POSTOPERATIVE CARE

Nasogastric Tubes

Some surgeons maintain nasogastric tube decompression of the stomach for a minimum of five days to avoid distension of the stomach. In the past, there was some concern that gastric distension might cause ligatures on short gastric vessels to slip off or increase the tendency to leak from that area if a portion of the stomach had been caught in a clamp or tied too tightly with a deep suture-ligature.[1] At present, most surgeons see little need for prolonged gastric decompression unless there are associated pancreatic or gastrointestinal injuries or ileus. Indeed, the pulmonary and other complications related to prolonged nasogastric decompression probably far outweigh whatever benefits it provides. Mucha et al[1] recommend nasogastric decompression for only 36-48 hours, unless dictated by other injuries.

Serial Platelet Counts

The practice of routinely checking platelet counts at specific intervals following a splenectomy to recognize significant thrombocytosis as a guide for institution of prophylactic anticoagulation has fallen into disrepute.[1] Nevertheless, if the platelet count exceeds $10^6/mm^3$, we will start the patient on one baby aspirin (75 mg) per day by mouth or by rectum.[84,183]

AXIOM Post-splenectomy thrombocytosis probably does not require any treatment unless the platelet count exceeds a million/mm³. Then, 75 mg of aspirin daily is probably adequate prophylaxis.

Although not proven, hypercoagulability due to thrombocytosis may partially explain a higher incidence of eventual ischemic heart disease and carotid-occlusive disease in splenectomized patients.

Prophylaxis Against OPSI

AXIOM All patients having a splenectomy for trauma should probably be given pneumovax before they leave the hospital.

Patients who have had a splenectomy probably have an increased lifetime likelihood of developing overwhelming infections, particularly in the lungs.[3] Streptococcus pneumoniae (the pneumococcus) is cultured in over half of the serious infections developed by asplenic

individuals. The currently available vaccines (Pneumovax 23, from Merck and Pnu-Immune 23, from Lederle) contain 23 serotypes of pneumococci which account for 90% of the pneumococcal infections.[184] The antibody response to vaccination of an otherwise normal asplenic patient is nearly equal that of controls, but the duration of elevated titers is unknown.[82,185] Additionally, the concept that an antibody level greater than 300 mg/ml is protective against pneumococcal disease has never been documented in asplenic patients.[186] Routine vaccination with pneumococcal vaccine, however, seems reasonable in light of its low toxicity.[187]

The question of the timing of the administration of the pneumovac is controversial. Caplan et al[188] and others[189] recommend immediate vaccination following splenectomy. In their experience the antibody response to vaccination was the same whether the inoculation was immediate or delayed. Our tendency is to give the pneumovax on the day of discharge from the hospital and warn the patients that they will probably have a reaction with some fever within 5-10 days.

The ability of the body to make appropriate antibodies to the pneumococcal vaccine following splenectomy has been questioned, and it is generally agreed that there is a suppression of antibody response following major trauma, even without a splenectomy.[190] The need for revaccination is also unclear. Reports of severe Arthus reactions with the newer 23 valent vaccines have tempered enthusiasm for booster injections.[1]

AXIOM All post-splenectomy children under 2 years of age should receive long-term penicillin prophylaxis, and older children and adults should receive such prophylaxis before any invasive procedure and with almost any upper respiratory infection.

Since pneumococcal sepsis can occur despite vaccination, long-term oral penicillin prophylaxis has been recommended, especially in children under 2 years of age. A number of investigators also recommend penicillin prophylaxis for adults.[1,4-6,60,84-89] Unfortunately, the documented compliance rate with penicillin prophylaxis programs is probably less than 50%.[191,192] The alternative is administration of antibiotics at the first signs of any respiratory infection which causes fever, sore throat, or a cough. This approach is supported in animal models;[193] however, corroborating clinical evidence is sparse.[1] In any event, the patient and family should be educated concerning the risks of OPSI. If available, a Medic-Alert bracelet should be worn by splenectomized patients to alert health care providers of the increased risk for OPSI.

OUTCOME

Mortality Rate

The overall mortality rate for splenic injury at Detroit Receiving Hospital in a 12-year period (1980-1992) was 18% (61/345) (Table 23-4). The mortality rate in patients having non-operative therapy (5%=2/43) or splenorrhaphy (8%=12/151) was much lower than for the patients requiring a splenectomy (31%=47/151). The mortality rate also rose with the grade of splenic injury from 10% (23/227) for grade 1-2 injuries, to 26% (21/82) for grade 3 injuries, to 47% (17/36) for grade 4-5 injuries. The mortality rate was also higher for GSW (24%=31/131) than for blunt injuries (15%=26/172) or stab wounds (10%=4/42).

The mortality rate was influenced greatly by the number and type of associated injuries. The mortality rate with up to two associated injuries was 6.4% (12/185), but for three or more associated injuries, the mortality rate was 30.6% (49/160) (Table 23-5). The more lethal associated injuries and their mortality rates were: major vessels—56% (31/55), small bowel—43% (12/28), liver—34% (34/101), pancreas—33% (26/80), and pelvic fractures—33% (8/24).

TABLE 23-4 Mortality Rate Correlated With Grade of Splenic Injury and Type of Treatment

Treatment of Spleen	1	2	3	4	5	Total
Non-operative Rx	2 (18) 11%	0 (25) 0%	—	—	—	2 (43) 5%
Splenorrhaphy	7 (54) 13%	3 (84) 4%	1 (12) 8%	1 (1) 100%	—	12 (43) 8%
Splenectomy	4 (10) 40%	7 (36) 19%	20 (70) 29%	14 (33) 42%	2 (2) 100%	47 (151) 31%
	13 (82) 16%	10 (145) 7%	21 (82) 26%	15 (34) 44%	2 (2) 100%	61 (345) 18%

Postoperative Complications

Early morbidity after splenectomy or splenorrhaphy may be due to local infection, acute gastric distention, gastric necrosis, recurrent splenic bed bleeding, or pancreatitis.

INFECTIONS

AXIOM Patients who have had a splenectomy should be watched carefully for development of delayed infections in the left subphrenic space.

Patients who have had splenic repairs or resections have an increased risk of developing intraabdominal infections in the area of the spleen.[1] This is particularly true if there has been enteric contamination and use of any foreign material for bolsters, pledgets, or wrapping. Huizinga and Baker,[194] however, found that removal of an injured spleen did not increase the incidence of serious infective complications in the early postoperative period in patients with injuries to the spleen alone (n=262), to the colon alone (n=50), or to both (n=91).

AXIOM Peritonitis following ligation of short gastric vessels may be due to necrosis of a portion of the stomach by one of the ligatures.

Devascularization of the greater curvature of the stomach occurs only rarely with suture ligature of the short gastric vessels;[195] however, if the ligatures include too much tissue and are tied too tightly, these areas may necrose leading to a gastric leak.

AXIOM Left subphrenic abscesses from isolated splenic injuries are uncommon and are generally due to concomitant hollow viscus injuries.

TABLE 23-5 Mortality Rate Associated With Number of Associated Injuries

Number of Associated Injuries	Blunt	Penetrating	Total
0	2 (43) 5%	2 (10) 20%	4 (53) 8%
1	2 (48) 4%	1 (22) 5%	3 (70) 4%
2	4 (31) 13%	1 (31) 3%	5 (62) 8%
3	6 (29) 21%	7 (43) 16%	13 (71) 18%
4+	12 (22) 55%	24 (67) 36%	36 (89) 40%

Broad spectrum antibiotics are usually given for at least five days after a splenic injury requiring repair or resection. Any evidence of sepsis which is not clearly due to some other cause should make one suspect an infection in this area. CT scans or ultrasound examinations of this area can be quite helpful. If a fluid collection is found, it can be tapped percutaneously with radiologic guidance; however, most such collections are sterile.

ACUTE GASTRIC DISTENTION

Acute gastric distention occurs more commonly in children following splenectomy, and is prevented by frequent checks of the position and function of the nasogastric tube. A nasogastric tube which is not functioning properly increases the chances of the patient aspirating gastric secretions.

RECURRENT BLEEDING

AXIOM Early postsplenorrhaphy bleeding is usually due to technical problems.[30]

Recurrent intraperitoneal bleeding following splenic surgery is usually due to failure to adequately secure short gastric or splenic hilar vessels. Any evidence of active bleeding is an indication for a prompt exploration. Any coagulation abnormality should be corrected simultaneously with platelets or FFP as needed. A mild-to-moderate, progressive drop in hemoglobin levels, however, is not unusual in patients who have had multiple blood transfusions and are not bleeding.

Although the overwhelming majority of splenic injuries are well healed by 4-6 weeks, delayed hemorrhage has been reported as late as 45 days after the repair.[3,195] Adults are at greater risk of delayed hemorrhage than children. Interestingly, animal studies have demonstrated that the strength of the postsplenorrhaphy wound at 3 weeks exceeds the breaking strength of the normal spleen.[160] In patients who have undergone celiotomy, the collagen formation for midline laparotomy incision is much slower than for the spleen, and, therefore, activity levels are determined largely by the healing of the abdominal incision.

POST-TRAUMATIC PANCREATITIS

Pancreatitis following splenic surgery may occur either from operative trauma or from the initial injury itself. Intraoperative pancreatic trauma can be minimized by ligating the hilar vessels near the splenic capsule and avoiding any blind clamping or suturing in that area. If a pancreatic injury is suspected, the area should be drained until the patient is on a full diet and there is little or no drainage.

POST-SPLENECTOMY THROMBOCYTOSIS

Postsplenectomy thrombocytosis can occur up to 6 weeks following splenectomy, but the platelet count rarely exceeds $10^6/mm^3$. If the platelet count does exceed a million, there may be an increased risk of thrombotic complications, such as deep venous thrombosis or arterial emboli, and antiplatelet therapy with aspirin or Persantin is often recommended.[1]

SPLENOSIS

Splenosis occasionally results from the implantation and subsequent growth of fragments of disrupted splenic tissue upon various peritoneal surfaces and organs. Although splenosis is usually harmless, intestinal obstruction may occur if the implants on adjacent loops of bowel become adherent.[92]

Return to Normal Activity and Follow-up Examination

Patients who have been managed nonoperatively should have a CT or scintigraphy 3-4 weeks postinjury. If the scan shows a normal spleen with no disruptions, the patient may resume normal activity. If the scan shows a persistent defect, re-scanning should be done at 6-8 weeks and then monthly as needed. Patients should not return to full activity until complete healing of the spleen is confirmed.

If the patient has been doing well for 4-6 weeks and the spleen is well healed, he/she should be encouraged to return to full activity gradually over the next 2-3 weeks. If an injured spleen has been left in place, no contact sports should probably be allowed for at least 6 months.[56] Moore et al, however, say that once the CT scan demonstrates a normal spleen, physical-contact sports are acceptable.[3]

Asplenic Registry

Mucha et al[1] have recommended that institutions caring for trauma victims maintain an "asplenic registry." This may help splenectomized patients to be aware of the potential long-term consequences of splenectomy. Such a listing may also help the trauma center keep splenectomized patients aware of recent developments and remind them of the importance of seeking early medical attention for any illness, even if it seems to only be a mild "cold". Several institutions also routinely provide Medic-Alert bracelets for splenectomized patients.[1]

⊘ FREQUENT ERRORS

In Managing Splenic Injuries

1. *Failing to mobilize the spleen gently and adequately when attempting surgery on an injured spleen.*
2. *Too brief a period of observation of an individual who may have a splenic injury.*
3. *Inadequate search for associated injuries in a patient who has splenic trauma and is hemodynamically stable.*
4. *Assuming that a CT scan can reliably rule out associated injuries to the pancreas and/or distal small bowel.*
5. *Transfusing more than two-three units of bank blood in an effort to continue non-operative management of a splenic injury.*
6. *Inadequate attempts to treat iatrogenic splenic injury without resection.*
7. *Prolonged efforts to save a mild-to-moderately-injured spleen in an adult with other life-threatening injuries.*
8. *Allowing an unreliable patient to leave the hospital after a splenectomy without first receiving pneumovax.*
9. *Inadequate attention to "minor" respiratory infections in patients who have a splenectomy.*

▼▼▼▼▼▼▼▼▼▼▼▼▼▼▼▼▼▼▼▼▼▼▼▼▼▼▼▼▼▼

SUMMARY POINTS

1. The spleen is an important immunological organ, especially in children less than 2 years of age.

2. Although the risk of OPSI is only about 1-2%, it is many times higher than in non-splenectomized individuals, and the risk of death from OPSI is very high.

3. Surgeons performing a splenectomy for hypersplenism must look carefully for accessory spleens, which may be present in more than a third of such cases.

4. The anatomical division of the spleen's vasculature into four to six segments facilitates the performance of partial splenectomy after trauma.

5. Although reimplanted slices of spleen can revascularize and develop some splenic function, it is not yet clear how beneficial they are.

6. Although it is often harder to repair the injured spleen or save part of it in patients with liver disease, it is particularly important in such patients.

7. Asplenic patients have low levels of IgM, properdin, and tuftsin, and these deficiencies contribute to an increased susceptibility to OPSI.

8. Patients with lower respiratory infections, particularly by encapsulated organisms, are particularly likely to develop overwhelming post-splenectomy infections (OPSI).

9. The incidence of severe sepsis after splenectomy is only about 0.5-2.0%, but this is up to 200 times more frequent than in patients with normal spleens.

10. Most early deaths in patients with splenic trauma are due to associated injuries.

11. An enlarged spleen is much more susceptible to accidental trauma than a normal spleen.

12. If there is evidence of a splenic injury, one must look carefully for associated intraabdominal injuries, especially in adults, before considering nonoperative treatment in hemodynamically stable adults.

13. Virtually all patients with acute penetrating splenic trauma should have a surgical exploration because of the high incidence of associated injury requiring treatment.

14. Delayed rupture of the spleen is usually only a delayed diagnosis of a significant splenic injury.

15. Any patient with an injured spleen that has been observed or repaired should be aware of the possibility of a delayed splenic rupture.

16. Children, in contrast to adults, may have a severe splenic injury with little or no evidence of chest or abdominal wall trauma.

17. Any patient who has had significant trauma to the abdomen should be observed for at least 24-48 hours, with frequent, careful examinations.

18. Splenic injury should be suspected in patients with abdominal trauma if the patient has a falling hematocrit and/or abruptly rising WBC or platelet count.

19. Delayed recognition of splenic injury is one of the most common causes of preventable death following blunt trauma.

20. An RBC count >100,000/mm^3 in the DPL fluid is positive for intraabdominal bleeding, but it does not necessarily mean that a laparotomy is required, especially in children.

21. DPL and CT scans should be viewed as complementary, and not competing, examinations in patients with suspected intraabdominal injuries.

22. Although plain chest and abdominal radiographs may be suggestive, they are only occasionally specific for splenic injury.

23. A properly performed CT scan with intravenous and upper GI contrast often provides the best anatomic description of a splenic injury.

24. CT scan can provide excellent information about most intraabdominal organ injuries, except the pancreas and distal small bowel.

25. Scintiscanning is probably the most convenient, accurate method for following the progress of healing in an injured spleen.

26. Trauma patients having an arteriogram for possible injuries in the thoracic aorta, pelvis, or extremities should also have a splenic arteriogram if there is any chance that the spleen has been injured.

27. Criteria for nonoperative management of pediatric splenic injuries documented by imaging techniques include: (a) hemodynamic stability, and (b) absence of serious associated intraabdominal injury.

28. Nonoperative management of adult splenic trauma appears to be most applicable to patients who have remained stable hemodynamically.

29. If more than 2 units of blood are needed to maintain hemodynamic stability in an adult, nonoperative management of an isolated splenic injury should be terminated.

30. Attempted nonoperative management of an injured spleen does not necessarily decrease the chances of splenic repair if surgery is required later.

31. In injured patients who remain in shock or have other life-threatening injuries, a bleeding splenic injury is an indication for splenectomy.

32. Gentle, adequate mobilization and exposure are the keys to safe and successful surgery on the spleen.

33. Whenever possible, repair rather than splenectomy should be the goal of surgery to control bleeding from the spleen.

34. After several weeks, an area of previous injury in the spleen appears to have more tensile strength than normal splenic tissue.

35. In the absence of other life-threatening problems, an injured spleen that cannot be repaired should be considered for partial splenectomy.

36. During partial splenectomies, one should attempt to save at least half the spleen.

37. A spleen without a patent splenic artery or intact short gastric vessels is probably of little immunologic use to the patient.

38. If bleeding is persistent, one should abandon prolonged efforts to repair or save a substantial part of an injured spleen, especially in older patients (> 55 years).

39. Every effort should be made to avoid damage to the tail of the pancreas while ligating the splenic artery and its major branches in the hilum of the spleen.

40. Although splenic implants may be viable and may grow, it is not completely clear that they are of an immunologic benefit to the patient.

41. Unless there is damage to the adjacent pancreas, splenic injuries should not be drained.

42. Postsplenectomy thrombocytosis probably does not require any treatment unless the platelet count exceeds a million/mm^3. Then, 75 mg of aspirin daily is probably adequate prophylaxis.

43. All patients having a splenectomy for trauma should probably be given pneumovax before they leave the hospital.

44. All postsplenectomy children under 2 years of age should receive long-term penicillin prophylaxis, and older children and adults should receive such prophylaxis before any invasive procedure and with almost any upper respiratory infection.

45. Any patient who has had a splenectomy should be watched carefully for development of delayed infections in the left subphrenic space.

46. Peritonitis following ligation of short gastric vessels may be due to necrosis of a portion of the stomach by one of the ligatures.

47. Left subphrenic abscesses from isolated splenic injuries are uncommon and are generally due to concomitant hollow viscus injuries.

48. Early postsplenorrhaphy bleeding is usually due to a technical error.

▲▲▲▲▲▲▲▲▲▲▲▲▲▲▲▲▲▲▲▲▲▲▲▲▲▲▲▲▲▲

REFERENCES

1. Mucha P Jr, Buntain WL. Spleen injuries. In Kreis DJ, Gomez GA, eds. Trauma management. Boston: Little, Brown & Co., 1989; 194-215.

2. Sherman R. Perspectives in management of trauma to the spleen: 1979 Presidential Address, American Association for the Surgery of Trauma. J Trauma 1980;20:1.

3. Moore FA, Moore EE, Abernathy CM. Injury to the spleen. In Moore EE, Mattox KL, Feliciano DV, eds. Trauma, 2nd ed. East Norwalk, CT: Appleton-Lange, 1991;30:465-483.

4. King H, Shumacker HB Jr. Splenic studies: I. susceptibility to infection after splenectomy performed in infancy. Ann Surg 1952;136:239.

5. Singer DB. Postsplenectomy sepsis. In Rosenberg HS, Bolande RP, eds. Perspectives in pediatric pathology. Chicago Year Book, 1973; 1:285.

6. Diamond LK. Splenectomy in childhood and the hazard of overwhelming infection. Pediatrics 1969;43:886.

7. O'Neal BJ, McDonald JC. The risk of sepsis in the asplenic adult. Ann Surg 1981;194:775.

8. Zarrabi MH, Rosner F. Serious infections in adults following splenectomy for trauma. Arch Intern Med 1984;144:1421.

9. Schwartz PE, Sterioff S, Mucha P, et al. Postsplenectomy sepsis and mortality in adults. JAMA 1982;248:2279.

10. Sekikawa T, Shatney CH. Septic sequelae after splenectomy for trauma in adults. Am J Surg 1983;145:667.

11. Malangoni MA, Dillon LD, Klamer TW, et al. Factors influencing the risk of early and late serious infection in adults after splenectomy for trauma. Surgery 1984;96:775.

12. Green JB, Shackford SR, Sise MJ, et al. A prospective analysis of late septic complications in adult patients following splenectomy for trauma. J Trauma 1986;26:999.

13. Powell RW, Blaylock WE, Hoff CJ, et al. The efficacy of postsplenectomy sepsis prophylactic measures: the role of penicillin. J Trauma 1988;28:1285.

14. Upadhyaya P, Simpson JS. Splenic trauma in children. Surg Gynecol Obstet 1968;126:781.

15. King DR, Lobe TE, Haase GM, et al. Selective management of injured spleen. Surgery 1981;90:677.

16. Kakkasseril JB, Steward D, Cox JA, et al. Changing treatment of pediatric splenic trauma. Arch Surg 1982;117:758.

17. Rothenberg S, Moore EE, Marx JA, et al. Selective management of blunt abdominal trauma in children. The triage role of peritoneal lavage. J Trauma 1987;27:1101.

18. Cogbill TH, Moore EE, Jurkovich GJ, et al. Nonoperative management of blunt splenic trauma. A multicenter experience. J Trauma 1989; 29:1312.

19. Hebeler RF, Ward RE, Miller PW, et al. The management of splenic injury. J Trauma 1982;22:492.

20. Malangoni MA, Levin AW, Droege EA, et al. Management of injury to the spleen in adults. Ann Surg 1984;200:702.

21. Mahon PA, Sutton JE. Nonoperative management of adult splenic injury due to blunt trauma: a warning. Am J Surg 1985;149:716.

22. Mucha P, Daly RC, Farnel MB. Selective management of blunt splenic trauma. J Trauma 1986;26:970.

23. Nallathambi MN, Ivatury RR, Wapnir I, et al. Nonoperative management versus early operation for blunt splenic trauma in adults. Surg Gynecol Obstet 1988;166:252.

24. Longo WE, Baker CC, McMillen MA, et al. Nonoperative management of adult blunt splenic trauma. Ann Surg 1989;210:626.

25. Elmore JR, Clark DE, Isler RJ, et al. Selective nonoperative management of blunt splenic trauma in adults. Arch Surg 1989;124:581.

26. Lucas CE. Splenic trauma: choice of management. Ann Surg 1991; 213:98.

27. Kram HB, Shoemaker WC, Clark SL, et al. Techniques of splenic preservation using fibrin glue. J Trauma 1990;30:97.

28. Morgenstern L, Shapiro S. Techniques of splenic conservation. Arch Surg 1979;114:449.

29. Millikan JS, Moore EE, Moore GE, et al. Alternative to splenectomy in adults after trauma. Am J Surg 1982;144:711.

30. Moore FA, Moore EE, Moore GE, et al. Risk of splenic salvage following trauma: analysis of 200 adults. Am J Surg 1984;148:800.

31. Feliciano DV, Bitondo CG, Mattox KL, et al. A four year experience with splenectomy versus splenorrhaphy. Ann Surg 1985;201:568.

32. Delany HM, Porreca F, Mitsudo S, et al. Splenic capping: an experimental study of a new technique for splenorrhaphy using woven polyglycolic acid mesh. Ann Surg 1982;196:187.

33. Pichardt B, Moore EE, Moore FA, et al. Operative splenic salvage in adults: a decade perspective. J Trauma 1989;29:1386.

34. Patel J, Williams JS, Shmigel B, et al. Preservation of splenic function by autotransplantation of traumatized spleen in man. Surgery 1981; 90:683.

35. Reigner O. Ueber einen fall von exstirpation der traumatisach zerrissenen milz. Berl Klin Wochenschr 1893;50:177.

36. Berger E. Die verletzunger der milz und ihre chirurgische behandling. Arch Klin Chir 1902;68:56.

37. Foster JM Jr, Prey D. Rupture of the spleen: an analysis of twenty cases. Am J Surg 1912;1:157.

38. Bland-Sutton J. Observation on the surgery of the spleen. Br J Surg 1912;1:157.

39. Morris DH, Bullock FD. The importance of the spleen in resistance to infection. Ann Surg 1919;70:153.

40. Huntley CC. Infection following splenectomy in infants and children. A review of the experience at Duke Hospital in infants and children during a twenty-two year period (1933-1954). Am J Dis Child 1958; 95:477.

41. Horan M, Colebatch JJ. Relation between splenectomy and subsequent infection: a clinical study. Arch Dis Child 1962;37:398.

42. Eraklis AJ, Filler RM. Splenectomy in childhood: a review of 1413 cases. J Pediatr Surg 1972;4:382.

43. Michels NA, ed. Blood supply and anatomy of the upper abdominal organs. Philadelphia: Lippincott-Raven, 1955; 210.

44. Nguyen HH, Person H, Hong R, et al. Anatomical approach to vascular segmentation of the spleen (lien) based on controlled experimental partial splenectomies. Anat Clin 1982;4:265.

45. Whitesell FB Jr. A clinical and surgical anatomic study of rupture of the spleen due to blunt trauma. Surg Gynecol Obstet 1960;110:750.

46. Campos CH. Segmental resections of the spleen. O Hospital (Rio de Janeiro) 1961;62:187.

47. Gupta CD, Gupta SC, Arora AK, Jeya SP. Vascular segments in the human spleen. J Anat 1976;12:613.

48. Silverstein ME, Chvapil M. Experimental and clinical experiences with collagen fleece as a hemostasis agent. J Trauma 1981;21:288.

49. Jalovec LM, Boe SB, Wyffels PL. The advantages of early operation with splenorrhaphy versus non-operative management for the blunt splenic trauma patient. Am Surg 1993;59:698.

50. Townsend MC, Flancbaum L, Choban PS, et al. Diagnostic laparoscopy as an adjunct to selective conservative management of solid organ injuries after blunt abdominal trauma. J Trauma 1993;35:647.

51. Clark ER. The spleen. In Schaeffer JP, ed. Morris' human anatomy, 11th ed. New York: The Blakiston Co., 1953; 892-897.

52. William PL, Warwick R. Gray's anatomy, 36th ed. Philadelphia: WB Saunders, 1980; 773-779.

53. Gross P. Zur kindlichen traumatischen milzruptur. Beitr Klin Chir 1965;208:396.

54. Mazel MS. Traumatic rupture of the spleen with special reference to its characteristics in young children. J Pediatr 1945;26:82.

55. Huu N, Person H, Hong R, et al. Anatomical approach to the vascular segmentation of the spleen (lien) based on controlled experimental partial splenectomies. Anat Clin 1982;4:265.

56. Buntain WL, Lynch FP, Ramenofsky ML. Management of the acutely injured child. In Maull KI, ed. Advances in trauma. Chicago Year Book, 1987;II:43-86.

57. Cooney DR, Swanson SE, Dearth JC, et al. Heterotrophic splenic autotransplantation in prevention of overwhelming postsplencetomy infection. J Pediatr Surg 1979;14:336.

58. Fasching MD, Cooner DR. Reimmunization and splenic autotransplantation: a long-term study of immunologic response and survival following pneumococcal challenge. J Surg Res 1980;28:449.

59. Scher KS, Scott-Conner C, Jones CW, et al. Methods of splenic preservation and their effect on clearance of pneumococcal bacteremia. Ann Surg 1985;202:595.

60. Sullivan JL, Ochs HD, Schiffman G, et al. Immune response after splenectomy. Lancet 1978;1:178.

61. Wilkelstein JA, Lambert GH. Pneumococcal serum opsonizing activity in splenectomized children. Pediatrics 1975;87:430.

62. Chaimoff C, Douer D, Pick IA, et al. Serum immunoglobulin changes after accidental splenectomy in adults. Am J Surg 1978;136:332.

63. Likhite VV. Opsonin and leukophilic gamma-globulin in chronically splenectomized rats with and without heterotopic autotransplanted splenic tissue. Nature 1975;253:742.

64. Najjar VA, Nishioka K. Tuftsin. A physiological phagocytosis-stimulating peptide. Nature 1970;228:672.

65. Constantopoulos A, Najjar VA, Smith JW. Tuftsin deficiency: a new syndrome with defective phagocytosis. J Pediatr 1972;80:564.

66. Carlisle HN, Saslaw S. Properdin levels in splenectomized patients. Proc Soc Exp Biol Med 1959;102:150.

67. Zoli G, Corazza GR, D'Amato G, et al. Splenic autotransplantation after splenectomy: tuftsin activity correlates with residual splenic function. Br J Surg 1994;81:716.

68. Amsbaugh DF, Prescott B, Baker PJ. Effect of splenectomy on the expression of regulatory T cell activity. J Immunol 1978;121:1483.

69. Ford WL, Smith ME. Lymphocyte recirculation between the spleen and the blood. In Role of the spleen in the immunology of parasitic diseases. Basel: Schwabe, 1979; 290-341.

70. Sy MA. Splenic requirement for the generation of suppressor T-Cells. J Immunol 1977;119:2095.

71. Wells WL, Basttisto JR. Splenic regulation of humoral and cellular immunological responses in other domains. In Role of the spleen in the immunology of parasitic diseases. Basel: Schwabe, 1979; 59-84.

72. Bogart D, Bigger WD, Good RA. Impaired intravascular clearance of pneumococcus type-3 following splenectomy. J Reticuloendothel Soc 1972;11:77.

73. Whitaker AN. Effect of pervious splenectomy on the course of pneumococcal bacteremia in mice. J Pathol Bacteriol 1968;95:357.

74. Church JA, Mahour GH, Lipsey AI. Antibody response after splenectomy and splenic autotransplantation in rats. J Surg Res 1981;31:343.

75. Herbert JC. Pulmonary antipneumococcal defenses after hemisplenectomy. J Trauma 1989;29:1217.

76. Hosesa SW, Brown EJ, Hamburger ML, et al. Opsonic requirements for intracellular clearance after splenectomy. N Engl J Med 1981;304:245.

77. Chu DZJ, Nichoika K, K El-Hagin T, et al. Effects of tuftsin on postsplenectomy sepsis. Surg 1985;97:701.

78. Constantopoulos A, Najjar VA, Wish JB, et al. Defective phagocytosis due to tuftsin deficiency in splenectomized subjects. Am J Dis Child 1973;125:663.

79. Downey EC, Catanzaro A, Ninnemann JC, et al. Long term depressed immunocompetence of patients splenectomized for trauma. Surg Forum 1980;29:41.

80. Durig M, Landmann RMA, Harder F. Lymphocyte subsets in human peripheral blood after splenectomy and autotransplantation of splenic tissue. J Lab Clin Med 1984;104:110.

81. Downey EC, Shackford SR, Fridlund PH, et al. Long-term depressed immune function in patients splenectomized for trauma. J Trauma 1987; 27:661.

82. Sullivan JL, Ochs HD, Schiff G. Immune response after splenectomy. Lancet 1987;1:181.

83. Sieber G, Breyer HG, Herrman F, et al. Abnormalities or B-cell activation and immunoregulation in splenectomized patients. Immunobiology 1985;169:263.

84. Gill PG, Deyoung NJ, Kiroff GK, et al. Monocyte antibody-dependent cellular cytotoxicity in splenectomized subject. J Immunol 1984;132: 1244.

85. Lau HT, Hardy MA, Altman RP. Decreased pulmonary alveolar macrophage bacterial activity in splenectomized rats. J Surg Res 1983;34:568.

86. Hull CC, Galloway P, Gordon NC, et al. Splenectomy and the induction of murine colon cancer. Arch Surg 1988;123:462.

87. Buntain WL, Could HR. Splenic trauma in children and technique of splenic salvage. World J Surg 1985;9:398.

88. Francke EL, Neu HC. Post splenectomy infection. Surg Clin North Am 1981;61:135.

89. Holschneider AM, Kreiz-klimeck H, Strasser B, et al. Complications of splenectomy in childhood. Z Kinerchir. 1982;35:130.

90. Llende M, Shumaker HB. Splenic studies: I. susceptibility to infection after splenectomy performed in infancy. Ann Surg. 1952;136:239.

91. Robinette CD. Splenectomy and subsequent mortality in veterans of the 1939-45 wars. Lancet 1977;2:127.

92. Walt AJ, Wilson RF. Specific abdominal injuries. In Management of trauma: pitfalls and practice. Walt AJ, Wilson RF, eds. Philadelphia: Lea & Febiger, 1975;23:348-374.

93. Naylor R, Coln D, Shires GT. Morbidity, mortality and injuries to the spleen. J Trauma 1974;14:773.

94. Schwartz SI. Spleen. In SI Schwartz, et al, eds. Principles of surgery. New York: McGraw-Hill, 1974; 1281.

95. Traub AC, Perry JR Jr. Injuries associated with splenic trauma. J Trauma 1981;21:840.

96. Fisher RP, Miller-Crotchett P, Reed RL. Gastrointestinal disruption: the hazard of nonoperative management with blunt abdominal injury. J Trauma 1988;28:1445.

97. Livingston CD, Sirinek KR, Levine BA, et al. Traumatic splenic injury: its management in a patient population with a high incidence of associated injury. Arch Surg. 1982;117:670.

98. Buckman RF Jr, Piano G, Dunham CM, et al. Major bowel and diaphragmatic injuries associated with blunt spleen or liver rupture. J Trauma 1988;28:1317.

99. Benjamin CI, Engrav LH, Perry JF. Delayed rupture or delayed diagnosis of rupture of the spleen. Surg Gynecol Obstet 1976;142:171.

100. Berlatzky Y, Shiloni E, Anner H, et al. "Delayed rupture of the spleen" or delayed diagnosis of the splenic injury? Isr J Med Sci 1980;16:659.

101. Kluger Y, Paul DB, Raves JJ, et al. Delayed rupture of the spleen—myths, facts, and their importance: case reports and literature review. J Trauma 1994;36:568.

102. Balance CA. On splenectomy for rupture without external wound. Practitioner 1898;60:347.

103. Baudet R. Ruptures de la rate. Medicine Practique 1907;3:565.
104. McIndoe AH. Delayed hemorrhage following traumatic rupture of the spleen. Brit J Surg 1931;20:249.
105. Olsen WR, Polley TZ Jr. A second look at delayed splenic rupture. Arch Surg 1977;112:422.
106. Zabinski EJ, Harkins NH. Delayed splenic rupture: a clinical syndrome following trauma. Arch Surg 1943;46:180.
107. Foster RP. Delayed hemorrhage from the ruptured spleen. Brit J Surg 1970;57:189.
108. Bonder E. Eim beitrag zur traumatischem zweizeitigen milzruptur. Zertralbl Clin 1973;98:150.
109. Benjamin CL, Engrav LH, Perry JF Jr. Delayed rupture or diagnosis of rupture of the spleen. Surg Gynecol Obstet 1976;142:171.
110. Ayala LA, et al. Occult rupture of the spleen. Ann Surg 1974;179:472.
111. Buntain WL, Could HR, Maull KI. Predictability of splenic salvage by computed tomography. J Trauma 1988;28:24.
112. Root HD, Houser CW, McKinley CR, et al. Diagnostic Peritoneal Lavage Surgery 1965;57:633.
113. Haertel M, Ryder D. Radiologic investigation of splenic trauma. Cardiovasc Radio 1979;2:27.
114. Federle MP, Crass RA, Jeffrey RB, et al. Computed tomography in blunt abdominal trauma. Arch Surg 1982;117:654.
115. Jeffrey RB, Laing FC, Federle MP, et al. Computed tomography of splenic trauma. Radiology 1981;141:729.
116. Marx JA, Moore EE, Jorden RC, et al. Limitations of computed tomography in the evaluation of acute abdominal trauma: prospective randomized study. J Trauma 1985;25:993.
117. Goldstein AS, Sclafani SJA, Kupferstein NH, et al. The diagnostic superiority of computerized tomography. J Trauma 1985;25:938.
118. Schurr MJ, Fabian TC, Woodman G, et al. Management of blunt splenic trauma: CT vascular blush predicts failure of nonoperative management. J Trauma 1994;37:164.
119. Hiraide A, Yamamoto H, Yahata K, et al. Delayed rupture of the spleen caused by an intrasplenic pseudoaneurysm following blunt trauma: case report. J Trauma 1994;36:743.
120. Fuchs WA, Robbotti G. The diagnostic impact of computed tomography in blunt abdominal trauma. Clin Radiol 1983;34:261.
121. Karp MP, Cooney DR, Berger PE, et al. The role of computed tomography in the evaluation of blunt abdominal trauma in children. J Pediatr Surg 1981;16:316.
122. Toombs BD, Lester RG, Ben-Menachem Y, et al. Computed tomography in blunt trauma. Radiol Clin North Am 1981;19:17.
123. Sutyak JP, D'Amelio LF, Chio W, et al. Economic impact and clinical predictors of successful non-operative treatment of adult splenic injury. J Trauma 1994;36:158.
124. Kohn JS, Clark DE, Isler RJ, Pope CF. Is computed tomographic grading of splenic injury useful in the nonsurgical management of blunt trauma? J Trauma 1994;36:385.
125. Little JM, McRae J, Smitananda N, et al. Radioisotope scanning of liver and spleen in upper abdominal trauma. Surg Gynecol Obstet 1967;125:725.
126. Gold RE, Redman HC. Splenic trauma: assessment of problems in diagnosis. Am J Radiol. 1972;116:413.
127. Mishalany HG, Miller JH, Woolley MM. Radioisotope spleen scan in patients with splenic injury. Arch Surg 1982;117:1147.
128. Wener L, Boyle CD. Splenic scintiscanning in the preoperative diagnosis of subcapsular hematoma. N Engl J Med. 1967;227:35.
129. Witek JT, Spencer RP, Pearson HA, et al. Diagnostic spleen scans in occult splenic injury. J Trauma 1974;14:197.
130. Nebesar RA, Rabinov KR, Potsaid MS. Radionuclide imaging of the spleen in suspected splenic injury. Radiology 1974;110:609.
131. O'Mara RE, Hall RC, Dombroski DL. Scintiscanning in the diagnosis of rupture of the spleen. Surg Gynecol Obstet 1970;131:1077.
132. Kaufman RA, Towbin R, Babcock DS, et al. Upper abdominal trauma in children: imaging evaluated. AJR 1984;142:449.
133. Uthoff LB, Wyffels PL, Adams CS. A prospective study comparing nuclear scintigraphy and computerized tomography in the initial evaluation of the trauma patients. Ann Surg 1983;198:611.
134. Haller JA. A new philosophy of pediatric splenic surgery: save our spleens. Surg Rounds 1980;3:23.
135. Howman-Giles R, Gilday DL, Venugopal S, et al. Splenic trauma: nonoperative management and long-term follow-up by scintiscan. J Pediatr Surg 1978;13:121.
136. Lutzker LG, Chun KJ. Radionuclide imaging in the nonsurgical treatment of liver and spleen trauma. J Trauma 1981;21:382.
137. Ward RE, Miller P, Clark DG, et al. Angiography and peritoneal lavage in blunt abdominal trauma. J Trauma 1981;21:848.
138. Fisher RG, Foucar K, Estrada R, et al. Splenic rupture in blunt trauma: correlation of angiographic and pathologic records. Radiol Clin North Am 1981;19:141.
139. Panetta T, Scalfani SJ, Goldstein AS, et al. Percutaneous transcatheter embolization for massive bleeding from pelvic fractures. J Trauma 1985;25:1021.
140. Goletti O, Ghiselli G, Lippolis PV, et al. The role of ultrasonography in blunt abdominal trauma: results in 250 consecutive cases. J Trauma 1994;36:178.
141. Salvino CK, Esposito TJ, Smith DK, et al. Laparoscopic injection of fibrin glue to arrest intraparenchymal abdominal hemorrhage: an experimental study. J Trauma 1993;35:762.
142. Shackford SR, Sise MJ, Virgilio RW, et al. Evaluation of splenorrhaphy: a grading system for splenic trauma. J Trauma 1981;21:538.
143. Buntain WL, Lynn HB. Splenorrhaphy: changing concepts for the traumatized spleen. Surgery 1979;86:748.
144. Moore EE, Shackford SR, Pacher HL, et al. Organ injury scaling: spleen, liver, and kidney. J Trauma 1989;29:1664.
145. Orland JC, Moore TC. Splenectomy for trauma in childhood. Surg Gynecol Obstet 1972;134:94.
146. Sherman NH, Asch MJ. Conservative surgery for splenic injuries. Pediatrics 1978;61:267.
147. Aronson DZ, Scherz AW, Einhorn AH, et al. Non-operative management of splenic trauma in children: a report of six consecutive cases. Pediatrics 1977;60:482.
148. Cohen RC. Blunt splenic trauma in children: a retrospective study of nonoperative management. Aust Paediatr J 1982;18:221.
149. Douglas GJ, Simpson JS. The conservative management of splenic trauma. J Pediatr Surg. 1971;6:565.
150. Ein SH, Shandling B, Simpson JS, et al. Nonoperative management of traumatized spleen in children: how and why. J Pediatr Surg 1978;13:117.
151. Weinstein ME, Govin GG, Rice CL, et al. Splenorrhaphy for splenic trauma. J Trauma 1979;19:692.
152. Wesson DE, Filler RM, Ein SH, et al. Ruptured spleen: when to operate? J Pediatr Surg 1991;16:324.
153. Brands W, Mennicken C, Beck M. Preservation of the ruptured spleen by gluing with highly concentrated human fibrinogen: experimental and clinical results. World J Surg. 1982;6:366.
154. Tibi P, Ouriel K, Schwartz SI. Splenic injury in the adult: splenectomy, splenorrhaphy, or nonoperative management. Contemp Surg 1985;26:73.
155. Luna GK, Dellinger EP. Nonoperative observation therapy for splenic injuries: a safe therapeutic option? Am J Surg 1987;153:462.
156. Derderian GP, Walshaw R, McGehee J. Ultrasonic surgical dissection in the dog spleen. Am J Surg. 1982;143:269.
157. Scheele J, Gentsch HH, Matteson E. Splenic repair by fibrin tissue adhesive and collagen fleece. Surgery 1984;95:6.
158. Dulchavsky SA, Geller ER, Maurer J, et al. Autologous fibrin glue: bactericidal properties in contaminated hepatic injury. J Trauma 1991;31:991.
159. Horton J, Ogden ME, Williams S, et al. The importance of splenic blood flow in clearing pneumococcal organisms. Ann Surg. 1982;195:172.
160. Dulchavsky SA, Ledgerwood AM, Lucas CE, et al. Wound healing of the injured spleen with and without splenorrhaphy. J Trauma 1987;27:1155.
161. Morgenstern L. The avoidable complications of splenectomy. Surg Gynecol Obstet 1977;145:525.
162. Hoivik B, Solheim K. Splenic artery ligation in splenic injuries. Injury 1983;15:1.
163. Keramidas DC. The ligation of the splenic artery in the treatment of traumatic rupture of the spleen. Surgery 1979;85:530.
164. Pabst R, Kamran D, Creutzig H. Splenic regeneration and blood flow after ligation of the splenic artery or partial splenectomy. Am J Surg 1984;147:382.
165. Lange D, Zaert PH, Merlotti GJ, et al. The use of absorbable mesh in splenic trauma. J Trauma 1988;28:269.
166. Oakes DD, Charters AC. Changing concepts in the management of splenic trauma. Surg Gynecol 1984;153:181.
167. Cooney DR, Dearth JC, Swanson SE, et al. Reactive merits of partial splenectomy, splenic reimplantation, and immunization in preventing postsplenectomy infection. Surgery 1979;86:561.
168. Steely WM, Satava RM, Brigham RA, et al. Splenic autotransplantation: determination of the optimal amount required for maximal survival. J Surg Res 1988;45:327.

169. Annexton M. Autotransplantation of spleen tissue after trauma: encouraging evidence. JAMA 1979;241:437.

170. Livingston CD, Levine BA, Sirinek KR. Site of splenic autotransplantation affects protection for sepsis. Am J Surg 1983;146:734.

171. Livingston CD, Levine BA, Sirinek KR. Site of splenic autotransplantation of the spleen following pneumococcal pneumonia. Surg Gynecol Obstet 1983;156:761.

172. Roth H, Waldherr R. Problems in spleen autotransplantation: comparative study of types of implantation in animal experiments. In Warnig P, ed. Progress in pediatric surgery. Berlin: Springer Verlag, 1985;18:182.

173. Traub A, Giebink GS, Smith C, et al. Splenic reticuloendothelial function after splenectomy, spleen repair and spleen autotransplantation. N Engl J Med 1987;317:1559.

174. Tavassoli M, Ratzan RJ, Crosby WH. Studies on regeneration of heterotrophic splenic autotransplants. Blood 1973;41:701.

175. Veleck FT, Kugaczewki JT, Jongco B, et al. Function of the reimplanted spleen in dogs. J Trauma 1982;22:502.

176. Sass W, Bergholz M, Kehl A, et al. Overwhelming infection after splenectomy in spite of some spleen remaining and splenosis: a case report. Klin Wochenschr 1983;61:1075.

177. VanWych DB, White MH, Witte CL, et al. Critical splenic mass for survival from experimental pneumococcemia. J Surg Res 1980;28:14.

178. Steely WM, Satava RM, Harris RW, et al. Comparison of omental splenic transplants to partial splenectomy: protective effect against septic death. Am Surg 1987;53:702.

179. Livingston CD, Levine BA, Sirineck KR. Preservation of splenic tissue prevents postsplenectomy pulmonary sepsis following bacterial challenge. J Surg Res 1982;33:356.

180. Schwartz AD, Goldthorn JF, Winkelstein JA. Lack of protective effect of autotransplant splenic tissue to pneumococcal challenge. Blood 1979;51:475.

181. Cohn LH. Local infections after splenectomy: relationship of drainage. Arch Surg 1965;90:230.

182. Pachter HL, Hofstetter SR, Spencer FC. Evolving concepts in splenic surgery: splenorrhaphy versus splenectomy and postsplenectomy drainage; experience in 105 patients. Ann Surg 1981;194:262.

183. Mucha P Jr. Changing attitude toward the management of blunt splenic trauma in adults. Mayo Clin Proc 1986;61:472.

184. The Medical Letter on Drugs and Therapeutics. New Rochelle, NY, November 1985;27:97.

185. Giebink GS, Foker JE, Kim Y, et al. Serum antibody and opsonic response to vaccination with pneumococcal capsular polysaccharide in normal and splenectomized children. J Infect Dis 1980;141:404.

186. Bolan G, Broome CV, Facklam RR, et al. Pneumococcal vaccine efficacy in selected populations in the United States. Ann Intern Med 1986;104:1.

187. Dunn DL. Vaccines and antibody immunotherapy in surgical patients. Am J Surg 1987;153:409.

188. Caplan ES, Boltansky H Snyder MJ, et al. Response of traumatized splenectomized patients to immediate vaccination with polyvalent pneumococcal vaccine. J Trauma 1983;23:801.

189. Barringer M, Meredith W, Sterchi M, et al. Effect of anesthesia and splenectomy on antibody response to pneumococcal polysaccharide immunization. Am Surg 1982;48:628.

190. Ertel W, Faist E, Nestle C, et al. Dynamics of immunoglobulin synthesis after major trauma. Arch Surg 1989;124:1437.

191. Dorgna-Pignatti C, DeStefano R, Barone F, et al. Penicillin compliance in splenectomized phalocemics. Europ J Pediatr 1984;142:83.

192. DePalma A, Buraschi G, Canpani G, et al. Compliance with oral penicillin prophylaxis in splenectomized phalocemic patients. Hematologica 1985;70:221.

193. Powell RW, Blaylock WE, Hoff CJ, et al. The efficacy of postsplenectomy sepsis prophylactic measures: the role of penicillin. J Trauma 1979;28:1285.

194. Huizinga W, Baker LW. The influence of splenectomy on infective morbidity after colonic and splenic injuries. Eur J Surg 1993;159:579.

195. Stiegmann GV, Moore EE, Moore GE. Failure of spleen repair. J Trauma 1979;19:698.

Chapter **24** Injury to the Stomach and Small Bowel

ROBERT F. WILSON, M.D.

ALEXANDER J. WALT, M.D.

HISTORIC PERSPECTIVE

According to Morgagni,[1,2,3] Aristotle was the first to recognize that intestinal injury could occur as a result of blunt abdominal trauma, and that this could occur without damage to the abdominal wall. Hippocrates was the first to report intestinal perforation from penetrating abdominal wounds.[2,4] In 1275, Guillaume de Salicet of Italy described the technique of lateral suture repair of intestinal injuries.[2,5]

The first report of gastric injury, as well as a resultant fistula, is credited to Schenk in the 16th century.[2,5] In 1685, Boneti[1,6] described a hunter who in 1648 was pinned to the trunk of a tree by a stag and then tossed into the air. A surgeon removed a piece of antler from the left buttock and bandaged a wound of the scrotum. The hunter had no obvious injury of his abdomen, but he complained of great pain and died the following day. An autopsy revealed severe peritoneal inflammation and multiple perforations of the ileum and cecum.[1,6]

The first operative repair of gastric injury was reported by Nolleson in the 18th century. At about the same time, Sachenus and, independently, Rambdohr described repair of completely divided intestine.[2,4]

In 1761 Morgagni[1,3] described the clinical features and autopsies of patients who died as a result of intestinal rupture following blunt abdominal trauma due to the kick of a horse or a blow from a stick.

Larrey,[1,7] the famous military surgeon of Napoleonic times, in his "Memoirs of a Military Surgeon" published in 1815, reported several cases of bowel perforation in soldiers who had no external marks on their bodies. Larrey surmised that these injuries resulted from the massive cannon balls striking at relatively low velocities producing no external abdominal signs of trauma.

In 1858 Poland,[1,8] in a discussion of several cases of contusion of the abdomen with injury to the stomach and intestines, noted a 95% mortality from non-operative management of these injuries. Longuet in 1875[1,9] and MacCormac in 1887[1,10] made similar observations and suggested the need for laparotomy and repair.

According to Poer and Woliver in 1889, Croft reported the first long-term survivor after operative repair of completely divided small bowel.[2,11] In 1890 Croft[1,12] reported two initially successful cases; his first patient died later from complications of the "artificial anus" he created at the site of the jejunal injury. The second patient survived a primary repair. Croft's experience was followed by reports by Motz in the French literature of several successful primary repairs.[1,13]

In the late 19th century, Theodore Kocher was the first surgeon to report successful repair of a gunshot wound to the stomach.[2] In the United States, the first notable case of a gunshot wound to the stomach was that of President McKinley in September, 1901. In spite of expeditious transport to the operating room (less than 75 minutes) and appropriate repair, a wound to the pancreas was overlooked, and McKinley died 1 week later of overwhelming sepsis.[1,14]

The routine modern use of exploratory laparotomy for suspected intestinal injury was not observed until late in World War I,[2] but exploratory laparotomy for intestinal perforation at that time carried a 75 to 80% mortality, almost equal to the mortality of nonoperative

management. With improvements in pre-hospital transport, resuscitation, and anesthesia and the development of antibiotics, the mortality rate from isolated injuries of the stomach or small bowel is probably less than 1%.[2,15]

INCIDENCE

Gastric and small bowel injuries collectively comprise the third most common type of blunt abdominal injury. Combined, they are the most common types of injury seen in penetrating abdominal trauma.[2] Injury patterns seen in blunt abdominal trauma range from simple perforation to complex crushes or tears, plus various mesenteric injuries producing ischemia.

The incidence of gastric injury from blunt abdominal trauma is very low and averages between 0.9% and 1.8%.[16] The incidence of small bowel injury due to blunt trauma ranges from 5% to 15%;[17,18] however, there generally are other injuries so that the incidence of isolated blunt small bowel disruption is only about 1-2%.[19] The incidence of intestinal injury secondary to penetrating trauma of the abdomen, especially from gunshot wounds, may exceed 80% and is sufficiently high to merit an exploratory laparotomy on all gunshot wounds of the abdomen. The incidence of hollow viscus injury secondary to stab wounds which have penetrated the peritoneum is about 30%.[21]

AXIOM Taken together, the stomach and small bowel are usually the most frequently injured organs in penetrating abdominal trauma[5] (Table 24–1).

Epidemiology

BLUNT TRAUMA

General

Today the most frequent causes of severe blunt trauma are motor vehicle accidents, and these account for about 80% of the trauma admissions to most medical centers.[1,22,23] Exceptions are the Third World countries[24] and the urban United States,[25] where intentional injuries predominate. Blunt abdominal trauma injures solid organs more than it does the stomach, small intestine, or colon,[27] but the incidence of blunt intestinal injuries is rising.[28,29] Stomach injuries from blunt trauma are extremely uncommon.

In a 12-year period (1980-1992) at Detroit Receiving Hospital, 573 patients had blunt intra-abdominal injuries. This included jejunum or ileum in 58 (10.1%) and stomach in only six (1.0%) (Table 24–1).

Motor Vehicle Accidents

At least part of the increase in small bowel injuries in MVAs appears to be related to the introduction of seat belts.[30-32] Harrison and Whelan[1] have noted that passengers with seat belts sustain bowel injury more frequently than pedestrians in motor vehicle accidents. They also observe that a seat belt without a proper shoulder harness is a major factor in causing these injuries. Williams and Ratliff[33] recently described four patients with gastrointestinal disruption and vertebral fractures associated with the use of seat belts.

TABLE 24–1 **Mortality Rates with Abdominal Injuries Seen in 12 Years at Detroit Receiving Hospital (1980-1992)**

		Type of Trauma		
Organ Injured	Blunt	GSW	Stabs	Total
Liver	(160)	(499)	(251)	(910)
	35%	22%	8%	20%
Small Bowel	(58)	(551)	(150)	(759)
	24%	14%	7%	13%
Colon	(43)	(462)	(122)	(627)
	16%	14%	6%	12%
Diaphragm	(28)	(273)	(119)	(420)
	25%	22%	8%	18%
Kidney	(145)	(229)	(45)	(419)
	7%	17%	13%	13%
Stomach	(6)	(241)	(93)	(340)
	50%	22%	11%	19%
Abd. Vessels	(23)	(257)	(53)	(333)
	70%	53%	32%	50%
Spleen	(172)	(131)	(42)	(345)
	15%	24%	10%	18%
Pancreas	(33)	(140)	(37)	(210)
	6%	24%	30%	22%
Duodenum	(10)	(124)	(33)	(167)
	30%	23%	21%	23%
Bladder	(44)	(84)	(6)	(134)
	18%	6%	17%	10%
Gallbladder	(3)	(59)	(19)	(81)
	100%	24%	5%	22%
Total	(573)	(1358)	(810)	(2741)
	16%	14%	5%	12%

AXIOM One should be suspicious of a characteristic tetrad of injuries caused by seat belts. These include abdominal wall contusion, small bowel rupture, mesenteric tears, and lumbar spine fractures.

Over a 12-year period (1980-1992) at Detroit Receiving Hospital, 2168 patients had abdominal organs injured by penetrating trauma. The small bowel was injured in 701 (32%) of these cases, and the stomach was injured in 334 (15%) (Table 24–2). Although the small bowel was the organ most frequently injured by gunshot wounds (551), the liver was injured much more frequently by stab wounds (251 versus 150).

Penetrating Trauma

As noted earlier, small bowel is the organ most frequently injured by penetrating abdominal trauma in most reported series. Because most assailants are right-handed, the left side of the abdomen is injured much more frequently by stab wounds than the right side. Gunshot wounds, in contrast, involve almost all parts of the abdomen equally.

PATHOPHYSIOLOGY

Perforations, contusions, and ligamentous or mesenteric avulsions of the stomach and small bowel have all been reported to occur after blunt abdominal trauma.[2,3,16-18,34,35] Most of the great disparity between the frequency and types of injury to the stomach and small bowel, especially with blunt trauma, can be explained by their anatomic dissimilarities in location, size, thickness, and fixation.[2]

The decompressed stomach, especially in a supine individual, is located largely in the intrathoracic abdomen and is protected to some degree by the lower chest wall.[2] When distended by swallowed food or liquid, the stomach expands inferiorly. Consequently, a greater portion of the stomach, particularly if the patient is erect, then lies in the

true abdomen, unprotected by the thoracic cage and more prone to injury.[36]

The stomach is fixed on its lesser curvature by the gastrohepatic ligament, cephalad by the crural attachments of the diaphragm, and distally by the retroperitoneal duodenum. The greater curvature is loosely bound to the transverse colon by the gastrocolic ligament and to the spleen by the short gastric arteries. In contrast to the small bowel, the stomach is rarely subject to burst injury because the esophageal and pyloric outlets can serve as relatively efficient safety valves in response to the sudden increases in intraluminal pressure that can be generated by blunt trauma.[2]

The small bowel occupies most of the true abdominal cavity and is protected anteriorly only by the abdominal wall musculature. For the most part, it is bound only by its mesentery. The characteristic convolutions of the small bowel predispose it to folding or kinking which can easily create closed loops.[2] Blunt trauma to the abdominal wall, especially over a loop of bowel fixed by adhesions or the natural ligaments at each end, may result in a burst type of injury. Another anatomic distinction is the mobility of the small bowel around fixed points (ligament of Treitz, adhesions, or cecum), predisposing the intestine at these points to avulsion injuries from shearing forces.

Mechanisms of Injury

PENETRATING INJURIES

Stab Wounds

Intestinal perforations caused by stab wounds are often singular and are seldom accompanied by any significant area of tissue damage. In many instances, the signs and symptoms may be minimal for a number of hours or days until peritonitis or abscess develops. If a DPL is done in less than three hours after the injury, the WBC response may not be adequate to raise the WBC in the effluent to $>500/mm^3$.

Gunshot Wounds

Gunshot wounds, in contrast, usually cause paired perforations and are often associated with some surrounding tissue damage. High velocity missiles can cause injury not only by direct contact, but also by the "blast effect" due to dissipation of energy lateral to its path. The extent of the injury zone surrounding a missile path will depend on the kinetic energy (KE) of the missile which is proportional to its mass (m) multiplied by the square of its velocity (v), (KE = ½ mv²).[37] Even without frank penetration, the blast effect generated, especially by high velocity missiles, may be powerful enough to necrose bowel wall several inches from its path. Perforation of the bowel may occur immediately or only after several days when the tissue begins to slough.

AXIOM One should assume that all gunshot wounds of the abdomen have injured some bowel.

TABLE 24–2 **Mortality Rates with Penetrating Injuries to Abdominal Organs**

	Types of Trauma		
Organ	GSW	Stab	Total
Liver	22% (499)	8% (251)	17% (750)
Small Bowel	14% (551)	7% (150)	12% (701)
Colon	14% (462)	6% (122)	12% (584)
Diaphragm	22% (273)	8% (119)	18% (392)
Stomach	22% (241)	11% (93)	19% (334)
Total	14% (1358)	5% (810)	11% (2168)

%=Mortality rate in each group
()=Number of patients in each group

The path of a missile that penetrates the body is variable and frequently is not in a straight line.[2] Two reasons for this phenomenon are: (a) the abdominal wall and intra-abdominal organs are not iso-dense, and missiles traveling through media of variable densities tend to change directions at such interfaces, and (b) missiles may ricochet off bone and continue in almost any direction.[38] In addition, the primary missile may hit bone and cause secondary bony missiles to go off at various angles.

AXIOM One should never assume that the path of a missile is a straight line between the entrance and exit wounds.

Shotgun Wounds

Shotgun injuries can pose unique problems in diagnosis and treatment.[2] Shotgun injuries from very close range (less than 15 feet) can be associated with massive destruction of the abdominal wall and intra-abdominal structures. Long-range shotgun blast injuries (greater than 50 feet) are characterized by a large scatter pattern and shallow pellet penetration.[39,40]

Foreign Bodies

Sharp foreign bodies that successfully leave the stomach and enter the duodenum probably cause perforation of the bowel in only a small percentage of cases. If a perforation does occur, it usually involves the more distal portions of the ileum and is often manifested as an abscess and/or bowel obstruction. If the perforation is walled off by surrounding small bowel, it may cause confusing signs and symptoms for days, weeks, or even months before it is diagnosed. Gerard et al[41] recently reported a duck bone perforation of the small bowel, but most of our foreign body perforations have been due to tooth picks.

BLUNT ABDOMINAL TRAUMA

Small Bowel

Small bowel rupture secondary to blunt abdominal trauma is uncommon, and the injury mechanisms remain controversial.[2] In 1890 the French surgeon Motz[1,13] postulated three possible mechanisms for injury to the bowel in blunt trauma: *écrasement, déchirure,* and *éclatement.* (Translation: *crushing* of the bowel against the bony prominences of the posterior abdominal wall; *shearing* of the bowel and mesentery from traction on their attachments or supports; and *bursting* of the bowel because of increased intraluminal pressure.)

DIRECT BLOWS. Several authors have reported that the duodenum, proximal jejunum, and terminal ileum are the areas of small bowel most likely to be injured by blunt trauma.[1,34,42,43] These are the areas where the small bowel is most likely to be crushed between the offending force and the spine or pelvic brim. Similarly, there is a propensity for blunt large bowel injuries to occur in the cecum, the midtransverse colon, and the sigmoid colon because the colon in these areas can be squeezed between the seat belt or shoulder harness and the spine or pelvic brim.[44] Experimental evidence indicates that a linear force strong enough to rupture intestine or gastric wall by this mechanism causes extensive damage to the bowel wall and also to the attached mesentery and adjacent structures.[45]

Since intestinal injuries secondary to blunt abdominal trauma are usually small (0.4-2.0 in diameter) and characteristically are not surrounded by large ecchymotic areas, direct blows or crushing does not appear to be the primary etiology.[45]

SHEARING FORCES. Violent torsions or rotational forces that can occur in automobile accidents are examples of shearing forces due to rapid deceleration in the lateral and horizontal planes.[2] Clinical examples of shearing force injuries are seen most frequently in automobile accidents and falls from great heights. It was formerly thought that most small bowel injuries from blunt trauma, especially with rapid deceleration, were due to shearing or tearing of mobile loops of bowel away from fixed points such as the ligament of Treitz or cecum.[11] It has now been shown, however, that the most common sites of intestinal rupture are the jejunum and ileum at least 30 cm from the points of fixation, such as the ligament of Treitz and cecum.[51]

PSEUDOCLOSED LOOP OBSTRUCTION. In the pseudoclosed loop obstruction or bursting types of injury, a segment of bowel partially filled with intestinal secretions, gas, or food can become entrapped between an external force and a firm anatomic object, creating a closed loop (Fig. 24–1).[2] In this setting, even small amounts of external force can generate the intraluminal bursting pressure of 140 mm Hg required to rupture the small intestine.[45,46] The lesions produced in experimental models are very similar to those found after blunt abdominal trauma.[47-51] Intestinal perforation is very difficult to produce as an isolated injury from blunt trauma unless there is intraluminal fluid and a functional closed loop at the time of impact.

Prior to the days of the automobile, most blunt injuries to the small bowel were single and resulted from a localized blow to the abdomen such as the kick of a horse.[1,52] This often produced a "blow out" perforation, usually on the antimesenteric border of the bowel.[53] Similar lesions have been found in sailors immersed near explosions of depth charges.[54] Kicks by horses occasionally have produced perforations remote from the blow[55] or even in several different sites in the intestine from one blow.[56] The third mechanism of Motz (bursting of a closed loop) has been invoked to explain these phenomena.

Sauerbruch[57] theorized that a temporary closed loop was formed by a peristaltic wave.[1] He believed that this type of injury was most apt to occur near the ligament of Treitz or the ileocecal valve where one end of the loop would be partially obstructed at all times. The resulting loop, when subjected to increased pressure, would rupture at its weakest point. This mechanism probably explains most ruptures of the stomach[16] and some ruptures of the duodenum from blunt trauma. Experimental evidence, however, has not confirmed that this is a significant cause of rupture of mobile small bowel. Surgically produced closed loops in mobile bowel in experimental animals have been shown to be resistant to rupture from blunt trauma.[58,59] When peritoneal and luminal pressures were simultaneously measured, the transmural pressures were generally much less than the bursting

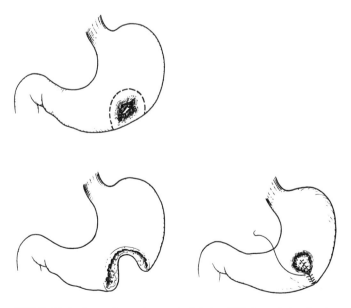

FIGURE 24–1 Large destructive gastric injuries. With large destructive lesions, all damaged tissue should be debrided and the stomach is then closed in two layers. The inner suture can be a continuous hemostatic layer of slowly absorbable suture. The outer layer is closed with nonabsorbable sero-muscular layer. (From Maull KI. Stomach, small bowel and mesentery injury. In Rob & Smith's Operative Surgery; Trauma Surgery, 4th ed. London: Butterworth, 1989;402.)

strength of the bowel, and sometimes the transmural pressures were actually negative.

AXIOM Severe blunt trauma can injure almost any part of the small bowel.

OTHER MECHANISMS. One mechanism that might explain antimesenteric blowout perforations from blunt trauma may be related to the properties of waves in an inhomogeneous fluid. Senn[55] hinted at this in 1904 when he said that bowel perforations from blunt trauma were caused by "violent momentary vibrations in a coil of intestine."[60] Such vibrations would tend to cause intestinal tears in areas of inherent weakness.[46,61] Histologically, the antimesenteric border is characterized by absence of large-diameter blood vessels and the presence of lymphoid aggregations, which may contribute to the observed weakness of this area. Another explanation may be the greater radius of curvature of a loop of bowel at the antimesenteric border. Applying the law of Leplace, this site would be subjected to greater wall tension. A similar argument could hold for the perforations at the greater curve of the stomach and the lateral aspect of the second portion of the duodenum.

SUMMARY. Thus, intestinal perforation, when small and occurring as an isolated injury from blunt trauma, is probably due to a blowout of a "pseudoclosed loop."[2] Larger perforations, frank disruptions, or perforations associated with large mesenteric hematomas are probably primarily due to direct blows. Large mesenteric tears may be due to shearing forces.

Blunt Stomach Injuries

Blunt rupture of the stomach is rare, unless it is distended with food and/or weakened by pre-existing pathology.[49] Blunt gastric perforations in adults most commonly occur on the lesser curvature. Presumably, this tissue has less elasticity, a limited muscular layer, and a paucity of mucosal folds.[16,50]

Recently Dupre et al[62] reported a traumatic rupture of the stomach secondary to a Heimlich maneuver performed on a patient who was choking. The patient was admitted some time later with abdominal pain caused by the stomach rupture. The authors found a total of four similar events in the literature.

CORROSIVE INJURIES

Various swallowed corrosive agents can damage the esophagus and stomach. In a recent report by Rappert et al,[63] 39 children were endoscoped because of suspected caustic ingestion, and 10 (26%) had caustic burns involving the stomach. Although the stomach only rarely becomes stenotic from such injuries, pooled caustic in the stomach can cause necrosis and rupture in the dependent area.

ELECTRICAL INJURIES

Electrical injuries involving the stomach are rare. Zhu et al[64] recently reported the first successful treatment of a child with a severe electrical injury of the stomach. The authors felt that their success was related to: (a) resection of the necrotic portion of the stomach immediately after admission, (b) excision of surrounding necrotic tissue while conserving all healthy or only partially damaged tissues, (c) early coverage of all exposed areas, (d) general comprehensive supportive therapy, and (e) local application of a saline solution containing chloromycetin and lidocaine.

MICROBIOLOGY OF THE GASTROINTESTINAL TRACT

Stomach

In the nondiseased state, the stomach contains relatively few microorganisms because of its acidity.However, any alteration that raises the luminal pH will enhance bacterial colonization and proliferation.

Therefore, although gastric perforation secondary to injury can cause severe peritonitis, initially the inflammation is due to chemical irritation and not bacterial contamination. Leakage of swallowed food and oral bacteria does not greatly increase the risk of infection if they are promptly removed at laparotomy; however, treatment with H_2 receptor blockers or antacids promotes bacterial overgrowth in the stomach and increases the risk of infection following traumatic perforation.[65]

AXIOM A stomach that has no acid or is full of blood can have a high bacterial content.

SMALL BOWEL

The small bowel has a relatively neutral pH, but it has relatively few bacteria, especially in its proximal portions. Therefore, extravasation of small bowel contents into the abdominal cavity causes relatively few clinical signs soon after injury; however, as the number of bacteria increase, the signs and symptoms of bacterial peritonitis grow progressively worse.

The predominant enteric flora vary depending on the point of injury. In the jejunum and proximal ileum, the organisms include grampositive, facultative organisms, predominately streptococcus species. Aerobic lactobacilli, diphtheroids, and fungi are also present, but the total concentration of organisms is usually only 10^4 per ml of fluid.

In the majority of patients, the terminal ileum is colonized with gram-negative microorganisms, such as the aerobic coliforms and anaerobic Bacteroides species. Nevertheless, when compared to the large bowel, the bacterial counts are still relatively low, with only about 10^5 to 10^8 organisms/ml of fluid. In the distal colon, the bacterial counts often exceed 10^{10} per gram of feces.[65]

AXIOM The colony count of bacteria in the distal small bowel can be extremely high and resemble that of colon.

DIAGNOSIS

General

Diagnosis of stomach or small bowel injury is no problem with gunshot wounds that clearly enter the abdomen because exploration is mandatory. With stab wounds and no signs of significant blood loss or peritoneal irritation, one may elect to explore the wound to see if the tract enters the abdomen. If it does, but the patient is essentially asymptomatic, one may elect to do a diagnostic peritoneal lavage (DPL) and explore the abdomen if it is positive. Diagnosis is even more difficult with blunt trauma and may require a number of diagnostic modalities.

History

Any history of trauma to the abdomen or lower thorax should alert the surgeon to the possibility of an intra-abdominal injury. Information about the severity of the trauma may help indicate the likelihood of intra-abdominal damage, but it is not specific for any organ.[34] Gastric and small intestinal injuries have been reported to occur from a variety of trauma, including blows with fists and other firm objects, low-voltage electrocution, aggressive cardiopulmonary resuscitation, and improper seat belt use.[66-68]

Increasing abdominal pain suggests irritation of the peritoneum by blood or gastrointestinal contents; however, the signs and symptoms with gastric or intestinal injury can be extremely variable. If the patient gives a history of passing out or dizziness, a significant blood loss is suspected. Vomiting of blood generally indicates the presence of upper gastrointestinal injury, but one must be sure that there is no evidence of swallowing blood from an injury of the mouth or nose. Passing blood per rectum also can indicate an intestinal injury, but such injuries usually involve the rectum or colon.

Physical Examination

Physical examination can be extremely helpful for diagnosing intra-abdominal injuries in patients who are awake and alert.[19] The early signs of intestinal perforation, however, are often variable and non-specific, and waiting for signs of peritonitis or sepsis can greatly increase morbidity and mortality rates.[11,42,56,58]

AXIOM Signs and symptoms of peritonitis after blunt intestinal trauma may be delayed for hours or days.

STOMACH INJURIES

Because of the acidity inside a normal stomach, the peritoneal signs and symptoms of a gastric tear will tend to be much more acute and severe than a laceration of the small bowel. After 6-12 hours, however, there is an increasing bacterial peritonitis by both types of injuries. Occasionally, a gastric injury can be suspected if the nasogastric aspirate is bloody.

SMALL BOWEL INJURIES

Mantovani et al[69] and Ford and Senac[70] have recently commented on the difficulties of diagnosing small bowel rupture after blunt trauma, especially in children.[70] If only the jejunum or ileum were injured, the authors found no characteristic signs, symptoms, laboratory studies, or radiologic findings. As a consequence, diagnosis and surgical treatment were often delayed.

AXIOM A high index of suspicion and serial abdominal examinations, coupled with serial laboratory and radiographic evaluations, is the most reliable method for identifying patients with isolated blunt intestinal injuries.

Isolated small bowel injuries tend to produce very subtle signs initially. The relatively neutral pH of the small bowel contents tends to cause slower and much less severe chemical peritonitis than gastric contents.[71] During this period, the relative absence of clinical signs and symptoms may lead to delays in diagnosis and treatment and alter the outcome significantly.[15,20,21,72] As the enteric microorganisms released into the peritoneal cavity multiply, however, endotoxins are synthesized and released, and an inflammatory response is initiated, producing increasing peritoneal irritation.[2]

Mesenteric avulsion and contusions resulting in segmental ischemia and subsequent necrosis of small bowel are notorious for presenting few, if any, early clinical signs of intra-abdominal injury.[2,73] Later, the necrotic bowel can leak intestinal contents, which can cause severe peritoneal irritation followed by increasing sepsis.[74] In some instances, the site of the perforation is sealed temporarily by omentum and/or adjacent loops of bowel so that only vague signs and symptoms are produced for days or even weeks. Sometimes, the injury is detected only much later, when the patient has surgery for a bowel obstruction. If the patient has a head or high-spinal-cord injury, or has impaired sensation because of alcohol or drugs, diagnosis can be especially delayed.

AXIOM One cannot rely on the physical examination of the abdomen to detect bowel injuries in patients with an altered sensorium.

There is a great deal of controversy about the value of bowel sounds in helping to diagnose intra-abdominal pathology. Although good bowel sounds will occasionally be heard in the presence of severe peritonitis, this is uncommon and the presence of good bowel sounds is somewhat reassuring. In contrast, if no bowel sounds are heard in spite of listening very carefully for at least 5 minutes in quiet surroundings, one should suspect an intraperitoneal injury.

Laboratory Studies

A progressive rise in serum amylase levels and the white blood cell count, especially with a shift to the left, should alert the surgeon to the possibility of an intra-abdominal injury to the pancreas or gastrointestinal tract.

Radiologic Studies

PLAIN FILMS

In general, plain radiographs of the abdomen are not helpful for diagnosing gastric or small bowel injuries, but occasionally, intraperitoneal air will allow one to see both sides of the bowel wall clearly. An erect chest radiograph or left lateral abdominal decubitus radiograph is much more apt to reveal the presence of free intraperitoneal air.[34] As a general rule, gastric injuries result in a detectable pneumoperitoneum much more frequently than injuries of the small intestine. Intramural air in the bowel wall itself may be an indication of local tissue necrosis due to a mesenteric injury.

AXIOM Intestinal injuries do not commonly cause free air to be visible on plain radiographs of the abdomen.

CONTRAST STUDIES

Gastrografin studies of the stomach and proximal small bowel will usually show a leak if one is present, but false-negative studies do occur. Occasionally, a contrast study will show occlusion of the small bowel lumen due to a hematoma or ischemic stenosis. Injuries to the distal small bowel generally require a barium follow-through study to demonstrate a leak or obstruction. Again, however, a falsely negative study is possible if the bowel injury has become sealed by clot, omentum, or other material.

CT SCANS

CT scans, in many cases, are replacing DPL in the diagnosis of intra-abdominal trauma, especially for retroperitoneal injuries.[2,75] A study by Goldstein et al,[76] in which CT scans compared favorably with DPL, had no cases of intestinal perforation. In contrast, a prospective trial done at Sunnybrook Medical Centre by Thadepalli et al[71] which included some intestinal injuries demonstrated a decreased sensitivity of CT scan when compared with DPL. In addition, the CT scan was less cost effective and was not possible in unstable patients. Furthermore, if there is renal impairment, it may be unwise to give intravenous contrast. In some centers, however, CT scanning has reduced the incidence of negative laparotomy by allowing the identification of certain injuries of solid organs, especially the spleen and liver, which can be treated non-operatively.[2] In addition, the scan can be tailored to include the bony pelvis, lumbosacral spine, and upper femurs.

The typical CT scan performed for possible abdominal trauma requires a combination of oral and intravenous contrast. About 15-30 minutes before the scan, 500 ml of a 2-3% solution of oral contrast is administered by mouth or via the nasogastric tube. Intravenous contrast, 2.0 ml/kg of methyl glutamine diatrizoate, is administered at the time of the CT scan. The patient is placed in the supine position with the arms raised over the head. If there is a nasogastric tube, it is withdrawn from the stomach to the level of the carina to prevent intraabdominal artifact. Sections are taken at 1-cm intervals from the top of the diaphragm to the bottom of the kidneys, and then at 2-cm intervals to the symphysis pubis.[70] In most centers, a special request must be made if one wishes to include the pelvis in the CT examination. If there is special interest in a particular area, the CT scan can be done with finer cuts through that area.

AXIOM One cannot rely on abdominal CT scans to detect injuries to the small intestine distal to the ligament of Treitz.

The specificity, sensitivity, and accuracy of CT scans for hollow viscus injury have yet to be established, since most reports are anecdotal and no center has sufficient experience with these rare cases.[75-77] Nevertheless, we agree with Fabian et al[78] that injuries to the small bowel distal to the ligament of Treitz are frequently missed on CT studies. Although reports from different centers vary,[76,77] the incidence of false-negative CT results appears to get lower as experience in radiographic interruption is gained.

Diagnostic Peritoneal Lavage (DPL)

AXIOM   DPL is the most reliable method for diagnosing injury to intraperitoneal hollow viscera; its timing, however, is a critical determinant of its accuracy.[1,2,19,69]

Using standard DPL criteria, Harrison and Whelan[1] have not missed a case of perforation or other serious injury to the stomach or small bowel in 77 patients. The DPL in such cases is generally positive because of an increased RBC or WBC count. Bile and food fibers are found so seldom in the DPL fluid in patients with intestinal perforation, that a good argument can be made for omitting these assays. Thus, the white cell count should never be omitted from effluent evaluation. Theoretically, the sensitivity of DPL could be improved by protein electrophoresis of the lavage fluid,[20] but Harrison and Whelan[1] have not found this to be necessary. Nevertheless, if the DPL is performed less than 3 hours after the injury, there may not be enough of a peritoneal inflammatory response to the intestinal contents to increase the WBC in the DPL above 500/mm^3.[77,79]

If one suspects a bowel injury and/or the initial lavage results are equivocal, the catheter can be left in place for a repeat DPL 3-6 hours later.[19] A white blood cell count equal to or greater than 500 cells/mm^3 is considered positive.[79]

Some authors have reported utilizing alkaline phosphatase levels in the lavage effluent as a means of diagnosing small-bowel injuries.[77,80] This assay is more costly than the white blood cell count, and because of the relative infrequency of isolated intestinal perforation in blunt trauma, it is difficult to prove that a routine alkaline phosphatase analysis significantly improves the diagnostic yield. This technique requires more controlled studies before it is recommended for routine application.[19]

Celiotomy

AXIOM   In suspicious cases, celiotomy is the safest course to follow, even in the face of little or no confirming data of an intra-abdominal injury.

Injuries to the stomach and small bowel are usually obvious at exploration, but there are several areas which can hide injuries and require particularly careful attention. These include the fat-infiltrated greater and lesser gastric curvatures, the proximal posterior gastric wall, the top of the gastric fundus, the posterior cardia, and the mesenteric border of the small bowel.[19] Injuries in these areas can easily may be overlooked unless one has an increased index of suspicion. In penetrating trauma, the discovery of an odd number of perforations should prompt the surgeon to make an increased effort to find additional injuries.[19]

TREATMENT

Indications for Laparotomy

As noted previously, any persisting suspicion of an injury to an intra-abdominal hollow viscus should prompt a laparotomy.[1,81] In addition, certain long-range shotgun or pellet injuries should also be explored. Gastric and small bowel injuries have been reported to occur after all types of penetrating trauma, including pellets from low-powered air rifles.[40,82,83] Several authors agree that penetration of the abdominal wall by more than four pellets, even in the absence of any peritoneal irritation, mandates an exploratory laparotomy.[40,82,83] Indeed, some surgeons will explore the abdomen if only a single pellet is thought to have violated the peritoneum.

With stab wounds of the abdomen, peritoneal penetration should make one strongly suspicious of gastric and/or intestinal injury.[82] In

general, evisceration of omentum or small bowel is also an indication for a prompt laparotomy.[84]

Initial Operative Management

AXIOM   The traditional techniques—prompt exploration, debridement, and repair of bowel, followed by irrigation and removal of any contamination—are still the cornerstones of the treatment of bowel injuries.

After the patient is given a dose of prophylactic antibiotics directed at enteric pathogens, including gram-negative aerobes (such as E. coli) and anaerobes (such as Bacteroides fragilis), the operative approach is through a generous midline incision.[1,2,19,85] The abdomen is opened expeditiously, and multiple injuries are usually managed in the following order: (a) control of hemorrhage; (b) control of contamination; and (c) thorough exploration for all possible injuries.

During the examination of the stomach, one should visualize the lesser curvature, the esophagogastric-gastric junction, lower third of the esophagus, and the top of the fundas. All injuries should be controlled as they are encountered to prevent continued contamination of the peritoneal cavity.

Placement of the Weinberg retractor enhances exposure of the left upper quadrant viscera, especially the esophagogastric junction.[2] The gastrohepatic and gastroduodenal ligaments are then inspected carefully.

The posterior wall of the stomach is inspected by division of the gastrocolic omentum along the greater curvature of the stomach up to the short gastric vessels. Care must be taken not to injure the middle colic artery, since it can pass very close to the stomach about midway along the greater curvature.

A more extensive exposure of the posterior stomach can be obtained, if needed, by mobilizing the stomach from the spleen by division of the short gastric vessels. This maneuver, however, is usually reserved for treatment of injuries high in the fundus or near the esophagogastric junction. Caution should be exercised in putting traction on the stomach while working in this area, because it can cause an avulsion injury of short gastric vessels or spleen with resultant troublesome hemorrhage.

AXIOM   Extensive mobilization of the gastric fundus or high greater curvature can easily damage the spleen or short gastric vessels.

EXAMINING THE SMALL BOWEL
The small bowel is eviscerated and inspected carefully throughout its entire length. Small non-expanding hematomas of the mesentery are carefully inspected at intervals throughout the operative procedure to assure their stability. If multiple adhesions are present and the patient has had blunt trauma, enough of the adhesions have to be lysed to be sure a leak is not present. With penetrating injuries, only the areas that may be involved need to be freed completely.

REPAIR OF THE STOMACH
If properly mobilized, the stomach is easily repaired. Its walls are generally thick, well vascularized, able to hold sutures well, and redundant in most areas, so that large defects usually can be closed primarily without tension. This contributes to quick healing and minimizes the chance of breakdown. Any tissue which is adjacent to a perforation and seems ischemic or has a tense hematoma should be excised. If the area in question is small, it can be inverted with the repair sutures.[1,86]

Gunshot wounds on the anterior wall of the stomach usually have an exit on the posterior surface.[2] If an exit wound cannot be found after complete exposure of the stomach, including the lesser curve, the posterior surface, and the fundus, the anesthesiologist can be asked to insufflate air into the stomach via the nasogastric tube. If the second hole still cannot be found, one should perform a gastrotomy to inspect the entire stomach thoroughly. One should look with particular care along the lesser curvature and the "bare area" high on the posterior wall of the stomach.

All gastric injuries should be debrided or inverted, then closed with absorbable, continuous, locking sutures for the inner layer, and non-absorbable or slowly-absorbable sutures for the seromuscular second layer (Fig. 24–1). All particulate matter and gastric juice that entered the peritoneal cavity should be removed and the surrounding area should be irrigated thoroughly. Particular attention should be given to the subhepatic and subphrenic spaces, the pelvis, and the lesser sac. Laparoscopy is being used increasingly to diagnose and treat a wide variety of traumatic and non-traumatic problems in the abdomen. Frantzides et al[87] recently described their use of laparoscopy to diagnose and treat two stab wounds of the anterior wall of the stomach. In a similar manner, Brams et al[88] used a new gasless laparoscopic technique to evaluate and repair a traumatic gastric perforation with success.

In the treatment of thoracoabdominal wounds with gross contamination of the thoracic cavity with gastric contents, Schwab et al[2] favor a separate thoracotomy incision for debridement of the chest, removal of contaminated material, lavage, and drainage. Extension of the abdominal midline incision across the avascular costochondral arch in contaminated cases exposes the patient to the risk of costal chondritis and a painful scar at the costal margin.[89]

Management of Small Bowel Injuries

Hematomas that obscure the bowel wall should be explored to rule out underlying perforations; this is especially true around the duodenum. Small perforations of the bowel wall are debrided as needed and closed primarily by lateral sutures. Adjacent intestinal perforations are joined to be sure the intervening bowel is not bleeding or ischemic (Fig. 24–2). Areas of necrosis are removed or, if small, they can be invaginated.[2] The use of either a single-layer or double-layer suturing technique is not crucial and is left to the discretion of the operating surgeon.[2]

AXIOM Several small bowel holes in close proximity are best treated by a segmental resection and primary anastomosis (Fig. 24–3).

The limits of resection are determined primarily by the injury and the vascular supply of the uninjured areas. Bowel wall hematomas are not routinely resected unless they are associated with a possible mucosal perforation or tissue of questionable viability.[1,2] Short segments of bowel of questionable viability should be resected; however, if most of the small bowel is of marginal viability, its color and peristalsis should be evaluated repeatedly. Intravenous fluorescein and examination under a Wood's light have also been used to clarify the condition of questionable areas.[90] If any doubt still exists at the end of the operation, a second-look operation should be performed within 24 hours.

Harrison and Whelan[1] feel that bowel of questionable viability should be left in situ only if the patient's survival may be threatened by "short-gut syndrome." They feel that the stress of an otherwise unnecessary second laparotomy can be detrimental to patients with multiple injuries.

There is little in the literature to support the superiority of any one of the three currently used anastomotic techniques (single-layer, double-layer, or stapled anastomosis) for injured bowel.[2] The single layer technique is an interrupted nonabsorbable seromuscular suture technique. Since there is no hemostatic inner layer suture, all submucosal bleeding must be controlled before starting the closure. The two-layer technique is performed with an absorbable running or interrupted suture on the inner layer, and this sutured area includes all layers of the bowel wall. The outer layer is closed with an inverting seromuscular suture, using non-absorbable sutures. The stapling techniques can use a combination of GIA and TA-55 or the EEA stapling devices. All mesenteric rents due to the injury or resection are closed with simple absorbable sutures to avoid potential internal hernias.

Recently Fansler et al[91] reported on the use of 25 biofragmentable anastomotic rings (BAR) to establish continuity between injured loops of bowel in 18 patients. Using a one-way analysis of variance, this group was compared to 63 historical examples of sutured or

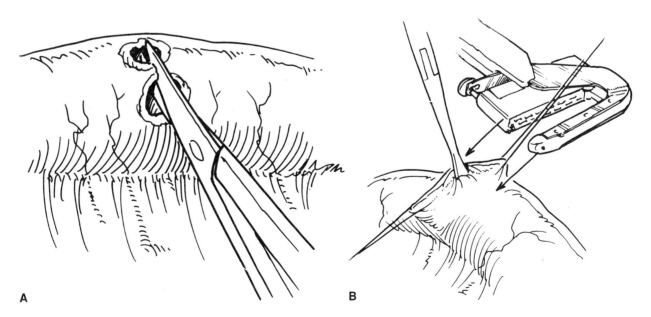

A   **B**

FIGURE 24–2 Intestinal perforations in close proximity should be joined, thereby producing a single larger perforation. The enterotomy exposes any bleeding or ischemic bowel that may lie between two wounds. In certain instances, if the defect in the intestinal wall does not exceed one-third of the circumference, a stapled closure can be effected very rapidly. (From Maull KI. Stomach, small bowel and mesentery injury. In Rob & Smith's Operative Surgery; Trauma Surgery, 4th ed. London: Butterworth, 1989;406.)

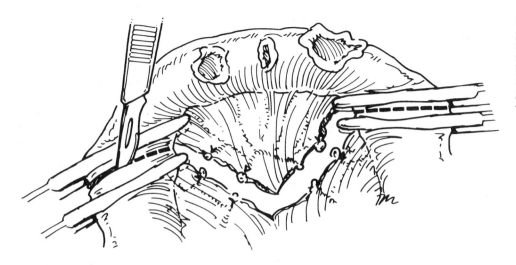

FIGURE 24–3 Multiple adjacent bowel perforations are best treated by segmental resection and primary end-to-end anastomosis. (From Maull KI. Stomach, small bowel and mesentery injury. In Rob & Smith's Operative Surgery; Trauma Surgery, 4th ed. London: Butterworth, 1989; 407.)

stapled anastomosis (SSA). There were no deaths due to the anastomotic technique in the SSA group (n=8) or in the BAR group (n=1). There was no significant difference (P=0.991) in the rate of postoperative intestinal obstruction between BAR (n=3) and SSA (n=8) groups, and none of the BAR patients required re-operation. The average length of time for return of bowel function was not significantly different between the BAR (4.3 days) and SSA (5.8 days) groups (P=0.197).

Mesenteric Injuries

Isolated mesenteric injuries are usually of little consequence, but they occasionally cause hemorrhage and/or late intestinal infarction.[19] The hemorrhage is usually detected at the time of surgery, but occasionally it may be delayed. Intestinal infarctions due to mesenteric hematomas can be very subtle and may cause few or no symptoms for 4 or 5 days.

AXIOM   Any deterioration in a patient with mesenteric trauma should be considered due to intestinal ischemia or perforation until proven otherwise.

The apparent viability of the bowel at the time of exploration can be very misleading, and the diagnosis of delayed intestinal ischemia should be suspected in all victims of blunt trauma who develop abdominal findings or sepsis several days after surgery. Under such circumstances, the best course is prompt reexploration of the abdomen. The intraoperative Doppler device can be very useful in determining the extent of devitalized bowel.[19] Marginally ischemic areas can be covered with warm moist towels and observed later.[1]

Small nonexpanding hematomas in the mesentery are generally not explored unless they are adjacent to bowel, are more than 3-4 centimeters in diameter or are expanding (Fig. 24–4). Nonexpanding hematomas are carefully inspected at intervals throughout the operation to be sure they are stable.

Injuries to the base of the mesentery associated with large hematomas should make one suspect a superior mesenteric artery (SMA) or vein (SMV) injury. Complete occlusion of the SMA distal to the middle colic artery can cause severe ischemia to the bowel, and such ischemia may extend from the ligament of Treitz down to the midtransverse colon. Collateral blood flow from the celiac and inferior mesenteric arteries is often inadequate to maintain viability of the entire bowel if the SMA becomes acutely occluded.[92] If the superior mesenteric vessels are injured, they should be repaired. In some instances, an interposition graft or patch graft may be necessary.

AXIOM   Access to the proximal SMA is best done from a lateral retroperitoneal approach after mobilizing the left-sided abdominal viscera to the right.

Access to the proximal portions of the SMA and SMV can be very difficult and is best gained by mobilizing the entire left colon and left-sided viscera to the midline so that the aorta and the origin of its major visceral branches can be visualized clearly. The entire suprarenal aorta, the celiac axis, and the proximal superior mesenteric artery should be identified and controlled. The involved vessels should then be dissected and repaired.[93]

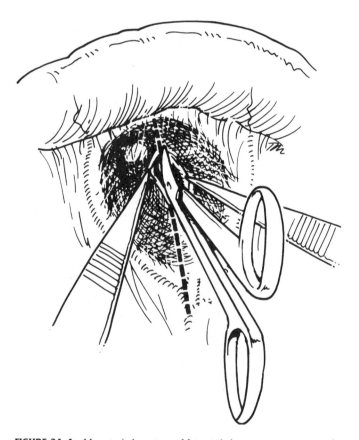

FIGURE 24–4 Mesenteric hematoma. Mesenteric hematomas are commonly found following penetrating and blunt trauma. A small stable hematoma is usually of no consequence unless it lies along the mesenteric wall of the intestine, in which case, the hematoma should be opened and the integrity of the bowel wall assessed. Expanding hematomas should be opened and direct vascular control established by suture ligatures. If the adjacent bowel appears dusky, the safest procedure is to resect the questionably viable bowel along with the haematoma, and perform an end-to-end anastomosis. (From Maull KI. Stomach, small bowel and mesentery injury. In Rob & Smith's Operative Surgery; Trauma Surgery, 4th ed. London: Butterworth, 1989;412.)

Avulsions of mesentery may cause adjacent bowel to become ischemic, resulting in later necrosis and leak or stenosis. Such areas should be resected and the remaining bowel joined by a primary anastomosis (Fig. 24–5). Some authors believe that only 50 cm of distal small bowel needs to be left to maintain near normal small bowel absorptive function,[5] but this appears to be highly variable from patient to patient, and it is probably much safer to leave at least 100 cm of distal small bowel.

Abdominal Closure

After the bowel repairs are completed, the abdomen should be irrigated copiously with warm saline to remove any remaining clots, foreign debris, and intestinal contents.[2] The use of antibiotics in the last liter of irrigant is controversial, but we believe that it may be beneficial.

> **AXIOM** Before closure, all patients with severe abdominal injuries should be considered for operative placement of an enteral feeding device.

Schwab et al[2] perform a needle catheter jejunostomy in virtually all patients with major abdominal injuries before closure except those who will be returning for relaparotomy within 24-48 hours. Ideally, these conduits are placed approximately 20-30 cm distal to the ligament of Treitz. The jejunum at the site of the jejunostomy is sutured securely and widely (6-8 cm) to the anterior abdominal wall to prevent twisting at that site. Accurate placement of the jejunal catheter can be confirmed postoperatively by injection of 10-20 ml of Gastrografin injected through the J-tube.[94]

Closure of the abdomen can be very difficult if the bowel becomes very dilated or edematous.[2] Dilatation of the bowel tends to occur more frequently if nitrous oxide is used as an inhalation agent. The bowel and its mesentery tend to become edematous if there has been prolonged hypotension or bowel ischemia, if the bowel has been displaced outside the abdomen for prolonged periods, or if large amounts of resuscitation fluids were given.[95] The bowel wall is particularly likely to swell after a major vascular injury because of reperfusion edema. Since most of the edema fluid is intramural or interstitial, an enterotomy to remove the fluid is seldom useful. Large intraluminal fluid or gas accumulations, however, can be removed by either retrograde milking of the fluid back into the stomach, where it may be aspirated via the nasogastric tube, or by passing a long intestinal tube.

In spite of these techniques, primary closure of the abdominal fascia may still not be possible. In such circumstances, one can sometimes close the skin and subcutaneous tissue and then repair the ventral hernia at a later date. Very large fascial defects may sometimes be bridged with Prolene or Marlex mesh.[96] If there has been much contamination, it is best to just pack the abdominal opening with moist dressings after covering the anterior bowel surfaces with silk or rayon cloth. These can be held in place with an abdominal binder or with retention-type sutures placed across the opening.

> **AXIOM** Closing the abdominal wall under tension increases the risk of abdominal wall and intestinal complications.

If large portions of the abdominal wall are missing, for example, as a result of close-range shotgun blast wounds, complex reconstructions involving rotational flaps and artificial materials are best delayed for at least several days, until repeat inspection under anesthesia ensures that there is no further necrosis of tissue or evidence of infection.[97]

Scheduled Relaparotomy

When the viability of large areas of bowel is in question because of a major vascular injury, it may become necessary to close the abdomen without 100% assurance that all the remaining bowel is viable. In such circumstances, the surgeon makes a commitment to perform a "second-look" operation 24-48 hours later. The relaparotomy should generally be done no matter how well the patient appears to be doing during the observation period.[5] If a relaparotomy is to be performed, ancillary procedures, such as a gastrostomy or a feeding jejunostomy, should usually be delayed until the time of the relaparotomy.

Postoperative Care

> **AXIOM** With gastric or intestinal injuries, gastric decompression should be continued until there is little or no threat of ileus.

Gastric decompression is generally continued until good bowel sounds are heard, the abdomen is not tender except at the incision, there is little or no distension, and the patient is passing flatus or has had a bowel movement. Jejunal feedings distal to any bowel injuries can often be begun as soon as tube placement has been confirmed by aspiration of bile stained intestinal contents or by radiologic contrast studies. Liberal and early use of the feeding jejunostomy has greatly reduced the use of parenteral hyperalimentation.[98] With distal small bowel injuries, however, it is probably wise to wait at least 4-5 days before beginning the jejunostomy feedings.

Although many surgeons start their tube feedings with a quarter-strength nutritional formula at 20-25 ml/hour,[2] isotonic feedings at about 10 ml/hour are generally tolerated well. The isotonic tube feedings can then be increased about 10 ml/hour every 12 hours as long as there is no bloating or cramping. Incremental advances are made until the patient's nutritional goal of at least 25-30 non-protein calories/kg/day are achieved.

Prophylactic preoperative antibiotics are continued for at least 24 hours if bowel perforation has occurred.[2] Wounds with low infectious potential (i.e., simple stomach or proximal small bowel perforations), may require only one or two doses of antibiotics. In patients who are a high risk for infection because of severe peritoneal contamination from the colon, multiple injuries, prolonged hypotension, and/or multiple blood transfusions, a full course of therapeutic antibiotics for at least 4-5 days may be warranted.[99] Although this is very controversial, intraperitoneal antibiotic irrigation may also be of some benefit in cases with severe peritoneal contamination.[100]

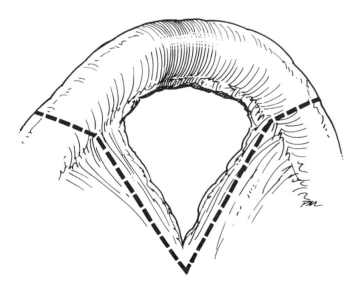

FIGURE 24–5 Mesenteric avulsion. Mesenteric avulsion refers to tearing of the mesentery from itself and from the small intestine. This usually occurs after blunt trauma. It can cause major bleeding and ischemia of the associated small bowel. In such cases, it is advisable to resect all questionably viable intestine and perform a primary anastamosis. (From Maull KI. Stomach, small bowel and mesentery injury. In Rob & Smith's operative surgery; trauma surgery, 4th ed. London: Butterworth, 1989;413.)

> **AXIOM**   Prophylactic antibiotics are usually needed for only one or two doses after gastric or small intestinal injuries.

COMPLICATIONS

The most important postoperative complications specific to gastric and small bowel injuries are bleeding, suture line disruption, and infection.[2,5] Metabolic or nutritional complications are rare, except in cases of massive small bowel resection, and even these have now become much more manageable with the use of modern alimentation techniques.

Hemorrhage

Postoperative bleeding complications are particularly apt to occur following a gastric repair if excess or prolonged traction was applied to the stomach to enhance exposure. Probably the single most common site of postoperative intra-abdominal bleeding after gastric surgery is an injury to the spleen. Bleeding into the gastric lumen can occur at suture lines or areas of bowel wall contusion.

> **AXIOM**   In critically ill or injured patients, the gastric ph should be monitored and kept above 4.5-5.0 until the patient is eating properly.

Postoperative gastric bleeding from the stomach may also be due to stress gastritis. Postoperative bleeding from injured small bowel is unusual, but bleeding from injured mesenteric vessels is not rare. Treatment consists of resuscitation and prompt re-exploration.

Bowel Obstruction

Small bowel obstruction is not unusual following intestinal injuries. Although the obstruction is usually due to adhesions, it can also be due to edema at an anastomosis or to an intussusception. Early postoperative small bowel obstruction can be difficult to differentiate from the usual postoperative ileus, and often is not diagnosed until there is clinical evidence of strangulated or leaking bowel.

> **AXIOM**   Early postoperative bowel obstructions tend to have a high mortality rate because they often are not diagnosed until strangulation or peritonitis occurs.

Suture Line Disruption

Suture line disruption is much more apt to occur in the small bowel than in the stomach; however, regardless of its source, it can be a catastrophic event. Large fluid shifts can occur as a result of the peritoneal contamination and third-space fluid sequestration. Prompt recognition is mandatory, and treatment consists of aggressive resuscitation, intravenous antibiotics, and prompt re-exploration and surgical correction. Any gastric anastomosis which leaks should be excised and reclosed. With small bowel leaks, the involved bowel should be resected and clean, uninvolved bowel can be re-anastomosed. If the distal ileum is the site of the leak and severe peritonitis is present, the proximal end of the involved bowel can be brought out as an ileostomy. The distal end can also be brought out, or simply stapled off and left in situ.

In polytraumatized patients, a leak at a suture line may be difficult to diagnose without reoperation. In some instances the only way to make the diagnosis is prompt exploration of patients who act septic or are not improving as they should. If the intra-abdominal infection is severe enough to warrant temporary diversion with an end-jejunostomy or ileostomy, total parenteral nutrition for metabolic support and meticulous stomal care are essential.

Occasionally, a suture line disruption is not recognized until there is an enterocutaneous fistula. If the patient is not septic, a small-volume enterocutaneous fistula without distal obstruction will usually heal spontaneously after 2-3 weeks of parenteral hyperalimentation and bowel rest.[2] If an enterocutaneous fistula is associated with a distal obstruction, operative repair is essential as soon as the patient's condition will allow it. Such obstructions may be caused by intestinal adhesions or interloop abscesses.

Metabolic Complications of Small Bowel Resection

Resection of large amounts of small bowel may lead to a malabsorption syndrome due to a loss of absorptive segments and alterations in bacterial flora.[101] Generally, at least half of the small bowel can be removed without serious disability.[2] Length for length, however, removal of the distal ileum leads to far more serious complications than removal of equal portions of the jejunum.

> **AXIOM**   If large amounts of small bowel must be removed, special efforts should be made to preserve the distal ileum.

Removal of jejunum may be associated with lactose intolerance, which is usually self-limited. Removal of the distal ileum often causes vitamin B_{12} and bile salt deficiencies, fat malabsorption, and bacterial overgrowth that compounds the other metabolic deficiencies. Interference with the absorptive capacity for fat leads to bile salt deficiencies, which can cause further reductions in the bowel absorption of vitamins A, D, K, and E. Vitamin B_{12} deficiencies will also tend to occur if the distal ileum is diseased or resected.

Functionally, the remaining small bowel can compensate to some degree for loss of absorptive area by increasing its absorptive capacity. Some experimental evidence notes a return of 60% of bowel absorptive capacity by the second month after resuscitation.[101]

In patients with short-bowel syndromes, the absorption of fat is usually a much greater problem than carbohydrate uptake. In spite of massive resections of small bowel, ingested disaccharides can induce changes in enzyme secretion in the remaining ileum or jejunum, so that after a relatively short time, intestinal adaptation occurs, and carbohydrate absorption may approach normal. Fluid and most electrolyte losses can be compensated to some degree by the kidneys, but large losses of calcium, magnesium, and zinc may be much more difficult to manage.[2]

An unusual syndrome, usually seen only with short bowel syndromes, is D-lactic acidosis, which can cause patients to exhibit bizarre behavior and various neurologic findings, including ataxia and confusion.[2] This problem is caused by an overgrowth of colonic bacteria that produce the D-isomer of lactic acid, which cannot be metabolized by the human body. The diagnosis of D-lactic acidosis should be suspected if the patient has an increased anion gap metabolic acidosis in the absence of usual causes such as uremia, ketoacidosis, or tissue ischemia. Treatment is directed at suppression of colonic bacterial overgrowth with appropriate enteral antibiotics.[102]

Gastric Stenosis

Postoperative stenosis in the cardia or body of the stomach is quite rare due to the generous lumen and the ability of the stomach to stretch;[2] however, if the injury is near the esophagogastric junction or the pylorus, stenosis can easily develop. Such injuries may require a pyloroplasty, gastric resection, Thal patch, or similar surgical maneuvers to assure patency and a secure closure.[2] With very large defects, gastric resection or an antrectomy and vagotomy may be necessary. Complex injuries at the esophagogastric junction can be extremely difficult to handle and may require proximal gastric resection with an esophagogastrostomy.

⊘ FREQUENT ERRORS

In the Management of Injuries to the Stomach or Small Bowel

1. *Inadequate exploration of the abdomen, because of an assumption that a particular organ could not possibly have been injured by a bullet apparently passing through another area of the abdomen.*
2. *Inadequate search for another hole if one can find only an odd number of openings in the bowel after a gunshot wound.*
3. *Assuming that an abdominal injury has not occurred because a CT scan and an early DPL are negative.*
4. *Inadequate debridement of small bowel injuries.*
5. *Failure to explore a hematoma at the base of the small bowel mesentery adequately.*
6. *Failure to consider placement of an enteral feeding tube in a patient who has severe injuries and is not apt to be eating by mouth within 4-5 days.*
7. *Closing the abdomen under tension and allowing an abdominal compartment syndrome to develop.*
8. *Delay in reoperating for a possible small bowel suture leak.*

▼▼▼▼▼▼▼▼▼▼▼▼▼▼▼▼▼▼▼▼▼▼▼▼▼▼▼▼▼▼▼

SUMMARY POINTS

1. Taken together, the stomach and small bowel are usually the most frequently injured organs in penetrating abdominal trauma.
2. One should be suspicious of a characteristic tetrad of injuries caused by seat belts which includes abdominal wall contusion, small bowel rupture, mesenteric tears, and lumbar spine fractures.
3. One should assume that all gunshot wounds of the abdomen have injured some bowel.
4. One should never assume that the path of a missile is a straight line between the entrance and exit wounds.
5. Severe blunt trauma can injure almost any part of the small bowel.
6. A stomach that has no acid or is full of blood can have a high bacterial content.
7. The colony count of bacteria in the distal small bowel can be extremely high and resemble that of colon.
8. Signs of peritonitis after blunt intestinal trauma may be delayed for hours or days.
9. One cannot rely on the physical examination of the abdomen to detect bowel injuries in patients with an altered sensorium.
10. Intestinal injuries do not commonly cause free air to be visible on plain radiographs of the abdomen.
11. One cannot rely on abdominal CT scans to detect injuries to the small intestine distal to the ligament of Treitz.
12. DPL is the most reliable method for diagnosing injury to intraperitoneal hollow viscera; its timing, however, is a critical determinant of its accuracy.
13. In suspicious cases, celiotomy is the safest course to follow, even in the face of little or no confirming data of an intra-abdominal injury.
14. The traditional techniques of prompt exploration, debridement, and repair of the bowel followed by irrigation and removal of any contamination are still the cornerstones of the treatment of bowel injuries.
15. Extensive mobilization of the gastric fundus or high greater curvature can easily damage the spleen or short gastric vessels.
16. Several small bowel holes in close proximity are best treated by a segmental resection and primary anastomosis.
17. Meticulous debridement and careful anastomosis of normal bowel are the keys to successful repair.
18. Any deterioration in a patient with mesenteric trauma should be considered due to intestinal ischemia or perforation until proven otherwise.

19. Access to the proximal SMA is best done from a lateral retroperitoneal approach after mobilizing the left-sided abdominal viscera to the right.
20. Before closure, all patients with severe abdominal injuries should be considered for operative placement of an enteral feeding device.
21. Closing the abdominal wall under tension increases the risk of abdominal-wall and intestinal complications.
22. With gastric or intestinal injuries, gastric decompression should be continued until there is little or no threat of ileus.
23. Prophylactic antibiotics are usually needed for only one or two doses after gastric or small intestinal injuries.
24. In critically ill or injured patients, the gastric pH should be monitored and kept above 4.5-5.0 until the patient is eating properly.
25. Early postoperative bowel obstructions tend to have a high mortality rate because they often are not diagnosed until strangulation or peritonitis occurs.
26. If large amounts of small bowel must be removed, special efforts should be made to preserve the distal ileum.

▲▲▲▲▲▲▲▲▲▲▲▲▲▲▲▲▲▲▲▲▲▲▲▲▲▲▲▲▲▲▲▲▲

REFERENCES

1. Harrison AW, Whelan P. Bowel injury from blunt abdominal trauma. In McMurtry RY, McLellan BA, eds. Management of blunt trauma. Baltimore: Williams & Wilkins, 1990;23:265-271.
2. Schwab CW, Shaikhra, Talucci RC. Injury to the stomach and small bowel. In Moore EE, Mattox KL, Feliciano DV, eds. Trauma. 2nd ed. Norwalk, CT: Appleton-Lange, 1991;31:485-497.
3. Morgagni. Epistola 1761;54:140-142.
4. Loria FL. Historical aspects of penetrating wounds of the abdomen. Int Abstr Surg 1948;89:521.
5. Blaisdell FW. General assessment, resuscitation and exploration of penetrating and blunt abdominal trauma. In Blaisdell FW, Trunkey DD, eds. Trauma management: abdominal trauma. New York: Thieme-Stratton, 1982; 1.
6. Boneti. Medicina Septertrionallis Collatita III, Sec XVII, Chap X. Geneva: Leonardi Choret Soc, 1685; 644-645.
7. Larrez DJ. Memoires de Chirurgie Militaire. Paris: Smith et Bruissan, 1815.
8. Poland A. A collection of several cases of contusion of the abdomen accompanied with injury of the stomach and intestines. Gray's Hosp Rep Series III 1858;4:123-168.
9. Longuet J. Remarques sur la rupture de l'intestin sans lesions des parois abdominales. Bull Soc Anat Paris 1875;3:799-823.
10. MacCormac Sir W. Abdominal section for the treatment of intraperitoneal injury. Br Med J 1887;1:975-1038.
11. Poer DH, Woliver E. Intestinal and mesenteric injury due to nonpenetrating abdominal trauma. JAMA 1942;118:11.
12. Croft J. Case of ruptured small intestine without external wound. Proc Clin Soc London 1890;23:141-149.
13. Motz. Etude sur les contusions de l'abdomen par coup de pied du cheval. Rev Chir 1890;10:875.
14. Wangensteen OH, Wangensteen SD. The rise of surgery from empiric craft to scientific discipline. Minneapolis, MN: University of Minnesota Press, 1978.
15. Surgery in World War II: general surgery. Washington, DC: Office of the Surgeon General, Department of the Army, 1955.
16. Yajko RD, Seydel F, Trimble C. Rupture of the stomach from blunt abdominal trauma. J Trauma 1975;15:177.
17. DiVincenti FC, Rives JD, Laborde EJ, et al. Blunt abdominal trauma. J Trauma 1968;8:1004.
18. Bosworth BM. Perforation of the small intestine from nonpenetrating abdominal trauma. Am J Surg 1948;76:472.
19. Fabian TC, Patterson CR. Injuries of the stomach, duodenum, pancreas, and small intestine. In Kreis DJ, Gomez GA, eds. Trauma management. Boston: Little, Brown & Company, 1989; 229-230.
20. Nance FC, Wennar MH, Johnson LW, et al. Surgical judgement in the management of penetrating wounds of the abdomen: experience with 2212 patients. Ann Surg 1974;179:639.
21. Lowe RJ, Boyd DR, Folk, FA, et al. The negative laparotomy for abdominal trauma. J Trauma 1972;12:853.

22. Bolton PM, Wood CB, Quarey-Papafio JB, et al. Blunt abdominal injury: a review of 59 consecutive cases undergoing surgery. Br J Surg 1973;60:657.

23. Karahaija EO. Blunt abdominal trauma in patients with multiple injuries. Injury 1972;4:307.

24. Robbs JV, Moore SW, Tially SP. Blunt abdominal trauma with jejunal injury: a review. J Trauma 1980;20:308.

25. Baker CC, Oppenheimer L, Stephens B, et al. Epidemiology of trauma deaths. Am J Surg 1980;140:144.

26. Perry JF, McClellan RJ. Autopsy findings in 127 patients following fatal traffic accidents. Surg Gynecol Obstet 1964;586.

27. Williams RD, Yarbo AA. Controversial aspects of diagnosis and management of blunt abdominal trauma. Am J Surg 1966;111:477.

28. Davis JJ, Cohn I Jr, Nance FC. Diagnosis and management of blunt abdominal trauma. Ann Surg 1976;183:672.

29. Denis R, Allard M, Atlas H, et al. Changing trends with abdominal injury in seat belt wearers. J Trauma 1983;23:1007.

30. Ryan P, Ragazzoni R. Abdominal injuries in survivors of road trauma before and since seat belt legislation in Victoria. Aust NZ J Surg 1979;49:200.

31. MacLeod JH, Nicholson DM. Seat belt trauma to the abdomen. Can J Surg 1969;12:202.

32. Dehner JR. Seatbelt injuries of the spine and abdomen. Radiology 1971;111:833.

33. Williams N, Ratliff DA. Gastrointestinal disruption and vertebral fracture associated with the use of seat belts. Ann R Coll Surg Engl 1993;75:129.

34. Cerise EJ, Schully JH. Blunt trauma to the small intestine. J Trauma 1970;10:46.

35. Dajee H, MacDonald AC. Gastric rupture due to seatbelt injury. Br J Surg 1983;69:436.

36. Murr P, Moore EE, Dunn EL, et al. Stabbed stuffed stomach syndrome. N Engl J Med 1979;300:625.

37. DeMuth WE. Bullet velocity and design as determinants of wounding capability: an experimental study. J Trauma 1966;6:222.

38. Jordan GL Jr, Beall AC Jr. Diagnosis and management of abdominal trauma. Curr Probl Surg 1971; 1-62.

39. DeMuth WE, Nicholas GG, Munger BL. Buckshot wounds. J Trauma 1976;18:53.

40. Flint LM, Cryer HM, Howard DA, et al. Approaches to the management of shotgun injuries. J Trauma 1984;24:415.

41. Gerard PS, Halpern D, Schiano T. Duck bone perforation of the small bowel (letter). J Clin Gastroenterol 1993;16:170.

42. Counseller VS, McCormack CJ. Subcutaneous perforation of the jejunum. Ann Surg 1935;102:365.

43. Thuck JM, Lowe RJ. Intestinal disruption due to blunt abdominal trauma. Am J Surg 1978;136:668.

44. Bergqvist D, Hedelin H, Karlsson G, et al. Intestinal trauma. Acta Chir Scand 1981;147:629.

45. Geoghegan T, Brush B. The mechanism of intestinal perforation from nonpenetrating abdominal trauma. AMA Arch Surg 1957;73:455.

46. Wagensteen OH. Intestinal obstruction. Springfield, IL: Charles C Thomas, 1955.

47. Reynolds BM, Balsano NA, Reynolds FX. Falls from heights: a surgical experience of 200 consecutive cases. Ann Surg 1971;174:304.

48. Lukas GM, Hutton JE, Lim RC, Mathewson C. Injuries sustained from high velocity impact with water: an experience from the Golden Gate Bridge. J Trauma 1981;21:612.

49. Rooney JA, Pesek IG. Transection of the stomach due to blunt abdominal trauma: review of previous reports and presentation of two cases. J Trauma 1968;8:487.

50. Glassman O. Subcutaneous rupture of stomach; traumatic and spontaneous. Ann Surg 1929;89:247.

51. Dauterive AH, Flancbaum L, Cox EF. Blunt intestinal trauma: a modern day review. Ann Surg 1985;201:198.

52. Berry J. Injuries of the intestines. Br Med J October 1921;22:643.

53. Vance BM. Traumatic lesions of the intestine caused by nonpenetrating blunt force. Arch Surg 1923;7:197.

54. Friedell MT, Ecblunt AM. Experimental immersion blast injury: preliminary report. US Navy Med Bull 1943;41:353.

55. Senn J. Traumatic intestinal rupture. Am J Med Sci 1904;127:968.

56. Massie G. Traumatic intestinal rupture. Lancet 1923;205:640.

57. Sauerbruch K. Die pathogenese de subcutanen rupturen des magerdarmtrabtus. Mitt Genzgeb Med Chir 1903;12:93.

58. Carter B, Farquhar. Contusion of the abdomen with rupture of the intestine. Am J Med Sci 1887;93:321.

59. Williams RD, Sargent FT. The mechanism of intestine injury in trauma. J Trauma 1963;3:288.

60. Sube J, Ziperman H, McIver WJ. Seatbelt trauma to the abdomen. Am J Surg 1967;113:346.

61. Cutting RA. The relative mechanical strength of enterostomies performed with and without clamps. Arch Surg 1928;17:666.

62. Dupre MW, Silva E, Brotman S. Traumatic rupture of the stomach secondary to Heimlich maneuver. Am J Emerg Med 1993;11:611.

63. Rappert P, Preier L, Korab W, Neubauer T. Diagnostic and therapeutic management of esophageal and gastric caustic burns in childhood. Eur J Pediatr Surg 1993;3:202.

64. Zhu ZX, Yu DC, Wang Y, Zhao L. Successful treatment of a severe electrical injury involving the stomach. Burns 1993;19:80.

65. Gorbach SL. Intestinal microflora. Gastroenterology 1971;60:1110.

66. Williams DB, Kark RC. Intestinal injury associated with low-voltage electrocution. J Trauma 21:246, 1981.

67. Aguilar JC. Fatal gastric hemorrhage: a complication of cardiorespiratory resuscitation. J Trauma 1981;21:573.

68. Backaitis SH. Injury patterns and injury sources of unrestrained and three point belt restrained car occupants in injury producing frontal collisions. 29th Proc Am Assoc Automotive Med 1985;365.

69. Mantovani M, Curi JC, Rizoli SB. Exclusive jejunal and ileal lesions due to blunt trauma. Rev Paul Med 1992;110:56.

70. Ford EG, Senac MO, Jr. Clinical presentation and radiographic identification of small bowel rupture following blunt trauma in children. Pediatr Emerg Care 1993;9:139.

71. Thadepalli H, Lou MA, Bach VT, et al. Microflora of the human small intestine. Am J Surg 1979138:845.

72. Freeark RJ. Penetrating wounds of the abdomen. N Engl J Med 1974; 291:185.

73. McBoyle MF, Schiller WR, Hurt AV. Massive gastrointestinal bleeding following blunt abdominal trauma: an unusual case presentation. J Trauma 1984;24:1057.

74. Schumer W, Burman SO. The perforated viscus: diagnosis and treatment. Surg Clin North Am 1972;52:231.

75. Davis RA, Shayne JP, Max MH, et al. The use of computerized axial tomography versus peritoneal lavage in the evaluation of blunt abdominal trauma. A prospective study. Surgery 1985;98:845.

76. Goldstein AS, Sclafani SJA, Kupferstein NH, et al. The diagnostic superiority of computerized tomography. J Trauma 1985;25:938.

77. Marx JA, Moore EE, Jorden RC, et al. Limitations of computed tomography in the evaluation of acute abdominal trauma. A prospective comparison with diagnostic peritoneal lavage. J Trauma 1985;25:933.

78. Fabian TC, Mangiante EC, White TJ et al. A prospective study of 91 patients undergoing both computed tomography and peritoneal lavage following blunt abdominal trauma. J Trauma 1986;26:602.

79. Mueller GL, Burney RE, Mackenzie JR. Leucocytosis in peritoneal lavage effluent after selected abdominal organ injury in an experimental model. Ann Emerg Med 1982;11:343.

80. Marx JA, Bar-Or D, Moore EE, et al. Utility of lavage alkaline phosphatase in detection of isolated small intestinal injury. Ann Emerg Med 1985;14:10.

81. Edwards J, Gaspard DJ. Visceral injury due to extraperitoneal gunshot wounds. Arch Surg 1974;108:865.

82. Moore EE, Marx JA. Penetrating abdominal wounds. Rationale for exploratory laparotomy. JAMA 1985;253:2705.

83. Morgan JC, Turner CS, Pennell TC. Air gun injuries of the abdomen in children. Arch Surg 1984;119:1437.

84. Granson MA, Donovan AJ. Abdominal stab wound with omental evisceration. Arch Surg 1983;118:57.

85. Walt AJ, Wilson RF. Specific abdominal injuries. In Walt AJ, Wilson RF, eds. Management of trauma: pitfalls and practice. Philadelphia: Lea & Febiger, 1975; 348-374.

86. Boyle D, Petregraw W. Postsplenectomy gastric perforation. Surgery 1967;61:239.

87. Frantzides CT, Ludwig KA, Aprahamian C, Salaymeh B. Laparoscopic closure of gastric stab wounds. A case report. Surg Laparosc Endosc 1993;3:63.

88. Brams DM, Cardoza M, Smith RS. Laparoscopic repair of traumatic gastric perforation using a gasless technique. J Laparoendosc Surg 1993; 3:587.

89. Talucci RC, Webb WR. Costal chondritis: the costal arch. Ann Thorac Surg 1983;35:318.

90. Bulkley GB, Perler BA, Zuidema GD. Mesenteric vascular disease. In Cameron JL, ed. Current surgical therapy, 5th ed. St Louis: Mosby, 1995:126.

91. Fansler RF, Mero K, Steinberg SM, et al. Utility of the biofragmentable anastomotic ring in traumatic small bowel injury. Am Surg 1994;60:379.

92. Lucas AE, Richardson JD, Flint LM, et al. Traumatic injury of the proximal superior mesenteric artery. Ann Surg 1981;193:30.

93. Mattox KL, McCollum WB, Jordan GL, et al. Management of upper abdominal vascular trauma. Am J Surg 1974;128:823.

94. Delany HM, Carnevale NJ, Garvey JW. Jejunostomy by a needle catheter technique. Surgery 1973;73:786.

95. Eger EI, Saidman LJ. Hazards of nitrous oxide anesthesia in bowel obstruction and pneumothorax. Anesthesiology 1965;26:61.

96. Larson GM, Vandertoll DJ. Approaches to repair of ventral hernia and full-thickness losses of the abdominal wall. Surg Clin North Am 1984; 64:335.

97. Shepard GH. High-energy, low velocity close-range shotgun wounds. J Trauma 1980;20:1065.

98. Moore EE, Jones TN. Benefits of immediate jejunostomy feeding after major abdominal trauma. J Trauma 1986;26:874.

99. Thadepalli H, Gorbach SL, Broido PW, et al. Abdominal trauma anaerobes and antibiotics. Surg Gynecol Obster 1973;137:270.

100. Ablan CJ, Olen RN, Dobrin, et al. Efficacy of intraperitoneal antibiotics in the treatment of severe fecal peritonitis. Am J Surg 1991; 1562:453.

101. Spiro HM. Primary structure disorders, short bowel syndrome. In Clinical gastroenterology. 3rd ed. New York: MacMillan, 1984.

102. Oh M, Phelps K, Traube M. D-Lactic acidosis in a man with a short bowel syndrome. N Engl J Med 1979;301:249.

Chapter 25 Injury to the Pancreas and Duodenum

ROBERT F. WILSON, M.D.

HISTORY

The first report of a pancreatic injury was provided in 1827 by Travers, who described a total transection of the pancreas found at necropsy in a patient who had been struck by the wheel of a stagecoach. By 1903, a collected series of pancreatic injuries reported only 45 patients. The mortality rate was 71% (17/24) for blunt injury, 75% (9/12) for gunshot wounds, and 11% (1/9) for stab wounds.[3] All the patients treated nonoperatively died regardless of the method of injury.

In 1905, Korte reported the first successful operation for an isolated traumatic transection of the pancreas. Although a fistula developed postoperatively, it closed spontaneously.[4] The first survivor of a pseudocyst developing after a blunt injury to the pancreas was reported by Kulenkampf in 1882,[5] and in a review of this problem by Moynihan in 1926,[6] a number of patients with traumatic pseudocysts were recorded.

Kocher in 1903 described his method for elevating the duodenum to evaluate both pancreatic and duodenal injuries.[7] Summers[8] credits Cachovie with performing a closure of the pylorus and then decompressing the stomach with a gastroenterostomy to treat duodenal fistulas. Summers also suggested occlusion of the pylorus with a pursestring suture and construction of a gastrojejunostomy to treat duodenal wounds.

ANATOMY

The pancreas and the duodenum are relatively well protected deep within the abdomen. Except for the first part of the duodenum, they are retroperitoneal and, therefore, protected anteriorly to some extent by the upper abdominal intraperitoneal organs. Posteriorly, they are protected by the thick paraspinal muscles. Consequently, these organs are usually injured only with deeply penetrating wounds or forceful blunt trauma.[1]

> **AXIOM** Associated injuries are the major cause of the high mortality rates seen with pancreatic and duodenal trauma.[1]

The first part of the duodenum lies at the level of the first lumbar vertebra (L1), the second or descending part parallels the second and third lumbar vertebrae (L2 and 3), and the third part crosses the midline at the level of L4 to end in the fourth or ascending part slightly to the left of the aorta.[9] In its various portions, the duodenum is in close proximity to the liver, common bile duct, portal vein, pancreas, right kidney, inferior vena cava, aorta, superior mesenteric artery and vein, the transverse colon, and the left kidney (Fig. 25–1). Any of these nearby structures may be injured concomitantly with the pancreas or duodenum, and these injuries can alter prognosis significantly.[9] Since the duodenum is predominantly a retroperitoneal structure, it lacks a complete serosal covering for most of its length. In the absence of a serosa, repairs of such bowel are generally less certain and have a relatively greater tendency to leak.[9] In addition, the pancreas has limited tensile strength, so that sutures tend to cut through it or pull out easily.[1] It is also difficult to penetrate the pancreas deeply at any point without passing through some ductal structures. For all of these reasons, injuries to the pancreas may be difficult to repair, and such repairs have an increased tendency to leak.

> **AXIOM** Pancreatic parenchymal injuries are difficult to repair and frequently leak for at least several days after injury.

The head of the pancreas is nestled into the curve of the duodenum and shares its blood supply.[1] There is dense adherence of these two structures throughout the second and most of the third portion of the duodenum, so that separating the two can be difficult. In addition, both of the pancreatic ducts (the ducts of Wirsurg and Santorini) penetrate the wall of the duodenum to allow pancreatic juices to enter the intestinal lumen. The tail of the pancreas nestles against the hilum of the spleen, and the spleen shares its blood supply with the body and tail of the pancreas.

> **AXIOM** Except for the dorsal pancreatic artery, which usually arises from the superior mesenteric artery, the pancreas has almost no independent arterial blood supply.[1]

The blood supply of the duodenum and the head of the pancreas include the superior and inferior pancreaticoduodenal arteries, which are branches of the gastroduodenal and superior mesenteric arteries, respectively.[9] The vascular arcades of these vessels are located in the pancreaticoduodenal groove, which parallels the medial wall of the second portion of the duodenum. Consequently, injury to one of these organs in this area is very likely to affect the other also.

PHYSIOLOGY

The pancreas and duodenum are closely related, not only because of their anatomic proximity and shared ductal system and blood supply, but also because of their physiologic responses. Since there is little absorption in the stomach, the duodenum receives virtually all of the ingested food as well as 1000-2500 ml of salivary and gastric secretions, 600-1000 ml of bile, 800 1500 ml of pancreatic juice, and some duodenal secretions. The total volume of these secretions may exceed 5-6 liters per day, and a large fistula in this area can cause serious fluid and electrolyte problems.

Stimuli to Secretion

Secretion of pancreatic juice occurs primarily in response to stimulation by the vagus nerves and by hormones formed in the duodenum. Secretin, which is secreted by duodenal mucosa primarily as a response to acid duodenal contents, stimulates secretion of pancreatic juice that is high in volume and bicarbonate and low in enzyme content. The other main secretagogue, cholecystokinin, is secreted in response to the breakdown products of food rather than acid, and this substances stimulates emptying of the gallbladder and passage of this bile into the duodenum. It also stimulates the exocrine pancreas to secrete a relatively low volume of pancreatic juice that has a high concentration of enzymes.

> **AXIOM** The secretin system is an important mechanism for preventing duodenal ulceration, and cholecystokinin (pancreozymin) is primarily for digestive purposes.[1]

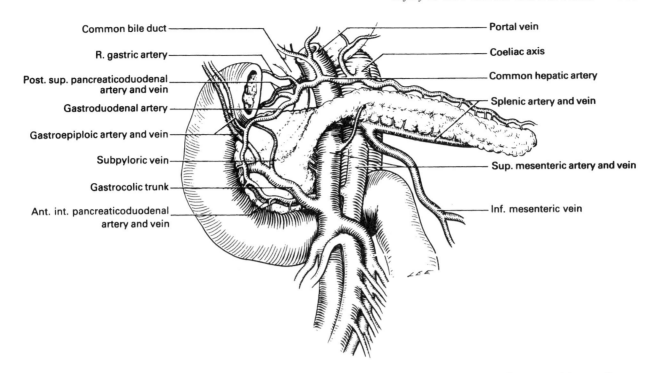

FIGURE 25–1 The pancreas and duodenum are closely associated with a large number of vessels, and the mortality rate for injuries to those organs is often determined by the associated vascular injuries (From Frey CF, Bodai BI. The surgical treatment of pancreaticoduodenal trauma. In Champion HR, Robbs JV, Trunkey DD, eds. Rob & Smith's operative surgery. London: Butterworths, 1989; 415.)

Activation of Enzymes

AXIOM Dehiscence of a duodenal suture line can be especially dangerous because of the large amounts of activated enzymes that may be rapidly liberated into the abdomen.

Dehiscence of any gastrointestinal suture line can have serious consequences, but duodenal leakage can be particularly devastating because the duodenum is the immediate common conduit for gastric, biliary, and pancreatic secretions. The components of these individual organ secretions include powerful digestive enzymes that are activated by their admixture. This combination has an autodigestive capacity that greatly exceeds that of its individual components, and makes the management of duodenal dehiscence a much more difficult problem than isolated injuries of the stomach, pancreas, or biliary system.

AXIOM Preventing leakage of the luminal contents is a major goal of treatment of duodenal injuries, and the nature and location of the injury may dictate diversion of those contents in addition to careful repair.

INCIDENCE AND MECHANISMS OF INJURY

Blunt trauma to the pancreas is rather uncommon. In one series of 839 patients with blunt abdominal trauma admitted to a hospital, there were only nine (1.1%) with pancreatic injury.[10] This is consistent with most reviews of blunt abdominal trauma.[11,12] In one collected series, penetrating pancreatic injuries out-numbered blunt damage four to one.[13]

In a 12-year period at Detroit Receiving Hospital ending June 30, 1992, 2,741 patients were noted to have abdominal injuries. Of these, 210 (7.7%) had pancreatic injury found on exploratory laparotomy or at laparotomy. Of these, 177 (84%) were caused by penetrating trauma and 33 (16%) were caused by blunt mechanisms (Table 25–1). The incidence of pancreatic injuries with blunt trauma, gunshot wounds, and stabs was 5.8%, 10.3%, and 4.6%, respectively.

TABLE 25–1 **Mortality Rates with Abdominal Injuries Seen in 12 Years at Detroit Receiving Hospital (1980-1992)**

	Type of Trauma			
Organ Injured	Blunt	GSW	Stabs	Total
Liver	(160)	(499)	(251)	(910)
	35%	22%	8%	20%
Small Bowel	(58)	(551)	(150)	(759)
	24%	14%	7%	13%
Colon	(42)	(498)	(122)	(662)
	16%	14%	6%	12%
Diaphragm	(28)	(273)	(119)	(420)
	25%	22%	8%	18%
Kidney	(145)	(229)	(45)	(419)
	7%	17%	13%	13%
Spleen	(172)	(131)	(42)	(345)
	15%	24%	10%	18%
Stomach	(6)	(241)	(93)	(340)
	50%	22%	11%	19%
Abd. Vessels	(23)	(257)	(53)	(333)
	70%	53%	32%	58%
Pancreas	(33)	(140)	(37)	(210)
	6%	24%	30%	22%
Duodenum	(10)	(124)	(33)	(167)
	30%	23%	21%	23%
Bladder	(44)	(84)	(6)	(134)
	18%	6%	17%	10%
Gallbladder	(3)	(59)	(19)	(81)
	100%	24%	5%	22%
Total	(573)	(1358)	(810)	(2741)
	16%	14%	5%	12%

In the first six decades of this century, the knife was a common wounding agent, but from 1960 to 1980 there was a steady increase in the incidence of gunshot wounds, so that now the gun is the most common weapon causing pancreatic injuries in the United States.[1] Of 177 penetrating pancreatic injuries seen at DRH, 128 (72%) were caused by pistols or rifles, 12 (7%) were caused by shotguns, and 37 (21%) were caused by knives.

Pancreas

BLUNT TRAUMA

During blunt trauma, the pancreas is injured primarily by direct impact or compression.[9] Direct impact is more likely to injure patients whose abdominal musculature is relaxed because of an altered sensorium or because of the suddenness and surprise of the blow.[13]

Of patients sustaining blunt intraabdominal injuries, pancreatic wounds are encountered in approximately 8% and duodenal damage in about 5%.[1] Because of the proximity of so many surrounding structures, multiple associated injuries are the rule rather than the exception.[14]

In blunt trauma, certain unique patterns of associated visceral damage are well recognized and must be looked for. Such injuries, which are often occult initially, may ultimately cause severe morbidity or death.[15] When the right upper quadrant is the epicenter of the blow, the organs situated in the area of the pancreatic head tend to be pushed upwards into the chest or downwards into the lower abdomen. As the liver is displaced upward and the duodenum and pancreas downward, the gastroduodenal artery and common bile duct may tear at their relatively fixed connection to the pancreas. In these circumstances, the liver is apt to tear along its suspensory ligaments while the downward movement of the transverse colon may cause disruption of its mesentery and vessels.

In the DRH series, the most frequent associated injuries with blunt pancreatic trauma were the liver (36%), spleen (30%), kidney (18%), colon (18%), and major vessels (9%) (Table 25–2). Jordan has also noted that injuries to major arteries and veins, which are the major cause of death in patients with pancreatic trauma, occur in about 9% of these patients.[1]

In a recent report by Henne-Bruns et al,[16] it was noted that of 68 patients who had an emergency laparotomy for severe blunt abdominal trauma, 8 (12%) had major vascular injuries which included portal vein (5), inferior vena cava (2), and mesenteric root (1). Injuries to the portal vein were always associated with a complete rupture of the pancreas, requiring a distal pancreatectomy in four cases and duodenum-preserving resection of the head of the pancreas in one.

PENETRATING INJURIES

The organs most frequently injured in association with penetrating wounds of the pancreas are the liver and stomach.[1] Of particular significance because of the high morbidity is the fact that up to 45% of patients with pancreatic wounds with penetrating trauma have associated injuries of major arteries or veins.[1] In the DRH series, the most frequent associated injuries with penetrating pancreatic trauma were the stomach (54%), liver (49%) and kidneys (44%) (Table 25–2).

Although pancreatic injury is relatively uncommon, the mortality rate can be high.[1] In 1971, Jones and Shires[11] reported a mortality of 20% in a large series. Most of the deaths occurred within the first 24 hours and were due to hemorrhage from associated injuries; however, a significant number of deaths occurred as a result of late complications from sepsis and multisystem organ failure. In a collected series that differentiated between early and late deaths, late deaths accounted for about 40% of the total mortality.[16-20]

In the DRH series (Table 25-3), the mortality rate with penetrating pancreatic injuries was 25% (45/177). This included a mortality rate of 23% (28/128) for gunshot wounds, 30% (11/37) for stab wounds, and 42% (5/12) for shotgun wounds. Deaths caused by gunshot wounds tended to occur early and were usually caused by prolonged hemorrhagic shock. Many of the deaths caused by stab wounds tended to be later deaths due to sepsis. Mortality rates were largely related to the number of associated injuries, and the patients with zero or 1 associated injuries had a mortality rate of only 4% (Table 25-3).

Duodenum

INCIDENCE

The duodenum is injured less frequently than the pancreas. In the DRH series, there were 167 patients with duodenal injuries and 210 with pancreatic trauma (Table 25–1).

BLUNT TRAUMA

In most series, blunt injuries to the duodenum occur as a result of motor vehicle accidents.[21-25] The duodenum is thought to be injured in one of three ways by such trauma: (a) by deceleration and the resulting shear forces produced at the junction of mobile and relatively fixed portions of the duodenum, (b) by direct compression against the vertebral column, or (c) by the production of high intraluminal

TABLE 25–2   Mortality Rates and Associated Injuries with Pancreatic Trauma

Organ Injured	Blunt	GSW	SGW	Stabs	Total
			Type of Injury		
Liver	(12)	(69)	(6)	(11)	(98)
	8%	26%	33%	36%	25%
Stomach	(1)	(68)	(8)	(20)	(97)
	100%	25%	38%	30%	29%
Kidney	(6)	(64)	(7)	(6)	(85)
	17%	23%	57%	50%	28%
Spleen	(10)	(52)	(5)	(12)	(79)
	10%	35%	60%	33%	33%
Duodenum	(1)	(49)	(6)	(9)	(65)
	0%	27%	33%	56%	31%
Abd. Vessels	(3)	(49)	(6)	(15)	(73)
	67%	41%	67%	60%	45%
Colon	(6)	(47)	(8)	(10)	(71)
	0%	21%	25%	30%	21%
Small Bowel	——	(40)	(6)	(7)	(53)
		30%	67%	43%	36%
Diaphragm	(1)	(39)	(3)	(5)	(48)
	0%	26%	67%	20%	27%
Total	(33)	(128)	(12)	(37)	(210)
	6%	23%	42%	30%	22%

TABLE 25–3   Mortality Rate of Pancreatic Injury Correlated with Number of Associated Injuries

Number of Associated Injuries	Blunt	GSW	SGW	Stabs	Total
			Type of Injury		
0	(14)	(5)	——	(13)	(32)
	0%	0%		8%	3%
1	(8)	(12)	——	(5)	(25)
	13%	0%		0%	4%
2	(4)	(25)	(1)	(7)	(37)
	0%	8%	0%	43%	14%
3	(3)	(32)	(6)	(5)	(46)
	0%	19%	17%	80%	24%
4	(4)	(54)	(5)	(7)	(70)
	25%	39%	80%	43%	41%
Total	(33)	(128)	(12)	(37)	(210)
	6%	23%	42%	30%	22%

pressures in the closed loop formed between the contracted pylorus and the angulation of the duodenum at the ligament of Treitz.[9]

The mortality rate from blunt duodenal injury has fallen from about 90% in 1910 to approximately 15% today, but this figure will probably be reduced even further if diagnosis and treatment are accomplished earlier and more systematically.[26] In the DRH series, the mortality rate from blunt duodenal trauma was 30% (Table 25–4). Unfortunately, at least 25% of patients with isolated blunt duodenal injuries present with relatively mild or vague symptoms. Duodenal injury itself seldom results in death if recognized and appropriately treated within 24 hours, but if the injury is not treated within 24 hours, the mortality rate rises precipitously.[27] In the DRH series all of the patients who died with blunt duodenal trauma had four or more associated injuries. Complications in patients with duodenal injuries who reach the hospital alive are most often from associated injuries, especially to the pancreas.

The relatively high incidence of duodenal injury in motor vehicle accidents has been ascribed to compression of the epigastrium by the steering wheel.[28] This can crush the duodenum against the vertebral column or cause blow out of the duodenal loop because it is partially closed at the pylorus and at the ligament of Treitz.[21] This would explain the propensity for blunt injuries to occur in the second part of the duodenum on the right lateral aspect.

Improperly applied seat belts can increase the incidence of duodenal injury.[23] Lap-type seat belts prevent ejection from the automobile but do not really protect against a blow to the epigastrium from the steering wheel. The addition of a shoulder harness helps prevent forward flexion of the body, reducing the possibility of steering wheel injury.[21] The wearing of seat belts and driving at lower speed limits are factors which are probably responsible for the reduced incidence of duodenal injuries in several large recent series of blunt abdominal trauma.[22,23,29] Certainly, the failure to use seat belts may explain the relatively high incidence of duodenal injuries from motor vehicle accidents reported in the 1960s and 1970s.[30,32]

The second most frequent mechanism of injury involves focal trauma to the epigastrium. The best example of this is damage caused by bicycle handlebars, and this is a common cause of duodenal injury in children. A special injury of the duodenum, rarely seen in blunt

TABLE 25–4 *Mortality Rates and Associated Injuries with Duodenal Trauma*

Organ Injured	Blunt	GSW	SGW	Stabs	Total
		Type of Injury			
Liver	(3) 100%	(67) 25%	(6) 17%	(12) 25%	(88) 27%
Abd. Vessels	(2) 50%	(62) 32%	(3) 67%	(16) 44%	(83) 36%
Small Bowel	(3) 33%	(59) 25%	(3) 33%	(16) 25%	(81) 26%
Colon	(4) 50%	(55) 25%	(6) 17%	(16) 25%	(81) 26%
Pancreas	(1) 0%	(49) 27%	(6) 33%	(9) 56%	(65) 48%
Stomach	(1) 100%	(48) 27%	(4) 0%	(8) 25%	(61) 26%
Kidney	(2) 50%	(38) 24%	(2) 50%	(6) 33%	(48) 27%
Gall-bladder	——	(23) 26%	(2) 50%	(2) 0%	(27) 26%
Diaphragm	(1) 0%	(18) 22%	——	(2) 0%	(21) 16%
Spleen	(1) 100%	(9) 56%	——	(1) 100%	(11) 64%
Total	(10) 30%	(116) 23%	(8) 25%	(33) 21%	(167) 23%

TABLE 25–5 *Mortality Rate of Duodenal Injury Correlated with Number of Associated Injuries*

Number of Associated Injuries	Blunt	GSW	SGW	Stabs	Total
		Type of Injury			
0	(5) 0%	(5) 0%	——	(7) 0%	(17) 0%
1	——	(14) 7%	(1) 0%	(9) 0%	(24) 4%
2	(1) 0%	(22) 27%	——	(7) 29%	(30) 27%
3	(1) 100%	(31) 13%	(3) 33%	(5) 60%	(40) 23%
4+	(3) 67%	(44) 36%	(4) 25%	(5) 40%	(52) 40%
Total	(10) 30%	(116) 23%	(8) 25%	(33) 21%	(167) 23%

trauma to any other abdominal organ, is an intramural hematoma producing partial or complete obstruction of the lumen.[1] Although 90-95% of patients with other types of duodenal trauma have associated intraabdominal and extraabdominal injuries, duodenal hematomas often occur in isolation.

Although blunt duodenal injuries are most common in the second part of duodenum, about 25% are found in the fourth part, close to the ligament of Treitz.[27] Consequently, this latter area must be carefully inspected by incising the peritoneum and working gently under the lower border of the pancreas. Unless this is done, a tear in this area can easily be missed. Most duodenal lacerations are traverse in direction and involve less than 50% of the diameter.[26]

AXIOM One should look very closely for an associated pancreatic injury whenever the duodenum is damaged.

About 40-50% of the patients with duodenal injuries have associated pancreatic damage of varying degrees, ranging from severe contusion to laceration or rupture.[26] Very occasionally, the pancreas itself may be intact, but it may be partially separated from the medial border of the duodenum, causing concern about the status of the common bile and pancreatic ducts. Associated pancreatic injuries increase the mortality rate of duodenal injuries from about 5-10% to almost 40%.[20] In the DRH series, none or only one associated injury resulted in a mortality rate of only 2.4%.

PENETRATING INJURIES

Of the 167 patients with duodenal injuries diagnosed at laparotomy at DRH in the 12-year period, 157 (94%) were due to penetrating trauma. These included 116 (74%) due to gunshot wounds, eight (5%) due to shotgun wounds, and 33 (21%) due to stab wounds.

Of the 167 patients with penetrating duodenal injuries, 92 (55%) had three or more associated injuries (Table 25–5), and of the 124 patients with gunshot or shotgun wounds, 82 (49%) had three or more associated injuries. Of the 33 patients with stab wounds, only 10 (30%) had three or more associated injuries.

The most frequent associated injuries in the 10 DRH patients with blunt duodenal trauma were the colon (40%), liver (30%), and small bowel (30%) (Table 25–4). With penetrating trauma, the most frequent associated injuries were the liver (54%), vessels (52%), small bowel (50%), and colon (49%). The mortality rates with the various associated blunt injuries were 60% for the spleen, 36% for abdominal vessels, and 31% for the pancreas.

The mortality rate with penetrating duodenal injuries was 23%. This included a mortality rate of 21% for stab wounds, 23% for gunshot wounds, and 25% for shotgun wounds. Of 36 patients with one or no associated injuries, only one (3%) died. Of 121 patients with two or more associated injuries, 35 (29%) died (P<0.005).

DIAGNOSIS

> **AXIOM**   The major principle in the diagnosis of blunt pancreatic or duodenal trauma is awareness of the initial subtlety of these injuries.[9]

Delay in diagnosis and treatment is uniformly recognized as the leading cause of morbidity and mortality in patients with blunt injuries of the pancreas or duodenum.[9,27,31,32] This circumstance is compounded by the lack of specific signs and symptoms for such injuries. Although trauma to the pancreas or duodenum is often accompanied by other significant organ injuries that prompt early exploration of the abdomen, the associated injuries are the major cause of death.[9,32,36]

History

> **AXIOM**   Injury to the pancreas or duodenum must be considered a possibility in all patients who sustain injury to the upper abdomen.[1]

The diagnostic approach to upper abdominal trauma varies with the wounding agent. For example, Fabian and Patterson[9] routinely explore all patients with suspected penetrating abdominal trauma, and the issue in such patients is one of intraoperative rather than preoperative diagnosis. Jordan, however, is more selective; for patients sustaining stab wounds of the upper abdomen, he believes that one should initially determine whether or not the peritoneum was penetrated. This is usually done by exploration of the wound under local anesthesia in the emergency room.[1] If the peritoneum is penetrated, but there are no obvious signs of intraperitoneal injury, he performs a diagnostic peritoneal lavage (DPL). If the DPL is positive, he explores the abdomen. He also explores all gunshot wounds of the abdomen unless there is conclusive evidence that the wound was tangential and could not have entered the peritoneal cavity.

Physical Examination

> **AXIOM**   The clinical changes in isolated pancreatic or duodenal injury may be extremely subtle until severe, life-threatening peritonitis develops.

The initial physical examination is notoriously inaccurate for determining the presence or absence of pancreaticoduodenal trauma; however, if there is evidence of peritonitis or intraperitoneal hemorrhage, the patient is taken to the operating room immediately.[1,9,35] If there is no evidence of such problems, DPL can be used for further evaluation.

In patients with other intraabdominal injuries, the associated injuries often dominate the clinical picture and serve as the main indication for exploration.[9] Although isolated retroperitoneal injuries occasionally can produce signs of frank peritonitis, the vast majority produce only a mild tenderness. Consequently, upper abdominal tenderness of any degree associated with an appropriate mechanism of trauma should raise suspicion of a pancreatic or duodenal injury.

> **AXIOM**   The best way to diagnose pancreatic or duodenal injuries is repeated careful reexamination of the patient combined with a high index of suspicion.[9]

Lucas[37] has described a transient diminution in abdominal tenderness in patients with pancreatic or duodenal injuries about 2 hours following admission. This is followed by an increased tenderness again about 4 hours later. Proper utilization of this characteristic profile requires, of course, serial examinations conducted by

the same physician throughout the early hours of the patient's hospitalization.

> **AXIOM**   A normal physical examination does not rule out significant pancreatic or duodenal injuries.

Differentiating between deep intraabdominal tenderness and the tenderness confined to the abdominal wall may be aided by asking the patient to raise his or her head up off the pillow.[9] Tightening of the abdominal musculature should reduce tenderness due to intraabdominal pathology, but tenderness due to abdominal wall injury should increase or remain essentially unchanged.

Laboratory Examinations

> **AXIOM**   Laboratory examinations are relatively insensitive and nonspecific for diagnosing duodenal or pancreatic injury.[9]

Serum amylase is probably the most widely discussed laboratory test for diagnosing pancreatic or duodenal injury. An elevated serum or urinary amylase can be helpful in making one suspect a pancreatic injury,[10,38-40] but a consistently elevated or rising serum or urinary amylase is a much stronger indicator of this problem. Northrop and Simmons[12] believe that an elevated urinary amylase is a much more sensitive indicator of pancreatic or duodenal injury than an elevated serum amylase.

Although an elevated serum amylase was found in 70% of the patients with duodenal injuries studied by Fabian et al,[32] and although Lucas[37] recommends rising amylase levels as an indicator of pancreatic injury, many investigators have found amylase to be an unreliable test.[34,41,42]

Jordan[1] has noted that serum amylase levels are elevated in only about 25% of patients sustaining penetrating injury to the pancreas; however, they may elevated in up to 80% of patients with blunt injury to the pancreas.[40] More specific studies of pancreatic and nonpancreatic isoenzymes have not been uniformly helpful.[43,44]

It should be remembered that perforation of the duodenum or any portion of the upper gastrointestinal tract may also lead to elevated serum amylase levels as a result of spillage of intraluminal amylase into the peritoneal cavity.[1] This is also true of elevated amylase levels found in intraperitoneal fluid aspirated by a peritoneal tap or after diagnostic peritoneal lavage.

> **AXIOM**   Monitoring serum amylase levels during the early postinjury phase seems prudent, but the clinician should regard normal levels as inconclusive.

The source of hyperamylasemia in patients with facial trauma or recent ethanol ingestion may be related to parotid injury or increased gastric permeability to salivary amylase.[9] In addition, pancreatic and/or duodenal injury occurs frequently without a rise in serum amylase levels.

Radiographic Studies

> **AXIOM**   The diagnosis of pancreaticoduodenal trauma is more often made by the astute clinician than by any laboratory test or radiograph.[9]

PLAIN FILMS

Plain films of the abdomen with the patient in the recumbent and upright positions are indicated, as in anyone suspected of having an intraabdominal injury; however, missed roentgenographic signs are frequently reported in retrospective series.[1,9] Flint et al[34] have emphasized the tendency of surgeons, and particularly radiologists, to overlook evidence that is present on plain films. Lucas[37] described scoliosis or obliteration of the right psoas shadow in 90% (18/20) of patients with duodenal rupture. In 50% of the patients, retroperitoneal air bubbles could be seen along the right psoas muscle or around the right kidney. The presence of retroperitoneal air is sufficient evidence to compel exploration, and Lucas[37] recommends an upper GI series with water-soluble contrast in patients with the less specific radiologic signs, such as of scoliosis or blurring of the psoas margin.

PITFALL ⊘

> *If an intent search for retroperitoneal air is not made on plain radiographs of the abdomen, the diagnosis of traumatic rupture of the duodenum will generally be delayed. Consequently, the mortality rate may be extremely high.[26]*

AXIOM   Plain films of the abdomen and upper GI contrast studies, like serum amylase determinations, should be used to prompt early exploration, not to dismiss the possibility of pancreaticoduodenal injury.

CONTRAST STUDIES

In individuals who do not have clinical evidence of peritonitis, an upper gastrointestinal series using water-soluble contrast material can provide positive results in 50% of patients with duodenal perforations.[45] Flint et al[34] reported two false-negative contrast studies in three patients with full thickness duodenal injury. Whenever possible, the gastrographin swallow should be done with the patient in the right lateral position. Some surgeons feel barium is more accurate and can provide more positive results, but it also tends to cause more peritoneal and retroperitoneal inflammation.[21]

AXIOM   A negative contrast study of the duodenum can be extremely dangerous because of the false sense of security it can inspire.[34]

Studies with contrast are also indicated in patients with a suspected hematoma of the duodenum, because these may demonstrate the classic "coiled-spring" appearance of complete obstruction by this mechanism.[1]

COMPUTED TOMOGRAPHY SCANS

Another examination that is of value in selected patients is the computed tomography (CT) scan. Many surgeons advocate more frequent use of this modality. Kunin et al,[46] for example, reported on seven patients with blunt trauma resulting in a duodenal hematoma in four and perforation in three. All seven were diagnosed correctly by the CT scan. Extraluminal gas or extravasated oral contrast was seen in the right anterior prerenal space in all three perforations and in one of the patients with only a hematoma.

Lane et al[47] recently reviewed the abdominal CT scans of 10 patients with pancreatic injury proven by surgery or autopsy after blunt abdominal trauma. The finding of fluid between the pancreas and the splenic vein was then studied, along with intraperitoneal fluid, pancreatic edema or hematoma, and thickening of the anterior renal fascia. The CT scans of all 10 patients showed abnormalities suggesting pancreatic injury, although only 40% of patients showed all the findings reported in the literature. Fluid between the splenic vein and the pancreatic parenchyma was seen on CT scans in 90% and was easy to recognize. Nelson et al[48] also found that, on the basis of their review of the CT scans of three patients with acute blunt pancreatic transection, a high index of suspicion combined with careful interpretation of the CT scan can usually provide the correct diagnosis.

Jordan,[1] however, does not use CT in the majority of his patients because of the time and expense required. Furthermore, he says the CT scan may be inaccurate in the diagnosis of pancreatic injury. His use of CT is restricted to patients in whom there is some suspicion of injury but surgical intervention will be deferred unless the test is positive. Harrison and Whelan[10] find that CT scanning is most useful in detecting late complications of pancreatic injury or surgery. However, CT scanning is unable to define the pancreatic duct consistently, and this decreases its value in the early assessment of injury.

Fabian and Patterson[9] have not found any convincing evidence that abdominal CT scanning is accurate in the early diagnosis of pancreatic or duodenal injuries. They admit that the CT may be capable of diagnosing pancreatic trauma reliably 24 hours after injury, but that is the time when clinical deterioration should be evident and should prompt exploration rather than performance of further diagnostic tests.

Contrast CT examinations may be more sensitive for duodenal injury than conventional radiologic studies, particularly for retroperitoneal air,[10] but the experience of Fabian and Patterson[9] with this technique indicates only that false-negative and false-positive results are possible. They currently employ CT in patients with a predisposing mechanism of injury, but without other evidence of retroperitoneal injury.

AXIOM   All techniques used to diagnose injuries of the pancreas or duodenum may be characterized as reliable only when they identify an injury; a "normal" study has relatively little negative predictive value.[9]

ULTRASONOGRAPHY

Potentially, ultrasonography can demonstrate changes in the size, shape, or consistency of the pancreas as well as a CT scan;[1] however, because of the limitations of ultrasound in the region of the body and tail (because overlying bowel gas is often present), a CT scan is generally the more useful modality. Nevertheless, an ultrasound may still be preferable for demonstrating large fluid collections surrounding the gland and for diagnosing pseudocysts.[1] In a recent case report, however, Gothi et al[49] described how they were able to demonstrate a fracture through the body of the pancreas along with disruption of the pancreatic duct using conventional ultrasound.

Diagnostic Peritoneal Lavage

Diagnostic peritoneal lavage (DPL) has been widely employed in the evaluation of blunt and, to a lesser extent, penetrating abdominal trauma; however, it is not reliable for detecting retroperitoneal injuries. While Flint et al[34] have been enthusiastic about DPL, the associated injuries in their series, rather than those involving the duodenum, were primarily responsible for its apparent sensitivity. Nevertheless, Fabian and Patterson[9] are convinced that DPL is the best ancillary means of evaluating victims of blunt abdominal trauma; however, they share the reservations of others concerning its efficacy in detecting retroperitoneal injuries.[36,37]

AXIOM   A DPL may be completely negative with isolated severe injuries of retroperitoneal organs, such as the pancreas and duodenum.

At some centers, a DPL is carried out on all patients with suspected intraabdominal injuries.[10] Amylase determinations are done on the lavage fluid, and the DPL amylase levels are elevated in many patients with significant pancreatic injury.[10] Although virtually all patients with blunt duodenal injury will eventually have elevated WBC and amylase levels in the peritoneal lavage fluid,[21,34] there have been several reports of a relatively low sensitivity of the DPL to duodenal perforation.[27,31,32,50] Interestingly, in only one of these reports were amylase levels determined in the lavage fluid.[50]

AXIOM   A negative peritoneal lavage finding does not rule out retroperitoneal duodenal perforation.[21]

Endoscopic Retrograde Cholangiopancreatography (ERCP)

There have been several reports of the use of endoscopic retrograde cholangiopancreatography (ERCP) for the diagnosis of pancreatic injury, particularly for the detection of major ductal disruption.[50] It can demonstrate injury to the main pancreatic ducts, which is an absolute indicator for laparotomy. It can also provide a helpful road map for the operative surgeon when the normal anatomy is obscured by hematoma or inflammation;[10] however, this technique has been used in relatively few cases, with the largest series containing only nine patients.[1]

AXIOM In an occasional patient with a suspected pancreatic ductal injury, an ERCP may be used to determine the need for surgery and to determine the exact site of a major ductal injury.

Whittwell et al[51] used ERCP to help make decisions concerning operation in blunt injuries. When no major ductal injury was identified, operation was not performed; however, if ductal disruption was noted, operative repair was indicated. In at least one patient, ERCP was used with success during an operation to investigate a possible ductal injury. Blind et al[52] recently reported similar success in two children with blunt pancreatic duct rupture.

Although ERCP can be very accurate, it is only rarely necessary in the management of pancreatic trauma.[1] In most instances, the indications for surgery are quite clear clinically, with or without peritoneal lavage. In questionable cases, if CT scan demonstrates no pancreatic injury, the patient can be observed clinically.[1]

Most of the suggestions to use ERCP are not derived from broad clinical experience. Fabian and Patterson,[9] for example, have not employed duodenoscopy in this manner, and their experience with endoscopic pancreatography has been restricted to patients with persistent hyperamylasemia or suspected pseudocysts following pancreatic trauma.

Golson et al[53] suggest that ERCP may be particularly helpful in evaluating patients with chronic abdominal pain and prior blunt trauma to the abdomen. The authors described three patients with chronic distal pancreatitis who had severe abdominal pain after an asymptomatic latent period of 3 months to 1 year after their blunt trauma. The ERCP showed ductal stenosis or obstruction in the midbody of the pancreas in all three patients, and in all three, distal pancreatectomy was curative.

Intraoperative Evaluation

AXIOM A "negative laparotomy" does not exclude the possibility of a delayed complication of pancreatic or duodenal injury.[9]

EXPOSING THE PANCREAS AND DUODENUM

The diagnosis of pancreatic or duodenal injury is often made in the operating room rather than in the preoperative period.[1,9,10,21] All patients with trauma to the upper abdomen should have a careful exploration of these organs, including opening of the lesser sac through the gastrocolic omentum to inspect the entire anterior surface of the pancreas, particularly if there is a hematoma overlying any portion of these structures.

AXIOM Upper midline retroperitoneal hematomas should be explored to rule out underlying duodenal, pancreatic, or vascular injuries.

There are many anecdotal reports of missed duodenal perforations at the time of laparotomy.[29] Missing such injuries at laparotomy can cause devastating complications, and consequently the exploration must be very careful and thorough.[9] A wide Kocher maneuver (opening the right lateral peritoneal reflection of the duodenum) will generally allow investigation of the first, second, and third portions of the duodenum.[21] The Kocher maneuver, if properly performed, also allows assessment of the posterior portion of the head of the pancreas over to the abdominal aorta, where it is crossed by the left renal vein.[9]

If the Kocher maneuver does not provide adequate exposure of the first three portions of the duodenum and head of the pancreas, one can add the Cattell maneuver.[54] This involves reflecting the right colon medially to the origin of its mesenteric vessels. This technique also allows full exposure of the duodenum except in its most distal portions. The Kocher maneuver can now usually be extended much further.

AXIOM A Kocher maneuver, with or without the additional mobilization possible after a Cattell maneuver, is recommended for complete inspection of the first three portions of the duodenum and the head of the pancreas.

The apparent path of a bullet or knife blade can be misleading, and close attention must be given to any indicators of injury. The cause of even minimal bile staining of paraduodenal tissues must be sought carefully. Some surgeons have even suggested performing needle cholecystocholangiogram if no duodenal or biliary tract injury is found on exploration.

AXIOM The presence of any bile staining or crepitation in the periduodenal area after trauma makes a very careful search of the bile ducts and duodenum mandatory.[21]

An overlying hematoma is the most common intraoperative indicator of pancreatic or duodenal injury. All upper central retroperitoneal hematomas should be explored, and if the hematoma is large, a major vascular injury should be suspected. It must also be noted that relatively small hematomas may be associated with fairly severe injuries of the duodenum or the pancreas.

The body and tail of the pancreas can generally be well visualized by opening the lesser sac and then reflecting the stomach superiorly and the traverse colon inferiorly.[10] The plane posterior to the superior margins of the pancreas can be entered bluntly along its entire length, thus allowing bimanual palpation of the entire organ. If indicated, the peritoneum along the entire inferior border of the pancreas may also be incised to allow elevation of the inferior margin of the body and tail of the pancreas to inspect the posterior surface.[1,55] In the process, active bleeding from the pancreas or from adjacent vascular structures can also be assessed and controlled. The fourth and distal third portion of the duodenum should already have been evaluated by mobilizing the ligament of Treitz.

AXIOM Severe edema, crepitance, or bile staining of periduodenal tissues implies a duodenal injury until proven otherwise.

After inspection of the entire duodenum, the common bile duct can be exposed by incision of the peritoneum and areolar tissue on the inferolateral border of the hepatoduodenal ligament; however, too extensive a dissection can devascularize the duct, and complete circumferential dissection should be avoided.[9]

If there is significant bleeding from the area of the head of the pancreas and duodenum, Fabian and Patterson[9] feel that the origin of the gastroduodenal artery from the common hepatic artery should be identified by exposing the common hepatic, the gastroduodenal, and the proper hepatic arteries. Confusion about the location of these three vessels and resultant ligation of the wrong vessel is usually due to an inadequate exposure of the relevant anatomy, particularly if the surgeon is inexperienced in dissections of this area.

The superior mesenteric artery (SMA) and vein (SMV) exit from behind the neck of the pancreas and cross the third portion of the duodenum.[9] The SMA is to the left and slightly posterior to the SMV. Full exposure of the SMA is rarely necessary in injuries of the pancreas and duodenum, but when necessitated by a proximal injury, it is usually preferable to approach it retroperitoneally. This involves reflection of the left colon, spleen, pancreas, and left kidney to the right.[9]

Exposure of the SMV is commonly required, usually as a prelude to pancreatic resection or transection of the pancreas for the control of portal vein injuries.[9] After opening up the gastrocolic ligament all the way to the right, the SMV is revealed by rotating the pancreas superiorly and incising the inferior peritoneal attachments of the pancreas in the region of its neck. Once the anterior perivenous plane is achieved, it can be extended superiorly by blunt dissection to separate the vein from the pancreas. Although the anterior surface of the SMV is generally free of branches, careful dissection is required to obtain circumferential control without damaging its thin-walled, high-flow lateral tributaries.[9] Indeed, circumferential control of the SMV is usually not necessary during operations for trauma.

METHYLENE BLUE

In unrevealing duodenal exploration in highly suspicious cases, Brotman et al[56] have recommended instillation of methylene blue through the nasogastric tube. The staining of periduodenal tissues with this blue-green dye is irrefutable evidence of an intestinal rupture in this area, and the lack of staining, in their hands, has proved reliable in ruling out full-thickness duodenal injury. Fabian and Patterson[9] have little experience with this technique, and are satisfied with dissection and irrigation of the duodenal hematoma. Detection of underlying injuries following dissection of pancreatic hematomas is more frequently equivocal than with duodenal hematomas. Nevertheless, the surgeon should try to decide whether or not there is major ductal injury.

AXIOM The major decision to be made at the time of exploration of a suspected pancreaticoduodenal injury is whether there is a tear in the duodenum or a major pancreatic duct injury.

PANCREATOGRAPHY

Identifying the integrity of the main ducts is of the utmost importance in patients with a suspected pancreatic injury.[10] Some surgeons feel that, if this cannot be accomplished by direct visualization, intraoperative pancreatography should be attempted by intubating the ampulla of Vater through a duodenotomy. A fine Fogarty catheter or a pediatric feeding tube can be used for this maneuver.[10] Some surgeons prefer to identify the duct for pancreatography by amputation of the tail of the pancreas.

AXIOM The use of intraoperative pancreatography in patients suspected of having injury to the major pancreatic duct may cause more harm than good and is controversial.[1,57]

The orifice of the pancreatic duct in the ampulla of Vater is usually distal and anteromedial to that of the bile duct, and care should be taken to avoid injury to this area.[9] The pancreatic duct angles cephalad and to the left from its origin at the ampulla. It courses more obliquely to the left near the junction of the upper and middle thirds of the pancreatic body and tail. The duct is relatively close to the anterior surface of the normal pancreas.

Although Fabian and Patterson[9] use intraoperative pancreatography in selected cases, Jordan has largely abandoned this procedure and relies more on careful examination of the pancreas and the type and the location of injury to determine whether a ductal injury is present.[1]

Some surgeons have used secretin to stimulate the pancreas intraoperatively with the hopes of finding leakage of pancreatic secretions from an otherwise undetected ductal injury; however, Jordan would consider doing this only in rare patients. Nevertheless, those who have used this technique indicate that after a secretin injection, the flow of pancreatic juice from a major ductal disruption is significantly greater than it is from torn smaller ducts.[1]

CHOLANGIOGRAPHY

Operative cholangiography can augment inspection of the extrahepatic biliary ducts, and is superior to dissection for evaluating the intrapancreatic portion of the common bile duct.[9] Intraoperative cholangiography can be accomplished by several techniques including: (a) direct needle into the common duct, (b) compression of a dye-filled gallbladder, or (c) cannulation of a transected cystic duct during cholecystectomy. The last method, however, should be used only if one is certain that the gallbladder will not be required for reconstruction.

Localization of the ampulla of Vater is occasionally possible by palpation through the wall of the intact duodenum.[9] It is generally located on the medial wall near the middle of the second portion of the duodenum. Intraoperatively many surgeons tend to look for it too far superiorly. If the ampulla cannot be identified, even with a duodenotomy, one can often locate it by passing a ureteral catheter through either the cystic duct or the supraduodenal common bile duct into the duodenum.

PANCREATIC WOUNDS

Grading Pancreatic Injuries

Determining the quality of care of pancreatic injuries at a particular trauma center may be facilitated by carefully grading and classifying the pancreatic injuries.[10] The organ injury scaling (OIS) Committee of the American Association for the Surgery of Trauma (AAST) has graded pancreatic injuries from I to V[58] (Table 25–6). A grade I injury is a simple contusion of the pancreas; a grade II injury is a major contusion or laceration without tissue loss or involvement of the main pancreatic duct; grade III includes a complete transection of the pancreas or a parenchymal injury with involvement of the major duct to the left of the SMV; grade IV involves ductal transection or a major parenchymal injury to the right of the SMV; grade V involves massive disruption of the head of the pancreas.

Preoperative Preparation

The initial approach to patients with pancreatic injuries is not different from that used for any serious abdominal wound.[1] Adequate upper extremity lines are essential, but preoperative time should not be wasted attempting to stabilize patients who are bleeding actively. The preparations for surgery, the number of diagnostic procedures performed, and the speed with which the patient should be taken to the operating room, will depend primarily on the hemodynamic stability of the patient.[1]

TABLE 25–6 Pancreatic Organ Injury Scale

Grade*		Injury Description[+]	AIS-90
I	Hematoma	Minor contusion without duct injury	1
	Laceration	Superficial laceration without duct injury	1
II	Hematoma	Major contusion without duct injury or tissue loss	2
	Laceration	Major laceration without duct injury or tissue loss	3
III	Laceration	Distal transection or parenchymal injury with duct injury	3
IV	Laceration	Proximal[a] transection or parenchymal injury involving ampulla	4
V	Laceration	Massive disruption of pancreatic head	5

[a] Proximal pancreas is to the patients' right of the superior mesenteric vein.
* Advance one grade for multiple injuries to the same organ
[+] Based on most accurate assessment at autopsy, laparotomy, or radiologic study
(From Moore EE, Cogbill TH, Malangoni MA, et al. Organ injury scaling II: pancreas, duodenum, small bowel, colon, and rectum. J Trauma 1990;30:11427.)

Priorities of Intraoperative Measures

AXIOM With any intraabdominal injury, the highest priorities are control of hemorrhage followed by control of bowel leaks.

The first intraoperative priority is control of active hemorrhage. Excessive bleeding is the most common cause of death following pancreatic injury.[10,26] Initially, such bleeding can be at least partially controlled with packs while the rest of the abdomen is explored rapidly. Persistent bleeding from the pancreas itself can usually be controlled with local pressure, fine suture ligatures, and/or fibrin glue.

The second priority in intraoperative management is prevention of further contamination of the peritoneal cavity from perforations of the gastrointestinal tract. When there are other serious injuries, the pancreas may be the last organ to be treated and, in most instances, is treated only with drainage.[1]

Management of Specific Pancreatic Injuries

The options for management of pancreatic injuries generally involve external drainage, internal drainage, resection, or a combination of these procedures.

INTACT DUCT

More than 88% of penetrating pancreatic wounds do not involve the main pancreatic duct,[59] and such wounds are generally successfully managed by external drainage alone.[9,12] Most blunt pancreatic injuries also do not involve the major ducts.

For a grade II pancreatic injury (lacerations without involvement of a major duct), several authors advocate the use of capsular sutures in addition to sump drainage.[12,19] Such sutures may also aid in hemostasis; however, if suturing is difficult because of a hematoma or loss of tissue in the area of the capsular tear, external drainage will usually be adequate.[10]

The type of sutures to be used is of some concern. Catgut rapidly dissolves in the presence of pancreatic juice, thus nonabsorbable sutures or those made of polyglycolic acid are preferable.[1] Other than catgut, there is no evidence to document that one type of suture is better than another in treating pancreatic wounds; however, monofilament sutures pass through pancreatic parenchyma with less trauma than do braided sutures.[1] Another important consideration is gentle approximation of the cut edges because sutures that are tied tightly may cut through the tissue as posttraumatic swelling occurs, and can be a cause of fistula formation.

DUCTAL INJURY

The most serious pancreatic wounds are those which transect a major pancreatic duct.[1] The major problem with such injuries is continued uncontrolled leakage of pancreatic exocrine secretions into the peritoneal cavity and retroperitoneum.[10] The resulting complications, which can include fistulas, pseudocysts, and sepsis, are the major causes of morbidity and mortality after 48 hours.

AXIOM Simple drainage of major pancreatic ductal injuries is frequently associated with major complications.

Drainage alone for major ductal injuries is generally inadequate.[60-61] These injuries have long been known to be the most significant factor determining the outcome of pancreatic injury.[10-11,19] Wounds involving the main duct in the distal body and tail of the pancreas can sometimes be treated by resection of the distal pancreas. In some instances, this can be done while leaving the splenic artery and vein intact; however, because of the multiple small short branches between the posterior surface of the pancreas and the splenic vein, this can be very difficult. If the short gastric vessels are intact, the splenic artery and vein should be ligated as far as possible away from the hilar vessels to increase the chances of preserving the spleen. In many instances, however, it is preferable to remove the spleen as a part of the pancreatic resection, especially in patients who are unstable or have multiple injuries.

On the basis of their experience with 24 patients with pancreatic trauma, Sukul et al[62] recommend that patients with pancreatic duct injury can be treated with debridement and external suction drainage. If the pancreatic duct lesion is located to the left of the superior mesenteric vessels, distal pancreatectomy and splenectomy with pancreaticojejunostomy, should be performed. If the pancreatic duct is injured to the right of the superior mesenteric vessels, treatment should consist of partial pancreatic resection and pancreatico-jejunostomy or a Whipple procedure.

TREATMENT OF PANCREATIC TRANSECTION

A total transection through the neck of the pancreas may exist as a single injury, but it is often associated with damage to other organs. It is these associated injuries which are the main determinant of the patient's outcome.[1,26]

Resection of Distal Pancreas

A review of the literature reveals that the most frequent operation performed for transection at the neck of the pancreas is resection of the distal portion (Fig. 25–2). From a technical standpoint, this is the most expeditious treatment in the majority of patients,[1,20] especially if there

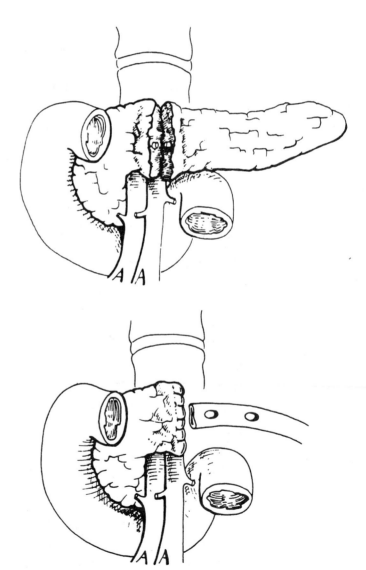

FIGURE 25–2 **A.** Traumatic division of the main pancreatic duct. **B.** Treatment with a distal pancreatectomy and drainage (From Wilson RH, Moorehead RJ. Current management of trauma to the pancreas. J Surg 1991;78:1196.)

is an associated injury of the spleen.[1,9] Usually the distal end of the remaining pancreas is simply closed, but it may be anastomosed to a Roux-en-Y loop of jejunum.[63]

Persistent postoperative diabetes mellitus or exocrine insufficiency following resection of the distal portion of an otherwise normal pancreas is uncommon.[10] A major theoretical disadvantage of this technique, especially in young patients, however, is that the spleen is usually lost. Preservation of the splenic vasculature is possible, but this can prolong the procedure significantly, and it is not usually clinically warranted, especially if there are multiple associated injuries.[63]

> **AXIOM** Splenic salvage should probably be attempted for traumatic rupture of the pancreas if the patient is young and hemodynamically stable and there are no other life-threatening injuries.

Severe associated injuries demand expeditious management of the pancreatic injury and prohibit the dissection often required to separate the tail of the pancreas from the splenic vessels and hilum.[9] During the usual resection of the distal pancreas, it is mobilized from the retroperitoneum, and the splenic vein and artery are identified and, individually, doubly ligated. A vascular clamp can be placed across the proximal pancreas if the traumatic transection has to be completed surgically; the bleeding that can result from incisions into normal pancreatic tissue can be truly alarming at times.

After completing the division of the pancreas, if that is required, a series of interlocking U-sutures of polypropylene are placed at close intervals in the distal end of the proximal pancreas to provide hemostasis.[9] If a vascular clamp was used, the sutures should be placed right against the clamp to avoid a large cuff of devitalized pancreas. After the sutures have been placed, the clamp is removed and an attempt is made to identify and ligate the main pancreatic duct separately. The pancreatic duct can usually be identified prior to tying the U-sutures. Any residual bleeding points are separately ligated as necessary to produce hemostasis.[9] An apron or tongue of viable omentum is then secured over the resected end of the pancreas to help prevent ligated vessels in adjacent tissues from being digested by leaking pancreatic enzymes. A closed suction drain is placed near, but not on, the resected edge of the pancreas. Pancreatic resection can also be accomplished with a GI stapling device.[9]

> **AXIOM** One should avoid Roux-en-Y jejunal anastomoses to the surface of damaged pancreas unless there is no other reasonable way to manage drainage from an injured major pancreatic duct.

Fabian and Patterson[9] feel that a pancreaticojejunostomy combined with resection of the distal pancreas is usually inadvisable. Resections of up to 80% of the distal pancreas usually result in no exocrine insufficiency in the otherwise healthy gland.[20,64]

Cogbill et al[65] found, in their multicenter experience with distal pancreatectomy for trauma, that five (71%) of seven patients treated in this manner had major complications, and three died of pancreatic infection. The authors describe two major problems that can contribute to the difficulties experienced with this procedure. The first problem is that normal pancreas does not hold sutures as well as a pancreas which has been chronically inflamed. Secondly, the jejunum supposedly can function as a "living vacuum," but these patients generally are severely injured, and they often have a severe ileus that persists for at least several days. This allows for colonization of the cut and/or injured pancreas by gastrointestinal flora, and this may result in pancreatic sepsis with or without disruption of the anastomosis.

Pancreatic Preservation Techniques

In an occasional patient in whom transection of the pancreas is the only major injury, attempts to preserve pancreatic tissue may be desirable.[66] A variety of techniques has been used to accomplish this.

REPAIR OF THE PANCREATIC DUCT USING A STENT. One of the earliest techniques used to preserve a transected pancreas was cannulation of the pancreatic duct from the duodenum and direct repair of the duct over the stent.[10] This had several disadvantages; the first was that it necessitated performing and repairing a duodenotomy, and the second was that there was a significant leak rate from the repaired duct in spite of the stent.[10]

> **AXIOM** Direct repairs of tears of the major pancreatic duct usually fail, even with a stent.

Another technique for preserving a transected pancreas involves reanastomosing the pancreatic substance and the duct over a stent and bringing the stent into the common bile duct and then out alongside a T-tube. This is a complicated procedure, and although Jordan has used it once, he does not advocate it.[1] In most cases, passing the stent from the pancreas into the common bile duct can be very difficult. In addition, the procedure may cause a later stricture in an otherwise normal common bile duct.

ROUX-EN-Y JEJUNUM. The most common procedure for treating pancreatic transections without a resection has involved anastomosis of the distal pancreas to a Roux en-Y loop of jejunum.[1] Strauch has also described anastomosis of the distal pancreas to the stomach.[67] Another technique described by Jones and Shires[11] includes anastomosis of both the proximal and distal ends of the transected pancreas to a Roux-en-Y loop of jejunum.

If an attempt must be made to preserve pancreatic tissue, Jordan[1,68] prefers closure of the transected proximal end of the pancreas and Roux-en-Y drainage of the distal pancreas as originally described by Letton and Wilson.[69] He had seen no deaths among several patients treated by this technique, and he had to reoperate on only one patient, and this was because of obstruction of the Roux-en-Y loop.[1] This was treated surgically with success, and the patient subsequently made an uneventful recovery.

> **AXIOM** If one feels that preservation of the distal portion of a transected pancreas is important, a Roux-en-Y loop is probably the best system for managing its exocrine secretions.

A few surgeons who have been greatly concerned about the need to preserve transected pancreatic substance have anastomosed the proximal pancreatic remnant to one side of a Roux-en-Y jejunal loop and the distal remnant to the opposite side, as mentioned previously. However, some authors see an increased risk of infection and leaks with this technique.[9,10] In addition, since the procedures are technically demanding and time-consuming, they are inappropriate in multiple trauma situations.[10,20]

> **AXIOM** Since 90% of the normal pancreas can generally be resected without significant endocrine or exocrine deficiency, complex preservation procedures are rarely indicated.[10]

CLOSURE OF BOTH TRANSECTED ENDS. If one desires to preserve as much pancreatic endocrine function as possible, closure of both ends of the transected pancreas is the simplest technique, but it has been associated with a significant incidence of pancreatic fistulas, especially from the distal end.

It is difficult to demonstrate that any one technique of closure of transected pancreas is better than the others.[1] Some surgeons use a stapler for such closures, since this is the quickest and most expeditious technique;[70] Jordan, however,[1] continues to prefer meticulous suture closures.

> **AXIOM** Closure of the transected ends of a divided pancreas will frequently fail, especially if the main duct is not identified and carefully ligated with sutures.

The first step in closure of both ends of a transected pancreas is identification of the main duct. Each end of the duct is then ligated with a mattress suture, including just enough pancreatic tissue to provide security when the suture is tied.[1] The ends of the pancreas are then closed with a series of horizontal mattress or figure-of-eight mattress sutures tied just tightly enough to approximate the gland and to provide hemostasis. A second row of running Prolene suture is often placed to complete the closure. Both ends should then be covered with a pedicle of omentum for additional security.[1]

AXIOM   All pancreatic injuries should be drained because there will be some leakage of pancreatic enzymes in almost all cases.

DAMAGE TO THE HEAD OF THE PANCREAS

Wounds to the head of the pancreas are usually the result of penetrating trauma.[9] Major associated vascular injuries are often present because of the proximity of the pancreas to the superior mesenteric vessels, portal vein, aorta, and inferior vena cava. A large portion of the operative effort in patients with trauma to the head of the pancreas is often directed at controlling the bleeding from associated vascular injuries, and such bleeding is the major reason for the high mortality rate.

Once the bleeding is controlled, one must decide whether there is damage to the major pancreatic duct.[1] If it can be ascertained that the duct is not injured, the treatment of wounds of the head of the pancreas is no different from that of wounds of the body and tail. If the main duct is injured, however, one is confronted with a major decision about the management of the patient.

Drainage With or Without Pyloric Exclusion

Fabian and Patterson[9] manage major injuries of the head of the pancreas by drainage, even if involvement of the main duct is suspected. If a pancreatic fistula develops, it is managed as a chronic fistula and treated at a second, elective exploration, if necessary.[9]

Some surgeons feel that one should anastomose a badly injured head of the pancreas to an onlay Roux-en-Y loop of jejunum. This may be done with or without a pyloric exclusion to direct gastric secretions away from the duodenum for at least three weeks. Drainage with a Roux-en-Y loop of jejunum conserves pancreatic tissue, and in theory it can also decrease the risk of external fistulas. Jordan's philosophy is conservation of pancreatic tissue whenever possible, and he reserves resection of the head of the pancreas for those instances in which the damage is so great that adequate drainage is impossible.[1]

Pancreaticoduodenectomy

Some surgeons think patients with injury to the main duct in the head of the pancreas require pancreaticoduodenectomy (Whipple procedure) and, rarely, a total pancreatectomy (Fig. 25–3).[71] This is controversial; however, in patients with severe complicated wounds of the head of the pancreas combined with a severe injury of the duodenum, there is relative agreement that one should perform a Whipple procedure. In some instances, this may have be done in two steps with the resection performed in the first stage, and the anastomoses performed 24-48 hours later. Delcare et al[72] reported on five patients in whom a pancreaticoduodenectomy followed by a pancreaticogastrostomy was performed in four patients and a distal pancreaticogastrostomy without resection of the head of the pancreas was performed in another patient (Fig. 25–4). This resulted in no leaks, infections, or other complications.

Torn Uncinate Process

Rarely, because of a sudden deceleration, the uncinate process is torn at the point where the mesenteric vessels emerge from behind the pancreas.[9] Fabian and Patterson[9] treated two such patients in two years. Both developed pseudocysts postoperatively, but did well following internal drainage procedures.

Drainage of Pancreatic Wounds

The most effective method for preventing complications following an injury to the pancreas is to control its exocrine secretions. In 75% of

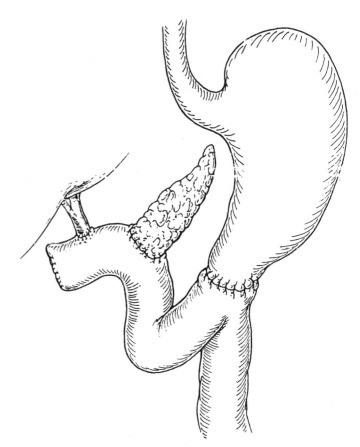

FIGURE 25–3   Reconstruction after a Whipple procedure. A single suction drain is placed through a right upper-quadrant stab wound and adjacent to the biliary and pancreatic anastomoses (From Carey LC. Pancreaticoduodenectomy. Am J Surg 1992;164:153.)

cases, external drainage with sump tubes and/or closed suction drains is adequate.[1,9,74] Several authors have shown the superiority of large soft sump drains over passive (Penrose) drainage systems because adequate dependent drainage cannot usually be obtained while the patient is lying supine in bed.[9,10] Although some surgeons feel that the use of sump drains decreases the incidence of pancreatic fistula, this is not a general observation.[59,74] Nevertheless, a much higher complication rate has been reported with Penrose drains than with sump drains.[59]

The disadvantage of all drainage systems is that, no matter which one is used, bacterial contamination from the environment occurs.[9] Such contamination occasionally produces a peripancreatic abscess; however, even without forming an abscess, drain tract infections can prolong hospitalization. Placing bacterial filters on the sump drains does not appear to reduce this problem.[9]

AXIOM   The incidence of infection of pancreatic drainage tracts is probably lowest when closed systems are used.

It is generally felt that closed suction drainage systems reduce the incidence of bacterial colonization, but such systems can become plugged very rapidly and require intermittent manipulation and/or irrigation.

AXIOM   Even if there is no evidence of a pancreatic leak, drains should be left in place until the patient is eating a fairly regular diet.

Pancreatic leaks often do not develop until the patient begins to eat.[10,59] If a pancreatic fistula develops, the drains are left in place until the fistula tract is well established, and this usually takes at least several weeks.

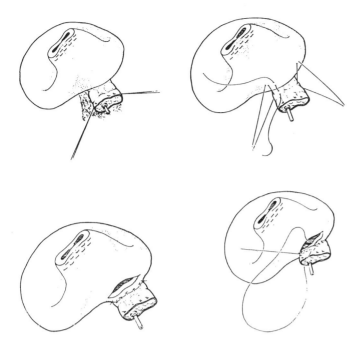

FIGURE 25–4 Technique of pancreatogastrostomy (From Delcore R, Thomas JH, Pierce GE, et al. Pancreato-gastrostomy: a safe drainage procedure after pancreatoduodenectomy. Surgery 1990;108:641.)

In spite of all the data to the contrary, Jordan[1] continues to use simple Penrose drains for pancreatic injuries. He feels that they are effective and are the least expensive drainage system. Most of his patients do not develop fistulas, and if a fistula does develop, it usually is small and closes spontaneously without complications. If a large fistula develops, the Penrose drains are removed and a suction drain is inserted.[1]

Complications of Pancreatic Injuries

The incidence of complications following pancreatic trauma in larger series ranges from 36% to 61%.[9,12,68] In a recent report by Moncure and Goins[75] on 44 patients with pancreatic or duodenal injuries, complications occurred in 61% of patients surviving longer than 24 hours. These included intraabdominal abscess in 31% of the patients (42% of whom required relaparotomy) and pancreatic fistulas in 16%.

In one series of six patients with pancreatic injuries, five (83%) of the patients had a total of six complications.[10] Although there were no deaths, the complications were serious and caused considerable morbidity and prolonged hospital stays.

Many of the intraabdominal complications seen with pancreatic injury are due to injuries to other organs, particularly the liver and colon; however, there is also a high incidence of problems resulting specifically from the pancreatic injury. The pancreatic complications are attributable to both the function and location of the gland.[9] The enzymes released from torn pancreatic tissue, if activated, can cause extensive autolytic tissue destruction. Because of the location of the pancreas in the upper abdomen and its close association with major vessels, such tissue destruction can cause multiple serious complications, such as sepsis with resultant multiple organ failure or severe bleeding.

Although they are never completely avoidable, pancreatic complications can be minimized by appropriate and expeditious operative management of both the pancreatic and associated injuries. The commonest pancreatic complications are pancreatitis, peripancreatic abscess, prolonged pancreatic drainage (fistula) drain tract infections, postoperative hemorrhage, pseudocysts, and pancreatic ascites.[61]

FISTULA

A fistula is the most common complication of pancreatic injury,[1,76] and it develops in nearly a third of patients with pancreatic wounds; however, a review of the literature reveals a wide variation in the incidence of fistula development depending upon the definitions used by the authors. Many surgeons expect some drainage from a pancreatic wound and do not consider it a complication unless the drainage is of large volume and/or persists for more than several days.[1] When such a definition is used, the incidence of pancreatic fistula is quite small.

AXIOM Mild drainage from peripancreatic drains during the first few days following trauma is seldom a serious problem.

Although it is anticipated that some leakage of pancreatic juice will occur after many pancreatic injuries, the majority of patients do not have drainage persisting for more than 2 or 3 days.[1] Jordan considers drainage of fluid with high amylase or lipase values that starts 3 or 4 days postoperatively or persists beyond that time as a pancreatic fistula.[1]

Fistulas are more likely to occur following wounds of the head of the pancreas than after wounds of the body and tail.[1] When the major pancreatic duct is injured, a fistula can be anticipated unless the ductal wound is repaired. In some series, the complication rate has been reduced by the use of intraoperative pancreatography to demonstrate ductal injuries.[10,57]

Classification

Pancreatic fistulas can be classified as minor, moderate, or major depending on the volume of drainage.[1] Minor fistulas drain less than 100 ml/day and usually heal relatively fast. Moderate fistulas drain from 200 to 700 ml/day, and major fistulas are those draining larger amounts. It is unusual to see a pancreatic fistula draining more than 1000 ml/day unless the major duct is involved and it has a proximal obstruction.

Diagnosis

If the source of an abdominal fistula is in doubt, the amylase concentration in the fluid should be determined.[1] Pure pancreatic juice usually has an amylase concentration of approximately 50,000 U/ml, but the amylase concentration in some fistulas exceeds 1,000,000 U/ml. Lesser values, for example, in the range of 5,000 to 10,000 U/ml can also indicate a pancreatic fistula with the pancreatic juice significantly diluted by intraperitoneal fluid.[1] Under these circumstances, the amount of pancreatic juice draining may be quite small, and such fistulas usually close relatively fast.[1]

Initial Treatment

AXIOM Initial treatment of ancreatic fistulas should be conservative because most of them heal spontaneously within 2-4 weeks.[1,9,10,26]

The principles of treatment of posttraumatic pancreatic fistulas include adequate drainage, prevention of infection, and protection of the skin.[1] Minor pancreatic fistulas are managed simply by leaving the drains in place. The enzymes are usually not activated and produce little problem with skin excoriation.[9]

AXIOM Peripancreatic drains should be left in place until the patient is eating a full diet and there is little or no drainage, or until the drainage tract is well-established.

Not infrequently, there may be little or no pancreatic fluid leak until the patient resumes eating by mouth. If the drains have already been removed, the pancreatic fluid leak can cause severe complications. Once a well-established tract has developed, however, the drains should be withdrawn 1 to 2 inches so that they do not lie against the pancreas. Drains left in juxtaposition to the pancreas may impede healing of the fistula. It is important, however, that a tract be maintained to an area near the pancreas so that any juice exiting from the gland will have a point of egress, preventing stagnation and activation of the juice.[1]

For treatment of fistulas that are moderate or large in size, the Penrose drains should be removed and a sump drain inserted as soon as a tract is established.[1] This will assure adequate evacuation of all drainage material and will serve also to protect the skin. Once a firm tract is established, a sinogram should be obtained to determine its size and course. If there are psuedopods from the tract or if there is a large cavity at the bottom of the tract, better drainage must be obtained. At times, this can be accomplished without reoperation, but occasionally a large cavity behind a long narrow drainage tract requires surgical creation of a larger, more direct drainage tract.[1]

When a single well-established tract exists, sump drainage may be discontinued, and the patient may be treated on an outpatient basis, particularly if adequate oral intake is possible.[1] A plastic or rubber catheter placed into the drainage tract about halfway between the skin surface and the estimated depth of the pancreas will allow collection of any fistula fluid into a bag, such as that used for ileostomies. This provides some protection of the skin. Elimination of suction on the drainage catheter will usually allow more rapid healing than if constant suction is applied. Although some large fistulas close relatively rapidly (within 2-3 weeks), it is not uncommon for the process to take 6-12 weeks or longer.[1]

Metabolic Support

> **AXIOM**   Fluid and electrolyte losses from large pancreatic fistulas can be very dangerous in malnourished patients.

Fluid, electrolyte, and nutritional balance should be maintained throughout the treatment of large pancreatic fistulas. In the early period, this is accomplished by intravenous fluids and intravenous hyperalimentation. Although some surgeons allow oral intake, the tendency of many surgeons is to keep patients with pancreatic or duodenal fistulas NPO for at least seven to 10 days and use jejunal tube feedings after bowel activity has resumed.[77]

Somatostatin

There are many agents that will decrease secretion from the pancreas. They include anticholinergic drugs, the use of high glucose concentrations in total parenteral nutrition, and somatostatin.[1] The agent that has been of greatest interest in recent years is somatostatin and its several analogs.[78] Somatostatin significantly decreases the volume of pancreatic secretions, and it may help provide a more rapid closure of some fistulas. Unfortunately, it is difficult to predict the natural course of a traumatic pancreatic fistula.[1] Some fistulas, even though very large, close within a short period of time, and others, though very small, many remain open for many weeks or even months. Nevertheless, most pancreatic fistulas close spontaneously within 4-6 weeks.[1,9,10] Patients who are doing well otherwise do not need to remain in the hospital during the entire period of healing of the fistula.

Operative Drainage

Rarely, a pancreatic fistula will persist for a long time and be so disabling that operative repair is indicated. In Jordan's entire series of pancreatic injuries, only two patients required another operation for management of pancreatic fistulas.[1] In such patients, there is usually an injury to the duct of Wirsung that can be demonstrated on fistulography.[9]

The surgical treatment of choice for a persistent pancreatic fistula is anastomosis of the fistula tract at the surface of the pancreas to a Roux-en-Y loop of jejunum.[1] This should not be done with an immature tract because anastomoses to such tissue are prone to leak. Once a chronic fistula develops and has been present for more than 4-6 weeks, there is usually enough fibrosis of the surrounding tissue so that it can be sutured to bowel safely. Deaths may occur in patients who develop fistulas, but the fistula is rarely the direct cause of death.[1]

PANCREATIC ABSCESSES

Intraabdominal abscesses develop in approximately 5% of patients with pancreatic injuries, but in most patients it is due primarily to associated injuries of the liver, colon, or small bowel.[1] A true pancreatic abscess is usually the result of inadequate debridement of necrotic pancreas at the time of surgery, resulting either from failure to operate, or an inadequate appreciation of the need for debridement at the time of operation.[1]

> **AXIOM**   The combination of a major bowel injury, necrotic pancreatic tissue, and a continuing pancreatic leak greatly increases the risk of intraperitoneal sepsis.

Hematomas and/or devitalized tissue contaminated by gastrointestinal contents are particularly apt to become infected.[9] Aerobic gram-negative rods and gram-positive cocci are the usual infecting organisms, and antibiotics covering these should be started as soon as possible after the trauma. Later adjustments can be made according to sensitivity testing of any bacteria recovered at surgery or from drainage sites. The risk of developing infection is particularly high in patients in whom inadequately drained pancreatic secretions damage local tissue, thereby providing an excellent culture medium. The resultant infections may develop as lesser sac abscesses, infected pseudocysts, or pancreatic phlegmons.[9]

Drain tract infections are seldom life-threatening, but they may require prolonged antibiotic therapy and hospitalization. Many of the organisms are the gram-negative enteric bacilli typically found in intensive care units and include *Escherichia coli* and various species of *Enterobacter, Acinetobacter, Pseudomonas,* and *Klebsiella.*[9] Proper management of the drains can reduce the incidence of these infections.

All sump drains will have some colonization at their bases.[9] Once the drainage tract is well established, a second drainage tube such as a sterile rubber or large Foley catheter should be reinserted in the tract. The secondary drain is gradually advanced over a period of several days as the tract heals, thereby reducing the risk of closed space infections. Using closed suction drains might prevent some of these infections, but only if they effectively drain any peripancreatic fluid that develops.

Early Diagnosis

> **AXIOM**   Pancreatic necrosis or an abscess should be suspected in anyone who becomes toxic or develops multiple organ failure after a major pancreatic injury.

An intraabdominal abscess should be suspected in any patient who develops fever, a prolonged ileus, or unexplained upper abdominal pain or tenderness in the postoperative period.[1] Mortality rates for a pancreatic phlegmon or abscesses may be particularly high, especially if there is a delay in diagnosis and treatment.

With the use of ultrasound and CT scans, the presence of pancreatic or peripancreatic abscesses or fluid collections can usually be confirmed or denied rapidly. Ultrasound performed by a competent ultrasonographer is a better diagnostic technique in most patients than is a CT scan because of the better differentiation of fluid collections from simple phlegmons.[1] In some areas, however, particularly in the region of the tail of the pancreas where gas-filled segments of the colon frequently distort the ultrasonographic image, a CT scan tends to be much more informative.

Antibiotics

As soon as a pancreatic abscess is strongly suspected, antibiotic therapy should be started with broad-spectrum coverage for gram-positive and gram-negative bacteria. If the abscess is drained or aspirated, the antibiotic coverage can be adjusted according to the Gram stain and culture and sensitivity results. Blood cultures can also sometimes help to document the presence or absence of bacteremia and the types of organisms present.[1]

Prompt Operation

If the presence of a pancreatic abscess is confirmed, prompt operation with adequate drainage is the treatment of choice; however, such collections are increasingly being drained percutaneously with CT or ultrasound guidance. If the percutaneous drainage does not improve the patient's condition rapidly, a laparotomy should be performed to provide improved drainage.

POST-TRAUMATIC PANCREATITIS

Many patients with pancreatic trauma develop abdominal or back pain with elevated serum and/or urine amylase levels.[1] If the patient is doing well clinically, he or she can be treated conservatively; however, an occasional patient can develop severe generalized inflammatory changes within the pancreas.

The presence of traumatic pancreatitis is usually not appreciated until at least the second or third day after injury. A persistent fever and a rise in serum amylase levels associated with increasing deep abdominal or mid-back pain should make one strongly suspect this possibility. When traumatic pancreatitis is diagnosed, the management is the same as for other types of pancreatitis.

Although traumatic pancreatitis can be very severe, and mortality rates reported in the surgical literature can be high,[59] it is generally a self-limited process and will usually resolve within a week or so with just symptomatic therapy.[9] Occasionally, the symptoms will completely resolve while serum amylase and lipase levels remain mildly to moderately elevated. Under such circumstances, the patients can often be fed without exacerbation of their pain.[9] If pain develops or if the amylase or lipase levels rise markedly, bowel rest can be reinstituted. If the patient is not eating adequately within five days, one should consider institution of total parenteral nutrition (TPN). In some patients, bowel rest and TPN will be required for a few weeks before the pancreatitis resolves.

AXIOM	Persistent posttraumatic pancreatitis is frequently the harbinger of complications such as a pseudocyst or pancreatic abscess.

Although acute traumatic pancreatitis usually resolves, a few patients will develop chronic recurrent pancreatitis.[1] Although it is not well documented, it is thought that such patients probably had an injury to the major pancreatic duct with resulting partial or complete obstruction.[1] Endoscopic retrograde pancreatography should be performed in these patients, and if ductal stricture is identified, the patient should be treated surgically by a Puestow operation or a resection of the pancreas beyond the stricture.[1,53]

PSEUDOCYSTS

Pseudocyst formation is uncommon after pancreatic trauma, but it is most likely to occur in patients who sustain moderate to severe blunt trauma without prompt operation or proper drainage, or have a major injury to the duct of Wirsuhung.[79] Although some series have reported an incidence of pseudocysts as high as 20%, for most series in which operation is undertaken promptly, the incidence is in the range of 1.5-5%.[1,68,80]

AXIOM	Development of a pancreatic pseudocyst should be suspected in anyone with an upper abdominal mass or a persistent elevation of serum amylase levels following pancreatic trauma.[1]

In the past, the diagnosis of a pancreatic pseudocyst was made primarily on the basis of upper gastrointestinal examinations with barium. Today, the most satisfactory and inexpensive procedure is ultrasound. Pseudocysts can also be diagnosed by CT scan, but this is more expensive, and it usually does not yield significantly more information.

The diagnosis of pseudocyst is not justified just because a simple collection of fluid is seen in the peripancreatic area in the early posttraumatic period. The term "pseudocyst" should be reserved for fluid collections with a fibrous capsule. When the diagnosis of a pancreatic pseudocyst is made, surgical drainage, preferably internal, should be instituted, even though success with percutaneous drainage has been reported.[81] If the pseudocyst is infected, it should be drained externally.[9] If the pseudocyst involves the distal pancreas, it can occasionally be resected.[9]

AXIOM	Endoscopic retrograde pancreatography should be performed prior to the treatment of pancreatic pseudocysts to aid in the selection of the most appropriate procedure.[9]

Portis et al[82] recently reported a case in which a previously healthy patient developed chronic hyperamylasemia and epigastric pain following blunt abdominal trauma. ERCP and CT examination revealed a pancreas divisum with traumatic disruption of the duct of Santorini and adjacent pseudocyst formation. Distal pancreatectomy with cystojejunostomy resulted in total recovery.

Although it is generally believed that posttraumatic pancreatic pseudocysts will need surgical drainage, Becmeur et al[83] recently reported three cases of posttraumatic pseudocyst in children that resolved with total parenteral nutrition and nonoperative management.

Lewis et al[84] recently reported on 15 patients who developed pseudocysts following pancreatic trauma. Pseudocysts developed in eight patients who had surgery within 48 hours of their abdominal trauma and in seven who were initially treated conservatively. In none was a duct injury diagnosed during initial management. In 14 patients, the diagnosis of a pseudocyst was confirmed by CT or ultrasound. Endoscopic retrograde pancreatography (ERCP) demonstrated the site and severity of the duct injury in eight of 11 patients.

Two patients with side duct injury on ERCP were treated successfully without surgery. Pseudocysts arising from distal duct injuries (four patients) were treated by percutaneous aspiration or catheter drainage, with one of these patients requiring subsequent distal resection for recurrent pancreatitis caused by a pancreatic duct stricture. Three patients with duct injuries in the neck or body with pancreatic disruption had distal pancreatectomies. Proximal duct injuries with mature pseudocysts (three patients) were drained internally. Three patients had pseudocyst complications (hemorrhage in one and sepsis in two) that necessitated emergency laparotomy and external drainage; one of these patients died from sepsis.

These authors[84] suggested that traumatic pancreatic pseudocysts that occur after peripheral duct injury may resolve spontaneously, and those associated with distal main duct injuries can be treated by percutaneous aspiration or catheter drainage. Proximal duct injuries, however, generally require surgical intervention with either resection or internal drainage, depending on the maturity of the cyst wall.

Pancreatic Sequestration

Another complication associated with pancreatic duct disruption is that of "pancreatic sequestrum," in which a portion of the pancreas is completely separated from the main pancreatic ducts. This condition has been described in patients long after a missed pancreatic injury.[85] Patients with a pancreatic sequestrum are among the few who develop a chronic pancreatitis or pseudocyst in the undrained portion of pancreas but do not develop the usual fulminant sequelae seen with untreated pancreatic injuries involving the major duct. The condition can be prevented by the identification of pancreatic injuries promptly. It should be suspected in patients presenting with continuing abdominal pain following remote trauma. Treatment usually requires resection or internal drainage of the disconnected pancreas.

DELAYED POSTOPERATIVE HEMORRHAGE

Pancreatic wounds seldom bleed massively in a delayed fashion after trauma; however, if a fistula or an abscess develops, erosion into a large adjacent vessel can cause delayed massive hemorrhage.[1] In some instances, the bleeding is so profuse that immediate emergency operation is needed. Such surgery, however, can be extremely difficult and dangerous. Once the bleeding site is controlled, wide pancreatic drainage is instituted, and the omentum is used to isolate the pancreas from the controlled bleeding site.[9]

Dissection in the presence of severe peripancreatic inflammation can be extremely difficult and dangerous. If time is available because the bleeding is not excessive, angiographic localization and occlusion of the bleeding site is generally preferable to surgery.

AXIOM   Delayed bleeding related to a pancreatic injury or its complications can often be treated more rapidly and more safely angiographically by an interventional radiologist than by surgery.

DIABETES MELLITUS

Diabetes mellitus is uncommon following pancreatic trauma, and Jones[33] reported this problem in only three (1.1%) of 274 patients surviving treatment of pancreatic trauma. All had resection of 80% or more of the pancreas. Two of the three patients required insulin, and one was treated by diet alone. Most surgeons have not encountered diabetes mellitus as a complication of pancreatic trauma except in patients undergoing total or near-total pancreatectomy.[1]

MALABSORPTION

Most patients sustaining pancreatic injury have a normal pancreas at the time of the traumatic episode, and exocrine insufficiency is unlikely to develop unless 80-90% or more of the pancreas is removed. Alcoholic patients or patients with recurrent pancreatitis may require administration of pancreatic enzymes with their food, especially after a major pancreatic resection.

PERIPHERAL FAT NECROSIS

Peripheral fat necrosis in an extremity is a rare complication of posttraumatic pancreatitis. Adams[86] recently reported a patient who developed severe peripheral fat necrosis after penetrating pancreatic trauma and as a result needed bilateral above-the-knee amputations.

Mortality Rates after Pancreatic Trauma

HISTORICAL TRENDS

The overall mortality rate for pancreatic wounds has decreased steadily in the past 50 years.[1] While the mortality rate in the American Civil War and World War I often exceeded 80%, the mortality rate decreased to 56% in World War II, and to 22% in the Korean conflict.[1,86] In the more recent reports of civilian injuries, the mortality rate has continued to improve. Although Wilson et al,[14] in a collected series published in 1967, found an average mortality rate of 26%, the average mortality rate in three large series from more recent literature was 16.5%.[14,33]

In 1983, 63 patients were treated for pancreatic injury at the Ben Taub General Hospital with a mortality rate of 12.8%, and in a random selection of 61 patients treated in 1984 and 1985, the mortality rate was 9.8%.[1] Unfortunately, this low mortality rate was not maintained in 1987, 1988, or 1989, and the mortality rate for pancreatic trauma remains above 15% in many series.

CAUSES OF DEATH

AXIOM   Most deaths in patients with pancreatic injuries are due initially to associated vascular injuries and later to sepsis.

The majority of deaths in patients sustaining pancreatic injury are due to hemorrhage and shock, and most of these deaths occur within the first 24-48 hours.[1] In earlier collected data, 58% of the patients died within 48 hours, and in a recent series, this figure rose to 75%.[76] The causes of late deaths are varied and include intraabdominal and systemic sepsis and pulmonary complications. Deaths specifically due to pancreatic injury have usually been caused by acute severe pancreatitis and/or pancreatic fistula, but the overall mortality rate that can be directly related to such problems is generally less than 2%.[1]

RISK FACTORS

Age

Age is an important risk factor for most diseases and for most types of trauma. In a study of patients with duodenal trauma, Webb et al[88] reported a mortality rate of 11% in patients under 20 years of age, 30% in patients 21-40 years of age, and 36% in older patients.

Children are more likely to sustain blunt injury, rather than penetrating trauma, and they usually have a lower mortality rate unless there is severe head trauma.[89] Of four deaths (8%) in one series of pancreatic injuries in children, two were due to cerebral injury.[84]

Associated Injuries

AXIOM   Mortality rates in pancreatic injuries are more closely related to the number and type of the associated injuries than to any other single factor.[1]

Because of the proximity to major vessels, severe hemorrhage can occur in patients with pancreatic or duodenal injuries. Indeed, there is an almost geometric rise in the mortality rate as the number of associated injuries increases.[1] The mortality rate is only 1-2% when only one organ is injured, but it often exceeds 30% in patients with five or more associated injuries.[68]

According to a recent report by Moncure and Goins[75] on 44 patients with pancreatic or duodenal injuries, six patients died, 83% within 8 hours of admission, all as a result of gunshot wounds. Increased mortality was seen in patients with higher blood transfusion requirements, higher penetrating abdominal trauma indices, shotgun wounds, the need for pancreaticoduodenectomy, hypotension on admission, and the presence of an associated major vascular injury. It appears that early operation and control of hemorrhage is of prime importance in decreasing the mortality rate associated with these injuries.

Shock

Shock is a significant risk factor for increasing mortality rate in all types of trauma.[60,68] Because the shock is usually due to blood loss, hemorrhage should be controlled rapidly. Jones,[33] in his series of patients with pancreatic trauma, noted a mortality rate of 38% in patients admitted in shock as compared with a mortality rate of only 4% in patients who were normotensive, regardless of other factors.[33]

Severity of Wounds

Single small wounds of the pancreas or duodenum, even through-and-through bullet wounds, rarely cause death; however, when severe contusion devitalizes portions of the pancreas or when major ductal injury occurs, pancreatic complications are much more likely to occur. There is also a significantly higher mortality rate in patients who require pancreatic resections than in those who do not.[1]

Location of Wound

Wounds of the head and neck of the pancreas are generally more serious than those of the body and tail.[1] This is partly because of the danger of associated serious injuries to the major vascular structures. Another important factor is the presence of larger pancreatic ducts in the head of the pancreas.

AXIOM   Through-and-through wounds of the head of the pancreas tend to have higher morbidity and mortality rates than more distal injuries.

If there is severe damage to the head of the pancreas and duodenum, a pancreatoduodenal resection (Whipple procedure) may be the simplest method for controlling the injured ducts and providing adequate debridement of devitalized tissues; however, this procedure has a higher mortality rate than any other technique for treating pancreatic wounds.[87] If one can ascertain that the major pancreatic duct is not injured, much smaller procedures can be used.

Wounding Agent

The mortality rate for pancreatic injury varies somewhat with the wounding agent.[26] In general, stab wounds cause a mortality rate of less than 10%, gunshot wounds have a mortality rate of about 25%, and close-range shotgun blasts have a mortality rate in excess of 60% because of the much more extensive damage they can cause to the pancreas and to adjacent structures.

DUODENAL WOUNDS

Classification

The serious consequences of improper or delayed treatment of leaking duodenal injuries make an organized approach essential;[21] however, comparing results with various types of treatment is possible only if the duodenal injuries are accurately classified. Useful systems have been proposed by a number of investigators, including Lucas and Ledgerwood.[27] More recently, the Organ Injury Scaling (O.I.S) Committee of the American Association for the Surgery of Trauma (AAST) developed a system which will probably be adopted by most investigators (Table 25–7).[58] Type I injuries include serosal tears or hematomas involving a single portion of the duodenum. Type II injuries include hematomas involving more than one portion of the duodenum or a laceration involving less than 50% of the circumference. Type III injuries include lacerations involving 50-75% of the circumference of the second part of the duodenum or a 50-100% disruption of any other part of the duodenum. Type IV injuries include disruptions involving more than 75% of the second part of the duodenum or lacerations involving the ampulla of Vater or the distal common bile duct. Grade V injuries include massive disruptions of both the duodenum and pancreas or pancreatic damage combined with devascularization of the duodenum.

TABLE 25–7 *Duodenum Organ Injury Scale*

Grade*		Injury Description+	AIS-90
I	Hematoma	Involving single portion of duodenum	2
	Laceration	Partial thickness, no perforation	3
II	Hematoma	Involving more than one portion	2
	Laceration	Disruption <50% of circumference	4
III	Laceration	Disruption 50-75% circumference of D2	4
		Disruption 50-100% circumference of D1, D3, D4	4
IV	Laceration	Disruption >75% circumference of D2	5
		Involving ampulla or distal common bile duct	5
V	Laceration	Massive disruption of duodenopancreatic complex	5
	Vascular	Devascularization of duodenum	5

D1 = 1st portion duodenum, D2 = 2nd portion duodenum, D3 = 3rd portion duodenum, D4 = 4th portion duodenum
* Advance one grade for multiple injuries to the same organ.
+ Based on most accurate assessment at autopsy, laparotomy, or radiologic study
(From Moore EE, Cogbill TH, Malangoni MA, et al. Organ injury scaling II: pancreas, duodenum, small bowel, colon, and rectum. J Trauma 1990;30:1427.)

Duodenal Hematomas

An uncommon but special type of duodenal injury following blunt trauma is an intramural hematoma, usually in the second or third portion, that results in partial or complete obstruction of the lumen. This problem is most frequently seen in children, but it has also been described in adults.[90-91]

Diagnosis of duodenal hematoma may be difficult. In many patients, this is the only injury, and the symptoms of abdominal pain and bilious vomiting may not be impressive early after injury. Touloukian[92] reported delays in hospital admission ranging from 18 hours to 7 days in several children with this problem.

The diagnosis may be suspected on the basis of a CT scan, but it is usually confirmed by an upper gastrointestinal study with barium. With such contrast studies, this lesion has a characteristic appearance resembling a "stack of coins" or a "coiled spring."[91] These studies usually also indicate a partial or complete obstruction to the flow of contrast material through the duodenum. Duodenal hematomas can also often be diagnosed by ultrasound or CT scan.[100]

AXIOM Duodenal obstruction due to an intramural hematoma can often be treated nonoperatively with success.

In the past, the treatment of duodenal hematomas was surgical, with either a simple incision into the wall of the duodenum and evacuation of the hematoma (without penetrating the mucosa) or a gastrojejunostomy.[1] Today, treatment with nasogastric suction and hyperalimentation is often employed, and resolution of the hematoma occurs in most patients within 1-3 weeks.[91,92] This technique is primarily used in children, even if the obstruction is complete, but it is also applicable in adults with partial obstruction.

Voss and Bass[93] recently reported that of 967 children presenting to their hospital with blunt abdominal trauma over a 15-year period, only nine (0.9%) had intramural duodenal hematomas. In the great majority of children, nonoperative management is successful. Laparotomy should be reserved for children with other intraabdominal injuries or where the diagnosis is in doubt.

Jordan recommends surgical therapy for adults if the duodenal occlusion is complete.[1] Although it is possible that gradual resolution might occur, one can generally anticipate a prolonged period of intravenous hyperalimentation in such individuals.

General Consideration in Operative Management

Fabian and Patterson[9] have pointed out two major considerations to take into account when deciding on the type of operative management for full-thickness duodenal injuries with spill. The first is the degree of tissue injury, and the second is whether the injury is intraperitoneal or extraperitoneal.[9] Wounds to portions of the duodenum which have a serosal surface can usually be managed successfully by simple primary closure with one or two layers of sutures;[21,27,34,45,50,88] however, the retroperitoneal duodenum has no serosal covering and is, therefore, at greater risk of leak from a primary repair.[9] Stab wounds and small-caliber, low-velocity weapons often produce relatively nondestructive wounds which tend to heal with little or no difficulty. Duodenal blunt trauma and high-velocity weapons, however, generally cause much more tissue injury.[9]

Dehiscence of duodenal suture lines is caused in part by the nature of duodenal contents.[9] These may include 1-3 liters of fluid rich in hydrochloric acid and pepsin from the stomach, 800-1200 ml of bile from the liver, and 600-1000 ml of enzyme-rich fluid from the pancreas.[9]

Operative Management of Duodenal Injuries

WOUND CLOSURES

Most duodenal injuries are simple lacerations, resulting from either penetrating or blunt trauma.[1,87] When a penetrating injury on the anterior surface of the duodenum is encountered, it is critical that the posterior and medial (pancreatic) surfaces also be examined very carefully.[1] Rarely, a simple perforation of the duodenum by a missile will occur, and the missile will then be found within the lumen of the bowel. A low-velocity bullet passing through one portion of the duodenum will usually continue to pass through the posterior wall as well. These wounds can be repaired by simple suture after adequate debridement.[1] Seventy of the 101 duodenal injuries reported by Kline et al[94] were treated with simple closure.

Debridement is usually not necessary for simple knife wounds, but with blunt injuries and high velocity missiles, some debridement is wise. Control of hemorrhage from the duodenal wound itself is rarely a problem, and management is usually no different than for a surgical wound made while performing a duodenotomy.[31]

AXIOM Gunshot wounds or blunt trauma to the duodenum should be repaired carefully after thorough debridement. The repaired area should also be buttressed with well-vascularized uninjured tissues.

High-velocity gunshot wounds of the duodenum and lacerations caused by blunt trauma are generally associated with much more tissue damage than knife or low-velocity bullet wounds, and simple repair of these more complex injuries may result in a very high incidence of complications.[95] Covering the completed repair with omentum or an onlay patch of jejunum should reduce the leak rate somewhat.

DUODENAL DECOMPRESSION

If primary repair of the duodenum is possible but there is significant concern about the wound closure, several special techniques have been advocated.[1] The simplest of these is the placement of a duodenal drainage catheter, as advocated by Stone and Fabian,[96] to keep the duodenum decompressed so that the suture line is less likely to be placed under tension.

AXIOM A simple duodenostomy drainage tube may be the most effective method for reducing the tendency to leak from the repair of a badly torn duodenum.

CORRECTION OF DUODENAL WALL LOSS

Wounds associated with loss of significant portions of the duodenal wall often require special repair techniques.[1] If the loss of tissue is only on the lateral wall, and the medial wall is intact, a transverse primary repair should be attempted, even though some narrowing of the duodenal lumen may occur. In some instances, however, primary repair is impossible without creating so much tension on the suture line that its security is in question. Several special techniques have been recommended for the management of such wounds.[1]

Side-to-side Duodenojejunostomy

A side-to-side duodenojejunostomy tends to produce a sound repair, and it is rare that reflux of jejunal contents through this anastomosis creates any problem.[1] A duodenojejunostomy can also be performed using a Roux-en-Y loop, and this can prevent reflux of jejunal contents into the duodenum. Patients with extensive damage to the third and fourth portions of the duodenum can be managed by distal duodenectomy and an end-to-end duodeno-Roux-en-Y-jejunostomy.[9] Injuries requiring such repairs are relatively rare because of the lethality of the associated vascular injuries that are usually seen with such trauma.[9]

Onlay Patch of Jejunum

Rather than making an anastomosis to the site of injury, the defect may be repaired by suturing the serosal surface of intact proximal jejunum as a patch over the defect.[1,9,31] This exposes the jejunal serosa to duodenal contents, resulting in a serositis that, at times, can result in a fistula between the duodenum and the jejunum;[1] however,

such a fistula rarely causes any more trouble than a purposely created duodenojejunostomy.

Reinforcement of Repairs with Jejunum or Omentum

Reinforcement of primary repairs of the duodenum by attaching jejunum over the duodenal suture line has not improved the results obtained with primary repair alone;[97,98] however, it is still probably wise to cover duodenal repairs with a patch of viable tissue. If omentum is used, it should be sutured firmly in place without impairing its blood supply.

Jejunal Patch

A vascularized pedicle of jejunum can be developed to replace a large portion of damaged duodenum, especially over the ampulla of Vater.[1] This can be used to treat some special duodenal problems, but it is a complicated procedure, since it requires creation of a jejunal patch, suturing of the patch to the duodenal opening, and an end-to-end jejunojejunostomy.

REPAIR OF DUODENAL TRANSECTIONS

When the duodenum is totally transected, the preferred treatment is usually a primary anastomosis of the two ends after appropriate debridement;[1] however, if a large amount of tissue is lost, approximation of the duodenum may not be possible without producing undue tension on the suture line. When such injuries occur distal to the ampulla of Vater, they should be repaired by resection or closure of the distal transected end and an anastomosis of the proximal end of the injured duodenum to a loop of jejunum.[1] The exact technique used depends on the anatomic configuration of the injury and the types and number of associated injuries.

If a total transection occurs in the first portion of the duodenum, an antrectomy should be performed, completing the procedure as a Billroth II gastrectomy and closure of the duodenal stump.[1] The most complicated injuries involve the ampulla of Vater. In an occasional patient, successful primary repair of the ampulla has been accomplished; however, more complicated procedures, including pancreatoduodenectomy, are often required.[1]

DUODENAL DIVERSION

Very severe injuries to the duodenum or combined injuries to both the duodenum and pancreas can be extremely difficult to treat and have a high incidence of complications, including sepsis and fistula formation. Fabian and Patterson[9] feel that nondevitalizing wounds of both the second and third portion of the duodenum and the head of the pancreas should be managed as though they had occurred separately.[9] The pancreatic wound is generally drained and the duodenal wound handled according to the extent of injury, often by duodenal diversion.

In patients with severe duodenal injuries, many surgeons[1,9,21,26] use some modification of the diverticulization procedure popularized by Berne et al in 1974 (Fig. 25–5).[36] This technique, as originally described, includes a distal gastrectomy, closure of the duodenal stump, closure of the duodenal wound, a gastrojejunostomy, and placement of a decompressive catheter into the duodenum. Two shortcomings of the procedure are the requirement for a gastric resection and the creation of two more gastrointestinal suture lines.

PYLORIC EXCLUSION

Jordan[1] devised a modification of the diverticulization technique similar to that suggested by Summers,[8] consisting of closure of the pylorus and creation of a gastrojejunostomy to divert the flow of gastrointestinal contents away from the injured duodenum. The closure of the pylorus originally was performed with a running suture of catgut through the opening in the stomach created for the gastrojejunostomy (Fig. 25–6). Currently, Prolene suture is used more commonly, and closure of the pylorus has also been performed with a stapler.[1]

The pylorus is closed so that duodenal mucosa will not be continuously exposed to gastric contents.[1] As originally designed, how-

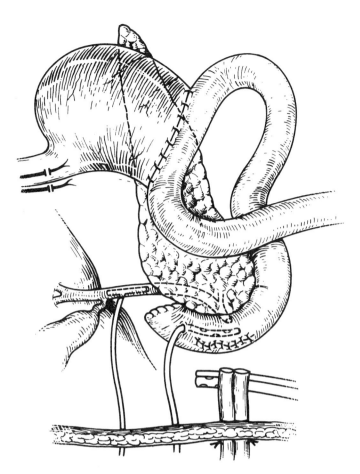

FIGURE 25–5 Duodenal diverticulization. For extensive injury of the duodenum and pancreas or severe injury of the duodenum alone, Berne et al described a duodenal diverticulization procedure which included: (a) suture repair of the primary injury, (b) antrectomy, (c) tube duodenostomy, and (d) generous drainable of the area. Truncal vagotomy and biliary decompression may also be advisable (From Thal ER. Duodenal injuries. In Champion HR, Robbs JV, Trunkey DD, eds. Rob and Smith's Operative Surgery. London: Butterworth, 1989;394.)

ever, it was anticipated that in a few weeks the catgut would dissolve and the pylorus would reopen with reinstitution of the flow of gastric contents into the duodenum. In fact, it has been found that it is very difficult to occlude the pylorus permanently by any technique.[1] In a report by Martin et al[99] in which absorbable polyglycolic acid or catgut suture was used for pyloric closure, 39 of 44 patients had reestablished flow through a patent pylorus within 3 weeks. In over 50 people who have been studied by Jordan,[1] the pylorus was open within 3 weeks, although two closures with polypropylene sutures were still closed at 37 and 53 days, and one closure with staples remained intact for several months.

A vagotomy is generally not performed at the time of the duodenal diverticulization.[1] These patients are severely injured, and the primary concern is salvage of the patient. Of equal importance is the fact that a properly constructed pyloric exclusion with a gastrojejunostomy is not an ulcerogenic operation, and one would not anticipate more marginal ulcers than spontaneously occurring duodenal ulcers in the normal population.[1] Jordan and his associates have used this technique in more than 135 patients, and the incidence of marginal ulcer is only about 3%.[1]

> **AXIOM** A gastrojejunostomy to divert gastric juice from an injured duodenum does not necessitate a vagotomy because a marginal ulcer develops only rarely in these circumstances.

Deglannis et al[100] recently reported on 74 patients with penetrating injuries of the duodenum, 63 of which were due to gunshot wounds. The increased incidence and severity of the gunshot injuries within the last few years resulted in increased use of pyloric exclusion with gradually improving results. When pyloric exclusion was added to the operative management of grade III duodenal injuries, the postoperative leakage rate fell from 43% to 12%. The authors suggest that pyloric exclusion be added to the treatment of most severe grade II and all grade III gunshot injuries of the duodenum.

On the other hand, Nassoura et al,[101] on the basis of their results with 100 patients with penetrating duodenal injuries (fistula rate of only 5% and duodenal mortality rate of 1.7%), feel that the vast majority of penetrating duodenal injuries should be managed by primary repair or resection and anastomosis. In their experience, complex duodenal decompression or diverticulization procedures are rarely necessary, but should be considered for patients with ATI >40, duodenal injury score >12, and associated injury to the head of the pancreas.

> **AXIOM** The type of duodenal exclusion performed is not as important as the care with which the procedure is performed.

As with complicated injuries of other organs, there is no uniform opinion about the choice of management techniques.[29] Jordan has continued to use pyloric exclusion and gastrojejunostomy in patients with severe duodenal wounds and considers his results to be excellent.[1] In his series of over 135 patients, there have been only two deaths attributable to the duodenal injury, and the incidence of fistula was only 6%.[1] In fact, the most recent incidence of fistula formation following duodenal trauma at Ben Taub Hospital has been only 2%.[95,99]

GASTROSTOMY PLUS DOUBLE JEJUNOSTOMY TUBE
Another approach, extensively used by Fabian and Patterson[9] for complex or retroperitoneal duodenal wounds, employs a retrograde jejunostomy tube for decompressing the duodenum, a prograde feeding jejunostomy and a gastrostomy tube to decompress the stomach (Fig. 25–7). After the duodenum is repaired, a proximal loop of jejunum is selected, and two Witzel jejunostomies are created for 16 F rubber catheters. One catheter is passed retrograde into the second portion of the duodenum and placed on gravity drainage to remove pancreatic and biliary secretions. The second jejunostomy is threaded distally for feeding and reinstallation of the pancreatic and biliary secretions. A gastrostomy is employed to reduce the problems of gastric reflux and the poor pulmonary toilet associated with prolonged nasogastric intubation.[1] This approach to management of duodenal wounds has produced excellent results, with only one (0.4%) duodenal leak in 237 patients so treated.[9]

PANCREATICODUODENECTOMY

General Considerations
Severe combined injuries to the head of the pancreas and duodenum are associated with high mortality and morbidity rates.[1,99,102-104] Patients with such trauma usually have a minimum of two other injuries, often with involvement of adjacent major vessels.[1]

Technical Considerations
A number of successful cases of primary pancreaticoduodenectomy have been described.[26] The indications are difficult to define exactly, but generally involve gross shattering of the head of the pancreas with severe injury to the duodenum, especially if there is disruption of their vascular supply and/or damage to the retropancreatic portal vein.[26]

> **AXIOM** Although a pancreaticoduodenectomy is a major operative procedure, if the injuries to the duodenum and head of the pancreas are very severe, it may be the simplest and safest approach.

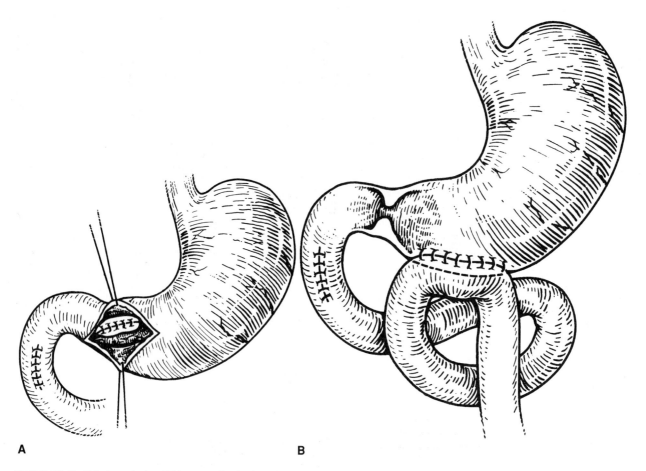

A   **B**

FIGURE 25–6   Pyloric exclusion. With severe duodenal or duodenal and pancreatic injuries, an alternative method of management is to obstruct the pylorus temporarily and perform a gastrojejunostomy without antrectomy. The duodenal wound is repaired primarily, followed by a gastrotomy on the greater curvature of the antrum at a site selected for gastrojejunostomy. Truncal vagotomy is not routinely performed although a small incidence of marginal ulcers has been reported (From Thal ER. Duodenal injuries. In Champion HR, Robbs JV, Trunkey DD, eds. Rob and Smith's Operative Surgery. London: Butterworth, 1989; 394.)

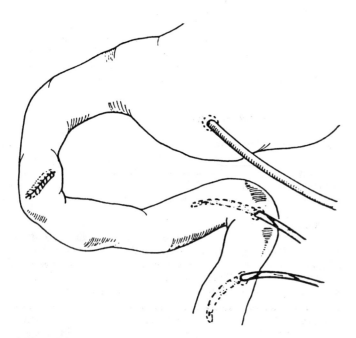

FIGURE 25–7   Use of gastric and jejunal decompression catheters, as well as a feeding jejunostomy for duodenal injury. (From Kelly G, Norton L, Moore G, et al. The continuing challenge of duodenal injuries. J Trauma 1978;18:160.)

In some cases of pancreaticoduodenal trauma, the pancreaticoduodenectomy is surprisingly easy because the original trauma has clearly defined the tissue planes for dissection.[105-107] The technique of the pancreaticoduodenectomy itself has been described in detail by Carey[105] in a recent publication. Anastomotic leaks occurred in less than 10% of his last 65 patients, and these resections were performed primarily for malignancies.

REPAIRS AROUND THE AMPULLA OF VATER

A very special type of combined pancreatoduodenal injury is severance of the major pancreatic duct and common bile duct in the region of the ampulla of Vater.[1] Jordan treated one such patient by direct repair.[109] The patient developed a fistula after this operation, but the fistula closed with conservative management, and the patient was known to be alive and well 10 years after the operation. Similar cases have been reported by others.[110,14] Kawarda et al[112] treated a case secondary to blunt trauma by anastomosing the ampulla to a Roux-en-Y limb of jejunum after removal of the remainder of the duodenum and a partial gastrectomy. The patient survived and was well 15 months later. A pyloric exclusion and drainage of the common bile duct with a T-tube may also be attempted (Fig. 25–8).

BILIARY DECOMPRESSION

Biliary decompression by means of a T-tube is occasionally used for injuries involving the common duct, but anastomosis to a Roux-en-Y loop of jejunum may be safer. A prospective study by Lucas and Walt[113] demonstrated the lack of utility of T-tubes for hepatic inju-

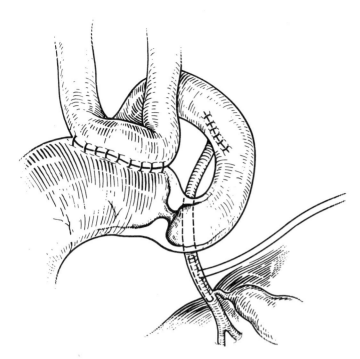

FIGURE 25–8 Pyloric exclusion with T-tube drainage of the common bile duct. For pancreatic duodenal injuries involving the ampulla of Vater, a pyloric exclusion can be performed and the common bile duct can be drained with a T-tube. If the bile duct has been avulsed, it can be reimplanted into a Roux-en-Y loop of jejunum. (From Thal ER. Duodenal injuries. In Champion HR, Robbs JV, Trunkey DD, eds. Rob and Smith's Operative Surgery. London: Butterworth, 1989; 394.)

ries and suggests that their placement in a normal common bile duct can cause many problems.

DRAINAGE OF DUODENAL INJURIES
Although pancreatic injuries should be drained, placing external drains in the vicinity of an isolated duodenal repair is not encouraged; indeed, a study by Stone and Fabian[96] reported a 23% duodenal leak rate when drains were used, compared with 8% when they were not.

AXIOM Placing a foreign body near an intestinal suture line increases the likelihood that it will leak.

Complications

There is a high incidence of complications following duodenal injuries. The complication rate for patients with combined pancreatoduodenal injury is particularly high. In one series of 118 patients, 99 (84%) survived more than 48 hours after injury, but a large number and variety of complications were recorded in the survivors.[1] The three most important complications relative to duodenal wounds include fistula formation, dehiscence, and obstruction.[1]

FISTULA FORMATION

Incidence and Mortality Rates
Fistula formation is the most feared complication of duodenal wounds.[1] In a collected series of 1563 patients with duodenal injuries, fistulas developed in 3-12%.[99] Without diverticulization or pyloric exclusion, these would all be lateral duodenal fistulas, which can be very difficult to treat. In the older literature, the mortality rate for lateral duodenal fistulas was 50-75%.[1] Currently, the mortality rate from duodenal fistulas is not nearly that high if the duodenal wounds are properly drained.

Treatment of Acute Fistulas

AXIOM Whether a duodenal fistula is an end-fistula or a side-fistula is not as important as the adequacy of the drainage of the fistula, the nutrition supplied, and the fluid and electrolyte replacement.

PROPER DRAINAGE. The primary objective in the management of duodenal fistulas should be their prevention; however, if a fistula does develop, and drains have been properly placed, the leaking duodenal contents will exit along the drain tract to the skin, and severe peritonitis will be avoided. The skin must be protected as much as possible, and sump drainage may be very helpful in this regard if there is a large amount of fluid draining from the fistula.[1]

FLUID AND ELECTROLYTE BALANCE. The amount of fluid loss through a side duodenal fistula may be very large, and careful fluid and electrolyte balance must be maintained. Scrupulous intake and output measurements, as well as analysis of the fistula fluid for its electrolyte and protein content, are important.

Some duodenal fistulas are well-tolerated, and in such patients, observation and parenteral nutrition can be expected to result in spontaneous closure.[9] "Tolerance" of duodenal or other high intestinal fistulas is generally defined as little or no pain, no signs of sepsis, no digestion of the abdominal wall, and the maintenance of adequate nutrition and fluid and electrolyte balance.[9]

METABOLIC SUPPORT
In patients who have had a duodenal diverticulization or pyloric exclusion procedure, oral alimentation is usually safe and inexpensive. Nevertheless, an increasing number of surgeons recommend the placement of a feeding jejunostomy tube at least 40 cm beyond the area of trauma at the initial operation if there is any concern about the formation of a duodenal fistula.

AXIOM Long-term nutritional support for duodenal fistulas is best provided by a jejunostomy tube that is at least 40 cm beyond the ligament of Treitz or any proximal anastomosis.

In selected patients, one may place a double-lumen tube through a gastrotomy incision, with one lumen opening into the stomach and the other segment of the tube passed through the gastroenteric stoma well into the jejunum.[1] This technique allows decompression of the stomach and instillation of food into the jejunum.[114] It also allows replacement of the aspirated material from the stomach so that fluid and electrolyte problems are less likely to occur.

Treatment of Persistent Fistulas
Once a duodenal fistula has become well established, a sinogram should be performed to determine whether there is a single track down to the opening into the duodenum and to determine whether the gastrointestinal tract is patent distal to the fistula.[1] When these two factors have been found to be present and the drainage tract has developed a strong fibrous wall (usually after 3-4 weeks), occlusion of the duodenal fistula may be performed as a final treatment modality.

A variety of materials have been used to occlude established duodenal fistula tracts. The simplest and most effective technique in Jordan's experience has been occlusion with bubble gum which has been chewed by the patient or made malleable by wetting and kneading.[1] Enough gum should be used to fill the length of the tract completely, and it is held securely in place by a pressure dressing.[109] Jordan has used this technique in the treatment of several well-established duodenal fistulas with prompt cessation of drainage and subsequent rapid healing.[1]

AXIOM Surgery to close well-established end duodenal fistulas is rarely required.

DUODENAL DEHISCENCE

The occurrence of a duodenal dehiscence may be signalled by a number of changes, including deterioration of the patient's general condition or by bile staining of the dressings.[9] If there is severe sudden deterioration, emergency reoperation is necessary, and the injury should be treated as a complex, retroperitoneal duodenal injury.[9] One should not attempt to close the opening by direct suture. Adequate drainage is essential, and if technically feasible, an attempt should be made to cover the dehiscence with a patch of jejunum.[1]

DUODENAL OBSTRUCTION

Obstruction may occur at any suture line in the gastrointestinal tract, but the duodenum is particularly at risk because one generally cannot simply resect the involved area of the closure. Even if an adequate duodenal lumen is available, swelling of the pancreatic head from associated trauma may occlude it. If this problem has been anticipated and a diverticulization procedure or even a simple gastroenterostomy has been performed, it may cause no difficulty; however, if the primary repair is performed without any protective secondary procedure, one should anticipate a possible duodenal obstruction and look carefully for evidence of its development.

AXIOM If obstruction appears to be present following a duodenal repair, an initial period of nonsurgical treatment is appropriate.

The initial approach to a duodenal obstruction should be prolonged nasogastric suction and intravenous nutritional support.[1] If there is no sign of improvement in 10 days or so, an upper gastrointestinal radiologic examination with barium should be performed to determine whether the obstruction is complete or whether there is some passage of barium beyond the point of the duodenal injury. If the obstruction is incomplete, further conservative therapy is indicated.

AXIOM Duodenal obstruction at a suture line, if persistent, should be bypassed surgically rather than treated with direct correction.

If the initial study shows complete obstruction at a site of duodenal repair and there is no improvement in 1 week, operative intervention is indicated.[1] If the obstruction is beyond the ampulla of Vater, it may be bypassed by a duodenojejunostomy or by a gastrojejunostomy. If the obstruction is proximal to the ampulla, a gastrojejunostomy is preferred.

Mortality

The mortality rates reported for duodenal wounds continue to be high and generally range from 10% to 25%.[21,29,32,34,45,50] The report by Adkins et al[115] of a mortality rate of 5.3% is the only one with a mortality rate below 12%;[98] however, these mortality rates include pancreatoduodenal injuries. The majority of the deaths are not due to the duodenal wound itself.[1] In fact, in a series of over 350 duodenal wounds, death was due to a complication of the duodenal wound itself in less than 1%.[1]

As with pancreatic wounds, most deaths in the first 24-48 hours are due to exsanguination.[1] Most late deaths are due to sepsis and the resulting multiorgan failure. Late complications associated with isolated duodenal wounds account for a very small number of deaths.[99]

Reported mortality rates after pancreatoduodenal wounds range from 16 to 100%, with an average of about 25%.[99,116] In one series of 129 patients treated in one institution, 38 (29%) died, and 21 (55%) of the deaths occurred in less than 48 hours due to hemorrhage and shock. Late deaths were primarily from sepsis with respiratory and/or renal failure. Less than 3% died of specific problems related to the pancreatic injury, including one patient who developed hemorrhagic pancreatitis.

⊘ **FREQUENT ERRORS**

In the Management of Pancreatic and Duodenal Injuries

1. *Assuming that an injury to the duodenum or pancreas can be ruled out by normal physical findings after severe trauma.*
2. *Relying on isolated serum amylase determinations to diagnose or rule out pancreatic injuries.*
3. *Failure to examine plain radiograph films of the abdomen closely for retroperitoneal air in patients with severe blunt trauma.*
4. *Assuming that a normal DPL and abdominal CT can accurately rule out pancreatic or duodenal injury.*
5. *Relying on a "negative" radiologic contrast study to rule out duodenal injury.*
6. *Failure to open retroperitoneal hematomas over the pancreas and duodenum.*
7. *Failure to adequately expose the pancreas if there is any suspicion that it may be injured.*
8. *Failure to adequately pursue the cause of any bile staining near the duodenum or head of the pancreas.*
9. *Attempting complex reconstruction of a transected pancreas in patients with other high-risk injuries.*
10. *Failure to provide efficient safe and continuing abdominal drainage to an injured pancreas.*

▼▼▼▼▼▼▼▼▼▼▼▼▼▼▼▼▼▼▼▼▼▼▼▼▼▼▼▼▼▼

SUMMARY POINTS

1. Associated injuries are the major cause of the high mortality rates seen with pancreatic and duodenal trauma.
2. Pancreatic parenchymal injuries are difficult to repair and frequently leak for at least several days after injury.
3. Except for the dorsal pancreatic artery, which usually arises from the superior mesenteric artery, the pancreas has almost no independent arterial blood supply.
4. The secretin system is an important mechanism for preventing duodenal ulceration, and cholecystokinin (pancreozymin) is primarily for digestive purposes.
5. Dehiscence of a duodenal suture line can be especially dangerous because of the large amounts of activated enzymes that may be rapidly liberated into the abdomen.
6. Preventing leakage of the luminal contents is a major goal of treatment of duodenal injuries, and the nature and location of the injury may dictate diversion of those contents in addition to careful repair.
7. One should look very closely for an associated pancreatic injury whenever the duodenum is damaged.
8. The major principle in diagnosis of blunt pancreatic or duodenal trauma is awareness of the initial subtlety of these injuries.
9. Injury to the pancreas or duodenum must be considered a possibility in all patients who sustain injury to the upper abdomen.
10. The clinical changes in isolated pancreatic or duodenal injury may be extremely subtle until severe, life-threatening peritonitis develops.
11. The best way to diagnose pancreatic or duodenal injuries is repeated careful reexamination of the patient combined with a high index of suspicion.
12. A normal physical examination does not rule out significant pancreatic or duodenal injuries.
13. Laboratory examinations are relatively insensitive and nonspecific for diagnosing duodenal or pancreatic injury.
14. Monitoring serum amylase levels during the early postinjury phase seems prudent, but the clinician should regard normal levels as inconclusive.

15. The diagnosis of pancreaticoduodenal trauma is more often made by the astute clinician than by any laboratory test or radiograph.

16. If an intent search for retroperitoneal air is not made on plain radiographs of the abdomen, the diagnosis of traumatic rupture of the duodenum will generally be delayed. Consequently, the mortality rate may be extremely high.

17. Plain films of the abdomen and upper GI contrast studies, like serum amylase determinations, should be used to prompt early exploration, not to dismiss the possibility of pancreaticoduodenal injury.

18. A negative contrast study of the duodenum can be extremely dangerous because of the false sense of security it can inspire.

19. All techniques used to diagnose injuries of the pancreas or duodenum are reliable only when they identify an injury; a "normal" study has relatively little negative predictive value.

20. A DPL may be completely negative with severe injuries of retroperitoneal organs, such as the pancreas and duodenum.

21. A negative peritoneal lavage finding does not rule out retroperitoneal duodenal perforation.

22. In an occasional patient with a suspected pancreatic ductal injury, an ERCP may be used to determine the need for surgery and to determine the exact site of a major ductal injury.

23. A "negative laparotomy" does not exclude the possibility of a delayed complication of pancreatic or duodenal injury.

24. Upper midline retroperitoneal hematomas should be explored to rule out underlying duodenal, pancreatic, or vascular injuries.

25. A Kocher maneuver, with or without the additional mobilization possible after a Cattell maneuver, is recommended for complete inspection of the first three portions of the duodenum and the head of the pancreas.

26. The presence of any bile staining or crepitation in the periduodenal area after trauma mandates a very careful search of the bile ducts and duodenum.

27. Severe edema, crepitance, or bile staining of periduodenal tissue implies a duodenal injury until proven otherwise.

28. The major decision to be made at the time of exploration of a suspected pancreaticoduodenal injury is whether there is a tear in the duodenum or a major pancreatic duct.

29. The use of pancreatography intraoperatively in patients suspected of having injury to the major pancreatic duct may cause more harm than good and is controversial.

30. With any intraabdominal injury, the highest priorities are control of hemorrhage followed by control of bowel leaks.

31. Simple drainage of major pancreatic ductal injuries is frequently associated with major complications.

32. Splenic salvage should probably be attempted for traumatic rupture of the pancreas if the patient is young and hemodynamically stable and there are no other life-threatening injuries.

33. One should avoid Roux-en-Y jejunal anastomoses to the surface of damaged pancreas unless there is no other reasonable way to manage drainage from an injured major pancreatic duct.

34. Direct repairs of tears of major pancreatic duct usually fail, even with a stent.

35. If one feels that preservation of the distal portion of a transected pancreas is important, a Roux-en-Y loop is probably the best system for managing its exocrine secretions.

36. Since 90% of the normal pancreas can generally be resected without significant endocrine or exocrine deficiency, complex preservation procedures are rarely indicated.

37. Closure of the transected ends of a divided pancreas will frequently fail, especially if the main duct is not identified and carefully and completely closed with sutures.

38. All pancreatic injuries should be drained because there will be some leakage of pancreatic enzymes in almost all cases.

39. The incidence of infection of pancreatic drainage tracts is probably lowest when closed systems are used.

40. Even if there is no evidence of a pancreatic leak, drains should be left in place until the patient has been eating for a few days.

41. Mild drainage from peripancreatic drains during the first few days following trauma is seldom a serious problem.

42. Pancreatic fistulas should be treated conservatively initially because most of them heal spontaneously within 2-4 weeks.

43. Peripancreatic drains should be left in place until the patient is eating a full diet and there is little or no drainage or until the drainage tract is well-established.

44. Fluid and electrolyte losses from large pancreatic fistulas can be very dangerous in malnourished patients.

45. The combination of a major bowel injury, necrotic pancreatic tissue, and a continuing pancreatic leak greatly increases the risk of intraperitoneal sepsis.

46. Pancreatic necrosis or an abscess should be suspected in anyone who becomes toxic or develops multiple organ failure after a major pancreatic injury.

47. Persistent posttraumatic pancreatitis is frequently the harbinger of complications such as a pseudocyst or pancreatic abscess.

48. Development of a pancreatic pseudocyst should be suspected in anyone with an upper abdominal mass or a persistent elevation of serum amylase levels following pancreatic trauma.

49. Endoscopic retrograde pancreatography should be performed prior to the treatment of pancreatic pseudocysts to aid in the selection of the most appropriate procedure.

50. Bleeding related to a pancreatic injury or its complications can often be treated faster and more safely angiographically, by an interventional radiologist, than by surgery.

51. Most deaths in patients with pancreatic injuries are due initially to associated vascular injuries and later to sepsis.

52. Mortality rates in pancreatic injuries are more closely related to the number and type of associated injuries than to any other single factor.

53. Through-and-through wounds of the head of the pancreas tend to have a higher morbidity and mortality than more distal injuries.

54. Duodenal obstruction due to an intramural hematoma can often be treated nonoperatively with success.

55. Gunshot wounds or blunt trauma to the duodenum should be carefully repaired after thorough debridement. The repaired area should also be buttressed with well-vascularized uninjured tissues.

56. A simple duodenostomy drainage tube may be the most effective method for reducing the tendency to leak from the repair of a badly torn duodenum.

57. A gastrojejunostomy to divert gastric juice from an injured duodenum does not necessitate a vagotomy because a marginal ulcer develops only rarely in these circumstances.

58. A pancreatic or duodenal fistula should not be closed until a firm fibrous track is present and one is assured that there is no proximal obstruction.

59. The type of duodenal exclusion performed is not as important as the care with which the procedure was performed.

60. Although a pancreaticoduodenectomy is a major operative procedure, if the injuries to the duodenum and head of the pancreas are very severe, it may be the simplest and safest approach.

61. Placing a foreign body near an intestinal suture line increases the likelihood that it will leak.

62. Whether a duodenal fistula is an end-fistula or a side-fistula is not as important as the adequacy of the drainage of the fistula, the nutrition supplied, and the fluid and electrolyte replacement.

63. Long-term nutritional support for duodenal fistulas is best provided via a jejunostomy tube that is at least 40 cm beyond the ligament of Treitz or any proximal anastomosis.

64. Surgery to close well-established end duodenal fistulas is rarely required.

65. If obstruction appears to be present following a duodenal repair, an initial period of nonsurgical treatment is appropriate.

66. Duodenal obstruction at a suture line, if persistent, should be bypassed surgically rather than treated with direct correction.

▲▲▲▲▲▲▲▲▲▲▲▲▲▲▲▲▲▲▲▲▲▲▲▲▲▲▲▲▲▲▲▲▲▲▲▲▲▲

REFERENCES

1. Jordan GJ Jr. Injury to the pancreas and duodenum (Chap 32). In Moore EE, Mattox KL, Feliciano DV, eds. Trauma, 2nd ed. Norwalk, CT: Appleton-Lange, 1991; 498-510.
2. Travers B. Rupture of the pancreas. Lancet 1827;12:384.
3. von Mikuliez-Radecki. Surgery of the pancreas with especial consideration of trauma and inflammatory processes. Ann Surg 1903;38:1.
4. Korte W. Quoted by Robson AWM, Cammidge PJ. The pancreas: its surgery and pathology. Philadelphia: WB Saunders, 1907.
5. Kulenkampff D. Ein fall von pancreas-fistel. Berl Klin Wochenschr 1882;19:102.
6. Moynihan B. Abdominal operations, vol II. Philadelphia: WB Saunders, 1926.
7. Kocher T. Mobilisierung des duodenum and gastroduodenostomy. Zentralbl Chir Leipz 1903;30:33.
8. Summers JE Jr. The treatment of posterior perforations of the fixed portions of the duodenum. Ann Surg 1904;39:727.
9. Fabian TC, Patterson CR. Injuries of the stomach, duodenum, pancreas, and small intestine. In Kreis DJ, Gomez GA, eds. Trauma management. Boston: Little, Brown & Co., 1989; 215-229.
10. Harrison AW, Whelan P. Retroperitoneal injuries. In McMurtry RY, McLellan BA, eds. Management of blunt trauma. Baltimore: Williams & Wilkins, 1990; 276-278.
11. Jones RD, Shires GT. Pancreatic trauma. Arch Surg 1971;102:424.
12. Northrop WF, Simmons RL. Pancreatic trauma: a review. Surgery, 1971;71:27.
13. Hendel R, Rustrals CH. Management of pancreatic trauma. Can J Surg 1985;28:359.
14. Wilson RF, Tagett JP, Pucelik JP, et al. Pancreatic trauma. J Trauma 1967;7:643.
15. Thal AP, Wilson RF. A pattern of severe blunt trauma to the pancreas. Surg Gynec Obstet 1964;119:773.
16. Henne-Bruns D, Kremer B, Lloyd DM, et al. Injuries of the portal vein in patients with blunt abdominal trauma. Surg 1993;6:163.
17. Smego DR, Richardson JD, Flint LM. Determination of outcome in pancreatic trauma. J Trauma 1985;25:771.
18. Herorejos A, Coehn DM, Mossa AR. Management of pancreatic trauma. Ann R Coll Surg Engl 1983;65:297.
19. Werschlay LR, Jordan GL. Surgical management of traumatic injuries to the pancreas. Am J Surg 1985;116:768.
20. Jones RC. Management of pancreatic trauma. Am J Surg 1985;150:698.
21. Harrison AW, Whelan P. Retroperitoneal injuries (Chap 24-Part C). In McMurtry RY, McLellan BA, eds. Management of blunt trauma. Baltimore: Williams & Wilkins, 1990;279-282.
22. Bergqvist D, Hedelin H, Karlsson G, et al. Upper gastrointestinal trauma. Acta Chir Scand 1981;147:637.
23. Dauterine AH, Flancbaum L, Cox EF. Blunt intestinal trauma: a modern day review. Ann Surg 1985;201:198.
24. Gifford SR, Hymes AC. Duodenal rupture after blunt abdominal trauma. Minn Med 1980;63:83.
25. Bergquist M, Hedelin H. Seat belt induced injury of the duodenum. J Trauma 1976;16:390.
26. Walt AJ, Wilson RF. Specific abdominal injuries. In Walt AJ, Wilson RF, eds. Management of trauma, pitfalls and practice. Philadelphia: Lea & Febiger, 1975; 23:348-374.
27. Lucas CE, Ledgerwood AM. Factors influencing outcome after blunt duodenal injuries. J Trauma 1975;5:839.
28. Donoval A, Hogan W. Traumatic perforation of the duodenum. Am J Surg 1966;111:341.
29. Vargish T, Urdaneta LF, Cram AE, et al. Duodenal trauma in the rural setting. Am Surg 1983;49:211-213.
30. Creise EF, Scully JH. Blunt trauma to the small intestine. J Trauma 1970;10:46.
31. Corley RD, Norcross WJ, Shoemaker WC. Traumatic injuries to the duodenum: a report of 98 patients. Ann Surg 1974;181:92.
32. Fabian TC, Mangianti EC, Miller M. Duodenal rupture due to blunt trauma: a problem in diagnosis. South Med J 1984;77:1078.
33. Jones RC. Management of pancreatic trauma. Am J Surg 1978;187:555.
34. Flint LM, McCoy M, Richardson JD, Polk HG. Duodenal injury: analysis of common misconceptions in diagnosis and treatment. Ann Surg 1980;191:697.
35. Friend PJ, Jamieson NV, MacFarland R. Blunt pancreatic injury: two case reports and a review of the literature. Injury 1985;16:391.
36. Berne CJ, Donoval AJ, White EJ, et al. Duodenal "diverticulation" for duodenal and pancreatic injuries. Am J Surg 1974;127:503.
37. Lucas CE. Diagnosis and treatment of pancreatic and duodenal injury. Surg Clin North Am 1977;57:49.
38. Olsen WR. The serum amylase in blunt abdominal trauma. J Trauma 1973;13:200.
39. White PH, Benfield JR. Amylase in the management of pancreatic trauma. Arch Surg 1972;187:555.
40. Morentz JA, Campbell DP, Parker DE, et al. Significance of serum amylase level in evaluating pancreatic trauma. Am J Surg 1975;130:739.
41. Davis JJ, Cohn I, Nance FC. Diagnosis and management of blunt abdominal trauma. Ann Surg 1976;183:677.
42. Talbot WA, Shuck JM. Retroperitoneal duodenal injury due to blunt abdominal trauma. Am J Surg 1975;130:659.
43. Bouwman DL, Weaver DW, Walt AJ. Serum amylase and its isoenzymes: a clarification of their implications in trauma. J Trauma 1984;24:573.
44. Greenlee T, Murphy K, Ram MD. Amylase isoenzymes in the evaluation of trauma patients. Am Surg 1984;50:637.
45. Adkins RB, Keyser JE. Recent experiences with duodenal trauma. Am Surg 1985;51:121.
46. Kunin JR, Korobkin M, Ellis JH, et al. Duodenal injuries caused by blunt abdominal trauma: value of CT in differentiating perforation from hematoma. Am J Roentgenol 1993;160:1221.
47. Lane MJ, Mindelzun RE, Sandhu JS, et al. CT diagnosis of blunt pancreatic trauma: importance of detecting fluid between the pancreas and the splenic vein. Am J Roentgenol 1994;163:833.
48. Nelson MG, Jones DR, Vasilakiz A, et al. Computed tomographic diagnosis of acute blunt pancreatic transection. W V Med J 1994;90:274.
49. Gothi R, Bose NC. Case report: ultrasound demonstration of traumatic fracture of the pancreas with pancreatic duct disruption. Clin Radiol 1993;47:436.
50. Levison MA, Petersen SR, Sheldon GF, et al. Duodenal trauma: experience of a trauma center. J Trauma 1984;24:475.
51. Whittwell AE, Gomez GA, Byers P, et al. Blunt pancreatic trauma: prospective evaluation of early endoscopic retrograde pancreatography. South Med J 1989;82:586.
52. Blind PJ, Mellbring G, Hjertkvist M, et al. Diagnosis of traumatic pancreatic duct rupture by on-table endoscopic retrograde pancreatography. Pancreas 1994;9:387.
53. Gholson CF, Sittig K, Favrot D, et al. Chronic abdominal pain as the initial manifestation of pancreatic injury due to remote blunt trauma of the abdomen. South Med J 1994;87:902.
54. Cattell RB, Brasch JW. Technique for exposure of the third and fourth portions of the duodenum. Surg Gynecol Obstet 1960;111:378.
55. Babb J, Harmon H. Diagnosis and management of pancreatic trauma. Am Surg 1976;42:390.
56. Brotman S, Cisternino S, Myers RA, Crowley RA. A test to help diagnosis of rupture in the injured duodenum. Injury 1981;12:464.
57. Berni GA, Bandyk DF, Oreskovich MR, et al. Role of intraoperative pancreatography in patients with injury to the pancreas. Am J Surg 1982;143:602.
58. Moore EE, Cogbill TH, Malangoni MA, et al. Organ scaling II: Pancreas, duodenum, small bowel, colon, and rectum. J Trauma 1990;30:1427.
59. Stone HH, Fabian TC, Satiani B, Turkleson ML. Experiences in the management of pancreatic trauma. J Trauma 1981;21:257.
60. Heitsch RC, Knutson CO, Fulton RL, et al. Delineation of critical factors in the treatment of pancreatic trauma. Surgery 1976;80:523.
61. Sims EH, Mandai AK, Schlater T, et al. Factors affecting outcome in pancreatic trauma. J Trauma 1984;24:125.
62. Sukul K, Lont HE, Johannes EJ. Management of pancreatic injuries. Hepatogastroenterology 1962;85:525.
63. Fitzgibbons TJ, Yellin AE, Maruyama MM, et al. Management of the transected pancreas following distal pancreatectomy. Surg Gynecol Obstet 1982;154:225.
64. Frey C. Trauma to the Pancreas and Duodenum. In Blaisdell FW, Trunkey DD, eds. Trauma management: abdominal trauma. New York: Thieme-Stratton, 1982; 87-94.
65. Cogbill TH, Moore EE, Morris JA Jr. et al. Distal pancreatectomy for trauma: a multicenter experience. J. Trauma 1991;31:1600.

66. Martin LW, Henderson BM, Welsch N. Disruption of the head of the pancreas caused by blunt trauma in children: a report of two cases treated with primary repair of the pancreatic duct. Surgery 1968;63:697.

67. Stauch GO. The use of pancreatogastrostomy after blunt traumatic pancreatic transection: a complete and efficient operation. Ann Surg 1972; 176:16.

68. Graham JM, Mattox KL, Jordan GL Jr. Traumatic injuries of the pancreas. Am J Surg 1978;136:744.

69. Letton AH, Wilson JP. Traumatic severance of pancreas treated by Roux-en-Y anastomosis. Surg Gynecol Obstet 1959;109:473.

70. Andersen DK, Bolman RM III, Moylan JA Jr. Management of penetrating pancreatic injuries: subtotal pancreatectomy using the auto suture stapler. J Trauma 1980;20:347.

71. Chambers RT, Norton L, Hinchey EJ. Massive right upper quadrant intraabdominal injury requiring pancreaticoduodenectomy and partial hepatectomy. J Trauma 1975;15:714.

72. Delcore R, Stauffer JS, Thomas JH, et al. The role of pancreatogastrostomy following pancreatoduodenectomy for trauma. J Trauma 1994; 37:395.

73. Anderson CB, Connors JP, Mejia DC, et al. Drainage methods in the treatment of pancreatic injuries. Surg Gynecol Obstet 1974;138: 587.

74. Sims EH, Lou MA, Schlater T, et al. Surgical management of pancreatic trauma. Am J Surg 1983;145:278.

75. Moncure M, Goins WA. Challenges in the management of pancreatic and duodenal injuries. J Nat Med Assoc 1993;85:767.

76. Jordan GL Jr. Pancreatic trauma In Howard JM, Jordan GL Jr, Reber HA, eds. Surgical diseases of the pancreas. Philadelphia: Lea & Febiger, 1986; 875.

77. Cogbill TH, Moore EE, Kashuk JL. Changing trends in the management of pancreatic trauma. Arch Surg 1982;117:722.

78. Pederzoli P, Bassi C, Falconi M, et al. Conservative treatment of external pancreatic fistulas with parenteral nutrition alone or in combination with continuous intravenous infusion of somatostatin, glucagon, or calcitonin. Surg Gynecol Obstet 1986;163:428.

79. Fraser GC. "Handlebar" injury of the pancreas: report of a case complicated by pseudocyst formation with spontaneous internal rupture. J Pediatr Surg 1969;4:216.

80. Tayiem AK. Pancreatic/duodenal trauma. J Kans Med Soc 1979;80: 247.

81. Bass J, DeLorenzo M, Desjardins JG, et al. Blunt pancreatic injuries in children: the role of percutaneous external drainage in the treatment of pancreatic psuedocysts. J Pediatr Surg 1988;23:721.

82. Portis M, Meyers P, McDonald JC, et al. Traumatic pancreatitis in a patient with pancreas divisum: clinical and radiographic features. Abdom Imaging 1994;19:162.

83. Becmeur F, Dhaoui R, Rousseau P, et al. Posttraumatic pancreatic pseudocyst: nonoperative conservative management—report on 3 cases. Eur J Pediatr Surg 1993;3:302.

84. Lewis G, Krige JE, Bornman PC, et al. Traumatic pancreatic pseudocysts. Br J Surg 1993;80:89-93.

85. Kudsk KA, Temizer D, Ellison EC, et al. Posttraumatic pancreatic sequestrum: recognition and treatment. J Trauma 1986;26:320.

86. Adams DB. Peripheral fat necrosis after penetrating pancreatic trauma: a case report. Am J Surg 1993;59:769.

87. Cameron AE, Southcott RD, Blake J, et al. Successful Whipple's operation for pancreatic injury. Injury 1985;16:233.

88. Webb HW, Howard JM, Jordan GL Jr, et al. Surgical experiences in the treatment of duodenal injuries. Surg Gynecol Obstet 1958;106:105.

89. Graham JM, Pokorny WJ, Mattox KL, et al. Surgical management of acute pancreatic injuries in children. J Pediatr Surg 1978;13:693.

90. Margolis IB. Intramural hematoma of the duodenum. Am J Surg 1983;132:779.

91. Foulandoran RJ. Protocol for the nonoperative treatment of obstructing intramural duodenal hematoma during childhood. Am J Surg 1983; 145:330.

92. Touloukian RJ. Protocol for the nonoperative treatment of obstructing intramural duodenal hematoma during childhood. Am J Surg 1983; 145:330.

93. Voss M, Bass DH. Traumatic duodenal haematoma in children. Injury 1994;25:227.

94. Kline G, Lucas CE, Ledgerwood AM, et al. Duodenal organ injury severity (OIS) and outcome. Am Surg 60:500, 1994.

95. Morton JR, Jordan GL. Traumatic duodenal injuries. J Trauma 1968; 8:127.

96. Stone HH, Fabian TC. Management of duodenal wounds. J Trauma 1979; 19:334.

97. Ivatury RR, Gudino J, Ascer E, et al. Treatment of penetrating duodenal injuries. Primary repair versus repair with decompressive enterostomy/ serosal patch. J Trauma 1985;25:337.

98. McInnis WD, Aust JB, Cruz AB, et al. Traumatic injuries of the duodenum: a comparison of primary closure and jejunal patch. J Trauma 1975;15:847.

99. Martin TD, Feliciano DV, Mattox, et al. Severe duodenal injuries. Arch Surg 1983;118:631.

100. Degiannis E, Krawczykowski D, Velmahos GC, et al. Pyloric exclusion in severe penetrating injuries of the duodenum. World J Surg 1993; 17:751.

101. Nassoura ZE, Ivatury RR, Simon RJ, et al. A prospective reappraisal of primary repair of penetrating duodenal injuries. Am Surg 1994;60:35.

102. Fanelli G, Nacchiero M. An interesting case of pancreaticoduodenal trauma. Am J Gastroenterol 1980;74:279.

103. Graham JM, Mattox KL, Vaughan GD III, et al. Combined pancreatoduodenal injuries. J Trauma 1979;19:340.

104. Moore JB, Moore EE. Changing trends in the management of combined pancreatoduodenal injuries. World J Surg 1984;8:791.

105. Yellin AE, Rosoff L. Pancreatoduodenectomy for combined pancreatoduodenal injuries. Arch Surg 1975;110:1177.

106. Oreskovich MR, Carrico CJ. Pancreaticoduodenectomy for trauma: a viable option? Am J Surg 1984;147:618.

107. McKone TK, Bursch LR, Scholten DJ. Pancreaticoduodenectomy for trauma: a life-saving procedure. Am Surg 1988;54:361.

108. Carey LC. Pancreaticoduondenectomy. Am J Surg 1992;164:153.

109. Jordan GL JR. Gastroenteric cutaneous fistula. Arch Surg 1964;88:540.

110. Lee D, Zacher J, Vogel TT. Primary repair in transection of duodenum with avulsion of the common duct. Arch Surg 1976;111:592.

111. Fish JC, Johnson GL. Rupture of duodenum following blunt trauma: report of a case with avulsion of the papilla of Vater. Ann Surg 1965;162:917.

112. Kawarda Y, Tani K, Yoshimine S, et al. Blunt injury of duodenum with avulsion of papilla of Vater: report of a case. Jpn J Surg 1984;14:499.

113. Lucas CE, Walt AJ. Analysis of randomized biliary drainage for liver trauma in 189 patients. J Trauma 1981;12:257.

114. Lee SM. The use of double-lumen tubes in upper gastrointestinal surgery. Am Surg 1980;46:363.

115. Adkins RB Jr, Keyser JE III. Recent experiences with duodenal trauma. Am Surg 1985;51:121.

116. Mansour A, Moore EE, Moore JB, et al. Management of pancreaticoduodenal injuries: a ten year experience. Am J Surg 1989;158:531.

Chapter **26** Injuries to the Colon and Rectum

ROBERT F. WILSON, M.D.

ALEXANDER J. WALT, M.D., CHB

SCOTT DULCHAVSKY, M.D.

"Ehud made a dagger—and came unto Eglan, King of Moab.—Ehud said unto him, I have a message from God unto thee,—and Ehud took the dagger—and thrust it unto his belly—and the 'dirt' came out." —Judges 3:16-22

INTRODUCTION

AXIOM Wounds of the colon and rectum can be lethal if they are not recognized and treated promptly.

Injuries to the colon and rectum can greatly increase the morbidity and mortality of patients with severe trauma. The presence of colon in all quadrants of the abdomen places it at risk with almost all penetrating abdominal wounds, and the high concentrations (10^9-10^{12} per ml) of bacteria in the colon make sepsis an ever-present threat in any patient in whom it is injured.

In spite of the frequency and potential of severe complications of colon and rectal injuries, the evolution of our management of these injuries clearly illustrates how slowly changes may occur in medicine. The conversion from yesterday's condemnation of primary repair of colon injuries to today's tendency to avoid colostomy whenever possible has been greatly influenced by our improved ability to treat shock and infection. Even more important, a willingness has emerged to challenge the traditional belief that all colon injuries should be treated with a colostomy.

Part of the slowness of the transition from performing colostomies to performing primary repairs for most colon injuries is the fact that the mortality rates seen with colon trauma have often been incorrectly attributed to the colon lesion rather than to the extensive associated injuries present in at least two-thirds of these cases.

Injuries of the colon and rectum, with current mortality rates often less than 6%, are being approached with greater confidence and less conservatism than in the past.[1-4] Although injuries to the large bowel continues to have a high morbidity, some of these are due to the colostomy or ileostomy and not the colon injury itself.

HISTORICAL PERSPECTIVES

From the time of the killing of Eglan, King of Moab, by Ehud, a deliverer of the children of Israel after 18 years of servitude, little was written on colon and rectal injuries for many centuries. Stone and Fabian[5] in 1979 noted that, although Lembert in 1827 was the first to record the successful closure of a small bowel perforation, repair of colon wounds failed consistently up until the time of World War I. Nance[2] has, however, mentioned Senn's hydrogen insufflation test of the 1890s to determine whether a wound involved the colon. Hydrogen gas was insufflated into the anus of the injured patient and a lighted taper was placed near the wound of entrance. A flaring blue flame or small explosion was considered a positive indication of a colon perforation.

Even elective operations on the colon were often attended by significant mortalities due to wound and intraperitoneal sepsis, as well as disruption of the bowel suture line. Closed techniques for bowel anastomosis, exteriorization of the site selected for reestablishing bowel continuity with a special clamp (e.g., Mickulicz, Rankin, etc.), and protection of such suture lines by creation of a proximal colostomy were among the various surgical maneuvers developed to deal with this problem.

As with most other injuries, the management of colon and rectal injuries in the wars of this century is an example of how improvements in the management of specific injuries can evolve over time as experience is gained with large numbers of cases.[6] Treatment of colonic injuries did not receive serious attention until World War I, when the practice of nonoperative management of military abdominal wounds began to be abandoned.[1]

In 1917, Cuthbert Wallace analyzed 1200 patients with gunshot wounds of the abdomen from World War I.[2] These included 252 patients with colonic injuries, of which 155 with isolated colonic injury were treated with primary repair. The mortality rate in 97 patients treated with a colostomy was 73%; and for those who had a primary repair, the mortality rate was almost 50%. Wallace felt that colostomy had its greatest application in the management of wounds of the extraperitoneal ascending and descending colon and the rectum.

The use of suture closure without colostomy for the treatment of most colonic wounds continued until 1944 during World War II.[2] Gordon-Taylor, in a monograph published in 1939 (based on World War I experience) advocated suture or resection for colonic injuries and gave little consideration to the role of colostomy.[2] In military surgical manuals prepared in 1942 for United States Army and Navy Medical officers, Storck advocated primary suture of colon injuries, suggesting that colostomy should be used primarily for flank and rectal injuries.[2] However, based on poor results with primary repair of colon injuries in North Africa, the Surgeon General in 1943 directed that all wounds of the large bowel should be exteriorized if possible, or otherwise treated by repair and proximal colostomy.[2]

Ogilvie in his 1944 report on experiences in the western desert of Africa noted that "the treatment of colon injury is based on the known insecurity of suture and dangers of leakage. Simple closure of a wound to the colon, however small, is unwarranted; men have survived such an operation, but others have died who would still be alive had they fallen into the hands of a surgeon with less optimism and more sense. Injured segments must either be exteriorized or functionally excluded by a proximal colostomy." Reliance on colostomy for treating injuries to the colon was credited with reducing the mortality rate from colon injury from approximately 70% to less than 35%. These lessons were brought back and incorporated into civilian practice, and following World War II, colostomy became the standard therapy for colonic injuries.[1]

Unfortunately, the environment in which this dogma developed is often unappreciated. In the desert and subsequently on the Italian front, there was usually a substantial delay between wounding and definitive operation at a field surgical unit. By the time the patient was operated upon, gross contamination and established infection of the peritoneal cavity were usually present. Antibiotics were not yet available. The patient was also treated by surgeons who were unschooled in the lessons of today's urban violence. Above all, Ogilvie[7] observed the disasters that occurred when these patients were cared for in understaffed and improvised units, and the deterioration that followed the transport of patients with freshly anastomosed colonic wounds over long distances on poor roads. The rapid establishment of a colostomy and early evacuation of the patient was shown to be much safer and more efficient from both clinical and military viewpoints. Fear of a leaking anastomosis and the resultant peritonitis became deeply ingrained in many combat surgeons. Continuing the practice of routine colostomy for colonic injuries in Korea and Vietnam produced further reductions in the mortality rate to 11-15%.[2]

By 1951, Woodhall and Ochsner[8] recognized that the enthusiasm for colostomy for all civilian colon and rectal injuries had gone too far. They noted that "the war time practice of exteriorization of colon wounds has been carried over into civilian practice too wholeheartedly for the patient's greatest good." They reported that at Charity Hospital in New Orleans, the use of colostomy for colon injuries had increased from 33% in 1941 to 80% by 1950. They also pointed out that since mortality and morbidity were considerably higher in patients whose injuries were managed by colostomy, a more selective approach, emphasizing primary suture in selected cases should be used. It was also pointed out that, with the use of antibiotics and modern supportive therapy, the more "radical" methods of treating major colon wounds would find greater applicability. Despite the pleas of Woodhall and Ochsner, and at least two subsequent papers[9-10] advocating primary suture, colostomy continued to be used in at least 50% of colon injuries treated at Charity Hospital.[1]

Unfortunately, the 1950s were interrupted by the Korean War, and the colostomy protocols of the campaigns which had ended just six years earlier were reinstituted. With this, a new generation of surgeons were again temporarily "immunized" against the concept of primary repair.

In 1957, Pontius et al[11] published the first of a series of papers from Baylor strongly advocating primary suture without colostomy for colon injuries. Although enthusiasm for primary suture of colon injury varied from time to time at Baylor, the most recent series of 914 patients published in 1986 strongly supported the use of primary suture in the majority of cases.[12] A similar conclusion was reached by Nance on his review of data from Charity Hospital.[2]

AXIOM Colon wounds due to high velocity missiles should be treated with a colostomy whereas most injuries due to stabs or low-velocity missiles can be closed primarily with safety.

In the 1960s, surgeons increasingly noted the differences between military and civilian colon injuries, and the safety of primary repair of most stab wounds and low velocity missile injuries;[1] however, increasing civilian use of guns, often of high velocity and causing extensive damage to multiple organs, reinforced the traditional tendency to treat most colon injuries with a colostomy. Consequently, conservative surgeons continued to promote the advantages of a defunctioning colostomy while ignoring its temporal, psychological, economic, and surgical disadvantages.

In the first randomized prospective study on the role of colostomy for colon injuries, Stone and Fabian[5] in 1979 concluded that, in properly selected patients, primary suture of colonic wounds was superior to colostomy. Their study, representing a milestone in the development of management protocols for colonic injury, nonetheless suffered from a number of defects, the most important of which was that almost 50% of patients were excluded from the study. Nevertheless, clinical research of this type, reinforced by improved training of residents in trauma centers, has led to increasing acceptance of primary repair as the appropriate treatment in most cases of colon injury. Stone and Fabian[17] also defined the contraindications to primary repair of colon injuries as: (a) shock with a preoperative blood pressure <80/60 mm Hg, (b) hemorrhage with intraperitoneal blood loss >1000 cc, (c) >2 intraabdominal organs injured, (d) significant peritoneal contamination by feces, (e) operation begun >8 hours after injury, (f) colonic wounds so destructive as to require resection, and (g) abdominal wall injury with major loss of substance requiring mesh replacement.

Nevertheless, firm prejudices against primary repair of colon injuries, especially those involving the left colon, continued. Left colon injuries are thought to be less likely to heal properly, partly because of the purported effects of increased collagenase in the descending colons of rabbits.[3] Thus, the concept of primary repair of left colon injuries remained, in the minds of many surgeons, outside the bounds of safe, surgical judgment.

AXIOM There is little or no difference between the healing capabilities of right and left colon wounds.

Continued studies in the 1980s extended the range of patients in whom primary repair of colon injuries came to be appropriate. Nehan and Lewis,[13] reporting on a series of patients from San Francisco General Hospital, concluded that a more aggressive employment of primary repair without colostomy was warranted. A similar conclusion was reached by Shannon and Moore from the Denver General Hospital.[14] George et al in 1989 reported on an unselected series of patients with colon injury, 93% of whom had a primary repair.[15] Although many trauma surgeons now believe a primary repair is applicable to the majority of colon injuries, until recently, some still considered colostomy appropriate in a significant number of colon injuries.[16] Nevertheless, it seems clear that the great majority of colonic injuries in hemodynamically stable patients can be repaired primarily by technically competent surgeons employing good clinical judgment.

An exteriorized primary repair, an alternative to colostomy or primary repair, has been advocated by Kirkpatrick and Rajpal.[17] This technique appears to represent an intermediate position between the two extremes. If the conditions are not quite ideal for a primary colon repair, the colon can still be repaired, but it is exteriorized on the anterior abdominal wall and is dropped back in the abdomen at 5-10 days if the repair heals well. If the repair breaks down, the exteriorized colon is converted to a colostomy.

AXIOM Although an extensive data base is now available to support the use of primary repair for most colon injuries, the temptation to perform primary repairs in unfavorable cases should be resisted.

MECHANISMS OF INJURY AND PATHOPHYSIOLOGY

Penetrating Trauma

About 90% of wounds of the colon and rectum in urban trauma centers are due to gunshots or stabs.[18] In the 12-year period 1980-1992, 2168 patients with gunshot, shotgun or stab wounds of abdominal organs were treated at Detroit Receiving Hospital. Of these, 620 (28.6%) involved the colon and 75 (3.5%) involved the rectum (Table 26–1).

Penetrating wounds of the colon can have a wide range of severity, from minute perforations to massive blowouts associated with close range shotgun blasts or high velocity missiles. Whenever the colon is injured, bowel content may leak from the lumen contaminating the peritoneum or retroperitoneal tissues. The concentration of bacteria in the large bowel averages 10^9-10^{12} organisms per gram of feces, making sepsis a frequent complication of severe colon injury. Anaerobes, particularly Bacteroides species, predominate in the colon, but large numbers of Clostridial species and anaerobic streptococci are also present. The gram-negative aerobes, such as E. coli, are also present, but in much lower concentrations of about 10^7-10^8 per gram. In the right colon, the stool is often liquid, permitting rapid contamination of the peritoneum, even from small perforations.

AXIOM Successful treatment of colonic injuries must include measures that restore the integrity of the bowel wall and control fecal spill.

TABLE 26-1 *Mortality Rates with Abdominal Injuries Seen in 12 Years at Detroit Receiving Hospital (1980-1992)*

	Type of Trauma			
Organ Injured	Blunt	GSW	Stabs	Total
Liver	56 (260) 35%	110 (499) 22%	19 (251) 8%	185 (251) 20%
Small Bowel	14 (58) 24%	75 (551) 14%	10 (450) 7%	85 (759) 13%
Colon	7 (42) 17%	69 (498) 14%	7 (122) 6%	83 (662) 13%
Diaphragm	7 (28) 25%	59 (273) 22%	10 (119) 8%	76 (420) 18%
Kidney	10 (145) 7%	40 (229) 17%	6 (45) 13%	56 (419) 13%
Spleen	26 (172) 15%	31 (131) 24%	4 (42) 10%	61 (345) 18%
Stomach	3 (6) 50%	53 (241) 22%	10 (93) 11%	66 (340) 19%
Abd. Vessels	16 (23) 70%	135 (257) 53%	17 (53) 32%	168 (333) 58%
Pancreas	2 (33) 6%	34 (140) 24%	11 (37) 30%	47 (210) 22%
Duodenum	3 (10) 30%	29 (124) 23%	7 (33) 21%	39 (167) 23%
Bladder	8 (44) 18%	5 (84) 6%	1 (6) 17%	14 (134) 10%
Gallbladder	3 (3) 100%	14 (59) 24%	1 (19) 5%	18 (81) 22%
Total	92 (573) 16%	192 (1358) 14%	40 (810) 5%	326 (2741) 12%

STAB WOUNDS

With stab wounds of the abdomen, the most common organs injured in order of frequency are the small bowel, liver, and colon, and colon injuries are found in approximately 5-10% of the patients explored.[1] Of 810 patients treated at Detroit Receiving Hospital over a 12-year period (1980-1992) for abdominal organ injuries caused by stab wounds, 122 (15.1%) had colon injuries (Table 26-1). The most frequent associated injuries in patients with stab wounds of the colon were the small bowel (39%), abdominal vessels (16%), and duodenum (13%) (Table 26-2). Only seven (6%) of the patients with stab wounds of the colon died, and of the 82 patients who did not have associated abdominal vascular injuries. only three (3.7%) died. These results are similar to those recently reported by Leppaniemi et al.[19]

Stab wounds usually produce clean incised wounds of the colon which are usually scaled as grade I or grade II injuries (Table 26-3). Injury is usually limited to the immediate area, spill is relatively minor, and primary repairs can be performed in almost all cases.

GUNSHOT WOUNDS

In patients with gunshot wounds of the abdomen, the incidence of colonic injury is 25%-30% in most series.[2] Of 1358 patients with abdominal organ or vessel injuries caused by gunshot or shotgun wounds, and treated at Detroit Receiving Hospital from 1980-1992, 498 (37%) had a colon injury. The most frequent associated injuries in these patients were small bowel (61%), liver (28%), and abdominal vessels (26%) (Table 26-2). Although the mortality rate for GSW of the colon was 14% (69/498), if the 118 patients with associated abdominal vessel injuries are excluded, the mortality rate was only 4.7% (18/380). Of the 38 patients who had only a colon injury, none died.

Of the 92 rectal injuries seen at DRH from 1980-1992, 71 (77%) were caused by GSW or SGW. The mortality rate was 7.0% (5/71) and if the 11 patients with associated abdominal vascular injuries are excluded, none of the remaining 60 patients died.

Gunshot wounds can produce extremely variable injuries. Small caliber, low-velocity gunshots produce injuries quite similar to those seen with stab wounds, and little or no debridement is required. Although high-velocity missile wounds are not frequent in civilian practice, if one occurs, the extent of the colon and tissue injury around the bullet tract can be very wide, and the amount of contamination may be great.

With any gunshot wound, efforts should be made to assure the viability of adjacent tissues before performing a primary repair, and debridement of the colon for 1 or 2 cm beyond the immediate area of injury may be necessary. Close-range shotgun injuries may destroy large amounts of the colon, and can also macerate and contaminate large quantities of adjacent tissues, greatly increasing the likelihood of myonecrosis and sepsis.

IMPALEMENTS AND IATROGENIC INJURIES

Impalements are a not-infrequent cause of rectal or colonic injuries. Thermometer perforations, enema injuries, and perforations during endoscopic procedures are well recognized. Injuries during rigid endoscopy usually occur when the tip of the instrument is pushed too forcefully against the bowel wall, especially when underlying disease is present. Deep biopsies or polypectomies, especially if the base is fulgurated, may also produce perforations, some of which may be delayed for several days.

In the past, endoscopic perforations were associated with a mortality rate as high as 50%,[2,18] and early recognition and prompt therapy are essential if one is to minimize the consequences of such accidents. Fortunately, the bowel has usually been cleansed prior to study. If operative repair is accomplished within 6 hours, virtually no complications should occur; however, if surgery is delayed for more than 24 hours, very high morbidity and mortality rates are apt to ensue.

Perforations caused by barium enemas are far more serious than purely instrumental perforations.[1] The combination of barium, blood, and feces can cause very severe infections. Subsequent granulomas and widespread dense adhesions with resulting intestinal obstruction often follow regardless of how much effort is made to wash out the

TABLE 26-2 *Associated Injuries and Mortality Rates with Colon Trauma*

	Type of Trauma				
Associated Injury	Blunt	GSW	SGW	Stab	Total
Small Bowel	2 (11) 18%	44 (279) 16%	4 (27) 15%	3 (48) 6%	53 (367) 14%
Liver	5 (15) 33%	26 (126) 21%	2 (12) 17%	0 (19) 0%	33 (173) 19%
Abd. Vessels	2 (4) 50%	51 (118) 43%	4 (10) 40%	4 (20) 20%	61 (152) 40%
Kidney	0 (5) 0%	17 (80) 21%	3 (14) 21%	3 (11) 27%	23 (110) 21%
Stomach	1 (2) 50%	12 (81) 15%	2 (13) 15%	0 (8) 0%	15 (104) 14%
Diaphragm	0 (5) 0%	8 (66) 12%	2 (6) 33%	1 (9) 11%	11 (86) 12%
Duodenum	2 (4) 50%	14 (55) 25%	1 (6) 17%	4 (16) 25%	21 (81) 26%
Pancreas	0 (6) 0%	10 (47) 21%	2 (8) 25%	3 (10) 30%	15 (74) 20%
Spleen	3 (8) 38%	8 (44) 18%	2 (8) 25%	0 (8) 0%	13 (69) 19%
Bladder	0 (10) 0%	2 (33) 6%	0 (4) 0%	1 (3) 33%	3 (50) 6%
Total	7 (43) 16%	62 (455) 14%	7 (43) 16%	7 (122) 6%	83 (661) 13%

TABLE 26-3 *Colon Organ Injury Scale*

Grade*		Injury Description+	AIS-90
I	Hematoma	Contusion or hematoma without devascularization	2
	Laceration	Partial thickness, no perforation	2
II	Laceration	Laceration <50% of circumference	3
III	Laceration	Laceration ≥50% of circumference without transection	3
IV	Laceration	Transection of the colon	4
V	Laceration	Transection of the colon with segmental tissue loss	4
	Vascular	Devascularized segment	4

* Advance one grade for multiple injuries to the same organ.
+ Based on the most accurate assessment at autopsy, laparotomy, or radiologic study.
From Moore EE, Cogbill TH, Malangoni MA, et al. Organ injury scaling II: pancreas, duodenum small bowel, colon, and rectum. J Trauma 1990;30:1427.

barium and feces at the time of surgery. Some of these injuries are caused by the large intrarectal balloon or the enema tip and may take the form of extensive lacerations, which are often extraperitoneal. It is highly questionable whether a barium enema that is performed gently can be held responsible for the perforation of a diverticulum, as is sometimes claimed.

AXIOM Immediate operation following perforation of the colon during a barium enema is essential to cleanse the peritoneal cavity and to prevent further contamination.

Perforation of the colon through a proximal colostomy by a carelessly employed catheter or enema tip is also an extremely dangerous event. Few victims survive, often because of delay in seeking surgical attention.

Blunt Trauma

Blunt trauma to the colon and rectum is unusual and causes only about 3-10% of the large bowel injuries treated in most centers.[20,21] Of 736 colon and rectal injuries seen from 1980 to 1992, only 51 (6.9%) were due to blunt trauma. Of the 51 patients with blunt injuries to the colon seen at DRH between 1980 and 1992, 34 (67%) were involved in automobile accidents either as pedestrians or passengers, while the remainder suffered falls or direct assaults.

A significant blunt force is required to produce a colonic injury; therefore, associated organ injury is noted in more than 90% of patients with blunt colonic injury. The liver and spleen are most frequently involved, and the mortality rates parallel the number and extent of the associated organ injuries. Injuries to the head, thorax and skeleton are also often present.

Non-penetrating trauma can cause colon injuries by three mechanisms: direct crushing, shearing forces, and burst injuries. Crush injuries to the colon occur most frequently and are usually due to a compression of the colon between the anterior abdominal wall and the lumbar spine. This may cause serosal tears, hematoma formation, or complete lacerations. Injuries of this nature occur most frequently in the transverse colon and must be suspected in patients sustaining significant blunt abdominal trauma, particularly if there is an anterior abdominal hematoma, rectus muscle injury, or spinal fractures.

Deceleration injuries of the colon involve shear stress at points of relative colonic fixation and mobility. Consequently, these injuries tend to occur at the splenic or hepatic flexures or in the distal sigmoid colon and may have associated mesenteric injuries due to the tearing forces.

Bursting injuries of the colon are similar to blunt duodenal and gastric injuries and involve a rapid increase in the intraluminal pressure, frequently against a competent ileocecal valve. Bursting injuries of the colon most commonly involve the cecum.

Overall, blunt colonic injuries most frequently involve the transverse colon followed by the right and left colon respectively. Transverse colonic injuries are most commonly serosal or mural hematomas; right and left colonic injuries are frequently full thickness.

The spectrum of injury varies widely. Serious injuries are almost equally divided between transections and perforations. Partial seromuscular tears, intramural hematomas, and contusions almost invariably heal spontaneously. A lurking threat is posed by an initially silent mesenteric tear. In this latter group, gradual ischemia of the associated colon wall may occur with development of subtle abdominal symptoms and an insidious peritonitis occurring some time between the fourth and eighth postinjury days when the now gangrenous bowel perforates.[22] In such cases, there may be little association between the severity of the injury and the subsequent degree of damage observed in the colon.

MOTOR VEHICLE AND SEAT BELT INJURIES
Although the small bowel and its mesentery are more frequently injured than the colon, the incidence of blunt colonic injury is increasing due in part to "seat belt injuries" and increased motor vehicle accidents. The presence of a "chance" (transverse) fracture through the body of a lumbar vertebra, especially in conjunction with a hematoma of the anterior abdominal wall, should serve as warning that the bowel may have been violently compressed between the two.

AXIOM Patients with "seat belt injuries" of the abdominal wall and vertebrae should be strongly suspected of having associated intestinal injuries.

The mechanism responsible for colon injuries in motor vehicle accidents is most often a shearing injury or increased intraluminal bursting tension, but in a few cases it seems to be a direct crush, especially when the patient is wearing a seat belt.[18] Seat belts, if not applied properly, can easily slip over the anterior superior iliac spines so that the full force of impact is transmitted to the viscera trapped between the seat belt and the spinal column. The resulting forces on the abdominal viscera may cause an acute perforation of the colon. Occasionally, a delayed leak can occur as a result of ischemia from either contusion, an extensive hematoma in the bowel wall or mesentery, or laceration or thrombosis of mesenteric vessels.

AXIOM Since contused and devitalized colon may extend beyond the area of obvious injury, primary repair of blunt colon injuries is risky.[18]

Large bowel injuries from blunt trauma usually occur in the ascending or descending colon, particularly if the injury is due to a misapplied seat belt.[2] Occasional patients develop hematomas of the colon wall that may perforate days or weeks after the injury. Consequently, hematomas over the colon should be evacuated so that one can be assured of an adequate blood supply to the underlying bowel wall.[2]

Several complications may arise from undiagnosed transmural colonic hematomas. While the vast majority of these hematomas resolve without complication, liquefaction will occasionally occur and result in a colocutaneous fistula and/or an intraabdominal abscess. Alternatively, colonic strictures may occur later due to localized ischemia or exuberant fibrosis. While the exact incidence of these complications is unknown, one should be aware of the possibility of such problems and look for them on follow-up examinations, especially if the patient has any symptoms.

AXIOM Even with evacuation of mesocolic hematomas, careful observation of the patient is essential for the early diagnosis of occult, but potentially lethal, delayed leaks.

Very occasionally, blunt trauma will cause the mesentery to be torn away from a segment of colon.[2] The resulting necrosis of the devascularized bowel may also cause a severe delayed peritonitis or abscess.

Perforation of the rectum by bone spicules from a fractured pelvis is an extremely hazardous complication because the hematoma associated with the fracture can make identification of the injury extremely difficult. In addition, the contaminated hematoma may cause severe sepsis and/or later osteomyelitis of the pelvis.

Severe implosion injuries at the anus are extremely rare but are thought to be related to a severe Valsalva maneuver at the time of the crush.[1] In this type of injury, the bowel tears at the anus and may be drawn up into the abdomen. This is most often seen when a pedestrian is run over by a car with a resultant tear of the pelvic sling.[23]

INSUFFLATION INJURIES

Insufflation injuries are often the result of a prank when an air pressure hose is pushed between the buttocks of the victim. Even though the end of the pressure hose may be several inches from the anus, very severe lacerations of the intraabdominal colon may result from the air pressure. It has been estimated that a pressure exceeding 4 lb/sq inch is needed to rupture bowel, and compressed air jets may generate up to 125 lb/sq in.[18] The laceration of the bowel usually occurs in the rectosigmoid area and may extend for 10 cm or more. Early operative treatment is essential.

AXIOM   Insufflation injuries of the colon can occur even without direct contact of the patient with the air hose.

ASSOCIATED INJURIES

One of the main factors influencing the outcome of colon and rectal injuries is the number and type of associated injuries. As pointed out earlier, the mortality rate of isolated colon and rectal injuries is extremely low. In the DRH series it was 1.6% (2/124). The most lethal associated injuries were those involving abdominal vessels with a mortality rate of 40.2% (66/164).

To establish the incidence of early postoperative infections after civilian injuries to the spleen, colon, or both and to assess the effect of splenectomy on outcome, Huizinga and Baker[24] studied 403 patients. Of these 353 had splenic injuries (91 with associated colonic injuries) and 50 were randomly selected patients with colonic injuries alone. Of these patients 45 had splenectomy and colonic injury (group 1), 46 had a colonic injury and the spleen conserved (group 2), 50 had colonic injury alone (group 3), 143 had splenectomy for injured spleen without colonic injury (group 4), and 119 had the spleen injured and conserved without colon injury (group 5). There were 68 (17%) deaths, more than half within 48 hours. Early mortality was highest in the groups in which the spleen was removed; however, after stratification by ISS and ATI, the differences were not significant. Late mortality (after 48 hours) associated with sepsis did not differ significantly between the groups, nor did the rate of infective complications. Thus, removal of an injured spleen did not have an adverse influence on the incidence of serious infectious complications in the early postoperative period in patients with colon injuries who also had a splenectomy.

DIAGNOSIS

Most colon injuries are diagnosed at laparotomy.[3] One of the biggest dangers in the present trend to treat hemodynamically stable adults with blunt trauma to the liver or spleen and hemoperitoneum non-operatively is the risk of missing an unsuspected colon injury.

AXIOM   Any abdominal injury from any direction can injure the colon.

Clinical Examination

Significant perforations of the colon or rectum may produce only modest symptoms until peritonitis or a pelvic cellulitis is present. Skin abrasions or tears of the rectus abdominous muscle which may be caused by a seat belt should be noted, especially because the underlying bowel lesions may have a prolonged and deceptive clinical course.[18] Most patients with bowel perforations, however, will eventually exhibit varying degrees of abdominal pain and tenderness.[1] The presence of peritoneal signs such as a guarding and rebound tenderness certainly aid in a decision to explore the patient. Shock may be present, but it is seldom caused by the colon lesion itself.

Bowel sounds may be present at the time of the initial evaluation following trauma, but they often disappear after a few hours if bowel perforation has occurred. There are many false-positive and false-negative correlations between the presence or absence of bowel sounds and the presence or absence of bowel injuries. Nance,[2] however, found that loss of bowel sounds is an ominous finding, and that it is frequently associated with bowel perforation or other serious abdominal injuries.

AXIOM   Loss of bowel sounds occasionally provides the earliest evidence of bowel injury after blunt trauma to the abdomen.

With penetrating wounds near the pelvis, the anal and gluteal regions should always be carefully inspected in a good light because small wounds may be hidden.[18] Even apparently minor penetrating wounds in this area may be associated with critical internal injuries.

PITFALL ⊘

Failure to examine the anal and gluteal areas closely may result in overlooking important penetrating injuries.

A rectal and pelvic examination should accompany the physical examination of all patients with blunt or lower abdominal penetrating injury. Gross blood found on the digital rectal exam strongly suggests a rectal or colonic injury, and an endoscopic evaluation should be performed preoperatively if the patient's clinical condition permits taking the time. Evaluation of sphincter tone should also be noted during the rectal examination.

AXIOM   Whenever possible, a proctosigmoidoscopic examination should be performed preoperatively in any patient suspected of having a rectal injury.

Occasionally, when a colon injury occurs during endoscopy, the patient immediately experiences acute abdominal or shoulder top pain, which is accentuated whenever air is insufflated into the colon.[18] In others, discomfort and subsequent peritonitis may not develop for a number of hours or even days. Early and persistent ileus may be an indicator of possible occult intraabdominal sepsis.[6]

In some patients with blunt trauma, symptoms and signs of serious intraabdominal injury may be delayed for a week or longer until ischemic bowel becomes necrotic and allows colonic contents to leak into the peritoneal cavity or retroperitoneal tissues.[18]

Intramural hematomas of the colon probably occur more often than has been recognized. Most of these probably regress spontaneously but, in a few cases, there may be either sudden rupture with intraperitoneal hemorrhage or chronic inflammatory changes leading to later colonic stenosis.[18]

Endoscopy

In stable patients with suspected rectal or colonic injury, anoscopy and/or cautious sigmoidoscopy may be of great value.[1] Some surgeons are reluctant to use enemas to clean out the feces before such endoscopy because of the potential risk of increasing contamination from rectal or low sigmoid injuries; however, a low careful Fleet's enema is not apt to cause much contamination and may greatly improve visibility. If positive findings are obtained, appropriate measures should be initiated promptly. A negative finding, i,e., the finding of an intact rectosigmoid mucosa and no blood, can greatly facilitate the decision-making process; however, occasionally, the endoscopy will miss a small tear, which may or may not heal spontaneously.

Radiological Examinations

PLAIN FILMS

Plain radiographs of the abdomen, with the entrance and exit wounds covered with opaque markers, may be very helpful in demonstrating the tract of a missile, the presence of free air, or associated fractures.[18] If no exit wound is visible, and the bullet is not seen, radiographs of the chest and limbs should also be obtained because missiles sometimes pursue very unpredictable courses or may even embolize in major vessels.

PITFALL ⊘

> *One should never assume that the path of a bullet is a straight line from its entrance to its exit wound or to its current position in the body.*

Loss of psoas shadows may suggest retroperitoneal injury, but this is not a reliable finding.[2] Abnormal air, either under the diaphragm (on an erect film) or in the flanks (on decubitus films), is usually a reliable sign of a perforated viscus, but it is seldom present with colon or rectal injuries. On the other hand, some free air may occasionally be present in the abdomen in the absence of bowel perforations because of the causative agent (especially large knives) or dissection of air from the chest because of injuries or excessive ventilatory pressures.[2] Since air is used to distend the colon lumen during colonoscopy, free intraperitoneal air is frequently present following endoscopic perforation of the colon. Demonstrating free air on radiographs is one of the most rapid ways to confirm the diagnosis in suspected cases.[2]

CONTRAST STUDIES

Cautious contrast roentgenographic studies are indicated in the evaluation of patients with a potential colonic injury, particularly when there is no other reason to explore the abdomen. Water-soluble contrast material should be used in most cases because free barium in tissues or the peritoneal cavity can greatly increase the tendency to severe infections and later fibrosis with scar contracture.

CT SCANS

Computed tomography (CT) can greatly assist in the selection of stable patients who can be treated non-operatively following abdominal trauma. Unfortunately, the diagnostic sensitivity of the CT scan for hollow viscus injuries is relatively poor, with a false-negative rate of up to 13%.

AXIOM The accuracy of CT scans in trauma is greatly influenced by the experience of the interpreter, and this must be factored into the decision making.

Triple-contrast CT examinations which include intravenous, gastric, and rectal (enema) instillation of water soluble contrast may greatly increase the likelihood of diagnosing a distal colonic injury; however, more proximal lesions may still escape diagnosis.

Recently, McAllister et al[25] reported on their prospective evaluation of the value of triple-contrast CT scans in the selective management of stab wounds to the back. Of 53 patients entered into the protocol, 31 had negative scans and 20 had scans showing injury, but not requiring exploration. In the two cases in which the triple-contrast CT was useful, it did not really alter the therapy, which was therapeutic celiotomy based on clinical findings anyway.

Peritoneal Lavage (DPL)

DPL has proved invaluable in the rapid evaluation of many patients with blunt abdominal trauma. Mesenteric or associated injuries may cause the lavage RBC count to exceed 100,000 cells/mm^3. Bacterial or fecal material on DPL allows the diagnosis of an intestinal injury to be made readily. The DPL WBC may not become elevated until 6-8 hours after injury. Consequently, if the DPL is performed soon after injury, one may wish to leave the catheter in place and repeat the procedure 4-6 hours later.

The precise value of diagnostic peritoneal lavage or CT scan of the abdomen in questionable patients is disputed. The criteria for a positive diagnostic peritoneal lavage in penetrating abdominal trauma ranges from 1,000-100,000 RBCs/mm^3 in various reports; using the lower figure results in a higher negative or non-therapeutic laparotomy rate whereas use of the higher number will cause an occasional significant injury to be missed. An RBC count of 10,000 /mm^3 for penetrating trauma is generally a reasonable compromise figure.

Although a DPL can be extremely helpful in detecting many intraperitoneal injuries, its value in colon trauma is somewhat controversial. Nance[2] feels that most patients with colonic injuries have sufficient physical findings to warrant early laparotomy without a lavage. Diagnosis of colonic injury by finding increased white cells, or even fecal fibers or bacteria, has been reported, but Nance[2] has never made the diagnosis of colonic injury on this basis alone. It should be noted that retroperitoneal colonic or rectal injuries are frequently associated with a false negative peritoneal lavage. In addition, it may take up to 6 hours for the peritoneum to react sufficiently to contamination by bowel contents to produce an increased WBC on DPL.

AXIOM A negative DPL does not reliably rule out gastrointestinal injuries, especially if the DPL is done soon after the trauma or if the injury is retroperitoneal.

Laparoscopy

The technique of laparoscopy is being used increasingly in trauma patients because it may allow early, organ-specific diagnosis following penetrating or blunt abdominal trauma. Furthermore, more advanced laparoscopic techniques may permit the repair of simple gastrointestinal and colonic injuries without laparotomy. Exquisite judgment needs to be exercised in these patients because complete laparoscopic visualization of the colon, especially its retroperitoneal portions, is not possible. Any suspicion of an injury in these areas mandates laparotomy. The ultimate role of laparoscopy in the management of patients sustaining abdominal trauma is still to be defined.

Laparotomy

The diagnosis of colonic injury, especially after blunt trauma, is often made during a laparotomy for associated organ injuries which have caused peritoneal signs or hypotension. Routine laparotomy is advocated for any gunshot wound that may have entered the abdominal cavity and for high velocity wounds coming close to the abdomen, so as not to overlook the blast effects of these missiles. In a series of patients with blunt colon injury seen at Detroit Receiving Hospital, concomitant injuries occurred in almost 90%.[13] The associated injuries included the spleen (26%), liver (23%), jejunum (17%), ileum (14%), blood vessels (11%), kidney (9%), and pancreas (9%). In addition, 46% of the patients with blunt colon trauma had major extremity fractures; 43% had head injuries; and 26% had associated chest trauma.

AXIOM Hemodynamically unstable patients with blunt abdominal trauma should undergo a prompt exploratory laparotomy, which generally uncovers any colon injuries that may be present.

Since colon injuries, per se, often produce little in the way of initial symptoms, patients who do not obviously need a prompt laparotomy are at much greater risk for late complications from an undiagnosed colonic wound.

AXIOM   The most reliable method for identification of colon injuries is exploratory laparotomy.

TREATMENT OF COLON INJURIES

Non-operative Management

IATROGENIC OR ACCIDENTAL INJURIES TO PREPARED COLON OR RECTUM

Partial-thickness colon injuries produced by endoscopy, enema tips, or thermometers can be cautiously observed.[2] In an extensive review of iatrogenic or accidental injuries in prepared bowel, Thomson et al[26] have noted that these patients generally do well by simply being kept NPO, given antibiotics, and carefully observed; however, the physician who elects this course of management bears a heavy responsibility for ensuring that the patient does not deteriorate or become septic. Some of these patients may not show any signs or symptoms for 2-3 days and then progress from minimal signs or symptoms to severe sepsis in 12-24 hours. If the perforation is caused by a biopsy or by fulguration of tissue, the lesion is best treated surgically as a stab wound.

STAB WOUNDS OF THE ABDOMEN

The treatment of knife wounds of the abdomen has undergone a transition from mandated laparotomy to selective observation in hemodynamically stable and alert patients. Any hemodynamically unstable patient without an extraabdominal cause, or one who has signs of peritoneal irritation, should undergo an emergency laparotomy. Clinically stable, alert, cooperative patients may safely be observed by the surgical team for development of any peritoneal signs.

PENETRATING WOUNDS OF THE FLANK OR BACK

Penetrating wounds to the flank or back may inflict occult injuries to the retroperitoneal right or left colon. Such injuries may initially seem to be innocuous due to the paucity of peritoneal findings.

AXIOM   As a general rule, stab wounds of the flank have a 15-25% incidence of causing an intraabdominal organ injury, whereas wounds in the back have a 5-10% incidence of such injuries.[2,3]

The lateral abdominal musculature affords little protection to the viscera, and the kidneys and colon are in relatively close approximation (2-3 cm) to the skin surface in non-obese individuals. Wounds in a more posterior location cause fewer problems because the spine and paraspinous muscles provide a thicker defense, and a wounding agent may have to penetrate 8 cm or more to cause significant organ damage. A selective approach to stab wounds of the back and flank may be safely adopted in cooperative patients. As with anterior stab wounds, development of any abdominal findings mandates laparotomy. During exploration for wounds of the back and flank, the retroperitoneal colon must be fully mobilized to allow careful examination in the region of the knife tract to exclude any posterior or intramesenteric injuries.

Indications for Operation

The usual indications for an exploratory laparotomy in patients with colon injuries include: (a) hemodynamic instability, (b) peritoneal signs or symptoms, (c) a high index of suspicion in blunt trauma, (d) patients with anterior penetrating wounds below the fifth intercostal space, and (e) patients with radiograph evidence of free air or bullets below the diaphragm.[6]

Patients with stable vital signs and abdominal stab wounds proven to penetrate into the peritoneal cavity can either have an immediate laparotomy, a DPL or simply careful observation for 24-48 hours for any evidence of peritonitis. If the DPL is positive because of the RBC count, one can still elect to observe the patient. If the DPL is positive for other criteria, the patient should be explored. With gunshot wounds of the abdomen, a laparotomy should be performed even if there is no evidence of organ injury.

AXIOM   Patients with gunshot wounds of the abdomen require routine laparotomy.

Preoperative Care

RESUSCITATION AND DIAGNOSTIC EFFECTS

Early operative therapy is required for the management of virtually all patients with evidence of a colon or rectal injury. The amount of time spent on insertion of large-bore intravenous lines, infusing fluid and blood, establishing an adequate urine output, and obtaining various diagnostic studies, all depend on the stability of the patient and the extent of the injuries.

AXIOM   ED resuscitation should be kept to a minimum in hemodynamically unstable patients with abdominal injuries. The bleeding needs to be controlled surgically as soon as possible.

Preoperative Antibiotics

Patients with suspected colon or rectal injuries should receive preoperative parenteral antibiotics to cover gram-negative aerobes (such as E. coli) and anaerobes (such as Bacteroides fragilis), so that adequate blood levels can be achieved by the time the laparotomy incision is made. Many surgeons use gentamicin or tobramycin plus clindamycin or metronidazole because most of the gut flora are covered by this combination. Addition of ampicillin to cover for possible enterococcus involvement is controversial and varies with each trauma center's experience. Some surgeons prefer single agents such as Cefoxitin, Timentin, Unasyn, Cefotetan, or Imipenem.

Most surgeons administer the antibiotics in the emergency room during the initial resuscitation. If there is much blood loss during the operation, the antibiotics should be administered again after the bleeding is controlled. If no hollow viscus injury is identified at operation, the antibiotics can be discontinued. If stomach or proximal small bowel is injured, one or two additional doses of the antibiotics can be given. If a colon perforation is identified, antibiotics are continued for 2-5 days according to the extent of the injury, the patient's host defenses, and the personal preferences of the surgeon. Appropriate monitoring of renal function and antibiotic levels should continue in the postoperative period as long as the antibiotics are administered.

Intraoperative Management

CONTROLLING BLEEDING AND CONTAMINATION

After appropriate wide preparation and draping from the chin to the knees, a standard midline incision is made and the abdomen is evaluated rapidly. If there is active bleeding, this must be controlled promptly. Once the bleeding has been controlled and hemodynamic stability established, a rapid examination of the bowel should be performed, looking for obvious intestinal perforations. Such injuries should be identified and controlled early with noncrushing clamps or running sutures to prevent further contamination. Nance[2] has found that a useful way to control spill is to grasp the edges of the open bowel with Allis forceps or Babcocks and applying a noncrushing clamp below them to close the defect. When an injury of such severity as will obviously require resection is found, proximal and distal occlusive clamping of the bowel with Kelly or Kocher clamps will help prevent further fecal contamination.[1]

SEARCHING FOR COLON INJURIES

If there are no associated injuries demanding immediate attention, all spilled material from the intestine should be removed at this time, followed by careful inspection of the entire abdomen, including the colon. If there is any suspicion or possibility of a retroperitoneal colon injury, it is mandatory that that portion of the colon be completely exposed by division of its lateral peritoneal attachments. Any hematoma, staining, or air in the retroperitoneum is an important indication of a possible retroperitoneal colonic injury.

AXIOM Retroperitoneal injuries of the large bowel are easily missed unless the colon is fully mobilized.

Care must be taken when evaluating the splenic flexure to avoid iatrogenic injury to the spleen. The vascular supply to the colon and its mesenteric attachments should also be examined. Generally the lesser sac should also be entered, and the entire length of the transverse colon should be examined carefully from all sides.

AXIOM Adhesions between the spleen and the splenic flexure of the colon should be carefully taken down before dissecting around these structures to perform a careful examination.

The examination of the colon should extend distally down to the peritoneal reflection; however, dissecting deeply into the pelvis to search for a rectal injury is generally not recommended and should only be performed after consideration of the possible risks and benefits. In the presence of a high rectal injury that has been previously seen on proctoscopy, it may be desirable to attempt a repair; however, extensively mobilizing the rectum can cause additional damage to the rectum, distal ureters, or other structures. If an injury to the lower rectum is suspected but not proven, endoscopy can be performed in the OR with the abdomen open. If that is not available, a proximal sigmoid loop colostomy may be the safest maneuver.

AXIOM Dissecting deep into the pelvis to look for possible rectal injuries may cause much more harm than good.

TEMPORARY LIGATION AND REPLACEMENT OF THE COLON (DAMAGE CONTROL)

In desperately ill patients with exsanguinating hemorrhage, coagulopathy, acidosis, and hypothermia, the colon can be stapled just proximal and distal to the injured areas. The colon can then be dropped back into the peritoneal cavity. The abdominal cavity is packed as needed for hemostatic control and then the incision can be closed very rapidly with multiple towel clips on the skin. Establishment of an end-colostomy at the initial operation would add relatively little time to the original operation and would have self-evident advantages; however, if one is attempting tamponade of intraabdominal bleeding, the colostomy opening would decrease the effectiveness of an otherwise watertight closure.

TREATING COLON INJURIES

After control of any bleeding sites and completion of the abdominal exploration, one can decide how to proceed further with the management of the colonic injuries. In general, the four options available for management of colon injuries include: (a) primary repair or right colectomy without a proximal colostomy or ileostomy, (b) primary repair with a proximal colostomy, (c) definitive colostomy at the area of injury, or (d) exteriorization of the repaired colon. The specific therapy chosen depends largely on the amount of damage to the colon, the patient's other injuries, and the hemodynamic stability of the patient.

The extensive literature on colon injuries provides a long list of factors that have been suggested as influencing the success or failure of primary colon repairs. The presence of shock, age of the patient, the extent of the colon injury, the number and types of associated injuries, the time interval from injury to surgery, and the degree of fecal contamination are mentioned most frequently. The anatomic,

physiologic, and bacteriologic differences between the right and left colon have been overemphasized as determinants of success of primary repair, and in fact, injuries of all segments of the colon can usually be managed primarily;[23] If a resection is performed, however, a colocolonic anastomosis, except in prepared bowel, is generally not recommended; small bowel-colonic anastomoses generally heal much better.

AXIOM The extent of the colon injury, the amount of contamination, the number and types of associated injuries, and the general condition of the patient are important factors in deciding on the most appropriate form of treatment.

Successful primary repair is possible in at least 60 percent of patients with colon injuries.[6] The majority of civilian colon injuries are caused by knives or low-velocity bullets that cause limited injuries, and most patients do not have severe associated injuries causing massive bleeding and persistent shock.

More difficult decisions occur when an extensive contusion is present or when there is bowel ischemia because of mesenteric trauma. In a previous Detroit Receiving Hospital study, all five patients who had right hemicolectomies because of extensive right colon or mesenteric injury with primary ileocolostomies did well;[1] however, other authors have reported occasional leaks with such a procedure. Special care must be taken with primary anastomoses in the presence of contusion. If there is any doubt regarding the blood supply of the involved bowel, resection and temporary colostomy or ileostomy are advisable.

Primary Repair

CONTRAINDICATIONS TO PRIMARY REPAIR. Primary repair of injured colon is the ideal goal, and rapid analysis of the many factors that militate against its success is vital to the treating surgeon. Ultimately, success depends on maintaining an adequate blood supply to the suture line, preventing local infection, and performing a technically correct anastomosis.

The ideal indications for a primary repair of a colon injury included: (a) a hemodynamically stable patient, (b) a wound involving less than a third of the circumference of the bowel, (c) no involvement of the mesentery of the bowel, (d) a good blood supply, (e) an injury less than 6-8 hours old, and (f) little or no contamination. In addition, the primary repair should not prolong the intraoperative management of patients with severe and/or multiple associated injuries.

Shock. Preoperative shock with a systolic BP of less than 80 mm Hg has been listed as a contraindication to primary repair of colon injuries.[5] The reduced blood flow associated with hypotension, if sustained, certainly may interfere with healing of the anastomosis. Any consideration of hypotension must, however, take into account its duration as well as its depth and the rapidity with which tissue perfusion is restored at the time of operation. In patients who are rapidly resuscitated to a normal BP and normal or supernormal cardiac output, the initial hypotension is not an absolute contraindication to primary repair.

AXIOM Transient hypotension is not a contraindication to primary repair of colon injuries.

Age. Advanced age is a factor in the outcome of most types of trauma. While this is intuitively understandable, old age should be defined by physiologic not chronological criteria. Nelkin and Lewis,[27] for example, found no correlation between age and the outcome after colon injury.

Thus, while aging tends to diminish the reserves of the cardiopulmonary, renal and other systems, these reductions, in the absence of significant established clinical deficits, are not likely to affect the outcome of a primary anastomosis. Nevertheless, in practice, we would prefer to perform a single operation, rather than staged multiple procedures, on older patients.

AXIOM   All things considered, older patients tend to do better with a single operation than with two or three separate procedures of similar cumulative duration.

Fecal Contamination.   The degree of fecal contamination tends to parallel the severity of the colon injury. This in turn is usually related to the destructive qualities of the causative agent, the number of associated injuries, and the amount of blood lost. There is uniform agreement that minor contamination has little effect on outcome, but continuing contamination may be associated with severe complications, including death. Patients with much fecal spillage, especially when cleansing of the peritoneal cavity is delayed beyond 6-8 hours, are certainly at an increased risk of septic complications. The influence of this factor on outcome has been examined by Nelkin and Lewis,[27] Burch et al,[12,28] Flint et al,[29] Atkins et al,[30] and George et al,[31] but no consensus has emerged. The important question is to what extent, if any, the initial surgical procedure selected can be correlated with the morbidity and mortality which is inevitable in severely injured patients.

Nance[2] has emphasized that there are no objective data to indict primary closure as producing greater morbidity than a colostomy with civilian injuries. As a result, a number of experienced surgeons contend that primary anastomoses in the face of gross contamination may not be associated with any higher mortality or morbidity; however, Nelin and Lewis disagree.[27]

Although there has been a shift in the management of penetrating injuries of the colon to primary repair without a protective diverting colostomy, relatively few patients with blunt trauma have been studied. In a retrospective review of 54,361 major blunt trauma patients admitted to nine regional trauma centers from January 1, 1986, through December 31, 1990, Ross et al[32] noted that only 286 (0.5%) of the patients suffered colonic injury; however, of patients undergoing laparotomy following blunt trauma, injury to the colon was found in more than 10%. Primary repair of full-thickness injuries or resection and anastomosis was generally performed without diversion. They also noted that gross fecal contamination was the strongest contraindication to primary repair. Delay of surgery, shock, and the timing of antibiotic administration were not associated with a significantly increased morbidity.

To a large extent, the condemnation of primary repair in the past seems to have been largely one of guilt by association. Nevertheless, the safety of primary repairs in marginal situations needs further testing, and until the validity of such an approach is definitively established, caution is still advisable.

AXIOM   Although the great majority of civilian colon injuries can be safely treated with a primary anastomosis, in the presence of severe contamination or overt peritonitis, a colostomy is probably the wisest choice.

Extent and Site of the Injury.   The extent of the colon or rectal injury is an important factor in determining whether to perform a primary repair or colostomy. Burch et al[28] defined "extensive" colonic injury as the tearing of more than 50% of the bowel circumference or the presence of overt ischemia; all other injury was defined as "routine." In their series, 252 of 1004 patients had "extensive" injuries and 752 did not. In the years 1985-89, primary repairs of "routine" injuries were performed in 98% for the right colon, 94% for the transverse colon, and 89% for the left colon. In contrast, primary repairs of "extensive" lesions were performed in 71% of the injuries of the right colon, but in only 12% of the transverse colon injuries and only 2% of the left colon injuries. The dramatic differences in these figures reflect the ease and perceived safety of right hemicolectomy as opposed to a left hemicolectomy.

Although the concept that the left colon heals less readily than the right colon is now seriously questioned by many, caution still prevails. Between 1980 and 1988 at Detroit Receiving Hospital, surgeons performed primary repair on 43 of 73 (59%) of the lesions of the right colon and only 23 of 88 (26%) of the lesions on the left colon.[3]

Moore et al,[33] and Nelkin and Lewis,[27] have found the penetrating abdominal trauma index (PATI) to be useful in predicting when a primary closure can be performed safely for colon injuries. The PATI was also found to be helpful in predicting costs and the incidence of complications.

The treatment of retroperitoneal colonic injuries is similar to that of wounds in other locations. If an injury to retroperitoneal colon is diagnosed late, the increased chance of subsequent sepsis mandates colostomy for maximal safety. There is also some feeling that closures of retroperitoneal bowel (which does not have a peritoneal covering) are more apt to leak.

It is generally accepted that most stab wounds of the colon can be repaired primarily whereas shotgun wounds or high velocity missile wounds are much more apt to cause extensive colon injuries. Lappaniemi et al[19] have confirmed that most stab wounds of the colon produce minor injuries that can be managed safely with early primary repair.

In a review he conducted at Charity Hospital in New Orleans, Nance[2] found that there were no absolute contra-indications to primary repair of colon injuries. In a series of 399 cases, 41 patients with left colon injuries presented in shock. The patients treated by a primary colon repair fared better than those managed with colostomy. Thompson et al[23] reported similar findings. Nance[2] also found that delay in surgery did not seem to affect suitability for primary suture unless peritonitis was well established at the time of surgery. Even when patients with three or more organ injuries were considered, patients managed with a primary repair did better than those who had a colostomy.

AXIOM   As a general rule, small bowel-colonic anastomoses heal better than colocolonic anastomoses on unprepared bowel.

A fundamental unresolved issue in colonic injury currently revolves around the role of a primary unprotected anastomosis following resection of a portion of the left colon. Even the trauma centers with the largest experience remain hesitant to perform primary L. colon-colonic anastomoses. Data on this decision are difficult to find, but when extractable, suggest that anastomotic complications following resection of the left colon have a significantly higher complication rate. Although Burch et al[28] had only 13 fecal fistulas in 592 primary repairs (2.2%), the incidence of fistulas with colocolostomy (3/14=21.4%) was 12 times higher than in the other 578 primary repairs.

AXIOM   In critically injured patients with persistent hypotension, primary repair of colon injuries is probably safer than a colostomy if it can be performed more rapidly.

Although no one specific type of associated injury is a contraindication to primary repair, in a severely traumatized patient a shorter operating time may be lifesaving. Consequently, if a primary repair can be performed more rapidly than a colostomy, that is what should be done.[6] For example, in some very obese patients with a short colon mesentery, performing a colostomy may be very difficult and much more time-consuming than a stapled repair or anastomosis.

With increasing confidence in primary colon repairs, the technique is now being used increasingly in war injuries where colostomy used to be considered mandatory. Moreels et al,[34] for example, in a series of 102 patients with penetrating intraperitoneal colon injuries during war surgery in Cambodia noted that the overall case fatality rate (CFR) was 26%. The primary repair CFR was 20% compared to 31% in the colostomy group, but the difference was not statistically significant (P=0.30). Adjustment for possible confounding factors in the two groups did not alter the results. Moreels et al[34] felt that considering the numerous advantages to the patient of a primary closure in the precarious situations where war surgery is often performed, this technique merits consideration.

It is clear that most of the factors determining the safety of primary closure of colon injuries are interrelated and difficult to disentangle from the literature with precision. In the last analysis, the surgeon's decision is driven by his or her clinical experience. This takes all of these factors into account and provides relative weights for each of them as they apply to a specific patient in the operating room.

TECHNIQUES OF PRIMARY REPAIR

Standard Techniques. Clean stab wounds and low velocity gunshots should have their edges debrided of any devitalized tissue as needed to assure a good blood supply to the repair. The anastomosis or repair should be tension-free. An inner row of running or interrupted 3/0 slowly absorbable sutures incorporating all layers of the bowel and providing hemostasis and an outer layer of inverting (Lembert) 3/0 or 4/0 interrupted silk sutures is used by most surgeons; however, a single layer of interrupted sutures can provide equally good results. A transverse orientation for the closure should be attempted whenever possible in order to reduce the tendency for the repair to narrow the lumen (Fig. 26–1). Many surgeons find it useful to connect through-and-through punctures and close the resulting single wound in two layers. Any readily available omentum may then be used to buttress the suture line.[2]

Stapling. In recent years, stapling devices have been used increasingly for expeditious closure of colonic injuries. The edges of the wound are brought together by three or more carefully placed Allis forceps, and a 30-, 55-, or 60-mm linear stapler is then placed beneath the Allis forceps, closed, and fired.[1] Excess tissue is trimmed with a knife. The closure is then carefully inspected for defects. Reinforcement of the staple line is seldom necessary. Occasionally, serosal defects without mucosal perforation are encountered. These can be most easily managed by superficially placed Lembert sutures.

Intraoperative Evacuation of Feces from the Colon. The presence of a substantial amount of feces in the bowel has been postulated as a mechanical cause of anastomotic disruptions. It is also suggested that intraluminal feces increases the likelihood of migration of organisms into the peritoneal cavity, which can then serve as a source of sepsis. Intraoperative irrigation to cleanse the bowel lumen to permit primary anastomosis in elective surgery has been advocated in the United Kingdom for some time.[35] This technique usually consists of insertion of a large tube into the distal end of the colon to be

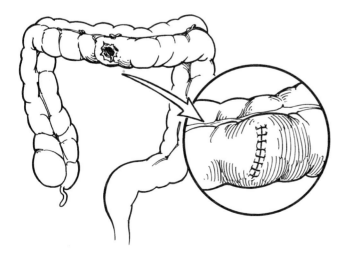

FIGURE 26–1 Repair of a simple perforation of the transverse colon. The repair has a transverse orientation to minimize narrowing of the lumen. From Nance FC. Injuries to the colon and rectum. In Trauma, 2nd ed. Moore EE, Mattox KL, Feliciano DV, eds.. Baltimore: Appleton-Lange, 1991; 525.

resected. The tube is connected to a sterile collection bag alongside the operating table. A large Foley catheter is inserted through the ileum about 5 cm proximal to the ileocecal valve. The end of the catheter is passed into the cecum where the balloon is inflated and drawn up against the ileocecal valve. Warm saline is then used to irrigate the colon in a prograde fashion. Solid feces is moved along by sequential manual manipulation as needed. This method was subsequently applied selectively to recently injured patients in Beirut and was thought to increase the feasibility and success of primary anastomosis.[35]

AXIOM Irrigation of feces from injured colon may increase the likelihood of a primary repair healing successfully.

Baker[36] has used an alternative method of removing feces from the colon by flushing it out in a prograde manner after the anastomosis has been completed. In a prospective randomized study of 172 patients, 91 had prograde colonic irrigation after a primary anastomosis; however, it did not reduce mortality or morbidity.[36]

Intracolonic Bypass Tube (ICBT). Recently, use of an intracolonic bypass tube (coloshield™) was extended from elective surgery to the definitive treatment of nine patients with colonic perforations which ordinarily would have been treated with a defunctioning colostomy.[37] Of the nine injuries, at least four had severe concomitant intraabdominal injuries, and all had gross contamination. No repair leaked, and the intracolonic bypass tube passed spontaneously in about 2 weeks.

Considerable resistance to the concept of intracolonic anastomotic stents exists, and no prospective randomized study has been done as yet. Until more experience has been gained, the use of the ICBT in trauma must be regarded as investigative.

Use of Fibrin Sealant. A number of methods to improve the safety of colonic anastomoses have been explored over the past century. The search for an effective glue to reinforce suture lines has not been completely successful as yet. Although fibrin sealant is readily available and biologically compatible, the results of animal experiments have not been promising.[38] Our own use of fibrin glue made from cryoprecipitate, however, seems to be successful.

RESECTION AND PRIMARY ANASTOMOSIS. Resection of injured colon and primary anastomosis is best used to manage extensive wounds of the right colon. A right colectomy with ileocolostomy can usually be performed rapidly with a very low leak rate in the majority of patients. A technique popularized by Ravitch and Steichen utilizing a GIA or Cutter staple can also be used to rapidly provide a so-called functional end-to-end anastomosis[2] (Fig. 26–2).

Although it is generally agreed that war injuries to the colon cause much more bowel damage and contamination then civilian injuries, Khayet[39] recently reported on 50 cases of war injury of the right colon. Complications included four infected wounds (8%), two patients with cellulitis of the abdominal wall (4%), and one patient (1%) with respiratory failure, bleeding stress ulcers, and an intraperitoneal abscess. Five patients (10%) died, but only two deaths were of causes related to their colonic injury. Although the author felt that this experience proves that right hemicolectomy with primary end-to-end anastomosis and perioperative antibiotic peritoneal lavage is a safe one-stage method for managing missile injuries of the right colon with peritoneal fecal soiling, diverting ileostomy might have prevented some of these complications.

Colostomy

GENERAL CONSIDERATIONS. With increased confidence in the safety of primary repair of colon injuries, colostomies are now established in less than 30% of patients with trauma to the large bowel.[4,40] With rectal injuries, however, colostomies continue to play a major role because primary repair is seldom feasible.

Colostomy is generally indicated: (a) with rectal injuries, (b) when a resection of the left colon is needed for an extensive injury,

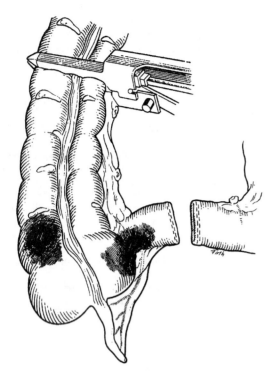

FIGURE 26–2 Resection and primary anastomosis without proximal diversion is usually performed for injuries of the right and transverse colon which are too extensive to close primarily. From Berne TV. Gastrointestinal tract. In Donovan AJ, ed. Trauma Surgery. St. Louis: Mosby, 1994; 100.

(c) where uncertainty exists about the quality of the colonic repair, (d) when an exteriorized repair breaks down or cannot be returned to the abdomen, or (e) in the presence of established peritonitis.

AXIOM Performing a colostomy is not always the safest way to manage a colon injury.

The use of colostomy for treating colon injuries has a number of potential drawbacks.[41] Among the obvious disadvantages are its aesthetic unpleasantness, the difficulty that many patients have in caring for it, associated complications, prolonged hospitalization, the need for readmission and another anesthetic for colostomy closure, the morbidity associated with both the establishment of the colostomy and the subsequent closure, the economic loss to the patient for time away from work, the prolonged convalescence, the cost to society of the hospitalizations, and the loss of productivity.

It is increasingly recognized that patients who have colostomies have an appreciably higher intraperitoneal and abdominal wound infection rate than do patients who have primary closure. For example, in a study reported by Nelkin and Lewis[27] the outcome of 37 patients treated with primary closure was compared with those of 39 similar patients on whom colostomies were performed. The injury severity score, penetrating abdominal trauma index, colon score, age, sex, degree of injury, shock, and delay between injury and operation were comparable. While major morbidity was much less in the primary closure group (11% versus 49%), the study was not randomized, and it is difficult not to suspect that patients were selected for the colostomy group because of disadvantageous clinical features at the time of laparotomy. Nevertheless, observations such as these suggest a critical need for careful review of the indications for colostomy in each individual case.

Until the early 1980s, colostomy was associated with a morbidity ranging up to 30% and an occasional mortality.[40] Results are much improved today in the hands of experienced surgeons. For example, Schultz et al,[42] reported on 100 consecutive patients with penetrating colon injuries which were repaired primarily in 57 (17 had a resec-

tion and anastomosis) and with a colostomy in 43. They noted that only two patients had severe colon-related morbidity. It appeared to the authors that the disadvantages of colostomy have been exaggerated somewhat, and this procedure should be regarded as one with a low morbidity provided that it is performed properly.

INDICATIONS FOR COLOSTOMY

After a Primary Repair. Primary colocolonic anastomoses after resections of left colon are generally considered to be more likely to leak than ileocolonic anastomoses. In ideal circumstances with minimal spill, left colon anastomoses can be performed, but in patients with extensive wounds, primary left colon anastomoses on unprepared bowel should probably be protected by a proximal colostomy. Although some surgeons believe that a right or left transverse colostomy is suitable for "protecting" a tenuous left colon repair, others say that a "protective" colostomy does not help a primary colonic anastomosis heal. However, diversion of the fecal steam does help seem to reduce the consequences of an anastomotic leak.[33]

After a Colon Resection. As a rule, when the conditions for a primary repair of a left colon injury do not seem optimal, it is considered safer to exteriorize the proximal bowel as an end colostomy. The distal bowel can then be brought out as a mucous fistula or it can be closed and returned to the abdominal cavity as a Hartmann's pouch.[3] Although colostomy has traditionally been employed to minimize septic complications, most series report a higher incidence of intraabdominal sepsis if a colostomy is performed.[1] This observation has also been noted by Moore,[14,23] Burch,[12] and Stone and Fabian.[5]

If a proximal colostomy is performed, one should avoid bringing it out through the midline wound.[1] A small transverse incision through the lateral border of the left or right rectus muscle is preferable.

Although an ileocolic anastomosis after a right colectomy is usually extremely safe, if there has been massive contamination or there is already established sepsis, a proximal ileostomy and end-colonic fistula is probably safer.

Colostomy as a Definitive Procedure. In patients with multiple severe injuries and/or prolonged hypotension, the injured segment of the colon can simply be exteriorized and the involved area can be resected outside the abdomen and stapled or clamped, and a definitive colostomy performed later. Even fixed portions of the colon can usually be mobilized for such a procedure fairly quickly.

TECHNICAL CONSIDERATIONS. Colostomies come in many forms. With the so-called Hartmann procedure, the proximal bowel is brought out as an end-colostomy and the distal bowel is closed after the involved segment of bowel has been resected. To reduce the difficulties with later re-anastomosis in the pelvis, one should leave as much sigmoid colon or rectum as possible, and the area of closure should be marked with a long Prolene suture so that it can be easily identified at the time of re-anastomosis. Insertion of a large rectal tube or a colonoscope through the anus before or during the laparotomy can also facilitate finding the end of the Hartmann's pouch.

To be sure that a colostomy is completely diverting, some surgeons favor a double-barrel colostomy with the two ends of colon separated (Fig. 26–3). The ideal distance between the two limbs has not been established, but placement of the two limbs within a few centimeters of each other can facilitate subsequent colostomy closure.

AXIOM Closure of a loop colostomy is often much safer and easier than a colostomy with a Hartmann's pouch, especially if there has been any intraperitoneal infection.

Sherman and Rehm[6] believe that the only colostomy that can reliably achieve complete diversion of colonic contents is an end colostomy. In emergency situations, the proximal involved colon can be brought out through a separate single colostomy incision and not "matured"; the distal colon can then be stapled off and left in the

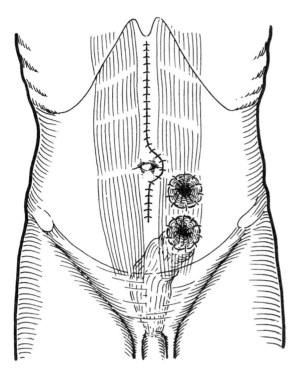

FIGURE 26–3 Colon injury managed by divided stoma double-barreled colostomy. Complete fecal diversion is assured, and the single-barreled colostomy is far easier for the patient to manage; however, later closure of the colostomy is more difficult. (From Ochsner MG Jr, Harviel JD, Champion HR. Diversion of the faecal stream. In Champion HR, Robbs JV, Trunkey DD, eds. Rob & Smith's operative surgery: trauma surgery; part I. 4th ed. Boston: Butterworths, 1989; 445).

abdomen. This leaves the patient with a colostomy with a single stoma, which is easier to manage than a loop. It has, however, the disadvantage of being much more difficult to close later. It may also be much more difficult to cleanse the distal colon mechanically.

It is sometimes convenient to close each exteriorized limb of colon with a DeMartel clamp or a line of staples. Opening or maturation of the proximal colostomy can then be deferred until the first or second postoperative day. Maturing a colostomy in an emergency situation may not be wise because postoperative abdominal distention can cause retraction of the stoma into the abdominal wall or peritoneal cavity.

A loop colostomy, while popular, has the disadvantage of being relatively bulky and more difficult for the patient to manage postoperatively (Fig. 26–4). Its advantage relates to the fact that when the colostomy is closed, only the anterior wall needs to be resutured and the loop can be gently replaced in the peritoneal cavity. Loop colostomy, with the distal limb closed by staples or sutures in order to remove the disadvantage of potential distal spillage, is advocated by some. In this case, resection of the colostomy with formal anastomosis of the two lumens is necessary. Cecostomy with a tube placed in the cecum in an attempt to keep it decompressed usually works poorly and is seldom of any help in "protecting" an anastomosis.

Exteriorized Primary Repair

An alternative to protecting a primary repair of injured colon with a proximal colostomy is a primary repair with exteriorization of the sutured segment of colon. This technique, in essence, seeks a middle ground between a colostomy and a primary repair.[2] To get optimal results with this procedure, the injured colon must be mobilized sufficiently to permit it to be brought out through the anterior abdominal wall with no tension.[43] The formal repair is then performed and the repaired bowel is kept exteriorized over a tongue of fascia.

The exteriorized colon is kept moist by saline-soaked gauzes or it may be covered by a colostomy bag. The exteriorized colon should be examined daily. If a leak occurs, the loop is converted to a colostomy with little risk of peritonitis. Otherwise, the patient is reoperated after 7-10 days and the repaired segment is dropped back into the abdomen.

Exteriorization of primary colon repairs was practiced briefly in World War II. Enthusiasm was rekindled in the 1970s when Kirkpatrick,[43] Lou et al,[44] and Robbs[45] were keen protagonists. The technique of performing exteriorized primary repairs is important, and Kirkpatrick and Rajpal[17] emphasized the need to avoid venous strangulation of the exteriorized segment. Care must also must be taken to prevent kinking of the bowel when, after successful healing, the bowel is put back into the abdomen.

Okies et al[46] in 1972 reported that they used this technique successfully (i.e., returned a healed colon repair to the abdomen) in 18 (49%) of 37 patients. In contrast, Schrock et al[47] reported a success rate of only 21%. In a prospective randomized study which included 29 cases in which the repaired colon was exteriorized for 10 days prior to return to the peritoneal cavity, Kirkpatrick and Rajpal in 1973[48] successfully avoided a colostomy in 55% of their cases; however, the length of hospitalization was not significantly reduced, due largely to delays in the healing of associated injuries. Mulherin and Sawyers[49] in 1975 expressed enthusiasm for exteriorized primary colon repairs, but a number of surgeons have had a large number of disruptions of the repair as well as obstruction of the colon at the site of the fascial closure.[2,47,50] Many surgeons feel that a colonic suture line inside the abdomen is surrounded and protected by omentum and loops of bowel and is far less likely to leak than when it is placed under dressings on the abdominal wall.

In a report by Ivatury et al[51], 252 patients with penetrating colon injuries were placed in a prospective protocol. Of 34 patients who had an exteriorized repair, largely because of delayed treatment, eight (23%) had a suture-link breakdown but the other 77% avoided a colostomy.

Thus, the success rate for an exteriorized primary repair varies between 20% and 77%, but a definite learning curve exists. Indeed, support for exteriorization dwindled in the 1980s, even among its previous enthusiasts, because of an increased tendency to perform primary anastomoses and leave them within the abdomen. This is demonstrated in Burch's series of 751 patients with "routine" colon injuries in whom exteriorization was performed in 72 of 465 patients between 1980 and 1984, but in only two of 286 patients between 1985 and 1989.[28]

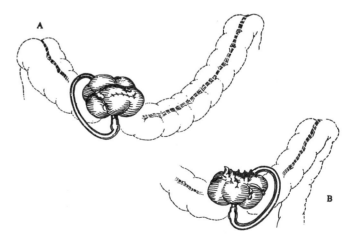

FIGURE 26–4 Exteriorized primary repair. It is important to have a bridge of fascia 5-7 cm wide supporting the exteriorized colon. At 5 days, if the repair is intact, the exteriorized colon anastamosis is dropped back into the abdomen. (From Shrock TR. Trauma to the colon and rectum. In Blaisdell FW, Trunkey DD, eds. Trauma management, vol. 1: abdominal trauma. 2nd ed. New York: Thieme-Stratton, 1982; 176).

The immediate appeal of exteriorization is easy to understand; if the repair heals, it can be dropped back into the peritoneal cavity in 7-10 days, and in the patients in whom it does not heal, a colostomy can be established easily at the bedside. Exteriorization is basically an exercise in caution when uncertainty exists about the future healing of a colonic anastomosis. Apart from this perceived advantage of guarding against an intraperitoneal leak, exteriorization in the 30-70% in whom the technique is successful obviates the need for a colostomy, often shortens the hospital stay, saves money, reduces discomfort, and permits an earlier return to work.

AXIOM   If a primary colon repair seems somewhat hazardous, one can still perform an exteriorized repair with relative safety.

Unfortunately, exteriorized primary repairs can have a number of problems. Because only mobile segments of the bowel lend themselves to this technique, attempts to exteriorize the right or left colon are often fraught with difficulty and are often associated with bulky and unsightly exteriorized bowel. Furthermore, if obstruction of the colon is to be avoided, there should be a gradual curve of the exteriorized segment of bowel over a 4-5 cm fascial bridge to avoid kinking and consequent high intraluminal pressures.[17] Local care of the exposed bowel includes regular moistening with saline, plus the application of petroleum gauze. A self-adhesive colostomy bag covering the exposed bowel helps preserve humidity.

In spite of these precautions, the exteriorized bowel often develops increasing edema and serositis with time. In fact, replacement of successfully healed bowel into the peritoneal cavity can be difficult if it is exteriorized for more than 7-10 days.

AXIOM   Because primary repair of colon injuries is feasible and will heal well in the great majority of patients, there seems to be little place for exteriorized primary anastomosis today.

Adjuvant Measures

DRAINS
Drains are now seldom employed in the management of intraperitoneal colonic wounds. Drains placed close to colonic suture lines are thought to lead to an increased number of anastomotic leaks.[6] Drains placed elsewhere in the abdominal cavity because of fecal contamination do not prevent infections and are not indicated.

AXIOM   Intraperitoneal drains are seldom indicated in patients with colonic injuries.

PERITONEAL LAVAGE
If extensive fecal soiling is encountered, copious saline lavage serves to remove or at least dilute the fecal matter and bacteria.[2] Bacterial contamination per se is handled fairly well by the peritoneal cavity, whereas gross fecal matter is a powerful adjuvant for bacteria to cause peritonitis and abscesses.

Some surgeons have worried that the irrigation may spread the contamination throughout the peritoneal cavity. Others have expressed concern that the saline lavage may impair normal peritoneal protective mechanisms. It is our impression, however, that the advantages gained by removal or dilution of the contamination far outweigh the disadvantages. The saline, however, should be warmed, and at least 6-8 liters are needed if there has been gross spill of feces.[1] The fluid should then be removed as completely as possible.

INTRAPERITONEAL ANTIBIOTICS
For many years, Nance[2] and others have employed a 1% kanamycin solution or a solution of 80 mg of tobramycin in 100 ml of saline to irrigate the peritoneal cavity after completion of a copious saline lavage. We have used a variety of antibiotic irrigants but currently use a liter of Neosporin irrigant. Most of the antibiotic irrigant is then aspirated, but some may be left behind. About 50 ml of the antibiotic solution is saved for lavage of the fascia and subcutaneous tissue just before closure.

Intraperitoneal anitbiotic irrigation was pioneered by Isidore Cohn Jr, and was shown by Noon et al[52] in a prospective randomized study to be effective in reducing the incidence of intraperitoneal infections following trauma. Other surgeons, however, feel that the efficacy of the antibiotic irrigant is doubtful when compared to the protective effect of adequate blood levels of appropriate antibiotics.[6]

NUTRITIONAL SUPPORT
Early and aggressive maintenance of nutrition is critical to survival of these potentially septic patients. A jejunostomy catheter for beginning early enteral feeding can be especially important.[53]

Wound Closure

The fascia of the midline incision may be closed in a wide variety of ways, but we tend to prefer interrupted, number 1 coated polyglycolic braided sutures or nonabsorbable monofilament sutures.[1] Retention sutures are seldom used unless extensive damage to the anterior abdominal wall has occurred.[2]

When there has been gross contamination of the peritoneal cavity, most surgeons feel that although the fascia can be closed, the skin and subcutaneous tissue should be left open. They can be closed by secondary suture or steri-strips between the fourth and seventh postoperative days if the wound appears to be healing well. Primary skin closure will probably be successful only if there is minimal contamination and adequate hemostasis has been achieved. If the skin and subcutaneous tissue are to be primarily closed, they should also be thoroughly irrigated prior to suturing.

Although most surgeons are rather selective about primary closure of skin in patients with colon injuries, Nance[2] and others close almost all their incisions primarily unless direct fecal contamination of the subcutaneous tissues has occurred. Nance[2] is, however, careful to close the skin with as few staples as needed to accomplish apposition. A colostomy or exteriorized repair is not a contraindication for primary wound closure, but they should be separated from the incision by an occlusive dressing or a well-fitting appliance.[3]

RECTAL INJURIES

Incidence and Significance

In civilian practice, rectal injuries represent only 3-5% of the total injuries to the colon[1]; however, because of its extraperitoneal location, injuries of the rectum are considered by many to be the most serious of all intestinal injuries.[52-54] In addition, the rectum is surrounded by poorly vascularized fatty tissue without fixed anatomic boundaries so that a perirectal infection can spread rapidly throughout the retroperitoneal pelvis and abdomen.

Impalements of the rectum by foreign objects are often the result of falls,[1] but a wide variety of foreign bodies have been inserted into the anus by the patient, friends, or assailants. These foreign bodies may produce very severe wounds of the anus and rectum and may penetrate deeply into the abdominal cavity. In today's society, rectal perforations may also result from a variety of perverse sexual activities.[55,56]

An uncommon form of rectal injury may occur in pedestrians run over by a vehicle when the intraabdominal pressure is raised and then suddenly released, resulting in rupture of the pelvic diaphragm.[18] The anorectal apparatus may be left intact, but it may be torn from the levator ani sling and pulled into the abdomen. Blast injuries from below have also been reported to produce similar lesions.

Perforations occurring during barium enemas can be extremely serious because the growth and multiplication of bacteria is potentiated by barium and the various substances found in feces, resulting in severe infections.[18] Most of these injuries are caused by manipulation or inaccurate placement of the enema tip or balloon and may take the form of extensive lacerations which are often extraperitoneal.

Associated Injuries

As pointed out earlier, the type and number of associated injuries have a great effect on outcome. The four most frequent associated injuries and their incidence in 92 patients with rectal injuries at DRH were small bowel (27%), colon (24%), bladder (21%), and abdominal vessels (13%). Excluding the 12 patients with associated abdominal vessel injuries, there were no deaths in the remaining 80 patients.

Franko et al[57] recently noted that patients who had combined penetrating rectal and genitourinary injuries had a very high incidence of complications which included retrovesical or rectourethral fistulas in 24% (4/17), abscesses in 18%, chronic urinary tract infections in 18%, bladder stones in 12%, and urethral strictures in 12%. Interestingly their incidence of bladder injuries with penetrating rectal injuries was only 6.5% (13/200). In contrast, at DRH the incidence of combined rectal and bladder injuries due to GSW was much higher (23%=17/75).

Diagnosis

Rectal injuries must be diligently sought in all patients with penetrating injuries of the pelvis or lower abdomen. Blunt rectal trauma should be suspected in anyone with severe pelvic fractures or perineal injuries. A meticulous examination of the anus, rectum, and vagina is essential in such patients. Any trauma patient with blood in the rectum should be assumed to have a rectal injury until it is clear that the blood has come from some other source. Sigmoidoscopy may be helpful when the rectum is clear of feces, but the examination is frequently hampered by an inability to adequately prepare the bowel.

The diagnosis of iatrogenic colon injury following colonic endoscopy is obvious if other intraabdominal organs are visualized through the endoscope.[58] Air insufflation during the examination can cause a large pneumoperitoneum that makes the diagnosis obvious roentgenographically. Colonic injury should also be suspected if there is sudden severe abdominal pain during the procedure or any time within the next several days. If one suspects a bowel perforation following endoscopy, a water soluble contrast enema is generally diagnostic, but a delayed perforation due to ischemia can still occur.

AXIOM Rectal injuries can easily be missed at laparotomy and should be diagnosed preoperatively whenever possible.

Since the rectum is extraperitoneal, routine exploration at laparotomy may fail to demonstrate some rectal injuries.[3] Consequently, patients with penetrating wounds of the perineum, buttocks, or lower abdomen need a careful preoperative examination of the retrosigmoid area. A careful digital examination of the rectum that shows any gross blood on the examining finger is highly suggestive of a rectal injury. Preoperative proctosigmoidoscopy can also be extremely important, and demonstration of gross blood in the rectum virtually confirms the diagnosis. Visualization of the injury itself is not always possible and is not necessary to make the diagnosis. In addition to proctosigmoidoscopy for any suspected rectal injury, a retrograde cystourethrogram should be obtained in males and a careful vaginal examination should be performed in females to rule out concomitant injuries to the urogenital system.

Blunt rupture of the pelvic diaphragm may be recognized by the retraction of the anus and rectum to a high position or by gross eccentric displacement of the anus in the perineum.[18] Patients with this type of injury will often be in shock and may have associated genitourinary injuries.

Treatment of Rectal Injuries

The treatment of rectal injuries generates little controversy. Diverting colostomy and presacral drainage are the cornerstones of management. Nance[2] notes that the management of rectal injuries rests on the three Ds: diversion, debridement and drainage. If a rectal injury

is suspected preoperatively in stable patients, endoscopic evaluation of the rectum should be performed. If any defect or gross blood from an unknown source is identified, a sigmoid colostomy should be part of the management.

REPAIR OF THE RECTUM

AXIOM Attempts to repair rectal injuries are generally ill-advised.

Repair of the rectal injury itself is not mandatory and should be done only if it can be visualized and performed easily, either transanally or at laparotomy without extensive dissection. Indeed, easily visualized, partial-thickness injuries of the rectum can be repaired without proximal diversion.[6] Usually, however, the extent of the damage is virtually impossible to assess adequately at the initial operation, and in many cases the situation is further complicated by associated genitourinary or sacral injuries. Thus, attempts to achieve initial definitive repair may be hazardous and may lead to excessive morbidity.[18] In a recent report by Bostick et al,[59] nine (32%) of 28 patients had a primary repair of the rectal injury, but all 28 had a proximal colostomy.

AXIOM Establishment of adequate drainage and fecal diversion are the keys to success with rectal injuries.

DIVERTING COLOSTOMY

A sigmoid loop colostomy is the preferred method of fecal diversion for rectal injuries for most surgeons[2] (Fig. 26–5) To ensure complete defunctionalizing of the colostomy, the proximal end of the rectum may be closed with a row of staples. An end sigmoid colostomy with a Hartmann's pouch is preferred by some surgeons to ensure complete diversion of fecal material away from the injured rectum.[6,60] Reestablishment of bowel continuity later, however, is more difficult than with a loop colostomy.

CLEANSING OF THE DISTAL RECTUM

Saline irrigation of the defunctionalized rectum to wash out the feces is not absolutely necessary, but in theory it should reduce the amount of continuing contamination of perirectal tissues.[6] This maneuver may be particularly important if the rectal vault is full of stool. Dilatation of the anus to three or four fingers may also be a useful adjunct at the conclusion of the case to allow any fluid in the rectum to come out through the anus rather than escape into perirectal tissues.

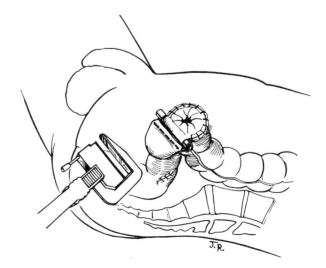

FIGURE 26–5 Sigmoid loop colostomy for rectal injury. A stapled closure of the distal limb assures complete fecal diversion. (Reprinted with permission from Burch JM, Feliciano DV, Mattox KL. Colostomy and drainage of civilian rectal injuries: is that all? Ann Surg 1989;209:600).

Jacobs and Plaisier[61] have recently described a technique of rectal irrigation which may reduce the amount of contamination that is usually caused by such procedures. The mucous fistula to the distal sigmoid colon and rectum is partly closed with a stapler around a 28-30 F Foley catheter. The balloon of the Foley catheter is inflated to ensure that the irrigation site does not leak. The anus is then dilated digitally as needed and standard corrugated plastic ventilator tubing is inserted into the rectum to direct the feces from the distal sigmoid colon and rectum into a bucket.

Although irrigation through the defunctioned rectal stump and a digitally dilated anus has many advocates and is customarily done for rectal injuries, the advantages are not unequivocally established. In a recent report by Bostick et al,[62] 53% of their patients with rectal injuries did not have distal rectal irrigation, and there was only one infection (3.6%) in the entire group.

AXIOM   If there is much feces in an injured rectum, it should be removed as carefully as possible to avoid increasing the contamination of the perirectal tissues.

PRESACRAL DRAINAGE

Adequate drainage of the presacral space posterior to the rectum is extremely important. Many surgeons prefer a sump or closed suction catheter placed in the retrorectal space and brought out just anterior to the coccyx. Some surgeons, however, will just insert a Penrose drain presacrally.

AXIOM   Presacral drainage is an integral part of the management of rectal injuries.

The insertion of presacral drains is usually done through a 3-4 cm semicircular incision made through the median raphe posterior to the anus. A blunt hemostat or finger is used to dissect just anterior to the coccyx and sacrum, through the pelvic sling, until the free presacral space is reached.[60] Sacral fractures or other pelvic bony defects should be avoided because of the risk of osteomyelitis.

If no significant leak is apparent at the end of 5 days, the presacral drain can usually be removed.[2] If a leak becomes apparent, closure of the fistula usually occurs spontaneously if fecal diversion was properly performed.

REPAIR OF ANAL DETACHMENTS

Patients with rupture of the pelvic diaphragm and internal retraction of the rectum and anus require early operation with a proximal colostomy, debridement and drainage of the perineum, repair of the bowel, and anchoring of the anal canal to the levator muscles and perineal skin.[18]

PERINEAL OR ANAL SPHINCTER WOUNDS

Occasional impalement injuries may produce extensive lacerations of the anus, its sphincters, and the pubic sling. Meticulous reapproximation of the tissues is critical to the repair of these lesions, and a proximal colostomy is desirable. Despite the frightening appearance of these wounds, incontinence seldom follows accurate reapproximation of the sphincter muscles; however, this assumes that fecal diversion with a colostomy plus presacral drainage prevents infection from developing.

RECTAL FOREIGN BODIES

Patients who present with retained foreign bodies of the rectum are nearly always males and are generally the subject of a deviant form of sexual practice.[63] Retained rectal foreign bodies are only rarely the result of violence. Patients usually seek medical attention late, after making multiple attempts of their own to remove the object. This can produce a great deal of edema in the adjacent tissues of the rectum and perianal region.[6]

The presence and location of the foreign body should be established by digital palpation, endoscopy, and/or roentgeno-graphic examination. The majority of these objects will be lodged in the sacral hollow, and they can usually be removed transanally once the anal sphincter has been relaxed.

Prior to removal of the foreign body, appropriate antibiotics and antitetanus prophylaxis should be administered.[6] In some patients, the foreign body can be removed in the emergency room under sedation and local anesthesia. If this is unsuccessful, removal in the operating room under general anesthesia will be required. A careful proctosigmoidoscopy should be performed following removal of the foreign body to rule out a perforation. Since most of these patients routinely give themselves enemas prior to inserting the foreign bodies, if a tear has occurred, the fecal spillage is usually not extensive. Nevertheless, a rectal perforation from a foreign body should be managed as a rectal injury from any other cause.

AXIOM   After a foreign body is removed from the rectum, endoscopy should be performed to rule out the presence of a perforation.

IMPALEMENT INJURIES

Rectal injuries as the result of violent insertion of a foreign body into the rectum are true impalement wounds.[3] Because of the anatomic relationship of the rectum and bladder, the impaling device often also penetrates the anterior rectal wall and enters the urinary bladder. Consequently, associated injury to the urinary bladder must always be searched for and ruled out in these patients.[6]

AXIOM   A careful search for a bladder perforation should be made in all patients with an impalement injury of the rectum.

Patients who present with perforation of the bowel secondary to sexual practices may give a history of an impalement injury to hide the true etiology; however, perforations due to deviant activity are nearly always above the peritoneal reflection and without urinary bladder injury.[6] Such perforations should be suspected in the presence of peritoneal signs, but can be confirmed by the presence of intraperitoneal free air on abdominal radiographs, by sigmoidoscopy, or with a water-soluble contrast enema.

Patients with an impalement injury of the rectum require a laparotomy. If a full-thickness rectal injury is present, it should be treated with a diverting colostomy and the distal sigmoid colon and rectum should be irrigated clean. If the tear is in the intraperitoneal colon, is small, and is without gross fecal spillage, a primary repair can be attempted.[3]

Small perianal and anal disruptions may bleed significantly initially but usually stop spontaneously. These can usually be handled like obstetrical injuries and may be primarily repaired without fecal diversion. If the anal and perianal injury is large or is seen after infection has developed, the wounds should be left open and protected from further soiling with a proximal colostomy. The injury can then be repaired secondarily if incontinence develops.[3]

OUTCOME FROM COLON AND/OR RECTAL INJURIES

Mortality

Although reported mortality rates for colon injuries range from 2-12% in most series, and although these mortality rates are substantially less than for pancreatic or duodenal injuries, patients with colon injuries die primarily because of hemorrhage from associated severe injuries. Even patients dying of sepsis usually have other injuries.[18] The patients dying of colon or rectal injuries at DRH had an average of two associated visceral injuries per patient, and those who died in the operating room received an average of 13 units of blood prior to death. During the past 12 years at DRH the mortality rate was 6% in patients with stab wounds, 14% in patients with gunshot wounds, and

16% in those with shotgun injuries of the colon (Table 26–2). Of the patients with none or only one associated injury, only 5% (15/318) died. Of those with two or more associated injuries, 20% (68/345) died (P<0.0001) (Table 26–4). If the patients with associated abdominal vessel injuries (who had a mortality rate of 40%) are excluded, the mortality rate was only 4% (22/509) (Table 26–2).

AXIOM Colonic or rectal wounds are seldom isolated injuries, and the mortality and morbidity generally reflects the number and severity of the extracolonic injuries.

The great majority (72%) of the 92 rectal injuries seen at DRH from 1980 to 1992 were due to gunshot wounds, and all of the deaths were in patients who had associated gunshot wounds to abdominal vessels (Table 26–5).

Complications

INCIDENCE OF COMPLICATIONS

Even with optimal therapy, colon and rectal injuries will be associated with a relatively high incidence of complications, including peritonitis or abscess formation, fever of unknown origin, fecal fistula, and wound infection. Abdominal abscesses may occur in 5-17% of these patients, and these usually occur with greater frequency among patients treated with colostomy.[2,51] Bostick et al,[62] however, reported a 25.2% incidence of septic complications in 231 patients with penetrating colon injuries. These included 36 (17%) wound infections and 18 (8%) abdominal abscesses; however, the method of surgical management of the colon injury was not a significant factor (P<0.39).

AXIOM Patients with colonic injuries and any visible fecal spill should generally not have the skin and subcutaneous tissues of their incisions or any wounds closed at the time of surgery.

Wound infections following rectal injuries have a frequency of about 5-15%, but can be avoided most of the time by leaving the skin and subcutaneous tissue open.[2] Fever is very common in patients with colon or rectal injuries and often eludes specific diagnosis. Fecal fistulas occur in 1-4% of these patients.[2]

In a recent report by Sasaki et al[64] on 154 patients with intraperitoneal colon wounds seen over a 6-year period in an urban trauma center, primary repair, including resection and anastomosis, was performed in 102 patients (66%) and diversion in 52 patients (34%). There were 11 (11%) septic-related complications in the diversion group and 10 (11%) septic-related complications in the primary re-

pair group. The probability for adverse outcome was significantly greater in the diversion group. The penetrating abdominal trauma index (PATI) had greater predictive value for determining morbidity and mortality than did colon injury scoring. Ivatory et al[51] also found the PATI to be the most significant factor associated with postoperative abdominal abscess (P<0.0001). The presence of a colostomy was also a highly significant factor (P<0.0004).

The role of retained bullets that have passed through the colon in the development of local sepsis has been studied by Demetriades and Charalambides.[65] Of 84 patients with gunshot wounds of the colon, the bullet was retained in the body in 40 and had exited or was removed from the body in 44. The groups were similar with regard to Revised Trauma Score, Injury Severity Score, Penetrating Abdominal Trauma Index and type of colonic trauma. The incidence of major local complications was 5% in patients with a retained bullet and 7% in those without. Nevertheless, we have noted an increased incidence of retroperitoneal abscesses at Detroit Receiving Hospital if the bullet is retained in the paravertebral muscles. Our neurosurgeons also believe that bullets that enter the spinal canal after passing through the colon should be removed.

COLOSTOMY CLOSURE

AXIOM The closure of a posttraumatic colostomy can be extremely difficult and may be associated with a number of serious complications.

Timing

A colostomy for colon or rectal trauma can be closed as soon as the injuries and all incisions and drainage sites have healed and the patient has achieved a positive nitrogen balance. This usually takes at least 4-8 weeks, but most surgeons prefer to wait at least 3 months. Endoscopy and/or barium enema is generally employed prior to the closure to be sure that the injured rectum and colon have healed and are of normal caliber.

The timing of colostomy closure may have some bearing on the complication rate. If closure is performed too early, complications appear to be more frequent than if it is delayed for 6 weeks or more.[66] On the other hand, patients seldom return to gainful employment until the colostomy has been closed. Thus, the risk of complications must be weighed against the patient's continuing disability.

In a series of patients seen at Detroit Receiving Hospital in 1978, the median interval from colostomy construction to colostomy clo-

TABLE 26–4 *Mortality Rates with Colon Injuries Correlated with Number of Associated Injuries*

Number of Associated Injuries	Type of Trauma				
	Blunt	GSW	SGW	Stab	Total
0	1 (7) 14%	0 (38) 0%	——	0 (34) 0%	1 (79) 1%
1	2 (9) 22%	8 (164) 6%	1 (9) 5%	3 (57) 5%	14 (239) 6%
2	1 (15) 7%	17 (102) 17%	1 (11) 9%	0 (16) 0%	19 (144) 13%
3	1 (6) 17%	19 (69) 28%	0 (10) 0%	1 (5) 20%	21 (90) 23%
4+	2 (6) 33%	18 (82) 22%	5 (13) 39%	3 (18) 30%	28 (111) 27%
Total	7 (43) 16%	62 (455) 14%	7 (43) 16%	7 (122) 6%	83 (663) 13%

TABLE 26–5   Associated Injuries and Mortality Rates with Rectal Trauma

Associated Injury	Type of Trauma				
	Blunt	GSW	SGW	Stab	Total
Small Bowel	—	2 (24) 8%	0 (1) 0%	—	2 (25) 8%
Colon	—	2 (21) 10%	0 (1) 0%	—	2 (22) 9%
Bladder	0 (2)	0 (17) 0%	—	—	0 (19) 0%
Abd. vessels	—	5 (13) 45%	—	0 (1) 0%	5 (12) 42%
Liver	—	1 (4) 25%	—	—	1 (4) 25%
Kidney	—	0 (2) 0%	—	—	0 (2) 0%
Duodenum	—	1 (2) 50%	—	—	1 (2) 50%
Stomach	—	1 (1) 100%	—	—	1 (1) 100%
Spleen	—	0 (1) 0%	—	—	0 (1) 0%
Diaphragm	—	0 (1) 0%	—	—	0 (1) 0%
Total*	0 (9) 0%	5 (66) 8%	0 (5) —	0 (4) 0%	5 (92)** 5%

*This does equal the total of the cases listed in each column because some patients had no associated injuries and many had more than one.
**Includes 8 other patients with other types of rectal trauma.

sure was 101 days.[41] In a study by Crass et al[67] in 1987, the median interval was 103 days with a range of 36-902 days. In the Louisville series,[40] the mean time was 122 days.

In a recent report by Renz et al,[68] 30 consecutive patient with rectal wounds (RW) (90% of which were due to gunshot wounds) were entered into a prospective study to determine if same admission colostomy closure (SACC) could be performed safely if the rectal wound was healed on contrast enema (CE). The first CE was performed 5-10 days after injury in 29 patients. The proportions of RWs radiologically healed at seven and 10 days after injury were 55% and 75% respectively. Sixteen patients with a normal CE underwent SACC 9-19 days after injury (mean, 12.4 days). There were two fecal fistulas (29%) after simple suture closure of seven of the colostomies, but there were no complications after resection of the stoma with end-to-end anastomosis in nine patients. The total mean hospitalization time was 17.4 days. Thus, CE confirmed healing of RWs in 75% of patients by 10 days after injury, and SACC was performed without complications in 88% of patients with radiologically healed rectal wounds. This report is very interesting, but the benefits of SACC need to be confirmed by other investigators before its use becomes more widespread.

Barium Enemas Before Colostomy Closures

Most surgeons examine the colon with a barium enema (BE) prior to scheduling closure of a colostomy performed for trauma. Atweh et al[69] suggested that this is particularly important for rectal injuries not visualized at the first operation. Sola et al[70] have recently questioned this practice. They reviewed 86 trauma patients who underwent colostomy closure during a 12-year period at their institution. In 95% the injuries were the result of penetrating trauma. Of 16 patients with rectal injuries, 15 had a BE more than 6 weeks after the trauma, and all showed healing of the injury. In the 70 patients with colonic injuries, 43 (group 1) had a BE prior to colostomy closure. Of these,

42 (98%) had negative studies. The only positive finding that was discovered did not affect the planned surgical procedure. The remaining 27 patients (Group 2) did not have a BE prior to colostomy closure. The overall complication rates were not significantly different between group 1 (18.6%) and group 2 (29.6%). Although the authors concluded that BE prior to colostomy closure for colonic injuries yields little useful information, most surgeons are probably not ready to abandon the use of barium enema to confirm colonic healing prior to colostomy closure at this time.

Techniques of Colostomy Closure

Once it has been decided that a colostomy can safely be closed, the colon and rectum must be completely cleaned preoperatively. Appropriate prophylactic parenteral antibiotics should be given about 30 minutes prior to the incision. After prepping and draping, the skin is carefully incised around the entire mucocutaneous junction of the colostomy stoma. Blunt dissection will then usually serve to mobilize the subcutaneous portion of the colostomy, but sharp dissection is usually required to free the colostomy from the fascia. If the posterior wall of a loop colostomy is intact, the anterior wall can sometimes be closed successfully with a stapler. Otherwise, a standard sutured or stapled anastomosis is performed. The closed colon can then be gently pushed below the fascia, which is then closed.[2]

Divided stoma colostomies and colostomies with a distal Hartmann's pouch require a formal laparotomy. The stomas are freed as with loop colostomies and then brought into the abdomen. The end of a Hartmann's pouch can be found easier with the use of a colonoscope. In many instances, the small bowel and colon to be used for the anastomosis have extensive adhesions which must be taken down very carefully. Once an adequate length of proximal and distal colon are freed up, they should be trimmed back to normal bowel and anastomosed in a standard fashion. Postoperatively these patients must be watched very carefully because it is not unusual to have leaks occur following colostomy closures.

Complications

Sola et al[71] have noted that the reported morbidity of colostomy closure in trauma patients varies from 5-27%. In order to assess the morbidity of colostomy closure, they reviewed all colonic injuries

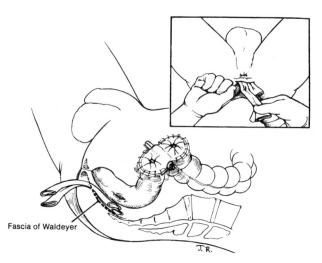

FIGURE 26–6   To obtain presacral drainage, the perineum is incised about half way between the anal verge and the tip of the coccyx. The presacral space is then bluntly dissected until one is certain that the space is opened up to the level of the rectal injury. (Reprinted with permission from Burch JM, Feliciano DV, Mattox KL. Colostomy and drainage of civilian rectal injuries: is that all? Ann Surg 1989;209:600).

Fascia of Waldeyer

from 1979 to 1991 at their institutions. In all, 86 trauma patients who underwent colostomy creation and closure were identified. There were no deaths after colostomy closure, but there was a total morbidity of 24%. There were 11 anastomotic complications (two of which required repeat laparotomy) and nine wound infections. The average length of stay was 10.4 days. Interestingly, these morbidities were most likely to occur in patients who had complications during their initial hospitalization. This was especially true if these patients underwent closure earlier tha 3 months after injury. Conversely, if the first operation was uncomplicated, waiting longer than 3 months to perform the colostomy closure did not improve the results. In a similar report, Taheri et al[72] studied 110 patients who underwent elective colostomy closure following trauma. These patients had a 9.1% intraabdominal complication rate and a 3.6% wound infection rate.

AXIOM   Fever, leukocytosis, or abdominal pain within two weeks of a colostomy closure should be considered due to a leaking anastomosis until proven otherwise.

If a colon leak occurs and the patient has any evidence of infection or intraperitoneal contamination, the anastomosis should be exteriorized as a colostomy; however, if the leak is small and relatively well contained, a proximal colostomy may suffice. The leaking anastomosis, however, has an increased chance of developing a stricture later. If a small colocutaneous fistula develops and there is no evidence of a distal obstruction or infection, the fistula will usually heal spontaneously without proximal colostomy.

SUMMARY

Colonic or rectal injury occurs in up to 10% of patients with penetrating or severe blunt abdominal trauma. The diagnosis should be suspected in patients with penetrating abdominal injury or with blunt trauma and any peritoneal signs. A very high index of suspicion is required to diagnose retroperitoneal or nontransmural injuries in a timely fashion. Diagnostic peritoneal lavage, computed tomography, and/or endoscopy may be helpful in selected patients, but the diagnosis of colonic injury is still made most frequently during an exploratory laparotomy for associated injuries.

Colonic injuries are amenable to careful primary repair in at least 60-70% of civilian injuries, and the trend toward avoiding colostomies whenever possible continues. The purported differences between the left and right colon are increasingly challenged. Colostomy is increasingly reserved for severe destructive colonic injuries and for rectal injuries. The mortality rates seen with colonic and rectal injuries are due primarily to the associated injuries.

⊘ FREQUENT ERRORS

Made in the Management of Injuries to the Colon and Rectum

1. *Failure to adequately examine the perineum and gluteal creases in patients with penetrating wounds of the lower abdomen, lower back, or pelvis.*
2. *Failure to completely examine all portions of the colon after gunshot wounds of the abdomen because the trajectory suggests that a colon injury would be extremely unlikely.*
3. *Failing to perform an early exploratory laparotomy if one suspects a colon injury.*
4. *Completely relying on a negative DPL to rule out a bowel injury.*
5. *Performing diagnostic techniques to rule out colon injuries on hemodynamically unstable patients.*

6. *Failing to perform a colostomy or ileostomy on patients who have colon injuries due to high-velocity missiles or close-range shotgun blasts.*
7. *Performing a primary colon repair on tissue that is not quite perfect just because all of the indications for a primary closure are present.*
8. *Assuming that peritoneal drains can help prevent peritonitis after diffuse contamination.*
9. *Closing the skin and subcutaneous tissue of the incision if there has been contamination from a colon injury.*
10. *Extensive dissection in the pelvis in an attempt to identify a suspected low rectal injury.*
11. *Failing to perform a diverting colostomy for a severe perianal or suspected rectal injury.*
12. *Delay in exploring a patient who is not doing well after a colostomy closure.*

▼▼▼▼▼▼▼▼▼▼▼▼▼▼▼▼▼▼▼▼▼▼▼▼▼▼▼▼▼▼

SUMMARY POINTS

1. Wounds of the colon and rectum can be lethal if they are not recognized and treated promptly.

2. Colon wounds due to high-velocity missiles should be treated with a colostomy, whereas most injuries due to stabs or low-velocity missiles can be closed primarily with safety.

3. There is little difference between the healing capabilities of right and left colon wounds.

4. Although an extensive data base is now available to support the use of primary repair for most colon injuries, the temptation to perform primary repairs in unfavorable cases should be resisted.

5. Successful treatment of colonic injuries must include measures that restore the integrity of the bowel wall and control fecal spill.

6. Immediate operation following perforation of the colon during a barium enema is essential to cleanse the peritoneal cavity and to prevent further contamination.

7. Patients with "seat belt injuries" of the abdominal wall and vertebrae should be strongly suspected of having associated intestinal injuries.

8. Since contused and devitalized colon may extend beyond the area of obvious injury, primary repair of blunt colon injuries is risky.

9. Even with evacuation of mesocolic hematomas, careful observation of the patient is essential for the early diagnosis of occult, but potentially lethal, delayed leaks.

10. Insufflation injuries of the colon can occur even without direct contact of the patient with the air hose.

11. Any abdominal injury from any direction can injure the colon.

12. Loss of bowel sounds occasionally provides the earliest evidence of bowel injury after blunt trauma to the abdomen.

13. Failure to examine the anal and gluteal areas closely may result in overlooking important penetrating injuries.

14. Whenever possible, a proctosigmoidoscopic examination should be performed perioperatively in any patient suspected of having a rectal injury.

15. One should never assume the path of a bullet is a straight line from its entrance to its exit wound or current position in the body.

16. The accuracy of CT scans in trauma is greatly influenced by the experience of the interpreter, and this must be factored into the decision making.

17. A negative DPL does not rule out gastrointestinal injuries reliably, especially if the DPL is done soon after the trauma or if the injury is retroperitoneal.

18. Hemodynamically unstable patients with blunt abdominal trauma should undergo a prompt exploratory laparotomy, which generally uncovers any colon injuries that may be present.

19. The most reliable method for identification of colon injuries is exploratory laparotomy.

20. As a general rule, stab wounds in the flank have a 15-25% incidence of causing an intraabdominal organ injury, whereas wounds in the back have a 5-10% incidence of causing such injuries.

21. Patients with gunshot wounds of the abdomen require routine laparotomy.

22. ED resuscitation should be kept to a minimum in hemodynamically unstable patients with abdominal injuries. The bleeding needs to be surgically controlled as soon as possible.

23. Retroperitoneal injuries of the large bowel are easily missed unless the colon is fully mobilized.

24. Dissecting deep into the pelvis to look for possible rectal injuries may cause much more harm than good.

25. The extent of the colon injury, the amount of contamination, the number and types of associated injuries, and the general condition of the patient are important factors in deciding on the most appropriate form of treatment.

26. Transient hypotension is not a contraindication to primary repair of colon injuries.

27. All things considered, older patients tend to do better with a single operation than with two-three separate procedures of similar cumulative duration.

28. Although the great majority of civilian colon injuries can be safely treated with a primary anastomosis in the presence of severe contamination or overt peritonitis, a colostomy is probably the wisest choice.

29. As a general rule small bowel-colonic anastomoses heal better than colocolonic anastomoses on unprepared bowel.

30. In critically injured patients with persistent hypotension, primary repair of colon injuries is likely to be safer if it can be performed much more rapidly than a colostomy.

31. Irrigation of feces out of an injured colon may increase the likelihood of a primary repair healing successfully.

32. Performing a colostomy is not always the safest way to manage a colon injury.

33. Closure of a loop colostomy is often much safer and easier than closure of a colostomy with a Hartmann's pouch, especially if there has been any intraperitoneal infection.

34. One should be certain that the remaining colon and the rectum are normal prior to attempting closure of a colostomy.

35. If a primary colon repair seems a bit hazardous, one can still perform an exteriorized repair with relative safety.

36. Because primary repair of colon injuries is feasible and will heal well in the great majority of patients, there seems to be little place for exteriorized primary anastomosis today.

37. Intraperitoneal drains are seldom indicated in patients with colonic injuries.

38. Rectal injuries can easily be missed at laparotomy and should be diagnosed preoperatively whenever possible.

39. Attempts to repair rectal injuries are generally ill-advised.

40. Establishment of adequate drainage and fecal diversion are the keys to success with rectal injuries.

41. If there is much feces in an injured rectum, it should be removed as carefully as possible so as to not increase the contamination of the perirectal tissues.

42. Presacral drainage is an important part of the management of rectal injuries.

43. After a foreign body is removed from the rectum, endoscopy should be performed to rule out the presence of a perforation.

44. A careful search for a bladder perforation should be made in patients with an impalement injury of the rectum.

45. Colonic wounds are seldom isolated injuries, and the mortality and morbidity generally reflect the number and severity of the extracolonic injuries.

46. Patients with colonic injuries and any visible fecal spill should generally not have the skin and subcutaneous tissues of their incisions or any wounds closed at the time of surgery.

47. The closure of a posttraumatic colostomy can be extremely difficult and may be associated with a number of serious, and even lethal, complications.

48. Fever, leukocytosis, or abdominal pain within 2 weeks of a colostomy closure should be considered due to a leaking anastomosis until proven otherwise.

▲▲▲▲▲▲▲▲▲▲▲▲▲▲▲▲▲▲▲▲▲▲▲▲▲▲▲▲▲▲▲▲▲▲▲

REFERENCES

1. Walt AJ. Injuries and iatrogenic disorders of the colon and rectum. In Berk JE, ed. Bockus Gastroenterology, 4th ed. Philadelphia: WB Saunders Co., 1985, 4:2575-2582.
2. Nance FC. Injuries to the colon and rectum. In Moore EE, Mattox KL, Feliciano DV, eds. Trauma, 2nd ed. Norwalk, Conn: Appleton-Lange, 1991;33:521-532.
3. Levison MA, Walt AJ. Colonic trauma in current therapy. In Faxio V, ed. Therapy in colon and rectal surgery. Philadelphia: BC Decker, 1989; 329-333.
4. Levison MA, Thomas DD, Wiencek RC, Wilson RF. Management of the injured colon: evolving practice at an urban trauma center. J Trauma 1990;30:247-253.
5. Stone HH, Fabian TC. Management of perforating colon trauma. Ann Surg 1979;190:430.
6. Sherman R, Rehm C. Injuries of the colon and rectum. In Kreis DJ Jr., Gomez GA, eds. Trauma management. Boston: Little, Brown & Co., 1989; 230-238.
7. Ogilvie WH. Abdominal wounds in the western desert. Surg Gynecol Obstet 1944;78:225.
8. Woodhal JP, Ochsner A. The management of perforating injuries of the colon and rectum in civilian practice. Surgery 1951;29:305.
9. Grablowsky OM, Gage JO, Ray JE, Hanley PH. Traumatic colonic and rectal injuries. Dis Colon Rectum 1973;16:296.
10. LoCicero J, III Tajima T, Drapanas T. A half century of experience in the management of colon injuries: changing concepts. J Trauma 1975; 15:575.
11. Pontius RG, Creech O Jr., DeBakey ME. Management of large bowel injuries in civilian practice. Ann Surg 1957;146:291.
12. Burch JM, Brock JC, Gevirtzman L, et al. The injured colon. Ann Surg 1986;203:701.
13. Nehan N, Lewis F. The influence of injury severity on complication rates after primary closure of colostomy for penetrating colon trauma. Ann Surg 1989;209:439.
14. Shannon FL, Moore EE. Primary repair of the colon: when is it a safe alternative? Surgery 1985;98:851.
15. George SM, Fabian TC, Voeller GR, et al. Primary repair of colon wounds. Ann Surg 1989;209:226.
16. Lucas CE Ledgerwood AM. Management of the injured colon. Curr Surg 1986;43:190.
17. Kirkpatrick JR, Rajpal SC. The injured colon: therapeutic considerations. Am J Surg 1975;129:187.
18. Walt AJ, Wilson RF. Specific abdominal injuries: colon, rectum, and anus. In Walt AJ, Wilson RF, eds. Management of Trauma: Pitfalls and Practice. Philadelphia: Lea and Fibiger, 1975;365-369.
19. Leppaniemi A, Karppinen K, Haapiainen R. Stab wounds of the colon. Ann Chir Gynaecol 1994;83:26.
20. Dauterive AH, Flanchbaum L, Cox EF. Blunt intestinal trauma. Ann Surg 1983;201:384-388.
21. Strate RG, Grieco JG. Blunt injury to the colon and rectum. J Trauma 1983;23:384-388.
22. Stahl KD, Geiss AC, Bordam DL, et al. Blunt trauma and delayed colon injury. Curr Surg 1985;4-9.
23. Thompson JS, Moore EC, Moore JB. Comparison of penetrating injuries of the right and left colon. Ann Surg 1981;193:414.
24. Huizinga WK, Baker LW. The influence of splenectomy on infective morbidity after colonic. Eur J Surg 1993;159:579.
25. McAllister E, Perez M, Albrink MH, et al. Is triple contrast computed tomographic scanning useful in the selective management of stab wounds to the back? J Trauma 1994;37:401.
26. Thomson SR, Fraser M, Stupp C, et al. Iatrogenic and accidental colon injuries; what to do? Dis Colon Rectum 1994;37:496.
27. Nelken N, Lewis F. The influence of injury severity on complication rates after primary closure or colostomy for penetrating colon trauma. Ann surg 1989;209:439-447.
28. Burch JM, Martin RR, Richardson RJ, et al. Evolution of the management of the injured colon in the '80s. Arch Surg 1991;126:979-984.
29. Flint LM, Vital GC, Richardson JD, Polk H. The injured colon. Ann Surg 1981;193:619-623.

30. Atkins RB, Zirkec PK, Waterhouse G. Penetrating colon trauma. J Trauma 1984;24:491-499.

31. George SM, Fabian TC, Mangiante EC. Colon trauma: further support for primary repair. Am J Surg 1988;156:16-20.

32. Ross SE, Cobean RA, Hoyt OB, et al. Blunt colonic injury—a multicenter review. J Trauma 1992;33:379.

33. Moore EE, Dunn EL, Moore JB. Penetrating abdominal trauma index. J Trauma 1989;21:438-445.

34. Moreels R, Pont M, Ean S, et al. Wartime colon injuries: primary repair or colostomy? J R Soc Med 1994;87:265.

35. Dudley HAF, Radcliffe AG, McGeehan. Intraoperative irritation of the colon to permit primary anastomosis. Br J Surg 1980;67:80-81.

36. Baker IW, Thomson SR, Chadwick SDJ. Colon wound management and prograde colonic lavage in large bowel trauma. Br J Surg 1990;77:872-876.

37. Ravo B. Colorectal anastomotic healing and the intracolonic bypass procedure. Surg Clin N Am 1988;68:1267-1294.

38. Van der Hamm AC, Kort WJ, Weijma IM, et al. Effect of fibrin sealant on the healing colonic anastomosis in the rat. Br J Surg 1991;78:49-53.

39. Khayat HS. Right hemicolectomy and peritoneal lavage in missile injuries of the right colon. J R Coll Surg Edinb 1994;39:23.

40. Livingston DH, Miller FB, Richardson JD. Are the risks after colostomy closure exaggerated? Am J Surg 1989;158:17-20.

41. Smit R, Walt AJ. The morbidity and cost of the temporary colostomy. Dis Col Rec 1978;8:558-561.

42. Schultz SC, Magnant CM, Richman MF, et al. Identifying the low-risk patient with penetrating colonic injury for selective use of primary repair. Surg Gynecol Obstet 1993;177:237.

43. Kirkpatrick JR. The exteriorized anastomosis: its role in surgery of the colon. Surgery 82:362-365, 1977.

44. Lou MA, Johnson AP, Atik M. Exteriorized repair in the management of colon injuries. Arch Surg 1981;116:926-929.

45. Robbs JV. The alternative to colostomy for the injured colon. S Afr Med J 1978;53:95-99.

46. Okies JE, et al. Exteriorized primary repair of colon injuries. Amer J Surg 1972;124:807.

47. Shrock TR, Christensen N. Management of perforating injuries to the colon. Surg Gynecol Obstet 1972;135:65.

48. Kirkpatrick JR, Rajpal FG. Management of a high-risk intestinal anastomosis. Amer J Surg 1973;125:312.

49. Mulherin JL, Sawyers JL. Evaluation of three methods for managing penetrating colon injuries: changing concepts. J Trauma 1975;15:575.

50. Thompson JS, Moore EE. Factors affecting the outcome of exteriorized colon repair. J Trauma 22:403, 1982.

51. Ivatury RR, Gaudino J, Nallathambi MN, et al. Definitive treatment of colon injuries: a prospective study. Am Surg 1993;59:43.

52. Noon GP, Beall AC, Jordon GL, et al. Clinical evaluation of peritoneal irrigation with antibiotic solution. Surgery 1967;62:73.

53. Kirkpatrick JR. Injuries of the colon. Surg Clin North Am 1977;57:767.

54. Vitale GC, Richardson JD, Flint LM. Successful management of injuries to the extraperitoneal rectum. Am J Surg 1983;49:159.

55. Witz M, Sphitz B, Zager M, et al. Anal erotic instrumentation. A surgical problem. Dis Colon Rectum 1984;27:331.

56. Bush RA, Owen WF. Trauma and other noninfectious problem in homosexual men. Med Clin North Am 1986;70:549.

57. Franko ER, Ivatury RR, Schwalb DM. Combined penetrating rectal and genitourinary injuries: a challenge in management. J Trauma 1993;34:347.

58. Christie JP, Marrazzo J. Miniperforation of the colon—not all postpolypectomy perforations require laparotomy. Dis Colon Rect 1990;34:132-135.

59. Bostick PJ, Johnson DA, Heard JF, et al. Management of extraperitoneal rectal injuries. J Natl Med Assoc 1993;85:460.

60. Barone JE, Yee J, Nealon TF. Management of foreign bodies and trauma of the rectum. Surg Gynecol Obstet 1983;156:453.

61. Jacobs LM, Plaisier BR. An efficient system for controlled distal colorectal irrigation. J Am Coll Surg 1994;178:305.

62. Bostick PJ, Heard JS, Islas JT. Management of penetrating colon injuries. J Natl Med Assoc 1994;86:378.

63. Crass RA, Trambaugh RF, Kudsk KA. Colorectal foreign bodies and perforation. Am J Surg 1981;142:85.

64. Sasaki LS, Mittal V, Allaben RD. Primary repair of colon injuries: a retrospective analysis. Ann Surg 1994;60:522.

65. Demetriades D, Charalambides D. Gunshot wounds of the colon: role of retained bullets in sepsis. Br J Surg 1993;80:772.

66. Parks SE, Hastings PR. Complications of colostomy closure. Am J Surg 1985;149:672.

67. Crass RA, Trambaugh RF, Kudsk KA. Colorectal foreign bodies and perforation. Am J Surg 1981;142:85.

68. Renz BM, Feliciano DV, Sherman R. Same admission colostomy closure (SACC). A new approach to rectal wounds: a prospective study. Ann Surg 1993;218:279.

69. Atweh NA, Vieux EE, Ivatury R, et al. Indications for barium enema preceding colostomy closure in trauma patients. J Trauma 1989;29:641-642.

70. Sola JE, Buchman TG, Bender JS. Limited role of barium enema examination preceding colostomy closure in trauma patients. J Trauma 1994;36:245.

71. Solo JE, Bender JS, Buchman TG. Morbidity and timing of colostomy in trauma patients. Injury 1993;24:438.

72. Taheri PA, Ferrara JJ, Johnson CE, et al. A convincing case for primary repair of penetrating colon injuries. Am J Surg 1993;166:39.

Chapter **27** Abdominal Vascular Trauma

ROBERT F. WILSON, M.D.

SCOTT DULCHAVSKY, M.D.

INTRODUCTION

AXIOM Prompt control of bleeding and aggressive resuscitation, including rewarming, are the keys to success with intraabdominal vascular injuries.

Penetrating trauma to major abdominal vessels occurs in only about 2-3% of soldiers who live long enough to have their wounds treated; however, civilians seem to have a much better prognosis.[1] In 1979, 15% of the patients with abdominal trauma treated at the Ben Taub General Hospital in Houston had injuries to major vascular structures.[2] Of 2741 patients treated at DRH from 1980-1992 for abdominal injuries, 333 (12%) had injuries to major abdominal vessels (Table 27–1).

It is estimated that patients with penetrating stab wounds to the abdomen will sustain major abdominal vascular injury about 10% of the time,[3] and patients with gunshot wounds to the abdomen will have injury to a major vessel about 25% of the time.[4] In the DRH series, the incidence of abdominal vessel injury in 1358 patients who had surgery for abdominal gunshot wounds was 18.9%. Of the 810 patients with injuries from abdominal stab wounds, 6.5% had vascular injuries (Table 27–1).

The large number of abdominal vascular injuries seen with penetrating trauma in civilian practice reflects the use of handguns with low-velocity missiles (which are less likely to cause rapid death than are high-velocity missiles from rifles or assault weapons) and the short prehospital transit times in most urban areas.

The incidence of injury to major abdominal vessels in patients sustaining blunt abdominal trauma is much lower, and is estimated at about 5-10%.[5,6] In the DRH series, it was 4.0% (23/573). While significant vascular injury occurs less frequently in blunt abdominal trauma, these injuries are frequently more complex and more likely to be fatal.[4,5] In the DRH series, the mortality rates with vascular injuries due to blunt trauma, gunshot wounds, and stabs were 70%, 53%, and 32% respectively.

PATHOPHYSIOLOGY

Penetrating Injuries

Penetrating trauma can create a wide variety of vascular injuries including perforations, intimal dissections, arterio-venous fistulas, and thrombosis. Knife wounds typically cause clean transections or lacerations amenable to arteriorrhaphy or venorrhaphy. Injuries created by gunshot wounds depend on the trajectory and energy transferred to the vessel, with the energy primarily related to bullet velocity. Since the energy transmitted to the tissues is proportional to the square of the velocity of the missile, high-velocity missiles ($>$ 2000 ft/sec) can cause 16 times more destruction than a similar bullet travelling at only 500 ft/sec. With high-velocity missiles, surgical debridement of a portion of the vessel is usually required to allow a safe repair. Even if the vessel appears to be grossly normal, it can be badly damaged for several centimeters beyond the bullet tract.

AXIOM Tissues damaged by high-velocity missiles may require extensive debridement to ensure that the remaining tissue is normal and will heal properly.

Diagnosis of an intimal flap or intramural dissection is best made by an arteriotomy at the site of the contusion or pre-operative arteriography. Treatment usually requires arterioplasty or resection with primary anastomosis.

Acute arteriovenous fistulas can occur following knife or bullet injuries. However, they may be difficult to detect preoperatively because they are rarely accompanied by the prominent bruit or thrill that is often present after several weeks or months.

The mortality rate with penetrating injuries varies greatly with the type of weapon used. In a recent series of 56 patients with penetrating injury to the abdominal aorta reported by Franc et al,[7] the mortality was 73%. The mortality rates were 78% for GSW, 67% for shotgun wounds and 43% for stab wounds. With the GSW, the mortality for bullets of 0.38 caliber or larger was 92% (36/39) and for 0.22 caliber bullets, it was 0% (0/7). However, since it is estimated that only 15% of the patients with penetrating injuries of the aorta reach the hospital alive, this is a highly selected group.

Associated injuries and the location of the injury in the major vessels also have an influence on outcome. Abdominal vascular injuries associated with splenic and/or diaphragmatic trauma tend to have an increased mortality rate (63% and 64% respectively) (Table 27–2). The abdominal vessel injuries with the highest mortality rates treated at DRH from 1980-1992 included the visceral portion of the aorta (100%), the retrohepatic IVC (90%), the diaphragmatic aorta (86%) and SMA (73%) (Tables 27–3, 27–4).

AXIOM In addition to the wounding mechanism, the most important factors determining survival are the initial blood pressure and its response to resuscitation.

Blunt Trauma

Blunt injuries damage blood vessels primarily by deceleration, shear injuries, and by crushing. Deceleration-type trauma such as those sustained in motor vehicle accidents can cause avulsion of branches off major vessels or intimal tears or flaps with secondary thrombosis of vessels, especially the superior mesenteric artery,[8] infrarenal abdominal aorta,[9,10] and iliac arteries.[11,12]

The aorta is frequently injured in its thoracic portion as a result of rapid deceleration; however, the fixed abdominal aorta is relatively well protected.[13] In a recent review of blunt trauma literature in English, Reisman and Morgan (1990) found only 37 cases of abdominal aortic injury.[14] Of 8710 post mortems on trauma victims, blunt injury to the abdominal aorta was found in only 0.18%.[11,12]

The usual mechanism of blunt abdominal aortic injury is compression against the lumbar spine by the steering wheel in a road traffic accident.[13] The infrarenal segment is most commonly involved (92% of reported cases) with the most common injury being intimal disruption with ensuing aortic thrombosis. Aortic contusion, dissecting intramural hematoma, pseudoaneurysm, and frank rupture have also been reported.

AXIOM Blunt aortic contusion may not cause signs and symptoms for days or weeks until the aorta becomes thrombosed.

Patients with blunt aorta injuries usually present with signs of an acute abdomen or arterial insufficiency; however, some of these in-

TABLE 27–1 Mortality Rates with Abdominal Injuries Seen in 12 Years at Detroit Receiving Hospital (1980-1992)

Organ Injured	Blunt	GSW	Stabs	Total
Liver	56 (160) 35%	110 (499) 22%	19 (251) 8%	185 (910) 20%
Small Bowel	14 (58) 24%	75 (551) 14%	10 (450) 7%	99 (759) 13%
Colon	7 (42) 17%	69 (498) 14%	7 (122) 6%	83 (662) 13%
Diaphragm	7 (28) 25%	59 (273) 22%	10 (119) 8%	76 (420) 18%
Kidney	10 (145) 7%	40 (229) 17%	6 (45) 13%	56 (419) 13%
Spleen	26 (172) 15%	31 (131) 24%	4 (42) 10%	61 (345) 18%
Stomach	3 (6) 50%	53 (241) 22%	10 (93) 11%	66 (340) 19%
Abd. Vessels	16 (23) 70%	135 (257) 53%	17 (53) 32%	168 (333) 58%
Pancreas	2 (33) 6%	34 (140) 24%	11 (37) 30%	47 (210) 22%
Duodenum	3 (10) 30%	29 (124) 23%	7 (33) 21%	39 (167) 23%
Bladder	8 (44) 18%	5 (84) 6%	1 (6) 17%	14 (134) 10%
Gallbladder	3 (3) 100%	14 (59) 24%	1 (19) 5%	18 (81) 22%
Total	92 (573) 16%	192 (1358) 14%	40 (810) 5%	326 (2741) 12%

symptoms consisting of claudication in 50%, decreased pulses in 42%, and an audible bruit in 42%. For the delayed presentation group, the average delay to operation was 21 months (range: 1 day to 9 years).

In their review of the literature, Reisman and Morgan[14] noted that only one of the 39 blunt aortic injuries was above the renal vessels. Twenty-two were between the renal vessels and inferior mesenteric artery, 13 were at the level of the inferior mesenteric artery, and three were at the aortic bifurcation. Although atherosclerosis has been thought to be a factor in this injury, it was present in only 44% of these cases.

Another cause of major abdominal vascular injuries is trauma associated with the wearing of seat belts.[15,16] The commonest site of damage is the aortic bifurcation; the pathology usually involved is an intimal tear with subacute thrombosis. There is a high incidence of associated bowel injury.

Severe, direct blows to the abdomen can also cause complete disruption of various vessels, especially the left renal vein where it crosses over the aorta,[17] and the abdominal aorta just distal to the renal vessels. These disruptions often lead to the development of false aneurysms.[15,19]

Iatrogenic injuries to major abdominal vessels are uncommon problems, but may occur during various diagnostic procedures (angiography, cardiac catheterization, or laparoscopy), abdominal operations, spinal operations (especially removal of herniated disks), cardiopulmonary bypass, and intraaortic balloon pumping.[20-22]

DIAGNOSIS

History

Penetrating wounds of the trunk between the nipple line and groin should be assumed to have penetrated the abdomen. Increasing abdominal pain and tenderness associated with hypotension should raise suspicion of bleeding within the abdomen. Similar symptoms and signs with blunt trauma should also make one suspect intra-abdominal vascular injury. Shoulder pain or pain with breathing may be referred pain from blood irritating the diaphragm.

juries do not become apparent until weeks, months, or even years later.[13]

In the series of abdominal aortic injuries reported by Reisman and Morgan,[14] 27 (73%) had an acute presentation, with 70% having neurologic findings and 96% having decreased peripheral pulses. Twelve (27%) had a delayed presentation with presenting

TABLE 27–2 Associated Injuries and Mortality Rates with Abdominal Vessel Injuries

	Blunt	Penetrating	SGW	Stab	Total
Liver	13 (17) 76%	66 (120) 55%	3 (4) 75%	8 (22) 36%	90 (163) 55%
Small Bowel	3 (4) 75%	51 (118) 43%	7 (10) 70%	7 (18) 39%	68 (150) 45%
Colon	1 (3) 33%	46 (92) 50%	4 (8) 50%	4 (11) 36%	55 (114) 48%
Duodenum	0 (1) 0%	20 (60) 33%	2 (3) 67%	7 (15) 47%	29 (79) 37%
Stomach	1 (1) 100%	30 (58) 53%	3 (5) 60%	4 (12) 33%	38 (76) 50%
Pancreas	2 (3) 67%	19 (45) 42%	4 (6) 67%	9 (15) 60%	34 (69) 49%
Kidney	4 (6) 67%	20 (44) 45%	4 (4) 100%	4 (5) 80%	32 (59) 54%
Diaphragm	3 (3) 100%	26 (42) 62%	1 (1) 100%	2 (5) 40%	32 (551) 63%
Spleen	6 (7) 86%	16 (28) 57%	2 (3) 67%	3 (4) 75%	27 (42) 64%
Total	16 (23) 70%	24 (241) 51%	11 (16) 69%	17 (53) 32%	68 (335) 50%

TABLE 27–3 *Abdominal Arterial Injuries and Mortality Rates*

Aorta			38/51 (75%)
	Diaphragmatic	6/7 (86%)	
	Visceral	18/18 (100%)	
	Pararenal	1/3 (33%)	
	Intrarenal	15/25 (60%)	
Iliac			34/58 (59%)
	Common	21/32 (60%)	
	External	8/18 (44%)	
	Internal	12/20(60%)	
Visceral			47/90 (52%)
	SMA	22/30 (73%)	
	IMA	2/4 (56%)	
	Mesenteric	1/8 (13%)	
	Colic	0/7 (0%)	
	Sup. Hemorrh.	1/2 (50%)	
	Celiac	4/8 (50%)	
	Splenic	4/10 (40%)	
	Gastric	3/18 (38%)	
	Hepatic	7/12 (58%)	
	Renal	7/16 (49%)	
Epigastric or Lumbar		2/9 (22%)	
Total Arteries			109/188 (58%)
Total Veins			118/249 (47%)
Total Abd. Vessels			168/335 (50%)

Fraction = number dead/total
( ) = Mortality rate

Physical Examination

AXIOM   Severe hypotension with a poor response to aggressive fluid resuscitation is usually due to continued bleeding which should be controlled rapidly in the OR.

Severe hypotension unresponsive to rapid fluid administration (2-3 liters in 10-15 minutes) with obvious abdominal trauma should make one suspect a major intraabdominal vascular injury. Loss of pulses to the legs may be seen with aortic injuries, whereas loss of the femoral pulses in only one leg occurs with an injury to the ipsilateral common or external iliac artery. A mass palpable within the abdomen, especially if it is pulsating and enlarging, may be seen with an enlarging hematoma from a major arterial injury.

Increasing abdominal distension, with persistent hypotension in spite of aggressive fluid resuscitation, implies massive continuing bleeding within the abdomen. Although this may occasionally be due to severe injury to the liver or spleen, it is more likely to be due to a major vascular injury.

Radiological Studies

FLAT PLATE OF THE ABDOMEN
The specific vessels injured by penetrating trauma may be inferred by the trajectory of the missile or knife wound. A flat radiograph of the abdomen with the entrance and exit marked or the location of a bullet within the abdomen may be of some predictive value. For example, injuries to the right upper quadrant may involve portal triad vessels, and midline injuries may involve the aorta or vena cava. However, the path of a bullet may be extremely capricious.

AXIOM   Injuries may occur to structures far outside the expected trajectory of bullets.

PELVIC FRACTURES
Continued bleeding in patients with pelvic fractures can be very difficult to manage. Although the superior and inferior gluteal arteries are the vessels most frequently found injured on arteriograms per-

formed for continued severe pelvic bleeding, the majority of blood loss is from injured veins and fractured cancellous bone.[23]

AXIOM   A laparotomy should not be performed just to control retroperitoneal bleeding from pelvic fractures.

It is much safer and effective to control the hemorrhage from pelvic fractures by application of a pneumatic antishock garment (PASG), or external stabilization of the pelvic fracture fragments. If significant bleeding continues, the involved arteries should be embolized by an interventional radiologist.

Intraabdominal bleeding sites outside the pelvis following blunt trauma are usually discovered during laparotomy because of a grossly positive diagnostic peritoneal lavage or other evidence of concomitant organ injury. In many instances, an interventional radiologist can also diagnose and control intraabdominal bleeding sites outside the pelvis.

IVP

Renal Vessels
Prelaparotomy suspicion of an injury to the renal vasculature usually comes from an intravenous pyelogram (IVP) or contrast-enhanced CT scan which shows nonvisualization or delay of visualization of one kidney. This implies renal artery or vein injury and is an indication for renal arteriography and/or surgical exploration.

AXIOM   Following trauma, nonvisualization of one kidney on IVP in a stable patient is usually an indication for renal arteriography or surgery.

CT SCAN
CT scans can demonstrate injuries to the solid intra-abdominal organs very effectively. It can also identify abnormal mass effects which may represent hematomas. Large amounts of free fluid in a patient who was hypotensive most likely represents blood. Use of intravenous contrast during the scan may demonstrate local collections of opacified blood, clots in vessels, or lack of opacification of some vessels.

Isolated injury to the infrarenal vena cava following blunt trauma is rare. In many patients with this injury, unstable vital signs preclude obtaining CT imaging prior to laparotomy. If a CT is performed, however, signs that should make one suspect caval injury are: (a) a retroperitoneal hematoma around the vena cava, (b) an irregular vena cava contour; and (c) extravasation of contrast-enhanced blood from the cava.[24]

TABLE 27–4 *Abdominal Venous Injuries and Mortality Rates*

Inf. Vena Cava			68/124 (55%)
	Intrarenal	28/58 (48%)	
	Pararenal	6/10 (60%)	
	Infrahepatic	19/40 (48%)	
	Retrohepatic	18/20 (90%)	
Iliac Veins			37/67 (55%)
	Common	19/37 (51%)	
	External	6/14 (43%)	
	Internal	20/34 (59%)	
Visceral			28/65 (43%)
	SMV	13/23 (57%)	
	IMV	4/7 (57%)	
	Mesenteric	1/8 (13%)	
	Splenic	5/10 (50%)	
	Renal	13/31 (42%)	
Total Veins			118/249 (47%)
Total Arteries			109/188 (58%)
Total Abd. Vessels			168/335 (50%)

Absence of both renal enhancement and excretion of intravenous contrast in the presence of a cortical rim sign is virtually diagnostic of blunt thrombosis of the renal artery, and arteriography is generally not necessary prior to corrective surgery if this radiological sign is present.[25]

ARTERIOGRAPHY

Preoperative abdominal aortography is seldom used to diagnose intraabdominal vascular injuries after penetrating trauma. However, it may be of some value in stable patients with other severe injuries. In patients with blunt trauma, aortography can be used to diagnose deep pelvic arterial bleeders associated with fractures[26] or to diagnose unusual injuries such as intimal tears with thrombosis in the infrarenal aorta,[8,13,15,16,18,19] iliac artery,[9,10,27] or renal artery.[28-30]

Diagnostic Peritoneal Lavage (DPL)

A diagnostic peritoneal lavage (DPL) will reveal gross blood in the majority of patients with significant abdominal vascular injury. The value of laparoscopy in abdominal trauma is unproven at this time, but it may be helpful in managing patients who are hemodynamically stable.

Laparotomy

AXIOM The diagnosis of abdominal vascular injury is most frequently made during a laparotomy for severe hemorrhagic shock.

During a laparotomy performed for trauma, control of active bleeding is of primary importance, and control is obtained initially with pressure applied digitally or with packs; later dissection can allow definitive treatment.[31] Not infrequently, major vascular injuries are well contained by a retroperitoneal hematoma or surrounding structures and will not be bleeding actively at exploration. In such instances, injuries to relatively large vessels can be missed quite easily.[32]

Patients with continued bleeding may be hypotensive on arrival at the hospital, but they often respond quite well to the initial fluid resuscitation. Later, if the patient does a Valsalva maneuver or if the retroperitoneum is opened before the surgeon is ready to handle such bleeding, the patient can rapidly exsanguinate.

PITFALL ⊘

Assuming that only a mild intraabdominal injury is present if the patient's initial hypotension is rapidly reversed by modest amounts of intravenous fluids.

RESUSCITATION

The majority of patients with significant intra-abdominal vascular injuries will be hypotensive on arrival to the emergency room. If the patient is moribund, the airway should be secured with endotracheal intubation and ventilation with 100% oxygen begun while two or three large intravenous lines are established. Evaluation of these patients should proceed rapidly following the advanced trauma life support guidelines, and the patient should be brought to the OR as expeditiously as possible.

ED Thoracotomy

AXIOM Resuscitative thoracotomy for cardiac arrest from abdominal bleeding is rarely successful; however, a prelaparotomy thoracotomy to cross-clamp the thoracic aorta can be lifesaving in patients who are severely hypotensive from intra-abdominal bleeding.

An emergency department (ED) resuscitative thoracotomy for a prehospital cardiac arrest due to intra-abdominal bleeding is rarely successful.[33] However, if cardiac arrest occurs in the ED or if the patient is about to have a cardiac arrest, an ED thoracotomy with cross-clamping of the descending thoracic aorta can be used to maintain cerebral and coronary flow until a celiotomy to obtain vascular control can be performed. This may provide the patient's only chance for survival.[34]

Fluid Resuscitation

Intravenous access should be accomplished rapidly by a minimum of two, and preferably three, large-bore intravenous catheters in upper extremity veins. If the patient does not have adequate extremity veins to permit this, central venous catheterization should be done rapidly. Insertion of large intravenous catheters into the internal jugular veins has been reported to cause less complications than insertion into subclavian veins; however, the intravenous routes chosen should be the ones with which the resuscitating physicians are most familiar.

Cutdowns or percutaneous intravenous line placement in the lower extremities may be of limited utility in patients with abdominal trauma. If there is an injury to the external or common iliac veins or to the inferior vena cava, the fluid that is given via lower extremity veins may extravasate from the injury and have relatively little resuscitative value, particularly after the injured vessel is clamped. Also, there is a theoretical risk of clot dislodgment in a venous injury if it is subjected to high intravascular pressures from lower extremity intravenous fluid resuscitation.[35] Finally, these lines can often be time-consuming to place and can have significant complications.

AXIOM Lower extremity intravenous access should be avoided whenever possible in patients with suspected major abdominal vascular injuries.

At the time of venous line placement, blood is drawn for routine analyses and blood typing and crossing. Resuscitation with warmed intravenous fluid should be begun at a minimum of 200 ml/min and should be infusing as the patient is being moved to the OR. A "Level One" or other similar fluid-warming devices should be utilized if available.

AXIOM If the patient remains in shock despite aggressive fluid resuscitation, severe active hemorrhage is generally present, and early control of the bleeding sites is essential.

If hypotension persists for more than 30 minutes in patients with trauma, mortality and complication rates are increased five- to tenfold.[36] Patients whose BP responds to the initial resuscitation, but who continue to require large amounts of fluid to maintain their blood pressure, probably have severe continuing blood loss. Type-specific blood can be given after the initial 2-3 liters of isotonic crystalloid, but when cross-matched blood becomes available, this is the resuscitative fluid of choice. Each unit of packed red cells should be given with approximately 500-1000 ml of isotonic fluid.

Prevention of Hypothermia

AXIOM Hypothermia is a major cause of morbidity and mortality in patients with abdominal vascular injury.

Patients requiring massive fluid resuscitation and blood transfusions will almost routinely have a core body temperature of less than 35°C. Hypothermia, particularly with core temperatures <32°C, is frequently associated with poor cardiac performance and myocardial irritability. Furthermore, hypothermia greatly contributes to the development of coagulopathies.

The etiology of trauma-associated hypothermia appears to be related to the temperature of the environment, the temperature of the resuscitative fluids, and the types and length of incision used. Warming the resuscitation fluids and the operating rooms and keeping the patient covered as much as possible in the ED and OR can be very helpful. A transfusion device with rapid warming capabilities is also very beneficial.

PITFALL ⊘

> *Hypothermia can be induced rapidly by infusion of room-temperature fluids and by using resuscitation and operating rooms which are inadequately warmed.*

Maneuvers to help prevent and correct hypothermia in the OR include: (a) covering the patient's head with transparent plastic; (b) placing the patient on a heating blanket; (c) covering the lower extremities with plastic bags or a "space" blanket; (d) irrigation of the nasogastric tube with warm (42°C) saline; (e) irrigation of thoracostomy tubes with warm saline; (f) irrigation of open body cavities with warm saline; and (g) use of a heating cascade on the anesthesia machine.[37]

Pneumatic Antishock Garment (PASG)

Laboratory studies and retrospective clinical reviews have suggested that application of a pneumatic antishock garment (PASG) in the field may be beneficial in patients with abdominal vascular injuries, particularly in patients with a long transit time to the hospital.[38,39] The large prospective study from Houston by Mattox et al[40] however, documented that survival was actually greater in patients who did not have the PASG applied. This may relate to an increase in blood pressure, causing increased bleeding and increased loss of the patient's own red cells, platelets, and coagulation factors.

AXIOM An inflated PASG can reduce bleeding from fractures in the lower extermities or pelvis, but prolonged administration can cause a compartment syndrome.

If the patient arrives in the emergency center with abdominal distention and continuing hypotension in spite of a inflated pneumatic antishock garment, the garment should remain inflated until the anesthesiologist and surgeons have completed their preparations and the surgeon is about to make the incision.

Prelaparotomy Thoracotomy

Although the results of an ED thoracotomy for cardiac arrest from intra-abdominal bleeding are poor,[33] there is a definite role for prelaparotomy thoracotomy in the OR for proximal aortic control in patients with massive hemoperitoneum and continued severe hypotension (systolic BP <70 mm Hg).[41] Patients with significant intra-abdominal bleeding from an abdominal vascular injury will have a tamponade effect produced by the intact abdominal wall. Release of the tamponade by the laparotomy incision may cause a hypovolemic cardiac arrest before the bleeding sites can be controlled.

AXIOM Patients with massive hemoperitoneum and continued severe hypotension should have a prelaparotomy thoracotomy with thoracic aortic cross-clamping.

In a recent study, prelaparotomy thoracotomy with thoracic aortic cross-clamping helped to keep shock duration <30 minutes and blood transfusions to less than 10.[42] In patients at high risk for dying or developing serious abdominal infections (admission systolic BP <70 mm Hg, four or more associated injuries, and/or a colon injury), if shock was kept to <30 minutes and blood transfusions to less than 10 units, the mortality rate was reduced from 92% (24/26) to 0% (0/12). Thus, in patients presenting to the OR with massive intraabdominal bleeding and systolic BP <70 mmHg, a prelaparotomy cross-clamping of the thoracic aorta should be considered.[43] If there is no response to thoracic aortic cross-

clamping, the patient has terminal cardiovascular failure and prolonged surgical efforts are futile.

Following laporatomy, the thoracic aortic clamp should be moved to the abdominal aorta as soon as possible. Care must be taken not to let the systolic BP in the proximal aorta exceed 150-160 mm Hg. If proximal hypertension develops, left ventricular dilation can cause acute cardiac failure to develop rapidly.

AXIOM If the aorta is cross-clamped, the proximal aortic pressure should not be allowed to exceed 160 mm Hg.

DEFINITIVE TREATMENT

Conduct of the Operation

ANESTHESIA AND PREPPING

Anesthesia is induced by a rapid sequence technique with esophageal compression at the cricoid to reduce the risk of aspiration of gastric contents. Type-specific or low-titer O-negative blood may be given as necessary until fully cross-matched blood is available. The patient is prepped from knees to chin to allow access to the chest, femoral vessels, and/or saphenous veins if necessary.

ABDOMINAL EXPLORATION

The abdominal exploration is performed through a long midline incision. The incision should not violate the peritoneum until the fascia is divided over the entire length of the incision. The peritoneum is then rapidly opened and an aortic occluder is applied over the supraceliac aorta if the patient is hypotensive or develops hypotension on opening the abdominal cavity.

As soon as the abdomen is opened, easily removed blood and clots are rapidly evacuated and lap pads are aggressively packed into the areas of suspected injury to tamponade the bleeding sites. Bleeding from solid organs and small-to-medium sized vessels can usually be controlled with this technique. Although proximal and distal control is often needed for major arterial injuries, venous bleeding, such as from the vena cava or portal vein, can usually be controlled with digital and/or sponge stick pressure. Continued bleeding despite packing usually indicates a major vascular injury requiring definitive control, often with proximal clamping of the aorta.

According to Veith and Daly,[44] to obtain exposure of the supraceliac aorta, the liver is pulled anteriorly and to the right using a 2-inch Deaver retractor. The left hand of the surgeon is then placed below the liver, and the lesser omentum is bluntly opened with a finger. This provides access to the posterior peritoneum and the crura of the diaphragm, which in turn overlie the aorta above the celiac axis. Using the left index or middle finger, the surgeon opens the posterior peritoneum between the esophagus and aorta (Fig. 27–1). Then, using blunt dissection with posterior directed pressure, the muscle fibers of the crura of the diaphragm are opened down to the periadventitial plane along the anterior wall of the aorta. This opening in the crura of the diaphragm is extended by pushing the index finger upward and downward along the aorta. This same motion is used in a posteromedial and posterolateral direction to clear off the anterior, lateral and medial walls of the aorta for distance of 2-3 cm.

The second and third fingers of the left hand, which are placed laterally and medially alongside the aorta, then apply traction downward creating a space on either side of the aorta. No attempt is made to dissect the aorta circumferentially. A large aneurysm clamp with slightly curved blades that parallel the fingers of the left hand is then placed on the aorta in a vertical direction.

Operative Exposure

Operative exposure of injured abdominal vessels must be rapid and effective. Since the best therapeutic intervention may not be known until the injury is exposed, flexibility with respect to reconstructive options is essential. To clarify what is often perceived as complex

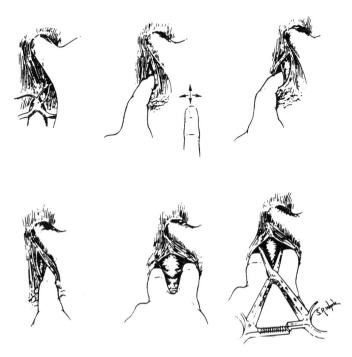

FIGURE 27–1 Exposure for clamping the supraceliac aorta through the abdomen. The heavy line in *(A)* indicates the location of the incision in the posterior peritoneum overlying the diaphragmatic crura. The muscle fibers of the diaphragmatic crura are digitally separated to gain access to the periadventitial plane of the aorta *(B)* The periaortic *(C and D)* plane is widened medial and lateral to the aorta. Inferior traction with the fingers creates a space on either side of the aorta, so that a totally occluding clamp can be applied *(E and F)*. (From Veith FJ, Gupta S, Daly V. Technique for occluding the supraceliac aorta through the abdomen. Surg Gyencol, & Obstet 1980; 151:427.)

anatomy and difficult operative exposure, several authors, including Fry et al,[45] have found it helpful to divide the abdominal arterial tree into four anatomic zones.

Zone 1

Zone 1 includes the suprarenal aorta, the celiac axis, the superior mesenteric artery, and the left renal artery (Fig. 27–2). Surgical exposure of these vessels can be achieved by dividing the peritoneal reflection of the descending colon, the splenic flexure and the peritoneum that attaches the spleen to the diaphragm and then moving all these viscera to the right side of the abdomen.

Zone 2

Zone 2 includes the entire infrahepatic IVC, right renal artery, the right side of the suprarenal aorta, the proximal right side of the superior mesenteric artery, and the common hepatic artery (Fig. 27–3). Exposure of these vessels involves incision of the peritoneal reflections of the right colon, hepatic flexure and the second and third parts of the duodenum with displacement of these structures to the left.

Zone 3

Zone 3 includes the infrarenal aorta and proximal common iliac arteries. The small bowel is rotated to the right upper quadrant to provide exposure in the mid-abdomen. The peritoneal reflection over the inferior aspect of the third and fourth portions of the duodenum is then incised and the duodenum and pancreas mobilized cephalad (Fig. 27–4). The incision into the retroperitoneum is made directly over the infrarenal aorta.

Zone 4

Zone 4 includes the common, external, and internal iliac arteries and veins. To expose the right iliac system, the cecum is mobilized cepha-

lad (Fig. 27–5). The bifurcation of the left common iliac artery is best exposed by reflecting the distal descending and sigmoid colon medially to the right.

GASTROINTESTINAL INJURIES

After major hemorrhage has been controlled with packs or vascular clamps, leaking gastrointestinal perforations are closed as quickly as possible with non-crushing clamps to avoid further contamination of the abdomen during the period of definitive vascular repairs. If only a few holes in the gastrointestinal tract are present, they may be closed rapidly with running sutures or with a stapler. Before any vascular repairs are performed, the abdomen is irrigated thoroughly. Following the vascular repairs, the injured vessels are covered with soft tissue, preferably omentum.

AXIOM Contained retroperitoneal hematomas should not be opened until actively bleeding vessels and gastrointestinal leaks are controlled.

If the patient has a contained retroperitoneal hematoma, the surgeon may have time to first perform the gastrointestinal repairs in the free peritoneal cavity, change gloves, and irrigate the abdomen with a warm saline solution. The surgeon can then expose and treat the retroperitoneal vascular injuries.[3]

PLANNED REOPERATION

Planned reoperations after an initial "damage control" operation are increasingly used in the management of critically injured patients.[46] The initial damage control operation includes measures to: (a) control bleeding, (b) prevent continued spillage of intestinal contents and urine, and (c) close the abdomen or chest. The patient is then warmed and resuscitated in the intensive care unit, until he or she is physi-

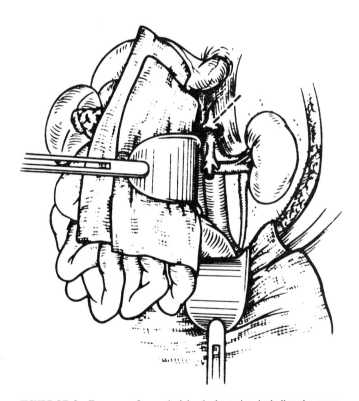

FIGURE 27–2 Exposure of zone 1 abdominal arteries, including the suprarenal and supraceliac aorta, the celiac axis, the superior mesenteric artery, and the left renal artery. To expose this zone adequately, the left colon, small bowel, and retroperitoneal gastric fundus are mobilized to the right. If the left kidney is mobilized to the right, the posterolateral surface of the aorta can also be visualized. (From Fry WR, Fry RE, Fry WJ. Operative exposure of the abdominal arteries for trauma. Arch Surg 1991;126:289.)

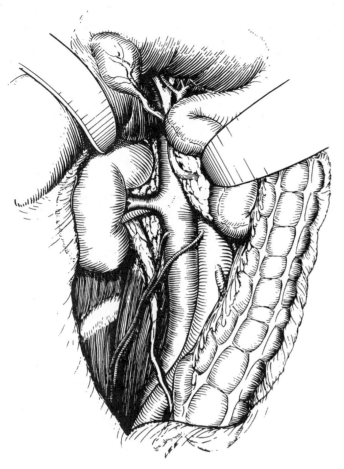

FIGURE 27–3 Exposure of zone 2 arteries, including the infrarenal aorta, inferior mesenteric artery and proximal iliac arteries, can be accomplished by mobilizing the right colon and hepatic flexure. A full Kocher maneuver is then performed to mobilize the duodenum and head of the pancreas medially to expose the orgins of the right renal artery and vein. This exposure also provides access to the inferior vena cava below the liver. (From Golocovsky M. Retroperitoneal vascular trauma. In Champion HR, Robbs JV, Trunkey DV, eds. Rob and Smith's operative surgery—trauma surgery, 4th ed. London: Butterworths, 1989; 556.)

ologically stable enough for a planned reoperation with definitive repair of the injuries.

There is increasing realization that some critically injured patients are unlikely to survive major definitive surgical procedures during the first operation. Prolonged operations and massive blood replacement in severely injured patients can lead to a triad of hypothermia, acidosis, and coagulopathy.

Hirshberg et al[46] recently reviewed the records of 124 patients treated over a two year period with planned reoperations. Penetrating injuries predominated (78%), and these primarily involved the abdomen or abdomen and chest. The initial precedure was terminated when direct hemostasis was impossible (102 patients), abrupt termination was required (56 patients), or the abdomen or chest could not be closed (20 patients). Some of the techniques employed at the initial operation included packing, rapid vascular control, gastrointestinal interruption, temporary urinary diversion, stapled lung resection, and plastic bag closures.

Seventy-three patients survived the initial procedure to undergo 101 reoperations. The first reoperation was planned in 52 patients and unplanned in 21 others who had their reoperation for bleeding or abdominal compartment syndrome. The overall mortality for patients having a planned reoperation was 58%. Survival was significantly better when the decision to abruptly terminate the initial procedure was made early.

Retroperitoneal Hematomas

Retroperitoneal hematomas are found in about 44% of patients who have a laparotomy for blunt abdominal trauma.[47] Since a significant vascular injury may be hidden in a retroperitoneal hematoma, no effort to open this should be made until proximal and distal control of the potentially involved vessels is obtained.

AXIOM   If a retroperitoneal hematoma is not expanding or actively bleeding, other intraabdominal injuries take precedence.

Feliciano has noted that hemorrhage from abdominal vascular injuries generally occurs in one of five locations:[48] midline supramesocolic, midline inframesocolic, lateral perirenal, lateral pelvic, and portal. If the hematoma or hemorrhage is superior to the transverse mesocolon, injury to the suprarenal aorta, celiac axis, proximal superior mesenteric artery, or proximal renal artery should be suspected. If the injury is in the midline below the mesocolon, one should suspect injury to the infrarenal aorta or inferior vena cava (IVC). Lateral perirenal hematomas occur with injury to the renal vessels or to the kidney. Lateral pelvic hematomas usually come from an injured iliac artery or vein. Major vascular injuries in the area of the portal triad below the liver usually involve the hepatic artery and/or portal vein.

Midline retroperitoneal hematomas above the pelvis are routinely explored (Fig. 27–6); however, lateral nonexpanding perirenal hematomas after blunt trauma are simply observed, unless the patient has been in shock or that kidney had not been visualized on IVP. Perire-

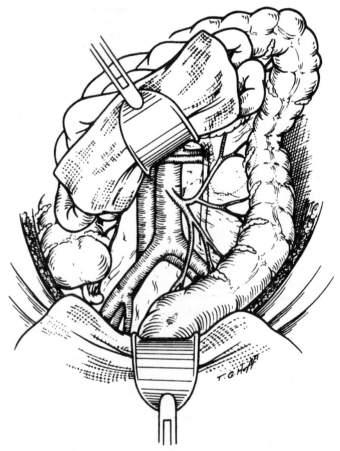

FIGURE 27–4 Exposure of zone 3 abdominal arteries, including the infrarenal aorta, the inferior mesenteric artery, and the proximal common iliac arteries. The ligament of Treitz is incised and the small bowel is rotated to the right upper quadrant. (From Fry WR, Fry RE, Fry WJ. Operative exposure of the abdominal arteries for trauma. Arch Surg 1991;126:289.)

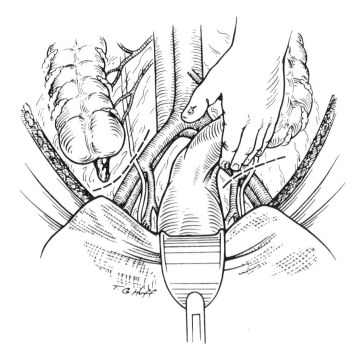

FIGURE 27–5 Exposure of zone 4 abdominal arteries. The arteries exposed include the distal common iliac, internal iliac, and external iliac arteries. (From Fry WR, Fry RE, Fry WJ. Operative exposure of the abdominal arteries for trauma. Arch Surg 1991;126:291.)

nal hematomas following penetrating trauma are routinely explored by some surgeons and explored only selectively by others. Routine exploration of these hematomas may lead to an increased nephrectomy rate; however, too selective a regimen may miss significant urinary leaks.

AXIOM   Pelvic hematomas following blunt trauma are usually due to bleeding from pelvic fracture sites and should not be opened.

If a pelvic retroperitoneal hematoma is expanding rapidly during exploratory laparotomy, the pelvis should be packed and the patient rapidly transported to the arteriography suite for embolization. Ligation of internal iliac arteries seldom, if ever, helps to control bleeding deep in the pelvis; however, injection of autologous clot into the internal iliac arteries may be effective.

Arterial Injuries

SUPRACELIAC AORTIC INJURIES
Penetrating injuries to the aorta as it enters the abdominal cavity carry a mortality exceeding 60% because of the difficulties in exposure and control of hemorrhage.[49] Injuries to this vessel should be suspected in patients with midline upper abdominal penetration and massive bleeding on exploration. A large midline, supramesocolic hematoma also suggests proximal aortic injury. Some surgeons believe that preoperative aortography is the procedure of choice for evaluating suspected abdominal aortic injuries due to blunt trauma in patients who are hemodynamically stable; however, it may be much easier and quicker to use CT to detect these injuries.

Surgical exposure of the suprarenal aorta, the celiac axis and the origins of the superior mesenteric artery and left renal artery (Fry, Zone 1) can be achieved by dividing the lateral peritoneal reflection over the descending colon, the splenic flexure, and the peritoneum that attaches the spleen to the diaphragm. The peritoneum is further divided as it reflects over the fundus of the stomach. This allows mobilization of the spleen, stomach, and left colon to the midline. The

left kidney can also be mobilized, but generally, the kidney should be left within Gerota's fascia. By dividing the splenorenal attachments, the left kidney can be left in its bed while the other organs are reflected. This exposes the posterior surface of the left colon, the pancreas, and the stomach. By dividing their loose areolar attachments posteriorly, these organs may be reflected beyond the midline.

AXIOM   Reflection of the left colon and abdominal viscera to the right is generally the best way to expose the supraceliac abdominal aorta rapidly.

The supraceliac aorta from the level of the superior mesenteric artery upward is covered with the left crus of the diaphragm. This can be divided in a radial fashion to provide exposure of the aorta from the left renal artery up to the eighth thoracic vertebra.[50] The spleen is mobilized until it is lying relatively free on the surface in the midline, but great care should be taken to avoid injury to this organ during the dissection.

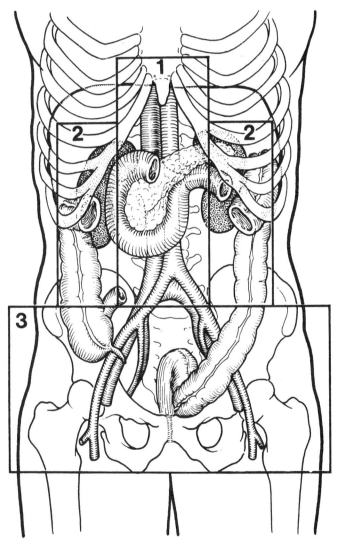

FIGURE 27–6 The retroperitoneum can be divided into three areas: zone 1 (the centromedial area), where hematomas are usually produced by injuries to the aorta, inferior vena cava, pancreas, duodenum or aortic or caval branches; zone 2, which contains the kidneys and suprapelvic ureters, and the right and left mesocolon and colon; and zone 3 (the pelvic area), which contains the rectum, posterior aspect of the bladder and distal ureters. (From Golocovsky M. Retroperitoneal vascular trauma. In Champion HR, Robbs JV, Trunkey DV, eds. Rob and Smith's operative surgery—trauma surgery, 4th ed. London: Butterworths, 1989; 556.)

To provide control of the thoracic aorta at a higher level, the midline laparotomy incision can be extended into the left chest along the seventh or eighth interspace. If the diaphragm is incised along its attachments to the ribs in a circumferential manner, the diaphragmatic blood supply and innervation are preserved.

If access to the left posterolateral surface of the lower supraceliac aorta is required, the kidney, along with its envelope of Gerota's fascia, may be reflected medially with the rest of the viscera. Disadvantages of this extensive mobilization include the time required to complete the maneuver, potential iatrogenic damage to the spleen, left kidney, or left renal artery during the maneuver, and the anatomic distortion that results when the left kidney is rotated anteriorly. If possible, one should leave the left kidney in its fossa, thereby eliminating potential distortion or twisting of the renal pedicle.

An alternative approach to provide added exposure to the suprarenal aorta is to divide the lesser omentum, retract the stomach and esophagus to the left, and split the crural muscle fibers digitally.[44] However, this procedure can be difficult if a large hematoma is present. Distal control is also difficult with this approach because the celiac and superior mesenteric arteries are in the way.

If active hemorrhage is coming from this area, the surgeon may attempt to control it by applying the aortic compressor high against the diaphragm.[51,52] If this does not control the hemorrhage, or if it does not allow dissection of the involved area, the abdominal incision should be extended into the chest so that the descending thoracic aorta can be clamped.

AXIOM The celiac artery can be ligated and divided at its origin to provide improved exposure of aortic injuries in that area.

On several occasions, when the injury was confined to the supraceliac aorta, Feliciano et al[3] have ligated the celiac axis to provide more space for their distal aortic clamp and subsequent vascular repair.

Following adequate exposure and control, the aorta should be debrided as needed and then repaired with 3-0 or 4-0 polypropylene suture. Stab wounds can usually be simply approximated with interrupted or running sutures without prior debridement; however, macerated or irregular vessel edges from gunshot wounds should be debrided prior to arteriorrhaphy. If the vessel is badly damaged or if the closure would result in significant narrowing, a patch graft or insertion of a vascular conduit is recommended. Farret et al[53] recently reported on the use of a saphenous vein spiral graft to reconstruct a gunshot wound of the suprarenal aorta.

Although concern exists regarding the placement of a prosthetic graft if there has been contamination by associated enteric injuries, septic complications are uncommon when Dacron grafts are used.[54] In a review of nine papers published between 1970 and 1987, Feliciano et al noted that only one of 40 Dacron interposition aortic grafts inserted for trauma with associated bowel injuries became infected.[3] Nevertheless, if an aortic prosthetic graft is required, exquisite care should be exercised not to allow contamination of the area of graft placement. The bowel injuries should be quickly isolated and packed away, and the operating team should change gloves prior to the vascular repair. Efforts to protect the completed anastomosis should include coverage with a pedicle of omentum, peritoneum or muscle.[55] Recently, fibrin glue containing antibiotics has been suggested to reduce graft sepsis in a contaminated animal model.[56] The retroperitoneum overlying the injury should then be closed in a watertight fashion.

If an aortic clamp has been in place for more than 30 minutes, the anesthesiologist should be warned at least 5-10 minutes prior to removing the clamp, so that additional fluid and blood can be given. The declamping should then be done very slowly so as to prevent central hypotension. Prophylactic administration of intravenous bicarbonate may be helpful to reverse the "washout acidosis" from the relatively ischemic lower limbs after the aorta is unclamped.[57]

The incidence of renal failure after aortic clamping is dependent on the aortic clamp time and also on the duration and severity of the pre-clamping hypotension.

AXIOM Great efforts should be made to limit aortic clamping to less than 30 minutes whenever possible.

Feliciano has noted that the survival rate of 151 patients with injuries to the suprarenal abdominal aorta in seven papers published between 1974 and 1987 was 36%.[3] However, associated injuries were major factors in outcome. According to a recent review from the Ben Taub General Hospital,[49] combined injuries to the suprarenal aorta and inferior vena cava had a 100% mortality rate.

CELIAC AXIS

AXIOM Celiac artery injuries should be ligated rather than repaired in patients with persistent shock and multiple injuries.

Injuries to the celiac axis and the proximal portions of its branches are difficult to repair because of the dense neural and lymphatic tissue in this area. Because of the technical difficulties of dissecting in this area and the excellent collateral blood supply of the branches of the celiac axis, prolonged efforts should not be made to repair isolated celiac, left gastric or splenic arterial injuries. The common hepatic artery can usually be identified by its larger diameter and its course toward the liver. Injuries to the hepatic artery proximal to the gastroduodenal artery generally can be ligated without incident. Although a simple lateral arteriorrhaphy may be possible with some arterial injuries in this area, complex procedures, including saphenous vein interposition or prosthetic graft insertion, should not be attempted. This is particularly pertinent in poor-risk patients; there is little or no benefit and there may be excessive blood loss and prolongation of operative time.

SUPERIOR MESENTERIC ARTERY (SMA)

The treatment of injuries to the SMA is dependent on the location of the injury.[58,59] Injuries at the aortic takeoff of the SMA may be approached by rotation of the left-sided abdominal viscera to the right to facilitate exposure of the aorta and the origin of the SMA and its proximal 2-3 cm. The left kidney, however, is left in its normal position. With injuries to the superior mesenteric artery beneath the pancreas (Fullen Zone 1) transection of the neck of the pancreas may be required to gain vascular control.[60]

In general, visceral arteries have excellent collateral circulation with the exception of the superior mesenteric, the renal and the proper hepatic arteries[61] (Fig. 27–7). Even the proper hepatic artery can be ligated safely, provided there is not an associated portal venous injury; however, the superior mesenteric and renal arteries should always be repaired.

It is usually safe to ligate the celiac axis provided its branches and the superior mesenteric artery are intact; however, ligation of the inferior mesenteric, left colic and distal superior mesenteric arteries can cause ischemic bowel which must be resected. Therefore, the collateral circulation to the bowel should be documented whenever possible. Prior to closure of the abdomen, the viability of the organs associated with the ligated vessels should be assessed carefully. If a saphenous vein interposition or prosthetic graft is required to repair an injury to the proximal SMA, it is safest to run the graft from the infrarenal aorta to the underside of the proximal SMA to avoid exposing the vascular anastomoses to secretions from the injured adjacent pancreas.

AXIOM Vascular anastomoses after abdominal trauma should be covered with omentum or other soft tissue to decrease the risk of infection and enteric fistulas.

The portion of the superior mesenteric artery at the base of the transverse mesocolon between the pancreaticoduodenal artery and the middle colic artery is known as Fullen's Zone 2.[60] Injuries in this area are difficult to repair because of the proximity of the pancreas and the usual large coexistent mesocolic hematoma. With severe in-

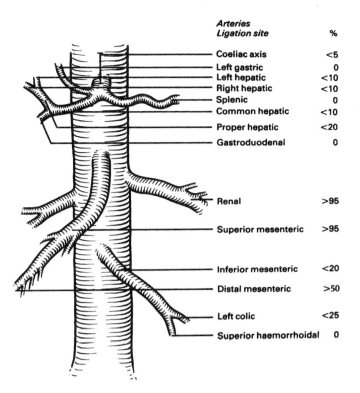

Arteries Ligation site	%
Coeliac axis	<5
Left gastric	0
Left hepatic	<10
Right hepatic	<10
Splenic	0
Common hepatic	<10
Proper hepatic	<20
Gastroduodenal	0
Renal	>95
Superior mesenteric	>95
Inferior mesenteric	<20
Distal mesenteric	>50
Left colic	<25
Superior haemorrhoidal	0

FIGURE 27–7 Risk of ischemic necrosis with interruption of branches of the abdominal aorta. (From Smith GJ, Holcroft JW. Mesenteric vascular trauma. In Champion HR, Robbs JV, Trunkey DV, eds. Rob and Smith's Operative Surgery—trauma surgery, 4th ed. London: Butterworths, 1989; 543.)

juries to the SMA in Fullen Zone 2, the SMA may be ligated.[61] However, the postoperative care of these patients should ensure adequate intravascular volume to maintain a good collateral blood flow to the intestines.

Injuries to the distal SMA beyond the middle colic branch (Fullen Zone 3) and at the level of the enteric branches (Fullen Zone 4) require repair because the injury is distal to the collateral blood supply. If the arterial injury cannot be repaired, a bowel resection may be required. If bowel of questionable viability is not resected, a "second look" within 24-48 hours is important. The survival rate of patients with penetrating injuries of the superior mesenteric artery from collected series averages about 58%.[3]

RENAL ARTERY

Diagnosis

Injuries of the renal artery may be identified preoperatively if angiography is performed. This is usually done if there is nonvisualization or delayed visualization of one of the kidneys on IVP or CT scan.

Authors of recent reports recommend CT as the initial diagnostic procedure of choice for the assessment of renal injury after blunt trauma.[62-63] Most authors agree that CT is of particular value for delineating renal parenchymal disruption, urine extravasation, renal and perirenal hematomas, and associated abdominal and retroperitoneal injuries. However, opinion is divided as to whether CT can be used accurately without angiography to detect post-traumatic occlusion of the main renal artery or a segmental branch.[64]

In 10 patients in whom post-traumatic occlusion of the main renal artery or one of its segmental branches was proven by angiography and/or surgery, Lopetin et al[63] found a termination of enhancement within the affected artery (renal artery cutoff sign) in one patient, and a thin, peripheral rim of renal cortical enhancement in an otherwise unenhanced renal segment (rim sign) in three patients. Thus, absence of a nephrogram on contrast-enhanced CT scans, particularly if a rim sign is present, is fairly good evidence of renal arterial oc-

clusion. At surgery, the first indication of a renal artery injury is usually a localized perinephric hematoma or a supramesocolic hematoma with lateral extension.[3]

Management

PERIRENAL HEMATOMAS

In patients who have suffered blunt abdominal trauma and have a normal preoperative IVP, renal arteriogram, or CT of the kidneys, there is no justification for exploring the kidney.[48] Although perirenal hematomas due to blunt trauma can often be observed, penetrating wounds of the kidney are generally explored unless it is clear by direct observation or CT scan that the pedicle is not involved. If a hematoma overlying a kidney is to be explored, it should not be opened until the surgeon has control of the proximal renal artery and vein.

AXIOM Hematomas overlying the kidneys may be due to renal parenchymal injuries which will heal spontaneously; an unnecessary nephrectomy may result if the hematoma is explored prior to control of the renal pedicle.

EXPOSURE

Exposure of the left renal artery is obtained by rotation of the left colon, spleen, and pancreas to the right, leaving the kidney in its retroperitoneal location (Fig. 27–8). If the renal artery injury is posterior, it may be visualized by mobilizing the kidney anteriorly.

Access to the left renal artery and vein may be improved by two maneuvers. Ligation of the adrenal, lumbar and gonadal tributaries markedly improves the cephalad and caudad mobilization of the left renal vein to expose the renal artery which lies posterior and cephalad to the vein. The second method to improve exposure involves li-

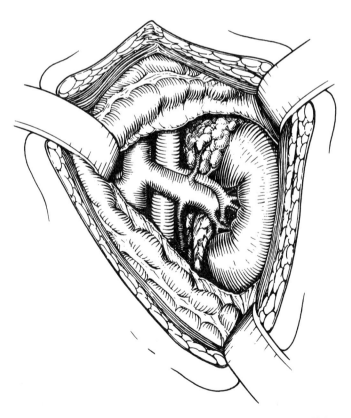

FIGURE 27–8 The left renal artery and vein can be exposed by mobilizing the left colon and small bowel to the right. (From Smith GJ, Holcroft JW. Mesenteric vascular trauma. In Champion HR, Robbs JV, Trunkey DV, eds. Rob and Smith's operative surgery—trauma surgery, 4th ed. London: Butterworths, 1989; 549.)

gation and division of the left renal vein at its junction with the inferior vena cava. The collateral drainage to the distal left renal vein is then provided by adrenal, lumbar, and gonadal veins.

Exposure of the right renal artery can be accomplished by incision of the peritoneal reflections of the right colon and hepatic flexure. The right colon is then reflected medially, exposing the duodenum. The peritoneal reflection over the second and third portions of the duodenum is then incised and a Kocher maneuver is performed to reflect the duodenum and the head of the pancreas to the midline. These maneuvers expose the inferior vena cava, the right renal vein, and the origin of the left renal vein. The origin of the right renal artery can now be exposed by mobilizing the inferior vena cava and proximal renal veins. The origin of the superior mesenteric artery may also be exposed with this technique.

AXIOM   The left renal vein may be ligated at its junction with the IVC to facilitate exposure of the right renal artery; however, the right renal vein must be spared to prevent venous infarction of that kidney.

Repairs

Renovascular injuries can be very difficult to manage, especially when the renal artery is involved. It is often deeply embedded in the retroperitoneum and closely surrounded by dense lymphatics, neural fibers and connective tissue. Repairs of the renal artery may be accomplished by lateral arteriorrhaphy or mobilization of the kidney with primary anastomosis.

Complex renal artery injuries requiring more than 30 minutes of vascular clamping require protection of the kidney from warm ischemia. Various maneuvers including ice packing and lavage, kidney excision with benchtop repair, and transposition to a pelvic location have been utilized to reduce the ischemic damage. Finally, nephrectomy may be required for severe renal arterial injuries or in patients with multiple injuries and excessive blood loss.

AXIOM   Before a nephrectomy is performed, one should try to ascertain that there is a functioning contralateral kidney.

Evidence that the contralateral kidney is functional includes visualization on IVP or continued good urine output if the vascular pedicle of the injured kidney has been clamped for some time.

Delayed Revascularization After Renal Artery Thrombosis

Controversy exists regarding the role of renal revascularization following delayed diagnosis of thrombosis of the renal artery from a contusion or intimal flap disruption.[64] These injuries are particularly apt to occur after high-speed deceleration motor vehicle accidents or falls from heights. Patients with renal artery occlusion may have few symptoms relative to the kidney, but some will have complaints of upper abdominal or flank pain from the ischemia.

The time interval from occlusion to revascularization appears to be a critical factor in the viability of a reperfused kidney. In one review of the problem, there was an 80% chance of restoring some renal function if the kidney was revascularized within 12 hours; however, this dropped to 57% if the kidney was not revascularized before 18 hours.[30] The low salvage rate and the 37% chance of delayed nephrectomy for postrevascularization complications, such as hypertension, have caused many surgeons to operate only if less than 12 hours have elapsed since injury.[28]

Once the area of the renal artery injury is visualized, mobilization of the injured renal artery will usually allow a limited resection of injured vessel and then an end-to-end anastomosis. Although some surgeons advocate perfusing the kidney with ice-cold fluid during the period of clamping, and some even recommend decapsulation of the ischemic kidney,[65] the value of these procedures is unclear. Most kidneys that have been ischemic for a few hours develop acute tubular necrosis, and it is usually not possible to determine if the revascularization was successful for at least 5-8 weeks.[29]

There are now five separate case reports in the literature that document either spontaneous revascularization and recovery of one or both kidneys after presumed blunt thrombotic occlusion of the renal artery.[66] These authors suggest that attempts at late revascularization may occasionally be rewarding, and they advise that early nephrectomy is unnecessary because of the low incidence of chronic hypertension.

AXIOM   Renal artery occlusions should be relieved within 6-12 hours; however, if this is not possible, immediate nephrectomy is usually not necessary.

INFRARENAL AORTA

Blunt Trauma

Abdominal aortic injury from blunt trauma is relatively rare and only one-twentieth that of blunt thoracic aortic injury.[67] Reisman and Morgan[68] found only 44 patients with abdominal aortic pathology secondary to blunt trauma in the literature since 1950. Their two patients brought that number to 46.

Both direct and indirect forces interact to cause blunt abdominal aortic injury.[68] Direct force on the abdominal aorta can occur from pressure against thoracolumbar fractures. Indirect forces can act in two ways: first, by transmitting the pressure of the initiating force through adjacent organs to the aortic wall with resultant increased intraaortic pressure. Complete rupture requires pressures of 1,000-2,500 mm Hg.[69] The second indirect effect is a shearing force caused by rapid deceleration.

Motor vehicle accidents cause the great majority of blunt abdominal aortic injuries. Some authors have focused on seatbelts as a cause of the aortic injury,[70,71] but only 41% of the patients reviewed were documented as wearing seatbelts at the time of injury. There is also some debate as to the importance of atheramotous disease in the injured vessels. Early reports concluded that arteriosclerosis was not related to the injury, but more recent literature seems to imply that the loss of elasticity and decreased compliance of the vessel may play an important role. Reisman and Morgan[68] found evidence of atherosclerotic disease in less than half of their patients.

AXIOM   The most controllable factor contributing to morbidity and mortality with blunt abdominal aorta injury is delay in diagnosis.

An awareness of the condition and a high index of suspicion are essential in making the diagnosis, and an abdominal aortic injury should be suspected in any patient with severe blunt abdominal trauma. Patients may complain of weakness or numbness of their lower extremities. Neurologic symptoms were noted in up to 70% of the patients reviewed.

The symptoms and signs of abdominal aortic injury are usually due either to ischemic peripheral neuropathy as described by Mozingo and Denton,[72] or to anterior spinal artery syndrome secondary to occlusion of the artery of Adamkiewicz. Objective findings suggesting an aortic injury may include abdominal or bilateral femoral bruits, diminished or absent femoral pulses, and coldness, cyanosis, or weakness of the lower extemities. If aortic injury is suspected, the patient should proceed to angiogram after being hemodynamically stabilized.

Blunt abdominal aortic injuries usually occur in the infrarenal aorta. This is due to the suprarenal aorta being somewhat protected from direct injury by the inferior bony thorax. The most common lesion is an intimal disruption, which can be partial or which can involve the entire circumference of the aorta. The inferior flap is then dissected downward by the blood flow. Thrombosis can then occur, causing acute arterial insufficiency. If all layers of the aorta are ruptured, this will lead to either false aneurysm formation or frank rupture.

The surgical treatment of this condition depends on the type and extent of the aortic injury. If the intimal dissection is not extensive, thromboendarterectomy with intimal flap suture can be performed, but if extensive injury has occurred, a prosthetic graft should be inserted.[68]

The high incidence of associated injuries emphasizes the need for thorough examination during the preoperative resuscitation. Recently, Shindo et al[73] described a patient who developed acute ischemia of both legs after an MVA due to occlusion of both popliteal arteries by atheroemboli from the abdominal aorta.

Penetrating Trauma

Access to Zone 3 of Fry et al, which includes the infrarenal aorta, the inferior mesenteric artery, and the proximal common iliac arteries can be gained by rotating the small bowel to the right upper quadrant (Fig. 27–4).[74] This exposes the third and fourth portions of the duodenum overlying the aorta. The midline retroperitoneum is opened directly over the aorta from the aortic bifurcation up to the left renal vein. The peritoneal reflection at the inferior aspect of the duodenum is then divided close to the duodenum where a relatively avascular plane exists. This is carried cephalad along the fourth portion of the duodenum with division of the ligament of Treitz. The duodenum and pancreas can then be mobilized cephalad to and above the left renal vein. This approach avoids injury to the inferior mesenteric vessels and left colonic mesentery.

The left renal vein can be divided at its origin from the IVC, if necessary, to gain more proximal exposure of the aorta. If the left renal vein is divided, it should be done as close to the vena cava as possible to avoid interrupting the collateral venous drainage of the left kidney. With this maneuver, several centimeters of the suprarenal aorta can be exposed and may be clamped as needed.

Injuries to the aorta in this area are repaired primarily whenever possible; occasionally a prosthetic graft is required. The retroperitoneal tissues are frequently thin in this location, making post-repair coverage difficult. Consequently, it may be worthwhile to cover an extensive aortic repair or aortic prosthetic graft by mobilized omentum if there are associated bowel injuries. The survival rate for 86 patients with infrarenal aortic injuries in five series quoted by Feliciano was 45%.[3]

INFERIOR MESENTERIC ARTERY

Injuries to the inferior mesenteric artery are less common than celiac axis or superior mesenteric arterial injuries.[75] Injuries to the IMA are suspected in patients with midline hematomas in an infrarenal location without aortic injury.[75] An injured IMA should generally be ligated as close to the aorta as possible.

ILIAC ARTERIES

Anatomy

The common iliac arteries arise at the bifurcation of the abdominal aorta, usually at the level of the L4 vertebra (Fig. 27–9).[76] The common iliac arteries bifurcate into an external iliac branch (which becomes the common femoral artery below the inguinal ligament) and the internal iliac arteries, which have multiple visceral and parietal branches. The collateral circulation in the pelvis is so extensive (Fig. 27–10) that ligating the internal iliac arteries generally has little effect on bleeding within the pelvis.

Blunt Trauma

AXIOM   Contained hematomas of the pelvis due to blunt trauma should not be disturbed unless the blood supply to the lower extremities is compromised.

An increasing number of iliac artery injuries due to major blunt abdominal trauma or pelvic fractures, particularly of the open type, have been described in recent years.[10,77] Nitecki et al[78] described two patients with seat belt injuries of the common iliac arteries. With blunt trauma, great efforts are made to not disturb the pelvic hematoma unless absolutely necessary to revascularize the lower extremities. If ad-

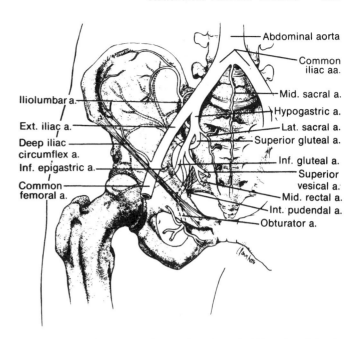

FIGURE 27–9   The common iliac arteries arise at the bifurcation of the abdominal aorta. The two major divisions are the external and internal (hypogastric) iliac arteries. The major branches are also shown. (From Rich NM, Spencer FC. Vascular trauma. Philadelphia: W.B. Saunders Co., 1978; 477.)

equate femoral pulses are present and the patient is hemodynamically stable, the pelvic hematoma is left undisturbed, and no further diagnostic or therapeutic efforts are required.

If the patient has intact femoral pulses but is bleeding excessively into the pelvis, and it is not controlled with external stabilization of the pelvis, arteriography is indicated. If the common and external iliac arteries are intact, the bleeding arteries, usually branches of the internal iliac artery, generally can be embolized radiographically.

If a common or external iliac artery is bleeding, it must be controlled. If these vessels cannot be repaired and must be ligated, an extraanatomic bypass, such as a cross-over femoral artery-femoral artery bypass or an axillary artery-femoral artery bypass, should be constructed. However, on rare occasions, the lower extremity may have to be sacrificed to save the patient's life.

Penetrating Trauma

Gunshot wounds which injure an iliac artery occasionally also cause severe pelvic fractures.[79] Iliac artery injury should be suspected in patients with large expanding pelvic hematomas or massive bleeding. Initial control of the hemorrhage during laparotomy is obtained by manual compression with laparotomy pads while proximal and distal control is accomplished.

Surgical access to this area (Zone 4 of Fry et al) may require no visceral mobilization (Fig. 27–4).[45] However, the ileocecal valve lies over the right iliac bifurcation, and it may be necessary to mobilize the cecum cephalad to gain adequate exposure to those vessels. The bifurcation of the left iliac artery is usually covered by the mesentery of the sigmoid colon. Rather than divide this mesentery, better exposure can usually be gained by reflecting the sigmoid colon and distal descending colon medially. This will also facilitate exposure of the left internal iliac artery as well as the left external iliac artery down to the level of the inguinal ligament.

Care must be exercised when looping the proximal common iliac artery to avoid iliac vein injury, especially in older individuals in whom vascular reaction to atherosclerosis may cause the common iliac artery and vein to be tightly adherent. Distal control is then attempted in the abdomen where the external iliac artery exits the abdomen. In external iliac artery injuries, distal control may have to be

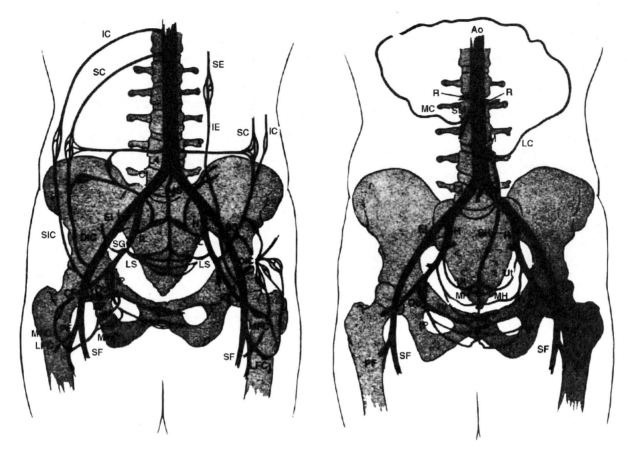

FIGURE 27–10   Branches of the iliac arteries form important potential collateral pathways: *(a)* parietal pathways and *(b)* visceral pathways. (From Rich NM, Spencer FC. Vascular trauma. Philadelphia: W.B. Saunders Co., 1978; 479.)

obtained on the common femoral artery or distal external iliac artery through an inguinal incision.

AXIOM   Isolation of a proximal common iliac artery can easily cause injury to an adherent iliac vein in older individuals.

The major difficulty in controlling iliac arterial bleeding is isolating the internal iliac artery to limit backbleeding. The internal iliac artery may be exposed by opening the retroperitoneum on the pelvic sidewall and placing traction on vascular loops around the proximal (common iliac) and distal (external iliac) arteries. The large branch dipping into the pelvis between the loops should be the internal iliac artery. This vessel may be looped at this point or ligated without ischemic sequelae.

Injuries to the common or external iliac artery should be repaired, preferably with a primary anastomosis. Ligation of either of these two vessels after trauma can result in a large number of amputations (40-50%).[80] If there is extensive pelvic contamination from associated bowel injuries, a prosthetic graft is at increased risk of becoming infected. If there is extensive contamination, the artery should be divided and the suture lines placed retroperitoneally. An extraanatomic graft may then be placed if the extremity appears to be in jeopardy at the completion of the procedure. In patients with prolonged lower extremity ischemia, the development of compartment syndrome must always be suspected.

AXIOM   Compartment syndrome should be suspected in any patient who has had lower extremity ischemia.

If a common or external iliac artery must be ligated to save a patient's life, particularly if the vein is also ligated, prophylactic lower extremity four-compartment fasciotomy is indicated. Prolonged ischemia to infrapopliteal tissues frequently causes muscle edema which leads to compartment syndrome. The availability of reliable systems to measure intracompartmental pressures has simplified early diagnosis and management of this problem.

The survival rate of patients with injuries to the iliac arteries will vary depending on the number of associated injuries to other major vessels. The survival rate in 189 patients in four recent large series collected by Feliciano was 61%.[79-82] If patients with other vascular injuries, especially to the iliac vein, were eliminated, the survival rate was 87%.[80,82] However, if the injury was large and there was free bleeding from the iliac artery into the peritoneal cavity during the preoperative period, the survival rate fell to about 45%.[80]

HEPATIC ARTERY

If a large hematoma or severe hemorrhage is present in the portal triad, injury to the hepatic artery or portal vein should be suspected. If there is continuing hemorrhage, a digital Pringle maneuver will often gain temporary control until some exposure can be obtained. After the proximal portion of the hepatoduodenal ligament is outlined, it should be looped with an umbilical tape or a noncrushing clamp should be applied to provide proximal control before opening the hematoma.

The common hepatic artery usually runs about 1-2 cm superior to the distal lesser curvature of the stomach and the first part of the duodenum. It can usually be exposed by reflecting the duodenum downward and incising the peritoneum in the lesser omentum.[45] In most instances, the gastroduodenal artery is the first branch and the right gastric artery is the second branch of the hepatic artery, but this order may be reversed. The gastroduodenal artery courses behind the first portion of the duodenum. The proper hepatic artery then courses cephalad toward the liver in the anteromedial portion of the hepatoduodenal ligament.

Because of the proximity of the common bile duct and portal vein, sutures should not be placed in the hepatic artery until precise identification of these structures and the arterial injury is attained. Lateral hepatic arteriorrhaphy can be difficult because the hepatic artery may be quite small in this area. Replacement of the artery with a substitute conduit is rarely indicated if portal flow is adequate, and ligation of the hepatic artery appears to be well tolerated, even beyond the gastroduodenal artery.[83-85] If the right hepatic artery is ligated proximal to the cystic artery, the gall bladder may become gangrenous and a "prophylactic" cholecystectomy should be performed.

AXIOM   If the proximal right hepatic artery is injured or ligated, the gall bladder should be removed.

Patients who have extensive liver injuries are at high risk of developing liver necrosis following hepatic artery ligation, especially if the liver is also packed to control bleeding.[86] Such packing can prevent portal venous collateral blood flow to the areas normally perfused by the ligated hepatic artery. Consequently, other methods to gain hemostasis for liver injuries should be used in these patients.

AXIOM   If the hepatic artery or one of its major branches is ligated, the liver should not be packed.

Venous Injuries

INFERIOR VENA CAVA (IVC)

Inferior vena caval injuries should be suspected in patients with retroperitoneal hematomas overlying the center of the abdomen. Hemorrhage from the vena cava can usually be controlled fairly easily by packing of the area or by manual pressure. As better exposure is obtained, more precise control can be provided by localized pressure with finger tips or with sponge sticks. The treatment of caval injuries depends on their severity and their location (Fig. 27–11).[87-89]

Retrohepatic IVC

Injuries to the retrohepatic IVC and/or hepatic veins are some of the most challenging vascular problems a surgeon can face. The short distance between the exit of hepatic veins from the liver and their entrance into the vena cava, coupled with the relative inaccessibility of the inferior vena cava and hepatic veins due to the diaphragm and liver, can make surgical treatment exceedingly difficult. A successful outcome depends on prompt volume restoration, a stratified selective management approach, and avoidance of hypothermia.[90]

Anatomically, there are usually two or three major hepatic veins (right, middle and left). In most patients, the left and middle hepatic veins merge to form a common channel before they enter the inferior vena cava.[91] There are also several short accessory veins that drain liver segments I and IV, and occasionally there is a short vein draining parts of the right lobe.[91-93]

The right hepatic vein runs between the anterior and posterior segments of the right lobe of the liver and enters the inferior vena cava anterolaterally.[93] It drains segments VI and VII, as well as part of segments V and VIII. The remainder of segments VIII and V is drained by the middle hepatic vein.[93,94]

In the majority of cases, the right hepatic vein runs outside the liver for approximately 1 cm and receives no branches in this part of its course. There is occasionally a superior or anterosuperior branch entering the right hepatic vein in its final centimeter.[91] With deceleration injuries of the right hepatic vein, there is usually avulsion of the vein from the vena cava or avulsion of the superior branch from the main right hepatic vein. Such injuries usually result in death from irreversible shock.[94,95]

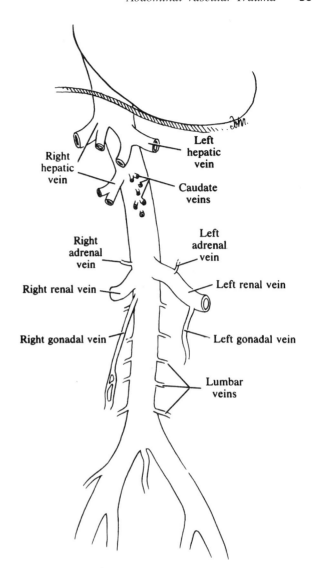

FIGURE 27–11   Anatomy of the inferior vena cava and its tributaries. (From Conti S. Abdominal venous trauma. In Blaisdell FW, Trunkey DD, eds. Abdominal trauma. New York: Thieme Medical Publishers, 1992;13:257.)

Major problems encountered in achieving hemostasis with torn hepatic veins are due to the difficulties with exposure of the retrohepatic vena cava, the risk of cardiac arrythmias or cardiac arrest if the cava is occluded, and the presence of small fragile caval branches that can be torn easily when the liver is rotated to improve exposure.[95]

AXIOM   Major retrohepatic venous injuries should be suspected in patients with severe bleeding posterior to the liver.

Attempts to visualize a major bleeding source in the retrohepatic area often result in more severe bleeding or enlargement of the vascular wound. Attempts to apply vascular clamps frequently results in further injury to the vessels; furthermore, once the site of injury is exposed, air embolism can occur.

If a retrohepatic caval injury is suspected and is not actively bleeding, it may be a good idea to avoid further dissection and judiciously pack the area to provide posterior liver compression.

Retrohepatic caval injuries which are bleeding actively can often be controlled by pressing the liver posteriorly digitally or with packs. The anesthesia team should be advised of the severity of the situation. The patient should receive warm blood in anticipation of further bleeding while control is accomplished. An intraoperative cell-saver can be very helpful in these situations. The midline laparotomy incision may be extended upward as a median sternotomy or as a right chest intercostal incision to provide access to the supradiaphragmatic vena cava. The retrohepatic IVC may then be controlled by vascular isolation or insertion of an atriocaval shunt. Caval isolation is accomplished by placing vascular clamps on the portal triad, the suprahepatic and infrahepatic vena cava and the abdominal aorta above the celiac artery.

AXIOM Clamping or accidentally compressing the IVC while the patient is hypovolemic can cause an almost immediate cardiac arrest.

Great care must be taken to avoid compression of the IVC at the diaphragm until or unless blood volume has been restored to greater than normal values or until the thoracic or upper abdominal aorta is occluded.

It is unclear how long the portal triad may be occluded without causing significant hepatic ischemia. Numerous clinical studies have documented the safety of occlusion times up to one hour without untoward effects. Induced surface hypothermia of the liver by application of iced slurry may be protective.

To visualize the retrohepatic cava adequately, the right lobe of the liver is fully mobilized. This usually allows visualization of injuries to the right hepatic vein as well as the anterior and lateral portions of the IVC. Depending on the number of tributaries communicating with the IVC, a substantial flow of blood may continue in the IVC despite vascular isolation. If bleeding is still substantial, one can improve visualization by inserted a Foley catheter or Fogarty balloon through the defect, inflating it and pulling the balloon up against the defect.

Initially the only survivors of major retrohepatic venous injuries were patients in whom a Satinsky clamp could be applied to control the bleeding and only partially occlude the inferior vena cava.[96] Some surgeons, such as Heaney and Jacobson,[97] have advocated complete caval occlusion to control the bleeding. Although this maneuver can be used relatively safely in elective hepatic surgery or transplantation,[98,99] it may reduce venous return so severely in a patient who is already hypovolemic that there is a high risk of cardiac arrest.[100,101]

In 1968, Shrock et al[92] recommended the use of an atriocaval catheter to control bleeding from the hepatic veins. They proposed inflow occlusion of the porta hepatis followed by atriocaval catheterization through a thoracic extension to the abdominal incision. Refinements in the technique have included exposure of the heart, usually through a median sternotomy, followed by insertion of a commercial atriocaval shunt through the right atrial appendage down to the suprarenal IVC.[102] A distal balloon is then inflated to provide secure hemostasis distally while a sidehole in the portion of the tube within the atrium allows venous return to the heart from the distal IVC to continue. If an atriocaval catheter is not available, a 34 F chest tube or large sterile endotracheal tube can be used.

AXIOM The decision to use atriocaval shunting should be made early because continued severe blood loss usually precludes a successful outcome.

To insert an atriocaval shunt, the pericardium is opened and a pursestring suture is placed in the right atrial appendage. The tip of the appendage is resected and the tube is gently inserted and directed downward into the suprahepatic inferior vena cava. The catheter is advanced down the IVC until the tip lies just superior to the renal veins. A distal balloon is inflated or a snare is tightened to secure the distal tube. The proximal side port should lie in the right atrial appendage. The pursestring on the atrium is then secured. Blood will now flow preferentially through the shunt from the infrahepatic IVC to the right atrium.

A properly functioning atriocaval shunt plus occlusion of the portal triad can greatly reduce blood loss from a torn retro-hepatic IVC. However, even then, back-bleeding from the superior vena cava and

phrenic veins may be difficult to control and may require snare occlusion of the suprahepatic vena cava around the shunt.

Occasionally, a hepatic venous injury can be approached directly through a deep central injury in the right lobe of the liver without resecting liver tissue. As the liver is opened directly down to the IVC, metal clips can be used on the larger bleeding vessels and cautery for the smaller vessels. After adequate exposure of the injured IVC or hepatic veins is obtained, the vascular defect can be repaired.

AXIOM With extensive lacerations of the liver, it may be safer and more effective at times to approach an injury to the retrohepatic cava transhepatically through an area of deep injury.

Difficulties in the expeditious insertion of an atriocaval shunt have led some surgeons[103,104] to attempt a transhepatic approach across uninjured liver to provide exposure of retrohepatic venous injuries. The liver is finger-fractured down to the injured vessels, which are then repaired. While Pachter et al[103,104] have reported some impressive patient survival statistics with this procedure, most surgeons do not use this technique unless a deep tear in the liver has already caused an almost complete right hepatectomy.

Shrock et al generally followed their atriocaval shunt with right hepatic lobectomy and repair of the hepatic vein and inferior vena cava. Even with atriocaval shunting, however, survival rates are poor. In one large report on atriocaval shunting in 18 patients,[105] only four (22%) survived and all four had penetrating liver injuries.

Another approach to the control of major retrohepatic venous bleeding is radiologically inserted balloon tamponade.[106] A balloon catheter can be inserted through the axillary artery into the upper abdominal aorta. Another balloon catheter, inserted through the internal jugular vein, could be placed in the retrohepatic inferior vena cava. During a subsequent, definitive laparotomy, both balloons can be inflated to control bleeding while the venous injury is repaired.

AXIOM In spite of multiple descriptions of methods to control blunt injuries to the retrohepatic vena cava or hepatic veins, mortality rates continue to be around 50-100%.[89,107,108]

Walt lamented in 1978 that there were probably more authors writing on the subject of juxtahepatic venous injuries than survivors.[109] Recent reports with atriocaval shunting for these injuries are somewhat more favorable. Burch et al[110,111] in 1988 reported a 19% survival in 31 patients with major juxtaheptic venous injuries treated with an atriocaval shunt.[108] However, technical problems related to the shunt were noted in 23% of their patients. Rovito reported a 50% survival rate in eight patients with blunt trauma requiring atriocaval shunting.[112]

In what appears to be the largest series of blunt hepatic venous injuries published, Holland et al[107] reported an overall mortality rate of 61% (25/41). With avulsion of the right hepatic vein from the IVC, the mortality rate was 80% (12/15) whereas avulsion of the upper branch of the hepatic vein was fatal in only 31% (4/13). The mortality rate with 13 other blunt hepatic venous injuries was 69% (9/13).

Despite occasional successes, there is general dissatisfaction with atriocaval shunts, and there are continuing efforts to develop alternative shunting methods for these injuries. Launois et al[113] for example, reported the successful use of extracorporeal circulation for the repair of a major juxtahepatic venous injury. However, this required systemic heparinization, which is usually hazardous in the multiple-trauma patient.

There has been a favorable experience using veno-venous bypass of the liver with a Bio-Medicus centrifugal pump both in human and animal hepatic transplantation. This active shunt consists of heparin-coated tubing draining the IVC and portal venous system with blood return to the heart assisted by a centrifugal pump. No significant clotting problems have been noted as long as bypass flow rates were maintained above 800 ml/min.[114]

The success of active shunting for liver transplantation stimulated Diebel et al[115] to construct a simplified version of this bypass using a pump to facilitate venous return from the infrahepatic IVC. Although this bypass was used successfully in animals, it caused significant splanchnic fluid sequestration as manifested by bowel edema and greatly increased fluid requirements during the study period. For prolonged portal vein occlusion, venous return from the portal circulation in the trauma setting could be provided by cannulating the inferior mesenteric vein.[116] Although shunt flow was increased markedly when both caval and portal venous blood was returned to the heart, this may not be necessary or practical in the trauma setting.

Suprarenal Cava

The IVC inferior to the liver and more than 1-2 cm superior to the renal veins is called either the suprarenal or infrahepatic IVC. Small injuries to the anterior surface of the IVC below the liver are usually easy to expose, control, and suture. However, care must be exercised to avoid occluding the IVC while controlling the bleeding because, even with hepatic venous flow continuing, complete occlusion of the infrahepatic IVC can cause hypovolemic patients to have a cardiac arrest.

Posterior wounds in the suprarenal IVC can be very difficult to expose and repair. If the posterior wound is not bleeding, occasionally it may be prudent to leave it undisturbed to heal spontaneously. Posterior wounds that are actively bleeding may be controlled by anterior pressure above and below the lesion while the anterior caval wound is enlarged enough to expose the posterior wound from inside. The repair can then be accomplished transcavally (Fig. 27–12A).[117] Alternatively, the IVC can be freed from surrounding tissue. Vascular clamps can then be placed in an anteroposterior plane and the IVC gently rotated until the posterior surface of the mid suprarenal cava is exposed (Fig. 27–12B).[117] In some cases, the right

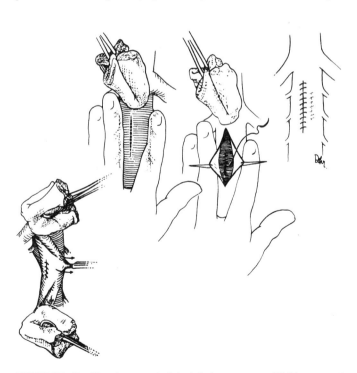

FIGURE 27–12 Vascular control of the inferior vena cava. *(A)* Management of a through-and-through wound of the inferior vena cava. Hemorrhage is controlled by direct pressure using sponge forceps proximally and distally and fingers on either side of the cava to compress the lumbar veins. The anterior wound is enlarged and the posterior wound is repaired from within. The anterior wound is then trimmed and closed. *(B)* The inferior vena cava can also be rotated for repair of a posterior wound after some lumbar veins have been divided and ligated. (From Conti S. Abdominal venous trauma. In Blaisdell FW, Trunkey DD, eds. Abdominal trauma. New York: Thieme Medical Publishers, 1992;13:273.)

kidney may have to be mobilized anteriorly out of its bed to be able to rotate the IVC adequately. Ligation and cutting of a few lumbar veins may also be necessary to provide enough mobility to expose and repair a posterior injury.

> **AXIOM** Ligation of the suprarenal IVC should not be done unless there is no other alternative to control bleeding.

If ligation of the suprarenal cava is contemplated, the portion to be ligated should be temporarily occluded with a vascular clamp to evaluate the degree of venous hypertension that will develop and the amount of renal function that will remain.[99] If urine output continues to be good (>0.5 ml/kg/hr) and the distal IVC pressure remains less than 30 cm H_2O, the IVC can be ligated relatively safely. Otherwise, ligation is contraindicated.

An alternative to suprarenal IVC ligation is a substitute vascular conduit. An externally supported PTFE graft may be very helpful. A portion of the inferior vena cava may also be utilized. Another technique involves a reversed inferior vena cava interposition. To accomplish this, the vena cava is divided just above the confluence of the common iliac veins. The lumbar veins are ligated and cut and the distal end of the IVC is swung up and anastomosed to the proximal end of the suprarenal IVC.

If an autogenous or prosthetic graft does not seem appropriate, the injury can be managed by a splenorenal or portocaval anastomosis. Another alternative is ligation with the idea that reoperation with reconstruction of this area can be performed as soon as the patient's condition has stabilized.[3]

Pararenal IVC

The portion of the IVC between the renal veins and 1-2 cm proximal and distal is sometimes referred to as the renal portion of the IVC. Injuries in this area are handled as are those in the suprarenal IVC, but control of the renal veins must usually also be obtained and the right kidney often must be mobilized from its bed to expose and repair posterior injuries.[110,111] The left renal vein can generally be ligated and cut at its junction with the IVC because it has an extensive collateral drainage.

> **AXIOM** Care must be taken to ligate, and not avulse, the first lumbar vein on the right, because in many cases it enters the junction of the right renal vein and inferior vena cava.

Infrarenal Cava

Attempts at visualizing the infrarenal IVC through the mesentery of the ascending colon can be difficult and dangerous. Optimal exposure of the infrarenal IVC is obtained by mobilizing the right colon, hepatic flexure, and duodenum towards the midline. This permits wide exposure of the IVC from the liver down to the iliac veins.

Care must be exercised when dissecting through the hematoma because the infrarenal cava is quite thin and easily injured. Direct pressure on the bleeding points generally provides acceptable hemostasis until vascular clamps can be applied carefully. Some authors have utilized Foley catheters inserted through the iliac vein to provide proximal and vistal control, but this is rarely necessary.

> **AXIOM** Injuries to the inferior vena cava can often be controlled better and more safely with digital pressure or with spongesticks than with vascular clamps.

It can be especially difficult to obtain proximal and distal control of the IVC at it junction with the common iliac veins.[3] Although sponge-stick compression can usually control the hemorrhage, exposure of posterior wounds can be extremely difficult. The distal IVC, and especially the proximal left common iliac vein are often obscured by the overlying aortic bifurcation. The aorta and iliac arteries usually have to be freed widely, and some lumbar arteries and the middle sacral artery must often be ligated and divided to provide adequate exposure. If there are no other significant injuries and the patient is very stable, the right common iliac artery can be divided to expose this area and then reanastamosed after the venous injury has been treated.

Another useful technique to control hemorrhage from the IVC is use of a Foley balloon catheter for tamponade.[118-119] The catheter is inserted into the IVC through the traumatic wound, the balloon is inflated in the lumen, and then pulled up to the hole to occlude it. A pursestring suture or a transverse venorrhaphy can then be formed. The balloon is deflated and the catheter removed as the sutures are tied.

Anterior wounds to the IVC can usually be repaired with a running suture of 5-0 or 6-0 polypropylene suture, preferably everting the edges. Everting the edges of veins when they are repaired ensures intima-to-intima approximation and should lessen the tendency to thrombosis at the suture line (Fig. 27–13).[117]

Transverse suture lines usually cause less narrowing than longitudinal repairs. Small posterior injuries that are not actively bleeding do not always require repair. However, if a posterior venorrhaphy is necessary because of bleeding, the IVC may be gently rolled after ligating and cutting the lumbar veins in the area of the injury. Alternatively, the anterior wound can be enlarged to allow an intraluminal repair, but this can be difficult because of continued venous return from lumbar veins.

AXIOM	Excessive efforts to mobilize the IVC to repair a small posterior wound may cause significantly more bleeding and damage than the original injury.

Ligation of the infrarenal IVC may be safer than repair in patients with complex injuries. Ligation of the infrarenal IVC is usually tolerated well hemodynamically unless the patient is hypovolemic. Consequently, the patient's intravascular volume should be assured before ligation, and a trial gradual occlusion with a vascular clamp should also be performed prior to ligation.

The long-term survival of these patients is largely determined by their associated injuries. Of 318 patients with penetrating injuries of infrarenal IVC collected from six papers by Feliciano, the survival rate was 75%.[3]

AXIOM	Long-term venous sequelae following infrarenal ligation of the IVC can usually be minimized by careful prevention of lower extremity edema and appropriate follow-up care.

The postoperative care of patients with IVC ligation should prevent excessive dilation of leg veins, which might render the values incompetent. This includes elevation of the legs for at least 5-7 days. Following this, the patient can ambulate with compressive wraps applied snugly to both lower extremities. If the patient develops lower extremity swelling or edema during ambulation despite the compressive wraps, full-length custom-made support hose are indicated upon discharge.

ILIAC VEINS

Iliac veins, after the IVC, are the most frequently injured of all the large veins in the abdomen. In a period of 12 years (1980-1992) at DRH, 37 patients had a total of 65 vein injuries with a mortality rate of 55%. In most instances, the iliac veins are injured by anterior trauma, but Feigenberg et al[120] recently reported on a patient with a life-threatening injury of an internal iliac vein caused by a stab wound of the gluteus.

Injured iliac veins are exposed using techniques similar to those described for injuries to the iliac arteries. It is not usually necessary to pass umbilical tapes around these vessels however, because they are readily compressible digitally or with spongesticks. Because the proximal left common iliac vein is somewhat inaccessible, transection and later reanastomosis of the right common iliac artery in hemodynamically stable patients has been suggested to improve exposure.[121]

Ligation and transection of an internal iliac artery can greatly improve exposure of an injured ipsilateral internal iliac vein.[122] Even if there is extensive bilateral injury, the internal iliac veins do not have to be repaired.

Injuries to the common or external iliac veins are best treated with either lateral or end-to-end repair using 5-0 or 6-0 everting polypropylene suture. In young patients, however, ligation of the common or external iliac veins is usually well tolerated if precautions are taken to prevent leg edema.[123] Nonetheless, repair rather than ligation is strongly recommended in many centers.[124]

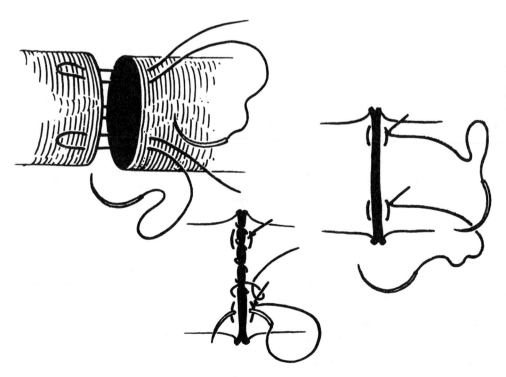

FIGURE 27–13 Horizontal mattress sutures ensure intima to intima approximation and should reduce the tendency toward thrombus formation at the suture line. (From Conti S. Abdominal venous trauma. In Blaisdell FW, Trunkey DD, eds. Abdominal trauma. New York: Thieme Medical Publishers, 1992;13:268.)

The amount of blood loss that can occur with iliac vein injuries can be extremely large. In many instances, the vascular injury in the pelvis that is the source of such massive and persistent blood loss may not be identifiable or accessible.[125] Ryan et al[80] were able to determine that 24 of their 97 patients with iliac vein injuries also had involvement of the presacral venous plexus, and these injuries can be extremely difficult to control.

Not infrequently, the initial attempts to control deep pelvic bleeding with packs is successful, and the BP comes up to normal levels with additional fluid and blood resuscitation. However, if the packs are removed to attempt more direct control of the bleeding sites, the BP often falls (usually to less than 80 mm Hg systolic).

> **AXIOM** If bleeding sites in the pelvis cannot be controlled during one or two inspections, and the patient becomes hypotensive during these inspections, one should pack the pelvis and close the abdomen.

Hemorrhage in the pelvis can usually be controlled adequately with careful packing. Such packs can then be removed in the OR under general anesthesia 1-3 days later, after the patient's hemodynamic and coagulation status have normalized. The injuries can then be reassessed more accurately and ligated or repaired as indicated and/or the pelvis can be repacked.

The survival rate of patients with injuries to the iliac veins is variable, but was 75% in 141 patients compiled by Feliciano[3] from three recent large series.[81-83] If patients with other vascular injuries, especially to the iliac artery, were excluded from the statistical analysis, the survival rate in 56 patients was 95%.

The mortality rate for iliac vein injuries in the series reported by Wilson et al[43] was much higher. Their mortality rate for injuries to the various veins were: common iliac vein 40% (6/15), internal iliac vein 65% (9/14), external iliac vein 29% (4/14), and two or more iliac veins 100% (6/6).

Although these patients obviously were severely injured, several deaths might have been prevented by earlier control of bleeding and a more rapid resuscitation, including restoration of core temperature to above 34° or 35°C. In several patients, early packing of the pelvis and closing of the abdomen, rather than persistent efforts to achieve definitive control of specific bleeding vessels, would probably have been better tolerated.

RENAL VEINS

It is difficult to differentiate renal vein injury from renal arterial damage prior to exposure of these vessels, which can be very difficult at times. Once the specific injury is identified, segmental renal veins may be ligated with few sequelae, but larger venous injuries should be repaired with fine vascular suture. The distal left renal vein may be ligated at the IVC if it is badly injured or to gain exposure to the proximal renal artery or aorta.[126] However, postoperative renal complications have increased in some series when this maneuver was used.[124]

Because the collateral venous drainage for the right kidney is limited, every effort should be made to repair injuries to the right renal vein. If the right renal vein must be ligated, and the left kidney is normal, a right nephrectomy is probably indicated.

The survival rate for patients with injuries to the renal veins from penetrating trauma has ranged from 42-88% in the recent literature, with the differences largely due to the magnitude and number of associated injuries.[35,127]

SUPERIOR MESENTERIC VEIN

The proximal superior mesenteric vein (SMV) lies just to the right of the SMA and injuries to this structure should be suspected when there is major bleeding at the base of the mesocolon. Treatment of proximal SMV injuries is complicated by the overlying pancreas, the proximity of the superior mesenteric artery, and its junction with the splenic vein. With some of the proximal SMV injuries, the pancreas may have to be transected to get adequate exposure for a repair.

Injuries to the more distal SMV can usually be sutured while the vein is compressed proximally and distally by the surgeon's fingers or non-crushing clamps. If multiple abdominal injuries are present, or the injury is impossible to repair, ligation may be the safest procedure. However, severe splanchnic congestion may develop postoperatively, and the patient's blood volume status must be watched carefully for at least three days.[128] In three recent series, ligation of the superior mesenteric vein was performed in 27 patients and 22 (82%) survived.[3,128-130]

> **AXIOM** In patients with extensive other injuries, ligation of an injured SMV may be much safer than a repair.

PORTAL VEIN (FIG. 27–14)

If a large hematoma or severe hemorrhage is present in the area of the portal triad, injury to the portal vein or hepatic artery must be suspected. Exposure should proceed as outlined for hepatic arterial trauma. Digital occlusion of the hepato-duodenal ligament, (Pringle maneuver) will usually control active bleeding until a vascular clamp can be applied. Mobilization of the common bile duct to the left, combined with an extensive Kocher maneuver, will usually provide adequate exposure of the majority of the portal vein.

Not infrequently, the neck of the pancreas must be divided to allow access to injuries to the retropancreatic portion of the portal vein (Fig. 27–15). In a recent series of 68 patients with blunt abdominal trauma reported by Henne-Bruns et al,[131] all five patients with portal vein injuries also had complete rupture of the pancreas.

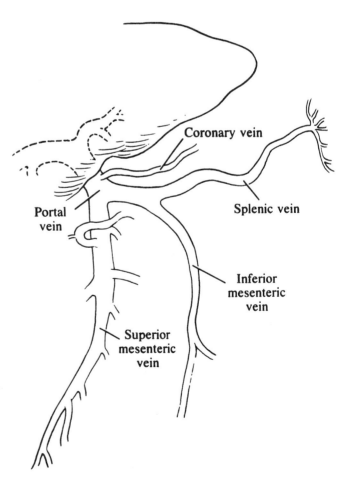

FIGURE 27–14 Portal venous anatomy. (From Conti S. Abdominal venous trauma. In Blaisdell FW, Trunkey DD, eds. Abdominal trauma. New York: Thieme Medical Publishers, 1992;13:259.)

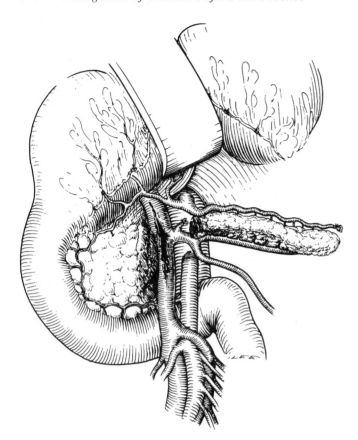

FIGURE 27–15 If uncontrolled bleeding is retropancreatic, the pancreas can be divided at its neck to expose the confluence of the splenic and superior mesenteric veins. If the venous injury is through the back wall as well, repair of the posterior wall can be accomplished through the anterior venotomy. One can then complete the procedure with a distal pancreatectomy, with or without a splenectomy. (From Smith GJ, Holcroft JW. Mesenteric vascular trauma. In Champion HR, Robbs JV, Trunkey DV, eds. Rob and Smith's operative surgery—trauma surgery, 4th ed. London: Butterworths, 1989; 549.)

With compression of the superior mesenteric vein below and a vascular clamp applied to the hepatoduodenal ligament above, the surgeon should gently open both ends of the retropancreatic tunnel over the anterior wall of the portal vein digitally or by a spreading motion with scissors.[3] If the gastroduodenal artery is in the way superiorly, it should be ligated and cut. When the tips of the surgeon's index fingers touch under the head of the pancreas, two straight noncrushing intestinal (Dennis) or slightly angled vascular (Glover) clamps or two large staplers are placed across the entire neck of the pancreas. The pancreas is divided between the clamps or staples and dissected and retracted away until the perforations in the portal vein can be adequately visualized.[3] One must be careful not to injure the many short, friable veins running from the posterior pancreas to the portal vein.

Injuries to the portal vein are frequently difficult to manage due to its posterior location, thin walls, and high flow rate. Techniques of repair vary, but lateral venorrhaphy with 5-0 polypropylene suture is preferred. End-to-end anastomosis, interposition grafting, transposition of the splenic vein, and portocaval shunting have been used because of concerns that portal vein ligation would cause venous infarction of the midgut.[130] However, all of these maneuvers take time, and if a portal-systemic shunt is performed, it can also cause postoperative hepatic encephalopathy.

AXIOM Ligation of a severe portal venous injury in an unstable patient may be much safer than a prolonged, complicated vascular repair.

Contrary to what was thought in the past, ligation of the portal vein is compatible with survival in many patients, as both Pachter et al[132] and Stone et al[128] have emphasized in recent years. In a review by Pachter et al,[132] only one of six survivors of ligation of the portal vein developed portal hypertension. The series in 1982 by Stone et al[128] included nine survivors out of 18 patients who underwent ligation of the portal vein. Thus, ligation of the portal vein can be a reasonable alternative if an extensive injury is present and the patient is hypothermic and acidotic. However, the surgeon must be prepared to infuse large amounts of fluids to reverse the central hypovolemia that will occur secondary to the splanchnic congestion and edema.[128] The survival rate of 134 patients with injuries to the portal vein collected by Feliciano was 50%.

HEMOSTATIC ADJUVANTS IN VASCULAR SURGERY

Hypothermia, thrombocytopenia, and dilutional coagulopathy frequently accompany major vascular injury and complicate hemostasis following successful vessel repair. By itself, hypothermia, particularly to core temperatures less then 32°C, can cause coagulopathies, and great efforts should be taken to prevent this problem.[133] Massive transfusions of bank blood increase the tendency to severe hypothermia, thrombocytopenia, and excessive bleeding. Finally, dilution and protein sequestration can lead to very low serum levels of factor VIII and XIII, further contributing to non-surgical bleeding.

Biologically based hemostatic agents can enhance native coagulatory mechanisms and improve local hemostasis.[134] Fibrin-based compounds have the added advantage of independence from the usual requirements for platelets or coagulation factors for hemostasis, and they can be effective during heparinization, thrombocytopenia, and various other coagulopathies.[135] In addition, the hemostatic effect may be tailored to the application site, avoiding unnecessary remote hypercoagulation risks and cost.

Fibrin Glue

AXIOM Localized bleeding in spite of surgical efforts can frequently be controlled by applying fibrin glue.

Fibrin glue mimics the last step in the natural coagulation cascade. Factor XIII and fibrinogen are activated by thrombin in the presence of calcium ion, converting fibrinogen to fibrin. Activated factor XIII polymerizes fibrin to form a stable clot. The thrombin in the glue is heterologously derived from bovine sources and is available in a variety of strengths. Although anaphylaxis to the bovine protein is a theoretical possibility, it is rarely of clinical importance, especially if care is taken to avoid intravascular application. The calcium ion serves both as a cofactor for the activation of factor XIII and to enhance fibrin crosslinking. Factor XIII and fibrinogen may be concentrated to provide increased adhesive strength; however, the hemostatic properties of the glue appear to be adequate without significant concentration.

The original fibrin glue described in European trials and in early United States experiences utilized pooled cryoprecipitate as the source of fibrinogen and factor XIII. Although the risk of hepatitis and AIDS transmission is apparent, none has been documented in over 3000 uses. Numerous methodologies, including predonation of blood, rapid concentration of native plasma, and solvent detergent treatment of donor plasma have been suggested as methods to decrease the potential viral transmission risk.[135,137]

Fibrin Gel

Fibrin gel is a physiologic variant of fibrin glue produced by rapid centrifugation of autologous plasma to provide the factor XIII and fibrinogen necessary for the preparation.[138] The resulting compound provides an effective hemostatic agent; however, the tensile strength and adhesive properties of the gel are less than fibrin glue because the fibrinogen concentration is lower. No cumbersome concentrating steps are necessary for the production of fibrin gel, thereby simplifying preparation and reducing cost. The fibrin gel may have the added benefit of a localized antibacterial effect secondary to activation of complement.

Vascular Surgical Uses

The majority of clinical reports involving fibrin glue or fibrin gel revolve around the hemostatic properties of the preparations. Fibrin glue and fibrin gel do not depend on native hemostatic mechanisms; therefore, their utility is greatest in situations where natural coagulation is defective or surgical control is difficult. Nevertheless, transient surgical control of the bleeding in these settings is essential; fibrin glue does not provide hemostasis during brisk bleeding.

AXIOM Fibrin glue and fibrin gel work best when bleeding from the area to which they are applied is temporarily controlled.

Fibrin glue may also be used to provide a hemostatic seal in knitted Dacron grafts to supplant preclotting.[139] An intriguing application of fibrin glue and gel involves the application of antibiotic-containing preparations to a contaminated field to allow subsequent placement of a prosthetic graft.[140] Several animal models have documented the antimicrobial efficacy of this approach to prevent localized sepsis, but clinical applicability remains to be defined.[140-141]

COMPLICATIONS OF INTRAABDOMINAL VASCULAR INJURIES

Hypothermia

Hypothermia is frequently seen in patients who have severe bleeding from abdominal vascular injuries, and this may contribute to coagulopathy and myocardial dysfunction. During the procedure, these patients should be placed on a warming blanket and receive warmed fluids and anesthetic gases. Once the bleeding is controlled, the abdomen should be irrigated with warm (42°C) fluid until the core temperature is at least 35°C.

AXIOM It is easier to prevent hypothermia than to correct it because of the impaired blood flow, acidosis and coagulation problems that accompany the lower temperatures.

Surgery in individuals with hypothermia should be performed rapidly, and every effort should be made to raise the core temperature to 35°C or higher as soon as possible. Once the vascular injuries are repaired or ligated, one can reduce OR time in patients with continued hypotension by perihepatic packing, single-layer closure of bowel injuries, colonorrhaphy instead of colostomy, and pyloric exclusion instead of resection.[4] Finally, towel clip closure of the skin of the abdominal wall or the use of a plastic silo sewn to the skin will allow more rapid wound closure and early transfer of the patient to the intensive care unit for continued resuscitation and warming.[37,142]

Maintenance of a normal arterial pH appears to be an important adjunct for survival.[3] In a patient who has remained hypotensive for some time, it may be difficult for normal compensatory mechanisms to correct an arterial pH under 7.10, and in many centers, supplemental infusions of bicarbonate are given until the pH is at least 7.20-7.25. It must be emphasized, however, that the PCO_2 must be kept in a range appropriate to arterial bicarbonate levels. The upper limit of acceptable $PaCO_2$ is equal to $[(1.5)(HCO_3) + 8]$. Giving bicarbonate and allowing hypercarbia to develop can greatly increase mortality rate.[36]

Coagulopathies

The majority of patients who arrive in the OR with active hemorrhage from a major abdominal vascular injury will require massive

transfusions. If more than 10 units of blood are required, the patient may develop a transfusion induced coagulopathy.[36] Although clinical coagulopathies often do not correlate well with laboratory clotting studies or platelet counts, any patient with significant bleeding and a low platelet count should receive platelet transfusions and fresh frozen plasma (FFP). The value of prophylactic fresh frozen plasma administration is unproven at this time and should be reserved for patients with clinical or laboratory coagulopathies.

PITFALL ⊘

Assuming that excess bleeding is due to a coagulopathy without first trying surgical control, especially if other areas are "dry."

Vascular Complications

The complications of vascular repairs in the abdomen include vessel thrombosis, ischemia to abdominal organs, dehiscence of suture lines, and infection. Vessel occlusion is not uncommon in the trauma situation when vasoconstricted vessels undergo lateral arteriorrhaphy or reanastomosis.

AXIOM If there is any question about a vascular repair, a completion arteriogram should be performed. If there is any question about intestinal viability, a second-look operation should be performed within 12-24 hours.[6]

Postoperatively, the diagnosis of ischemic bowel should be suggested by excessive abdominal pain or tenderness, an increased arterial lactate, or excessive uptake of intravenous fluids. Biorck and Hedberg[143] have suggested that tonometric monitoring of intramucosal pH (pH_i) in the sigmoid colon may provide early warning of gastrointestinal ischemia after aortic surgery. A gastric pH_i below 7.20 predicted major complications with a sensitivity of 100%, and a colonic pH_i below 6.86 predicted endoscopically detectable ischemic colitis.

A substitute vascular conduit placed in the area of the pancreas may be disrupted at any time if a pancreatic leak develops, and one must be prepared for this possibility. Vascular-enteric fistulas may develop after weeks, months or years if a vascular anastamosis is performed near bowel. The incidence of this problem can be reduced by covering the vascular suture lines with omentum, mesentery, or retroperitoneal tissues.

Infections

The high incidence of infection following intraabdominal vascular injury is probably related to the frequent occurrence of three main factors: (a) prolonged shock, (b) massive transfusions, and (c) associated bowel injuries. Thus, the incidence of infections is determined largely by the competence of the patient's host defenses, which in turn depend on the extent of the injuries and may be reflected by the patient's condition on arrival.[144]

The importance of colon injuries, particularly those requiring a colostomy, in causing an increased risk of infection after abdominal trauma has been noted in a number of reports.[145-148]

AXIOM The combination of massive transfusions, prolonged shock and intestinal spill will result in serious postoperative infections in at least a third of the patients who survive more than 48 hours.

In a recent series of 210 patients with abdominal vascular injuries, the incidence of serious infection in those who survived 48 or more hours was 37% (41/111).[42] Of the 41 patients with infections, 23 (50%) were intra-abdominal, and the mortality rate in the patients with abdominal infections was 35% (8/23).

Regardless of the patient's initial condition, the surgeon may be able to reduce the rate of infection somewhat by more aggressive fluid and blood resuscitation and by earlier intraoperative control of blood loss. A very strong correlation between mortality rate and duration of shock has also been reported in several other studies.[40-42,89,145,147]

AXIOM Patients with prolonged shock tend to be anergic, and consequently are more apt to become infected and less likely to show the usual signs of infection.

Blood loss should obviously be kept to a minimum. The strong correlation between the number of blood transfusions and mortality rates has been noted frequently.[40-42,89,149-151] Surgeons are becoming increasingly aware of the effects of massive transfusions on host defenses. Transfusions appear to decrease the incidence of rejection of solid organ transplants, inhibit the lymphocyte response to mitogens, and increase suppressor T-cell activity.[149] Nichols et al[145] also noted an increased risk of infection with massive transfusions, even when one factored out the presence of shock. In one recent study, all of the patients receiving more than 20 units of blood in 24 hours developed infections.[36]

SUMMARY

Abdominal vascular injuries are frequently seen in patients with penetrating wounds of the abdomen. The injuries may present with large hematomas and/or active bleeding. When a hematoma with tamponade of the bleeding vessels is present, proximal and distal control should be obtained prior to opening the hematoma. If active hemorrhage is present, direct compression with a finger, sponge stick, or lap pad at the site of injury is necessary until proximal and distal vascular control can be attained.

Vascular repairs, generally performed with polyproplyene sutures, can range from simple arteriorrhaphy or venorrhaphy to insertion of substitute vascular conduits. If hemorrhage can be quickly arrested, and the patient does not have significant associated injuries, most patients with major abdominal vascular injuries will survive.

AXIOM One should not hesitate to ligate important vessels if the vessel is not critical for survival, especially if a repair is apt to increase blood loss and prolong operating time.

⊘ FREQUENT ERRORS

In the Management of Abdominal Vascular Injuries

1. *Delaying surgery needed to control intraabdominal bleeding in an attempt to restore a normal blood pressure preoperatively.*
2. *Delaying surgery needed to control intraabdominal bleeding in order to perform urologic studies for hematuria.*
3. *Relying on only one or two standard-size intravenous lines or on lower-extremity veins for intravenous access when an abdominal injury with hypotension is present.*
4. *Opening a pelvic retroperitoneal hematoma following blunt trauma if the femoral pulses are satisfactory.*
5. *Assuming that the intraabdominal injury is mild if the patient's hypotension is rapidly corrected preoperatively with intravenous fluids.*
6. *Failure to take active early steps to prevent hypothermia.*
7. *Failure to rapidly correct hypothermia after the major bleeding sites are controlled.*
8. *Allowing proximal aortic pressure to rise above 160-170 mm Hg after the thoracic or abdominal aorta is cross-clamped.*
9. *Taking time to repair nonvital injuries when bleeding or other major trauma is present.*
10. *Inadequate debridement of tissue following a high-velocity missile injury.*

11. *Failure to interpose adequate tissue between vascular and intestinal repairs.*
12. *Exploring a perirenal hematoma without adequate prior control of the renal vessels at the hilum.*
13. *Failure to look for elevated lower extremity compartment pressures after temporary aortic or iliac artery occlusion.*
14. *Compressing or clamping the retrohepatic IVC in a hypovolemic patient without first clamping the abdominal or lower thoracic aorta.*
15. *Waiting until the patient is acidotic and cold before inserting an atriocaval shunt to bypass a severe retrohepatic venous injury.*
16. *Packing the liver to control bleeding from an area that has already had its major hepatic artery branch ligated.*
17. *Attempting a complicated portal vein repair in a patient with prolonged severe hypotension.*

▼▼▼▼▼▼▼▼▼▼▼▼▼▼▼▼▼▼▼▼▼▼▼▼▼▼▼▼▼▼▼

SUMMARY POINTS

1. Prompt control of bleeding and aggressive resuscitation, including rewarming, are the keys to success with intraabdominal vascular injuries.
2. Tissues damaged by high-velocity missiles may require extensive debridement to ensure that the remaining tissue is normal and will heal properly.
3. In addition to the wounding mechanism, the most important factors determining survival are the initial BP and its response to resuscitation.
4. Blunt aortic contusion may not cause signs or symptoms for days or weeks until the aorta becomes thrombosed.
5. Severe hypotension with a poor response to aggressive fluid resuscitation is usually due to continued bleeding which should be controlled rapidly in the OR.
6. Injuries may occur to structures far outside the expected trajectory of bullets.
7. A laparotomy should not be performed just to control retroperitoneal bleeding from pelvic fractures.
8. Following trauma, nonvisualization of one kidney on IVP in a stable patient is usually an indication for renal arteriography or surgery.
9. The diagnosis of abdominal vascular injury is most frequently made during a laparotomy for severe hemorrhagic shock.
10. Assuming that only a mild intra-abdominal injury is present if the patient's initial hypotension is rapidly reversed by modest amounts of intravenous fluids.
11. Resuscitative thoracotomy for cardiac arrest from abdominal bleeding is rarely successful; but prelaparotomy thoracotomy to cross-clamp the thoracic aorta can be life-saving in patients who are severely hypotensive from intraabdominal bleeding.
12. Lower extremity intravenous access should be avoided whenever possible in patients with suspected major abdominal vascular injuries.
13. If the patient remains in shock despite aggressive fluid resuscitation, severe active hemorrhage is generally present, and early control of the bleeding sites is essential.
14. Hypothermia is a major cause of morbidity and mortality in patients with abdominal vascular injury.
15. Hypothermia can be induced rapidly by infusion of room-temperature fluids and by using resuscitation and operating rooms which are inadequately warmed.
16. An inflated PASG can reduce bleeding from fractures in the lower extremities or pelvis, but prolonged administration can cause compartment syndrome.
17. Patients with massive hemoperitoneum and continued severe hypotension should have a prelaparotomy thoracotomy with thoracic aortic cross-clamping.
18. If the aorta is cross-clamped, the proximal aortic pressure should not be allowed to exceed 160 mm Hg.

19. Contained retroperitoneal hematomas should not be opened until actively bleeding vessels and gastrointestinal leaks are controlled.

20. If a retroperitoneal hematoma is not expanding or actively bleeding, other intraabdominal injuries take precedence.

21. Pelvic hematomas following blunt trauma are usually due to bleeding from the pelvic fracture sites and should not be opened.

22. Reflection of the left colon and abdominal viscera to the right is generally the best way to rapidly expose the superceliac abdominal aorta.

23. The celiac artery can be ligated and divided at its origin to provide improved exposure of aortic injuries in that area.

24. Great efforts should be made to limit aortic clamping to less than 30 minutes whenever possible.

25. Celiac artery injuries should be ligated rather than repaired in patients with persistent shock and multiple injuries.

26. Vascular anastomosis after abdominal trauma should be covered with omentum or other soft tissue to decrease the risk of infection and enteric fistulas.

27. Hematomas overlying the kidneys may be due to renal parenchymal injuries which will heal spontaneously. An unnecessary nephrectomy may result if the hematoma is explored prior to control of the renal redicle.

28. The left renal vein may be ligated at its junction with the IVC to facilitate exposure of the right renal artery; however, the right renal vein must be spared to prevent venous infarction of that kidney.

29. Before a nephrectomy is performed, one should try to ascertain that there is a functioning contralateral kidney.

30. Renal artery occlusions should be relieved within 6-12 hours; however, if this is not possible, immediate nephrectomy is usually not necessary.

31. Contained hematomas of the pelvis due to blunt trauma should not be disturbed unless the blood supply to the lower extremities is compromised.

32. Isolation of a proximal common iliac artery can easily cause injury to an adherent iliac vein in older individuals.

33. Compartment syndrome should be suspected in any patient who has had lower extremity ischemia.

34. If the proximal right hepatic artery is injured or ligated, the gall bladder should be removed.

35. If the hepatic artery or one of its major branches is ligated, the liver should not be packed.

36. Major retrohepatic venous injuries should be suspected in patients with severe bleeding posterior to the liver.

37. Clamping or accidentally compressing the IVC while the patient is hypovolemic can cause an almost immediate cardiac arrest.

38. The decision to use artiocaval shunting should be made early because continued blood loss usually precludes a successful outcome.

39. With extensive lacerations of the liver, it may be safer and more effective at times to approach an injury to the retrohepatic cava transhepatically through an area of deep injury.

40. In spite of multiple descriptions of methods to control blunt injuries to the retrohepatic vena cava or hepatic veins, the mortality rates continue to be around 50-100%.

41. Ligation of the suprarenal IVC should not be done unless there is no other alternative to control bleeding.

42. Injuries to the inferior vena cava can often be controlled better and more safely with digital pressure or with sponge sticks than with vascular clamps.

43. Excessive efforts to mobilize the IVC to repair a small posterior wound may cause significantly more bleeding and damage than the original injury.

44. Long-term venous sequelae following infrarenal ligation of the IVC can usually be minimized by careful prevention of lower extremity edema and appropriate follow-up care.

45. If bleeding sites in the pelvis cannot be controlled during one or two inspections, and the patient becomes hypotensive during each inspection, one should simply pack the pelvis and close the abdomen.

46. In patients with extensive injuries, ligation of an injured SMV may be much safer than a repair.

47. Ligation of a severe portal venous injury in an unstable patient may be much safer than a prolonged, complicated vascular repair.

48. Localized bleeding in spite of surgical efforts can frequently be controlled by applying fibrin glue.

49. Fibrin glue or fibrin gel work best when bleeding from the area to which they are applied is temporarily controlled.

50. It is easier to prevent hypothermia than correct it because of the impaired blood flow, acidosis and coagulation problems that accompany the lower temperatures.

51. One should not assume that excessive bleeding is due to a coagulopathy without first trying to obtain surgical control, especially if other areas are "dry."

52. If there is any question about a vascular repair, a completion arteriogram should be performed. If there is any question about intestinal viability, a second-look operation should be performed within 12-24 hours.

53. The combination of massive transfusions, prolonged shock and intestinal spill will result in serious postoperative infections in at least a third of the patients who survive more than 48 hours.

54. Patients with prolonged shock tend to be anergic, and consequently are more apt to become infected and less likely to show the usual signs or infection.

55. One should not hesitate to ligate important vessels if the vessel is not critical for survival, especially if a repair is apt to increase blood loss and prolong operating time.

▲▲▲▲▲▲▲▲▲▲▲▲▲▲▲▲▲▲▲▲▲▲▲▲▲▲▲▲▲▲▲▲▲▲▲▲▲▲▲

REFERENCES

1. Hughes CW. Arterial repair during the Korean War. Ann Surg 1958; 147:555.
2. Rapaport A, Feliciano DV, Mattox KL. An epidemiologic profile of urban trauma in America Houston style. Tex Med 1982;78:44.
3. Feliciano DV, Burch JM, Graham JM. Abdominal vascular injury. Ch. 34. In Moore EE, Mattox RL, Feliciano DV, eds. Trauma. 2nd ed. East Norwalk, CT: Appleton-Lange, 1991; 533-552.
4. Feliciano DV, Burch JM, Spjut-Patrinely V, et al. Abdominal gunshot wounds: an urban trauma center's experience with 300 consecutive patients. Ann Surg 1988;208:362.
5. Fischer RP, Miller-Crotchett P, Reed RL II. Gastrointestinal disruption: the hazard of nonoperative management in adults with blunt abdominal injury. J Trauma 1988;28:1445.
6. Cox CF. Blunt abdominal trauma. A 5-year analysis of 870 patients requiring celiotomy. Ann Surg 1984;199:467.
7. Frame SB, Timberlake GA, Rush DS, et al. Penetrating injuries of the abdominal aorta. Am Surgeon 1990;56:651.
8. Lock JS, Huffman AD, Johnson RC. Blunt trauma to the abdominal aorta. J Trauma 1987;27:674.
9. Smejkal R, Izant T, Born C, et al. Pelvic crush injuries with occlusion of the iliac artery. J Trauma 1988;28:1479.
10. Buscaglia LC, Matolo N, Macbeth A. Common iliac artery injury from blunt trauma: case reports. J Trauma 1989;29:697.
11. Strassman G. Traumatic rupture of the aorta. Am Heart J 1947;33:508.
12. Parmley LF, Mattingly TW, Manion WC, et al. Non-penetrating traumatic injury of the aorta. Circulation 1958;17:1086.
13. Lassonde J, Laurendeau F. Blunt injury of abdominal aorta. Ann Surg 1981;194:745.
14. Reisman JD, Morgan AS. Analysis of 46 intra-abdominal aortic injuries from blunt trauma: case reports and literature review. J. Trauma. 1990; 30:1294.
15. Dajee H, Richardson JW, Iype MO. Seat belt aorta: acute dissection and thrombosis of the abdominal aorta. Surgery 1979;85:263.
16. Warrian RK, Shoenut JP, Lannicello CM, et al. Seatbelt injury to the abdominal aorta. J Trauma 28:1505, 1988.
17. Feliciano DV. Abdominal vascular injuries. Surg Clin North Am 1988; 68:741.
18. Matsubara J, Seko T, Ohta T, et al. Traumatic aneurysm of the abdominal aorta with acute thrombosis of bilateral iliac arteries. Arch Surg 1983;118:1337.
19. Bass A, Papa M, Morag B, et al. Aortic false aneurysm following blunt trauma of the abdomen. J Trauma 1983;23:1072.
20. Rich NM, Hobson RW II, Fedde CW. Vascular trauma secondary to diagnostic and therapeutic procedures. Am J Surg 1974;128:715.

21. McDonald PT, Rich NM, Collins GJ Jr, et al. Vascular trauma secondary to diagnostic and therapeutic procedures: laparoscopy. Am J Surg 1978;135:651.

22. Kozloff L, Rich NM, Brott WH, et al. Vascular trauma secondary to diagnostic and therapeutic procedures: cardiopulmonary bypass and intraaortic balloon assist. Am J Surg 1980;140:302.

23. Moreno C, Moore EE, Resenberger A, et al. Hemorrhage associated with major pelvic fracture: a multispecialty challenge. J Trauma. 1986; 26:987.

24. Parke CE, Stanley RJ, Berlin AJ. Infrarenal vena caval injury following blunt trauma: CT findings. J Comput Assist Tomogr 1993;17:154.

25. Sclafani SJA. The diagnosis of bilateral renal artery injury by computed tomography. J Trauma 26:295, 1986.

26. Panetta T, Sclafani SJA, Goldstein AS, et al. Percutaneous transcatheter embolization for massive bleeding from pelvic fractures. J Trauma 1985; 25:1021.

27. McConnell DB, Trunkey DD. Pelvic vascular injuries. In Bongard FS, Wilson SE, Perry, MO, eds. Vascular injuries in surgical practice. East Norwalk, CT: Appleton-Lange, 1991;17:195-205.

28. Spirnak JP, Resnick MI. Revascularization of traumatic thrombosis of renal artery. Surg Gynocol Obstet 1987;164:22.

29. Barlow B, Gandhi R. Renal artery thrombosis following blunt trauma. J Trauma 1980;20:614.

30. Maggio AJ Jr, Brosman S. Renal artery trauma. Urology 1978;11:125.

31. Feliciano DV. Approach to major abdominal vascular injury. J Vasc Surg 1988;7:730.

32. Martella AT, Coomaraswamy M. Delayed presentation of a penetrating suprarenal aortic injury: case report. J Trauma 1993;34:148.

33. Washington BC, Wilson RF, Steiger Z. Emergency thoracotomy for penetrating trauma. J. Trauma, 1983;23:672.

34. Feliciano, DV, Mattox KL. Indications, technique, and pitfalls of emergency center thoracotomy. Surg Rounds 1981;4:23.

35. Accola KD, Feliciano DV, Mattox KL, et al. Management of injuries to the superior mesenteric artery. J Trauma 1986;26:313.

36. Wilson RF, Dulchavsky SA, Soullier G, Beckman B. Problems with 20 or more transfusions in 24 hours. Am Surgeon 1987;53:410.

37. Feliciano DV, Patcher HL. Hepatic trauma revisited. Curr Probl Surg 1989;26:453.

38. Traverso LW, Lee WP, DeGuzman LR, et al. Military antishock trousers prolong survival after otherwise fatal hemorrhage in pigs. J Trauma 1985; 25:1054.

39. Aprahamian C, Thompson BM, Towne JB, Darin JC, et al. The effect of a paramedic system on mortality of major open intra-abdominal vascular trauma. J Trauma 1983;23:687.

40. Mattox KL, Bickell W, Pepe PE, et al. Prospective MAST study in 911 patients. J Trauma 1989;29:1104.

41. Ledgerwood AM, Kazmers M, Lucas CE. The role of thoracic aortic occlusion for massive hemoperitoneum. J Trauma 1976;16:610.

42. Wiencek RG, Wilson RF. Injuries to the abdominal vascular system: how much does aggressive resuscitation and prelaparotomy thoracotomy really help? Surgery, 1987;102:731.

43. Wilson RF, Wiencik RG Jr, Balog M. Factors affecting mortality rate with iliac vein injuries. J Trauma 1990;30:320.

44. Veith FJ, Gupta S, Daly V. Technique for occluding the supraceliac aorta through the abdomen. Surg Gyencol & Obstet 1980;151:427.

45. Fry WR, Fry RE, Fry WL. Operative exposure of the abdominal arteries for trauma. Arch Surg 1991;126:289.

46. Hirshberg A, Wall MJ, Mattox K. Planned reoperation for trauma: a two year experience with 124 consecutive patients. J Trauma 1994: 37:365.

47. Henao F, Aldrete JS. Retroperitoneal hematomas of traumatic origin. Surg Gynecol Obstet. 1985;161:106.

48. Feliciano DV. Management of traumatic retroperitoneal hematoma. Ann Surg 1990;211:109.

49. Accola KD, Feliciano DV, Mattox KL, et al. Management of injuries to the suprarenal aorta. Am J Surg 1987;154:613.

50. Buchness MP, LoGerfo FW, Mason GR. Gunshot wounds of the suprarenal aorta. Ann Surg 1978;42:1.

51. Conn J Jr, Trippel OH, Bergan JJ. A new atraumatic aortic occluder. Surgery 1968;64:1158.

52. Mahoney BD, Gerdes D, Roller B, et al. Aortic compressor for aortic occlusion in hemorrhagic shock. Ann Emerg Med 1984;13:29.

53. Farret A, da Ros CT, Fisher CA, et al. Suprarenal aorta reconstruction using a saphenous spiral graft: case report. J Trauma 1994;37:114.

54. Rich NM, Hughes GW. The fate of prosthetic material used to repair vascular injuries in contaminated wounds. J Trauma. 1972;12:459.

55. Bunt TJ, Doerhosff CR, Haynes JL. Retrocolic omental pedicle flap for routine application to abdominal aortic grafts. Surg Gynecol Obstet 1984; 158:802.

56. Ney AL, Kelley PH, Tutu R, Tsukayama DT, Bubrick MP. Fibrin glue antibiotic suspension in the prevention of prosthetic graft infection. J Trauma 1990;30:1000.

57. Oyama M, McNamara JJ, Suehiro GT. The effects of thoracic aortic cross-clamping and declamping on visceral organ blood flow. Ann Surg 1983;197:459.

58. Accola KD, Feliciano DV, Mattox KL, et al. Management of injuries to the superior mesenteric artery. J Trauma 1986;26:313.

59. Lucas AE, Richardson JD, Flint LM, Polk HC. Traumatic injury of the proximal superior mesenteric artery. Ann Surg 1981;196:30.

60. Fullen WD, Hunt J, Altemeir WA. The clinical spectrum of penetrating injury to the superior mesenteric arterial circulation. J Trauma 1972; 12:656.

61. Smith GJ, Holcroft JW. Mesenteric vascular trauma. In Champion HR, Robbs JV, Trunkey DV, eds. Rob and Smith's operative surgery—trauma surgery, 4th ed. London: Butterworths, 1989; 539.

62. Cass AS, Viera J. Comparison of IVP and CT findings in patients with suspected severe renal injury. J Urol 1987;29:484.

63. Lopetin AR, Mainwaring BL, Deffner RH. CT diagnosis of renal artery injury caused by blunt abdominal trauma. AJR 1989;153:1065.

64. Brewster DC, Darling RC. Renal artery reconstruction. Surg Rounds 1978;1:18.

65. Stothert JC Jr. Renal blood flow and intrarenal distribution of blood flow after decapsulation in the postischemic kidney. Am surg 1980; 191:456.

66. Greenholz SK, Moore EE, Peterson NE, et al. Traumatic bilateral renal artery occlusion: successful outcome without surgical intervention. J Trauma 1986;26;941.

67. Lock JS, Huffman AD Johnson RC. Blunt trauma to the abdominal aorta. J Trauma 1987;27:674.

68. Reisman JD, Morgan AS. Analysis of 46 intra-abdominal aortic injuries from blunt trauma: case reports and literature review. J Trauma 1990; 30:1294.

69. Bergquist D, Takolander R. Aortic occlusion following blunt trauma of the abdomen. J Trauma 1981;21:319.

70. Randhawa MP Jr, Menzoian JO. Seat belt aorta. Ann Vasc Surg 1990; 4:370.

71. Dajee H, Richardson JW, Iype O. Seat belt aorta: aorta dissection and thrombosis of abdominal aorta. Surgery 1979;85:263.

72. Mozingo JR, Denton IC Jr. The neurologic deficit associated with sudden occlusion of abdominal aorta due to blunt trauma. Surgery 1975; 77:118.

73. Shindo S, Okamoto H, Nagai M, et al. Acute ischemia of the lower legs from blunt abdominal trauma: an unusual cause of atheroembolism—case report. J Trauma 1994;36:451.

74. Julian OC, Grove WJ, Dye WS, et al. Direct surgery of arteriosclerosis: resection for abdominal aorta with homologous aortic graft replacement. Ann Surg. 1953;138:387.

75. Graham JM, Mattox KL, Beall AC, et al. Injuries to the visceral arteries. Surgery 1978;84:835.

76. Rich NM, Spencer FC. Vascular trauma. Philadephia: WB Saunders Co. 1978; 475.

77. Rothenberger DA, Fischer RP, Perry JF Jr. Major vascular injuries secondary to pelvic fractures: an unsolved clinical problem. Am J Surg 1978;136:660.

78. Nitecki S, Karmeli R, Ben-Arieh Y, et al. Seatbelt injury to the common iliac artery: report of two cases and review of the literature. J Trauma 1992;33:935.

79. Mattox KL, Rea J, Ennix CL. Penetrating injuries to the iliac arteries. Am J Surg 1978;136:663.

80. Ryan W, Snyder W, Bell T. Penetrating injuries to the iliac vessels. Am J Surg 1982;144:642.

81. Sirinek KR, Gaskill HV III, Root HD, et al. Truncal vascular injury—factors influencing survival. J Trauma 1967;7:7.

82. Millikan JS, Moore EE, Man Way CW III, et al. Vascular trauma in the groin: contrast between iliac and femoral injuries. Am J Surg 1981; 142:695.

83. Mays ET, Wheeler CS. Demonstration of collateral arterial flow after interruption of hepatic arteries in man. N Engl J Med 1974;290:993.

84. Mays ET, Conti S, Fallahzadeh H, et al. Hepatic artery ligation. Surgery 1979;86:536.

85. Flint LM Jr, Polk HC Jr. Selective hepatic artery ligation: limitations and failures. J Trauma 19:319, 1979.

86. Lucas CE, Ledgerwood AM. Liver necrosis following hepatic artery transection due to trauma. Arch. Surg 1978;113:1107.

87. Weichardt RF, Hewitt RL. Injuries to the inferior vena cava: report of 35 cases. J Trauma 1970;10:649.

88. State DL, Bongard FS. Abdominal venous injuries. In Bongard FS, Wilson SE, Perry MO, eds. Vascular injuries in surgical practice. East Norwalk, CT: Appleton-Lange, 1991;16:185.

89. Wiencek RG, Wilson RF. Abdominal venous injuries. J Trauma 1986;26:771.

90. Klein SR, Baumgartner FJ, Bongard FS. Contemporary management strategy for major inferior vena caval injuries. J Trauma 1994;37:35.

91. Nakamura S, Tusuzuki T. Surgical anatomy of the hepatic veins and the inferior vena cava. Surg Gynecol Obstet 1981;152:43.

92. Schrock T, Blaisdell FW, Mathewson C. Management of blunt trauma to the liver and hepatic veins. Arch Surg 1968;96:698.

93. Bismuth H. Surgical anatomy and anatomical surgery of the liver. World J Surg 1982;6:3.

94. Waltuck TL, Crow RW, Humphrey LJ, Kauffman HM. Avulsion injuries of the vena cava following blunt abdominal trauma. Ann Surg 1970;171:67.

95. Millikan JS, Moore EE, Cogbill TH, Kashuk JL. Inferior vena caval injuries: a continuing challenge. J Trauma 1983;23:207.

96. Hansen JG. Avulsion of hepatic veins with survival. Am J Surg 1970;120:388.

97. Heaney JP, Jacobson A. Simplified control of upper abdominal hemorrhage from the vena cava. Surgery 1975;78:138.

98. Heaney JP, Stantion WK, Halbert DS, et al. An improved technic for vascular isolation of the liver: experimental study and case reports. Ann Surg 1966;163:237.

99. Starzl TE, Groth CG, Brettschneider L, et al. Extended survival in three cases of orthotopic homotransplantation of the human liver. Surgery 1968;63:549.

100. Doty DB, Berman IR. Control of hepatic venous bleeding by transvenous balloon catheter. Surg Gynecol Obstet 1970;131:449.

101. Yellin AE, Chaffee CB, Donavan AJ. Vascular isolation in treatment of juxtahepatic venous injuries. Arch Surg 1971;102:566.

102. Bricker DL, Morton JR, Okiec JE, et al. Surgical management of injuries to the vena cava: changing patterns of injury and newer techniques of repair. J Trauma 1978;11:725.

103. Pachter HL, Spencer FC, Hofstetter SR, et al. The management of juxtahepatic venous injuries without an atriocaval shunt: preliminary clinical observations. Surgery 1986;99:569.

104. Pachter HL, Spencer FC, Hofstetter SR, Coppa GF. Experience with the finger fracture technique to achieve intrahepatic hemostasis in 75 patients with severe injuries of the liver. Ann Surg 1983;197:771.

105. Kudsk KA, Sheldon GF, Lim RC. Atrio-caval shunting (ACS) after trauma. J Trauma 1982;22:81.

106. Little JM, Fernades A, Tait N. Liver trauma. Aust NZ J Surg 1986;56:613.

107. Holland MJ, Little JM. Hepatic venous injury after blunt abdominal trauma. Surg 1990;107:149.

108. Buechter KJ, Sereda D, Gomez G, et al. Retrohepatic vein injuries: experience with 20 cases. J Trauma 1989;29:1698.

109. Walt AJ. The mythology of hepatic trauma or Babel revisited. Am J Surg 1978;135:12.

110. Burch JM, Feliciano DV, Mattox KL, et al. Injuries of the inferior vena cava. Am J Surg 1988;156:548.

111. Burch JM, Feliciano DV, Mattox KL. The atriocaval shunt: facts and fiction. Ann Surg 1988;207:555.

112. Rovito, PF. Atrial caval shunting in blunt hepatic vascular injury. Ann Surg 1987;205:318.

113. Launois B, deChateaubriant P, Rosat P, et al. Repair of suprahepatic caval lesions under extracorporeal circulation in major liver trauma. J. Trauma 1989;29:127.

114. Griffith BP, Show BW, Hardesty RL, et al. Venovenous bypass without systemic anticoagulation for transplantation of the human liver. S.G.O. 1985;160:271.

115. Diebel LN, Wilson RF, Bender J, et al. A comparison of active and passive shunting for bypass of the retrohepatic IVC. J Trauma 1991;32:987.

116. Sloof MJH, Bams JL, Slueter WJ, et al. A modified cannulation technique for veno-venous bypass during orthotopic liver transplantation. Trans Proced 1989;21:2328.

117. Conti S. Abdominal venous trauma. In Blaisdell FW. Trunkey DD, eds. Abdominal trauma. New York: Thieme Medical Publishers, 1992;13:257.

118. Ravikuma S, Stahl WM. Intraluminal balloon catheter occlusion for major vena cava injuries. J Trauma 1985;25:458.

119. Feliciano DV, Burch JM, Mattox KL, et al. Balloon catheter tamponade in cardiovascular wounds. Am J Surg 1990;160:583.

120. Feigenberg Z, Ben-Baruch D, Barak R, et al. Penetrating stab wound of the gluteus—a potentially life-threatening injury: case reports. J Trauma 1992;33:776.

121. Salam AA, Stewart MT. New approach to wounds of the aortic bifurcation and inferior vena cava. Surgery 1985;98:105.

122. Vitelli CE, Scalea TM, Phillips TF, et al. A technique for controlling injuries of the iliac vein in the patient with trauma. Surg Gynecol Obstet 1988;166:551.

123. Mullins RJ, Lucas CE, Ledgerwood AM. The natural history following venous ligation for civilian injuries. J Trauma 1980;20:737.

124. Agarwal N, Shah PM, Clauss RH, et al. Experience with 115 civilian venous injuries. J Trauma 1982;22:827.

125. Owen DR, Hodgson PE. Control of hemorrhage following missile wound to the pelvis. J Trauma, 1980;20:906.

126. James EC, Fedde CW, Khuri NT, et al. Division of the left renal vein: A safe surgical adjunct. Surgery 1978;83:151.

127. Brown MF, Graham JM, Mattox KL, et al. Renovascular trauma. Am J Surg 1980;140:802.

128. Stone HH, Fabian TC, Turkleson ML. Wounds of the portal venous system. World J Surg 1982;6:335.

129. Kashuk JL, Moore EE, Millikan JS, et al. Major abdominal vascular trauma—a unified approach. J Trauma 1982;22:672.

130. Graham JM, Mattox KL, Beall AC Jr. Portal venous system injuries. J Trauma 1978;18:419.

131. Henne-Bruns D, Kremer B, Lloyd DM, et al. Injuries of the portal vein in patients with blunt abdominal trauma. HPB Surg 1993;6:163.

132. Pachter HL, Drager S, Godfrey N, et al. Traumatic injuries of the portal vein. Ann Surg 1979;189:383.

133. Patt A, McCroskey BL, Moore EE. Hypothermia induced coagulopathy in trauma. Surg Clin No Amer 1988;68:775.

134. Gestrin GF, Lerner R. Autologous fibrinogen for tissue adhesion, hemostasis, and embolization. Vasc Surg 1983;17:294.

135. Siedentop KH, Harris DM. Autologous fibrin tissue adhesive. Laryngoscope 1985;95:1074.

136. Durham LH, Willatt DJ, Yung MW, et al. A method for preparation of fibrin glue. J Laryngol Otol 1987;101:1182.

137. Lerner L, Binuer NS. The current status of surgical adhesives. J Surg Res 1990;48:165.

138. Dulchavsky SA, Geller ER, Maurer J, et al. Autologous fibrin gel: bactericidal properties in contaminated hepatic injury. J Trauma 1991;31:991.

139. Jones RA, Schoen FJ, Ziemer G, et al. Biologic sealants and knitted Dacron conduits: comparison of collagen and fibrin glue pretreatments in circulatory models. Ann Thorac Surg 1987;44:283.

140. Ney AL, Kelly PH, Tutu T, et al. Fibrin glue antibiotic suspension in the prevention of prosthetic graft infection. J Trauma 1990;30:1000.

141. Ing RD, Saxe J, Hendrick S, et al. Antibiotic primed fibrin gel improves outcome in contaminated splenic injury. J Trauma 1992;33:118.

142. Feliciano DV. Abdominal trauma. In Schwartz SI, Ellis H, eds. Maingot's abdominal operations. East Norwalk, CT: Appleton-Lange, 1989;457.

143. Bjorck M, Hedberg B. Early detection of major complication after abdominal aortic surgery: predictive value of sigmoid colon and gastric intramucosal pH monitoring. Br J Surg 1994;81:25.

144. Polk HC, George DC, Wellhausen S, et al. Study of host defense processes in badly injured man. Ann Surg 1986;204:282.

145. Nichols RL, Smith JW, Klein DB, et al. Risk of infections after penetrating abdominal trauma. N Engl J Med 1984;311:1065.

146. Shannon, FL, Moore EE. Primary repair of the colon: when is it a safe alternative? Surgery 1985;98:851.

147. Stone HH, Fabian TC. Management of perforating colon trauma. Ann Surg 1979;190:430.

148. Fry DE, Pearlstein L, Fulton RL, et al. Multiple systems organ failure: the role of uncontrolled infection. Arch Surg 1980;115:136.

149. Graves TA, Cioffi WG, Mason AD, et al. Relationship of transfusion and infections in a burn population. J Trauma 1989;29:948.

150. Jones RC, Thal ER, Johnson NA, et al. Evaluation of antibiotic therapy following penetrating abdominal trauma. Ann Surg 1985;201:576.

151. Wilson RF, Mammen E, Walt AJ. Eight years of experience with massive blood transfusions. J Trauma 1971;11:275.

Chapter 28 Pelvic Fractures

ROBERT F. WILSON, M.D.

JAMES TYBURSKI, M.D.

GREGORY M. GEORGIADIS, M.D.

INCIDENCE AND SEVERITY

Pelvic fractures are quite common in patients with severe multisystem trauma. They account for at least one of every 1,000 hospital admissions,[1,2] and represent 3% of all fractures.[3] They are the third most frequent type of injury found at autopsy in victims of motor vehicle crashes.[4]

> **AXIOM** Next to fractures of the skull, pelvic fractures make up the commonest type of skeletal injury associated with death in patients with multiple injuries.

The overall incidence of pelvic fractures in the U.S. is 37 per 100,000 person-years, with a gradual increase with age to a maximum incidence of 446 per 100,000 person-years in females aged 85 years or more.[5] These elderly women often have pelvic fractures with minimal falls because of an underlying severe osteoporosis.[5]

Although pelvic fractures are often considered to be severe injuries, over 80% are relatively minor. In one series, 30% of the patients with pelvic fractures did not even require admission, and of 533 patients with pelvic fractures in one series, there were only four (0.75%) deaths directly attributable to the pelvic injury.[6]

Most of the mortality and disabling morbidity with pelvic fractures occurs in a relatively small number of patients because of their association with major trauma involving adjacent major blood vessels and nerves and the genitourinary and distal gastrointestinal tract.

> **AXIOM** The main cause of death in patients with pelvic fractures is uncontrolled bleeding, usually from associated injuries.[1]

Late mortality from pelvic fractures is usually caused by pelvic or generalized sepsis and multiorgan failure resulting from contamination of large retroperitoneal hematomas from associated intestinal, genitourinary, or soft tissue injuries.

Mortality rates in excess of 80% were reported for pelvic fractures treated before 1900.[1] By the early 1900s, less than 40% of the patients died. By the 1930s, the mortality rate with pelvic fractures was reduced to 10-30%. During the past two decades, mortality rates in most reported series have ranged from 5-20% with morbidity rates of 33-74%.[5]

> **AXIOM** The outcome for patients with pelvic fractures is largely determined by the associated injuries.

Variations in the outcome of recently reported series primarily reflect the types of pelvic fractures seen and the severity of the associated injuries. If all fractures, including simple avulsions and isolated single breaks, are included, mortality rates average around 5%. With complex injuries, mortality rates range around 18-39%.[1,6]

In trauma victims with rapid access to modern-day comprehensive care, an isolated pelvic fracture should be an uncommon cause of death. However, the potential for long-term disability is great because of the frequent involvement of the lumbosacral plexus and pelvic nerves which control lower extremity, bladder, anorectal, and sexual function.

ANATOMY

The pelvis includes the sacrum and paired pubic, ischial and iliac bones. The pelvic ring consists of two innominate bones which represent fusion of the ilium, ischium, and pubis at the acetabulum.[1] Anteriorly, the pubic bones of the pelvis are joined at the pubic symphysis by a fibrocartilaginous disc. Posteriorly, the innominate bones articulate with the sacrum at the sacroiliac joints.

The articulation of the lateral surfaces of the sacrum with the iliac bones is held together by strong dorsal (posterior) sacroiliac ligaments, which together with the sacrotuberous and sacrospinous ligaments stabilize the sacrum and prevent posterior rotation of the pelvis. The anterior sacroiliac ligaments are thin, and their only real function is that of a joint capsule.

The major function of the pelvis is to serve as a weight-bearing structure for the trunk and lower extremities.[1] It also serves to protect lower abdominal viscera and act as an anatomic "trough" or "conduit" through which many structures pass. Structures in the pelvis include the lower genitourinary tract, reproductive organs, the distal small intestine, the distal colon, and the rectum. It also contains the iliofemoral vessels and lumbosacral plexus bilaterally.

Brotman et al[7,8] have described the arterial network of the pelvis as four interconnected collateral loops: one posteromedian, one anteromedian and two lateral. The posteromedian loop is made up of the segmental vertebral plexus which joins with the lumbar, medial sacral, and posterior division of the internal iliac artery (including the iliolumbar, lateral sacral, and gluteal branches) (Fig. 28–1). Some of these vessels traverse the posterior wall of the bony pelvis, others pass through the sacral foramina. This explains the frequent occurrence of arterial damage associated with fracture or dislocation of the sacroiliac joint, sacrum, or ilium. The superior gluteal artery and vein exit the pelvis very close to the bone in the greater sciatic notch. These structures are at high risk of injury when displaced pelvic fractures extend into the sciatic notch.

The anteromedian vascular loop is formed by branches of the anterior division of the internal iliac artery. These interconnect with the gonadal, superior epigastric, and superior rectal arteries and with tributaries of the external iliac and femoral vessels. This loop supplies blood to the pubis, ischium, perineum, and pelvic viscera. It is most apt to be injured in pubic fractures and wide separations of the symphysis pubis. The lateral loop of pelvis vessels on each side is formed by collaterals between the femoral and internal iliac arteries. This vascular loop is most apt to be injured with severe crushing of the lateral pelvis.

Veins accompanying the arteries in the four pelvic vascular systems are also at great risk of being injured directly in pelvic fractures.[7] In particular, the link between the superior rectal vein and the valveless portal venous system can contribute to the excessive bleeding which can occur from torn pelvic veins. Indeed, pelvic venous injury can result in reversal of portal blood flow away from the liver and toward the pelvis.[8]

> **AXIOM** The rich interconnection of the pelvic vessels explains why occlusion of a single trunk, such as the hypogastric (internal iliac) artery, does little to decrease hemorrhage after pelvic trauma.[7,9,10]

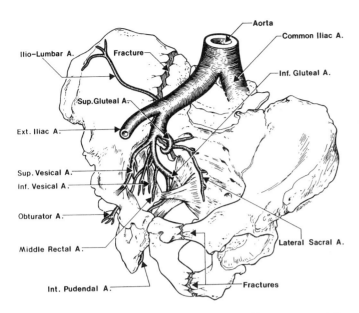

FIGURE 28–1 The posterior division of the internal iliac artery, especially the superior gluteal artery and its branches, are vulnerable to injury from pelvic fractures (From Brotman S, Soderstrom CA, Cranite MO, et al. Management of severe bleeding in fractures of the pelvis. Surg Gynec Obstet 1981;153:823.)

Single-vessel injury in blunt trauma to the pelvis is rare. Pelvic fractures are usually associated with damage to multiple small vessels; only 6-18% of pelvic hemorrhage is primarily from the arterial system.[11,12]

AXIOM The pelvis can be described as a vascular sink because it is a distensible reservoir for blood flowing antegrade from the aorta and retrograde from the legs and portal circulation.[7,8]

The retroperitoneal space can accommodate several liters of blood before any appreciable tamponade of bleeding sites occurs.[10] Consequently, the main factor limiting the extent of hemorrhage from pelvic fractures is the tamponading effect of the bony pelvis and its associated tissues. As high pressures are capable of overcoming this effect, bleeding from large arteries is more apt to be severe than bleeding from pelvic veins. In open pelvic fractures, however, both arterial and venous systems may bleed profusely because of a relative lack of resistance to outflow.[13]

MECHANISMS OF INJURY

The mechanism and force of the trauma determine the type and magnitude of the pelvic injury,[1] and are major factors in the classification of these injuries.[14,15,16] The major forces applied to the pelvic girdle can be divided into anteroposterior compression, lateral compression, vertical shear, and combined patterns.[15] The most common mechanism of injury for pelvic fractures in multiple trauma patients is lateral compression. Major differences in mortality and associated organ injury have also been found when pelvic fractures are classified in this way. For example, associated head trauma is more commonly found in lateral compression injuries than in anterior compression injuries.[15]

The majority of pelvic fractures are due to simple falls or direct blows to bony prominences, such as the anterior superior or inferior iliac spines, the ischial tuberosities, or the superior pubic rami.[4] Fractures may also occur from avulsions of muscular attachments to the pelvis (Fig. 28–2). The more severe fractures usually result from forces which disrupt the pelvic ring by: (a) opening the ring at the symphysis pubis, (b) crushing the pelvis in anteroposterior or lateral directions, or (c) disrupting the sacroiliac joints with forces applied from the perineum upward. Although sacroiliac joint dislocation can cause significant vascular and skeletal problems, the associated disruption of nerves and blood vessels in the area of the sacral foramina is usually of much greater importance.[1]

Direct-impact injuries occurring anteriorly or posteriorly tend to produce inward axial compression of the pelvic ring. This tends to cause fractures of the pubic symphysis and dislocations of the sacroiliac joints. This can result in a classic "open book" diastasis at the pubic symphysis, which is often seen in pedestrians struck by high-speed motor vehicles[17] (Figs. 28–3, 28–4). Associated pelvic injuries include external rotation of the iliac bones and disruption of the sacroiliac joints posteriorly.

Certain types of trauma striking the pelvis at an angle can cause vertical shearing forces which can produce unilateral anterior and posterior disruptions of the pelvic ring known as Malgaigne fractures[1,18] (Figs. 28–5, 28–6). Such fracture patterns tend to be seen with falls from heights, motorcycle accidents, and high-speed deceleration motor vehicle crashes.

Forceful outward splaying of the thighs or direct blows to the perineum, as with straddle injuries, can cause bilateral superior and inferior pubic rami fractures[1] (Fig. 28–7). These fractures have a high incidence of associated lower urinary tract injuries.

Acetabular fractures with femoral head dislocations tend to occur when force is applied to the hip from the front or the rear. This injury can occur when an unrestrained motorist hits the dashboard with his knees in a deceleration injury. The force is transmitted along the femur, causing fracture of the posterior lip of the acetabulum and dislocation of the hip posteriorly. Central acetabular fracture and dislocation can occur when the hip is hit from a lateral direction and is much less common. Lateral compression can also cause fractures involving the acetabulum, sacrum, and pubic rami (Figs. 28–8, 28–9).

Iliac wing fractures, although painful, can generally be ignored unless they also involve the acetabulum or sacroiliac joint. Fractures

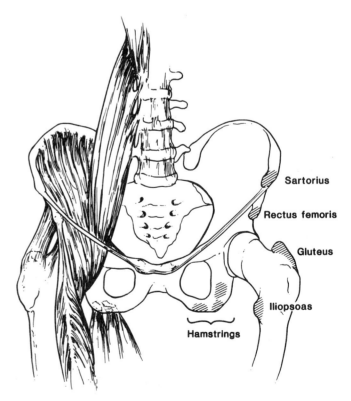

FIGURE 28–2 Illustration of the muscle insertions and origins of the pelvis and hips relative to the sites of common avulsion fractures. (From Berquist TH, Coventry MB. The pelvis and hips. In Berquist TH, ed. Imaging of orthopedic trauma, 2nd ed. New York: J.B. Lippincott, 1992; 232.)

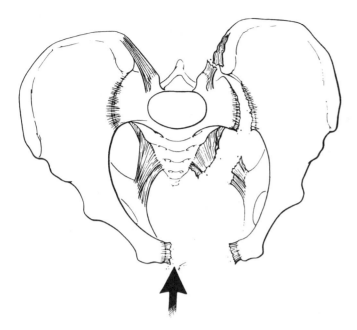

FIGURE 28–3 Pelvic fracture from anterior compression with wide diastasis of the symphysis and disruption of the anterior and posterior sacroiliac ligaments. (From Berquist TH and Coventry MB. The pelvis and hips. In Berquist TH, ed. Imaging of orthopedic trauma, 2nd ed. New York: J.B. Lippincott, 1992; 230.)

that primarily involve the posterior portion of the pelvic ring are more commonly associated with concomitant organ, nerve and vessel injuries, massive hemorrhage, and late complications. Consequently, they tend to have much higher mortality and morbidity rates than pure anterior pelvic fractures.[19]

AXIOM Forceful crushing, axial compression, or vertical shear injuries have a high incidence of associated injuries to adjacent structures.

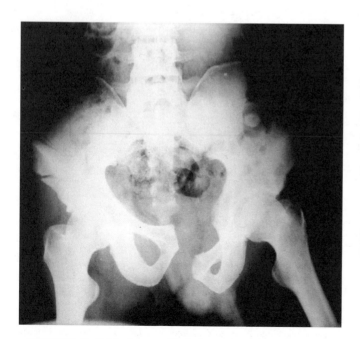

FIGURE 28–4 Pelvic fracture with displacement of left anterior pelvis.

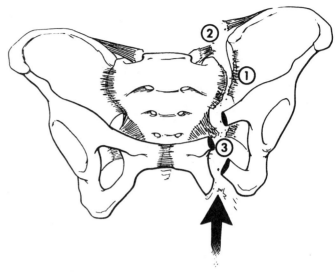

FIGURE 28–5 Pelvic fracture due to vertical shearing injury with disruption of the anterior and posterior ring on the left. (From Berquist TH and Coventry MB. The pelvis and hips. In Berquist TH, ed. Imaging of orthopedic trauma, 2nd ed. New York: J.B. Lippincott, 1992; 231.)

FRACTURE TYPES

Classification of Fracture Patterns

Numerous classification systems have been proposed for pelvic fractures. Many consider the mechanism of injury and the forces exerted on the pelvic ring. The simple classification of Tile and Pennal (Table 28–1) includes anteroposterior compression, lateral compression, and vertical shear.[14,20] This classification has been expanded extensively by other authors[15,16,21] (Table 28–2). Letourneal has proposed a classification based on the site of injury.[22] Bucholtz developed his classification based on autopsy studies.[23]

Classification systems have also been used to alert physicians to the problems involved in acute patient resuscitation. For example, in the system of Young and Burgess,[16] anteroposterior compression and

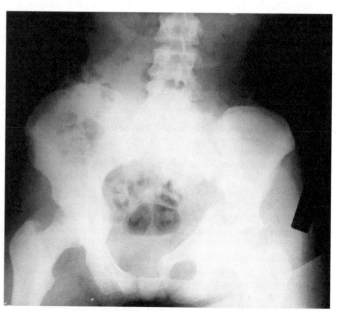

FIGURE 28–6 Malgaigne fracture of the pelvis involving the pubic rami and acetabulum plus reverse sacroiliac joint diastasis.

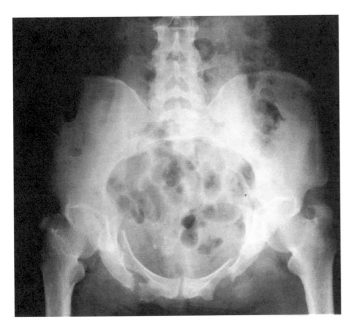

FIGURE 28–7 Straddle type of pelvic fracture.

lateral compression injuries are divided into three grades depending on the amount of displacement. Anteroposterior patterns tend to have a high incidence of intraabdominal visceral injuries, shock, sepsis, and respiratory distress. More severe associated injuries are seen with more severe fracture displacements. Lateral compression injuries have a high incidence of associated brain, lung, and upper abdominal visceral injuries. Cryer and al, using Pennal's classification, found that the amount of displacement of the pelvic fracture correlated with the amount of blood that was required in the acute resuscitation of their patients.[11]

Pelvic stability is an important concept. A stable pelvis is one that can withstand normal forces without abnormal displacement. The pelvis can be thought of as a ring consisting of the sacrum and the two innominate bones. The bony structures themselves have no real inherent stability, and thus it is the ligamentous attachments of the pelvis that provide stability. These include the iliolumbar, posterior and anterior sacroiliac, interosseous sacroiliac, sacrospinal and sacrotuberous ligaments, and the symphysis pubis. Of these the posterior structures are by far the strongest and most important. They hold the posterior pelvis together and transmit the forces of the vertebral spine through the sacrum and sacroiliac joints, transmitting most of the weight of the body through this posterior weight-bearing arch.[24] Sectioning studies have shown that if the symphysis alone is cut, the resulting pubic diastasis does not exceed 2.5 cm.[25] If the sacrospinous, sacrotuberous, and anterior sacroiliac ligaments are also cut, a significant diastasis can occur with external rotation, but there is no vertical displacement. Only additional sectioning of the posterior sacroiliac ligaments can produce significant vertical displacement.

These observations have lead to the concepts of rotational and vertical stability that have been used in the classification system of Tile.[21] In this system, pelvic fractures are divided into rotationally and vertically stable injuries (type A), rotationally unstable but vertically and posteriorly stable injuries (type B), and rotationally and vertically unstable injuries (type C). These major categories can then be further subdivided, and the system is illustrated in Table 28–1.[21,26]

Open Versus Closed Fractures

Patients with open pelvic fractures, especially if they are compounded through the perineum, have had massive forces acting on the pelvic ring, causing severe damage and shearing of associated soft tissues. These open pelvic fractures usually result from one of two different mechanisms of injury:

1. crushing injuries, which cause compression and shattering of the pelvic girdle, with the soft tissues tending to crack open across the perineum and into the rectum.
2. hyperabduction of a lower extremity, whereby it is almost torn off the pelvis.

Open pelvic fractures may involve skin, urogenital system, rectum, and major blood vessels. Those with extensive perineal, rectal, or vaginal involvement have a 40-50% mortality rate if not treated properly.[1,2,13]

With closed pelvic fractures, there may be a large blood loss from the bone and adjacent vessels into the retroperitoneal space, but it is usually not exsanguinating. In open pelvic fractures, however, the tamponading effect of the peritoneum is lost and a much more severe

FIGURE 28–8 Type I, Pelvic fracture from lateral compression with pubic rami fractures plus crush injury to the sacrum, ilium and/or sacroiliac joint. (From Berquist TH and Coventry MB. The pelvis and hips. In Berquist TH, ed. Imaging of orthopedic trauma, 2nd ed. New York: J.B. Lippincott, 1992; 231.)

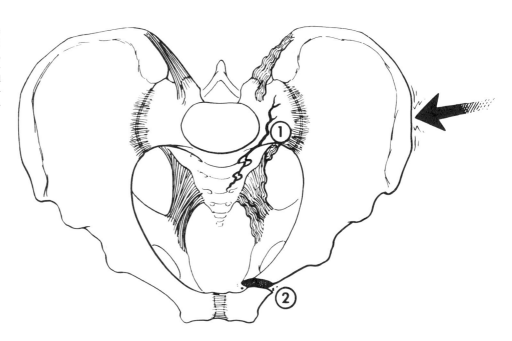

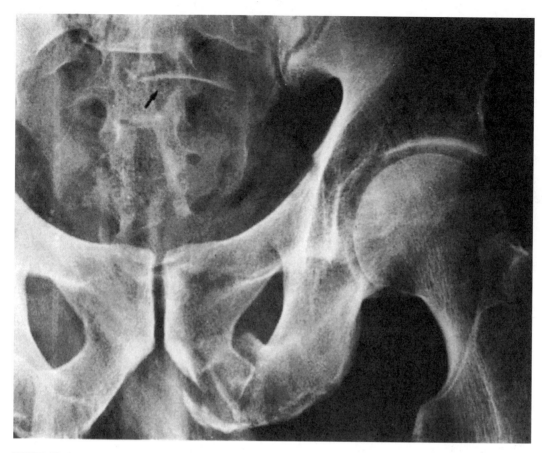

FIGURE 28–9 Lateral compression injury with fractures of the left acetabulum, sacrum, and pubic ramus. (From Berquist TH and Coventry MB. The pelvis and hips. In Berquist TH, ed. Imaging of orthopedic trauma, 2nd ed. New York: J.B. Lippincott, 1992;5:230.)

blood loss can occur, contributing to the high mortality rates seen with this injury.

Hemodynamic Status

From the standpoint of initial management and prognosis, major pelvic fractures can be separated into those in which: (a) the patient has little or no bleeding and is hemodynamically stable, (b) there is significant bleeding, but vital signs can be maintained with transfusion, and (c) the patient is exsanguinating and is hemodynamically unstable.

Approximately 75-85% of pelvic fracture victims are hemodynamically stable and have a relatively uncomplicated course, requiring initial emergency department evaluation, admission to the orthopedic surgery service, and pain relief.[7] Later in the course of their hospitalization, some of these patients may require surgery for repair of bony and ligamentous pelvic disruptions.[27,28]

TABLE 28–1 *Pelvic Fracture Classifications*[14,20]

Tile-Pennal
1. Anteroposterior compression
   Open book
   Straddle fractures
2. Lateral compression
   Ipsilateral double fractures
   Bucket handle fractures
   Straddle fractures with posterior disruption
3. Vertical shearing fractures

Approximately 15-25% of the patients with pelvic fractures are in an intermediate hemodynamic group, usually presenting in a critical condition with varying degrees of hypotension and overall injury severity.[7] Associated extrapelvic injuries involving the head, thorax, abdomen, and long bones are often significant factors affecting outcome in this group of patients.[6,29] These patients usually respond to aggressive infusions of crystalloid initially, but subsequently they may require relatively large amounts of blood and other fluid to maintain a normal blood pressure and urine output.

Severe external bleeding from open fractures or severe retroperitoneal bleeding from closed fractures occurs in about 0.5-1.0% of patients with pelvic fractures.[7,30,31] These patients usually arrive in the hospital with severe hypotension and respond poorly to resuscitative measures, including aggressive intravenous fluids.

AXIOM Failure to respond to an initial aggressive fluid resuscitation implies severe active bleeding, which must be controlled rapidly if the patient is to survive.

With this third group, one must determine rapidly if there is intraperitoneal blood loss from associated injuries which requires immediate surgical control. If the bleeding sites are all in the pelvis, the responsible vessels must be compressed or embolized rapidly.

DIAGNOSIS

History and Physical Examination

A preliminary diagnosis of a fractured pelvis can usually be made clinically from the history and physical examination.[1] Frequently, a description of the events and the mechanism of injury, provided

TABLE 28–2 Classification of Pelvic Ring Disruptions[21]

Type A Stable
    A1 Fractures not involving ring; avulsion injuries
        A1.1 Anterior superior spine
        A1.2 Anterior inferior spine
        A1.3 Ischial tuberosity
    A2 Stable, minimal displacement
        A2.1 Iliac wing fractures
        A2.2 Isolated anterior ring injuries (4-pillar)
        A2.3 Stable, undisplaced or minimally displaced fractures of the pelvic ring
    A3 Transverse fractures of sacrum and coccyx
        A3.1 Undisplaced transverse sacral fractures
        A3.2 Displaced transverse sacral fractures
        A3.3 Coccygeal fracture
Type B Rotationally Unstable, Vertically and Posteriorly Stable
    B1 External rotation instability; open-book injury
        B1.1 Unilateral injury
        B1.2 Less than 2.5 cm displacement
        B1.3 Greater than 2.5 cm displacement
    B2 Internal rotation instability; lateral compression injury
        B2.1 Ipsilateral anterior and posterior injury
        B2.2 Contralateral anterior and posterior injury
            Bucket-handle fracture
        B3.3 Bilateral rotationally unstable injury
Type C Rotationally, Posteriorly and Vertically Unstable
    C1 Unilateral injury
        C1.1 Fracture through ilium
        C1.2 Sacroiliac dislocation and/or fracture dislocation
        C1.3 Sacral fracture
    C2 Bilateral injury, one side rotationally unstable, one side vertically unstable
    C3 Bilateral injury, both sides completely unstable

either by the patient or prehospital personnel, can clearly indicate the diagnosis.

AXIOM Suprapubic pain, low back pain or lower extremity shortening, weakness, and/or diminished sensation after trauma suggest the presence of a pelvic fracture.[11]

Careful physical examination of the pelvis and its contents is imperative in every major trauma victim. One must also look particularly carefully for the various physical signs that tend to be associated with pelvic fractures (Table 28–3).

Swelling in the suprapubic and groin areas may be a sign of massive blood loss. Such blood loss can also cause ecchymosis in the external genitalia, medial thigh and flanks. Inspection may also reveal abrasions and contusions over bony prominences. Ecchymosis about the pubis, perineum, or scrotum or the presence of blood in the urethral meatus is highly suggestive of lower genitourinary trauma.

AXIOM Part of the examination of an injured pelvis is determination of the stability of the major fragments.

Pelvic instability occurs when there is abnormal displacement of the bony pelvis. An immediate clinical assessment is very important. A quick inspection for obvious limb length inequalities should be made, as well as the position and neurovascular status of the lower extremities. Bilateral pressure on the anterior iliac spines or iliac crest, looking and feeling for opening and closing of the pelvis, can detect rotational instability. Pushing and pulling gently on a leg may reveal vertical or gross instability. More precise determination of injury patterns requires special radiographic studies. Another extremely important part of the physical exam of an injured pelvis is a check for hematuria or blood in the vagina or rectum.

AXIOM Lacerations of the perineum, groin, or buttock after blunt trauma indicate an open pelvic fracture until proven otherwise.

An unsuspected urethral laceration in men is potentially devastating.[1] Even when treated optimally, urethral stricture, incontinence and impotence commonly follow such injuries. Although the initial trauma is the major determinant of the extent of the urethral injury, a partial urethral tear can be converted to a complete disruption by forceful insertion of a urethral catheter. A careful search for signs of urethral injury during the initial examination, before a urethral catheter is inserted, is very important. These signs include: (a) blood at the urethral meatus, (b) a perineal hematoma, or (c) a displaced or "floating" prostate found on rectal examination. Although these can be very helpful signs, their absence does not exclude injury.

In the female, the pelvic examination should also include palpation of the posterior pubis and lateral pelvic walls. The presence of rectal blood is usually considered to be diagnostic of a rectal injury. A lax anal sphincter and lack of a response to perianal pain or to a request to tighten the anal sphincter often indicates a major neurologic injury or extensive anorectal damage.

AXIOM In all major pelvic fractures one must look carefully for rectal, genitourinary, or perineal injuries.

The elasticity of the rectal wall makes it less susceptible to tearing than the perineal skin.[1] When the rectum does tear, the tear is most commonly just inside the anus where the rectum is fixed and less distensible. The rectum and vagina may also be injured by forceful compression against the sacral promontory or by perforation from bony spicules.

AXIOM A full bladder is much more susceptible to injury than one that is empty.

Bladders can be injured in a variety of ways. A full bladder may shear off the urethra at the pubis with a severe deceleration or it may burst because of excessive compression. Management of bladder ruptures is determined to some extent by whether they occur intraperitoneally or extraperitoneally.

Crushing forces applied to the pelvis can cause severe damage to the skin and muscles. If the skin is stripped from its underlying fascia, it may lose its blood supply and undergo necrosis. The severity of muscle crushing in the lower abdominal wall, buttocks or upper thighs is rarely completely evident at the initial examination.

Neurological injuries to the cauda equina or the sciatic or femoral nerves are easily missed in patients with severe trauma. Performing an adequate neurological examination may be extremely difficult initially and may lead to delayed diagnosis with a greater chance for permanent neurological defects.

Radiologic Evaluation

A minimum radiographic examination of the pelvis is the anteroposterior view, which provides a rapid survey of the problem and is a standard study taken in all seriously injured patients.[32] More precise evaluation of the problem requires further radiographs and a CT scan of the pelvis. Routine CT scanning is not needed for every pelvic

TABLE 28–3 Physical Signs of Pelvic Fracture

1. Groin and/or suprapubic swelling
2. Severe point tenderness over the pubis, iliac wings, and/or ischial tuberosity
3. Swelling and ecchymosis of the upper medial thigh, groin, or genitalia
4. Instability of the pelvis
5. Neuropathy in lower extremity

fracture, but it does provide invaluable information for assessment of the sacroiliac joints and fractures of the acetabulum. It should be performed in more severe injuries, when there are concerns about pelvic stability or the extent of the injury, and before elective pelvic procedures. The additional anatomic information obtained by CT scans can often change the interpretation of the extent of injury as assessed by the original radiographs.[33]

The possibility of early pregnancy in women of child-bearing age should be considered before undertaking extensive radiological examinations after low-energy trauma. However, radiographs for evaluation and management of serious pelvic injuries should not be delayed.

PLAIN FILMS

AXIOM   A radiograph of the pelvis should be obtained on all patients with major blunt trauma.

A simple anteroposterior (AP) view of the pelvis will detect most pelvic fractures, and it can determine pelvic ring stability in the great majority of cases. In fact, Gillott et al[32] and many other centers now advocate routine initial radiographs of the lateral cervical spine, AP chest and AP pelvis on all patients with severe blunt trauma; however, Civil et al[34] have questioned the need for routine pelvic radiography in awake, alert, and asymptomatic patients.

Patients with established pelvic fractures should have inlet and outlet views of the pelvis.[14] These views are taken without moving the patient from the supine position. The inlet view is performed by directing the radiograph beam from the head to the mid-pelvis at an angle of 40 degrees. It is useful for assessing the pelvic brim and sacral ala. The outlet view is taken similarly, but with the beam beginning at the feet and directed 40 degrees to the mid-pelvis. If the acetabulum is involved, two oblique views,

the so-called Judet views, should be preformed.[22] These views involve rolling the patient on his or her side at an angle of 45 degrees.

STUDIES OF THE GU TRACT

Traditionally, associated injuries to the genitourinary system were assessed by intravenous pyelography, cystography and urethrography. However, CT scans of the abdomen and pelvis with intravenous contrast can provide much better delineation of the kidneys and bladder. Retrograde contrast urethrography is performed if there is any clinical evidence of urethral injury. This study should also be considered if the pelvis is fractured at the symphysis.

With a large pelvic hematoma, cystography frequently discloses a characteristic "teardrop" deformity of the urinary bladder due to compression and elevation by the surrounding blood. Empty ("washout") views are important and sometimes provide the only clear evidence of a bladder injury. The washout views should be obtained in the anteroposterior and oblique projections to detect small tears.

CT SCANS

AXIOM   A CT scan is usually needed to define the extent of a pelvic fracture accurately.

CT scans of the pelvis can be particularly helpful because they allow three-dimensional assessment of the posterior sacroiliac elements (Fig. 28–10), the weight-bearing acetabulum and the pelvic contents.[1,33,35-37] Indeed, Gill and Bucholz[33] reported that more than a third of their pelvic fractures which were classified on routine radiographs had to be reclassified on the basis of additional information provided by CT scans. However, the patient's clinical status will dictate whether such sophisticated tests can be done safely.

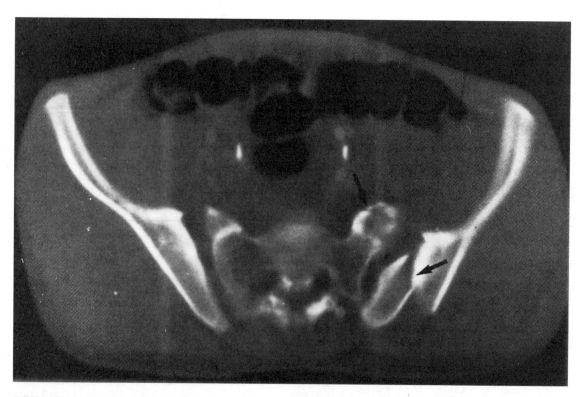

FIGURE 28–10   CT scan at the level of the sacrum showing separation of both sides of the sacroiliac joint as well as fractures through the ilium and body of the sacrum on the left side (arrows). The extent of these injuries were not as apparent on the plain films. (From Daffner RH. Pelvic trauma. In McCort JJ. Trauma radiology. 1990;7:357.)

In some patients, full hemodynamic monitoring and constant physician and nurse attendance should be maintained during the radiologic evaluations. However, if the patient is restless and will not hold still, the radiological studies may be suboptimal and can be very difficult to interpret.

AXIOM	The results of a CT scan or any other radiologic procedure are only as good as the quality of the films obtained and their interpretation.

ANGIOGRAPHY

Angiography may be extremely helpful in determining the site of continued severe blood loss in the pelvis or abdomen.[37] Posterior branches of the internal iliac artery are a common location for persistent bleeding in these patients (Fig. 28–11). If a specific site of arterial hemorrhage is found, it can usually be embolized radiologically. Because of the excellent collateral blood flow, there is little or no concern about the adequacy of the blood supply to the pelvic structures if a branch or even one entire iliac artery is embolized and occluded.

AXIOM	Angiography of the abdominal aorta and iliac arteries can be used to diagnose and treat continued intraabdominal or pelvic bleeding.

Occasionally external trauma will cause a compression injury with occlusion of the external iliac artery at or just above the inguinal ligament (Fig. 28–12). With this injury, there is usually relatively little blood loss, and there may be relatively little evidence of ischemia in the lower extremity.

DIAGNOSTIC PERITONEAL LAVAGE

If there is concern about intraperitoneal bleeding or intestinal injury in a patient with a fractured pelvic bone, a diagnostic peritoneal lavage (DPL) may be performed. In the presence of a pelvic fracture, the DPL should be performed as an open procedure above the umbilicus.[38,39] Ideally, it should be performed in the OR so that one can go directly ahead with a laparotomy and/or external fixation of the pelvis as indicated.

AXIOM	In a patient with a pelvic fracture, a negative DPL is generally a highly accurate indicator that significant intraperitoneal injury is not present;[1,11] however, the DPL is often false-positive if a pelvic hematoma is present.

The main difficulty with DPL in pelvic fractures is the high false positive rate, which may exceed 28%. Further complicating the problem is the increased mortality rate (up to 30%) for patients undergoing an unnecessary laparotomy in the presence of a pelvic fracture.[1,7,40] Some surgeons say that the number of red blood cells for a positive DPL in patient with pelvic fractures should be raised to 200,000/mm^3. Others believe that severe bleeding from an intraperitoneal source is probably not present unless gross blood is aspirated.

TREATMENT

In 1964, McLaughlin described three pitfalls in the management of patients with a fractured pelvis.[1,41] He felt that the most common catastrophic pitfall is to treat an obvious fracture and overlook occult associated visceral injuries until there were problems from infection or hemorrhage. The second pitfall was overtreatment of a stable pelvic fracture. His third pitfall involved treatment of an unstable pelvic fracture without recognizing its potential for producing permanent disability and/or anatomical deformity.

The initial management of any patient with a complicated pelvic fracture is similar to that of any other seriously injured patient. A systematic approach with simultaneous resuscitation and evaluation is recommended.

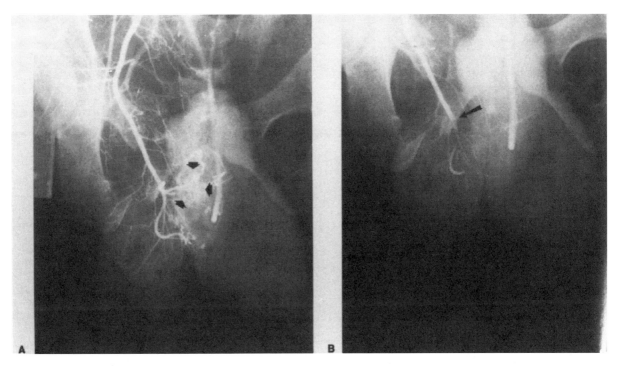

FIGURE 28–11 Arteriogram showing extravasation from several branches of the hypogastric artery in a patient with a pelvic fracture. (From Schwarcz TH. Therapeutic angiography in the management of vascular trauma. In Flanigan DP, ed. Civilian vascular trauma. 1992;32:340.)

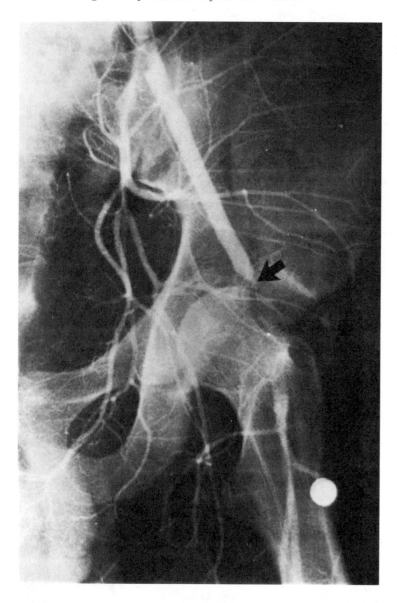

FIGURE 28-12   Arteriogram showing complete occlusion of the external iliac artery at the level of the acetabulum (arrow). The vessel reconstitutes from collaterals at the level of the greater trochanter. (From Daffner RH. Pelvic trauma. In McCort JJ. Trauma radiology. 1990;7:374.)

Resuscitation and Control of Bleeding

INCIDENCE OF HEMODYNAMIC INSTABILITY

AXIOM   The hemodynamic status of the patient at the time of presentation to the ED is the single most important predictor of his outcome.[1]

Mucha has noted that the mortality rate for pelvic fractures in patients who were hypotensive on admission was 42%, but in patients who were hemodynamically stable, the morbidity rate was only 3%.[42] Although 10-15% of patients with pelvic fractures are hemodynamically unstable initially, in almost two-thirds of these, spontaneous tamponade of the pelvic fracture hemorrhage occurs, and the patient can be stabilized by the usual resuscitation.[6]

AXIOM   The foremost consideration with pelvic fractures is rapid resuscitation and control of exsanguinating hemorrhage.

In many series, over 50% of the patients with pelvic fractures require blood; 10-20% require 1-3 units, 10-20% require 4-9 units, and 10-20% require 10 or more units of blood.[1,7] In one study of 72 pelvic fracture patients who were in shock on admis-

sion, the average number of blood transfusions was 16 units per patient.[1]

AXIOM   One should always anticipate significant blood loss with major pelvic fractures.

INTRAVENOUS LINES

At least two large-bore (12- to 14-gauge) peripheral intravenous lines should be established, and blood and component therapy should be started early. In patients with a systolic blood pressure less than 80 mm Hg on admission, insertion of sterile intravenous extension tubing via a basilic vein cutdown or insertion of an 8.5-French subclavian catheter via a wire guide vein-dilatation technique can greatly facilitate rapid blood and fluid administration. As a general rule, lower extremity routes for fluid administration should be avoided in patients with suspected pelvic fractures because of the possibility of associated iliac or femoral vein injury. If fluids are administered rapidly (2-3 liters in 10-15 minutes) and there is little or no hemodynamic improvement or it is only transient, a PASG should be applied and inflated to try to reduce bleeding from the lower extremities and pelvic area while one arranges for more definitive control of the bleeding.

Monitoring

Continuous monitoring of the vital signs of patients with pelvic fractures from the time of injury through definitive treatment and for the first 24-48 hours postoperatively is essential.[1] Central venous pressure monitoring and urinary bladder catheterization (if not temporarily contraindicated pending contrast evaluation of the lower genitourinary tract) are also advisable, especially in older individuals.

Recognition that hemorrhage is occurring in a patient with a pelvic fracture is usually not difficult. Hypotension, acute reduction of the hematocrit, increased heart rate, and a decrease in central venous pressure in spite of vigorous administration of fluids and blood are important signs of continuing significant blood loss.[7] Difficulty can arise, however, in determining whether the site of bleeding is the pelvic fracture or associated injuries.

The most common extrapelvic sources of hemorrhage in patients with pelvic fractures include long bone fractures and intrathoracic and abdominal organ injuries.[7] Diagnosis of long bone fractures and intrathoracic injuries requires only physical examination and skeletal and chest radiographs.

> **AXIOM**   Diagnostic peritoneal lavage (DPL) is the initial test of choice for diagnosis of bleeding from intraperitoneal organs.

Pneumatic Antishock Garments

Temporary packing of all external bleeding wounds is carried out in the emergency department (ED). If there is evidence of continued blood loss, apposition of the disrupted pelvic fracture fragments by the application of a pneumatic antishock garment (PASG) can reduce external and internal bleeding.[31-33] This may allow the patient's general condition to improve enough with fluid resuscitation to allow diagnostic procedures, such as arteriography, outside the ED.

Although controversy exists about the role of the pneumatic antishock garment (PASG) in trauma care, many feel that it can be useful for the initial management of pelvic fractures.[43,44,45] The PASG, according to some authors, should be applied to all hemodynamically unstable patients with pelvic fractures in the prehospital phase, especially if transport time exceeds 10 minutes.[6,46] The PASG can provide temporary stabilization of the pelvic fracture and associated lower extremity injuries and some degree of counterpressure tamponade of torn small vessels.

If a patient with severe blunt trauma is not already in a PASG on arrival, some physicians recommend, it should be applied to any patient with a pelvic fracture who is hypotensive.[1,43] After a brief examination of the genitalia, rectum and lower extremities, the PASG may be inflated. This may result in dramatic reduction in blood loss and improvement in hemodynamics.[6,46,47] Even in hemodynamically stable patients, low-pressure inflation of the PASG provides some splinting of the pelvis and lower extremity fractures while the patient's evaluation is continuing.

The effect of PASG on hemodynamics can sometimes be dramatic, but it is not consistent. Optimal results have been achieved with inflation pressures of about 25-40 mm Hg applied to each of its three compartments.[44] Prolonged high inflation pressures (exceeding systemic diastolic pressure) should be avoided to prevent underlying pressure necrosis and lower extremity compartment syndromes.[48]

Some padding with bath towels, foam rubber or similar material over the iliac crests, greater trochanters, knees, and ankles is advised before the PASG is inflated.[1] Once the patient is hemodynamically stable, sequential decompression of the abdominal compartment first, then each of the legs should be performed while carefully monitoring the patient's vital signs. If the systolic BP falls by more than 5 mm Hg, the compartment is reinflated and more fluid given before another PASG decompression is attempted. Rapid deflation of the PASG must be avoided, especially in patients who may still be hypovolemic.

If the pressures in the PASG are only 30-40 mm Hg, they have been left in place for as long as 24-48 hours.[7,46,47] However, such patients are at high risk for compartment syndromes, especially if they are hypotensive, and the duration of suit application should be no longer than clinically needed. If major pelvic bleeding cannot be controlled quickly, external fixation of the pelvis and/or pelvic angiography should be attempted.[49,50,51]

Although a PASG can be of great benefit in some patients with pelvic fractures, it can also cause a number of problems. It prevents observation of and ready access to the patient's abdomen, groin, and perineum. It also causes difficulty in performing selective angiography.[9,52] Deflation of the garment in the operating room or at the time of angiography may result in sudden hypotension.

> **AXIOM**   An inflated PASG should be deflated only one segment at a time while constantly monitoring the blood pressure.

In open pelvic fractures or in those with associated lacerations of the thigh, buttocks, or perineum, deflation of the device may be followed by profuse bleeding. Inflation of the PASG may also increase intracranial pressure, and this may be deleterious in a patient who has a closed head injury. Since cephalad displacement of intraabdominal organs by the inflated PASG may compromise the patient's ventilation, endotracheal intubation and controlled ventilation should be given serious consideration after application of the PASG.

> **AXIOM**   A patient who has marginal ventilation should be intubated and provided with ventilatory support prior to inflation of the abdominal component of the PASG.

Definitive Management of Soft Tissue Injuries

CONTROL OF HEMORRHAGE

> **AXIOM**   Only about 5-10% of patients with pelvic fractures remain hemodynamically unstable in spite of the initial resuscitation; however, these are the patients most apt to die.[1]

Postmortem injection studies in trauma victims with severe pelvic fractures suggest that 90-95% of the blood loss occurs from lacerations of small vessels which bleed into the soft areolar tissue of the retroperitoneum.[53] This potential space can extend from the respiratory diaphragm down to the mid-thigh and may accommodate several liters of blood. In addition, lacerations of major branches of the internal iliac arteries occur in approximately 5-10% of patients with pelvic fractures.[53]

Exsanguinating Patients

In patients with pelvic fractures and a systolic BP persistently less than 60 mm Hg in spite of aggressive fluid resuscitation, an immediate operation may offer the only chance for survival.[1] However, many of these patients do not have surgically accessible bleeding points, and those who do frequently exsanguinate before adequate exposure can be obtained.

PRELAPAROTOMY THORACOTOMY.   If the patient reaches the OR with a systolic BP less than 70 mm Hg in spite of aggressive fluid resuscitation, a prelaparotomy thoracotomy with cross-clamping of the descending thoracic aorta just above the diaphragm should be considered.[54,55] This can improve coronary and cerebral artery perfusion threefold and reduce bleeding below the diaphragm.

> **AXIOM**   If the patient's systolic BP does not rise to at least 90 mm hg within 5 minutes of thoracic aorta cross-clamping, the patient is in terminal cardiovascular failure.

Since all of the patients not responding to thoracic aortic cross-clamping have died in the operating room despite multiple units of blood and many hours of surgery, some physicians say that one should not continue aggressive resuscitation and perform prolonged surgery under such circumstances.[37]

OPERATION. In the operating room, patients with pelvic fractures and persistent hypotension should be placed in the lithotomy position as for an abdominoperineal resection. This will allow the perineum and abdomen to be explored simultaneously by two teams if needed. In females, the vagina should also be cleansed for careful examination.

Perineal Team. If lacerations in the perineum were previously packed, the packs are removed and the perineal wounds thoroughly inspected. Major hemorrhage is controlled surgically with ligatures, sutures, or cautery wherever possible. Debridement of devitalized tissues should not be attempted until the bleeding, hypothermia and coagulopathies are controlled and the patient's vital signs are stable. Widespread bleeding from small vessels is best controlled by immediate repacking. Any laboratory or clinical coagulopathy is corrected rapidly with platelet packs and fresh frozen plasma or cryoprecipitate.

After the patient is hemodynamically stable, the vagina is examined carefully. Any vaginal injury is debrided as needed and loosely approximated with absorbable sutures. The anus is then closely inspected for injury. The rectum is manually emptied of formed feces and thoroughly cleansed by irrigation. The rectum is then thoroughly examined using hemorrhoid retractors, an anoscope and a sigmoidoscope.

Lacerations of the anus or rectum are repaired in two layers with absorbable sutures, first in the underlying muscle and then in the mucosa. If the anal sphincter is completely disrupted, it should have a primary repair in two layers unless the wound needs packing to control bleeding and/or appears marginally viable. After a repeat sterile preparation, a presacral drain should be inserted and the laparotomy team should perform a sigmoid colostomy.

Laparotomy Team. The abdominal operation is performed through an upper midline incision long enough to allow adequate inspection of all intraabdominal structures. Any area which is bleeding actively should be packed to control the bleeding. Packing of the pelvis with laparotomy pads or sterile towels can often reduce pelvic bleeding and allow direct control of other bleeding sites.[46] After the extrapelvic bleeding sites are controlled, the patient can be transferred to the angiography suite for embolization as needed to control continued pelvic bleeding.

If the initial packing does not control the pelvic bleeding and the systolic BP remains less than 60 mm Hg, the aorta should be clamped or compressed, if this has not already been done. Once the patient is reasonably resuscitated, any extrapelvic bleeding should be controlled.

If the pelvic peritoneum is found to be intact and the hemorrhage can be controlled by perineal packing, the retroperitoneal space should not be opened. Intraabdominal opening of a retroperitoneal tamponade may result in torrential bleeding from multiple intrapelvic sites with no possibility of achieving surgical control before the patient exanguinates. However, if there is direct bleeding into the peritoneal cavity from the pelvis, this must be controlled, usually with packing. Cross-clamping of the aorta below the origin of the renal arteries can often decrease the rate of bleeding in the pelvis while packing is inserted.

If bleeding from a specific portion of the internal iliac vessels can be recognized (which is unusual), it should be ligated. If a small tear in the common or external iliac artery is recognized, it should be repaired using 4/0 or 5/0 monofilament polypropylene sutures as necessary.

Internal iliac artery ligation to control pelvic bleeding was used fairly frequently in the past to control massive pelvic bleeding. However, this technique is rarely successful, and the dissection required to expose the internal iliac arteries for ligation can cause even more bleeding to occur.

In a preliminary report by Saueracker et al,[31] intraoperative embolization of a severely bleeding internal iliac artery vessel, using a slurry of autologous blood clot (30 ml) combined with microfibrillar collagen, thrombin, and calcium, successfully controlled internal iliac artery hemorrhage. Although the complications of operative embolization may exceed those of the angiographic approach, its risks may be acceptable in exsanguinating patients. Intraluminal balloon tamponade accomplished by passage of Fogarty catheters into the hypogastric arteries through an infrarenal aortotomy has been described,[56] but few surgeons have experience with this technique.

AXIOM If a rapidly expanding or ruptured pelvic hematoma is found at laparotomy, it should be packed and arrangements made for immediate bony pelvic fixation and/or angiographic embolization of the bleeding vessels.

During laparotomy, pelvic packing through the abdominal incision is probably the best way to achieve control of pelvic bleeding. Gauze rolls should be packed in as tightly as possible, preferably with a nonporous material between the gauze packs and the bleeding vessels. This may allow the surgeon to control other life-threatening injuries and correct any hypothermia or coagulopathy which has developed.

AXIOM Following pelvic packing, a second-look operation in 24-48 hours is recommended if the patient's coagulation and bleeding studies can be returned to normal.

With an almost complete traumatic hemipelvectomy, the transected vessels often contract, and bleeding may stop or slow down when the systolic BP falls below 50-60 mm Hg; however, an increase in blood pressure caused by painful manipulations or fluid resuscitation may result in sudden exsanguination.[7] These patients should be taken to the operating room immediately; the pelvic vessels should be ligated, and the hemipelvectomy completed.[30,57,58]

AXIOM Hemipelvectomy for pelvic bleeding should be performed only if most of the dissection has already been accomplished by the trauma.

An emergency hemipelvectomy or hemicorpectomy should probably be done only when the trauma itself has done most of the dissection. If one is dealing with an already devitalized hemipelvis, this is the only reasonable management. However, the psychologic implications of removing an otherwise potentially viable hindquarter to salvage a life usually prevents its timely application.[30]

Continuing Pelvic Bleeding

DEFINITION AND CAUSE. Significant ongoing pelvic bleeding is defined as bleeding which persists after the initial resuscitation is complete.[1] This may be recognized by recurrent hypotension, external bleeding, or hematocrit levels which continue to fall or fail to rise with continuing blood transfusions. If the only injury is a pelvic fracture, and if more than 4-6 units of blood are required in the 6-8 hours following an initially adequate resuscitation, additional measures to control the bleeding are required.

PASG. Bleeding from closed pelvic fractures can often be treated effectively with external compression and immobilization using the three-compartment pneumatic anti-shock garment (PASG).[1] The leg compartments are inflated to 40 mm Hg and the abdominal compartment to 30 mm Hg. Support of ventilation is often necessary because of the presence of the severe injury and the tendency of the inflated PASG to reduce tidal volume.

The PASG also has some diagnostic value. Failure of pelvic bleeding to cease within 4-6 hours of PASG placement usually indicates laceration of a major artery which may be detected and controlled angiographically.

PELVIC FRACTURE STABILIZATION. Immediate external fixation of the pelvic fracture, preferably in the OR, has been increasingly recommended. Ideally there should be no indication for a laparotomy, and the pelvis should be the only site of continuing significant blood loss.[49-51,59-62]

Use of external fixation of pelvic fractures has gained increasing popularity in recent years. These devices limit pelvic hemorrhage by several mechanisms. They reduce the volume of the pelvic retroperitoneal space by approximating the displaced fracture fragments. Thus, the volume at which bleeding is tamponaded is reduced. Since, in the majority of patients, bleeding is mainly from small vessels on the edges of the fractured bones, patient movement promotes additional bleeding. External fixators reduce this effect by stabilizing the fracture fragments.[63] Proper external fixation may also approximate and occlude exposed bleeding bone. However, if there is a reasonable likelihood of associated intraperitoneal hemorrhage, laparotomy should precede external fixation of the pelvis.

There are many advantages of external fixation over PASG.[7] First, it permits easy access to the lower part of the body, facilitating the performance of peritoneal tap, urethrography, cystography, and femoral angiography. Second, it enables early mobilization of the patient. Third, it does not affect ventilation and intracranial pressure. External fixators are generally easy to use; they can often be applied in the emergency department or under local anesthesia in the operating room in about 10-20 minutes.

The classical external fixator is an excellent means of obtaining stability of an unstable pelvic injury in an emergency situation (Figs. 28–13, 28–14). It can be applied quickly. Simple frame designs are adequate for initial treatment.[64] Recently, a new external fixation device has been described, the antishock pelvic clamp[65] (Fig. 28–15). More clinical information however, is needed about this new fixator.

AXIOM The most important disadvantages of external fixators are that they do not stabilize posterior pelvic fractures adequately and they introduce the possibility for pin tract infections.

External fixation of the anterior pelvis may not have much affect on posterior bleeding vessels. However, recent advances in pelvic fracture management have demonstrated that early open reduction and internal fixation of pelvic fractures (within 12-36 hours of trauma) is possible in many instances, and provides better results than external fixators.[27] Posterior fixation generally cannot be used for the initial management of pelvic hemorrhage, but it may be useful for situations in which pelvic bleeding persists for several hours in spite of all other therapy.

DIAGNOSTIC AND THERAPEUTIC ANGIOGRAPHY. Successful percutaneous angiographic localization of pelvic fracture hemorrhage followed by therapeutic embolization has been reported by several institutions over the past decade.[6] However, timely application of this sophisticated technology requires preplanning and organization. If a patient has a pelvic fracture and responds poorly to resuscitation because of significant ongoing pelvic fracture hemorrhage (greater than 4-6 units within 6-8 hours following an initially adequate resuscitation), many consider emergency angiography to be the diagnostic and therapeutic procedure of choice.

Several centers advocate routine diagnostic DPL before angiography.[9,30,38] Others tend to favor selective application of DPL to those patients in whom there is a strong clinical suspicion of associated intraperitoneal injury.[30,46]

If the patient has had an exploratory laparotomy, and a ruptured, expanding, or pulsating hematoma in the pelvis was found, this is an indication for angiographic embolization.[7] If the patient has had a DPL and it is negative, the decision to perform diagnostic angiography is based on the rate of bleeding; a transfusion requirement greater than 4-6 units within the first 12-24 hours is, according to many authors, an indication for angiography and embolization if there is arterial bleeding.[6]

Some centers rely on an initial aortic injection of contrast at the diaphragm to angiographically identify significant associated intraabdominal bleeding sites.[1] If a rapidly bleeding intraperitoneal injury is found and it cannot be controlled angiographically, immediate operative intervention is indicated. However, if the patient is in the angiography suite, operative management of mild-to-moderate intraperitoneal bleeding can usually be deferred until the pelvic hemorrhage has been controlled by embolization.

Angiography also enables definitive assessment of possible thoracic aortic, peripheral vascular, and renal trauma.[1] Although visualization of the bladder is often possible after the patient's kidneys excrete the angiographic contrast material, accurate appraisal of the urethra and bladder is best afforded by retrograde studies. However, cystourethrography is a secondary priority and can usually be delayed until the hemorrhage is controlled.

When pelvic bleeding is demonstrated angiographically, successful embolization can be achieved in nearly all patients, and reported long-term survival rates with this technique usually exceed 80%.[1,6] These results are far superior to the 10-15% survival rates previously seen with direct operative attempts at controlling severe hemorrhage from pelvic fractures.[66,67]

AXIOM Most pelvic arterial and venous injuries can be controlled by appropriate arterial embolization.

If the pelvic bleeding is diffuse, and it is felt that occlusion of a proximal internal iliac artery is indicated, the collateral vasculature of the normal pelvis is so good that bilateral embolization of the major internal iliac arterial branches will usually be necessary to control the bleeding. However, such an extensive disruption of the arterial blood supply to a severely traumatized pelvic area can cause significant ischemia. Ischemic mucosal injury to the rectum and sloughing of pelvic tissues have been reported after bilateral internal iliac artery occlusion.[6,37,42] Impotency in males has also been noted. However, this is difficult to ascribe solely to angiographically induced ischemia because severe associated lumbosacral nerve plexus injuries are usually also present in these patients.[1]

Because of these and other inherent complications, unnecessary angiographic embolization should be avoided. In general, angiography should be reserved for pelvic fracture patients with clinical evidence of significant ongoing hemorrhage. Overall, angiography may be indicated in only about 2% of all pelvic fractures.[6,46]

EXTERNAL WOUNDS. External bleeding via a laceration which communicates with a fracture is best controlled by gauze packing or suturing the laceration shut. In many instances, fibrin glue can help control the bleeding.

LAPAROTOMY. If severe external hemorrhage continues in spite of all these measures, a formal laparotomy with intermittent occlusion of the abdominal aorta during pelvic packing may be required to help control the bleeding.

Intraperitoneal rupture of a massive pelvic hematoma is frequently lethal. If this is encountered, little can be accomplished by searching for individual bleeding points which may include fracture sites and/or the presacral venous plexus. Occlusion of the distal abdominal aorta can reduce bleeding while the pelvis is packed tightly with gauze rolls. The gauze pack tends to work better if there is a watertight layer of plastic or preclotted sponge between the packs and the bleeding tissue. A pneumatic anti-shock garment (PASG) or external pelvic fixation may be applied after the abdomen has been closed.

Management of Associated Injuries

Constant evaluation for other injuries is extremely important in the successful management of pelvic fractures.

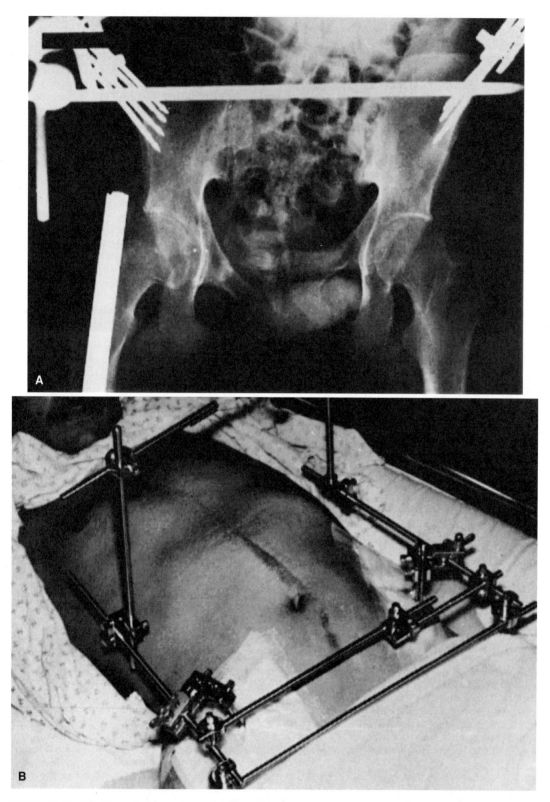

FIGURE 28–13 **(A).** Hoffman-Vidal apparatus used as an external fixater for an unstable vertical fracture of the left side of pelvis. **(B).** The patient in bed with the external fixator in place. (From Berquist TH, Coventry MB. The pelvis and hips. In Berquist TH, ed. Imaging of orthopedic trauma, 2nd ed. New York: J.B. Lippincott, 1992;5:247.)

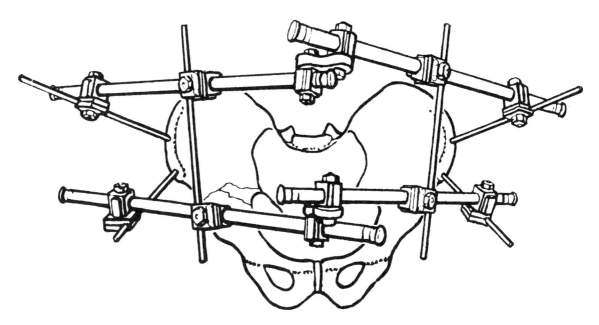

FIGURE 28–14 A simple anterior frame utilizing four Shanz screws (two in each iliac wing). (From Behrens F. External fixation. In: Muller ME, Allgower M, Schneider R, Willenegger H (eds). Manual of Internal Fixation. Techniques recommended by the AO-ASIF Group, 3rd ed. Berlin 1991;5:395.)

AXIOM Almost 90% of patients with major pelvic fractures have injuries to other body regions.[3,6,68]

The immediate threats of concomitant head, thoracic, or abdominal injuries may postpone definitive management of the pelvic fracture. Associated injuries to the lower extremities have been reported in over 60% of patients with major pelvic fractures,[1] and these can seriously complicate orthopedic management of the pelvis. Any of these associated injuries can also adversely affect outcome and result in prolonged disability if not properly treated in a timely fashion.

GENITOURINARY TRACT

Because of its close anatomic relationship to the bony pelvis, the genitourinary tract is the site of injury in at least 5-10% of patients with pelvic fractures admitted to a trauma center. The bladder and urethra are injured in about 4% and 2% of cases respectively (Table 28–4).[69,70] Of those with genitourinary tract injuries associated with pelvic fractures, Clark and Prudencio[71] have noted posterior urethral injury in 58% (Fig. 28–16), bladder injury alone in 32%, and combined urethral and bladder injury in 10%.

Findings suggestive of urethral or bladder injury include urethral blood, perineal hematomas, abnormal location of the prostate, and

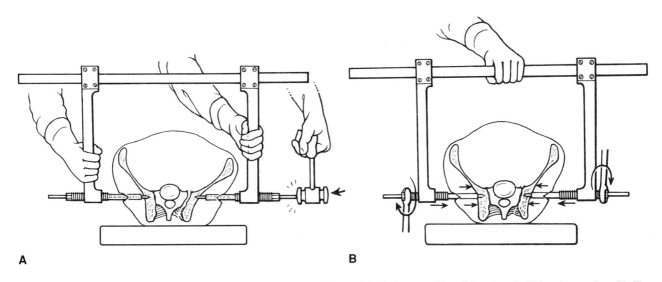

A **B**

FIGURE 28–15 **(A).** The Steinmann pins of the antishock clamp are driven 1.0 cm into the ilium with a mallet. **(B).** The sidearms are then pushed medially along the crossbar. This results in the threaded bolts sliding over the Steinmann pins until the end of the bolts contact the wall of the ilium. The threaded bolts are advanced further medially with a wrench, resulting in compression of the ilium and stabilization of the posterior fracture-diastasis. (From Ganz R, Krushell RJ, Jacob RB, Kuffer. The antishock pelvis clamp. Clin Orthopaedics 1991;267:71.)

TABLE 28–4   Abdominal Injuries in a Collective Review of 2,422 Patients with Pelvic Fractures

	Number	*%*
Bladder	89	3.7
Urethra	49	2.0
Spleen	46	1.9
Liver	31	1.3
Mesentery	24	1.0
Intestine	24	1.0
Kidney	24	1.0
Pancreas	7	0.3
Diaphragm	6	0.3
Gallbladder	1	0.04

gross hematuria. Pubic arch fractures and straddle or butterfly pattern fractures are particularly apt to involve the genitourinary tract and indicate the need for a complete evaluation of the bladder and urethra. However, up to 57% of men with urethral injury will have no suggestive physical signs.[69] In males with a possible urethral injury, retrograde urethrography is indicated. The female urethra is very short and seldom has an injury that requires emergency repair.

Severe bladder injuries can occur in either sex and should be ruled out by retrograde cystography if there is hematuria or a severe anterior fracture. Initially, a small volume of contrast permits assessment of the urethrovesical junction. Next, a retrograde stress cystogram us-

ing at least 300 ml of a 20-30% contrast agent is performed to dislodge any clot or fat that may be sealing a tear of the bladder. Finally, a postvoid radiogram enables identification of posterior bladder injuries that might have been concealed by a full bladder on the AP view. Following the retrograde studies, intravenous pyelography (IVP) or a CT scan with intravenous contrast can be performed.[3,42,69]

More than 75% of bladder ruptures seen with pelvic fractures are extraperitoneal[71] (Fig. 28–17). Intraperitoneal bladder tears usually produce signs of peritonitis and are generally managed at laparotomy (Fig. 28–18). The bladder repair is performed in 2-3 layers using absorbable sutures. Continuous drainage of the bladder in men and some women is then provided with a suprapubic catheter. In contrast, small extraperitoneal bladder injuries can often be managed simply with bladder drainage, which usually involves insertion of a large suprapubic catheter in males and a Foley catheter in females.

Urethral injuries are usually treated initially with suprapubic drainage and later repair. Injuries to the vagina, uterus and adnexa are treated with debridement, repair and drainage as needed.

ABDOMINAL VISCERA

Injuries to the liver, spleen, mesentery, intestine or kidneys are seen in at least 5-10% of patients with severe pelvic fractures. Hemodynamic instability is the usual clinical presentation if the patient has severe spleen, liver or mesenteric injuries.

In hemodynamically stable patients with pelvic fractures, many centers now use contrast-enhanced CT scans for assessment of both the pelvic and intraabdominal contents. If one relies on CT, however, injuries to the intestine are easily missed, even with intestinal con-

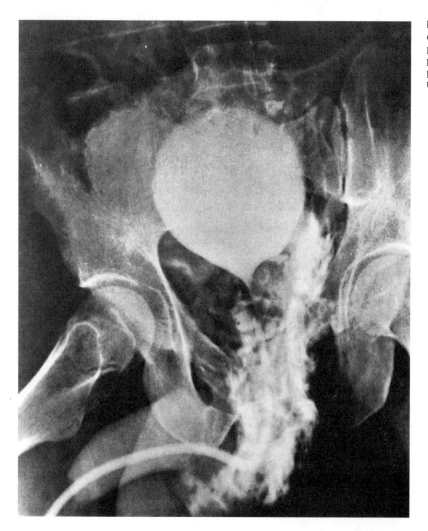

FIGURE 28–16   Type III rupture of the posterior urethra with extravasation of contrast above and below the urogenital diaphragm. There is a marked elevation of the bladder due to a pelvic hematoma. (From Berquist TH and Coventry MB. The pelvis and hips. In Berquist TH, ed. Imaging of orthopedic trauma, 2nd ed. New York: J.B. Lippincott, 1992;5:257.)

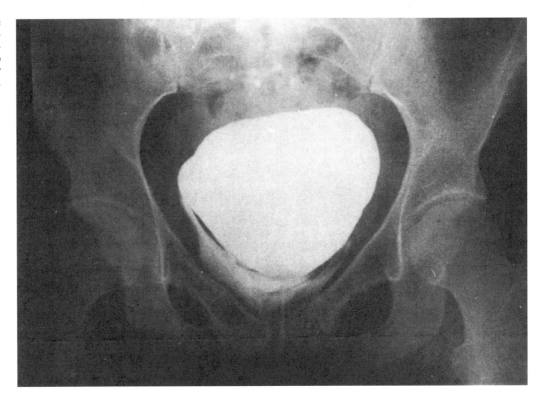

FIGURE 28–17 Bladder rupture secondary to pelvic fractures. Cystogram shows extraperitoneal rupture of the bladder secondary to pelvic fractures. (From Daffner RH. Pelvic trauma. In McCort JJ. Trauma radiology. 1990;7:377.)

trast given orally or into the stomach 30-60 minutes before the CT examination. Consequently, even if there are negative findings on CT, frequent abdominal examinations looking for evidence of increasing peritoneal irritation are necessary.

Intestinal injuries, if untreated, will usually produce signs and symptoms of peritonitis within a few hours. Except for surgery, the most objective means of excluding this problem is DPL. A positive DPL for bowel injury is usually interpreted as greater than 500 white blood cells (WBC)/mm³ or evidence of bowel content in the lavage aspirate. The longer the time between intestinal injury and DPL, the more likely the DPL is to show an increased WBC. Consequently, in cases of suspected bowel injury and an early negative DPL, the DPL catheter should be left in place and a repeat lavage performed 6 hours later.

Although determining amylase levels in DPL fluid is often not considered to be cost-effective, an early elevated DPL amylase may be an indication of intestinal injury.[72] Some authors have also used an elevated alkaline phosphatase in DPL fluid to diagnose intestinal injury.

RECTUM

Despite the close anatomic relationship, rectal injuries are uncommon following pelvic fractures. Extensive perineal and buttock lacerations are much more frequent.

AXIOM If the patient with a pelvic fracture has a rectal or extensive perineal wound, the fecal stream should be diverted with a colostomy.

Fecal diversion for a rectal injury or severe perineal lacerations is best accomplished by an end-sigmoid colostomy and mucous fistula.[1] It is also worthwhile to extract and irrigate out any feces present in the defunctionalized rectum because it might act as an ongoing source of bacterial contamination. Irrigation of the distal colon with broad-spectrum antibiotic solutions (neomycin 0.5% or Betadine 5%) has also been recommended.[42]

Colostomy closure to provide intestinal continuity is restored only after (a) all the rectal and perineal wounds have healed, (b) the patient is ambulating well, and (c) the patient has reached an optimal

nutritional state, usually in 9-12 weeks.[1] Prior to colostomy closure, it is important to perform proctoscopic and/or rectal contrast studies to ensure that rectal healing is complete. Manometric studies may also be done preoperatively if the adequacy of anal sphincter function is questionable.

NEUROLOGIC INJURY

Associated neurologic injuries, particularly to the lumbosacral plexus, are usually of relatively little concern in the immediate management of the severe pelvic fractures. However, they may have very important long-term consequences.[1,73,74] Once bleeding has been controlled, a complete neurologic examination of the lower extremities should be performed. Neuropathies secondary to hematoma compression, unrelated to pelvic fractures, may be alleviated by early operative decompression.[75] However, diagnosing such a problem and determining the optimal time for decompression can be extremely difficult.

With persistent neurologic deficits, electromyography (EMG) is recommended 3 weeks after injury to serve as a baseline for determining eventual prognosis. Even in the absence of clinically apparent neurological signs, injury to the lumbosacral plexus is demonstrated by electromyographic abnormalities in up to 64% of patients with sacral fracture and sacroiliac joint separation.[76] An aggressive rehabilitation program with early attention to passive range of motion and maintenance of motor tone offers the patient the best chance for a functional return to society.

Orthopaedic Management of Pelvic Fractures

The vast majority of pelvic injuries are stable, and can be adequately treated by closed means. The treatment goals are to rehabilitate the patient as soon as possible. This most often means bed rest until comfortable, and then standing up as tolerated with crutches. However, some fractures that are widely displaced, or known to be unstable from the previously described radiographic work-up, should undergo operative intervention. Unstable fractures not only preclude early mobilization and weight bearing, but may also result in leg length inequality, nonunion, neurologic injuries, and chronic pain.[25]

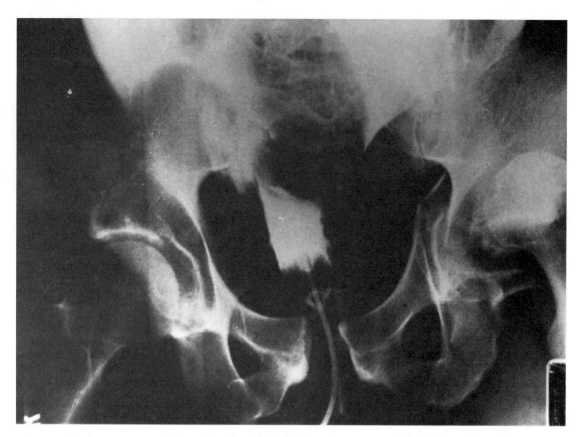

FIGURE 28–18 Intraperitoneal rupture of the bladder as a result of severe pelvic fractures and symphaseal diastasis. The cystogram shows contrast that has extravasated intraperioneally surrounding loops of bowel. (From Daffner RH. Pelvic trauma. In McCort JJ. Trauma radiology. 1990;7:377.)

AXIOM An important orthopaedic question with pelvic fractures is pelvic stability, since this often determines subsequent care and the need for operative intervention.

TYPES OF PROCEDURES FOR PELVIC FRACTURE MANAGEMENT

External Fixation (Figs. 28–14, 28–15)

External fixation has an important role to play in the management of acute pelvic fractures and may be required during the acute resuscitation.[49-51,64] External fixation of the pelvis consists of inserting fixation pins between the tables of the iliac crest and connecting them with anterior external bars. Many different frame designs have been proposed, but there are no significant biomechanical differences between them, and simple constructs (i.e., anterior half frames) are usually recommended.

No anterior external fixation frame can control a vertically unstable pelvis adequately. Thus, some other modality (open reduction and internal fixation, traction, or spica casting) must also be used for these injuries.

External fixation has the inherent advantage of being a closed treatment modality; however, pin tract infection can be a problem, especially if the frame is left for a prolonged period of time. Therefore, meticulous pin site care is recommended.

Internal Fixation

Open reduction and internal fixation of pelvis fractures is increasing in popularity.[77,78] Because a thorough preoperative evaluation and plan is required, as well as a medically stable patient, it is rarely performed acutely. External fixation, traction or bed rest are the usual provisional treatments until internal fixation can be performed. Typi-

cal indications for internal fixation are widely displaced anterior lesions, unstable posterior lesions, and acetabular fractures. Potential complications include iatrogenic neurovascular injury and the risk of postoperative infection.

Traction/Pelvic Slings

Skeletal traction is a frequently used provisional modality in patients with unstable pelvic or acetabular fractures. It is usually applied through a femoral pin and is discontinued when the definitive treatment is performed. Rarely is prolonged bed rest in traction, with its many potential complications, indicated as definitive treatment.

Pelvic slings were once advocated in the treatment in anterior lesions, but have now been largely abandoned.

OPERATIVE MANAGEMENT OF VARIOUS FRACTURES

Fractures of the Iliac Crest or Pubic or Ischial Rami

Most isolated fractures of the ilium or of pubic or ichial rami can be treated nonoperatively. These are typically minimally displaced and stable. Occasionally, however, open reduction will be needed for widely displaced fractures. This is especially true in the injuries close to the perineum, where dyspareunia can develop.

Disruptions of the Symphysis Pubis (Anterior Lesions)

Symphysis pubic disruptions where the diastasis is over 2.5 cm can be treated operatively. This can be done in a number of different ways, including application of a small two hole plate.[79] Larger plates, or double plates can be used to provide increased stability,[25,78] but as with external fixation, anterior plates alone cannot adequately control unstable posterior lesions (Fig. 28–19). Application of anterior plates is typically performed on a delayed basis, but may be performed

FIGURE 28–19 Complex pelvic fracture involving the pubic symphysis and left sacroiliac joint requiring internal fixation to achieve stability. (From Berquist TH and Coventry MB. The pelvis and hips. In Berquist TH, ed. Imaging of orthopedic trauma, 2nd ed. New York: J.B. Lippincott, 1992;5:248.)

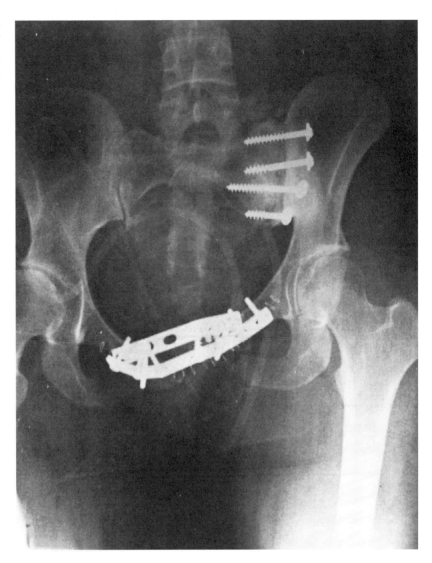

acutely in open injuries, or when the surgical exposure is performed for emergency treatment of another injury (e.g., acute repair of a ruptured bladder).

Anterior lesions can also be managed definitively with external fixation.[61] Pin tract infections and the relative inconvenience of the frame are factors to be considered. If the soft tissues anteriorly are less than optimal for internal fixation (i.e. previous infection or extreme swelling) then external fixation should be used.

Unstable Posterior Vertical Shear/Sacroiliac Joint Disruptions

Posterior unstable lesions are indications for operative intervention once the patient is medically stable. Sacroiliac joint disruptions can be approached anteriorly and plated,[80] or can be approached posteriorly and fixed with bars[25] or screws.[78,81] Sacroiliac joint fixation with fluoroscopically assisted screw placement into the body of the sacrum is a demanding technique that is being employed increasingly (Fig. 28–20).

Sacral Fractures

Sacral fractures are frequently undiagnosed and untreated, and they can have many late complications including neurological deficits, and urinary, rectal and sexual dysfunction. Denis' classification of sacral fractures based on direction, location and level is useful.[82] Surgical decompression in cases of neurologic injury may be beneficial in selected cases.

Acetabular Fractures

Acetabular fractures represent extremely complex injuries, and thorough review of the subject is beyond the scope of this text. In the past, satisfactory results were reported with nonoperative treatment.[83] However, many different fracture types were often lumped together, and the nature of these injuries, their classification and the anatomical approaches had not been well worked out. There has been much recent interest and work in this field.[22,25,84-86] Today, if technically possible, displaced acetabular fractures are treated with the same principles as other intraarticular joint fractures-that is, open anatomic reduction, stable internal fixation, and early motion.

These procedures are technically difficult and often lengthy, and require significant preoperative planning. Considerable resources, equipment, assistants and an experienced surgeon are needed. Therefore they are not performed acutely, but rather at some point in the early postinjury period. Appropriate preoperative studies include an anteroposterior radiograph of the pelvis and the involved hip, and Judet views.[22,84] A CT scan should also be performed.

The preoperative radiographs allow for classification of the fracture pattern. The most commonly used classification system among acetabular surgeons is that of Letournel.[22,84] It divides these injuries into two large groups. There are five elementary patterns (posterior wall, posterior column, anterior wall, anterior column, and transverse fractures) and five associated patterns which include at least two of the elementary forms (posterior wall and posterior column, anterior

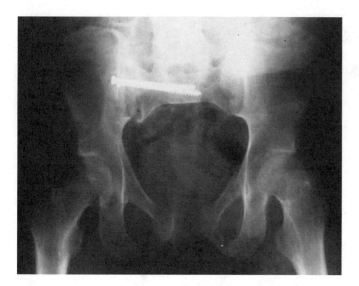

FIGURE 28–20 Posterior fixation of the pelvis is accomplished with two threaded screws.

wall and posterior hemi-transverse, transverse and posterior wall, T-type, and both column fractures). Once the fracture pattern has been studied and classified, the appropriate surgical approach and fixation can be planned.

Operative indications include incongruency of the weight-bearing acetabulum and instability of the hip joint. These include posterior or anterior wall fractures with instability, displaced dome, transverse or column fractures. Intraarticular osteochondral fractures and femoral head fractures are also indications for surgery.

The results of open reduction of these injuries are good if an anatomical reduction can be achieved.[84,85] However, there is a definite learning curve for surgeons performing these procedures, and numerous postoperative complications and problems can occur. These include excessive blood loss, infection, nerve injury, heterotopic bone, thromboembolic disease, nonunion, malreduction, and posttraumatic arthritis.

MANAGEMENT OF COMPLICATIONS

Complications of particular concern with pelvic fractures include pelvic sepsis, posttraumatic pulmonary insufficiency, deep venous thrombosis, hyperbilirubinemia, impotency, and prolonged postinjury convalescence.

Pelvic Sepsis

AXIOM The most common cause of death more than 48 hours after a pelvic fracture is sepsis.[10,68,87]

Efforts to prevent pelvic sepsis are extremely important. Appropriate debridement and irrigation of all open wounds and diversion of the fecal stream, when indicated, are extremely important. The antibiotics used should be effective against gram-negative enteric bacilli (such as E. coli) and anaerobes (such as Bacteroides fragilis). Although it is not clear how long such antibiotics should be given, unless there is continued contamination, 4-6 days should be adequate.

Retroperitoneal abscess formation resulting from direct extension of a local infection or hematogenous seeding of a pelvic hematoma with bacteria can be a highly lethal complication.[88] Liberal use of CT scans can assist in the early recognition of infected pelvic and retroperitoneal collections. Percutaneous aspiration for diagnosis of suspected infection in these collections and definitive catheter drainage can sometimes be accomplished by CT guidance. If this is not possible or adequate, surgical drainage is often possible via an extra-

peritoneal approach. Very rarely, severe life-threatening infections involving large areas of devitalized tissue in the pelvis may require a hemipelvectomy.[13]

Hyperbilirubinemia

AXIOM Jaundice before the 8th day after a pelvic fracture is usually due to hematomas and blood transfusions; jaundice beginning after the 8th day is usually due to sepsis.

Hyperbilirubinemia during the first 5 days after trauma is fairly common in patients with severe pelvic fractures requiring massive blood transfusions. Clinical jaundice with total serum bilirubin levels in the 5-12 mg/dl range was reported in 26 patients with pelvic fractures who received 10 or more units of blood and survived for at least 5 days.[6,42] Since these patients often have a significant fraction of conjugated (direct) bilirubin, the differential diagnosis must include biliary tract obstruction due to associated injury to the head of the pancreas, the second portion of the duodenum, or the extrahepatic bile ducts. Jaundice developing after the 8th day is more likely to be due to sepsis, particularly from an intraperitoneal infection by multiple organisms, including Bacteroides fragilis.

Impotence

Impotence is a well-established complication of membranous urethral injury which commonly occurs in association with anterior pelvic disruptions.[1] Impotence has also been described in association with pelvic fractures without vesicourethral injury in patients with severe pelvic hemorrhage treated by angiographic embolization.[89] In such cases, the associated injuries to the lumbosacral nervous plexus seem far more likely to have caused the impotence.

AXIOM Evidence of impotence should be sought in all sexually active males with pelvic fractures so that the psychosocial aspects of this problem can be dealt with as early as possible.

Deep Vein Thrombosis

The incidence of deep vein thrombosis (DVT) after pelvic fractures is not well-defined, although, it is probably around 15-20%.[90] Pelvic fracture patients often are immobilized, and the fragment and associated soft tissue injury may lead to a hypercoagulable state locally. Eight of 60 patients with pelvic fractures developed a DVT diagnosis by duplex ultrasound in a recent series.[91] One of these patients suffered a pulmonary embolism. In light of the high incidence of DVT, duplex ultrasonography of the lower extremities should be routinely employed in pelvic fracture patients. This noninvasive technique can be employed at the bedside with a high degree of accuracy.

DVT prophylaxis in these patients is difficult. Early ambulation is desirable in all patients for both its circulatory and pulmonary benefits. However, many patients cannot undergo early ambulation secondary to multiple injuries. It is also difficult to administer subcutaneous heparin to trauma patients at risk for bleeding. Sequential compression stockings should have no increased risk of bleeding and have been liberally employed by the authors in this setting. Treatment for DVT in patients with pelvic fractures is anticoagulation if possible; however, many times it is not, and placement of a vena caval filter is appropriate.[92,93]

Physical Disabilities

Patients with severe pelvic fractures often have severe disabilities and require extensive physical therapy and rehabilitation.[1,94] Even with rather simple avulsion fractures, patients often require hospitalization for weeks, and physical disability persists for an average of 19 weeks.[1] Thus, patients with more complex fractures involving the pelvic ring or the acetabulum can be hospitalized for prolonged periods, especially if there are other associated injuries or complications. Major disabilities usually last for more than 6-9 months, or can be permanent. Late complications of pelvic fractures includes chronic pain from malunion or nonunion, posttraumatic sacroiliac arthritis, and permanent nerve root injuries. Accurate reduction of posterior vertical shear injuries and sacroiliac joint disruptions appears to have decreased the incidence of late chronic pain.[25,90] Decompression of sacral fractures with nerve root involvement should also be considered.[82]

SUMMARY

About 80-90% of pelvic fractures are minor and are primarily an orthopedic concern. However, the severe pelvic fractures in the remaining 10-20% have a high mortality and morbidity rate from pelvic bleeding and associated injuries.

Although simultaneous involvement of several specialties is important, the initial emphasis is on resuscitation, control of hemorrhage, and prevention or treatment of delayed sepsis. Massive retroperitoneal bleeding in the pelvis is often extremely difficult to control and can be lethal. Hypotension due to bleeding from associated intraperitoneal injuries should either be rapidly ruled out with open DPL or controlled at laparotomy.

If there is severe persistent pelvic bleeding, external fixation of the pelvis and/or angiographic localization and embolization of the major sites of hemorrhage are increasingly performed with success.

All major pelvic fracture victims should be carefully evaluated for occult injuries to the genitourinary tract or rectum. Earlier ambulation with either external or internal stabilization and aggressive physical therapy can greatly reduce the length of convalescence and the amount of permanent disability. Repeated examination of the patient and anticipation of the potential complications of serious pelvic injuries are essential in optimizing the patient's chances of recovery and early functional return to society.

⊘ FREQUENT ERRORS

1. *Failure to look carefully for associated injuries.*
2. *Failure to be aggressive in determining and controlling the cause of persistent or recurrent hypotension or continuing large fluid and blood requirements.*
3. *Reliance on plain radiographs to rule out pelvic fractures in patients with symptoms suggesting this injury.*
4. *Failure to consider a pelvic fracture as one which is open in patients with perineal lacerations.*
5. *Rapid removal of an inflated PASG without carefully evaluation of associated BP changes.*
6. *Opening a pelvic hematoma due to blunt trauma.*
7. *Failure to perform a diverting sigmoid colostomy in a patient with a pelvic fracture and a laceration in or very near the rectum.*
8. *Failure to thoroughly evaluate the lower genitourinary tract in patients with hematuria or severe anterior fractures.*

▼▼▼▼▼▼▼▼▼▼▼▼▼▼▼▼▼▼▼▼▼▼▼▼▼▼▼▼▼▼

SUMMARY POINTS

1. Next to fractures of the skull, pelvic fractures are the commonest skeletal injuries associated with death in patients with multiple injuries.
2. The main cause of death in patients with pelvic fractures is uncontrolled bleeding, usually from associated injuries.
3. The outcome of patients with pelvic fractures is largely determined by the associated injuries.
4. The rich interconnection of the pelvic vessels explains why occlusion of a single trunk, such as the hypogastric (internal iliac) artery, does little to decrease hemorrhage after pelvic trauma.

5. The pelvis can be described as a vascular sink because it is a distensible reservoir for blood flowing antegrade from the aorta and retrograde from the legs and portal circulation.
6. Forceful crushing, axial compression, or vertical shear injuries have a high incidence of associated injuries to adjacent structures.
7. Failure to respond to the initial fluid resuscitation implies severe active bleeding which must be controlled rapidly if the patient is to survive.
8. Suprapubic pain, low back pain or lower extremity shortening, weakness, or diminished sensation after trauma should suggest the presence of a pelvic fracture.
9. Part of the examination of an injured pelvis is determination of the stability of the major fragments.
10. Lacerations of the perineum, groin or buttock after blunt trauma indicate an open pelvic fracture until proven otherwise.
11. In all major pelvic fractures one must look carefully for rectal, genito-urinary, or perineal injuries.
12. A full bladder is much more susceptible to injury than one which is empty.
13. An AP radiograph of the chest and pelvis and a lateral radiograph of the cervical spine should be obtained on all patients with major blunt trauma.
14. A CT scan is usually needed to define the extent of a pelvic fracture accurately.
15. The results of a CT scan or any other radiologic procedure are only as good as the quality of the films obtained and their interpretation.
16. Angiography of the abdominal aorta and iliac arteries can be used to diagnose and treat continued intraabdominal or pelvic bleeding.
17. A negative DPL in a patient with a pelvic fracture is generally a highly accurate indicator that significant intraperitoneal injury is not present; however, the DPL is often falsely positive.
18. The hemodynamic status of the patient at the time of presentation to the ED is the single most important predictor of the outcome.
19. The foremost consideration with pelvic fractures is rapid resuscitation and control of exsanguinating hemorrhage.
20. One should always anticipate significant blood loss with pelvic fractures.
21. Diagnostic peritoneal lavage (DPL) is the initial test of choice for diagnosis of bleeding from intraperitoneal organs.
22. An inflated PASG should be deflated only one segment at a time while constantly monitoring the blood pressure.
23. A patient who has marginal ventilation should be intubated and provided with ventilatory support prior to inflation of the abdominal component of a PASG.
24. If the patient's systolic BP does not rise to at least 90 mm Hg within 5 minutes of thoracic aorta cross-clamping, the patient is in terminal cardiovascular failure.
25. If a rapidly expanding or ruptured pelvic hematoma is found at laparotomy, it should be packed and arrangements made for external pelvic fixation and/or angiographic embolization of the bleeding vessels.
26. Following pelvic packing, a second-look operation 24-48 hours later is recommended if the patient's coagulation and bleeding studies can be returned to normal.
27. Hemipelvectomy for pelvic bleeding should be performed only if most of the dissection has already been accomplished by the trauma.
28. With the exception of trauma to the common and external iliac arteries, most pelvic arterial and venous injuries can be controlled by appropriate arterial embolization.
29. Almost 90% of patients with major pelvic fractures have injuries to other body regions.
30. If the patient with a pelvic fracture has a rectal or extensive perineal wound, the fecal stream should be diverted with a sigmoid colostomy.
31. An important initial orthopedic consideration with a pelvic fracture is stability. This can be assessed clinically, but usually requires radiographic studies.

32. The most common cause of death more than 48 hours after a pelvic fracture is sepsis.

33. Jaundice before the 8th day after a pelvic fracture is usually due to hematomas and blood transfusions; jaundice beginning after the 8th day, is usually due to sepsis.

34. Evidence of impotence should be sought in all sexually active males with pelvic fractures so that the psychosocial aspects of this problem can be dealt with as early as possible.

▲▲▲▲▲▲▲▲▲▲▲▲▲▲▲▲▲▲▲▲▲▲▲▲▲▲▲▲▲▲▲

REFERENCES

1. Mucha P. Pelvic fractures. In Moore EE, Mattox KL, Feliciano DV, eds. Trauma, 2nd ed. Norwalk, CT: Appleton-Lange, 1991; 553.
2. Rothenberger DA, Velaseo R, et al. Open pelvic fractures: a lethal injury. J Trauma 1978;18:124.
3. Kane WJ. Fractures of the pelvis. In Green DP, Rochwood CA, eds. Fractures. Philadelphia: JB Lippincott, 1984; 1093.
4. Perry JE Jr, McClellan RJ. Autopsy findings in 127 patients following fatal traffic accidents. Surg Gynecol Obstet 1964;47:581.
5. Melton LJ 3rd, Sampson JM, et al. Epidemiologic feature of pelvic fractures. Clin Orthop 1981;155:43.
6. Mucha P Jr, Farnell MB. Analysis of pelvic fracture management. J Trauma 1984;24:379.
7. Patel KP, Capan LM, Grant GJ, Miller SM. Musculoskeletal injuries. Capan LM, Miller SM, Turndorf H, eds. Trauma—anesthesia and intensive care. Philadelphia: J.B. Lippincott, 1991; 525-536.
8. Brotman S, Soderstrom CA, Oster-Granite M, et al. Management of severe bleeding in fractures of the pelvis. Surg Gynecol Obstet 1981;153:823.
9. Patterson FP, Morton KS. Neurological complications of fractures and dislocations of the pelvis. J Trauma 1972;12:1013.
10. Siebel RW, Border JR, Flint LM. Pelvic trauma. In Richardson JD, Polk HC, Flint LM, eds. Clinical care and pathophysiology. Chicago: Year Book, 1987; 421.
11. Cryer HM, Miller FB, Evers BM, et al. Pelvic fracture classification: correlation with hemorrhage. J Trauma 1988;28:973.
12. Gilliland MG, Ward RE, Flynn TC, et al. Peritoneal lavage and angiography in the management of patients with pelvic fractures. Am J Surg 1982;144:744.
13. Richardson JD, Harty J, Amin M, Flint LM. Open pelvic fractures. J Trauma 1982;22:533.
14. Pennal GF, Tile M, Waddell JP, Garside H. Pelvic disruption: assessment and classification. Clin Orthop 1980;151:12.
15. Dalal SA, Burgess AR, Seigel JH, Young JW, Brumback RJ, Poka A, Dunham GM, Gens D, Bathon H. Pelvis fracture in multiple trauma: classification by mechanism is key to pattern of organ injury, resuscitative requirements, and outcome. J Trauma 1989;29:981.
16. Young JWR, Burgess AR. Radiological management of pelvic ring fractures. Baltimore: Urban & Schwarzenberg, 1987.
17. Rodstein M. Accidents among the aged: incidence, causes, and prevention. J Chron Dis 1964;17:515.
18. Peltier LF. Historical note: Joseph Francois Malgaigne and Malgaigne's fractures. Clin Orthop 1980;151:4.
19. Gilliland MD, Ward RE, Barton RM, et al. Factors affecting mortality in pelvic fractures. J Trauma 1982;22:691.
20. Tile M, Pennal GF. Pelvic disruption: principles of management. Clin Orthop 1980;151:56.
21. Tile M. Pelvic ring fractures: should they be fixed? J Bone Joint Surg 1988;70B:1.
22. Letournel E. Acetabular fractures, classification and management. Clin Orthop 1980;151:81.
23. Bucholz RW. The pathological anatomy of the Malgaigne fracture-dislocations of the pelvis. J Bone Joint Surg 1981;63-A:400.
24. Burgess AR, Tile M. Fractures of the pelvis. In Rockwood CA, Green DP, Bucholtz RW, eds. Fractures in adults. 3rd ed. Philadelphia: J.B. Lippincott, 1991; 1399-1479.
25. Tile M. Fractures of the pelvis and acetabulum. Baltimore: Williams & Wilkins, 1984; 26.
26. Kellum JF, Browner BD. Fractures of the pelvic ring. In Browner BD, Jupiter JB, Levine AM, Trafton PG, eds. Skeletal trauma. Philadelphia: WB Saunders, 1992; 857.
27. Goldstein A, Phillips T, Sclafani SJA, et al. Early open reduction and internal fixation of the disrupted pelvic ring. J Trauma 1986;26:325.
28. Ward EF, Tomasin J, Vander Griend RA. Open reduction and internal fixation of vertical shear pelvic fractures. J Trauma 1987;27:291.
29. Trunkey DD. Pelvic injuries. In Najarian JS, Delaney JP, eds. Trauma and critical care surgery. Chicago: Year Book, 1987; 147.
30. Moreno C, Moore EE, Rosenberger A, et al. Hemorrhage associated with pelvic fracture: a multispecialty challenge. J Trauma 1986;26:987.
31. Saueracker AJ, McCroskey BL, Moore EE, Moore FA. Intraoperative hypogastric artery embolization for life-threatening pelvic hemorrhage: a preliminary report. J Trauma 1987;27:1127.
32. Gillott A, Rhodes M, Lucke J, et al. Utility of routine pelvic x-ray during blunt trauma resuscitation. J Trauma 1988;28:1570.
33. Gill K, Bucholz RW. The role of computerized tomographic scanning in the evaluation of major pelvic fractures. J Bone Joint Surg 1989;66A:34.
34. Civil ID, Ross SE, Botehlo G, et al. Routine pelvic radiography in severe blunt trauma: is it necessary? Ann Emerg Med 1988;17:488.
35. Berquist TH, Coventry MB. The pelvis and hips. IN Berquist TH, ed. Diagnostic imaging of the acutely injured patient. Munich: Urban & Schwarzenberg, 1985; 181.
36. Buckley SL, Burkus JK. Computerized axial tomography of pelvic ring fractures. J Trauma 1987;27:496.
37. Panetta T, Sclafani SJA, Goldstein AS, et al. Percutaneous transcatheter embolization for massive bleeding from pelvic fractures. J Trauma 1985;25:1021.
38. Moore JB, Moore EE, Markovehick VJ. Diagnostic peritoneal lavage for abdominal trauma—superiority of the open technique at the infraumbilical ring. J Trauma 1981;21:570.
39. Pachter HL, Hofstetter SR. Open and percutaneous paracentesis and lavage for abdominal trauma: a randomized prospective study. Arch Surg 1981;116:318.
40. Hubbard SG, Vivins BA, Sachatello CR. Diagnostic errors with peritoneal lavage in patients with pelvic fractures. Arch 1979;114:844.
41. McLaughlin HL. Fractures of the hips. In Mosely MF, ed. Accident surgery. East Norwalk, CT: Appleton-Lange, 1964.
42. Mucha P Jr. Pelvic fractures. IN McIlrath DC, Farnell MB, eds. Problems in general surgery. Philadelphia: J.B. Lippincott, 1984; 154.
43. Batalden DJ, Wickstrom PH, et al. Value of the G suit in patients with severe pelvic fractures. Arch Surg 1974;109:326.
44. Hoffman JR. External counterpressure and the MAST suit: current and future roles. Ann Emerg Med 1980;9:419.
45. Gaffney FA, Thal ER, Taylor WF, et al. Hemodynamic effects of medical anti-shock trousers (MAST garment). J Trauma 1981;21:931.
46. Mucha P Jr, Welch TJ. Hemorrhage in major pelvic fractures. Surg Clin North Am 68:757, 1988.
47. Dove AF, Poon WS, Weston PA. Haemorrhage from pelvic fractures: dangers and treatment. Injury 1982;13:375.
48. Aprahamian C, Towne JB, Thompson BM, et al. Effect of circumferential pneumatic compression devices on digital flow. Ann Emerg Med 1984;13:1092.
49. Kellum JF. The role of external fixation in pelvic disruptions. Clin Orthop 1989;241:66.
50. Wild JJ, Hanson GW, Tullos HS. Unstable fractures of the pelvis treated by external fixation. J Bone Joint Surg 1982;64A:1010.
51. Gylling SF, Ward RE, Holcroft JW, Bray TJ, Chapman MW. Immediate external fixation of unstable pelvic fractures. Am J Surg 1985;150:721.
52. Naam NH, Brown WH, Hurd R, et al. Major pelvic fractures. Arch Surg 1983;118:610.
53. Huittinen VM, Slatis P. Postmortem angiography and dissection of the hypogastric artery in pelvic fractures. Surgery 1973;73:454.
54. Wiencek RG Jr, Wilson RF. Injuries to the abdominal vascular system: how much does aggressive resuscitation and prelaparotomy thoracotomy really help? Surg 1987;102:731.
55. Wilson RF, Wiencek RG, Balog M. Factors affecting mortality rate with iliac vein injuries. J Trauma 1990;30:320.
56. Sheldon GF, Winestock DP. Hemorrhage from open pelvic fractures controlled intraoperatively with balloon catheter. J Trauma 1978;18:68.
57. Moore WM, Brown JJ, Haynes JL, Vaimontes L. Traumatic hemipelvectomy. J Trauma 1987;27:570.
58. Rodriguez-Morales G, Phillips T, Conn AK, Cox EF. Traumatic hemipelvectomy: report of two survivors and review. J Trauma 1983;23:615.
59. Carbolona P. Contribution of the external fixation in disjunctions of the pubis and of the sacroiliac articulation. Montpellier Chir 1980;19:61.
60. Karaharju EO, Slatis P. External fixation of double vertical pelvic fractures with a trapezoid compression frame. Injury 1978;10:142.
61. Slatis P, Karaharju EO. External fixation of unstable pelvis fractures: experience in 22 patients treated with a trapezoidal frame. Clin Orthop 1980;151:73.

62. Mears DC, Fu F. External fixation in pelvic fractures. Orth Clin North Am 1980;11:465.
63. Trafton PG, Herndon JH. External fixators in fracture management. In Maull KI, Cleveland HC, Stauch GO, Wolfert CC, eds. Advances in trauma. Chicago: Year Book, 1986; 257-260.
64. Sanders R, DiPasquale T. External fixation of the pelvis: application of the resuscitation frame. Techniques Orthop 1990;4(4):60.
65. Ganz R, Krushell RJ, Jacob RP, Kuffer J. The antishock pelvic clamp. Clin Ortho 1991;267:71.
66. Ravitch NM. Hypogastric artery ligation in acute pelvic trauma. Surgery 1964;56:601.
67. Seavers R, Lynch J, et al. Hypogastric artery ligation for uncontrollable hemorrhage in acute pelvic trauma. Surgery 1964;55:516.
68. Peltier LF. Complications associated with fractures of the pelvis. J Bone Joint Surg 1965;47A:1060.
69. Mucha P Jr. Recognizing and avoiding complications with pelvic fractures. Infect Surg 1985;11:53.
70. Emerman CE. Abdominopelvic injury associated with pelvic fracture. J Am Coll Emerg Phys 1979;8:312.
71. Clark SS, Prudencio RF. Lower urinary tract injuries associated with pelvic fractures. Diagnosis and management. Surg Clin North Am 1972; 52:183.
72. Alyono D, Perry JF Jr. Value of quantitative cell count and amylase activity of peritoneal lavage fluid. J Trauma 1981;21:345.
73. Conway RR, Hubbell SL. Electromyographic abnormalities in neurologic injury associated with pelvic fracture: case reports and literature review. Arch Phys Med Rehabil 1988;69:539.
74. Patterson FP, Morton KS. Neurological complications of fractures and dislocations of the pelvis. J Trauma 1972;12:1013.
75. Mastroianni PP, Roberts MP. Femoral neuropathy and retroperitoneal hemorrhage. Neurosurgery 1983;13:44.
76. Weis EB Jr. Subtle neurological injuries in pelvic fractures. J Trauma 1984;24:983.
77. Letournel E. Pelvic fracture operations. In Rob C, Smith R, eds. Operative surgery: accident surgery. London: Butterworths, 1978.
78. Helfet DL. Open reduction internal fixation of the pelvis. Techniques Orthop 1990;4(4):67.
79. Webb LX, Gristina AG, Wilson JR, Rhyne AL, Meredith JH, Hansen ST Jr. Two-hole plate fixation for traumatic symphysis pubis diastasis. J Trauma 1988;28:813.
80. Simpson LA, Waddell JP, Leighton RK, Kellam JF, Tile M. Anterior approach and stabilization of the disrupted sacroiliac Joint. J Trauma 1987;27:1332.
81. Matta JM, Saucedo T. Internal fixation of the pelvic ring. Clin Orthop. 1989;242:83.
82. Denis F, Davis S, Comfort T. Sacral fractures: an important problem. Clin Orthop 1988;227:67.
83. Rowe CR, Lowell JD. Prognosis of fractures of the acetabulum. J Bone Joint Surg 1961;43A:30.
84. Letournel E, Judet R. Fractures of the actabulum. 2nd ed. Berlin: Springer-Verlag, 1993.
85. Matta JM, Merritt PO. Displaced acetabular fractures. Clin Orthop 1988;230:83.
86. Mayo KA. Fractures of the acetabulum. Orthop Clin North Am 1987;18:43.
87. Trunkey DD, Chapman MW, Lim RC Jr, et al. Management of pelvic fractures in blunt trauma injury. J Trauma 1974;14:912.
88. O'Keefe TJ. Retroperitoneal abscess: a potentially fatal complication of closed fracture of the pelvis. J Bone Joint Surg 1978;60A:1117.
89. Ellison M. Timberlake GA, Kerstein MD. Impotence following pelvic fracture. J Trauma 1988;28:695.
90. Consensus Development Conference. National Institutes of Health. Prevention of venous thrombosis and pulmonary embolism. JAMA 1986;256:744.
91. White RH, Goulet JA, Bray TJ, et al. Deep-vein thrombosis after fracture of the pelvis. Assessment with serial duplex-ultrasound screening. J Bone Joint Surg 1990;72A:495.
92. Webb LX, Rush PT, Fuller SB, Meredith JW. Greenfield filter prophylaxis of pulmonary embolism in patients undergoing surgery for acetabular fracture. J Orthop Trauma 1992;6:139.
93. Buerger PM, Peoples JB, Lemmon GW, McCarthy MC. Risk of pulmonary emboli in patients with pelvic fractures. Am Surg 1993; 59:505.
94. Henderson RC. The long-term results of nonoperatively treated major pelvic disruptions. J Orthop Trauma 1989;3:41.

Chapter 29 Trauma to the Urinary Tract

ROBERT F. WILSON, M.D.

JAMES B. SMITH, M.D.

KATHLEEN A. MCCARROLL, M.D.

The urinary tract may be damaged by a wide variety of blunt or penetrating trauma to the chest, abdomen or pelvis. Urologic injuries occur in approximately 3-4% of trauma cases.[1] The kidney is injured 80-90% of the time, and 80-90% of these injuries are due to the blunt trauma.[2,3] Overall, the bladder and urethra are injured about 5-10% of the time but most of the urethral injuries occur in adult males. For example, in one series of 200 patients with a fractured pelvis, there were urethral injuries in 17 of the 121 men but in none of the 79 women.[4] Ureteral trauma is usually iatrogenic, although it occurs occasionally as the result of a knife or gunshot wound.[2,3]

Although some of the more frequent complications of trauma involve the genitourinary (GU) tract, few GU injuries are immediately life-threatening.[2] Thus, one must resist the temptation to perform a retrograde urethrogram in a male patient with a fractured pelvis until it is clear that pelvic angiography will not be needed. Patients do not die immediately of a ruptured urethra, but they can die rapidly from a torn internal iliac artery. Angiography and embolization, which may be required to treat continued arterial bleeding with pelvic fractures, will be difficult or impossible to perform if the pelvis is filled with contrast medium from urologic studies.[5,6] Nevertheless, urinary tract trauma is often associated with other serious injuries, and the combined injuries may contribute significantly to increased morbidity and mortality.[7]

PITFALL ⊘

If the physician concentrates his attention on obvious genitourinary damage, other injuries which are more likely to be lethal may cause sudden deterioration.

RENAL INJURIES

Although the kidneys are well protected by the ribs, vertebrae, back muscles and abdominal viscera, they are among the most commonly injured abdominal organs in blunt trauma. Blunt trauma accounted for 94% of the renal trauma in one series;[1] furthermore, in many cases of blunt renal trauma (83% in one series)[1] there were other injuries. In up to 30% of cases, the other non-renal injuries are serious.[8] The presence of fractures of the vertebral processes or the 11th or 12th rib are also common.

Abnormal kidneys, such as those with congenital anomalies, tumors, or hydronephrosis, are much more susceptible to injury than normal kidneys. Indeed, in some children, rupture of Wilms' tumor after a seemingly minor injury is the first sign of the tumor's presence.[2]

Types of Injury

Blunt injuries to the kidneys range from cortical lacerations and subcapsular hematomas to deep lacerations involving the collecting system and major vessels. With penetrating trauma, the extent of renal damage cannot be estimated from the appearance of the wound or the amount of hematuria present.[3] Nevertheless, since 20% of the cardiac output goes to the kidneys, blood loss from a renal pedicle injury can be massive.

Five types of renal injury are generally recognized[9] (Fig. 29–1). In increasing order of severity they are:

1. Contusions: bruises or minor tears of the renal parenchyma without capsular tears.
2. Minor lacerations: parenchymal disruptions with capsular damage without involvement of the collecting system.
3. Major lacerations: Deep lacerations of the renal parenchyma or fragmentation with or without urinary extravasation.
4. Vascular injuries: tears or occlusion of the renal arteries or veins.
5. Combinations of parenchymal and vascular injuries.

In the series of McAninch et al,[9] about half of the cases were major lacerations and 7% were vascular injuries. The Organ Scaling Committee of the American Association for the Surgery of Trauma has also graded the various types of renal injuries (Table 29–1).

Diagnosis

HISTORY

The keystone to the diagnosis of renal injuries is a high index of suspicion based on the type of trauma and its location.[7] Penetrating wounds anywhere near the kidney are suspect. With blunt abdominal, pelvic or lower thoracic trauma, the presence of flank or abdominal pain should make the physician suspicious of a genitourinary tract injury. Flank contusions and fractures of lower ribs or lumbar vertebrae are frequent associated injuries. The pain of serious renal injury is often described as a "dull ache."[2] Retroperitoneal bleeding may also cause nausea, vomiting, and paralytic ileus.

PHYSICAL EXAMINATION

After the patient has been completely examined and while careful monitoring of vital signs is continued, a more specific search can be made for possible renal injury. Flank or upper abdominal tenderness is a frequent finding after renal injury, and in some patients, a flank mass may be palpable. An expanding mass may indicate that the renal injury is severe enough to cause extravasation of blood or urine into perirenal tissues, and perhaps through Gerota's fascia.

PITFALL ⊘

If the physician fails to auscultate over the lower back following severe blunt trauma, important renal vascular injuries may be missed.

Occasionally a bruit heard in the posterior midline near the first and second lumbar vertebrae may be the only indication of damage to renal vessels.[7] In penetrating injuries in the upper abdomen or flank, a bruit suggests the presence of an arterial injury or acute arteriovenous fistula involving the renal artery and either the renal vein or inferior vena cava.

LABORATORY STUDIES

Urinalysis

If the patient can void, a midstream urinalysis should be obtained and, ideally, it should be examined by either the physician seeing the patient or the urology consultant.[7]

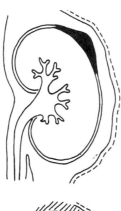
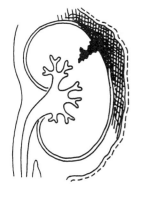
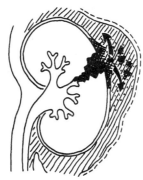
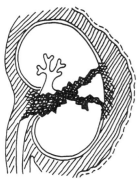

FIGURE 29–1 Types of renal injuries. **(A).** subcapsular hematoma, **(B).** shallow cortical laceration with perirenal hematoma, **(C).** deep parenchymal laceration into collecting system with extravasation, **(D).** fracture with avulsion of the lower pole. (From Herschron S, Kodoma A, Abara ED. Genitourinary trauma. In McMurty RY, McLellan BA, eds. Management of blunt trauma. Baltimore: Williams & Wilkins, 1990;25:285.)

AXIOM Although hematuria strongly suggests the presence of a urologic injury and is an indication for complete urologic examination, the absence of hematuria is of little diagnostic value.

Hematuria is present in 90% of renal injuries; however, if the vascular pedicle or ureter has been transected, the urinalysis may be completely normal.[7] Indeed, up to 30% of major renal injuries may exist with a normal urinalysis,[3,10,11] and up to one-third may have only microscopic hematuria.[12] Krieger found that 40% of patient with gross hematuria had only contusion or simple lacerations of the kidney, whereas three of the 22 patients with severe injuries had only microhematuria.[1] Federle[12] found no correlation between the severity of the renal injury and the presence and amount of hematuria in patients with deep stab wounds of the back and flank. Only 25% of patients with gross hematuria have had serious renal damage.[12,13] In patients with only microscopic hematuria, that figure drops to 1-2%.[13,14]

AXIOM In most centers, the presence of >40-50 RBC/HPF in the injured patient warrants complete radiologic investigation of the urinary tract.

Microscopic hematuria with more than 40-50 RBC/HPF suggests a possible urinary tract injury. Except for renal pedicle injuries, a lesser degree of hematuria tends to rule out serious urinary tract damage.[7]

PITFALL ⊘

Insertion of a Foley catheter before obtaining a urine specimen greatly reduces the value of the urinalysis.

Since the insertion of a urethral catheter can cause hematuria, the urine to be examined should, whenever possible, be collected without catheterization. Unfortunately, seriously injured patients often cannot urinate within the first 15-30 minutes, and a Foley catheter must be inserted so that the urine output can be monitored properly. In addition, in menstruating females, a catheterized specimen is usually much more accurate than a spontaneously voided specimen.

AXIOM Creatinine clearance is a much more accurate test of renal dysfunction than the BUN or serum creatinine.

BUN and Creatinine

A rising blood urea nitrogen (BUN) or serum creatinine may indicate impaired renal function following trauma. These changes, however are not usually apparent for at least 24-48 hours. The BUN, moveover, may rise without renal disease or damage. Blood in the intestinal tract, for example, may increase the BUN up to 50 mg/dl. The serum creatinine varies far less; it is less influenced by diet; and is affected very little by blood in the gut, but normal values vary widely depending on muscle mass and activity. Furthermore, creatinine clearance may fall long before serum creatinine values rise above normal.

TABLE 29–1 *Renal Injury Scale*[a]

	Grade[b]	Injury Description[b]	AIS 90[d]
I	Contusion	Microscopic or gross hematuria; urologic studies normal	2
	Hematoma	Subcapsular, nonexpanding without parenchymal laceration	2
II	Hematoma	Nonexpanding perirenal hematoma confined to renal retroperitoneum	2
	Laceration	<1.0 cm parenchymal depth of renal cortex without urinary extravasation	2
III	Laceration	>1.0 cm parenchymal depth of renal cortex with collecting system rupture or urinary extravasation	3
IV	Laceration	Parenchymal laceration extending through the renal cortex medulla, and collecting system	4
	Vascular	Main renal artery or vein with contained hemorrhage	4
V	Laceration	Completely shattered kidney	5
	Vascular	Avulsion of renal hilum which devascularizes kidney	5

[a]This classification scheme for acute renal injury has been devised by the Organ Injury Scaling Committee of the American Association for the Surgery of Trauma.
[b]Advance one grade for multiple injuries to the same organ.
[c]Based on most accurate assessment at autopsy, laparotomy, or radiologic study.
[d]AIS 90=1990 version of the Abbreviated Injury Score.

RADIOLOGIC STUDIES

Problems with Unstable Patients

AXIOM The patients who are usually in most need of complete radiological evaluation are often those who can least tolerate it because of multiple other injuries.

Patients with severe genitourinary injuries are often unstable and in need of immediate resuscitation and/or operation. In such cases, there is no time for a detailed radiologic GU evaluation. Nevertheless, it is important to assess the integrity of the urinary tract before major renal surgical intervention. Although not optimal, excretory urography can be performed in the resuscitation suite or on the operating table to evaluate the presence and function of the contralateral kidney prior to removal of a severely damaged kidney. The information gained will not be detailed but will be fundamentally accurate in the face of a surgical emergency.

INDICATIONS FOR RADIOLOGICAL STUDIES

The majority of patients are stable and not in need of immediate radiological studies in the emergency department or operating room, and thus a wide array of imaging procedures is available to them. Indications for imaging the kidneys in stable patients include: (a) hematuria, (b) multiple injuries, (c) rapid deceleration, and (d) posterior penetrating injuries.

All patients with gunshot wounds of the abdomen and many patients with anterior stab wounds will have an exploratory laparotomy. The urinary tract of these patients may be evaluated with an emergency department of intraoperative IVP depending upon the patient's hemodynamic condition and the urgency of surgery. There is, however, a trend toward conservative management of patients with penetrating injuries of the back and flank if there is no evidence of significant blood loss or intraabdominal injury. The safety of this approach is enhanced if there is reliable CT evidence that there is no intraperitoneal or retroperitoneal organ injury.[15]

Patients who have undergone rapid deceleration injury deserve special consideration in the radiological assessment of renal trauma. This is the mechanism by which renal pedicle avulsion occurs, and these patients, regardless of the presence or absence or hematuria, warrant further investigation.

AXIOM If there is any suspicion of renal damage, a CT or intravenous urogram (IVP) should be performed.

Types of Radiological Studies

Radiological imaging is the most accurate means for evaluating renal injuries. The techniques used include plain film radiography, intravenous urography (IVU/IVP) with or without nephrotomography, computed tomography (CT), ultrasonography (US), retrograde pyelography, renal angiography and, in special circumstances, radionuclide scintigraphy.

PLAIN FILMS OF THE ABDOMEN

The so-called kidney-ureter-bladder (KUB) study may provide important information concerning the retroperitoneum and associated skeletal structures.[8] The films should be examined for fractures of the lower ribs, lumbar spine (especially L1-3 transverse processes) and pelvis, which may suggest possible adjacent urinary tract injury.

AXIOM A normal-appearing plain radiograph of the abdomen is of little or no value for ruling out kidney damage.

A soft-tissue mass, loss of the psoas shadow (especially upper third) and scoliosis suggest the presence of blood, urine, or pus in the retroperitoneum.[7] A large perinephric fluid collection may elevate the ipsilateral hemidiaphragm. Displacement or abnormal size of the kidneys may indicate trauma or a pre-existing abnormality or disease process. Hessel[16] found only 30% of patients with renal injuries to have plain film findings which correlated well with the type and extent of renal damage present. Thus, while plain films may be invaluable for initial evaluation, especially for skeletal fractures or foreign body detection, they are relatively insensitive for identification of intrinsic urinary tract injury.

The localization of foreign bodies or bullets in or near the urinary tract is vital. With penetrating wounds, particularly those caused by bullets, radiopaque markers should be placed over the entrance and exit wounds. However, the path or the missile should never be presumed from the location of the entrance and exit wounds.

INTRAVENOUS UROGRAPHY

The IVP has been the mainstay of urologic imaging since its inception over 60 years ago. It has functioned as the initial screening examination with adequate sensitivity for safe patient management. Lang[17] reported that urography excluded significant renal injury in 87% of cases. However, his reported high accuracy rates were dependent upon the use of sufficiently high doses of contrast, optimal technique, and the use of nephrotomography. This is often not the type of study obtained in a busy urban ER, and the accuracy of urography must be understood to be highly dependent upon the quality of the examination. Other authors do not believe urography to be reliable in the evaluation of renal injury.[18,19,20]

AXIOM IVPs done under emergency circumstances may provide very little information about the kidneys.

It is now widely accepted that CT provides significantly more detailed and reliable information about renal injuries with less variability in technique and quality. Nevertheless, it seems wasteful and inappropriate to utilize expensive modalities for patients deemed to be at minor risk of significant renal trauma. Likewise, it is not always possible to obtain a CT scan for a variety of reasons including instability of the patient, presence of more urgent cases or nonfunction of the scanner.

Excretory urography is indicated if there is (a) hematuria (gross or microscopic >40-50 RBC/HPF), (b) flank or lateral abdominal pain, tenderness, or a mass; (c) fractures of transverse processes of the lumbar vertebrae; (d) a severe deceleration injury; or (e) a perirenal hematoma found at laparotomy.[7] It may also be indicated in patients with fractures of lower posterior ribs. However, radiographic assessment of renal trauma might not always be necessary.

AXIOM Excretory urography is usually not needed in blunt trauma victims who have no associated major intraabdominal injuries, no microscopic hematuria, and no hypotension.

Intravenous urography may be used as a screening tool in low-risk patients. A normal IVP with tomography can reliably exclude a major renal injury although renal contusions and small lacerations will probably not be seen. However, if the patient is going to CT for another study, consideration should be given to urinary tract CT imaging at the same time instead of doing an IVP.

The recommended adult trauma IVP dose is greater than the standard 1 cc/kg used for a routine, prepped IVP. Bolus administration of 100-150 cc (1 cc/lb up to 150 cc) of standard 60% iodinated contrast is necessary to compensate for intravenous fluid hemodilution and possible decreased renal perfusion. Systolic pressures of less than 80-90 mm Hg often result in very poor glomerular filtration and nondiagnostic levels of contrast excretion.

Drip infusion pyelography is preferred by some and may still be used with satisfactory results. The information obtained is similar to the high-dose trauma urogram, but the lower concentration of iodinated contrast (60% iodinated contrast medium diluted with an equal amount of water) results in a lower peak plasma concentration of iodine and, thus, decreased glomerular filtration and excretion of radiopaque iodine. The result is decreased opacification of the renal parenchyma and urine, making parenchymal injuries and small leaks more difficult to see. For the truly emergency study, in which the presence and function of the kidneys is the only desired information, virtually any technique works.

The recommended technique for the so-called "one-shot IVP" calls for bolus administration of 60% urographic contrast in a dose of 1 cc/lb and a single abdominal film taken three to five minutes after injection. If at all possible, a flat plate of the abdomen should be obtained prior to the IVP. Thus, any changes in the radiograph after the intravenous contrast is given can be assumed to be due to the excreted contrast material. An extra 50 ml of 60% contrast should probably be given to get good renal visualization if: (a) a great deal of intravenous fluid has been given, (b) renal function appears to be good and (c) urine output is greater than 1.0 ml/kg/hr. In a recent evaluation of 239 "one shot" IVPs done because evaluation in the radiology suite was felt to be unsafe, it was found that 8% of the patients with a normal one-shot IVP had renal injuries, and 26% with an abnormal one-shot IVP had no intraoperative evidence of renal injury.[21] The authors felt that delaying definitive therapy to obtain a preoperative one-shot IVP in an unstable patient is not warranted.

AXIOM Failure of both kidneys to visualize on a "one-shot IVP" is usually due to inadequate renal perfusion, inadequate intravenous contrast, or other technical factors.

If a history of allergy (especially to iodine or prior intravenous contrast agents) is elicited, caution is in order. The preliminary "test-dose" of 1.0 cc of iodinated contrast can cause anaphylaxis, shock and death as reliably as the full urographic dose in the susceptible patient. In "allergic type" patients (asthma, food allergies, etc.) who have no known iodine sensitivity, a low-osmolality, non-ionic agent (e.g., iohexol) is recommended.

The history of a previous allergic reaction (urticaria, edema, etc) to iodinated contrast or iodine-containing foods (e.g., shellfish) should contraindicate the use of iodinated contrast agents unless the benefit clearly outweighs the risk. Non-contrast CT, ultrasound, or radionuclide imaging may be satisfactory substitutes in such high risk patients. If nothing but iodinated contrast will do, steroid pretreatment protocols are available in most radiology departments. For complicated imaging problems in allergic patients, consultation with the radiologist is strongly suggested.

RETROGRADE PYELOGRAPHY

In an occasional case, the IVP or CT scan indicates that an injury to a ureter or the collecting system may be present.[2] In such instances cystoscopy with insertion of catheters into the ureters and retrograde urography may be needed to delineate a rupture of the collecting system. However, in many instances, a CT scan will adequately delineate the injury.

Computed Tomography

AXIOM An abdominal CT scan with intravenous contrast is the most accurate technique for visualizing a kidney that may be injured.

The majority of multiply injured patients can be stabilized enough to permit relatively complete radiographic evaluation. In such circumstances, CT is the modality of choice (Fig. 29–2). There are several inherent benefits to CT including: (a) identification of both major and minor injuries heretofore impossible with IVP, (b) good visualization of the relationship of the injury to the collecting system, (c) quantification of the extent of hematoma, (d) detection of even minimal amounts of contrast extravasation from anywhere in the urinary tract and (e) evaluation of multiple other organ systems simultaneously. The latter is of particular benefit in the patient with multiple injuries.

In addition, CT scanning is noninvasive and provides unparalleled imaging detail of renal anatomy and function. Properly performed, CT may provide information previously available only by arteriogra-

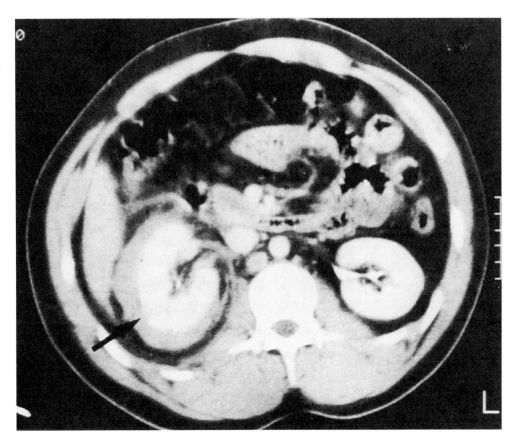

FIGURE 29–2 CT scan showing a perirenal hematoma surrounding the right kidney and a small renal cortical laceration (arrow). (From Harris JH Jr, Harris WH, Novelline RA. The radiology of emergency medicine. Baltimore: Williams & Wilkins, 1993; 670.)

phy. Furthermore, CT evaluation of the kidneys also allows a detailed evaluation of other intraabdominal injuries with up to a 98% accuracy for both intraperitoneal and extraperitoneal blunt injuries.[22]

AXIOM CT is recommended for evaluation of the urinary tract in any stable patient who is felt to have a significant risk of renal injury and in any patient who has an equivocal IVP.

CT is the preferred imaging modality in penetrating back and flank trauma, obviating the need for surgical exploration in a significant number of patients.[12] CT is also helpful as a postoperative baseline study for the patient who was too ill to tolerate the study preoperatively but who will need follow-up.

In patients who have had an IVP, a CT scan is indicated if excretory urography shows distortion of the calices, incomplete collecting-system filling, or delayed opacification.[2]

In most institutions, "CT of the abdomen" extends only to the iliac crests. If evaluation of the pelvis is also desired, it must usually be ordered separately. In trauma, however, abdominal CT should ideally include screening of the pelvis because a large hematoma may be present in the bony pelvis with relatively little or no identifiable injury in the upper abdomen. The study is usually performed by obtaining images every 10 mm from the lung bases through the iliac crests and every 20 mm from the iliac crests to the symphysis. However, if there is any question of direct injury to the pelvis, 10 mm or smaller cuts should be used as appropriate.

AXIOM Whenever possible, abdominal CT examinations should be done with intravenous and gastrointestinal contrast.

Dilute contrast should be administered by mouth or by nasogastric tube. For visualizing the upper abdomen, including the kidneys, 300 cc of oral contrast is given 30 minutes and again 5 minutes before scanning. If an injury to the ureters or bladder is suspected, 300 cc of oral contrast is also given 1 hour prior to scanning. Scans are obtained through the kidneys prior to administration of the intravenous contrast for detection of high density collections of fresh blood (contusions or hematomas). The entire postcontrast study from diaphragm to symphysis is performed during dynamic intravenous contrast injection.

If an IVP has been performed, a CT scan of the abdomen should not be performed for at least 3–4 hours. If a CT scan must be performed before the IVP contrast has cleared, it is done after only a 50 cc intravenous contrast bolus. While more information will be gained with the post-IVP CT than with the IVP, a CT will yield significantly more information if it is done as the primary examination. It should be remembered that injured kidneys tend to retain contrast longer than the noninjured kidney, and contrast may still be visible in some injured kidneys up to 24 hours later. Consequently, a CT scan done up to 24 hours after an IVP may still show significant injury even without additional contrast material being administered. In a recent study of the value of triple contrast CT scanning for guiding selective management of stab wounds to the back in 53 patients, the CT was either negative (in 31) or showed injuries not requiring exploration (in 20). In the remaining two, the CT was not really needed because other factors indicated a need for surgery.[23]

For isolated or predominantly pelvic injuries, a CT cystogram can be performed. For this study, CT of the pelvis is performed following retrograde bladder opacification without oral or intravenous contrast.

Renal Arteriography

If no renal function is apparent on urography or CT, arteriography may be indicated.[2,8] In patients who have sustained other injuries, it may be possible to embolize a bleeding vessel during the same procedure, thereby obviating the need for an operation.

In the past, renal angiography was often used to help assess se-

---

vere renal injury, but following the addition of CT scanning to the imaging armamentarium, its use has been largely curtailed. While some authors feel that CT is very reliable in the evaluation of major renal vascular injury,[22,23] others believe it merely consumes valuable time without adding significant information.[24] Finding of major vascular injury on CT usually warrants immediate surgical intervention rather than delaying surgery to get an arteriogram.

PITFALL ⊘

The 4-6 hours of warm ischemia that a kidney can tolerate can be lost while waiting for an arteriogram.

In the stable patient with evidence of vascular injury, a preoperative angiogram may be desirable and can provide valuable information (Fig. 29–3); however, it can also delay needed surgery. Indications for renal angiography include: (a) penetrating trauma where the likelihood of vascular injury is high, (b) possible use of embolization to treat persistent bleeding,[24] and (c) pre-op "road mapping." Later, arteriography may be necessary in the work-up of posttraumatic hypertension, persistent hematuria, or a suspected AV fistula.

Ultrasound

There are several potential uses for renal sonography (US) in the trauma setting. Acute parenchymal, perinephric or pelvic hematomas and urinomas may present as anechoic collections on ultrasound, but injured parenchyma and hematoma may be isoechoic and very difficult to distinguish from normal parenchyma and perinephric fat.[25] Sonography may also assess the integrity of the kidney by identification of separated renal fragments. Clots may also be seen in the collecting system or bladder. The presence of the two kidneys and their sizes may also be assessed. Doppler studies can evaluate flow in the major renal vessels.[26,27] Although the utility of ultrasound in acute GU trauma is limited, it may be a useful clinical adjunct when intravenous contrast is contraindicated. Certainly sonography provides significantly more information than plain films and may clarify confusing findings on noncontrast CT scans. If the CT is normal and only microscopic hematuria is present, Jaske[26] believes no further work-up is necessary; however, this philosophy is not unanimously held.

Radionuclide Imaging

Scintigraphy can provide both anatomic and physiologic evaluation of the urinary tract. It is rarely used now for acute trauma because of the improved resolution of CT. This fact is so widely accepted that there are few studies comparing the accuracy of radionuclide scanning with other modalities.[17,28] However, some studies have shown three-phase renal scintigraphy to be significantly more sensitive than IVP.[29] Additionally, the nuclear medicine department may be able to provide critical information in the iodine allergic patient. Technetium-99m glucoheptonate is the agent of choice and can be used to assess perfusion, parenchymal integrity and function. Radionuclide imaging is also an appropriate method for assessing the continued viability of renal fragments.

Treatment

GENERAL APPROACH

AXIOM Most renal injuries heal well without surgical intervention.

Contusions and superficial lacerations make up the majority of renal injuries. Even lacerations extending through the renal capsule usually heal very well without surgical intervention. Nevertheless, some surgeons believe that all deep lacerations and all penetrating injuries require exploration.[2] However, if the collecting system and pedicle are intact and there is no ongoing bleeding, we are usually content to observe kidneys with penetrating injuries. Utilizing the same philoso-

FIGURE 29–3 Traumatic renal artery occlusion after a motor vehicle accident. The digital subtraction arteriogram performed shortly afterward shows complete occlusion of the left renal artery just distal to the early origin of a left renal artery branch supplying the inferior hilar lip. (From Harris JH Jr, Harris WH, Novelline RA. The radiology of emergency medicine. Baltimore: Williams & Wilkins, 1993; 683.)

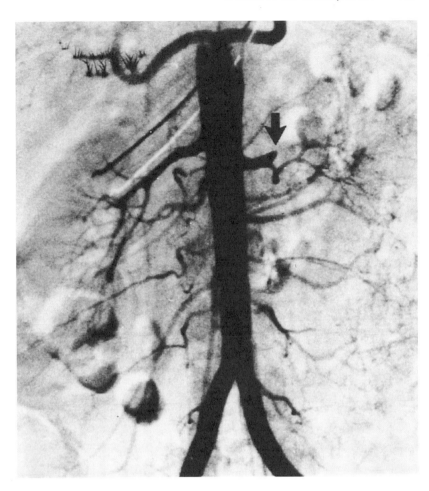

phy, Cheng et al[30] were able to treat 13 of 16 type III renal injuries non-operatively.

Later surgery may be necessary if: a) uncontrollable sepsis develops, b) the involved kidney becomes functionless or, c) the patient develops severe hypertension. When the patient has only one kidney, treatment should be even more conservative, and every effort should be made to salvage the solitary kidney, even if it is severely damaged or bleeding.

Although multiple severe renal lacerations usually require nephrectomy, sometimes a severely lacerated kidney may be treated with a partial nephrectomy. However, this may add 1-2 hours to the surgery, and a partial nephrectomy should not be attempted in critically injured patients with an intact contralateral kidney.

PITFALL ⊘

If it is assumed that persistent hypotension in an injured patient is due to bleeding from a damaged kidney, more life-threatening injuries are apt to be missed.

Bleeding

Bleeding from a badly injured kidney may occasionally cause severe shock, but this is unusual, and blood loss from other structures is much more likely.[8] The perirenal fascia usually provides an excellent tamponading effect, and most bleeding from the kidney subsides very rapidly as the perirenal space fills. Therefore, if the hemoglobin and blood pressure continue to fall, the patient must be carefully checked for other possible sites of blood loss.

Hypotension following blunt trauma to the left or right kidneys is often due to associated splenic, liver or mesenteric injuries. However,

even if such injuries are found, exploration of the kidney is indicated if there is evidence of an enlarging perirenal hematoma.

AXIOM If time is available and if the patient to be explored specifically for severe renal trauma is hemodynamically stable, it may be helpful to obtain a renal arteriogram prior to surgery.

Renal Vascular Injury

A renal arteriogram can give the surgeon an excellent concept of the location and extent of the injury as well as the status of any collateral circulation. If a devascularized kidney is to be saved, its blood supply should be restored within 4-6 hours of the injury, and the amount of functional recovery is usually inversely proportional to the duration of normothermic ischemia.[31-33] The decision as to whether a devascularized kidney can be salvaged depends largely on the appearance of the kidney at the time of exploration and how easily the bleeding is controlled. If the kidney is very dark, it is probably infarcted, and nephrectomy is usually necessary.

UPJ Disruption

Complete disruption of the ureteropelvic junction occasionally occurs. If an IVP or CT scan is performed, extravasation of contrast material into the retroperitoneal space is often seen. In some instances, the kidneys may appear relatively normal; however, contrast material may not be seen in the involved ureter. Patients with this injury require emergency exploration and rapid reestablishment of the continuity of the ureter.

Rupture of the Renal Pelvis

Rupture of the renal pelvis from blunt trauma is rare if the tissue in that area is normal; however, if the patient has preexisting disease, such as hydronephrosis, this type of injury is not uncommon.[2,7] Failure to recognize a rupture of a part of the urinary collecting system, particularly the renal pelvis or ureter, generally leads to development of a urinoma. This pseudoencapsulated enlarging sac of urine usually develops inferior and medial to the kidney and tends to push the kidney superiorly and laterally. Urinomas are sometimes not identified until 4-6 weeks after the injury and can become quite large. A possible post-traumatic urinoma is best evaluated by computed tomography but can also be well-visualized by ultrasonography.

If a retrograde ureterogram indicates a leak from the renal pelvis but the ureteropelvic junction (UPJ) is intact, simple drainage of the perirenal space with a Jackson-Pratt or similar catheter is generally the easiest and most effective method of management in acute situations when a laparotomy is required for other injuries.[7] However, if a laparotomy is not indicated for other injuries or if the diagnosis is made later, cystoscopy with insertion of a ureteral stent should be attempted. Alternatively, percutaneous, image-guided drainage, rather than an operative approach, may be used unless there is another surgical indication. If the UPJ is not intact, it should be repaired and a ureteral stent and/or nephrostomy catheter inserted.

> **AXIOM**   In severe trauma, unless the ureter and kidney are seen on an IVP or another imaging study prior to emergency surgery, these structures should be examined at laparotomy. Ureteral injuries are easily missed and can lead to significant morbidity.

Surgical Examination of the Kidneys

Examination of the kidney at the time of operation can sometimes be extremely difficult, particularly if there is a large amount of blood in the area. Consequently, preoperative radiological evaluation of the kidney can be extremely helpful whenever the patient's condition allows. This is particularly true if there is any thought that a nephrectomy might have to be performed. If the patient was so hemodynamically unstable that there was no time for a preoperative IVP, CT or angiogram, once the bleeding is controlled, an excretory urogram should be done in the operating room before the kidney is removed.

> **AXIOM**   The function of a kidney cannot be evaluated by its size or appearance or by the way it feels on palpation.

If an expanding retroperitoneal hematoma is overlying the kidney, or the patient is hypotensive for no other apparent reason, the peritoneum over the perirenal hematoma should not be opened until the renal vessels are controlled.[7] When the retroperitoneal space around the kidney is opened, the tamponading effect of the perirenal fascia is lost and severe bleeding is apt to develop unless the renal vessels can be clamped promptly.

> **PITFALL** ⊘
>
> *Failure to control the renal vessels before opening a perirenal hematoma can result in severe bleeding and a possibly unnecessary nephrectomy.*

APPROACH TO THE RENAL VESSELS

Exploration of the abdomen and an acutely traumatized kidney should be carried out through a midline abdominal incision. This usually provides the best exposure to associated intraabdominal injuries and the other kidney. Sometimes the perirenal hematoma is so large that difficulty is encountered in approaching the renal vessels. If there is little or no bleeding, a Kocher maneuver followed by dissection and retraction of the ascending and right transverse colon to the left can expose the right renal artery between the vena cava and the aorta;

however, one must be careful not to disturb the perirenal hematoma until the renal vessels have been controlled.

If there is ongoing bleeding from the kidney, it is usually safer to get control of the renal arteries by incising the peritoneum over the aorta at the base of the transverse mesocolon and then dissecting upwards along the aorta until the renal arteries are found[9] (Fig. 29–4). The right renal artery can usually be found going posterior to the inferior vena cava. The inferior vena cava above and below the renal veins can usually be controlled with local pressure until the renal veins are found.

The left renal artery can usually be found by entering the lesser sac and incising the posterior peritoneum over the aorta. If the bleeding is too great to be controlled by any of these techniques, occlusion of the aorta at the diaphragm should be considered. If this still does not adequately control the bleeding, a left thoracotomy and occlusion of the aorta just superior to the diaphragm should be considered.

If the patient goes into shock while the renal vessels are being secured, pressure over the pedicle area with sterile packs will usually control the bleeding until the blood volume can be restored to a safe level and any associated hypothermia corrected. Following this, attempts to expose and control the renal vessels can be begun again.

REPAIRS OF THE KIDNEY

After the renal vessels are controlled, the hematoma can be opened and evacuated and the kidney carefully inspected. After all ischemic or macerated tissue has been debrided, the collecting system, if open,

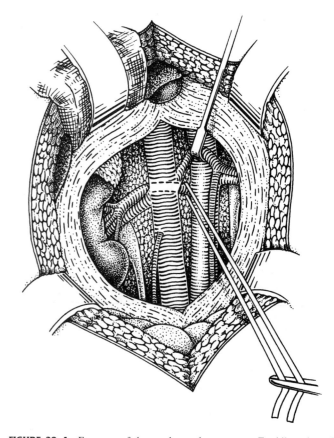

FIGURE 29–4   Exposure of the renal vessels at surgery. For bilateral renal pedicle control, the small intestine is eviscerated and held to the right, and the posterior peritoneum from the cecum to the ligament of Treitz is incised. The origins of the left and right renal artery are posterior to the junction of the left renal vein with the inferior vena cava. (From Chambers RJ Jr, Champion HR, Edson M. Ureteric and renal trauma. In Champion HR, Robbs JV, Trunkey DV, eds. Rob and Smith's operative surgery—trauma surgery, 4th ed. London: Butterworths, 1989; 472.)

is closed with continuous slowly absorbable suture material. The remaining portions of the kidney are then carefully closed to control hemorrhage and decrease the risk of leakage of urine. Horizontal mattress sutures tied over Teflon pledgets, to reduce the chance of tearing the capsule, may be very useful for this purpose. Perirenal fat or omentum can also be used.

RENAL VASCULAR REPAIRS

Renovascular injuries can be very difficult to manage, especially when the renal artery is involved. The renal arteries are often deeply embedded in the retroperitoneum and closely surrounded by dense lymphatics, neural fibers and connective tissue. Repairs of the renal artery may be accomplished by lateral arteriorrhaphy or mobilization of the kidney with primary anastomosis.

Complex renal artery injuries requiring more than 30 minutes of vascular clamping require protection of the kidney from warm ischemia. Various maneuvers including ice packing and lavage, kidney excision with benchtop repair, and transposition to a pelvic location have been used to reduce the ischemic damage. Finally, nephrectomy may be required for severe renal arterial injuries or in patients with multiple injuries and excessive blood loss.

> **AXIOM** Before a nephrectomy is performed, it is important to know that there is a functioning contralateral kidney. Evidence that the contralateral kidney is functional includes visualization on IVP or CT or continued good urine output after the pedicle of the injured kidney is occluded.

Management of the Renal Injury

> **AXIOM** A severely injured kidney should not be removed unless one is certain that the other kidney is functional.

Unless the vascular injury to the kidney is so great that no repair can be done and the bleeding cannot be controlled, a nephrectomy should not be done unless it is certain that the contralateral kidney is adequate to support life. If the right renal vein cannot be repaired or grafted, the kidney may have to be removed. On the left, however, the renal vein can generally be ligated near the inferior vena cava and an adequate venous return will be maintained by its rich collateral drainage.

Bench Surgery

In certain rare instances, if preservation of an injured kidney is important because of absence or poor function of the opposite kidney, a surgeon with special skill and facilities can remove the kidney from the patient and repair it while it is cooled with an ice-cold physiologic salt solution. This so-called bench surgery requires experience and optical magnification. The kidney can then be returned to the patient as an autotransplant, usually into the contralateral iliac fossa. Since these patients often go into renal failure, at least temporarily, and since they are not usually candidates for peritoneal dialysis, hemodialysis must be readily available.

Partial Nephrectomy

If the upper or lower pole of the kidney has been so badly torn from the rest of the kidney that it is no longer viable, but the rest of the kidney appears normal, a partial nephrectomy may be performed (Fig. 29–5). The decision to perform this procedure is much easier to make if the patient has had a preoperative renal arteriogram. However, if the patient has severe associated injuries and has developed a coagulapathy, hypothermia or hypotension, it is probably better to terminate the operation rapidly than spend an extra hour or two saving a part of a kidney.

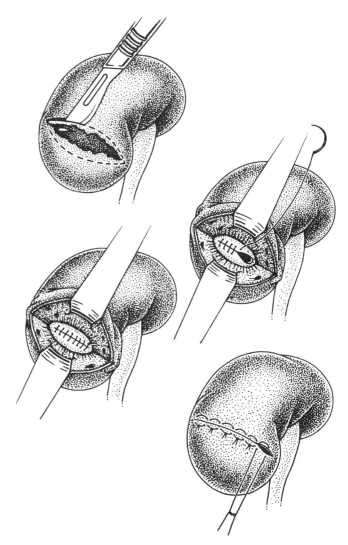

FIGURE 29–5 Repair of deep lacerations into the renal pelvis. Once complete exposure and vascular control are obtained, Gerota's fascia may be opened. All devitalized tissue should be resected back to bleeding tissue. Segmental renal arteries and veins are suture-ligated with 4/0 and 5/0 chromic catgut. Tears in the collecting system are closed and then the margins of resection are approximated with the renal capsule using mattress sutures of 4/0 chromic catgut. (From Chambers RJ Jr, Champion HR, Edson M. Ureteric and renal trauma. In Champion HR, Robbs JV, Trunkey DV, eds. Rob and Smith's operative surgery—trauma surgery, 4th ed. London: Butterworths, 1989; 473.)

> **AXIOM** If the patient has a contralateral functioning kidney, a partial nephrectomy should only be considered if the patient is hemodynamically stable and will not be jeopardized by 1-2 hours of additional surgery.

If a partial nephrectomy is performed, the raw renal surface can be covered with omentum, and the kidney is replaced in Gerota's fascia. Retroperitoneal drains are placed to remove any blood or urine that might leak from the open surface of the kidney.

DELAYED DIAGNOSIS OF RENAL ARTERY THROMBOSIS

Controversy exists regarding the role of renal revascularization following delayed diagnosis of thrombosis of the renal artery from contusion or intimal flap disruption.[31] These injuries are particularly apt to occur after high-speed deceleration motor vehicle accidents or falls from heights. Patients with renal artery occlusion may be relatively asymptomatic relative to the kidney, but some will complain of upper abdominal or flank pain from the ischemia. The time interval from occlusion to repair appears to be a critical factor. In one review of the problem, there was an 80% chance of restoring some renal function if the kidney was revascularized before 12 hours. However, this dropped to 57% if the kidney was not revascularized before 18 hours. The low salvage rate and the 37% chance of delayed nephrectomy for postrevascularization complications, such as hypertension, have caused may surgeons to operate only if less than 12 hours have elapsed since injury.[32] Chambers et al[3] note that delay in revascularization beyond 3 hours is often associated with severe tubular necrosis.

AXIOM An ischemic kidney should be revascularized within 3-6 hours if at all possible.

Once the area of the renal artery injury is visualized, mobilization of the injured renal artery will usually allow a limited resection with an end-to-end anastomosis. Although some surgeons advocate perfusion of the kidney with ice-cold fluid during the period of clamping, sometimes with decapsulation of the ischemic kidney, the value of these procedures is unclear. Most kidneys that have been ischemic for a few hours develop acute tubular necrosis, and it is usually not possible to determine if the revascularization was successful for at least 5-8 weeks.[33]

There are now five separate case reports in the literature that document spontaneous revascularization or recovery of one or both kidneys after presumed blunt thrombotic occlusion of the renal artery.[34] These authors suggest that attempts at late revascularization may occasionally be rewarding, and they advise that early nephrectomy is unnecessary because of the low incidence of chronic hypertension.

AXIOM If renal artery occlusion cannot be relieved within 6-12 hours, an immediate nephrectomy is not necessary because occasional spontaneous revascularization can occur.

Postoperative Management

Following any surgery on the kidney for trauma, the perirenal space should be adequately drained, preferably with closed drains, such as a Jackson-Pratt drain brought out through a stab wound in the flank. These drains should be left in place for at least 5-7 days. If urine leakage persists beyond 5-7 days, an intravenous pyelogram or CT should be obtained to rule out obstruction of the collecting system or ureter.

Once the gross hematuria has resolved, the patient may be mobilized.[2] Hourly urine output and daily serum creatinine levels should be monitored.

Complications of Renal Injury

Severely injured kidneys are subject to a number of complications. Some of the more immediate problems that may develop in the first few days following injury include recurrent hemorrhage, urinary fistulas or urinomas, infection and nonfunction. Some of the delayed problems occurring weeks, months or even years later include hydronephrosis (resulting from obstruction of the ureteropelvic junction), renal calculi, renovascular hypertension, and arteriovenous fistulas.

Occasionally, a perirenal hematoma is not properly absorbed and becomes infected or forms a perirenal cyst.[2] Fibrosis in response to extravasation of blood or urine may obstruct the kidney or ureter, leading to hydronephrosis. Perinephric abscesses can be drained surgically or percutaneously. Atrophy or hydronephrosis may necessitate nephrectomy or repair.

To facilitate early diagnosis of these complications, all patients with renal trauma should have frequent serial evaluations of their vital signs plus daily blood counts, urinalyses and serum creatinine determinations for the first few days. Later, after the patient appears to have recovered from the acute injury, a follow-up CT scan, intrave-

nous urogram or radionuclide study should be performed before the patient leaves the hospital.

Follow-up examinations after serious renal injuries should include urinalysis, blood pressure, and an imaging procedure every 3-6 months for at least 2 years.[7] Late postoperative hypertension occurs in less than 5% of patients and is a result of renal artery stenosis or partial renal infarction.[3]

AXIOM Hypertension due to an injured kidney may not develop until 1-2 years after the initial trauma.

It is important to consider in advance the type of information being sought from follow-up imaging and, therefore, the type of study necessary to best provide that specific information. The prediscarge baseline and all follow-up exams should be of the same type to allow meaningful comparison. For example, while CT and US are both reliable for diagnosis of urinoma, use of one test as the baseline and the other for follow-up makes accurate comparison for progression or regression of the fluid collection exceedingly difficult. Planning the posthospital management of the patient will also increase the information gained from the diagnostic studies obtained and avoid major imaging pitfalls.

INJURIES TO THE URETER

Etiology

The depth and mobility of the ureters protect them from most types of injury, and many ureteral injuries are iatrogenic in origin.[2] Ureteral injuries are said to occur in 2.5-3.0% of abdominal hysterectomies and have been reported in about 1% of patients from whom renal or ureteral stones were removed percutaneously.[35-37]

Traumatic ureteral injuries are usually the result of gunshots or stabs.[2] Blunt abdominal trauma rarely involves the ureter, and when it does, there usually is disruption at the ureteropelvic junction. Associated intraabdominal injuries must always be suspected when there is penetrating trauma to the ureters.

Pathology

IATROGENIC INJURIES

During any intraabdominal operation, a ureter may be severed, lacerated, ligated, kinked, crushed, or devitalized. Such injuries are especially likely to occur in patients with pelvic tumors, infection, or prior radiation.[38] If the injury is not identified and repaired immediately, the incidence of hydronephrosis, peritonitis, cellulitis, a retroperitoneal mass, urinary fistula, or extravasation can be greatly increased. Ureteral catheterization or endourologic procedures such as ureterorenoscopy and stone basketing may cause ureteral perforation, avulsion, or (rarely) separation.[36,39]

EXTERNAL TRAUMA

External trauma to the ureters can be classified as penetrating or blunt. Penetrating injuries are usually caused by knives or gunshot wounds and may produce lacerations, contusions, or complete severance. Gunshot wounds can cause contusions, and the blast effect can severely damage the intima of the small blood vessels in the ureteral wall. In severe cases, thrombosis, ischemia, necrosis, and leakage can occur.[40]

Blunt injuries of the ureter usually take the form of rupture or avulsion of the ureteropelvic junction or of a renal pelvic tear. They may be caused by hyperextension injury in a child or by traffic accidents. Occasionally, they can be caused by relatively minor falls and, in such instances, may be diagnosed only by later radiologic studies.[41] Not infrequently, the problem may not be diagnosed for several days.[42]

AXIOM Injuries of the ureteropelvic junction are often associated with fractures of the lower ribs, and make up the most common type of ureteral injury in children.[7]

Diagnosis

IATROGENIC INJURIES

If an iatrogenic injury of a ureter is not recognized intraoperatively, one should suspect it in the postoperative period in patients with flank or abdominal pain and unexplained fever, vomiting, and paralytic ileus.[8] Pyelonephritis or peritonitis may also develop and complicate the picture. If the injury is bilateral, anuria is possible. Occasionally, the first evidence of a urinary tract injury is urine leaking from the incision.

Slight extravasation of contrast medium is common after endourologic stone removal, and probably indicates small tears.[2] However, if the kidney and ureters are adequately drained, these leaks are usually transient. If it is not clear intraoperatively whether the ureter has been injured, indigo carmine can be given intravenously.[2] Appearance of the blue dye in the operating field indicates leakage from the urinary tract.

Postoperatively, an IVP may show that extravasation is present, and cystoscopy with retrograde pyelography can identify the site of leakage more clearly. Injuries during endourologic procedures are usually identified by nephroscopy or ureteroscopy during the procedure or by a post-procedure nephrostogram.

EXTERNAL INJURIES

A ureter lacerated or severed by a gunshot produces the same signs and symptoms as one injured by a scalpel. These may include a mass, abdominal distention, extravasation, vomiting, paralytic ileus, and cellulitis.[2] In contrast, a contusion will often show no immediate signs except some hematuria. Microscopic hematuria is present in 90% of patients with ureteric trauma. However, if the ureter is completely ruptured and the blood and urine are draining into the retroperitoneum, hematuria is usually absent.[43,44]

The diagnosis of ureteral damage is frequently made on the basis of extravasation of contrast material on an IVP or CT; however, this injury should also be suspected if one of the kidneys is not functioning due to injury to the main renal vessels. In a recent report on 12 ureter injuries caused by penetrating trauma, the IVP missed the ureteral injury in all nine cases in which it was used.[44] If ureteral injury is suspected and the IVP and/or CT are nondiagnostic, it may be necessary to make the diagnosis with a retrograde ureteropyelogram.

Not infrequently the diagnosis of ureteral damage from accidental trauma can be made at the time of surgery. However, sometimes the surgeon will have difficulty finding the ureter if there is a great deal of surrounding hematoma.

PITFALL ⊘

Failure to visualize the ureters clearly on IVP or CT scan or at laparotomy when there is a penetrating wound in the vicinity of these structures.

During exploratory laparotomy, 5 ml of indigo carmine injected intravenously will demonstrate lacerations of the ureter by extravasation of the dye.

Treatment

Early operative repair of an injured ureter is generally considered to be essential to prevent serious complications and possible loss of the associated kidney.

PRESERVATION OF URETERAL VESSELS

PITFALL ⊘

Excessive mobilization of the ureter or disturbance of its adventitia during dissection may result in necrosis of the ureter by interfering with its blood supply.

The ureter obtains its blood supply from the renal artery and from segmental vessels from the aorta, common iliac and hypogastric vessels. The segmental vessels can be sacrificed as long as the longitudinal vessels running in and along the adventitia coming from either the lower or upper ureter are intact. If more than 1-2 cm of the adventitia is disturbed during the dissection or trauma, a segment of the ureter may necrose and form a ureteral fistula.

UPPER URETERAL INJURIES

With injuries involving the upper two-thirds of the ureter, the ends of the ureter should be freshened until they bleed properly, spatulated for about 1 cm, and then sutured end-to-end (Fig. 29–6). The ureteral repair is usually performed with two running 5-0 absorbable sutures. It is important to try to obtain a watertight anastomosis. It is particularly important that no tension be allowed on the suture line because this almost invariably leads to a breakdown of the anastomosis.[43,44] The ureter is then stented.

LOWER URETERAL INJURIES

Although the lacerated end of the middle and upper third of the ureters can generally be reanastomosed directly, such repairs can be difficult in the lower third. If the ureter is damaged just above or near the bladder, it usually has to be reimplanted in the anterolateral bladder, preferably employing an antireflux type of insertion. If the ureter is injured somewhat higher, near the pelvic rim, it may be necessary to use a pedicled flap of bladder known as a Boari or Ockerblad flap.

It may be possible to obviate the need for a bladder flap by mobilizing the bladder and fixing it to the psoas muscles and the pelvic rim.[3,7] The ureter can then be reimplanted into the mobilized bladder. This operation is known as a psoas-hitch type of ureteral reimplantation.

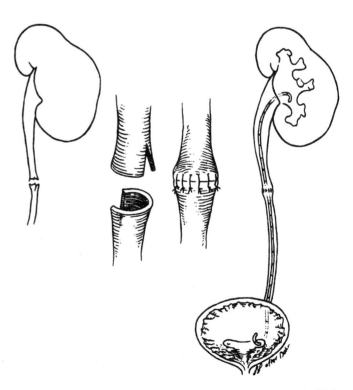

FIGURE 29–6 Repair of a mid ureteral injury. The upper and middle thirds of the ureter are best repaired with a primary ureteroureterostomy. The injured ends of the ureter should be adequately debrided and should be dissected proximally and distally to make the anastomosis tension-free. The ends of the ureter are spatulated to prevent stenosis at the site of the repair, which is performed with fine interrupted absorbable sutures. A silicone stent of the double J type can be passed via a guidewire from the site of the repair proximal to the renal pelvis and distal to the bladder. (From McAninch JW. Injuries to the urinary system. In Blaisdell WF, Trunkey DD, eds. Trauma management: abdominal trauma. New York: Thieme-Stratton, 1982; 216.)

Autotransplantation of the kidney from the lumbar fossa to the iliac fossa occasionally may be another method of handling the short ureter.[7] The use of a transureteroureterostomy (suturing the lacerated end of the proximal ureter into the side of the other ureter) may also be considered in selected instances when the lower ureter is severely injured and no other treatment seems adequate (Fig. 29–7). Cutaneous ureterostomy may be used as a last resort if it is impossible to provide ureterobladder continuity, and especially if the functional status of the other kidney is in question. If it is certain that the contralateral kidney and urinary tract are normal, removal of the kidney and the injured ureter is generally preferred to a cutaneous ureterostomy.

URETERAL STENT

Whenever possible, a ureteral stent should be used with all ureteral injuries.[2,7,43] The stent should be small enough so that it will not cause pressure on the ureter walls, and it should extend from the renal pelvis down into the bladder, where it can later be retrieved by cystoscopy.

AXIOM Ureteral stents greatly improve the chances for a ureteral repair to heal without complications.

DRAINS

With all ureteral injuries, a drain should be left in the periureteral area and brought out through a stab wound in the flank to remove any urine or blood that may leak into that area.[43,44]

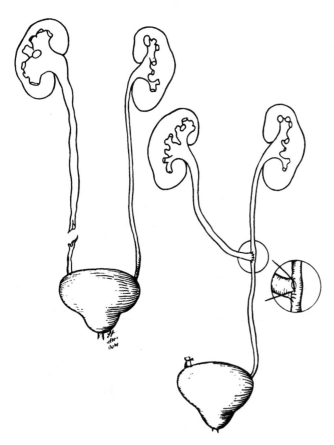

FIGURE 29–7 Technique of transureteroureterostomy. A short segment of the intact ureter is mobilized and a short linear incision is then made on its medical aspect so that an end-to-side ureteroureterostomy can be created using interrupted absorbable sutures. With all ureteric surgery, dissection should be kept to a minimum to ensure an adequate blood supply, and all anastomoses should be tension-free and watertight. (From McAninch JW. Injuries to the urinary system. In Blaisdell WF, Trunkey DD, eds. Trauma management: abdominal trauma. New York: Thieme-Stratton, 1982; 216.)

DELAYED RECOGNITION OF URETERAL INJURIES

Most ureteral injuries that are missed initially are picked up on a later IVP or CT scan with intravenous contrast. Ureterectasis, pyelectasis, a dense nephrogram, or delayed or absent opacification of the collecting system indicates obstruction, whereas extravasation or a mass effect suggests leakage.[8]

Ultrasonography can be a useful screen for hydronephrosis or a urinoma. Although CT scanning is probably unnecessary in most cases, it can often precisely locate a urine collection and suggest its cause. Retrograde pyelography can also usually reveal the site of the injury. If a complete obstruction or a complete tear of the ureter is found, a percutaneous nephrotomy tube can be inserted to drain the kidney while the treatment approach is being selected.[45]

Stents can be very helpful in managing ureteral injuries. Most endourologic ureteral injuries heal well if the ureter is stented and the urine is thoroughly diverted. Contusion of the ureter secondary to gunshot wounds usually also does well with simple stenting.[2]

Ureteral or ureteropelvic junction avulsions and ruptures generally occur in conjunction with other severe injuries that take precedence. As a result, optimal management of the ureter injured at the initial operation is often impossible. Percutaneous nephrostomy may be advisable as a temporizing measure and should reduce the number of cases in which nephrectomy becomes the only option. In some cases, percutaneous antegrade ureteral stenting can successfully treat complicated ureteral injuries.[46]

INJURIES OF THE BLADDER

Etiology

Bladder injuries can occur with blunt or penetrating trauma, and are often associated with fractures of the pelvis and long bones.[1,47] Predisposing factors include bladder distention, fixation by tumor or scar, and obstruction. Interestingly, children are more susceptible to blunt bladder injury than adults.

AXIOM The bladder is much more easily ruptured when it is full.

When the bladder is empty, it is extremely well-protected against most types of trauma. However, when it is distended with urine, not only is it much more likely to be ruptured by blunt trauma, but it also presents a bigger target for penetrating wounds.[7] Occasionally, a full bladder may be ruptured by a minor fall, such as on the ice.

Types of Bladder Injuries

Bladder injuries can be classified as ruptures or contusions.[2] Intraperitoneal and extraperitoneal ruptures occur with approximately equal frequency, and approximately 10% of patients with bladder ruptures have both types. Intraperitoneal ruptures usually occur on the posterior superior wall as a result of blunt trauma to a full bladder. Extraperitoneal ruptures are usually on the anterior or anterolateral bladder wall near the bladder neck and are almost always associated with pelvic fractures.[47] It has been estimated that about 5% of patients with pelvic fractures have an extraperitoneal rupture of the bladder. Extraperitoneal ruptures are generally caused by spicules of bone from the pelvis or, less often, the femur. A few cases are caused by knives or guns which cause pelvic hematomas that compress the bladder and cause an obstructive uropathy.[48]

Pathophysiology

In the infant and young child, the bladder is primarily intraabdominal; in the adult it is more of a pelvic organ.[49] Its relationship to the pubis and pelvis walls anteriorly and the rectum posteriorly make it very susceptible to injury when pelvic bones or the rectum are injured. Superiorly and over a small area posteriorly, the bladder is covered by peritoneum. The bladder base is fixed and does not move with filling.

Intraperitoneal rupture of the bladder leads to peritonitis, which is worse if the urine is infected.[2] Extraperitoneal extravasation of infected urine can lead to spreading pelvic cellulitis and sepsis.

Diagnosis

Associated injuries tend to mask the signs and symptoms of a bladder injury and are responsible for many of the fatalities.[49]

AXIOM Bladder injuries should be suspected with any trauma to the lower abdomen or pelvis, especially if there is a fracture of the pubic rami or separation of the pubic symphysis.

CLINICAL

The classic triad of symptoms and signs of bladder injury includes lower abdominal pain, gross hematuria, and inability to void.[7] If the bladder rupture is intraperitoneal, the patient may also have signs and symptoms of peritonitis, including pain, tenderness and rebound. Pain referred to the top of the shoulder (Kehr's sign) suggests the presence of blood or urine irritating the diaphragm or a diaphragmatic hernia.

With any possible bladder injury, careful rectal and vaginal examination should be done in search of an enlarging pelvic mass or an injury extending into the vagina or rectum.

URINALYSIS

Although examination of a voided urine specimen is an important part of the initial work-up, if there is a high index of suspicion of bladder injury and the patient is unable to void, retrograde urethral or suprapubic catheterization must be done. However, retrograde urethral catheterization generally should not be attempted until retrograde urethrography excludes a urethral tear.

CYSTOGRAPHY

Sometimes the extravasated contrast material from a ruptured bladder can be seen on an IVP, but there are many false-negatives. Excretory urography is not a substitute for cystography;[47] in one series, IVP revealed only five (21%) of 23 proven bladder ruptures.[47]

When injuries of both the upper and lower urinary tracts are suspected, determining the order of the CT, IVP and retrograde cystourethrogram may be difficult. There is significant debate in the literature as to the preferred order, and the examination performed first in each patient should be determined by the site with the highest index of suspicion.[2,3] Nevertheless, oral contrast (e.g., for CT) should not be given before an IVP or cystogram because extravasation may be obscured by the GI contrast.

RETROGRADE CYSTOGRAMS

Cystography is an accurate method for diagnosing injury to the bladder and is customarily performed following a retrograde urethrogram. CT cystography may be preferred when there is no suspected urethral injury.

Cystograms are usually done through an indwelling catheter. However, in patients with known or suspected urethral ruptures, a retrograde urethrogram is first performed. If an injury is found, conventional catheter passage is ill-advised. In some of these patients, it may be appropriate to perform cystography through a suprapubic puncture.

Retrograde cystograms are obtained by emptying the bladder with a catheter and then filling it by gravity with at least 300-400 ml of a standard cystographic contrast medium.[7] Full bladder distension with contrast is imperative to avoid false-negative studies.[2] Filling must be performed under fluoroscopic control to avoid filling the entire peritoneal cavity through a tear.

AXIOM The "post-evac" cystogram film is the view most apt to show small bladder injuries.

The cystogram should include films taken in the AP, lateral, and both posterior oblique projections, before and after contrast enters the bladder. This is followed by post-drainage films of the pelvis, occasionally after the bladder is "rinsed" with saline.[2] The "post-evac" film may be the only film to demonstrate a small amount of extravasation, particularly posteriorly, and should not be omitted.

Intraperitoneal rupture is characterized radiologically by (a) failure of the bladder to fill on cystography or during intravenous urography,[49] and (b) contrast material between loops of intestine above the bladder. The typical cystography findings in extraperitoneal rupture are a flame-like extravasation of contrast outside the bladder and a teardrop appearance to the bladder because of compression by hematoma.

If there is no extravasation of contrast, evidence of a pelvic hematoma should be sought. Large pelvic hematomas elevate and narrow the bladder concentrically at its base, causing it to assume the shape of an inverted pear, thus the name "pear-shaped" bladder.[7] The sensitivity of CT for diagnosing pelvic hematomas is far greater than that of cystography.

PITFALL ⊘

Large, tense pelvic hematomas can temporarily prevent extravasation of contrast from a bladder injury and can thereby cause the cystogram to be falsely negative.

If there is no extravasation on the cystogram and a pelvic hematoma is present, the patient may still have a ruptured bladder with tamponade of the tear by blood clot. Of 25 cases with a ruptured bladder proven at surgery following blunt trauma, two (8%) had a cystogram which looked normal.[7] In another series of patients with penetrating wounds to the bladder, only a third (33%) had an abnormal cystogram. With penetrating wounds to the bladder, it is not uncommon for a hematoma in the pelvis or wall of the bladder to tamponade off the hole. In some instances, tears up to 2-4 cm in length may be sealed by hematoma.

AXIOM Patients with pelvic fractures should be watched carefully for delayed extravasation from a missed bladder injury after the Foley catheter has been removed.

Treatment

INTRAPERITONEAL BLADDER RUPTURE

Foley catheter drainage may be the treatment of choice for a bladder injury if there is minimal extravasation, no infection or disruption of visceral structures, and no other abdominal injury.[49] However, most patients with penetrating or blunt injuries to the bladder should undergo exploration.

The patient is explored through a vertical midline lower abdominal incision and the peritoneal cavity is inspected for blood or injury to the bowel or other intraperitoneal organs. After repair of any associated intraabdominal injuries, the injured bladder can be repaired.

The entire bladder is inspected, and then the mucosa and muscle are closed with a running 4-0 or 5-0 absorbable suture, followed by a second or even a third layer closing the muscle and serosa over this to seal the bladder further. Postoperatively, the bladder and the perivesical space are drained until it has been shown that the bladder has healed.

EXTRAPERITONEAL BLADDER INJURIES

AXIOM Small extraperitoneal bladder injuries can often be treated by simple catheter drainage of the bladder.

Most extraperitoneal bladder injuries can be handled nonsurgically by inserting a Foley catheter and attaching it to a closed drainage system. These injuries usually seal quite readily with only Foley catheter drainage.[1,49,50] Only extraperitoneal injuries which are extremely large or associated with bony fragments will not seal in this fashion. Because the injury is extraperitoneal, peritonitis is rarely a problem.

If the bladder rupture is extraperitoneal and is large enough to require repair, the injury is best repaired from within the bladder. After opening the peritoneum and inspecting the contents of the peritoneal cavity, the peritoneum is closed. The bladder is then entered anteriorly through a midline incision and the area of rupture located. The muscularis is closed with either an interrupted or a running 4-0 absorbable suture. The mucosa is then closed with a running 5-0 absorbable suture.

The midline incision in the bladder is then closed in three layers. A 4-0 or 5-0 absorbable suture is used on the mucosal lining of the bladder; the muscularis and serosa are then closed as a second layer with a running 3-0 or 4-0 absorbable suture, and a third layer, consisting of an inverting serosa-muscular suture of running 3-0 or 4-0 is used to seal the bladder cystotomy site further.[7]

PARAURETHRAL INJURIES

If a penetrating wound of the urinary bladder is near a ureteral orifice, the ureteral insertion into the bladder may be severely damaged or blown off. Treatment of the bladder damage alone without proper attention to an associated ureteral injury can cause considerable morbidity and pelvic infection and may result in loss of the associated kidney. If there is any possibility of a ureter injury, cystoscopy and a retrograde ureterogram can be performed on the table. If further investigation is not possible at that time, passage of a ureteral stent through the area of ureter in question may facilitate healing.[43]

BLADDER DECOMPRESSION

AXIOM   Adequate drainage of a mildly-to-moderately injured bladder is best done with a urethral Foley catheter. With severe trauma, one should drain the bladder with a suprapubic cystostomy in males; however, a large Foley catheter is usually adequate in females.

Complete bladder drainage is important following any bladder injury. If the patient is a male, a Pezzar cystostomy tube is placed into the bladder through a stab wound through the abdominal wall, halfway between the umbilicus and symphysis pubis, at least 2-3 cm from the incision. Once it is clear, postoperatively, that the cystostomy tube drains the bladder adequately, the Foley catheter can be removed. If

the bladder injury is small and there has been minimal adjacent injury or contamination, or if the patient is a female, an 18 F Foley catheter can be left in place without a cystostomy tube.

If a cystostomy tube has been used, this should be left in place for at least 8-10 days and then clamped if there is no evidence of a urine leak.[23] If there are no complications after it has been clamped for 24 hours and the patient can empty the bladder well, the cystostomy tube can be removed. However, if there is any question about bladder integrity, a cystogram should be performed prior to removal of the cystostomy tube.

DRAINAGE OF THE PERIVISCERAL SPACE

AXIOM   Patients with surgery on the kidneys, ureters, or bladder should have the adjacent tissue drained in the event of a postoperative urine leak.

Following all bladder surgery, a Penrose or Jackson-Pratt type drain is left in the perivesical space and brought out through a stab wound separate from the incision.[8] If healing is proceeding satisfactorily, this drain can usually be removed in 4-5 days, but it should not be removed prior to cessation of urinary leakage.

INJURIES TO THE PROSTATIC OR MEMBRANOUS URETHRA

Anatomy (Fig. 29–8)

The male urethra is divided anatomically by the urogenital diaphragm into three parts: (a) the prostatic urethra between the bladder and the superior leaf of the urogenital diaphragm, (b) the membranous urethra which traverses the urogenital diaphragm, and (c) the anterior urethra distal to the inferior leaf of the urogenital diaphragm.[23] The anterior urethra may be further subdivided into the bulbous or perineal urethra (extending to the penoscrotal junction) and the distal penile or pendulous urethra.

Etiology

Urethral injuries almost always occur in male patients and are extremely rare in females. Serious urethral injuries are most often associated with pelvic fractures, especially anterior arch fractures with displacement. The incidence of urethral and bladder injury accompa-

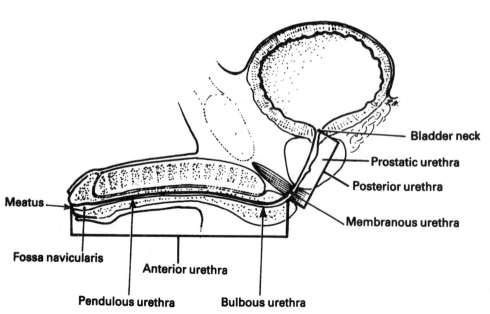

FIGURE 29–8 Urethral anatomy. The urethra can be divided into the anterior and posterior urethra. The anterior urethra extends from the inferior edge of the urogenital diaphragm to the external urethral meatus. The posterior portion of the urethra extends from the bladder neck to the inferior edge of the urogenital diaphragm. (From Edson M. Injuries to the urethra. In Champion HR, Robbs JV, Trunkey DV, eds. Rob and Smith's operative surgery—trauma surgery, 4th ed. London: Butterworths, 1989; 476.)

Bladder neck
Prostatic urethra
Posterior urethra
Membranous urethra

Meatus
Fossa navicularis
Pendulous urethra
Anterior urethra
Bulbous urethra

nying pelvic fractures ranges from 0.7-25%.[2,6,50,51] In approximately half of these lower urinary tract injuries, only the urethra is injured. However, 95% of the patients with urinary tract injuries have other significant injuries.[50] In female patients, pelvic fractures are seldom associated with urethral injuries. When these do occur, vaginal lacerations are generally also present. Most instances of trauma to the female urethra are secondary to obstetric complications, vaginal operation, or foreign bodies.

Injuries of the male urethra may affect the membranous (posterior) (Fig. 29–9) portion or the bulbous and penile (anterior) portion (Fig. 29–10), with the former outnumbering the latter approximately three to one.[47] Severe blunt trauma to the lower abdomen and pelvis, causing fractures of the pubic rami, characteristically tears the prostatic urethra just above the superior leaf of the urogenital diaphragm. Sometimes the urogenital diaphragm itself is torn as it is avulsed off an ischial ramus. Rarely, the tears may extend into the membranous urethra.

Injuries of the membranous urethra occur because it is enclosed and immobilized by the urogenital diaphragm.[2,7] With tears of the prostatic urethra, blood or urine extravasates into the periprostatic and perivesical spaces, and, if the urogenital diaphragm is badly damaged, also into the perineum. Continued extravasation of urine can lead to cellulitis and sepsis, and urethral stricture is a common long-term problem no matter what is done immediately after the injury. Urinary incontinence may also occur if the urinary sphincter is injured. Approximately one-third of patients will suffer erectile impotence, probably as a result of pelvic nerve injury.[49]

Penetrating wounds may damage any portion of the urethra. Blunt trauma, however, causes certain characteristic lesions. The classic straddle injury is one in which the male patient falls astride a bar such as a crossbar on a bicycle or a fence and sustains a severe blow to his perineum. In this injury, the bulbous urethra, just below the urogenital diaphragm, is crushed against the ischial rami and may rupture.

INJURIES OF THE BULBOUS OR PENILE URETHRA

Etiology

Injuries of the bulbous or penile urethra (Fig. 29–10), below the urogenital diaphragm, are usually caused by direct blows, straddle accidents, or urethral instrumentation.[2]

AXIOM If there is a suspicion of a urethral injury, a urethral catheter should not be passed until a retrograde urethrogram has excluded a tear.

Vigorous or repeated attempts to catheterize a damaged urethra may further injure the urethra, particularly in its membranous portion, and greatly compound the problems of healing.

PITFALL ⊘

Persistent attempts to pass a urethral catheter, especially after a pelvic injury, can cause severe complications.

Diagnosis

Urethral injury should be suspected with any severe blunt trauma to the pelvis or perineum. If the patient has a perineal hematoma and there is blood coming out of his urethral meatus, there is a very strong likelihood of rupture of the bulbous urethra with an associated perineal hematoma. If the patient has voided since the injury, there may also be extravasated urine in the perineum.

In blunt trauma, the nature of the pelvic fracture can be a valuable guide to the nature of the urethral injury. For example, Blandy and King[53] have noted that "spring-back fractures" of the rami of the pubic or ischial bones which are in their normal positions usually cause only a bruise, kink or partial tear of the urethra. However, if

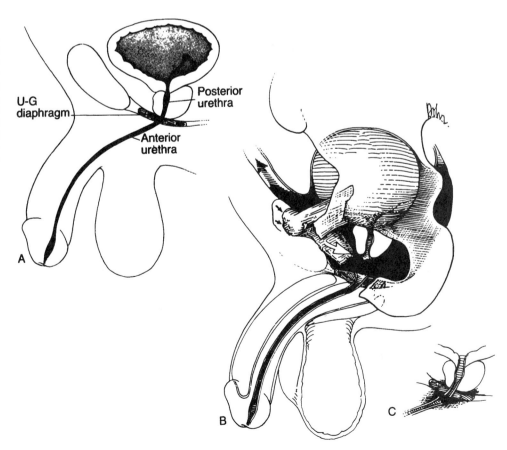

FIGURE 29–9 Posterior urethral rupture. **A.** The normal anatomic portions of the urethra. **B.** Prostatomembranous disruption just superior to the urogenital diaphragm, allowing the prostate to be displaced superiorly by hematoma. **C.** Rupture at the inferior surface of the urogenital diaphragm. (From McAninch JW. Assessment and diagnosis of urinary and genital injuries. In McAninch JW, ed. Trauma management: urogenital trauma. New York: Thieme-Stratton, 1985;2:1.)

U-G diaphragm

Posterior urethra

Anterior urethra

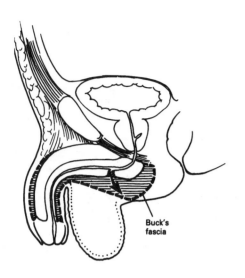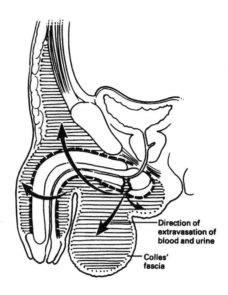

FIGURE 29–10 Extravasation of blood and urine after urethral tears. If Buck's fascia remains intact, there will be discoloration and edema of the penis and the extravasation of blood and urine will be contained between Buck's fascia and the corpora of the penis. If Buck's fascia is disrupted, the extravasation is only confined by Colles's fascia and may be extensive. (From Edson M. Injuries to the urethra. In Champion HR, Robbs JV, Trunkey DV, eds. Rob and Smith's operative surgery—trauma surgery, 4th ed. London: Butterworths, 1989; pg 477.)

large portions of the pelvic girdle are displaced, the patient generally has a disrupted membranous urethra, with the extent of the bony displacement indicating the extent of the tearing of the soft tissues, including the urethra.

The symptoms of urethral injury are pain in the perineum and lower abdomen and inability to void. Frequent signs include urethral bleeding and gross hematuria.[2] A tender suprapubic mass may represent a distended bladder or extravasated blood and urine.

If Buck's fascia around the corpora of the penis remains intact, only discoloration and edema of the penis will be seen. If Buck's fascia is disrupted, the extravasation of urine and blood can be extensive and is contained only by Colles' fascia. Colles' fascia extends posteriorly around the anterior half of the anus and only a short distance laterally to the fascia lata of the thighs. Anteriorly, the blood can spread up over the entire abdomen and chest.

If both the urethra and Buck's fascia are torn, blood and urine can extravasate into the perineum initially and then into the scrotum, penis, and abdominal wall. Serious infection often follows such extravasation, and a stricture may form.

Tears of the penile urethra can cause severe pain. Attempts to micturate are painful, and they also can cause increased perineal or penile swelling. Urethral bleeding and a tender perineal mass are common. Swelling and discoloration of the skin of the scrotum, penis, and lower abdomen tend to be late signs.

On rectal examination of the patient who has had a separation of the prostatic urethra from the membranous urethra, the prostate may be felt to be riding higher than usual. However, not infrequently, rectal examination can identify only a large boggy mass of extravasated fluid. In such instances, upward displacement of the prostate, even if it is free-floating, can be difficult to identify. In addition, a periprostatic and perivesical hematoma may make the prostate feel as though it is higher than normal, although no separation is actually present.

AXIOM Any patient with a pelvic crushing injury who is unable to void or has bloody urine should have a retrograde urethrogram prior to catheter insertion.

Although patients with significant urethral or bladder injuries generally have gross hematuria,[4] this must not be assumed. A retrograde urethrogram is indicated in any patient who has blood at the urethral meatus or any other finding suggesting a possibility of urethral injury.

Plain films of the abdomen can show the nature and extent of larger pelvic fractures. Lateral views are often important in identifying spring-back fractures of the pubis, because these fractures can have a nearly normal appearance on anteroposterior views.[52]

AXIOM If there is any suspicion of a urethral injury, a Foley catheter should not be inserted until a urethrogram has been performed.

If there has been a partial urethral laceration with an incomplete separation and a Foley catheter is passed into the bladder, the injury may be completely missed, and the catheter is apt to be removed before urethral healing is adequate. The catheter may also enter the tear and be advanced submucosally, turning a small, unobstructing tear into a large, obstructing injury.

PITFALL ⊘

Whenever a Foley catheter is inserted into a patient with severe pelvic or perineal trauma before a urethrogram is performed, a urethral injury may be missed or made worse. In such circumstances, it is wise to obtain a urethrogram alongside the Foley catheter before it is removed.

If a patient with a urethral tear has had a Foley catheter in place for some time, the possibility of a ureteral injury may be forgotten. If the patient does have a urethral injury and the Foley catheter is removed, when the patient urinates, infected urine may extravasate into the adjacent pelvic tissues, and it can cause a severe pelvic cellulitis.

A retrograde urethrogram is obtained by gentle injection of 10-25 cc of sterile 30% iodinated contrast material into the urethra with a bulb syringe or soft catheter.[7] If a Foley catheter is already in place, it should not be removed as it may be difficult or impossible to reinsert. A small catheter can be placed alongside it, at the urethral meatus, to obtain the urethrogram. The patient should be placed in a posterior oblique position, with the contrast instillation and filming performed under direct fluoroscopic guidance. Areas of extravasation from the urethra should be noted and the study terminated as soon as the necessary information is obtained. Special efforts should be made to determine whether the extravasation is below or above the urogenital diaphragm. This question can usually be answered on the hard x-ray copies with only a small amount of contrast extravasation. The use of excess contrast will not make a difficult determination easier, and it may obscure important anatomic landmarks.

Treatment

MEMBRANOUS OR PROSTATIC URETHRA (FIG. 29–10)

Posterior urethral injuries are usually a result of severe blunt trauma to the pelvis with fractures of the pubic and/or ischial rami in 90%

of cases.[53-56] They carry a very high incidence of complications, including stricture of the urethra (which is often obliterative), sexual impotence, and chronic urinary infection (from prolonged drainage with catheters).

The proper treatment of posterior (membranous and prostatic) urethral injuries is still controversial because the results are often unsatisfactory no matter what is done. Blandy and King[52] have offered a useful listing of the goals one should seek as a guide to selecting treatment procedures:

1. Save the patient's life.
2. Prevent strictures.
3. If it is not possible to prevent a stricture, ensure that the stricture can be managed by the simplest and least invasive means.
4. If the stricture cannot be managed simply, ensure that only a simple urethroplasty will be needed.
5. Prevent other complications such as incontinence, impotence, deformity, and pelvic instability.

In most patients with multiple trauma and complete urethral rupture, other injuries take precedence, and the urologist's efforts may be confined to inserting a suprapubic cystostomy tube. Further approaches to the urethral injury may have to be delayed until the orthopedic surgeons have reduced the pelvic fractures and, as a consequence, brought the severed ends of the urethra closer together.[52]

Opinion is divided on whether urethral continuity should then be restored by open end-to-end anastomosis or use of interlocking sounds or catheters passed through the urethra and the bladder neck simultaneously or whether suprapubic drainage with later urethroplasty is optimal.[51,53,54]

Delayed urethroplasty has become more appealing with the demonstration that urethral continuity can often be reestablished by a combination of transurethral and endoscopic means without open operation.[55] In the experiences of Cass and others,[2] most of these patients require pelvic surgery to exclude bladder rupture and to insert a suprapubic tube. At the same time, one can realign the urethra after cutting the puboprostatic ligaments, if necessary.

The patient's long-term problems, such as impotence, are determined primarily by the nature of the injury rather than by anything the urologist does.[2,22] However, one can cause ischemic necrosis of the bladder neck, and consequent incontinence, if overenthusiastic traction is applied to a Foley catheter in an effort to align the torn ends of the urethra.[52]

Thus, at the very least, patients with injuries to the membranous or prostatic urethra should have a suprapubic cystostomy. If possible, an attempt should be made to pass a catheter gently in an antegrade fashion from the bladder into the urethra.[7] If this is successful, a urethral catheter can be sutured to its end and pulled into the bladder in a retrograde manner, to function as a urethral stent. Although this stent can be very helpful, vigorous attempts to insert the catheter should not be undertaken. If a urethral catheter cannot be passed easily in an antegrade manner, a suprapubic cystostomy, using a 30 F Pezzar catheter, should be performed. A drain should also be left in the perivesical area.

Recently, Corriere et al[57] reported on the voiding and erectile function in 50 patients who had suffered a total disruption of the posterior urethra in conjunction with a fractured pelvis. These patients were treated with immediate suprapubic cystostomy and a delayed one-stage urethroplasty. Of the 50 patients, 38 (76%) voided normally after surgery and were continent. However, 16 (32%) were still not having erections, and 16 others had less than optimal erections.

Partial ruptures of the posterior urethra are managed by a combination of suprapubic cystostomy and perivesical drainage or by urethral catheter drainage.[7] Only an experienced urologist should attempt to pass a urethral catheter in these patients, as there is considerable risk of converting a partial rupture into a complete one.

AXIOM   If a transection of the urethra is incomplete, it is important not to increase the extent of the injury by passing a Foley catheter or performing excessive operative manipulations.

If one side of the urethra is intact, the autonomic nerves to the penis which pass through the urogenital diaphragm from the pelvis along the course of the urethra may also be intact, and if they are not damaged by further manipulation, the patient may not be rendered impotent.[2,3] Occasionally, especially in young boys, the edge of the urethra can be sewn together. Attempts to do this, however, should be pursued only by a surgeon with extensive experience in this area.

ANTERIOR URETHRA

Incomplete Tears
If the rupture of the anterior urethra is incomplete, and it is confined by the fascial covering of the corpus spongiosum so that there is no extravasation of blood and urine into the perineum, treatment may involve only splinting of the urethra with a urethral catheter for 5-7 days. If a urethral catheter cannot be passed, a suprapubic cystostomy with a 30 F Pezzar catheter should be performed.[8]

If a Foley catheter is left in place, its management is extremely important. The catheter should be taped onto the anterior abdominal wall or medial thigh and cleansed frequently at the point where it enters the urethra. This cleansing is extremely important because one of the complications of urethral catheter drainage is purulent urethritis, which can cause urethral stricture, and occasionally can lead to septic shock. Mechanical cleansing of the catheter with soap and water or betadine solution five or six times a day is very effective. The bladder drainage system should be kept completely closed to reduce the chance of contamination.

Complete Tears
Complete ruptures of the anterior urethra are repaired by end-to-end anastomosis with evacuation of the hematoma, suprapubic cystostomy drainage, and adequate antibiotic coverage. If there is evidence of extravasation into the perineum and/or anterior abdominal wall, it may also be necessary to open and drain the involved areas for at least 5-7 days.

If the urethral injury is extensive and more than 2 cm of urethra has been destroyed, the distal and proximal ends as well as other areas involved are sutured to the penile skin with 4/0 polyglycolic acid sutures.[57]

If the patient's condition is precarious, urethral surgery is delayed and only suprapubic cystostomy is indicated. If the tear and extravasation are minimal and the patient is not undergoing laparotomy for other injuries, a suprapubic cystostomy can be performed percutaneously. If the patient is undergoing abdominal exploration, a No. 28 Malecot catheter is placed suprapubically at the time of open surgery. These patients should have suprapubic drainage of the bladder for at least three or four weeks. If a Foley catheter has passed easily, it can act as a stent, but if urethritis develops, the Foley catheter must be removed.

At the end of 3-4 weeks, the suprapubic catheter can be clamped and the patient given a trial of voiding, after a cystourethrogram has been performed and has shown no leaks.[2,3] If the patient voids well for 24 hours, the cystostomy tube is removed. It is imperative that these patients be followed for at least a year to make sure that they are not developing a urethral stricture.

STRICTURES
For most types of urethral injury, the resulting strictures can often be corrected by cold-knife urethrotomy. If the stricture is less than 2 cm long, this technique is successful in more than 90% of patients, obviating the need for repeated urethral dilatations.[58]

INJURIES OF THE FEMALE URETHRA
Complete ruptures of the female urethra produce much the same signs and symptoms as do those of the male urethra.[2] These injuries are frequently accompanied by pelvic fractures and lacerations involving the vagina and/or perineum. The female patient with a significant urethral injury is often hemodynamically unstable, and vaginal repair to control bleeding plus placement of a suprapubic catheter without dis-

turbance of the pelvic hematoma is indicated.[56] Planned second-stage surgery is performed when the patient has recovered from her other injuries.

Severe distal urethral injuries may be approached transvaginally, with catheterization of the distal segment and suturing of the vaginal incision around the neomeatus. The bladder is kept empty and the torn urethra is splinted with a Foley catheter.

If the urethra has been detached from the bladder, it can be reconstructed over a catheter by a retropubic approach. Any associated vaginal lacerations should also be repaired to reduce the incidence of fistula formation. Suprapubic cystostomy drainage is generally used postoperatively.

AXIOM   Overenthusiastic traction on a urethral catheter can cause damage to the bladder neck with resulting incontinence.

URETHRAL INJURIES IN CHILDREN

Anterior urethral injuries in children are uncommon.[56] The usual cause of a bulbous urethral rupture is a straddle injury such as may occur in bicycle accidents or falls onto fences. Pendulous urethral injuries may occur secondary to penetrating trauma. Management is similar to that described for adults.

Posterior injuries in children tend to occur at the bladder neck rather than in the prostatomembranous region. Indwelling urethral catheters should be avoided in the management of the male child, because of the small calibre of the urethra and the resultant high rate of stricture formation.

INJURIES OF THE PENIS

Blunt Penile Injuries

Injuries to the penis are usually due to direct trauma and are generally diagnosed quite readily.[2] Many of these injuries occur because excessive stress has been placed on the penis in the erect state.[59,60] The patient will often report a loud cracking sound and immediate pain and detumescence. Swelling of the entire penile shaft is usually also noted.

Urethral injury is present in approximately 20% of cases and is usually evidenced by a small amount of bloody urethral discharge.[56,60] Urethrography is indicated with all major penile injuries and operative repair should be undertaken. The most common severe injury is penile fracture (rupture of the corpora cavernosa), frequently with an associated rupture of the suspensory ligaments.[61] Other less frequent injuries include strangulation (tourniquet syndrome), severe mechanical suction (e.g., by a vacuum cleaner), amputation, and burn or zipper injuries to the skin.

There are two schools of thought on the appropriate treatment of penile fracture. One school advocates conservative measures including urethral catheter or suprapubic cystostomy drainage, ice pack, anti-inflammatory and sedative drugs (i.e., oxyphenbutazone and diazepam),[62] and oral streptokinase.[63] The other school advocates immediate surgical evacuation of the hematoma and primary repair of the torn structures.[61,64] This approach appears to produce better long-term results, because conservative management may lead to infection of the hematoma, painful penile lumps, permanent deformity, suboptimal erections, and difficulty with coitus.[62,65-68]

AXIOM   As a general rule, penile injuries with lacerations of the tunica albuginea should be repaired.

Traumatic rupture of the suspensory ligament can result from ventral lacerations of the erect penis or from severe anterior pelvic fractures. Pain and swelling occur at the base of the penis. To prevent abnormal erections later, Pryor and Hill[69] recommend open repair with nylon sutures between the symphysis pubis and the tunica albuginea. The penis is then inflated with saline, and if the

resulting erection is not normal, additional sutures are placed as needed.

Penetrating Penile Injuries

Penetrating penile injuries from gunshots or stab wounds require urethrography and operative exploration.[70,71] Debridement should be minimal because of the excellent blood supply of the penile tissues. Injuries to the glans penis are carefully reconstructed, and bullet openings are simply managed by approximation of the wound edges.

Strangulation Injuries

The patient with penile tourniquet syndrome may present early (with pain and swelling distal to the constricting device) or late (with urethral fistula or partial amputation).[2] Necrosis of the glans penis may not occur because slow constriction may allow some deep collateral circulation to develop.

AXIOM   A hair strangulation of the penis should be suspected in any circumcised boy with a swollen glans penis.

Human hair is a particularly common cause of penile strangulation.[2] Because human hair is stretchable when wet, it may become buried in the swollen penile skin to the point of near invisibility. If the condition is untreated, the hair may cut dorsally into the shaft, sparing the urethra but damaging the neurovascular bundle, or it may transect the urethra but spare sensation to the glans.

A single-stage repair is usually adequate for the milder injuries; however, for more severe injuries, a staged repair is advisable because the blood supply may be precarious.

Vacuum Cleaner Injuries

Vacuum cleaner injuries to the penis are not uncommon.[2] Eleven of the first 13 cases reported by Cass had multiple lacerations of the glans, shaft, prepuce, or urethral meatus, and only suturing was needed.[2] In two patients the corpora was also involved. However, five patients had extensive injury of the glans with loss of 1-2 inches of the urethra.

Traumatic Amputation

The treatment of choice in traumatic amputation is reattachment if the distal segment is in good condition, if the ischemia time is less than 12-18 hours, and if expertise in microneurovascular repair is available.[2,3]

The dismembered part is cleansed and placed in iced saline. Microsurgery should be undertaken immediately, with sequential repair of the urethra and tunica albuginea. At least one major artery and two veins should be repaired microscopically with 10/0 vascular sutures. However, the results with replantation are usually less than optimal. As a result some urologists favor repairing the remaining tissues and suturing the urethral mucosa to the skin to form a neourethrostomy.

The proper management of the penile skin after a reattachment is controversial. Some authorities advocate reapproximation, but there is a high incidence of skin necrosis if the amputation was complete.[2] Other authorities suggest removing the skin and burying the penis in the scrotum, although it has been argued that this maneuver causes tension on the corporal and urethral suture lines and reduces corporal blood flow. Patients who have had a penile amputation require the cooperative efforts of the urologist, plastic surgeon, and psychiatrist or psychologist.

In patients with other severe injuries, the preferred initial treatment of an amputated penis in most instances is to obtain hemostasis, oversew the ends of the corporal bodies and then spatulate the urethra and suture it to cover the end of the remaining penis.[7]

Major Skin Loss

Major skin loss can occur from avulsion injuries, necrotizing infection, burns and massive penetrating injuries.[70,72] With such injuries the deep structures of the penis, spermatic cord, testicles and urethra must also be evaluated.

SKIN AVULSION INJURIES

Penile skin trapped in a zipper can sometimes be freed by manipulation under local anesthesia. Alternatively, the zipper can be destroyed by applying bone-cutting pliers to the median bar or diamond.[73]

Avulsed skin may often be locally reconstructed.[72] Any skin that remains attached to the penis or has been brought with the patient should be thoroughly cleaned and replaced to reduce the amount of skin grafting that will be necessary. However, some surgeons feel that avulsed skin should not be reattached because it is very likely to become necrotic and infected.[2]

Significant adipose tissue attached to the avulsed skin should be removed before replacement; this facilitates more rapid neovascularization of the skin and its subsequent survival. Subcutaneous drainage should be used under large flaps of tissue to prevent serous fluid collections and infection. The portion of the penis without skin can be temporarily protected with moist sterile dressings until it can be covered definitively with skin grafts.

BURNS

Burns can create massive edema of the skin, and at times this may cause urethral obstruction.[59] A urethral catheter, inserted during the initial resuscitation, should be maintained or replaced by suprapubic cystostomy. When possible, deep third-degree burns should have immediate full-thickness skin excision, followed by split-thickness skin grafting to the penile shaft.[70] First- and second-degree burns should have local care and subsequent split-thickness skin grafting if needed.

INJURIES TO THE TESTES

Etiology and Pathology

Testicular rupture usually results from massive blunt scrotal trauma, most often caused by assaults, sports injuries and auto-pedestrian accidents. The actual mechanism is usually a direct blow with impingement of the testis against the symphysis pubis. The mobility of the testes, cremaster muscle contraction, and the tough capsule of the testis (tunica albuginea) are responsible for its infrequent injury, even in patients with multiple other injuries.

Diagnosis

Patients with testicular injuries usually have a large scrotal hematoma on the injured side and severe pain due to the swelling and intracapsular testicular edema. The surrounding hematoma often prevents palpation of the testicle, but real-time ultrasonography can be extremely reliable in detecting testicular rupture.[70,74] US is preferred due to the direct testicular radiation dose inherent in scrotal CT scans.[8] However, if there is a large scrotal hematoma, significant testicular ruptures can be missed by US, CT or physical examination.

AXIOM All large traumatic scrotal hematomas should be explored.

Scrotal trauma associated with a large hematoma can mask a ruptured testicle on physical exam and on imaging modalities. This can result in loss of an injured, but untreated, testicle.

Treatment

If the tunica albuginea of the testis is not ruptured, the initial treatment should include bed rest, scrotal support, analgesics and cold ap-

plications for 24-48 hours. If the tunica vaginalis sac is filled with blood (Hematocele) resulting in a large, swollen, tender, blue scrotal mass, the testicle should be explored, the hematoma evacuated, the area debrided, and the tunica albuginea reapproximated with sutures (Figure 29–11).[2,8]

Nonoperative management of testicular injury may be complicated by significant pain and secondary infection of the hematocele or the injured testis. The pressure effect of a tense hematocele can also result in atrophy of the testis after the hematocele resolves.

Postoperatively, if the testicle maintains its normal size, it has probably maintained its viability.[59] However, hormonal and spermatogenic function is difficult to assess if the contralateral testicle is nor-

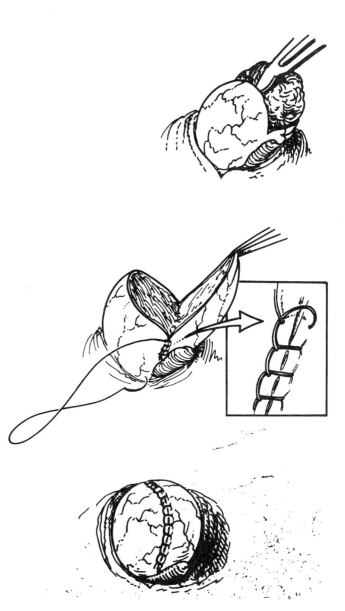

FIGURE 29–11 Evacuation of a testicular hematoma. A transverse scrotal incision is made over the midpoint of the hematoma, which is opened and evacuated to expose the testicle completely. The testicular parenchyma will be seen extruding through a transverse laceration of the tunica albuginea. The extruding parenchyma is removed by sharp dissection, and the entire tunica albuginea is preserved for final reconstruction. Hemostasis must be carefully maintained. The edges of the tunica albuginea are approximated with a running 4/0 absorbable suture, which maintains hemostasis and reconstructs the external portion of the testicle. (From McAninch JW. Genital injury. In Champion HR, Robbs JV, Trunkey DV, eds. Rob and Smith's operative surgery— trauma surgery, 4th ed. London: Butterworths, 1989; 491.)

mal. Orchidectomy is seldom necessary if diagnosis and reconstruction are prompt.

Penetrating testicular and scrotal injuries require operative exploration, debridement, and reconstruction of any damaged parts. Lacerations of the vas deferens and epididymis are best repaired by microsurgical techniques.[60]

Scrotal Avulsion

If at all possible, the remaining scrotal skin should be reconstructed around the testes, even if the closure is under considerable tension.[2] The scrotum usually regains nearly normal size within a few months. If scrotal reconstruction is impossible, the testicles should be placed in thigh pockets superficial to the subcutaneous fat, where the temperature is similar to that inside the scrotum.

As healing occurs, the regenerating scrotal skin develops hair and rugation resembling that of the normal scrotum.[59] If the medial thighs have also been severely injured, a split-thickness skin graft can be applied directly to the testicles to provide coverage and create a new scrotum. However, this procedure results in a less desirable cosmetic appearance. a significant incidence of contracture, and failure of hair to develop.

AXIOM Following healing of a scrotal avulsion, serum testosterone levels are usually normal; however, fertility may be altered because of increased temperature of the testicle under the tissue flap.

SUMMARY

Injury to the urinary tract should be suspected with any blunt or penetrating trauma to the lower chest, abdomen or pelvis. Any patient with hematuria, difficulty in voiding or severe pain or swelling in the flank should have the urinary tract investigated completely. Unless the mechanism of the injury is known to be localized either to the kidney or bladder, computed tomography and retrograde urethrocystography should be performed. An IVP is less reliable.

The great majority of renal injuries are best treated nonoperatively unless there is severe continued bleeding or urine extravasation. Injuries of the ureters or bladder are generally best treated by early operation. Severe prostatomembranous urethral injury is usually treated with cystostomy and perivesical drainage. Subsequent urethral stricture, which is likely to occur, can be treated electively at a later date.

⊘ FREQUENT ERRORS

In the Management of Trauma to the Urinary Tract

1. *Neglect of the patient's general condition and other injuries while investigating the urinary tract.*
2. *Failure to give a hemodynamically stable patient an opportunity to void spontaneously before a Foley catheter is inserted.*
3. *Failure to obtain an early IVP or CT scan in patients who might have renal injury. (If the patient is hemodynamically stable, a CT scan is preferred).*
4. *Failure to obtain a CT or an arteriogram promptly if a kidney is not visualized on IVP.*
5. *Exploring all renal injuries, even if the patient is hemodynamically unstable.*
6. *A conservative surgical approach to lower urinary tract injuries.*
7. *Assuming that the uninjured kidney is normal because it looks and feels normal.*
8. *Failure to obtain control of the renal vessels before opening a perirenal hematoma.*
9. *Excessive mobilization of the ureter while examining or repairing it.*
10. *Vigorous attempts to pass a Foley catheter in a patient who may have a urethral or bladder injury.*

▼▼▼▼▼▼▼▼▼▼▼▼▼▼▼▼▼▼▼▼▼▼▼▼▼▼▼▼▼▼

SUMMARY POINTS

1. If the physician concentrates his attention on obvious genitourinary trauma, other injuries which are more likely to be lethal may cause sudden deterioration.
2. If the physician fails to auscultate over the lower back following severe blunt trauma, he may miss important renal vascular injuries.
3. Although hematuria strongly suggests the presence of a urologic injury and is an indication for complete urologic examination, the absence of hematuria is of much less diagnostic value.
4. In most centers, the presence of >40-50 RBC/HPF in the injured patient's urine warrants complete radiologic investigation of the urinary tract.
5. Insertion of a Foley catheter before obtaining a urine specimen greatly reduces the value of the urinalysis.
6. Creatinine clearance is a far better test of renal function than the BUN or serum creatinine.
7. The patients who are usually in most need of complete radiologic evaluation are often those who can least tolerate it because of multiple other injuries.
8. If there is any suspicion of renal damage, a CT scan or intravenous urogram (IVP) should be performed.
9. A normal-appearing plain radiograph of the abdomen is of little or no value for ruling out kidney damage.
10. IVPs done under emergency circumstances may provide very little information about the kidneys.
11. Excretory urography is usually not needed in blunt trauma victims who have no associated major intraabdominal injuries, no microscopic hematuria, and no hypotension.
12. Failure of both kidneys to visualize on a "one-shot IV" is usually due to inadequate renal perfusion, inadequate intravenous contrast, or other technical factors.
13. An abdominal CT scan with intravenous contrast is the most accurate technique for visualizing a kidney that may be injured.
14. CT is recommended for evaluation of the urinary tract in any stable patient who is felt to have a significant risk of renal injury as well as in any patient who has an equivocal IVP.
15. Whenever possible, abdominal CT examination should be done with intravenous and gastrointestinal contrast.
16. The 4-6 hours of warm ischemia that a kidney can tolerate can be lost while waiting for an arteriogram.
17. Most renal injuries heal well without surgical intervention.
18. If it is assumed that persistent hypotension in an injured patient is due to bleeding from a damaged kidney, injuries that are more life-threatening are apt to be missed.
19. If time is available and if the patient to be explored specifically for severe renal trauma is hemodynamically stable, it may be helpful to obtain a renal arteriogram prior to surgery.
20. In severe trauma, unless the ureter and kidney are seen on an IVP or another imaging study prior to emergency surgery, these structures should be examined at laparotomy. Ureteral injuries are easily missed and can lead to significant morbidity.
21. The function of a kidney cannot be evaluated by its size or appearance or by the way it feels on palpation.
22. Failure to control the renal vessels before opening a perirenal hematoma can result in severe bleeding and a possibly unnecessary nephrectomy.
23. Before a nephrectomy is performed, it is important to know that there is a functioning contralateral kidney. Evidence that the contralateral kidney is functional includes visualization on IVP or CT or continued good urine output after the pedicle of the injured kidney is occluded.
24. A severely injured kidney should not be removed unless one is certain that the other kidney is functional.

25. If the patient has a contralateral functioning kidney, a partial nephrectomy should only be considered if the patient is hemodynamically stable and will not be jeopardized by 1-2 hours of additional surgery.

26. An ischemic kidney should be revascularized within 3-6 hours if at all possible.

27. If renal artery occlusion cannot be relieved within 6-12 hours, an immediate nephrectomy is not necessary because occasional spontaneous revascularization can occur.

28. Hypertension due to an injured kidney may not develop until 1-2 years after the initial trauma.

29. Injuries of the ureteropelvic junction are often associated with fractures of the lower ribs and are the most common type of ureteral injury in children.

30. It is important to visualize the ureters clearly (either on IVP or CT scan or at laparotomy) if there is a penetrating wound in the vicinity of these structures.

31. Excessive mobilization of the ureter or disturbance of its adventitia during dissection may result in necrosis or the ureter by interfering with its blood supply.

32. Ureteral stents greatly improve the chances for a ureteral repair to heal without complications.

33. The bladder is much more easily ruptured when it is full.

34. Bladder injuries should be suspected with any trauma to the lower abdomen or pelvis, especially if there is a fracture of the pubic rami or separation of the symphysis pubis.

35. The "post-evac" cystogram film is the view most apt to show small bladder injuries.

36. Large tense pelvic hematomas can temporarily prevent extravasation of contrast from a bladder injury and thereby cause a cystogram to be falsely negative.

37. Patients with pelvic fractures should be watched carefully for delayed extravasation from a missed bladder injury after the Foley catheter has been removed.

38. Small extraperitoneal bladder injuries can often be treated by simple catheter drainage of the bladder.

39. Adequate drainage of a mildly-to-moderately injured bladder can be provided with a urethral Foley catheter. With severe bladder trauma, one should drain the bladder with a suprapubic cystostomy in males; however, a large Foley catheter is usually adequate in females.

40. Patients with surgery on the kidney, ureters, or bladder should have the adjacent tissue drained in the event there is a postoperative urine leak.

41. If there is a suspicion of a urethral injury, a urethral catheter should not be passed until a retrograde urethrogram has excluded a tear.

42. Persistent attempts to pass a urethral catheter, especially after a pelvic injury, may cause severe complications.

43. Any patient with a pelvic crushing injury who is unable to void or who has bloody urine should have retrograde urethrogram prior to catheter insertion.

44. If there is any suspicion of a urethral injury, a Foley catheter should not be inserted until a urethrogram has been performed.

45. Whenever a Foley catheterization is performed, a urethral injury may be missed or made worse. In such circumstances, it is wise to perform a urethrogram alongside the Foley catheter before it is removed.

46. If a transection of the urethra is incomplete, it is important not to increase the extent of the injury by passing a Foley catheter or performing excessive operative manipulations.

47. Overenthusiastic traction on a urethral catheter can cause damage to the bladder neck with resulting incontinence.

48. As a general rule, all penile injuries with lacerations of the tunica albuginea should be repaired.

49. A hair strangulation of the penis should be suspected in any circumcised boy with a swollen glans penis.

50. All large trauma scrotal hematomas should be explored.

51. Following healing of a scrotal avulsion, serum testosterone levels are usually normal; however, fertility may be altered because of the increased temperature of the testicle under the tissue flap.

▲▲▲▲▲▲▲▲▲▲▲▲▲▲▲▲▲▲▲▲▲▲▲▲▲▲▲▲▲▲▲▲

REFERENCES

1. Kreiger JN, Algood CB, Mason JT, et al. Urological trauma in the Pacific Northwest: etiology, distribution, management and outcome. J Urol 1984;132:70.
2. Cass AS. Genitourinary trauma. In Kreis DJ, Gomez GA, eds. Trauma management. Boston: Little, Brown & Co., 1989;11:265-280.
3. Chambers RJ Jr, Champion HR, Edson M. Ureteric and renal trauma. In Champion HR, Robbs JV, Trunkey DV, eds. Rob and Smith's operative surgery—trauma surgery, 4th ed. Boston: Butterworths, 1989; 466-475.
4. Fallon B, Wendt JC, Hawtrey CE. Urological injury and assessment in patients with fractured pelvis. J Urol 1984;131:712.
5. Ben-Menachem Y. Logic and logistics of radiography, angiography, and angiographic intervention in massive blunt trauma. Radiol Clin North An 1981;19L:9.
6. Ben-Menachem Y, Handel SF, Ray RD, et al. Embolization procedures in trauma: a matter of urgency. Semin Intervent Radiol 1985;1:107.
7. Wilson RF, Pierce JM Jr. Trauma to the urinary tract. In Walt AJ, Wilson RF, eds. Management of trauma: pitfalls and practice. Philadelphia: Lea & Febiger, 1975;14:375-392.
8. Campbell JE. Urinary tract trauma. J Can Assoc Radiol 1983;34:237.
9. McAninch JW, Carroll PR, Armenakas NA, et al. Renal gunshot wounds: methods of salvage and reconstruction. J Trauma 1993;35:279.
10. Stables DP, Fouche RF, Devilliers VN, et al. Traumatic renal artery occlusion: 21 cases. J Urol 1979;115:229.
11. Guerriero WG, Carlton CE, Scott R, Beall AC. Renal pedicle injuries. J Trauma 1971;11:53.
12. Federle MP, Brown TR, McAninch JW. Penetrating renal trauma: CT evaluation. J Comput Assist Tomogr 1987;11:1026.
13. Hardeman SW, Husmann DA, Chinn HKW, Peters PC. Blunt urinary trauma: identifying those patients who require radiological diagnostic studies. J Urol 1987;138:99.
14. Cass AS, Luxenberg M, Gleich P, Smith CS. Clinical indications for radiographic evaluation of blunt renal trauma. J Urol 1986;136:370.
15. Phillips T, Sclafani SJA, Goldstein A, et al. Use of the contrast-enhanced CT enema in the management of penetrating trauma to the flank and back. J Trauma 1986;26:593.
16. Hessel SJ, Smith EH. Renal trauma: a comprehensive review and radiologic assessment. CRC Crit Rev Clin Radiol Nucl Med 1974;5:251.
17. Lang EK, Sullivan J, Frentz G. Renal trauma: radiological studies. Comparison of urography, computed tomography, angiography and radionuclide studies. Radiology 1985;154:1.
18. Erturk E, Sheinfeld J DiMarco PL, Cockett ATK. Renal trauma: evaluation by computerized tomography. J Urol 1985;133:946.
19. Carroll PR, McAninch JW. Operative indications in penetrating renal trauma. J Trauma 1985;25:587.
20. Wilson RF, Ziegler DW. Diagnostic and treatment problems in renal injuries. Am Surg 1987;53:399.
21. Stevenson J, Battistella FD. The one-shot intravenous pyelogram: is it indicated in unstable trauma patients before celiotomy? J Trauma 1994;36:828.
22. Peitzman AB, Makaroun MS, Slasky BS, Ritter P. Prospective study of computed tomography in initial management of blunt abdominal trauma. J Trauma 1986;26:585.
23. McAllister E, Perez M, Albrink MH, et al. Is triple-contrast computed tomographic scanning useful in the selective management of stab wounds to the back? J Trauma 1994;37:401.
24. Fisher RG, Ben-Menachem Y, Whigham C. Stab wounds of the renal artery branches: angiographic diagnosis and treatment by embolization. AJR 1989;152:1231.
25. Furtschegger A, Egender G, Jaske G. The value of sonography in the diagnosis and follow-up of patients with blunt renal trauma. Br J Urol 1988;62:110.
26. Jaske G, Furtschegger A, Egender G. Ultrasound in patients with blunt renal trauma managed by surgery. J Urol 1987;138:21.
27. Martin KW, McAlister WH, Shackelford GD. Acute renal infarction: diagnosis by Doppler ultrasound. Pediatr Radiol 1988;18:373.
28. Berg BC. Nuclear medicine and complementary modalities in renal trauma. Semin Nucl Med 1982;12:280.
29. Chopp RT, Hekmat-Ravan H, Mendez R. Technetium-99m glucoheptonate renal scan in diagnosis of acute renal injury. Urol 1980;15:201.

30. Cheng DL, Lazan D, Stone N. Conservative treatment of type III renal trauma. J Trauma 1994;36:491.
31. Dean RH. Management of renal artery trauma. J Vasc Surg 1988;8:89.
32. Spirnak JP, Resnick MI. Revascularization of traumatic thrombosis of renal artery. Surg Gynecol Obstet 1987;164:22.
33. Barlow B, Gandhi R. Renal artery thrombosis following blunt trauma. J Trauma 1980;20:614.
34. Greenholz SK, Moore EE, Paterson NE, et al. Traumatic bilateral renal artery occlusion: successful outcome without surgical intervention. J Trauma. 1980;26:941.
35. Reddy PK, Hulbert JC, Lange PH, et al. Percutaneous removal of renal and ureteral calculi: experience with 400 cases. J Urol 1985;134:662.
36. Segura JW, Patterson DE, LeRoy AJ, et al. Percutaneous removal of kidney stones: review of 1,000 cases. J Urol 1985;134:1077.
37. Lee WJ, Smith AD, Cubelli V, et al. Percutaneous nephrolithotomy: analysis of 500 consecutive cases. Urol Radiol 1986;8:61.
38. Smith AD. Ureteral obstruction in the female. In Raz S, ed. Female urology. Philadelphia: WB Saunders. 1983; 394.
39. Winfield HN, and Clayman RV. Complications of percutaneous removal of renal and ureteral calculi. World Urol Update Series 1985;2:37.
40. Cass AS. Ureteral contusion with gunshot wounds. J Trauma 1984;24:59
41. Cross JJL, Wong V, Irving HC, et al. Ureteric rupture in an elderly patient following minor trauma: case report. J Trauma 1994;36:594.
42. Whitesides E, Kozlowski D. Ureteral injury from blunt abdominal trauma: case report. J Trauma 1994;36:745.
43. Rober PE, Smith JB, Pierce JM. Gunshot injuries of the ureter. J Trauma 1990;30:83.
44. Brandes SB, Chelsky MJ, Buckman RF, et al. Ureteral injuries from penetrating trauma. J Trauma 1994;36:766.
45. Demos TC, Churchill R, Flisak ME, et al. The radiologic diagnosis of complications following gynecologic surgery: radiography, computed tomography, sonography, and scintigraphy. CRC Crit Rev Diagn Imaging 1984;22:43.
46. Toporoff B, Sclafani S, Scalea T, et al. Percutaneous antegrade ureteral stenting as an adjunct for treatment of complicated ureteral injuries. J Trauma 1992;32:534.
47. MacMahon R, Hosking D, Ramsey EW. Management of blunt injury to the lower urinary tract. Can J Surg 1983;26:415.
48. Kluger Y, Altman GT, Deshmukh R, et al. Acute obstructive uropathy secondary to pelvic hematoma compressing the bladder: report of two cases. J Trauma 1993;35:477.
49. Edson M. Injury to the bladder. In Champion HR, Robbs JV, Trunkey DV, eds. Rob and Smith's operative surgery—trauma surgery, 4th ed. London: Butterworths, 1989; 481-484.
50. Palmer JK, Benson GS, Corriere JN Jr. Diagnosis and initial management of urological injuries associated with 200 consecutive pelvic fractures. J Urol 1983;130:712.
51. Devine PC, Devine CJ Jr. Posterior urethral injuries associated with pelvic fractures. Urology 1982;20:467.
52. Blandy JP, King JB. Management of the fractured pelvis with urethral injury in the male. World Urol Update Series 1983;1:2.
53. Webster GD, Mathes GL, Selli C. Prostatomembranous urethral injuries: a review of the literature and a rational approach to their management. J Urol 1983;130:898.
54. Al-Ali IH, Husain J. Disrupting injuries of the membranous urethra: the case for early surgery and catheter splinting. Br J Urol 1983;55:716.
55. Gonzales R, Chiou RK, Hekmat Km et al. Endoscopic re-establishment of urethral continuity after traumatic disruption of the membranous urethra. J Urol 1983;130:785.
56. Edson M. Injuries to the urethra. In Champion HR, Robbs JV, Trunkey DV, eds. Rob and Smith's operative surgery—trauma surgery, 4th ed. London: Butterworths, 1989; 476-480.
57. Corriere JN Jr, Rudy DC, Benson GS. Voiding and erectile function after delayed one-stage repair of posterior urethral disruptions in 50 men with a fractured pelvis (abstract). J Trauma 1993;35:160.
58. Clayman RV. Diagnostic and therapeutic applications of outpatient cystourethroscopy. In Kays KW, ed. Outpatient urologic surgery. Philadelphia: Lea & Febiger. 1985; 111.
59. McAninch JW. Genital injury. In Champion HR, Robbs JV, Trunkey DV, eds. Rob and Smith's operative surgery—trauma surgery, 4th ed. London: Butterworths, 1989; 486-491.
60. Mansi MK, Emran M, El-Mahrouky A, et al. Experience with acute penile fractures in Egypt: long-term results of immediate surgical repair. J Trauma 1993;35:67.
61. Nymark J, Kristensen JK. Fracture of the penis with urethral rupture. J Urol 1983;129:147.
62. Julla A, Wani NA, Rashid PA. Fracture of the penis. J Urol 1980;123:285.
63. Creecy AA, Beazlie F Jr. Fracture of the penis: traumatic rupture of corpora cavernosa. J Urol 1967;78:620.
64. Gross M, Arnold TL, Peters P. Fracture of the penis with associated laceration of the urethra. J Urol 1977;117:725.
65. Farah R, Cerny JC. Penis tourniquet syndrome and penile amputation. Urology 1973;2:310.
66. Walton JK. Fracture of the penis with laceration of the urethra. Br J Urol 1979;51:308.
67. Pryor JP, Hill JT, Packham DA, et al. Penile injuries with particular reference to injury to the erectile tissue. Br J Urol 1981;53:42.
68. Bergner DM, Wilcox ME, Frentz GD. Fracture of the penis. Urology 1982;20:278.
69. Pryor JP, Hill JT. Abnormalities of the suspensory ligament of the penis as a cause of erectile dysfunction. Br J Urol 1979;51:402.
70. McAninch JW, Kahn RI, Jeffrey RB, et al. Major traumatic and septic genital injuries. J Trauma 1984;24:291.
71. Engelman ER, Polito G, Perley J, et al. Traumatic amputation of the penis. Urology 1974;112:774.
72. Clup DA. Genital injuries: etiology and initial management. Urol CL North Am 1977;4:143.
73. Saraf P. Zipper injury of the foreskin. Am J Dis Child 1982;136:556.
74. Anderson KA, McAninch JW, Jeffrey RB, et al. Ultrasonography for the diagnosis and staging of blunt scrotal trauma. J Urol 1983;130:933.
75. Cass AS. Testicular trauma. J Urol 1983;129:299.

Chapter 30 Gynecologic and Obstetrical Trauma

ROBERT F. WILSON, M.D.

CHARLES VINCENT, M.D.

GYNECOLOGICAL INJURIES IN THE NONPREGNANT FEMALE

With the exception of sexual assault and domestic violence, injury to female reproductive organs in the nonpregnant state is uncommon. Blunt trauma rarely injures the internal genitalia unless the organs are previously enlarged or diseased.

> **AXIOM** Gynecologic injuries are important, and yet they are easily missed because of the patient's modesty or the doctor's reluctance to examine the perineum (unless there is severe pain, bleeding or an obvious wound).[1]

In addition to the usual early complications of any tissue injury, such as pain, infection or hemorrhage, certain delayed sequelae of gynecological injuries may be extremely important. These include infertility, pelvic contraction or distortion (necessitating abdominal fetal delivery), rectovaginal or vesicovaginal fistulas, and vaginal and uterine synechiae.

Vulvovaginal Injuries

Because the history is often inaccurate or frankly deceptive, accurate diagnosis of vulvovaginal injuries depends primarily on careful complete examination.

> **PITFALL** ⊘
>
> *If general anesthesia is not used to obtain a complete pelvic examination in uncooperative patients, severe gynecologic injuries are easily missed.*

If there is any difficulty obtaining full patient cooperation, there should be no hesitancy in using general anesthesia to obtain an adequate examination. Severe injuries of the perineum, vagina, urethra, bladder, and rectum can easily be overlooked during the initial examination of a struggling, anxious patient. This is especially true with children, who are more likely to have serious associated injuries and are less likely to cooperate than adults.

The vulva and vagina, which are considered contaminated areas, and all associated wounds should be carefully cleaned prior to any examination. Since the bladder, if partially distended, can interfere with a proper pelvic examination, it should be emptied with a sterile catheter prior to the examination, and the urine submitted for urinalysis. In the adult, digital and speculum examination is mandatory, especially if the vagina may be injured; in the child, a rectal examination plus vaginal endoscopy will usually suffice. If there is a possibility of rectal damage, proctosigmoidoscopy is also indicated.

Additional information may be obtained by flat and upright radiographs of the abdomen. Free air, foreign bodies, and displaced loops of bowel all may have diagnostic value. If there is any suspicion of lower urinary tract injury, urethrograms and cystograms should also be performed.

HEMATOMAS

Before menopause, the vulva and vagina have a copious blood supply, and this rich plexus of veins is easily torn. Furthermore, since there is little resistance in this area to the expansion of hematomas, they may dissect deeply and rapidly into the perineum and ischiorectal fossa. Nevertheless, a nonpregnant woman with a large pelvic hematoma after only minimal trauma should be investigated for coagulopathies and platelet disorders.

> **PITFALL** ⊘
>
> *Failure to obtain immediate complete coagulation and platelet studies on any patient with excessive bleeding or a large hematoma may delay accurate therapy, and surgery may be undertaken in a patient in whom reasonable hemostasis is impossible.*

Pain is the most common symptom of a pelvic hematoma, and it is usually directly proportional to the distension and disruption of the tissues.

> **AXIOM** Ecchymoses about the perineum may be the only evidence of severe concealed hemorrhage into the ischiorectal fossa.

Occasionally, excessive distension of a vulvar hematoma may either obliterate the vagina or cause a rupture of the overlying skin with external bleeding. Rarely, the hematoma will continue to expand in spite of conservative treatment and cause hypovolemic shock. Although the presence of a vulvar hematoma is usually obvious, outlining its full extent often requires careful vaginal and rectal examination under general anesthesia.[2]

Most vulvar hematomas are less than 5 cm in diameter and resolve spontaneously without surgical intervention. However, hematomas which are progressively enlarging or are greater than 5 cm in diameter require incision of the overlying mucosa or skin and evacuation of the clots.[1] If specific bleeding vessels are not found (and they usually are not), the hemorrhage can often be controlled by multiple figure-of-eight sutures around the periphery of the hematoma followed by tight packing of the hematoma cavity. Concomitant packing of the vagina may also facilitate hemostasis. If bleeding and coagulation studies are normal, the pack can generally be removed after 24-48 hours. The hematoma cavity will usually gradually disappear over the next 2-3 weeks. In rare instances, a progressively enlarging subperitoneal hematoma may require laparotomy to achieve control of the bleeding.

LACERATIONS

Early thorough cleansing, debridement and generous irrigation of all vulvovaginal wounds is essential. Additional treatment depends on the duration of the injury, the amount of inflammation and necrosis present, and the presence of associated injuries to the urethra, bladder, rectum or peritoneal cavity. If the injuries are less than 12 hours old and there is minimal tissue reaction, rectovaginal and vesicovaginal fistulas can be closed and injuries to the anal sphincter carefully repaired. However, a proximal colostomy is usually recommended if a large perineal or rectal laceration or rectovaginal fistula is present.[2]

RAPE AND COITUS

PITFALL ⊘

> *Failure to perform a complete initial examination on an alleged rape victim increases not only the risk of complications but also the possibility of gross injustice.*

Rape is not always easily confirmed. The examining physician can only describe specific areas of obvious trauma and the presence or absence of spermatozoa or prostatic fluid. Any material in the vagina obtained during the speculum examination should be studied microscopically as a wet-mount and analyzed for acid-phosphatase. If the vagina is empty, it can be irrigated with saline which can then be removed and examined microscopically.

Coital trauma is not always evident, but if tissue damage is present, it is usually in the form of lacerations rather than a hematoma. If the vagina is atrophic or the assault occurs in a woman with vaginismus, the lacerations are likely to be longitudinal. If the victim is a virgin, the rape or coitus may cause multiple hymenal and vaginal lacerations with severe bleeding. Occasionally, the arterial bleeding following initial coitus is so severe that ligation of the bleeding vessels and blood replacement are required.

In addition to the pelvic evaluation, all rape victims should have a thorough general physical examination in search of extrapelvic injury. The level of consciousness and sobriety should be noted, and a blood alcohol level and drug screen should also be drawn.

All suspected or proven victims of rape should be protected from pregnancy by the oral administration of some form of estrogen. Ovral is extremely effective and has a low incidence of side effects when taken in the usual dose of 2 tablets within 72 hours (preferably 12-24 hours) of coitus and 2 tablets again 12 hours later.[3]

FOREIGN BODIES

AXIOM Vaginal drainage in a child is due to a foreign body until proven otherwise.

Trauma to the vulva or vagina from foreign bodies is most common in young children. Hemorrhage may occur immediately after insertion of the foreign body if it is sharp and causes a penetrating injury. However, there is often a delay of days or weeks before the child is brought to the physician because of the purulent vaginal discharge. Rectal examination with simultaneous insertion of a uterine sound into the vagina may detect a metallic foreign body. Because of the associated pain, general anesthesia is often necessary to perform an adequate examination and to remove the foreign body. In some instances, special radiologic techniques may be required to find the foreign body.[4]

If the foreign body is removed early, before there is severe infection, no additional therapy besides several days of antibiotics may be required. In all other instances, packing the vagina with vaseline gauze is important to prevent adhesive vaginitis and later vaginal atresia, dyspareunia, or infertility. It should also be remembered that vaginal foreign bodies are often associated with child sexual abuse.[5]

Pelvic Fractures

The rising number of high-speed automobile accidents has resulted in a marked increase in the incidence of severe pelvic fractures in females. Since the pelvis is a rigid ring, great force is usually required to cause bony displacement, and this will occur only if the ring is disrupted in at least two places.

BLEEDING

Pelvic fractures may cause severe bleeding and extensive gynecologic and urologic injuries.[6] Often, over 2000 ml of blood is lost into the resulting retroperitoneal hematomas. Torn branches of an internal iliac artery are the most likely sources of continued severe bleeding under these circumstances.

PITFALL ⊘

> *Direct surgical intraabdominal attempts to control hemorrhage from pelvic fractures usually results in much more severe bleeding and complications.*

If at all possible, pelvic hematomas due to fractures from blunt trauma should not be opened. Once the tamponading effect of the overlying peritoneum is lost, the bleeding may be almost impossible to control. Sutures and other methods of direct hemostasis are usually unsatisfactory in this area. If the hematoma is progressively expanding at the time of laparotomy and the bleeding cannot be controlled, the area should be packed. Further therapy may include external fixation of the pelvis and/or radiological embolization of the bleeding vessels. If a pelvic pack is inserted to control bleeding, it should usually be removed after 24-48 hours, but only after any coagulopathy has been corrected.

EXTERNAL GYNECOLOGICAL INJURIES

Pelvic fractures are associated with the majority of blunt injuries to the external genitalia, and these most commonly involve the vagina and perineum.[7] Indeed, simultaneous injury to the lower urinary and genital tracts is not an uncommon complication of pelvic fractures. There have also been some reports of vaginal injuries as a result of water-skiing.[8]

AXIOM Patients with vaginal tears secondary to pelvic fracture have, by definition, compound fractures and an increased incidence of pelvic abscess and septic complications.

Vaginal lacerations associated with pelvic fractures may be extensive and may involve the perineum, vaginal canal, or fornices. Rupture into the bladder or urethra may produce urethral-vaginal or vesicovaginal fistulas. Osteomyelitis has also been reported.[9] Vaginal tears may result from direct penetration from bony fragments, diastasis of the pubis, or shearing forces associated with bilateral ischiopubic rami fractures, the so-called butterfly fracture. Vaginal bleeding is the most common clinical finding; however, it may be obscured by vaginal spasm.

Diagnosis

Blood coming from the vagina should serve as a warning of a possible open pelvic fracture into the genital tract. In patients with displaced bilateral pubic rami or Malgaigne variant fractures, the pelvic exam must be be done very gently.

AXIOM If the pelvic examination in a patient with a pelvic fracture is not performed very gently, a closed pelvic fracture can easily be converted into an open one.

With the patient in a lateral position and using a Sims speculum, the physician can often gain some impression of the extent of injury, which may involve the base of the bladder, the vesical neck and the urethra. Injection of 2 ml of methylene blue into the bladder may help identify a traumatic fistula into the vagina. Use of radiopaque material may also be used to demonstrate openings into the peritoneal cavity.

Treatment

Under most circumstances lower urinary tract injuries should be repaired immediately, especially if intraperitoneal rupture of the bladder has been confirmed on cystography. The risk of pelvic abscess increases if a vaginal laceration is not recognized. Vaginal lacerations should be closed transvaginally with slowly-absorbable suture after the vagina is gently but thoroughly cleansed with an antiseptic solution. Deep perineal tears, with or without rectal injury, usually require a proximal diverting colostomy plus irrigation of the distal defunctionalized segment of bowel.[10] Preoperative and perioperative antibiotics are indicated.

INTERNAL GYNECOLOGICAL INJURIES

In a case report and review of the literature, Doman and Hoekstra found that internal gynecological injuries with blunt trauma are extremely rare if the patient is not pregnant and is otherwise normal.[11] If an exploratory laparotomy is performed on a female with pelvic fractures, the gynecological structures should be evaluated carefully. If a fallopian tube, an ovary, or the uterus is lacerated, it should be repaired if possible; however, considerable caution should be taken not to release an associated retroperitoneal hematoma.

LATE COMPLICATIONS OF PELVIC FRACTURES

Bilateral pubic rami fractures can result in severe obstetrical sequelae, including infertility and obstetrical difficulty. The incidence of cesarean section is much higher in women with pelvic fractures who subsequently become pregnant due to a contracted pelvis. However, because elective cesarean section is a reliable and safe procedure with a mortality of less than 0.1%, this possibility alone is not a sufficient reason to perform open reduction and internal fixation of complex pelvic fractures.

Uterine Injuries

IATROGENIC INJURIES

Perforation of the myometrium from within the endometrial cavity with a curette, ovum forceps or uterine sound occurs about once in every 350 cases.[2] Similarly, the uterine wall may be perforated during insertions of radioactive material in the treatment of endometrial cancer.

AXIOM When recognized immediately, perforation of the nonpregnant uterus in the operating room can usually be managed non-operatively, but the patient must be observed carefully for evidence of hemorrhage or infection.

In questionable cases, culdocentesis can be performed to rule out intraperitoneal hemorrhage. Whenever uterine perforation is suspected, further attempts at curettage should be abandoned, except in cases of suspected malignancy, when they can be continued if care is taken to avoid the site of perforation. Similarly, curettage of an incomplete abortion may be continued carefully with removal of large fragments of placental tissue if the perforation was caused by a uterine sound or small curette.

Although most iatrogenic perforations of the uterus can be treated nonoperatively, any evidence of omentum or bowel within the perforated uterus demands immediate laparotomy. When the laparotomy is carried out, the bowel, omentum and all adjacent intraperitoneal structures must be carefully examined for injury. Parametrial bleeding may also occur and sometimes will require hypogastric artery ligation.

CONTRACEPTIVE DEVICES

Intrauterine contraceptive devices such as the "coil" may be pushed through the uterine wall by various types of trauma. Such devices in the peritoneal cavity can result in bowel obstruction, especially if the device contains a loop.[12] Hysterography in such instances can confirm the extrauterine location of the device, which should then be removed.

CRIMINAL ABORTIONS

Perforation of the uterine wall can easily occur as a result of attempts to induce abortion. Repeated insertions of rigid instruments into the uterus can result in multiple uterine wounds. These patients often delay in reporting to a physician or until signs and symptoms of severe infection appear. Most of these patients will also deny having attempted to cause the abortion. However, the combination of vaginal bleeding, fever, and a tender uterus should lead the physician to suspect instrumentation and the need for vigorous emergency measures.

AXIOM Attempted abortion should be suspected when septic shock occurs in young women of childbearing age.

Prompt treatment to combat shock and infection must be initiated. The uterus should be evacuated after: (a) hypovolemia has been corrected, (b) the patient's condition is stabilized, (c) proper cultures have been obtained, and (d) full doses of broad-spectrum antibiotics have been started. Administration of the correct antibiotics to these patients is vital. The organisms most frequently involved are a combination of aerobic gram-negative enteric bacilli and anaerobic bacteria, especially peptostreptococcus and bacteroides and clostridial species. Clostridium welchii infection is rare but often fatal.

Pelvic abscesses bulging into the cul-de-sac of Douglas should be confirmed by culdocentesis and then drained from below. Unless bleeding is active, oxytocic drugs are contraindicated in patients with septic abortions because the severe vasoconstriction they produce impairs circulation and local natural defenses.

AXIOM All patients suspected of having a criminal abortion should have radiologic studies to search for an extrauterine foreign body. However, radiographs do not always rule out foreign bodies, especially those made of plastic.

When uterine perforation or rupture is suspected in a patient with a criminal abortion, exploratory celiotomy is indicated. If the uterus is found to be perforated and infected, a hysterectomy should be performed.

AXIOM An extensive laceration of a grossly infected uterus is best managed by hysterectomy.

Patients with severe pelvic infections, especially those with Bacteroides fragilis, tend to develop septic pelvic thrombophlebitis. In patients who develop multiple septic pulmonary emboli, the inferior vena cava and both ovarian veins should be ligated.

BLUNT TRAUMA TO THE UTERUS

The non-pregnant uterus is usually well protected by the bony pelvis. However, it may occasionally be so badly damaged by pelvic trauma that hysterectomy may be necessary. This is most apt to be required in a woman of high parity, whose uterus is usually less able than others to contract and control bleeding.

Blunt injury to the uterus may also occur from seat belts following sudden deceleration. Signs of seat belt injuries include lower abdominal contusions, abrasions, and ecchymoses, which may be associated internally with mesenteric lacerations, transection of the rectus abdominis muscles and bowel, traumatic thrombosis of iliac vessels and Chance fractures of lumbar vertebrae.[13]

EXTERNAL PENETRATING INJURY

Penetrating gynecological trauma follows the pattern seen with penetrating injuries to other intraabdominal organs, with the likelihood of injury directly related to the size and surface area of the involved structures.[14] Thus, penetrating wounds occur in descending order of frequency to the uterus, tubes, ovaries, and cervix. Associated injuries most frequently involve the intestine, but vascular injuries are also common and may be life-threatening.

Reproductive function should be preserved in young women unless the extent of injury demands immediate resection of internal genitalia. Injuries to already diseased structures may require excision but must be managed on an individual basis. The associated non-genital injuries are usually more severe, and initial attention is directed to the control of bleeding and the avoidance of further contamination.

Treatment of extensive penetrating uterine injury in young women depends on whether or not the uterus can be reconstructed well enough to make a future pregnancy reasonably safe. If this cannot be accomplished, hysterectomy is the treatment of choice. However, in the critically injured patient, it is unwise to insist on total hysterectomy unless there is bleeding from an injury to the cervix and unless it can be accomplished as rapidly as a subtotal hysterectomy.

Because blunt injury to the tubes and ovaries is usually restricted to organs with preexisting disease, the decision to repair or resect is usually obvious. In penetrating trauma, adnexal injuries should be repaired if possible; however, resection may be safer if there are severe associated injuries and the organs on the opposite side are normal.

CHEMICAL INJURIES TO THE UTERUS

Severe chemical injury to the uterus and vagina with ulceration and bleeding due to the use of agents, such as potassium permanganate, for criminal abortions is quite rare now. However, if it occurs, the initial chemical damage may be followed by fistula formation, extensive scarring and vaginal atresia. Treatment consists of careful irrigation with large quantities of saline, control of infection, and, in some instances, loose packing with Vaseline gauze to prevent vaginal synechiae.[2]

Adnexa Injuries

Penetrating injury to uterine adnexa may be associated with extensive hemorrhage, usually resulting from disruption of the ovarian or ascending uterine arteries. The extent of the deprivation of ovarian blood supply will determine the amount of ovarian tissue which can be preserved.

Occasionally, minimal trauma may lead to torsion or rupture of adnexal structures, especially when ovarian cysts are present. The patient may have so much pain and tenderness that diagnosis can be accomplished only by examination under anesthesia. Rarely, a ruptured ovarian cyst may be fatal because of severe hemorrhage or severe chemical peritonitis resulting from rupture of a dermoid cyst or tubo-ovarian abscess.

TRAUMA TO PREGNANT WOMEN

General Considerations

Approximately eight million women become pregnant each year in the United States. The ages at which a woman is most likely to become pregnant coincides with the ages (14-40 years) when women are also likely to sustain trauma. Trauma is the leading cause of death in women during their reproductive years[15] and accounts for more than twice as many deaths in women as the total annual maternal mortality. It is estimated that about 6-7% of all pregnancies are complicated by trauma.[16] A successful outcome for the severely injured obstetrical patient depends on a concerted, cooperative effort on the part of emergency physicians, surgeons, and obstetrical consultants in order to expedite resuscitation, diagnostic studies, and operative intervention as needed.

In a review of major trauma in pregnant women admitted to Tampa General Hospital Regional Trauma Center, Drost et al[17] found that gravid patients represented only 0.3% of 8000 trauma admissions in a 5-year period. Approximately 64% of the pregnant trauma patients were injured in motor vehicle accidents, 16% were burn victims, 8% were assaulted, 8% were victims of penetrating injuries, and 4% were injured in falls.

The average injury severity score (ISS) in mothers with fetal or neonatal deaths was 30. In those who delivered, the contributions of material hypoxia and shock to adverse fetal outcome cannot be overstated. The fetus is unable to protect itself from shock and anoxia and responds with bradycardia.[18] In a review of 103 cases of blunt maternal trauma reported by Rothenberger et al, eight of 10 women who presented in shock had an unsuccessful pregnancy outcome. Other factors contributing to fetal loss included prematurity, specific pelvic visceral injuries, and direct fetal injury.[19] Among mothers who survive their injuries, placental abruption is the most common cause of fetal loss.[20]

AXIOM Maternal death is the most frequent cause of fetal death after trauma.

Among pregnant women who die as a result of trauma, head injury and hemorrhagic shock account for most deaths.[19,21] There are no data suggesting that serious injuries result in a higher mortality rate in pregnant than in nonpregnant women. However, increased risks of splenic rupture[22] and retroperitoneal hemorrhage[23] due to blunt abdominal trauma during pregnancy have been reported. Conversely, the bowel is reported to be less frequently injured when the victim is pregnant.[24]

Approximately 6-7% of all pregnancies are complicated by some type of trauma,[7] and 0.3-0.4% of all pregnant women require hospitalization for trauma.[17,25] Pregnant women in the third trimester tend to have balance difficulties and gait instability. These contribute to an increased likelihood of falls at home and in the workplace. Consequently, the incidence of minor trauma increases from the first to the third trimester, when it is more common than at any other time during adulthood.[26,27]

AXIOM For all injured pregnant women, the possibility of chemical dependency must be considered in the initial assessment.

At Detroit Receiving Hospital, a Level I trauma center in the Detroit Medical Center, the female trauma victims, whether pregnant or not, increasingly cite the cause of their problems as related to drugs, usually to cocaine or heroin. In 80% of the serious female trauma victims seen at DRH, one of these substances is present in the blood and/or urine at the time of admission. The Wayne County Medical Examiners Office reported that 50% of the homicide victims between the ages of 20 and 50 test positive for cocaine.

Physiologic Changes

CARDIOVASCULAR

Blood volume increases steadily during pregnancy from 20-25% at the end of the first trimester to 30-50% above normal near term (Table 30–1).[28] There is a greater increase in plasma volume, and this results in a slight-to-moderate decrease in hematocrit from a normal mean of 40% to an average of about 32-34% by the 32nd-34th week.

Cardiac output increases by 30-40% from a normal average of 4.5 L/min to 6-7 L/min from the 10th week until the end of the pregnancy. This occurs in spite of a drop in the average central venous pressure from 9 mm Hg in nonpregnant females to about 4 mm Hg in the third trimester. This is accompanied by a modest increase in the heart rate by about 10-15 beats per minute throughout pregnancy. The high diaphragms and the other cardiovascular changes of pregnancy tend to shift the axis of the heart about 15 degrees to the left, resulting in Q waves in leads II and AVF.

There is a modest drop in systolic and diastolic blood pressure (10-15 mm Hg) from an average normal of 110/70 to about 102/55 at the end of the second trimester. At term, the BP often returns to normal.[29]

PITFALL ⊘

One cannot assume that fetal-placental blood flow is adequate if an injured pregnant woman is normotensive.

It is important to realize that the increased intravascular volume may delay the signs of shock in the traumatized pregnant patient. As much as 1500 ml of blood may be lost with little change in maternal vital signs, but there may be a severe reduction in placental blood flow causing fetal distress or death.

HEMATOLOGIC

In addition to a progressive drop in hematocrit to about 32% during pregnancy, a relative leukocytosis occurs raising the white blood

TABLE 30–1 *Physiologic and Anatomic Changes of Pregnancy*

Cardiovascular	Plasma volume increases by 40-50%
	Hct decreases from a mean of 40% down to 32%
	Cardiac output increases by 30-40%
	Heart rate increases by 10-15 beats/min
	Sys blood pressure decreases slightly (10-15 mm Hg)
	Peripheral vascular resistance decreases
	CVP falls from a mean of 9 down to 4 mm Hg
	EKG shows L. axis deviation (10-15°)
Respiratory	Minute ventilation increases by 40-50%
	Tidal volume increases by 40-50%
	Respiratory rate is unchanged
	P_aCO_2 decreases to 30-32 mm Hg
	Functional residual capacity decreases 20%
	Oxygen reserve decreases
Hematologic	Hematocrit decreases to about 32%
	A white blood cell count of 12,000 per mm³ may be normal
	Fibrinogen increases to 400 mg/dL
	Coagulation factors VII, VIII, IX, X, and XII all increase
	Coagulation times decrease
Anatomic	Pituitary gland doubles in size
	Heart is pushed upward and rotates
	Diaphragm elevates 4 cm
	Uterus becomes the largest intraabdominal organ
	Bladder is displaced into the abdominal cavity
	Pelvic joints loosen

Pimentel L Mother and child, trauma in pregnancy. Emer Medical Clin of N A 1991;9:549.

cell count (WBC) from a previous mean of 7200/mm³ to about 9800/mm³ in the third trimester.[30] A WBC up to 12,000-15,000/mm³ is often "normal" in pregnant women, and counts up to 20,000/mm³ are not uncommon during labor. The differential count is usually unaffected.

During pregnancy, blood becomes "hypercoagulable" with increases in factors VII, VIII, IX, X and XII. Plasma fibrinogen levels tend to rise, and the plasma levels of plasminogen activator tend to fall. Indeed, fibrinogen levels may rise to 400-450 mg/dl, which are about double those found in the nonpregnant state.[31,32] All of these changes increase the speed and tendency to clot. In addition, plasminogen activator levels gradually decrease throughout pregnancy so that the clots are slower to be lysed.[31,33] Indeed, clotting times tend to be reduced so consistently in pregnancy that even if DIC is present, the PT and PTT may be normal.

AXIOM Normal concentrations of coagulation factors in a critically injured pregnant woman should make one suspicious of the presence of DIC.

The erythrocyte sedimentation rate (ESR) rises progressively to a high of about 78 mm/hour at term because of increased plasma levels of globulins and fibrinogen. All of these hematologic changes in pregnancy can compound the difficulty in interpreting the clinical picture, especially if there is suspected hemorrhage or intraabdominal injury with peritonitis.

PULMONARY

As the uterus enlarges and encroaches on the upper abdomen, the diaphragms rise about 4 cm and the functional residual capacity of the lungs is reduced about 20%. Nevertheless, the tidal volume and minute ventilation rise approximately 50%. The increase in tidal volume and metabolic rate tend to cause a chronic state of compensated respiratory alkalosis and reduced buffering capacity. The resultant fall in $PaCO_2$ to a mean of 31 mm Hg combined with a decrease in serum bicarbonate to a mean of 21 mEq/L results in an increase in arterial pH to a mean of 7.45. However, the reduced buffering capac-

ity, largely due to decreased hemoglobin and bicarbonate levels, may aggravate the effects of shock and lactic acidosis.

GASTROINTESTINAL

AXIOM Although all trauma patients are at increased risk for vomiting and aspiration of gastric contents, pregnant women are especially susceptible because of the decreased gastrointestinal motility that accompanies pregnancy.

Combined with decreased gastroesophageal sphincter competency, the traumatized pregnant patient is at significant risk of aspiration of gastric contents. Compression by the gravid uterus and an overall reduction in smooth muscle tone is a further cause for delays in gastric emptying and prolonged intestinal transit times.

AXIOM Since the peritoneum has a decreased sensitivity during pregnancy, there is less pain and tenderness, and it can be much more difficult to diagnose intraabdominal injury or disease.[31]

URINARY TRACT

As with the gastrointestinal tract, the urinary tract is affected by the compression of the gravid uterus and the increased progesterone. IVP studies show ureteral dilation that is physiological, but which can be increased by compression by ovarian vessels and the uterus.

There is increased bladder capacity and delayed urinary bladder emptying that can lead to urinary stasis, bacteremia, and even pyelonephritis. The urinary stasis may persist for up to six weeks after delivery.

ENDOCRINE CHANGES

The pituitary gland gets 30-50% heavier during pregnancy. As a consequence, shock may cause necrosis of the anterior pituitary, resulting in postpartum pituitary insufficiency (Sheehan's syndrome).

UTERUS AND PLACENTA

The uterus grows from a 7-cm long, 70-gm organ in the adult nonpregnant state to a 36-cm, 1000-gm organ at term, and the combined weight of the uterus, fetus, placenta, and amniotic fluid at term is about 4500 gm. The larger the uterus, the greater its risk of injury with trauma. Blood flow to the uterus increases from 1 ml per second (60 ml per minute) to 10 ml per second (600 ml per minute) at term. This predisposes pregnant women to massive blood loss if the uterine vasculature is disrupted.[34]

The pregnant uterus remains an intrapelvic organ until the 12th week of gestation, when it begins to rise out of the bony pelvis and encroach on the peritoneal cavity, reaching its maximum supraumbilical extent at 36 weeks.

AXIOM At about 26 weeks, when the delivery of a viable fetus is possible, the top of the uterus is about halfway from the umbilicus to the xiphoid process.

The enlarging uterus reduces the confines of the intraperitoneal space and tends to push the intestines to the upper abdomen. The uterine enlargement is accompanied by marked congestion and dilation of the pelvic veins with increased blood flow in the uterine arteries. During the last four weeks of gestation, the fetus slowly descends as the fetal head engages in the pelvis.

During maturation of the fetus, the intrauterine environment gradually changes from one which is very protected to one which is very vulnerable. During the first trimester, the uterus is a thick-walled structure confined within the safety of the bony pelvis. During the second trimester, the uterus leaves its protected intrapelvic location, but the small fetus is still relatively well protected because it remains mobile and is cushioned by a relatively large amount of amniotic fluid. By the third trimester, the uterus is large and thin walled.

The placenta reaches its maximum size at 36-38 weeks and is virtually devoid of elastic tissue. The placental vasculature exists in a state of maximum vasodilatation throughout gestation, but it is exquisitely sensitive to catecholamine stimulation so that mild maternal vasoconstriction may be associated with severe placental vasoconstriction and hypoperfusion. Direct trauma to the placenta or uterus can release high concentrations of placental thromboplastin (a plasminogen activator) from the myometrium into the circulation and can cause disseminated intravascular coagulation.[6]

Ligaments of the symphysis pubis and sacroiliac joints are increasingly loosened as term approaches. Consequently, before one can make a diagnosis of a symphysial diastasis following trauma, one must consider that the symphysis pubis may widen to 31-38 mm by the seventh month of pregnancy. The laxity of the pelvic ligaments contributes to gait instability. By the third trimester, there is also marked venous congestion in the pelvis, thereby increasing the potential for severe hemorrhage with pelvic injuries.

HYPONATREMIA

The normal expansion of the extracellular fluid volume during pregnancy may result in a significant dilutional hyponatremia.[35] During late pregnancy, this hyponatremia may be made even worse by restriction of sodium intake.

SUPINE HYPOTENSION

> **AXIOM** At least 10% of women in late pregnancy will develop hypotension if placed in the supine position.

Hypotension from compression of the inferior vena cava by the gravid uterus may falsely suggest extensive internal damage following trauma, and the physician may dangerously overload the patient with fluid or blood.[22] Turning the patient about 10-15 degrees to the left or displacing the uterus to the left will usually restore a normal blood pressure rather promptly. The vena caval compression which occurs in the supine position also increases venous pressure in the lower part of the body and may increase bleeding from injuries to the pelvis and lower extremities.

> **PITFALL** ⊘
>
> *If a woman who is injured during late pregnancy is not turned to her left side, hypotension unrelated to the trauma may develop.*

Mechanisms of Injury

BLUNT TRAUMA

The automobile is the leading nonobstetric cause of maternal and fetal mortality.[37] Rothenberger reviewed 103 cases of blunt maternal trauma and found successful outcome for the pregnancy in only 39% of cases associated with major trauma.[38] The most common fetal injuries from blunt trauma are skull fracture and intracranial hemorrhage.[39]

Pelvic ligamentous laxity and the protuberant abdomen contribute to gait instability and the increased incidence of falls. Assaults, especially from domestic violence, are the third most common cause of maternal blunt trauma.[2,7]

> **AXIOM** Placental separation is the leading cause of fetal death when the mother survives.

Abruptio placentae from direct trauma is caused by maldistribution of shearing forces between the elastic and flexible uterine wall and the inelastic placenta. Placental separation may also follow sudden deceleration.[40] Disruption of 25% or less of the placenta from the uterus is compatible with fetal survival but often produces external bleeding and premature labor. Disruption of 50% or more of the placenta is almost always fatal to the fetus.

Pelvic fracture is the most common injury to the mother that results in intrauterine death which may be due to three mechanisms: maternal shock, placental separation, and direct fetal injury. Of the direct fetal injuries, skull fracture with intracranial bleeding is the leading cause of death. Other injuries that are encountered frequently after blunt trauma in the adult, especially spleen and liver damage, may also be found in the fetus.[41,42] Extremity fractures have also been reported.[43]

Uterine rupture after blunt trauma most often occurs at the site of a previous cesarean section.[44] Without prior operation, the most likely site of rupture is the posterior uterine wall.[45] Forces that can rupture the uterus can also damage the bladder. The urinalysis frequently shows hematuria because of concomitant bladder injury, and it may also show meconium.[46]

Distension of the maternal spleen and liver with blood during gestation, as well as displacement and compression by the gravid uterus, makes them much more susceptible to rupture by minor trauma during the later stages of pregnancy.[47] Occasionally, there is catastrophic hemorrhage due to rupture of the liver when no history of trauma can be obtained.

The advisability of the use of seat belt restraints for pregnant automobile passengers was questioned in a case report in 1964 by Rubuvits[48] who attributed the uterine rupture to compression by a lap belt worn by the patient. Furthermore, experimental impact studies have shown that use of lap belts on pregnant baboons results uniformly in fetal death as a result of 40-mph head-on impacts.[49] However, a retrospective review of rural automobile collisions by Crosby and Costiloe[50] showed that ejection from the vehicle (due to not using a seat belt) substantially increased the risk of death for accident victims. Indeed, the maternal death rate in pregnant women was 33% in ejected victims versus 5% in the absence of ejection. Likewise, fetal loss decreased from 47% in ejected victims to 11% in nonejected victims.

When the combined lap/shoulder restraints became available on a widespread basis, Crosby et al[51] conducted a controlled randomized comparison of lap belts and lap/shoulder retraints using near-term baboons. None of the baboon mothers was injured in this study, and there was a statistically significant reduction in fetal loss from 50% when only lap belts were used to 12.5% when the lap belt/shoulder harness system was used. Based on these data, this combined system is now recommended. The lap belt portion of the system should be placed under the pregnant woman's abdomen, and the shoulder harness should be as snug as is comfortably possible.[52]

PENETRATING INJURY

Gunshot Wounds

Gunshot wounds are the most common cause of penetrating trauma to pregnant women and may result from domestic or other intentional violence. Rarely, they may be incurred accidentally. They may even be self-inflicted in an effort to produce abortion.[53]

Penetrating wounds to the abdomen during the late second and third trimester are very likely to involve the uterus and its contents. However, if they miss the enlarged uterus, they tend to cause vascular injury and multiple intestinal perforations.

The usual guidelines for surgical exploration of abdominal gunshot wounds also apply to pregnant patients. When the uterus is damaged, there is a 19-38% incidence of associated visceral injuries.[54] The incidence of gunshot wounds that miss the uterus and penetrate the upper abdomen is unknown.

Fetal survival after penetrating uterine trauma is determined by fetal maturity, the site of fetal injury, and the availability and timeliness of tertiary care. Gunshot wounds to the gravid uterus involve the fetus 60% of the time and have a fetal mortality approaching 80% if wounding is sustained preterm vs 40% if the fetus is near term.[55]

In Koback and Hurwitz's report of 14 patients with gunshot wounds of the pregnant uterus, spontaneous fetal delivery occurred within 17 days, and the majority within 48 hours.[56] All delivered vaginally, eight after laparotomy and uterine repair and six without laparotomy. No cases of uterine rupture occurred in these women. One mother delivered within an hour of injury without repair of the gunshot wound to the uterus. In this group of 14 women, three delivered live fetuses, but all three infants had sustained injury from bullets. Thus, if the fetus is less than 26 weeks gestation or is dead and the uterine injury is small, the uterus can be sutured and the mother left to deliver the fetus vaginally. In such cases, potential complications, such as abruptio placenta and amnionitis, are managed expectantly. Although fetal mortality is high with low-velocity gunshot wounds of the uterus, maternal mortality from such trauma is uncommon. This is related to the high density of the uterine contents and the rapid dissipation of kinetic energy by the muscular uterine wall, the fetus, and the amniotic fluid. In contrast, high-velocity missiles are frequently lethal to both the mother and the fetus.

Stab Wounds

Two-thirds of abdominal stab wounds occur in the upper abdomen above the umbilicus.[30] In stable patients, local exploration of an upper abdominal wound can usually determine whether penetration into the peritoneal cavity has occurred. However, this technique is not applicable to injuries of the lower chest where such exploration can cause a pneumothorax. Patients in whom local wound exploration demonstrates peritoneal entry, or in whom the technique cannot be performed, should undergo open diagnostic peritoneal lavage (DPL). A positive DPL with a penetrating abdominal wound is often defined by the same criteria as in blunt trauma. However, with stab wounds of the lower chest, the RBC criterion is often lowered to 5,000/mm^3 to increase the sensitivity of the DPL for diaphragmatic injuries.[30]

Lower abdominal stab wound management is controversial. Careful local wound exploration can identify superficial injury, and peritoneal lavage is helpful in ruling out significant intraperitoneal bleeding or bowel injury; however, if the mother is hemodynamically stable, the penetration usually involves only the uterus and/or the bladder. Retrograde cystography can generally rule out a bladder injury, and external fetal monitoring will establish fetal stability. Indeed, several case reports demonstrate that mothers and fetuses who are stable after stabs to the lower abdomen frequently do well with nonsurgical management.[54]

AXIOM   If a full evaluation rules out life-threatening injuries to both the mother and the fetus, pregnant women with lower abdominal stab wounds are managed with careful observation instead of immediate laparotomy.

BURNS

Burns severe enough to warrant hospitalization occur in less than 0.1% of all pregnant women.[57] Schmitz found that burns affecting less than one third of the total body surface area did not affect the pregnancy. Larger burns resulted in termination of the pregnancy within one week,[58] especially if they occurred during the second trimester.[31] Fetal loss can be expected with a severe burn injury during the third trimester unless delivery or cesarean section occurs within 5 days. The harmful effects of the burn on the fetus are related to stress, catecholamine release, maternal shock, and decreased uterine blood flow.[32]

Amy et al,[59] in a review of 30 pregnant burn patients at one burn center, found that there were no fetal or maternal deaths in patients with burns of less than 20% body surface area. In mothers with 20-50% burns, all survived, but four fetuses aborted spontaneously coincident with maternal complications of infection, hypotension, or hypoxia.[59] In patients with burns of greater than 50% body surface area, 10 of 10 mothers died, but one fetus at 36 weeks of gestation survived.[59]

In a similar manner, Taylor found that all mothers with burn areas greater than 60% died; however, before dying, each mother delivered spontaneously, and the majority of children were delivered alive.[60] Fetal survival was primarily based on maturity. Mothers with less than 60% burns tended to live, and 83% had a viable pregnancy at the time of discharge.

It has been suggested that abortions and premature deliveries occurring within a week of injury are secondary to inadequate resuscitation. In such cases, the fetus was probably damaged by decreased uterine blood flow, even when the maternal shock may seem to have been adequately corrected.

Resuscitation of pregnant burn victims must rapidly correct maternal hypoxia and hypotension. Supplemental oxygen and ventilatory support, if needed, are indicated early in the management scheme. Using standard burn formulas as a guide, enough fluid should be administered to maintain normal maternal blood pressure and a urine output of 30-50 ml per hour.[60]

AXIOM   Fetal monitoring is important during maternal resuscitation because fetal heart rate abnormalities are often the first indication of inadequate resuscitation.

Sterile technique while caring for burned pregnant patients is extremely important. Sepsis correlated with fetal death in all cases in one study.[59] One should also avoid the topical antibiotic, silver sulfadiazine, because it may cause increased icterus in the neonate.[61]

NONCATASTROPHIC TRAUMA

Several studies and multiple case reports have documented fetal injury and death as a result of relatively minor trauma.[61] In a study of pregnancy-related complications which included premature labor, separation of the placenta, direct fetal injury, and fetal death, two significant associations with adverse fetal outcome included: (1) the presence of any abnormal obstetric findings on presentation, including vaginal bleeding, uterine tenderness, or uterine contractions or (2) domestic violence as the etiology of the trauma.[62]

AXIOM   Occult placental abruption is the most common cause of fetal death in patients with noncatastrophic trauma.

The high pressures that can be generated during deceleration injuries may cause relatively little extrauterine damage, but may create marked uterine distortion and a shearing effect on the placental insertion site. Consequently, abruption and fetal injury can occur with little or no external sign of trauma to the abdominal wall.[63-65] Vaginal bleeding is likewise often absent, and fetal distress is frequently the initial presentation.[66]

AXIOM   Cardiotocographic monitoring after the 20th week of pregnancy is very sensitive at predicting adverse outcome[63] and can predict abruptio placentae at any early stage, allowing for timely diagnosis and intervention.[34]

Management of Injured Pregnant Women

GENERAL CONSIDERATIONS

AXIOM   The initial approach to severely injured pregnant women should probably be more aggressive than for nonpregnant women.

As in all injured patients, prehospital information can be critical; the more severe the injury mechanism, the more concerned and aggressive the physician should be. Even if the initial vital signs are normal, the physician should remain concerned about significant visceral injury. The mother's prenatal history is also important, and the trauma physician should be particularly concerned about the presence of diabetes mellitus, preeclampsia, or vaginal spotting prior to the accident. The last time of food consumption is more significant than usual because of the prolonged gastric emptying times during pregnancy.

FIELD MANAGEMENT

AXIOM   Oxygen may be of benefit in all injured patients, but especially for the fetus in pregnant women.

Supplementation of maternal oxygen does little for the normal mother since the hemoglobin in arterial blood is usually almost completely saturated at room air; however, fetal blood functions on a different oxygen hemoglobin dissociation curve and an increased placental PO_2 can significantly improve fetal hemoglobin saturation.[67,68] The more oxygen reserve a distressed fetus has, the better the APGAR scores and the fetal outcome are likely to be.[67]

Early intravenous access for volume resuscitation is important. Uterine blood flow to the fetus can be severely compromised by the vasoconstrictive effect of maternal hypovolemia. Hemorrhage can reduce fatal blood flow 10-20% before maternal blood pressure is affected.[69] Vasopressors are to be avoided because they further decrease uterine blood flow.

AXIOM   Hypovolemia must be rapidly corrected, and vasopressors should be avoided in pregnant women.

TRANSPORTATION

Because of the physiologic changes during pregnancy, both mother and fetus are particularly vulnerable during transport and require special precautions.[70] As much oxygen as possible should be given to the mother, and i.v. fluids should be running rapidly if the mother may be hypovolemic. Maternal vital signs and fetal heart tones must be checked frequently en route to the hospital. During the second and third trimesters, the pregnant patient should be transported on her left side or with the right hip elevated and the uterus manually displaced to the left side of the vertebral column to prevent compression of the inferior vena cava.

AXIOM   During the second and third trimesters, gravid patients should not be allowed to lie supine, especially after trauma.

If there is a possibility of a spine injury, the gravid patient would be immobilized properly on a long backboard and the backboard tilted 15 degrees to the left. The supine position should be avoided whenever possible because it tends to increase the incidence of hypotension, placental abruption, and uterine vascular shunting.

The value of pneumatic anti-shock garments (PASG) during prehospital management of injured gravid women is unknown. No prospective studies have been done to determine if pregnancy is a relative contraindication to the use of the abdominal part of the PASG, but currently it seems to be wise not to inflate the abdominal compartment after the first trimester. Indeed, during the third trimester, the patient's girth may anatomically preclude closure of the abdominal compartment.[30]

ED RESUSCITATION

Resuscitation priorities for pregnant patients are essentially the same as for other trauma patients.

AXIOM   Resuscitation of the mother takes priority over all other considerations, including that of the fetus.[52]

Oxygen, Airway, and Ventilation

Fetal blood normally has a low PO_2. This baseline fetal hypoxemia provides the gradient for oxygen to diffuse from the uterus to the placenta, and this gradient also gives the fetus a certain tolerance for transient maternal hypoxemia.[7] In sheep, fetal O_2 consumption does not decrease until the delivery of oxygen is reduced by about 50%.[71] However, a persistently low PO_2 in the mother will greatly compromise the fetus, and correction of hypovolemia and hypoxemia generally takes priority over all other considerations during resuscitation. Patency of the maternal airway should be determined first. Oxygen supplementation is clearly indicated in all injured obstetrical patients, and endotracheal intubation and ventilatory support should be considered if an airway problem is suspected.

PITFALL ⊘

Injured pregnant women with a marginal airway or ventilation must be rapidly intubated, ventilated, and oxygenated.

Correcting Hypovolemia and Hypotension

There are several important concepts to keep in mind during the initial cardiovascular resuscitation of an injured pregnant patient.

AXIOM   The physiologic hypervolemia of pregnancy can mask the extent of bleeding in the mother, who may lose 1500 ml or more blood without manifesting any hypotension.

The release of endogenous maternal catecholamines may help maintain the mother's blood pressure, but it can cause profound placental vasoconstriction.

AXIOM   Even if an injured mother appears stable, the fetus may have dangerously inadequate perfusion.

Volume replacement, therefore, should be vigorous and prompt to prevent maternal and fetal hypoperfusion. If not already inserted, two large bore peripheral intravenous lines are started, preferably above the diaphragm. If there is any question at all about the adequacy of the fluid resuscitation, a central venous pressure (CVP) or pulmonary artery line should be inserted to monitor the response to further fluid-loading.

PITFALL ⊘

If transfusion to a moderately hypovolemic but normotensive injured pregnant woman is delayed, severe fetal distress may develop.

After trauma, both maternal and fetal homeostasis should be restored as soon as possible by rapidly replacing deficits in blood volume and red cell mass with crystalloids and blood transfusions. The hematocrit should probably be kept above 30%. Colloids and crystalloids may restore the circulating blood volume, but they are not as effective as packed cells for improving fetal oxygenation.[72,73] Vasopressors should be avoided since these drugs can cause severe decreases in uterine blood flow.

Use of the Pneumatic Antishock Garment (PASG)

Use of a pneumatic antishock garment in the ED on a pregnant woman's legs may be considered for persistent hypovolemia and to reduce blood loss from fractures of the lower extremities. However, pregnancy requires extra caution in the use of PASG.[7]

AXIOM   Inflation of the abdominal portion of the PASG is usually contraindicated in the pregnant patient after the first trimester because it might damage the fetus and compromise maternal venous return.

Although fetal loss attributed to PASG has not been substantiated, this policy appears prudent. The only exception may be the mother in extremis with major pelvic fractures.

Other Measures

A nasogastric tube (or an orogastric tube if major facial trauma is present) is passed to empty the stomach and reduce the chances of later aspiration of gastric contents. A urinary catheter should be passed to record urinary output as an additional guide to the adequacy of tissue perfusion. It may also help to assess for the possibility of urinary tract trauma.

Cesarean Section

> **AXIOM** If the fetus is viable but in distress despite resuscitative measures, or if the mother is not considered to be salvageable, urgent cesarean section is recommended.

The benefit of cesarean section to allow repair of intrauterine fetal injuries must be weighed against the risk of prematurity. Unfortunately, the benefits of surgery are hard to estimate because the severity of the fetal injury is difficult to predict. Nevertheless, a non-viable fetus (less than 26 weeks gestation) in distress should be treated conservatively in utero by optimizing fetal oxygenation and uterine blood flow.

Likewise, if the mother's condition is poor but viable, primary repair of all maternal wounds is the best course, even at the expense of a distressed fetus.

> **AXIOM** The best protection for the fetus after trauma is an early and aggressive restoration of normal maternal oxygenation and perfusion.

Cesarean section usually prolongs a laparotomy done for other injuries by about an hour and increases blood loss by at least 1000 ml.[74] In contrast, the critically injured mother who has her injuries treated and then delivers vaginally within 24 hours will generally tolerate the stress of vaginal delivery better than emergency prolonged surgery right after admission.[56] Vaginal delivery in the early postoperative period has not been shown to have any deleterious effect on the mother, fetus, or uterus.[45] However, if the fetus continues to be distressed and it is felt that the mother can withstand the extra operating time at the initial operation, a cesarean section should be done. Other reasons for cesarean section include uterine rupture and situations in which the uterus mechanically limits repair of maternal injuries (Table 30–2).

> **AXIOM** Fetal death is not an indication for cesarean section.

POSTMORTEM CESAREAN SECTION

Numa Pompilus of Rome (715-673 BC) decreed that if any pregnant woman died, the infant was to be cut from her abdomen immediately.[75] Since Julius Caesar was delivered through an abdominal incision, this procedure has come to be known as a cesarean section.

Deciding when the mother becomes nonviable and the fetus remains viable can be very difficult. Clinical judgement is the most applicable tool available in the emergency department. However, before stopping maternal resuscitation, one should check to make sure that the patient has been in the left lateral decubitus position. Once the decision is made to pronounce the mother dead, salvage of the fetus must be considered. The likelihood of fetal survival with postmortem cesarean delivery depends on fetal maturity and the time since the mother's death.

TABLE 30–2 Indications for Cesarean Section after Trauma

Fetal
Placental separation
Uterine rupture
Fetal malposition during premature labor
Severe unstable pelvic or lumbosacral spine fractures*
Maternal
Inadequate exposure for control of other injuries
Disseminated intravascular coagulation, if vaginal delivery is not feasible

*Pimentel L. mother and child, trauma in pregnancy. Emer Medi Clin of N A 1991;9:549.

TABLE 30–3 Variables Favoring Successful Perimortem Cesarean Section

Fetal age greater than 28 weeks
Prompt and aggressive attempts at resuscitation
Fetus delivered within 15 minutes of maternal arrest
Continous maternal resuscitation during Cesarean section
Neonatal intensive care support
Staff preparedness

Weber CE. Postmortem Caesarean section: review of the literature and case reports. Am J Obstet Gynecol 1971;110:158.

> **AXIOM** If the fundus of the uterus is palpable midway between the umbilicus and the xyphoid, a viable fetus is usually present.[76]

Ritter's review of 250 years of literature documented 120 successful postmortem cesarean sections.[75] Of all the children who survived postmortem cesarean section from 1900-1985, 70% were delivered within 5 minutes of the mother's death, and all of these infants were neurologically normal; 13% had their C-sections within 5-10 minutes, but 13% had mild neurologic sequelae; 12% were delivered in 10-15 minutes, but 17% had severe neurologic sequelae. After 15 minutes the survival rate was only 2-3% and 67-100% had severe neurological sequelae.[76]

In their review, Katz et al[77] vigorously advocated perimortem cesarean delivery as a critical procedure in maternal resuscitation if standard CPR is unsuccessful in the first 4 minutes. They noted that chest compressions in the pregnant patient in the third trimester generate only 30% of the stroke volume of the nonpregnant patient due to compression of the inferior vena cava. Pushing the uterus off of the inferior cava makes the compressions much more effective. Brain damage in the fetus is estimated to occur between 6 and 10 minutes following maternal arrest.[77] Strong and Lowe[78] have noted that the amount of time that passes from the death of the mother to the delivery of the infant is the single most important fetal prognostic factor (Table 30–3).

> **AXIOM** If fetal delivery is accomplished within 5 minutes of maternal cardiac arrest, the likelihood of survival of a mature fetus without neurologic sequelae is 69%.[78]

Weber noted that there is no authentic record of any fetal survival from C-section when the mother has been dead for more than 25 minutes.[79] Although a live fetus may be delivered after the mother has been dead for more than 10 minutes, ultimate survival rates may be very low. Behney[80] reported an overall 53% survival rate from postmortem sectioning in 72 cases, but only 15% were discharged home alive.

> **AXIOM** Cesarean section should be performed in the emergency department if the mother is dead or about to die, if uterine size is greater than 26 weeks gestation, and if the fetus may be alive.

If other evidence of fetal viability is not available, an ultrasound during the maternal resuscitation should be positive or at least indeterminate for fetal life.[30] No time should be wasted obtaining consent for a postmortem C-section. The most readily available physician should perform the procedure immediately. A pediatric consultation should be obtained as soon as possible.

The cesarean section should be done while CPR or open heart massage (without aortic cross-clamping) is continued on the mother. A classic midline vertical incision is made from the epigastrium to the symphysis pubis and rapidly carried down through all layers of the abdomen to the peritoneal cavity (Fig. 30–1). A vertical incision is

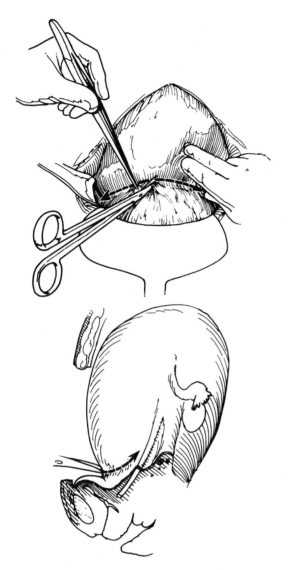

FIGURE 30–1 For an elective cesarean section, one can use a low transverse incision in the abdomen and in the uterus. Under emergency circumstances, a vertical incision in the abdominal wall and in the uterus is used. **(A).** A-P view. **(B).** Lateral view, In elective situations, the loose peritoneum overlying the bladder and uterus is grasped with forceps and incised close to its uterine attachments. A short uterine flap and long vesicular peritoneal flap are created as the front of the uterus is dissected bluntly from the back of the bladder to expose the lower uterine segment just above the cervix. From Fischer RP, Hefner JD. The gravid uterus. In Champion HR, Robbs JV, Trunkey DV, eds. Rob and Smith's Operative Surgery—Trauma Surgery, 4th ed. Boston: Butterworths. 1989; 462.

then made in the anterior uterus from the fundus to the upper bladder reflection (Fig. 30–2). Assistants and additional surgical instruments are helpful but are not required. If, when the uterus is entered, an anterior placenta is encountered, it should be incised in other to reach the fetus promptly. The umbilical cord should be promptly clamped and cut following delivery of the child (Fig. 30–3).

Diagnosis of Injuries in Pregnant Women

HISTORY

While instituting immediate life-saving resuscitation procedures and monitoring vital signs, a complete history should be elicited, if possible, from the mother, family members, or others. Prior medical records should be obtained whenever possible. The date of the last menstrual period, the expected date of confinement (from Nagele's

rule, which calculates the predicted day of labor by subtracting three months from the first day of the last menstrual period and adding seven days), the first perception of fetal movement, and the most recent maternal perception of fetal movement are all important. The status of the current as well as previous pregnancies should be determined as well as a history of previous serious illness and current medications.

> **AXIOM**   Nagele's rule calculates the predicted day of labor by subtracting three months from the first day of the last menstrual period and adding seven days.

PHYSICAL EXAMINATION

With respect to physical examination, it is important to emphasize that the traditional external manifestations of shock and vital sign changes are often delayed in gravid patients. In addition, traditional signs of peritoneal irritation may be delayed or absent because the parietal peritoneum is displaced. The vascularity of the pelvis in pregnancy may result in massive concealed retroperitoneal bleeding, which may manifest itself as shock only late in the patient's presentation.[81] As part of the complete physical examination, there should be an early determination of the fetal heart tones and a vaginal speculum examination to detect any dilatation of the cervix or bleeding from the cervical os.

> **AXIOM**   Vaginal bleeding is absent in 20% of patients with abruptio placentae, and the uterus may fill with as much as 2000 ml of blood with little external evidence of exsanguination.[7]

Following the initial evaluation and stablization of the mother, attention is directed to the fetus. Physical examination, except for absence of fetal heart tones on Doppler evaluation, is a poor predictor of fetal outcome.[17] Fetal compromise is manifested by a baseline fetal tachycardia, loss of accelerations, and prolonged or late decelerations.[81] Fetal monitoring is also of benefit to the mother because the fetal heart rate is a more sensitive indicator of decreases in maternal blood flow and oxygenation than maternal changes.[20]

Laboratory Tests (Table 30–4)

The initial laboratory studies should include: (a) a complete blood count with a differential, (b) type and cross-match, (c) arterial blood gases, (d) serum electrolytes, (e) serum amylase, (f) blood alcohol and toxicology studies, (g) urinalysis, and (h) indirect Coombs test. The indirect Coombs test is included so that Rh sensitization may be detected and prevented. If blood is needed immediately, Type O blood with negative Rh antigen can be used. However, crystalloids can usually provide an adequate resuscitation for the 10 minutes that it takes to get type-specific blood.

Nitrazine paper pH analysis of any vaginal discharge is also done. Normal amniotic fluid has a pH of about 7, whereas normal vaginal fluid has a pH of about 5.[2,7] Vaginal bleeding from the fetus is identified by using the Kleihauer-Betke stain.[82,83] If this test is strongly positive and the fetus is alive and of appropriate gestational age, immediate cesarean section may be indicated.

> **AXIOM**   Falling fibrinogen levels are the most sensitive indicator of DIC in the pregnant woman with a placental injury.

Disseminated intravascular coagulation (DIC) may be another reliable indicator of severe fetal injury. Development of a clinical coagulopathy in the mother generally suggests placental separation or amniotic fluid embolization and a need for a full set of coagulation studies, including PT, PTT, fibrinogen, platelet count, bleeding time, fibrin-split products, and D-dimers.

> **AXIOM**   DIC in an otherwise stable injured pregnant woman is an indication for prompt induction of labor.

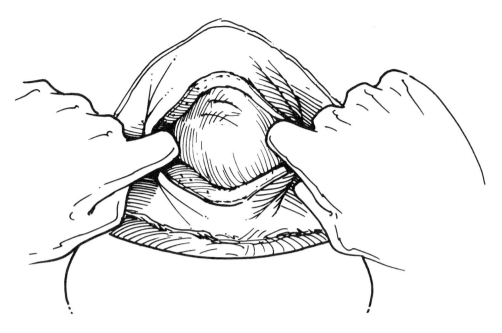

FIGURE 30–2 In elective situations, a small transverse incision is made with a scalpel in the lower uterine segment just above the uterocervical junction. In emergency circumstances, a vertical incision is used over the anterior midline of the uterus. The incision is enlarged to permit passage of the baby's head by hooking the index fingers in the incision and retracting laterally. If the placental attachment is beneath the incision, the placenta is manually swept aside to expose the baby's head. From Fischer RP, Hefner JD. The gravid uterus. In Champion HR, Robbs JV, Trunkey DV, eds. Rob and Smith's Operative Surgery—Trauma Surgery, 4th ed. Boston: Butterworths. 1989; 463.

If delivery does not follow within 6-8 hours of diagnosis of a suspected DIC or if the maternal condition worsens, evacuation of the uterine contents is required and should be performed promptly to avoid additional bleeding problems. Abdominal delivery via a C-section should be reserved as a last resort, with adequate quantities of fresh frozen plasma, packed red cells, platelets, and cryoprecipitate available.

AXIOM There is no such thing as being a little bit pregnant. Any pregnancy, regardless of how early it is, requires special concern for two individuals.

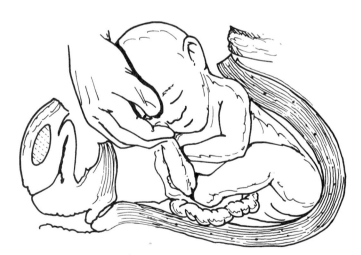

FIGURE 30–3 A hand is placed beneath the baby's head for support while gentle fundal pressure assists the delivery. After delivery, the baby's oropharynx is cleared using a bulb syringe, the midportion of the umbilical cord is clamped and divided, and methylergometrine maleate (Methergin) and/or oxytocin (Pitocin) is administered to the mother. The placenta is then expressed or removed manually, and the endometrial surface is inspected to ensure complete removal of all membranes. A three-layer closure of the uterus is accomplished with the minimum number of 2/0 chromic catgut sutures necessary for hemostasis. The deep suture line evenly approximates the inner half of the myometrium. These sutures should not penetrate the decidual lining of the uterus. From Fischer RP, Hefner JD. The gravid uterus. In Champion HR, Robbs JV, Trunkey DV, eds. Rob and Smith's Operative Surgery—Trauma Surgery, 4th ed. Boston: Butterworths. 1989; 463.

If the patient is not obviously pregnant (i.e., does not have a uterus greater than 16-20 weeks in size), a qualitative (rapid) pregnancy test should be performed immediately. Pregnancy tests use serum or urine to detect human chorionic gonadotrophin (HCG) produced by the trophoblastic cells of the placenta. This can be detected within two days after implantation, which may be up to 2 weeks before the first missed menstrual period. The qualitative test will detect levels of the beta fragment (Bhcg) as low as 10 mIU/ml within 30 minutes of beginning the test. The quantitative test will detect levels as low as 2.5 mIU/ml, but it is a 2-hour test. HCG levels should double in amount every 2 days during the first 2 months of pregnancy if the products of conception are normally implanted.

AXIOM A quantitative Bhcg performed every 2 days can assist in predicting the health of an existing pregnancy.

One can comfortably rule out pregnancy if the Bhcg radioimmunoassay is below a specific laboratory's level for pregnancy.

RADIOLOGICAL TESTS

Risk of Irradiation

AXIOM A diagnostic modality considered necessary for proper evaluation of an injured gravid woman should not be withheld for fear of potential hazard to the fetus.

The likelihood of fetal radiation damage depends on the dose of radiation and the gestational age of the fetus. The highest death rate

---

TABLE 30–4 *Initial Laboratory Studies Obtained During ED Resuscitation of Injured Pregnant Women*

1. CBC with differential
2. Type and cross-match
3. Arterial blood gases
4. Electrolytes, including calcium and magnesium
5. Amylase and lipase
6. Alcohol and toxicology screen
7. PT, PTT, platelet count, and fibrinogen
8. Urinalysis
9. Indirect Coombs
10. Tests for fetomaternal hemorrhage

from radiation exposure occurs during the preimplantation phase. Because of a multiplicity of factors, the actual absorbed radiation dose varies a great deal with each radiological study. Generally speaking, however, 30% of the dose absorbed by the mother is transmitted to the fetus.[2]

AXIOM   The fetus is most vulnerable to developing deformities if more than 10-15 rads of irradiation are given during the period from the 10th day through the 10th week after conception.

The risk of congenital defects below a 10-rad exposure to the fetus at any stage of pregnancy is minimal when compared to the 4-6% incidence of congenital defects seen with no history of irradiation.[30] The risk of malformation is increased when the radiation dose is above 10-15 rads. Diagnostic radiographic studies should, therefore, be performed with due regard for fetal protection, but necessary diagnostic studies should not be withheld out of concern for fetal radiation. When medically appropriate, consideration should be given to minimizing potential fetal irradiation by limiting the scope of the examination. Fetal irradiation can also be reduced by technical means, such as shielding and collimation.[84] Nevertheless, children with solid tumors or leukemia are 2-3 times more likely to have been exposed to radiation in utero.[85]

Routine Radiographs in Severe Blunt Trauma

A lateral cervical spine and chest radiograph are usually indicated in patients with blunt multisystem trauma. However, cervical spine films are not needed in the patient who is wide awake, has no distracting injuries, and has no neck signs or symptoms.[86] If the physical examination suggests a pelvic fracture, radiologic evaluation is essential.

Urological Studies

The presence of bloody urine may indicate urinary tract injury and mandates cystography as well as evaluation of the upper urinary tracts, preferably through contrast-enhanced computed tomography (CT). Computed tomography of the abdomen may obviate multiple studies, such as intravenous pyelography (IVP), and consultation with the radiologist can help minimize the number of radiation exposures of injured pregnant patients. The advantage of the abdominal CT over most other modalities, such as DPL, is its ability to also examine retroperitoneal structures, such as the kidneys, pancreas, duodenum, and major vessels.

Ultrasound

AXIOM   Ultrasound of the abdomen, uterus, and fetus should be performed on all gravid patients with moderate-to-severe abdominal trauma.

The ultrasound can be very beneficial at determining the presence of a pregnancy, fetal viability, placental position, and the presence of a moderate or large abruption or other obstetrical problems.[17] With proper use and experience, pregnancy as early as 5 weeks can be viewed. However, ultrasound may miss a small abruption, and it gives only limited information regarding maternal trauma with the exception of fluid in the cul-de sac of Douglas.

DIAGNOSTIC PERITONEAL LAVAGE (DPL)

AXIOM   If a DPL is indicated in an injured pregnant woman after the 12th week, it should be done as an open technique above the umbilicus and uterus.

Because of the relative insensitivity of abdominal examination in pregnant trauma victims, early consideration should be given to performing DPL. Injured pregnant women have as much risk for bleeding from other viscera as the nonpregnant patient, and confirmation of internal bleeding is just as important.

Some authors believe that DPL is contraindicated in pregnancy.[87,88] However, DPL can be done with reasonable safety if it is performed in a supraumbilical location superior to the enlarged uterus with inspection of the peritoneum and opening of the peritoneum under direct vision.[7] DPL usually has an accuracy rate exceeding 95% in evaluating blunt abdominal trauma and the usual parameters of more than $100,000/mm^3$ red blood cells or more than $500/mm^3$ white blood cells are the same as for the nonpregnant patient. Rothenberger et al[87] in a study of DPL in 12 pregnant patients with blunt abdominal trauma found that the precedure was safe and 100% sensitive and specific. Esposito et al[88] documented a 92% accuracy for DPL in 13 pregnant blunt trauma patients. The single patient with a false-negative result had an equivocal red blood cell count of $76,000/mm^3$.

FETAL EVALUATION

AXIOM   Fetal monitoring is essential in all pregnant women with severe trauma.

Fetal evaluation includes checking fetal heart rate, fetal movement, uterine size and irritability, and observing the vagina for amniotic fluid or blood. As noted previously, early signs of fetal distress include decreased variability of heart rate, bradycardia of 110 beats per minute or less,[69] and late fetal deceleration.[89] Where available, continuous monitoring strips are preferable to frequent auscultation of the fetal heart for identifying early fetal distress.

Determining fetal age and maturity is critical to deciding whether and when to deliver the fetus of a severely injured woman; however, such determinations can be very difficult. Fifteen percent of patients do not remember the date of their last menstrual period and another 15% misidentify their last period.[90] Measuring fundal height by palpation of the abdomen is probably the quickest way to estimate fetal age. If the top of the uterus is more than halfway from the umbilicus to the xiphoid process, the fetus may be viable.

AXIOM   Ultrasonography can be invaluable in the emergency department if fetal heart tones are inaudible, fundal height is questionable, or vaginal bleeding is present.

If neonatal facilities are available, the fetus should be considered viable at approximately 26 weeks. At this age, extrauterine survival is about 50%. Generally, before 30 weeks gestation, weight is a more important parameter for survival than is estimated age.[90] Infants weighing less than 750 gm have a 10% chance for extrauterine survival, whereas with infants weighing 750-1000 gm, the probability of survival increases to 60%.[90,91]

Fetal Injuries

AXIOM   Severe fetal injury can result from blunt trauma with minimal uterine damage.[92]

Direct fetal injury is infrequent after trauma, since the maternal soft tissues, uterus, and amniotic fluid absorb much of the energy and diminish the force delivered to the fetus. Several studies have shown that minor trauma is rarely the cause of fetal loss early in pregnancy; such loss is usually due to congenital abnormalities.[61] Nevertheless, the more severe the maternal injury, the greater the likelihood of fetal death.[21,38] However, even minor maternal injuries can result in death of the fetus.[23,93,94,95] Except for maternal death, the most common cause of fetal death after major organ trauma is abruptio placentae.[38] Fetal deaths due to direct injury or uterine rupture have also been described, but they are much less common.[38,96,97]

Cranial injuries are the most frequently reported category of direct fetal damage after blunt abdominal trauma.[23,98,99] Most cranial injuries occur in the third trimester, when the engaged fetal head is particularly vulnerable to injury if the maternal pelvis is fractured.[38,98] Other fetal injuries from blunt trauma include clavicle and long bone fractures. Skin lacerations may also heal slowly in utero. Unhealed fractures and skin lacerations have been reported up to three months after injury.[100]

Penetrating uterine trauma can be devastating and is frequently fatal to the fetus. In late pregnancy, the enlarged uterus becomes the largest intraabdominal organ[18] and bears the brunt of most penetrating abdominal injuries.[101] Estimates of fetal mortality from such wounds range from 47-71%,[102] with the higher figure due primarily to gunshot wounds to the uterus.[81] Fetal mortality in such instances is secondary to both direct injury to the uterus, placenta, or fetus and/or an ill-timed premature delivery.[76,103]

Although the severity of the external force is extremely important in determining fetal outcome, the duration of gestation is also a critical factor. During early gestation, the uterus is shielded by the bony pelvis, and fetal loss from trauma during the first trimester is very unusual.[13] Later, as the uterus enlarges up and out of the pelvis, the protective effect of the amniotic fluid is all that remains. Although the total volume of amniotic fluid continues to increase until about the 38th week of pregnancy, the amount present in relation to the size of the uterus falls as the pregnancy progresses. Thus, the risk of fetal injury increases with gestational age and is particularly great after the fetal head has become fixed in the maternal pelvis. This fixation of the fetal head may explain the high incidence of skull fractures and intracranial hemorrhage resulting from blunt trauma.[45]

Many fetal injuries, including multiple fractures, will heal partially or completely by the time of birth. Surprisingly, however, fetal wounds tend to heal slowly in utero. Fractures or skin lacerations of the fetus which have not healed after up to three months have been reported.[39] In the traumatized pregnant patient, regardless of whether or not fetal heart tones are heard, continuous electronic fetal heart rate monitoring and uterine pressure with contractile monitoring should be instituted as early as possible, along with mandatory obstetrical consultation. If the fetus is viable, continuous monitoring for at least 24-48 hours is essential because fetal distress can occur at any time during that period without warning. One can also detect fetal hypoxemia or marginal placental oxygen reserve by measuring the fetal heart rate in response to uterine contractions.

Pearlman et al[63] found that there was frequent uterine activity within the first few hours following trauma in virtually all patients in whom abruption was subsequently diagnosed. On the basis of their data, Goodwin and Breen[62] recommended only 30 minutes of monitoring in the patients without obstetric findings. Although Esposito et al[88] recommended a 24- to 48-hour monitoring period, only one of their 40 blunt abdominal trauma patients had a cesarean section for fetal distress, and the distress was noted within the first 4 hours of monitoring. After reviewing nine cases of fetal death following motor vehicle accidents, Agran et al[104] recommended 24 hours of continuous monitoring. They described two cases in which patients were discharged from emergency departments after evaluation and subsequently had placental abruptions diagnosed. In neither case, however, was there documentation of any ongoing monitoring.

Several case reports have noted placental abruptions occurring 5-7 days after minor trauma.[105] In one report, the authors point out that trauma is the cause of abruption in less than 2% of all cases. It has been estimated that nontraumatic abruption complicates between 0.4% and 3.5% of all pregnancies.[106] In the rare instances of abruption 5-7 days after minor trauma, it has been suggested that etiologies other than trauma must be considered.[105]

AXIOM Based on the available literature, monitoring for 4 hours after an episode of minimal trauma to a pregnant woman with no other criteria for admission and no obstetric findings appears to be a safe and acceptable practice.

Fetomaternal Hemorrhage

The incidence of fetal hemorrhage into the maternal circulation following trauma is about 26% compared to 6% for controls.[30] The amount of blood lost from the fetus varies from 5-40 ml, represent-

ing up to 14-34% of the fetal blood volume. Neither the nature of the trauma nor the gestational age is related to the frequency or volume of fetomaternal hemorrhage.[107] However, fetomaternal hemorrhage is more common if the placenta has an anterior location[108,109] or if there is uterine tenderness after the trauma.[108]

AXIOM Fetal hemorrhage into the maternal circulation is common after trauma and can cause significant complications.

As little as 0.01-0.03 ml of fetomaternal hemorrhage will sensitize 70% of Rh-negative mothers.[110] The Kleihauer-Betke acid elution assay[111] is one method used to detect fetomaternal hemorrhage. An acid phosphate buffer is used to elute adult hemoglobin from red blood cells in a sample of maternal venous blood. After staining, maternal ghost cells (ruptured maternal red blood cells) and cells containing fetal hemoglobin are counted. The ratio of fetal cells to ghost cells is recorded, enabling prediction of the volume of fetal blood that has leaked into the maternal circulation. This test is recommended in all cases of maternal trauma to determine the need for Rh immunoglobulin in Rh-negative mothers and as a guide for identifying abruptial bleeding that potentially could lead to fetal distress.[83,107]

Interestingly, in a 1990 report of pregnancy outcome and fetomaternal hemorrhage after noncatastrophic trauma, Goodwin and Breen[62] pointed out that the amount of fetomaternal hemorrhage sufficient to sensitize certain Rh-negative mothers is far below the sensitivity of the Kleihauer-Betke test. Consequently, they recommend routine treatment of all Rh-negative mothers who present with abdominal trauma.[62] Goodwin and Breen, however, used the Kleihauer-Betke test to determine who might require Rho (D) immune globulin in excess of the standard dose (0.6%, 30 ml).

Another reason for quantifying fetomaternal hemorrhage is detection of the rare but massive bleeding that can occur in the absence of other significant pregnancy-related injuries. Although the incidence of fetomaternal hemorrhage is high in pregnant trauma patients, occasional case reports have been published documenting massive hemorrhage resulting in fetal distress.[112,113] For this reason, investigators recommend Kleihauer-Betke testing in all patients more than 11 weeks pregnant with evidence of physical trauma.[61]

The treatment of a viable injured fetus should be approached much as that of any newborn infant. After rapid delivery of the fetus by cesarean section, a second team of physicians should immediately begin treatment of the fetus. The umbilical vein provides rapid access to the fetal circulation, but great care must taken not to overload the cardiovascular system with fluids.

Some rather bizarre fetal injuries have been reported following penetrating trauma. In one instance, an infant died shortly after birth as a result of severe hemorrhage from a gunshot wound of the femoral artery.[114] In another instance, the fetus swallowed the bullet and, following birth, developed an intestinal obstruction which was cured spontaneously by passage of the bullet in the stool.[115]

Placental Injury

INCIDENCE AND ETIOLOGY

AXIOM One should look for placental injury in all traumatized pregnant women, especially if there is any fetal distress.

The second most common cause of fetal death from trauma (after maternal death) is placental abruption. Abruptio placentae after blunt abdominal trauma complicates about 1-5% of minor injuries. In reviews of "severe" trauma to pregnant women, the incidence of abruption is between 7 and 66%.[40,105] However, in one study of over 200 women in minor automobile accidents, there were no cases of abruption.[26] If more than half of the placental surface separates from the uterus, the fetal mortality rate approaches 100%. Placental separation results from shearing forces between the elastic uterus and the more rigid placenta. Direct injury to the uterus is not needed for abruption to occur; sudden deceleration forces provide enough energy for shearing. The substantial simultaneous increase in intraamniotic pressure can cause even more placenta to shear away from the uterus.[116]

Factors that increase the risk of traumatic abruption include hypertension, abuse of drugs such as cocaine,[117] preeclampsia/eclampsia, smoking, diabetes mellitus, advanced maternal age, and multiparity. Decidual necrosis from reduced blood flow to the uterus is thought to be the underlying pathologic mechanism behind these risk factors.

PHYSIOLOGICAL SIGNIFICANCE

Because gas exchange between the pregnant woman and the fetus takes place across the placenta, the separation of the placenta from the underlying decidua decreases the delivery of oxygen to the fetus and causes carbon dioxide to accumulate in the fetal circulation. This may lead to fetal hypoxia, acidosis, or death.[34] Fetal mortality from abruption ranges from 30-68%.

AXIOM	Disruption of 25% or less of the placental-uterine surface is compatible with fetal survival but separations greater than 50% generally result in fetal death.

Although maternal mortality from abruptio placenta is said to be less than 1%, injury to the placenta can cause severe morbidity by release of its thromboplastin and development of a consumptive coagulopathy. The injured gravid uterus may also release large amounts of plasminogen activator and cause severe, rapid fibrinolysis.[118] Consequently, all cases of suspected abruption should have complete clotting studies performed. In true DIC, D-dimer levels (which are formed only if there is increased cross-bridging of fibrin) will be elevated. In primary fibrinolysis without prior excessive intravascular clotting, fibrin-split products will be increased, but D-dimer levels will be relatively normal.

DIAGNOSIS

Clinical

Pregnant women with major injuries and a viable fetus should be monitored closely for at least 48 hours. If the fetus is doing well after 48 hours, it is unlikely that a significant placental separation is present or that it will affect the pregnancy.[14] Although there are rare reports of abruption producing fetal distress 5-6 days after the initial injury, these cases involved extremely severe mechanisms of injury to the gravid abdomen.[26] Obviously, such situations demand extra caution and warrant fetal monitoring beyond 48 hours. Patients with minor injuries probably need only 12-24 hours of monitoring.

Clinical findings of abruption can include vaginal bleeding, uterine tenderness (from blood extravasation between myometrial muscle fibers), abdominal pain or cramps, amniotic fluid leakage, maternal signs of hypovolemia out of proportion to visible bleeding, a uterus larger than expected for the gestational age, increasing uterine size, or a change in the fetal heart rate.[38,119,120] If the placenta is implanted posteriorly, the uterus may not be tender, but the patient may complain of severe backache.[21]

A small number of cases have been reported involving full-thickness tearing of the placenta instead of separation. With full-thickness tearing of the placenta, blood collects retroplacentally. Consequently, no pain, tenderness or rigidity of the uterus may develop. Fetal exsanguination in 10 minutes was reported in one such case.[122]

Cardiotocographic Monitoring

Confirming the diagnosis of abruptio placentae can be difficult, but cardiotocographic monitoring after trauma beyond the 20th week of pregnancy can apparently predict abruptio placentae early and accurately.[108,109] Since abruptio placentae usually becomes manifest shortly after injury, monitoring should begin as soon as possible after the patient arrives at the hospital.

AXIOM	Cardiotocographic monitoring is probably the best way to make an early diagnosis of abruptio placentae after trauma.

Both components of cardiotocographic monitoring-Doppler measurement of fetal cardiac activity and measurement of uterine activity-appear to be useful in the evaluation of pregnant women after trauma. Changes in the fetal heart rate due to fetal hypoxia from abruptio placentae, such as late decelerations and the loss of beat-to-beat variability, are more easily detected with continuous monitoring than with intermittent auscultation. Tonometry, the second component of electronic monitoring, can predict abruptio placentae early in its course. In Pearlman's study, no instance of abruptio placentae was identified unless frequent uterine activity was noted in the first four hours of monitoring.[108] In another study with a minimum of 30 minutes of cardiotocography after life-threatening maternal trauma, more than 25% of the patients with at least three uterine contractions in a 20-minute period had abruptio placentae or preterm labor.[109] In the opinion of Pearlman et al,[108] four hours of cardiotocographic monitoring is sufficient to predict which patients will have abruptio placentae as a consequence of the trauma. In addition, women in whom complications do not develop during the four hours of monitoring can be expected to have pregnancy outcomes similar to those of uninjured controls.[108]

Ultrasonography

The use of ultrasonography after trauma during pregnancy has also been advocated to assist in the diagnosis of abruptio placentae and to evaluate fetal well-being,[123,124] but cardiotocographic monitoring appears to be superior. Ultrasonography is not sensitive in making the diagnosis of abruptio placentae because a large portion of the placenta must be separated before it can be visualized.[90] In general, abruption will cause clinical fetal distress before ultrasound can visualize it. However, ultrasonography may be useful for: (a) the establishment of gestational age if it is uncertain; (b) determination of fetal well-being if the results of cardiac monitoring are equivocal; (c) verification of fetal cardiac activity in the presence of maternal tachycardia or if the death of the fetus is suspected; and (d) estimation of the volume of amniotic fluid if it is uncertain whether the amniotic membranes have ruptured.

AXIOM	If no fetal heart sounds or activity are identified after trauma, fetal nonviability should be confirmed by real time and B-mode ultrasonography.

TREATMENT

If the fetus is doing well and there is no bleeding, the patient can be watched. If the fetus is dead, spontaneous evacuation of the uterus can be anticipated within one week.[125] However, if DIC or sepsis seems to be developing, the uterus should be evacuated promptly.

Placental Laceration

In a recent case report and literature review by Civil et al,[126] the rarity of placenta laceration, rather than abruption, was emphasized. The value of the CT scan for diagnosing this problem was emphasized. Although radiation dosage is a concern in early pregnancy, the estimated absorbed dose of 2 mGy with a CT scan is about half that of standard pelvimetry. In addition, while the use of CT in early pregnancy for screening purposes may not be justified, in the near-term fetus with suspected trauma, it may have a very important role.

The development of coagulopathy is common following uteroplacental abruption or amniotic fluid embolism, but it may also occur following placental laceration, probably as a result of activation of the fibrinolytic system.

AXIOM In patients with possible placental injury, development of a coagulopathy is generally an indication for immediate evacuation of the uterus.

In the absence of maternal complications, spontaneous labor should be awaited to deliver a dead fetus, as this is associated with the fewest long-term problems; however, if the patient develops a coagulopathy, urgent evacuation of the uterus is indicated. If induction of labor is not rapidly successful, cesarean section may be required.

Post-traumatic Abortion

AXIOM The presence or absence of symptoms immediately after injury is not totally predictive of whether the pregnancy will or will not require termination.

Because the incidence of spontaneous premature labor in pregnancy with or without trauma is similar (10%), a definite cause-and-effect relationship between injury and abortion can be difficult to confirm. For confirmation of a posttraumatic abortion, it is essential that the fetus be known to be developing normally and abort within hours of the traumatic incident.

In selected cases, amniocentesis can provide useful information about the maturity and possible distress of the fetus. If the amniotic fluid surrounding the fetus is bloody, mahogany-colored, or meconium-stained, this may indicate imminent fetal death. An aliquot should also be studied for lecithin-sphingomyelin (L-S ratio) and the level of phosphatidyl glycerol (PG). If PG is present, the fetus is mature, and forced or elective intervention is less likely to result in death or complications due to prematurity.[31]

Premature Labor

Premature labor is a common complication of maternal truama. In a prospective controlled study of outcome after varying degrees of trauma during pregnancy, 41% of the patients studied had frequent contractions during the initial 4 hours of evaluation.[69] Postulated etiologies include placental abruption, uterine contusion, membrane ischemia, and membrane ruptures.

AXIOM If there is evidence of uterine contractions and progression of cervical dilatation in an injured mother who is not at term, tocolysis should generally be employed to allow time for full fetal evaluation.

Premature labor generally should be stopped if the fetus is viable but premature. There is, however, some controversy on the indications for and methods of producing tocolysis. Neufeld et al[30] feel that beta-2 sympathomimetics (e.g., terbutaline in 0.25 mg doses SC or IV) relax smooth muscle in lung and uterine tissue and have relatively little effect on the heart.

Lee et al[127] recommend tocolysis for premature labor, with magnesium sulfate being the drug of choice. They discourage use of beta-adrenergics due to concerns about maternal hemodynamic instability and fetal shock and death in the bleeding fetus.[20] Pearlman et al[63] discourage tocolysis for premature labor after trauma because they believe that these contractions are indicative of placental abruption until proven otherwise. The decidua cells involved in the process of abruption release prostaglandins, which cause most victims in late pregnancy to have uterine contractions. They found in their study that 90% of the premature contractions stopped without tocolysis. The other 10% either had placental abruptions or were at or near term.[63]

It is generally agreed that contraindications to tocolysis include: (a) active vaginal bleeding, (b) suspected placental abruption (because blood will further accumulate inside a relaxed uterus), (c) preeclampsia or eclampsia, (d) uncontrolled diabetes mellitus, (e) serious cardiac disease, (f) maternal hyperthyroidism, and (g) cervical dilatation

greater than 4 cm.[30] However, even with advanced cervical dilatation, exceptions can be made when there is fear of fetal immaturity or an urgent need to transfer the patient.

Intrauterine Fetal Death

With intrauterine death, labor usually ensues within 48 hours and is rarely delayed beyond 3 weeks. If the treatment plan includes observation until labor ensues, clotting studies (PT, PTT, fibrinogen, and fibrin-split products) should be followed closely. Abruption and fetal demise can cause maternal disseminated intravascular coagulation through the release of tissue thromboplastin into the maternal circulation.[4] Once DIC develops, maternal shock and death can occur with startling speed. Consequently, the uterus should be emptied as rapidly as possible in such patients.

INJURIES TO GRAVID PATIENTS

Specific pregnancy-related injuries occur primarily in the second and third trimesters. Reproductive organ damage or fetal loss requires a very severe blunt injury to the mother, which usually includes disruption of the pelvis.[128] The risk of uterine injury in the face of a pelvic fracture increases with the length of gestation.[127] Other injuries associated with pelvic fractures in the mother include retroperitoneal hemorrhage, urinary tract injuries, and uterine rupture.[102] Stable pelvic fractures do not usually interfere with vaginal delivery. Unstable fractures, however, may predispose the patient to bony displacement and urinary tract injuries if vaginal delivery is attempted.[129]

Uterine rupture from trauma usually occurs in mid to late pregnancy. Previous cesarean section is a predisposing factor, and rupture under such circumstances most commonly occurs at the site of the old scar. Without prior surgery, the posterior uterine wall is the most common site, and it is associated with pelvic fractures.[30] Uterine rupture also occurs late in gestation if a direct blow to the abdomen presses the uterus against the spine. Because so much blood flows to the gravid uterus, uterine rupture can precipitate catastrophic hemorrhage. Although it is not a strict contraindication to vaginal delivery, severe coagulopathy may accompany this injury.[126]

Management

AXIOM Withholding needed surgery is poorly tolerated by both mother and fetus.

The presence of a gravid uterus should not be a deterrent to needed operative intervention after trauma, and the surgery itself is unlikely to lead to premature labor unless extensive manipulation of the uterus is required.

Anesthesia

AXIOM General anesthesia is preferred for all pregnant patients with multisystem injuries requiring operative management.

Premature labor is related more to the injuries and the gestational age than to the anesthetic agent or technique used.[130] The risk of spontaneous abortion is greatest during the first trimester and least toward the end of the second trimester.

AXIOM The main anesthetic risks for the gravid patient are related to the gastrointestinal, cardiovascular, and pulmonary changes that occur with pregnancy.

Gastric atony makes aspiration a frequent danger with general anesthesia, and a rapid-sequence induction is essential for safe intubation. This includes the infusion of rapid intravenous induction agents and muscle relaxants, cricoid pressure to block reflux of gastric contents, and endotracheal intubation under direct visualization. Although insertion of a Foley catheter should always be done under sterile conditions, extra precautions should be taken in gravid women because of the high risk of bladder and renal infection during pregnancy.

Higher concentrations of oxygen should be given to all severely injured pregnant patients. Intraoperative fetal monitoring is imperative, and it is even more important than usual to maintain an adequate blood volume, blood pressure, and oxygen saturation.

MATERNAL THORACIC INJURIES

It has been speculated that tension pneumothorax or lung damage may cause much more dramatic changes in pregnant women because of the elevation of the diaphragms and the pulmonary hyperventilation which are already present.[131] A missed diaphragm laceration may produce a delayed herniation at the time of delivery because of the greatly increased intraabdominal pressures that can develop during labor. Mortality from this injury ranges from 16-20% and increases to 25-66% if bowel becomes strangulated.[54]

There is an increased risk of spontaneous aortic dissection during pregnancy. 50% of dissecting aneurysms in women less than 40 years of age occur during pregnancy. The increased cardiac output and larger circulating blood volume of pregnancy and the hypertension of preeclampsia may be predisposing factors.[132] Whether these factors also place the pregnant woman at greater risk for developing traumatic aortic tears is unknown.

MATERNAL ABDOMINAL INJURIES

It is generally felt that the indications for laparotomy for trauma in pregnancy are similar to those in nonpregnant females and include evidence of significant intraabdominal bleeding or injury to a hollow viscus. Others however, feel that management of penetrating abdominal trauma to the gravid patient may differ from that of the nonpregnant patient.[61] For example, maternal mortality is lower late in pregnancy because the uterus shields the other intraabdominal organs from injury. If the uterus is involved, selective observation can be advocated if: (a) the entry wound is below the fundus of the uterus, (b) the mother is hemodynamically stable with a fetus that is either dead or without injury or compromise, or (c) there is no evidence of injury to the genitourinary or gastrointestinal tracts.[103]

> **AXIOM**   If a penetrating wound is above the uterus or lateral to it, celiotomy is indicated for repair of other injuries.

Abdominal Incision and Exposure

The standard vertical midline incision is employed as in other trauma patients so that adequate exposure of the entire peritoneal cavity and retroperitoneum may be accomplished. Adequate visualization is mandatory, and the pregnant uterus should not be allowed to interfere with exploration or repair of intraabdominal injuries. However, celiotomy is not a license for cesarean section, even if there is an injury to the uterus.[7]

Specific Injuries

SPLEEN.   Although the spleen and liver are not usually significantly enlarged in pregnancy, the gravid state is thought by some to predispose them to rupture with trauma. Sparkman reviewed 28 cases of spontaneous splenic rupture and 16 cases due to trauma in pregnant women.[133] Women with toxemia and malaria were most susceptible to spontaneous rupture. Of the 16 trauma cases, 10 occurred from trivial injuries that are not ordinarily associated with visceral injury. Sparkman postulated that the spleen is more prone to rupture in pregnancy because of increased maternal blood volume or intrasplenic vascular anomalies.[133] Buchsbaum[47] feels that splenic rupture from minimal trauma in pregnancy is probably actually a biphasic bleeding problem. He speculates that an earlier injury to the spleen, without clinical consequence, causes an expanding subscapular hematoma

or a clotted laceration. At a later time, increasing hematoma pressure ruptures the splenic capsule or the clot is dislodged by mild trauma.

LIVER.   The incidence of liver injury may be increased in pregnancy, but there is little or no evidence for spontaneous hepatic rupture.[30] The liver may have an increased risk of spontaneous rupture during eclampsia, but unrecognized trauma cannot be ruled out in most of these cases.

UTERUS

Blunt

> **AXIOM**   Uterine rupture following blunt trauma usually occurs in women with previous cesarean sections.

Auto accidents are an increasingly frequent cause of severe pelvic trauma and are now the most common cause of nonobstetric uterine rupture. Although the seat belt may prevent some severe injuries, it is not entirely harmless and has been increasingly incriminated as a cause of abdominal injuries, especially tears of the small intestine.[48,134]

Uterine rupture due to blunt trauma is an injury unique to pregnancy, but it complicates only about 0.6% of injuries occurring during pregnancy.[2,6,15] Uterine rupture tends to occur only in the most serious accidents involving direct abdominal trauma. With traumatic rupture of the uterus, fetal mortality approaches 100%, whereas maternal mortality is less than 10%.[2,15] In fact, most maternal deaths involving uterine rupture are due to concurrent injuries.[2,15]

It can be extremely difficult to make the diagnosis of uterine rupture following blunt abdominal trauma. Vaginal bleeding is not always present and abdominal tenderness and guarding may be minimal and easily confused with damage to the anterior muscles of the abdominal wall.

> **AXIOM**   Uterine rupture must be ruled out whenever labor seems to be precipitated by trauma.

In some instances, the pain of uterine rupture may closely resemble the pain of parturition.[2] When faced with this dilemma, it is important to follow the fetal heart tones closely. If they slow or become inaudible, severe uterine damage or blood loss must be suspected.

Uterine injury, whether by blunt or penetrating forces, is best treated by repair; it is much faster than a hysterectomy, and it allows future pregnancies. The performance of cesarean section prolongs the operative procedure and usually increases blood loss by at least 1000 ml. Even in patients with pelvic fractures, provided there is no gross pelvic deformity, vaginal delivery is safe and should be encouraged following repair of the uterus.[135]

Penetrating Uterine Trauma

> **AXIOM**   With penetrating abdominal wounds during pregnancy, a "conservative," "watching and waiting" approach is not usually indicated; exploratory laparotomy should be performed as soon as the patient's condition permits.

Stab wounds of the gravid uterus are the second most common penetrating injury to the uterus after gunshot wounds. Degefu et al recently found 22 cases of stab wounds of the pregnant uterus in the literature.[136] The typical patient is between 18 and 28 years of age and is usually in the third trimester.[14,28] All of the patients who were stabbed in the abdomen had uterine wounds varying from 2-5 cms in length. The angle of the penetration and the length of the knife have a direct correlation with the depth of injury inflicted. Even if the patient sustains a stab wound of the chest, possible extension through the diaphragm extending into the gravid uterus should be suspected.

AXIOM	Superficial uterine wounds can usually be closed primarily, even in advanced pregnancy.

Superficial wounds should be repaired as long as it has been ascertained that there was no penetration into the placenta or uterine lumen. If the gravid uterus is in the way of proper exploration of serious maternal wounds, the uterus should be emptied regardless of the maturity of the fetus.

AXIOM	Under no circumstances should consideration for maintaining a pregnancy compromise management of maternal wounds.

In 20% of patients with injury to the gravid uterus, there will be significant associated visceral damage.[7] Hemorrhage from large adjacent intrapelvic vessels can be severe and life-threatening. Rapid control of such bleeding is particularly important if there is to be any chance of salvaging the fetus. Once the severe bleeding is controlled, exploration and repair or removal of other injured viscera should be deferred until the infant is delivered. Recent reports suggest that penetrating wounds of the uterus in which there is no evidence of fetal or maternal hemorrhage or bowel injury can be treated nonoperatively.[137] Even with high-velocity penetrating war injuries, Awwad et al[138] noted that laparatomy may be used selectively in anterior lower abdominal injuries.

Cesarean Section. If the penetration extends through the uterine wall and if the gestation is greater than 32 weeks, prompt delivery by cesarean section is generally indicated. Amniocentesis, pelvic and abdominal ultrasound, and fetal monitoring should be utilized to ensure fetal safety, but this may be difficult. When in doubt, the physician should err on the side of cesarean delivery of term fetuses to avoid fetal loss. Although the fetus will occasionally survive after the death of the mother, it is much more likely to die than the mother as a result of shock and decreased placental perfusion.[139] Even relatively mild injuries to the mother may cause severe fetal hypoxia and alter the subsequent course of the pregnancy or delivery. Removal of a premature infant by cesarean section is not warranted when the uterus appears to be intact.

Dead Fetus. If the fetus is dead, if the entrance wound is below the fundus, and if the missile can be confirmed radiologically to lie within the uterine cavity, exploration may be avoided.[39] If uterine damage is extensive or if there has been gross contamination of the uterus, hysterectomy should be performed.

Fetal death is best managed by repair of the uterus and induction of labor postoperatively after the mother is stable; however, spontaneous labor often occurs within 48 hours.[76] Labor and delivery are usually tolerated quite well even a few hours after celiotomy.

Prevention of Infection
Prevention of infection following trauma to pregnant women is best accomplished by maintaining good tissue perfusion and appropriate debridement and cleansing of any open or contaminated wounds. Antibiotics can be helpful, but one should generally avoid using aminoglycosides, amphotericin B, tetracyclines, chloramphenicol, quinolones, nitrofurantoin, and sulfanamides because of their possible harmful effects on the fetus. Antibiotics which are relatively safe include the penicillins, cephalosporins, clindamycin and erythromycin. Tetanus toxoid and immune globulin have no apparent detrimental effect on the fetus.

Prognosis
Interestingly, the prognosis following pelvic wounds during pregnancy is surprisingly good. Gunshot wounds of the abdomen in the nongravid female have a mortality rate four times greater than that found during pregnancy. The enlarging uterus apparently displaces other viscera and serves as a protective shield.[39,140] The uterine wall

and amniotic fluid provide a cushioning effect, diminishing the force of any penetrating missile. In addition, force applied to the uterus, in contrast to a solid organ, is distributed equally in all directions.

A stab wound of the gravid uterus with proper intervention has a good prognosis for the mother. However, the fetus frequently suffers. Of the cases reported in the literature, the mothers have had 100% survival.[141] However, out of 15 fetuses whose status was reported, only 10 survived. Four of the five fetuses that died were stillborn. Nine of the 15 patients had vaginal delivery with 77% fetal survival. One of the stillbirths was a 900 gram fetus. The high associated perinatal mortality is due to premature delivery as well as direct injury to the fetus, placenta and umbilical cord.[141]

PELVIC FRACTURES
Yosipovitch et al[142] and others[143] have noted that when a pelvic fracture occurs in a woman of childbearing age, a deformed pelvis can complicate subsequent pregnancy and parturition. Furthermore, such a fracture can interfere with the well-being of the fetus. There is also increased difficulty in assessing pelvic fractures by roentgenograms because of the risk of fetal exposure to the radiographs. There is also a general unwillingness to treat pregnant women surgically because of a fear of inducing labor prematurely or of causing death of the fetus by shock or operative manipulation. Thus, pelvic fractures are usually managed conservatively.

Speer and Peltier,[144] in a large review of women who became pregnant after suffering pelvic fractures, noted that 54% delivered vaginally, 36% delivered by cesarean section, and 10% miscarried. Other authors, however, have found that a previous pelvic fracture causes obstetric complications in only a limited number of patients.[143] Moreover, at the present time, cesarean section is a safe and reliable procedure with a mortality rate of 0.2% or less when performed electively. Thus, it is generally felt that open reduction or prophylactic osteotomies should not be performed in pregnant or potentially pregnant women with pelvic fractures. However, if the fracture of the pelvis is such that it will inevitably cause posttraumatic arthritis of the hip joint because of a severe involvement of the weight-bearing portion of the acetabulum, open reduction and internal fixation are warranted.[145] Furthermore, with present techniques of modern anesthesia and fetal monitoring, the risks to the mother and fetus are minimal.[142,146]

General Complications of Trauma in Pregnancy
ECLAMPSIA

AXIOM	Any traumatized pregnant patient presenting with seizures or coma may have a trauma-induced intracerebral bleed, but these CNS changes may also be due to preeclampsia or eclampsia.

The incidence of eclampsia in pregnancy is variably reported as 0.05-0.2% of all deliveries.[147] It has a predilection for the young primigravida, the older multigravida, diabetics and women with chronic hypertension.[148] Hypertension, edema, proteinuria and hyperactive reflexes are usually present, but they may not be prominent. Postpartum eclamptic seizures can occur more than 15 days after delivery, but they usually occur within the first 48 hours.

In any suspected eclamptic, intravenous magnesium sulphate ($MgSO_4$) should be started promptly, and immediate cesarean section considered.[30] Eclamptic patients have died while waiting for CT scans or other diagnostic procedures. A loading dose of 4 grams of 20% $MgSO_4$ solution is given intravenously, followed by either 2-3 grams IV per hour or 5 grams IM in each buttock immediately after the loading dose, and then every 4 hours as long as the deep tendon reflexes are still present. Since administration of $MgSO_4$ can cause vasodilation and hypotension, careful monitoring is essential, especially in the traumatized patient. The $MgSO_4$ treatment should continue for at least 24 hours postpartum or 24 hours after the last seizure.

ARRHYTHMIAS

Cardioversion, electively and emergently, for cardiac dysrhythmias has been performed safely in all three trimesters of pregnancy. Energies up to 300 watt-seconds have been used without fetal heart rhythm disruption or induction of premature labor.[149] Although the amount of electrical current reaching the fetal heart during cardioversion is small, fetal monitoring is essential. Experimental studies have shown that fetal hearts can be made to fibrillate only with difficulty, and the fibrillation is usually self-limited.[149]

THROMBOPHLEBITIS

AXIOM The three main risk factors for thromboembolic disease are stasis, hypercoagulability, and vascular damage, and all three are present during pregnancy.[30]

The first factor, stasis, is potentiated in pregnancy by increased venous capacitance, compression of the IVC by the gravid uterus and decreased mobility. The second risk factor, increased coagulability, is present throughout the pregnancy and may be important for reducing bleeding when the placenta separates from the uterus at the time of birth.[150] The third risk factor, vascular damage, can occur with the trauma of delivery or because of venous hypertension.

Overall, pregnancy is associated with a 5.5-fold increase in the risk of thromboembolism, especially in the postpartum period.[151] Aaro et al found that 81% of deep venous thrombosis and 75% of pulmonary embolism in pregnant women occurs postpartum.[152] Increasing age and parity are two important risk factors associated with an increased risk of fatal pulmonary embolism during or following pregnancy.[153]

DISSEMINATED INTRAVASCULAR COAGULATION

Separation (abruptio) of the placenta from the uterine wall can cause a sudden release of thromboplastin-rich material from the placenta into the circulation. This can produce disseminated intravascular coagulation (DIC) with lethal hemorrhage unless the uterus is emptied rapidly and the clotting defects are corrected.[154] Fibrinogen levels in late pregnancy are generally two to three times those found in nonpregnant patients. Consequently, fibrinogen levels which would be normal in a nonpregnant female often reflect a serious deficit in a patient near term.

AXIOM Normal fibrinogen levels at term should make one suspicious of DIC.

MEDICOLEGAL PROBLEMS

The medicolegal implications of injuries during pregnancy are protean. If pregnancy continues normally for several weeks following trauma, subsequent abortion or premature labor is probably not due to the injury. Indeed, traumatic abortions of normal pregnancies are rare.[155] Hertig[156] suggests that a prima facie case for traumatic abortion must include evidence that the abortus was anatomically normal up to the time of the trauma.

Outcome

The pregnant trauma victim is actually two patients,—both in need of expert care. Initial management should always be done as a team effort with early obstetrical consultation. If the pregnancy is near term or if delivery is anticipated, both a perinatologist and a neonatologist should be alerted. The ABCs of resuscitation must be followed in the pregnant patient, just as they are in every other traumatized patient, and the gravid uterus should not cause undue alarm or distraction. Diagnostic studies necessary for evaluation of the mother should be performed judiciously. Timely operative intervention, combined with continuous fetal monitoring and maintenance of maternal normotension and oxygenation, constitute the keys to successful maternal and fetal outcome.

In their study of 103 gravid patients with blunt abdominal trauma, Rothenberger et al[19] felt that 21 had major injuries because of shock, skull fracture, cerebral contusion, intracranial hemorrhage, spinal column fracture, spinal cord injury, chest or genitourinary injury requiring operative intervention, and pelvic fractures. Five (24%) of the 21 mothers died with their fetuses. In addition, there were six fetal deaths among the 16 surviving mothers for a total fetal loss of 52% in the patients sustaining major trauma.[19] Buchsbaum noted that 25% of pregnant patients with major injuries died and 60% of fetuses were lost. He also noted that pregnancy as an independent variable did not adversely affect maternal survival and that pregnancy may actually improve survival from penetrating trauma.[101]

SUMMARY

Accurate diagnosis of gynecologic and obstetric injuries requires careful pelvic examination, often using general anesthesia when the patient cannot or will not cooperate. Injuries due to blunt trauma, especially retroperitoneal hematomas, can often be treated conservatively, whereas most penetrating wounds should have early surgical exploration.

Since even mild hypovolemia in the pregnant woman may greatly reduce uterine blood flow, any delay in administering needed fluid or blood can cause severe fetal distress. If a penetrating injury to the pregnant uterus cannot be repaired well enough to make subsequent delivery safe, hysterectomy should be performed after delivering the mature fetus by cesarean section. If vaginal bleeding or labor pains develop after blunt trauma, uterine rupture should be suspected and oxytocic drugs are contraindicated. If a pregnant woman with a mature fetus dies suddenly, immediate postmortem cesarean section should be considered.

⊘ FREQUENT ERRORS

In Managing Gynecologic and Obstetrical Trauma

1. *Any reluctance to thoroughly examine the perineum of a woman with severe trauma, especially if there is any suggestion of pelvic trauma.*
2. *Failure to use general anesthesia to examine a girl's or woman's vagina or perineum if that is the only way a needed proper examination can be performed.*
3. *Failure to perform a complete physical examination and obtain all proper specimens in an alleged rape victim.*
4. *Failure to pursue the etiology of a perineal hematoma after trauma.*
5. *Failure to look carefully for a foreign body and sexual abuse in a young girl with a vaginal discharge.*
6. *Failure to consider an attempted abortion in a young woman with septic shock.*
7. *Failure to consider a possible ectopic pregnancy in a young woman who has fainted or is hypotensive.*
8. *Failure to correct hypovolemia adequately and promptly in pregnant women, even if they are not hypotensive.*
9. *Failure to turn an injured pregnant woman to the left promptly to move the uterus off the inferior vena cava.*
10. *Failure to monitor the fetus adequately in a pregnant woman who has experienced trauma.*
11. *Failure to appreciate adequately the physiologic changes that occur with pregnancy.*
12. *Failure to provide prompt ventilatory assistance to pregnant women with marginal ventilator or blood gases.*
13. *Failure to obtain a needed radiologic test because of its possible effect on the fetus.*
14. *Failure to perform, or delay in performing, needed surgery in a pregnant woman because of the possibility of causing an abortion or premature delivery.*

▼▼▼▼▼▼▼▼▼▼▼▼▼▼▼▼▼▼▼▼▼▼▼▼▼▼▼▼▼▼

SUMMARY POINTS

1. Gynecologic injuries are important, and yet they are easily missed because of the patient's modesty or the doctor's reluctance to examine the perineum (unless there is severe pain, bleeding or an obvious wound).

2. If general anesthesia is not used to obtain a complete pelvic examination in uncooperative patients, severe gynecologic injuries are easily missed.

3. Failure to obtain immediate complete coagulation and platelet studies on any patient with excessive bleeding or a large hematoma may delay accurate therapy, and surgery may be undertaken in a patient in whom reasonable hemostasis is impossible.

4. Ecchymoses about the perineum may be the only evidence of severe concealed hemorrhage into the ischiorectal fossa.

5. Failure to perform a complete initial examination on an alleged rape victim increases not only the risk of complications but also the possibility of gross injustice.

6. Vaginal drainage in a child is due to a foreign body until proven otherwise.

7. Direct surgical intraabdominal attempts to control hemorrhage from pelvic fractures usually results in much more severe bleeding and complications.

8. Patients with vaginal tears secondary to pelvic fractures have, by definition, compound fractures and an increased incidence of pelvic abscess and septic complications.

9. If the pelvic examination in a patient with a pelvic fracture is not performed very gently, a closed pelvic fracture can easily be converted into one which is open.

10. When recognized immediately, perforation of the nonpregnant uterus in the operating room can usually be managed nonoperatively, but the patient must be observed carefully for evidence of hemorrhage or infection.

11. Attempted abortion should be suspected when septic shock occurs in young women of childbearing age.

12. All patients suspected of having a criminal abortion should have radiologic studies to search for an extrauterine foreign body. However, radiographs do not always rule out foreign bodies, especially those made of plastic.

13. An extensive laceration of a grossly infected uterus is best managed by hysterectomy.

14. Maternal death is the most frequent cause of fetal death after trauma.

15. For all injured pregnant women, the possibility of chemical dependency must be considered in the initial assessment.

16. One cannot assume that fetal-placental blood flow is adequate if an injured pregnant woman is normotensive.

17. Normal concentrations of coagulation factors in a critically injured pregnant woman should make one suspicious of the presence of DIC.

18. Although all trauma patients are at increased risk for vomiting and aspiration of gastric contents, pregnant women are especially susceptible because of the decreased gastrointestinal motility that accompanies pregnancy.

19. At about 26 weeks, when the delivery of a viable fetus is possible, the top of the uterus is about halfway from the umbilicus to the xiphoid process.

20. At least 10% of women in late pregnancy will develop hypotension if placed in the supine position.

21. If a woman who is injured during late pregnancy is not turned to her left side, hypotension unrelated to the trauma may develop.

22. Placental separation is the leading cause of fetal death when the mother survives.

23. Fetal monitoring is important during maternal resuscitation because fetal heart rate abnormalities are often the first indication of inadequate resuscitation.

24. Occult placental abruption is the most common cause of fetal death in patients with noncatastrophic trauma.

25. Cardiotocographic monitoring after the 20th week of pregnancy is very sensitive at predicting adverse outcomes and can predict abruptio placentae at any early stage, allowing for timely diagnosis and intervention.

26. The initial approach to severely injured pregnant women should probably be more aggressive than for nonpregnant women.

27. Oxygen may be of benefit in all injured patients, but especially for the fetus in pregnant women.

28. Hypovolemia must be corrected rapidly, and vasopressors should be avoided in pregnant women.

29. During the second and third trimesters, gravid patients should not be allowed to lie supine, especially after trauma.

30. Resuscitation of the mother takes priority over all other considerations, including that of the fetus.

31. Injured pregnant women with a marginal airway or ventilation must be rapidly intubated, ventilated, and oxygenated.

32. The physiologic hypervolemia of pregnancy can mask the extent of bleeding in the mother, who may lose 1500 ml or more blood without manifesting any hypotension.

33. Even if an injured mother appears stable, the fetus may have dangerously inadequate perfusion.

34. If transfusion to a moderately hypovolemic but normotensive injured pregnant woman is delayed, severe fetal distress may develop.

35. Inflation of the abdominal portion of the PASG is usually contraindicated in the pregnant patient after the first trimester because it might damage the fetus and compromise maternal venous return.

36. If the fetus is viable but in distress despite resuscitative measures, or if the mother is not considered to be salvageable, urgent cesarean section is recommended.

37. The best protection for the fetus after trauma is an early and aggressive restoration of normal maternal oxygenation and perfusion.

38. Fetal death is not an indication for cesarean section.

39. If the fundus of the uterus is palpable midway between the umbilicus and the xyphoid, a viable fetus is usually present.

40. If delivery is accomplished within 5 minutes of cardiac arrest, the likelihood of survival of a mature fetus without neurologic sequelae is 69%.

41. Cesarean section should be performed in the emergency department if the mother is dead or about to die, if uterine size is greater than 26 weeks gestation, and if the fetus may be alive.

42. Vaginal bleeding is absent in 20% of patients with abruptio placentae, and the uterus may fill with as much as 2000 ml of blood with little external evidence of exsanguination.

43. Falling fibrinogen levels are the most sensitive indicator of DIC in the pregnant woman with a placental injury.

44. DIC in an otherwise stable injured pregnant woman is an indication for prompt induction of labor.

45. There is no such thing as being a little bit pregnant. Any pregnancy, regardless of how early it is, requires special concern for two individuals.

46. A quantitative Bhcg performed every 2 days can assist in predicting the health of an existing pregnancy.

47. A diagnostic modality considered necessary for proper evaluation of an injured gravid woman should not be withheld for fear of potential hazard to the fetus.

48. The fetus is most vulnerable to developing deformities if more than 10-15 rads of irradiation are given during the period from the 10th day through the 10th week after conception.

49. Ultrasound of the abdomen, uterus, and fetus should be performed on all gravid patients with moderate-to-severe abdominal trauma.

50. If a DPL is indicated in an injured pregnant woman after the 12th week, it should be done as an open technique above the umbilicus and uterus.

51. Fetal monitoring is essential in all pregnant women with severe trauma.

52. Ultrasonography can be invaluable in the emergency department if fetal heart tones are inaudible, fundal height is questionable, or vaginal bleeding is present.

53. Severe fetal injury can result from blunt trauma even if there is only minimal uterine damage.

54. Based on the available literature, monitoring for 4 hours after an episode of minimal trauma to a pregnant woman with no other criteria for admission and no obstetric findings appears to be a safe and acceptable practice.

55. Fetal hemorrhage into the maternal circulation is common after trauma and can cause significant complications.

56. One should look for placental injury in all traumatized pregnant women, especially if there is any fetal distress.

57. Disruption of 25% or less of the placental-uterine surface is compatible with fetal survival, but separations greater than 50% generally result in fetal death.

58. Cardiotocographic monitoring is probably the best way to make an early diagnosis of abruptio placentae after trauma.

59. If no fetal heart sounds or activity are identified after trauma, fetal nonviability should be confirmed by real time and B-mode ultrasonography.

60. In patients with possible placental injury, development of a coagulopathy is generally an indication for immediate evacuation of the uterus.

61. The presence or absence of symptoms immediately after injury is not totally predictive of whether the pregnancy will or will not require termination.

62. If there is evidence of uterine contractions and progression of cervical dilatation in an injured mother who is not at term, tocolysis should generally be employed to allow time for full fetal evaluation.

63. Withholding needed surgery is poorly tolerated by both mother and fetus.

64. General anesthesia is preferred for all pregnant patients with multisystem injuries requiring operative management.

65. The main anesthetic risks for the gravid patient are related to the gastrointestinal, cardiovascular, and pulmonary changes that occur with pregnancy.

66. If a penetrating wound is above the uterus or lateral to it, celiotomy is indicated for repair of other injuries.

67. Uterine rupture following blunt trauma usually occurs in women with previous cesarean sections.

68. Uterine rupture must be ruled out whenever labor seems to be precipitated by trauma.

69. With penetrating abdominal wounds during pregnancy, a "conservative", "watching and waiting" approach is not usually indicated; exploratory laparotomy should be performed as soon as the patient's condition permits.

70. Superficial uterine wounds can usually be closed primarily, even in advanced pregnancy.

71. Under no circumstances should consideration for maintaining a pregnancy compromise management of maternal wounds.

72. Any traumatized pregnant patient presenting with seizures or coma may have a trauma-induced intracerebral bleed, but these CNS changes may also be due to preeclampsia or eclampsia.

73. The three main risk factors for thromboembolic disease are stasis, hypercoagulability, and vascular damage, and all three are present during pregnancy.

74. Normal fibrinogen levels at term should make one suspect DIC.

▲▲▲▲▲▲▲▲▲▲▲▲▲▲▲▲▲▲▲▲▲▲▲▲▲▲▲▲▲▲▲▲▲▲▲

REFERENCES

1. Stone NN, Ances IG, Brotman S. Gynecologic injury in the nongravid female during blunt abdominal trauma. J Trauma 1984;24:626.
2. Evans TN, Teshima J. Gynecologic and obstetric trauma. In Walt AJ, Wilson RF, eds. Management of trauma: pitfalls and practice. Philadelphia: Lea & Febiger. 1975, 25:393-402.
3. Yuzpe A, Smith R, Rademaker A. A multicenter clinical investigation employing ethinyl estradiol combined with dl-norgestrel as a postcoital contraceptive agent. Fertil Steril 1982;37:508.
4. Wittich AC, Murray JE. Intravaginal foreign body of long duration: a case report. Am J Obstet Gynecol 1993;169:211.
5. Herman-Giddens ME. Vaginal foreign bodies and child sexual abuse. Arch Pediatr Abolesc Med 1994148:195.
6. Miller WE. Massive hemorrhage in fractures of the pelvis. South Med J 1963;56:933.
7. Maull KI, Pedigo RI. Injury to the female reproductive system. In Moore EE, Mattox KL, Feliciano DV, eds. Trauma, 2nd ed. Norwalk, CT: Appleton-Lange. 1991; 587-595.
8. Gray HH. A risk of water-skiing for women (letter). West J Med 1982;136:169.
9. Niemi TA, Norton LW. Vaginal injuries in patients with pelvic fractures. J Trauma 1985;25:547.
10. Maull KI, Sachatello CR, Ernst CB. The deep perineal laceration—an injury frequently associated with open pelvic fractures: a need for aggressive surgical management. J Trauma 1977;17:685.
11. Doman AN, Hoekstra OV. Pelvic fracture associated with severe intra-abdominal gynecologic injury. J Trauma 1988;28:118.
12. Shimkin PM, Siegel HA, Seaman WB. Radiographic aspects of perforated intrauterine contraceptive devices. Radiology 1969;92:353.
13. Doerch KB, Dozier WE. The seat belt syndrome. The seat belt sign, intestinal and mesenteric injuries. Am J Surg 1968;116:831.
14. Quast DC, Jordan GL Jr. Traumatic wounds of the female reproductive organs. J Trauma 1964;4:839.
15. Fildes J, Reed L, Jones N, et al. Trauma: the leading cause of maternal death. J Trauma 1992;32:643.
16. Patterson RM. Trauma in pregnancy. Clin Obstet Gynecol 1984;27:32.
17. Drost TF, Rosemurgy AS, Sherman HF, et al. Major trauma in pregnant women: maternal/fetal outcome. J Trauma 1990;30:574.
18. Franaszek JB. Trauma in pregnancy. Top Emer Med 1985;7:51.
19. Rothenberger D, Quattlebaum FW, Perry JF, et al. Blunt maternal trauma. A review of 103 cases. J Trauma 1978;18:173.
20. Crosby WM. Trauma in the pregnant patient. Conn Med 1986;50:251.
21. Crosby WM, Costiloe JP. Safety of lap-belt restraint for pregnant victims of automobile collisions. N Engl J Med 1971;284:632.
22. Sparkman RS. Rupture of the spleen in pregnancy: report of two cases and review of the literature. Am J Obstet Gynecol 1958;76:587.
23. Lane PL. Traumatic fetal deaths. J Emerg Med 1989;7:433.
24. Crosby WM. Automobile injuries and blunt trauma. In Buchsbaum HJ, ed. Trauma in pregnancy. Philadelphia: WB Saunders. 1979;27.
25. Lavin JP, Polsky SS. Abdominal trauma during pregnancy. Clin Perinatol 1983;10:423.
26. Crosby WM. Trauma during pregnancy: maternal and fetal injury. Obstet Gynecol Surv 1974;29:683.
27. Fort AJ, Harlin RS. Pregnancy outcome after non-catastrophic maternal trauma during pregnancy. Obstet Gynecol 1970;35:912.
28. Hytten FE, Leitch I. The Physiology of human pregnancy, 2nd ed. Oxford, England: Blackwell Scientific Publications. 1971;18.
29. Cruikshank DP. Anatomic and physiologic alterations of pregnancy that modify the response to trauma. In Buchsbaum HJ, ed. Trauma in pregnancy. Philadelphia: WB Saunders. 1979;21.
30. Neufeld JDG, Moore EE, Marx JA, et al. Trauma in pregnancy. Emerg Med Clin N Am 1987;5:623.
31. Lavin JP, Polsky SS. Abdominal trauma during pregnancy. Clin Perinatol 1983;10:423.
32. Biland L, Duckert F. Coagulation factors of the newborn and his mother. Thromb Diath Haemorrh 1973;29:644.
33. Hytten FE, Lind T. Diagnostic indices in pregnancy. Basel, Switzerland: Ciba-Geigy. 1973;48.
34. Pearlman MD, Tintinalli JE, Lorenz RP. Blunt trauma during pregnancy. N Engl J Med 1990;373:1609.
35. Rhodes P. The volume of liquor amnii in early pregnancy. J Obstet Gynec Brit Comm 1966;73:23.
36. Marx GF. Shock in the obstetric patient. Anesthesiology 1965;26:423.
37. Crosby WM. Traumatic injuries during pregnancy. Clin Obstet Gynecol 1983;26:902.
38. Rothenberger DA, Quattlebaum FW, Zabel J, et al. Blunt maternal trauma: a review of 103 cases. J Trauma 1978;18:173.
39. Buchsbaum HJ. Accidental injury complicating pregnancy. Am J Obstet Gynecol 1968;102:752.
40. Higgins SD, Garite TJ. Late abruptio placenta in trauma patients: implications for monitoring. Obstet Gynecol 1984;63:10S.
41. Amine ARC. Spinal cord injury in a fetus. Surg Neurol 1976;6:369.
42. Rothenberger DA, Horrigan TP, Sturm JT. Neonatal death following in utero traumatic splenic rupture. J Pediatr Surg 1981;16:754.
43. Timms MR, Boyd CR, Gongaware RD. Blunt and penetrating trauma during pregnancy: four cases. J Med Assoc Ga 1985;74:158.

44. Schrinsky DC, Benson RC. Rupture of the pregnant uterus: a review. Obstet Gynecol Surv 1978;33:217.

45. Dyer I, Barclay DL. Accidental trauma complicating pregnancy and delivery. Am J Obstet Gynecol 1962;83:907.

46. Raghavaiah NV, Devi AI. Bladder injury associated with rupture of the uterus. Obstet Gynecol 1975;46:573.

47. Buchsbaum JH. Splenic rupture in pregnancy. Report of a case and review of the literature. Obstet Gynecol Surv 1967;22:381.

48. Rubovits FE. Traumatic rupture of the pregnant uterus from seat belt injury. Am J Obstet Gynecol 1964;90:828.

49. Crosby WM, Snyder RG, Snow CC, et al. Impact injuries in pregnancy. I. Experimental studies. Am J Obstet Gynecol 1968;101:100.

50. Crosby WM, Costiloe JP. Safety of lap belt restraints for pregnant victims of automobile collisions. N Engl J Med 1971;284:632.

51. Crosby WM, King AI, Stout LC. Fetal survival following impact: improvement with shoulder harness restraint. Am J Obstet Gynecol 1972;112:1101.

52. Attico NB, Smith RJ, FitzPatrick MB, et al. Automobile safety straints for pregnant women and children. J Reprod Med 1986;31:187.

53. Buchsbaum HJ, Stables PP Jr. Self-inflicted gunshot wound to the pregnant uterus: report of two cases. Obstet Gynecol 1985;65:32S.

54. Buchsbaum HJ. Penetrating injury of the abdomen. In Buchsbaum HJ, ed. Trauma in pregnancy. Philadelphia: WB Saunders. 1979;82.

55. Iliya FA, Hajj SN, Buchsbaum HJ. Gunshot wounds of the pregnant uterus: report of two cases. J Trauma 1980;290:90.

56. Kobak AJ, Hurwitz CH. Gunshot wounds of the pregnant uterus. Obstet Gynecol 1954;4:383.

57. Haycock CE. Burns and other trauma in pregnancy. In Haycock CE, ed. Trauma and pregnancy. Littleton, MS: PSG Publishing Co. 1985;6:57.

58. Schmitz JT. Pregnancy patients with burns. Am J Obstet Gynecol 1971;110:57.

59. Amy BW, McManus WF, Goodwin CW, et al. Thermal injury in the pregnant patient. Surg Gynecol 1985;161:209.

60. Taylor JW, Plunkett GD, McManus WF, et al. Thermal injury during pregnancy. Obstet Gynecol 1976;47:434.

61. Pimental L. Mother and child. Trauma in pregnancy. Emerg Med Clin North Am 1991;9:549.

62. Goodwin TM, Breen MT. Pregnancy outcome and fetomaternal hemorrhage after noncatastrophic trauma. Am J Obstet Gynecol 1990;116:665.

63. Pearlman MD, Tintinalli JE, Lorenz RP. A prospective controlled study of outcome after trauma during pregnancy. Am J Obstet Gynecol 1990;162:1502.

64. Schoenfeld A, Ziv E, Stein L, et al. Seat belts in pregnancy and the obstetrician. Obstet Gynecol Surv 1987;42:275.

65. Fakhoury GW, Gibson JRM. Seat belt hazards in pregnancy: case report. Br J Gynacol 1986;93:395.

66. Kettel LM, Branch DW, Scott JR. Occult placental abruption after maternal trauma. Obstet Gynecol 1988;71:449.

67. Marx GF, Mateo CV. Effects of different oxygen concentrations during general anaesthesia for elective Caesarean sections. Can Anaesth Soc J 1971;18:587.

68. Shaw DB, Wheeler AS. Anesthesia for obstetric emergencies. Clin Obstet Gynecol 1984;27:112.

69. Morkovin V. Trauma in pregnancy. In Farrell RG, ed. Ob/gyn emergencies. Rockville, MD: Aspen Systems. 1986;71.

70. Katz VL, Hansen AR. Complications in the emergency transport of pregnant women. South Med J 1990;83:7.

71. Wilkening RB, Meschia G. Fetal oxygen uptake, oxygenation, and acid-base balance as a function of uterine blood flow. Am J Physiol 1983;244:H749.

72. Boba A, Linkie DM, Plotz EJ. Effects of vasopressor administration and fluid replacement on fetal bradycardia and hypoxia induced by maternal hemorrhage. Obstet Gynec 1966;27:408.

73. Greiss FC Jr. Uterine vascular response to hemorrhage during pregnancy, with observations on therapy. Obstet Gynec 1966;27:549.

74. Buchsbaum HJ. Diagnosis and management of abdominal gunshot wounds during pregnancy. J Trauma 1975;15:425.

75. Ritter JW. Postmortem Caesarean section. JAMA 1961;175:715.

76. Vanderver Veer JB. Trauma during pregnancy. Top Emerg Med 1984;6:72.

77. Katz VL, Dotters DJ, Droegemueller W. Perimortem Caesarean delivery. Obstet Gynecol 1986;68:671.

78. Strong TH, Lowe RA. Perimortem Caesarean section. Am J Emerg Med 1989;7:489.

79. Weber CE. Postmortem Caesarean section: review of the literature and case reports. Am J Obstet Gynecol 1971;110:158.

80. Behney CA. Caesarean section delivery after death of the mother. JAMA 1961;176:135.

81. Shere DM, Schenkier JF. Accidental injury during pregnancy. Obstet Gynecol Surv 1989;44:330.

82. O'Brien JA, Coustan DR, Singer DB, et al. Prepartum diagnosis of traumatic fetal-maternal hemorrhage. Am J Perinatol 1985;2:214.

83. Bickers RG, Wennberg RP. Fetomaternal transfusion following trauma. Obstet Gynecol 1983;61:258.

84. National Council on Radiation Protection and Measurements. Medical Radiation Exposure of Pregnant and Potentially Pregnant Women, no 54, July 15, 1979.

85. Harvey EB, Boice JD, Homenay M, et al. Prenatal x-ray exposure and childhood cancer in twins. N Engl J Med 1985;312:541.

86. Fischer RP. Cervical radiographic evaluation of alert patients following blunt trauma. Ann Emerg Med 1984;13:905.

87. Rothenberger DA, Quattlebaum FW, Zabel J, et al. Diagnostic peritoneal lavage for blunt trauma in pregnant women. Am J Obstet Gynecol 1977;129:479.

88. Esposito TJ, Gens DR, Smith LG, et al. Evaluation of blunt abdominal trauma occurring during pregnancy. J Trauma 1989;29:1628.

89. Freeman RK, Gartie TJ. Fetal heart rate monitoring. Baltimore: Williams & Wilkins. 1981;69.

90. Hobbins JC. Ultrasound in obstetrical emergencies. In Taylor KJW, ed. Ultrasound in emergency medicine. New York: Churchill Livingstone. 1981;156.

91. Dornan KJ, et al. Fetal weight estimation by real-time ultrasound measurement of biparietal and transverse trunk diameter. Am J Obstet Gynecol 1982;142:652.

92. Theurer DE, Kaiser IH. Traumatic fetal death without uterine injury. Report of a case. Obstet Gynec 1963;26:477.

93. Agran PF, Dunkle DE, Winn DG, et al. Fetal death in motor vehicle accidents. Ann Emerg Med 1987;16:1355.

94. Stafford PA, Biddinger PW, Zumwalt RE. Lethal intrauterine fetal trauma. Am J Obstet Gynecol 1988;159:458.

95. Parkinson EB. Perinatal loss due to external trauma to the uterus. Am J Obstet Gynecol 1964;90:30.

96. Elliott M. Vehicular accidents and pregnancy. Aust NZ J Obstet Gynaecol 1966;6:279.

97. Williams JK, McClain L, Rosemurgy AS, et al. Evaluation of blunt abdominal trauma in the third trimester of pregnancy: maternal and fetal considerations. Obstet Gynecol 1990;75:33.

98. Pepperell RJ, Rubinstein E, MacIsaac IA. Motor-car accidents during pregnancy. Med J Aust 1977;1:203.

99. Varner MW. Maternal mortality in Iowa from 1952-1986. Surg Gynecol Obstet 1989;168:555.

100. Buchsbaum HJ. Accidental injury complicating pregnancy. Am J Obstet Gynecol 1968;102:752.

101. Haycock CE. Injury during pregnancy: saving both mother and fetus. Consultant 1982;269.

102. Dudley DJ, Cruikshank DP. Trauma and acute surgical emergencies in pregnancy. Semin Perinatol 1990;14:42.

103. Franger AL, Buchsbaum HF, Peaceman AM. Abdominal gunshot wounds in pregnancy. Obstet Gynecol 1989;160:1124.

104. Agran PF, Dunkle DE, Winn DG, et al. Fetal death in motor vehicle accidents. Ann Emerg Med 1987;16:1355.

105. Higgins SD, Garite TJ. Late abruptio placenta in trauma patients: implications for monitoring. Obstet Gynecol 1984;63:10S.

106. Sher G, Statland BE. Abruptio placentae with coagulopathy: a rational basis for management. Clin Obstet Gynecol 1985;28:15.

107. Rose PG, Strohm PL, Zuspan FP. Fetomaternal hemorrhage following trauma. Am J Obstet Gynecol 1985;153:844.

108. Pearlman MD, Tintinalli JE, Lorenz RP. A prospective controlled study of outcome after trauma during pregnancy. Am J Obstet Gynecol 1990;162:1502.

109. Goodwin TM, Breen MT. Pregnancy outcome and fetomaternal hemorrhage after noncatastrophic trauma. Am J Obstet Gynecol 1990;162:665.

110. Mollison PL. Clinical aspects of Rh immunization. Am J Clin Pathol 1973;60:287.

111. Maile JB. Laboratory medicine hematology, 6th ed. St. Louis: CV Mosby. 1982;885.

112. Rose PG, Strohm PL, Zuspan FP. Fetomaternal hemorrhage following trauma. Am J Obstet Gynecol 1985;153:844.

113. Towery R, English TP, Wisner D. Evaluation of pregnant women after blunt injury. J Trauma 1993;35:731.

114. Bryant JF, Moore MD. Gunshot wound of gravid uterus with simulta

neous exploration of mother and fetus: report of a case. Am Surg 1964;30:207.

115. Buchsbaum HJ, Caruso PA. Gunshot wound of the pregnant uterus. Case report of fetal injury deglutition of missile and survival. Obstet Gynecol 1969;33:673.

116. Crosby WM, Snyder RG, Snow CC, et al. Impact injuries in pregnancy. I. Experimental studies. Am J Obstet Gynecol 1968;101:100.

117. Acker D, Sachs BP, Tracey KJ, et al. Abruptio placentae associated with cocaine use. Am J Obstet Gynecol 1983;146:220.

118. Philips LL, Skroedelis V, Taylor HC. Hemorrhage due to fibrinolysis in abruptio placentae. Am J Obstet Gynecol 1962;84:1447.

119. Goplerud CP. Bleeding in late pregnancy. In Danforth DN, Scott JR, eds. Obstetrics and gynecology, 5th ed. Philadelphia: Lippincott-Raven. 1986;433.

120. Weinstein L. Lightning: a rare cause of intrauterine death with maternal survival. South Med J 1979;72:632.

121. Notelovitz M, Bottoms SF, Dase DF, et al. Painless abruptio placentae. Obstet Gynecol 1979;53:270.

122. Peyser MR, Toaff R. Traumatic rupture of the placenta. Obstet Gynecol 1969;34:561.

123. Sherer DM, Schenker JG. Accidental injury during pregnancy. Obstet Gynecol Surv 1989;44:330.

124. Drost TF, Rosemurgy AS, Sherman HF, et al. Major trauma in pregnant women: maternal/fetal outcome. J Trauma 1990;30:574.

125. Bondurant S, Boehm FH, Fleischer AC, et al. Antepartum diagnosis of fetal intracranial hemorrhage by ultrasound. Obstet Gynecol 1984;63(3 Suppl):25S.

126. Civil ID, Talucci RC, Schwab CW. Placental laceration and fetal death as a result of blunt abdominal trauma. J Trauma 1988;28:708.

127. Lee RB, Wudel JH, Morris JA Jr. Trauma in pregnancy. J Tenn Med Assoc 1990;83:74.

128. Haycock CE. Emergency care of pregnant traumatized patient. Emerg Med Clin North Am 1984;2:843.

129. Schoenfeld A, Ziv E, Stein LB, et al. Vehicular trauma in pregnancy: an algorithm for diagnosis and fetal therapy. Fetal Therapy 1987;2:51.

130. Erian M, Wu WH. Anesthetic management of the traumatized patient. In Haycock CE, ed. Trauma and pregnancy. Littleton, MS: PSG Publishing Co. 1985;8:80.

131. Najafi JA, Gunzman LG. Spontaneous pneumothorax in labor: case report. Milit Med 1978;143:341.

132. Pedowitz P, Perell A. Aneurysms complicated by pregnancy. Am J Obstet Gynecol 1957;73:720.

133. Sparkman RS. Rupture of the spleen in pregnancy. Am J Obstet Gynecol 1958;76:587.

134. Fish J, Wright RH. The seat belt syndrome . . . does it exist? J. Trauma, 1965;5:746.

135. Madsen LV, Jensen J, Christensen ST. Parturition and pelvic fracture: follow-up of 34 patients with a history of pelvic fracture. Acta Obstet Gynecol Scand 1983;62:617.

136. Degefu S, O'Quinn AG, Pernoll ML, et al. Stab wound of the gravid uterus: a case report and literature update. J La State Med Soc 1988;140:39.

137. Grubb DK. Nonsurgical management of penetrating uterine trauma in pregnancy: a case report. Am J Obstet Gynecol 1992;166:583.

138. Awwad JT, Azar GB, Seoud MA, et al. High-velocity penetrating wounds of the gravid uterus: review of 16 years of civil war. Obstet Gynecol 1994;83:259.

139. Romney SL, Gabel PV, Takeda, Y. Experimental hemorrhage in late pregnancy. Effects on maternal and fetal hemodynamics. Am J Obstet Gynecol 1963;87:636.

140. Beatie JF, Daly RF. Gunshot wound of the pregnant uterus. Am J Obstet Gynecol 1960;80:772.

141. Wright CH, Posner AC, Gilchrist J. Penetrating wounds of the gravid uterus. Am J Obstet Gynecol 1954;67:1085.

142. Yosipovitch Z, Goldberg I, Ventura E, et al. Open reduction of acetabular fracture in pregnancy. A case report. Clin Orthop 1992; 282:229.

143. Madsen LV, Jensen J, Christensen ST. Parturition and pelvic fracture. Follow-up of 34 obstetric patients with a history of pelvic fracture. Acta Obstet Gynecol Scand 1983;62:617.

144. Speer DP, Peltier LF. Pelvic fractures and pregnancy. J Trauma 1972;12:474.

145. Matta JM, Mehne DK, Roff R. Fractures of the acetabulum: early results of a prospective study. Clin Orthop 1986;205:241.

146. Pals SD, Brown CW, Friermood TG. Open reduction and internal fixation of an acetabular fracture during pregnancy. J Orthop Trauma 1992;6:379.

147. Sibai BM, McCubbin JH, Anderson GD. Eclampsia: I. Observations from 67 recent cases. Obstet Gynecol 1981;58:609.

148. Willson JR, Carrington, ER. Bleeding during late pregnancy. In obstetrics and gynecology. St. Louis: CV Mosby. 1979; 358.

149. DeSilva RA, Graboys TB, Podrid PJ, et al. Cardioversion and defibrillation. Am Heart J 1980;100:881.

150. Bonnar J, McNicol GP, Douglas AS. Fibrinolytic enzyme system and pregnancy. Br Med J 1969;3:387.

151. Bolan JC. Thromboembolic complications of pregnancy. Clin Obstet Gynecol 1983;26:913.

152. Aaro LA, Johnson TR, Juergens JL. Acute deep venous thrombosis associated with pregnancy. Obstet Gynecol 1966;28:553.

153. DeSwiet M. Thromboembolism. Clin Hematol 1985;14:643.

154. Beller FK. Hemorrhagic disorders in pregnancy. Clin Obstet Gynecol 1964;7:269.

155. Javert CT. Role of the patient's activities in the occurrence of spontaneous abortion. Fertil Steril 1960;11:550.

156. Hertig AT. Symposium on problems relating to law and surgery: minimal criteria required to prove prima facie case of traumatic abortion or miscarriage; analysis of 1000 spontaneous abortions. Ann Surg 1943;117:596.

Chapter **31** Musculoskeletal Trauma

GREGORY M. GEORGIADIS, M.D.
ROBERT F. WILSON, M.D.

FRACTURES AND DISLOCATIONS IN ADULTS

PRIORITIES

AXIOM The most obvious injuries are often not the most important.

In patients with multiple injuries, severe deformities of the extremities are often so striking that they tend to receive much of the initial attention with consequent neglect of other, more serious, injuries. Maintenance of an adequate airway and ventilation, control of hemorrhage, and correction of hypovolemia take priority over injured bones. Nevertheless, open fractures are surgical emergencies and should receive operative intervention within 6 hours of injury to have the best chance for a favorable outcome.[1] In similar fashion, fractures and dislocations, when associated with neurovascular compromise, are true surgical emergencies requiring prompt attention.[2]

DIAGNOSIS

After the initial resuscitative measures have been accomplished, a thorough evaluation of the patient can be made.

History

In relation to musculoskeletal injuries, special attention should be given to the mechanism of injury, location of pain, limitation of motion, and neurovascular function. It is important to remember that pain from fractures is occasionally referred to more distal portions of the extremity; hip fractures, for example, commonly cause pain in the thigh and knee.

The history is especially important in managing open fractures. Identification of the source and extent of contamination is critical, as is a knowledge of the extent of bony injury, i.e., if the bone was exposed and then retracted into the tissues.

The history is also critical in assessing the true zone of injury, as soft tissue damage in both open and closed fractures can be much greater than first realized.[3] If not appreciated this can result in inadequate debridement, inappropriate procedures, and wound problems. Potential tissue damage is proportional to energy dissipation by the body, as described by the formula:

$$K = \tfrac{1}{2}\, mv^2$$

where K = Kinetic energy, m = mass and v = velocity.[4] For example, the energy disrupting tissues is 1,000 times greater after a bumper injury at 20 miles per hour, than from a fall at a curb (Table 31–1).[3,5]

If the extent of the injury is inconsistent with the history, a pathologic fracture should also be considered. For example, an elderly patient should not sustain a fracture about the hip from turning over in bed. Although pathologic fractures should be suspected in patients with known malignant or metabolic disease, they may also occur in completely asymptomatic patients.

In a child, multiple fractures in various stages of healing are characteristic of child abuse.[6] Skull fractures and long bone fractures in children less than 3 years of age are also unusual and should raise a suspicion of abuse.[7,8]

AXIOM Child abuse should be suspected whenever the history is inconsistent with the physical examination or radiographs, or when there are multiple fractures at different stages of healing.

Physical Examination

The physical examination should include, in addition to a complete examination of all potentially injured bones and joints, a careful evaluation of the motor and sensory nervous function and distal pulses and blood flow.

AXIOM An extremity cannot be adequately evaluated if it is covered.

Any obvious deformities of the extremities should be recorded, as should the location and size of any contusions, abrasions, swellings, or lacerations. All extremities should be gently palpated, noting the location and severity of any tenderness. In comatose patients, areas of deformity or abnormal motion may not be apparent and crepitation, elicited gently, may be the only objective evidence of a fracture. The joints should be evaluated for range of motion, tenderness or effusion.

Radiographs

After any immediate life-threatening problems have been controlled and appropriate dressings and splints have been applied, the patient may be taken to the x-ray department. The radiograph request should contain as much pertinent information about the injury as possible, and should list all areas that might require x-rays. The physician examining the patient must carefully review the radiographs and correlate them with the physical findings. Ideally, the patient's history should be discussed with a radiologist who may be able to organize the radiological procedures most efficiently, but this is often not possible in the acute trauma setting.

PITFALL ⊘

Accepting poor-quality radiographs.

Assuming the patient is otherwise stable, poor quality radiographs should not be accepted regardless of the time and effort it takes to get the proper films. Some fractures are missed either due to inadequate physical examination, poor quality radiographs, or both. Despite a conscientious initial evaluation, however, it is perhaps inevitable that some injuries will be missed. In a recent study from a busy Level I trauma center, as many as one in five severe multiple trauma victims had at least one occult orthopaedic injury that was not initially appreciated.[9] Only regular, repeated and comprehensive orthopaedic examinations after admission with appropriate radiographs will result in rapid detection and treatment of these missed injuries.

AXIOM A regular orthopaedic reexamination is mandatory in the early hospital course of all trauma patients to detect possible occult fractures.

TABLE 31–1   Energy Dissipation After Selected Injuries[3]

Mechanism	Energy (foot-pounds)
Fall from curb	100
Skiing injury	300-500
High velocity gunshot wound	2,000
Automobile bumper injury (20 mph)	100,000

GENERAL CONSIDERATIONS

Describing Fractures

This is an area that is often quite confusing. There are numerous fracture eponyms, and in general their use is now discouraged. There are also numerous classification schemes in use, with no universally accepted system. The need for a systematic and orderly approach to this problem has recently led the AO group (Arbeitsgemeinshaft fur Osteosynthesefragen) to develop a new classification of long bone fractures.[10] However, the reliability of many classification systems in orthopaedics is currently being questioned.[11,12]

Any description of a fracture must include the bone involved, the location within the bone (i.e epiphyseal, metaphyseal, diaphyseal), a description of any articular involvement, the fracture pattern (i.e., transverse, oblique, segmental, comminuted) and any bone loss if present. Whether the fracture is open (any loss of skin integrity near the fracture) or closed is critical information. The older terminology of "compound fracture" to describe open fractures is now becoming obsolete. Newer classification systems now emphasize the degree of injury to the soft tissues (skin, muscle, tendons, nerves arteries) in addition to the fracture.[3,13]

Splinting

EMERGENCY SPLINTING

Any splints that were applied before the patient reached the hospital must be inspected carefully and adjusted to assure that they are adequate, are not causing excessive pressure, and are not hiding any neurovascular problems or open fractures.

AXIOM   Fractures which have not already been immobilized should be splinted as soon as possible after arrival at the hospital.

UPPER EXTREMITY INJURIES

Shoulder and Arm

The extremity is placed in a sling, with the elbow usually at a right angle, and is bound to the chest with a bandage or a sling and a swathe. Humeral fractures may also be immobilized with a coaptation splint.[14] The coaptation splint is formed with plaster placed over the shoulder, down along the lateral aspect of the arm, around the elbow and then up along the medial side of the arm into the axilla. This splint must be well padded to prevent irritation of the axilla and chest wall.

Elbow

If an injured elbow can be placed easily at a right angle, adequate emergency splinting may be provided as described above for the shoulder and arm. If, however, an injured elbow is in extension, no attempt should be made to flex it to a right angle, as this may cause excessive pain or serious neurovascular compromise. A posterior splint may be used for fractures about the elbow. An inflatable air splint may also be useful.

Forearm and Wrist

Padded commercial metal splints or inflatable air splints may be used. For forearm fractures, a sugar tong splint can be applied easily

in the emergency department (ED).[14] It consists of a well-padded length of plaster that extends dorsally from just proximal to the metacarpal heads to around the elbow and then back to the palmar surface of the hand at the proximal crease. This splint is applied with an elastic bandage. The addition of a sling with the elbow at a right angle often adds to the patient's comfort. Alternatively, volar or separate volar and dorsal splints can be applied in a similar manner.

LOWER EXTREMITY INJURIES

Hip, Thigh, and Knee

Fixed traction splinting in a Thomas or hinged half-ring splint, using a hitch about the foot and ankle, is the most effective. The hitch may be applied over a shoe if it is not easily removed.

The Hare splint is easier to apply than a Thomas splint. The Hare splint provides slings with Velcro grips and a special windlass attached to the distal end of the splint for providing and adjusting traction.

An alternative to fixed traction is the use of padded board splints. A long board extending to the lower thorax is placed on the lateral side and a shorter board is placed on the medial side of the extremity. Bandages securely bind the splints to the extremity and the long board to the lower thorax and pelvic area. For injuries about the knee, a long inflated air splint may be used.

Leg and Ankle

An inflated air splint can provide excellent emergency splinting. Effective alternatives include a posterior molded plaster splint or padded board splints extending to the mid-thigh. For fractures at the ankle, a pillow wrapped securely with tape around the lower leg, ankle and foot can be effective. The foot must always be included to prevent rotation during transport.

SPLINTING OPEN FRACTURES

A bone fragment protruding through an open wound should be covered with a sterile dressing and left undisturbed until definitive care is provided. With traction splinting, one should not pull extruded bone back into the wound unless the distal circulation is compromised. With neurovascular impairment, severe angular and rotary deformities should be corrected by traction, even if a protruding fragment is pulled back into the wound.

VERTEBRAL INJURIES

Neck

The patient should be supine on a firm surface such as a long spine board. A rigid collar should be applied with the head and neck in the neutral midline position. The neck should not be flexed, extended or rotated.

Thoracic and Lumbar

The patient should be on a firm surface such as a long spine board in the supine position with a small roll under the lumbar spine. Flexion, extension or rotation of the spine is to be avoided. If turning is necessary, the patient should be rolled "like a log" by two or three individuals.

Healing of Fractures

Fracture healing is unique because it occurs with the reconstitution of normal tissue (i.e., bone) as opposed to scar tissue. An adequate review of this process is beyond the scope of this discussion, but the most important prerequisites for healing are close proximity of the fracture fragments with adequate stability and maintenance of good blood supply. Local impairment of circulation due to fracture location (i.e., certain fractures have a tenuous blood supply like the femoral or talar neck) or soft tissue stripping (i.e., from injury or surgery) may interfere with bony union. Inadequate apposition of fragments, loss of stability, soft tissue interposition or infection can all adversely affect bony healing.

OPEN FRACTURES

Most classification systems for open fractures attempt to grade the degree of injury to soft tissue associated with the fracture. The most popular classification system used in North America is that of Gustilo and Anderson,[15] with its later modification[16] (Table 31–2). Grade I fractures are those with a wound less than 1 cm long and without any significant soft tissue damage. Grade II fractures have larger wounds or more underlying tissue damage. Grade III fractures have been subdivided: grade IIIA has significant wounds due to high-energy trauma, often with extensive lacerations and soft tissue flaps, but such that after final debridement, adequate local soft tissue coverage is not lost and delayed primary closure is feasible. Grade IIIB includes major wounds with considerable devitalized soft tissue, foreign material, or both. Bone is exposed in the wound, and extensive periosteal avulsion may be present. Coverage of the soft tissue defect usually requires a local or free microvascular tissue transfer. Grade IIIC includes open fractures with an associated arterial injury that requires repair (Table 31–2). Recently, the interobserver reliability of the Gustilo and Anderson classification system has been questioned.[12]

Reported infection rates range from 0-9% for grade I fractures, 1-12% for grade II fractures, and 9-55% for grade III fractures.[1,15,17,18] Grade III fractures with associated vascular injuries have an infection rate three times higher than those without an ischemic component.[18]

The management of grade IIIC tibia fractures is both difficult and controversial. One issue is whether such patients are better off with early amputation rather than complex attempts at salvage.[19,20] At present, the complication and ultimate amputation rate for grade III open fractures remains high.[21]

The goals in the treatment of open fractures include prevention of infection, achieving bony union, and restoring function. Prevention of infection in soft tissue wounds begins when they are first examined by medical personnel. Manipulation of wounds should be limited to whatever is necessary to control major hemorrhage or relieve neurovascular impairment until definitive treatment can be carried out in the operating room. Additional contamination should be kept to a minimum. Tscherne et al have shown that the infection rate following open fractures was four times lower in patients who had a sterile dressing in place from the scene of the accident to the operating room, compared with those who did not.[22] The earliest possible treatment of open fractures should be provided. Quantitative wound cultures reveal an increasing frequency of bacterial contamination and risk of wound infection as the duration from injury to definitive wound care increases.[23] Quantitative tissue cultures are generally not useful in the management of acute open fractures, but may be helpful in deciding when to close contaminated open wounds.

TABLE 31–2 *Gustilo Classification of Open Fractures*[15,16]

Grade I:	Skin opening of 1 cm or less, quite clean, Most likely from inside to outside. Minimal muscle contusion. Simple transverse or short oblique fractures.
Grade II:	Laceration more than 1 cm long, with extensive soft tissue damage, flaps, or avulsion. Minimal to moderate crushing component. Simple transverse or short oblique fractures with minimal comminution.
Grade III:	Extensive soft tissue damage including muscles, skin, and/or neurovascular structures. Often a high-velocity injury with a severe crushing component.
IIIA:	Extensive soft tissue laceration, but adequate bone coverage. Segmental fractures, gunshot injuries.
IIIB:	Extensive soft tissue injury with periosteal stripping and bone exposure. Usually associated with massive contamination.
IIIC:	Vascular injury requiring repair.

Parenteral antibiotics have played a key role in reducing infection rates in open fractures.[15,24,25] Ideally they should be started as soon as possible in the emergency room. Pretreatment wound cultures are often obtained, although there is controversy as to their usefulness, with some surgeons preferring to obtain deep wound cultures in the operating room.[26] The precise specificity and sensitivity of routine perioperative cultures in open fractures is also unclear.[27] It is important, however, to realize that since the majority of open fractures are contaminated on presentation, antibiotic therapy represents treatment, and not simply prophylaxis.

The antibiotic of choice is a cephalosporin, typically one or two grams of cefazolin every 6-8 hours. For grade III injuries, an aminoglycoside is added. Because of the increasing number of gram-negative infections that are being encountered, a cephalosporin/aminoglycoside combination is increasingly used. For clostridia-prone wounds (i.e., farm injuries), 3-4 million units of penicillin every 4 hours should be added. The duration of antibiotic therapy remains controversial, but current recommendations call for treatment for 3 days.[24] Antibiotics should also be given during any subsequent procedures such as wound closures or open reduction and internal fixation.

AXIOM Antibiotics by themselves do not prevent wound infections.

A thorough surgical debridement is essential in the treatment of any open fracture. It is important that all crushed or devitalized skin and soft tissue should be excised. An inadequately excised wound is prone to infection, regardless of how much antibiotic is used. The skin incisions must be long enough to examine the wounds and zone of injury adequately, as the extent of the injury may be far more severe than initially appreciated. Careful debridement removes nonviable tissue and also homogenized fat, hemoglobin, and foreign materials that can promote and nourish bacterial growth.[28,29] In many cases muscle compartments should be opened to examine the muscle for injury and as a prophylactic measure for compartment syndrome. High energy open fractures are at risk for compartment syndrome, and the open nature of the injury often does not provide for adequate decompression.[30,31]

Muscle which does not bleed when cut or twitch when pinched is dead and should be removed. Muscle which bleeds but does not twitch when pinched may be alive, but it should be trimmed of lacerated ends and separated fibers. The viability of muscle, or any other questionable tissue, can be assessed at the time of future debridement. All foreign bodies, with the exception of inaccessible missile fragments, should be removed. All bleeding points should be controlled.

Essential structures such as nerves, tendons, large blood vessels, and ligaments should be cleansed mechanically with voluminous irrigation under pressure. This is especially helpful for a wound in which all tissue is viable but dirt or other foreign material is present. The appropriate irrigation force may be obtained using one of the available commercial irrigation devices or a 35-ml syringe with a 19-gauge needle. Rubber bulb syringes or irrigation by gravity from intravenous bags are much less effective.[32]

High pressure irrigation should not be used indiscriminately but should be reserved for dirty or contaminated wounds that cannot be adequately debrided. In these wounds the removal of dirt and bacteria is beneficial and offsets any adverse effects of irrigation.[33] It is also clear that the fluids used to irrigate or clean a wound should be balanced electrolyte solutions. Various antiseptic solutions, such as Betadine are often used for killing bacteria in open wounds or abscess cavities, but they may damage the natural host-defense mechanisms in the wound even more.[34,35]

Frayed ends of tendons and ligaments should be trimmed economically, and the structures left in place. Bone fragments completely free of any soft tissue attachment should be removed. Whether large avascular fragments that are important for stability should be replaced in the wound is controversial. Current trends involve discarding all avascular fragments, with later reconstructive procedures for bone loss.

Dirty bone ends must be thoroughly cleansed, if necessary by a brush or curette, to remove any embedded dirt.

Following debridement and wound cleansing, the fracture should be stabilized. This can be done in a number of different ways. In general, casts are not recommended for open fractures, as they do not provide for easy wound access, cannot accommodate swelling that may cause ischemia or compartment syndrome, may result in significant cast window edema if openings are made, and do not provide for anatomic reduction.[3] External fixation is often a good option, as it can stabilize the fracture without adding more foreign material to the wound. Internal fixation can also be used, and may be preferred for certain articular injuries. Some types of internal fixation (i.e., plates and screws for severe open tibial fractures) have been associated with increased infection rates, consequently, use of internal fixation in open fractures should be considered carefully.

AXIOM Although early fixation of fractures of the lower extremity permits earlier mobilization and results in fewer pulmonary complications, if infection develops at the fracture site, the result can be disastrous.

After debridement and stabilization of open fractures, proper wound management is important. Dead space should be eliminated and any large collections of fluid avoided.[36-44] Parenteral antibiotics have greatly decreased wound infection rates, and primary wound closure may be done in some open fractures with minimal tissue damage and contamination.[24,25,26] However, primary closure of open fractures is associated with an increased risk of infection, especially from clostridial myonecrosis ("gas gangrene"). For this reason, leaving the wound open, with later delayed primary closure, is always a safer option.[45,46,47]

AXIOM Delayed wound closure is safer than primary closure in most grossly contaminated open fractures.

After the initial surgery, plans should be made to return patients with grade II or III open fractures to the operating room within 24-72 hours for further debridement. Delayed primary closure should be performed when possible within 3-5 days. Skin grafting, local muscle flaps or free tissue transfers may be needed if delayed primary closure is not possible. Rates of infection and other complications increase if soft tissue coverage cannot be accomplished in this time period after injury.[48,49,50]

In severe open fractures, local antibiotics can be delivered in polymethylmethacrylate (PMMA) beads impregnated with gentamicin or tobramycin.[51,52] These are typically used in addition to intravenous antibiotics. The PMMA beads can be removed at the time of wound closure. Alternatively, they can be retained and used as tissue spacers after bone loss. Soft tissue coverage, often with local or free flaps, is then performed over the beads. Osseous reconstruction is accomplished at a later date (often 6-8 weeks after the injury) when the skin wounds are completely healed. This is performed by cancellous bone grafting, and the antibiotic beads can be removed at the same time.[53]

Finally, the attending physician must determine for each patient what prophylaxis for tetanus is required. Regardless of the active immunization status of the patient, meticulous surgical care, including removal of all devitalized tissue and foreign bodies, should be provided immediately to all wounds. With tetanus-prone injuries, human tetanus immune globulin and antibiotics should be given in addition to a tetanus toxoid booster.

Associated Nerve Injuries

All injured extremities must be examined carefully initially for neurologic damage. This is particularly important since many of these extremities may require further procedures like manipulations or surgeries that may place neurovascular structures at further risk.

AXIOM The neurovascular status of an injured extremity should be evaluated both before and after any manipulation.

Trauma to peripheral nerves is relatively common and can produce devastating loss of function. Up to 12% of humeral shaft fractures are accompanied by paralysis of the radial nerve,[54,55] and up to 18% of knee dislocations have accompanying injuries to nerves.[56]

The most common mechanism of peripheral nerve injury is blunt trauma to tissue overlying the nerves; however, penetrating injuries that do not clearly lacerate the nerve occur with nearly equal frequency. Peripheral nerves also can be injured by stretching, or compression by fractures and hematomas. Because of their high susceptibility to ischemic damage, peripheral nerves can also be injured when surrounding tissue pressure is high, such as in compartment syndromes in the upper or lower extremities.

FREQUENT NEURAL INJURIES

Upper Extremities

About 95% of peripheral nerve injuries occur in the upper extremities, the most common being injury to the radial nerve in humeral-shaft fractures, especially at the junction of its middle and distal thirds.[14] Other neurologic lesions frequently seen with musculoskeletal injuries in the upper extremities include: (a) lacerations, contusions, or stretching of the axillary nerve or brachial plexus in dislocations of the shoulder, (b) injuries to the median or ulnar nerve in supracondylar fractures and posterior dislocations of the elbow, and (c) injuries to the median nerve in fractures about the wrist.

Lower Extremities

In the lower extremity, injury to the sciatic nerve, especially its peroneal portion, can be seen in up to 13% of posterior dislocations of the hip. Nerve injuries have been reported in 18% of knee dislocations.[6,55] The peroneal nerve is especially apt to be involved when there are tears of the lateral collateral ligament or fractures of the proximal fibula.

TREATMENT

AXIOM Closed fractures and dislocations seldom disrupt nerves completely, and contusion or stretching is the usual cause of neurologic deficits.

It is often impossible to identify accurately the functional or anatomic extent of the damage to a nerve on first examination.[55] In addition, complete functional loss at the time of injury does not preclude a complete, spontaneous recovery without intervention. Consequently, it is not wise to make a great effort to explore peripheral nerves which may be injured for possible early repair.

If a well-localized nerve injury is found at the time of the initial wound exploration, it can often be repaired. However, if there is much contamination, if the extent of the nerve damage is not clear, or if the surgeon does not feel capable of performing an accurate anastomosis, nerve repair should be delayed until the wound has healed.

After the fracture has been treated and is healed, nerve function can be evaluated both clinically and by electromyo-graphic and conduction studies. If there is no evidence of reinnervation after 6-8 weeks, the nerve should be explored.

Associated Vascular Injuries

A wide variety of combined bone and vascular injuries can occur with gunshot wounds, and these are covered in the chapter on vascular injury.

MOST FREQUENT INJURIES

Upper Extremities

The blunt upper extremity injuries most apt to damage major vessels include dislocations of the shoulder compressing or contusing the axillary artery, mid-shaft humeral fractures bruising or tearing the brachial artery, and dislocations of the elbow or supracondylar fractures of the humerus compressing the brachial artery, particularly if the elbow is flexed to bring about a reduction of the fragments.

Lower Extremities

Blunt lower extremity injuries particularly apt to involve major vessels include fractures of the mid-distal femoral shaft (tearing or contusing the superficial femoral artery) and dislocations of the knee (causing intimal flaps in the popliteal artery). Fractures of the tibia and fibula can produce compartment syndromes compressing distal branches of the popliteal artery.

TREATMENT

In many instances, reduction of a dislocation will relieve neurovascular embarrassment in an extremity, but an arteriogram should still be performed. Otherwise a large intimal flap which may cause later occlusion may be missed. With fractures of the shafts of large bones, traction will realign the fragments and often will restore normal pulses. If a position of extreme flexion is needed to reduce a fracture, such as supracondylar fracture of the humerus, compression of the artery because of surrounding soft tissue swelling can occur. Such a position should be abandoned, and treatment should involve internal fixation and immobilization in a position which will not cause any vascular problems.

Early Post-reduction Care

The first 24-72 hours after fracture reduction is a period of increasing swelling and danger of soft tissue complications. Immediately after reduction and recovery from any anesthesia used, the integrity of the circulation and peripheral nerve function should be checked. Radiographs confirming the reduction should be taken.

Splints are often used for the initial immobilization, and the circulatory status of the injured part must be kept under close surveillance. This may necessitate hospitalization for observation. If a circular cast is used for immobilization, it should be bivalved or removed if the patient complains of pain or if there is any question of vascular embarrassment. No patient should be allowed to leave the hospital without receiving specific instructions to return immediately if: (a) the fingers or toes distal to a cast or splint become white, blue, cold, or insensitive, or (b) if there is severe, intractable pain.

> **AXIOM** A well reduced and immobilized fracture should not cause severe pain.

Increasing or excessive pain often indicates tissue pressure or ischemia that requires urgent correction. Splinting or casting a fracture should make the patient more comfortable. If it does not, then this must be thoroughly investigated. In general, patients who are complaining of increasing pain should not be given more analgesics, as this may prevent the diagnosis of a serious complication.

> **PITFALL** ⊘
>
> *Failing to promptly investigate excessive or increased pain under a cast.*

Constant localized pain under a plaster cast or constricting bandage is often indicative of tissue ischemia or a pressure point which should be investigated and decompressed immediately. Severe pain which gradually decreases to no pain at all may be a bad sign, because once compressed tissues begin to necrose, they become relatively insensitive. A large and deep "pressure sore" may then develop silently and remain unrecognized until exudate seeps through and stains the plaster or becomes malodorous.

The patient with a cast should be given advice concerning elevation of the injured part and detailed instructions in finger or toe exercises to be carried out for short periods at frequent intervals. For injuries to the hand, forearm and elbow, it may be useful to instruct the patient to keep the arm and forearm elevated by holding it up with the opposite hand rather than carrying it dependent in a sling for the first few days.

The patient should be reexamined the day after reduction and the splints or casts checked for comfort, efficiency, and absence of constriction or unwanted pressure. From time to time, until tissue swelling is past its peak, plaster splints may have to be rebandaged.

If there is any suggestion of excessive tissue swelling or pressure, circular casts should be split longitudinally down to skin and spread to decompress the tissues. As the tissue swelling recedes with time, the split cast can be rebandaged more securely or replaced.

Circumferential casts can also be a cause of compartment syndrome. In such a situation, the extremity should not be elevated because it further reduces tissue perfusion. If a compartment syndrome is suspected, the cast should be immediately removed, and a thorough neurovascular examination performed. If the pain and swelling persist, direct tissue pressure measure-ments are indicated, and the patient may require a fasciotomy.

SPECIFIC INJURIES

Spine (See Chapter 11)

Shoulder Girdle

SCAPULA

> **PITFALL** ⊘
>
> *Failure to look carefully for intrathoracic injuries in patients with a fractured scapula.*

Fractures of the scapula usually require great force and are generally of relatively little significance compared to the damage to underlying ribs and thoracic viscera. Displacement of fracture fragments is usually minimal because the powerful muscles attached to the scapula tend to hold the fragments in place.

The fractures themselves can usually be treated symptomatically with a "sling-and-swath" for a few days, followed by early motion of the arm in a sling so that a frozen shoulder does not result. Fractures of the neck of the scapula and fractures extending into the glenoid fossa should be treated as shoulder injuries. If the displacement is minimal, simple partial immobilization is all that is needed. If there is marked displacement or comminution into the joint, open reduction may be required.

CLAVICLE

Fractures of the clavicle may occur with direct or indirect trauma. These occur most frequently in the middle third and allow the shoulder to drop downward, forward and inward. Sling application is suggested for all age groups until range of motion of the shoulder is painless. A figure-of-eight dressing is popular for use in children; however, these bandages seldom reduce the overriding fragments, and the use of a sling is more hygienic.[6] In bedridden patients, a rolled towel placed vertically between the shoulders may relieve discomfort from these injuries. In children, healing is usually accomplished in 3-4 weeks, whereas in adults it may take 6-12 weeks. Indications for operative treatment of clavicular fractures are few, and include associated injuries to the subclavian artery or brachial plexus, open injuries, and closed fractures with marked displacement which interferes with the integrity of the skin.

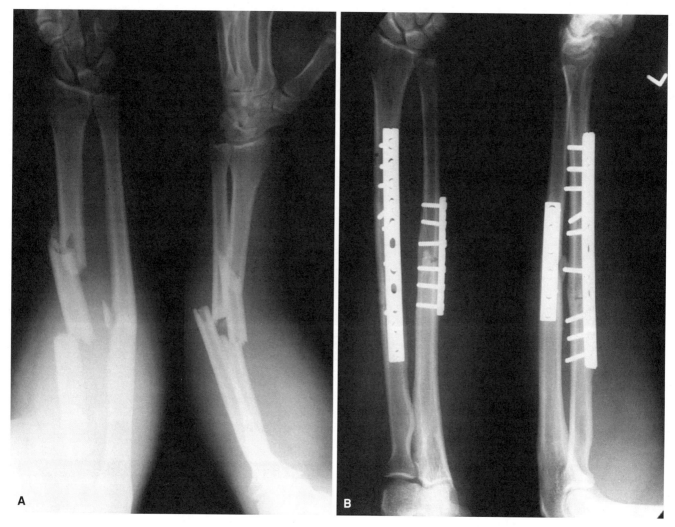

FIGURE 31–1   A. Displaced both bone forearm fracture in an adult. **B.** This injury is best treated with open reduction and internal fixation. Both the radius and ulna have been plated in this patient.

DISLOCATION OF THE STERNOCLAVICULAR JOINT

These injuries are frequently missed during the initial evaluation of patients with multiple injuries because they are so uncommon. Pain, tenderness and asymmetry over the sterno-clavicular joint should alert one to this injury; however, a radiographic diagnosis is often difficult to make. The dislocation may be anterior or posterior, and computed tomography (CT) scanning can be very helpful in making an accurate diagnosis.[57]

Posterior dislocations are managed by closed reduction, frequently under general anesthesia. Sling immobilization is the preferred post-treatment.[14] Closed reduction must be performed with care because of the proximity of large vessels immediately posterior to the sternoclavicular joints. Anterior dislocations can be managed conservatively. In general, open reduction and internal fixation of these injuries is not indicated, and the use of pins in these locations has been associated with numerous complications.[58]

ACROMIOCLAVICULAR SEPARATIONS

Acromioclavicular separations or dislocations are often associated with athletic or industrial accidents and result from a direct blow to the shoulder or a fall on the point of the shoulder. The extent of this injury may range from a slight subluxation, with only a tear of the acromioclavicular capsule, to a complete dislocation, with complete tearing of the coracoclavicular ligaments and stripping

of the deltoid and trapezius muscles from the outer third of the clavicle.

The patient will be tender directly over the acromioclavicular joint, and the outer third of the clavicle may be prominent on physical examination. A radiograph of the shoulder may not demonstrate the injury clearly because the acromioclavicular joint may be underpenetrated. Therefore, specific acromioclavicular views are usually required.

A grade I separation of the acromioclavicular joint is one in which tenderness to palpation is present but no radiographic abnormalities are seen. Grade II injuries are subluxations, and grade III injuries represent a true dislocation of the acromioclavicular joint and disruption of the coracoclavicular ligaments with obvious gross deformity on physical examination. With grade IV injuries, the distal clavicle is dislocated posteriorly and embedded in the trapezius. Grade V injuries involve a more marked version of the grade III injury with the distal clavicle lying subcutaneously. Grade VI injuries are inferior dislocations and are very rare.[59]

Treatment of grade I and II acromioclavicular separations is immobilization in a sling, until the patient is asymptomatic (1 or 2 weeks). Initial treatment of grade III injuries is also immobilization in a sling. Surgery for these injuries is controversial, as the results of operative treatment have not always been superior to conservative management. Surgical intervention, however, is indicated for gradeIV, V and VI injuries.

DISLOCATIONS OF THE SHOULDER

Dislocation of the glenohumeral joint is the most common dislocation of a major joint. They are usually due to forced abduction and external rotation of the arm until the humeral head is levered downward out of the glenoid cavity. After it has torn through the inferior portion of the capsule of the shoulder joint, the head of the humerus usually is located anteriorly beneath the coracoid process (subcoracoid dislocation). In one series, up to 98% of all traumatic shoulder dislocations were in an anterior direction.[60] Dislocation with the head of the humerus lying behind the glenoid (posterior or subspinous dislocation) is much less common and is most likely to occur with seizure disorders or in alcoholics. A third type, subglenoid dislocation, is quite rare. After anterior shoulder dislocation, the acromion is prominent and there is a visible and palpable absence of the subacromial fullness normally produced by the head of the humerus. The long axis of the arm points to the base of the neck. Pain is severe and little movement of the shoulder is possible. The displaced humeral head may be palpated deep to the pectoral mass. The elbow cannot be made to touch the side and the hand cannot be placed on the opposite shoulder unless there is an associated fracture of the humerus.

While these signs often permit accurate clinical diagnosis, one should generally obtain a prereduction radiograph to rule out complicating fractures. Three views, the so-called shoulder trauma series, are recommended: an anteroposterior and lateral (Y) view in the plane of the scapula, and an axillary view.[61]

Damage to the axillary nerve by the humeral head as it leaves the shoulder joint occurs in as many as 15% of dislocations. The nerve injury can cause anesthesia over the outer shoulder and paralysis of the deltoid muscle. Fortunately, this usually represents a traction injury, so that spontaneous recovery may be anticipated.

Occasionally, signs of trauma to the axillary vessels and large nerves of the brachial plexus are present. The motor and sensory nerve deficits may be expected to disappear spontaneously, but if signs of impaired arterial flow are present, immediate angiography is indicated. If an abnormality is found, the axillary artery should be repaired as soon as possible, particularly if the hand is ischemic.

Reduction of the dislocation can usually be accomplished using only intravenous analgesia. General anesthesia makes the reduction easier and minimizes the risk of producing a fracture of the surgical neck of the humerus or further soft tissue damage, and may sometimes be needed if reduction under sedation is unsuccessful. Recently, intraarticular injection of lidocaine has been proposed as an effective anesthetic method for reducing anterior shoulder dislocations.[62]

Techniques for shoulder reduction typically involve either traction or leverage. Leverage or manipulative techniques are associated with an increased incidence of complications, especially neurovascular injury and fracture. Therefore, they generally are not recommended. Traction techniques often involve traction-counter-traction methods using two sheets.[61] Gravity reduction with the patient lying prone can be attempted, although this is sometimes difficult due to patient discomfort. Numerous other shoulder reduction techniques are described in the literature.[61]

Once the shoulder dislocation has been reduced, it is typically immobilized in a sling. Pendulum exercises can be started when the patient is comfortable, but external rotation should be avoided, as it can lead to re-dislocation. The primary risk factor for repeat dislocation is the age of the patient, with younger patients having higher recurrence rates. The length of time the shoulder should be immobilized is controversial, with 4-6 weeks often recommended in young patients. In individuals over 35 years of age, the risk of recurrence is much less. Shorter periods of immobilization, with early range of motion exercises should be employed in elderly patients to prevent shoulder stiffness.

Recurrent shoulder dislocation may require late operative repair. The personality of the patient, as well as etiology, direction and nature of the dislocation must first be determined. For example, posttraumatic, involuntary, anterior dislocations in young, motivated patients respond well to surgical repair of the anterior structures.[63] In contrast, voluntary or atraumatic, multidirectional dislocations are less well suited to surgical intervention.

Arm and Forearm

FRACTURES OF THE PROXIMAL HUMERUS

Fractures of the proximal end of the humerus usually result from a fall on the outstretched hand or elbow in elderly individuals. The majority of these fractures involving the anatomic or surgical neck are impacted. With almost all impacted cases, the position of the fragments should be accepted, and efforts to disengage the fragments and improve their position are not recommended. Better and more prompt functional results will usually be obtained by accepting the position of impaction and beginning early motion.

Pain can often be alleviated by supporting the extremity in a sling, with or without a swathe, for a few days. Relaxed circumduction or pendulum exercises in and out of the sling should be initiated less than a week after injury and carried out energetically during the entire course of treatment. Unimpacted fractures of the proximal end of the humerus in satisfactory position are managed similarly.

Fractures of the proximal humerus may involve four major component fragments: the humeral head, shaft, and greater and lesser tuberosities.[64] Unstable fractures in which there is complete displacement between the head and shaft fragments may require operative intervention, especially if there is more than 1 cm of displacement of the tuberosity fragment or more than 45° of angulation the humeral head. Three-part and four-part fractures, or fracture-dislocations (head, shaft and one or more tuberosities) usually require operative treatment. Plates and screws can occasionally be used in young patients, but current trends are toward tension band wiring.[65] Four-part fractures are at high risk for both nonunion and avascular necrosis and may require prosthetic replacement of the humeral head, especially in elderly patients.

FRACTURES OF THE GREATER TUBEROSITY

Isolated fractures of the greater tuberosity of the humerus are not uncommon. They may occur after a fall on the point of the shoulder or forcible abduction so that the greater tuberosity impinges on the acromion. They are often associated with shoulder dislocation, and most reduce with reduction of the dislocation. Undisplaced or minimally displaced fractures require only a sling for comfort and early active exercises. However, if there is upward displacement of the tuberosity more than 1 cm, open reduction and internal fixation of the fragment may be indicated.[66]

FRACTURES OF THE SHAFT OF THE HUMERUS

The humeral shaft extends from about two inches below the shoulder to about two inches above the elbow. Fractures of the humeral shaft may be caused by a direct blow, excessive torsion, or undue leverage on the arm when the shoulder is relatively fixed.

Several strong muscles tend to cause obvious displacement and angulation of fractures of the humeral shaft. The pectoralis major muscle adducts, and the deltoid muscle abducts the fragments to which they are attached. The forearm muscles may also cause angulation of the lower fragment.

The radial nerve in the spiral groove of the humerus is particularly susceptible to injury by fractures of the shaft. As in all extremity injuries, the physician must determine at the first examination whether any deficit in the sensory or motor function of the major peripheral nerve trunks is present. If the nerve palsy was there prior to any manipulations, it will usually recover spontaneously over the course of 2-3 months. If recovery is not seen at that point, electromyographic (EMG) studies should be performed.

The majority of humeral shaft fractures respond to conservative management. Options include a sling, hanging arm cast, coaptation splints and functional braces. Early use of functional bracing allows movement of adjacent joints and has had a high success rate.[67] Indications for operative stabilization of humeral shaft fractures include radial nerve palsy that occurs after manipulation of a fracture, polytrauma, vascular injury, open fracture, ipsilateral forearm or articular injury, and pathologic fracture.

FRACTURES OF THE LOWER END OF THE HUMERUS

Transverse Supracondylar Fractures
Supracondylar fractures of the humerus occur most often in children and usually result from a fall on an extended, outstretched arm, resulting in posterior displacement of the distal fragment. The patient usually has a grossly swollen elbow shortly after injury. Because there is a high association of injuries to the median, radial, or ulnar nerves or brachial artery with these fractures, it is important to carefully assess the neurovascular status of the arm prior to any manipulation. The brachial artery may also be trapped in the fracture site or even transected. Often, an absent pulse can be restored by extending the arm, but if this fails, arteriography should be considered. If arteriography cannot be obtained in a timely fashion, and the extremity is ischemic, prompt closed or open reduction of the fracture with internal fixation plus surgical exploration of the brachial artery is appropriate.

Since even slight malunion in the coronal plane can result in a significant elbow deformity (typically a cubitus varus or "gunstock" deformity), even minimally displaced fractures are often reduced under general anesthesia. In children, closed reduction followed by percutaneous pinning has the advantage of allowing for accurate reduction and obviates the need for an excessively flexed position postoperatively. Elbow flexion in children with supracondylar fractures of the humerus can lead to "Volkmann's" ischemic contracture which is an extremely serious complication. In general, severely displaced fractures about the elbow are treated with closed reduction and percutaneous pinning, but children can also be treated by various forms of skin or skeletal traction. Occasionally open reduction may be required.[68] In adults, true supracondylar fractures are rare. A satisfactory reduction of these fractures generally requires a formal open reduction with internal fixation. This may help prevent late complications, such as malunion, and will allow for early motion.

T-or Y-shaped Fractures of the Lower Humerus
These intercondylar or bicondylar fractures result from a blow or a fall directly on the elbow. Adults with this injury have a painful, swollen elbow and varying degrees of comminution in the distal humerus. Marked displacement is common. Satisfactory joint function cannot be expected unless the fragments are accurately reduced.

Even with extensive comminution, if the patient is young or middle-aged, open reduction and internal fixation with screws and plates is recommended to obtain the best possible result.[69] If the patient is elderly or the fracture is so badly comminuted that adequate reduction and fixation are impossible even with operation, continuous traction using a Kirschner wire through the olecranon with the arm elevated anteriorly may be preferable.

Condyle Fractures in Children
In children, fractures of the lateral condyle are not uncommon. Undisplaced fractures require only a plaster cast or posterior splint for a few weeks; however, careful follow-up is important because late displacement can occur. If adequate closed reduction of displaced fractures of either condyle cannot be obtained readily, open reduction and internal fixation are advisable.

Fractures of the Medial Epicondyle in Adults
Fractures of the medial epicondyle in the adult are rare. Generally they occur from a direct blow on the inner side of the elbow. Unless the fragment is widely displaced, the best treatment is support of the extremity in a sling for 7-10 days. If the fragment is widely displaced, operative fixation is done to reanchor the origin of the flexor muscles of the forearm.

Fractures of the Capitellum
These fractures usually involve the anterior half of the capitellum, and therefore the fragment is partly covered with articular cartilage. Frequently the line of fracture extends medially into the lateral aspect of the trochlear process. Options include excision of the fragments if they are small and extensively stripped of soft tissue, and open reduction and internal fixation for larger fragments.[70]

FRACTURES OF THE OLECRANON
Olecranon fractures usually result from falls or blows on the back of the elbow, but they occasionally occur because of a violent contraction of the triceps muscle. On physical examination there is local pain and swelling, and a defect along the olecranon can often be felt. The elbow joint tends to become filled with blood and may be quite painful. In undisplaced fractures, the extensor power of the elbow is not lost.

The best treatment of an undisplaced fracture of the olecranon is immobilization of the elbow in moderate extension with a posterior molded splint for 7-14 days. Thereafter, a sling may be substituted and removed frequently for active exercise. Full return of function may be anticipated.

When the fracture fragment is separated from the ulna, the fascial expansions of the triceps tendon are also usually torn on one or both sides, and the elbow cannot be extended actively against gravity. Therefore, displaced olecranon fractures are reduced anatomically and fixed internally. If the fragment is comminuted or cannot be reduced, it can be excised and the triceps mechanism can be reattached more distally on the ulna.

DISLOCATIONS OF THE ELBOW
Elbow dislocations occur from a fall on the outstretched hand with the elbow extended. With posterior dislocations, the upper radius and ulna are displaced posteriorly and laterally. The coronoid process may be fractured or intact depending upon the angle of the elbow at the time of injury. Anterior dislocations do not occur without an accompanying fracture of the olecranon.

Loss of length of the extremity and painful motion at the elbow, with deformity, are hallmarks of a posterior dislocation. Although an obvious deformity at the elbow is apparent early, later swelling may obliterate the deformity. Circulation and nerve function should be checked and recorded before reduction is attempted. Radiographs, including oblique views, should be taken to rule out fractures, particularly of the radial head.

After careful assessment of the neurovascular status of the hand, reduction should be attempted. This can sometimes be accomplished without formal sedation, but intravenous sedation, relaxants, or general anesthesia are often needed. Reduction can generally be accomplished by applying steady traction at the wrist while an assistant provides counter-traction to the arm. After traction has led to some relaxation, the forearm is levered medially (as needed) and forward. If the reduction is not complete, it is impossible to flex the elbow freely.

Radiographs should be made immediately to verify reduction, and there should be frequent careful checks on the circulation. Since a great amount of swelling usually occurs with this injury, vascular complications due to compression of the vessels must be watched for closely.

The elbow should not be immobilized for longer than 7-10 days at about 90° in a posterior molded splint and sling. Thereafter, only a sling is required. Some even advocate a sling immediately postreduction if the elbow is stable. Longer periods of immobilization can lead to loss of joint motion. Active flexion exercises should be carried out daily. Early, forceful passive manipulation in an effort to increase the range of motion is contraindicated, as it can further damage the elbow, risk redislocation, and cause heterotopic ossification.

FRACTURE-DISLOCATION OF THE ELBOW
Dislocation of the ulna with an associated fracture or dislocation of the head of the radius can be a devastating injury and may severely

compromise function of the elbow. Patients with these injuries have an extremely painful and swollen elbow. After careful assessment of the neurovascular status, reduction can usually be accomplished by application of longitudinal traction under regional or general anesthesia. The fracture of the head of the radius may be treated nonoperatively, excised, internally fixed or replaced with a silastic implant depending on the anatomy of the fracture. Even with optimal treatment of fracture-dislocations of the elbow, loss of motion of the joint is frequent.

FRACTURE OF THE HEAD OF THE RADIUS
Radial head fractures are usually caused when an adult falls on an outstretched hand. Clinically, a fracture of the radial head should be suspected if there is localized tenderness, and restricted supination. The joint may also be distended with blood, producing considerable pain. However, the injury can often be missed even with careful evaluation. Because of the difficulty in making an radiographic diagnosis if there is an undisplaced fracture, two oblique views should be obtained in addition to an AP and lateral views. A posterior fat pad sign indicates intraarticular swelling and can be present when there are nondisplaced fractures about the elbow, such as radial head fractures.

If a fracture is not seen, treatment may include aspiration of the elbow joint and rest in a sling for about 48 hours followed by gradually increasing active exercises. Radiographs made 2-3 weeks later may then demonstrate a fracture line.

With minimal displacement of the fracture fragments or with a fragment of less than one third of the articular surface of the proximal radius, a brief period of immobilization in a sling or posterior splint is usually all that is indicated. This should be followed by active range of motion exercises of the elbow, which will generally lead to satisfactory results.

If the fracture of the radial head involves more than a third of the articular surface, if there is significant comminution, or a block to pronation and supination is present, then excision may be indicated. Insertion of a silastic radial head spacer is an alternative that may prevent late proximal translation of the radius. Certain radial head fractures may be amenable to open reduction and internal fixation.

FRACTURES OF THE FOREARM

Monteggia Fracture
In 1814 Monteggia described this fracture, which involves the ulnar shaft plus a dislocation of the head of the radius. These are usually due to direct trauma. The forearm is painful and swollen after a fall on the outstretched extremity. If angulation or overriding is present, the ulna is shortened and, consequently, the radial head will tend to dislocate in the direction of the apex of the angular deformity of the ulna. The radial head usually dislocates anteriorly, but can also dislocate laterally or posteriorly. If the radial head subluxes posteriorly, a fracture of the anterior lip of the radial head is common.

PITFALL ⊘

> *Failure to examine the elbow carefully in all fractures of the shaft of the ulna.*

When a fracture of the ulna is suspected, radiographs must include the elbow joint in order to ascertain the position of the radial head. On a lateral radiograph, an imaginary line drawn down the shaft of the proximal radius should pass through the middle of the capitellum if the elbow is properly reduced.

Monteggia fractures in children are best treated by closed reduction of the ulna. The radial head dislocation will usually reduce spontaneously with reduction of the ulnar fracture. Reduction is accomplished by full forearm supination, followed by elbow flexion of 90° or more. The arm is then casted or splinted in this position.

In adults, closed reductions of the ulna are unlikely to prevent redislocation of the radial head. The preferable treatment is open reduction of the ulnar fracture by plating to provide rigid fixation. Reduction of the ulna usually leads to reduction of the head of the radius.

If the dislocated radial head cannot be reduced through closed techniques, an open reduction may be required.

Isolated Fractures of the Shaft of the Ulna
Isolated fractures of the shaft of the ulna are usually the result of a direct blow to the forearm and are sometimes referred to as "nightstick fractures." There is usually localized pain and swelling over the fracture but little deformity. Fractures of the shaft of the ulna without a complicating fracture or dislocation of the radius are usually undisplaced or minimally displaced.

In the past, treatment of an isolated ulnar shaft fracture involved immobilization in a short or long arm cast. Nonunion was not rare. Increasingly, these fractures are now being treated with brief periods of short arm splinting or functional bracing, which lead to union in several months.[71] Fractures that are significantly displaced may still require internal fixation.

FRACTURE OF THE SHAFT OF THE RADIUS
Solitary nondisplaced or minimal fractures of the shaft of the radius are usually a result of direct trauma or a fall on an outstretched arm. Local tenderness, deformity, or swelling is usually present in the area of injury, which is most commonly the junction of the middle and distal thirds of the radial shaft. However, there is almost always an associated distal radioulnar joint injury with significantly displaced radius fractures if the ulna is intact. Therefore careful examination of the wrist is necessary. Galeazzi's fracture is the eponym used for a radial shaft fracture combined with dorsal or volar dislocation of the distal ulna. Although closed reduction can be attempted, open reduction and internal fixation of the radius is almost always required in order to obtain a satisfactory outcome. The radius is typically plated, and the distal radioulnar joint disruption can be treated by closed reduction and casting or pinning.

COMBINED FRACTURES OF THE SHAFTS OF THE RADIUS AND ULNA
Fracture of both bones of the forearm is a high-energy injury that may occur secondary to direct or twisting trauma. The forearm usually will have an obvious angular deformity with associated tenderness and swelling. Radiographically, one may see a transverse fracture of the radius and the ulna at the same level or oblique fractures at disparate levels.

In children, one or both of the fractures may be incomplete (greenstick). If a greenstick fracture is present, completion of the fracture is sometimes required to prevent recurrent angular deformity after closed reduction. Children are usually treated by closed reduction and casting. Careful early follow-up is required because the reduction can shift in the cast and require remanipulation and repeat casting.

In adults, the treatment of displaced radius and ulna fractures is operative with internal fixation for the best functional results (Fig. 31–1). Supplementary bone grafting at the time of open reduction and internal fixation may be indicated if the fractures are comminuted.

AXIOM   Anatomic reduction and fixation of both bone fractures of the forearm is needed to maintain the interosseus space to allow normal pronation and supination.

Fractures and Dislocations about the Wrist

FRACTURES OF THE DISTAL RADIUS
Fractures of the distal radius are the most frequent fractures of the upper extremity. They may be associated with a fracture of the ulnar styloid or distal end of the ulnar shaft. Even if a fracture of the ulna is not present, the ulnar collateral ligament is often injured. Eponyms such as Colles', Smith's or Barton's fracture continue to be commonly used to denote specific fracture patterns. Numerous classification systems have been described and are in use for these fractures. Recently a comprehensive classification has also been proposed by the AO group.[10]

Closed reduction by manipulation is the initial method by which displaced distal radius fractures are managed. Several important radiographic landmarks should be evaluated.[72] These include the palmar slope of the distal radius on the lateral radiograph (average 11-12°), the radial inclination on the anteroposterior radiograph (the line from the tip of the radial styloid to the ulnar border of the articular surface, average 22-23°), radial length (the perpendicular distance from the tip of the radial styloid to the distal articular surface of the ulna, average 11 to 12 mm), and the radial width (distance between the longitudinal axis through the center of the radius and the lateral tip of the radial styloid). For any given fracture these parameters can be compared to the contralateral uninjured side.

Once a reduction is achieved, closed management in a cast for 5-6 weeks is necessary. The so-called Cotton-Loder position of the wrist in a cast (extreme flexion) has led to complications of median nerve compression and digital stiffness and should not be used.

For widely displaced fractures, or fractures at risk for loss of fixation in a cast, percutaneous fixation of the distal fragment is an option. Another option for comminuted or open fractures is external fixation across the wrist from the radius to the metacarpals. Anatomic reduction of any intraarticular extension into the distal radius is important, especially in young, active patients.[73] If it cannot be achieved by the above methods, open reduction may be required.

AXIOM   With all wrist fractures, exercise of the fingers to maintain range of motion throughout the period of immobilization is extremely important.

FRACTURES OF THE CARPUS

The most important and common fracture of the carpus is that of the carpal navicular (scaphoid). Fractures involving the other carpal bones are much less common. Scaphoid fractures often occur in young adult males. The scaphoid usually has a precarious blood supply which enters the bone distally. When a displaced fracture is sustained across the waist or proximal pole of the scaphoid, the proximal fragment loses most of its blood supply so that it may develop avascular necrosis.

The diagnosis of a scaphoid fracture can be very difficult. Clinically, there is pain and swelling in the wrist with moderate-to-severe tenderness in the anatomic snuff box. In such an instance, added radiographs, in addition to the usual anteroposterior and lateral views (i.e., oblique or ulnar deviation projection) may be required to see the fracture. Some fractures will not be visible on any initial radiographs.

AXIOM   A "wrist sprain" which does not resolve quickly may represent a scaphoid fracture.

In some instances the fracture line in the scaphoid is not visible until 10-14 days after injury when enough bone resorption has occurred on either side of the fracture. If a diagnosis of a sprain is made originally, good practice calls for plaster immobilization for 10-14 days and then repeat roentgenograms after the cast is removed.

As a rule, when the fracture is nondisplaced, treatment is by immobilization in a long- or short-arm thumb spica cast. Initial long-arm immobilization may be beneficial.[74] If the fragments are displaced, then surgical intervention is generally required.

AXIOM   The majority of nondisplaced scaphoid fractures will unite if the fragments are properly immobilized for a long enough period.

Immobilization for 3 months and sometimes longer may be required for fracture union. Some orthopedic surgeons feel that if progress toward healing is not evident by 6-10 weeks, open reduction and bone grafting may significantly speed union (Fig. 31–2).

Even if avascular necrosis of the proximal fragment occurs, union of the fracture may still be possible with prolonged immobilization. However, nonunion is common, and posttraumatic arthritis of the wrist joint is the end result. Once this occurs, late salvage procedures may be needed to restore a painless and functional wrist.

DISLOCATIONS OF THE CARPUS

Dislocations of the wrist result primarily from forced hyperextension of the hand. Although one can often determine clinically that a significant wrist injury has occurred, the exact diagnosis is made only by radiographic examination. Anteroposterior and lateral views usually are sufficient, but oblique views and films of the normal uninjured wrist may be helpful.

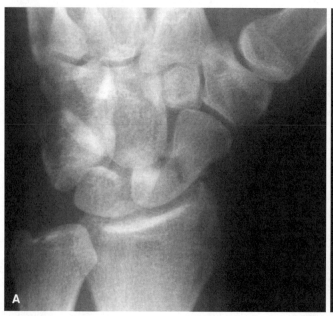 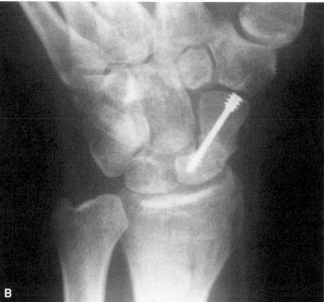

FIGURE 31–2 **A.** This patient had a painful scaphoid non-union that did not heal with immobilization. **B.** Treatment with open bone grafting and internal fixation.

Dislocation of the Lunate

When the lunate dislocates, its dorsal ligamentous attachments are torn, causing it to rotate and be extruded anteriorly so that it lies deep to the flexor tendons and the volar carpal ligament. Its only remaining ligamentous attachment is to the anterior lip of the radius. Median nerve hyperesthesia and impaired finger flexion may occur as a result of impingement of the dislocated bone on the nerve and tendons.

On the lateral radiograph the dislocated lunate does not articulate with the radius as it normally does, and it is displaced anteriorly. The capitate appears to articulate with the radius. In the AP view, the dislocated lunate appears elongated and square rather than its usual round shape.

Closed reduction, should be attempted as soon as possible. Reduction should be confirmed by radiographic examination before application of the cast. Percutaneous pin fixation, in addition to cast treatment, is also an option.

If efforts at closed reduction are not successful or do not yield a satisfactory radiographic appearance, open reduction is indicated. A high incidence of avascular necrosis is associated with this injury.

Perilunate Dislocation

The term perilunate dislocation represents a radiographic picture in which the lunate retains its normal relationship with the radius but the remaining carpal bones are displaced. It is treated in the same manner as lunate dislocation. However, there is a high association with scaphoid fracture, hence the term "trans-scaphoid, perilunate, fracture dislocation." In this situation the injury is treated operatively with open reduction and internal fixation of the scaphoid plus stabilization of the rest of the carpus in an anatomic position.

Midcarpal Dislocation

As the hand is forcibly hyperextended, the distal row of carpal bones may be dislocated dorsally on the proximal row. The correct diagnosis is frequently missed, because the relationships of the carpal bones are often not clearly seen on the lateral view. This is a serious injury which can result in severe permanent limitation of hand function, particularly if it is not reduced promptly.

Early closed reduction under anesthesia is usually feasible. Reduction is best maintained by immobilization in a plaster cast with the hand in slight palmar flexion for a period of 3 or 4 weeks. If efforts at closed reduction are unsuccessful, early open reduction is indicated.

Fractures of the Pelvis (See Chapter 28)

Fractures and Dislocations about the Hip

HIP FRACTURES

Fractures about the hip comprise the single largest group of serious fractures in elderly patients. The incidence of these fractures appears to be increasing. They usually occur after a fall, which is often provoked by one of the patient's medical problems. Not infrequently, however, a patient will have the sensation that the hip broke because of a misstep or stumble before the actual fall occurred.

The dominant complaint is severe pain in the hip, but in some instances the pain is referred to the knee. The injured lower extremity typically appears shortened and falls into external rotation. Radiographs in two planes are necessary to confirm and identify the type of the fracture. A satisfactory lateral roentgenogram is not obtained easily, but it is essential for adequate fracture assessment.

High mortality rates have been associated with hip fractures. These patients tend to have a significant number of complications, including progression of cardiovascular and renal disease, pneumonia, and pulmonary embolism. Mortality in trochanteric fractures is higher than with intracapsular fractures (30% versus 15%), even though fractures of the trochanteric region almost always unite and fractures of the femoral neck often result in nonunion.

Hip fractures in the elderly, even if the patient survives, usually results in a drastic lifestyle change for the patient and his or her family.[75] It often signals the end of that person's independent life and the beginning of some form of institutionalization.

Fractures of the Neck of the Femur

Intracapsular fractures of the hip have been called "the unsolved fractures" because they often result in nonunion and vascular necrosis. The blood supply to the femoral head comes primarily from small vessels on the femoral neck, and it is easily disrupted when a displaced fracture occurs.

Several classification systems exist for femoral neck fractures, but they can be broadly divided into minimally displaced or impacted fractures versus displaced fractures.

NONDISPLACED, MINIMALLY DISPLACED, OR IMPACTED FEMORAL NECK FRACTURES. The prognosis for these fractures is generally good. Nonoperative treatment may be an option in some settings. Generally, however, internal fixation with multiple pins or screws is recommended. This lessens the possibility of further displacement.

DISPLACED FEMORAL NECK FRACTURES. Almost all of these fractures are treated operatively unless the patient is nonambulatory. In younger patients, early anatomic reduction by closed or open means, followed by multiple pin or screw fixation, is mandatory. The complication rates of nonunion and avascular necrosis remain high (Fig. 31–3). In older patients, excision of the femoral head and prosthetic hemiarthroplasty replacement is another treatment option (Fig. 31–4).

> **AXIOM** As a general rule, the earlier a fractured hip is stabilized, the less likely the patient is to develop cardiopulmonary complications.

Although patients with fractures of the femoral neck are often relatively poor surgical risks, early internal fixation may greatly reduce hospital morbidity and mortality rates. However, appropriate preoperative medical evaluation is mandatory.

Intertrochanteric Fractures of the Femur

The fragments in intertrochanteric (IT) fractures have an excellent blood supply and almost always unite. The high mortality rate with these fractures is due to the advanced age (70-85 years) of these patients and their preexisting cardiopulmonary dysfunction. In addition, these patients can lose a considerable amount of blood at the fracture site. It is estimated that about a liter is lost into the tissues with most IT fractures, and more blood is lost during operative fixation of IT fractures than occurs with operation for fractures of the femoral neck.

Most IT fractures should be treated by internal fixation. Although different operative techniques are available, the sliding hip screw is most commonly used (Fig. 31–5). To achieve a stable reduction, there should be good bony contact between the proximal and the distal fragment, especially posteromedially.

Subtrochanteric Fractures

Subtrochanteric fractures are less common than intertrochanteric or femoral neck fractures.[76] There are two distinct patient populations in whom these injuries occur. One is the younger age group, as a result of high-energy trauma, and the other is older individuals who may have fractures with relatively little trauma.

Controversy exists about the best means of fixation of these fractures. Most will unite after prolonged traction, but only younger patients will tolerate this form of treatment because it precludes early mobilization. Surgical treatment using interlocking nails with screws inserted into the femoral neck and head ("reconstruction nails") has shown great promise in these difficult fractures. Screws and sideplates, conventional intramedullary nails, flexible nails, and fixed angled blade plates (Fig. 31–6) have all been used to treat these difficult fractures.[76,77,78]

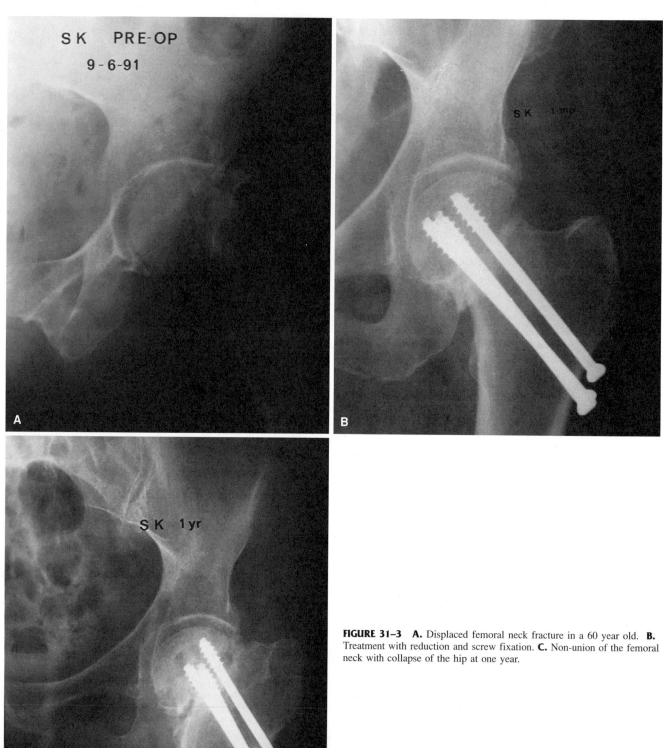

FIGURE 31–3   A. Displaced femoral neck fracture in a 60 year old. **B.** Treatment with reduction and screw fixation. **C.** Non-union of the femoral neck with collapse of the hip at one year.

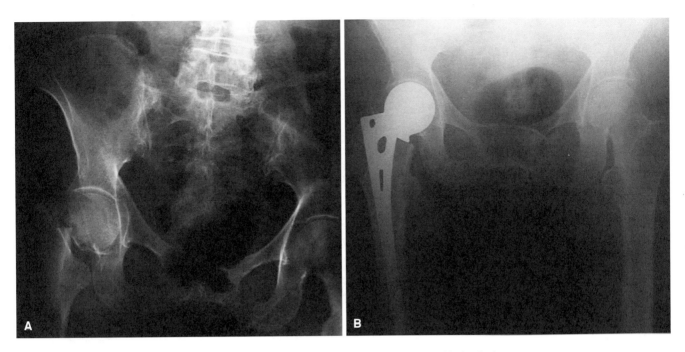

FIGURE 31–4 **A.** Eighty year old with displaced femoral neck fracture. **B.** Treatment with immediate hip hemiarthroplasty.

DISLOCATIONS OF THE HIP

Dislocations of the hip occur only with severe trauma. In the majority, approximately 90%, the head of the femur comes to rest posterior to the acetabulum. Posterior dislocations often have an associated fracture of the posterior acetabular wall or a portion of the femoral head. Anterior dislocations in which the femoral head comes to rest in front of the acetabulum are fairly rare and are less commonly associated with fractures. Avascular necrosis of the femoral head may be a late complication of hip dislocation.

> **AXIOM** Hip dislocations are orthopaedic emergencies, and should be reduced as soon as possible.

Posterior Dislocation of the Hip Without Fracture

Posterior dislocation of the hip is usually sustained while the thigh is flexed and adducted, as in an automobile collision when the knee strikes the dashboard. The posteriorly dislocated hip remains flexed, adducted and internally rotated, and the extremity appears shortened. The peroneal portion of the sciatic nerve may be injured by either the dislocated femoral head or a fragment of acetabulum, resulting in inability to dorsiflex the foot actively. Therefore, careful motor and sensory examination of the extremity should be made before reduction is attempted.

Reduction of a posterior dislocation of the hip must be done as soon as possible. This injury represents a true orthopaedic emergency. Studies have shown that if a dislocated hip is not reduced within 6-12 hours the rate of avascular necrosis increases significantly.[79] Gentle closed reduction under intravenous sedation or general anesthesia should be performed as soon as possible. If a closed reduction cannot be achieved, an open reduction must be performed.

After reduction, a gentle examination should be done to ensure that the hip is stable from 0-90° of flexion. Radiographs should confirm a concentric reduction of the high joint. A nonconcentric reduction may represent fracture debris trapped inside the hip joint. There is a very high incidence of osteochondral fractures with hip dislocations (Fig. 31–7), and significant intraarticular fragments are an indication for open reduction. Therefore, many surgeons routinely use computerized tomography to look for this after the initial emergency closed reduction has been accomplished. Any associated posterior acetabular wall fracture can also be more fully evaluated in this manner.

Management protocols after reduction vary greatly from prolonged traction to early mobilization. The prognosis after hip dislocations is variable. Patients with high energy injuries and prolonged time to reduction generally have a poorer prognosis. Major complications include neurovascular injures, avascular necrosis and posttraumatic arthritis.

Posterior Dislocations of the Hip with Fractures of the Acetabulum

Fracture of the posterior portion of the acetabulum frequently complicates a posterior dislocation of the hip.[80] Reduction of the hip can usually be achieved by traction in the long axis of the thigh. A defect in the posterior acetabular well may allow the hip to repeatedly dislocate or subluxate. While there is no consensus on how large the posterior wall fragment must be before surgery is required, large fragments should be reduced and fixed. Computerized tomography of the hip is especially helpful in evaluating this area.[81,82]

Anterior Dislocation of the Hip

Anterior dislocation of the hip is uncommon, but it may occur when the thigh is forced into extreme abduction and external rotation. The head of the femur usually comes to rest in the obturator foramen. The extremity goes into abduction, external rotation, and some flexion, and appears longer than the uninjured limb. While the position of the extremity resembles that assumed with a fracture of the hip, it may be distinguished clinically because of the increased rather than decreased length and the mild flexion. Obliteration of the femoral pulse may accompany this injury, and prompt reduction is imperative under such circumstances.

Reduction of anterior dislocation of the hip can usually be achieved rather easily, often without anesthesia, by traction in the axis of the thigh, followed by internal rotation and adduction. Only a few days of bed rest (with avoidance of abduction, external rotation and hyperextension), followed by about 4 weeks on crutches are needed. Avascular necrosis of the femoral head is not as common following anterior dislocation of the hip, particularly if reduction is performed within a few hours of injury.

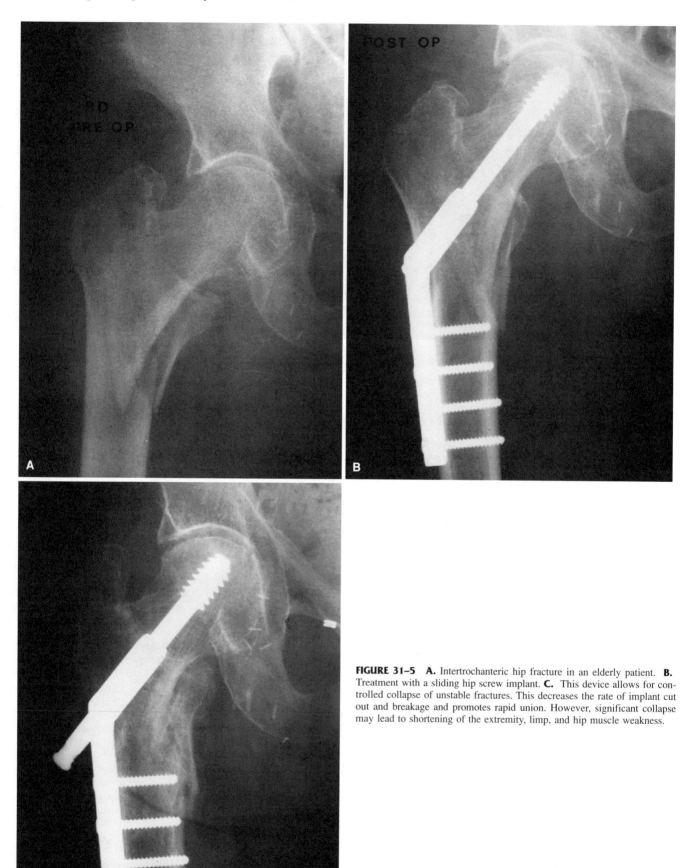

FIGURE 31–5 **A.** Intertrochanteric hip fracture in an elderly patient. **B.** Treatment with a sliding hip screw implant. **C.** This device allows for controlled collapse of unstable fractures. This decreases the rate of implant cut out and breakage and promotes rapid union. However, significant collapse may lead to shortening of the extremity, limp, and hip muscle weakness.

FIGURE 31–6 **A.** Subtrochanteric femur fracture. **B.** Treatment with fixed angle blade plate.

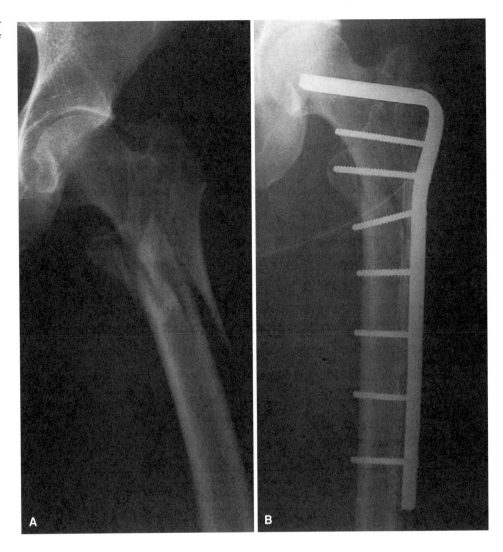

FRACTURES OF THE SHAFT OF THE FEMUR

The shaft of the femur extends distally from about 1 inch below the lesser trochanter to the supracondylar area. Its blood supply is good, and although powerful muscles attach to the femur and tend to cause angulation and overriding, nonunion is rare unless the fracture is not adequately reduced or immobilized.

Because considerable violence is required to break the femoral shaft, local blood loss exceeding 1.0-1.5 liters often accompanies this injury. In addition, the bone fragments can easily injure large adjacent blood vessels. As a consequence, a compartment syndrome of the thigh may occur.

Complete fractures of the femoral shaft are usually easily diagnosed because contracture of the powerful thigh muscles results in an obvious deformity with severe angulation and overriding.

> **AXIOM** If the knee or hip is not evaluated carefully in patients with femoral-shaft fractures, serious problems may not be appreciated until they are very difficult to treat.

Examination of the knee is extremely difficult when the shaft of the femur is fractured, not only because of the instability of the distal femur but also because of the pain. Consequently, associated knee injuries can easily be missed. In addition to antero-posterior and lateral radiographs of the femur, radiographs of the pelvis should be taken to rule out hip or pelvic involvement. If immediate surgical intervention is not undertaken, the patient is typically placed in skeletal traction with a femoral or tibial traction pin.

Femur fractures in children are most often treated closed with immediate or early hip spical casting. They can also be treated with skin or skeletal traction. Older children or adolescents can be treated with conventional reamed nailing or flexible nails.[83,84] External fixation has been less commonly used for stabilization of children's fractures, but can be used in certain settings, such as open fractures or polytrauma.

In adults, various treatment options are possible in the treatment of femoral shaft fractures, including skeletal traction and cast bracing. These, however, are not indicated for multiple trauma patients and are essentially obsolete. These fractures today are treated surgically to allow for early mobilization and better fracture alignment. A number of flexible nails, plates and screws, and external fixators have been described for treating these fractures, but closed, reamed intramedullary nailing is now the most commonly used technique.[85,86] Interlocking nails have expanded the indications for intramedullary nailing to include comminuted shaft fractures, and fractures from just distal to the lesser trochanter to just proximal to the condyles. Fractures of the distal shaft that do not involve the articular surface (infraisthmal fractures) are best treated with an interlocking, intramedullary nail. Closed intramedullary nailing, correctly done, has been shown to have a higher rate of success than any other method of treatment yet described for the majority of adult femoral fractures (Fig. 31–8).

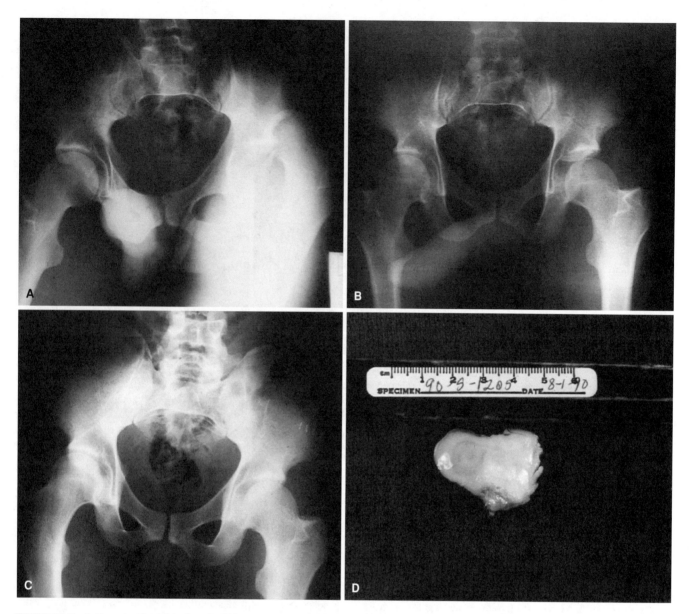

FIGURE 31–7   A. Posterior hip dislocation.   **B.** Closed reduction reveals nonconcentric reduction with bony fragment in hip joint.   **C.** Concentric reduction of the hip after arthrotomy for removal of intraarticular bone fragments.   **D.** Osteochondral fracture fragment from acetabulum removed from the hip joint.

Open femur fractures can be treated by debridement followed by intramedullary nailing.[87,88] The infection rates after grade I or II open fractures appear to be low.[89] In severe contaminated fractures (grade III, or in critically ill patients with extensive soft tissue injury), external fixation can be used.[90,91] This treatment modality carries with it the problems of pin tract infection and knee stiffness. There is no consensus as to the optimal treatment for grade III open femur fractures. In isolated injuries, debridement followed by traction and delayed nailing after the wounds are clean and closed is a reasonable option. In the polytrauma setting, where immediate fixation and mobilization are essential, either external fixation or nailing can be used. More complications can be expected with these injuries.[92]

Nonoperative treatment of femoral fractures should be reserved for children. Rarely, adults with skin lesions over the proposed incision site, very poor general medical condition, previous osteomyelitis, preexisting surgical implants, or highly comminuted and complex fracture patterns not easily amenable to internal fixation are managed by traction or a cast brace.

Injuries about the Knee

FRACTURES OF THE DISTAL END OF THE FEMUR

Displaced supracondylar fractures of the femur are best treated by reduction and internal fixation. This restores the anatomical alignment of the knee joint and allows for early motion. Blade plates or dynamic condylar screws are often used.[93,94] However, these fractures can sometimes be managed by intramedullary nailing if the technique is pushed to its limits.[95]

Displaced intracondylar fractures require an anatomic reduction of the joint surface. Any supracondylar component is then addressed. Postoperative management consists of early passive and active motion and delayed weight leaning until bony healing is present.

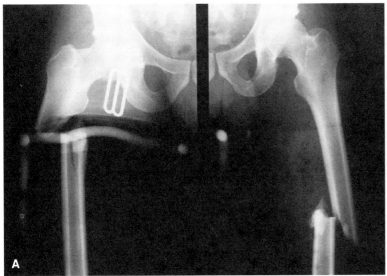

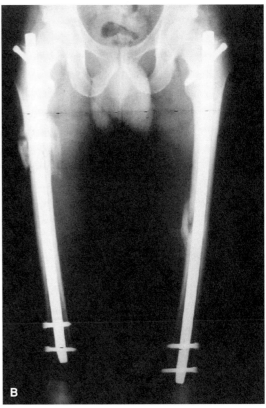

FIGURE 31–8 A. Bilateral femoral shaft fractures. **B.** Treatment with bilateral locked intramedullary nailing.

DISLOCATIONS ABOUT THE KNEE

Patellar Dislocations

Dislocations about the knee may occur either at the patellofemoral or at the tibiofemoral joint. Patellofemoral (patellar) dislocations are relatively common and may occur secondary to a congenital deformity, usually in adolescent girls, or as a result of relatively mild trauma to the knee from the side, usually with no other complications.[6]

Patellar dislocations are typically lateral and often occur during sudden straightening up from a squatting position. There is a palpable lateral deformity, and the knee cannot be actively extended. Reduction is accomplished by direct pressure over the deformity with the knee passively extended, followed by 4-6 weeks of immobilization. Spontaneous reduction before being seen by a physician is not uncommon. Postreduction radiographs should be carefully examined for the presence of osteochondral fractures which may need treatment. Recurrent dislocations may require surgical reconstruction.

Knee Dislocations

AXIOM Knee dislocations are orthopaedic emergencies. They require immediate reduction and assessment of the vascular status of the extremity.

Tibiofemoral (knee) dislocations are much less common but are associated with extensive ligamentous disruption and an increased incidence of severe neurologic and vascular injuries. They are caused by a combination of indirect forces to the knee during violent trauma. There is usually obvious deformity, and radiographs will confirm the dislocation. Dislocations of the knee may occasionally reduce spontaneously. In such instances, the only clues to the true nature of the injury may be the history, a gross instability of the knee, a hemarthrosis, and not infrequent neurovascular injury.

The classification of knee dislocations is based on the relationship of the tibia to the femur and the resultant forces applied to the knee. Hence, knee dislocations can be posterior, anterior, medial, lateral, or rotational. The majority are either anterior or posterior. For the knee to dislocate, both collateral ligaments and cruciate ligaments are often torn. In complete dislocation of the knee, the tibia is displaced so that it no longer articulates with the femur.

A complete dislocation of the knee represents a surgical emergency. It should be reduced immediately, and this is usually easily accomplished by traction and manipulation. Postreduction orthopaedic management may consist of either immobilization or early ligament repair.[96] Current trends have been toward early surgical intervention to repair the damaged ligaments.[97,98]

Complications of complete dislocation of the knee include damage to the popliteal artery and to the peroneal or posterior tibial nerves behind the knee. The peroneal nerve is injured in dislocation of the knee more often than the posterior tibial nerve. Although complete examination of motor and sensory nerve function of the lower leg and foot should be performed before and after any attempts at reduction, early exploration for a damaged peripheral nerve trunk is not indicated. If a major neurologic defect with no evidence of recovery persists for more than 6-12 weeks, surgery may be considered after appropriate electro-myography studies have been performed. The prognosis for recovery is poor, however, and bracing or tendon transfers are usually necessary.

The incidence of popliteal artery injury can be quite high (25-30%) and may include contusions, tears, or intimal flaps with or without thrombosis. Even if normal pedal pulses return following reduction, early arteriography is indicated to rule out a large intimal flap or other lesions that can result in thrombosis. If anything worse than a small intimal tear is found, the vascular injury should be repaired urgently. Once this has been completed, repair or reconstruction of the ligaments may be carried out immediately or up to 2 weeks after injury.[6]

AXIOM   An arteriogram of the knee should be considered in all patients with a knee dislocation.

INTERNAL DERANGEMENTS OF THE KNEE
Internal derangement of the knee is a poor but commonly used "wastebasket" term that refers to intraarticular meniscal or ligamentous injuries.

Meniscal Injuries
The medial and lateral menisci of the knee are relatively avascular structures that receive much of their nutrition from joint fluid. Only the outer rim near the joint capsule has a consistent blood supply. The menisci have an essential role in stress distribution across the knee joint; however, with certain twisting motions they can be torn. The medial meniscus is torn far more frequently than the lateral.

In the classic syndrome of a torn medial meniscus, which occurs in only a few patients, the patient gives a history of a twisting injury accompanied by a painful snapping sensation on the inner side of the knee. The knee joint is usually locked in slight flexion. In a truly locked knee, the leg cannot be extended completely because of a mechanical block, but it can be flexed fairly well. Pain persists and considerable effusion develops. Tenderness, which is fairly well localized, is found over the medial joint line. This clinical syndrome, however, occurs in only a small number of patients.

In the majority of instances, the diagnosis of a torn meniscus is made on the history of a twisting injury to the knee, and subsequent repeated episodes of painful, slipping, catching and near-locking sensations on the inner side of the knee. So that the medial meniscus can be evaluated specifically, the patient lies supine and the involved knee is fully flexed. The tibia is then externally rotated on the femur and the knee is slowly extended, and this tends to force the torn segment of meniscus into the joint. On extension of the knee, a pop or click may be heard and the patient may feel pain as the femur and tibia catch the torn fragment. To evaluate the lateral meniscus, the knee is flexed but the tibia is kept in internal rotation.

Physical examination, however, may not be completely reliable to diagnose meniscal injury, and confirmatory tests are sometimes needed. These may include noninvasive studies like CT scans or magnetic resonance imaging or invasive procedures such as diagnostic arthroscopy.[99,100,101]

AXIOM   The meniscus cartilages of the knee have a poor blood supply, and tears frequently do not heal.

The presence of a meniscal tear per se is not an indication of surgery. True mechanical locking, or chronic pain and effusion, should be present. Complete excision of a torn cartilage is to be avoided if possible, as it will lead to late degenerative arthritis. An arthroscopic partial meniscectomy, leaving a smooth and stable rim of cartilage, is generally performed. Occasionally a meniscal tear can be successfully repaired. This depends on the location and type of tear. A high rate of healing has been obtained only in tears near the meniscal rim, where the blood supply is much better than in the remainder of the meniscus.[102]

Torn Collateral Ligaments
Tears of the collateral ligaments result from varus or valgus forces on the extended knee. A tear of a collateral ligament of the knee on one side and fracture of the tibial plateau on the other side may result from the same trauma. Tears of the medial collateral ligament are much more common than those of the lateral collateral ligament.

Tears of the collateral ligaments are acutely painful and cause immediate disability. In all but minor injuries, the patient cannot tolerate weight-bearing. Pain and tenderness are localized over the torn collateral ligament, and a hemarthrosis can develop rapidly. Within

12-24 hours, the skin overlying the torn ligament is likely to become discolored from subcutaneous hemorrhage seeping toward the surface.

The diagnosis is confirmed on physical examination. The injured knee should be stressed in a varus and valgus direction in both the fully extended and a 30° flexed position. Any increased laxity should be compared with similar testing of the contralateral uninjured knee. Lack of a firm endpoint or gross instability often indicates complete ligament tears. The optimal time to examine the patient is immediately after the injury, before extreme pain, swelling and muscle spasm make the examination much more difficult. When that occurs, demonstration of increased laxity may require local or general anesthesia. Stress radiographs may document abnormal mobility and should be obtained when possible.

Many collateral ligament injuries can be treated by a hinged knee brace that provides for medial to lateral support but allows for knee motion. Good results have been reported with nonoperative treatment of medial collateral ligament tears.[103] Operative treatment may be considered for complete tears of the lateral ligament complex, or when multiple ligamentous injuries are present.

Torn Cruciate Ligaments
The anterior cruciate ligament runs from the posterior portion of the lateral femoral condyle to the anterior aspect of the tibial spines and prevents anterior displacement of the tibia on the femur. Conversely, the posterior cruciate ligament runs from the anterior aspect of medial femoral condyle to the posterior tibial spine and prevents posterior displacement of the tibia on the femur.

The cruciate ligaments are stretched or torn in injuries which cause excessive movement of the tibia on the femur in the anteroposterior direction. The anterior cruciate ligament, which limits hyperextension, is often torn in twisting hyperextension injuries. The posterior cruciate ligament, which prevents backwards displacement of the tibia on the femur, is torn when the upper portion of the flexed tibia is driven backward on the femur. The diagnosis of torn cruciate ligaments begins with the history. For example, the anterior cruciate is often torn as a result of a decelerating or hyperextension injury to the knee. There is typically an associated hemarthrosis. After any traumatic knee hemarthrosis, a cruciate ligament injury or osteochondral fracture should be suspected. In addition, after fixation of long bone fractures of the lower extremity, an examination of the knee should be performed to rule out an associated knee ligament injury.[104,105]

On physical exam, there is excessive movement of the tibia on the femur. For anterior cruciate tears, the most reliable test is the Lachman maneuver. It is performed with the knee flexed about 20° and the tibia directed straight ahead. The femur is held steady with one hand, while the other attempts to translate the tibia forward. Any excessive laxity is noted and can be compared with the other knee. Knees with torn anterior cruciate ligaments can also demonstrate rotational instability as gauged by a number of different "pivot shift" test. In the lateral pivot shift test, the knee is held in extension and gently rotated internally while a valgus stress with axial load is applied. This subluxes the knee. As the knee is then flexed, a reduction occurs that can be both visible and palpable. The so-called anterior drawer sign, in which the knee is flexed to 90° and anterior translation of the tibia on the femur is tested, is considered a much less reliable test for anterior cruciate insufficiency. The posterior drawer sign can be used to detect posterior cruciate ligament tears. This is performed with the knee flexed to 90°, looking for excessive posterior displacement of the tibia on the femur on manual testing.

In many instances, swelling and pain can make a good clinical evaluation impossible. An examination under anesthesia or an arthroscopic exam of the knee can than be considered. Magnetic resonance imaging is also emerging as a means for diagnosing ligamentous injuries to the knee.[100,101]

The treatment of anterior cruciate tears must be individualized. Primary repair of this ligament has not been shown to be successful. Thus, treatment is usually conservative or performed with surgical reconstruction. Older, low-demand patients may be treated without surgery in many cases, whereas younger, higher-demand or athletic patients often have surgical reconstruction. One should also be very wary of the "isolated" anterior cruciate tear. These injuries have a very high association with other knee injuries, especially meniscal tears.

Posterior cruciate ligament tears are more likely to be treated nonoperatively, if isolated, than anterior cruciate ligament injuries. However, surgical repair or reconstruction may be needed if multiple ligamentous injuries are present. Occasionally the posterior cruciate is avulsed with attached bony fragments from the posterior proximal tibia. This injury is an excellent indication for surgical intervention, as the ligament itself is intact and bony fixation restores knee stability.

Osteochondral Fractures

Osteochondral fractures are pieces of articular cartilage with accompanying subchondral bone that can be broken off inside the knee. They typically originate from the femoral condyles, but can also come from the patella, especially after patellar dislocations. An osteochondral fracture should be suspected in any patient with a traumatic knee hemarthrosis, and the radiographs should be examined carefully for any signs of bony fragments in the joint. Unrecognized osteochondral fractures can result in painful loose bodies inside the knee and severe post-traumatic arthritis. When loose bodies are detected in the knee joint, arthrotomy or arthroscopy is indicated. The fragments should either be fixed, if possible, or excised.

FRACTURES OF THE PATELLA

The patella is a large sesamoid bone in the extensor mechanism of the thigh at the knee. Fractures of the patella can occur indirectly from contracture of the quadriceps mechanism, or from a direct blow to the flexed knee. They are characterized clinically by a hemarthrosis, and when they are displaced there is a palpable defect and an inability to actively extend the knee. The radiographs show varying degrees of separation of the bony fragments. This indicates that the extensor mechanism of the knee has been disrupted.

If there is a patellar fracture without separation, aspiration of the hemarthrosis and a compression dressing and splinting is often all that is needed. The use of crutches for several weeks will usually serve as an adequate safeguard against sudden uncontrolled flexion at the knee. Undisplaced fracture of the patella may also be treated by short periods of casting in extension.

Fractures with separation require accurate open reduction and fixation, often with a tension band wiring technique and repair of the defects of the quadriceps expansion on both sides of the patella. A well fixed fracture allows for immediate active motion of the knee. If the fracture is extensively comminuted, a partial patellectomy[106] or complete patellectomy may be performed. Some loss of extensor strength can be expected after a complete patellectomy, and therefore this should be avoided if possible.

FRACTURES OF THE PROXIMAL END OF THE TIBIA

Fractures of the proximal tibia occur from a direct blow to the lateral side of the knee or to the foot, from hyperextension, or from an axial load.[6] There is usually massive hemarthrosis and deformity. Neurovascular injury may also occur and must be identified early. Detailed radiographs, tomograms, and/or CT scans are usually necessary to identify the configuration of the fracture.

The lines of fracture usually extend into the knee joint through articular cartilage. The objectives of management are to restore a smooth articular surface over the proximal tibia, to establish stability of the joint, and to reestablish the normal mechanical axis of the extremity. These fractures may be diagnosed only by adequate radiographic studies. In addition to plain radiographs, tomography or CT scans are often used to better define the intraarticular fracture.

Fractures of the Tibial Spine

An undisplaced fragment of the tibial spine (or one which drops into perfect position with moderate extension of the knee) requires merely aspiration of blood from the joint and a long leg plaster cast for 4 weeks. Displaced fragments usually require an open procedure to fix the fragment in perfect position.

Fractures of the Lateral Tibial Plateau

Fractures of the lateral tibial plateau result from force applied to the lateral side of an extended knee. This may be associated with a tear of the medial collateral ligament and/or the lateral meniscus. Large displaced fractures require open reduction and internal fixation. For certain depressed fractures, elevation of the tibial plateau and autologous bone grafting in addition to internal fixation may be required. Stable internal fixation should allow for immediate continuous passive motion and early active range of knee motion. Non-weight-bearing, progessing slowly to protected weight-bearing, is required for 2-3 months.

Fractures of the Medial Tibial Plateau

Medial tibial plateau fractures are much less common than those on the lateral side. These fractures usually result from forces applied to the medial side of an extended knee, and such trauma can also cause tears of the lateral collateral ligament. Treatment of these fractures is analogous to those of the lateral plateau. These fractures may have a worse prognosis, however, especially if associated with high energy trauma or a "fracture-dislocation" of the knee.

Fractures of the Tibial Shaft

Fractures of the shafts of the tibia and fibula are among the most common extremity injuries. They can result from direct trauma, such as impact with an automobile bumper, or from indirect trauma such as severe rotation or leverage strain caused by a person stepping into a deep hole while running. Because the tibia is entirely subcutaneous on its anterior and medial surfaces, open fractures of this bone are common.

Diagnosis of fractures of both the tibia and fibula are usually established easily by the clinical symptoms and signs. Adequate radiographs, however, help identify the characteristics of the fracture and are mandatory for definitive management. It is important that the entire shafts of both the tibia and fibula be well visualized. If the fibula is also broken, its splinting effect on the tibia is lost. This typically represents a higher energy injury then if the tibia alone is involved.

CLOSED FRACTURES

When a stable reduction of a closed tibial shaft fracture can be achieved, closed treatment can be satisfactory. It should involve early weight-bearing. For example, long leg casting followed by early conversion to a short leg walking cast or weight-bearing function brace has produced excellent results.[6,107,108]

Closed management, however, is not without problems. For example, prolonged immobilization in a cast may result in permenent ankle or subtalar stiffness. Some shortening or malalignment of the fracture site many be inevitable for certain unstable fractures. The amount of acceptable deformity remains controversial.[109] Angular malunions outside the usual plane of motion may also have detrimental long term effects on adjacent joints.[110]

Which closed tibia fractures should be treated surgically still depends largely on the judgement and treating philosophy of the attending physician. Situations which are excellent indications for internal fixation include fractures with significant shortening or malalignment, associated compartment syndrome, or the polytrauma setting.

Although many techniques for fixation are available, intramedullary nailing, if technically possible, is generally preferred. The introduction of interlocking nails (Fig. 31–9) has greatly increased the spectrum of fractures that can be stabilized with intramedullary techniques and has decreased the need for postoperative immobilization.[111]

Most closed tibia fractures will heal within 12-20 weeks. Factors that are likely to increase the risk of delayed union or nonunion are significant initial fracture displacement, comminution, associated soft tissue wounds, infection, and distraction.[112]

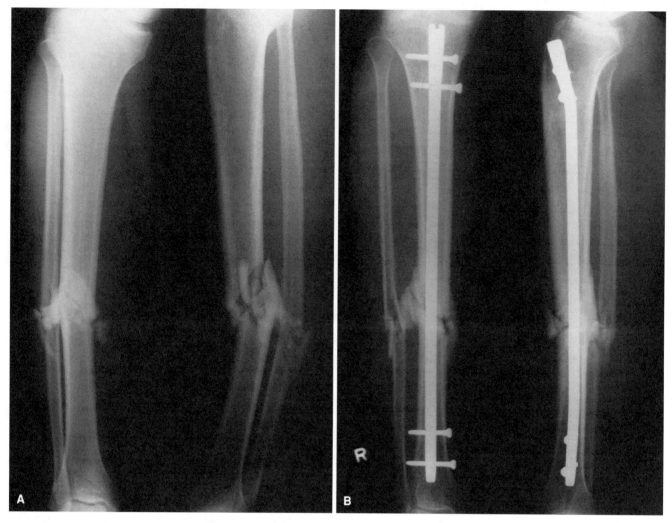

FIGURE 31–9 **A.** High energy tibial shaft fracture. **B.** Treatment with locked intramedullary nailing.

OPEN FRACTURES

Open tibia fractures are the most common open fractures in the lower extremity. There may be only a tiny puncture wound from a spike of bone penetrating the relatively thin skin and subcutaneous tissue, or there may be massive injury with avulsed flaps, loss of bone, and irreparable neurovascular injury.[16] The most important factor in achieving successful healing is prompt surgical debridement of all necrotic and devitalized tissue. Antibiotics are an addition to, and not a substitute for, adequate surgical treatment. Many of the treatment principles involved are outlined in the section on open fractures in this chapter.

Primary stabilization of the fracture is usually necessary to protect otherwise precarious wound edges and to facilitate mobilization of the multiply injured patient. Less severe open fractures can be stabilized with intramedullary nails. In fact, in some situations, this technique has fewer complications than external fixation.[113,114] Because reaming of the endosteal canal can result in further disruption of the blood supply to the bone in an already injured and infection-prone extremity, there has been interest in unreamed nailing for open fractures. The addition of locking screws for unreamed nails has also expanded their use.[115,116] Current trends are toward the use of unreamed locked nails in grade I, II, and IIIA open tibia fractures. The role of intramedullary nailing in grade IIIB and IIIC open tibial fractures is less well defined, and external fixation still remains the treatment of choice for many physicians.

Once bony stability has been acheived, early soft tissue coverage is essential to decrease the rates of infection and complications.[48,49,50] Grade III injuries often cannot be closed with local tissues. In such instances, local or distant soft tissue transfers are necessary.

If open reduction appears preferable but is contraindicated because of the injured skin, poor general condition of the patient, or inadequate equipment, one can use continuous traction via a pin or Kirschner wire through the os calcis or lower tibia until the conditions for surgery improve.

Bony union after open tibial fractures may be delayed or may not occur at all due to the severe injury to the soft tissues, devascularization of the bone ends, comminution, or bone loss. In some situations, prophylactic autogenous cancelleous bone grafting, usually at 6 weeks or once the soft tissues have healed, has resulted in high union rates for open tibia fractures.[117] Techniques to bridge large bony defects include massive cancellous bone grafting or vascularized bone transfer (i.e., free vascularized fibula). Recently, bone transport involving corticotomy and traction osteogenesis has also been popularized as a method to treat tibial bone loss.[118]

SEVERE OPEN FRACTURES

Severe open tibial fractures, especially with arterial injuries where adequate debridement cannot be accomplished without major tissue loss, may benefit from immediate amputation.[6,19,20,119,120] A viable perfused foot after successful vascular repair does not necessarily indicate a salvageable extremity. The main indications that suggest that primary amputation may be the optimal initial procedure is irreparable injury to nerves, resulting in a patient with an anesthetic foot.

Modern rehabilitation techniques with a below-knee prosthesis will often allow a patient to have a normal gait and a cosmetically acceptable limb. Amputation following trauma should not be a salvage procedure or a surgical defeat, but rather a primary treatment and rehabilitation option in the patient with a mangled extremity. Ideally the decision to recommend amputation and prosthetic fitting should be made as early as possible in the patient's postinjury management.[19,21,121,122]

COMPARTMENT SYNDROME

AXIOM   With fractures of the shaft of the tibia, one should look for a compartment syndrome, especially after high energy injuries.

A compartment syndrome may follow closed or open fractures of the tibia, particularly when there has been a significant crushing component or a period of ischemia. If this problem develops and is not corrected promptly, irreparable damage to the lower leg muscles and nerves may occur. Details of the diagnosis and management of compartment syndromes are presented in Chapter 33.

Fractures and Dislocations about the Ankle

GENERAL CONSIDERATIONS

Displaced open or closed fractures and fracture-dislocations of the ankle may cause severe deformity and extensive swelling. They commonly result from rotational or indirect injuries. Direct or crushing injuries, however, may cause pilon fractures of the distal tibia. Radiographs in several planes are necessary and should clearly demonstrate the "mortise," which is the relationship between the medial and lateral malleolus and the portion of tibia between them sitting on the talus.

Many classification systems have been developed for ankle fractures. The Danis-Weber (A-O) classification is simple and is based on the level of the fibular fracture. The Lauge-Hansen classification is based on cadaver studies and refers to forces required to create the fracture pattern.[123]

Assessment of the fractured ankle begins with the history and physical examination. The mechanism of injury helps distinguish direct from indirect fractures and gives the physician an idea of the magnitude of the force needed to create the fractures. A thorough physical examination should assess the neurovascular status, skin, tendons and muscles about the ankle as well as bony and ligamentous structures. Once this has been performed, three radiographic projections (AP, lateral and mortise views) are obtained.

Best results after displaced ankle fractures have been associated with accurate open reduction of the malleoli (Fig. 31–10). Initially, the importance of accurate reduction of the medial malleolus was emphasized, but there is now increasing recognition that an accurate reduction of the lateral malleolus is also essential.[124] Increasingly, displaced posterior malleolar fragments (the posterior portion of the distal tibial articular surface as seen on the lateral radiograph) are also being reduced and fixed.

Fixation of the fibula is usually accomplished with a small plate and screws. Screws are also used to fixate the medial and posterior malleoli. Smaller bony fragments can be secured with tension band wire techniques. A less-than-perfect reduction will result in changes in tibiotalar contact area and can lead to late degenerative arthritis.[125] Even patients with an excellent surgical reduction can have poor results if there has been significant articular damage.[126]

When a displaced ankle fracture is first evauated, any subluxation or dislocation should be promptly reduced and splinted. Delays in reducing these injuries place significant pressure on the soft tissues and can lead to fracture blisters or other skin problems. Early operative treatment of ankle fracture dislocations (less than 24 hours after injury) has been associated with fewer wound problems.[127]

PITFALL ⊘

> *Delayed reduction of ankle fracture-dislocations will result in an increased incidence of skin and neurovascular complications.*

Occasionally high-risk or elderly patients are treated with closed reduction and casting. This is often not optimal, but it is necessary because of the medical problems. Typically, a long leg cast is required. Further displacement and loss of reduction in the cast is not uncommon. Therefore, close follow-up of such patients at weekly intervals is advisable, and repeat reductions and castings are not uncommon.

SPECIAL PROBLEMS

Pilon Fractures

The tibial "pilon" or "plafond" refers to the weight-bearing articular surface of the distal tibia. Fractures in this location can involve all three malleoli, as well as considerable comminuation of the joint surface. These injuries are extemely difficult to treat, and represent a significant surgical challenge.[128] Optimal care involves surgical reconstruction of the articular surface of the distal tibia and early motion. Unfortunately, open reduction and internal fixation for high energy fractures can be associated with significant complications.[129,130] While open reduction with internal fixation is still the treatment method of choice, there are trends toward minimal internal fixation to restore the articular surface and external fixation for high energy fractures.

Open Ankle Fractures

Open ankle fractures should be treated with debridement, and immediate open reduction and internal fixation.[131] Higher complication rates can be expected, but the alternatives are poor.

Ankle Fractures in the Elderly

Soft osteoporotic bone is difficult to hold securely with internal fixation devices, and higher complication rates can be expected in elderly patients.[132] Operative treatment, however, produces more predictable and satisfactory results and is preferred whenever possible.[133]

SOFT TISSUE INJURIES

Soft tissue injuries are frequently encountered about the ankle. "Sprains" are usually injuries to the lateral collateral ligament complex. The anterior talofibular ligament is more frequently injured, followed by the calcaneofibular and rarely the posterior talofibular ligament. Most injuries are treated nonoperatively initially, even for acute tears. Occasionally, chronic posttraumatic instability will require a late operative reconstruction.

Tendon injuries are less common than ankle ligament injuries. A careful physical examination should be performed for proper assessment. For example, Achilles' tendon ruptures can be missed if this injury is not suspected, and the Thompson test (gastrocnemius squeeze) is not used to look for plantar flexion of the foot.

Fractures of the Bones of the Foot

Injuries to the foot may result from direct blows to the plantar or dorsal surfaces (which may lead to severe skin injury) or from severe flexion-extension trauma.[6] Foot injuries are often unrecognized or underestimated in multiply injured patients. As a consequence, definitive therapy may be delayed, resulting in increased disability.

A swollen foot following trauma should be assumed to be fractured until proven otherwise. Radiographs should be obtained to detect all suspected fractures and to locate possible foreign bodies. Major injuries, such as tarsometatarsal dislocations, may have subtle radiograph findings; however, most fractures arc obvious.

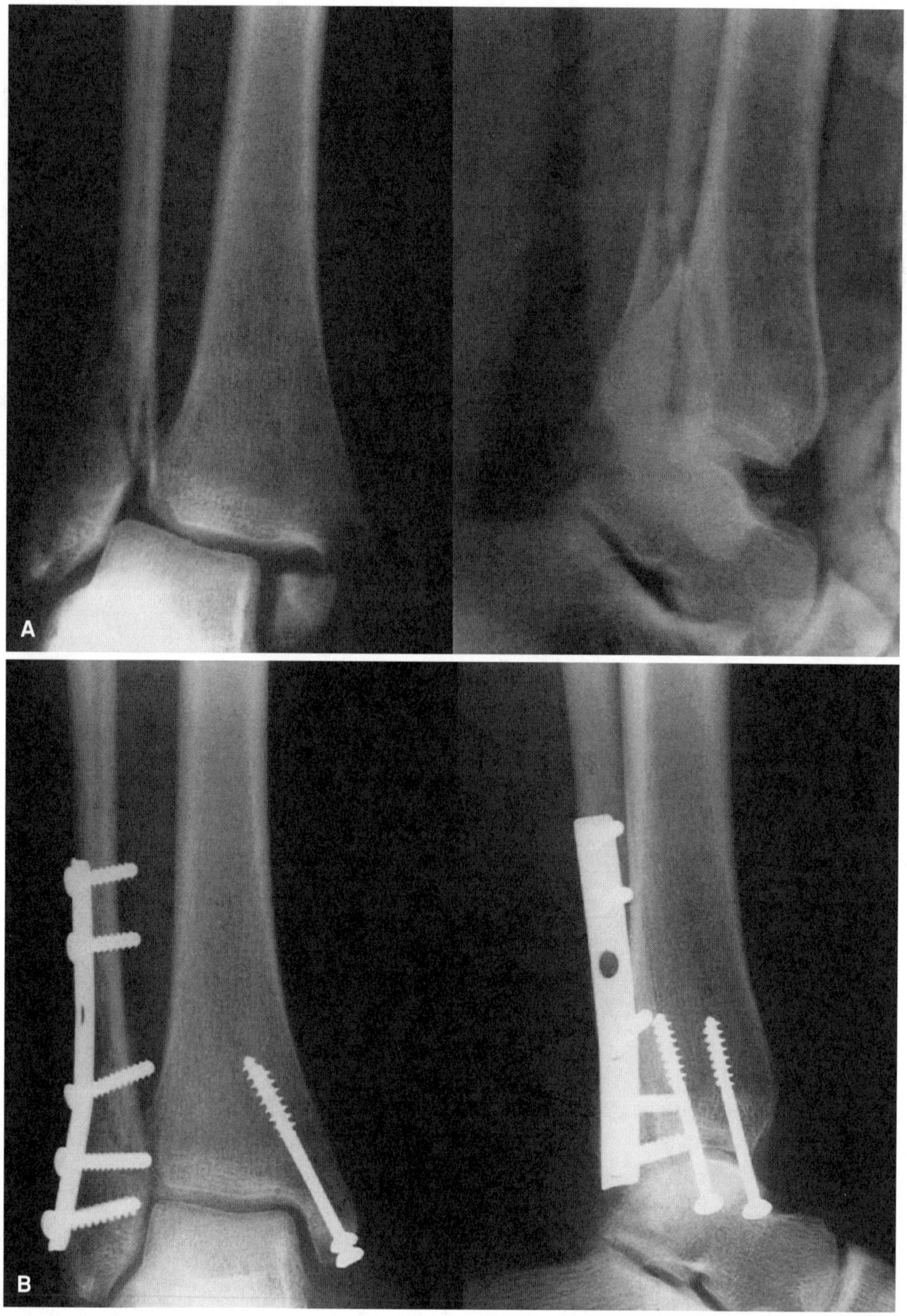

FIGURE 31–10 A. Fracture dislocation of the ankle. **B.** Treatment by open reduction and internal fixation of the medial and lateral melleoli.

FRACTURES OF THE CALCANEUS

Fractures of the calcaneus are usually due to severe blows to the plantar surface of the heel, usually because of a fall from a height. These fractures are often associated with compression fractures of the lumbar spine. The presence of either indicates a special need for thorough examination and radiographic visualization to see if the other fractures are also present. Fractures of the calcaneus often result in severe pain and marked swelling and discoloration as a result of hemorrhage. The swelling may become severe enough to cause massive bleb formation and even spotty necrosis of the skin on the sides of the heel.

Special radiographic views are often needed to confirm the presence of a fracture and to determine its type and extent. In addition to a standard lateral view, an anteroposterior view of the calcaneus along with special views of the subtalar joint are often required. Computerized tomography is increasingly used to identify the three-dimensional nature of these fractures. Such studies have led to increasing interest in surgical treatment aimed at restoring the congruity of the subtalar joints.[134] However, this is still a controversial area, and there is no uniform consensus as to the classification of these fractures, indications for surgery, type of operative approach, or postoperative care.[134]

Calcaneus fractures can be divided into intraarticular and extraarticular fractures. Extraarticular fractures typically do not need surgical intervention.

Treatment of displaced intraarticular fractures of the calcaneus include: (a) reduction of swelling prior to efforts at reducing the fracture, (b) restoration of the articular surface of the posterior facet and the contour of the body of the calcaneus (c) early mobilization of the foot and ankle in order to minimize any permanent restriction of motion, (d) avoidance of weight-bearing until mature bony healing has taken place, (e) minimizing of postimmobilization edema by adequate elastic support, and (f) early mobilization of the foot and subtalar joint.

Early surgical intervention is often not possible due to severe soft tissue swelling. Patients are typically treated with bed rest and elevation until the swelling resolves and wrinkles return to the skin (wrinkle test). This often takes 7-14 days. In some severely comminuted fractures, where surgical intervention is not thought to be technically possible or prudent, satisfactory results may be obtained by omitting immobilization altogether and starting non-weight-bearing and active exercises immediately.

Considerable permanent disability can occur from fractures of the calcaneus because of pain on weight-bearing from subtalar arthritis, loss of inversion and eversion of the foot, restricted ankle motion at the ankle joint, peroneal tendon impingement, sural nerve irritation and shoe wear problems.

FRACTURES OF THE TALUS

Fractures of the talus usually result from trauma which produces excessive dorsiflexion of the foot. Incomplete dislocations or subluxations of the talus are easily overlooked. Surgical intervention usually is indicated for displaced fractures, since an anatomic reduction gives the best chance for recovery after the injuries.

With fractures of the neck of the talus, avascular necrosis of the proximal fragment (the body of the talus) is the most important complication. The major nutrient arteries for the talus enter through the distal portion of the bone. A fracture through the neck of the talus destroys the major blood supply to the proximal bone. Avascular necrosis is uncommon in undisplaced fractures, but it is rather common when the fracture has been displaced, especially if there is any delay in reduction.

Aseptic necrosis in the body of the talus may result in disabling traumatic arthritis of the ankle. This problem may occur after any fracture of the talus or calcaneus communicating with the joint, even when early, accurate surgical restoration of the articular surfaces can be accomplished.

FRACTURES OF THE MIDTARSAL BONES

Midtarsal fractures involving the navicular, cuboid, and/or cuneiforms result from side-to-side crushes or from a heavy weight falling on the foot. After these fractures have healed, there is often considerable disability from loss of motion in the midtarsal joints and from pain and soreness on twisting. Fragments can usually be reduced by manual manipulation, but open reduction and some form of internal fixation is advantageous in many cases.

Open fractures of the foot are treated with debridement, repair of critical structures, and fixation of fractures as necessary to prevent further loss of skin.[6] Loss of dorsal or plantar skin is a serious complication. The dorsal skin contains virtually all of the venous drainage of the foot, and the weight-bearing plantar skin is unlike any other skin in the body and cannot be fully replaced. Free, composite tissue transfers have been used with some early, limited success in managing skin loss on the foot.

TARSOMETATARSAL (LISFRANC) FRACTURE DISLOCATIONS

Fracture dislocation of the tarsometatarsal joint (Lisfranc's) are either a result of a dorsiflexion stress to the foot or are associated with a high energy trauma and other foot injuries. Open reduction and internal fixation is usually required for best results.[135]

FRACTURES OF THE METATARSALS

Fractures of the metatarsals may be grouped into: (a) fractures of the shafts or necks of the metatarsals, (b) fractures of the base of the fifth metatarsal, and (c) stress fractures. Undisplaced fractures of the shafts or necks of the metatarsals require only a compression dressing and crutches for 4-6 weeks. A walking boot cast with a long plantar slab

to protect the toes may be preferable because it makes the patient ambulatory without crutches. Displaced fractures of the first and fifth metatarsals require accurate reduction so that the weight-bearing heads of these bones are in their normal position.

Undisplaced fractures of the base of the fifth metatarsal require little active treatment. An elastic bandage may suffice, and weight-bearing as tolerated is permitted. Proximal diaphyseal fractures of the fifth metatarsal ("Jones fracture") typically occur in young male athletes. These have a higher propensity for non-union. Treatment should be a non-weight bearing cast for 6-8 weeks, particularly in high performance athletes.

A stress (fatigue or "march") fracture of the second, third, or fourth metatarsal results from prolonged strain. Unconditioned military personnel who have been subjected to long fatiguing hikes are prone to this injury. In many instances, it can be managed with only a metatarsal pad in the shoe combined with restricted activity. If pain or disability is excessive, a walking cast for several weeks may be required.

FRACTURES OF THE TOES

The only treatment necessary for undisplaced fractures of the toes, including the great toe, is protection from additional injury. Strapping of the injured toe to the adjacent toe or toes with small strips of adhesive tape affords some protection and tends to minimize discomfort. Crutches may be used as needed for comfort during the first 7-10 days. A metatarsal bar applied to the shoe may permit patients to resume activity more quickly. In displaced fractures of the great toe, particularly in the proximal phalanx, reduction is necessary.

Traumatic amputations in the foot may occur in industrial or home accidents. The tissue is usually severely crushed and heavily contaminated, requiring thorough surgical debridement.[3] Mangling injuries of the toes are usually treated with primary amputation, and more extensive amputations often require primary and later revisions of the amputation. Replantation is almost never indicated in the foot.

FRACTURES IN CHILDREN

Fractures in children are unique in many ways. Their bones have many anatomic, physiologic, and biomechanical differences compared with adults. For example, incomplete or greenstick fractures are much more common in children. The periosteum is much thicker, making initial displacement less, and allowing for easier reductions on periosteal sleeves. In addition, the blood supply from this thick periosteum makes nonunions uncommon. Certain fractures (such as displaced femoral neck fractures), however, still have a high risk of avascular necrosis, just as in their adult counterparts.

The presence of intact growth plates means that the immature skeleton is constantly changing, and introduces special problems. Fractures involving growth plates can cause abnormal growth, limb length inequality, or angular deformities. In addition, because the bones in the joints may not be completely ossified, special studies or comparison films with the contralateral extremity are often needed for accurate evaluation of joint injuries.

The majority of pediatric fractures can be treated by closed means. In certain cases, however, especially for displaced intraarticular injuries and certain growth plate fractures, an open reduction will be needed. A detailed review of this subject is beyond the scope of this book. Only a brief overview and certain selected fractures are presented. Recent textbooks can provide an excellent review of the subject.[136,137]

Remodeling and Growth

AXIOM In children, angulation and overriding of fracture fragments will often be corrected by growth, but rotation will not.

The younger the child and the closer the fracture is to the growth center of the bone, the greater the degree of remodeling that will take place, and the greater the degree of deformity and angulation that can be accepted. This is especially true if the fracture angulation is in the plane of motion of that joint. Overriding with bayonet apposition is also acceptable in a child. The shortening that occurs will usually correct itself because of overgrowth of the involved extremity. It must be remembered, however, that rotation is not affected by remodeling and must be corrected at the time of the reduction of the fracture.

Epiphyseal Injuries

TYPES OF EPIPHYSES

Pressure Epiphyses
Epiphyses at the ends of the long bones are subjected to pressure, may be considered as articular epiphyses, and through their epiphyseal plates contribute to longitudinal growth.

Traction Epiphyses (Apophyses)
Traction epiphyses (apophyses) are the sites of origin or insertion of major muscles and are subjected to traction rather than pressure. They are nonarticular and do not contribute to the longitudinal growth of bone. Examples are the greater and lesser trochanters of the femur.

EPIPHYSEAL LESIONS
When an epiphysis is separated from the rest of the bone by injury, the plane of separation tends to occur through the weakest area of the epiphyseal plate which is the zone of calcifying cartilage. The main problem is not the mechanical damage to the plate itself, but whether or not the separation will interfere with the blood supply to the epiphysis. In long bone epiphyses, the blood vessels penetrate the side of the epiphysis at a point remote from the epiphyseal plate. These vessels usually are not injured by epiphyseal separation. A notable exception is the proximal femoral epiphysis where the blood vessels enter the epiphysis by traversing the rim of the plate. These vessels are often ruptured at the time of epiphyseal separation with subsequent avascular necrosis of the epiphysis.

INJURIES INVOLVING PRESSURE EPIPHYSES
Of injuries to the long bones during childhood, approximately 15% involve an epiphyseal plate.

Age and Sex Incidence
Although injuries to epiphyseal plates may occur at any age during childhood, they are more common in periods of rapid skeletal growth especially during the prepubertal growth spurt (9-12 years for girls and 12-14 for boys). The growth spurt for the distal humerus, however, is 4-5 years for girls and 5-8 years for boys. Epiphyseal injuries are more frequent in boys than in girls.

Sites
The lower radial epiphyseal plate is by far the most frequently separated. Other frequent sites of epiphyseal injuries are the distal humerus (including the epicondyles), proximal radius, distal femur and distal tibia.

Clinical Diagnosis

AXIOM   Any injury near a joint in a child should be assumed to involve the epiphysis until proven otherwise.

An epiphyseal injury should be suspected clinically in any child who shows evidence of pain, swelling, tenderness, and spasm at a joint. Sprains in children are uncommon. A fairly secure clinical diagnosis may be established by demonstrating focal tenderness exactly at the epiphyseal plate.

Roentgenographic Diagnosis
Accurate interpretation of radiographs for epiphyseal injuries requires a knowledge of their normal appearance at various ages. Two views at right angles to each other are essential, and comparable views of the opposite uninjured extremity can be invaluable. Tenderness exactly at an epiphysis usually indicates a separation of the epiphysis, possibly without displacement, in which case the roentgenogram may be negative.

AXIOM   A positive radiograph confirms the diagnosis, but a negative radiograph does not exclude epiphyseal injury in a child.

Possible Effect on Growth
Fortunately, epiphyseal plate injuries are not usually associated with disturbance of growth unless there is severe crushing or separation. If the entire epiphyseal plate ceases to grow, the result is progressive shortening, usually without angulation. However, if the involved bone is one of a parallel pair (such as tibia and fibula or radius and ulna), progressive shortening of one bone can produce an increasingly severe angular deformity. A similar problem can occur if growth ceases in one part of the epiphyseal plate but continues in the rest of the plate.

Classification of Epiphyseal Plate Injuries
The Salter-Harris classification of epiphyseal plate injuries is the most accepted system used today.[138] It is a radiographic classification that is based on the relationship of the fracture line to the growing cells of the epiphyseal plate, and it is correlated with potential disturbances of growth.

TYPE I.   With a type I injury, the epiphysis is separated from the metaphysis without a bone fragment. The growing cells remain with the epiphysis. This type is more common in birth injuries and in early childhood when the epiphyseal plate is relatively thick. Wide displacement is uncommon because the periosteal attachment is usually intact. Reduction is not difficult, and the prognosis for future growth is usually excellent.

TYPE II.   With type II injuries, the epiphysis is separated along the epiphyseal plate and out through the metaphysis, leaving a characteristic triangular fragment attached to the epiphysis (the "Thurston-Holland" fragment). This is the most common type of epiphyseal injury. The growing cartilage cells remain with the epiphysis, the circulation remains intact, and the prognosis is usually good.

TYPE III.   With type III injuries, there is an intraarticular fracture through the epiphysis, extending from the articular surface to the weak zone of the epiphyseal plate and then along the plate to its periphery. This results from an intra-articular shearing force and occurs usually at the upper or lower tibial epiphysis. Accurate reduction is essential and open reduction may be necessary.

TYPE IV.   With type IV fractures, an intraarticular fracture extends from the joint surface across the full thickness of the epiphyseal plate and through a portion of the metaphysis to produce a complete split. It most commonly occurs at the lateral condyle of the humerus. Perfect reduction is essential both to prevent growth disturbances and to provide a smooth joint surface.

TYPE V.   With type V injuries, a severe force crushes the epiphysis at one area of the plate. It may result in growth retardation or premature closure by mechanical derangement of the plate. Initial diagnosis is based on clinical suspicion from a knowledge of the forces applied and the clinical findings of epiphyseal tenderness with joint motion restriction. Treatment consists of splinting and no weight-bearing for 3 weeks or until the epiphyseal tenderness disappears.

General Considerations in the Treatment of Children's Fractures

CLOSED METHODS

Most children's fractures can be treated with manipulative reduction and a plaster cast with excellent results. Alignment is the chief requirement. The fracture should not remain malrotated or grossly angulated.

Angulated Greenstick Fractures

With greenstick fractures, one cortex remains unbroken but there is often some angulation. This type of fracture is seen more frequently in the forearm bones of older children. The fracture must often be completed to allow for accurate reduction.

A torus fracture (usually in or near the distal third of the radius) is a form of greenstick fracture in which neither cortex appears broken on radiograph examination; the bone is merely bent slightly from an impacting force. No attempt at reduction should be made. Only 2-3 weeks of protection by a splint or plaster cast is required.

Epiphyseal Fractures

In general, epiphyseal fractures are best treated by closed methods. Exceptions are: (a) fractures at the proximal end of the femur, and (b) joint fractures, particularly at the elbow, if an accurate reduction cannot be obtained. The initial injury may cause damage to the epiphyseal plate, but manipulations are also a risk, with increasing likelihood of further damage with each successive manipulation. The need for periodic follow-up examinations should be explained to the parents. Such visits permit early recognition of growth disturbances and an opportunity to provide timely remedial measures if necessary.

Immobilization

Children are active; consequently, it is wise to immobilize one or more joints on either side of the fracture until the callus is solid. Permanent stiffness of joints due to such immobilization is virtually unknown in children.

Physical Therapy

Physical therapy is seldom necessary in the management of children's fractures. However, manipulative reduction should be gentle to avoid soft tissue damage, and there must be no obstruction to circulation by casts, splints, bandages, or traction. Swelling at the injury may be minimized by applying ice carefully during the first 24 hours and elevating the part. At the proper time, active motion in unlimited quantities is supplied by the healthy child.

AXIOM Passive joint motion or manipulation should be avoided in children. It usually does more harm than good.

OPEN REDUCTION AND INTERNAL FIXATION

In children, the treatment of fractures is usually nonoperative. Operative reduction may be followed by infection and osteomyelitis. Internal fixation may be lost as a result of the metal loosening or breaking, and additional operative procedures may be required. Improperly applied metal plates may cause distraction of the fragments. In addition, internal fixation devices left in situ can become permanently embedded in the growing bone. After fracture union, hardware removal is often recommended to prevent refracture at the end of a plate or screw, and to decrease the possibility for late infections.

AXIOM Open reduction and internal fixation (ORIF) is rarely indicated in long bone fractures in children.

Although ORIF is rarely needed for long bone fractures in children, open reduction may be necessary in certain epiphyseal injuries to restore a smooth joint surface and to lessen the possibility of growth disturbance. The elbow is the joint most commonly involved with injuries requiring open reduction (i.e., lateral humeral condyle, medial humeral epicondyle, or proximal radial epiphysis with displacement). Other joint injuries which involve an epiphysis and which may require open reduction are separation of a proximal femoral epiphysis, and rare intraarticular fractures.

In older children who may be approaching epiphyseal closure and bone maturity, the indications for open reduction of long bone fractures more nearly approximate those of adults. In addition, certain special clinical situations in injured children, like polytrauma or head injury, may best be treated with internal or external fixation.

Selected Injuries in Children

SUPRACONDYLAR FRACTURES OF THE HUMERUS

Supracondylar fracture of the humerus is the most frequent elbow fracture in children. The fracture is sustained by a fall on the outstretched hand with the force transmitted through the radius and ulna to the lower end of the humerus, which becomes fractured through or just above the broadest portion of the condyles. The most common deformity is posterior angulation or displacement of the distal fragment. In addition, there is often lateral or medial displacement and rotation of the distal fragment. The bony deformity may vary considerably from none to extreme.

Diagnosis

The bony landmarks at the elbow posteriorly are helpful in clinically differentiating between a displaced supracondylar fracture and a dislocation of the elbow, however, radiographs are necessary to properly diagnose this injury.

Complications

This is one of the most potentially serious of all childhood fractures. Hemorrhage, swelling, and displacement of the distal fragment may cause compression, kinking, or stretching of the brachial artery, and can be a serious threat to the circulation of the forearm and hand. If improperly treated and unrelieved, the circulatory embarrassment may rapidly lead to ischemic muscle damage and then Volkmann's contracture.

Nerve injuries are not infrequent with elbow fractures, with the radial nerve or its motor branch (posterior interosseous) being the most frequently injured. The median nerve, especially its anterior interosseous branch, also may be injured. Ulnar nerve deficits are rare. In most cases, impairment of nerve function is the result of contusion or stretching rather than laceration, and complete spontaneous recovery of nerve function usually occurs within a few weeks.

Angular elbow deformities, especially cubitus varus, are common complications of elbow fractures. They can best be avoided by an accurate initial reduction of the fracture.

Treatment

Minimally displaced supracondylar fractures are treated with splinting or casting. Severely displaced fractures can be treated by either skin or skeletal traction, but this is not popular today; manual reduction is usually performed. The reduction often cannot be maintained, however, unless the elbow is flexed more than 90°. This position places the acutely swollen extremity at risk for vascular compromise. Consequently, closed reduction followed by percutaneous pinning is a popular treatment modality. It allows for an accurate reduction, maintains this reduction without extreme flexion, decreases the risk of vascular problems, and reduces hospital stay. The limb is immobilized in a posterior splint for 3 weeks. The pins are then removed and active motion is begun.

FRACTURE OF THE DISTAL HUMERAL CONDYLES

Fractures of the medial or lateral condyles in children represent epiphyseal injuries, which carry late complications of malunion, nonunion, arrest of normal growth, and late ulnar nerve palsy.[14] The incidence of fractures of the lateral condyle far exceeds that of the medial side. These injuries are seen more frequently in younger children, in whom the elbow is predominantly cartilaginous. The elbow is swollen and painful on initial evaluation. Routine radiographs of the elbow, even when compared to the child's normal side (a procedure suggested in all epiphyseal fractures), may be difficult to analyze. If there is any doubt about the extent of the injury, arthrography of the elbow is suggested.

For minimally displaced or nondisplaced fractures, careful observation over the first several weeks of treatment is important. Closed reduction of displaced fractures is extremely difficult, and anatomic open reduction by direct visualization with smooth pins placed across the epiphysis should be performed. Pin removal at 3-4 weeks, followed by early motion, is suggested if radiographs show healing.

SUBLUXATION OF THE RADIAL HEAD ("PULLED ELBOW")

Dislocation of the head of the radius, often called "pulled elbow" or "nursemaid's elbow," is a very common injury in children between the ages of 2 and 6 years. The mechanism of the injury is a sudden pull, jerk, or lift on the child's wrist or hand by someone trying to hurry the youngster across a street or up steps. Sometimes while holding the parent's hand, the child stumbles, and the parent, in an attempt to protect the child from the fall, pulls up quickly on the hand and wrist.

The pathology is not definitely understood, but either the radial head is pulled distally and jammed into the annular ligament which grips it tightly, or the ligament is split and a portion is caught between the radial head and capitellum.

The child usually has a history of not moving the arm for several hours or days and is apprehensive during the examination of the arm. The main symptoms are pain and refusal to use the elbow and arm. The history of a jerk on the arm is invaluable. Flexion and extension at the elbow are usually not limited but are painful. Supination is definitely limited. The child holds the arm extended, but little swelling or deformity is seen. There is no characteristic palpable deformity. Radiographic examination is of no value except to rule out other bony injury.

Reduction is accomplished with the patient's elbow flexed and with the examiner's thumb placed over the radial head. The forearm is slowly supinated and thumb pressure applied to the radial head. A snap or click is usually heard. The forearm is again tested to make certain that full supination has been regained. The elbow should then be moderately flexed and rested in a sling. The child will usually begin to use the arm spontaneously within a few hours. The prognosis is excellent; however, this injury may be recurrent up to the age of 4-5 years.

SLIPPED CAPITAL FEMORAL EPIPHYSIS

An acute slipped capital femoral epiphysis represents a traumatic separation of the growth plate of the proximal femur. It is, therefore, a displaced Salter I facture. It usually requires accurate reduction, either open or closed, followed by internal fixation. Unfortunately, the rate of avascular necrosis after such an injury, no matter how well or how early it is treated, is extremely high.

A chronic slipped capital femoral epiphysis results in an abnormal tilting of the proximal femur that is typically seen in overweight boys who are 10-12 years of age and in certain hormonal deficiencies. This problem is due to shearing forces on the immature hip causing a slowly increasing deformity at the unfused growth plate. Clinically, a chronic slipped capital femoral epiphysis can present with either a limp, hip pain, or knee pain. It is usually differentiated from an acute slip in that symptoms have been present for at least 3 weeks. Treatment involves promoting fusion of the the growth plate in order to prevent further deformity. Pinning of the hip with a single cannulated pin under image intensification is a popular technique that is currently used.

⊘ FREQUENT ERRORS

In the Management of Musculoskeletal Trauma

1. *Concentrating on the most obvious injuries first in patients with multiple trauma.*
2. *Failing to provide proper early immobilization of extremities with possible fractures.*
3. *Sending patients for radiographs of possibly fractured limbs before one is certain that the airway, ventilation, and circulation are properly secured.*
4. *Failing to accurately document a careful and complete neurovascular examination on all possibly injured extremities.*
5. *Failing to check carefully for frequent associated injuries, such as the lumbar spine with calcaneus fractures or the pelvis with severe lower extremity fractures.*
6. *Accepting radiographs that are of poor quality or which do not completely show both ends of a possibly fractured bone.*
7. *Failing to perform a complete orthopedic reexamination within 24-48 hours of admission.*
8. *Failure to properly protect open fracture wounds prehospital and in the ED prior to adequate cleaning and debridement.*
9. *Not promptly seeking the cause of increased pain after splinting or casting a fracture.*
10. *Failure to obtain accurate reduction of fractures involving joint surfaces of the legs.*
11. *Prolonged immobilization of joints, especially in the upper extremities, particularly in elderly patients.*
12. *Failure to ensure adequate motion of fingers or toes when the limb is casted.*
13. *Failure to watch for development of compartment syndromes with elbow and tibial fractures, especially if there has been any ischemia to the limb.*
14. *Failure to radiograph the opposite uninjured limb in children.*

▼▼▼▼▼▼▼▼▼▼▼▼▼▼▼▼▼▼▼▼▼▼▼▼▼▼▼▼▼▼▼▼

SUMMARY POINTS

1. The most obvious injuries are often not the most important.
2. The saving of life comes first. Asphyxia, hemorrhage, shock, and other life-endangering conditions are controlled before treating fractures.
3. An extremity cannot be adequately evaluated if it is covered.
4. The injured part should be examined for signs of vascular and nerve injuries, particularly before and after any manipulations, and the findings should be recorded completely and accurately.
5. One should make certain that the obvious fractures are the only injuries.
6. One should not be deceived by the absence of deformity and disability; with many fractures, some ability to use the limb persists.
7. Fractures which have not already been immobilized should be splinted as soon as possible after arrival at the hospital.
8. Always radiograph the pelvis if there is major lower limb trauma.
9. Always check the spine in the presence of calcaneus fractures.
10. Radiographs should always show both ends of a possibly involved bone.
11. One should not accept poor-quality radiographs.
12. Most fractures are missed either because the patient was examined improperly or because the radiographs were of poor quality.
13. A complete orthopaedic re-examination is mandatory in the early hospital course of all trauma patients to detect possible occult fracture.
14. Most ligamentous joint injuries will have normal radiographs, and diagnosis depends primarily on physical examination.

15. In patients with multiple severe trauma, reduction and immobilization of lower extremity fractures within 24 hours tends to reduce cardiorespiratory complications, especially in older individuals.

16. Open fractures are contaminated wounds and are orthopaedic emergencies. The risk of infection can be reduced by emergent and thorough debridement, fracture immobilization, antibiotics, and delayed closure of the wound.

17. Delayed wound closure is safer than primary closure in grossly contaminated open fractures.

18. Antibiotic agents by themselves do not prevent wound sepsis.

19. Continued severe pain, especially under a cast or splint, often indicates circulatory impairment and requires immediate attention.

20. The chief aim in the treatment of fractures of the upper extremity is to ensure the proper functioning of the hand and other joints.

21. The chief aim in the treatment of fractures of the lower extremity is to ensure painless, stable weight-bearing. Malalignment must be prevented, and maintenance of length is desirable.

22. Throughout the treatment of a fracture, attention should be focused on the patient as a whole rather than just the injured part.

23. Limbs in continuous traction should be checked frequently.

24. All joints that are not immobilized for treatment of the fracture should be encouraged to undergo early active motion.

25. Failure to look carefully for intrathoracic injuries in patients with a fractured scapula.

26. Failure to carefully examine the radial head in all fractures of the shaft of the ulna.

27. Anatomic reduction of both bone fractures of the forearm is needed to maintain the interosseous space to allow normal pronation and supination.

28. With all wrist fractures, exercise of the fingers throughout the period of immobilization is extremely important.

29. A "wrist sprain" which does not quickly resolve may represent a scaphoid fracture.

30. As a general rule, the earlier a fractured hip is reduced and fixed, the less likely the patient is to develop cardiopulmonary complications.

31. If the knee is not evaluated closely in patients with femoral-shaft fractures, serious injuries may be missed.

32. Hip dislocations are orthopaedic emergencies, and should be reduced as soon as possible.

33. Knee dislocations are orthopaedic emergencies. They should be reduced and the vascular status of the extremity evaluated as soon as possible.

34. Tibia fractures, both open and closed, are at special risk for compartment syndrome. One should maintain a high index of suspicion for this condition in these injuries.

35. Fracture-dislocation of the ankle should be reduced and definitively treated as soon as possible to decrease complication rates.

36. Child abuse should be suspected whenever the history is inconsistent with the physical examination or radiographs, or whenever there are several fractures at different stages of healing.

37. Children's fractures are unique and different from adult fractures. Most can be treated closed, but some will require surgery, especially intraarticular fractures or certain growth plate injuries.

38. Any injury near a joint in a child should be assumed to involve the epiphysis until proven otherwise.

39. A positive radiograph confirms the diagnosis, but a negative radiograph does not exclude epiphyseal injury in a child.

40. Passive joint motion or manipulation should be avoided in children. It usually does more harm than good.

41. Open reduction and internal fixation (ORIF) is rarely indicated in long bone fractures in children.

▲▲▲▲▲▲▲▲▲▲▲▲▲▲▲▲▲▲▲▲▲▲▲▲▲▲▲▲▲▲▲▲

REFERENCES

1. Dellinger EP. Prevention and management of infection. In Moore EE, Mattox KL, Feliciano DV, eds. Trauma, 2nd ed. East Norwalk, CT: Appleton-Lange. 1989;15:236.
2. Dellinger EP, Miller SD, Wertz MJ, et al. Risk of infection after open fracture of the arm or leg. Arch Surg 1988;123:1320.
3. Behrens F. Fractures with soft tissue injuries. In Browner BD, Jupiter JB, Levine AM, Trafton PG, eds. Skeletal trauma. Philadelphia: WB Saunders. 1992;14:311-336.
4. Chapman, MW. Open fractures. In Rockwood CA, Green DP, Bucholz RW, eds. Fractures in adults, 3rd ed. Philadelphia: J.B. Lippincott. 1991;3:223-264.
5. Chapman MW. Role of bone stability in open fractures. In Instructional course lectures, The American Academy of Orthopaedic Surgeons, St. Louis: CV Mosby. 1982;31:75.
6. Rosenthal RE. Lower extremity fractures and dislocations. In Moore EE, Mattox KL, Feliciano DV, eds. Trauma, 2nd ed. East Norwalk, CT: Appleton-Lange. 1989;40:623-638.
7. Thomas SA, Rosenfield NS, Leventhal JM, Markowitz RI. Long-bone fractures in young children: distinguishing accidental injuries from child abuse. Pediatrics 1991;88:471.
8. Loder RT, Bookout C. Fracture patterns in battered children. J Orthop Trauma 1991;5:428.
9. Ward WG, Nunley JA. Occult orthopaedic trauma in the multiply injured patient. J Orthop Trauma, 1991;5:308.
10. Muller ME, Nazarian S, Koch P, Schatzker J. The comprehensive classification of fractures of long bones. Berlin: Springer Verlag. 1990.
11. Burnstein AH. Fracture classification systems: do they work and are they useful? J Bone Joint Surg 1993;75A(12):1743.
12. Horn BD, Rettig ME. Interobserver reliablity in the Gustilo and Anderson classification of open fractures. J Orthop Trauma 1993;7:357.
13. Muller ME, Allgower M, Schneider R, Willenegger H. Manual of internal fixation. Techniques recommended by the AO-ASIF Group, 3rd ed. Berlin: Springer Verlag. 1991;17:683.
14. Kearns RJ, Gartsman GM. Upper extremity fractures and dislocations. In Moore EE, Mattox KL, Feliciano DV, eds. Trauma, 2nd ed. East Norwalk, CT: Appleton-Lange. 1989;38:597-605.
15. Gustilo RB, Anderson JT. Prevention of infection in the treatment of one thousand and twenty-five open fractures of long bones. J Bone Joint Surg 1976;58A:453.
16. Gustilo RB, Mendoza RM, Williams DN. Problems in the management of type III (severe) open fracture. A new classification system of type III open fractures. J Trauma 1984;24:742.
17. Chapman MW, Mahoney M. The role of early internal fixation in the management of open fractures. Clin Orthop 1979;138:120.
18. Dellinger EP, Caplan ES, Seaver LD, et al. Duration of preventive antibiotic administration for open extemity fractures. Arch Surg 1988;123:333.
19. Hansen ST. The type IIIC tibial fractures: salvage on amputation. J Bone Joint Surg 1987;69A:799.
20. Fairhurst MJ. The function of the below-knee amputee versus the patient with salvaged Grade III tibial fracture. Clin. Orthop 1994;301:227.
21. Caudle RF, Stern PJ. Severe open fractures of the tibia. J Bone Joint Surg 1987;69A:801.
22. Tscherne H, Oestern HJ, Sturm J. Osteosynthesis of major fractures in polytrauma. World J Surg 1983;7:80.
23. Robson MC, Duke WF, Krizek TJ. Rapid bacterial screening in the treatment of civilian wounds. J Surg Res 1973;14:426.
24. Patzakis MT. Management of open fractures wounds. In Instructional course lectures, The American Academy of Orthopaedic Surgeons, St. Louis: CV Mosby. 1987;36:367.
25. Patzakis MJ, Harvey P Jr, Ivler D. The role of antibiotics in the management of open fractures. J Bone Joint Surg 1974;56A:532.
26. Chapman MW. Open fractures. In Chapman MW. Operative orthopaedics. Vol II. Philadelphia: J.B. Lippincott. 1988;173-179.
27. Kreder HJ, Armstrong P. The significance of perioperative cultures in open pediatric lower extremity fractures. Clin Orthop 1994;302:206.
28. Haury B, Rodeheaver G, Vensko JA, et al. Debridement: an essential component of traumatic wound care. In Hunt TK, ed. Wound healing and wound infection. New York: Appleton-Century-Crofts. 1980;229.
29. Dhingra U, Schauerhamer RR, Wangensteen OH. Peripheral dissemination of bacteria in contaminated wounds; role of devitalized tissue: evaluation of therapeutic measures. Surgery 1976;80:535.

30. Blick SS, Brumback RI, Poka A, Burgess AR, Ebraheim NA. Compartment syndrome in open tibial fractures. J Bone Joint Surg 1986;68A: 1348.

31. DeLee JC, Steihl JB. Open tibia fractures with compartment syndrome. Clin Orthop 1981;160:175.

32. Brown LL, Shelton HT, Bornside GH, Cohn I Jr. Evaluation of wound irrigation by pulsatile jet and conventional methods. Ann Surg 1978; 187:170.

33. Wheeler CB, Rodeheaver GT, Thacker JG, et al. Side effects of high pressure irrigation. Surg Gynecol Obstet 1976;143:775.

34. Custer J, Edlich RF, Prusak M, et al. Studies in the management of the contaminated wound. An assessment of the effectiveness of phisohex scrub and betadine surgical scrub solutions. Am J Surg 1971;121:572.

35. Rodeheaver G, Bellamy W, Kody M, et al. Bactericidal activity and toxicity of iodine-containing solutions in wounds. Arch Surg 1982;117:181.

36. Polk HC Jr, Lopez-Mayor JF. Postoperative wound infection: a prospective study of determinant factors and prevention. Surgery 1969;66:97.

37. Krizek TJ, Davis JH. The role of the red cell in subcutaneous infection. 1965;J Trauma 5:85.

38. Alexander JW, Korelitz J, Alexander NS. Prevention of wound infection: a case for closed suction drainage to remove wound fluids deficient in opsonic proteins. Am J Surg 1976;132:59.

39. Niinikoski J. The effect of blood and oxygen supply on the biochemistry of repair. In Hunt TK, ed. Wound healing and wound infection. New York: Appleton-Century-Crofts. 1980;56.

40. Hohn DC. Host resistance to infection: established and emerging concepts. In Hunt TK, ed. Wound healing and wound infection. New York: Appleton-Century-Crofts. 1980;264.

41. deHoll D, Rodeheaver G, Edgerton MT, Edlich RF. Potentiation of infection by suture closure of dead space. Am J Surg 1974;127:716.

42. Edlich RF, Rodeheaver G, Golden GT, Edgerton MT. The biology of infections: sutures, tapes, and bacteria. In Hunt TK, ed. Wound healing and wound infection. New York: Appleton-Century-Crofts. 1980;214.

43. Magee C, Rodeheaver GT, Golden GT, et al. Potentiation of wound infection by surgical drains. Am J Surg 1976;131:547.

44. Cerise EJ, Pierce WA, Diamond DL. Abdominal drains: their role as a source of infection following splenectomy. Ann Surg 1970;171:764.

45. Edlich RF, Rogers W, Kaspar G, et al. Studies in the management of the contaminated wound. I. Optimal time for closure of contaminated open wounds. II. Comparison of resistance to infection of open and closed wounds during healing. Am J Surg 1969;117:323.

46. Gottrup F, Fogdestam I, Hunt TK. Delayed primary closure: an experimental and clinical review. J Clin Surg 1982;1:113.

47. Edlich RF, Smith QT, Edgerton MT. Resistance of the surgical wound to antimicrobial prophylaxis and its mechanisms of development. Am J Surg 1973;126:583.

48. Byrd HS, Spicer TE, Cierny G. Management of open tibial fractures. Plast Reconstr Surg 1985;76:719.

49. Cierny G, Byrd HS, Jones RE. Primary versus delay soft tissue coverage for severe open tibial fractures. A comparison of results. Clin Orthop 1983;178:54.

50. Godina M. Early microsurgical reconstruction of complex trauma of the extremities. Plast Reconstr Surg 1986;78:285.

51. Henry SL, Ostermann PAW, Seligson D. The prophylactic use of antibiotic impregnated beads in open fractures. J Trauma 1990;30:1231.

52. Henry SL, Ostermann PAW, Seligson D. The antibiotic bead pouch technique. The management of severe compound fractures. Clin Orthop 1993;295:54.

53. Christian EP, Bosse MJ, Robb G. Reconstruction of large diaphyseal defects, without free fibular transfer, in Grade-IIIB tibial fractures. J Bone Joint Surg 1989;71A:994.

54. Pitts LH, Rosegay H. Peripheral nerve injury. In Moore EE, Mattox KL, Feliciano DV, eds. Trauma, 2nd ed. East Norwalk, CT: Appleton-Lange. 1989;42:663-673.

55. Gurdjian ES, Smathers HM. Peripheral nerve injury in fractures and dislocations of long bones. J Neurosurg 1945;2:202.

56. Kennedy JC. Complete dislocations of the knee joint. J Bone Joint Surg 1963;45A:889.

57. Weingarten MJ, Tash R, Klein RM, et al. Posterior dislocation of the sternoclavicular joint. NY State J Med 1985;85:225.

58. Rockwood CA. Injuries to the sternoclavicular joint. In Rockwood CA, Green DP, Bucholz RW, eds. Fractures in adults, 3rd ed. Philadelphia: J.B. Lippincott. 1991;15:1253.

59. Rockwood CA, Williams GR, Young DC. Injuries to the acromioclavicular Joint. In Rockwood CA, Green DP, Bucholz RW, eds. Fractures in adults. Philadelphia: J.B. Lippincott. 1991;14:1181.

60. Rowe CR. Prognosis in dislocations of the shoulder. J. Bone Joint Surg 1956;38A:957.

61. Rockwood CA, Thomas SC, Matsen FA. Subluxations and dislocations about the glenohumeral joint. In Rockwood CA, Green DP, Bucholz RW, eds. Fractures in adults, 3rd ed. Philadelphia: J.B. Lippincott. 1991;13: 1021.

62. Lippitt SB, Kennedy JP, Thompson TR. Intra-articular lidocaine versus intravenous analgesia in the reduction of dislocated shoulders. Orthop Transactions 1991;15:804.

63. Thomas SC, Matsen FA. An approach to the repair of avulsion of the glenohumeral ligaments in the management of traumatic anterior glenohumeral instability. J Bone Joint Surg 1988;71A:506-513.

64. Neer CS. Displaced proximal humeral fractures: classification and evaluation. J Bone Joint Surg 1970;52A:1077.

65. Hawkins RJ, Kiefer GN. Internal fixation techniques for proximal humerus fractures. Clin Orthop 1987;223:77.

66. Flatow EL, Cuomo F, Maday MG, Miller SR, McIlveen SJ, Bigliani LU. Open reduction and internal fixation of two-part displaced fractures of the greater tuberosity of the proximal humerus. J Bone Joint Surg 1991;73A:1213.

67. Sarmiento A, Kinman PB, Calvin EG et al. Functional bracing of fractures of the shaft of the humerus. J Bone Joint Surg 1977;59A: 596.

68. Wilkins KE. Fractures and dislocations of the elbow region. In Rockwood CA, Wilkins KE, King RE, eds. Fractures in children. Philadelphia: Lippincott-Raven. 1991;6:526-617.

69. Waddel JP, Hatch J, Richards R. Supracondylar fractures of the humerus—results of surgical treatment. J Trauma 1988;28:1615.

70. Mosheiff R, Liebergall M, Elyashuv O, Mattan Y, Segal D. Surgical treatment of fractures of the capitellum in adults: a modified technique. J Orthop Trauma 1991;5:297.

71. Pollock FH, Pankovich AM, Prieto JJ, et al. The isolated fracture of the ulnar shaft: treatment without immobilization. J Bone Joint Surg 1983; 65A:339.

72. Jupiter JB. Current concepts reveiws. Fractures of the distal end of the radius. J. Bone Joint Surg 1991;73A:461.

73. Knirk JL, Jupiter JB: Intra-articular fractures of the distal end of the radius in young adults. J Bone Joint Surg 1986;68A:647.

74. Gellman H, Caputo RJ, Carter V, Aboulafia A, McKay M. Comparison of short and long thumb spica casts for non-displaced fractures of the carpal scaphoid. J Bone Joint Surg 1989;71A:354.

75. Sexson SB, Lehner JT. Factors affecting hip fracture mortality. J Orthop Trauma 1987;1:298.

76. Seinsheimer F. Subtrochanteric fractures of the femur. J Bone Joint Surg 1976;60A:300.

77. Zuckerman JD, Veith RG, Johnson KD, et al. Treatment of unstable femoral shaft fractures with closed interlocking intramedullary nailing. J Orthop Trauma 1987;1:209.

78. Kinast C, Bolhofner BR, Mast JW, Ganz R. Subtrochanteric fractures of the femur. Results of treatment with the 95° condylar blade-plate. Clin Orthop 1989;238:122.

79. Hougaard K, Thomsen PB. Coxarthrosis following traumatic posterior dislocation of the hip. J Bone Joint Surg 1987;69A:679.

80. Rosenthal RE, Coker WL. Posterior fracture-dislocation of the hip. An epidemiologic review. J Trauma 1979;19:572.

81. Keith JE, Brashear R, Guilford WB. Stability of posterior fracture-dislocations of the hip: quantitative assessment using computed tomography. J Bone Joint Surg 1988;70A:711.

82. Calkins MS, Zych G, Latta L, et al. Computed tomography evaluation of stability in posterior fracture dislocation of the hip. Clin Orthop 1988;227:152.

83. Fein LH, Pankovich AM, Spero CM, et al. Closed flexible intramedullary nailing of adolescent femoral shaft fractures. J Orthop Trauma 1989; 3:133.

84. Kirby RM, Winquist RA, Hansen ST Jr. Femoral shaft fractures in adolescents: a comparison between traction plus cast treatment and closed intramedullary nailing. J Pediat Orthop 1981;1:193.

85. Browner BD, Cole JD. Current status of locked intramedullary nailing: a review. J Orthop Trauma 1987;1:183.

86. Bucholz RW, Jones A. Current concepts review. Fractures of the shaft of the femur. J Bone Joint Surg 1991;73A:1561.

87. Lhowe DW, Hansen ST Jr. Immediate nailing of open fractures of the femoral shaft. J Bone Joint Surg 1988;70A:812.

88. Murphy CP, D'Ambrosia RD, Dabezies EJ, et al. Complex femur fractures: treatment with the Wagner external fixation device or the Gross-Kempf interlocking nail. J Trauma 1988;28:1553.

89. Brumback RJ, Ellison PS, Poka A, Lakatos R, Bathon GH, Burgess AR. Intramedullary nailing of open fractures of the femoral shaft. J Bone Joint Surg 1989;71A:1324.

90. Alonso J, Geissler W, Hughes JL. External fixation of femoral fractures: indications and limitations. Clin Orthop 1989;241:83.

91. Rooser B, Bengtson S, Herrlin K, Onnerfalt R. External fixation of femoral fractures: experience with 15 cases. J Orthop Trauma 1990;4:70.

92. Green A, Trafton PG. Early complications in the management of open femur fractures: a retrospective study. J Orthop Trauma 1991;5:51

93. Sanders R, Regazzoni P, Reudi TP. Treatment of supracondylar-intracondylar fractures of the femur using the dynamic condylar screw. J Orthop Trauma 1989;3:214.

94. Siliski JM, Mahring M, Hofer HP. Supracondylar-intercondylar fractures of the femur. Treatment by internal fixation. J Bone Joint Surg 1989; 71A:95.

95. Leung KS, Shen WY, So WS, Mui LT, Grosse A. Interlocking intramedullary nailing for supracondylar and intercondylar fractures of the distal part of the femur. J Bone Joint Surg 1991;73A:332.

96. Shields L, Mital M, Cave E. Complete dislocation of the knee: experience at the Massachusetts General Hospital. J Trauma 1969;9: 192.

97. Meyers MH, Moore TM, Harvey PJ. Follow-up notes on articles previously published in the journal. Traumatic dislocation of the knee joint. J Bone Joint Surg 1975;57A:430.

98. Sisto DJ, Warren RF. Complete knee dislocation: a follow-up study of operative treatment. Clin Orthop 1985;198:94.

99. Manco LG, Kavanaugh JH, Lozman J, et al. Diagnosis of meniscal tears using high-resolution computed tomography: correlation with arthroscopy. J Bone Joint Surg 1987;69A:498.

100. Fisher SP, Fox JM, Del Pizzo W, et al. Accuracy of diagnoses from magnetic resonance imaging of the knee. J Bone Joint Surg 1991;73A:2.

101. Raunest J, Oberle K, Loehnert J, Hoetzinger H. The clinical value of magnetic resonance imaging in the evaluation of meniscal disorders. J Bone Joint Surg 1991;73A:11.

102. DeHaven KE, Black KP, Griffiths HT. Open meniscus repair technique and two to nine year results. Am J Sports Med 1989;17:788.

103. Indelicato PA. Non-operative treatment of complete tears of the medial collateral ligament of the knee. J Bone Joint Surg 1983;65A:323.

104. Moore TM, Patzakis MJ, Harvey JP. Ipsilateral diaphyseal femur fractures and knee ligament injuries. Clin Orthop 1988;232:182.

105. Templeman DC, Marder RA. Injuries of the knee associated with fractures of the tibial shaft. Detection by examination under anesthesia. A prospective study. J Bone Joint Surg 1989;71A:1392.

106. Saltzman CL, Goulet JA, McClellan RT, Schneider LA, Matthews LS. Results of treatment of displaced patellar fractures by partial patellectomy. J Bone Joint Surg 1990;72A:1279.

107. Sarmiento A. A functional below knee cast for tibial fractures. J Bone Joint Surg 1970;52A:295.

108. Sarmiento A, Gersten LM, Sobol PA. et al. Tibial shaft fractures treated with functional braces. Experience with 780 fractures. J Bone Joint Surg 1989;71B:602.

109. Merchant CT, Dietz FR. Long term follow-up after fractures of the tibial and fibular shafts. J Bone Joint Surg 1989;71A:599.

110. Puno RM, Vaughan JJ, Stetten ML, Johnson JR. Long term effects of tibial angular malunion on the knee and ankle joints. J Orthop Trauma 1991;5:247.

111. Olerud S, Karlstrom G. The spectrum of intramedullary nailing of the tibia. Clin Orthop 1986;212:101.

112. Nicoll EA. Fractures of the tibial shaft. A survey of 705 cases. J Bone Joint Surg 1964;46B:387.

113. Holbrook JL, Swiontkowski MF, Sanders R. Treatment of open fractures of the tibial shaft: ender nailing versus external fixation. J Bone Joint Surg 1989;71A:1231.

114. Whitelaw GP, Wetzler M, Nelson A, et al. Ender rods versus external fixation in the treatment of open tibial fractures. Clin Orthop 1990; 253:258.

115. Whittle AP, Russell TA, Taylor JC, Lavelle DG. Treatment of open fractures of the tibial shaft with the use of interlocking nailing without reaming. J Bone Joint Surg 1992;74A:1162.

116. Tornetta P, Bergman M, Watnik N, et al. Treatment of grade III B open tibial fractures. A prospective randomised comparison of external fixation and non-reamed locked nailing. J Bone Joint Surg 1994;76-B:13.

117. Blick SS, Brumback RJ, Lakatos R, et al. Early prophylactic bone grafting of high energy tibial fractures. Clin Orthop 1989;240:21.

118. Paley D, Catagni MA, Argnani F, et al. Ilizarov treatment of tibial nonunion with bone loss. Clin Orthop 1989;241:146.

119. Pozo JL, Powell B, Andrews BG, et al. The timing of amputation for lower limb trauma. J Bone Joint Surg 1990;72B:288.

120. Georgiadis GM, Behrens FF, Joyce MJ, et al. Open tibial fractures with severe soft tissue loss: limb salvage versus below knee amputation. J Bone Joint Surg 1993;75A:1431.

121. Bondurant FJ, Cotler HB, Buckle R, et al. The medical and economic impact of severly injured lower extremities. J Trauma 1988;28:1270.

122. Clark JD, Malchow D. How to avoid errors in limb salvage decisions. Orthop Rev 1984;13:197.

123. Lindsjo U. Classifcation of ankle fractures. The Lauge Hansen or A-O system? Clin Orthop 1985;199:12.

124. Yablon IG, Heller FG, Shouse L. The key role of the lateral malleolus in displaced fractures of the ankle. J Bone Joint Surg 1977;59A:169.

125. Ramsey PL, Hamilton W. Changes in tibiotalar area of contact caused by lateral talar shift. J Bone Joint Surg 1976;58A:356.

126. Lantz BA, McAndrew M, Scioli M, Fitzrandolph RL. The effect of concomitant chondral injuries accompanying operatively reduced malleolar fractures. J Orthop Trauma 1991;5:125.

127. Carragee EJ, Csongradi JJ, Bleck EE. Early complications in the operative treatment of ankle fractures. Influence of delay before operation. J Bone Joint Surg 1991;73B:79.

128. Mast JW, Spiegel PG, Pappas JN. Fractures of the tibial Pilon. Clin Orthop 1988;230:68.

129. Dillin L, Slabaugh P. Delayed wound healing, infection, and nonunion following open reduction and internal fixation of tibial plafond fractures. J Trauma 1986;26:116.

130. McFerran MA, Smith SW, Boulas HJ, Schwartz HS. Complications encountered in the treatment of pilon fractures. J Orthop Trauma 1992; 6:195.

131. Wiss DA, Gilbert P, Merritt PO, Sarmiento A. Immediate internal fixation of open ankle fractures. J Orthop Trauma 1988;4:265.

132. Beauchamp CG, Clay NP, Thexton PW. Displaced ankle fractures in patients over 50 years of age. J Bone Joint Surg 1983;65B:329.

133. Ali MS, McLaren CAN, Rouholamin E, et al. Ankle fractures in the elderly: non-operative or operative treatment. J Orthop Trauma 1987; 1:275.

134. Sanders R. Intra-articular fractures of the calenueus: present state of the art. J Orthop Trauma 1992;6:252.

135. Arntz CT, Veith RG, Hansen ST. Fractures and fracture-dislocations of the tarsometatarsal joint. J Bone Joint Surg 1988;70A:173.

136. Ogden JA. Skeletal injury in the child. Philadelphia: WB Saunders. 1990.

137. Rockwood CA Jr, Wilkins KE, King RE, eds. Fractures in children. Philadelphia: J.B. Lippincott. 1991.

138. Bright RW. Physeal injuries. In Rockwood CA Jr, Wilkins KE, eds. Fractures in children. Philadelphia: J.B. Lippincott. 1991;2:87-186.

Chapter 32 Amputations After Trauma

ROBERT F. WILSON, M.D.

GREGORY M. GEORGIADIS, M.D.

In the not too distant past, amputation was the only treatment for a severely mangled extremity. Today, many patients can have their severely injured limbs salvaged. Thus, trauma surgeons can be faced with difficult decisions as to which extremities to amputate primarily, and which to attempt to save. In cases of complete traumatic amputations, irreparable major peripheral neurologic injury, and/or severe crush injuries in combination with prolonged ischemia or life-threatening injuries, primary amputation is indicated.[1,2,3,4] In patients below the age of 55, almost half of all amputations are related to some type of trauma.[5]

> **AXIOM** It is improper to amputate a severely injured limb unless there is no reasonable alternative; however, one should not attempt to save a marginal limb if it will be of little or no use to the patient and salvage will be achieved only at great cost.

There are some trauma victims in whom, because of a combination of surgical or technical enthusiasm, clinical misjudgment, and/or wishful thinking, an unwarranted salvage of an unretrievable limb has been attempted when, in fact, such efforts are doomed to failure.[1] Although a limb may initially seem viable, intractable pain, infection, or ischemia can supervene, resulting in a nonfunctional, useless extremity with late amputation as the only reasonable remedy. Such patients have a substantial risk of morbidity and mortality from the efforts to preserve the badly injured limb, and their hospital costs are significantly increased.[4,6]

All too often, physicians have considered an amputation as a last resort and as an acknowledgment of failure; however, in some instances, early amputation is preferred because it can greatly speed up the rehabilitation of severely injured patients.[2] In addition, outcome studies have shown that the quality of life of traumatic below-knee amputees is comparable to that of many patients with salvaged, but abnormal, limbs.[7,8,9] Therefore, amputation surgery can be viewed as a reconstructive procedure, and not a destructive, mutilating event.

> **AXIOM** Although no prosthesis can ever function as well as a normal extremity, most prostheses function better than mangled, painful, insensate limbs.

Before the surgeon embarks on a prolonged series of complicated procedures to save a severely injured limb, he should consider numerous factors.[10,11] Long hospitalizations and numerous surgeries can have negative medical, economic, social, and psychological effects on patients. The patient may easily become a disabled, nonproductive citizen afterwards.[2] Thus, the amount of time lost from work, number of procedures, pain and inconvenience, probability of success, and final functional outcome of the salvaged limb all need to be considered. An independent review by an orthopaedic and plastic surgeon, with the aim of establishing a prognosis for successful salvage, may also be useful.[6] Ideally, the patient should be involved in and make the final decision,[11] but this will not always be possible in life-threatening multiple trauma situations.

> **PITFALL** ⊘
>
> *When a surgeon attempts to reconstruct a severely injured limb that will probably have no function, he places the patient's life and the function of the remainder of the extremity in unnecessary jeopardy.*

INDICATIONS FOR AMPUTATION

The main indications for amputation include loss of tissue viability and loss of function. Unfortunately, the status of the viability and function of an injured extremity is not always clear, especially in the early post-trauma period.

Early (Within Hours of Injury)

AVULSION OR TRAUMATIC AMPUTATIONS
With complete avulsion or traumatic amputations, bleeding is controlled and wound toilet is performed with the aim of producing a useful viable stump. However, in children, a relative clean, noncrushing amputation, especially of the upper extremity, can often be replanted successfully.

SEVERE CRUSH AND DEGLOVING INJURIES ('MANGLED LIMB')
Considerable judgment is required in the management of mangled extremities. As a general rule, the combination of multiple fractures, nerve disruption, warm ischemia time greater than 6 hours, and/or extensive crush injury involving muscle and skin is not compatible with restoration of useful function. Similar pathology may be created by shotgun or high velocity missile wounds.

> **AXIOM** Scoring systems for determining need for primary amputation of mangled extremities provide only guidelines, not mandates.

A number of scoring systems have been developed in an effort to help predict the need or lack of need for amputation of a severely injured limb.[12-15] Each of these studies with its various scoring system, however, has crucial shortcomings. For example, several of them combined mangled upper and lower extremities even though the salvage implications of these are significantly different.[16,17] Some studies used "functional" limb salvage as the end point. However, a number of disparate issues, such as patient motivation, delayed appearance of chronic causalgia or dystrophy, and development of overwhelming infections, complicate such attempts at functional assessment, and none of these factors are predictable at the time of initial evaluation. Finally, several of these scoring systems are quite complex and use many variables based only on retrospective data (Table 32–1).

Johansen et al noted that certain issues that are crucial to lower extremity function (preservation of protective sensation, anatomic continuity of major nerves, and avoidance of limb length discrepancy) are of less importance in upper extremities.[18,19] Furthermore, prosthetic limbs (especially for below-knee amputations) are much more advanced for lower extremities than for upper extremities.[1] The authors also mention that a badly injured lower extremity with division of the sciatic or posterior tibial nerve in adults should have immediate amputation.

The MESS (mangled extremity severity scoring) system developed by Johansen has four components: (a) skeletal/soft tissue injury with 1-4 points, (b) limb ischemia with 1-6 points, (c) shock with 0-2 points, and (d) age with 0-2 points. Johansen et al found in both retrospective and prospective studies that all limbs with a MESS of 6 or less were salvaged while all limbs with a MESS of 7 or higher were amputated (Table 32-2).[1]

Although, all of these scoring systems may provide helpful guidelines, they cannot be followed blindly, and many surgeons find them

TABLE 32–1 Some Factors Determining if a Limb is Salvageable[1]

I. Patients' General Condition
  1. Age
  2. Coexisting medical conditions
  3. Shock; need for vasopressors
  4. Hypothermia, audosis, coagulopathy
II. Preexisting Condition of Extremity
  1. Skin
  2. Muscle
  3. Vessels, especially preexisting atherosclerosis
III. Local Trauma
  1. Nerve disruption, especially protective sensation
  2. Vessels arterial and/or venous injuries
    a. Site of damage
    b. Vein ligation
    c. Duration of ischemia
  3. Fractures; location, comminution
  4. Loss of skin
  5. Loss of muscle; compartment syndrome
IV. Trauma to Other Organs
  1. Life-threatening versus extent of tissue damage
  2. Priorities, blood loss, brain, etc.

unreliable.[20] For example, trauma victims with mangled limbs may have concurrent life-threatening craniocerebral, thoracic, abdominal, or pelvic injuries that must be managed first. Primary amputation may be indicated to minimize operative time or to facilitate intraoperative or postoperative management.[2,3] However, advances in free tissue transfer and other techniques might make occasional trauma victims candidates for attempts at limb salvage even with extremely high mangled extremity scores.[21]

GRADE III-C LEG INJURIES

AXIOM   Severe open leg fractures with prolonged warm ischemia should have a primary amputation.

Several investigators have pointed out the poor general prognosis of grade III-C injuries of the leg (severe open tibia fractures combined with acute arterial insufficiency).[15,16,22,23] With open crush injuries combined with warm ischemia exceeding 6 hours, limb salvage is virtually unprecedented, and primary amputation seems warranted.[2]

NEUROLOGIC INJURIES

As a general rule, when four of the five main components or structures of a limb (skin, bone, muscles, vessels, nerves) are injured, but there is little or no nerve injury, efforts to reconstruct and salvage the extremity can be considered. If the nerve injury is so severe that it is unlikely that the extremity will have any function or protective sensation, the most prudent course to follow is immediate amputation and early fitting with a prosthesis. Even if the nerves are intact, "every effort" should not always be made to salvage the extremity if the other four components, especially the major vessels, are badly damaged.

AXIOM   If protective nerve function to an extremity is permanently lost, that limb has a poor prognosis.

Restoration of protective nerve function is usually the primary factor determining the success of replantation or reconstruction of a severely injured extremity. Since the first successful replantation of an extremity 20 years ago, it has become increasingly apparent that the final result is measured primarily by the degree of nerve regeneration. Amputation of an anaesthetic flail limb may even be requested by the patient.

Unfortunately, a detailed neurologic assessment (e.g., sciatic or brachial plexus) at the time of acute injury may be difficult, espe-

cially in patients with impaired levels of consciousness or severe pain and anxiety. It also can be difficult to clearly identify nerve integrity at operation in the presence of severe associated soft tissue trauma. Under such circumstances, it is advisable to treat the vascular and soft tissue injuries and defer final assessment of the extent of the nerve injury and the possible reconstruction and recovery of the limb.

IRREVERSIBLE ISCHEMIA

AXIOM   Severe tissue damage with a warm ischemia time exceeding 6 hours as a result of vascular injury is generally an indication for a primary amputation.[24]

With severe multiple injuries to a limb involving bone and major vessels, insertion of a temporary vascular shunt may maintain viability of the distal extremity while other injuries are treated.[25]

Frank gangrene with fixed skin staining obviously mandates early amputation. Muscle rigidity involving all fascial compartments with fixed equinus deformity of the ankle also indicates irreversible muscle ischemia or damage. However, rigidity confined to the extensor compartment of the leg or anaesthesia of only the dorsum of the foot often warrants an attempt at fasciotomy and revascularization.

ENTRAPMENT

An amputation at the scene of injury may be required to free a patient trapped beneath fallen rubble. An additional consideration under such circumstances is the possible development of life-threatening crush syndrome if the irreversibly damaged limb is still in place when the entrapped limb is finally freed.

OTHER INJURIES

The presence of life-threatening injuries involving the head and torso take precedence over limb-salvage. In such individuals, prolonged efforts to save a limb may significantly increase the risk of death or major complications, and a primary amputation may be indicated.

Later Indications for Amputation

SEPSIS

If severe infection develops in a limb that has been severely injured or has had prolonged ischemia, extensive debridement may make return of useful function almost impossible. In some instances, the patient may become so septic from the infected limb, that an early amputation may be needed to save the patient's life.

TABLE 32–2 MESS (Mangled Extremity Severity Score) Variables

A. Skeletal/soft-tissue injury	
Low energy (stab, simple fracture, "civilian" GSW)	1
Medium energy (open or multiple Fxs, dislocation)	2
High energy (close-range shotgun or "military" GSW, crush injury)	3
Very high energy (above + gross contamination, soft-tissue avulsion)	4
B. Limb ischemia	
Pulse reduced or absent but perfusion normal	1*
Pulseless, parasthesias, diminished capillary refill	2*
Cool, paralyzed, insensate, numb	3*
*score doubled for ischemia >6 hrs	
C. Shock	
Systolic BP always >90 mm Hg	0
Hypotensive transiently	1
Persistent hypotension	2
D. Age (yrs)	
<30	0
30-50	1
>50	2

CAUSALGIA

If conventional measures fail to control the severe pain and discomfort of causalgia, the patient may occasionally request amputation to control the symptoms.

DEFORMITIES AND DYSFUNCTION

Development of severe, fixed flexion deformities, repeated breakdown of extensive skin-grafted areas, or poor limb function resulting from extensive debridement may eventually require amputation to allow proper rehabilitation of the patient.

PRINCIPLES CONCERNING AMPUTATION

Once a decision to amputate has been made, all subsequent steps must be aimed toward rehabilitation and return of the patient to an active and productive life. To do this, one can be guided by several principles.[12]

1. One should amputate as little tissue as possible initially; the first procedure need not be definitive.
2. One should consider the patient's potential ability to use a prosthesis.
3. One should know the level of residual limb that will allow optimal prosthetic use.
4. Rehabilitation, both mental and physical, begins at the time of amputation.
5. One should not close the amputation wound if infection is present or likely to occur.

AXIOM A surgeon should not perform an amputation without completely considering the future goals of rehabilitation and without a clear understanding of the type of prosthesis which will provide optimal function.

The surgeon's responsibility to the patient does not end with the amputation; he must be prepared to make all efforts to restore the patient to maximal function using appropriate prosthetic devices.

AXIOM For best results, an amputation should be considered as part of a total rehabilitation program.

The optimal approach toward amputees is as a team, including physical therapy, occupational therapy, and limb-fitting. Rehabilitation starts virtually from the moment of recovery from the anaesthetic.[26] Active, positive psychological support and encouragement are of paramount importance.[10]

OPEN AND CLOSED AMPUTATIONS

Open (Guillotine) Amputations

AXIOM It is generally ill-advised to attempt a primary definitive amputation on a severely injured or infected extremity.

Open amputations are interim lifesaving procedures in which no attempt is made to close or approximate any of the tissues. One should not close an amputation site if nonviable or contaminated tissue is present. However, full evaluation of skin and soft tissue viability and neurologic integrity may be difficult in the presence of crush injury, blast wounds, shotgun injuries, or high velocity missile wounds.[27] It can also be difficult to define the level of irreversible ischemia when there is no clear line of demarcation. The situation may be further complicated when foreign bodies are present or the tissues are discolored by road dirt.

AXIOM During initial surgery, guillotine or open amputation should be performed at a level at which tissues are assessed to be viable, but not through the level at which a definitive amputation would be made.

A guillotine amputation should provide maximal open drainage of the tissues while preserving as much length as possible. The wound should be covered with a sterile dressing and viability reassessed within 24-48 hours, using general or regional anaesthesia if needed. Further debridement is done as necessary. The amputation site is reassessed at 24-48 hour intervals until the wound is clean and stable. At that time, a definitive, closed amputation can be performed. If further operative procedures, including a closed proximal amputation, are not possible, gradual skin traction applied via a stockinette glued to the skin just proximal to the amputation site can often lengthen the skin flap enough to provide coverage. Alternatively, in the lower extremity, a rolled flap technique may be applied to the skin edges. This improves retention of bone length and skin flaps. These flaps can be taken down later to allow a delayed primary closure.[28]

Closed (Flap) Amputations

In the absence of infection and nonviable tissue, primary closure of the amputation may be performed. The incisions are made to produce two flaps of skin, attempting, except perhaps with above-knee amputations, to keep the scar from the end or weight-bearing portion of the stump. The flap with the tougher skin and better blood supply is fashioned longer. Ideally, large arteries and veins should be ligated separately to prevent A-V fistula formation. Hemostasis is achieved with fine ligatures. Cautery is avoided as much as possible. The nerves are divided under traction so they will not adhere to the scar and produce stump pain. The deep fascia is sutured to allow proper muscle attachment to the bone and to prevent muscle ends from adhering to the skin.

Requirements for the ideal amputation stump include:

1. The stump must be durable, adequately perfused, and capable of wear over pressure areas. Partial-thickness skin grafts are incapable of withstanding such wear and tear and should be avoided over pressure areas. Residual full-thickness flaps that may result in "unconventional" placing of the scar may be employed provided the scars can be kept away from pressure areas.
2. There should be neither neuromas nor areas of tenderness at pressure areas.
3. Bone should be covered with muscle or fascia without residual prominent spicules or protuberances.
4. Proximal joints should retain full mobility with strong balanced muscle action. It is important to attach opposing muscle groups to help avoid fixed flexion deformities.
5. The length and shape of the stump should allow placement into a prosthetic socket and application of sufficient leverage to produce motion without the stump disengaging or "popping out."

AXIOM Exercise to strengthen and prevent contracture of the muscles of the extremity at the amputation site should be begun early, even before the extremity has healed completely.

LOWER EXTREMITY AMPUTATIONS

The main goals in rehabilitation of the patient with a lower extremity amputation include: (a) preservation of the knee, whenever possible, (b) salvage of an end-weight-bearing stump, and (c) reliance, if possible, on full-thickness covering of the stump.

As a general rule, the energy cost of walking in lower extremity amputees is related to the level of amputation. The lower the amputation, the lower the energy cost and the better the performance. Thus, every effort should be made to amputate at the lowest possible level.[29]

AXIOM With amputations, every effort should be made to salvage a functional knee or elbow.

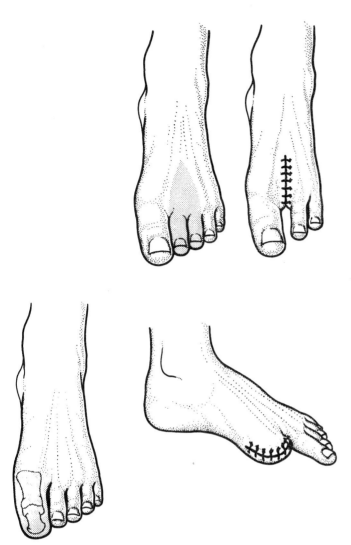

FIGURE 32–1 Toe amputations. When a single toe requires removal, a ray amputation is generally advised. The metatarsal should be divided approximately midshaft. When the great toe is amputated, it should be disarticulated at the metatarsophalangeal joint and the cartilage cap removed because keeping the metatarsal head helps maintain balance for ambulation. (From: Robbs JV. Amputation for trauma. In: Champion HR, Robbs JV, Trunkey DD, eds. Rob and Smith's operative surgery: trauma surgery, part 2. London: Butterworths, 1989; 597.)

Digital (Toe) Amputations (Fig. 32–1)

Toe amputation is indicated when gangrene, infection, or unreconstructible trauma is limited to a digit or digits distal to the metatarsophalangeal joint. However, infection of the foot itself, especially in the plantar space, may be a contraindication to this procedure. In patients with proximal vascular disease or trauma, distal perfusion pressures should be determined.[24,30] An ankle-brachial systolic BP index (ABI) below 0.45 (0.55-0.60 in a diabetic) generally indicates that perfusion will not be adequate to heal an open wound adequately.

Observation of dry gangrene with eventual autoamputation may be appropriate, especially if there is proximal vascular disease or a marginal blood supply. However, although this technique may be effective in the long run, it is a long process and often objectionable to the patients. It is generally preferable to perform amputations as soon as convenient after demarcation is complete.

Amputation of a digit begins with a circumferential incision made distal to the metatarsophalangeal skin crease and carried down to bone. The bone is preferentially transected through the proximal phalanx. However, the distal head of the metatarsal bone may be removed

to allow a tension-free closure. Amputation through the metatarsophalangeal joint should be avoided, except with the great toe, because of the poor blood supply of the cartilage. If the great toe must be amputated, preservation of its metatarsal head helps preserve balance for ambulation. Terminal joint cartilage should be excised because it heals poorly.

A loose skin closure is performed with interrupted monofilament sutures or steri-strips. If there appears to be any dead space, it is obliterated with a firm bandage.

Sutures are generally left in place for at least 3 weeks. Individual sutures that appear to be too tight can be removed and replaced with well-anchored steri-strips. Ambulation is begun in 3 to 5 days with partial weight bearing. Full weight bearing can often begin at about 10 to 14 days.

Toe amputations in general cause little disturbance of gait.[31] Amputation of the great toe typically produces loss of push-off strength and causes instability of the medial longitudinal arch of the foot, but results in little functional disability.[32] If multiple toes are involved, consideration should be given to a transmetatarsal amputation.

Transmetatarsal (Forefoot) Amputations (Fig. 32–2)

This is a useful amputation site. Some spring and resilience of the foot is lost, but there is little disability in routine gait. It is the highest level of amputation at which no special prosthesis is required.

> **AXIOM** A good plantar flap is necessary for a successful and useful transmetatarsal amputation.

In the usual situation, almost no dorsal flap is used, and the plantar flap begins at the metatarsophalangeal skin crease. Although exposed tendons should be sharply excised, it is important to keep the plantar flap as thick as possible. The dorsal skin incision is 1.0 to 1.5 cm distal to the point at which the bones are divided, which is usually at the midmetatarsal level. If there is some involvement of the distal plantar skin, this may not be possible. In such cases, division of the metatarsal bones at a more proximal level and use of a short dorsal flap (a "fishmouth" type incision) may allow a reasonable tension-free closure.

Postoperatively, the extremity should be kept horizontal or slightly elevated for at least 3 to 5 days, and then partial weight bearing can be begun. Some surgeons apply a short leg cast at or soon after the initial surgery to facilitate early ambulation. To enhance long-term rehabilitation, a small prosthesis or shoe mold is useful but not necessary.

Midfoot Amputations (Lisfranc's, Chopart's, Boyd's, Pirogoff's) (Fig. 32–3)

A number of different midfoot amputations have been described.[33] They have the advantage of preserving length and a weight-bearing stump. However, they are seldom used in most trauma settings because of other damage in the injured foot and the problem of equinus deformity.[34] Lisfranc's amputation is performed at the tarsometatarsal level, and Chopart's amputation is performed at the midtarsal joint. Boyd's amputation involves talectomy and calcaneotibial fusion. Pirogoff's amputation is similar, but involves calcaneotibial fusion after rotation and vertical sectioning of the calcaneus.

Syme's Amputation (Ankle Disarticulation) (Fig. 32–4)

> **AXIOM** Syme's amputation is considered a reasonable alternative to below-knee amputation if there is a good heel pad to use as a base.

Syme's amputation involves disarticulation of the ankle with preservation of the heel pad. Unlike a classic below-knee amputation, it offers an end-bearing stump. It may be attempted whenever the talus

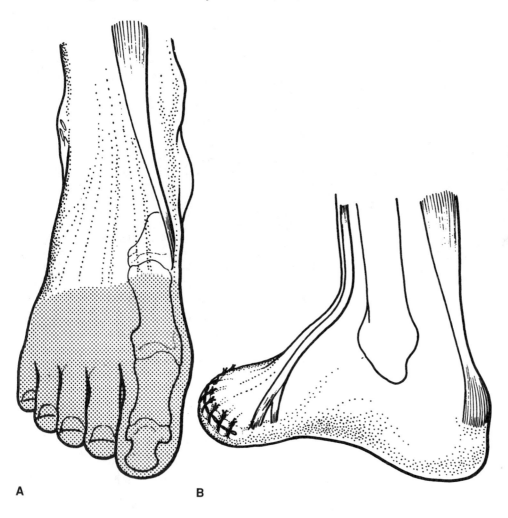

A   **B**

FIGURE 32–2 Transmetatarsal amputation. In the presence of severe injury to multiple toes in which a forefoot amputation is necessary, consideration should be given to maintaining the attachment of the tibialis anterior tendon which provides dorsiflexion at the ankle. This tendon is inserted into the medial cuneiform bone and the adjoining part of the base of the first metatarsal. (From: Robbs JV. Amputation for trauma. In: Champion HR, Robbs JV, Trunkey DD, eds. Rob and Smith's operative surgery: trauma surgery, part 2. London: Butterworths, 1989; 598.)

and calcaneus and the overlying soft tissue are normal. The major advantage is that short distances (such as to the bathroom at night) can be covered without the necessity of a prosthesis. It can also provide a better cosmetic result in females than a below-knee amputation.

Some surgeons feel that Syme's amputation is too difficult to perform and use it only rarely. One of the biggest problems with this amputation is the mobility of the heel pad; however, immediate application of a short leg cast after surgery can decrease this. Other techniques to decrease excessive heel pad mobility include removal of the distal articular surface of the tibia and fibula, or attaching the plantar fascia to the distal tibia using sutures through holes drilled in the distal bone.

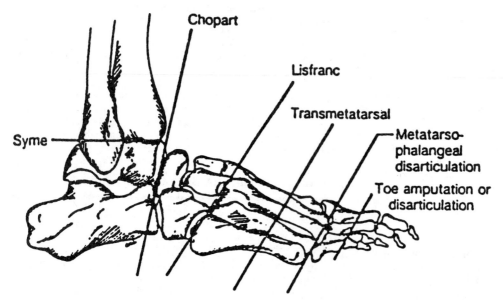

FIGURE 32–3 Midfoot amputation sites. With amputations through the metatarsal-tarsal joint, one should try to preserve the insertion of the tibialis anterior on the medial cuneiform and distal first metatarsal to allow dorsiflexion at the ankle. Chopart's amputation at the junction of the tarsal bones and the talus and calcaneus is rarely used now. (From: Robbs JV. Amputation for trauma. In: Champion HR, Robbs JV, Trunkey DD, eds. Rob and Smith's operative surgery: trauma surgery, part 2. London: Butterworths, 1989; 599.)

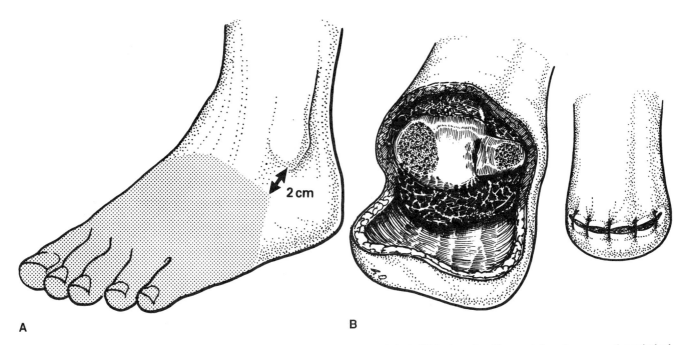

A

B

FIGURE 32–4 Syme's amputation (ankle disarticulation). While through-ankle amputations have many theoretical advantages, rehabilitation is often poor, and many patients require proximal revision because of the development of equinus/adduction displacement of the heel pad so that end-bearing is often not tolerated. (From: Robbs JV. Amputation for trauma. In: Champion HR, Robbs JV, Trunkey DD, eds. Rob and Smith's operative surgery: trauma surgery, part 2. London: Butterworths, 1989; 599.)

Disadvantages to Syme's amputation can include poor rehabilitation resulting from a bulbous stump, difficulties with prosthetic fitting, and heel pad migration and contracture preventing adequate end bearing. These problems can be diminished by careful surgical techniques. If they occur, they can be addressed with a prosthesis designed to relieve some end bearing, or formal revision to a classic below-knee amputation.

For Syme's amputation, a dorsal incision is made across the front of the ankle joint about 2 cm distal to the tips of the malleoli. The second incision crosses the sole of the foot across the anterior end of the heel pad. After division of all anterior soft tissue, the neck of the talus is exposed. With firm plantar flexion of the joint, the medial and lateral ligaments are divided by sharp dissection and the talus peeled forward out of the ankle mortise.

The calcaneus is now seen, and the Achilles' tendon is divided as close as possible to its insertion. By continued firm plantar flexion and forward traction on the foot, the calcaneus is shelled out of the heel pad by sharp dissection. The plane of dissection must remain as close as possible to the calcaneus to avoid buttonholing the skin and to preserve a well-vascularized, substantial heel pad.

A saw is now used to trim the malleoli flush with the tibia, and the tibial cartilage is excised by sharp dissection. It is vital that this weight-bearing surface be horizontal in relation to the ground to ensure even distribution of weight. Some surgeons prefer to leave the tibial cartilage intact. The skin is loosely approximated after hemostasis and irrigation of the wound.

A "two-stage" Syme's amputation has been described in cases in which there is gross infection in the forefoot. It involves disarticulation of the ankle, with incisions slightly more distal than the one-stage procedure. The second stage involves trimming the malleoli through separate medial and lateral incisions.

Below-Knee Amputations (Fig. 32–5)

When an amputation must be performed above the ankle, the site should provide a stump that extends 5 to 7 inches below the knee joint. Longer stumps are difficult to fit to a prosthesis.

AXIOM Rehabilitation with a below-knee prosthesis is much better than with an above-knee prosthesis.

Despite marked improvements in above-knee prosthetic devices, it is virtually impossible for an above-knee amputee to achieve anything resembling complete rehabilitation unless he is a young, healthy individual and a hydraulic knee is used. However, with a below-knee amputation, it is possible for many rehabilitated persons to achieve an active lifestyle.[8,35] If the viability of below-knee tissue is in question, transcutaneous measurements of PO_2 or xenon-clearance studies may be helpful.[36,37] In doubtful cases, the "gamble" to preserve a below-knee stump is usually worthwhile.

Whenever possible, the patient should be evaluated preoperatively by a physiatrist and a prosthetist. In the absence of significant contamination or a marginal stump in patients who are candidates for a prosthesis, some surgeons prefer immediate casting and application of a prosthesis with early ambulation. This can greatly speed up the patient's mental, psychological, and physical rehabilitation.[38,39]

Below-knee amputations are usually done with the patient in the supine position under spinal anesthesia. However, if general anesthesia is used, excellent exposure can be provided with the patient in the prone position.

AXIOM One should make a great effort to keep below-knee amputation incisions away from pressure and weight-bearing areas.

To appreciate the implications of wound placement with below-knee amputations, it must be understood that the pressure and weight-bearing areas concerning prosthetic fitting are the patellar tendon and proximal tibia and fibula. Considerable pressure and friction occur over the anterior border of the tibia during walking with a prosthesis as this area is largely responsible for providing the leverage to "kick" the prosthesis forward before placing the heel ("heel strike"). It is extremely important to avoid placing wounds or skin grafts over these pressure areas. This must also be carefully

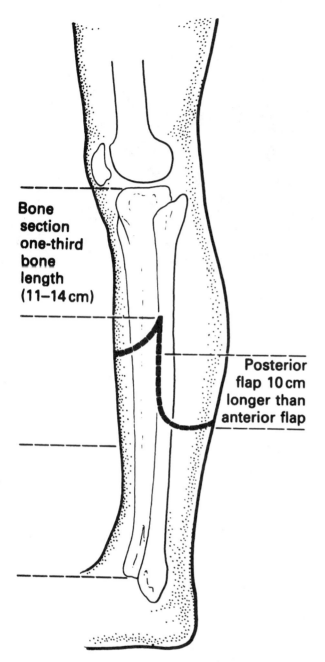

**Bone
section
one-third
bone
length
(11–14 cm)**

**Posterior
flap 10 cm
longer than
anterior flap**

FIGURE 32–5 Skin flaps for definitive below-knee amputations. Considerable pressure and friction occur over the anterior border of the tibia during walking with a below-knee prosthesis because this area is largely responsible for providing the leverage to "kick" the prosthesis forward before the "heel strike." It is, therefore, extremely important to avoid placing wounds or skin grafts over this area. To avoid this problem, the posterior flap should be made approximately 10 cm longer than the anterior flap. The anterior flap is made at a level about one cm behind the posterior tibial border, curving the incision cephalad. (From: Robbs JV. Amputation for trauma. In: Champion HR, Robbs JV, Trunkey DD, eds. Rob and Smith's operative surgery: trauma surgery, part 2. London: Butterworths, 1989; 600.)

considered if residual full-thickness flaps are used after initial debridement.

Posteriorly, a long skin flap that incorporates the gastrocnemius muscle is developed.[40] Anteriorly, the skin is transected 8 to 9 cm distal to the tibial tuberosity, and the incision is carried directly posteriorly one-half the diameter of the calf, to join the beginning of the posterior flap. The posterior flap should be approximately 10 cm longer than the anterior flap. No flap is needed anteriorly, but a small

flap is acceptable if gangrene or prior trauma limits the amount of skin available posteriorly (Fig. 32–5).

Deeper dissection is begun anteriorly (Fig. 32–6). The anterior tibial muscles are divided, and the tibia is isolated and transacted with a Gigli's saw 6 to 7 cm distal to the tibial tuberosity or 10–12 cm distal to the knee joint. Slightly longer stumps are acceptable in most cases and certainly preferable to ones that are too short. Stumps shorter than 8 cm provide insufficient leverage for standard prostheses.

The anterior half of the tibia is beveled at a 45° angle. The fibula is divided just slightly shorter than the tibia.[41] This ensures a more cylindrical shape to the stump (instead of a conical shape if too much fibula is resected) that enhances prosthetic fitting (Fig. 32–7). Once the tibia and fibula have been transected, posterior displacement of the distal extremity will usually expose the neurovascular structures rather well. The arteries and veins are ligated separately with nonabsorbable sutures. The nerve is mobilized and transacted under tension so that it retracts. The nerve may be ligated with absorbable suture, but this is rarely necessary.

The posterior flap with gastrocnemius muscle is then developed, and the remaining calf muscles are transected at the level of tibial transection. In many young trauma patients, the calf is bulky and it is often advisable in such patients to debulk the posterior flap muscles by shaving them down somewhat. However, care must be taken to avoid overgenerous excision and possible devitalization of the flap. Hemostasis is secured with absorbable sutures, and use of the cautery is kept to a minimum. Using absorbable sutures, gastrocnemius muscle tendon is approximated to the periosteum of the tibia, and then the fascial and subcutaneous layers are closed. Tension-free skin approximation is done with interrupted monofilament sutures or staples.

Unfortunately, in many traumatic situations the severe soft tissue injury does not allow for the ideal techniques of closed amputations with long posterior muscle flaps. Many patients will require immediate open or guillotine amputations, with closure after debridements.

Techniques for closure may vary depending on available tissues, and may range from fishmouth type incisions in the anteroposterior or sagittal planes, to nontraditional local tissue rotations. The principles of not placing wounds or skin grafts over pressure areas are important as outlined earlier. Occasionally, unconventional techniques have been used to salvage the below-knee level, including free tissue transfer,[8] tissue expanders,[42] foot "fillet" flaps,[43] or "composite bone" flaps.[44]

AXIOM   It is worthwhile to attempt to preserve the knee in "doubtful" cases in young trauma victims.

Through-knee Amputations

Amputations through the knee joint are unpopular with many prosthetists because the added length of femur hinders construction of a cosmetically-pleasing functional knee prosthesis. Many prosthetists prefer a long above-knee stump that provides adequate space for the knee joint mechanism, and hence provides a better cosmetic and functional result. However, amputation through the knee provides for a weight-bearing stump that is functionally superior to an above-knee amputation.

A number of different skin incisions have been recommended, including equal anterior-posterior flaps, long anterior flaps, or equal sagittal flaps[45] (Fig. 32–8). After flap mobilization, the knee is disarticulated by division of the cruciate and collateral ligaments. This is facilitated by flexion of the knee joint. The popliteal vessels are then ligated. The patella need not be excised, although it can be removed if there is patellofemoral pathology. The patellar tendon is then sewn to the cruciate stump, followed by the hamstring tendons (Fig. 32–9). This provides for stability of the thigh muscles. The skin and subcutaneous tissues are then closed. Rehabilitation is similar to that for below-knee amputations.

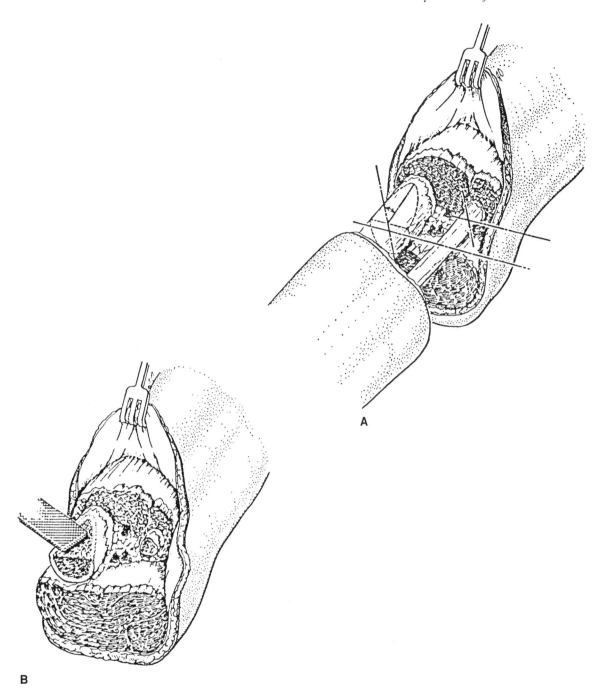

A

B

FIGURE 32–6 Deeper dissection in below-knee amputations. It is advisable to divide all soft tissues before dividing the bone. The tibial and peroneal vessels are ligated with nonabsorbable suture, and the nerves are gently distracted and allowed to retract proximally after division. The muscles are divided at the level of the distal extent of the flaps. The front half of the tibia is beveled about 45°, and the end of the tibia must be filed smooth. The fibula is divided about 2 to 3 cm proximal to the end of the tibia. If the calf is bulky, it is advisable to shave some of the posterial muscle down to allow a tension-free closure. The deep fascia of the calf should be approximated to the anterior deep fascia without tension using interrupted absorbable suture material. The tibial periosteum should be included in the central portion of the wound. It is important that the skin be closed without any tension using subcutaneous fascial sutures as needed. Some surgeons leave gaps between the skin sutures to allow adequate drainage, but we feel that total skin coaptation improves healing. (From: Robbs JV. Amputation for trauma. In: Champion HR, Robbs JV, Trunkey DD, eds. Rob and Smith's operative surgery: trauma surgery, part 2. London: Butterworths, 1989; 602.) *Continued.*

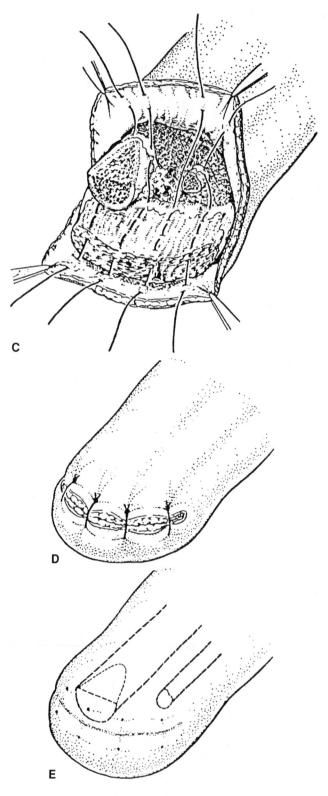

C

D

E

FIGURE 32–6   (continued.)

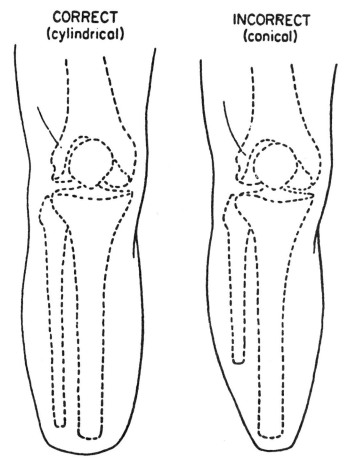

CORRECT (cylindrical)   INCORRECT (conical)

FIGURE 32–7 Closure and shaping of below-knee amputation stumps. Ideally, the stump should be shaped like a cylinder rather than like a cone. (From: Moore WS. Below-knee amputation. In: Moore WS, Malone JM, eds, Lower Extremity amputation. WB Saunders 1989;126.)

Above-knee Amputations

Above-knee amputation should be reserved for patients who have: (a) traumatic amputations above the level of the knee, (b) frank gangrene extending above the knee, and/or (c) documented nonambulation before the injury.

If the patient is a candidate for a prosthesis, as much femur as pos-

sible is maintained. The optimum length is approximately two-thirds the length of the femoral shaft as measured from the greater trochanter. This is approximately 35-40 cm in the average individual. If circumstances dictate a more proximal amputation, a femur length of 10-12 cm from the greater trochanter is the shortest that allows use of a conventional prosthesis. Shorter stumps require the use of the cumbersome "tilting table" prosthesis. Prosthetic weight bearing is mainly on the ischium with some weight distributed to the sides because of the cone-shape of the stump. If ambulation is not thought likely, midfemur amputation provides better healing than more distal sites.

A fishmouth incision with equal anterior and posterior flaps is generally used; however, there may occasionally be an advantage in placing them medially and laterally (Fig. 32–10). The muscles should be divided at the level of the distal end of the flaps and no attempt is made to debulk or shape them. The femoral vessels are individually transfixed and ligated with nonabsorbable material. The sciatic nerve is pulled down gently, but with some tension, and divided so that it retracts to a position well above the suture line. The bone is transected at the level of the apex of the wound and the edges are filed smooth. A multiple-layer closure over the bone is important. To ensure adequate balanced muscle action, it is important to oppose muscle groups. An effective technique involves drilling the bone and using the drill holes to firmly attach the muscles to the bone (myodesis). It is easier to drill the holes before dividing the femur. Six to eight equally-spaced holes around the circumference are drilled with a 2-3 mm diameter bit about 3-4 mm from the eventual bone end.

The stump is thoroughly irrigated with normal saline until all bone and loose muscle fragments have been removed. The muscle groups are then sutured to the bone end by threading the suture through the layers of deep fascia in a radial fashion using heavy absorbable sutures. This is done so that once the sutures have been tied, the muscle ends will overlap the bone end. The other muscle groups can then be approximated with interrupted sutures to form a further cushion over the bone end. The skin edges should be loosely approximated with interrupted monofilament sutures or staples. If there is any tendency for oozing from the proximal cut tissues, a closed drain, such as a hemovac, can be left in for a day or two.

A temporary prosthesis is of some value. Early periodic placement of the patient in a prone position may help to prevent a flexion contracture at the hip.

Hip Disarticulation (Fig. 32–11)

True hip disarticulation is rarely required in the trauma patient except with severe avulsions in pedestrian accidents or when a patient

FIGURE 32–8 Standard incisions for through-knee amputations. In general, equal anteroposterior flaps or sagittal flaps are preferred. (From: Burgess EM. Knee disarticulation and above-knee amputation. In: Moore WS, Malone JM, eds. Lower extremity amputation. WB Saunders Co., 1989; 136.)

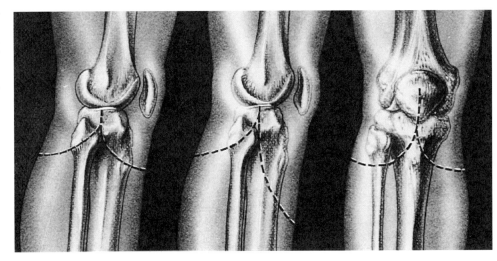

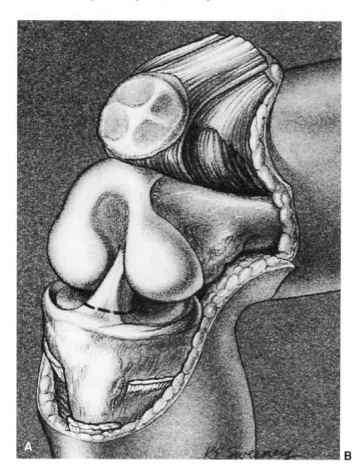

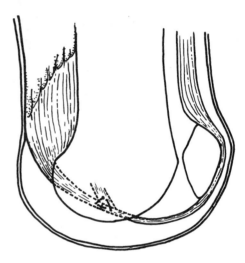

FIGURE 32–9   Knee disarticulation with the patella sewn to the ends of the cruciate ligaments. (From: Burgess EM. Knee disarticulation and above-knee amputation. In: Moore WS, Malone JM, eds. Lower extremity amputation. WB Saunders Co., 1989; 137.)

develops severe synergistic or gas gangrene. Even when disarticulation of the hip seems necessary, one should still try to make do with a high above-knee amputation. The femoral head and proximal femur should be retained whenever possible because they help preserve buttock contour and provide for better sitting balance and comfort.

UPPER LIMB AMPUTATIONS

General Principles

Weight bearing is not an issue in upper extremity amputation stumps, and more use can be made of residual unconventionally based flaps to obtain soft tissue cover of bone ends. However, there is no advantage in producing a strange shaped stump of unusable length because the ultimate goal is to provide a viable stump suitable for the fitting of a conventional prosthesis. It is, however, important to have protective sensation. Partial-thickness skin grafts should be avoided whenever possible because of their friability.

The usual trauma causing an upper extremity injury requiring an amputation is that of severe crush, bomb blast, or shotgun injury. Initial management includes debridement of dead tissue and removal of foreign material and debris. This should be followed within 24-48 hours by repeat wound inspection and debridement as needed. When the tissue is clean, definitive closure or formal amputation can be performed at a higher level. Conventional levels of upper limb amputation above the hand are disarticulation at the wrist, through the forearm, and above the elbow. Shoulder disarticulation is virtually never indicated for trauma. Amputations through the elbow joint offer no

advantage as the bulky stump makes fitting of a prosthesis quite difficult. In addition, the prosthetic joint would have to be placed either at a level below the normal elbow joint or on the sides of the socket, making the area rather bulky. Both situations are cosmetically unacceptable.

Finger and Hand Amputations

Amputations of fingers and the hand and possible replantation are discussed in the chapter on hand injuries.

Wrist Disarticulation (Fig. 32–12)

If the hand is unreconstructible, preservation of any part of the wrist confers no advantage because the added length makes prosthetic fitting difficult. Skin incisions are begun about 1 cm distal to the styloid process, and the flaps designed to provide a long volar and short dorsal flap. After proximal reflection of the flaps, the radiocarpal joint is disarticulated. Sufficient length of long flexor and extensor tendons should be retained to allow them to be sutured together over the bone end to provide a cushion. The joint cartilages and radial and ulnar styloid processes should be excised.

Forearm Amputations (Fig. 32–13)

Amputations through the forearm are performed with the extremity in supination. The optimum length is at the junction of the middle and distal thirds of the forearm. This allows adequate leverage and

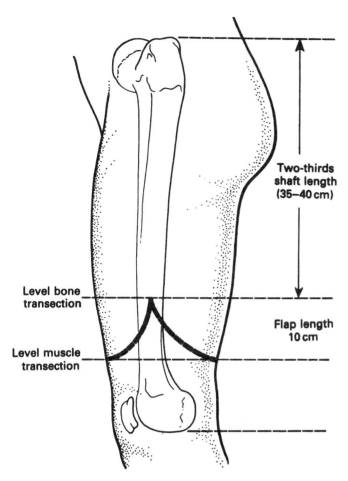

FIGURE 32–10 Above-knee amputation skin incisions. The optimum length is approximately two-thirds the length of the femoral shaft as measured from the greater trochanter to the knee. If circumstances require a more proximal amputation, a length of 10-12 cm from the greater trochanter is generally the shortest that allows proper use of a conventional prosthesis. The flaps are of equal length so that the scar is placed over the end of the stump. The flaps should be approximately 10 cm long, as measured from the "angle" of the wound of each side of the thigh. (From: Robbs JV. Amputation for trauma. In: Champion HR, Robbs JV, Trunkey DD, eds. Rob and Smith's operative surgery: trauma surgery, part 2. London: Butterworths, 1989; 603.)

space to accommodate the usual prosthesis. In addition, there is sufficient muscle at this level to provide good soft tissue coverage of the bone ends.

Equal anterior and posterior skin and muscle flaps are made about 3-4 cm longer than the proposed site of bone section, so that the sutured wound lies transversely across the end of the stump. Nerves should be cut under gentle traction to allow them to retract an adequate distance from the bone ends. The major vessels are then individually ligated. After division of the bones, the ends should be carefully filed and rounded. Opposing muscle groups are sutured over the bone ends with absorbable sutures. The skin is loosely closed to allow drainage.

Above-elbow Amputations (Fig. 32–14)

AXIOM The primary concerns with above-elbow amputations are obtaining healing and preserving shoulder function.

The optimum length of humerus to accommodate a prosthetic elbow is provided by an amputation site about 9 cm above the medial and lateral humeral epicondyles. This leaves a stump approximately two-thirds the length of the humerus. The shortest stump that will

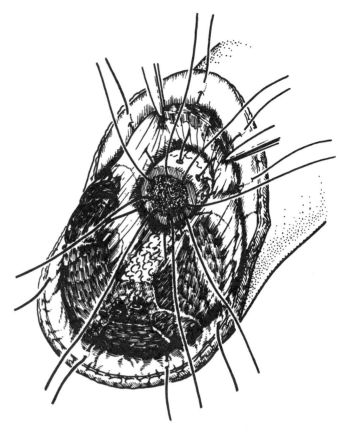

FIGURE 32–11 Technique of above-knee amputation. To help ensure adequate balanced muscle action, one can drill the bone to facilitate reattachment of the hip flexors and extensor muscles. In most instances, however, the muscles are sutured together securely over the end of the bone without drilling the bone. (From Robbs JV. Amputation for trauma. In: Champion HR, Robbs JV, Trunkey DD, eds. Rob and Smith's operative surgery: trauma surgery, part 2. London: Butterworths, 1989; 602.)

allow some useful function with a prosthesis is 6 cm below the anterior axillary fold.

On occasion, it may prove necessary to amputate proximal to the ideal prothesis level, particularly if there is a severe crush injury or if the patient has an avulsed brachial plexus with a flail anaesthetic limb. Under these circumstances, it is important to not disarticulate the humerus, but to divide the bone through its neck. This preserves the shoulder contour and enables the patient to wear a cosmetic prosthesis with some comfort.

Equal anterior and posterior flaps comprising skin and subcutaneous and muscle tissue are made approximately 4-5 cm longer than the proposed site of bone section. After gentle distraction and section of the nerves, adequate ligation of the individual brachial vessels is secured. The humerus is divided and the bone end filed smooth. Opposing muscle groups are sutured over the bone end with absorbable sutures in order to provide a suitable cushion. The skin is loosely approximated.

IMMEDIATE POSTSURGICAL PROSTHESIS

Complete wound healing of a lower-extremity amputation was often prerequisite to the fitting of prosthetic devices. For many years now, however, the early application of a temporary prosthesis has been used in many centers.

For practical purposes, the term "immediate postsurgical prosthesis fitting" is synonymous with below-knee amputations because: (a) below-knee amputations are the most common type of amputations in which this technique is used, (b) the rigid dres-

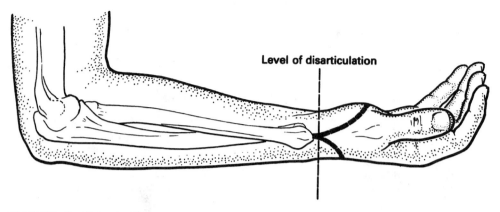

FIGURE 32–12 Wrist disarticulation. The skin incision is begun about 1 cm distal to the styloid processes. The flaps are designed to provide a long volar and a short dorsal flap so that the sutured incision lies dorsally. After proximal reflection of the flaps, the radiocarpal joint is disarticulated. Sufficient length of long flexor and extensor tendons should be retained to allow them to be sutured together over the bone ends. The radial and ulnar styloids should be excised. (From: Robbs JV. Amputation for trauma. In: Champion HR, Robbs JV, Trunkey DD, eds. Rob and Smith's operative surgery: trauma surgery, part 2. London: Butterworths, 1989; 606.)

sing is easiest to apply at this level, and (c) early ambulation is best achieved in the below-knee amputee.[39] Amputation is completed, a rigid dressing is applied to the stump, and then a walking pylon is added to the dressing. Early and immediate postsurgical prosthetic fitting has also been successfully employed in the upper extremity amputee.[46]

Early Ambulation

Early ambulation is the most controversial part of the immediate prosthesis program; indeed, many centers have modified their approach and are delaying ambulation on the prosthesis for a few days. However, many highly motivated patients can begin crutch walking the night of surgery. By the first or second postoperative day, all patients are encouraged to begin crutch walking, applying up to 25 pounds of weight bearing on the amputated side. By the fifth day, they are walking between parallel bars with increasing weight bearing. Progress from this point is individualized.

Delayed Ambulation

With delayed ambulation, the extremity is kept horizontal or slightly elevated for 3 to 5 days. Ambulation with partial weight bearing begins at 5 to 7 days, and full weight bearing is delayed until 10 to 14 days.

COMPLICATIONS OF AMPUTATION

Whenever extensive areas of necrotic or mangled tissue have been present for more than 6 hours or when there is residual tissue of doubtful viability, anticipated complications include sepsis and crush syndrome.

Local Complications

Infected amputation sites with gross pus should be opened as soon as possible for incision, drainage, and debridement as needed. If there is any delay in opening an infected wound, the pus may track be-

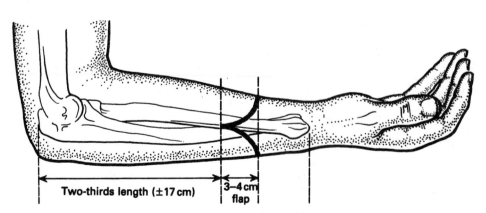

FIGURE 32–13 Below-elbow amputation. The optimum length of a forearm amputation is at approximately the junction of the middle and distal thirds of the forearm. This allows leverage and space to accommodate the prosthesis. In addition, there is sufficient soft tissue at this level to provide adequate cover for the bone ends, which is lacking at more distal levels. Equal anterior and posterior skin and muscle flaps should be made 3 to 4 cm longer than the proposed site of bone section, so that the sutured wound lies transversely across the end of the stump. (From: Robbs JV. Amputation for trauma. In: Champion HR, Robbs JV, Trunkey DD, eds. Rob and Smith's operative surgery: trauma surgery, part 2. London: Butterworths, 1989; 607.)

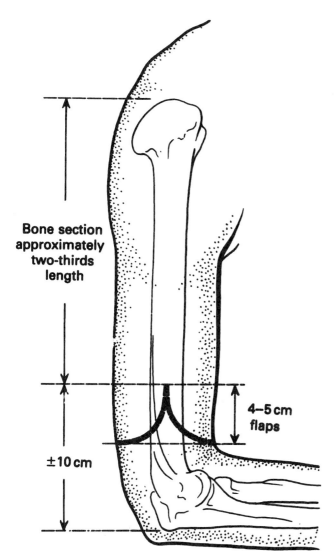

**Bone section
approximately
two-thirds
length**

**4–5 cm
flaps**

±10 cm

FIGURE 32–14   Above-elbow amputation. The optimum length to accommodate a prosthetic elbow is provided by an amputation 10 cm above the joint (1 cm above the medial and lateral humeral epicondyles), which leaves a stump approximately two-thirds the length of the humerus. The shortest stump that will give some useful function with a prosthesis is 6 cm below the anterior axillary fold. Equal anterior and posterior flaps of skin and subcutaneous and muscle tissue are made approximately 4-5 cm longer than the proposed site of bone section. (From: Robbs JV. Amputation for trauma. In: Champion HR, Robbs JV, Trunkey DD, eds. Rob and Smith's operative surgery: trauma surgery, part 2. London: Butterworths, 1989; 602.)

tween the muscles, increasing the likelihood of deep tissues becoming involved and exposing the end of the bone which may then have to be resected further.

Other local complications after amputation include wound hematomas and skin necrosis which may require reoperation. Later stump problems may include neuromas, phantom pain, chronic sores or stump pain, and problems with prosthetic fit which may require formal late stump revision.

Crush Syndrome

Crush syndrome generally refers to the systemic signs and symptoms resulting from the products of devitalized tissue entering the circulation. These problems can include sudden severe hyperkalemia with possible arrhythmias and acute oliguric renal failure resulting from myoglobinuria, with or without hemoglobinuria.

Maintenance of a high urine output, of at least 100 and preferably 200 ml/hr, will help prevent renal failure. Maintaining an alkaline urine by infusing sodium bicarbonate IV (1-2 mEg/kg/hr) to increase the urine solubility of myoglobin and hemoglobin may reduce the likelihood of these pigments precipitating and occluding renal tubules. The formation of ferrihemate, which is toxic to tubule cells, is also reduced if the patient is alkalemic.

⊘ FREQUENT ERRORS

In Traumatic Amputations

1. *Amputating an extremity without considering possible alternatives.*
2. *Making exceptional efforts to salvage a marginal, nonfunctional extremity, particularly in an elderly individual.*
3. *Amputating an extremity without considering the goals of rehabilitation and the optimal prosthesis.*
4. *Performing a definitive amputation on a badly mangled or infected extremity.*
5. *Amputating through an area with marginal blood supply.*
6. *Closing amputation tissues when the extremity has been badly contaminated.*
7. *Delaying physical therapy and rehabilitation of a patient with an amputation.*

▼▼▼▼▼▼▼▼▼▼▼▼▼▼▼▼▼▼▼▼▼▼▼▼▼▼▼▼▼

SUMMARY POINTS

1.   It is improper to amputate a severely injured limb unless there is no reasonable alternative; however, one should not attempt to salvage a marginal, nonfunctional extremity.

2.   Although no prosthesis can ever function as well as a normal extremity, most prostheses function better than mangled, painful, insensate limbs.

3.   When a surgeon attempts to reconstruct a severely injured limb that will probably have no function, he places the patient's life and the function of the remainder of the extremity in unnecessary jeopardy.

4.   If protective nerve function to an extremity (especially the foot) is permanently lost, that limb is essentially useless.

5.   A surgeon should not perform an amputation without completely considering the future goals of rehabilitation and without a clear understanding of the type of prosthesis which will provide optimal function.

6.   For best results, an amputation should be considered as part of a total rehabilitation program.

7.   It is generally ill-advised to attempt a primary definitive amputation on a severely injured or infected extremity.

8.   During initial surgery, guillotine or open amputation should be performed at a level at which tissues are assessed to be viable, but not through the level at which a definitive amputation would be made.

9.   Exercises to strengthen and prevent contracture of the muscles of the extremity at the amputation site should be begun early, even before the extremity has healed completely.

10.   With amputations, every effort should be made to salvage a functional knee or elbow.

11.   Syme's amputation can be considered a reasonable alternative to below-knee amputation if there is a good heel pad to use as a base.

12.   Rehabilitation with a below-knee prosthesis is much better than with an above-knee prosthesis.

13.   An attempt should be made to preserve the knee in "doubtful" cases of severe lower extremity trauma.

14.   One should make a great effort to keep below-knee amputation incisions away from pressure and weight-bearing areas.

15.   The primary concerns with above-elbow amputations are obtaining healing and preserving shoulder function.

▲▲▲▲▲▲▲▲▲▲▲▲▲▲▲▲▲▲▲▲▲▲▲▲▲▲▲▲▲

REFERENCES

1. Johansen K, Daines M, Howey T, et al. Objective criteria accurately predict amputation following lower extremity trauma. J Trauma 1990; 30:568.
2. Hansen ST Jr. The type III-C tibial fracture: salvage or amputation. J Bone Jt Surg 1987;69-A:799.
3. Lange RH, Bach AW, Hansen ST Jr, et al. Open tibial fractures with associated vascular injuries: prognosis for limb salvage. J Trauma 1985;25:203.
4. Bondurant FJ, Cotler HB, Buckle R, et al. The medical and economic impact of severely injured lower extremities. J Trauma 1988;28:1270.
5. Robbs JV. Amputation for trauma. In: Champion HR, Robbs JV, Trunkey DD, eds. Rob and Smith's operative surgery: trauma surgery. 4th ed. London: Butterworth & Co., Ltd., 1989;595-607.
6. Pozo JL, Powell B, Andrews BG, et al. The timing of amputation for lower limb trauma. J Bone Joint Surg 1990;72B:288.
7. Fairhurst MJ. The function of below-knee amputee versus the patient with salvaged grade III tibia fracture. Clin. Orthop 1994;301:227.
8. Georgiadis GM, Behrens FF, Joyce MJ, et al. Open tibial fractures with severe soft-tissue loss: limb salvage compared with below-the-knee amputation. J Bone Joint Surg 1993;75-A:1431.
9. Lerner RK, Esterhai JL, Polomano RC, et al. Quality of life assessment of patients with post-traumatic fracture nonunion, chronic refractory osteomyelitis and lower extremity amputation. Clin Orthop 1993; 295:28.
10. Bradway JK, Malone JM, Racy J, et al. Psychological adaptation of amputation: an overview. In: Moore WS, Malone JM, eds. Lower extremity amputation. Philadelphia: WB Saunders, 1989.
11. Clark JD, Malchow D. How to avoid errors in limb salvage decision. Orthopedic Review 1984;13:197.
12. Kirkpatrick Jr, Wilson RF. Amputations following trauma. In: Walt AJ, Wilson RF, eds. Management of trauma: pitfalls and practice. Philadelphia: Lea & Febiger, 1975;270-284.
13. Gregory RT, Gould RJ, Peclet M, et al. The mangled extremity syndrome (MES): a severity grading system for multisystem injury of the extremity. J Trauma 1985;25:1147.
14. Howe HR, Poole GV, Hansen KJ, et al. Salvage of lower extremities following combined orthopedic and vascular trauma: a predictive salvage index. Am Surg 1987;53:205.
15. Seiler JG, Richardson JD. Amputation after extremity injury. Am J Surg 1986;152:260.
16. Shah PM, Ivatury RR, Babu SC, et al. Is limb loss avoidable in civilian vascular injuries? Am J Surg 1987;154:202.
17. Rosenthal RE. Letter to the editor. J Trauma 1986;26:579.
18. Zhong-wei C, Meyer VE, Kleinert HE, et al. Present indications and contraindications for replantation as reflected by long-term functional results. Orthop Clin N Am 1981;12:849.
19. Oreskovich MR, Howard JD, Copass MK, et al. Geriatric trauma: injury patterns and outcome. J Trauma 1984;24:565.
20. Bonanni F, Rhodes M, Lucke JF. The futility of predictive scoring of mangled lower extremities. J. Trauma 1993;34:99.
21. Melissinos EG, Parks DH. Post-trauma reconstruction with free tissue transfer—analysis of 442 consecutive cases. J Trauma 1989;29:1095.
22. Caudle RJ, Stern PJ. Severe open fractures of the tibia. J Bone Jt Surg 1987;69-A:801.
23. Gustilo RB, Mendoza RM, Williams DN. Problems in the management

of type III (severe) open fractures: a new classification of type III open fractures. J Trauma 1984;24:742.
24. Miller HH, Welch CS. Quantitative studies on the time factor in arterial injuries. Ann Surg 1949;130:428.
25. Johansen K, Bandyk D, Thiele B, et al. Temporary intraluminal shunts: resolution of a management dilemma in complex vascular injuries. J Trauma 1982;22:395.
26. Malone JM, Moore WS, Leal JM, et al. Rehabilitation for lower extremity amputation. Arch Surg 1981;116:93.
27. Simper LB. Below-knee amputation in war surgery: a review of 111 amputations with delayed primary closure. J Trauma 1993;34:96.
28. Vanden Brink KD, Waring TL. A new technique of open amputation: use of the rolled flap. Clin Orthop Rel Res 1977;123:70.
29. Waters RL, Perry J, Antonelli EE, et al. Energy cost of walking of amputees: the influence of level of amputation. J Bone Joint Surg 1976;58-A:42.
30. Schwartz JA, Schuler JJ, O'Connor RJA, et al. Predictive value of distal perfusion pressure in healing of the digits and the forefoot. Surg Gynecol Obstet 1982;154:865.
31. Tooms RE. Amputations of lower extremity. In: Crenshaw AH, ed. Campbell's operative orthopedics. 7th ed. St. Louis: CV Mosby, 1987.
32. Mann RA, Poppen NK, O'Konski M. Amputation of the great toe: a clinical and biomechanical study. Clin Orthop Rel Res 1988;226:192.
33. Wagner WF. Amputations of the foot. In: Chapman MW, ed. Operative orthopaedics. Philadelphia: JB Lippincott, 1988.
34. Lieberman JF, Jacobs RL, Goldstock L. Chopart amputation with percutaneous heel cord lengthening. Clin Orthop 1993;296:86.
35. Purry NA, Hannon MA. How successful is below-knee amputation for injury? Injury 1989;20:32.
36. Burgess EM, Matsen FA, Wyss CR, et al. Segmental transcutaneous measurements of PO2 in patients requiring below-the-knee amputation for peripheral vascular insufficiency. J Bone Joint Surg 1982;64A:378.
37. Moore WS, Henry RE, Malone JM, et al. Prospective use of xenon-133 clearance for amputation level selection. Arch Surg 1981;116:86.
38. Malone JM, Moore WS, Goldstone J, et al. Therapeutic and economic impact of a modern amputation program. Ann Surg 1979;189:798.
39. Zette JH. Immediate postoperative prosthesis and temporary prosthesis. In: Moore WS, Malone JM, eds. Lower extremity amputation. Philadelphia: WB Saunders, 1989;177-214.
40. Roon AJ, Moore WS, Goldstone J. Below-knee amputation: a modern approach. Am J Surg 1977;134:153.
41. Moore WS. Below-knee amputation. In: Moore WS, Malone JM, eds. Lower extremity amputation. Philadelphia: WB Saunders, 1989.
42. May JW, Sheppard J. Reconstruction of the stump after below-the-knee amputation, soft tissue expansion and local muscle rotation flaps: a case report. J Bone and Joint Surg 1987;69A:1240.
43. Sanders WE. Amputation after tibial fracture: Preservation of length by use of a neurovascular island (fillet) flap of the foot. J Bone Joint Surg 1989;71A:435.
44. Younge D, Dafniotis O. A composite bone flap to lengthen a below-knee amputation stump. J Bone Joint Surg 1993;75-B:330.
45. Burgess EM. Knee disarticulation and above-knee amputation. In: Moore WS, Malone JM, eds. Lower extremity amputation. Philadelphia: WB Saunders, 1989.
46. Burkhalter WE, Mayfield G, Carmona LS. The upper-extremity amputee: early and immediate post-surgical prosthetic fitting. J Bone Joint Surg 1976;58A:46.

Chapter 33 Compartment Syndrome

ROBERT F. WILSON, M.D.

GREGORY M. GEORGIADIS, M.D.

INTRODUCTION

Compartment syndrome has been defined by Matsen "as a condition in which increased pressure within a limited space compromises the circulation and function of the tissues within that space."[1] Although Dietrich et al[2] have noted that Malgaigne was the first to describe compartment syndrome, the first medical reference to it was probably by von Volkmann.[3] In 1882, Rudolph von Volkmann first described a contracture of forearm musculature that he attributed to tight bandaging of an arm after a supracondylar fracture of the distal humerus. In 1926, Jepsen,[4] in an experimental study, reported that the devastating sequelae of compartment syndrome could be prevented by prompt decompression of the compartment.

Although compartment syndrome may occur anywhere that muscles are enclosed by fascia, it is most common in the lower leg. The forearm is the next most common site and the thigh is a distant third.[5,6,7] There has also been increasing awareness of abdominal compartment syndrome.[8,9]

ETIOLOGY

Most compartment syndromes are associated with fractures and related bleeding or muscle damage (Table 33-1). However, compartment syndromes can also be seen with any condition that interferes with blood flow or damages muscle enclosed within a fascial space.[10] It may also occur spontaneously. Bourne and Rorabeck[11] have noted that compartment syndromes may be acute (as after ischemia or fractures) or chronic (as after repeated episodes of compartment pain with physical exertion in athletes).

Sheridan et al[12] reported on infections occurring in compartment syndromes in patients with large burns. A multi-institution review of 1171 burn admissions identified five patients (0.4%) who developed intracompartment sepsis with fever and purulent drainage or fever, erythema, and swelling. Contributing factors may have included high-volume resuscitation, delayed escharotomy, extravasated intraosseous infusions, cannulation-related arterial injury, and splinting or positioning difficulties. The authors stressed that a high index of suspicion and an aggressive surgical approach facilitate successful management of this unusual problem.

Lower Extremity

Compartment syndrome of the lower leg is most frequent and most severe in the anterior compartment. It is particularly likely to occur after fractures of the tibia, combined arteriovenous injuries at the knee, prolonged compression, or severe muscle contusions. Other problems that can cause compartment syndrome include proximal venous ligation, infection, inadvertent intra-arterial injection of drugs, and localized pressure by casts, circular dressings, burn eschar, or pneumatic antishock garments (PASG). Occasionally, it can result from lying down in an unusual way for prolonged periods because of altered consciousness after drug ingestion or injury to the brain.[5,7] Overuse of muscles, such as with prolonged marching in military recruits or strenuous excercise,[13] may also cause this syndrome. A decrease in compartment size secondary to suturing fascial defects, closed reduction of fractures, or intramedullary nailing can increase local pressure and lead to compartment syndrome.[14]

AXIOM Any prolonged compression of an extremity can cause compartment syndrome.

A report of 27 cases of compartment syndrome after application of a pneumatic antishock garment, suggests that systemic hypotension and increased external pressure may be important factors in etiology.[15]

Upper Extremities

Development of compartment syndrome in the upper extremities, especially the forearm, has been attributed to a multitude of causes including: supracondylar fractures, fractures of the forearm, brachial artery puncture for arterial blood gases or for arteriography, subfascial intravenous infiltrations, hemophilia, crush injuries, drug overdose, replantations, and gunshot wounds.[5-7] The deep volar compartment of the forearm is particularly vulnerable because it is nourished by the anterior interosseous artery which has no significant collateral flow.

Much attention has been given to the relationship between supracondylar fractures of the humerus and the development of compartment syndrome in the forearm. Severe swelling can develop rapidly around the elbow with these injuries, and the brachial artery can be compressed if the elbow is flexed too much in an effort to provide an accurate reduction of the distal fragment. If the forearm muscles are ischemic for too long a period, they will necrose. The resulting fibrosis, particularly of the volar muscles, can result in severe flexion deformities of the hand and wrist, a condition often called Volkmann's ischemic contracture.

AXIOM Hand injuries, especially metacarpal fractures, occasionally cause compartment syndrome localized to the hand.

Compartment syndrome of the hand should be suspected if the hand is severely swollen and the fingers are in the intrinsic minus position (i.e., extended at the metacarpophalangeal joints and flexed at the interphalangeal joints).

Abdominal Compartment Syndrome

DEFINITION

Abdominal compartment syndrome (ACS), sometimes referred to as intra-abdominal hypertension, exists when there is abdominal organ dysfunction because of increased intra-abdominal pressure.

HISTORIAL ASPECTS

Eddy et al[9] have noted that Coombs[16] discussed the mechanisms of the regulation of intra-abdominal pressure in an article in 1920. Coombs wrote that Marey in 1863 and Burt in 1870 were the first to demonstrate the association between respiratory function and intra-abdominal pressures. In 1890, Coombs also noted that Heinricius showed that intra-abdominal pressures of 27 to 46 cm H_2O were fatal in cats and guinea pigs. Heinricius attributed the deaths to "prevention of respiration by interference with thoracic expansion." In 1911, Emerson implicated cardiovascular factors as the cause of death in cats, dogs, and rabbits subjected to intra-abdominal hypertension. The association between ACS and anuria was first described by Wendt in 1913.[16]

ETIOLOGY

Multiple clinical problems can increase intra-abdominal pressure. The most common are probably ruptured aneurysms or any problem in which there is continued intra-abdominal bleeding, such as when the abdomen is packed for microvascular bleeding after trauma. Closing the abdomen tightly may cause bowel to become ischemic, and ischemic tissues will continue to accumulate third space fluid and further increase intra-abdominal pressure.

INCIDENCE

The reported incidence of lower limb compartment syndrome after skeletal and/or vascular injury is extremely variable. Patmen et al[17] reported an incidence of 32% with arterial injuries and 14% with venous injuries.

Contrary to the impressions of some clinicians, compartment syndrome can occur in open tibia fractures, despite opening one or more compartments. Indeed, the incidence with open tibial fractures has been reported to be between 6% to 9%.[18,19] This is probably related to the high energy involved in open fractures. With open fractures, some compartments may be inadequately decompressed, and others may not be decompressed at all.

The incidence of compartment syndrome in closed fractures has been reported as 1%.[18] However, the true incidence may be much higher, especially since some of the late sequelae of compartment syndrome in the leg can be quite subtle. These can include varying degrees of joint stiffness, claw toes, and cavus or equinus deformities. Some studies note that the high rates of residual disability after tibia fractures may result primarily from sequelae of ischemic contracture.[20,21]

AXIOM   Delayed repair of combined injuries to the popliteal or lower femoral artery and veins is likely to cause compartment syndrome, especially if the vein is ligated.

The incidence of compartment syndrome of the leg in patients with combined popliteal arterial and venous injuries is quite high. Indeed, over 50% of our patients with combined popliteal artery and vein injuries have required a fasciotomy.[22] The incidence of abdominal compartment syndrome is unknown, but Morris et al[23] note a 15% incidence in high risk trauma patients.

PATHOPHYSIOLOGY

Ischemic or damaged muscle and other tissues tend to swell. If the muscle or tissue is confined to a tight fascial space, the resultant increased intracompartment pressure can retard venous return and capillary blood flow, causing even more ischemia.

AXIOM   Cessation of capillary blood flow can occur at tissue pressures of 25-30 mm Hg, which is much less than normal arterial pressure.

Reperfusion injury plays a major role in many cases of compartment syndrome,[24] and compartment pressure often begins to rise precipitously only after the blood supply has been reestablished in ischemic muscles. Heppenstall et al[25] experimentally demonstrated that elevated tissue pressures combined with tissue ischemia produced much greater tissue destruction than ischemia alone.

PITFALL ⊘

Allowing hypotension to develop or persist in a patient with possible compartment syndrome.

More recent work by Heppenstall et al[26] emphasizes the importance of the compartmental perfusion pressure (CPP), which is the mean arterial blood pressure (mBP) minus the compartment pressures (CP). An increasing compartment pressure and decreasing systemic pressure can quickly lower the compartment perfusion pressure to

ischemic levels. Perfusion pressures to muscles that might be developing compartment syndrome should be kept above 70-80 mm Hg, if possible, without causing fluid overload.

In a study of dogs reported by Matava et al,[27] the critical pressure threshold for the arterolateral muscle compartment in the hindlimb was 20 mm Hg less than the diastolic BP. Although this study looked at the amount of muscle necrosis present at 14 days, it appeared that peripheral nerves were much more sensitive to ischemia than muscle was.[28,29]

Holden[30] has suggested that the "vicious cycle" of compartment syndromes begins with vascular damage or tissue hemorrhage. Vascular damage causes ischemia and increased intracellular and interstitial edema, and this plus any tissue hemorrhage increases local pressure and reduces capillary blood flow. The enclosed muscle becomes ischemic and swells even more, further reducing compartment blood flow. As the vicious cycle continues, intracompartment pressures rise higher and higher.

Development of compartment syndrome with MAST (military antishock trousers), a type of pneumatic antishock garment (PASG), suggests that systemic hypotension and increased pressure on muscles may be important factors. The application of MAST to normal volunteers increases compartment pressure[31] and decreases perfusion and transcutaneous oxygenation in the underlying tissues.[32]

PITFALL ⊘

Failure to consider the possible need for a fasciotomy on an extremity that has had severe blunt trauma, prolonged ischemia, or compression.

Peripheral nerves and muscles have less resistance to ischemia than skin, and muscle and other deep tissue can die even though there are little or no skin changes.

The outcome after a period of ischemia varies not only with the tolerance of the tissue to hypoxia, but also with the extent of local changes, such as tissue damage or hematomas, that may impair restoration of normal blood flow after correction of the inciting causes.

Ames and his coworkers described "the no-reflow phenomenon" occurring after a period of severe ischemia.[33] Although there is a transient period of increased perfusion to most tissues, after the circulation is restored over the next 30-60 minutes, blood flow to the ischemic tissues often falls almost to zero. They ascribed the delayed but progressively worse hypoperfusion to narrowing of the lumens of arterioles and capillaries by various factors including swollen endothelial cells. These workers also demonstrated a secondary type of capillary narrowing associated with formation of intravascular blebs on the capillary endothelium.[34] Others have demonstrated that trapping of red cells in the narrowed capillaries can contribute to the impaired reflow. More recent studies show that clumps of leukocytes can also plug capillaries in skeletal muscle and the lung during and after prolonged hemorrhagic shock.[35,36]

AXIOM   Compartment pressures are apt to rise most precipitously shortly after blood flow is reestablished to ischemic tissues.

Some of the accelerated tissue changes with reperfusion may result from the formation of increased quantities of free radicals. These free radicals can cause lipid peroxidation of cell membranes and many other intracellular and extracellular structures.

Originally it was thought that mannitol was of benefit in compartment syndrome because its osmotic and diuretic effects reduced cell swelling and "pulled" fluid from edematous tissue into the vascular space from which it could be rapidly excreted in the urine. However, it is now recognized that mannitol is also a scavenger of toxic oxygen-derived hydroxyl radicals. This may prevent some of the cellular damage that leads to increased capillary and cell membrane permeability.[37,38]

Interestingly, it now appears that partial ischemia is capable of causing more cell damage than that caused by complete ischemia.[39] Partial ischemia prevents adequate ATP production for normal cell function, but it provides enough oxygen to allow the formation of free radicals.

In the abdomen, ischemic bowel and mesentery can take large quantities of fluid into their tissues, and the bowel lumen can dilate. After major trauma, coagulopathies or inadequate control of injured vessels can also cause intra-abdominal pressure to rise to levels that can interfere with capillary and venous blood flow. Diebel et al[8] showed that intra-abdominal pressures above 20-30 mm Hg could drastically reduce renal, hepatic, and intestinal mucosal blood flow.

Of 2500 ICU admissions during a six-year period, Widergren and Battistella[40] reported on 46 patients with abdominal compartment syndrome. The overall mortality was 41%. The most important physiologic changes occurring after relieving the intra-abdominal pressure were a decline in peak inspiratory pressure from 52 ± 12 to 44 ± 11 cm H_2O, and a rise in the PaO_2/FiO_2 ratio from 159 ± 105 to 215 ± 119 mm Hg. It is interesting, however, that the patients were not really oliguric and had a urine output of 79 ± 55 ml/hr before decompression. After decompression, bladder pressures were still somewhat elevated (22 ± 11 cm H_2O).

DIAGNOSIS

> **AXIOM** The initial clinical signs of compartment syndrome are often subtle. Early diagnosis requires a high index of suspicion.

Problems in Making an Early Diagnosis

It can be extremely difficult at times to make an early diagnosis of compartment syndrome. The surgeon's attention may be diverted by more immediately life-threatening injuries. The patient's central nervous system may be compromised by injury, anesthesia, or substance abuse, making it difficult to assess pain, motion, and sensation. The patient may be uncooperative, and this is most likely to occur in the very young and very old and in patients with substance abuse.

The three earliest symptoms and signs of compartment syndrome in the extremities are severe increasing pain, parasthesias, and pain on passive stretch. The pain from an early compartment syndrome is often more severe than one would expect from the injury, and it continues to get worse despite increased narcotic usage and splinting. Parasthesias are subtle but important early signs, because the sensory nerves in a compartment are especially sensitive to ischemia. However, a proximal nerve injury or an unconscious patient may mask both these signs. Pain on passive motion is an important sign of early compartment syndrome, but the examination must be done carefully. Distinguishing ischemic pain from the pain of muscle injury, fracture, or contusion can be extremely difficult.

TABLE 33–1 *Etiologies of Compartment Syndrome*

Trauma
   Crush
   Wringer injury
   Fractures
   Burns (eschar)
Arterial insufficiency, especially from trauma
Deep vein thrombosis or ligation
Internal pressure
   Casts
   Pneumatic antishock garment
Snakebite
Bleeding disorders
Eclampsia
Vigorous exercise (may also produce a chronic compartment syndrome)

From: Rhodes RS. Compartment syndrome. In: Cameron JL, ed. Current surgical therapy-3. Toronto: BC Decker Inc., 1989; 692-695.

> **AXIOM** Compartment syndrome may be present even if circulation to distal tissues appears adequate. Palpable distal pulses do not rule out the presence of compartment syndrome.

In patients requiring major vascular surgery, the prolonged anesthesia can make physical examination unreliable for several hours postoperatively. However, after recovery from anesthesia, the clinical findings may be obvious, necessitating a second anesthetic for fasciotomy. Feliciano et al[41] emphasized this fact and pointed out that 19% of the fasciotomies performed at Houston's Ben Taub Hospital were done at reoperation.

In certain patients who are at continued risk for 24 to 48 hours after surgery, careful and continuous monitoring may be impractical or impossible, and prophylactic fasciotomies may be indicated. Prophylactic fasciotomies are recommended if: (a) the arterial supply to a limb is interrupted for more than 4 to 6 hours, (b) the patient is unconscious or has peripheral nerve injuries, and (c) an open fracture reduction is being carried out near a compartment at risk.

Martin et al[42] reported on 188 patients with lower extremity arterial injuries: 31 iliac, 105 femoral, 40 popliteal, and 14 tibial. Lower extremity fasciotomies were performed in 58 patients. Forty-two were done at the time of the initial repair and 16 were performed later because a compartment syndrome was suspected clinically or because compartment pressures were increased. Three complications occurred because of delays in performing fasciotomies. Two patients had some muscle loss in the anterior compartment, and one patient had some muscle loss in the posterior deep compartment because of an inadequate initial fasciotomy.

Clinical Features

HISTORY

Predisposing Conditions

A history of severe trauma to the lower leg, thigh, or forearm should raise suspicion of this injury, particularly if fractures were present and if blood flow to the muscles in those areas was reduced for prolonged periods by proximal vessel injury or external pressure.

> **PITFALL** ⊘
>
> **Not diagnosing compartment syndromes until the six Ps of ischemia are present.**

The early findings of compartment syndrome involving the anterior tibial compartment have been described by Mubarak and Rorabeck as the six Ps: increased compartment pressure, pulselessness, paresis or paralysis, paraesthesias or anesthesia, loss of a normal pink color, and pain with stretch.[14] Pulselessness and paralysis are frequently late signs of compartment syndrome.

> **AXIOM** The potential for development of compartment syndrome after vascular trauma should be kept in mind, and the diagnosis should be relentlessly pursued, especially in high risk patients.

It can be difficult at times to distinguish between compartment syndrome, arterial injury, and nerve injury (Table 33-2). These conditions frequently coexist and their clinical findings often overlap. All three problems may have associated motor or sensory deficits and pain. However, arterial injury is usually associated with absent pulses, poor skin color, and decreased skin temperature. In contrast, compartment syndrome usually presents with intact peripheral pulses, at least initially. Nerve injuries often cause relatively little pain, and the diagnosis is frequently made by the exclusion of the other two entities. Doppler flow determinations, arteriography, and tissue intracompartment pressure measurements may be required to differentiate between these three conditions.

TABLE 33–2 Features That Distinguish Between Compartment Syndrome, Arterial Injury, and Nerve Injury

	Compartment syndrome	Arterial injury	Nerve injury
Pressure increased in compartment	+	–	–
Pain with stretch	+	+	–
Paraesthesia or anaesthesia	+	+	+
Paresis or paralysis	+	+	+
Pulses intact	+	–	+

From: Muburak SJ, Rorabeck CH. Treatment of compartment syndrome. Operative surgery. Trauma surgery. 4th ed. London: Butterworths, 1989; 585–594.

In the abdomen, major vascular injuries, coagulopathies, prolonged ischemia, or prolonged evisceration of bowel can cause increased intra-abdominal pressure, especially if the abdomen is closed under tension at the end of the procedure.

Symptoms

AXIOM Excessive pain is often the first indication of compartment syndrome.

The most characteristic symptom of developing compartment syndrome is deep, throbbing, unrelenting pain in the area in question (Table 33–3). The pain is usually much greater than expected from the physical signs.[1,43] Unfortunately, most patients with abdominal compartment syndrome have an endotracheal tube or are too sick or too sedated to complain.

PHYSICAL SIGNS

AXIOM Frequent and thorough sensory and motor examinations are required on any extremity that may develop compartment syndrome.

Leg Signs

PAIN ON PASSIVE EXTENSION OF THE TOES OR FOOT. Increased pain on gentle passive extension of the toes or foot can be a valuable clinical finding. However, such signs may also be seen with direct trauma.

TENSE CALF MUSCLES. Increased tenseness and swelling of the calf on palpation can be helpful signs. However, these symptoms are subjective and may be relatively late signs because they only assess the superficial posterior compartment, and this is the least likely compartment to be involved. Some surgeons feel that a thorough examination of the muscle can sometimes permit them to distinguish those patients who have scattered areas of dead muscle from those who just have a diffusely tender muscle group.[5]

NEUROMUSCULAR FUNCTION. It is important to understand the cross-sectional anatomy of the leg (Fig. 33–1). There are four compartments

TABLE 33–3 Clinical Features of Acute Compartment Syndrome

1. Pain out of proportion to the clinical situation
2. Weakness and pain on passive stretching of muscles
3. Hypesthesia in the distribution of the nerves in the compartment
4. Tenseness of fascial boundaries of the compartment

Modified from: Matsen FA, Winquist RA, Krugmire RB. Diagnosis and management of compartmental syndromes. J Bone Joint Surg (Am) 1980;62:286.

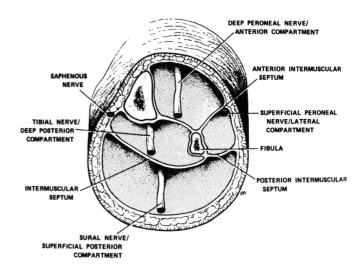

FIGURE 33–1 Cross-section at junction of middle and distal thirds of the leg, illustrating the four fascial compartments and their respective nerves. (From: Mubarak SJ, Owen CA. J Bone Joint Surg 1977;59A:184.)

(anterior, lateral, superficial posterior, and deep posterior). Each compartment contains important neurovascular structures.

In the leg, the deep peroneal (anterior tibial) nerve runs the length of the anterior compartment. It innervates the muscles of that compartment and supplies sensation to the dorsal web space between the first and second toes. Because the anterior compartment is the most frequently involved, if the examiner only tests plantar sensation, anterior compartment involvement could be missed.[5] Likewise, when checking for extension of the toes, the patient may be able to plantarflex the toes and then return them to the neutral position on relaxation. At times, the return of the toes to the neutral position can be erroneously interpreted as attempted extension of the toes; therefore, an active effort at extension must be confirmed by feeling the tightened tendons of the extensor hallucis longus and extensor digitorum longus muscles.

The superficial peroneal (musculocutaneous) nerve traverses the lateral compartment and innervates the peroneus longus and brevis muscles. It also supplies sensation to the dorsum of the foot, except for the first web space.

The tibial nerve lies within the deep posterior compartment of the calf and supplies motor branches to the posterior muscles of the lower leg and sensation to the plantar surface of the foot. Because the deep posterior compartment is smaller and less accessible, its involvement can be missed very easily.[44]

PITFALL ⊘

Depending on fullness or hardness of the calf to diagnose compartment syndrome.

The superficial posterior compartment is the largest compartment of the lower leg, and it is the least likely to be involved. The sural nerve traverses the proximal portion of this compartment and perforates the fascia to supply sensation to the lateral border of the foot. It has no muscular branches.

DISTAL PULSES. Assessment of distal arterial pulses is an important part of the examination. However, loss of distal pulses is usually a late sign because the compartment pressures required to compress major arteries far exceed those needed to stop capillary blood flow to the muscles in the compartment. Thus, severe muscle damage can occur in the calf despite palpable pulses in the feet.

CUTANEOUS ERYTHEMA. Cutaneous erythema, reflecting an inflammatory response in underlying ischemic muscle, is a very late sign.[2] It is most likely to be noticed over the anterior and/or lateral compartments, and it almost always is associated with the presence of underlying necrotic muscle.

Forearm

The same general principles used to detect early compartment syndrome in the leg also apply to the forearm.

Hand

A crushed, swollen, painful hand held in an intrinsic minus position (metacarpophalangeal joints in extension and interphalangeal joints in flexion) plus pain on passive abduction and adduction of the fingers suggest the presence of interosseous compartment syndrome in the hand.[45]

Abdomen

In the abdominal compartment syndrome, the abdomen is usually distended and tight. Examination of the chest usually reveals that the diaphragms are high. If the patient is on a ventilator, peak inspiratory pressures tend to increase as intra-abdominal pressure rises.

Laboratory Studies

> **AXIOM** High and/or rising CPK levels may reflect extensive muscle damage and may indicate the presence of an otherwise unsuspected compartment syndrome.

Severely elevated levels of creatine phosphokinase (CPK) often reflect severe muscle trauma or ischemia.[46] High levels that continue to rise suggest increasing muscle ischemia, as in compartment syndromes. Initially, CPK levels that are not quite as high and tend to decline can be characteristic of uncomplicated muscle trauma. However, CPK levels may also decline after there is complete loss of circulation to an involved compartment.

In abdominal compartment syndrome, urine output tends to decrease, and the urine tends to have the changes usually seen with a prerenal oliguria.

Compartment Pressures

> **AXIOM** Compartment syndromes are often detected by repetitive, careful clinical evaluation, but in patients with equivocal clinical findings, measurements of compartment pressures are essential.

To circumvent the diagnostic problems associated with physical examination, especially in obtunded patients, several techniques have been developed to directly measure compartment pressures.

> **AXIOM** Measurement of compartment pressure is the most accurate technique for diagnosing compartment syndrome, especially in the early phases when a fasciotomy produces the best results.

Measurement of intracompartment pressure by saline injection through needles was first done by French and Price in 1962,[47] and was also described by Renaman in 1968[48] and Whitesides et al in 1975.[49] Later, Matsen et al[50] described a variation of the needle technique that employed a continuous infusion of saline.

WATER MANOMETER

Patman described the use of a central venous pressure manometer, which is filled with sterile saline and attached to an extension tube and a regular 18-gauge needle that is inserted directly into the muscle compartment, with the extremity positioned level with the heart.[51] The manometer is positioned so that initially the top of its fluid level is slightly below the compartment being tested. The stopcock is then opened and the manometer gradually raised until the meniscus falls. Matsen proposed using a small needle catheter with a continuous slow infusion for long-term surveillance.[1]

To measure intra-abdominal pressure, one can use a nasogastric tube, but a Foley catheter in the urinary bladder is usually preferred. The usual technique, first described by Kron et al[52] in 1984, involves clamping the Foley catheter just distal to the aspiration port. A variable amount of sterile saline (30-90 ml) is then instilled into the urinary bladder via a needle in the catheter proximal to the clamp on the collection tubing. The needle is then connected to an electric transducer or a filled water manometer with the midaxillary line of the patient or the pubic tubercle as the zero joint. The water level in the manometer falls until the pressure in the bladder (which is essentially the same as the intra-abdominal pressure) equals the pressure reflected by the water level in the manometer.

WICK CATHETER

The wick catheter uses strands of polyglycolic acid and an electronic pressure sensor to monitor compartment pressures. This was modified for clinical use by Mubarak et al.[53] The principal advantage of the wick catheter is that injection or continuous infusion of saline is not necessary to measure compartment pressures.

SLIT CATHETER

The slit catheter developed by Rorabeck et al[54] combines the advantages of several clinical techniques for measuring intracompartment pressure. Five 3 mm long slits in the tip of a polyethylene tube inserted into the muscle maintain continuity between the tissue fluids and the saline within the catheter without injections or flushing. The catheter is connected to a pressure transducer and recorder to monitor intracompartment pressures.

SIDE-PORTED NEEDLE

A side-ported needle provides rapid and facile measurements of multiple muscle compartments.[55] It is an 18-gauge steel needle with a small side-hole close to the beveled opening of the needle.

COMPARISON OF CATHETER AND NEEDLE TECHNIQUES

In an experimental animal study, Moed and Thorderson[56] found that both the side-ported needle and slit catheter gave accurate compartment pressure measurements. A simple 18-gauge needle, however, gave consistently higher values than the other two methods.

SOLID-STATE TRANSDUCER

The recent development of a solid-state transducer small enough to fit in a catheter tip has simplified measurements of compartment pressures.[43] This handheld, inexpensive solid-state transducer (Stryker Surgical of Kalamazoo, Michigan) allows rapid, repeatable, or continuous pressure monitoring[2] (Fig. 33–2). Normal intracompartment pressures are usually less than 10 mm Hg.

CRITICAL COMPARTMENT PRESSURE LEVELS

> **AXIOM** One of the major problems with using compartment pressures to make surgical decisions is the lack of agreement on a critical level of pressure.

The critical pressure for a compartment may be altered by low perfusion states, patient positioning, and the duration of compartment hypertension. There are also concerns about the reproducibility of measurements within a given patient or with different techniques. Furthermore, it is not known whether compartment pressures should be measured continuously or intermittently or whether just one or all suspected compartments should be monitored.

> **PITFALL** ⊘
>
> *Failure to perform a clinically indicated fasciotomy just because compartment pressures are less than 30-45 mm Hg.*

Muscle compartment pressures in the leg are normally about 5-10 mm Hg. With absent or equivocal clinical signs, Patman and others suggest that fasciotomy be performed if the pressure exceeds 40 mm Hg.[1,43,51] However, there is no consensus regarding these measure-

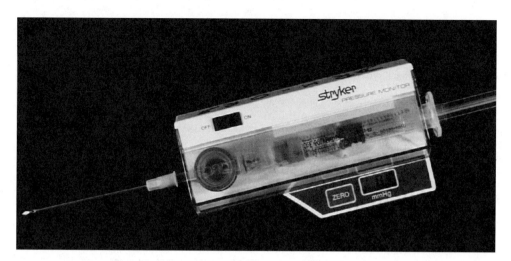

FIGURE 33–2   Portable hand held compartment pressure monitor (Stryker, Kalamzoo, MI).

ments, and Matsen et al[1] and Russell and Burns[43] in separate reports described patients in whom compartment pressure exceeded 40 mm Hg, yet no untoward effects resulted from continued observation.[1,43] Matsen et al[1] subsequently suggested that a tissue pressure in excess of 45 mm Hg is only a relative indication for surgical decompression, assuming a normal blood pressure, an adequate blood volume, and a normal peripheral vascular system. However, we agree with Perry et al[57] that compartment pressures above 30 mm Hg, when associated with appropriate clinical findings, are a firm indication for fasciotomy; yet, totally asymptomatic, alert, and cooperative patients with compartment pressures of 30-40 mm Hg can probably continue to be observed without fasciotomy.[6] Based on animal studies, Heckman et al[58] suggest that fasciotomies be performed if compartment pressures rise to a level that is within 10-20 mm Hg of the diastolic blood pressure.

> **AXIOM**   If unequivocal signs of compartment syndrome are present, one should proceed with fasciotomy without waiting for measurements of compartment pressures.

Other Diagnostic Techniques

TRANSCUTANEOUS DOPPLER MEASUREMENT OF VENOUS FLOW

In studies on 10 patients, Perry and associates noted a correlation between elevation of anterior compartment pressures in the leg and interference with tibial venous blood flow as determined by transcutaneous Doppler techniques.[57] When tissue pressure exceeded venous pressure (approximately 7 to 16 mm Hg), spontaneous and augmented tibial venous blood flow ceased. Thus, in patients with equivocal signs of compartment syndrome, sequential examination of tibial venous flow with a Doppler flow probe may be helpful. Loss of spontaneous venous flow may be an early indication of a dangerous rise in tissue pressure.

NERVE CONDUCTION

Measurements of nerve conduction velocity as described by Matsen et al may also be of some assistance in diagnosing compartment syndrome, particularly in patients who cannot cooperate or who have sustained direct extremity trauma.[1] If the patient is unable or unwilling to contract the muscles in a compartment voluntarily, the motor nerves to the muscles in the compartment can be stimulated using surface or needle electrodes.

ARTERIOGRAPHY

> **PITFALL** ⊘
>
> *Assuming that compartment syndrome is not present because distal pulses are present.*

In patients with vascular injury, a preoperative arteriogram may help pinpoint the exact cause and site of the circulatory problem. Arteriography may also be helpful when there are disturbances in motor function or perception of light touch. However, if the arteriogram is not absolutely necessary, it can sometimes cause the revascularization of an extremity to be delayed beyond the initial 4 hours when the results of vascular surgery are the best. In patients with established muscle necrosis in the lower extremity, an arteriogram may demonstrate patent tibial arteries but fail to opacify muscular branches. Failure to opacify any muscular branches is usually a grave prognostic indication of tissue death.[59]

NONINVASIVE METHODS

Palpation of muscle compartments is a qualitative clinical method to evaluate interstitial pressure. Experimental studies in animals have been performed in an attempt to quantitate the hardness of various muscle compartments by noninvasive surface probes.[60] Field et al,[61] however, emphasize that selective fasciotomy should be based on well-defined criteria and measurement of compartment pressures rather than serial physical examinations. The authors noted a 22% (4/18) infection rate when possibly unnecessary fasciotomies were performed.

PREVENTION OF COMPARTMENT SYNDROME

> **AXIOM**   Compartment syndrome is best treated by prevention.

Maintaining Vascular Inflow

Any vascular problem causing distal ischemia must be corrected promptly. Warm ischemia time must be kept to a minimum, preferably less than 4 hours. Cardiac output and blood pressure should be kept at the upper limits of normal or slightly higher to maintain the best possible collateral circulation.

With supracondylar fractures of the humerus, if there is any question at all about circulation to the forearm or hand, after attempts at closed reduction, the arm should be taken out of flexion and closely observed. If circulatory embarrassment persists, arteriography should be performed. However, immediate fracture stabilization followed by formal surgical exploration may be more appropriate if the extremity is clearly ischemic and an arteriogram cannot be done promptly.

> **AXIOM**   If any evidence of ischemia persists distal to a fracture after attempts at traction or closed reduction, immediate arteriography or surgical exploration is indicated.

Minimizing External Pressure

AXIOM One should look for compartment syndrome in any patient who has had external compression or a PASG inflated for more than 30 minutes.

With patients who have had external compression or a PASG inflated for more that 30 minutes, one should provide aggressive volume resuscitation and remove the external compression or decompress the PASG as soon as possible. Aggressive volume resuscitation should be provided as the PASG is decompressed to prevent a systolic BP drop greater than 5 mm Hg. The thighs and calves should then be evaluated clinically and/or with compartment pressures to identity the presence of compartment syndrome. If the PASG has been inflated for more than 30-60 minutes, one should continue to monitor the calves for development of compartment syndrome for at least 24 hours after PASG removal, particularly if there are any suspicious clinical signs.

Preventing Excess Venous Pressures

Although BP and cardiac output should probably be kept at levels slightly-moderately above normal to maintain optimal perfusion to injured or ischemic tissues, the central venous pressure should not be allowed to rise above normal. In patients treated with diuretics, compartment pressures have fallen about 25% over 24 hours, with a 40% decrease by the third day.[62] This suggests that overhydration tends to increase tissue and compartment pressures.

TREATMENT

Initial Steps

If compartment syndrome is suspected, one should remove any potential constricting circumferential dressing (i.e., release any bivalve circular bandages or casts). The extremity should probably not be elevated because this may reduce compartment perfusion. Repeated detailed neurovascular examinations are essential, along with palpation of the compartments and gentle stretching of the muscles that may be involved. Narcotic pain relief should not be increased because it can interfere with the assessment. Direct measurement of compartment pressures is generally the best way to make an early diagnosis of compartment syndrome.

Tissue Perfusion

AXIOM If compartment pressures are marginally elevated, hypotension can cause severe ischemic damage to intracompartmental muscles.

In patients with marginal ischemia of compartment muscles, the difference between the mean BP and the intracompartment pressure is probably the most important determinant of blood flow to the involved muscles. Consequently, efforts should be made to keep systemic BP and cardiac output as high as possible in patients with an increased risk of compartment syndrome. If possible, this increased perfusion should be accomplished without increasing the CVP above 5-10 mm Hg.

AXIOM In patients with a warm ischemia time of more than 4-6 hours distal to a vascular injury, a fasciotomy should be performed before the vascular repair.

When the warm ischemia time to muscle distal to injured blood vessels exceeds 4-6 hours, compartment pressures may rise rapidly after reperfusion.[63]

INDICATIONS FOR FASCIOTOMY

Extremities

Experienced trauma surgeons can often make an appropriate decision on the need for fasciotomy based solely on the patient's preoperative history, physical findings, or proximal vessel involvement.

Many surgeons feel that a prophylactic fasciotomy should be carried out when: (a) there has been a significant delay between the onset of ischemia or injury and reperfusion, (b) there has been prolonged hypotension, (c) massive tissue swelling occurs before or during the operative procedure, (d) there is combined proximal arterial and venous injury, (e) the major veins in the popliteal area or distal thigh are ligated, or (f) there is a severe crush injury.

PITFALL ⊘

Delaying fasciotomy to obtain compartment pressures when there is already clear clinical evidence of compartment syndrome.

Although the threshold level of compartment hypertension necessitating fasciotomy is quite controversial, it is generally agreed that a compartment pressure of more than 25-30 mm Hg is abnormal and requires either fasciotomy or, at least, continuous monitoring. Few would disagree that fasciotomy should be performed before arterial exploration if obvious compartment syndrome exists or if intracompartment pressures are significantly elevated (above 30-45 mm Hg) before reperfusion. In such instances, fasciotomies in the distal extremity can often be performed in 10-20 minutes and may be invaluable in preventing subsequent neuromuscular disability.

PITFALL ⊘

Delaying fasciotomy when there is clinical evidence of compartment syndrome but the compartment pressures appear to be less than 30-45 mm Hg.

Abdomen

Although peak inspiratory ventilatory pressures may rise early in abdominal compartment syndrome, many other factors are usually responsible for these changes, thus one may not immediately suspect abdominal hypertension. However, a decline in urine output in spite of normal or higher cardiac output and blood pressure should make one suspect abdominal compartment syndrome. If measured intra-abdominal pressures are 20 mm Hg or higher and there is oliguria in spite of a good BP and cardiac output, the abdomen should be opened. If intra-abdominal pressure is above 30 mm Hg, one should probably open the abdomen even if the urine output has been relatively well-maintained.

TECHNIQUES OF FASCIOTOMY

Lower Leg

Most authorities suggest that a four-compartment fasciotomy should be performed in the calf in almost all patients with suspected compartment syndrome, even though symptoms, signs, or elevated pressures may be confined to the anterior compartment. However, some surgeons limit decompression to the anterolateral compartments if they are the only ones with elevated pressures. If this is done, the pressures in the posterior compartments should be observed closely for at least 24 hours.

FIBULECTOMY FASCIOTOMY. Some surgeons favor doing a four-compartment fasciotomy in the lower leg through a single incision anterolaterally with excision of the mid and upper shaft of the fibula.[64] Removing most of the shaft of the upper fibula plus its periosteum and fascial connections provides relatively good access to and decompression of all four compartments. However, this procedure not only entails a relatively large amount of surgery, but for complex open tibia fractures, an intact fibula can be extremely important for initial stabilization and later bony reconstructive procedures.

SINGLE INCISION FASCIOTOMY WITHOUT FIBULECTOMY. Rollins and coworkers describe a single incision four-compartment fasciotomy without fibulectomy.[1,65] This involves a long lateral incision made directly over the fibula, extending from just below the neck of the fibula to a point 3-4 cm above the lateral malleolus. The lateral compartment containing the peroneal muscles lies directly beneath the incision and can be opened simply by deepening the skin incision. An anterior flap of skin and subcutaneous tissue is then raised to gain access to the anterior compartment.

A transverse incision is made just through the exposed fascia to identify the intermuscular septum that separates the anterior from the lateral compartment. While this is being done, one should identify the superficial peroneal nerve because it lies in the lateral compartment near the septum.[2] A second long fascial incision is then made through the anterior fascia of the anterior compartment, with care taken to avoid the superficial peroneal nerve as it exits from the fascia in the distal third of the leg near the septum.

A flap of skin and subcutaneous tissue over the posterior compartment is then raised in a similar fashion, and the fascia overlying the full length of the gastrocnemius and soleus muscles is divided. Finally, the attachments of the soleus to the fibula are divided. This allows retraction of the gastrocnemius-soleus muscle group in order to visualize the deep posterior compartment. The fascia of this compartment is then incised, taking care to avoid injury to the adjacent peroneal and posterior tibial vascular bundles.

TWO-INCISION FASCIOTOMY. Most trauma surgeons use the two-incision, four-compartment fasciotomy popularized by Mubarak and Owen[66] because it can be performed quickly and safely. Although it is often possible to decompress all four compartments fairly well through limited skin incisions, the skin itself can sometimes cause significant constriction, and a small incision does not allow one to adequately evaluate the entire muscle mass within those compartments.[67]

AXIOM The skin incisions for decompressive fasciotomies should be long enough to ensure that none of the underlying muscle is still compressed.

If needed, this type of fasciotomy can be carried out at the bedside under local anesthesia. The anterior and lateral compartments can be exposed by an anterolateral incision that begins between the fibular shaft and the crest of the tibia at midleg level (Fig. 33–3). The intermuscular septum can be identified by making a transverse incision through the fascia. The compartments are then released by longitudinal incisions with scissors. Care should be taken to avoid the superficial branch of the peroneal nerve, especially when extending the fascial incision proximally in the lateral compartment. The course of this nerve can be quite variable.[68]

AXIOM During anterior and lateral compartment fasciotomies, the superficial peroneal nerve should be visualized in order to avoid injuring it.

The superficial and deep posterior compartment can be decompressed through a posteromedial incision approximately 2 cm posterior to the posterior margin of the tibia. The greater saphenous vein and nerve can usually be protected by keeping them with the tissues anterior to the incision (Fig. 33–4).

The superficial posterior compartment is decompressed first. The posterior fasciotomy should extend the entire length of the compartment proximally and distally to a point behind the medial malleolus.

The deep posterior compartment is released distally and then proximally under the soleus. If the soleus muscle is attached to the tibia more than halfway down the shaft, this attachment should be released before performing the deep posterior compartment fasciotomy. Occasionally, the soleus muscle extends almost to the ankle,

completely covering the fascia of the deep posterior compartment. In such cases, the deep posterior compartment will not be seen until the superficial posterior fascia has been opened and the soleus is freed from the edge of the tibia.

RESPONSE TO DECOMPRESSION. After decompression of a compartment, it can be useful to quantify and document the changes in compartment pressures, thereby verifying adequate decompression.[69] This can be performed using any of the techniques described earlier. A method that involves readily available equipment in most operating rooms uses a 20-gauge spinal needle or intravenous catheter, long sterile extension tubing, a three way stopcock and a precalibrated intra-arterial pressure transducer of the type that anesthesiologists typically use for arterial pressure monitoring.[70] Care should be taken to place the transducer at the level of the injured extremity. Once the anesthesiologist has calibrated the system, both pre- and postfasciotomy compartment pressures can be documented on the monitor. The surgeon remains scrubbed and there is little disruption of the operative procedure. Gentle pressure on the compartment will produce visual increases in pressure that return to a baseline after release, thus confirming appropriate needle insertion. If the compartment pressures are still elevated because of inadequate skin or fascial incisions,[67] appropriate measures should be taken.

MANAGEMENT OF ASSOCIATED TIBIAL FRACTURES

AXIOM The most common cause of acute compartment syndrome in the lower leg is tibial fracture.

If compartment syndrome develops in a patient with a fractured tibia, fixation of the tibial fracture using plates and screws has been helpful in managing the bone and soft tissues and accomplishing later skin closure.[71] Plate fixation can be applied through the incision generally used for decompressing the anterior and lateral compartments.

Recently, the locked unreamed tibial nail has been used for stabilization of both closed and open tibia fractures with compartment syndrome.[72] However, if there is an open fracture with significant contamination, an external fixation device may still be preferred for bone immobilization. Stable internal or external fixation is desirable in these injuries instead of casting, as it allows for better care of the fasciotomy wounds and facilitates rehabilitation.

Thigh

Compartment syndromes in the thigh are unusual except with severe crushing injuries. A fracture of the femur is often present, and this can cause loss of more than 1 to 2 liters of blood into the deep tissues. The principles of management are similar to those in the leg, and all three of the compartments should be opened if indicated by clinical examination or measurement of compartment pressure. In most instances, only the quadriceps compartment must be decompressed, but the adductor and flexor compartment pressures should also be checked and followed.[73-76] After MAST application, thigh compartment syndrome rarely can occur in the absence of lower extremity trauma.[77]

Foot

Patients with calcaneus fractures or other severe foot trauma can develop foot compartment syndromes. Surgical techniques for decompression typically involve dorsal or medial incisions, or a combination, to adequately decompress the foot.[78,79]

Forearm

In the forearm, the volar and dorsal compartments are the major confined areas (Fig. 33–5). The compartment containing the mobile wad, which includes the brachioradialis and extensor carpi radialis longus and brevis muscles, can be approached through the volar incision.[2]

VOLAR INCISION. The volar incision for decompressing the muscle compartments of the forearm begins proximal to the antecubital fossa

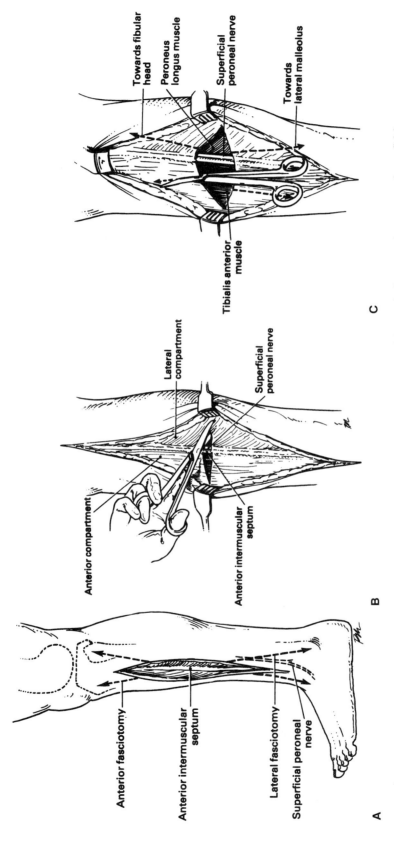

FIGURE 33-3 **(A)**. Lateral fasciotomy incision in the leg. **(B)**. Initial transverse incision with identification of the anterior intermuscular septum and superficial peroneal nerve. **(C)**. Longitudinal releases of the anterior compartment. (From: Muburak SJ, Rorabeck CH. Treatment of compartment syndrome. Operative surgery. Trauma surgery. 4th ed. London: Butterworths, 1989; 592.)

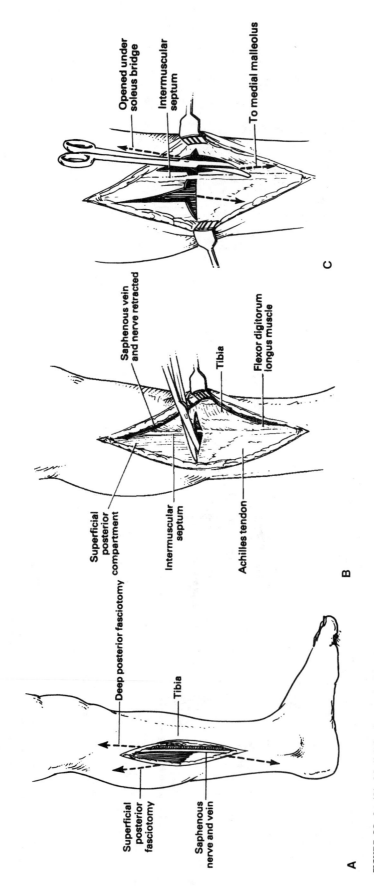

FIGURE 33–4 **(A).** Medial fasciotomy incision in the leg. Skin incision with identification of saphenous neurovascular bundle. **(B).** Initial transverse fasciotomy incision. **(C).** Longitudinal compartment release. (From: Muburak SJ, Rorabeck CH. Treatment of compartment syndrome. Operative surgery. Trauma surgery. 4th ed. London: Butterworths, 1989; 593.)

FIGURE 33–5 Fasciotomy incisions in the forearm. **(A).** Volar fasciotomy incision. **(B).** Volar-ulnar fasciotomy incision. **(C).** Dorsal fasciotomy incision. (From: Moore EE, Eisman B, Van Way CW. Critical decisions in trauma. St. Louis: CV Mosby Co., 1984.)

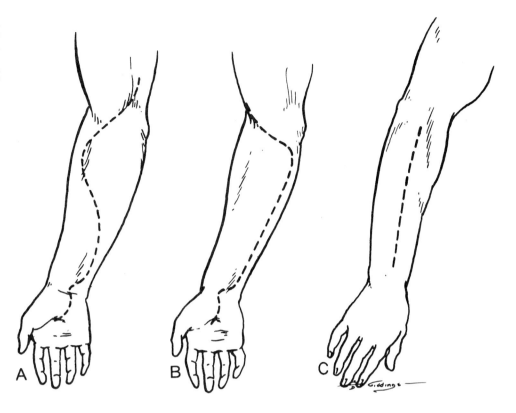

and extends to the midpalm. The incision allows division of the volar and brachial fascia and the transverse carpal ligament, as well as exposure of the arteries and nerves of the forearm and the mobile wad.[69,80] The incision is generally in the form of a "lazy" double S (Fig. 33–5). It should start near the medial epicondyle at the elbow and then course distally and obliquely toward the pronator teres insertion at the radial margin of the forearm at the junction of the middle and proximal thirds. The incision should then gently curve back toward the ulnar border of the forearm at the junction of the distal and middle thirds of the forearm. Then it gently curves in a radial direction again to the midportion of the wrist flexion crease and into the palm.

Skin flaps are then raised. A complete fasciotomy of all compartments should be performed from elbow to wrist. The superficial flexors are decompressed, and then the space between the flexor carpi ulnaris and the flexor digitorum sublimis is opened up to expose the deep flexor compartment muscles. Some feel that the individual muscles within each compartment should also be decompressed (Fig. 33–6A–D).

AXIOM A complete forearm fasciotomy may require decompression of each nerve and muscle.

Some surgeons believe that the median and ulnar nerves should also be carefully explored and freed from any constrictions when performing a fasciotomy. This may be especially important with the median nerve in four places: (a) the lacertus fibrosus (which is always released as part of the fasciotomy), (b) the pronator teres, (c) the proximal yoke of the flexor digitorum superficials, and (d) the carpal tunnel.[43] The ulnar nerve is most apt to be constricted as it passes between the two heads of the flexor carpi ulnaris.

If the mobile wad is involved clinically or by pressure measurements, this can be approached through the volar incision.

DORSAL INCISION. If it is necessary to open the dorsal compartment, this is usually done through a separate longitudinal incision directly over the extensor muscles. The dorsal skin incision begins 2 cm lat-

eral and 2 cm distal to the lateral epicondyle, and extends approximately 10 cm distally toward the wrist. The skin edges are undermined and the dorsal fascia incised throughout the length of the forearm. Individual muscles are freed as needed.

FASCIOTOMY IN THE PRESENCE OF FRACTURES. If acute compartment syndrome is associated with fractures of the radius and ulna, bone fixation should be undertaken at the time of fasciotomy. However, the plates should not be exposed in the fasciotomy wounds. If there has been severe contamination, external fixators may be preferred for stabilization of the fractures.

Hand

There is some controversy over the need for decompressing the hand if there is forearm compartment syndrome; however, if there is any question about the status of the hand, the volar incision in the forearm should be extended into the palm and the carpal tunnel should be released. In addition, the four interosseous muscle compartments should be opened via incisions on the dorsum of the hand over the second and fourth metacarpals.[45]

Abdomen

When the abdomen has been closed tightly to control a coagulopathy, the patient should be warmed to a core temperature of 35° or higher and the platelet count, PT, and PTT corrected with infusion of platelet concentrates and/or fresh frozen plasma as needed before reopening it.

Ideally, the abdominal fascia should be opened in the operating room so that any residual bleeding sites can be controlled with cautery or ligatures. The bowel is then protected with moist rayon or nylon, and moist dressings are applied and held in place with retention sutures or with an abdominal binder over the dressings.

DEBRIDEMENT OF NONVIABLE TISSUE

If may be extremely difficult to decide how much nonviable or marginally viable tissue to debride at the time of fasciotomy. Certainly, all obviously necrotic or nonviable tissue should be removed. Tissue that looks relatively healthy and bleeds when cut but does not con-

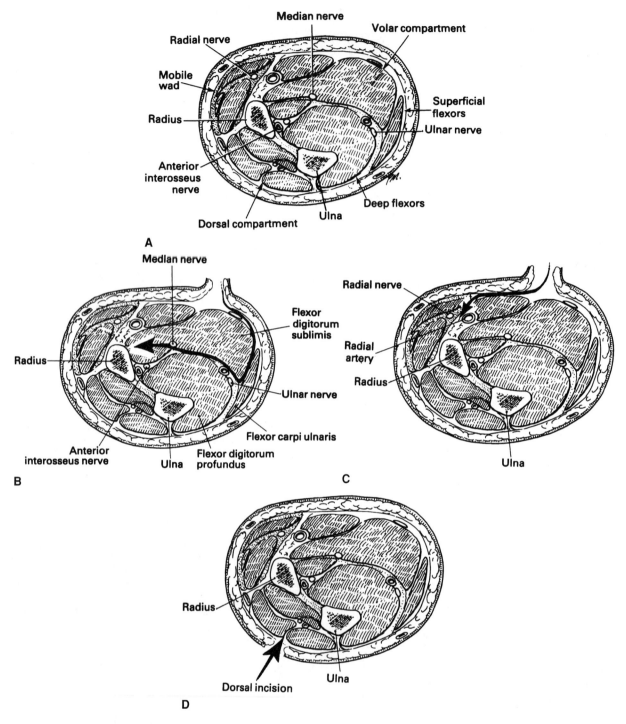

FIGURE 33–6   Forearm fasciotomy. (A) Cross sectional anatomy. (B and C) Volar decompression. (D) Dorsal decompression. (From: Muburak SJ, Rorabeck CH. Treatment of compartment syndrome. Operative surgery. Trauma surgery. 4th ed. London: Butterworths, 1989; 585-594.)

tract when stimulated can probably be left behind and observed closely. However, in an open wound, exposed marginally viable or ischemic tissue often becomes necrotic or infected over the next few days. Consequently, this tissue must be examined carefully, preferably in the OR, at least every 24-48 hours.

AXIOM   If the patient is becoming septic, any marginally ischemic tissue should be removed.

Hemostasis must be virtually perfect because use of compressive wraps to try to decrease bleeding may compromise tissue perfusion.

POST-FASCIOTOMY CARE

Fasciotomy incisions are packed open with saline-soaked dressings and covered with a dry, bulky bandage. The limb is kept elevated. If there is any question about muscle viability, the wound is examined carefully in the operating room every 24-48 hours. If any of the muscle is necrotic, further debridement is carried out as needed, and the compartments are reexplored every 1-2 days until the granulating bed is healthy.

Once the edema resolves, which usually takes at least 5-10 days, a delayed primary closure can be accomplished in most patients. However, if the skin edges have been widely separated, the large central portion of the fasciotomy wound may require a split-thickness skin graft. In some instances, progressive wound edge approximation as described by Patman may be used.[51] Multiple relaxing incisions may be another method of wound closure.

> **AXIOM** Early physical therapy is essential to prevent contractures after a fasciotomy.

After fasciotomy, passive and active exercises with the leg or arm elevated are maintained throughout convalescence to ensure joint mobility and to improve venous and lymphatic drainage. If a split-thickness skin graft is applied, the exercises are discontinued for 5-7 days and then reinstituted.

CONTROVERSIES AND CONCERNS ABOUT FASCIOTOMY

A number of controversial issues have been raised regarding fasciotomy.[5] Some surgeons are concerned that fasciotomy increases the risk of infection, particularly in patients with open fractures. Actually, the opposite is probably true. It is unlikely that healthy tissues exposed by an early fasciotomy will become infected, whereas necrotic tissue associated with a late fasciotomy will almost certainly become infected and can be extremely difficult to manage.

Concerns about prolonged hospitalization and cosmetic appearance after fasciotomy also seem unwarranted. The multiple operative procedures, disability, and appearance associated with an inappropriately delayed fasciotomy far outweigh any potential problems that might result from a "premature" fasciotomy.

Some orthopaedic surgeons have expressed concern that a fasciotomy will convert a closed tibial fracture into an open one and increase the risk of osteomyelitis. There are no reported data to support this concern, and the risks of infection are greater if ischemic tissue is overlooked.[5]

When fibulectomy was advocated as a technique for fasciotomy, there were concerns that it destabilized the tibial fracture. However, the declining use of the fibulectomy fasciotomy and the increasing use of internal or external fixation devices have significantly reduced concern over this issue.

COMPLICATIONS OF FASCIOTOMY

Infection

Proponents of fasciotomy for the treatment of compartment syndromes stress the importance of providing decompression before tissue death occurs. If muscle dies because of a delay in treatment and then is exposed by a fasciotomy, infection is almost certain to develop unless adequate debridement is obtained. Unfortunately, in some cases, adequate debridement, especially if infection becomes established, may involve amputation.

Patients requiring a fasciotomy should be given broad-spectrum antibiotics at the time of the procedure, and for at least 24-48 hours postoperatively, especially if any marginally viable tissue is present. Although some believe that the incidence of infection may be reduced if the fasciotomy incisions are closed early, early closure may cause death of additional tissue if the closure is tight and there is any residual marginally ischemic muscle.

Nerve Injury

Accidental injury to nerves is always a risk when performing fasciotomies. On occasion, causalgia follows compartment syndrome, but this is usually a result of the initial trauma or ischemic nerve damage rather than operative injury during the fasciotomy.

Some patients have viable muscle but become disabled because of neuropraxia from the initial injury or compartment syndrome. This usually resolves over 1-3 months, and in the meantime, these patients need optimal physical therapy to prevent muscle atrophy and contracture.

Adjunctive Therapy

The major, immediate complications of compartment syndrome result from the presence of devitalized muscle and include hyperkalemia, renal failure (secondary to myoglobinuria), infection, and limb loss. Efforts to prevent these must be begun early and pursued aggressively.

PREVENTING RENAL FAILURE

Studies on patients with muscle necrosis may reveal elevated levels of creatine phosphokinase (CPK),[81] hyperkalemia,[63] and myoglobinuria.

> **AXIOM** "Hemoglobinuria" on a urinary dipstick examination without microscopic hematuria is myoglobinuria until proven otherwise.

In patients with myoglobinuria, restoration of normal or increased blood volume and blood pressure and administration of mannitol to enhance urine flow to at least 100-200 ml/hr are important to improve intrarenal blood flow and prevent acute renal failure. Alkalinization of the urine to a pH of 7.0-8.0 with intravenous sodium bicarbonate (0.5-2.0 mEq/min) may help prevent the precipitation of myoglobin within the renal tubules.[57] Serum creatinine and BUN may be deceptive, and urine creatinine and urine and serum osmolality should be determined to calculate creatinine clearance and free water clearance, which are much more sensitive guides and accurate indicators of renal function.

FREE RADICAL SCAVENGERS

Mannitol

Many surgeons advocate the use of mannitol in patients who may develop a compartment syndrome. Buchbinder and coworkers demonstrated that reperfusion syndrome can be prevented in some patients by the administration of mannitol.[82] The salutary effects of mannitol were initially thought to be a result of osmotic activity, but it is now clear that mannitol is also a potent scavenger of toxic hydroxyl ions.[34,37,83]

Other Free Radical Scavengers

Other scavengers of free radicals (superoxide dismutase, catalase, and dimethyl sulfoxide) may be of some benefit in the treatment of compartment syndromes. Intracellular free radical scavengers, such as dimethyl thiourea, may be particularly helpful.[84]

Pentafraction

Pentafraction (PF) has been shown to seal abnormally large clefts in the leaking capillaries associated with scald burns as evidenced by a decrease in albumin leakage.[85] In addition, it has been shown to limit myocardial infarction size following ischemia reperfusion injury in dogs.[86] Hakaim et al[87] reported the effects of PF on ischemia reperfusion-induced compartment syndrome in rabbits that underwent bilateral femoral artery occlusion after ligation of branches from the terminal aorta to the popliteal artery. After 7 hours of ischemia, reperfusion was established. In the control group, anterior compartment pressure significantly increased from 10.8 ± 4.1 mm Hg at the end of the ischemic interval to 36.4 ± 9.9 mm Hg after 1 hour of reperfusion to 44.6 ± 15.4 mm Hg after 2 hours of reperfusion (P less than 0.007). The compartment pressures in the PF group went from 10.6 ± 2.6 at the end of the ischemic period to 11.4 ± 12.9 mm Hg and 7.4 ± 2.8 mm Hg after 1 and 2 hours of reperfusion.

PROBLEMS WITH INADEQUATE OR DELAYED TREATMENT

Problems in the Limb

The final clinical state of the untreated limb with compartment syndrome is a replacement of the involved muscle with scar tissue. In the forearm, this can produce a severe flexion contracture of the wrist and fingers (Volkmann's contracture). A "strangulation neuropathy" of the median and ulnar nerve can also occur where the nerves pass through the fibrous tissue, resulting in a hand that has no intrinsic muscle function and is completely numb over the median and ulnar nerve distributions.

AXIOM   Muscle death and/or ischemic nerve damage may result from compartment syndrome; the severe contractures that usually result can only be prevented by early, continued, vigorous physical therapy.

If muscle death has occurred, delayed repair of nerves often can not be accomplished because of severe scarring and because the injury to the nerve often extends over a long segment.[5]

AXIOM   Restoration of normal limb function without extensive reconstructive surgery is virtually impossible once muscle contracture has developed.

Reconstructive surgery after scarring or loss of muscle tissue usually includes excision of all fibrotic muscle, multiple tendon transfers, and neurolysis and epineurolysis of the entrapped nerves. When wide debridement of muscle is required, some disability is inevitable; however, physical therapy and proper splinting and bracing can help preserve function of the limb.

Renal Failure

A low urine output, hypotension, and increased release of myoglobin into the blood stream and urine can precipitate oliguric renal failure. If the patient is elderly or large doses of intravenous contrast have been given, the risk of renal failure is even greater. If oliguric renal failure develops, prophylactic hemodialysis or continuous arteriovenous hemodialysis (CAVH) should be considered.

Hyperkalemia

Hyperkalemia may develop with or without renal failure if enough muscle is damaged. Even 2-4 weeks later, succinylcholine can cause acute severe hyperkalemia in patients with paraplegia or extensive muscle injury.

⊘ **FREQUENT ERRORS**

In the Management of Compartment Syndrome

1. *Failure to recognize that compartment syndrome can occur with any type of compression of an extremity, even with a pneumatic antishock garment.*
2. *Failure to recognize that compartment syndrome can be confined to a hand.*
3. *Failure to anticipate the development of compartment syndrome in a limb that has been rendered acutely ischemic, especially after reestablishment of perfusion.*
4. *Allowing a patient with possible compartment syndrome to become marginally hypotensive.*
5. *Assuming compartment syndrome is not present in the lower leg if the calf feels soft, compartment pressures are less than 25-30 mm Hg, or if a distal pulse is present.*

6. *Failure to repeatedly check deep peroneal nerve function (sensation in the first dorsal web space and extension of the big toe) in a patient at risk for developing compartment syndrome in the lower leg.*
7. *Failing to adequately assess the reason for excessive or increasing lower leg pain after trauma or ischemia.*
8. *Failure to adequately incise skin and fascia to completely relieve the pressures in all possible compartments in a patient with either diagnostic clinical findings or elevated compartment pressures.*
9. *Failure to check for and treat myoglobinuria in a patient with suspected or proven compartment syndrome.*
10. *Failure to promptly and adequately debride nonviable muscle resulting from compartment syndrome.*

▼▼▼▼▼▼▼▼▼▼▼▼▼▼▼▼▼▼▼▼▼▼▼▼▼▼▼▼▼

SUMMARY POINTS

1.   Any prolonged compression of an extremity can cause compartment syndrome.
2.   Delayed repair of combined injuries to the popliteal or lower femoral artery and veins is likely to cause compartment syndrome, especially if the vein is ligated.
3.   Hand injuries, especially metacarpal fractures, occasionally cause compartment syndrome localized to the hand.
4.   Cessation of capillary blood flow can occur at tissue pressures of 20-30 mm Hg, which is much less than normal arterial pressures.
5.   One should not allow hypotension to develop or persist in a patient with possible compartment syndrome.
6.   One should carefully consider the possible need for fasciotomies on an extremity which has had severe blunt trauma, prolonged ischemia, or compression.
7.   Compartment pressures are apt to rise most precipitously shortly after reestablishing blood flow to an ischemic limb.
8.   Early diagnosis of compartment syndrome is contingent upon an alert physician with a high index of suspicion. The early clinical signs are often subtle.
9.   Compartment syndrome may be present even if circulation to distal tissues appears adequate. Palpable distal pulses do not rule out the presence of compartment syndrome.
10.   One should diagnose compartment syndrome before the six Ps of ischemia develop.
11.   The potential for development of compartment syndrome after vascular trauma should be kept in mind and the diagnosis should be relentlessly pursued, especially in high risk patients.
12.   Excessive pain in an injured or previously ischemic extremity is often the first indication of compartment syndrome.
13.   A thorough sensory and motor examination is required on any extremity that may develop compartment syndrome.
14.   One should not depend on fullness or tension of tissues in an extremity to diagnose compartment syndrome.
15.   Compartment syndromes are often detected by repetitive, careful clinical evaluation, but in patients with equivocal clinical findings, measurements of compartment pressures can offer valuable information.
16.   Measurement of compartment pressure is invaluable when doubt exists about the diagnosis, especially if the physical examination is unreliable or cannot be performed.
17.   One of the major problems with using compartment pressures to make surgical decisions is lack of agreement by experts as to what constitutes critical levels of compartment pressure.
18.   If definite clinical signs of compartment syndrome are present, one should perform a fasciotomy without waiting until compartment pressures exceed 30-45 mm Hg.
19.   Compartment syndrome is best treated by prevention of muscle ischemia and compression.

20. If any evidence of ischemia persists distal to a fracture after attempts at traction or closed reduction, immediate arteriography and/or surgical exploration is indicated.

21. One should look for compartment syndrome in any patient who has had a PASG inflated for more than 30 minutes.

22. When compartment pressures are marginally elevated, even mild hypotension can cause severe ischemic damage to intracompartment muscles.

23. In patients with a warm ischemia time of more than 4-6 hours distal to a vascular injury, a fasciotomy should be performed before the vascular repair.

24. The presence of any neuromuscular dysfunction in a patient with possible compartment syndrome is an indication for urgent fasciotomy.

25. The skin incisions for decompressive fasciotomies should be long enough to ensure that none of the underlying muscle is still compressed.

26. During anterior and lateral compartment fasciotomies, the superficial peroneal nerve should be visualized in order to avoid injuring it.

27. The most common cause of acute compartment syndrome in the lower leg is tibial fracture.

28. A complete forearm fasciotomy may also require decompression of each nerve and muscle.

29. If the patient is becoming septic, any marginally ischemic tissue should be removed.

30. Early physical therapy is essential to prevent contractures after a fasciotomy.

31. Despite the limitations in function imposed by muscle debridement, removal of all obviously necrotic tissue is essential.

32. "Hemoglobinuria" on dipstick examination of urine from a trauma victim without microscopic hematuria should be considered myoglobinuria until proven otherwise.

33. Muscle death and/or ischemic nerve damage may result from compartment syndrome; severe contractures can only be prevented by early, continued, vigorous physical therapy.

▲▲▲▲▲▲▲▲▲▲▲▲▲▲▲▲▲▲▲▲▲▲▲▲▲▲▲▲▲▲▲▲▲▲

REFERENCES

1. Matsen FA, Winquist RA, Krugmire RB. Diagnosis and management of compartmental syndromes. J Bone Joint Surg 1980;62-A:286.
2. Dietrich D, Paley KJ, Ebraheim NA. Spontaneous tibial compartment syndrome: case report. J Trauma 1994;37:138.
3. Von Volkmann R. Die ischaemischen kontuckturen. Zentralbl Chir 1991; 8:801.
4. Jepson P. Ischemic contracture, experimental study. Ann Surg 1926; 84:785.
5. Mubarak SJ, Rorabeck CH. Treatment of compartment syndrome. Operative surgery. Trauma surgery. 4th ed. London: Butterworths, 1989; 585.
6. Perry MO. Compartment syndromes and reperfusion injury. Surg Clin N Am 1988;68:853.
7. Rhodes RS. Compartment syndrome. In: Cameron JL, ed. Current surgical therapy-3. Toronto: BC Decker Inc., 1989;692.
8. Diebel LN, Wilson RF, Dulchavsky SA. Effect of increased intra-abdominal pressure on hepatic arterial, portal venous and hepatic microcirculatory blood flow. J Trauma 1992;33:279.
9. Eddy VA, Key SP, Morris JA. Abdominal compartment syndrome: etiology, detection, and management. J Tenn Med Assoc 1994;87:55.
10. Mubarak SJ, Hargens AR. Acute compartment syndromes. Surg Clin N Am 1983;63:539.
11. Bourne RB, Rorabeck CH. Compartment syndromes of lower legs. Clin Orthop 1989;240:97.
12. Sheridan RL, Tompkins RG, McManus WF, et al. Intracompartmental sepsis in burn patients. J Trauma 1994;36:301.
13. Kahan JS, McClellan RT, Burton DS. Acute bilateral compartment syndrome of the thigh induced by exercise. J Bone Joint Surg 1994;76-A:1068.
14. Tischenko GJ, Goodman SB. Compartment syndrome after intramedullary nailing of the tibia. J Bone Joint Surg 1990;72-A:41.
15. Aprahamian C, Gessert G, Banoyk DF, et al. MAST-associated compartment syndrome (MACS): a review. J Trauma 1989;29:549.
16. Coombs HC. The mechanism of regulation of intra-abdominal pressure. Am J Physiol 1920;61:159.
17. Patman RD. Compartmental syndromes in peripheral vascular surgery. Clin Orthop 1975;113:103.
18. DeLee JC, Stiehl JB. Open tibia fracture with compartment syndrome. Clin Orthop Rel Res 1981;160:175.
19. Blick SS, Brumback, Poka A, Burgess AR, Ebraheim NA. Compartment syndrome in open tibial fractures. J Bone Joint Surg 1986;68-A:1348.
20. Ellis H. Disabilities after tibial shaft fractures: with special reference to Volkmann's ischaemic contracture. J Bone Joint Surg 1958;40-B:190.
21. Owen R, Tsimoukis B. Ischaemia complicating closed tibial and fibular shaft fractures. J Bone Joint Surg 1967;49-B:268.
22. Thomas DD, Wilson RF, Wiencek RG. Vascular injury about the knee: improved outcome. Am Surg 1989;55:370.
23. Morris JA Jr, Eddy VA, Blinman TA, et al. The staged celiotomy for trauma: issues in unpacking and reconstruction. Am Surg 1993;217:576.
24. McCord JM. Oxygen derived free radicals: a link between reperfusion injury and inflammation. Adv Free Biol Med 1986;2:235.
25. Heppenstall RB, Scott R, Sapega A, et al. A comparative study of the tolerance of skeletal muscle to ischemia. J Bone Joint Surg 1986;68-A:820.
26. Heppenstall RB, Sapega AA, Scott R, et al. The compartment syndrome: an experimental and clinical study of muscular energy metabolism using phosphorous nuclear magnetic resonance spectroscopy. Clin Orthop Rel Res 1988;226:138.
27. Matava MJ, Whitesides TE, Seiler JG, et al. Determination of the compartment pressure threshold of muscle ischemia in a canine model. J Trauma 1994;37:50.
28. Gelberman RH, Szabo RM, Williamson RV, et al. Sensibility testing in peripheral nerve compression syndromes: an experimental study in humans. J Bone Joint Surg 1983;65A:632.
29. Szabo RM, Gelberman RH, Williamson RV, et al. Effects of increased systemic blood pressure on the tissue fluid pressure of peripheral nerve. J Orthop Res 1983;1:172.
30. Holden CE. Compartment syndromes following trauma. Clin Orthop 1975;113:95.
31. Chisholm CD, Clark DE. Effect of the pneumatic antishock garment on intramuscular pressure. Ann Emerg Med 1984;13:581.
32. Aprahamian C, Towne JB, Thompson BM, et al. Effect of circumferential pneumatic compression devices on digital flow. Ann Emerg Med 1984;13:1092.
33. Ames A 3rd, Wright RL, Kowada M, et al. Cerebral ischemia: the no-reflow phenomenon. Am J Pathol 1968;52:437.
34. Fischer EG, Ames A 3rd. Studies on mechanisms of impairment of cerebral circulation following ischemia: effect of hemodilution and perfusion pressure. Stroke 1972;3:538.
35. Bagge U, Amundson B, Lauritzen C. White blood cell deformability and plugging of skeletal muscle capillaries in hemorrhagic shock. Acta Physiol Scand 1980;108:159.
36. Ernst E, Hammerschmidt DE, Bagge U, et al. Leukocytes and the risk of ischemic diseases. JAMA 1987;257:2318.
37. Bulkley GB. Pathophysiology of free radical-mediated reperfusion injury. J Vasc Surg 1987;5:512.
38. McCord JM. Oxygen-derived free radicals in postischemic tissue injury. N Engl J Med 1985;312:159.
39. Roberts JP, Perry MO, Hariri RJ, et al. Incomplete recovery of muscle cell function following partial but not complete ischemia. Circ Shock 1985;17:253.
40. Widergren JT, Battistella FD. The open abdomen: treatment for intra-abdominal compartment syndrome. J Trauma 1994;37:158.
41. Feliciano DV, Cruse Pa, Spjut-Patrinely V, et al. Fasciotomy after trauma to the extremities. Am J Surg 1988;156:533.
42. Martin LC, McKenney MG, Sosa JL, et al. Management of lower extremity arterial trauma. J Trauma 1994;37:598.
43. Russell WL, Burns RP. Acute upper and lower extremity compartment syndromes. In: Bergen JJ, Yao JST, eds. Vascular surgical emergencies. Orlando: Grune and Stratton, 1987;203.
44. Matsen FA 3rd, Clawson DK. The deep posterior compartmental syndrome of the leg. J Bone Joint Surg 1975;57A:34.
45. Wolfort FG, Cochran TC, Filtzer H. Immediate interossei decompression following crush injury of the hand. Arch Surg 1973;106:826.
46. Haimovici H. Metabolic complications of acute arterial occlusions. J Cardiovasc Surg 1979;20:349.
47. French EB, Price WH. Anterior tibial pain. Brit Med Journal 1962;ii:1291.

48. Reneman RS. The anterior and the lateral compartment syndrome of the leg. The Hague: Mouton, 1968.

49. Whitesides TE, Haney TC, Morimoto K, Hirada H. Tissue pressure measurements as a determinant for the need of fasciotomy. Clin Orthop 1975;113:43.

50. Matsen FA 3rd, Mayo KA, Sheridan GW, Krugmire RB Jr. Monitoring of intramuscular pressure. Surgery 1976;79:702.

51. Patman RD. Fasciotomy: indications and technique. In: Rutherford RR, ed. Vascular surgery. Philadelphia: WB Saunders, 1984;513.

52. Kron IL, Harman PK, Nolan SP. The measurement of intra-abdominal pressure as a criterion for abdominal re-exploration. Ann Surg 1984;199:28.

53. Mubarak SJ, Hargens AR, Owen CA, et al. The wick catheter technique for measurement of intramuscular pressure: a new research and clinical tool. J Bone Joint Surg 1976;58-A:1016.

54. Rorabeck CH, Castle GS, Hardie R, et al. Compartmental pressure measurements: experimental investigation using the slit catheter. J Trauma 1981;21:446.

55. Awbrey BJ, Sienkiewicz PS, Mankin HJ. Chronic excercise-induced compartment pressure elevation measured with a miniatured fluid pressure monitor: a laboratory and clinical study. Am J Sports Med 1988;16:610.

56. Moed BR, Thorderson PK. Measurement of intracompartmental pressure: a comparison of the slit catheter, side ported needle, and simple needle. J Bone Joint Surg 1993;75-A:231.

57. Perry MO, Shires GT III, Albert SA. Cellular changes with graded limb ischemia in reperfusion. J Vasc Surg 1984;1:536.

58. Heckman MM, Whitesides TE Jr, Grewe SR, et al. Histologic determination of the ischemic threshold of muscle in the canine compartment syndrome model. J Orthop Trauma 1993;7:199.

59. Tompkins GS, Hiatt Jr. Compartment syndrome and fasciotomy. In: Bongard FS, Wilson SE, Perry MO, eds. Vascular injuries in surgical practice. Norwalk, CT: Appleton & Lange, 1991;231.

60. Steinberg BD, Gelberman RH. Evaluation of limb compartment with suspected increased interstitial pressure: a noninvasive method for determining quantitative hardness. Clin Orthop 1994;300:248.

61. Field CK, Senkowsky J, Hollier LH, et al. Fasciotomy in vascular trauma: is it too much, too often? Am Surg 1994;60:409.

62. Christenson JT, Wulff K. Compartment pressure following leg injury: the effect of diuretic treatment. Injury 1985;16:591.

63. Shackford SR, Rich NH. Peripheral vascular injury. In: Moore EE, Mattox KL, Felicano DV, eds. Trauma. 2nd ed. Norwalk CT: Appleton & Lange, 1991; 653.

64. Ernst CB, Kaufer H. Fibulectomy fasciotomy: an important adjunct in the management of low extremity arterial trauma. J Trauma 1971;11:365.

65. Rollins DL, Bernhard VM, Towne JB. Fasciotomy: an appraisal of controversial issues. Arch Surg 1981;116:1474.

66. Mubarak SJ, Owen CA. Double-incision fasciotomy of the leg for decompression in compartment syndromes. J Bone Joint Surg Am 1977; 59A:184.

67. Cohen MS, Garfin SR, Hargens AR, Mubarak SJ. Acute compartment syndrome. Effect of dermotomy on fascial decompression in the leg. J Bone Joint Surg 1991;73B:287.

68. Adkison DP, Bosse MJ, Gaccione DR, Gabriel KR. Anatomical variations in the course of the superficial peroneal nerve. J Bone Joint Surg 1991;73A:112.

69. Matsen FA, Mubarak SJ, Rorabeck CH. A practical approach to compartment syndromes in instructional course lectures. American Academy of Orthopaedic Surgeons. St. Louis: CV Mosby, 1983;32:83-113.

70. Smith M. An intraoperative technique for measuring compartmental pressures. Ortho Rev 1989;28:1316.

71. Gershuni DH, Mubarak SJ, Yaru NC, Lee YF. Fracture of the tibia complicated by acute compartment syndrome. Clin Orthop Rel Res 1987; 217:221.

72. Hak DJ, Johnson EE. The use of the unreamed nail in tibial fractures with concomitant preoperative or intraoperative elevated compartment pressure or compartment syndrome. J Orthop Trauma 1994;8:203.

73. Schwartz JT, Brumback RJ, Lakatos R, et al. Acute compartment syndrome of the thigh. A spectrum of injury. J Bone Joint Surg 1989;71A:392.

74. Gorman PW, McAndrew MP. Acute anterior compartmental syndrome of the thigh following contusion. A case report and review of literature. J Orthop Trauma 1987;1:68.

75. Foster RD, Albright JA. Acute compartment syndrome of the thigh: case report. J Trauma 1990;30:108.

76. Tarlow SD, Achterman, Hayhurst J, Ovadia D. Acute compartment syndrome in the thigh complicating fracture of the femur. J Bone Joint Surg 1986;68A:1439.

77. Kunkel JM. Thigh and leg compartment syndrome in the absence of lower-extremity trauma following MAST application. Am J Emerg Med 1987;5:118.

78. Manoli A 2nd, Weber TG. Fasciotomy of the foot: an anatomical study with special reference to release of the calcaneal compartment. Foot Ankle 1990;10:267.

79. Bonutti PM, Bell GR. Compartment syndrome of the foot. J Bone Joint Surg 1986;68A:1449.

80. Gelberman RH, Zakaib GS, Mubarak SJ, et al. Decompression of forearm compartment syndromes. Clin Ortho 1978;134:225.

81. Chiu D, Wang HH, Blumenthal MR. Creatine phosphokinase release as a measure of tourniquet effect on skeletal muscle. Arch Surg 1976; 111:71.

82. Buchbinder D, Karmody AM, Leather RP, et al. Hypertonic mannitol: its use in the prevention of revascularization syndrome after acute arterial ischemia. Arch Surg 1981;116:414.

83. Flores J, DiBona DR, Beck CH, et al. The role of cell swelling in ischemic renal damage and the protective effect of hypertonic solute. J Clin Invest 1972;51:118.

84. Rutherford RB. Nutrient bed protection during lower extremity arterial reconstruction. J Vasc Surg 1987;5:529.

85. Zikria BA, King TC, Stanford J, et al. A biophysical approach to capillary permeability. Surgery 1989;105:625.

86. Zikria BA, Subbarao C, Goldberg G, et al. Reduction of ischemia-reperfusion injury of the myocardium by hydroxyethyl starch macromolecules. Circ Shock Suppl 1988;78:4.

87. Hakaim AG, Corsetti R, Cho SI. The pentafraction of hydroxyethyl starch inhibits ischemia-induced compartment syndrome. J Trauma 1994;37:18.

Chapter **34** Fat Embolism Syndrome

ROBERT F. WILSON, M.D.

GREGORY M. GEORGIADIS, M.D.

INTRODUCTION

Post-traumatic fat embolism syndrome (FES) is a clinical condition characterized by pulmonary and/or central nervous system dysfunction resulting from fat microemboli to the lungs, brain, skin, and other tissues, usually after fractures of long bones or the pelvis. It is a poorly understood entity, and there is no clear consensus as to the incidence, pathophysiology, morbidity, mortality, and optimal treatment of this disease.[1] The symptoms may develop rapidly but classically begin approximately 24 to 48 hours after injury.

> **AXIOM** The main clinical findings in FES include tachypnea with respiratory failure, mental confusion, and petechiae.

There are four main causes of pulmonary complications following musculoskeletal trauma. These include: (a) atelectasis with pneumonia, (b) fat embolism syndrome (FES), (c) adult respiratory distress syndrome (ARDS) as a result of nonpulmonary sepsis or severe inflammation, and (d) deep venous thrombosis with pulmonary emboli.[2]

HISTORY

The first description of the pathology of fat embolism at autopsy was given by Zenker in 1862.[3] He described fat emboli in the lungs of a patient who been crushed between two railroad cars, suffering multiple rib fractures and a ruptured liver and stomach. Scriba, in an extensive review of the subject in 1880, included the observation that fat appeared in the urine of these patients. This was the first diagnostic test for this injury. He also concluded that there was not enough fat in the larger long bones to cause significant fat embolism if one of those bones was fractured.

The first clinical diagnosis of fat embolism was made by Ernst von Bergmann in 1873.[3] He arrived at this diagnosis because of the similarity of a patient's symptoms with those of cats into which he had injected oil intravenously for his doctoral thesis 10 years previously. His patient, a 38-year-old blacksmith, fell from a roof, incurring a comminuted femoral fracture. Sixty hours later, the patient developed hemoptysis, dyspnea, cyanosis, and coma, culminating in death 79 hours after injury. Autopsy revealed massive pulmonary fat embolism.

The clinical diagnosis of fat embolism was first made in the United States at Cook County Hospital, Chicago by Fenger and Salisbury in 1879.[3] The patient was a 45-year-old housewife who fell from a roof and fractured her femur. Forty-eight hours later the patient developed tachypnea, dyspnea, cyanosis, bubbling rales, and then coma, followed by death 96 hours after injury. Autopsy revealed pulmonary fat embolism.

CLINICAL SETTING AND INCIDENCE

> **AXIOM** A subclinical form of fat embolism with a reduced platelet count and increased P(A-a)O$_2$ occurs after almost all fractures.[4]

Classic fat embolism syndrome occurs most frequently as an early complication of traumatic fractures of the pelvis and large long bones, particularly the shaft of the femur.[1] The syndrome develops in 1 to 25% of persons with fresh long fractures, and averages about 2 to 4%, depending on the criteria for the diagnosis and the selection of patients at risk.[2]

In an extensive review of FES, Muller et al[5] concluded that FES is encountered in about 0.9 to 2.2% of patients with long bone fractures. During intramedullary manipulations, such as prosthetic stem insertion or reaming, the incidence is typically lower (0.5 to 0.8%). In a study by Robert et al,[6] the incidence of FES in patients with fractures of the pelvis, femur, and/or tibia was only 0.26%, but increased with the number of "at risk" fractures.

In contrast, Ganong,[1] in a study of healthy young skiers, found an incidence of FES of 23% in patients with a fractured tibia and 75% in those with a fractured femur. In the 44 cases of FES that he described, the mean PO$_2$ was 45 mm Hg, and 40% of the patients had petechiae. However, no patient required mechanical ventilation, and no one died.

> **AXIOM** Despite the fact that fat droplets are found in venous blood as much as 90% of the time after long bone fractures, the incidence of full-blown FES is relatively rare.

FES is rare after elective orthopaedic procedures. It has been noted in procedures that involve pressurization of the intramedullary canal, such as arthroplasty of the hip and knee.[7-13] Intramedullary guides of modern total knee systems are now designed to avoid canal pressurization,[8] and intramedullary aspiration and lavage during total joint surgery may also decrease the incidence of pulmonary emboli.[14]

The incidence of clinical fat embolism syndrome after intramedullary nailing of long bone fractures is also low. It is postulated that reaming in the presence of a fracture may decompress the medullary canal, minimizing fat release into the circulation.[15] However, intramedullary nailing has also been linked with the development of fat embolism.[16] Recently, transesophageal echocardiography has been used to detect intracardiac embolization during reamed intramedullary nailing,[17,18] and suggests that fat emboli may be more prevalent than previously realized. Intramedullary reaming and pressurization of intact long bones, such as during prophylactic nailing of femoral metastasis, may result in a much higher risk of fatal FES.[19]

FES has occasionally been noted in many other traumatic and nontraumatic conditions. These include diabetes mellitus, burns, severe infections, inhalation anesthesia, chronic pancreatitis, chronic alcoholism, cardiopulmonary bypass, sickle cell anemia, renal transplantation, renal infarction, steroid-induced fatty liver, acute decompression sickness, liposuction, and parenteral lipid infusion.[20]

PATHOPHYSIOLOGY

Source of Fat Emboli

> **AXIOM** The two main theories to explain the source of the fat in FES are mechanical and biochemical.

The sources of fat emboli in the fat embolism syndrome are still debated. The mechanical theory has been proposed since the time of Zenker and von Bergmann, when it was assumed that fat emboli came from the marrow of fractured long bones. For fat to embolize from a fracture site, two conditions are necessary: (a) concurrent injury to the marrow and local vessels, and (b) a transient increase in extravascular pressure that favors movement of the fat into the intravascular compartment. Fat then embolizes to the lung and causes capillary obstruction, often subclinically. Early systemic and cerebral embolization can subsequently occur as the fat traverses the capillary bed and arteriovenous shunts in the lung.

The mechanical theory began to be questioned when Lehman and Moore in 1927 calculated that the fat content of the marrow cavity of an adult femur was only 65 ml. They believed that this amount was insufficient to account for the pathological findings in fat embolism.[3] They concluded that there must be an alternate source for the embolic fat, which was probably chylomicrons in the circulating blood. This led to the concept of agglomeration of chylomicrons, fibrin, platelets, and other blood elements as the source of fat emboli.

The biochemical theory assumes that increased intravascular fat results from mobilization of lipids from fat depots (Fig. 34–1). This, with loss of chylomicron emulsion stability, results in coalescence and formation of fat globules.[21] The driving force for these initial biochemical changes is assumed to be trauma induced catecholamine release. Neutral fats (triglycerides) that embolize to the lung are converted to free fatty acids by the action of pulmonary lipase.

The first laboratory evidence that biochemical processes might be involved in fat embolism was reported by Struppler in 1940, who noted that patients with fat embolism often had elevated serum lipase levels.[3] The free fatty acids that are formed by the lipase are toxic to the lung and disrupt capillary epithelium, leading to interstitial edema and hemorrhage and then atelectasis.

The release of thromboplastin that occurs with orthopaedic and other types of trauma induces platelet aggregation on any abnormal

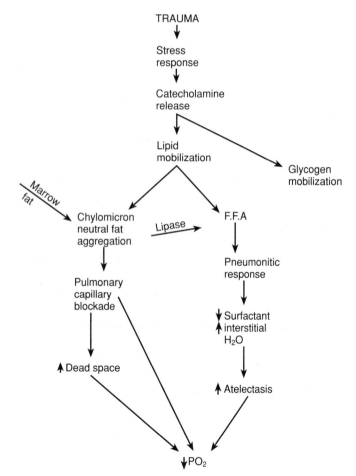

FIGURE 34–1 The fat content of the blood may increase after trauma by marrow fat entering torn veins at fracture sites and by increased lipid mobilization by catecholamines. The neutral fat can cause mechanical pulmonary capillary blockade, and the free acids formed later from the neutral fat can cause chemical pneumonitis. (From Shier MR, Wilson RF. Fat embolism syndromes. Surg Ann 1980;12:139.)

surface (i.e., fat globules) and accelerates the coagulation cascade. The latter process may be the mechanism responsible for the diffuse systemic and CNS microvascular thromboses and for the petechiae of fat embolism.

For many years, Hardaway emphasized that there was evidence of disseminated intravascular coagulation (DIC) in many severely injured patients suffering from shock.[3] Although a clear association between DIC and fat embolism syndrome has never been demonstrated, patients with fat embolism tend to have a consumption of coagulation factors and platelets. In fact, the thrombocytopenia is so consistent that it is an important diagnostic criterion.[22]

Although the chemical changes described and the small amount of free fat found in the marrow of large long bones favored a chemical source for fat emboli, Peltier concluded on the basis of extraction of fat from entire human tibial and femurs that most of the fat was contained within the metaphyseal sponge of these bones rather than their diaphyseal tubes.[23] He noted that the combined quantities from the diaphyseal tube plus the metaphyseal sponge were far in excess of those previously estimated. Experiments performed in animals demonstrated that the majority of tagged neutral fat given intravenously became sequestered in the lungs.[24,25] In addition, trauma-induced depression of reticuloendothelial function and of fibrinolytic activity along with catecholamine-induced mobilization of lipids greatly increased free fatty acid levels in the blood and aggravated the process.[26]

Additional data indicating the fat emboli came primarily from fractured bone was provided by chemical studies of the fat emboli. The chemical composition of fat emboli was similar to that of fat extracted from human bones. It consisted almost entirely of neutral fat, of which 65 to 80% has unsaturated fatty acids, with oleic acid the most important.[27]

When lipase acts on a neutral fat, the fat is broken down into glycerol, which is an innocuous water-soluble substance, and fatty acids, which can rapidly cause severe pulmonary changes. Peltier's classic studies showed that intravenous injection of neutral fat did not cause pulmonary changes for at least 24 to 48 hours. However, intravenous injection of fatty acids produced immediate effects on the lung closely resembling those of clinical fat emboli. This included extensive disruption of the capillary network in the lung and confluent hemorrhages.[28] It is unknown why certain patients develop this syndrome, when others with similar trauma and the presence of fat emboli do not.

AXIOM Both mechanical and biochemical mechanisms are probably involved in the development of most cases of fat embolism syndrome.

Platelets Changes

Severe trauma causes a massive release of tissue thromboplastin and other platelet activators, which results in platelet adhesion to any abnormal surface, particularly exposed collagen and fat droplets. These platelets release vasoactive amines, which can cause pulmonary vascular dysfunction, and cause the formation of thrombin, which can result in intravascular coagulation, all of which can cause hypoxemia (Fig. 34–2).

Platelet changes can be divided into three phases: (a) release of various chemicals in response to contact with connective tissue in vessel walls, (b) adhesion and aggregation induced by adenosine diphosphate (ADP) released from platelets or other injured cells, and (c) increased aggregation with stabilization of platelet aggregates by blood coagulation.

Exposure of platelets to collagen, particularly beneath disrupted endothelium, causes platelets to adhere to the collagen and react with it. Normally, platelets have osmophilic granulations that contain serotonin, histamine, and adenine nucleotides (ATP and ADP). When platelets interact with exposed collagen, these amines and nucleotides are discharged from these granules as the platelet-release reaction.

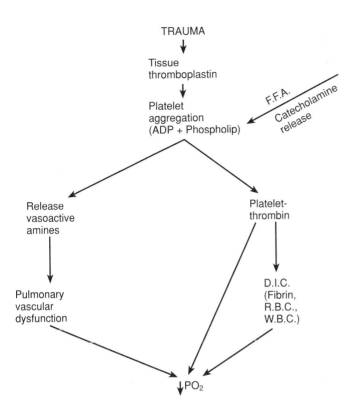

FIGURE 34–2 One of the main factors in the pathogenesis of fat embolism syndrome is platelet activation by tissue thromboplastin. The platelet aggregation, in turn, causes a release of vasoactive amines, especially serotonin, and thrombin formation, producing intravascular coagulation, all of which impair pulmonary function. (From Shier MR, Wilson RF. Fat embolism syndromes. Surg Ann 1980;12:139.)

Platelets also have granules that contain enzymes, such as beta-glucuronidase, acid phosphatase, and cathepsin, that may be released upon exposure to collagen. Platelets also release a permeability factor similar to that found in leukocyte granules. The enzymes and amines elaborated during the release reactions are probably responsible for many of the pathophysiologic changes of fat embolism syndrome.

Platelet aggregation and ADP can cause changes in the shape of platelets from that of a disc, which is characteristic of the resting or inactive state, to a more active form with pseudopods. In the presence of calcium and mechanical stimulation, the altered platelets are then able to adhere to one another. As aggregation proceeds, phospholipids on the platelet membrane accelerate the clotting interactions between factors IX and VIII and between factors X and V. Thrombin generated in the area of the platelet aggregation further releases platelet constituents, accelerates the clotting process, and activates the fibrin-stabilizing factor, factor XIII.

Epinephrine and norepinephrine, which are released during stress, particularly if shock develops, can also cause or increase platelet aggregation. In addition, epinephrine potentiates the action of ADP and thrombin in causing platelets to aggregate.

Coagulation Changes

Within minutes of experimental fractures, there is an abrupt decline in the plasma concentrations of fibrinogen and factors V and VIII,[29] reflecting an increase in intravascular clotting. Some of this clotting obviously occurs at the site of the fracture where multiple vessels are torn. However, the clotting at the fracture site is not adequate to explain the tremendous consumption of these factors.

Increasingly, it appears that the platelet activation caused by tissue thromboplastin and the subsequent platelet aggregation occurring at multiple sites in the body, particularly in the pulmonary capillar-

ies, may stimulate the intrinsic clotting pathway. As thrombin is released in areas where blood flow is impaired, clotting may increasingly accelerate.

Although it is believed that disseminated intravascular coagulation is an important component of fat embolism syndrome, its exact role is unknown. Nevertheless, there appears to be a definite correlation between the severity of intravascular coagulation and blood gas changes. It seems reasonable to assume that intravascular clots add to the obstructive problem in the small vessels of the lungs and that substances, such as serotonin, released from the clot further impair lung function.

Phases of Fat Embolism

All of the specific mechanisms leading to fat embolism syndrome are not fully understood, but it is clear that the syndrome involves more than early mechanical obstruction of small vessels by fat droplets. An important aspect of the pathogenesis of FES appears to be the delayed endothelial injury caused by fatty acids released by lipoprotein lipase from impacted fat droplets. The fatty acids increase microvascular permeability and fluid leakage into the interstitial spaces.

AXIOM Fat embolism syndrome can be divided into two phases: (a) an initial phase in which the mechanical obstruction of capillaries and other small vessels by neutral fat emboli is most important, and (b) a later chemical phase, as fatty acids are formed from neutral fat.[3]

Pulmonary Changes

The vast majority of the fat emboli released from fractured bone lodge in the lung. Initially, the pulmonary microemboli mechanically block small pulmonary vessels. The resulting engorgement of pulmonary capillaries and arterioles causes the lung to become more rigid, and increases the afterload for the right heart.[3]

The lung responds to the presence of neutral fat particles by secreting lipase which hydrolyzes the neutral fat into free fatty acids and glycerol. The free fatty acids damage the local capillaries and alveoli and inactivate surfactant.[25] Both the mechanical and chemical effects of the fat emboli on the lung can seriously reduce the ability of the lung to oxygenate blood.

Although the effects of fatty acids on pulmonary capillary endothelium appear to be important in initiating the lung injury, the pathogenesis of full-blown respiratory failure may be far more complex. Other tissue components besides fat may be liberated from fracture sites, and these, as well as the injured pulmonary capillary endothelium, may activate clotting, complement, and other contact systems.[3]

Cerebral Changes

Hypoxemia resulting from lung injury explains the brain dysfunction of fat embolism syndrome in many cases, but not all.[30] In some fatal cases, cerebral symptoms occur early and seem to reflect direct brain injury. Histological examination of the brain may reveal many fat emboli and associated hemorrhage and necrosis. In such cases, the neurologic changes are often much worse than would be expected from the degree of hypoxemia.[21] In patients with a patent foramen ovale, the cerebral symptoms and signs may be particularly severe.[31]

Petechiae

The reason for the petechiae in fat embolism syndrome is not known. Damage to the skin capillaries by fatty acids and thrombocytopenia may be important factors. In some patients, the thrombocytopenia may be quite severe and appears to be associated with other laboratory evidence of disseminated intravascular coagulation.[3] There is also no explanation for the striking localization of the petechiae to the pectoral regions, axillae, and conjunctivae.

Bone Changes

In an examination of patients with femoral head fractures after trauma, Jones noted a trend toward intravascular coagulation and osteonecrosis.[32] He found an absolute overload of subperiosteal and subchondral fat emboli that could produce osteonecrosis by progressive fibrin platelet thromboses.

DIAGNOSIS

AXIOM   FES should be suspected in all patients with major fractures, and it is a frequent cause of pulmonary or CNS changes that develop 24-48 hours after trauma.

Clinical

TYPE OF TRAUMA

Fat embolism syndrome is most likely to occur in patients with multiple severe long bone fractures and hypovolemic shock.[3] Other predisposing factors include preexisting cardiac or pulmonary disease. Damage to a fatty liver can also be a source of fat emboli. Indeed, it is not unusual to find emboli of bone marrow or liver in the lungs at autopsy in patients who have died of severe blunt trauma.

DIAGNOSTIC CRITERIA

There should be a high level of suspicion for the development of FES within the first 48 to 72 hours after trauma that has caused fractures of major long bones. Gurd's criteria are often used for the diagnosis, and they are divided into major and minor criteria.[33] Major criteria are axillary or subconjunctival petechia, hypoxemia (PaO_2 less than 60 mm Hg or an FiO_2 of 0.4), central nervous system depression disproportionate to the hypoxemia or head injury, and pulmonary edema. Minor criteria are tachycardia (more than 110 beats per minute), pyrexia (temperature more than 38.5°), retinal changes on fundoscopic exam (fat or petechia), urinary changes (anuria, oliguria, fat globules), sudden drops in hemoglobin or platelet levels, high erythrocyte sedimentation rate, and fat globules in the sputum.

At least one sign from the major criteria and at least four from the minor criteria have been used by Gurd to make the diagnosis of fat embolism syndrome.[33] Other authors have questioned the reliability of Gurd's criteria, stressing the need for detection of a sustained PaO_2 of less and 60 mm Hg, or other signs of respiratory distress.[34] Indeed, it appears that many patients can develop significant hypoxemia without developing clinical signs. This has been referred to as subclinical fat embolism syndrome.[35]

Organ Changes

PULMONARY CHANGES

The characteristic clinical pulmonary changes with FES include an initial tachypnea and increased minute ventilation.[3] There are usually some rales and rhonchi at the bases, but these are usually not as severe as with atelectasis and pneumonia. X-ray changes usually appear after 24 to 48 hours and are typically a diffuse microatelectasis and congestion.[35,36]

AXIOM   In spite of the hyperventilation and low arterial PCO_2 usually present in FES, the arterial PO_2 in young adults with fat emboli tends to be 70 mm Hg or less.

Because the PCO_2 is often 25-35 mm Hg, the alveolar-arterial PO_2 differences ($P[A-a]O_2$) on room air tend to be 40 mm Hg or more. A $P(A-a)O_2$ of 55 mm Hg or more on room air indicates severe pulmonary dysfunction.[4,35]

NEUROLOGICAL CHANGES

AXIOM   Up to two-thirds of patients with FES have an encephalopathy without any focal neurological changes.

Neurological manifestations are common in FES, and may occur in up to 84% of patients.[26,37] Many with encephalopathy develop CNS changes before there is any clinical evidence of pulmonary failure. These patients tend to be delirious, and their mental status usually does not improve until the hypoxemia is corrected. However, once the pulmonary disorder has resolved, the encephalopathy usually improves rapidly.

One-third of the patients with CNS changes have focal neurological abnormalities that tend to occur at the same time as the most severe impairment of the level of consciousness.[37] Some of the more common focal features include apraxia, hemiplegia, scotomata, anisocoria, and conjugate eye deviation.[38] Occasionally, fat emboli can be seen on fundoscopic examination of the eyes of these patients.[3]

PITFALL ⊘

Failure to examine the optic fundi in patients with CNS changes after multiple trauma.

Although most patients develop fat embolism within 24 to 48 hours of the initial trauma, Silverstein reported that three of his eight patients with CNS abnormalities resulting from fat embolism developed neurologic changes 5 or more days after the trauma.[39] Murray and Racz[40] reported some cases developing neurological manifestations 11 days after trauma.

The differences between the groups with and without focal CNS findings are interesting but difficult to explain. All patients who developed focal neurologic signs initially presented with cerebral rather than pulmonary symptoms.[37] There also was a trend for the patients with focal features to develop neurological changes earlier than the patients with encephalopathy alone. This suggests that patients with focal features have a more fulminant disorder. However, in one study, two of the four patients with focal neurological changes had no pulmonary manifestations or fever. There also have been several other documented cases of fat embolism syndrome with neurologic disorders but with no apparent pulmonary abnormality or fever.[30,41]

PETECHIAE

AXIOM   A transient petechial rash may develop in 50 to 60% of patients with FES.

Petechiae usually occur on the skin of the chest, axilla, and neck, and on the conjunctivae. However, petechiae can easily be missed because they are often transient and may be present for less than 4 to 6 hours.[21]

Laboratory Changes

There are no specific laboratory tests that are diagnostic of fat embolus syndrome. However, there are a number of tests that can help confirm a clinical diagnosis.

AXIOM   A combination of thrombocytopenia and low PaO_2 (or high $P[A-a]O_2$) occurring relatively suddenly within 24-48 hours of major fractures is almost diagnostic of fat embolism syndrome.

ABG

Arterial blood gases (ABG) should be measured soon after admission and every 12 to 24 hours during the next 48 to 72 hours in all patients with major fractures. The characteristic ABG changes of FES on room air include a $PaCO_2$ of 25 to 35 mm Hg, a PaO_2 of 55 to 75 mm Hg, and a $P(A-a)O_2$ of 35 to 65 mm Hg.[4,35,36] However, similar changes in patients with fractures but without clinical signs of FES may represent subclinical FES.[36]

Although it is generally assumed that the blood gas changes associated with fractures are largely related to fat entering the blood stream and becoming converted to free fatty acids, Blitzer and Hamilton[42] found no statistically significant decreases in oxygen saturation during reaming and intramedullary nailing of 15 femoral fractures.

It has been suggested by Moed et al[43] that pulse oximetry is an effective technique to screen for FES in patients with fractures of long bones and/or the pelvis. Of 43 such patients, 15 (35%) had a pulse oximetry saturation of less than 94%. These patients were managed with an intensive pulmonary care regimen, and the hypoxemia resolved in all patients within 48 hours of initial therapy.

PLATELET COUNTS

> **AXIOM** A normal platelet count after long bone fractures generally rules out the presence of FES.

Platelet counts should be performed on admission and then daily during the first 3 to 4 days after injury. An early thrombocytopenia below $100,000/mm^3$ is almost diagnostic for fat embolus if the patient has not had massive transfusions or severe prolonged shock.[35,36] The drop in the platelet count is usually associated with an increased $P(A-a)O_2$ on room air (Fig. 34–3).

EXAMINATIONS FOR FAT

> **AXIOM** Increased fat in blood, sputum, and urine is a relatively nonspecific finding after major trauma.

Other tests that might be helpful in diagnosing FES include examinations of urine, sputum, CSF, and blood for fat. However, lipuria occurs in about half of all patients with significant bony injury, most of whom have no other findings suggestive of FES. Examination of frozen peripheral blood via a cryostat test for fat droplets may also be too sensitive to be of clinical value.[44] Adolph et al,[45] however, have shown that frozen sections of blood aspirated from a pulmonary artery catheter in patients with FES show greatly increased microvascular fat.

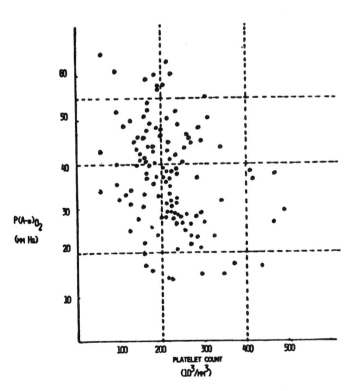

FIGURE 34–3 Correlation between alveolar-arterial oxygen differences and platelet count the first day after uncomplicated extremity fractures. Patients with the lowest platelet counts tended to have the highest alveolar-arterial oxygen differences (r = 0.186, P less than 0.05). (From: Shier MR, Wilson RF. Fat embolism syndrome: traumatic coagulopathy and respiratory distress. Surg Ann 1980;12:139.)

Gitin et al,[46] however, found a relatively poor correlation between the amount of pulmonary microvascular fat in blood drawn through a wedged pulmonary capillary catheter and the FiO_2 required, the levels of the PCO_2, and the mixed venous oxygen saturations.

Benzer et al[47] were able to perform an automated semiquantitative analysis of fat within alveolar macrophages obtained by bronchoalveolar lavage (BAL) in patients with suspected FES. The percentage of fat in alveolar macrophages in two patients with FES was 40 and 53%. A third similar patient who did not develop FES had only 4% fat in the alveolar macrophages.

Stanley et al,[48] however, found that 25 of 34 patients with suspected pulmonary disease but no trauma had more than 5% of their BAL cells laden with lipid. Consequently, they concluded that staining of BAL cells for lipids is not a specific test for FES.

SERUM LIPASE

Serum lipase is elevated after 5 to 6 days in about half of all patients with fractures. Thus, this test is also too insensitive by itself to be of clinical value.

CBC

Hemoglobin levels may decline by as much as 3 to 5 grams/dl with FES. However, one should look carefully for other injuries before attributing this change to fat embolism syndrome.

COAGULATION STUDIES

Complete coagulation studies in full-blown cases of FES may reveal a consumptive coagulopathy with low levels of platelets, fibrinogen, prothrombin, factor V, and factor VIII.

> **AXIOM** Almost all of the laboratory tests for FES are too sensitive and nonspecific to be of great diagnostic value; however, if multiple tests are positive in the appropriate clinical setting, the diagnosis is likely.

Radiological Examinations

PLAIN CHEST X-RAYS

> **AXIOM** The chest x-ray findings of FES tend to lag at least 12 to 24 hours behind the clinical, blood gas, and platelet changes.

The plain chest x-ray with uncomplicated FES is usually normal for at least 12 to 36 hours, and the clinical and ABG changes usually become clinically obvious at least 12 to 24 hours before any radiological abnormalities appear.[35,36] When x-ray changes become apparent, they resemble those of other types of ARDS and include early congestion and diffuse microatelectasis. Later, the infiltrates may become more confluent and may even produce a complete whiteout of the lung in the most severe cases. If the radiological changes occur before clinical respiratory changes, one should suspect pulmonary contusion.

> **AXIOM** Before it is assumed that the neurologic changes occurring after major trauma are a result of FES, a CT scan of the head is needed to rule out space-occupying lesions.[49]

MRI AND SPECT

In studying a patient with cerebral fat embolism, Erdem et al[50] found that the brain CT showed no abnormality. However, an MRI performed after recovery from trauma, when the patient had aphasia and quadraparesis, demonstrated multiple abnormalities in the white matter. A SPECT exam showed left-sided hypoperfusion that resolved parallel to the clinical improvement one month later.

Transesophageal Echocardiography

Pell et al[51] have used transesophageal echocardiography to monitor perioperative cardiac function in high-risk surgical patients. In their experience, echocardiographically detectable fat emboli may be observed in approximately 40% of patients undergoing major orthopaedic procedures. More recently, they described a patient with a fracture of the femoral shaft who, several seconds after a guide wire was inserted into the medullary cavity of the proximal femur, had a shower of small (1 to 2 mm) echogenic masses appearing in his right atrium and ventricle.[52] Further manipulation of the fracture increased the quantity of echogenic material in the right heart. The flap valve of the fossa ovalis then opened, and large quantities of the echogenic emboli passed into the left atrium. At that time the arterial O_2 saturation fell to 75%. The end-tidal CO_2 fell to 9 mm Hg, and the PA pressure went from 45/20 to 72/40.

PREVENTION OF FAT EMBOLISM SYNDROME

Several approaches have been used in attempts to prevent FES.[3,4,35,36] These include: (a) early aggressive correction of hypovolemia and hypotension, (b) early fixation of fractures, (c) reduction of platelet aggregation with corticosteroids and/or aspirin, (d) administration of albumin, and (e) early nutrition.

Correction of Hypovolemia and Hypotension

AXIOM Rapid correction of hypotension and hypovolemia in all patients with long bone fractures may reduce the incidence and severity of FES.

It has been known for some time that the incidence of FES increases in patients with hypovolemic shock.[3] Nevertheless, one should be careful to not overload the circulation and cause cardiogenic pulmonary edema, especially if there has been coincident chest trauma. In a prospective randomized study of patients with extremity fractures admitted to a hospital, Shier et al found that early aggressive fluid administration did not reduce the incidence of thrombocytopenia or improve blood gas changes; however, none of these patients was in shock.[4]

Early Fixation of Fractures

AXIOM Early fixation of long bone fractures is one of the best ways to prevent or treat FES.

It has been postulated that the formation of fat emboli requires fragmentation of the bony tissue plus access to the circulation. This involves intravasation of tissue fragments into relatively large vascular sinusoids in bone. Early operation on the fracture and decompressing and evacuating the associated hematoma should reduce the amount of fat entering the circulation. Indeed, early open reduction and internal fixation of fractures significantly reduce the risk of fat embolism.[53,54] Thus, prevention of fat embolism may include: (a) gentle handling, proper splinting, and careful transport of fracture patients and (b) immediate open reduction and internal fixation of multiple long bone fractures.[53-55]

Reduction of Platelet Aggregation

At one time or another, 5% ethyl alcohol, heparin, and low molecularweight dextran (LMWD) have been advocated for the prevention of FES.[3] Heparin, in particular, was recommended for its lipolytic and anticoagulant properties;[2] however, heparin may actually increase the formation of free fatty acids.

The use of corticosteroids has been extremely controversial since first reported beneficial for the treatment of FES by Ashbaugh and Petty in 1966.[56] Indeed, most authors state that there is no evidence that corticosteroids are of value in preventing or treating FES. Experimental support for the use of corticosteroids in FES was furnished by Wertsberger and Peltier two years later.[57]

The treatment of patients with fat embolism with corticosteroid hormones was popularized by Fischer et al.[58] Their value for prophylaxis in high risk patients was further established by numerous authors.[4,59,60,61] When corticosteroids are given, it is usually as methylprednisolone in doses of 30 mg/kg. This may be given in 2 to 3 doses about 6 to 12 hours apart, or it may be given in doses of 7.5 mg/kg every 6 hours for 3 days, but it must be started within 6 hours of the injury. Some evidence suggests than even lower doses of methylprednisolone (9 mg/kg) may also be effective.[62]

Shier et al also found that aspirin (300 mg every 6 hours during the first 24-48 hours by mouth or by rectum) also caused less platelet aggregation and maintained a significantly higher platelet count and lower $P(A-a)O_2$ on room air than controls.[4]

Albumin Administration

The amount of lung damage in FES appears to be related primarily to the levels of free fatty acids (FFA). Fatty acids are bound primarily by albumin, and the more the plasma albumin levels decrease, the higher the FFA levels rise.[78] Although low albumin levels are associated with a poor prognosis, giving albumin does not usually improve pulmonary function or prognosis. Furthermore, excessive administration of albumin can increase the tendency to heart failure and ARDS.

Early Nutrition

Inadequate caloric intake increases the mobilization of fat from tissue stores, and hypertonic glucose has been reported to reduce the incidence and severity of FES.[59] However, in a prospective randomized study, early aggressive administration of glucose did not alter the platelet count or ABG changes from those in control patients.[4]

TREATMENT OF FAT EMBOLUS SYNDROME

Ventilatory Assistance

AXIOM Because most of the symptoms of FES appear to be the direct or indirect result of respiratory failure, ventilator assistance should be instituted early.

An important observation in patients with FES is the high incidence of hypoxemia, which often is not detected by clinical examination.[3,35] Consequently, it is essential that early arterial blood gas analysis and/or monitoring with a pulse oximeter be performed in patients who are at risk for fat embolism. With such studies, it has become increasingly evident that fat embolism is largely a pulmonary problem and that ventilatory support should be begun early to maintain the PO_2 at about 80 to 90 mm Hg. The PCO_2 should probably be kept around 30 to 35 mm Hg if CNS changes are present. Indeed, early ventilatory support has resulted in a significant decrease in mortality.[2]

Positive end-expiratory pressure (PEEP) may reduce the need for high concentrations of inspired oxygen and should be considered if an FiO_2 greater than 0.4 or 0.5 is needed. However, increased PEEP may increase the ICP in patients with severe CNS changes. Restricting fluid intake if an adequate O_2 delivery can be maintained may reduce fluid accumulation in the lungs. In some cases, use of diuretics may also have to be considered.

Management of Neurological Dysfunction

The initial approach to patients with post-traumatic neurologic dysfunction should be to exclude intracranial hemorrhage and intercurrent toxic, metabolic, or infectious CNS problems.[37] If these problems are ruled out in patients with long bone fractures, the CNS changes should be considered a result of fat embolism syndrome until proven otherwise. In such patients, early aggressive ventilation and maintenance of normal or increased cerebral perfusion with well-oxygenated blood should provide the best overall results.

OUTCOME

Reported mortality rates for FES have been as high as 29%, but these data are difficult to interpret because many of the patients in these series had associated injuries to the head, chest, and abdomen. Robert et al,[6] for example, found that the mortality rate of FES was directly related to the injury severity score (ISS). More recent studies have tried to exclude patients with associated injuries, and under such circumstances, the mortality rate from FES itself is probably less than 10%. It is certainly much lower than the 40-50% or greater mortality rate for most other causes of adult respiratory distress syndrome.[2,36]

⊘ FREQUENT ERRORS

In the Management of Fat Embolism Syndrome

1. *Failing to consider the possible presence of fat emboli in a patient with major fractures, especially if there are any pulmonary or neurologic changes not clearly due to direct trauma.*
2. *Failure to promptly and adequately resuscitate patients with major fractures.*
3. *Failure to examine the optic fundi in patients with CNS changes after trauma.*
4. *Failure to check the platelet count in patients with hypoxemia after major fractures.*
5. *Delay of ventilatory support in patients with hypoxemia after major fractures.*
6. *Delaying rigid fixation of major fractures in trauma patients, especially if there is evidence of pulmonary dysfunction.*
7. *Failure to obtain CT scans of the head in trauma victims with impaired CNS function because other evidence of fat embolism is present.*

▼▼▼▼▼▼▼▼▼▼▼▼▼▼▼▼▼▼▼▼▼▼▼▼▼▼▼

SUMMARY POINTS

1. The main clinical findings in FES include tachypnea with respiratory failure, mental confusion, and petechiae.
2. A subclinical form of fat embolism with a reduced platelet count and increased $P(A-a)O_2$ occurs after almost all fractures.
3. Despite the fact that fat droplets are found in venous blood as much as 90% of the time after long bone fractures, the incidence of full-blown FES is relatively rare.
4. The two main theories to explain the source of the fat in FES are mechanical and biochemical.
5. Both mechanical and biochemical mechanisms are probably involved in the development of most cases of fat embolism syndrome.
6. Fat embolism syndrome can be divided into two phases: (a) an initial phase in which the mechanical obstruction of capillaries and other small vessels by neutral fat emboli is most important, and (b) a later chemical phase, when fatty acids are formed from the neutral fat.
7. FES should be suspected in all patients with major fractures, and it is a frequent cause of pulmonary or CNS changes that develop 24-48 hours after trauma.
8. In spite of the hyperventilation and low arterial PCO2 usually present in FES, the arterial PO2 in young adults with fat emboli tends to be 70 mm Hg or less.
9. Up to two-thirds of patients with FES have an encephalopathy without any focal neurological changes.

10. A combination of thrombocytopenia and low PaO_2 [or high $P(A-a)O_2$] occurring within 24-48 hours of major fractures is almost diagnostic of fat embolism syndrome.
11. A normal platelet count after long bone fractures generally rules out the presence of FES.
12. Increased fat in blood, sputum, and urine is a relatively nonspecific finding after major trauma.
13. Almost all of the laboratory tests for FES are too sensitive and nonspecific to be of great diagnostic value; however, if multiple tests are positive in the appropriate clinical setting, the diagnosis is likely.
14. The chest x-ray findings of FES tend to lag at least 12-24 hours behind the clinical, blood gas, and platelet changes.
15. Before it is assumed that the neurologic changes occurring after major trauma are a result of FES, a CT scan of the head is needed to rule out space-occupying lesions.
16. Rapid correction of hypotension and hypovolemia in all patients with long bone fractures may reduce the incidence and severity of FES.
17. Early fixation of long bone fractures is one of the best ways to prevent or treat FES.
18. Because most of the symptoms of FES appear to be the direct or indirect result of respiratory failure, ventilator assistance should be instituted early.

▲▲▲▲▲▲▲▲▲▲▲▲▲▲▲▲▲▲▲▲▲▲▲▲▲▲▲▲▲▲▲▲

REFERENCES

1. Ganong RB. Fat emboli syndrome in isolated fractures of the tibia and femur. Clin Orthop 1993;291:208.
2. Bolhofner BR, Spiegel PG. Prevention of medical complications in orthopedic trauma. Clin Orthop 1987;222:105.
3. Peltier LF. Fat embolism: a perspective. Clin Orthop 1988;232:263.
4. Shier MR, Wilson RF. Fat embolism syndromes: traumatic coagulopathy with respiratory distress. Surg Ann 1980;12:139.
5. Muller C, Rahn BA, Pfister U, et al. The incidence, pathogenesis, diagnosis, and treatment of fat embolism. Orthop Rev 1994;23:107.
6. Robert JH, Hoffmeyer P, Broquet PE, et al. Fat embolism syndrome. Orthop Rev 1993;22:567.
7. Caillouette JT, Anzel SH. Fat embolism syndrome following the intramedullary alignment guide in total knee arthroplasty. Clin Orthop 1990;251:198.
8. Dorr LD, Merkel C, Mellman MF, Klein I. Fat emboli in bilateral total knee arthroplasty: predictive factors for neurologic manifestations. Clin Orthop 1989;248:112.
9. Monto RR, Garcia J, Callaghan JJ. Fatal fat embolism following total condylar knee arthroplasty. J Arthroplasty 1990;5:291.
10. Orsini EC, Richards RR, Mullen JM. Fatal fat embolism during cemented total knee arthroplasty: a case report. Can J Surg 1986;29:385.
11. Spengler DM, Costenbader M, Bailey R. Fat embolism syndrome following total hip arthroplasty. Clin Orthop 1976;121:105.
12. Watson JT, Stulberg BN. Fat embolism associated with cementing of femoral stems designed for press-fit application. J Arthroplasty 1989;4:133.
13. Hall TM, Callaghan JJ. Fat embolism precipitated by reaming of the femoral canal during revision of a total knee replacement. J Bone Joint Surg 1994;76A:899.
14. Byrick RJ, Bell RS, Kay JC, et al. High-volume, high-pressure pulsatile lavage during cemented arthroplasty. J Bone Joint Surg 1989;71(A):1331.
15. Manning JB, Bach AW, Herman CM, Carrico CJ. Fat release after femur nailing in the dog. J Trauma 1983;23:322.
16. Talucci RC, Manning J, Lampard S, et al. Early intramedullary nailing of femoral shaft fractures: a cause of fat embolism syndrome. Am J Surg 1983;146:107.
17. Pell AC, Christie J, Keating JF, et al. The detection of fat embolism by transesophageal echocardiography during reamed intramedullary nailing. J Bone Joint Surg 1993;75B:921.
18. Wozasek GE, Simon P, Redl H, et al. Intramedullary pressure changes and fat extravasation during intramedullary nailing: an experimental study in sheep. J Trauma 1994;36:202.
19. Kerr PS, Jackson M, Atkins RM. Cardiac arrest during intramedullary nailing for femoral metastases. J Bone Joint Surg 1993;75B:972.
20. Levy D. The fat embolism syndrome: a review. Clin Orthop 1990;261:281.

21. Gossling HR, Pellegrini VD. Fat embolism syndrome: a review of the pathophysiology and physiological basis of treatment. Clin Orthop 1982; 164:68.
22. Innes D, Sevitt S. Coagulation and fibrinolysis in injured patients. J Clin Pathol 1964;17:1.
23. Peltier LF. Fat embolism I: the amount of fat in human long bones. Surgery 1956;40:657.
24. Cobb CA Jr, Lequire VA, Gray ME, et al. Therapy of traumatic fat embolism with intravenous fluids and heparin. Surg Forum 1958;9:751.
25. Parades S, Comer F, Rubin S, et al. Fat embolism: distribution of fat tagged with ^{131}I within the body of the rat at various times following intravenous injection. J Bone Joint Surg 1965;47A:216.
26. Nixon JR, Brock-Utne JG. Free fatty acid and arterial oxygen changes following major injury. J Trauma 1978;18:23.
27. Peltier LF, Wheeler DH, Boyd HM, et al. Fat embolism II: the chemical composition of fat obtained from human long bones. Surgery 1956; 40:662.
28. Peltier LF. Fat embolism III: the toxic properties of neutral fats and fatty acids. Surgery 1956;40:665.
29. Bergentz SE, Nilsson IM. Effect of trauma on coagulation and fibrinolysis in dogs. Aceta Chir Scand 1961;122:21.
30. Scopa M, Magatti M, Rossitto P. Neurologic symptoms in fat embolism syndrome: case report. J Trauma 1994;36:906.
31. Etchells EE, Wong DT, Davidson G, et al. Fatal cerebral fat embolism associated with a patent foramen ovale. Chest 1993;104:962.
32. Jones JP Jr. Fat embolism, intravascular coagulation, and osteonecrosis. Clin Orthop 1993;292:294.
33. Gurd AR. Fat embolism: an aid to diagnosis. J Bone Joint Surg 1970; 52B:732.
34. Lindeque BG, Schoeman HS, Dommisse GF, et al. Fat embolism and the fat embolism syndrome: a double-blind therapeutic study. J Bone Joint Surg 1987;69B:128.
35. Wilson RF, McCarthy B, LeBlanc LP, et al. Respiratory and coagulation changes after uncomplicated fractures. Arch Surg 1973;106:395.
36. Shier MR, Wilson RF. Fat embolism syndrome: traumatic coagulopathy and respiratory distress. Surg Annual 1980;12:139.
37. Jacobson DM, Terrence CF, Reinmuth OM. The neurologic manifestations of fat embolism. Neurology 1986;36:847.
38. Thomas JE, Ayyar DR. Systemic fat embolism: a diagnostic profile in 24 patients. Arch Neurol 1972;26:517.
39. Silverstein A. Significance of cerebral fat embolism. Neurology 1952; 2:292.
40. Murry DG, Racz GB. Fat embolism syndrome. J Bone Joint Surg 1974; 56:1338.
41. Findlay JM, DeMajo W. Cerebral fat embolism. Can Med Assoc J 1984; 131:755.
42. Blitzer CM, Hamilton L. Oxygen saturation during reaming and intramedullary nailing of the femur. Orthop 1992;15:1403.
43. Moed BR, Boyd DW, Andring RE. Clinically inapparent hypoxemia after skeletal injury: the use of the pulse oximeter as a screening method. Clin Orthop 1993;293:269.
44. Cross HE. Examination of CSF in fat embolism. Arch Int Med 1965; 115:470.
45. Adolph MD, Fabian HF, el-Khairi SM, et al. The pulmonary artery catheter: a diagnostic adjunct for fat embolism syndrome. J Orthop Trauma 1994;8:173.
46. Gitin TA, Seidel T, Cera PJ, et al. Pulmonary microvascular fat: the significance? Crit Care Med 1993;21:673.
47. Benzer A, Ofner D, Totsch M, et al. Early diagnosis of fat embolism syndrome by automated image analysis of alveolar macrophages. J Clin Monit 1994;10:213.
48. Stanley JD, Hanson RR, Hicklin GA, et al. Specificity of bronchoalveolar lavage for the diagnosis of fat embolism syndrome. Am Surg 1994; 60:537.
49. Sakamota T, Sawada Y, Yukioka T, et al. Computed tomography for diagnosis and assessment of cerebral fat embolism. Neuroradiology 1983; 24:283.
50. Erdem E, Namer IJ, Saribas O, et al. Cerebral fat embolism studied with MRI and SPECT. Neuroradiology 1993;35:199.
51. Pell ACH, Keating JF, Christie J, et al. Use of tranesophageal echocardiography to predict patients at risk of the fat embolism syndrome following traumatic injuries. J Am Coll Cardio 1993;21(Suppl):264A.
52. Pell AC, Hughes D, Keating J, et al. Fulminating fat embolism syndrome caused by paradoxical embolism through a patent foramen ovale. N Engl J Med 1993;329:926.
53. Allardyce DB, Meek RN, Woodruff B, et al. Fat embolism: a prospective study of 43 patients with fractured femoral shafts. J Trauma 1974;14:955.
54. Riska EB, von Bonsdorff H, Hakkinen S, et al. Prevention of fat embolism by early internal fixation of fractures in patients with multiple injuries. Injury 1976;8:110.
55. Riska EB, Myllynen P. Fat embolism in patients with multiple injuries. J Trauma 1982;22:891.
56. Ashbaugh DG, Petty TL. The use of corticosteroids in the treatment of respiratory failure associated with massive fat embolism. Surg Gynecol Obstet 1966;123:493.
57. Wertzberger JJ, Peltier LF. Fat embolism: the effect of corticosteroids on experimental fat embolism in the rat. Surgery 1968;64:143.
58. Fischer JE, Turner RH, Herndon JH. Massive steroid therapy in severe fat embolism. Surg Gynecol Obstet 1971;132:667.
59. Stoltenberg JJ, Gustilo RB. The use of methylprednisolone and hypertonic glucose in the prophylaxis of fat embolism syndrome. Clin Orthop 1979;143:211.
60. Schonfeld SA, Ploysongsang Y, DiLisio R, et al. Fat embolism prophylaxis with corticosteroids. Ann Int Med 1983;99:438.
61. Alho A, Saikku K, Eerola P, et al. Corticosteroids in patients with a high risk of fat embolism syndrome. Surg Gynecol Obstet 1978;147:358.
62. Kallenbach J, Lewis M, Zaltzman M, et al. Low-dose corticosteriod prophylaxis against fat embolism. J Trauma 1987;27:1173.

Chapter 35 Vascular Injuries

ANNA M. LEDGERWOOD, M.D.

CHARLES E. LUCAS, M.D.

INTRODUCTION

Many isolated vascular injuries, particularly in the extremities, can be easily managed; however, correct diagnosis and successful treatment of vessel damage associated with multiple trauma can be extremely challenging. During initial resuscitation and definitive management, the trauma team must remember that life takes priority over limb. Patients must be fully resuscitated and life-threatening injuries controlled before a nonlife-threatening vascular injury is fully treated. Also, when treating limb injuries, the maintenance of function is a high priority.

AXIOM Maximal limb function is maintained after vascular injury by minimizing the ischemic insult and protecting neural function.

Technical advances, particularly the increased use of arteriography, Doppler ultrasound, autogenous grafts, and peripheral arterial balloon catheters, have revolutionized the management of vascular injuries. Unfortunately, limbs may still be lost or crippled when investigation of a limb injury is superficial and vascular damage is overlooked.[1]

PITFALL ⊘

Delay in definitive repair of an arterial injury beyond 4 to 6 hours increases the incidence of severe complications.

Prolonged ischemia in a limb may cause irreversible tissue damage with consequent loss of limb or impairment of function as a result of replacement of muscle by fibrous tissue. In addition, hypotension combined with toxemia resulting from tissue necrosis may cause renal, respiratory, and cardiac failure.

HISTORIC PERSPECTIVE

In 1896, Murphy performed the first successful end-to-end anastomosis in a human.[2] Since then, the principles of treatment of vascular trauma have evolved during military conflicts.[3,4,5] Although Makins[6] had noted the high amputation rate associated with ligation of an injured popliteal artery, ligation was still the usual treatment for major arterial injuries well into World War II. DeBakey and Simeone reported a 49% amputation rate in American troops during World War II.[7] This included a 75% amputation rate in soldiers with femoral-popliteal injuries. The need to rapidly control hemorrhage without resuscitative fluids, banked blood, or antibiotics influenced this approach. Preservation of life superseded limb salvage.

The advent of antibiotics and better resuscitation fluids encouraged a more aggressive approach to arterial injury during the Korean conflict. Vascular reconstruction, even when performed under less than ideal circumstances, was associated with an overall amputation rate of only 13%.[8,9] This contrasted an amputation rate of 50% when ligation was employed. There was a similar success rate after primary vascular repair during the Vietnam conflict despite the more frequent exposure to high-velocity missiles and antipersonnel devices.[10] Long-term follow-up of these soldiers was made possible by the Vietnam Vascular Injury Registry established and maintained at the Walter Reed Army Hospital.[10-13]

Valuable lessons learned from these experiences included the benefit of rapid transport and improved prehospital care, intravascular shunts to decrease warm ischemia time, aggressive soft tissue coverage, and liberal use of fasciotomy to reduce compartment pressures.[14-19]

EPIDEMIOLOGY

Types of Trauma to Vessels

The incidence of civilian arterial and venous injuries treated in hospitals continues to increase.[3,20] Factors contributing to this include increasing personal violence, high-speed transport, and invasive diagnostic and therapeutic vascular procedures. Most patients with vascular injuries have extremity trauma, and the brachial and superficial femoral artery are the most frequently injured peripheral vessels.

AXIOM One must carefully assess vascular compromise after percutaneous angiography, especially in older or smaller patients.

Iatrogenic vascular injury from percutaneous arterial catheterization is being documented more frequently.[20-23] Femoral artery thrombosis, the most frequent complication of retrograde aortic catheterization, has been noted in 1.2 to 7.0% of patients.[24] A low cardiac output and increased arteriosclerosis may contribute to this complication in older patients.

Characteristics of Various Types of Trauma

PENETRATING INJURIES
The high-velocity rifle bullet with a muzzle velocity of 3000 feet per second creates a cavitational effect on impact. This causes massive destruction of soft tissues, including vessels. The tissue may be severely contused several centimeters around the visible missile tract, and extensive contamination of such wounds is common.[25] In contrast, low-velocity missiles (500 to 1000 feet/sec), typically from handguns, usually cause far less adjacent soft-tissue injury.

AXIOM High-velocity missiles can severely damage tissues up to several centimeters beyond the missile tracts.

Close-range shotgun blasts can also cause extensive soft-tissue damage.[1] Furthermore, the wad and plastic caps used to separate the powder charge from the shot may deeply penetrate the wound. When not recovered, severe infection may ensue.

PITFALL ⊘

Failure to look for and locate the plastic wad in close-range shotgun blasts.

BLUNT TRAUMA
Arterial injury often results from automobile accidents and athletic injuries. Such injuries are associated with long bone fractures or severe dislocations, especially at the knee.[1] The adjacent vessel may be contused, stretched, torn, or perforated by the fracture fragments. Vascular damage can also occur after prolonged compression without a fracture or dislocation when the leg is pinned or crushed.

The more common sites of combined vascular and orthopaedic trauma include: (a) fractured femoral shaft and superficial femoral artery injury, (b) knee dislocation and popliteal artery injury, (c) fractured clavicle and subclavian artery injury, (d) dislocated shoulder and axillary artery injury, and (e) supracondylar fracture of the humerus and brachial artery injury.[1] Brachial artery injury associated with supracondylar fractures of the humerus occurs primarily in children.[1] Frequent and careful examination of the radial pulse and the circulation to the hand is essential, especially when the fracture is reduced and maintained in a position of flexion. Prolonged ischemia to the forearm muscles may cause necrosis and later Volkmann's ischemic contracture.

PATHOPHYSIOLOGY

Vascular trauma can lead to a variety of systemic, regional, and local pathophysiologic disturbances. The systemic effects and treatment of acute blood loss are discussed elsewhere. The regional and local consequences vary according to the sensitivity of the tissues to ischemia, the type of trauma, and the type of vessel damage.

Sensitivity of Tissues to Ischemia

Acute cessation of arterial flow can produce regional ischemia to the organ or limb perfused by the artery. The vulnerability of tissue to ischemic insult depends on its basal energy requirement and substrate stores. The central nervous system is extremely vulnerable to any cessation of arterial flow because of a high basal energy requirement and an absence of glycogen stores.[26] Hence, 4 minutes of brain ischemia can cause irreversible damage. Peripheral nerves and skeletal muscle, in contrast, are much more tolerant to ischemia. Malan and Tattoni[27] have noted that extremity tissues can survive without nutrient blood flow up to 4 hours without developing any of the histologic changes of ischemia. Although some investigators have found that changes caused by ischemia for more than 6 hours can be reversed with reperfusion,[27] others have found that the ischemic changes in skeletal muscle are not always reversed by reperfusion.[28]

> **AXIOM**   A limb that has been ischemic for 6 hours or longer is at risk for sustaining histologic changes that may not be reversible with reperfusion.[28]

Types of Trauma

The extent of vascular damage is usually determined by the mechanism of injury. Gunshot wounds, especially from high-velocity missiles, produce more severe injury than stab wounds because of the greater kinetic energy imparted to the tissues. Blunt trauma may compress the vessel causing intramural contusion, intimal tear, or full-thickness necrosis. Prolapse of a flap of torn intima may occlude the lumen and cause distal thrombosis.

Types of Vessel Damage

LACERATIONS
A laceration is the most frequent injury to both arteries and veins.[3] Knives can cause punctures, extensive tears, or complete transection. Gunshot wounds tend to cause slightly irregular holes that may be tangential or through-and-through. After complete transection, severed arterial ends retract and thrombosis occurs before the onset of extensive blood loss. Exsanguination is more likely with partial transections which prevent vessel retraction. Blood loss may also be reduced if the bleeding is contained within the perivascular tissues. Such blood may clot and lead to a pulsatile hematoma, often called a false aneurysm. If there are contiguous wounds to both the artery and the vein, an arteriovenous fistula may develop.

CONTUSION
Direct trauma to a vessel may cause hemorrhage or edema in the wall of the vessel, producing narrowing or partial occlusion of the lumen.[1]

> **AXIOM**   Narrowing of the arterial lumen at an injury site is seldom a result of spasm. Failure to correct or closely observe such areas can result in late occlusion with rapid ischemic necrosis of distal tissue.

Although narrowing of an arterial lumen after trauma may occasionally result from spasm, such areas usually represent damage to the vessel wall and can cause occlusion. Obstruction is particularly apt to occur if an intimal flap develops from a crack in the vessel or if thrombosis develops on the surface of injured intima. At the time of exploration, vessels suffering significant contusion usually have a mottled external appearance because of subadventitial hemorrhage.

FALSE ANEURYSMS
When the lumen of a partially lacerated artery does not become occluded, the resultant perivascular hematoma may develop a cavity in continuity with the arterial lumen and become a "pulsating hematoma." Later, this cavity becomes lined with endothelial cells and becomes a "false" aneurysm. Distal blood flow usually continues unless there is excessive pressure on the true lumen by the aneurysm.

ARTERIOVENOUS FISTULAS
A traumatic arteriovenous (AV) fistula develops when a penetrating injury causes laceration in an artery and its adjacent vein. The high arterial pressure allows blood to flow continuously into the adjacent hematoma and then into the vein. Later, as the hematoma wall becomes fibrotic and retracts, the holes in the artery and vein are often brought into direct continuity.

A large AV fistula can produce a significant increase in pulse rate, pulse pressure, and cardiac output.[29,30] If the fistula is large enough, high-output cardiac failure may result. This is associated with an increased incidence of bacterial endocarditis. Compression of the fistula often causes a characteristic decrease in pulse rate (Nicoladoni's/Branham's sign).[1]

SPASM

> **PITFALL** ⊘
>
> *If distal ischemia persists after reduction of fracture or dislocation, vessel damage or thrombosis should be suspected.*

On rare occasions, severe sustained contraction of vascular smooth muscle, associated with little or no apparent external damage to the vessel, may partially obliterate the lumen. Such spasm is usually self-limiting and generally disappears within a few minutes following relief or removal of local compression.

Attempts to correct vessel narrowing with proximal nerve blocks, such as lumbar, epidural, or stellate ganglion blocks, can be hazardous.[3] Attempts to relieve spasm with these indirect methods can cause dangerous delays in the exploration and repair of injured vessels.

> **AXIOM**   Nerve blocks to correct spasm after trauma to a vessel should generally be condemned because the time lost with such procedures may allow the distal ischemia to become irreversible.

For a short time after an injured artery has been repaired, some degree of spasm may persist, not only at the site of the injury, but also in the distal vessels.[1] Under these circumstances, local stripping of the adventitia 1 to 2 cm above and below the repair, with the local application of papaverine or Xylocaine, may improve flow. Injection of dilute papaverine or Xylocaine into the vessel lumen with temporary inflow occlusion may also improve distal blood flow. One should also be sure that the patient is not hypovolemic. Systolic blood pressure should be maintained in the normal range after vessel repair.

If blood flow distal to the repair still seems inadequate, an arteriogram should be performed in the operating room. Any evidence of partial or complete blockage at the site of injury mandates correction, even if a new end-to-end anastomosis must be done or an autologous vein graft inserted.

PREHOSPITAL CARE

EMTs at the scene of any trauma should control active external bleeding as completely and rapidly as possible. This is usually best accomplished by digital pressure or a compression dressing directly over the bleeding site. If refractory bleeding occurs, the compression dressing should be reapplied with or without the adjuvant use of a sphygmomanometer cuff placed proximal to the injury and inflated above the systolic pressure.

When a vascular injury is associated with suspected long bone fractures, the limb should be splinted using either inflatable splints or MAST in order to reduce the likelihood of further neurovascular injury during transport to the nearest emergency facility.

EMERGENCY DEPARTMENT CARE

When recurrent bleeding from an injured limb occurs after removal of splints in the emergency department, reapplication of the splints and dressings with precise pressure over the vascular injury will usually provide hemostasis.

AXIOM Blind placement of clamps in the depths of an actively bleeding wound should be condemned.

Blind clamping in a wound in an attempt to control bleeding may lead to irreparable damage to the artery or adjacent nerves. Direct digital pressure or reapplication of a well-placed compression dressing is much safer and more apt to be successful.

Patients with dislocations or fracture-dislocations often have absent distal pulses. When possible, immediate reduction and splinting or traction on the injured limb should be done in an attempt to relieve arterial kinking, compression, or entrapment. Patients presenting with 90° eversion dislocations of the ankle often have poor circulation to the foot. Restoration of pedal circulation can usually be accomplished quite simply by putting the foot back into its proper position.

AXIOM Failure to promptly reduce a dislocation to restore the circulation to an extremity may result in extensive tissue necrosis and need for a later amputation.

Other dislocations that can lead to temporary loss of arterial circulation include anterior dislocations of the shoulder and posterior dislocations of the knee. Early reduction of these dislocations often leads to rapid restoration of perfusion to the distal extremity. If possible, an immediate x-ray of the involved joint should be done to identify any associated fractures before attempting to reduce the joint.

AXIOM Whenever possible, x-rays should be taken before attempting to reduce a dislocation.

DIAGNOSIS

Any delay in diagnosing and treating a major vascular injury increases the risk of developing irreversible ischemia or dysfunction.[3] The workup should be expeditious with the goal to reestablish perfusion of the ischemic limb in less than 4-6 hours. Although there is no absolute 4-6 hour "golden period" that applies to all vascular injuries in extremities, the results are less successful if restoration of arterial flow cannot be secured within that interval.

History

A history of pulsatile, bright red blood spurting from a wound strongly suggests arterial injury, while the history of a steady flow of dark blood from the wound usually indicates a venous injury.[3] If the patient is not able to cooperate, it is important to try to obtain such information from anyone who might have been present when the injury occurred.

AXIOM Because peripheral pulses may be present in up to 25% of the patients with extremity arterial injuries,[31,32] a history suggesting vascular injury may be the most important diagnostic indicator at the time of the initial evaluation.

The amount of blood loss from a wound may be estimated from a description of blood found at the scene, the necessity for a tourniquet, or a history of hypotension or syncope. Such information can be helpful because penetrating wounds involving major vessels may appear relatively minor when first seen in the hospital.

Physical Examination

Evaluation of the circulation in hypotensive patients can be difficult because the peripheral pulses are diminished and capillary refill is delayed.[32,33] Indeed, it may not be possible to determine whether or not an arterial or venous injury is present until shock has been corrected by infusion of fluids and the peripheral pulses in the uninjured limbs have returned.

AXIOM Many patients with penetrating arterial injury have a palpable distal pulse although it is often weaker than in the contralateral limb.

In dealing with penetrating wounds, particular attention should be given to the type of bleeding, the location and direction of the wound, the size of the surrounding hematoma, and the presence or absence of a thrill or bruit.[3] A large, pulsatile hematoma is virtually diagnostic of an arterial injury. Venous bleeding can also create a relatively large, tense hematoma.

A bruit or thrill over a site of injury indicates the presence of an arteriovenous fistula which may be the only evidence of a major vascular injury.[1]

AXIOM Careful auscultation over the area of trauma is an important part of the physical examination.

The seven Ps that may suggest a vascular injury include pulselessness, pain, pallor, poikilothermia, paresthesias, paralysis, and paresis. The neurologic signs of paresthesias and paralysis are particularly important because peripheral nerves tend to be relatively tolerant of ischemia for up to 6 hours.[3] There is relatively little risk of gangrene if neurologic function is intact; however, once neurologic function is lost as a result of ischemia, gangrene is more likely unless circulation is quickly restored.

PITFALL ⊘

If the diagnosis of an arterial injury is not made until motor function in the distal extremity becomes impaired, the delay in treatment may be disastrous.

Loss of distal motor function is a late sign of ischemia to muscles and nerves and, therefore, of relatively little value for diagnosing vascular injuries early, when repair is most apt to be successful.[1] With concomitant injuries to peripheral nerves, neurologic function as an index to the severity of the ischemia is of little use. However, ischemia tends to produce stocking or glovelike neurologic deficits of the involved extremity, while injuries to peripheral nerves tend to produce deficits that are limited to specific dermatomes or muscle groups.

Signs directly indicative of ischemia or severe bleeding are commonly referred to as "hard signs" of vascular injury.[3] These include pulsatile bleeding, expanding hematoma, palpable thrill, audible bruit, severe rest pain, pallor, paralysis, paresthesia, poikilothermia, and pulselessness (Table 35–1). These usually indicate an urgent need for surgery.

Signs suggestive of vascular injury, but without definite evidence of ischemia or hemorrhage, are called "soft signs." These include a history of moderate hemorrhage, injury (fractures or penetrating wounds) in proximity to major vessels, diminished but palpable pulses, diminished ankle-brachial index (ABI), abnormal flow velocity waveforms, peripheral nerve deficits, and knee dislocation. These soft signs indicate a need for further investigation. In such patients, diagnostic imaging and/or noninvasive studies of flow and pressure can help to either confirm or exclude arterial injury.

Major fractures or dislocations frequently cause vascular injuries in extremities.[3] Although the deformity produced by a fracture or dislocation is usually obvious, spontaneous reduction can occur before the patient is seen by a physician. If the patient is not questioned in detail about any deformities that were present, even if only temporarily, or if the joint is not examined carefully for severe laxity, the dislocation may never be suspected.

Although many patients presenting with injury to a major extremity vessel will have ischemic pain, pallor, pulselessness, paresthesia, paralysis, active bleeding, coolness, or a thrill or bruit, some patients with such injuries will have none of these signs and symptoms. Likewise, some patients with the above signs and symptoms will have injuries to structures near the artery and vein but have no vascular injury. Consequently, one often has to rely on noninvasive or angiographic studies to identify the presence and nature of peripheral vascular injuries.

Noninvasive Studies

Doppler techniques for the determination of segmental blood pressures and for arterial waveform analysis have been used increasingly to diagnose peripheral vascular trauma.[14,34] Shah et al[14] consider any decrease in ankle pressure greater than 20 torr (compared to the uninjured limb) or an abnormal waveform to be indicative of arterial injury. Others[34] have suggested that an ankle-brachial index of 0.9 or less should arouse suspicion of an arterial injury.

The combination of ultrasound imaging with spectral analysis (duplex scanning) may be useful in the diagnosis of traumatic arterial or venous thrombosis, arterial pseudoaneurysm, and arterial fistula.[3] Image resolution is not sufficient to display intimal injury unless the disruption is severe enough to produce a major disturbance in flow. Duplex studies are hampered by associated injury to bone or soft tissue severe enough to interfere with proper positioning.

Angiography

EMERGENCY SURGERY

AXIOM   Unstable patients with suspected vascular injury or threatened limbs should be taken directly to the operating room.

The decision to circumvent diagnostic angiography for a suspected vascular injury must be made on the basis of the clinical findings

TABLE 35–1   Signs and Symptoms Suggesting Vascular Injury

Massive bleeding
Shock
Hematoma (large or pulsating)
Thrill or bruit
Pain
Pulseless
Paresthesia
Paralysis/paresis
Pallor
Paralysis
Poikilothermia

TABLE 35–2   Guidelines for Arteriography

Penetrating Wounds
1. Signs or symptoms of arterial injury
2. Threatened or ischemic limb
Blunt Trauma
1. Signs or symptoms of arterial injury
2. Long bone fracture with large hematoma
3. Threatened or ischemic limb
4. Posterior knee dislocation by history or physical exam

and the duration and severity of distal ischemia. When a patient has a threatened distal extremity, immediate transportation to the operating room for exploration of the involved vessel is appropriate.[35] When threatened ischemia from inadequate circulation is reversed, intraoperative angiography can be used as needed,[23,36,37] especially if there are multiple possible sites of vascular injury.

Another alternative in marginally perfused limbs is "single-stick" arteriography in the resuscitation area in which anteroposterior projections can usually be obtained and reviewed in 15 minutes.[3]

"HARD SIGNS" OF VASCULAR INJURY

Patients with "hard signs" of vascular injury can usually be taken directly to surgery without the delay of formal arteriography.[38] Exceptions to this policy include stable patients with multiple possible sites of injury, high risk patients, and patients with vascular injury that is easily accessible to the angiographer, but difficult for the surgeon to expose.[39,40]

Patients with clinical signs and symptoms of an arterial injury without threatened ischemia are candidates for angiography which is used to identify the site of the injury and to provide a road map for the surgeon to facilitate operative intervention (Fig. 35–1A and 35–1B). Another indication of arteriography is altered or absent distal pulses associated with long bone fractures, even if the pulses return to normal with reduction and splinting (Table 35–2).

Spasm should never be diagnosed just on the basis of the clinical findings in a patient with proximal penetrating wounds or long bone fractures from blunt trauma (Fig. 35–2).

Another indication for arteriography is severe fractures or fracture-dislocations about the knee even though the peripheral pulses are present. There is a high incidence of associated arterial damage with such injuries.

"SOFT SIGNS" OF VASCULAR INJURY

Arteriography is quite reliable for excluding arterial injury in patients with "soft signs" of vascular injury.[3] In addition, many such patients will have an abnormal arteriogram.[32,35] An abnormal arteriogram means that the arteriogram revealed occlusion, extravasation, pseudoaneurysm, arteriovenous fistula, intimal flap, intimal irregularity, spasm, or extraluminal compression. Occlusion of a small branch of the main artery is an abnormal finding, but does not require operative intervention and has no clinical significance.

AXIOM   The significance of any abnormal findings on arteriography is determined by the surgeon who coordinates the clinical and roentgenographic findings.

Arteriography in patients with only soft signs of vascular injury has a sensitivity of 97-100%, a specificity of 90-98%, a negative predictive value of 99-100%, and an overall accuracy of 92-98%.[35,41-45] Virtually all of the errors are a result of false positive readings, which occur in 2-8% of patients.

PROXIMITY INJURIES

Before the general availability of arteriography, operative exploration was advocated for patients with injuries near major vessels.[31] This

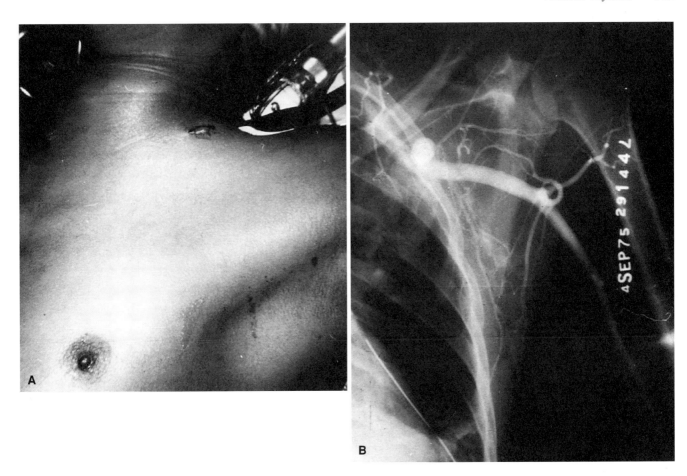

FIGURE 35–1 **A.** This patient sustained a gunshot wound that appeared to enter over the left clavicle and exited the left posterior chest causing a hemopneumothorax. He had no hematoma and pulses were present. He did have an incomplete median and ulnar nerve deficit. **B.** Arteriography demonstrated a false aneurysm arising from the axillary artery. This was resected with end-to-end anastomosis with a good result.

resulted in a high negative exploration rate. Use of arteriography to exclude vascular injury in proximity wounds decreased the negative exploration rate.[31,35] Nevertheless, certain patients should go directly to surgery without waiting for angiography.

The need for arteriography in patients with a penetrating wound in proximity to a neurovascular bundle and no hard signs of vascular injury are somewhat controversial. Arteriography in this setting will identify a certain small number of patients who have intimal tears with maintained distal blood flow (Fig. 35–3) and patients with small arterial wounds causing perivascular hemorrhage without occlusion (Fig. 35–4A and 35–4B).

Proximity as a sole indication for angiography has an extremely low yield for revealing a clinically significant injury.[41-45] The incidence of arterial injury in patients in whom proximity of either a fracture or a penetrating wound to a major artery was the sole indication for arteriography ranged from 0 to 6.7%. Frykberg et al[43] found only 16 arteriographic abnormalities in major arteries in 152 proximity wounds (10.5%). They concluded that arteriography was not cost-effective in evaluating patients who had penetrating proximity wounds but no clinical evidence of arterial injury. The likelihood for misinterpretation of arteriograms also increases when performed in the emergency setting.[38,40]

COMPLICATIONS OF ANGIOGRAPHY

Angiography is not without risks; complications occur in about 2 to 4% of patients.[45] Most are minor, such as groin hematomas, and do not compromise patient care. Major complications, such as embolic occlusion or pseudoaneurysm, occur infrequently.[24,45]

Digital Contrast Studies

Intra-arterial digital subtraction arteriography (IADSA) has a sensitivity and specificity similar to arteriography and has several advantages, including a shorter time to complete the examination, less exposure to radiation, reduced cost, reduced dye load, and less discomfort.[41,46] Because a smaller catheter is used, IADSA may lessen the chances of an iatrogenic injury. Its usefulness is limited, however, in shotgun injuries in which metallic fragments may distort the images.

Digital angiography after intravenous injection of the contrast agent has also been used successfully in vascular trauma,[47] but the resolution is less than with IADSA, and small intimal injuries can be missed. Furthermore, digital venous studies require longer patient cooperation since any movement of the limb during the study will make the images unreadable.

Other Invasive Studies

The sensitivity and specificity of radionuclide imaging with 99mTc-pertechnetate in the diagnosis of acute arterial injury has a sensitivity and specificity similar to arteriography.[3,48] The study can be completed in 10 minutes as it requires only a venipuncture and little in the way of experienced support staff. However, this technique has limited resolution and may miss small injuries.

Venography may be useful in certain circumstances for identifying reparable venous injuries.[49] Probably the main indication for preoperative venography after trauma is signs and symptoms of arterial injury in a nonthreatened distal limb with a normal arteriogram. Such

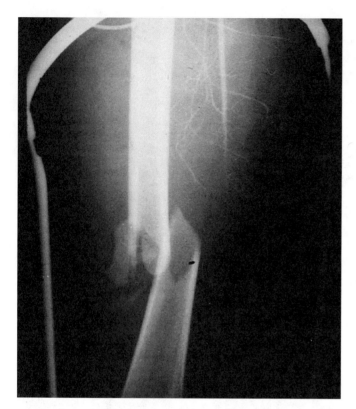

FIGURE 35–2 This patient sustained blunt injury to the right thigh. He had massive swelling in the thigh and an unstable fracture of the right femur. There were no pulses. Arteriography demonstrates flow in small collateral vessels distal to the main femoral artery. This indicates occlusion of the superficial femoral artery resulting from thrombosis.

patients may have a perivenular hematoma causing symptoms that can mimic arterial injury (Fig. 35–5A and 35–5B). Venography may also be important in identifying the pathway of bullets embolized within the venous systems. However, most life- or limb-threatening venous injuries are either clinically apparent or are associated with significant arterial injuries.[3]

AXIOM Venography is seldom helpful and may be hazardous if it delays treatment of more severe injuries.

NONOPERATIVE MANAGEMENT

The treatment of some angiographic defects, such as intimal irregularity, focal narrowing, and small pseudoaneurysms, is controversial.[3,43] Until recently, the management of these injuries was routine operation.[50] Recent experience, however, suggests that these injuries have a benign course and can be safely observed. Frykberg et al[43,51] followed 20 cases of such injuries documented arteriographically and found that 53% resolved, 16% improved, and 26% remained unchanged. One patient required operation for enlargement of a brachial artery pseudoaneurysm. Rose and Moore[42] reported no sequelae in five patients with intimal injuries observed an average of 11 months. Indeed, there is little likelihood that these lesions progress or present precipitously.[43]

The experience in Korea and Vietnam suggested that asymptomatic pseudoaneurysms could be safely observed for at least 3 months.[8] In fact, some pseudoaneurysms will resolve within that time.[52] Similarly, arteriographic demonstration of segmental spasm or focal narrowing, but persistent distal flow, has been demonstrated to cause no morbidity on long-term follow-up.[53]

AXIOM Nonoperative management of selected cases of clinically occult focal narrowing, pseudoaneurysm, or intimal irregularities is safe, practical, and cost-effective.[43]

Follow-up of any vascular injury should include frequent physical examinations and objective assessment of both the anatomy and the flow characteristics of the injured artery and the distal arterial bed with duplex imaging. Similarly, observation can be advocated in asymptomatic injuries of arterial segments that are difficult to expose or control, such as high lesions in the carotid or vertebral arteries.[52]

OPERATIVE MANAGEMENT

General Principles

CONTROL OF BLEEDING

External bleeding must be controlled with digital pressure or compressive bandages until the involved vessels can be controlled proximally and distally. Occasionally, one can expose the involved area and directly control the bleeding site with a single curved vascular clamp, but such efforts should generally be done in the operating room.

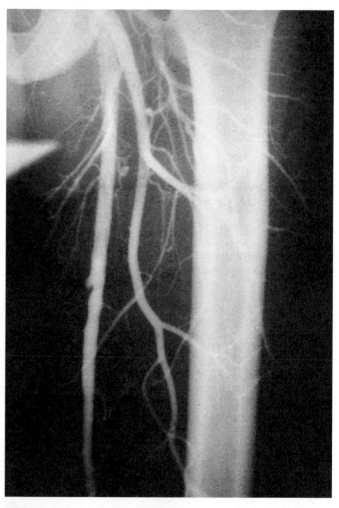

FIGURE 35–3 Arteriography done for a gunshot wound that transversed the left thigh in the region of the femoral vessels demonstrates an intimal flap in the midportion of the left superficial femoral artery. There were no signs of arterial injury and pulses were present. The area of injury was resected with an end-to-end anastomosis. This injury can be treated nonoperatively as long as a pulse is maintained.

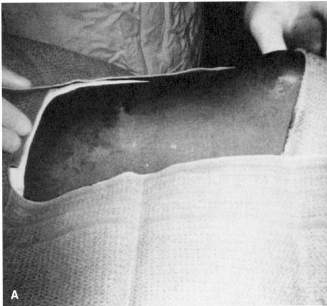

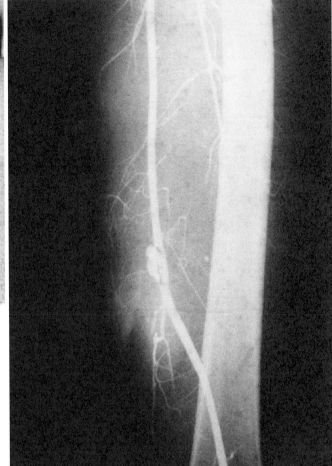

FIGURE 35–4   A. This patient presented with a stab wound to the left anterior thigh. Pulses were present, but there was a history of red blood squirting from the wound after injury. **B.** The arteriogram done because of proximity demonstrates extravasation from the left superficial femoral artery with good flow distally. Repair was achieved with resection and end-to-end anastomosis.

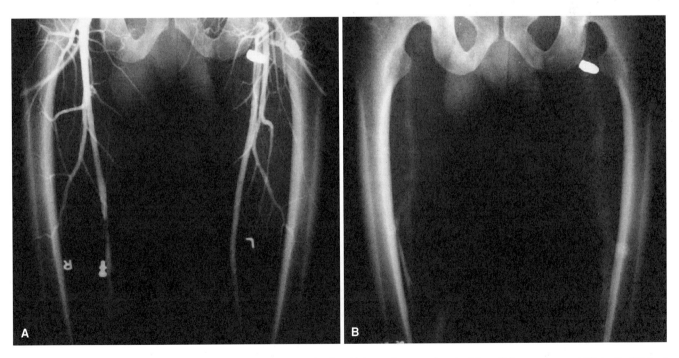

FIGURE 35–5   A. This patient sustained multiple gunshot wounds to both legs. Pulses were present bilaterally. Bilateral arteriograms done with percutaneous puncture in the emergency department revealed both femoral systems to be intact. Unfortunately, the obturator for the arteriogram needle was left in the field. **B.** A venogram done on the same patient demonstrates normal flow through the left system, but the right system appears to be occluded with reconstitution. At operation, he had injury to the right common femoral vein which was ligated.

RESTORATION OF PERFUSION

Rapid restoration of perfusion is the goal of treatment of injuries to major peripheral arteries. In some instances, a temporary shunt can be used while other procedures, such as reduction and fixation of fractures, are performed.

PREVENTION OF INFECTION

Broad spectrum antibiotics should be started as soon as possible after injury and continued through the first postinjury day.[3] Extensive soft tissue injury or contamination may require extensive debridement and aggressive irrigation and may necessitate longer therapy. Patients with contamination resulting from open fractures or gunshot wounds should also receive tetanus prophylaxis.

PREPARATION FOR AUTOLOGOUS VEIN GRAFT

Preparation of the skin and draping of the uninjured extremity permits harvesting a segment of superficial vein, usually the greater saphenous vein in the thigh, for potential use as a vascular conduit.[3] Incorporating the hand or foot of the injured extremity allows the surgeon to evaluate pulses and color changes when an arterial repair is complete.

Immediate Amputation

In some patients, the bone, vessels, nerves, and soft tissue are so badly injured that primary amputation is indicated. These "mangled limbs" are associated with a high morbidity and a poor return of function; thus the amputation rate is high (Table 35-3).[54-56]

AXIOM Selected patients with mangled extremities will benefit from primary amputation, particularly if the nerves have been completely severed.[3]

Bondurant et al[55] noted that 43 patients undergoing primary amputation for mangled lower limbs averaged 22.3 days of hospitalization, 1.6 surgical procedures to the involved limb, and an average of $28,964 in hospital charges. Those having delayed amputation averaged 53.4 days of hospitalization, 6.9 surgical procedures on the involved limb, and $53,462 in hospital charges. In addition, six patients with delayed amputation developed sepsis from the injured lower extremity and died, while no patient with a primary amputation developed sepsis or died. Johansen and associates[56] have described similar experiences.

The decision to amputate primarily, especially with the upper extremity is often difficult. The extent of soft tissue damage is seldom appreciated during the initial examination. Distal perfusion also may be difficult to assess, especially while the patient is hypotensive. Moreover, the neurologic evaluation may be compromised in patients with associated intracranial injury or limb ischemia.

Gregory and coworkers[54] and Johansen et al[56] have developed objective scoring systems that assist in predicting final outcome. Both systems combine an assessment of the soft tissue, bone, vascular, and nerve injury with an evaluation of premorbid factors (including age more than 40 years and associated illness) and an estimate of systemic and regional perfusion. There are, however, many gray zones;

TABLE 35-3 Factors Increasing the Likelihood of Early Amputation after Vascular Trauma

Severe blunt trauma
Delay in diagnosis or operation
Ligation of major venous drainage
Late fasciotomy for compartment syndrome
Severe adjacent soft tissue injury
Wound infection
Inadequate soft tissue coverage of vessels

thus, relying on the mangled limb scoring systems to make decisions concerning early amputation has drawbacks.[56]

Importance of Early Intervention

Prompt diagnosis and therapy not only reduce bleeding, but also increase the likelihood of successful arterial repair. The time from vascular injury until definitive reconstruction can strongly affect outcome. If the delay exceeds 4-6 hours, the potential for ischemic complications from the vascular injury increases. This relative urgency in providing vascular reconstruction, however, should not interfere with proper resuscitation and treatment of other life-threatening injuries that have higher priority. Control of arterial bleeding has a high priority whereas definitive reconstruction of that artery may have a lower priority than care of other injuries.

AXIOM Life takes precedence over limb throughout resuscitation and treatment.

Intraoperative Management of Fluids

Depending upon the extent of injury and the amount of blood loss, two or three large intravenous catheters should be inserted in the ED. After initial blood samples are drawn for a blood count and type and cross-matching, fluid and blood should be infused rapidly until the vital signs are restored to normal. If it appears that the patient is still bleeding, he or she should be rushed to the OR. Once the bleeding sites have been controlled, enough fluid and blood should be given to raise the systolic blood pressure to improve collateral blood flow and to maintain a urine output of at least 1.0 ml/kg/hr. Efforts should also be made to keep the core temperature above 35° C.

Prepping and Draping

AXIOM The position and draping for emergency vascular surgery should allow rapid securing of proximal and distal control of the injured vessels and an autologous vein graft if needed.

In the operating room, the extremity and adjacent trunk should be prepared and draped so that the surgeon can readily secure proximal and distal control of the injured vessels and also evaluate the blood flow and pulses distally without risking contamination of the wound. Provision should also be made for obtaining an autologous vein graft. If the trauma involves one leg, the opposite groin, thigh, and lower leg should be prepared and draped so that a saphenous vein graft can be readily obtained. If there is a chance that the saphenous veins will not be suitable or available, one arm and shoulder should be prepared and draped so that the cephalic vein can be used. Whenever a vascular patch or graft is needed, the injured patient's own veins generally provide the most suitable material.

Intraoperative Surgery

HEMOSTASIS

The first priority during operation is control of bleeding. Techniques for controlling active external bleeding preoperatively often are compromised during transit to the operating room and preparation for surgery. When digital pressure is used, the operative prep should be done around the gloved finger which is left within the operative field through the period of draping until a member of the operative team can take over (Fig. 35-6).

AXIOM Refractory external bleeding from leg or forearm injuries can often be controlled by a sphygmomanometer inflated well above systolic pressure on the proximal thigh or arm.

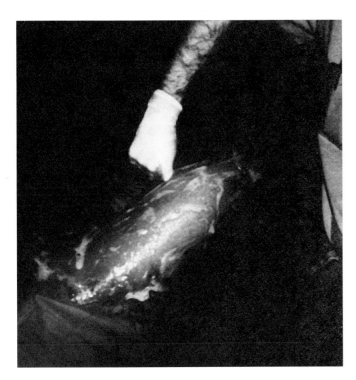

FIGURE 35–6 This patient presented with a single gunshot wound that entered the left medial thigh. There was massive hematoma and blood squirting from the wound. A gloved finger was placed in the wound and the patient was taken directly to the operating room. The leg was prepped and draped with the finger tamponading the bleeding. This was continued through exposure of the vessel at the site of injury.

The incision in most patients with extremity wounds should follow the course of the neurovascular bundle and remain between natural anatomic planes to reduce the chance of causing inadvertent injury to adjacent structures. When the injury is at the junction of anatomic compartments, the incision may have to be carried into the more proximal compartment to achieve proper exposure and control of the vessels. When the injury involves the femoral triangle and proximal compartment control is needed, the longitudinal incision extending from the anterior thigh superior to the inguinal ligament can then be curved laterally in an oblique manner to a point two finger widths superior to the ipsilateral anterosuperior iliac supine. This extension permits ready retroperitoneal access to the external iliac vessels and even more proximal vessels if the need arises.

> **AXIOM** In approaching injured vessels, the surgeon should try to stay within anatomic planes, and thereby avoid injury to important adjacent structures.

When the injury occurs at the shoulder and more proximal vascular control is needed, the incision can be carried along the deltopectoral groove to the level of the clavicle and then along the superior margin of the clavicle to the suprasternal notch (Fig. 35–7). Control of the subclavian artery can be obtained immediately superior to the clavicle before unroofing the site of injury. This is facilitated by keeping the upper extremity at the side of the patient so that the lateral portion of the clavicle moves inferiorly (Fig. 35–8).

When the site of injury is at the junction of the subclavian and axillary arteries, excision of a portion of the clavicle facilitates taking down the muscular attachments along the inferior border of the clavicle and thereby exposing this area. Further exposure of the axillary artery can be achieved by dividing the pectoralis major insertion on the humerus and rotating this muscle medially and inferiorly to unroof the insertion of the pectoralis minor into the coracoid pro-

cess. When the pectoralis minor is detached from the coracoid process and rotated medially and inferiorly, the entire axillary artery is exposed (Fig. 35–9).

The same principles of proximal exposure along anatomic planes apply when the injury involves the thoracic outlet. The medial portion of the supraclavicular incision is extended from the suprasternal notch to the xiphoid as a median sternotomy. This exposes the innominate artery and the origins of the common carotid arteries and left subclavian artery.

PROXIMAL AND DISTAL CONTROL

PITFALL ⊘

> *Failure to obtain proximal and distal control before exposing the site of injury of a large vessel may convert a careful anatomic dissection into a frantic attempt to stop massive hemorrhage.*

Having both proximal and distal vascular control decreases the risk of hemorrhage when the injury site is exposed. After obtaining control with vascular tapes, one can gradually dissect along the vessel toward the site of injury and at the same time replace the vascular tapes closer to the injury until the distance between the proximal and distal tapes is reduced to the area of injury plus one or two centimeters at each end. Dissection of these last few centimeters of soft tissue covering the injured vessel is greatly facilitated by knowledge of the preoperative arteriogram and normal anatomy to prevent inadvertent injury to collateral branches coursing through the perivascular hematoma.

As the remaining portions of the injured vessels are dissected out, there will often be a sudden rush of blood as the protective soft tissues and clot are dislodged from the arterial injury. Direct digital pres-

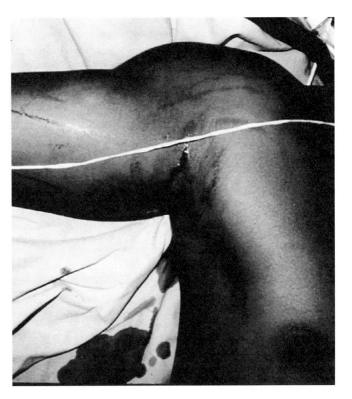

FIGURE 35–7 The umbilical tape outlines the site of the incision in this patient with a gunshot wound in the area of the right shoulder. The incision follows the deltopectoral groove. It is often easier to proceed from distal to proximal, taking down the pectoralis major from the humerus as the initial step in exposure of the axillary artery.

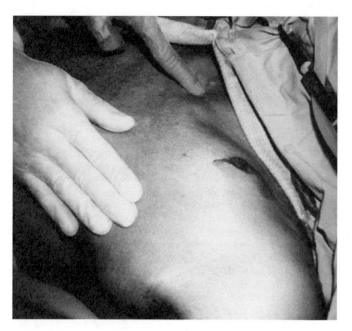

FIGURE 35–8 This patient presented with a gunshot wound overlying the left clavicle with a huge hematoma in the left axilla. The proximal subclavian artery can be exposed superior to the clavicle by taking down the sternocleidomastoid muscle. The site of the subclavian artery superior to the clavicle is identified in this photograph by the index finger.

sure is applied immediately while the last few millimeters above and below the injury are unroofed. At this time, the dissection is carried out in the subadventitial plane in order to free up the vessel for appropriate resection or repair.

INTRALUMINAL SHUNTS

After achieving proximal and distal control, extraction of any intravascular clots with a Fogarty catheter, and regional heparinization, a decision must be made as to whether the vascular reconstruction can be accomplished immediately or whether care of other injuries has a higher priority. If the vascular repair is to be delayed for more than

30 minutes, temporary restoration of blood flow can be achieved with a Javid or similar shunt placed in the proximal and distal ends of the vessel and secured while other injuries are treated (Fig. 35–10).[57-60]

While the Javid shunt is in place, the vascular surgeon should remain on the scene to check the circulation and prevent inadvertent kinking or compression of the shunt while the orthopaedic surgery team treats the associated long bone fracture. The integrity and patency of the shunt can be monitored by checking the distal pulses.

Johansen et al[59] have documented shunt "dwell" times for these temporary intraluminal shunts of up to 6 hours with an average of 3.7 hours without morbidity. The experiences of Shackford and Rich[3] are similar, and shunts have occasionally been left in place for 36-48 hours without thrombosis. According to Eger et al[57] and Nichols et al,[60] early use of an intraluminal shunt may reduce the amputation rate resulting from injury to the popliteal artery.

THROMBOSIS

Before definitive arterial repair, one must be assured that any clots that may have formed proximally or distally are removed. Proximal extraction of clot can often be achieved by releasing the proximal vascular clamp and allowing fresh blood to flow through the vascular wound.

AXIOM Good back-bleeding from the distal artery does not ensure the absence of intravascular thrombus beyond the first patent collateral vessel.

The distal extraction of clots is best achieved with Fogarty balloon catheters passed distally until resistance is met. As the catheter is being slowly extracted, the balloon is inflated just enough to cause a slight resistance to its withdrawal. Overinflation must be avoided since it can produce arterial injury. The Fogarty balloon catheter is passed as many times as necessary to ensure that the last passage produces no clot.

HEPARINIZATION

After clot extraction, the authors prefer local heparinization with a heparin solution containing 100 units/ml. A Fogarty irrigating catheter is used to instill 10-20 ml of this solution distally and 3-5 ml proximally.

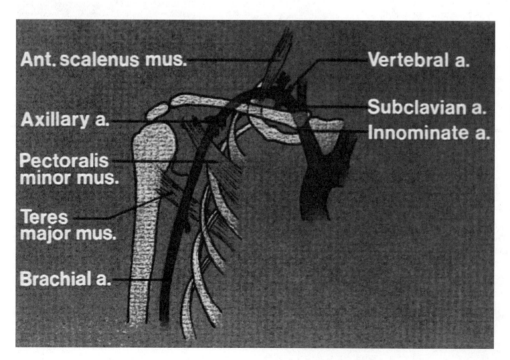

Ant. scalenus mus.

Axillary a.

Pectoralis minor mus.

Teres major mus.

Brachial a.

Vertebral a.

Subclavian a.

Innominate a.

FIGURE 35–9 This diagram of the subclavian-axillary vessels indicates the site at which the proximal subclavian and vertebral arteries and the vertebrae can be identified superior to the clavicle. It also identifies the pectoralis minor muscle that can be detached from the coracoid process to provide complete exposure of the axillary artery.

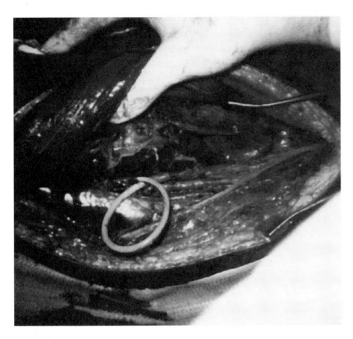

FIGURE 35–10 This patient, shown previously in Figure 4 with blunt trauma causing femur fracture and occluded right superficial femoral artery, has now had the artery exposed and the site of injury resected. Thrombectomy with a Fogarty catheter was done followed by placement of a Javid shunt. Orthopaedic surgeons repaired the fracture with the shunt in place. The vessel was then repaired with end-to-end anastomosis.

Systemic heparinization with 50-100 units heparin/kg body weight has the advantage of producing a more complete and effective anticoagulation; however, if there is little or no distal blood flow, additional heparin will have to be injected beyond the injury to prevent distal thrombosis. Local heparinization is also much safer if the patient has other injuries that can bleed during systemic heparinization.

When vascular anastomosis is completed, the heparin is allowed to metabolize. Giving protamine to counteract the remaining heparin effect is generally unnecessary and probably unwise because it may cause rebound hypercoagulability.

VESSEL DEBRIDEMENT
Grossly damaged portions of the vessel should be sharply debrided.[3] Visible areas of contusion should be excised. Avulsed or transected arteries usually have stretched the adventitia, which may be prolapsed several millimeters over the edges of the intima and media. This damaged tissue should be thoroughly debrided to avoid incorporating it into the suture line. Debridement, however, should not extend beyond the point of gross injury. There is no data showing that extensive resection of grossly normal artery improves the ultimate success of the repair.[11,12] Recent experiments and our clinical observations suggest that microscopic changes in the normal artery immediately adjacent to a grossly damaged segment do not affect the ultimate outcome of the vascular repair; thus, removal of a large segment of normal vessel is not warranted.[61]

VESSEL REPAIR
When arterial repair is performed, small vascular clamps and fine synthetic monofilament sutures on small atraumatic needles should be used. This includes 5-0 polypropylene sutures for the femoral, axillary, popliteal, and brachial arteries.

The type of repair varies with the extent of injury. When a simple primary closure of a transverse laceration is performed, the sutures can be started at each end and brought toward the middle with each bite placed one millimeter from the previous stitch. Alternatively, with larger arteries, a single suture begun at one end and finished at the opposite end will usually achieve excellent results.

When a stab wound causes a through-and-through arterial injury, a simple running closure of both perforations may cause excessive narrowing. This injury is best treated by resection of the injured segment and end-to-end anastomosis.

AXIOM Resection of the site of injury with end-to-end anastomosis is indicated in several circumstances including gunshot wounds, lacerations caused by bone fragments, and arterial wall contusions with an associated intimal tear.

At least 2 and sometimes 3 centimeters of most named extremity arteries can be resected and enough proximal and distal artery mobilized to permit a relatively tension-free primary anastomosis. Before suturing, the adventitia is freed from the underlying media about 3 millimeters from each end.

To help achieve the desired length of proximal and distal vessel, major collaterals can be dissected free of surrounding tissue, but they should not be interrupted just to achieve sufficient length for a primary anastomosis. If flexion of the joint is used during exposure of the vascular injury, the extremity should be returned to a straight position before repair to ensure adequate proximal and distal length to perform an end-to-end anastomosis without undue tension. However, during the actual repair, the extremity can be flexed to easily suture the ends of the vessel.

End-to-end reconstruction can then be achieved by placing two lateral sutures that are run respectively from one side to the other to approximate the posterior and anterior walls. The most critical technical aid in performing the anastomosis is keeping the two ends of the artery approximated without tension. Consequently, the greatest attention to detail is accomplished by the second assistant who holds the two vascular clamps to perfectly approximate the ends of the vessel while the first assistant provides the precise tension and the correct position to properly expose the artery. The authors prefer to run the anterior wall, after which the artery is carefully turned 180° to facilitate a running closure of the posterior wall.

Contrary to popular practice, the authors do not vent the artery of air until the last suture has been placed. When the last suture has been tied and one is assured that each suture is supporting the same amount of tension, the distal clamp can be released to allow blood to flow retrograde through the anastomosis, at which time the air will also be vented. When this has been accomplished, the proximal clamp is removed. A nonbleeding anastomosis requires no additional sutures. Oozing through needle holes or between sutures can usually be satisfactorily controlled by gentle digital pressure placed immediately over the site of oozing for 5 minutes. This patience usually obviates the need for "fixer" sutures.

AXIOM Properly placed digital pressure on small bleeding points at a completed vascular anastomosis, with a little patience, will usually obviate the need for repair sutures.

The technique of end-to-end anastomosis varies with surgical preference. With smaller vessels, especially those less than 5 mm in diameter, some surgeons prefer to use the spatulated technique in which the artery on each end is cut in an elongated "spatulated" manner with the length of the spatulated extension approximately twice the diameter of the distal vessel.[61-63] The spatulated extension is made on the proximal artery which is then anastomosed to the distal segment which has been appropriately slit longitudinally in order to accommodate the spatulated extension.

The authors prefer the end-to-end technique with the proximal and distal arterial segments cut at right angles without spatulation. Comparing the two techniques in animal studies of small arterial injuries, both techniques provide comparable long-term patency rates and flow rates.[63]

INTERPOSITION GRAFTS
Close-range shotgun blasts, rifle wounds, some blunt injuries, and deep avulsion injuries often cause extensive arterial disruption,

thereby precluding end-to-end anastomosis after appropriate debridement of the damaged vessel. Reconstruction after large segment arterial disruption must be accomplished by means of interposition grafting. The saphenous vein, taken from an uninjured lower extremity, usually provides the most readily available and safest graft for arterial interposition.[22,31,15-17,64,65]

If autologous vein is not available or is of inadequate luminal size or quality, both Dacron and polytetrafluoroethylene (PTFE) have been used successfully as synthetic vascular conduits.[14,15,17,22] While the long-term patency rate is less than with autologous vein, previous concerns about the potential for infection with prosthetic grafts have not been realized in civilian reports.[19,66]

VENOUS REPAIR

The relative importance of venous repair in an extremity with an arterial injury has been questioned.[67] Although it is important to restore arterial flow to relieve distal ischemia as soon as possible, it may be advantageous to repair the injured vein first in circumstances in which compromised venous return may cause rapid thrombosis of the arterial repair. Hobson et al[68] have shown experimentally that ligation of major veins in the hindlimb can cause a significant reduction in arterial flow and a significant increase in both venous pressure and peripheral arterial resistance.

AXIOM Repair of major veins helps circumvent the problems of venous hypertension.

If the ischemia time is already long, an intraluminal shunt can be placed in the artery to reestablish perfusion before repairing the vein. The only satisfactory conduit for peripheral venous repair is autogenous vein.

VESSEL REPAIR EVALUATION

After vascular reconstruction, excellent distal flow should be apparent by the restoration of normal peripheral pulses. If there is any question about the successful restoration of flow, as may occur in patients

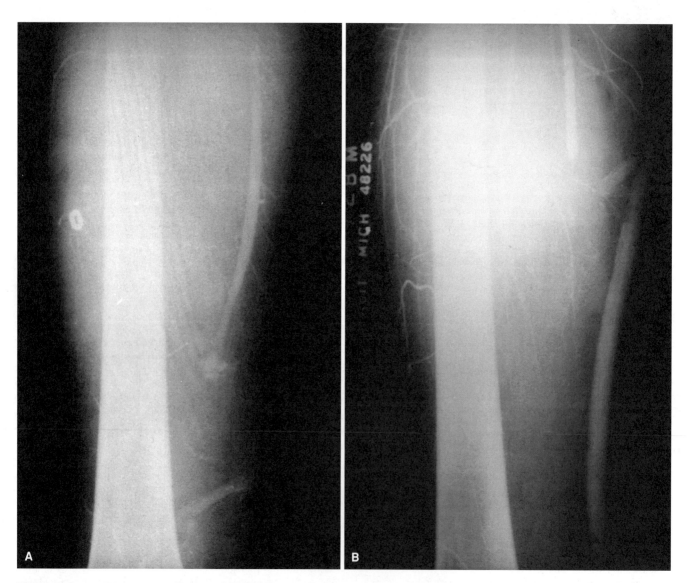

FIGURE 35–11 A. This patient sustained a gunshot wound through the right thigh. There were no pulses and the patient had occlusion of the superficial femoral artery with extravasation of contrast at the site of injury. He was promptly taken to the operating room where resection of 1½ cm of injured artery and end-to-end anastomosis were performed. **B.** Postoperatively, there was no pulse in the foot in the recovery room and a repeat arteriogram demonstrated occlusion of the artery more proximal to the previous repair. He was taken back to the operating room for thrombectomy. Heparin was not instilled proximal to the occluding clamp at the initial procedure.

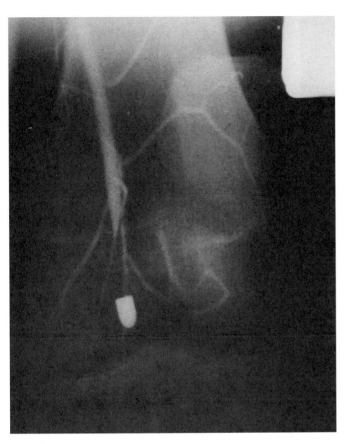

with peripheral vasoconstriction from prolonged ischemia, intraoperative arteriography is needed (Fig. 35–11A and 35–11B). If an anatomic problem is noted at the site of injury, the anastomosis should be redone or bypassed as needed. Occasionally, the most distal pulses are absent immediately after repair as a result of hypothermia and vasoconstriction. Once the extremities are warmed, distal pulses should be present. If pulses are absent, arteriography should be obtained (Fig. 35–12).

IRRIGATION AND WOUND CLOSURE

After successful vascular repair, all devitalized tissue and foreign material should be debrided to reduce the risk of postoperative infection.[3] Unusually dirty wounds may require sharp debridement of devitalized tissue and extensive irrigation with sterile saline using a pulsatile, low-pressure spray.

After adequate debridement and irrigation, the authors approximate the soft tissue with interrupted absorbable sutures to allow egress of blood and fluid from associated soft tissue injury and hematoma. With severe soft tissue injury, temporary drainage with a sump catheter for 12-36 hours may be used.

SPECIAL PROBLEMS WITH VESSEL TRAUMA

Massive Soft Tissue Injury

EXTRA-ANATOMIC BYPASS

Successful vascular repair mandates that the repaired vessel be safely covered by viable soft tissue. When arterial injury is associated with massive soft tissue loss, the muscle and subcutaneous tissue normally overlying the neurovascular bundle may be gone. If a vein graft is exposed or covered only by ischemic or contaminated muscle, it will necrose and rupture.[13] If a prosthetic graft becomes infected, a false aneurysm can develop at the site of repair or sometimes in the artery just proximal or distal to the anastomosis.[68]

One technique that may be utilized to preclude the need for primary amputation in such patients is rerouting the vascular bypass graft through an extra-anatomic plane (Fig. 35–13A and 35–13B). Patients with massive groin injuries involving the femoral artery and vein and

FIGURE 35–12 This patient was admitted hypotensive with a gunshot wound to the abdomen. Laparotomy revealed a single perforation of the abdominal aorta. His femoral pulses were palpable postoperatively. He complained of left leg pain 3 days after injury at the time of extubation. There were no palpable pulses in the left foot. An arteriogram demonstrated a bullet embolus in the left popliteal artery that was subsequently removed with return of pulses.

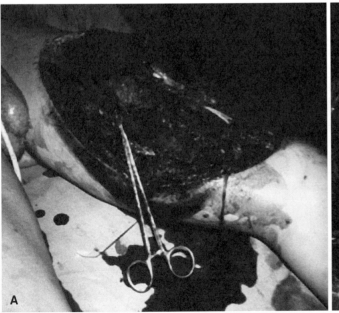
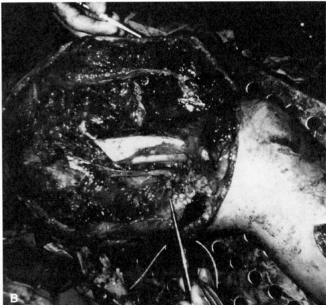

FIGURE 35–13 **A.** This patient sustained a massive injury to his right thigh with loss of skin, subcutaneous tissue, muscles, fractured femur, and lacerated femoral artery. The clamp is occluding the proximal artery. At operation, a Javid shunt was placed and then the muscles were debrided. **B.** The wound has been irrigated and a vein graft from the opposite leg passed through the healthy posterior muscle groups and then anastomosed proximally and distally with a good result. This allowed coverage of the entire vein graft in an extra-anatomical plane through healthy tissue.

adjacent soft tissue may be reconstructed by placement of an extra-anatomic graft from the external iliac artery through the obturator foramen down the posterior medial muscle compartment to the proximal portion of the popliteal artery.[33] This protects the bypass graft while the area of injury is allowed to heal by second intent. Likewise, reconstruction of massive leg injuries involving the deep and superficial posterior compartments may be accomplished by rerouting an extra-anatomic bypass graft through the anterior or lateral compartments.[69]

BIOLOGIC DRESSINGS TO COVER BYPASS GRAFTS

When safe extra-anatomic bypass is precluded because the injury involves all the muscle compartments of the involved limb, the bypass graft will, perforce, be exposed on one wall or more. When a vein graft is thus exposed, the wall of the vein that touches the covering dressing will be deprived of moisture and oxygen, become necrotic, and perforate causing massive hemorrhage. Oxygenation to a vein graft is provided not from the red cells that flow through the lumen, but from oxygen dissolved in the interstitial fluid bathing the bypass vein. Consequently, some technique must be utilized to permit oxygen-containing fluid to bathe all portions of the walls of the vein[70] (Fig. 35–14A). This can be achieved by the placement of biological dressings, such as split-thickness porcine skin grafts, over the exposed arterial or vein graft wall.[71-75] This will succeed as long as one wall of the vein is lying on healthy muscle with oxygenated interstitial fluid that flows by capillary action between the exposed vein wall and the covering split-thickness porcine graft (Fig. 35–14B). The porcine graft can be changed every 48 hours at the bedside if the patient has no associated long bone fractures and does not require general anesthesia to facilitate the dressing change.

Over a period of 4-6 weeks, the exposed vein graft will gradually become covered with pink granulation tissue, after which the vein wall can no longer be seen (Fig. 35–14C). At this time, the vein graft and the covering granulation tissue will accept an autologous split-thickness skin graft. This technique has been associated with dramatic success and long-term patency confirmed by subsequent arteriography. In theory, other biologic dressings, such as placenta or commercially produced dressings, should achieve the same excellent results; however, the successful experience of the authors has been limited to split-thickness porcine skin grafts.

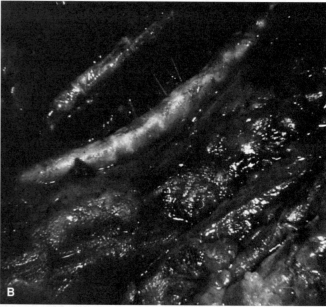

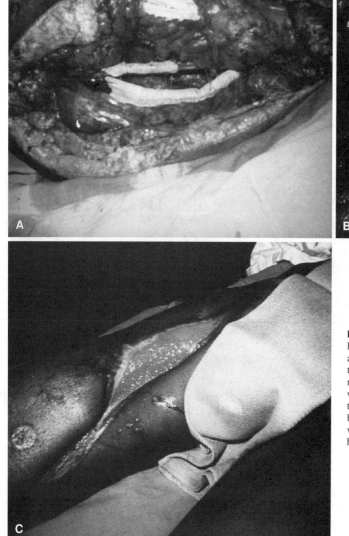

FIGURE 35–14 A. This patient sustained a massive shotgun wound to his right thigh with superficial femoral artery, vein, and nerve injury. The artery was replaced with a 15 cm segment of saphenous vein graft from the opposite thigh. The vein graft was placed before complete debridement. This left insufficient tissue to cover the vessel. Absorbable sutures were placed through the viable muscle groups to approximate the muscle to the vein graft. Pigskin covered the vein graft and exposed vessel as a biological dressing. **B.** This demonstrates a close-up of one wall of the vein graft firmly adherent to the underlying viable muscle. **C.** The wound has essentially healed 2 months after injury and is now ready for skin graft.

Combined Orthopaedic and Vascular Injuries

Vascular trauma occurs in only 0.2-1.7% of lower extremity fractures.[3,76-78] Successful arterial reconstruction can be difficult in the presence of an associated long bone fracture. This is especially true for midshaft femur fractures which tend to be unstable and have a potential for sudden angulation and disruption of any associated vascular repair. Prior use of mind-altering agents, such as alcohol, street narcotics, or other medicines, increases the potential for sudden inadvertent movement of the leg with disruption of vascular repair. Consequently, these patients are best treated by some sort of rigid fixation of the fracture to protect the vascular reconstruction. Patients with combined midshaft femur fractures and superficial femoral artery disruption are excellent candidates for this combined approach, especially if it is a closed fracture.

Open fracture, in which the skin has been punctured by the fractured femoral shaft, increases the potential for bone infection, therefore one must weigh the risks and benefits of a combined repair.[79] However, in conjunction with the orthopaedic surgical team, the authors have used this combined approach on a number of patients with penetrating wounds with good results (Fig. 35–15A, 35–15B, and 35–15C).

When this combined approach is used, temporary restitution of distal blood flow is accomplished by a Javid shunt while the orthopaedic surgical team fixes the fracture. This sequence ensures that the desired amount of tension will be present on the vein graft when it is anastomosed because no further manipulation of the bone will be needed.

Occasionally, the soft tissue injury around the associated fracture is too extensive for definitive internal fixation and stabilization. Although such patients may be treated with balanced skeletal traction, the potential for subsequent injury to the vascular repair is great and has lead to sudden catastrophes. Better protection to the vascular repair is afforded by the use of external skeletal fixators that will keep the bone fragments from inadvertently disrupting the vascular repair. Application of the external skeletal fixators must be precise so that the pins themselves do not cause injury or kinking of the vessels or associated interposition vein graft.

Compartment Syndrome

ETIOLOGY AND PATHOPHYSIOLOGY

Patients with extensive soft tissue disruption, associated venous injury, or prolonged shock or distal ischemia are candidates for developing a compartment syndrome, in which tissue pressure within a muscle compartment exceeds capillary perfusion pressure, leading to increasing ischemia of the enclosed tissues.[80]

Classical clinical findings are usually absent before vascular repair and appear after the extremity has been reperfused.

AXIOM One should watch for compartment syndrome after restoration of blood flow to an extremity especially if it has been ischemic for more than 4-6 hours.

The normal hydrostatic capillary pressure approximates 35 mm Hg or about 45 cm H_2O. Consequently, compartment decompression is indicated whenever the muscle compartment pressure exceeds 30 mm Hg (40 cm H_2O).

The likelihood for development of compartment syndrome is much greater in the leg than in the forearm, and compartment syndromes are rare in the thigh and upper arm. Consequently, the presence of poor blood flow to the thigh or arm after trauma should be assumed a result of injury to named arteries rather than adjacent soft tissue pressure.

DIAGNOSIS

The potential for development of compartment syndrome after vascular trauma should be kept in mind and the diagnosis relentlessly pursued, especially in high risk patients.[3] While history and physical examination are helpful, the common clinical findings of anesthesia and/or paralysis are not sensitive, and when present, may indicate irreversible neuromuscular damage.

If there is associated intracranial injury or drug ingestion, physical examination can be unreliable. In addition, if the patient needs prolonged anesthesia after vascular repair in an extremity to treat associated injuries, repetitive physical examination may be difficult or impossible; however, after recovery from anesthesia, the clinical findings may become obvious, necessitating a second anesthetic for fasciotomy. Feliciano et al[81] have underscored this fact by pointing out that 19% of the fasciotomies performed at Ben Taub Hospital were done at reoperation.

AXIOM Prophylactic fasciotomy should be considered in patients who are a high risk for developing compartment syndrome and will require prolonged general anesthesia.

Compartment syndrome may be confirmed by several techniques.[82] Arteriography may show a gradual narrowing of named arteries to the point where no further blood flow exists as a result of compression by the surrounding muscle; or the main vessel may be intact, but shows no flow in the muscular branches.

AXIOM The most reliable technique for early diagnosis of compartment syndrome is sequential direct measurements of compartment pressure.

The measurement of compartment pressure is invaluable when doubt exists about the diagnosis or when physical examination is unreliable or cannot be performed. Tissue pressures, as measured with a wick catheter or by needles placed in the involved muscle compartment, are considered positive for the presence of compartment syndrome if they exceed 30 mm Hg. The recent availability of a hand-held, inexpensive solid state transducer (Stryker Surgical, Kalamazoo Michigan) allows rapid, repeatable or continuous pressure monitoring.[3,83] Normal intracompartment pressures are usually less than 10 torr.

While the threshold level of compartmental hypertension necessitating fasciotomy is argued, the authors recommend fasciotomy whenever compartment pressure exceeds 30 torr. Radioactive isotopes of xenon or krypton may also be used to show slowed disappearance from the involved muscle compartment.

When exact compartment pressures are not available and other more sophisticated techniques for identifying compartment syndrome cannot be performed, the diagnosis can often be made on the basis of the history and clinical findings. Items in the history that suggest the need for fasciotomy include a prolonged delay between injury and arterial repair and an episode of significant preoperative hypotension.

Physical findings suggesting the presence of compartment syndrome include swelling, tightness, paresthesias, impaired motor function, altered calf contour, and pallor. Operative findings suggesting the need for fasciotomy include severe preoperative swelling of the calf, associated crush injury, combined arterial and venous injuries, and ligation of the major venous drainage in the popliteal or distal femoral area.[3]

Fasciotomy should be performed before arterial exploration when obvious compartment syndrome exists or when intracompartment pressures are significantly elevated (greater than 30-35 torr) before reperfusion.[3] In such instances, fasciotomies in the distal extremity can often be performed in 10-20 minutes and may be invaluable in preventing subsequent neurologic disability.

The technique of compartment decompression varies with the extent of the compartment syndrome.[84] Since access to the deep posterior compartment is best obtained at the junction of the middle and distal third of the leg, excision of the fibula to facilitate the decompression has been advocated.[85,86] With a fibulectomy-fasciotomy, the middle two-quarters of the fibula are excised. The head of the fibula is preserved proximally so that the lateral deep pe-

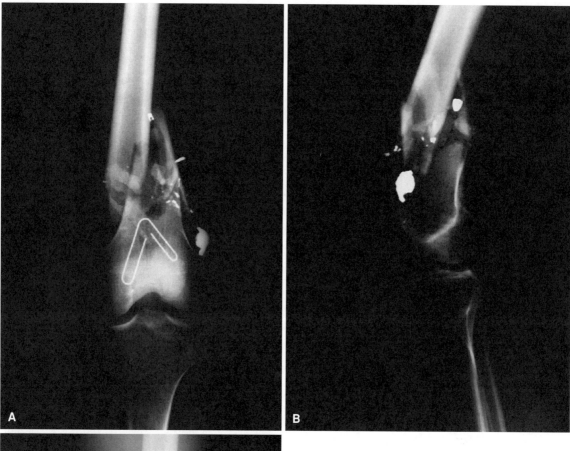

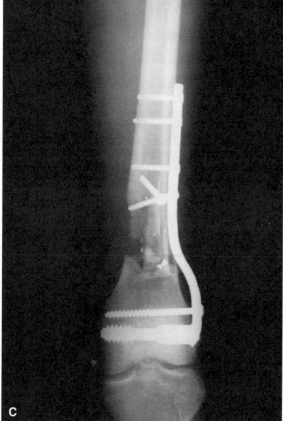

FIGURE 35–15   A. This 32-year-old patient presented with a close-range gunshot wound to his left posterior thigh just proximal to the knee. He had severe deformity of the leg and massive bleeding from the wound. The roentgenograms demonstrated the site of entrance at the area of the paper clip and a severely comminuted fracture of the distal femur. He had no distal pulses. Digital control of bleeding from the wound was done while the leg was prepped and draped in the operating room. The distal superficial femoral artery was exposed and a Javid shunt placed.   **B.** The orthopaedic service provided internal fixation of the femur fracture and the artery was repaired with a vein graft with a good result. The wounds healed without infection.   **C.** Postoperative stability was good, thus protecting the vascular repair.

roneal nerve will not be damaged, and the lower end is preserved to maintain the mortise of the ankle joint. This fibulectomy-fasciotomy may be of particular value in decompressing the deep compartments that contain the peroneal and posterior tibial arteries and veins.

Some surgeons prefer the two-incision, four-compartment fasciotomy popularized by Mubarak and Owen[87] because it can be performed quickly and safely. This includes a long anterolateral incision made about 2 cm anterior and parallel to the fibula and a posteromedial incision about 2 cm posterior to the tibia. The medial incision is kept posterior to the greater saphenous vein and extends through the skin, subcutaneous tissue, and fascia. Decompression of the deep posterior compartment may not be optimal with this method. Subcutaneous fasciotomy, whereby a small skin incision is made and the underlying fascia slit with a long knife, is not recommended. The skin incision should extend down to just above the tendons, and up to the lower portion of the head of the fibula.

The anterior compartment containing the dorsal extensors of the ankle and foot and the lateral compartment containing the peroneal muscles are effectively decompressed by one long incision between these two compartments extending anterior to the fibula. The superficial posterior compartment containing the gastrocnemius and soleus muscles, and the deep posterior compartment containing the flexors of the foot and ankle can be decompressed through a long medial incision about 2 cm posterior to the tibia and extending to the fascia covering the deep posterior compartment (Fig. 35–16). Confirmation of effective compartment decompression can be made by intraoperative measurement of tissue pressures, which will be less than 20 mm Hg for those muscles that have been adequately decompressed.

If the skin incision is small, patients with compartment syndrome may rapidly show signs of the skin acting as the entrapping organ after the underlying fascia has been incised. The underlying volume of fluid and pressure that has accumulated in the muscles and surrounding soft tissues may cause the muscle to bulge out significantly and may separate the incised skin more than 3 or 4 inches.

Vessel Damage in the Lower Leg

When arteriography is performed in patients with major fractures of the tibia, injuries to major collaterals or accessory vessels will often be found. It is not uncommon to find injuries to one of the tibial arteries and/or the peroneal artery, but if one of the remaining arteries is uninjured and communicates with the pedal arch, the leg and foot will usually have adequate circulation. Although some surgeons have explored and repaired the second vessel,[88] this is not mandatory[89] unless there is active bleeding. If the limb is viable, immediate repair of one of the injured vessels will add nothing and surgical exploration may convert an associated closed fracture into an open fracture with a greatly increased risk of osteomyelitis. The authors do not advocate repair of an injured infrapopliteal vessel if there is no bleeding and circulation to the foot is intact because the likelihood of later claudication is low, and if claudication does develop, it can be treated with less risk to the patient at that time.[88,90]

Persistent Vasoconstriction

When disruption of vascular collaterals below the knee and persistent arterial spasm coexist, ischemia of the foot may occur.[3] Some have suggested that lumbar sympathectomy in this setting may be helpful.[91] An alternative approach is to continuously infuse a mixture of 1000 mL of normal saline containing 1000 units of heparin and 500 mg tolazoline into the proximal artery at about 30 mL/hour.[92] This can be done by introducing the infusion catheter through a small side branch of the superficial femoral artery at the time of operation.[93] The infusion may have to be continued for up to 48 hours to obtain optimal results.

Pediatric Vascular Injuries

The incidence of pediatric vascular trauma is increasing as a result of more invasive diagnostic and therapeutic procedures and because children are more frequently the victims of domestic violence.[3,94] Iatrogenic injury is also common, accounting for 50-95% of cases in some series.[95,96] Attempts at diagnosis should initially be made noninvasively as arteriography has the potential of further injury, especially if the vessels are small.[97] Even if the extremity is viable, injured major arteries should be repaired.

POSTOPERATIVE CARE

AXIOM The immediate aims of postoperative management after repair of a vascular injury are to maintain intravascular volume and to rewarm the patient.

FIGURE 35–16 This cross-sectional view of the lower leg indicates the location of the vessels and nerves in the deep posterior and anterior compartments. The anterior and lateral compartments can be decompressed with one incision along the lateral aspect of the leg, incising the fascia between the anterior and lateral compartments. The superficial and deep posterior compartments can be decompressed by an incision along the medial aspect of the lower leg, including opening the fascia just posterior to the tibia.

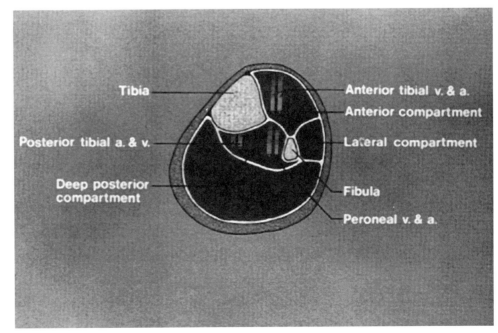

Prompt replacement of all blood and fluid losses will help maintain flow through the vascular repair and ensure adequate perfusion of the injured extremity.[31] Hypothermia, which frequently accompanies prolonged operative procedures, can cause peripheral vasoconstriction, making it difficult to assess the distal pulses.

> **AXIOM** Frequent reassessment of the distal circulation in an injured extremity is essential.

Frequently, peripheral pulses are not immediately palpable in either the injured or uninjured extremity. In such instances, the distal circulation can be evaluated by examining capillary refill or by comparing segmental Doppler pressures or transcutaneous PO_2 in the injured and uninjured limbs.[98]

If distal blood flow becomes impaired, reoperation may be required, even if the anastomosis is patent on arteriography. However, if the skin temperature is only slightly reduced and motor and nerve function are adequate, the limb may be carefully observed while attempting to improve blood flow by infusing additional fluids, blood, or low molecular weight dextran. If the limb is edematous, its circulation may be improved by elevating it. If the limb muscle becomes tense, a fasciotomy should be performed. If all of these efforts fail to provide adequate distal blood flow, repeat arteriograms should be performed. If any obstruction or significant narrowing is noted, reoperation is indicated.

> **AXIOM** If the survival of a limb begins to appear doubtful any time after vascular repair, immediate arteriography and reoperation should be performed with correction of any anastomotic problem and distal thrombectomy with Fogarty catheters.

Use of postoperative heparin may increase the tendency to local hematomas which can occasionally occlude smaller vessels. In addition, patients with multiple injuries may develop bleeding in other locations.

COMPLICATIONS

Thrombosis

Thrombosis of the site of repair is the most immediate and potentially dangerous complication after vascular injury.[3] Disappearance of a pulse suggests the development of thrombus at the site of arterial repair, whereas the rapid development of severe edema in the extremity may be associated with venous occlusion. In either instance, the patient should be returned immediately to the operating room to restore flow. If an arterial repair thromboses several days postoperatively and if it is obvious that there is sufficient collateral blood flow to maintain viability of the extremity, revascularization may be performed at a later time.[75]

Infection

Infection of the site of vascular repair is a dreaded complication that may require ligation of the involved vessels and an extra-anatomic bypass to maintain the viability of the distal tissues. Attempts at local repairs of a vessel that may be infected generally only lead to future disruptions and occasionally may result in exsanguinating hemorrhage. If ligation is required and the distal extremity is compromised, an extra-anatomic bypass should be attempted unless such a procedure would represent a high risk in that patient.[69,99]

When performing an extra-anatomic bypass, it is essential that the proximal and distal artery be dissected well away from the site of infection, which should be draped out of the surgical field. The graft,

preferably autologous vein, can be placed subcutaneously or brought through a viable muscular tunnel.

Delayed Complications

Delayed complications of repaired vascular injuries include stenosis, late thrombosis, and infections. Delayed complications of saphenous vein grafts include aneurysmal changes and intimal hyperplasia.[8] In addition, some injuries, such as pseudoaneurysms or arteriovenous fistulas, can be missed at the initial evaluation and become symptomatic later.[88,90,100]

> **AXIOM** The potential for late complications and symptomatic missed injuries underscores the need for prolonged follow-up of patients with vascular injuries.

The use of less invasive diagnostic methodologies, such as duplex scanning, flow and waveform analysis, radionuclide scanning, and digital venous angiography, have lessened patient discomfort and allow rapid and objective assessment of the morphology and dynamics of flow at the area of injury.[3]

OUTCOME

Mortality

The mortality rate after isolated peripheral vascular trauma is low, and some series report no mortalities.[14-17,64,99] Feliciano et al[65] reported a mortality rate of 2.7% in a series of 220 patients with vascular injuries of the lower extremities. Four of the six deaths occurred within 72 hours and were attributed to complications of hemorrhagic shock. Of the two late deaths, one was a result of sepsis and the other, pulmonary embolus.

Amputations

The amputation rate after peripheral vascular trauma continues to decrease.[3,14,16,17,65] Shah et al[14] and Lim and associates[16] reported no amputations in 61 patients with injury to the popliteal artery. Pasch et al[15] reported a single amputation (0.7%) in 139 patients with a variety of peripheral vascular injuries, and Menzoian and colleagues[17] had an amputation rate of 1.5% in 386 patients.

> **AXIOM** Poor outcome after peripheral vascular injury is usually a result of prolonged ischemia, shock, or severe damage to other structures.

Early postoperative amputation appears to be primarily related to prolonged ischemia. Late amputation is primarily done for disability or continued infection.[65,101] Virtually all vascular repairs can achieve temporary technical success as determined by immediate postoperative patency. Immediate technical success, however, does not necessarily imply that the limb will be salvaged or have satisfactory functional outcome.[3] Although most reported series have low early rates of amputation, there is little data on return of function, late amputations, or long-term complications. This paucity of data mainly results from the young and transient nature of much of the trauma population.[68]

CAROTID ARTERY INJURY

The indications for primary reconstruction of injuries to the carotid or innominate artery deserve special attention. The decision to perform primary reconstruction is influenced by several factors, including the neurological status of the patient, arteriographic findings, and the flow status. Patients presenting with normal neurologic function are best treated by primary vascular repair without the use of a shunt.

Patients with normal preoperative neurological function should not have a neurological deficit postoperatively.

When the patient presents in an awake state with normal hemodynamics, but has the appearance of a stroke, the decision to do primary vascular reconstruction versus primary ligation is controversial. Although experience is limited, the authors have identified that the incidence of postoperative stroke is high in these patients regardless of how the injured artery is treated. The authors prefer primary vascular reconstruction in this setting with the hopes and expectation that it may improve the patient's rehabilitation.

If the patient is stable hemodynamically, but has deep coma, the outcome has been uniformly fatal regardless of how the involved arterial injury is treated.[102-105] Such patients should not have vascular repair.

If the patient is in shock, the depressed sensorium precludes proper assessment for localized neurological deficits. Primary vascular reconstruction is recommended in such patients with the hope that this will prevent stroke in some patients and prevent death in others. About half of the patients in this subgroup will have normal neurological status after primary repair.

AXIOM Patients with severe shock and coma may have normal neurological function after carotid repair.

The likelihood for a good result after reconstruction of the carotid system is higher in patients with flow beyond the point of injury as judged by the preoperative arteriogram and in those patients who have good back-bleeding at the time of surgical exploration (Fig. 35–17A, 35–17B, and 35–17C). Every effort should be made to prevent and rapidly correct hypovolemia or hypotension in patients with carotid injuries.

AXIOM Although a number of factors may help predict the postoperative result in patients undergoing carotid artery reconstruction, definitive repair is advocated in all patients except those who have preoperative deep coma and a normal cardiovascular state.

The hesitancy to perform primary vascular reconstruction in patients with acute carotid artery injury and stroke largely reflects the clinical experience of many surgeons with patients who develop acute carotid occlusion from vascular occlusive disease.[106] Early carotid reconstruction in patients with a stroke resulting from occlusive disease may cause hemorrhagic infarction and death. However, after acute arterial injury, strokes have not been well-documented to progress to hemorrhagic infarction after early reconstruction.[107] Our studies suggest that patients who succumb after carotid reconstruction have diffuse cerebral edema.

VENOUS INJURIES

Venous injury is usually diagnosed during surgical exploration for a known arterial injury or by venography obtained in patients with signs and symptoms of a vascular injury but a normal arteriogram. Because reports from large urban trauma centers uniformly show a greater incidence of arterial injury than venous injury after penetrating wounds, and because the incidence of venous and arterial injury should be similar after penetrating wounds, one must conclude that many venous injuries go unrecognized and untreated.

AXIOM Venous injuries usually do not have to be repaired unless there is persistent bleeding, an A-V fistula, or compression of other structures by the hematoma.

Although some patients with untreated venous injuries may subsequently develop late sequelae of venous thrombosis, the paucity of such patients reflects the benignity of isolated venous thrombosis in most patients. This should be remembered when one observes the continuing controversy regarding the relative merits of primary venous repair versus venous ligation.

During the 1960s, most injured veins identified at the time of surgery for proven arterial injury were ligated because it was believed that primary repair would cause early thrombosis and subsequent pulmonary embolization. Many centers, including our own, challenged this wisdom since studies of organ function in canine models requiring multiple venous cutdowns over a period of several weeks showed that the previously repaired veins would be patent at the time of subsequent explorations.[108] Also, pulmonary embolization after primary venous repair in our patients was not seen. By the mid 1960s, all of our patients with easily repairable penetrating venous injuries underwent primary venorrhaphy.

The type of venous repair used varies with the extent of the injury. Most stab wounds of veins only need a simple primary closure. Patients with small caliber through-and-through gunshot wounds often can be treated by combining the entrance and exit sites into one larger opening which is then repaired in a transverse manner by simple venorrhaphy using a running suture of 5-0 polyethylene suture.

With moderately severe venous injuries, a primary repair should be attempted if the patient is stable, the overall operative time is relatively short, and the venous repair can be accomplished with reasonable likelihood for long-term patency.[108-111] When patients with moderately severe venous injury do not meet these criteria, primary venous ligation is recommended. Patients with extensive injury to a vein are best treated by venous ligation as the likelihood for a long interposition vein graft or a long suture line staying patent is not high. Furthermore, the increased time to perform such surgery adds insult to the involved limb, particularly if an ipsilateral saphenous vein is used.

AXIOM Whenever venous ligation is deemed necessary, care must be taken to minimize the sequelae of venous interruption and to prevent the development of postphlebitic limb syndrome.

When venous ligation is needed in patients with a concurrent arterial injury and significant ischemic time, compartment syndrome may develop. However, continuous postoperative elevation of the involved limb will circumvent the need for fasciotomy in 80% of patients with venous ligation. Fasciotomy in the remaining 20% of patients, however, may be limbsaving.

Whether or not fasciotomy is needed, the limb needs to be elevated until the postoperative edema has resolved completely.[112] Once this edema-free state has been achieved with elevation, the patient may be started on trials of ambulation to see if the increased hydrostatic pressure causes the edema to return. Recurrent edema with ambulation necessitates rest and elevation of the leg for another 3 days before another trial at ambulation. Once the patient can ambulate without edema, discharge is planned. If the patient has refractory edema in spite of elevation, support hose designed to maintain tissue pressure at 35 mm Hg is applied before discharge.

AXIOM After venous ligation, every effort should be made to keep the involved limb from becoming edematous.

A compulsive approach to postvenous ligation edema minimizes long-term problems with venous insufficiency and prevents postphlebitic limb syndrome. When this program has been followed, less than 10% of our patients had edema after venous ligation, and only 2% had severe edema. Furthermore, none of our patients developed skin ulcerations from venous insufficiency and none developed venous

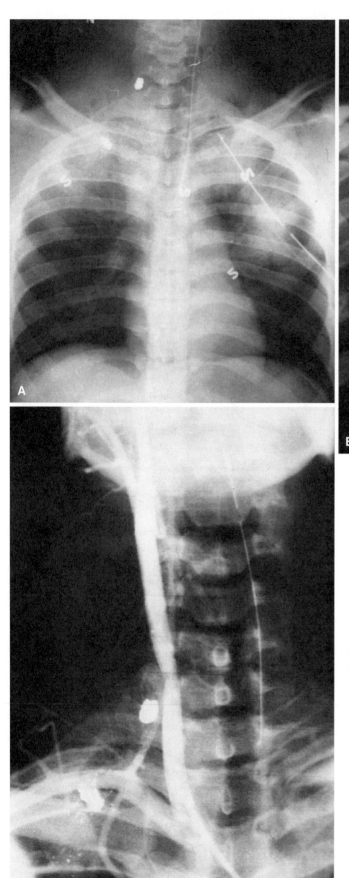

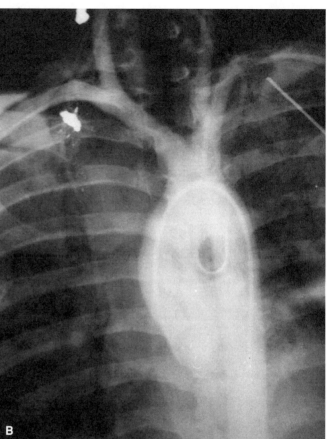

FIGURE 35–17 A. This 18-year-old patient presented with multiple gunshot wounds (represented by numbers on the roentgenogram). There was a left lung contusion and a left hemopneumothorax, and a chest tube was placed. He had a left hemiparesis. A single bullet was located in the right neck and the trachea was deviated to the left. **B.** An aortic arch study was done to determine the presence and site of any vascular injury. The aorta and proximal arch vessels were normal. **C.** A closer view of the right carotid demonstrates a narrowed area in the lower third adjacent to the bullet fragment. At operation, he had a through-and-through wound of the carotid artery with the bullet in the carotid sheath. This was repaired with an end-to-end anastomosis in spite of his neurological deficit as he had excellent flow distal to the site of injury. He recovered from hemiparesis.

gangrene requiring amputation. In addition, when the venous ligation was performed in conjunction with primary arterial repair, all arterial repairs remained patent. Thus, at least in our experience, venous ligation does not compromise an associated arterial repair.

ILLICIT NARCOTIC AND SEPTIC VASCULAR EMERGENCIES

Arterial Mycotic Aneurysms

The widespread use of illicit narcotics that are "mainlined" into veins has created a whole new group of vascular emergencies.[113,114] The incidence of arterial mycotic aneurysms rose spectacularly during the two decades when the use of heroin mixed with various diluents became a trendy form of social entertainment.[115] Although most mainliners are hard-core addicts, many are weekend users gainfully employed on weekdays.

Arterial mycotic aneurysm is really a misnomer for an infected pseudoaneurysm resulting from both needle trauma to the artery and bacterial contamination of the periarterial hematoma by the diluent used to "cut" the heroin. More recently, the identification of intravenous heroin use with a high risk of transmitting the human immunodeficiency virus (HIV) has lead to reduced mainlining as many narcotic users have switched to crack cocaine which can be inhaled. Before this change of preference, we excised mycotic aneurysms frequently.

Patients presenting with an infected pseudoaneurysm often give a history of having "hit the pink," indicating direct arterial puncture instead of the desired venous puncture. The most frequent early symptom is painful swelling at the site of injection. Physical examination usually reveals a tender pulsatile mass. Fever, leukocytosis, and anemia often coexist and a bruit is heard in about half of the patients. Severe distal ischemia or gangrene is unlikely.

Based on this history and the physical findings, a correct diagnosis of infected pseudoaneurysm can be made clinically about 80% of the time. The most common missed diagnoses include associated abscesses or cellulitis. Once the diagnosis is suspected, preoperative arteriography provides a road map to the exact site of arterial rupture and the location of important collateral vessels, particularly when the infected pseudoaneurysm is close to the bifurcation of the common femoral artery (Fig. 35–18).

Recommended therapy includes aneurysmectomy with proximal and distal ligation immediately adjacent to the resected aneurysm.[116] Although the area of surrounding cellulitis and pulsation often is extensive, one can usually excise these aneurysms without going into a more proximal body compartment. Indeed, most groin aneurysms can be excised without extending the incision above to the inguinal ligament to obtain proximal control of the external iliac artery.

One should excise only the aneurysm and not the surrounding cellulitis since the surrounding cellulitis contains collateral vessels that keep the distal limb alive. Severe ischemia or gangrene after aneurysmectomy is uncommon unless the aneurysm involves the femoral artery at its bifurcation, necessitating excision of a portion of the common femoral, superficial femoral, and profunda femoral arteries. When these three vessels are ligated, approximately half of these patients with ischemic symptoms or signs will progress to gangrene if some type of emergency reconstruction is not performed.[116]

Because these patients uniformly have severe cellulitis throughout the anterior femoral triangle, successful reconstruction is best accomplished by means of an extra-anatomic bypass graft extending from the external iliac artery through the obturator foramen to the popliteal artery.[117,118] These addicts generally have no usable veins, and a prosthetic interposition graft is needed. If the associated cellulitis circumferentially involves the entire thigh and its muscle compartments, vascular reconstruction is contraindicated.

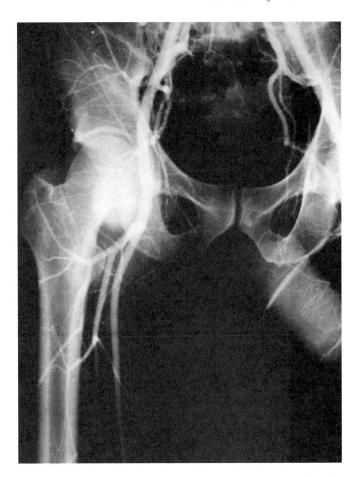

FIGURE 35–18 This patient presented with a pulsatile mass in the right groin after injection of illicit drugs. An arteriogram showed the vessel intact with extravasation of dye at the site of the bifurcation of the common femoral artery. At operation, there was an infected false aneurysm of the right common femoral artery that required ligation. Limb salvage was achieved without vascular reconstruction.

Infected Venous Aneurysms

Although the venous system is the site for injection of "cut" heroin or "mixed jive," the incidence of infected venous aneurysms is quite low compared to arterial mycotic aneurysms.[119] Multiple venipunctures with infected needles and injectate certainly contaminate the perivenous tissue, but the greater likelihood of perivascular hematoma after an arterial hit plus higher arterial pressure makes arterial pseudoaneurysms far more frequent.

Occasionally, a mycotic venous aneurysm is recognized at the time that a mycotic arterial aneurysm is being excised. When this occurs, any associated venous communication with the infected arterial pseudoaneurysm necessitates venous ligation immediately above and below the site of communication. Other patients present with venous pseudoaneurysms without an arterial component. The diagnosis in these patients often is difficult since septic phlebitis is a common complication of mainlining and can easily be confused with infected venous aneurysm.[119] The most common initial diagnosis is septic phlebitis, cellulitis, or a combination of both.

Antibiotics designed to cover methicillin-resistant Staphylococcus aureus and gram-negative coliform bacilli should be instituted as soon as the diagnosis is made. When septic venous phlebitis and surrounding cellulitis coexist without venous aneurysm, appropriate antibiotic therapy and elevation of the limb will usually lead to gradual resolution of the infectious process.

Often the area of apparent cellulitis harbors an abscess that needs to be drained. If bloody pus is present when the abscess is incised, the surgeon should be aware that there is probably an underlying venous communication. Careful, gentle exploration of the abscess cavity will usually identify the venous communications that should be ligated and the aneurysm excised. Once the involved venous aneurysm has been excised, the wound should be packed open and allowed to heal by second intent. Any residual clot at the site of venous transections should be extracted because it will usually contain bacteria.

Other problems of infected venous pseudoaneurysms include postphlebitic limb syndrome and pulmonary infections, probably resulting from the dislodgement or migration of tiny fragments of infected clots as septic emboli. Heparin therapy is not recommended after resection of infected venous pseudoaneurysms because of the bleeding complications that may occur and because of the potential for bacterial embolization to other organs.

Postligation venous insufficiency results from both excision of the infected venous pseudoaneurysm and associated soft tissue infections that develop around the multiple injection sites in the soft tissue of the distal thigh and leg. This "skin popping" causes venous and lymphatic infection with scarring, fibrosis, and vascular insufficiency. This can cause severe leg edema, even when the deep venous system is patent.

Bacteriology of Mycotic Aneurysms

Mycotic aneurysms in hard-core addicts tend to have organisms that are resistant to many antibiotics. Most of these patients with positive wound and blood cultures are infected with Staphylococcus aureus organisms of which about 90% are penicillin-resistant and 70% are methicillin-resistant.[116] Approximately 25% of the cultures will grow Pseudomonas aeruginosa. The probability of a mixed infection with multiple bacteria is great.

AXIOM Initial antibiotic therapy for mycotic aneurysms should cover gram-negative aerobes, such as pseudomonas, and methicillin-resistant Staphylococcus aureus.

Initial antibiotic therapy, which is begun before the results of culture and sensitivity data are available, should include an aminoglycoside, such as gentamicin, for gram-negative aerobes, and vancomycin to cover the methicillin-resistant Staphylococcus aureus. Intravenous antibiotics should continue until the area of surrounding cellulitis has resolved. Antibiotic coverage for more than 10-14 days is not indicated unless the patient has a secondary problem, such as bacterial endocarditis or cellulitis, that does not respond to excision of the infected pseudoaneurysm.

After excision of the infected pseudoaneurysm, the wound is packed open and allowed to heal by second intent. Muscle flap coverage or later split-thickness skin graft coverage of these open wounds is meddlesome and does not shorten the time for healing. Once the wound has a good bed of granulation tissue, no antibiotic coverage is needed. The patient is taught self wound care and then discharged for weekly follow-up visits.

Intra-arterial Injection Injuries

Drug addicts occasionally will inadvertently inject narcotics or amphetamines intra-arterially. Intra-arterial methamphetamine, alone or in combination with heroin, can cause severe necrotizing angiitis.[119] This usually occurs in the upper extremity; the radial artery at the wrist is the most common site. However, arteritis leading to progressive arterial occlusion of the lower extremities has been reported in young Moroccans who were heavy smokers of cannabis extracts.[120] The classic clinical syndrome of an intra-arterial injection at the wrist includes sudden, constant, burning pain in the hand, particularly in the thumb, index finger, and long finger. Blanching of the involved fingers is also often seen.

The pathophysiology leading to this complex appears to be a combination of arterial spasm and small vessel occlusion by injected particulate matter. Frequently, the syndrome is not adequately appreciated until the patient returns for a second or third emergency department visit. The end result of such an injection often is ischemic dry gangrene of the thumb and one or more adjacent fingers.[22] Some patients may develop a secondary infection with severe cellulitis and myositis that may, in some patients, progress to wet gangrene of the entire hand or forearm necessitating amputation at either the wrist or elbow.

Early treatment for this syndrome includes elevation of the limb and antibiotics for methicillin-resistant Staphylococcus and gram-negative coliform bacilli. Treatment with intra-arterial injection of vasodilators, sympathetic blocking agents, or anticoagulants have not been helpful in palliating this syndrome in our patients; however, in patients who present with marginal ischemia and severe constant pain, a stellate ganglion block or a dorsal sympathectomy will usually improve the ischemic insult and decrease the pain. This approach, however, seldom completely alleviates the pain that usually persists for many weeks. Occasionally, late amputation of a viable distal phalanx is the only way to control refractory pain so that patient can be restored to normal function.

SUMMARY

Success in the management of vascular injuries depends on early, accurate diagnosis, followed by immediate repair with restoration of blood flow (Table 35-4). Preoperative arteriography is important if the patient is stable and the clinical picture is equivocal. Ischemia distal to a vascular injury is virtually never a result of spasm, and attempts to correct spasm nonsurgically generally cause delays that can jeopardize the patient's life and limb.

Continued ischemia after vascular repair often results from unsatisfactory anastomosis or distal thrombosis, and early reoperation is usually indicated. Increased use of arteriography, Doppler ultrasonography, autogenous vein grafts, Fogarty catheters to remove distal thrombi, and early complete fasciotomy if tissue ischemia has been prolonged has greatly improved the prognosis for most arterial injuries.

TABLE 35-4 Factors Associated with Improved Limb Salvage after Vascular Trauma

Rapid prehospital transport
Penetrating injury
Minimal soft tissue injury
Prompt diagnosis and treatment
Early reperfusion using intraluminal shunts
Early stabilization of fractures
Venous repairs
Aggressive wound debridement
Prompt tissue coverage of arterial repairs
Liberal early fasciotomy
Complete arteriography
Aggressive reoperation for technical failures

⊘ **FREQUENT ERRORS**

IN THE MANAGEMENT OF PERIPHERAL VASCULAR INJURIES

1. *Failing to look for vascular injuries in patients with fractures and dislocations.*
2. *Assuming that inadequate circulation after trauma or vascular catheterization is a result of spasm rather than mechanical occlusion of the vessel.*
3. *Delaying definitive repair to obtain arteriography when the need for vascular exploration is obvious.*

4. *Failing to prepare and drape the entire involved extremity and to make provisions for obtaining an autologous vein for grafting from an uninvolved leg if needed.*

5. *Failing to obtain adequate proximal and distal control before exposing the site of a major vascular injury.*

6. *Failing to explore an artery with persistent severe spasm.*

7. *Failing to perform an adequate thrombectomy after vascular repair because there is "good back-bleeding."*

8. *Failing to adequately heparinize the proximal and distal portions of an injured vessel while it is occluded during vascular repair.*

9. *Delay in performing an adequate fasciotomy in patients with compartment syndrome.*

10. *Failing to look for and excise an associated infected pseudoaneurysm if drainage of an abscess near major vessels uncovers significant bleeding.*

▼▼▼▼▼▼▼▼▼▼▼▼▼▼▼▼▼▼▼▼▼▼▼▼▼▼▼▼▼▼

SUMMARY POINTS

1. Maximal limb function is maintained after vascular injury by minimizing the ischemic insult and protecting neural function.

2. Vascular complications may occur after percutaneous angiography, especially in older or smaller patients.

3. High-velocity missiles can severely damage tissues up to several centimeters beyond the missile tracts.

4. A limb that has been ischemic for 6 hours or longer is at risk for sustaining histologic changes that may not be reversible with reperfusion.

5. Narrowing of the arterial lumen at an injury site is seldom a result of spasm. Failure to correct or closely observe such areas can result in late occlusion with rapid ischemic necrosis of distal tissue.

6. Nerve blocks to correct spasm after trauma to a vessel should generally be condemned because the time lost with such procedures may allow the distal ischemia to become irreversible.

7. Blind placement of clamps in the depths of an actively bleeding wound should be condemned.

8. Failure to promptly reduce a dislocation to restore the circulation to an extremity may result in extensive tissue necrosis and need for a later amputation.

9. Whenever possible, x-rays should be taken before attempting to reduce a dislocation.

10. Peripheral pulses may be present in up to 25% of the patients with extremity arterial injuries; a history suggesting vascular injury may be the most important diagnostic indicator at the time of the initial evaluation.

11. Patients with penetrating arterial injury may have a palpable distal pulse although it is often weaker than in the contralateral limb.

12. Careful auscultation over the area of trauma is an important part of the physical examination.

13. Hemodynamically unstable patients with suspected vascular injury or threatened limbs should be taken directly to the operating room.

14. The significance of any abnormal findings on arteriography is determined by the surgeon who coordinates the clinical and roentgenographic findings.

15. Venography is seldom helpful and may be hazardous if it delays treatment of more severe injuries.

16. Nonoperative management of selected cases of clinically occult focal narrowing or intimal irregularities is safe, practical, and cost-effective.

17. Selected patients with mangled extremities will benefit from primary amputation, particularly if the nerves have been completely severed.

18. Life takes precedence over limb throughout resuscitation and treatment.

19. The position and draping for emergency vascular surgery should allow rapid securing of proximal and distal control of the injured vessels and for obtaining an autologous vein graft if needed.

20. Refractory external bleeding from leg or forearm injuries can often be controlled by a sphygmomanometer inflated well above systolic pressure on the proximal thigh or arm.

21. In approaching injured vessels, the surgeon should try to stay within anatomic planes, and thereby avoid injury to important adjacent structures.

22. Failure to obtain proximal and distal control before exposing the site of injury of a large vessel may convert a careful anatomic dissection into a frantic attempt to stop massive hemorrhage.

23. Good back-bleeding from the distal artery does not ensure the absence of intravascular thrombus beyond the first patent collateral vessel.

24. Resection of the site of injury with end-to-end anastomosis is indicated in several circumstances including gunshot wounds, lacerations caused by bone fragments, and arterial wall contusions with an associated intimal tear.

25. Properly placed digital pressure on small bleeding points at a completed vascular anastomosis, with a little patience, will usually obviate the need for repair sutures.

26. Repair of major veins helps circumvent the problems of venous hypertension.

27. One should watch for compartment syndrome after restoration of blood flow to an extremity, especially if the limb has been ischemic for more than 4-6 hours.

28. Prophylactic fasciotomy should be considered in patients who are a high risk for developing compartment syndrome and will require prolonged general anesthesia.

29. The most reliable technique for early diagnosis of compartment syndrome is sequential direct measurements of compartment pressures.

30. The immediate aims of postoperative management after repair of a vascular injury are to maintain intravascular volume and to rewarm the patient.

31. Frequent reassessment of the distal circulation in an injured extremity is essential.

32. If the survival of a limb begins to appear doubtful any time after a vascular repair, immediate arteriography and/or reoperation should be performed to correct any anastomotic problem and perform distal thrombectomy with Fogarty catheters.

33. The potential for late complications and symptomatic missed injuries underscores the need for prolonged follow-up of patients with vascular injuries.

34. Poor outcome after peripheral vascular injury is usually a result of prolonged ischemia, shock, or severe damage to other structures.

35. Patients with severe shock and coma after a carotid injury may have normal neurological function after carotid repair.

36. Although a number of factors may help predict the postoperative result in patients undergoing carotid artery reconstruction, definitive repair is advocated in all patients except those who have preoperative deep coma and a normal cordiovascular state.

37. Venous injuries usually do not have to be repaired unless there is persistent bleeding, an A-V fistula, or compression of other structures by the hematoma.

38. Whenever venous ligation is deemed necessary, care must be taken to minimize the sequelae of venous interruption and to prevent the development of postphlebitic limb syndrome.

39. After venous ligation, every effort should be made to keep the involved limb from becoming edematous.

40. Initial antibiotic therapy for mycotic aneurysms should cover gram-negative aerobes, such as Pseudomonas, and methicillin-resistant Staphylococcus aureus.

▲▲▲▲▲▲▲▲▲▲▲▲▲▲▲▲▲▲▲▲▲▲▲▲▲▲▲▲▲▲

REFERENCES

1. Yao J, Plant J, Wilson RF. Peripheral vascular injuries. In: Walt AJ, Wilson RF, eds. Management of trauma: pitfalls and practice. Philadelphia, Lea and Febiger, 1975; 403.
2. Murphy JB. Resection of arteries and veins injured in continuity: end-to-end suture. Exp Clin Res Med Rec 1987;51:73.
3. Shackford SR, Rich NH. Peripheral vascular injury. In: Moore EE, Mattox KE, Feliciano DV, eds. Trauma. 2nd ed. Norwalk, CT. Appleton Lange 1991; 639.
4. Soubbotitch V. Military experiences of traumatic aneurysms. Lancet 1913;2:720.
5. Rich NM, Clagett CP, Salander JM, et al. The Matas/Soubbotitch connection. Surgery 1983;93:17.
6. Makins GH. Gunshot injuries to the blood vessels. Bristol, England: John Wright and Sons, 1919.
7. DeBakey ME, Simeone FA. Battle injuries of arteries in World War II: an analysis of 2,471 cases. Ann Surg 1946;123:534.
8. Hughes CW, Jahnke EJ Jr. The surgery of traumatic arterovenous fistulas and aneurysms: a five-year follow-up study of 215 lesions. Ann Surg 1958;148:790.
9. Hughes CW. Arterial repair during the Korean War. Ann Surg 1958; 147:555.
10. Rich NM, Hughes CW. Vietnam vascular registry: a preliminary report. Surgery 1969;62:218.
11. Rich NM, Manion WC, Hughes CW. Surgical and pathological evaluation of vascular injuries in Vietnam. J Trauma 1969;9:279.
12. Rich NM. Vascular trauma in Vietnam. J Cardiovasc Surg 1970;11:368.
13. Rich NM, Baugh JH, Hughes CE. Acute arterial injuries in Vietnam: 1,000 cases. J Trauma 1970;10:359.
14. Shackford SR, Hollingsworth-Fridlund P, Cooper GF, et al. The effect of regionalization upon the quality of trauma care assessed by concurrent audit before and after institution of a trauma system: a preliminary report. J Trauma 1986;26:812.
15. Shah DM, Naraynsingh V, Leather RP, et al. Advances in the management of acute popliteal vascular blunt injuries. J Trauma 1985; 25:793.
16. Pasch AR, Bishara RA, Lim LT, et al. Optimal limb salvage in penetrating civilian vascular trauma. J Vasc Surg 1986;3:189.
17. Lim LT, Michuda MS, Flanigan DP, et al. Popliteal artery trauma. Arch Surg 1980;115:1307.
18. Menzoian JO, Doyle JE, Cantelmo NL, et al. A comprehensive approach to extremity vascular trauma. Arch Surg 1985;120:801.
19. Feliciano DV, Bitondo CG, Mattox KL, et al. Civilian trauma in the 1980s: a 1-year experience with 456 vascular and cardiac injuries. Ann Surg 1984;199:717.
20. Mattox KL, Feliciano DV, Burch J, et al. Five thousand seven hundred sixty cardiovascular injuries in 4459 patients. Ann Surg 1989; 209:698.
21. Youkey JR, Clagett GP, Rich NM, et al. Vascular trauma secondary to diagnostic and therapeutic procedures: 1974 through 1982. Am J Surg 1983;146:788.
22. Rich NM, Hobson RW II, Fedde CW. Vascular trauma secondary to diagnostic and therapeutic procedures. Am J Surg 1974;128:715.
23. O'Gorman RB, Feliciano DV, Bitondo CG, et al. Emergency center arteriography in the evaluation of suspected peripheral vascular injuries. Arch Surg 1984;119:568.
24. Kloster FE, Bristow JD, Griswold HE. Femoral artery occlusion following percutaneous catheterization. Amer Hosp J 1970;79:175.
25. Amato JJ, et al. High velocity arterial injury: a study of mechanism of injury. J Trauma 1971;11:412.
26. Siesjo BK. Cerebral circulation and metabolism. J Neurosurg 1984; 60:883.
27. Malan E, Tattoni G. Physio- and anatomopathology of acute ischemia of the extremities. J Cardiovasc Surg 1963;4:214.
28. Sanderson RA, Foley RK, McIvor GW, et al. Histological response of skeletal muscle to ischemia. Clin Orthop Rel Res 1975;113:27.
29. Elkin DC, Warren JV. Arteriovenous fistulas, their effect on the circulation. JAMA 1947;134:1524.
30. Holman E. The anatomic and physiologic effects of arteriovenous fistula. Surgery 1940;8:362.
31. Perry MO, Thal ER, Shires GT. Management of arterial injuries. Ann Surg 1971;173:403.
32. Drapanas T, Hewitt RL, Weichert RF III, et al. Civilian vascular injuries: a critical appraisal of three decades of management. Ann Surg 1970;172:351.
33. Morris GC Jr, Beall AC Jr, Roof WR, et al. Surgical experience with 220 acute arterial injuries in civilian practice. Am J Surg 1960;99:775.
34. Bliss B, Bradley JWP, Fairgrieve J, et al. Vascular injuries. J Bone Joint Surg 1989;71:738.
35. Snyder WH, Thal ER, Bridges RA, et al. The validity of normal arteriography in penetrating trauma. Arch Surg 1978;113:424.
36. O'Gorman RB, Feliciano DV. Arteriography performed in the emergency center. Am J Surg 1986;152:323.
37. McDonald E, Goodman P, Winestock D. The clinical indications for arteriography in trauma to the extremity: a review of 114 cases. Radiology 1975;116:45.
38. Mufti MA, et al. Diagnostic value of hematoma in penetrating arterial wounds of the extremities. Arch Surg 1970;101:562.
39. Dillard BM, Nelson DL, Norman HG Jr. Review of 85 major traumatic arterial injuries. Surgery 1968;63:391.
40. Lain KC, Williams GR. Arteriography in acute peripheral arterial injuries: an experimental study. Surg Forum 1970;21:179.
41. Howard CA, Thal ER, Redman HC, et al. Intra-arterial digital subtraction angiography in the evaluation of peripheral vascular trauma. Ann Surg 1989;210:108.
42. Rose SC, Moore EE. Trauma angiography: the use of clinical findings to improve patient selection and case preparation. J Trauma 1988;28:240.
43. Frykberg ER, Vines FS, Alexander RH. The natural history of clinically occult arterial injuries: a prospective evaluation. J Trauma 1989;29:577.
44. Gomez GA, Kreis DJ, Ratner L, et al. Suspected vascular trauma of the extremities: the role of arteriography in proximity injuries. J Trauma 1986;26:1005.
45. Reid JD, Weigelt JA, Thal ER, et al. Assessment of proximity of a wound to major vascular structures as an indication for arteriography. Arch Surg 1988;123:942.
46. Goodman PC, Jeffrey RB Jr, Brant-Zawadzki M. Digital subtraction angiography in extremity trauma. Radiology 1984;153:61.
47. Fabian TC, Reiter CB, Gold RE, et al. Digital venous angiography: a prospective evaluation in peripheral arterial trauma. Ann Surg 1984; 199:710.
48. Rudavsky AZ, Moss CM. Radionuclide evaluation of peripheral vascular injuries. Semin Nucl Med 1983;13:142.
49. Gerlock AJ Jr, Thal ER, Synder WH. Venography in penetrating injuries of the extremities. Am J Roentgenol 1976;126:1023.
50. Gryska PF. Major vascular injuries: principles of management in selected cases of arterial and venous injury. New Engl J Med 1962;266:381.
51. Frykberg ER, Crump JM, Vines FS, et al. A reassessment of the role of arteriography in penetrating proximity trauma: a prospective study. J Trauma 1989;29:1041.
52. Hiatt JR, Martin NA, Machleder HI. The natural history of a traumatic vertebral artery aneurysm: case report. J Trauma 1989;29:1592.
53. McCorkell SJ, Harley JD, Morishima MS, et al. Indications for angiography in extremity trauma. Am J Roentgenol 1985;145:1245.
54. Gregory RT, Gould RJ, Peclet M, et al. The mangled extremity syndrome (MES): a severity grading system for multisystem injury of the extremity. J Trauma 1985;25:1147.
55. Bondurant FJ, Cottler HB, Buckle R, et al. The medical and economic impact of severely injured lower extremities. J Trauma 1988;28:1270.
56. Johansen K, Daines M. Howie T, et al. Objective criteria accurately predict amputation following lower extremity trauma. J Trauma 1990; 30:568.
57. Eger M, Golcman L, Goldstein A, et al. The use of a temporary shunt in the management of arterial vascular injuries. Surg Gynecol Obstet 1971; 132:67-70.
58. Nunley JA, Koman LA, Urbaniak JR. Arterial shunting as an adjunct to major limb revascularization. Ann Surg 1981;193:271.
59. Johansen K, Bradyk D, Thiele B, et al. Temporary intraluminal shunts: resolution of a management dilemma in complex vascular injuries. J Trauma 1982;22:395.
60. Nichols JG, Svoboda JA, Parks SN. Use of temporary intraluminal shunts in selected peripheral arterial injuries. J Trauma 1986;26:1094.
61. Denis R, Benishek DJ, Ledgerwood, et al. Spatulated versus end-to-end anastomosis for small vessel injury. J Trauma 1986;26:556.
62. Brener BJ, Raines JK, Darling RC. The end-to-end anastomosis of blood vessels of diverse diameters. Surg Gynecol Obstet 1974;138:249.
63. Eisenhardt HJ, Hennecken H, Klein PJ, et al. Experience with different techniques of microvascular anastomosis. J Microsurgery 1980;1:341.
64. Keeley SB, Synder WH, Weigelt JA. Arterial injuries below the knee: 51 patients with 82 injuries. J Trauma 1983;23:285.
65. Feliciano DV, Herskowitz K, O'Horman RB, et al. Management of vascular injuries in the lower extremities. J Trauma 1988;28:319.

66. Feliciano DV, Mattox KL, Graham JM, et al. Five-year experience with PTFE grafts in vascular wounds. J Trauma 1985;25:75.

67. Timberlake GA, O'Connell RC, Kerstein MD. Venous injury: to repair or ligate. J Vasc Surg 1986;4:553.

68. Hobson RW, Howard EW, Wright CB, et al. Hemodynamics of canine femoral venous ligation: significance in combined arterial and venous injuries. Surgery 1973;74:824.

69. Feliciano DV, Accola KD, Burch JM, et al. Extra-anatomic bypass for peripheral arterial injuries. Am J Surg 1989;158:506.

70. Artz CP, Rittenbury MS, Yarbrough DR III. An appraisal of allografts and xenografts as biological dressings for wounds and burns. Ann Surg 1972;175:934.

71. Bromberg BE, Song IC, Mohn MP. The use of pigskin as a temporary biological dressing. Plast Reconstr Surg 1985;36:80.

72. Carrasquilla C, Watts J, Ledgerwood, et al. Management of massive thoraco-abdominal wall defect from close range shotgun blast. J Trauma 1971;11:715.

73. Ledgerwood AM, Lucas CE. Biological dressings for exposed vascular grafts: a reasonable alternative. J Trauma 1975;15:567.

74. Ledgerwood AM, Lucas CE. Massive thigh injuries with vascular disruption: role of porcine skin grafting of exposed arterial vein grafts. Arch Surg 1973;107:201.

75. Ledgerwood, Lucas CE. Split-thickness porcine graft in the treatment of close range shotgun wounds to extremities with vascular injury. Am J Surg 1973;135:690.

76. Drost TF, Rosemurgy AS, Proctor D, et al. Outcome of treatment of combined orthopedic and arterial trauma to the lower extremity. J Trauma 1989;29:1331.

77. Howe HR, Poole GV, Hansen KJ, et al. Salvage of lower extremities following combined orthopedic and vascular trauma: a predictive salvage index. Am Surg 1987;53:205.

78. Ashworth EM, Dalsing MC, Glover, et al. Lower extremity vascular trauma: a comprehensive, aggressive approach. J Trauma 1988;28:329.

79. Rich NM, Metz CW, Hutton JE. Internal versus external fixation of fractures with concomitant vascular injuries in Vietnam. J Trauma 1971;11:463.

80. McCord JM. Oxygen derived free radicals: a link between reperfusion injury and inflammation. Adv Free Biol Med 1986;2:235.

81. Feliciano DV, Cruse PA, Spjut-Patrinely V, et al. Fasciotomy after trauma to the extremities. Am J Surg 1988;156:533.

82. Mubarak SJ, Owen CA, Hargens AR, et al. Acute compartment syndromes: diagnosis and treatment with the aid of the wick catheter. J Bone Joint Surg 1978;60A:1091.

83. Matsen FA III, Winquist RA, Kruguire RB. Diagnosis and management of compartment syndrome. J Bone Joint Surg 1980;62:286.

84. Patman RD, Thompson JE. Fasciotomy in peripheral vascular surgery: report of 164 patients. Arch Surg 1970;101:663.

85. Ernst CB, Kaufer H. Fibulectomy-fasciotomy: an important adjunct in the management of lower extremity arterial trauma. J Trauma 1971;11:365.

86. Patman RD, Thompson JE. Fasciotomy in peripheral vascular surgery: report of 164 patients. Arch Surg 1970;101:663.

87. Mubarak SJ, Owen CA. Double-incision fasciotomy of the leg for decompression in compartment syndromes. J Bone Joint Surg 1977;59A:184.

88. Kelly G, Eiseman B. Management of small arterial injuries: clinical and experimental studies. J Trauma 1976;16:681.

89. Hollerman JH, Killebrew LH. Tibial artery injuries. Am J Surg 1982;144:362.

90. Rich NM, Hobson RW II, Collins GJ Jr. Elective vascular reconstruction after trauma. Am J Surg 1975;130:712.

91. Williams GD, Crumpler JB, Campbell GS. Effect of sympathectomy on the severely traumatized artery. Arch Surg 1970;101:704.

92. Dickerman RM, Gewertz BL, Foley DW, et al. Selective intra-arterial tolazoline infusion in peripheral arterial trauma. Surgery 1977;81:605.

93. Peck JJ, Fitzgibbons TJ, Gaspar MR. Devastating distal arterial trauma and continuous intra-arterial infusion of tolazoline. Am J Surgery 1983;145:562.

94. Shaker IJ, White JJ, Singer RD, et al. Special problems of vascular injuries in children. J Trauma 1976;16:863.

95. Whitehouse WM, Coran AG, Stanley JC, et al. Pediatric vascular trauma. Arch Surg 1976;111:1269.

96. LeBlance J, Wood AE, O'Shea MA, et al. Peripheral arterial trauma in children. J Cardiovasc Surg 1985;26:325.

97. Flanigan DP, Keifer TJ, Schuler JJ, et al. Experience with iatrogenic pediatric vascular injuries. Ann Surg 1983;198:430.

98. Kram HB, Wright J, Shoemaker WC, et al. Perioperative transcutaneous O2 monitoring in the management of major peripheral arterial trauma. J Trauma 1984;24:443.

99. Meyer JP, Lim LT, Castronuovo JJ, et al. Peripheral vascular trauma from close-range shotgun injuries. Arch Surg 1985;120:1126.

100. Feliciano DV, Cruse PA, Burch JM, et al. Delayed diagnosis of arterial injuries. Am J Surg 1987;154:579.

101. Gustilo RB. Open fractures with arterial and nerve injuries: management of open fractures and their complications. Philadelphia: WB Saunders, 1982; 118.

102. Liekweg WG Jr, Greenfield LJ. Management of penetrating carotid arterial injury. Ann Surg 1978;188:587.

103. Monson DO, Saletta JD, Freeark RJ. Carotid and vertebral trauma. J Trauma 1969;9:987.

104. Rubio PA, Reul GJ, Beall AC Jr, et al. Acute carotid injury: 25 years' experience. J Trauma 1974;14:967.

105. Thal ER, Snyder WH, Hays RJ, et al. Management of carotid artery injuries. Surgery 1974;76:955.

106. Bradley EL. Management of penetrating carotid injuries: an alternative approach. J Trauma 1973;13:248.

107. Cohen A, Brief D, Mathewson C Jr. Carotid artery injuries. Am J Surg 1970;120:210.

108. Rich NM, Hobson RW, Wright CB, et al. Repair of lower extremity venous trauma: a more aggressive approach required. J Trauma 1974;14:639.

109. Rich NM, Collins GJ, Anderson CA, et al. Autogenous venous interposition grafts in repair of major venous injuries. J Trauma 1977;17:512.

110. Sullivan WG, Thornton FG, Baker LH, et al. Early influence of popliteal vein repair in the treatment of popliteal vessel injuries. Am J Surg 1971;122:528.

111. Sullivan WG, Thornton FG, Baker LH, et al. Early influence of popliteal vein repair in the treatment of popliteal vessel injuries. Am J Surg 1971;122:528.

112. Mullins RJ, Lucas CE, Ledgerwood AM. The natural history following venous ligation for civilian injury. J Trauma 1980;20:737.

113. Huebl HC, Read RC. Aneurysmal abscess. Minn Med 1966;49:11.

114. Ledgerwood AM, Lucas CE. Mycotic aneurysm of the carotid artery. Arch Surg 1974;109:496.

115. Anderson CB, Butcher HR, Ballinger WR. Mycotic aneurysms. Arch Surg 1974;109:712.

116. Johnson JE, Ledgerwood AM, Lucas CE. Mycotic aneurysm: new concepts in therapy. Arch Surg 1983;118:577.

117. Fromm SH, Lucas CE. Obturator bypass for mycotic aneurysm in the drug addict. Arch Surg 1970;100:82.

118. Guida PM, Moore SW. Obturator bypass technique. Surg Gynecol Obstet 1969;128:1307.

119. Johnson JE, Lucas CE, Ledgerwood AM. Infected venous pseudoaneurysm: a complication of drug addiction. Arch Surg 1984;119:1097.

120. Baker CC, Peterson SR, Shelden GF. Septic phlebitis: a neglected disease. Am J Surg 1979;138:97.

Chapter **36** Injuries to the Hand

PAUL ZIDEL, M.D.

ROBERT F. WILSON, M.D.

INTRODUCTION

The hand is a uniquely specialized organ. It contains what may be the largest number and variety of integrated structures found in the body.[1] It is capable of perception and a wide variety of movements with strength and precision.

Injuries to the hand and upper extremity account for almost one-third of all trauma emergency room visits in many hospitals, making them one of the most common injuries seen by physicians.[1,2] Consequently, all individuals caring for trauma victims should be capable of properly examining the injured hand and determining what type of definitive care should be administered.

AXIOM The quality of the initial management of a hand injury is a major determinant of outcome.

The key to success in the management of hand injuries is the initial evaluation and treatment of the patient. Above all else, this helps determine the patient's ability to regain function of his or her injured hand.

FUNCTIONAL ANATOMY AND BIOMECHANICS

Nomenclature

A thorough knowledge of the functional anatomy of the hand is essential to optimize care of hand injuries, and standard nomenclature should be used. Rather than numbering the fingers, the digits should be referred to by their common names: thumb, index, middle, ring, and small or little fingers (some physicians think of the hand as having five fingers and others think of the hand as having a thumb and four fingers). The sides of a digit should be described as "radial" or "ulnar" rather than "medial" and "lateral" to further reduce confusion. "Flexion" and "extension" of the thumb refer to motion occurring at the metacarpophalangeal (MP) or interphalangeal (IP) joints. "Adduction" of the thumb occurs when the extended thumb moves toward the palm, and with "abduction" the extended thumb moves away from the hand. "Opposition" is the rotational motion of the extended thumb toward the tip of the other fingers so that the thumbnail approaches parallel position to the nail plate of the fingers.

Muscles

The muscle-tendon units that produce motion in the hand are divided into intrinsic and extrinsic groups.

EXTRINSIC MUSCLES

The origins of the extrinsic muscles are proximal to the wrist, and most of these muscles are either flexors or extensors of the hand and/or digits.

Flexors

IN THE FOREARM. The extrinsic flexor muscles lie on the volar side of the forearm and are arranged in three layers (Fig. 36–1). The most superficial group consists of the pronator teres, flexor carpi radialis (FCR) and ulnaris (FCU), and the palmaris longus (PL). The intermediate group consists of the flexor digitorum superficialis (FDS), the four tendons of which move independently to flex the proximal interphalangeal (PIP) joints. The deep group of flexors contains three

muscles. The flexor pollicus longus (FPL) lies on the radius and flexes the interphalangeal (IP) joint of the thumb. The flexor digitorum profundus (FDP) lies on the ulna, and it has a common muscle belly to the middle, ring, and little fingers in the forearm, whereas the index finger is usually independent. These muscles produce flexion of the distal interphalangeal (DIP) joints. The deepest muscle in this compartment, the pronator quadratus, is not a flexor muscle, and it lies between the radius and the ulna. All of the key structures, except the FCR, FPL, and the radial artery and nerve, lie in the "ulnar" half of the distal forearm.

AT THE WRIST. The tendons of the hand on the flexor or volar surface at the wrist are classically arranged in three layers as they enter the carpal canal (Fig. 36–2). Starting on the radial side and moving to the ulnar side, the most superficial layer includes the flexor carpi radialis, palmaris longus, and flexor carpi ulnaris. The middle layer includes the tendons of the flexor digitorum superficialis with the middle and ring finger tendons lying superficial to those of the tendons to the index and small fingers. The deepest layer includes the tendons of the four flexor digitorum profundus muscles and the flexor pollicis longus on the radial side. On dissection, the flexor pollicis longus can be differentiated from the flexor carpi radialis by its distal muscle belly.

Extensors

IN THE FOREARM. The extrinsic extensor muscles are located dorsally in the forearm and may be divided into three subgroups (Fig. 36–3). The most radial (lateral) subgroup of extensors consists of three muscles often termed the "mobile wad." Two of these, the brachioradialis and extensor carpi radialis longus, originate from the lateral shaft of the distal humerus, whereas the extensor carpi radialis brevis originates from the lateral epicondyle of the humerus. The extensor carpi radialis longus and brevis muscles extend and deviate the wrist to the radial side. The brachioradialis produces flexion at the elbow and supination in the forearm.

The second subgroup of extensors forms a superficial layer originating from the lateral epicondyle. The extensor carpi ulnaris extends and deviates the wrist to the ulnar side. The extensor digitorum communis acts primarily to extend the metacarpophalangeal joints of all of the fingers except the thumb. The extensor digiti quinti minimi causes a similar action, but only in the little finger.

The deep subgroup of extensors consists of five muscles, all of which act on the thumb and index finger. Those acting on the thumb include the abductor pollicis longus, extensor pollicus brevis, and extensor pollicus longus. The index finger receives the extensor indicis proprius. The supinator, arising from the lateral epicondyle of the humerus and inserting on the proximal radius, assists in supination of the wrist and hand, but the biceps brachii muscle is the chief supinator.

AT THE WRIST. On the dorsal aspect of the wrist are six extensor compartments (Fig. 36–4). The first compartment contains the extensor pollicis brevis and the abductor pollicus longus. Tendonitis in this compartment is called "de Quervain's disease." The second compartment contains the extensor carpi radialis longus and brevis. The third compartment has the extensor pollicus longus which wraps around a bony prominence on the radius called "Lister's tubercle." The fourth compartment has the four tendons of the

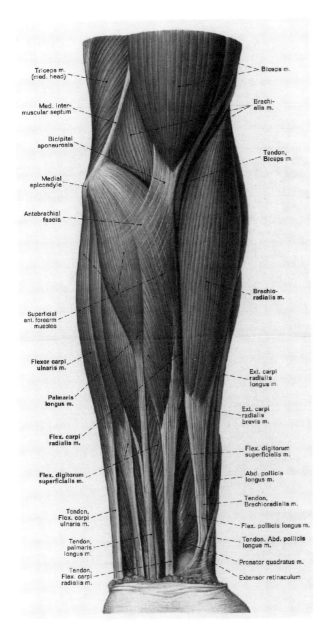

FIGURE 36–1 The flexor muscles of the forearm. The superficial anterior forearm muscles arise from the medial epicondyle of the humerus and include the pronator teres, flexor carpi radialis, palmaris longus, and flexor carpi ulnaris. Beneath these is the flexor digitorum superficialis. The median nerve lies deep to the flexor digitorum superficialis throughout much of its course in the forearm, but just above the wrist it usually becomes visible between the tendons, with the flexor pollicis longus and flexor carpi radialis on its radial side and the tendons of the palmaris longus and flexor digitorum superficialis on its ulnar side. The three muscles of the deep group include the flexor digitorum profundus, the flexor pollicis longus and the pronator quadratus. (From: Clemente CD. Anatomy: a regional atlas of the human body. 3rd ed. Philadelphia: Lea & Febiger, 1987.)

extensor digitorum communis as well as the tendon of the extensor indicis proprius which inserts on the ulnar side of the communis tendon on the index finger. This arrangement allows harvesting of the extensor indicis proprius for a tendon transfer if needed. The fifth compartment contains the extensor digiti quinti (minimi) which inserts into the extensor mechanism of the little finger on the ulnar side of the communis tendon. In the sixth compartment is the extensor carpi ulnaris, the sheath of which also provides support for the wrist.

INTRINSIC MUSCLES

The intrinsic muscles arise at or distal to the wrist. Those that activate the thumb make up the thenar eminence, and those that move the little finger form the hypothenar eminence.

Lumbrical Muscles

The lumbricals originate from the flexor digitorum profundi tendons and proceed distally, volar to the metacarpophalangeal joint axis, and then move dorsally to insert on the radial side of the extensor mechanism, providing flexion at the metacarpophalangeal joint and extension at the proximal and distal interphalangeal joints (Fig. 36–5). The first and second lumbricals on the radial side of the hand are innervated by the median nerve. The third and fourth lumbricals on the ulnar side of the hand are innervated by the ulnar nerve. The lumbrical muscles help the hand grasp large objects.

Interosseous Muscles

There are four dorsal interosseous muscles which originate from the sides of the metacarpal bones and insert on the sides of the extensor mechanisms so that the other fingers can be abducted away from the middle finger. The three volar interosseous muscles insert on the other sides of the extensor mechanism so that the fingers can be adducted or brought towards the middle finger. All of the interosseous muscles are innervated by the ulnar nerve. They assist the lumbricals in flexing the digits at the MP joints and extending at the PIP and DIP joints.

Nerves

ANATOMY[3]

Radial Nerve

As the radial nerve travels between the brachioradialis and the extensor carpi radialis longus and brevis muscles, it supplies innervation to the supinator muscle and then divides into the posterior interosseous and the superficial radial nerves.[4] The posterior interosseous nerve is motor to the long extensors of the hand and sensory to the wrist joint. The superficial radial nerve runs subcutaneously along the radial side of the forearm and can often be palpated in the distal one-third of the forearm over the bone. It provides sensation to the skin of the dorsum of the thumb, the proximal radial three digits, and the associated portion of the dorsum of the hand (Fig. 36–6).

Ulnar Nerve

The ulnar nerve enters the forearm through the cubital tunnel at the elbow. In the forearm, it provides motor innervation to the flexor carpi ulnaris and the two ulnar flexor digitorum profundi muscles. Proximal to the wrist crease, it gives off a dorsal sensory branch that innervates the ulnar side of the dorsum of the hand. The main portion of the ulnar nerve enters Guyon's canal between the pisiform and hamate bones and divides into motor and sensory branches. The motor branches supply the hypothenar and a number of other intrinsic hand muscles. A sensory branch supplies the little finger and the ulnar side of the ring finger. There is also a small sensory branch to the ulnar side of the palm.

In the hand, the deep motor branch of the ulnar nerve innervates the two ulnar lumbricals, the three volar interossei (which adduct the fingers), and the four dorsal interossei (which abduct the fingers). It also innervates the adductor pollicus longus and the deep head of the flexor pollicis brevis of the thumb, as well as the three hypothenar muscles (abductor, opponens, and flexor brevis digiti minimi).

Median Nerve

The median nerve has a branch in the upper forearm called the anterior interosseous nerve that is motor to the flexor pollicis longus, pronator quadratus, and the radial half of the flexor digitorum profundus. One of the signs of damage to this nerve is the inability to make an "O" with the thumb and index finger; this motion requires the function of the flexor pollicis longus to the thumb and the flexor digitorum profundus to the index finger. The main portion of the median

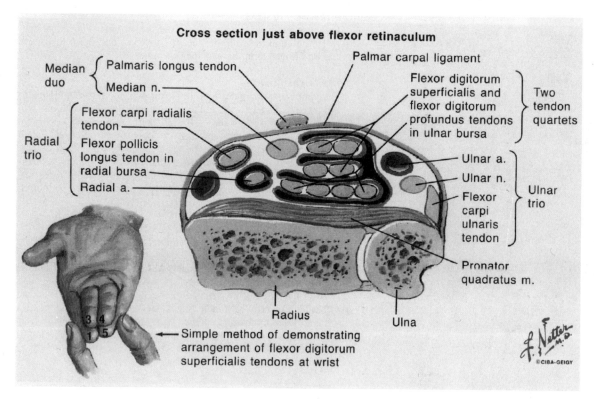

Cross section just above flexor retinaculum

FIGURE 36–2   The flexor tendons at the wrist. The tendons of the flexor pollicis longus, flexor digitorum superficialis, and flexor digitorum profundus muscles pass through the carpal tunnel. The tendons of the flexor digitorum superficialis muscle destined for the ring and middle fingers lie superficial to the tendons for the index and little fingers. Still deeper in the compartment are the four tendons of the flexor digitorum profundus muscle, lined up side by side. The tendon of the flexor pollicis longus muscle passes through the carpal tunnel deeply on the radial side. The median nerve passes into the hand through the carpal tunnel radial to the superficial row of flexor tendons. (From: Netter FH. The CIBA collection of medical illustrations. Vol. 8: musculoskeletal system. Part I: anatomy, physiology, and metabolic disorders. New Jersey: Ciba-Geigy Corp., 1987; 61.)

nerve continues with a palmar cutaneous branch arising approximately 7 centimeters proximal to the volar carpal ligament. This innervates the base of the palm.

The median nerve passes into the palm through the carpal canal with the flexor tendons and divides into a motor branch to the thenar muscles and into common (sensory) digital nerves. The first branch off the median nerve in the hand is motor to the thenar muscles, including the abductor pollicus brevis, opponens pollicus, and superficial head of the flexor pollicus brevis. The next branches include two digital sensory nerves to the thumb, branches to the two radial lumbricals, and digital sensory nerves. The digital sensory branches supply sensation to the palmar skin, flexor surfaces of the digits, and the dorsal digital skin distal to the DIP joint on the index, middle, and radial half of the ring finger.

Arteries

The two main blood supplies to the hand are the radial and ulnar arteries (Fig. 36–7). Variations exist so that either of the two may be the sole source of blood to major portions of the hand. In most instances, the branches of each vessel communicate so well with the other that excellent hand perfusion is maintained even if one of the two vessels is completely occluded. There may also be a persistent median artery, but this artery is usually small.

The ulnar artery enters the palm of the hand through Guyon's canal on the ulnar side of the wrist. The artery then forms the superficial palmar arch that gives off digital arteries to the fingers. The superficial arch is deep to the palmar fascia but superficial to the nerves and the tendons. A deep branch of the ulnar artery then communi-

cates with the deep palmar arch formed from the deep branch of the radial artery.

The radial artery branches at the wrist into superficial and deep branches. The superficial branch crosses the thenar muscles and gives off a princeps pollicis branch to the thumb and then anastomoses with the superficial arch from the ulnar artery. The deep branch first courses dorsally to pass between the first and second metacarpals and then moves in a palmar direction to form the deep palmar arch. The deep palmar arch crosses the palm proximal to the superficial arch and beneath the flexor tendons and joins the deep branch of the ulnar artery. The deep palmar arch is the dominant arterial supply to the thumb and fingers. The common digital arteries to the fingers usually arise from the deep palmar arch which is the dominant blood supply. Branches from the common digital arteries supply the fingers as well as give off branches into mesenteries called "vincula" which supply the flexor tendons. There are two vincula (longus and brevis) to each flexor profundus tendon and two vincula (longus and brevis) to each flexor superficialis tendon.

Bones

The bones of the fingers are the distal, middle, and proximal phalanxes to the index, middle, ring, and small fingers, and a distal and proximal phalanx to the thumb. There is little motion in the second and third metacarpal, so they provide a fixed unit for the hand with which the thumb and ulnar digits can grasp various objects. The distal carpal bones, radial to ulnar, consist of the trapezium (greater multangulum), trapezoid (multangulum), capitate, and hamate. The proxi-

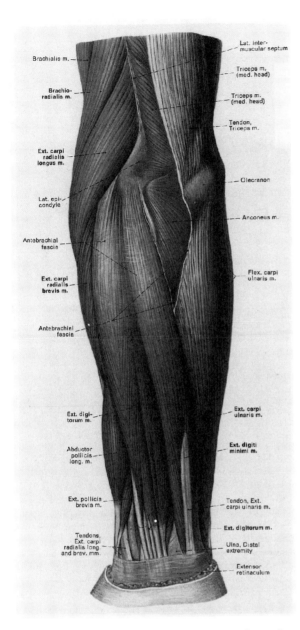

FIGURE 36–3 The extensor muscles of the forearm. The six muscles of the superficial layer of extensors, in order from the radial to the ulnar side, include the brachioradialis, extensor carpi radialis longus, extensor carpi radialis brevis, extensor digitorum communis, extensor digiti minimi, and extensor carpi ulnaris. The muscles of the deep layer of extensors include the supinator, abductor pollicis longus, extensor pollicis brevis, and extensor pollicus longus, but some of their tendons and parts of their fleshy bellies may become more superficial just above the wrist. (From: Clemente CD. Anatomy: a regional atlas of the human body. 3rd ed. Philadelphia: Lea & Febiger, 1987.)

mal row consists of the scaphoid (navicular), lunate, triquetrum, and pisiform, all held with a complex of ligaments.[5]

Ligaments

The ligaments of the joints of the fingers are the collateral and accessory collateral ligaments. When the fingers are extended, the ability to abduct at the MCP joint is increased because laxity of these ligaments allows a wider grasp. When the metacarpophalangeal joints are flexed, the collateral ligaments are tightened to stabilize the grasp.

Nail Plate[6]

The nail plate of each nail is a small but important structure (Fig. 36–8). It helps stabilize the soft tissues of the finger pulp to allow picking up of small objects. The nail plate is cornified epithelium that originates in the nail matrix proximal to the epinychial nail fold.

Biomechanics of the Hand

The biomechanics of the hand basically involve a fixed central unit (index and middle rays) opposed by mobile units (thumb, ring, and small) (Fig. 36–9). Also intrinsic to the function of the units are the flexor tendon sheaths that not only provide nutrition for the flexor tendons but also the thickenings of which form a pulley system for the flexor tendons.

> **AXIOM** If the pulley system is not restored after repair of a flexor tendon, the tendon tends to bowstring, decreasing flexion.

Of particular interest are the flexor tendon sheaths, originating at the distal palmar crease and extending to the distal interphalangeal joint. There are a number of annular thickened areas of this bilaminar sheath that function like pulleys. The three most important pulleys for each finger are the Λ1 pulley at the proximal end of the tendon sheath, where trigger finger deformities occur, the A2 pulley in the proximal phalanx, and the A4 pulley in the midportion of the middle phalanx. These latter two key pulleys provide support and prevent bowstringing of the tendons during flexion. There are also other annular and cruciate thickenings of the tendon sheath or pulleys in the hand, but they are less important.

DIAGNOSIS

> **AXIOM** Not performing a careful systematic examination of the hand, even with apparently minor injuries, can lead to disaster.

History

The history of the type of trauma coupled with direct observation of the injured area will often lead to a fairly accurate diagnosis. For example, a fall directly on the palm of the hand while the wrist is extended and which is associated with numbness in the small finger should lead one to consider a fracture of the hook of the hamate with injury to the underlying ulnar nerve.

> **AXIOM** Awareness of the preinjury use of the hands and the expectations of the patient after treatment can be of great importance in planning treatment.

The history should include the age of the patient, the nature of the accident, hand dominance, occupation, hobbies, prior injuries, and co-morbid factors. One should also ask specific questions regarding the mechanisms of injury. Some examples of questions to ask with various types of trauma are:

1. Lacerations: The position of the fingers (flexed or extended) at the time of injury; the length of the penetrating weapon; the amount of force against the hand; the amount of initial pulsatile bleeding; was loss of sensation immediate?
2. Crush injury: The amount and kind of force; the type of surface and length of time under pressure; was there associated heat from a machine?
3. Injection: The type of material injected; what was the amount of pressure or force of the injection?
4. Amputation: What type of machine was responsible; what was done with the amputated part; what is the pertinent medical history?

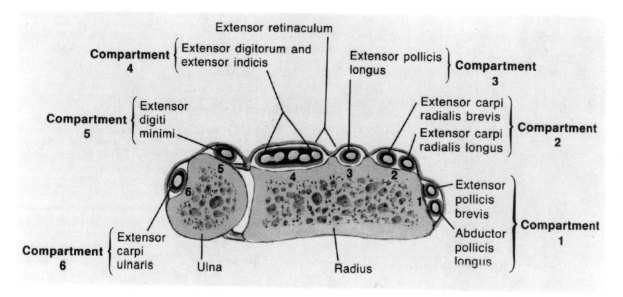

FIGURE 36–4 The extensor tendons at the wrist. The extensor tendons at the wrist are arranged in six separate compartments. The tendons of the abductor pollicis longus and extensor pollicis brevis muscles occupy the first (radialmost) compartment, which is located at the styloid process of the radius. The second compartment, which lies over the rather smooth area of the radius, radial to its dorsal tubercle, contains the tendons of the extensor carpi radialis longus and extensor carpi radialis brevis. The third compartment is occupied by the tendon of the extensor pollicis longus. This tendon, passing obliquely to its insertion in the distal phalanx of the thumb, forms the prominent dorsal border for the anatomic snuffbox. The fourth compartment, over the smooth ulnar third of the dorsum of the radius, contains the four tendons of the extensor digitorum muscle and the tendon of the extensor indices. The small fifth compartment is located directly over the distal radioulnar joint and transmits the tendon of the extensor digiti minimi muscle. The sixth compartment, which overlies the head of the ulna, contains the tendon of the extensor carpi ulnaris. (From: Netter FH. The CIBA collection of medical illustrations. Vol. 8: musculoskeletal system. Part I: anatomy, physiology, and metabolic disorders. New Jersey: Ciba-Geigy Corp., 1987; 60.)

5. Fractures: Any previous fractures; what was the previous function of the extremity?

The pertinent medical history also includes previous surgery on the extremity, cigarette use, medical disorders, and medications.

> **AXIOM**   With hand injuries, one should perform a full assessment before taking off the bandage or manipulating the wound. The function of the hand is as informative as the wound itself.

Physical Examination

SYSTEMATIC EVALUATION

Testing each system of the hand in a specific order will help ensure thoroughness and completeness.

> **PITFALL** ⊘
>
> *Letting a dramatic or gory wound distract the physician from performing a complete exam of all the other structures that may be injured.*

As a general rule, the injured area should be examined last. This helps one to perform a more complete and systematic examination. A systematic examination of the hand might involve answering the following questions:[1]

1. General appearance of the hand: Is the hand or finger viable? Is there active bleeding, swelling, cyanosis, pallor, deformity, abnormal position of digits, or old scars?
2. Location of the wound: Which deep structures may be involved?
3. Nature of the wound: Is the wound clean or crushed? Does it have

avulsion of skin? Are skin flaps present and viable? What is the condition of the underlying soft tissues? Is there any deep contamination?

> **AXIOM**   Sharp lacerations of a tendon in the hand often also involve other structures, such as vessels or nerves.

4. Palpation: Is there any suggestion of occult fractures as evidenced by localized tenderness, crepitus, abnormal contours, or instability?
5. Circulation: Are the digits pink with good capillary refill? Are any digits cyanotic or pallid? Is there pulsatile bleeding?
6. Sensation: Is two-point discrimination intact? It is hard to assess two-point discrimination in patients who are intoxicated, have multiple injuries, are very young, or have crush injuries. If the digital artery is lacerated from a palmar surface injury, the digital nerve is usually also cut.
7. Tendons: What is the posture or position of the fingers or hand? Is there any evidence of impaired finger or thumb movement? The differential action of the flexor digitorum profundus and the flexor digitorum superficialis is important and more difficult to assess in a painful hand, especially if there are associated fractures.

INSPECTION AND SURFACE ANATOMY

> **AXIOM**   The function of each tendon should be evaluated separately, but it must be remembered that a partially lacerated tendon that needs repair may seem to function relatively well.

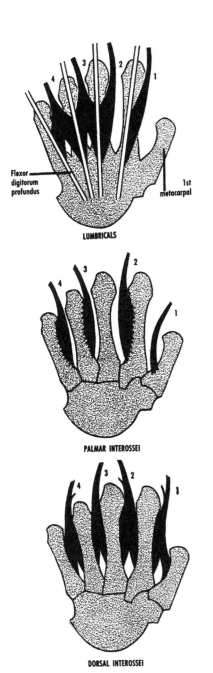

FIGURE 36–5 The deep muscles of the hand. The deep muscles of the hand include lumbrical and interosseus muscles and the muscles of the thenar and hypothenar eminences. The central compartment of the hand contains four slender lumbrical muscles arising from the flexor digitorum profundus tendons. The interosseus muscles are located in the intervals between the metacarpal bones. The median nerve supplies the abductor pollicis brevis, opponens pollicis, the superficial head of the flexor pollicis brevis, and the radialmost two lumbrical muscles; the ulnar nerve supplies all the other intrinsic muscles of the hand. (From: Gardner E, Gray DJ, O'Rahilly R. Anatomy: a regional study of human structure. 4th ed. Philadelphia: WB Saunders Co., 1975; 146.)

Observation is important to diagnosis. In most cases, only one hand is injured, and if there have been no prior injuries, the uninjured hand can be used for comparison.

The position of the bones in the hand relative to the surface anatomy are often not well-known to most physicians. For example, the distal palmar crease overlies the metacarpal heads while the volar crease at the proximal end of each finger is actually at the midpoint of the proximal phalanx.

Partial tendon lacerations should be suspected when the patient has weakness or pain with attempted motion against resistance. Consequences of unrecognized partial tendon lacerations include rupture, adhesions, and triggering.

Each tendon should be evaluated separately. The flexor digitorum profundus provides flexion at the distal interphalangeal joint. Since the superficialis and profundus tendons have a common origin, the flexor digitorum superficialis can only be evaluated if the profundus muscle bellies are blocked. Therefore, the superficialis tendons are evaluated by blocking (holding) three of the four fingers with their distal interphalangeal joints extended. This only will allow flexion at the proximal interphalangeal joint of the unheld finger by the superficialis. One can also have the patient oppose the distal pulp of the finger to the thumb and look for flexion at the PIP joint.

The flexor digitorum profundus is tested by blocking the other fingers in extension at the PIP joint and asking the patient to flex the DIP joint of the finger in question. The flexor pollicis longus is tested by blocking the MP joint in extension and asking the patient to flex the interphalangeal joint of the thumb.

Evaluating the long extensors can be accomplished by testing each compartment. For dual extensors (i.e., the indicis proprius and digiti minimi), the patient makes a fist while one looks for greater extension of the index and small fingers (to zero degrees), compared to the middle and ring fingers.

AXIOM Painful extension against resistance may be the only clinical evidence of partial extensor tendon lacerations.

High risk areas for partial extensor tendon lacerations are over the dorsum of the MP joints. Fingers with lacerations in these areas should have x-rays and be splinted prophylactically.

NERVES
The motor and sensory function of the three main nerves of the hand should be evaluated in a systematic manner after any upper extremity injury.

Sensation
The sensory component of the radial nerve can be evaluated in the relatively autonomous area it innervates in the first dorsal web space between the thumb and index finger. Sensory function of the median nerve is best tested over the distal pulp of the index finger. For the ulnar nerve, the best area to test sensation is over the distal pulp of the small finger.

Various techniques are used to evaluate sensation. The simplest is lightly touching a non-sharp instrument, such as a cotton swab or paper clip, to the area, barely blanching the skin. An injection needle should not be used. The patient is asked to determine whether the sensation with similar testing of the other hand is similar or different. Differentiating between "sharp" and "dull" may also be helpful.

AXIOM Sensation on the hand is ideally evaluated by two-point discrimination testing.

Weber's two-point discrimination test is a more reliable and reproducible method to diagnose sensory deficits. When two blunt points are lightly touched against the skin of the fingertip, healthy persons can discriminate two points 3 to 5 mm apart. Comparison with the uninjured hand provides corroboration of identified sensory deficits. Factors that limit the value of this test include severe pain, crush injuries, and ischemia.

In children, a more reliable sign of sensory nerve damage is loss of sweating of the skin in the distribution of the nerve. If neural func-

Cutaneous Innervation of Wrist and Hand

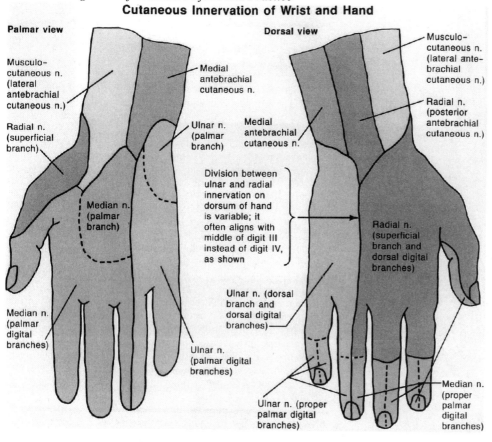

Palmar view

Musculo-
cutaneous n.
(lateral
antebrachial
cutaneous n.)

Radial n.
(superficial
branch)

Median n.
(palmar
branch)

Median n.
(palmar
digital
branches)

Medial
antebrachial
cutaneous n.

Ulnar n. (palmar
branch)

Ulnar n.
(palmar digital
branches)

Dorsal view

Medial
antebrachial
cutaneous n.

Division between
ulnar and radial
innervation on
dorsum of hand
is variable; it
often aligns with
middle of digit III
instead of digit IV,
as shown

Ulnar n. (dorsal
branch and
dorsal digital
branches)

Ulnar n. (proper
palmar digital
branches)

Musculo-
cutaneous n.
(lateral ante-
brachial
cutaneous n.)

Radial n.
(posterior
antebrachial
cutaneous n.)

Radial n.
(superficial
branch and
dorsal digital
branches)

Median n.
(proper
palmar
digital
branches)

FIGURE 36–6 Sensory innervation of the hand. There is much overlap of the sensory innervation of the hand. The most autonomous areas are the first dorsal web space for the radial nerve, the volar pad of the index finger for the median nerve, and the ulnar side of the little finger for the ulnar nerve. (From: Netter FH. The CIBA collection of medical illustrations. Vol. 8: musculoskeletal system. Part I: anatomy, physiology, and metabolic disorders. New Jersey: Ciba-Geigy Corp., 1987; 58.)

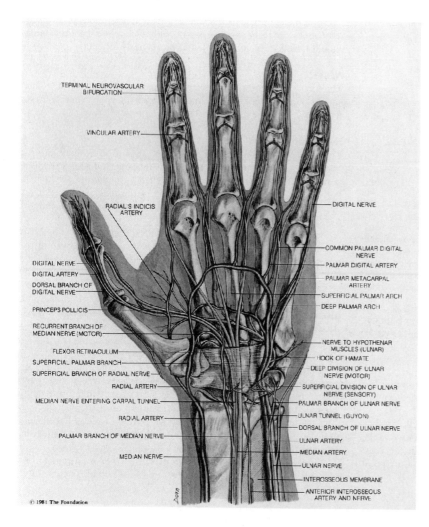

TERMINAL NEUROVASCULAR
BIFURCATION

VINCULAR ARTERY

RADIALIS INDICIS
ARTERY

DIGITAL NERVE
DIGITAL ARTERY
DORSAL BRANCH OF
DIGITAL NERVE

PRINCEPS POLLICIS

RECURRENT BRANCH OF
MEDIAN NERVE (MOTOR)

FLEXOR RETINACULUM
SUPERFICIAL PALMAR BRANCH
SUPERFICIAL BRANCH OF RADIAL NERVE
RADIAL ARTERY
MEDIAN NERVE ENTERING CARPAL TUNNEL
RADIAL ARTERY
PALMAR BRANCH OF MEDIAN NERVE
MEDIAN NERVE

DIGITAL NERVE

COMMON PALMAR DIGITAL
NERVE
PALMAR DIGITAL ARTERY
PALMAR METACARPAL
ARTERY
SUPERFICIAL PALMAR ARCH
DEEP PALMAR ARCH

NERVE TO HYPOTHENAR
MUSCLES (ULNAR)
HOOK OF HAMATE
DEEP DIVISION OF ULNAR
NERVE (MOTOR)
SUPERFICIAL DIVISION OF ULNAR
NERVE (SENSORY)
PALMAR BRANCH OF ULNAR NERVE
ULNAR TUNNEL (GUYON)
DORSAL BRANCH OF ULNAR NERVE
ULNAR ARTERY
MEDIAN ARTERY
ULNAR NERVE
INTEROSSEOUS MEMBRANE
ANTERIOR INTEROSSEOUS
ARTERY AND NERVE

© 1981 The Foundation

FIGURE 36–7 The blood supply to the hand. The two main arteries to the hand are the radial and ulnar arteries. The superficial palmar branch of the radial artery to the hand leaves the radial artery just before it turns from the radial border of the wrist onto the back of the hand. It descends over or through the muscles of the thumb and joins the superficial branch of the ulnar artery to form the superficial palmar arterial arch. The ulnar artery at the wrist lies deep to the flexor carpi ulnaris muscles and enters the hand in company with the ulnar nerve. It forms the deep palmar arterial arch. (From: Beasley RW, Brown HG, Meyer VE, Rabischong P. Atlas of surgical anatomy of the hand and forearm. The Foundation for Hand Research, 1981;Plate 5:164.)

FIGURE 36–8 The anatomy of the fingernail. The fingernail is a horny plate composed of closely welded, horny scales or cornified epithelial cells. The nail adheres to the subjacent nail bed where strong fibers pass to the periosteum of the distal phalanx, providing a firm attachment. The nail is formed from the proximal part of the nail bed, where the thick epithelium extends as far distally as the whitened lunula. Developing from the nail matrix, the nail moves out over the longitudinal dermal ridges of the nail bed at a growth rate of approximately 1 mm/wk. (From: Beasley RW. Surgical anatomy of the hand. In: Beasley RW, ed. Hand injuries. Philadelphia: WB Saunders Co., 1981.)

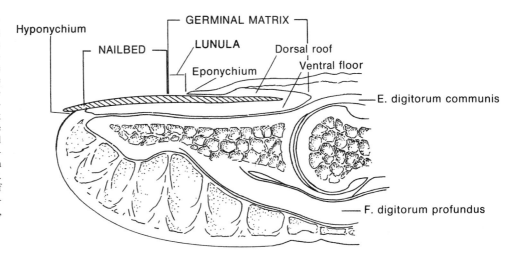

tion to an area of skin is intact, beads of sweat can be readily seen through an ophthalmoscope. With the wrinkle test, the area in question is immersed under water for 10-20 minutes; normal skin tends to wrinkle, whereas denervated skin will not.

Additional testing includes evaluation of vibratory and position sense, two-point discrimination testing, and use of the Semmes-Weinstein monofilament hairs that bend at specific forces.[7]

Motor Function

For the evaluation of motor function, abduction by the abductor pollicis brevis so that the thumb is at right angles to the palm is an action unique to the median nerve. The ability to spread the

fingers apart while they are extended at the IP and MP joints uses the dorsal interosseus muscles innervated solely by the ulnar nerve. Simultaneous extension at the wrist and MP joints is an action specific to the radial nerve. In a similar manner, the ability to cross the fingers requires ulnar nerve function, and snapping of the fingers requires median nerve function. One can also palpate the hypothenar muscles for contraction during attempted finger motion to check for ulnar innervation of intrinsic muscles. Even though some of the deep muscles of the thenar eminence are supplied by the ulnar nerve, palpation of the thenar muscles may help determine if median nerve innervation to the hand is intact.

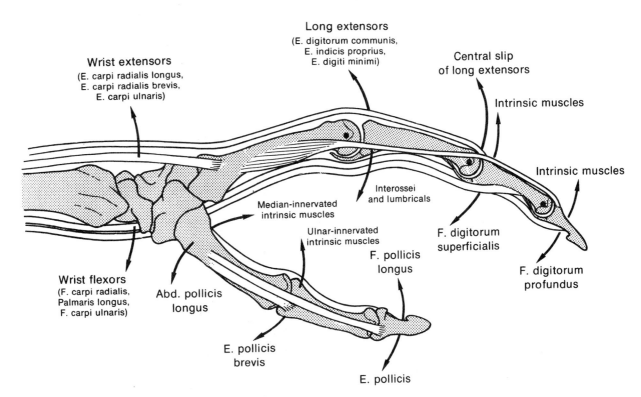

FIGURE 36–9 Muscle balance in the hand and fingers. Muscle balance in the hand and fingers is provided by opposing muscle forces acting across each joint in a protagonist-antagonist relationship. These forces acting across the joint are also compressive. Unless controlled, imbalance across one joint will be followed by reciprocal deformity at the next joint in a zigzag configuration. (From: Beasley RW. Surgical anatomy of the hand. In: Beasley RW, ed. Hand injuries. Philadelphia: WB Saunders Co., 1981; 13.)

BLOOD VESSELS

Preoperative evaluation for blood vessel injury should include assessment of the amount of bleeding and evidence of distal ischemia. For example, pallid skin suggests an arterial defect, whereas edema with dusky skin suggests venous occlusion.

The patency of the radial and ulnar arteries at the wrist can be determined by Allen's test[8] which involves the patient raising an arm and hand. The fist is clenched several times, and then clenched again firmly while the examiner occludes the ulnar and radial arteries. The patient's hand is then lowered and the fist opened. The hand should look quite pale. The pressure on the ulnar artery is then released. If the hand does not pink up within 3 seconds, Allen's test is considered positive, and there is some concern about the adequacy of ulnar artery blood flow to the hand. The hand can then be raised and the test repeated for the patency of the radial artery.

> **AXIOM**   A false-positive Allen's test can occur if the patient is hypovolemic, is hypotensive, has a low cardiac output, is receiving vasoconstrictor drugs, or overextends the fingers.

Iatrogenic injury to a radial artery proximal to a hand in which the ulnar artery is not dominant can lead to a devastating effect. Because the neurovascular bundles on each side of each finger are just volar to the topmost crease of the flexed digit, accurate assessment of an injury can be determined by the location of the laceration and knowledge of the anatomic relationship of the artery just dorsal to the nerve. This neurovascular bundle is encased in two ligaments, the volar ligaments of Grayson and the dorsal ligaments of Cleland. More proximal neurovascular injuries, such as thoracic outlet syndrome, also need to be evaluated.[9]

DIAGNOSTIC AIDS[1]

1. X-rays: Three views of any bone thought to be fractured are mandatory. If there is an amputated part, it should also be x-rayed. Soft tissue films, ultrasound, and/or MRI may be helpful in determining the presence and location of other lesions (Fig. 36–10).[2]
2. Arteriography: Arteriography may be useful in a few patients, including those with previous severe hand injuries, prior or present shunts for dialysis, or congenital deformities.

> **AXIOM**   If emergent exploration of an injured hand is warranted, one should not delay the surgery to obtain arteriography.

3. Doppler: Doppler ultrasound can be used to assess arterial patency rapidly; however, excessive edema may preclude a satisfactory examination. A Doppler flow probe may also be useful in determining the site of a vascular injury and the competency of the collateral circulation.[10]
4. Measurements of compartment pressure: Commercial units for monitoring compartment pressures are available in most hospitals. Such pressures should be measured if there is a question about the presence of compartment syndrome,[11,12] even with low-velocity gunshot wounds to the forearm.[13]
5. Anesthetic blocks: After a thorough evaluation, local anesthetic blocks can be used under special conditions to further define certain injuries.

> **AXIOM**   Anesthetic blocks for diagnostic purposes should not be performed except by the surgeon who will be providing the definitive care of the hand injury.

TREATMENT

Basic Principles of Surgical and Nonsurgical Care

ULTIMATE GOALS

The basic principles of care, both surgical and nonsurgical, of an injured hand involve restoration of viability and maximization of func-

tion and aesthetic appearance. If complete evaluation reveals no injuries to deeper structures, skin lacerations can be closed with appropriate sterile technique, often with local anesthesia or a proximal regional nerve block.

> **AXIOM**   Ideally, hand injuries should be repaired in an operating room where the wounds can be examined completely and the environment is completely sterile.

PRIORITIES IN HAND CARE

In general, the priorities in surgical care of hand injuries are: (a) provision of an adequate blood supply, (b) establishment of a clean wound, (c) skin coverage, especially over bones, joints, and tendons, (d) bone alignment and stability, (e) tendon repairs, and (f) nerve repairs.

ANESTHESIA

Many procedures on the digits can be performed under local anesthesia. The most commonly used form of local anesthesia is the digital block, which is both widely applicable and extremely effective. Marcaine (bupivacaine hydrochloride, 0.25-0.50%) or 1-2% lidocaine, without epinephrine, is injected through a 27- or 30-gauge needle. The needle is introduced into the dorsal aspect of the hand approximately 1-2 cm proximal to the web. A small weal of Mar-

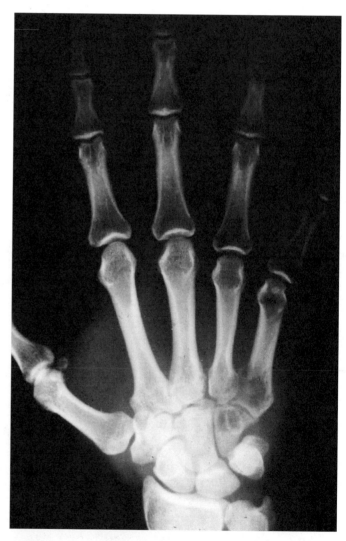

FIGURE 36–10   Coincidental malignancy of the bones of the hand. The need to be thorough in evaluation of any injury is evident in this case in which the original x-ray, taken for minor trauma overlooked a coincident malignancy involving the base of the fifth metatarsal bone and the hamate.

caine may be introduced at the site of the skin penetration, but this is not essential. The tip of the needle is advanced proximally and volarly just dorsal to the palmar fascia on either side of the metacarpal bone of that finger (Fig. 36–2). The syringe is aspirated to avoid an intravascular injection. Approximately 2.0 ml of lidocaine or Marcaine, without adrenaline, are then injected. Because rapid distension of the tissues with anesthetic solution is extremely uncomfortable, the discomfort experienced by the patient will be minimized if the anesthetic solution is injected slowly. The adjacent web space is infiltrated in a similar manner, and if surgery is required to the dorsum of the finger, then a small amount of anesthetic can be injected over the extensor tendon to block the terminal branches of the nerves. If this technique is used, satisfactory anesthesia can be obtained with minimal discomfort to most patients.

> **AXIOM** An excessive volume of anesthesia can cause venous congestion and vascular compromise in a finger.

EXPLORATION

Skin lacerations usually will not indicate the presence or extent of deeper injuries, especially in lacerations from a piece of glass or sharp knife. Closed injuries, such as fractures associated with vascular deficits or irreducible fragments, will also need exploration.

> **AXIOM** Most penetrating wounds of the hand should be thoroughly explored in the operating room with a proximal tourniquet applied to provide maximum visibility of all structures.

Unnecessary probings of hand wounds in the emergency room should be discouraged. Adequate surgical exposure frequently requires proximal and distal extension of wounds and may also require a proximal counterincision for tendon retrieval. Basic principles of extending incisions include: (a) preservation of local circulation, (b) extension along non-pinch surfaces whenever possible, and (c) crossing flexion creases at angles less than 90° in order to avoid scar-related flexion contractures.

TETANUS TOXOID AND ANTIBIOTICS

Routine initial management of open hand wounds includes appropriate prophylaxis against tetanus. Tissue smears and cultures should be performed whenever open wounds are explored and there appears to be significant contamination. These studies can provide definitive information on the extent of contamination and can help guide later antibiotic use, if needed. The use of antibiotics in hand wounds is influenced primarily by the surgeon's experience and philosophy, but a short course begun as soon as possible after the injury is appropriate when the wounds are contaminated.

DEBRIDEMENT

> **AXIOM** There is no substitute for thorough surgical debridement and lavage for preventing wound infections after trauma.

All devitalized and severely contaminated tissues should be debrided, and a thorough irrigation of exposed structures must be performed. Controlled pulsating lavage with pressure can be quite effective for removing surface contamination. Safe debridement requires a tourniquet.

FASCIOTOMY

Fasciotomies in the forearm and hand are often indicated after severe roller injuries, crush injuries, high pressure injection injuries, and prolonged ischemia.[2]

> **AXIOM** If there is any question about the need for a fasciotomy, it should either be done or serial compartment pressures should be performed. Open fractures can still have compartment syndrome.

Common Injuries

SKIN WOUNDS

Proper inspection of a hand wound requires adequate anesthesia, instruments, light, and hemostasis by a tourniquet. On the upper arm, padding is placed under a wide blood pressure cuff, the arm is elevated, blood is squeezed out of the arm with an elastic bandage, unless infection or tumor is suspected, and the cuff pressure is then raised to 100 mm Hg above the systolic pressure, usually to at least 250-280 mm Hg. The cuff should be deflated for 15-20 minutes every 1.5-2.0 hours and the process repeated as needed. Thorough hemostasis must be accomplished with the cuff removed before skin closure.

The importance of thorough cleansing by copious irrigation, removal of any foreign objects, and sharp debridement of devitalized tissue cannot be overstressed. Most untidy wounds can be cleansed to the point at which primary closure is reasonable and repair of underlying structures is possible.

> **AXIOM** Hand wounds caused by contact with another individual's teeth have a high risk of severe infection and should not be closed; they should be explored, debrided, and irrigated.

Although most hand wounds can be closed primarily, if there is suspected contamination from human or animal bites, or obvious contamination from soil or grease, it is best to leave the wound open after thorough sharp debridement. When there are no underlying injuries to tendon or bone, these wounds can be allowed to heal by second intent. The skin and subcutaneous tissue of contaminated wounds can be left open and then closed several days later if the wound is clean.

X-ray examinations are part of the wound assessment in any case in which there may be fractures or retained foreign bodies. Stone, tooth, metal, and many forms of glass are radiopaque. Most wood and some types of glass are radiolucent.

FRACTURES

General Principles

STABLE VERSUS UNSTABLE FRACTURES. Fractures of the hand can often be accurately classified by clinical and x-ray studies as stable or unstable. Because of the complex insertions of multiple tendons, once a fracture is displaced, there is a high likelihood of continued instability, and such injuries usually require some form of stabilization after accurate reduction.

Nondisplaced fractures are often stable, but they should be carefully evaluated for subtle rotational deformities. This can be done by passive motion of the wrist and fingers thereby allowing the tenodesis effect to show malrotation. The digits are then accurately splinted or casted to prevent any movement of the fragments. Follow-up physical examination and timely x-rays are essential.

> **AXIOM** Unstable hand and wrist fractures need fixation, not an aluminum splint.

TYPES OF FRACTURES. An accurate radiological description of all fractures is essential to determine the type of trauma involved and optimal therapy. Simple descriptions, such as "an oblique nondisplaced midshaft fracture of the index metacarpal," are generally the best. Often the pattern of the fracture indicates the nature of the deforming forces. For example, a spiral fracture is usually a result of an angular or twisting injury. In children, the Salter classification for epiphyseal injuries should also be used.

OPEN FRACTURES. Open fractures generally require antibiotics and surgical exploration as soon as possible. Extensive cleansing, irrigation, and meticulous debridement are mandatory. Small devitalized fragments of floating bone should be removed. If cancellous bone is present on such fragments, it can be separated and used as material for grafting at the fracture site. Unless the patient is going to the operating room immediately, open fracture wounds should be loosely closed with a few tacking sutures in the emergency department to reduce the contamination of deeper tissues.[15]

Always be aware that an open fracture on the hand may be due to the patient striking another individual in the mouth. Human bites usually require intravenous antibiotics to prevent what can be serious infections caused by virulent mouth flora, including Eikenella corrodens. Cephalosporins may not be adequate to prevent infection in severely contaminated wounds. A combination of penicillin plus an antistaphylococcal antibiotic may be adequate for many wounds; however, one should not hesitate to use a combination of high doses of penicillin with an aminoglycoside and clindamycin, especially if there is evidence of severe infection.

> **AXIOM** Patients with open hand fractures should receive antibiotics against gram-positive cocci (including streptococci and Staphylococcus aureus), aerobic gram-negative bacilli (such as Escherichia coli), and mouth anaerobes.

For unstable fractures of small bones, such as phalanges, crossed Kirschner wire fixation is usually satisfactory. Condylar fractures especially need stabilization.[16] In larger bones, minicompression plates or rigid internal fixation can often be used, and these allow early motion.[17] With badly contaminated open fractures, the use of external fixators or percutaneous fixation proximal and distal to the wound itself can prevent fracture motion and help diminish the potential for infection.[18] Tissue smears and cultures should be taken at the time of surgery, and perioperative prophylactic antibiotics use is routine.[19,20]

REDUCTION OF FRACTURES. Fractures should be treated closed whenever possible to lessen the risk of infection. However, accurate reduction is essential for intra-articular fractures if good joint motion is to be preserved. One should also attempt to correct any angulation and malrotation. This can be assessed by passive flexion and extension of the wrist using the tenodesis effect to demonstrate any finger malposition. If closed efforts cannot provide an accurate reduction of joint surfaces, open reduction and internal fixation (ORIF) is indicated.

FIXATION OF FRACTURES. Fixation of fractures is indicated if a satisfactory and stable reduction cannot be maintained with a cast or splint. Spiral, oblique, or displaced fractures are often quite unstable without rigid fixation by small rods.

IMMOBILIZATION. Immobilization maintains reduction of the fracture, promotes healing of bone, and protects adjacent soft tissue. Whenever the hand will be immobilized for more than a few days, it should be placed in the "safe position," also called the "intrinsic plus position." In this position, the wrist is neutral or slightly extended, and there is MP joint flexion and interphalangeal joint extension. A stiff hand in the intrinsic plus position is easier to mobilize than a stiff hand in a claw or intrinsic minus position.

> **AXIOM** Immobilization is important in fracture healing and rigid internal fixation can be used to maintain proper joint function.

Immobilization for fractures should include one joint above and one joint below the fracture. Three weeks of immobilization usually allows adequate healing of most phalangeal and metacarpal fractures, and protected motion can begin at that time. Rigid internal fixation with plates and screws will allow early mobilization within the first few days postoperatively.

ELEVATION. The entire injured extremity should be elevated to reduce edema. If the patient is hospitalized, the extremity can be secured to an intravenous pole or a Carter foam pillow. At home, the extremity can be elevated above the heart using pillows at night and a sling during the day. Ace wraps, if used, should not be applied tightly, es-

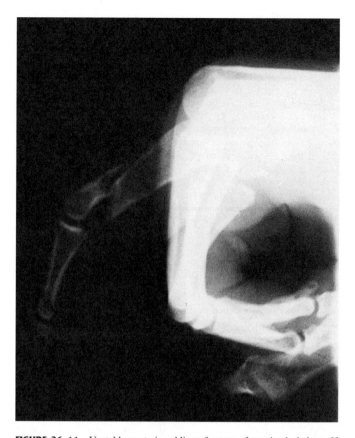

FIGURE 36–11 Unstable posterior oblique fracture of proximal phalanx. If the reduction of a phalangeal shift fracture seems stable, it can be treated by application of a splint or a cast. Most phalangeal fractures, however, especially those that are oblique, need to be stabilized with crossed Kirschner wires because of the deforming tendon forces.

pecially proximally, because this could cause swelling from venous occlusion.

Special Fractures

PHALANGEAL SHAFT FRACTURES. If a fracture of the shaft of a phalanx is stable and is not displaced, splinting in the "safe position," followed by protected motion for 2 to 3 weeks with a "buddy splint" (i.e., securing it to an adjacent, uninjured finger) will usually provide a good result. If the reduction of a phalangeal shaft fracture seems stable, it can be treated by application of a splint or a cast. Most phalangeal fractures, however, especially those that are oblique, need to be stabilized with internal fixation because of the deforming tendon forces (Fig. 36–11). This can usually be readily accomplished with crossed Kirschner wires, screws, or plates.

METACARPAL FRACTURES. Metacarpal fractures are extremely common. It is reasonable to cast nondisplaced fractures and reevaluate them within a week for displacement; however, one must be certain that there is no subtle rotation by noting if the plane of motion of each finger as it is flexed and extended is the same as in the noninvolved hand. Spiral and oblique fractures usually require open reduction and fixation with Kirschner wires or minicompression plates.

The common boxer's fracture involving the head of the fourth or fifth metacarpal can often be treated with closed reduction (Fig. 36–12). However, if there is more than 30 to 45° of volar angulation of the distal fragment that is not corrected, there will be: (a) volar loss of the knuckle contour, (b) pain in the palm at the metacarpal head with grasp, and (c) a zigzag deformity of the finger. Fractures of the heads of the third and fourth metacarpals require accurate reduction to prevent a prominent lump in the palm.

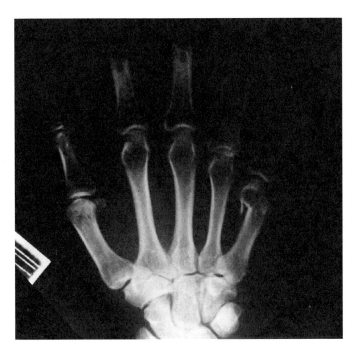

FIGURE 36–12 A boxer's fracture of the distal portion of the fifth metacarpal. A boxer's fracture involving the head of the fourth or fifth metacarpal can often be treated with closed reduction. However, if there is more than 30 to 45° of volar angulation of the distal fragment that cannot be corrected, there will be: (a) volar loss of the knuckle contour, (b) pain in the palm at the metacarpal head with grasp, and (c) a zigzag deformity of the finger. Fractures of the heads of the third and fourth metacarpals require accurate reduction to prevent a prominent lump in the palm.

Fractures of the base of the first metacarpal are usually classified as Bennett's or Rolando's fractures, depending upon the degree of comminution and the pattern of the fracture. These often require internal fixation.

CARPAL FRACTURES. One of the most common fractures within the carpus (wrist) is that of the scaphoid (navicular) bone. The scaphoid bone, which is in the proximal row of carpal bones, is a key element in the wrist, and it has a precarious distal and dorsally based blood supply. Scaphoid fractures frequently are not apparent on x-ray until there is resorption of bone on either side of the fracture line, and this usually takes at least 2 weeks.

AXIOM If pain and tenderness are present over the carpal scaphoid ("snuffbox" area) after trauma but the x-rays are negative, the hand and forearm should be immobilized with a splint or cast and repeat x-rays should be obtained in 2 weeks.

Significant pain or tenderness in the anatomical snuffbox should increase one's suspicion enough to immobilize that area within a well-molded spica cast or splint from the IP joint of the thumb to above the elbow, with the wrist slightly pronated and radially deviated. The cast should limit pronation and supination, but can allow flexion and extension at the elbow. Reevaluation with x-rays at 2 weeks is essential, and immobilization is continued until healing is assured.[21]

Open reduction with bone grafting may be necessary if there is displacement of the fragments. Sometimes scaphoid fractures are associated with lunate dislocations, producing what has been called a "transcaphoid perilunate dislocation."[22]

AXIOM Improper restoration of anatomical alignment and stability of the carpal bones can result in severe osteoarthritis, with pain and dysfuntion at the wrist.

Another common carpal fracture occurring from a fall on an outstretched hand involves the hook of the hamate, resulting in tenderness over the palm of the hand. The fracture is readily diagnosed on radiographs with a carpal tunnel view. A bone scan is also sensitive, particularly if the patient has clinical signs of a fracture but negative x-rays.[23]

AXIOM Carpal fractures are frequently associated with significant ligamentous injury and carpal instability that also need treatment.[24,25]

INTRA-ARTICULAR FRACTURES. Intra-articular fractures, especially if they are comminuted, can be difficult to treat.[26] Open reduction for significantly comminuted intra-articular fractures can make the joint surface worse, but if the fragments are large enough, one should attempt to reestablish a smooth articular surface. If this is not possible, an external traction device that will pull the finger out to adequate length and allow early range of motion exercises may be helpful. In some instances, this will allow a pseudoarthrosis to form, and this is preferable to a fixed deformity.[27]

AXIOM Improper immobilization of intra-articular fractures can lead to severe stiffness and deformity of the involved joints.

Whenever possible, early motion should be provided, without disturbing the fracture fragments. This generally provides the best functional result.

PHYSEAL INJURIES

AXIOM Physeal injuries can result in growth deformities, particularly if the reduction is not accurate.

A Salter I fracture, which is a separation of the epiphysis from the metaphysis, can usually be reduced rather easily. A type II Salter fracture is a fracture that passes through the epiphysial plate and then through the metaphysis, resulting in a triangular fragment of bone attached to the epiphysis. This fracture is usually easily reduced by closed techniques because the periosteum is generally intact. A type III fracture is an intra-articular fracture extending from the joint through the growth plate. A type IV fracture is an intra-articular fracture extending through the epiphysis, the growth plate, and metaphysis. Accurate reduction of type III and IV fractures is essential, even if it must be done surgically. A type V fracture is a crush injury.

AXIOM With any epiphyseal fracture, the patient and family must be warned about the likelihood of future growth disturbances and resultant deformities.

JOINT INJURIES WITHOUT FRACTURE. Joint injuries can be caused by trauma, infections, tumors, synovitis, and degenerative arthritis. When there is a mechanical disruption of the supporting ligaments, including the volar plate and collateral and accessory collateral ligaments, the injury may be either a dislocation or a fracture-dislocation (Fig. 36–13).

Dislocations. Most dislocations of digits, when seen early (under 12 hours after injury), can be reduced under local anesthesia. Whenever possible, x-rays should be taken before reduction to determine the presence of associated fractures, and postreduction x-rays are necessary to determine the adequacy of reduction.

Dorsal dislocation of the PIP joint of a finger is by far the most common dislocation in the hand, and it usually results from a combination of hyperextension and axial compression. It is common in athletic games that require handling of balls or tackling. With complete dislocation, the volar plate is torn, and the collateral ligament mechanism is torn to some degree. The status of the collateral ligaments determines the difficulty of closed reduction and the stability

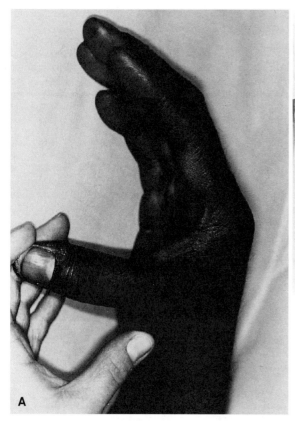

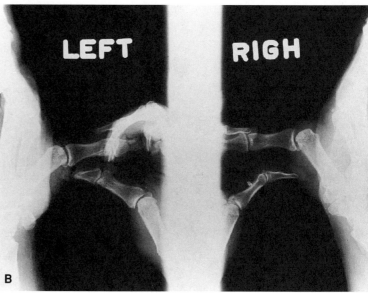

FIGURE 36–13   (A) Injury involving the ulnar collateral ligament of the metacarpophalangeal joint of the right thumb (gamekeeper's thumb) showing abnormal motion and (B) comparison stress x-rays views of right and left first MP joint with instability of the right MP joint.

after reduction. The more severely torn joints are easy to reduce, but they are unstable after reduction.

Manipulative reduction is accomplished by longitudinal traction on the finger and digital pressure distally against the dislocated joint surface. A proper digital anesthesic block usually renders this procedure painless and allows unimpeded testing of stability in anteroposterior and lateral planes after reduction. Because the volar plate is ruptured, there is almost always some hyperextension instability.

After reduction, the stability of the collateral ligaments and the palmar plate should be assessed by applying lateral and medial tension against the joints. If the ligaments are unstable, they should be repaired; this is especially important for an unstable thumb, but it is not as necessary for unstable PIP collateral ligaments. Unstable carpal-metacarpal joint dislocations require percutaneous Kirschner wire fixation.

AXIOM   Dislocations associated with severe distal ischemia should be reduced immediately without waiting for x-rays.

Failure of the circulation to return promptly after reduction of a dislocation requires emergency surgical exploration of the vessels that may be involved. Irreducible dislocations must also be treated operatively. Irreducible dislocations of phalangeal joints are most apt to occur with complete dorsal dislocations and interposition of the volar (palmar) plate. This problem is suspected when a skin dimple is present on the palmar aspect of the involved joint. Forceful attempts at reduction by just pulling on the finger can cause the volar (palmar) plate to move into the joint and make the joint irreducible. If gentle efforts at reduction with good anesthesia are not successful, the patient should be prepared for reduction in the OR. Strenuous efforts at reduction can cause severe injury to already traumatized tissues.

PITFALL ⊘

Improper reduction or prolonged immobilization of a dislocated phalanx can result in severe stiffness, deformity, and/or arthritis.

Once the joint is reduced, the digit can be moved immediately, but it should be protected with buddy taping. It can also be splinted in 30° of flexion for approximately 2 weeks, after which a guided motion therapy program can be instituted. Flexion contractures occur with prolonged immobilization. Radial and ulnar support with a dorsal blocking type splint, such as a silver ring splint, is excellent for this problem. It allows flexion of the finger and radial and ulnar stability without allowing excessive extension.

Lacerations into Joints

AXIOM   All dorsal lacerations of metacarpophalangeal joints should be assumed to be of human bite origin until proven otherwise.

Lacerations extending into joints can cause severe problems, especially if the joint becomes infected. Any laceration suspected to be from a fist fight is assumed to be a human bite. As mentioned previously, virulent human mouth flora, including peptostreptococcus and Eikenella corodens, can cause severe, invasive infections.

TENDON INJURIES

Whenever primary healing of skin lacerations can be expected, one should strive for primary tendon repairs. If large soft-tissue defects are present, the use of free or local flaps for coverage may also allow primary tendon repair. When this is not possible, delayed tendon repair, up to 4 weeks later, can provide satisfactory results.[28,29] Segmental tendon defects may be managed by tendon grafts or staged reconstruction.

AXIOM   Vital factors for success with tendon repairs are the patient's awareness of his postoperative restrictions and the importance of continuing occupational and physical therapy.

Extensor Tendons

GENERAL PRINCIPLES. There is a common misconception that extensor tendon injuries are repaired with ease and heal uneventfully. Although circulation to the extensor mechanism is good, factors conspiring against a good outcome are: (a) the flat, thin tendon distal to the metacarpophalangeal joint is easily frayed with improper handling, (b) the repaired tendon is easily ruptured by the much stronger flexors, and (c) the structure of the extensor system is quite complex, particularly at the level of the proximal interphalangeal joints.

The level of the injury to the extensor tendons will determine the deformity produced and the type of surgery required. Lacerated tendons at the wrist usually retract several centimeters, and a relatively long or separate incision is often required to find the proximal ends. If the injury is located over the distal half of the hand, the tendon ends separate minimally because of the fibrous (juncturae tendinum) connections between these tendons. At the level of the interphalangeal joints, the extensor tendons are intimately associated with the joint capsule, and injuries here often also involve the joint.

Extensor tendons should be repaired in the operating room with proper anesthesia and vascular control with a tourniquet. The wound is extended sufficiently to expose the ends of the tendon and accomplish repair. For lacerations involving the extensor mechanism on the fingers, additional exposure can be obtained with angled longitudinal incisions on the dorsum of the finger.

Minimal handling of the tissue, especially the ends and surface of the tendon, decreases subsequent scarring and adhesions. The tendons are repaired with 4-0 nonabsorbable suture using a modified Kirchmayr (Kessler), figure-of-eight, or other techniques.[30] The area of repair can be tidied up with interrupted or continuous finer sutures in the epitenon. Another technique uses the epitenon suture first.[31]

Postoperative care includes immobilization in a position that minimizes tension on the repair (i.e., wrist in extension, MP joints in slight flexion, and IP joints in full extension) for approximately 3 weeks, followed by 2 to 3 weeks of dynamic splinting and protected digital motion.[32]

BOUTONNIERE DEFORMITY. The extensor mechanism on the digits not only involves the long extensor tendons but also intrinsic contributions from the lumbrical and interosseus muscles. Disruption of the central portion of the extensor mechanism without proper repair can result in a boutonniere deformity. This deformity occurs if the lateral bands of the extensor mechanism are allowed to become volar to the moment arm of the proximal interphalangeal (PIP) joint. This causes flexion at the PIP joint and a compensatory hyperextension at the distal interphalangeal (DIP) joint.

An early boutonniere deformity resulting from a closed injury may be corrected by dynamic splinting of the PIP joint in extension, allowing the DIP joint to flex. This is best achieved by 4 weeks of immobilization in a Capener splint. The finger is monitored closely during that time to avoid worsening of the deformity. This is followed by intermittent removal of the splint and active and passive exercises for an additional 3 weeks.

MALLET FINGER. A mallet finger is an acute interruption of the extensor tendon at its insertion into the distal phalanx, resulting in an inability to extend the DIP joint. The joint is held flexed by the unopposed pull of the flexor profundus tendon even when the proximal IP joint is extended. Treatment requires immobilization with the DIP joint in slight hyperextension for 6 to 8 weeks.

If an associated avulsion fracture involves >33% of the joint surface or produces instability of such a magnitude that palmar subluxation of the distal segment is apparent on x-ray, open reduction is required. A mallet finger resulting from a laceration should be repaired by suture of the tendon and fixation of the associated fracture. Postoperatively, the DIP joint is splinted in extension for 6 to 8 weeks.

Flexor Tendons

GENERAL PRINCIPLES

AXIOM Tendons should be repaired as soon as possible.

The choices for repair of flexor tendons include primary repair within 18 to 24 hours of injury or delayed repair performed 3 to 10 days later when wound inflammation has subsided and there is no risk of infection. However, when the condition of the wound allows, it is preferable to perform a primary repair of the flexor tendons, followed by immediate controlled mobilization. This usually provides the best chance for a good functional recovery.[33-34] It is recommended that a protective splint be applied while the patient is waiting to go to the OR. This helps prevent contamination, tendon retraction, and conversion of an incomplete tear to one that is complete.

Relative contraindications to primary tenorrhaphy include evidence of infection or severe contamination, severe crush injuries with loss of skin and soft tissue, and segmental tendon defects. Secondary reconstruction is also preferable in injuries in which primary stabilization of associated fractures is difficult.

Flexor tendons are repaired in the operating room under adequate extremity anesthesia, using magnification as needed, and vascular control with a tourniquet. Flexor tendons are usually repaired with nonabsorbable 3-0 or 4-0 material, using a modified Kirchmayr (Kessler) suture (Fig. 36–14). This suture is employed because it tightens the pull on the tendon in a transverse manner and is not likely to pull through the longitudinally oriented fibers. This is followed by a running 6-0 suture in the epitenon to accurately coapt the tendon edges and to provide a smoother surface for gliding of the tendon within the sheath.[33] Now, four core sutures and a running circumferential suture are recommended.

Associated injuries to nerves and vessels are repaired at the same time whenever possible. Tissues are kept moist with lactated Ringer's solution during the operation, and satisfactory hemostasis must be assured before closure of the wound.

SITE OF INJURY. Injuries to the flexor tendons in the forearm and the hand are classically divided into five zones (Fig. 36–15):

Zone 1: Injuries to the profundus tendon distal to the insertion of the flexor digitorum superficialis on the middle phalanx should have a primary repair whenever possible. Lacerations in which the distal portion is more than 1.0 cm long can be repaired end-to-end. Alternatively, the distal sutures can be placed directly into the bone and then supported with a pull-out wire. Sutures directly into bone are more reliable, but they may result in a slight flexion deformity at the DIP joint.

Zone 2: Zone 2 extends from the insertion of the flexor digitorum superficialis to the start of the flexor tendon sheath at the distal palmar crease. This is often referred to as "no-man's-land" for flexor tendon injuries because of the poor results obtained in the past with primary tendon repairs. The profundus and superficialis tendons are closely held in a tight tendon sheath, and because of the adhesions that tend to form between these structures, most hand surgeons in the past only repaired the profundus tendon in this area if both tendons were cut. Only recently have surgeons routinely repaired both the superficialis and profundus tendons in this area.

Repair of the flexor tendons in no-man's-land demands careful technique and experience, and it is better to leave the tendons unrepaired than to proceed without expertise. If delayed repair is elected, it should be done within 2 weeks.

AXIOM Tendons lacerated in no-man's-land can be repaired early, but the procedure must be done carefully.

The tendon sheath is opened between the annular pulleys as needed to effect the repair. If insufficient distal tendon is present at the level of the laceration, a distal window in the sheath may facili-

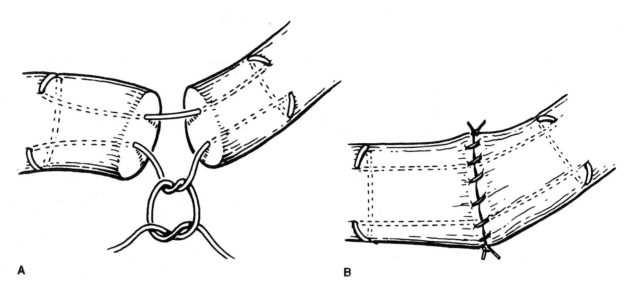

A   **B**

FIGURE 36–14 Flexor tendon repairs. Flexor tendon repairs are accomplished with intratendinous placement of a core 4-0 nylon modified Kessler suture when there is adequate length of the distal stump. A running, shallow epitendinous suture of 6-0 nylon is added to smooth the surface of the repair so that the tenorrhaphy site can glide freely within the tendon sheath system. (From: Markison RE. Tendon injuries in the hand. In: Champion HR, Robbs JV, Trunkey DD, eds. Rob and Smith's operative surgery: trauma surgery, part 2. 4th ed. Boston: Butterworths, 1989; 735.)

tate exposure and repair. Both the profundus and superficialis tendons are repaired in a similar fashion. There are several suture techniques for this, but the general principles are intratendinous suture without exposed knots, preservation of the pulley systems to whatever extent is possible, and early controlled passive mobilization. If the superficialis is cut at the level of its decussation or just distal to it, each slip should be repaired with a carefully placed, buried, nonabsorbable figure-of-eight suture or a modified Kirchmayr suture.

The tendon repairs in zone 2 must be performed meticulously, and the sutures are placed volar in the tendon to avoid the dorsal blood supply from the vinculum. The synovial sheath is also accurately repaired. This provides support and enhances nutrition of the tendons.

AXIOM   Proper tendon repairs include careful reconstruction of the tendon sheath pulleys.

If the flexor pulleys are destroyed, primary repair can be carried out in many ways, especially to repair the A2 pulley. If residual pulley is present at the periosteal attachment, multiple perforations are made in the fibrous periosteal attachment and a piece of tendon graft or extensor retinaculum is then woven through the holes in a lacing fashion and then over the flexor tendon. If the pulleys are not repaired, severe bowstringing of the tendon can occur later.

Zone 3: Zone 3, which extends from the carpal tunnel to the distal palmar crease, is also known as the lumbrical area in the palm. Primary tendon repair is always recommended at this level. The ends of the profundus tendon are tethered by the lumbrical muscles that originate from them and usually prevent proximal migration beneath the carpal ligament. In deep penetrating injuries in this area, one should also check the deep motor branch of the ulnar nerve. If this nerve is injured, its repair precedes that of the more anterior tendons.

Zone 4: Zone 4 is the carpal tunnel. Although all nine of the extrinsic flexors of the hand are relatively tightly collected in this area, primary repair usually provides excellent results. Excision of blood-soaked tenosynovium may be necessary before the repair. Part of the transverse carpal ligament should be left intact or repaired using Z-plasty if needed. Otherwise, the tendons may dislocate out of the canal when the wrist is flexed postoperatively.

Zone 5: Proximal to the carpal tunnel, primary repairs are indicated for all tendon lacerations in the forearm.

AXIOM   Early motion of repaired tendons without tension is important to maintain optimal function.

Recent developments in the research of tendon healing have shown that the eventual motion of the finger is improved when limited active extension and passive flexion by the use of rubber band traction is begun under close supervision within 2-3 days of repair. Absolute patient reliability and close personal follow-up by the surgeon are essential to this form of rehabilitation.

AXIOM   A change in the position of a finger during rubber band exercises should make one suspect disruption of a tendon repair.

If rubber band traction is used, two rubber bands are sewn to the fingernail or to a hook glued on the involved digit(s) at the end of the operation. A circumferential short-arm plaster dressing is then applied past the PIP joints, keeping the wrist in 30° of flexion and the metacarpophalangeal joints in 45° of flexion to allow relaxation of the repaired tendons. A safety pin is fixed in position at the level of the scaphoid (Fig. 36–16).

AXIOM   PIP flexion contractures are the most common complications of rubber band therapy.

Two to three days postoperatively, an ellipse is removed from the palmar surface of the dressing, and the rubber bands are attached to the safety pin. This draws the finger(s) into flexion and allows motion of the tendon juncture(s) within the sheath(s). The patient is instructed to extend the finger actively to the limits of the extensor splint and then allow the rubber band to bring the finger back into flexion. No active flexion is permitted for 3-4 weeks. The exercise is repeated 50 times, three to four times

After 3-4 weeks, the dressing is removed, and the patient is encouraged to gently squeeze an ordinary sponge in warm water for 5-10 minutes, three to four times a day. No power gripping is permitted for a further 2-3 weeks. Between exercises, a splint holding the wrist and hand in a position of function is applied for an additional week or two. The pull-through buttons and tie-over sutures are removed at 6 weeks.

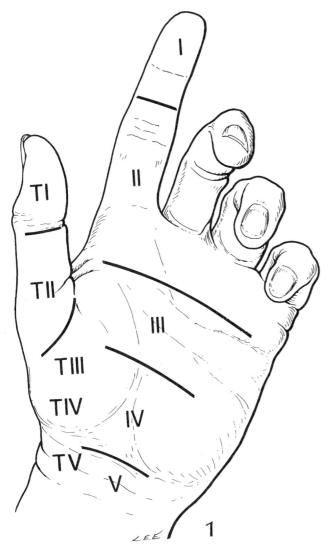

FIGURE 36–15 Zones of flexor tendon injuries. International agreement among hand surgeons has resulted in a standard nomenclature to describe the zones of flexor tendon injury. The region of the fibro-osseous sheath through which both the deep and superficial flexor tendons travel to the finger was previously called "no-man's-land" and is now referred to as zone II. (From: Markison RE. Tendon injuries in the hand. In: Champion HR, Robbs JV, Trunkey DD, eds. Rob and Smith's operative surgery: trauma surgery, part 2. 4th ed. Boston: Butterworths, 1989; 734.)

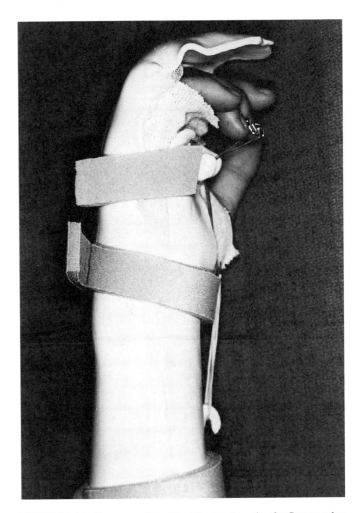

FIGURE 36–16 Extensor splint with rubber band traction for flexor tendon repairs in the fingers. An excellent result with flexor tendon repairs depends upon the injury, the repair, patient motivation, and compliance with appropriate postoperative therapy. Tendon healing research has shown that the eventual motion of the finger is improved when limited active extension and passive flexion by the use of rubber band traction is begun under close supervision within 2 to 3 days of repair. The rubber bands draw the finger into flexion and allow motion of the tendon within the sheath. The patient is instructed to extend the finger actively to the limits of the extensor splint and then allow the rubber band to bring the finger back into flexion. No active flexion is permitted for 3 to 4 weeks. The exercise is repeated 50 times, three times a day.

The patient's progress is objectively recorded as total active motion ([PIP + DIP] flexion - [PIP + DIP] extension deficit) divided by 175 and then multiplied by 100 equals the percent of normal active (PIP + DIP) motion. The patient's ability to approximate the tip of each finger to the proximal palmar crease should also be noted, and any deficiency should be measured. Both hands are compared. Unreliable patients with flexor tendon injuries are either kept fully immobilized for 3 weeks or treated by gentle passive motion of the injured finger(s) twice weekly, beginning 2-5 days postoperatively.

Another type of flexor tendon pathology is a trigger finger, due to stenosing tenosynovitis at the A1 pulley (Fig. 36–9).[35]

VASCULAR INJURIES

Revascularization of an injured hand is rarely necessary, but if the hand is ischemic, an experienced surgeon and hand center are needed. Some hands will survive despite transection of both the radial and ulnar arteries, and fingers may survive despite transection of both digital arteries. However, it is best to repair these paired structures, if the surgeon is technically able to do so.

AXIOM   Major arteries in the hand, wrist, and forearm should be repaired to maintain optimal blood flow to the hand.

With increasing sophistication in vascular microsurgery, improved results have been obtained in the repair of injuries to small vessels in the wrist and hand. Prior reports indicated only a 50% patency rate with such repairs. Because of the high occlusion rate and the excellent distal backflow which is usually present when either the radial or ulnar artery are lacerated at the wrist or in the hand, many surgeons felt it was not worthwhile to repair them. Now, with newer techniques, there is at least a 70% success rate with such repairs, and this results in much less cold intolerance.[36,37]

Proper repair of vascular injuries in the hand requires magnification and the use of microsurgical techniques. Before repair, the condition of the vessels must be carefully evaluated. Intimal separation (as may be reflected by a coiled appearance of the vessel) and hemorrhage along the path of the vessel indicate a severe stretch injury. With such an injury or when a primary anastomosis produces significant tension, it is best to resect the injured segment of the involved vessel and insert a reversed vein graft using veins from the dorsum of the hand or distal volar forearm.[38]

AXIOM   If a displaced fracture is associated with vascular compromise, the fracture should be promptly reduced. If the blood flow is still inadequate, prompt exploration with or without a preoperative arteriogram should be performed.

Occasionally, a displaced proximal fracture will impair blood flow to the hand. If the fracture cannot be reduced promptly or if reduction of the fracture fragments do not improve distal blood flow, it may be prudent to insert a temporary vascular shunt until the fracture can be reduced. Good proximal flow must be assured before anastomosis is performed. The retrograde bleeding is usually fairly good because of the excellent collateral circulation that is generally present. The adventitia of the vessels to be anastomosed is debrided 1 to 2 mm from the cut vessel ends, and after approximation with a double clamp, the anastomosis is performed. In general, digital vessels are repaired with 10-0 microsuture, and vessels in the distal forearm level may be repaired with 6-0 to 8-0 suture. Distal flow should occur immediately after release of the clamp. Most small leaks at the anastomosis will close with topical maneuvers such as gentle pressure and/or application of thrombin-soaked Gelfoam. With larger persistent leaks, additional (repair) sutures are often needed.

Anticoagulation is not used routinely postoperatively unless there has been a crush or stretch injury or the ischemia time was prolonged and collaterals are likely to thrombose. Under such circumstances, aspirin, 75 mg daily, plus low molecular weight dextran, 500 ml over the first 24 hours, is usually adequate. Color, capillary refill, and bleeding are fairly good indicators of satisfactory distal flow beyond the anastomosis or vein graft. Postoperative surveillance with Doppler flow probes and temperature probes can help assess continued patency of the vessels.

AXIOM   Crush injuries should be treated with early fasciotomy unless hand function and compartment pressures are normal and can be measured frequently.

After crush injuries or delayed revascularization of proximal vascular injuries, fasciotomy may be indicated to relieve increases in intracompartment pressures. If compartment pressures rise above the closing pressure of veins, secondary occlusion of capillary inflow can produce irreversible damage to muscles and nerves. Fasciotomy of the forearm flexor compartments and hand should be performed whenever this problem is suspected.[39,40]

AXIOM   The first symptom of compartment syndrome is often a subjective decrease in sensation or pain with passive stretch.

NERVE INJURIES AND NEUROPATHIES

Blunt injuries and closed fractures commonly reduce sensory perception and motor function for a few weeks, but permanent injury to the nerves is unlikely. Such deficits may be watched without surgery for up to 12 weeks, and recovery of sensation may occur quickly as the traumatic edema subsides.[41]

Neuropathies

ULNAR NERVE.   Common compressive neuropathies for the ulnar nerve include cubital tunnel syndrome at the elbow and Guyon's canal syndrome in the palm. Electrodiagnostic studies are helpful in determin-

ing the severity of these neuropathies. Initial treatment of ulnar neuropathies is conservative and includes keeping the elbow from being flexed or held overhead when asleep and avoidance of increased pressure on the elbow, such as when driving or sitting. If symptoms persist, surgery consists of the anterior subcutaneous or submuscular transposition of the ulnar nerve.

MEDIAN NERVE.   The median nerve is subject to multiple neuropathies, such as anterior interosseous, pronator, and carpal tunnel syndromes (Fig. 36–10). Physical findings should be confirmed by electrodiagnostic studies, including electromyographic and motor and sensory nerve conduction. Phalen's test is the timed reproduction of symptoms with the fully flexed wrist. Tinel's sign refers to paresthesias that occur distally when tapping over the median nerve at the volar carpal ligament. Inability to make an "O" sign by flexion of the index DIP and thumb IP joints is pathognomonic for an anterior interosseous syndrome.

RADIAL NERVE.   Compression radial neuropathies are rather uncommon. From an anatomic standpoint, the radial nerve is most vulnerable to compression at the junction of the upper and middle third of the arm where it passes in the musculospiral groove of the humerus. The nerve can be compressed by a displaced fraction of the humerus. It can also be occluded with "Saturday night palsy," in which an intoxicated individual sleeps with his head lying on his upper arm for prolonged periods.

Posterior interosseous nerve compression occurs where the radial nerve courses around the neck of the radius and enters the supinator muscle. Repetitive actions may cause hypertrophy of the supinator muscle which can compress the nerve, or a constant rotary effect of the radius against the nerve may result in direct flattening of the nerve and limited conduction. Radial nerve compression will lead to progressive loss of wrist and finger extension. Treatment of the posterior interosseous nerve compression syndrome requires decompression of the nerve. Incision of the supinator muscle is usually required. Improvement tends to occur if the compression is not severe, if the nerve is released relatively early, and if repetitive physical activities are not resumed.

Hypesthesia, paresthesias, or hyperesthesia on the dorsum of the thumb and index finger may be related to compression of the cutaneous branch of the radial nerve where it is compressed between the sheath of the brachioradialis and the shaft of the radius. A similar problem can also occur if the nerve is compressed by a swollen inflamed abductor pollicis longus at the wrist. Trauma about the wrist or the base of the thumb may also cause compression. Treatment usually involves release of the nerve from its fibrous canal under the tendon of the brachioradialis. If this nerve is compressed distally by adhesions to the annular ligament or by external compression, the etiologic factor should be removed.

Acute Neuronal Injuries

BLUNT.   Acute nerve injuries resulting from blunt trauma can be divided into neuropraxia (in which there is functional impairment but no anatomic disruption of the nerve), axontmesis (in which the axons, but not the nerve sheaths, are torn), and neurontmesis (in which both the axons and nerve sheaths are torn). It is also possible to have nerve injury at more than one site, as in "double crush syndrome."[42] Electrodiagnostic studies are usually postponed for 3 weeks after the initial trauma to be more accurate. They are then repeated at 3 months as indicated.

AXIOM   If there is a reasonable likelihood that injury to a nerve is only functional (neuropraxia), early exploration is not required; however, careful follow-up exams are extremely important.

PENETRATING NERVE INJURIES. Penetrating injuries with nerve dysfunction require examination of all possibly involved nerves at the time of surgery. Nerve repair is the last priority in emergency treatment, but it is important to reestablish nerve integrity by repair or grafting during the first 2 weeks because the hand cannot function optimally without sensation. In some instances, a nerve graft is needed to provide a tension-free repair.

When time and the wound permit, it is probably best to repair nerves primarily. Later repair involves mobilization of nerve ends, resection of neuromas, and, occasionally, repair under a bit more tension than would have been necessary initially. However, this is preferable to immediate repair of nerves that have contused or are in a badly contaminated wound.

AXIOM Lacerated nerves to the hand should have a grouped fascicular repair performed under an operating microscope whenever possible.

Nerve repair demands experience, meticulous technique, and proper instrumentation, including visual magnification. Sharply divided nerves are directly repaired, whereas crushed segments of nerve should be excised and grafted. Neural repair should be performed so that there is no tension at the repair site.

A nerve is composed of a number of fascicles; thus, neurorrhaphy should include a fascicular approximation followed by tension-free repair of the outer epineurium as a second layer. Even partial nerve lacerations can be repaired.[43] Sutures of 9-0 to 10-0 nylon are used. Accurate coaptation of the motor and sensory fascicles is important and can be aided with various vital stains, topographical aids, and nerve charts.[44]

If it is not possible to repair an injured nerve without tension, primary grafting is preferred.[45-47] The sural nerve provides adequate length (up to 30 cm) for procedures requiring multiple interfascicular grafts. Also, bilateral sural nerves may be harvested if needed. For defects in digital nerves, the lateral antebrachial cutaneous nerve at the elbow and the posterior interosseous nerve at the wrist are suitable donor choices;[28,29] however, the patient must be warned preoperatively about the sensory loss that results from taking the donor nerve. One must also be aware of the reconstruction options, such as neurovascular islands, that are available for correcting sensory dysfunction (Fig. 36–17).

NAIL INJURIES

AXIOM Aggressive, precise, early repair of an injured nail bed is the key to optimal healing.

Although seemingly trivial, nail bed injuries can cause great concern because of the severe nail deformities that can develop. Injury to the germinal and/or sterile matrix is virtually assured if there is a subungual hematoma associated with a distal tuft fracture from a crush injury. Because the nail bed is so important for adherence and conformity of the nail, it is essential with these injuries to remove the nail plate and accurately repair the nail bed. The nail plate can then be replaced to protect the nail bed.

If the eponychium and nail bed are both cut, they should be sutured separately (Fig. 36–11). A small wick of paraffin mesh or vaseline gauze should then be inserted under the eponychium to ensure that no adhesions develop between it and the nail bed. Such adhesions may produce a split nail. The paraffin mesh or vaseline gauze wick is extruded from under the eponychium as the fresh nail advances.

In children, dislocations of the nail matrix commonly occur with a slip of the distal phalangeal epiphysis, and the nail matrix may remain dislocated when the epiphyseal injury is reduced. In such cases, it may be necessary to suture the nail matrix back to its original place under the eponychium. Again, it is useful to insert a small paraffin

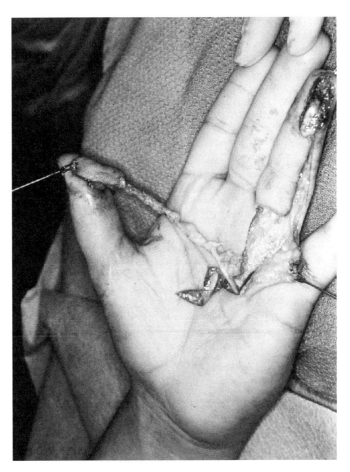

FIGURE 36–17 Neurovascular island transferred to an insensate thumb. If it is not possible to repair an injured nerve without tension, primary grafting is preferred, using either the sural nerve, the lateral antebrachial cutaneous nerve at the elbow, or the posterior interosseous nerve at the wrist. In some instances, transfer of an intact neurovascular island may be the best option.

mesh wick to hold the eponychium off the nail bed in the early phases of healing.

If nail matrix has been lost, a split matrix graft obtained from the great toe can be applied. Alternatively, a reversed dermal graft can be used, but the secondary adherence of the nail with this technique is much less reliable.[48-50]

SOFT TISSUE INJURIES ON THE FINGERTIPS

Fingertip injuries are a common problem. If the loss of skin is less than 1 cm^2, the pulp can be allowed to granulate and heal by secondary intention with good results. Larger defects without exposed bone can be covered with full-thickness skin grafts. Various deformities, such as a hook nail, can occur, but they can usually be corrected.[51]

AXIOM Whenever possible, one should try to maintain finger length after amputations. Excising bone to close the soft tissue at the tip is often easier, but generally it is not optimal therapy.

Large defects with exposed bone may be covered by a variety of techniques depending on the shape of the defect and the experience of the surgeon.[52,53] If bony length is desirable for function, especially when the distal interphalangeal joint or fingernail can be preserved, flap reconstruction is indicated. Two of the more common techniques are: (a) V-Y flap advancement from the volar surface or sides of the finger for closure of traverse and oblique dorsal amputations, and (b) cross-finger flaps for oblique amputations with loss of the volar pad. If bone protrudes from the soft tissue wound and flap coverage will not be used, the bone should be rongeured to a level below the wound surface, soft tissue mobilized over the bone, and a skin graft applied.

Most transected nerves in fingertip amputations that are untreated will form a terminal neuroma and can cause much pain unless cushioned by surrounding soft tissue. The tendency to form neuromas may be reduced by bipolar coagulation of the proximal end of the nerve while longitudinal traction is applied. The nerve is then severed just distal to the site of coagulation and allowed to retract into undamaged tissues.

AXIOM With proximal digital amputations, the tendon ends should not be secured over the end of the bone.

If an amputation occurs sufficiently proximal for the flexor and extensor tendons to be divided, these should be left retracted and should not be sutured over the stump of the phalanx. Incorrect tension of the flexor-extensor mechanism of the finger will not only impair movement of the affected finger, but may also affect the function of the digits next to it. The bone ends of the amputated stump should be rounded with bone instruments. If disarticulation through a joint is performed, the condyles and flexor aspect of the epicondyles should be beveled so that the stump is not bulbous.

Major soft tissue loss is a category of injury in which either a simple skin graft is inadequate or the recipient bed is unable to sustain a skin graft. If the epitenon is gone or the periosteum is compromised in a clean wound, a viable tissue flap should be used for coverage. If there is major skin loss with contamination, "aggressive" debridement and topical and intravenous antimicrobials are used to achieve a clean wound. Before later coverage with a graft or flap, one should confirm the presence of a clean wound by follow-up quantitative tissue cultures. It is important to not compromise hand function and positioning when one plans the subsequent coverage, whether it be with local flaps, regional flaps, tube flaps, free flaps, or artificial, synthetic, or autogenous skin.

ROLLER AND OTHER CRUSHING INJURIES

When the hand or separate digits are crushed between rollers, such as those found in bakeries or industrial settings, severe injury to multiple structures frequently results. Crushing of bone, nerves, and vascular structures can occur in combination and may be associated with degloving as the trapped part is forcibly withdrawn. Late loss of skin resembling a third-degree burn is not uncommon, and coverage with pedicle or free flaps is often necessary.

Massive swelling of the hand may result in compartment syndrome, and fasciotomy of the intrinsic muscles may be required. This should be performed early, especially if there will be any delay in definitive treatment. Vascular reconstruction is often difficult because of shearing and stretching of the vessels, and vein grafting is usually needed to repair the larger occluded vessels.

RING AVULSION INJURIES

Severe avulsion of skin and soft tissue may occur when a finger ring becomes caught on a stationary object, such as a nail or hook, as the individual is jumping or falling. The magnitude of injury ranges from a skin laceration to complete degloving or amputation. A useful classification divides the injuries into four categories.[54]

Class I: Circulation adequate
Class II: Circulation inadequate, no fracture
Class III: Circulation inadequate, with injury to bone or joints
Class IV: Amputation

Class I circumferential injuries may require a Z-plasty to prevent late contracture. Attempts to salvage digits with class II to IV injuries often require multiple or lengthy microsurgical operations. The

decision to proceed with salvage depends on the surgeon's experience and a thorough understanding of the problems by a motivated patient anxious to salvage the digit.[55]

REPLANTATIONS AND REVASCULARIZATIONS

Replantation is the restoration of viability to a totally amputated part of the body. Revascularization refers to restoration of the blood supply of an organ or limb that is incompletely amputated.[56]

AXIOM Replantation should only be attempted if experienced surgeons are available, if the wound ends are optimal, and microsurgical technique and careful follow-up care can be provided.

Microsurgery has made possible the replantation of a wide variety of amputated structures.[56] With proper indications, useful restoration of hand function may be accomplished in many instances. Surgical judgment is important, as the presence of an amputated part does not, in and of itself, provide an indication for replantation. Important considerations include the type and location of the trauma, associated injuries, age of the patient, health, occupational needs, and smoking history.

AXIOM Preservation of life should not be jeopardized to try to save a limb.

As the techniques of replantation have advanced, there have been fewer and fewer contraindications; however, life-threatening injuries always take precedence. Other significant contraindications to replantation include multiple-level amputations in the hand or digits, the "red line sign" along both neurovascular bundles (which indicates shearing in avulsion injuries),[38,57] and severe crushing of the amputated part, destroying the microcirculation. Relative contraindications include advanced age, chronic severe illness, single-digit amputations except the thumb, especially at levels proximal to the insertion of the sublimis tendon, prolonged ischemia (12 hours warm or 40 hours cold), and heavy contamination.

AXIOM With subtotal amputations, one should not generally salvage the part unless the ultimate outcome will be better than an amputation with a prosthesis.

Some of the more common indications for replantation include multiple amputations of digits and amputation of the thumb, especially in children.[57-60] If replantation seems feasible, the patient should be counseled preoperatively on the long-term effects of the operation. Some patients are better served in terms of function with a primary amputation than with multiple subsequent operations, decreased sensation, and pain and cold intolerance.[61] In order of importance, the priorities for replantation of amputated digits are the thumb, middle, ring, small, and index finger.

AXIOM The best time to do an amputation is at the first operation; otherwise, there can be greatly increased morbidity and anguish on the part of the patient.

Clean amputations at the level of the lunula (moon-shaped area at the base of a nail) may be able to be salvaged by a "cap" nonmicrosurgical technique or, preferably, at the level of the eponychium by a skilled microsurgeon.[62-64] If a surgical team skilled in replantation is not available, transfer to an appropriate facility should be arranged.[65] Limb survival rates greater than 90% can be expected in centers where the care of these complex injuries is routine.[59] Obviously, the promptness and quality of the initial care provided to the proximal wound and to the amputated parts are major determinants of the success of replantations. Immediate cooling of the amputated part is essential as well as rapid transport to an adequate facility that has a microvascular team.

Cooling of the amputated part is accomplished by completely covering it with a sterile sponge that has been lightly moistened with lactated Ringer's solution. It is then placed in a sealed, plastic, watertight envelope in a large container of regular ice. Dry ice should not be used.

AXIOM Because ischemic tissue easily develops frostbite, amputated parts should not come directly into contact with ice.

During replantation, the proximal and distal wounds are carefully explored and debrided. After this, all nerves, arteries, and veins are labeled with sutures. Bony fixation is then accomplished, often with about 5 mm of shortening. With hand replantations, the flexor tendons are usually repaired first. The hand is then turned over, and the extensor tendons are repaired. Lastly, the veins, arteries, nerves, and skin are repaired in that order. The replanted parts are then covered with a dressing and noncompressive protective casting or splinting.

The replanted part must be constantly watched for several days for the adequacy of perfusion. The surgeon(s) undertaking replantation must be prepared to reexplore the hand if vascular compromise becomes evident. Some anticoagulation, preferably with aspirin and/or dextran, may be indicated if the amputation was produced by means other than a clean cut. Full dose heparin may increase the incidence of hematomas which in themselves can compress smaller vessels.

INJURIES FROM PRESSURE INJECTIONS

Pressure injection injuries can cause severe tissue loss, dysfunction, and deformities and must be treated as an emergency. The nature of the injected substance must be ascertained because methods to remove the substance from the tissues and the prognosis will vary. Immediate exploration and meticulous debridement are required.[66-68]

AXIOM One should assume that all injection injuries are severe and that they require extensive debridement and exploration in the OR.

The main pitfall with injection injuries lies in the initial evaluation. Often there will be minimal pain and edema and only a small puncture wound at the injection site. Thus, there may be little clinical evidence of the amount of underlying injury; however, if the material injected is radiopaque, plain x-rays may indicate the extent of the injection. The severity of these injuries must be recognized, and emergency surgical exploration and debridement must be undertaken to obtain maximal tissue survival with the least risk of later infection and deformities. Extravasation injuries, depending on the substances in the tissues, may also need immediate attention.[69]

LOSS OF SKIN

Loss of skin frequently accompanies trauma to the hand. Because tendons, bones, joints, nerves, and vessels tend to desiccate if they are left exposed, some type of coverage of these tissues is important. If infection or swelling precludes primary closure, temporary coverage with moist dressings or skin grafts may be satisfactory.

AXIOM Exposed tendons, vessels, nerves, and bone should be kept moist and covered as soon as possible.

Small skin defects on the dorsum of the hand or fingers can often be closed primarily after mobilization of the skin. If a large defect is present but the tendon sheaths are still present, a split-thickness skin graft can often be used successfully. If bare tendon is exposed, rota-

tional or transposition flaps are indicated. Occasionally, a reverse cross-finger flap can be used.[70]

Skin grafts on the volar surface of the fingers or palm should be of similar color and texture, especially for patients with darker pigmented skin. Potential donor sources are the hypothenar eminence and the non-weight bearing aspect of the foot.

Avulsed skin flaps that have been defatted may be used as full-thickness skin grafts as long as minimal crush occurred during the injury. Skin flaps with an attachment at the proximal base and intact venous drainage may simply be replaced. The skin color and evidence of capillary bleeding and refill help determine what level of the flap may be preserved. Distally attached flaps generally do not have intact venous drainage and are best detached, defatted, and reapplied as free full-thickness skin grafts.

Large defects with exposed tendon, bone, joint, and blood vessels require flap coverage. Local pedicle flaps may be sufficient if the size and the location of the wounds permit.[71] However, a microvascular free flap transfer may be preferred for several reasons: the limb is not dependent, a second operative procedure is not required, the hospital stay is shorter, and a flap similar to the recipient site can be selected more readily.[14] With large open wounds, an abdominal flap may be helpful.

THERMAL INJURIES

The severity of thermal injuries varies with the temperature and duration of application. These injuries can be divided into those that will usually heal without operative intervention and those that require surgery. First-degree and superficial second-degree burns will usually heal within 14 days unless they become infected. Deep second-degree and full-thickness burns are best treated with prompt excision and grafting and an aggressive rehabilitation program.

If there is possible vascular compromise to the hand by a circumferential burn, one should also make sure that the circulating volume is adequate for good tissue perfusion. This includes checking the proximal axillary, brachial, radial, and ulnar pulses.

AXIOM The first sign of vascular compromise to the hand after a deep proximal circumferential burn is usually a subjective change in the sensation of the fingers.

Loss of pulses tends to occur quite late and escharotomies are performed before this occurs. Escharotomies are begun on the "nondominant" sides of the fingers. Properly performed escharotomies of just the burned skin and subcutaneous tissue usually restore an adequate circulation and also decrease compartment pressures. If there is still any evidence of vascular compromise, however, formal fasciotomies, including digital fasciotomies of the Grayson and Cleland ligaments around the neurovascular bundles, may be required.

Much controversy exists regarding optimal treatment of superficial partial-thickness burns characterized by blistering. Some feel that the blister fluid is protective because analysis of the blister fluid has revealed increased levels of IgG and IgM. If penicillin had been administered, this is also found in the blister fluid. However, blister fluid analysis has also shown increased levels of thromboxane, which causes platelet aggregation and vasoconstriction and can be deleterious to local blood flow and healing.

Clinical studies looking at infection rates, duration of pain, and time of healing suggest that one should not debride blisters. They should either be left intact or simply aspirated. However, other considerations in determining what to do with burn blisters include the potential for proper follow-up and the materials available to cover the blister site. For example, if synthetic coverings, such as

Biobrane gloves, are applied over debrided blisters, the patients can usually move their fingers quite freely and relatively little care is needed afterwards. Nevertheless, there should be careful follow-up to make sure that the patient is following instructions and that no infection has developed. Such outpatient follow-up should continue until the skin is well-healed, which usually takes at least 10-14 days.

Postinjury Therapy

To achieve optimal results after major hand injuries, one needs to communicate closely with the physical or occupational therapists who are part of the hand-care team. It is also essential to thoroughly educate the patient on: (a) the relationship between the ultimate function of the hand and the program of physical and occupational therapy and (b) the time that will be lost from work. Since the therapists often spend large amounts of time with these patients, they should be in close communication with the surgeon and tell him of any changes in the status of the patient.

AXIOM   Recovery of hand function is often only as good as the postinjury occupational and physical therapy.

COMPLICATIONS OF HAND INJURIES

Complications may be defined as unexpected results from injury or treatment. These should be differentiated from the inability to restore function which is primarily a result of the injury itself. The quality of the initial treatment is a major factor in determining outcome, and complications from unforeseen factors can best be prevented by constant vigilance and prompt changes in therapy as needed.

PITFALL ⊘

> *With hand infections, one should not assume that swelling of the back of the hand is a result of a dorsal process.*

Any hand injury may become infected. There are multiple spaces in the hand that can become involved (Fig. 36–18). One needs to be familiar with these to provide adequate drainage of the deeper hand infections. Volar infections in the hand can often cause significant dorsal swelling, and one may be fooled into thinking that the process is actually dorsal rather than volar in origin. Individuals who are intravenous drug abusers may also be prone to special types of infections at the sites of injection.[72]

Infections around the nail (paronychia) need to be drained early and adequately. If the nail bed needs to be removed, care must be taken to avoid injury to the germinal matrix. Felons need to be drained thoroughly because residual bacteria may infiltrate into the septa, but one should avoid a fish mouth incision through the end of the finger.[73]

Kanavel described four classic signs of tenosynovitis in the fingers: flexed position, fusiform swelling, tenderness along the flexor tendon sheath, and pain on passive extension. These infections usually require surgical drainage of the tendon sheath plus intravenous antibiotics.

SUMMARY

Repair of hand injuries is an exciting field of surgery, and it is technically demanding if optimal function and appearance are to be obtained. The goal of every surgeon treating hand injuries should be to restore normal anatomy and function as soon as possible and to provide the best possible rehabilitative therapy. This also involves treating not just the hand injury but the patient as a whole human being.

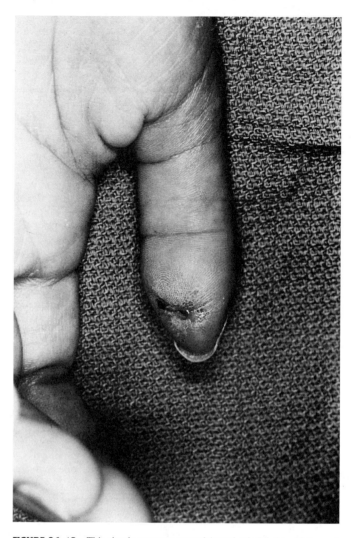

FIGURE 36–18   This simple puncture wound (now healed) led to a felon and then to osteomyelitis. Puncture wounds of the distal volar pad of the finger may be particularly dangerous because any resultant infection involving the closed spaces can rapidly lead to osteomyelitis.

⊘   **FREQUENT ERRORS**

1. *Believing that secondary reconstructions of the hand can make up for suboptimal primary care.*
2. *Assuming a tendon is not injured because the finger moves properly.*
3. *Repairing tendon or deep soft tissue injuries of the hand outside the OR.*
4. *Exploring hand injuries without a proximal tourniquet or adequate anesthesia.*
5. *Inadequately debriding a hand wound because the tissue in question might be helpful in coverage of underlying structures.*
6. *Attempting to fixate unstable finger fractures with splints.*
7. *Not warning the patient or family about subsequent growth abnormalities that may occur with hand injuries in children.*
8. *Immobilizing joints for a prolonged period after tendon repairs, fractures, or dislocations, especially in elderly patients.*
9. *Failure to accurately repair nail bed lacerations.*
10. *Failing to rapidly determine the cause of excessive pain or decreased sensation in a hand after trauma.*
11. *Failure to perform primary amputation on a viable but unsalvageable extremity.*

12. *Not suspecting human bite wounds, chemical burns, or compartment syndrome.*
13. *Not checking skeletal alignment clinically.*
14. *Not checking sensation before giving an anesthetic block.*

▼▼▼▼▼▼▼▼▼▼▼▼▼▼▼▼▼▼▼▼▼▼▼▼▼▼▼▼▼▼▼▼▼

SUMMARY POINTS

1. The quality of the initial management of a hand injury is a major determinant of outcome.
2. If the pulley system is not restored after repair of a flexor tendon, the tendon tends to bowstring and flexion is impaired.
3. Not performing a careful systematic examination of the hand, even with apparently minor injuries, can lead to disaster.
4. Awareness of the preinjury use of the hands and the expectations of the patient after treatment can be of great importance in planning treatment.
5. With hand injuries, one should perform a full assessment before taking off the bandage or manipulating the wound. The function of the hand is as informative as the wound itself.
6. Sharp lacerations of a tendon in the hand often also involve other structures, such as vessels or nerves.
7. The function of each tendon should be evaluated separately, but it must be remembered that a partially lacerated tendon that needs repair may seem to function relatively well.
8. When there is a finger laceration, tenderness over a flexor tendon sheath may indicate a partial tendon tear, even if the finger can move properly.
9. Painful extension against resistance may be the only clinical evidence of partial extensor tendon lacerations.
10. Sensation on the hand is ideally evaluated by two-point discrimination testing.
11. A false-positive Allen's test can occur if the patient is hypovolemic, is hypotensive, has a low cardiac output, is receiving vasoconstrictor drugs, or overextends the fingers.
12. If emergent exploration of an injured hand is warranted, one should not delay the surgery to obtain arteriography.
13. Anesthetic blocks for diagnostic purposes should not be performed except by the surgeon who will be providing the definitive care of the hand injury.
14. Ideally, hand injuries should be repaired in an operating room where the wounds can be examined completely and the environment is more sterile.
15. An excessive volume of anesthesia can cause venous congestion and vascular compromise in a finger.
16. Most penetrating wounds of the hand should be thoroughly explored in the operating room with a proximal tourniquet applied to provide maximum visibility of all structures.
17. There is no substitute for thorough surgical debridement and lavage for preventing wound infections after trauma.
18. If there is any question about the need for a fasciotomy, it should either be done or serial compartment pressures should be performed. Open fractures can still have compartment syndrome.
19. Hand wounds caused by contact with another individual's teeth have a high risk of severe infection and should not be closed; they should be explored, debrided, and irrigated.
20. Unstable hand and wrist fractures need fixation, not an aluminum splint.
21. Patients with open fractures should receive antibiotics against gram-positive cocci (such as streptococci, Staphylococcus aureus), aerobic gram-negative bacilli (such as Escherichia coli), and mouth anaerobes.
22. Immobilization is important in fracture healing and rigid internal fixation can be used to maintain proper joint function.
23. If pain and tenderness are present over the carpal scaphoid ("snuffbox" area) after trauma but the x-rays are negative, the hand and forearm should be immobilized with a splint or cast and repeat x-rays should be obtained in 2 weeks.

24. Improper restoration of anatomic alignment and stability of the carpal bones can result in severe osteoarthritis at the wrist.
25. Carpal fractures are frequently associated with significant ligamentous injury and carpal instability that also need treatment.
26. Improper immobilization of intra-articular fractures can lead to severe stiffness and deformity of the involved joints.
27. Physeal injuries can result in growth deformities, particularly if the reduction is not accurate.
28. With any epiphyseal fracture, the patient and family must be warned about the likelihood of future growth disturbances and resultant deformities.
29. Dislocations associated with severe distal ischemia should be reduced immediately without waiting for x-rays.
30. Improper reduction or prolonged immobilization of a dislocated phalanx can result in severe stiffness, deformity, and/or arthritis.
31. All dorsal lacerations of metacarpophalangeal joints should be assumed to be of human bite origin until proven otherwise.
32. Vital factors for success with tendon repairs are the patient's awareness of his postoperative restrictions and the importance of continuing occupational or physical therapy.
33. Tendons should be repaired as soon as possible.
34. Tendons lacerated in no-man's-land can be repaired early, but the procedure must be done carefully.
35. Proper tendon repairs include careful reconstruction of the tendon sheath pulleys.
36. Early motion of repaired tendons without tension is important to maintain optimal function.
37. A change in the position of a finger during rubber band exercises should make one suspect disruption of a tendon repair.
38. PIP flexion contractures are the most common complications of rubber band therapy.
39. Major arteries in the hand, wrist, and forearm should be repaired to maintain optimal blood flow to the hand.
40. If a displaced fracture is associated with vascular compromise, the fracture should be promptly reduced. If the blood flow is still inadequate, prompt exploration with or without a preoperative arteriogram should be performed.
41. Crush injuries should be treated with early fasciotomy unless hand function and compartment pressures are normal and can be measured frequently.
42. The first symptom of compartment syndrome is often a subjective decrease in sensation or pain with passive stretch.
43. If there is a reasonable likelihood that injury to a nerve is only functional (neuropraxia), early exploration is not required; however, careful follow-up exams are extremely important.
44. Lacerated nerves to the hand should have a grouped fascicular repair performed under an operating microscope whenever possible.
45. Aggressive, precise, early repair of an injured nail bed is the key to optimal healing.
46. Whenever possible, one should try to maintain finger length after amputations.
47. With proximal digital amputations, the tendon ends should not be secured over the end of the bone.
48. Replantation should only be attempted if experienced surgeons are available, if the wound ends are optimal, and if microsurgical technique and careful follow-up care can be provided.
49. Preservation of life should not be jeopardized to try to save a limb.
50. With subtotal amputations, one should not generally salvage the part unless the ultimate outcome will be better than an amputation with a prosthesis.
51. The best time to do an amputation is at the first operation; otherwise, there can be greatly increased morbidity and anguish on the part of the patient.
52. Because ischemic tissue easily develops frostbite, amputated parts should not come directly into contact with ice.
53. One should assume that all injection injuries are severe and that they require extensive debridement and exploration in the OR.

54. Exposed tendons, vessels, nerves, and bone should be kept moist and covered as soon as possible.

55. The first sign of vascular compromise to the hand after a deep proximal circumferential burn is usually a subjective change in the sensation of the fingers.

56. Recovery of hand function is often only as good as the postinjury occupational and physical therapy.

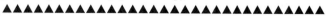

REFERENCES

1. Kleinert HE, Freund RK. Hand Injury. In: Moore EE Mattox KL, Feliciano DV, eds. Trauma. 2nd ed. Norwalk, CT: Appleton & Lange, 1991; 607-621.
2. Angermann P, Lohmann. Injuries to the hand and wrist: a study of 50,272 injuries. J Hand Surg 1993;18B:642.
3. Matlous HS, Yousif NJ. Peripheral nerve anatomy and innervation pattern. Hand Clin 1992;8:201.
4. Prasartritha T, Liopolvanish P, Rojanakit A. A study of the posterior interosseous nerve (PIN) and the radial tunnel in 30 Thai cadavers. J Hand Surg 1993;18A:107.
5. Viegas SF, Patterson RM, Hokanson JA, et al. Wrist anatomy: incidence of distribution and correlation of anatomic variations, tears and arthrosis. J Hand Surg 1993;18:463.
6. Zook EG. Anatomy and physiology of the perionychium. Hand Clin 1990; 6:1.
7. Dellon AL, Mackinnon SE, Brandt KE. The marking of the Semmes-Weinstein nylon monofilaments. J Hand Surg 1993;18A:756.
8. Levinsohn DG, Gordon L, Sessler D. The Allen's test: analysis of four methods. J Hand Surg 1991;16A:279.
9. Novak CB, Mackinnon SE, Patterson GA. Evaluation of patients with thoracic outlet syndrome. J Hand Surg 1993;18A:292.
10. Rothkopf DM, Chu B, Gonzalez F, et al. Radial and ulnar artery repairs: assessing patency rates with color Doppler ultragonographic imaging. J Hand Surg 1993;18A, 626.
11. Mubarak SJ, Hargens SAR, Owens CA, et al. The wick catheter technique for measurement of intramuscular pressure. J Bone Joint Surg 1976; 58A:1016.
12. Whitesides TE, Haney TC, Morimoto K, et al. Tissue pressure measurements as a determinant for the need of fasciotomy. Clin Orthop Rel Res 1975;113:43.
13. Moed BR, Fakhouci AJ. Compartment syndrome after low-velocity gunshot wounds to the forearm. J Orthop Trauma 1991;5:134.
14. Lister, GD. Injury. In: Lister GD, ed. The hand: diagnosis and indications. New York: Churchill Livingstone, 1984; 34, 59, 82.
15. Duncan RW, Freeland AE, Jubaley ME, et al. Open hand fractures: an analysis of the recovery of active motion and of complications. J Hand Surg 1993;18A: 387.
16. Weiss APC, Hasting H. Distal unicondylar fractures of the proximal phalanx. J Hand Surg 1993;18A:594.
17. Gonzalez MH, McKay W, Hall RF. Low-velocity gunshot wounds of the metacarpal: treatment by early stable fixation and bone grafting. J Hand Surg 1993;18A:267.
18. Piemer CA, Smith RJ, Leffert RD. Distraction-fixation in the primary treatment of metacarpal bone loss. J Hand Surgery 1981;6:111.
19. Gustilo RB, Anderson JT. Prevention of infection in the treatment of 1025 open fractures of long bones. J Bone Joint Surg 1976;58A:453.
20. Patzakis MJ, Harvey JP, Ivler D. The role of antibiotics in the management of open fractures. J Bone Joint Surg 1974;56A:532.
21. Herndon JH, ed. Scaphoid fractures and complications. American Academy of Orthopaedic Surgeons Monograph Series 1994.
22. Herzberg G, Comtet JJ, France L, et al. Perilunate dislocations and fracture-dislocation: a multicenter study. J Hand Surg 1993;18A: 768.
23. Lacser CF, Brondum V, Wienholtz G, et al. An algorithm for acute wrist trauma. J Hand Surg 1993;18B:207.
24. Dobyns JH, Linschied RL. Fractures and dislocations of the wrist. In: Rockwood CA, Green DP, eds. Fractures. Philadelphia: Lippincott, 1984; 1:411.
25. O'Brien ET. Acute fracture and dislocations of the carpus. In: Lichtman DM, ed. The wrist and its disorders. Philadelphia: Saunders, 1988; 129.
26. Stern PJ, Roman RJ, Kiefhaber TR, et al. Pilon fractures of the proximal interphalangeal joint. J Hand Surg 1991;16A:844.
27. Shibata T, O'Flanagan SJ, Ip FK, et al. Articular fracture of the digits: a prospective study. J Hand Surg 1993;18B:225.
28. Schneider LH, Hunter JM, Norris TR, et al. Delayed flexor tendon repair in no man's land. J Hand Surg 1977;2:452.
29. Tsuge K, Ikuta Y, Matsuishi Y. Repair of flexor tendons by intratendinous suture. J Hand Surg 1977;2:436.
30. Greenwald DP, Hong HZ, May JW. Mechanical analysis of tendon suture techniques. J Hand Surg 1994;19A:641.
31. Sanders WE. Advantages of epitenon first suture placement technique in flexor tendon repair. Clin Orthop 1992;280:198.
32. Karlander LE, Berggren M, Larsson M, et al. Improved results in zone 2 flexor tendon injuries with a modified technique of immediate controlled mobilization. J Hand Surg 1993;18B:26.
33. Lister GD, Kleinert HE, Kutz JE, et al. Primary flexor tendon repair followed by immediate controlled mobilization. J Hand Surg 1977; 2:441.
34. Kleinert HE, Verdan C. Report of the committee on tendon injuries. J Hand Surg 1983;8:794.
35. Patel MR, Bassini L. Trigger fingers and thumb: when to splint, inject, or operate. J Hand Surg 1992;17A:110.
36. Pichora DR, Masear VR. Efficacy of direct repair to partial arterial lacerations. J Hand Surg 1994;19A:552.
37. Panetta TF, Hunt JP, Buechter KJ, et al. Duplex ultrasonography versus arteriography in the diagnosis of arterial injury: an experimental study. J Trauma 1992;33:627.
38. VanBeek AL, Kutz JE, Zook EG. Importance of the ribbon sign, indicating unsuitability of the vessel in replanting a finger. Plast Reconst Surg 1979;61:689.
39. Brooker AF, Pezeshki C. Tissue pressure to evaluate compartment syndrome. J Trauma 1979;19:689.
40. Matson FA, Winquist RA, Krugmire RB. Diagnosis and management of compartmental syndromes. J Bone Joint Surg 1980;62A:286.
41. Kline DG. Timing for exploration of nerve lesions and evaluation of the neuroma-in-continuity. Clin Ortho Rel Res 1982;163:42.
42. McKinnon SE. Double and multiple "crush" syndrome: double and multiple entrapment neuropathy. Hand Clinics 1992;8:369.
43. Hurst LC. Partial lacerations of median and ulnar nerves. J Hand Surg 1991;16A 207.
44. Deutinger M, Girsch W, Burggasser G, et al. Peripheral nerve repair in the hand with and without motor sensory differentiation. J Hand Surg 1993;18A:426.
45. Millesi H, Meissl G, Gerger A. The interfascicular nerve-grafting of the median and ulnar nerves. J Bone Joint Surg 1972;54A:727.
46. Terzis JK, Strauch B. Microsurgery of the peripheral nerve: a physiological approach. Clin Orthop Rel Res 1978;133:39.
47. Hentz VR. The nerve gap dilemma: a comparison of nerves repaired end to end under tension with nerve grafts in a primate model. J Hand Surg 1993;16A:417.
48. Shepard GH. Treatment of nail bed avulsions with split-thickness nail bed grafts. J Hand Surg 1983;8:49.
49. Zook EG, Guy RJ, Russel RC. A study of nail bed injuries: causes, treatment and prognosis. J Hand Surg 1984;9A:247.
50. Van Beek AL, Kassan MA, Adson MH, et al. Manangement of acute fingernail injuries. Hand Clin 1990;6.23.
51. Kuman VP, Satku K. Treatment and prevention of "hook nail" deformity with anatomic correlation. J Hand Surg 1993;18A:617.
52. Atasoy E, Ioakimidis E, Kasdan ML, et al. Reconstruction of the amputated fingertip with a triangular volar flap. J Bone Joint Surg 1970; 52A:921.
53. Kleinert HE, McAlister CG, MacDonald CJ, et al. A critical evaluation of cross finger flaps. J Trauma 1974;14:756.
54. Kay S, Werntz J, Wolff TW. Ring avulsion injuries: classification and prognosis. J Hand Surg 1989;14A:204.
55. McGeorge DD, Stilwell JH. The management of the complete ring avulsion injury. J Hand Surg 1991;16B:413.
56. Axelrod TS, Buchler U. Severe complex injuries to the upper extemity: revascularization and replantation. J Hand Surg 1991;16A:574.
57. Sixth People's Hospital of Shanghai. Replantation of severed fingers: clinical experience in 162 cases involving 270 severed fingers. Chinese Med J 1973;1:3.
58. Kleinert HE, Tsai TM. Miscrovascular repair in replantation. Clin Orthrop Rel Res 1978;133:205.
59. Kleinert HE, Jablon M, Tsai TM. An overview of replantation and results of 347 replants in 245 patients. J Trauma 1980;20:390.
60. Stevenovic MV, Vucetic C, Bumbasirevic M, et al. Avulsion injuries of the thumb. Plast Reconstr Surg 1991;87:1099.

61. Chow Sp, Ng C. Hand function after digital amputation. J Hand Surg 1993;18B:125.

62. Rose EH, Norris MS. The "cap" technique: nonmicrosurgical reattachment of fingertip amputations. J Hand Surg 1989;14A:513.

63. Goldner RD, Stevanovic MV, Nunley JA, et al. Digital replantation at the level of the distal interphalangeal joint and the distal phalanx. J Hand Surg 1989;14A:214.

64. Foucher G, Norris RW. Distal and very distal digital replantations. Br J Plast Surg 1992;45:199.

65. Yamano Y. Replantation of fingertips journal 1993;18B:157.

66. Gelberman R, Posch JL, Jurist JM. High-pressure injection injuries of the hand. J Bone Joint Surg 1975;57A:935.

67. Schoo MJ, Scott FA, Boswick JA. High-pressure injection injuries of the hand. J Trauma 1980;20:229.

68. Pinto MR, et al. High-pressure injection injuries of the hand: review of 25 patients managed by open wound technique. J Hand Surg 1993;18A:125.

69. Gault DT. Extravasation injuries. Br J Plast Surg 1993;46:91.

70. Atasoy E. Reversed cross-finger subcutaneous flap. J Hand Surg 1982;7:481.

71. Meland NB, Lincenberg SM, Cooney WP III, et al. Experience with the island radial forearm flap in local hand coverage. J Trauma 1989;29:489.

72. Gonzalez MH, Garst J, Nourbash P, et al. Abscesses of the upper extremity from drug abuse by injection. J Hand Surg 1993;18A:868.

73. Canales FL, Newmeyer WL, lll, Kilgore ES Jr. The treatment of felons and paronychias. Hand Clin 1989;5:515.

Chapter **37A** Thermal Injuries

R. RUSSELL MARTIN, M.D.

WILLIAM K. BECKER, M.D.

WILLIAM G. CIOFFI, M.D.

BASIL A. PRUITT, JR., M.D.

INTRODUCTION

Of the two million people burned each year in the United States, approximately 70,000 require hospital treatment. Of these, 80% can be managed in a general hospital setting; however, the remaining 20% should receive care at a burn center. The American Burn Association has established the following guidelines for determining which patients will benefit from burn center care:[1]

1. Greater than 10% total body surface area (TBSA) burns in patients less than 10 or greater than 50 years of age.
2. Greater than 20% TBSA burns in patients 10 to 50 years of age.
3. Significant burns of the face, hands, feet, genitalia, perineum or skin overlying major joints.
4. Full-thickness burns greater than 5% TBSA.
5. Significant electric injury, lightning injury, and chemical burns.
6. Inhalation injury.
7. Burns associated with significant preexisting illness.
8. Burns associated with a need for special social or emotional support, rehabilitation, and cases involving child abuse or neglect.

The management of such burns in specialized centers permits an organized approach to treatment and ensures the availability of the expertise needed to address the multisystem effects of these severe injuries. Advances in treatment at burn centers have resulted in a significant decrease in mortality. When the United States Army Institute of Surgical Research began studying burns in 1947, a 43% TBSA burn in the young adult (15-40 years) age group was associated with only a 50% survival. The LD-50 for a burn in the same age group during the last decade rose to 75% TBSA.

PREHOSPITAL CARE

Burn Wounds

Burn wounds (other than those caused by chemical agents) require minimal early care. At the scene, the patient should be removed from the source of heat or flame. Clothing should be promptly removed from the involved areas because garments may continue to smolder or retain sufficient heat to extend the area or depth of the wound. If the patient is seen immediately after injury, application of cool or cold water or cold towels affords relief of pain and may lessen the degree of injury. However, after several minutes the heat will have dissipated from the wound and further application of cold water or compresses will not prevent further damage and may result in systemic hypothermia. Covering the patient with a clean dry sheet will decrease pain from convection of air over the surface of the burn. No other specific early wound care is required. More elaborate dressings or topical agents will interfere with assessment and treatment of the wound at the burn center.

PITFALL ⊘

Wet dressings and cold compresses applied to large burn wounds for prolonged periods may cause hypothermia.

Chemical Burns

Chemical exposure is a special situation in which prompt appropriate care of the wound is essential to prevent additional direct tissue injury and systemic toxicity resulting from continued absorption of the chemical.[2] The victim's shoes, gloves, and other clothing should be removed immediately, but care should be taken to not spread or splash the chemical on caregivers or bystanders. Identification of the offending agent is important to determine proper decontamination procedures. For instance, white phosphorus, which most often causes burns in a military setting, is a special hazard. Any retained phosphorus particles may ignite when exposed to oxygen, thereby causing additional tissue damage and possibly injuring caregivers.[3]

AXIOM Cutaneous damage from chemicals results in an injury that may continue to progress long after the initial exposure, especially if the irritant remains in contact with the skin.

Prompt recognition of a chemical burn and copious, early skin irrigation may reduce the area and depth of injury. Such lavage, with water or saline solution, should be initiated at the scene. The duration of irrigation depends on the agent that caused the injury. Irrigation until pain in the wound relents (which may require several hours) is a useful endpoint.

AXIOM One should not irrigate chemical burns with neutralizing acid or alkali solutions because the heat of reaction that can occur may cause further tissue damage.

For chemical injuries to the eyes, irrigation with water should be initiated immediately at the scene and continued with saline at the site of definitive care until a physician experienced in the treatment of such eye injuries sees the patient.[5] Acid or alkali injury to the eyes requires irrigation until the pH is neutral by litmus test.

AXIOM Removal of the offending agent by removal of clothing and irrigation is the mainstay of early treatment of chemical injury.

The depth of a chemical injury may be difficult to assess. A full-thickness burn caused by strong acid may have a silky texture and the bronzed appearance of a deep suntan.

In addition to local destruction caused by direct contact with a chemical, systemic toxicity resulting from cutaneous absorption may occur, especially with phenol, formate, or nitrate exposure. Immediate lavage and cleansing of the wound reduce the risk of systemic absorption and toxicity.

Hydrofluoric acid is unique among agents that cause chemical burns in that therapy consists of immediate decontamination by water lavage or a quaternary ammonia solution followed by specific treatment to detoxify the fluoride ion absorbed through the skin into the subcutaneous tissues.[4] Topical application of 2.5% calcium gluconate gel forms an insoluble calcium salt with the fluoride ion and is a treatment option, but its efficacy is controversial. Alternatively, a 5% solution of calcium gluconate may be injected into the exposed area at a dose not to exceed 0.05 mL/cm². Some investigators have reported immediate relief of pain with such injections. Recurrence of pain is an indication that additional injections may be necessary. Intra-arterial calcium gluconate has also been used in the treatment of hydrofluoric acid burns of an extremity, but the effectiveness of this therapy is unconfirmed. Failure to recognize hydrofluoric acid exposure and institute appropriate treatment can lead to extensive tissue loss and, if the burn is extensive, it can also cause significant hypocalcemia and hyperkalemia.

AXIOM Chemical burns may be complicated by systemic toxicity if the agent is absorbed. A history that identifies the causative agent allows specific treatment of systemic effects.

INITIAL HOSPITAL MANAGEMENT

Indications for Early Endotracheal Intubation

When the patient arrives at the site of definitive care, the airway should be secured and fluid therapy instituted. In patients with burns of the head and neck, marked facial edema often occurs during fluid resuscitation. Although initially the airway may be normal, supraglottic and glottic edema can develop rapidly, resulting in upper airway obstruction. Patients burned by steam or ingestion of scalding liquids may also rapidly develop upper airway edema. It may then be difficult or impossible to intubate the patient, and an emergency cricothyrotomy or tracheostomy may be required. Thus, patients who have major burns involving the head and neck and will require large volumes of fluid for resuscitation and patients with oropharyngeal burns should be intubated, preferably via the nasotracheal route before significant edema develops.

Extubation can usually be performed safely when the edema of the head and neck has receded, usually 3 or 4 days later.

PITFALL ⊘

In patients with severe facial burns, increasing pharyngeal edema can result in airway compromise and extremely difficult intubation as resuscitation proceeds.

Cleansing the Wound

Because the presence of soot and debris can lead one to overestimate the extent of burn, all involved areas should be cleansed gently with a mild soap or detergent. The wounds should also be debrided to remove loose, nonviable epidermis and bullae greater than 2 cm in diameter. Hair should be removed from the wound and shaved from a generous margin of adjacent unburned skin. Once this is accomplished, the extent of the burn can be accurately assessed.

Estimating the Depth and Extent of the Burn

Mortality from burn wounds is primarily determined by the extent of burn and the age of the patient. The depth and extent of the tissue injury also determines the type of wound care required, the need for grafting, and the fluid requirements. Consequently, thermal burns are usually classified on the basis of estimated depth of injury.

First-degree injury, such as a sunburn, consists of epidermal damage alone. Second-degree burns involve the entire epidermal layer and part of the underlying dermis. They are often divided into superficial or deep partial-thickness injuries. Superficial partial-thickness injuries are usually quite painful and have an erythematous appearance with blebs and bullae. In deep partial-thickness burns, sensation is impaired to a variable degree.

Third-degree or full-thickness thermal injury implies destruction of all epidermal and dermal elements. The skin is often charred or leathery and has a pearly-white sheen. Although it is anesthetic, there are typically intermixed areas of full and partial-thickness injury, thus, sensation in the wound is not a reliable discriminating feature.

Severe scald injuries, particularly in the very young and very old, may initially appear bright red and may be classified as superficial partial-thickness burns even though the damage is full-thickness. Failure of erythematous deep scald burns to blanch with pressure also helps differentiate them from partial-thickness injuries.[6]

The size of the patient (body weight) and the area of burned body surface are the main determinants of the amount of resuscitation fluid required.[7] Inaccurate assessment of the extent of burn can result in failure to refer the patient to a burn center when such referral is warranted and can also lead to inappropriate fluid resuscitation.

AXIOM Accurate determination of the extent of the burn wound is essential for properly estimating the initial resuscitation fluid needs.

The patient must be weighed and the percentage of body surface involved accurately estimated. Initially, in the adult, the size of the burn wound can be estimated using the "rule of nines" (Fig. 37A–1). Subsequent to this, a more exact determination should be made using a surface area diagram, such as the Lund-Browder chart (Fig. 37A–

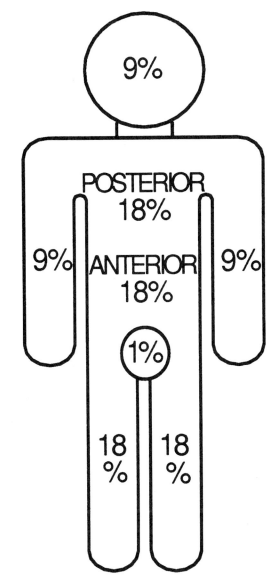

FIGURE 37A–1 The rule of nines assigns major anatomic divisions of the body a percent surface area in intervals of 9. This allows a rapid first approximation of burn size.

2), because the proportion of the body surface area of certain body parts is significantly different in children compared to adults. These body surface diagrams for the pediatric age groups should be readily available in all emergency departments and burn units.

The fact that the surface of the patient's hand represents approximately 1% of the total body surface area can be used to estimate the extent of irregular areas of burn injury. When calculating the extent of a burn, only second- and third-degree injuries are included. First-degree injuries do not usually require fluid resuscitation, unless they are extensive.

The extent of injury is often difficult to assess in patients with electric injury.[8] Although there may be a significant thermal component to an electric injury as a result of ignition of clothing or arcing of electric current, it is not uncommon for the cutaneous injury to be minor in the presence of extensive destruction of underlying muscle and other soft tissue.

PITFALL ⊘

Electric injuries are often much more extensive than estimated by the extent of the surface injury.

Further Resuscitation

Primary concerns during the first 48 hours following thermal injury are maintenance of an adequate airway, pulmonary gas exchange, circulating volume, and tissue perfusion. Although airway obstruction takes precedence in evaluation and treatment, this problem usually does not develop until later in the resuscitation period; however, treatment of carbon monoxide poisoning is an immediate concern. Fluid resuscitation should also be initiated as soon as possible. Other considerations during this initial phase of care include monitoring for vascular and ventilatory compromise from constrictive burn eschar.

Carbon Monoxide Poisoning

Failure to recognize and rapidly treat carbon monoxide poisoning may result in significant cardiac and neurological impairment and even death.[9] A history of smoke exposure in an enclosed space and disproportionate obtundation should always alert one to the possibility of carbon monoxide intoxication. Other clinical findings, such as cherry-red skin coloration, are inconsistent, and their absence does

FIGURE 37A–2 The Lund-Browder diagram allows accurate assessment of burn size and accounts for the different anatomic relationships in pediatric patients.

BURN ESTIMATE AND DIAGRAM
AGE vs AREA

Area	Birth 1 yr	1–4 yr	5–9 yr	10–14 yr	15 yr	Adult	2°	3°	Total	Donor Areas
Head	19	17	13	11	9	7				
Neck	2	2	2	2	2	2				
Ant Trunk	13	13	13	13	13	13				
Post Trunk	13	13	13	13	13	13				
R Buttock	2½	2½	2½	2½	2½	2½				
L. Buttock	2½	2½	2½	2½	2½	2½				
Genitalia	1	1	1	1	1	1				
R U Arm	4	4	4	4	4	4				
L.U. Arm	4	4	4	4	4	4				
R L Arm	3	3	3	3	3	3				
L L Arm	3	3	3	3	3	3				
R Hand	2½	2½	2½	2½	2½	2½				
L Hand	2½	2½	2½	2½	2½	2½				
R Thigh	5½	6½	8	8½	9	9½				
L. Thigh	5½	6½	8	8½	9	9½				
R Leg	5	5	5½	6	6½	7				
L Leg	5	5	5½	6	6½	7				
R. Foot	3½	3½	3½	3½	3½	3½				
L Foot	3½	3½	3½	3½	3½	3½				
						TOTAL				

BURN DIAGRAM

AGE_____

SEX_____

WEIGHT_____

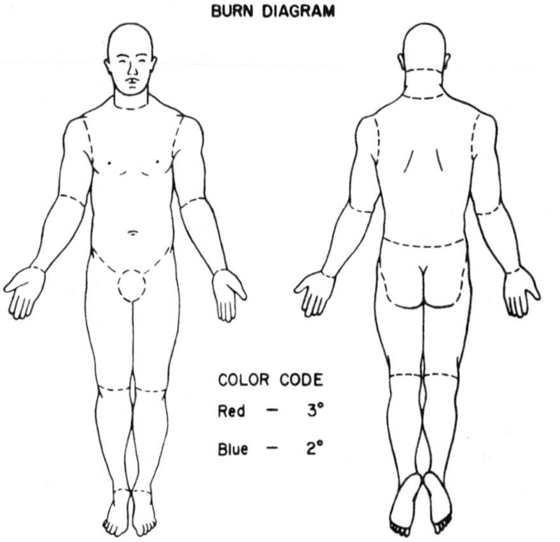

COLOR CODE

Red — 3°

Blue — 2°

BAMC Form 299 NS
1 May 74

not exclude the possible presence of a clinically significant level of carboxyhemoglobin.

Measurement of arterial blood gases by the conventional techniques often used for pulmonary monitoring will not exclude carbon monoxide poisoning. PaO_2 levels of 80 torr on room air may indicate adequate amounts of dissolved oxygen in the blood, even when carboxyhemoglobin levels exceed 40%. Direct measurement of the level of carboxyhemoglobin and oxyhemoglobin is the only reliable way to evaluate patients for carbon monoxide poisoning.

PITFALL ⊘

> *Carbon monoxide poisoning should be suspected with a history of a burn injury in a closed space or findings of obtundation, even if the PaO_2 is normal.*

The treatment for patients suspected of carbon monoxide poisoning is administration of 100% oxygen via a tight fitting nonrebreathing face mask or endotracheal tube. This reduces the half-life of carboxyhemoglobin from 4 hours while inspiring room air to approximately 40 minutes. Rapid reduction in carboxyhemoglobin levels is the main mechanism by which hypoxic injury may be avoided, and treatment should be continued until the carboxyhemoglobin level decreases to less than 10%.

AXIOM   The use of hyperbaric oxygen (HBO) therapy for carbon monoxide poisoning is generally unnecessary.

Not only is hyperbaric oxygen generally not needed for the treatment of carbon monoxide poisoning, but it may place the thermally injured patient at additional risk for complications. No published study has documented reduction in neurological impairment after the use of hyperbaric oxygen for carbon monoxide poisoning. Theoretically, the immediate institution of normobaric 100% oxygen results in the reduction of carboxyhemoglobin levels by at least 50%, long before the patient could be prepared for the hyperbaric chamber. This means that in a patient with an initial carboxyhemoglobin level of 80%, the level probably would be reduced to less than 40% before institution of HBO. Most importantly, HBO therapy entails a period of at least 90 minutes during which the ability to monitor the patient's resuscitation and general condition is severely limited.

Fluid Resuscitation

Significant burn injury (greater than 20% of the total body surface area) results in an obligatory loss of substantial amounts of fluid into the burn wound and a subsequent decrease in cardiac output and vital organ perfusion.[10] This state of burn shock, if left untreated, can result in oliguria that may progress to anuria and acute tubular necrosis. Prompt infusion of adequate volumes of resuscitation fluid into patients with significant burn injuries can almost universally prevent acute renal failure and has revolutionized the care of burn patients.[11]

AXIOM   The size of the patient and the extent of the burn injury are the most important determinants of the volume of resuscitation fluid required.

Fluid resuscitation should begin as early as possible after the burn injury using a large bore peripheral intravenous line, preferably placed in an area of unburned skin. If unburned sites are not available, a cannula can be placed into a vein underlying burned tissue. Central venous and pulmonary artery catheters are usually unnecessary in the initial resuscitation of burn patients.

Lactated Ringer's solution is our fluid of choice for burn resuscitation in the first 24 hours.[12] The fluid needs for adults can be calculated as 2 ml per kilogram body weight per percent body surface area burned. In children weighing less than 30 kilograms, the usual fluid needs are 3 ml per kilogram per percent body surface area burned (Table 37A–1). Half of this volume is usually administered within the first 8 hours after injury and the remainder over the subsequent 16 hours.

TABLE 37A–1   USAISR Formula for Estimation of Fluid Resuscitation Needs in Burn Patients

First 24 hours postburn:
  Adults and children ≥30 kg
    Lactated Ringer's solution—2 ml/kg/% burn
      half given in first 8 hours
      half given in remaining 16 hours
  Children <30 kg
    Lactated Ringer's solution—3 ml/kg/% burn + maintenance fluids*
Second 24 hours postburn
  5% albumin in lactated Ringer's solution
    30-50% burn—0.3 ml/kg/% burn
    50-70% burn—0.4 ml/kg/% burn
    >70% burn—0.5 ml/kg/% burn
  5% dextrose in water to maintain urine output at 30-50 ml/hr‡

* Frequent adjustments to maintain a urine output of 0.5-1.5 ml/kg/hr are necessary in children. Increasing the rates calculated above will be necessary in about 50% of patients.[13]
‡ D5 ½ NS is substituted for 5% dextrose in water for maintenance fluids in children <30 kg.

AXIOM   The initial calculated rate of fluid administration is used only as a guide to begin resuscitation.

Thus, an 80 kg adult with a 50% second- and third-degree burn would theoretically require 8000 ml of isotonic crystalloid in the first 24 hours. About 4000 ml should be given in the first 8 postburn hours at a rate of about 500 ml/hr. The adequacy of resuscitation is then determined by frequent examination of the patient and evaluation of tissue perfusion. Urine output is the most clinically useful and readily available means of judging central organ perfusion.

AXIOM   Burn resuscitation formulas provide an estimation of fluid requirements, and adjustments are made as required by frequent assessment of the clinical response, especially urine output.

In adult patients, the usual goal is to infuse fluid at a rate that will result in a urine output of 30-50 ml per hour. In children weighing less than 30 kg, the desired urine output is 1 ml per kilogram per hour. Conditions that may result in fluid requirements above those initially calculated include: (a) a delay in resuscitation, (b) drug or alcohol intoxication, (c) inhalation injury, and (d) electric injury in which the exact extent of tissue damage is difficult to assess.

If urine output fails to meet the stated goal of 30-50 ml per hour, the volume of infusion should be incrementally increased until the desired urine output is achieved. Bolus administration of fluid is discouraged because its effect is short in duration compared with increasing the volume infusion by fixed amounts on a continuous basis. If fluid requirements appear to exceed greatly the amount initially calculated, a specific reason for this, such as occult intracavitary hemorrhage from an associated mechanical injury, should be sought.

AXIOM   Occult hemorrhage from associated mechanical trauma should be suspected when fluid requirements are much greater than those calculated from the apparent extent of the burn.

If no additional injuries can be found to explain fluid needs that are much greater than expected, invasive monitoring and measurements of cardiac output and pulmonary artery wedge pressure (PAWP) should be performed. Use of inotropic agents is only justified when a benefit can be anticipated and demonstrated by such measurements. If cardiac output has been restored, but anuria or oliguria persist despite the administration of fluid that significantly exceeds estimated requirements, it may be reasonable to administer diuretics cautiously in small amounts.

Although inadequate fluid infusion resulting in burn shock and organ failure should be avoided, excessive administration of fluid can also be detrimental and can cause peripheral and pulmonary edema. Increased peripheral edema can cause tissue damage and may precipitate a need for escharotomy in circumferentially burned extremities. In patients with preexisting cardiovascular disease, the resulting pulmonary edema can also result in severe respiratory failure. Consequently, when urine output exceeds the stated goal, the fluid infusion rate should be reduced by approximately 10% per hour.

PITFALL ⊘

> *Edema from excessive fluid administration may precipitate ischemia in circumferentially burned extremities and predispose the patient to pulmonary edema, particularly during the edema resorption period.*

Fluid Needs During the Second 24 Hours

Approximately 24 hours after injury, the resuscitation fluid should be changed in the adult from Ringer's lactate to a colloid-containing solution. This can be given as 5% albumin in a balanced salt solution in an amount equivalent to 0.3 to 0.5 ml per kilogram body weight per percent body surface area burn. Thus, an 80 kg man with a 50% burn would require 1200-2000 ml of 5% albumin in the second 24 hours. This is infused to replenish the plasma volume deficit that usually persists at the end of the first 24 hours postburn. In adults, electrolyte-free fluid should also be infused fast enough to maintain a urine output of 30 to 50 ml per hour. In children weighing less than 30 kilograms, salt-free water is not used. Instead, a fluid such as 5% dextrose in ½ normal saline is administered to maintain a urine output of 1 ml per kilogram per hour.

At the completion of resuscitation, serum sodium levels are often decreased to approximately 130 to 132 mEq per liter as a reflection of the sodium concentration of the large volume of Ringer's lactate the patient has received. Despite this hyponatremia, total body sodium is generally markedly increased by the sodium content of the resuscitation fluids. Consequently, additional salt-containing solutions should not be infused in an attempt to increase serum sodium concentrations. Mild hyponatremia usually does not cause any symptoms and it is readily corrected by reducing the fluid infusion rate and allowing evaporative water loss to occur from the surface of the burn wound.

AXIOM   Modest hyponatremia is expected after resuscitation with lactated Ringer's solution;, and because total body sodium generally is increased, fluid restriction, not sodium administration, is indicated later to restore serum sodium levels to normal.

Significant evaporative water loss from open burn wounds will facilitate the correction of hyponatremia, but it can also cause dehydration. If postresuscitation fluid therapy does not take evaporative water loss into account, hypernatremia as a consequence of dehydration can develop rapidly.

The formula for estimating insensible water loss (in ml/hr) is 25 + percent body surface burned multiplied by total body surface area in m^2. Thus, a 50% burn in a patient with a total body surface area of 2.0 m^2 would have an insensible water loss of about $(25 + 50) (2)$ or 150 ml/hr.

After resuscitation, fluid administration should be reduced because edema resorption will occur, and the fluid and salt administered during resuscitation will be "off-loaded." A daily loss of 10 to 12% of the weight gained during resuscitation should be permitted until the patient returns to his or her preburn weight by the 7th to 10th postburn day. The best way to monitor fluid balance in this period is to maintain an accurate log of the patient's intake and output and get daily weights and serum sodium concentrations. Departure of a patient from the desired weight trajectory mandates careful review of the fluid management regimen and adjustment as necessary.

Adult burn patients do not generally require glucose infusions during the first 24 hours postinjury. In fact, hormonally mediated glycogenolysis and gluconeogenesis generally results in hyperglycemia. Children, however, because of their limited glycogen stores, are prone to develop hypoglycemia if dextrose-free intravenous fluids are infused for prolonged periods.

Many burn formulas fail to account for maintenance fluid needs which are higher in proportion to body weight in children than in adults.[13] Fluid requirements for small children with small to moderate size burns, when estimated by burn formulas, may not be sufficient to meet basal maintenance requirements. Maintenance fluids should be administered to pediatric patients less than 30 kg in the form of D5 ½ normal saline at a rate of 1500 ml/m^2 body surface area (in addition to the burn resuscitation fluids), a rate that will produce a urine output of 1 ml per kilogram per hour.

Children are also far more susceptible than adults to cerebral edema as a result of overhydration and rapid shifts in serum sodium. Consequently, the serum sodium should be monitored frequently, and rapid shifts in serum sodium should be prevented by avoiding or strictly limiting the use of salt-free solutions such as D5W.

PITFALL ⊘

> *Adult resuscitation formulas do not take into account the infant's need for glucose, higher maintenance fluid needs, and increased sensitivity to hyponatremia.*

Escharotomy

As resuscitation proceeds, vascular compromise may occur in an upper or lower extremity with a circumferential full-thickness thermal injury. Formation of edema in the tissue beneath the inelastic eschar can result in elevation of interstitial pressure to levels that exceed venous and capillary pressures, and can thereby result in tissue ischemia and subsequent muscle necrosis. The Doppler ultrasonic flow probe is useful in assessing the vascular status of burned limbs. Throughout the resuscitation period, peripheral pulses (i.e., the radial, ulnar and posterior tibial, the palmar arch and digital pulses) should be evaluated hourly using the Doppler flow probe. As the resuscitation progresses and tissue edema forms, diminution of the Doppler signal indicates impaired tissue perfusion and the potential need for escharotomy.[14] Since the loss of a Doppler signal can also be caused by hypovolemia, the adequacy of resuscitation should always be assessed prior to performing escharotomies. Since capillary blood flow may cease before peripheral pulses are lost, any neurological changes should make one promptly measure subescharatomy pressures.

Close attention to the perfusion status of circumferentially burned limbs is needed to not only avoid tissue necrosis but also to prevent unnecessary escharotomies. Continuous elevation of the extremities and active exercise of the involved limbs for 5 minutes every hour can reduce the need for escharotomy in patients with circumferential limb burns.[15]

PITFALL ⊘

> *Before performing an escharotomy, one should ascertain that absence of peripheral pulses or loss of Doppler signals is not a result of inadequate fluid resuscitation.*

TECHNIQUE OF ESCHAROTOMY

Escharotomy should be performed in the midmedial and/or midlateral lines of the involved limb with the patient in the anatomic position (Fig. 37A-3). Escharotomy can be performed at the bedside using a knife or electrocautery and does not require anesthesia because the incision is generally made through insensate full-thickness burn injury.

The burn eschar should be incised only down to the superficial subcutaneous fat. It is not necessary to incise deep into the subcutaneous fat or to the level of investing fascia because excessive bleeding may occur and the deeper tissues will be unnecessarily exposed

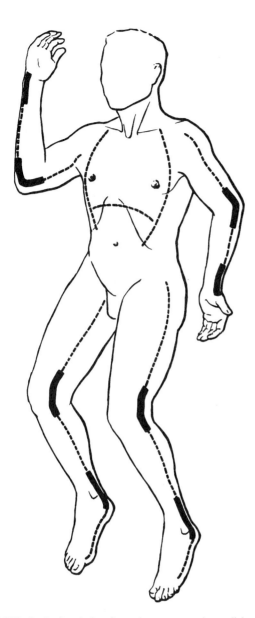

FIGURE 37A–3 Preferred sites for escharotomy are the medial and lateral aspects of the extremities.

to an increased risk of infection. The escharotomy incision should be carried across the entire length of the full-thickness injury and extend across involved joints. Pulses, neurological function, and compartment pressures should be rechecked after the escharotomy to ensure that blood flow has been restored.

FASCIOTOMY

In patients with high voltage electric injury, those with associated soft tissue mechanical trauma, and patients with deep thermal injury in whom escharotomy fails to restore tissue blood flow, fasciotomy of the involved compartments should be performed.

AXIOM   Although escharotomy alone is generally adequate to restore perfusion to circumferentially burned extremities, if the thermal injury is deep or if the patient had an electrical injury, a fasciotomy may also be indicated.

In general, a fasciotomy is a procedure that should be performed in the operating room with appropriate anesthesia. After fasciotomy, pulses should be rechecked to ensure that blood flow has been restored.

CHEST WALL ESCHAROTOMIES

Circumferential deep thermal injury of the chest and abdomen may impair chest wall excursion to the point that ventilation is impaired and respiratory failure ensues. If the blood gases are deteriorating or if peak airway pressures on a ventilator are rising to levels where barotrauma is likely, chest wall escharotomies should be performed.

AXIOM   Blood gas or ventilatory impairment in patients with circumferential deep chest wall burns indicates a need for escharotomy.

For circumferential chest burns, the eschar is incised to the level of the subcutaneous fat in the anterior axillary lines. If the eschar continues onto the abdomen, the lateral chest incisions should be connected by another escharotomy at the level of the costal margins to free the anterior chest wall plate. This procedure should result in an immediate increase in chest wall excursion, decrease in peak inspiratory pressure, and improvement in ventilation.

Inhalation Injury

Inhalation injury is most commonly caused by entry of products of incomplete combustion into the trachea, lower airways, and pulmonary parenchyma. Except for inhalation of steam under high pressure, there is no direct thermal injury to the lungs. A history of being burned in an enclosed space, the presence of facial burns, or an extensive burn should raise the suspicion of inhalation injury. The presence of soot in the nares and mouth, inflammatory changes in the oropharyngeal mucosa, and carbonaceous sputum are consistent with but not diagnostic of inhalation injury. Patients in whom there is any suspicion of inhalation injury should be treated with high fractions of inspired oxygen at the scene because of the potential for concomitant carbon monoxide poisoning. Oxygen administration is continued until the patient receives definitive care.

When the patient arrives at the hospital, arterial blood gases and carboxyhemoglobin levels should be promptly obtained. If there is severe hypoxemia or other evidence of respiratory distress, the patient should be intubated, preferably by the nasotracheal route. Fiberoptic bronchoscopy in combination with xenon-133 scanning is the most reliable means of diagnosing inhalation injury. Positive findings on bronchoscopy include carbonaceous material below the true vocal cords. Concomitant erythema and/or ulceration in the tracheobronchial mucosa indicate moderate to severe injury.

Because inhalation of fine particulate matter less than 0.05 microns may only affect terminal bronchioles and lung parenchyma, bronchoscopy does not detect all injuries. Therefore, patients suspected of having inhalation injury who have a negative bronchoscopic exam should have xenon-133 ventilation/perfusion lung scanning.[16] Positive findings consist of unequal lung field radiation density and retention of xenon-133 longer than 90 seconds. A positive scan with normal bronchoscopic findings usually defines a mild inhalation injury.

Early in the resuscitative period, vasoconstriction and poor perfusion may prevent development of inflammatory erythema in the bronchial mucosa and yield false-negative bronchoscopic findings. The xenon-133 scan may also be inaccurate in patients who are heavy smokers, those who have chronic bronchitis, and when performed after the first 48 hours postburn (resulting from hyperventilation). The combination of positive bronchoscopy and lung scan is 93% specific for the diagnosis of inhalation injury.[17]

AXIOM   Bronchoscopy plus xenon-133 lung scanning is the most reliable method for establishing the diagnosis of inhalation injury.

The pathophysiology of inhalation injury includes occlusion of small, distal airways by inflammatory exudate and sloughed debris. The resulting atelectasis causes ventilation-perfusion mismatch. The collapsed alveoli are further compromised by epithelial damage and changes in the capillary endothelium. The damaged bronchial mucosa and the associated impairment of mucociliary clearance further predispose the airways to bacterial colonization, as manifested by a 38% incidence of pneumonia, which usually occurs early.

The presence of an inhalation injury increases the mortality rates associated with burns by as much as 20%.[18] The combination of inhalation injury with pneumonia is particularly dangerous and can increase mortality as much as 60%. Therefore, maintaining good pulmonary toilet and complete expansion of affected lung segments is critical. Prophylactic antibiotics do not prevent pneumonia and are contraindicated. Corticosteroid use has been associated with an increased incidence of infectious complications and should be avoided.[19] The treatment of choice for patients with documented inhalation injury includes provision of humidified air, adequate oxygen to prevent hypoxemia, and aggressive pulmonary toilet. Frequent bronchoscopy to remove sloughed mucosal debris is often also necessary.

AXIOM   Treatment of inhalation injury consists of providing adequate humidified oxygen and aggressive pulmonary toilet; prophylactic antibiotics and steroids are contraindicated.

If endotracheal intubation is required, conventional ventilation techniques may further impair clearance of secretions and barotrauma may compound the injury, particularly if high peak ventilatory pressures are used.

High frequency percussive ventilation is currently used at the United States Army Institute of Surgical Research for patients with inhalation injury, and this generally provides adequate ventilation and oxygenation at lower peak airway pressures and inspired oxygen concentrations. This mode of ventilatory support has also been associated with a decreased incidence of pneumonia and decreased mortality when compared with historical and concurrent controls.[20]

Patients with inhalation injury should undergo routine microscopic examination and surveillance cultures of tracheobronchial secretions to identify the predominant bacterial organisms. When the tracheobronchial aspirate reveals greater than 20 to 25 white blood cells and less than 10 squamous cells per high power field, a diagnosis of tracheobronchitis is made and antibiotic therapy based on previously obtained surveillance cultures and sensitivity results is begun. By the same token, if pneumonia develops, as diagnosed by a new or increasing pulmonary infiltrate on chest roentgenogram in association with fever and tracheobronchial leukorrhea, antibiotics should be started on the basis of the previously obtained cultures. Antibiotic therapy is later adjusted, as necessary, to conform to the results of culture and sensitivity tests obtained at the time of diagnosis.

Tetanus Prophylaxis

Although tetanus is a rare complication after burn injury, it has been reported in patients who have not received adequate primary immunization.[21] Elderly patients, the very young, and patients who reside in developing countries are most likely to be unprotected against tetanus. An adequate history of tetanus immunization should be obtained when the patient is evaluated initially. If the patient has never been immunized or the immunization status is uncertain, tetanus toxoid should be administered along with tetanus immune globulin. Subsequent doses of toxoid should be given at appropriate intervals to complete active immunization. If the patient has already received a primary series of immunizations, a booster of tetanus toxoid may be required depending on the nature of the wound and the time that has elapsed since the last dose of toxoid.

AXIOM   Proper tetanus immunization should be provided to all burn patients.

BURN WOUND CARE

Treatment of the burn wound must be carefully planned and executed to maximize survival and optimize rehabilitation. Pharmacologic measures include tetanus immunization and topical chemotherapy to control bacterial proliferation. Early excision and grafting of the wound must be staged and planned to minimize complications and maximize yield from limited donor sites. This regimen should result in early wound closure with a low incidence of burn wound infection.

Topical Antimicrobial Agents

The denatured proteins in the avascular eschar of a full-thickness burn provide a hospitable environment for proliferating bacteria that can penetrate the eschar and invade deeper viable tissues. Such bacterial proliferation in the eschar should be suppressed by topical antibiotics until excision and grafting can be performed.

Mafenide acetate (Sulfamylon) is an N' unsubstituted sulfonamide that is water-soluble and penetrates eschar well. It is effective against gram-negative organisms, including Pseudomonas aeruginosa. The main problems with its use are its inhibition of carbonic anhydrase, which can result in a metabolic acidosis, and the fairly severe pain it causes when applied to partial-thickness wounds with intact sensation.

Silver sulfadiazine (1%) is also effective against gram-negative bacilli, but resistance tends to develop with time. It is painless when applied to partial-thickness burns, and it does not disturb acid-base homeostasis. However, diffusion of this agent into the eschar is limited, so treatment must begin immediately before bacteria have invaded the wound. Continued application of silver sulfadiazine may cause leukopenia, and neutrophil counts should be monitored. Alternate application of these two agents on a 12-hour schedule reduces the incidence of side effects and realizes the benefits of both.

Silver nitrate (0.5%) soaked dressings can be applied to wounds of patients with allergies to sulfa derived agents; however, silver nitrate can leach sodium and chloride from the wound, and it discolors everything with which it comes in contact. The dressings also must be kept moist.

Excision and Grafting

Excision and grafting of full-thickness burns and deep partial-thickness burns that will take longer than 3 weeks to heal is begun as soon as resuscitation is complete and mobilization of "third space" fluid is evidenced by decreasing daily weights. Early excision and grafting may decrease hospital stay (especially in patients with small full-thickness burns), decrease infectious complications, and improve cosmetic and functional results. However, excision of a burn wound may be associated with massive blood loss ranging from one-half to one unit of blood per percent body surface area excised depending on the anatomic location and maturity of the wound. Because transfusion of blood products is associated with a risk of disease transmission as well as immunosuppression and increased infections, their use should be minimized.[27]

In patients with extensive full-thickness burn wounds, excision to the level of the investing fascia results in less blood loss than tangential excision. For burns on an extremity, the blood loss caused by tangential excision can be reduced by using a tourniquet applied proximal to the operative site. However, this complicates assessment of the adequacy of excision because the major criterion used is the presence of uniformly distributed fine punctate bleeding over the excised wound bed. In areas not amenable to tangential excision under tourniquet control, limited areas of the burn can be excised sequentially. After excision of each small section, a topical hemostatic solution, such as thrombin, is applied to the wound surface and covered with warm laparotomy pads to minimize blood loss.

PITFALL ⊘

Excision of large burn wounds should be carefully planned to prevent massive blood loss and hypothermia.

For burns without evidence of infection, operative procedures are staged and limited to 20% of the body surface or that which can be accomplished in 2 hours to avoid massive transfusion and hypothermia. Hypothermia is also minimized by placing the patient on a warming blanket, maintaining the operating room at 85-90° F with a relative humidity of 40-60%, and warming the blood, intravenous fluids, and inspired gases.

Availability of donor sites is often the limiting factor in the closure of extensive burn wounds. It is essential that each autografting procedure have the best opportunity for success. Loss of graft not only leaves the burn wound open but also increases the total area of open wound. Since the donor site is also a partial-thickness injury, it increases physiologic stress and the risk of infection.

In patients with extensive full-thickness burns, it is often advantageous to perform the initial excision on large flat surfaces such as the chest, abdomen, or back at the level of the investing fascia. This not only minimizes blood loss but also provides a bed of unequivocally viable tissue for grafting. The excised area can then be autografted with available donor sites using a 3:1 to 4:1 expanded "mesh" graft. Cutaneous allografts are placed over the meshed autogenous tissue to protect the open interstices. Once the large planar surfaces have been successfully grafted, attention can be directed to other areas as donor sites become available for reharvesting.

Expansion of the graft to ratios greater than 4:1 is frequently associated with desiccation of the recipient bed and failure to obtain closure with autograft. Also, closure of the graft interstices is prolonged and the cosmetic and functional results are often poor. As an alternative to the use of excessively expanded grafts, cutaneous allografts may be used to cover excised areas temporarily until the donor sites become mature enough for repeat harvesting.

To ensure successful take of cutaneous autografts, it is essential that all nonviable tissue in the areas to be grafted be completely excised. When performing tangential excision, this is assured when there is uniformly distributed fine punctate bleeding from the entire surface of the excised burn wound.

Postoperative loss of graft as a result of mechanical shearing secondary to patient movement can be prevented by totally immobilizing the body part grafted. A bulky dressing consisting of fine mesh gauze placed directly over the graft, covered with laparotomy pads, and wrapped in a gauze dressing that is stapled in place will help maintain the graft in apposition to the wound bed and protect the graft from avulsion.

In patients requiring grafting to the back and/or buttocks, use of a large bulky dressing and positioning of the patient on an air fluidized bed for 7 to 10 days minimizes loss as a result of shearing and pressure. Extremities should be splinted one joint above and one joint below the site of grafting and held immobile for a period of 5 to 10 days. Hands are an exception; they should be splinted only briefly and mobilized in 3 days.

Another cause of graft loss is infection, the incidence of which can be decreased by several techniques. Complete excision of the burn wound helps prevent the infection and graft loss which almost invariably occur if the burn wounds are inadequately excised.

PITFALL ⊘

Inadequate excision of burn wounds invariably results in loss of skin grafts that are applied.

Keeping meshed grafts moist with a topical antimicrobial agent reduces the proliferation of bacteria in the graft interstices. The dressings of wounds covered with meshed grafts should be kept moist by application of an antimicrobial solution. The authors prefer to apply a 5% solution of mafenide acetate every 2-3 hours, but that agent is not generally available. In addition, the take of autograft skin placed immediately adjacent to unexcised burn wounds may be compromised by the organisms and suppuration from the intact eschar. If inadequate autograft skin is available to cover the entire area, the adjacent burn wound should be excised completely and those areas that cannot be autografted should be covered with allograft skin or another biological dressing.

Burn Wound Infection

Definitive burn wound treatment by excision and grafting is accomplished as rapidly as possible, and the effectiveness of topical antimicrobial agents allows this to proceed in a deliberate, planned fashion. Nevertheless, invasive burn wound infection remains a risk until all eschar has been excised and the wounds are healed. As a consequence, the burn wound is examined daily for signs of infection, which include focal dark discoloration of the wound, conversion of a partial-thickness injury to full-thickness injury, green discoloration of subcutaneous tissue, early separation of eschar, and vesicular eruption in healing or recently healed partial-thickness injuries. These changes mandate biopsy of the most suspicious areas of the burn wound along with adjacent deep viable tissue. Part of the specimen is sent for culture and the rest is processed by frozen and rapid section technique for examination by the pathologist.[23]

The microbial status of the wound and adjacent viable tissue is characterized by histologic criteria (Table 37A–2)[24] and the finding of organisms in viable tissue. Serial biopsies demonstrating progressive eschar colonization indicate loss of microbial control and mandate change in the wound care regimen. Quantitative cultures of the burn wound are not reliable in diagnosing invasive burn wound infection. Most burn wounds will be colonized with bacteria within several days of admission to the hospital, and these microorganisms commonly proliferate in the nonviable eschar without invading adjacent viable tissue.[25]

AXIOM Histologic examination of a burn wound biopsy is the mainstay in the diagnosis of invasive burn wound infection.

Invasive burn wound infection is treated immediately with systemic antibiotics appropriate for the organisms identified by specific culture or surveillance procedures. For gram-negative bacterial infection, clysis of the subeschar space with a broad spectrum penicillin is performed 6 to 12 hours before urgent surgical excision of the wound.[26] Invasive fungal wound infections are excised immediately, and systemic amphotericin B is administered. Early identification of such infections by biopsy and aggressive local surgical control is the only way to improve survival in these patients.[27]

Critical Care Issues

Burn patients are subject to all of the complications experienced by severely injured patients receiving aggressive, invasive care. However, there are certain aspects of critical care that are unique to burn patients, and these must be given special consideration.

TABLE 37A–2 *Criteria for Histologic Grading of Burn Wound Biopsy*

I. Wound colonization: microorganisms limited to burned, nonviable tissue
  A. Superficial—organisms on wound surface
  B. Penetration—organisms in eschar
  C. Proliferation—organisms in subeschar space
II. Invasion: microorganisms in unburned tissue
  A. Microinvasion—organisms in viable tissue immediately adjacent to subeschar space
  B. Generalized—penetration of organisms deep into viable tissue
  C. Microvascular—organisms in blood vessels and lymphatics

Anesthesia and Analgesia

The administration of general anesthesia early after a major injury may result in cardiovascular collapse; thus, during the initial period of resuscitation, general anesthesia should be avoided if possible. Procedures such as wound debridement and escharotomy can generally be performed safely in the intensive care unit using small doses of intravenous narcotics titrated to the patient's needs. If a patient with a significant burn (i.e., greater than 30% total body surface area) requires general anesthesia because of concomitant mechanical trauma, a Swan-Ganz catheter should be placed and invasive cardiac monitoring employed to guide fluid therapy and other hemodynamic support measures.

The use of succinylcholine should be avoided in patients with extensive burns and tissue damage. This drug may precipitate a rapid release of potassium from damaged tissue, causing hyperkalemia of sufficient magnitude to induce asystole. Even small doses of this drug may be injurious in the small percentage of the population that has a defect in cholinesterase.

Pain medication given subcutaneously or intramuscularly during the early postburn period may be ineffective because perfusion of these tissues may be significantly decreased. If repeated intramuscular or subcutaneous doses are administered in an attempt to relieve pain, as resuscitation proceeds and perfusion of the soft tissues improves, this large depot of unabsorbed analgesic may rapidly enter the systemic circulation and cause hypotension or respiratory depression. Therefore, after major thermal injury, all pain medication should be given intravenously. Morphine is the preferred analgesic in these circumstances, and it is generally quite safe when given in small intravenous doses titrated to the patient response.

PITFALL ⊘

Intramuscularly or subcutaneously administered narcotics in the early postburn period often result in inadequate pain control initially and/or overdose later.

Gastrointestinal Complications

In patients with burns of 25% or more of the body surface area, ileus is virtually universal, and a nasogastric tube is placed to prevent emesis and aspiration. The nasogastric tube can also be used to monitor intragastric pH. Bleeding from gastric erosions or duodenal ulcerations in burn patients can be virtually eliminated by adequate buffering of gastric acid.[28,29] An H_2 antagonist, such as cimetidine, should be started soon after admission in a dose appropriate for the patient's weight and renal function. The drug should be given intravenously at first, but it can be given orally once normal bowel function has been restored. Gastric pH should be monitored every hour, and if less than 5, sufficient antacids should be administered to raise the pH. If the gastric pH is maintained above 5, bleeding from gastric or duodenal erosions or ulcers is uncommon.

AXIOM Serious gastrointestinal bleeding from erosive gastritis or duodenal ulcers can generally be prevented by maintaining the gastric pH above 5.

Unfortunately, maintenance of the gastric pH above 5 may not be without some adverse effects. Bacterial overgrowth in an acid-neutralized stomach has been proposed as a significant risk factor leading to nosocomial pneumonia. Consequently, nonbuffering cytoprotective agents such as PGE_2 or sucralfate, which do not promote bacterial overgrowth in the stomach, have been proposed for use in stress ulcer prophylaxis. However, a randomized study in burn patients showed no difference in the incidence of pneumonia when sucralfate was compared with a regimen of antacids and H_2 blocker prophylaxis.[30]

AXIOM The resumption of oral intake as soon as possible is probably the best prophylaxis against upper gastrointestinal stress ulcers.

Intra-abdominal inflammatory conditions, such as acute cholecystitis, appendicitis, pancreatitis, and lower gastrointestinal ulceration and perforation, are infrequent but potentially lethal occurrences in burn patients. Indeed, burn patients may develop severe peritonitis without the usual signs and symptoms because of multiple factors, including burns of the abdominal wall, obtundation, and injury-induced immunosuppression. Careful, repeated abdominal examinations and a high index of suspicion are necessary to make a timely diagnosis. Even minimal abdominal complaints should be fully investigated because they may be the only evidence of an intra-abdominal catastrophe. Peritoneal lavage has been reliable in predicting pathology if the leukocyte count is greater than 500/mm^3 or a Gram's stain of the effluent shows bacteria.[31]

If a laparotomy is necessary in the burn patient, complications can be expected. One of the more common and serious complications is dehiscence of the abdominal wound. The incidence of this problem can be minimized by the use of interrupted nonabsorbable sutures in the fascial layer and retention sutures. If the skin and subcutaneous tissues are packed open and allowed to close by secondary intention, the incidence of wound infection is greatly reduced.

Pseudo-obstruction of the colon (Ogilvie's syndrome) is not uncommon in extensively burned patients, especially the elderly or debilitated.[32] The typical x-ray appearance is that of isolated colonic distention, usually most marked at the cecum. Colonoscopic decompression is indicated if the cecum is greater than 10-12 cm in transverse diameter and there is no evidence of perforation. Multiple recurrences of pseudo-obstruction or evidence of bowel ischemia and perforation will require operative intervention for tube decompression or resection of the involved portion of the colon.

Diagnosing Infection

Septic complications are common in burn patients, but the fact that systemic and local responses characteristic of infection are also evoked by the burn injury per se makes diagnosing infection much more difficult.[33] Following resuscitation, burn patients tend to develop a hyperdynamic, hypermetabolic response similar in many respects to the systemic response that occurs with infections. This response is characterized by an increased cardiac output, oxygen delivery, and oxygen consumption, and a low calculated systemic vascular resistance. The presence of these findings in resuscitated burn patients is normal and does not imply systemic sepsis. Indeed, failure to develop this response is often associated with a poor outcome. Hyperthermia is also an unreliable indicator of infection because most burn patients will have core temperatures in the range of 100 to 101.5° F, even in the absence of an infection.

AXIOM Fever, leukocytosis, and a hyperdynamic circulatory response are part of the physiologic response to thermal injury and are not reliable indicators of infection.

Although invasive burn wound infection is not unusual in patients with extensive burns, its prevalence is much less than it was 10 to 20 years ago. Indeed pneumonia, often in association with tracheobronchitis, is now the most common septic complication in burn patients.[34] In addition, a number of other septic processes, such as suppurative thrombophlebitis, sinusitis, endocarditis, and cystitis, can also occur in critically ill burn patients. Alterations in mental status, glucose intolerance, metabolic acidosis, oliguria, rising serum creatinine levels, and jaundice may be the first signs of systemic sepsis in burn patients.

If systemic sepsis is suspected, a thorough evaluation of the patient should be made to identify the site of infection. The entire burn wound should be examined closely. Areas of the wound showing changes characteristic of infection should be promptly evaluated by biopsy and histopathologic examination. If a diagnosis of invasive burn wound infection is made on the basis of histopathologic examination of the wound, prompt treatment is necessary.

If invasive burn wound infection has been excluded, further detailed evaluation of the patient is necessary. A careful physical examination and appropriate laboratory and diagnostic tests should be undertaken to search for a septic process. Blood, urine, and tracheobronchial aspirates should be sent for Gram's stain and culture. Antibiotics should be reserved for treatment of specific infections, and the selection of the agents to be used should be guided and modified by the results of appropriate cultures. Blood cultures with polymicrobial growth or serial blood cultures showing growth of different organisms are not always attributable to contamination of the specimen. In critically ill burn patients, these results should be regarded as a reflection of the polymicrobial flora of the burn wound against which host defenses have failed. Consequently, antibiotic therapy must include agents effective against all of the organisms found on properly obtained cultures.

Nutrition

The magnitude of the catabolic response after thermal injury is proportional to the burn size. In patients with burns of 50% or more of the body surface, the elevation of the metabolic rate plateaus at approximately one and a half to two times the predicted resting energy expenditure. Catecholamines appear to be one of the mediators of the exaggerated metabolic response, and their excretion correlates well with burn size and the increased metabolic rate. In addition, the catabolic pattern is also characterized by increased circulating levels of glucagon and cortisol.

Insulin levels are initially depressed, but they gradually return to normal as catabolism decreases and anabolism increases. Hyperglycemia results from increased tissue resistance to insulin and increased gluconeogenesis.[35] Increased glucose demands are generated by the wound which uses carbohydrates in an obligatory fashion via anaerobic metabolism.[36] The resulting lactate then serves as a 3-carbon skeleton for hepatic gluconeogenesis. Protein from muscle or vital organs is also broken down to provide the liver with substrate for glucose production, resulting in erosion of lean body mass. The net effect of this response is increased glucose flow, increased excretion of urea nitrogen, and a negative nitrogen balance.

To prevent the erosion of lean body mass that would otherwise occur in unalimented burn patients, nutritional support should provide adequate protein and calories to match the elevated metabolic needs. Both glucose and protein are necessary so that visceral and muscle protein synthesis are supported and lean body mass is maintained. Formulas based on estimations of calorie needs derived from earlier studies tend to significantly overestimate calorie needs determined by more accurate techniques.[37] Because of improvements in burn care, predictive formulas should be based

TABLE 37A–3 *Formula for Predicting Caloric Requirements Based on Burn Size*[37]

$$EER = BMR \times [0.891 + (0.013 \times TBS)] \times M^2 \times 24 \times AF$$
$$BMR\ (males) = 54.3 - 1.2\ age + 0.025\ age^2 - 0.00018\ age^3$$
$$BMR\ (females) = 54.7 - 1.5\ age + 0.036\ age^2 - 0.00026\ age^3$$

EER = estimated energy requirements (kcal/day)
BMR = basal metabolic rate (kcal/m^2/hr)
TBS = total burn size (fraction)
M^2 = body surface area (m^2)
AF = activity factor (1.25)

This equation predicts caloric needs based on burn size, age, and sex and is based on regression analysis of indirect-calorimetry data from 1987-1989. Predictive equations based on older data may overestimate requirements.

on recent data and used only as an estimate (Table 37A–3). The bulk of calorie needs is supplied with glucose; however, the capacity for glucose metabolism is limited to 4-5 mg/kg/min in most patients, and at higher infusion rates, hyperglycemia can become a problem. The remaining calorie needs must be met with lipids. Nitrogen requirements can be estimated as 1 gram of nitrogen per 150 kilocalories. Alternatively, nitrogen losses may be measured in the burn wound exudate, urine, and feces and replaced accordingly.

Calorie requirements change as the burn wounds are closed and activity increases, therefore, nutritional support must be adjusted periodically. Serum visceral proteins have not been reliable indicators of nutritional status.[38] Severely burned patients should have nitrogen balance and resting metabolic expenditure measured by 24-hour urine collections and indirect calorimetry at weekly or twice weekly intervals to monitor nutritional requirements. Adjustments in nutritional support can then be made as indicated.

PITFALL ⊘

Estimates of calorie needs in severely burned patients should be based on indirect calorimetry rather than derived formulas.

Enteral feeding is possible in nearly all patients and eliminates the risks of central venous catheters, helps maintain gut mucosal integrity, and ameliorates some of the metabolic consequences of the acute inflammatory and hypermetabolic phase. Even though a higher survival has been demonstrated in burn patients maintained on enteral nutrition, parenteral nutrition should be used to prevent excessive erosion of the lean body mass if adequate nutritional support cannot be provided by the enteral route.[39]

Hypothermia

Failure to maintain extensively burned patients in a warm environment can lead to hypothermia and can greatly increase the stress placed upon homeostatic mechanisms. The normal response to cold stress includes an increase in catecholamine secretion and heat production in an attempt to maintain core body temperature. In burn patients, this compensatory response may be impaired. Patients who are already at the limits of their metabolic reserve cannot adapt to further stress, and circulatory collapse may be precipitated if they attempt to maintain body temperature in a cooler environment.

AXIOM Patients with major burns should be kept in a warm environment that will maintain a core temperature of 100.0 to 100.5° F.

The ideal core temperature of patients with major burns is 100.0 to 100.5° F. This can usually be accomplished by maintaining the ambient temperature at 84° F with a relative humidity at 40-50%. Heat lamps and heat shields may also be necessary, especially in small children and in the early postoperative period.

Thromboembolism Prophylaxis

Thromboembolic complications in burn patients have been reported to occur with a frequency of 0.4% to 7%. Over a 10-year period at the United States Army Institute of Surgical Research, the incidences of deep venous thrombosis and fatal pulmonary embolism were 0.9% and 0.14%, respectively.[40] This low incidence of thromboembolism does not justify the risks of routine low dose heparin prophylaxis which is associated with a 0.6% to 5% incidence of complications including bleeding, thrombocytopenia, and arterial thrombosis. However, the high incidence of pulmonary embolism in morbidly obese burn patients, even in the face of heparin prophylaxis, may justify the use of vena cava filter placement for prophylaxis.[41]

Disclaimer

The opinions or assertions contained herein are the private views of the authors and are not to be construed as reflecting the view of the Department of the Army or the Department of Defense.

⊘ FREQUENT ERRORS

In Burn Care

1. *Failure to promptly remove a patient's garments that may still be hot or contaminated with chemicals.*
2. *Failure to promptly intubate patients with major burns that also involve the face.*
3. *Underestimating or overestimating burn size by failure to use a burn chart.*
4. *Underestimating the extent of underlying tissue damage in electrical burns.*
5. *Excessive reliance on burn formulas to determine the quantity and speed of fluid resuscitation.*
6. *Failure to adequately and promptly explain excessive fluid requirements in a burn patient.*
7. *Failure to anticipate the need for escharotomy in patients with deep circumferential burns involving the upper chest and/or extremities.*
8. *Failure to supply adequate glucose during fluid resuscitation of children with major burns.*
9. *Failure to anticipate the presence of an inhalation injury in patients with flame burns in a closed environment.*
10. *Use of prophylactic antibiotics in patients with a major inhalation injury.*
11. *Excessive blood loss during burn wound excision.*
12. *Relying on clinical criteria to diagnose and treat invasive burn wound infection.*
13. *Underfeeding or overfeeding patients with severe burns.*
14. *Maintaining patients with severe burns in an environment with a temperature less than 84° F.*

▼▼▼▼▼▼▼▼▼▼▼▼▼▼▼▼▼▼▼▼▼▼▼▼▼▼▼▼

SUMMARY POINTS

1. Wet dressings and cold compresses applied to large burn wounds for prolonged periods may cause hypothermia.
2. Cutaneous damage from chemicals results in an injury that may continue to progress long after the initial exposure, especially if the irritant remains in contact with the skin.
3. One should not irrigate chemical burns with neutralizing acid or alkali solutions because the heat of reaction that can occur may cause further tissue damage.
4. Removal of the offending agent by removal of clothing and irrigation is the mainstay of early treatment of chemical injury.
5. Chemical burns may be complicated by systemic toxicity if the agent is absorbed. A history that identifies the causative agent allows specific treatment of systemic effects.
6. In patients with severe facial burns, increasing pharyngeal edema can result in airway compromise and an extremely difficult endotracheal intubation as resuscitation proceeds.
7. Accurate determination of the extent of the burn wound is essential for properly estimating initial resuscitation fluid needs.
8. Electric injuries are often much more extensive than estimated by the extent of the surface injury.
9. Carbon monoxide poisoning should be suspected with a history of burn injury in a closed space or finding of obtundation, even if the PaO_2 is normal.
10. The use of hyperbaric oxygen (HBO) therapy for carbon monoxide poisoning is generally unnecessary.

11. The size of the patient and the extent of the burn injury are the most important determinants of the volume of resuscitation fluid required.
12. The initial calculated rate of fluid administration is used only as a guide to begin resuscitation.
13. Burn resuscitation formulas provide an estimation of fluid requirements, and adjustments are made as required by frequent assessment of the clinical response, especially urine output.
14. Occult hemorrhage from associated mechanical trauma should be suspected when fluid requirements are much greater than those calculated from the apparent extent of the burn.
15. Edema from excessive fluid administration may precipitate ischemia in circumferentially burned extremities and predispose the patient to pulmonary edema, particularly during the edema resorption period.
16. Modest hyponatremia is expected after resuscitation with lactated Ringer's solution;, and because total body sodium generally is increased, fluid restriction, not sodium administration, is indicated later to restore serum sodium levels to normal.
17. Adult resuscitation formulas do not account for the infant's need for glucose, higher maintenance needs, and increased sensitivity to hyponatremia.
18. Before performing an escharotomy, one should ascertain that absence of peripheral pulses or loss of Doppler signal is not a result of inadequate fluid resuscitation.
19. Although escharotomy alone is generally adequate to restore perfusion to circumferentially burned extremities, if the thermal injury is deep or if the patient had an electrical injury, a fasciotomy may also be indicated.
20. Blood gas or ventilatory impairment in patients with circumferential deep chest wall burns indicates a need for escharotomy.
21. Bronchoscopy plus xenon-133 lung scanning is the most reliable method for establishing the diagnosis of inhalation injury.
22. Treatment of inhalation injury consists of providing adequate humidified oxygen and aggressive pulmonary toilet; prophylactic antibiotics and steroids are contraindicated.
23. Proper tetanus immunization should be provided to all burn patients.
24. Excision of large burn wounds should be carefully planned to prevent massive blood loss and hypothermia.
25. Inadequate excision of burn wounds almost invariably results in loss of the skin grafts that are applied.
26. Histologic examination of a burn wound biopsy is the mainstay in the diagnosis of invasive burn wound infection.
27. Intramuscularly or subcutaneously administered narcotics in the early postburn period often result in inadequate pain control initially and/or overdose later.
28. Serious gastrointestinal bleeding from erosive gastritis or duodenal ulcers can generally be prevented by maintaining the gastric pH above 5.
29. The resumption of oral intake as soon as possible is probably the best prophylaxis against upper gastrointestinal stress ulcers.
30. Fever, leukocytosis, and a hyperdynamic circulatory response are part of the physiologic response to thermal injury and are not reliable indicators of infection.
31. Estimates of calorie needs in severely burned patients should be based on indirect calorimetry rather than derived formulas.
32. Patients with major burns should be kept in a warm environment that will maintain a core temperature of 100.0 to 100.5° F.

▲▲▲▲▲▲▲▲▲▲▲▲▲▲▲▲▲▲▲▲▲▲▲▲▲▲▲

REFERENCES

1. Resources for optimal care of the injured patient. Committee on Trauma, American College of Surgeons, 1993; 64.
2. Mozingo DW, et al. Chemical burns. J Trauma 1988;28:642.
3. Pruitt BA Jr. The burn patient: I. Initial care. Curr Probl Surg 1979;16:1.

4. Chemical burns and white phosphorus injury. In: Emergency war surgery. Washington, DC: US Government Printing Office, 1975.
5. Kohnlein HE, Merkle P, Springorum HW. Hydrogen fluoride burns: experiments and treatment. Surg Forum 1973;24:50.
6. Heimbach MD, Engrav L, Grube B, et al. Burn depth: a review. World J Surg 1992;16:10.
7. Pruitt BA Jr. Advances in fluid therapy and the early care of the burn patient. World J Surg 1978;2:139.
8. Frank DH. Evaluation and treatment of special types of skin injury. In: Wachtel TS, Kahn V, and Frank HA, eds. Current topics in burn care. Rockville: Aspen Publication, 1983.
9. Shirani KZ, Pruitt BA Jr, Moylan JA Jr. Diagnosis and treatment of inhalation injury in burn patients: In: J Loke, ed. Pathophysiology and treatment of inhalation injuries. Marcel Dekker, Inc., 1988.
10. Pruitt BA Jr, Mason AD Jr, Moncrief JA. Hemodynamic changes in the early postburn patient: the influence of fluid administration and of a vasodilator (hydralazine). J Trauma 1971;11:36.
11. Cope O. Fluid and electrolyte requirements in burns. Symposium on burns. Washington, DC: National Academy of Sciences, National Research Council, 1951; 33-39.
12. Pruitt BA Jr, Goodwin CW. Thermal injuries. In: Davis JH, ed. Clinical surgery. St. Louis: CV Mosby Co., 1987.
13. Graves TA, et al. Fluid resuscitation of infants and children with massive thermal injury. J Trauma 1988;28:1656.
14. Moylan JA, Inge WW Jr, Pruitt BA Jr. Circulatory changes following circumferential extremity burns evaluated by the ultrasonic flowmeter: an analysis of 60 thermally injured limbs. J Trauma 1971;11:763.
15. Salisbury RE, Loveless S, Silverstein P. Postburn edema of the upper extremity: evaluation of present treatment. J Trauma 1973;13:857.
16. Moylan JA Jr, Wilmore DW, Mouton DE, et al. Early diagnosis of inhalation injury using xenon-133 lung scan. Ann Surg 1972;176:477.
17. Pruitt BA Jr, Cioffi WG, Shimazu T, et al. Evaluation and management of patients with inhalation injury. J Trauma 1990;30:S63.
18. Shirani KZ, Pruitt BA Jr, Mason AD Jr. The influence of inhalation injury and pneumonia on burn mortality. Ann Surg 1987;205:82.
19. Robinson MD, Hudson MD, Riem M, et al. Steroid therapy following isolated smoke inhalation injury. J Trauma 1982;22:876.
20. Cioffi WG, Rue LW, Graves TA, et al. Prophylactic use of high-frequency percussive ventilation in patients with inhalation injury. Ann Surg 1991;213:575.
21. Amy BW, McManus WF, Pruitt BA Jr. Tetanus following a major thermal injury. J Trauma 1985;25:654.
22. Graves TA, et al. Relationship of transfusion and infection in a burn population. J Trauma 1989;29:948.
23. Kim SH, et al. Frozen section technique to evaluate early burn wound biopsy: a comparison with the rapid section technique. J Trauma 1985;25:1134.
24. Pruitt BA Jr. Biopsy diagnosis of surgical infection. N Engl J Med 1984;310:1737.
25. McManus AT, Seung HK, McManus WF, et al. Comparison of quantitative microbiology and histopathology in divided burn-wound biopsy specimens. Arch Surg 1987;122:74.
26. McManus WF, Goodwin CW, Pruitt BA Jr. Subeschar treatment of burn-wound infection. Arch Surg 1983;118:291.
27. Spebar MJ, Walter MJ, Pruitt BA Jr. Improved survival with aggressive surgical management of noncandidal fungal infections of the burn wound. J Trauma 1982;22:867.
28. Czaja AJ, McAlhany JC, Pruitt BA Jr. Acute gastroduodenal disease after thermal injury: an endoscopic evaluation of incidence and natural history. N Engl J Med 1974;291:925.
29. McElwee HP, Sirinek KR, Levine BA. Cimetidine affords protection equal to antacids in prevention of stress ulceration following thermal injury. Surgery 1979;86:620.
30. Cioffi WG, McManus AT, Rue LW III, et al. Comparison of acid neutralizing and non-acid neutralizing stress ulcer prophylaxis in thermally injured patients. J Trauma 1994;36:544.
31. Mozingo DW, Cioffi WG, McManus WF, et al. Peritoneal lavage in the diagnosis of acute surgical abdominal thermal injury. J Trauma 1995; 38:5.
32. Lescher TJ, Teegarden DK, Pruitt BA Jr. Acute pseudo-obstruction of the colon in thermally injured patients. Dis Colon Rectum 1978; 21:618.
33. Pruitt BA Jr. Infection: cause or effect of pathophysiologic change in burn and trauma patients. In: M. Paubert-Braquet, ed. Lipid mediators in the immunology of shock. Plenum Publishing Corporation, 1987.
34. Pruitt BA Jr, McManus AT. The changing epidemiology of infection in burn patients. World J Surg 1992;16:57.
35. Jahoor F, Herndon DN, Wolfe RR. Role of insulin and glucagon in the response of glucose and alanine kinetics in burn-injured patients. J Clin Invest 1986;78:807.
36. Wilmore DW, Aulick LH, Mason AD, et al. Influence of the burn wound on local and systemic responses to injury. Ann Surg 1977;186:444.
37. Carlson DE, Cioffi WG, Mason AD, et al. Resting energy expenditure in patients with thermal injuries. Surg Gynec Obstet 1992;174:270.
38. Carlson DE, Cioffi WG, Mason AD, et al. Evaluation of serum visceral protein levels as indicators of nitrogen balance in thermally injured patients. J Parenter and Ent Nutr 1991;15:440.
39. Herndon DN, Barrow RE, Stein M, et al. Increased mortality with intravenous supplemental feeding in severely burned patients. J Burn Care Rehabil 1989;10:309.
40. Rue LW III, Cioffi WG, Rush R, et al. Thrombo-embolic complications in thermally injured patients. World J Surg 1992;16:1151.
41. Sheridan RL, Rue LW III, McManus WF, et al. Burns in morbidly obese patients. J Trauma 1992;33:818.

Chapter 37B Temperature-related (Nonburn) Injuries

ROBERT F. WILSON, M.D.

Now King David was old and stricken in years; and they covered him with clothes, but he gat no heat. Wherefore his servants said,—let there be sought—for the king a young virgin; and let her—cherish him and—lie in his bosom, that my lord the king may get heat. —1 Kings 1:1-2

INTRODUCTION

Adverse environmental temperatures and conditions can cause a wide variety of temperature-related injuries and syndromes. Nonfreezing cold injuries and frostbite are induced by exposure to cold and freezing temperatures, respectively. A variety of heat overload syndromes secondary to exposure to hot environments may also occur.[1] These problems develop when the environment overwhelms the body's homeothermic defenses.[1,2,3]

Homeothermic Regulation

Homeothermic (warm-blooded) animals tend to maintain a relatively constant internal (core) temperature that allows free mobility through hostile ambient temperatures, but the body temperature of poikilothermic (cold-blooded) animals tends to take on that of the environment.[1]

The thermoneutral air temperature for unclothed humans is about 27° C (81° F).[1] Extreme precautions become necessary only under extreme or prolonged thermal adversity because the insulation of the body and the homeothermic mechanisms allow maintenance of a constant body core temperature when exposed, unclothed, to dry air from 13-60° C (55-140° F).[4] Humans respond to low temperatures by increasing physical activity and retarding heat loss with protective clothing. At higher temperatures, humans limit physical activity and shed excess clothing.[1]

AXIOM Impairment of mental or cardiovascular function greatly increases the risk of patients developing accidental heat or cold injury.

Homeothermic regulation begins with detection of the ambient (external) temperature by peripheral thermal receptors and the core temperature by central receptors.[1] The skin is richly supplied with thermal receptors that are especially sensitive to cold. Signals from these receptors pass to the hypothalamic areas for temperature regulation along pathways in the spinal cord identical to those traversed by signals for pain. Thermal receptors in the central nervous system (CNS), especially the preoptic hypothalamus, track directly to the hypothalamic areas concerned with temperature regulation.[1]

The posterior hypothalamus initiates heat production by increasing muscle tone and by increasing secretion of thyroxine and catecholamines, especially epinephrine.[5] The shivering that results from increased muscle tone is perhaps the most important of these effects because it can increase the basal metabolic rate two to five times above its normal 40-60 kcal/hr.[6,7]

Responses to a Cold Environment

The homeothermic responses to a cold environment include: (a) physical thermogenesis (shivering and increased muscle tone), (b)

metabolic thermogenesis, (c) vasoconstriction, and (d) conscious responses such as increased physical activity (Table 37B–1).[1] Thus, the responses to hypothermia are designed to increase heat production and decrease heat loss. Chemical (metabolic) thermogenesis (60%) and physical thermogenesis (40%) account for all heat production in the body. Heat production is increased with increasing levels of skeletal muscle metabolic activity. At basal levels, total heat production generally ranges from 65-85 kcal/hr, but may rise up to 300, 600, or even 900 kcal/hr under situations of increasing exertion or shivering[6-9] (Table 37B–2).

Responses to a Hot Environment

Besides a basal heat production of approximately 70-80 kcal/hr, up to 150 kcal/hr may result from irradiation from the sun.[10] To this load is added the heat produced by any work being performed (Table 37B–1).

AXIOM The body's responses to hyperthermia are limited and include cutaneous vasodilation, sweating, and decreased physical activity.

Once the ambient temperature exceeds that of the skin, heat loss can only occur by evaporation of insensible water or sweat. Mechanisms to dissipate heat include evaporation of insensible water and sweat and cutaneous vasodilation, which increases heat loss through radiation, conduction, and convection. Unfortunately, however, when the ambient temperature (temperature of the external environment) exceeds body temperature, heat can only be lost through evaporation. Even at maximum efficiency, sweating may result in only 400-650 kcal/hr of heat dissipation.[2] Furthermore, increased humidity and/or pooling of sweat reduces the efficacy of evaporation as a means of heat loss.

AXIOM Heatstroke syndrome is more likely to occur if there is increased activity and the person is poorly acclimatized.

The physiologic process whereby an individual adapts to work in a hot environment is often referred to as acclimatization.[8] The changes involved in acclimatization include decreased sweat production, decreased sodium concentration in sweat, increased aldosterone secretion, and a decreased maximal cardiac output, stroke volume, and heart rate. Additionally, acclimatized subjects are noted to drink greater quantities of water spontaneously and have baseline increases in their calculated extracellular fluid volumes. The metabolic efficiency of these individuals also increases, thereby decreasing the net heat production for a given unit of work. All of these factors substantially reduce the risk of exertional heatstroke developing as a result of demanding physical work in high ambient temperatures.[2]

The magnitude of the homeothermic responses is generally proportional to the magnitude of the thermal challenge.[1] An example of this response is the regulation of heat loss via blood flow to the skin. Heat conduction from the core of the body to the skin increases linearly eightfold from its vasoconstricted state at an ambient temperature of 24° C (75° F) to its maximally vasodilated state at 43° C (110° F).[4] Sweating can increase heat loss up to ten times that of basal heat production.[4] Shivering, however, can increase heat production fourfold to fivefold.[4]

TABLE 37B–1 *Physiologic Responses to Maintain Homothermia*[10]

	Environment	
	Cool	Warm
Physical thermogenesis	Increased activity Shivering Increased muscle tone	Decreased activity
Metabolic rate	Increased	Decreased
Skin	Vasoconstriction	Vasodilation Sweating

There are a number of conditions that predispose a patient to homeothermic failure. Any circumstances that adversely affect sensation, the hypothalamic areas of temperature regulation, or the end organ(s) can reduce or abolish the protective homeothermic responses. For example, transection of the spinal cord abolishes shivering and reduces muscular activity, skin vasoconstriction, and sweating distal to the level of injury.[1] Protective homeothermic mechanisms are also seriously impaired if the core temperature exceeds 41° C (106° F) or falls below 34° C (94° F).

AXIOM The homeothermic responses to cold are virtually nonexistent at core temperatures below 28° C (83° F).[1]

NONFREEZING COLD INJURY

Introduction

Nonfreezing cold (NFC) injury primarily afflicts military personnel.[1,10,11] This problem was recognized as distinct from frostbite during the first winter of the Crimean War (1854-1855).[11] The temperature rarely fell below freezing that winter, yet 1924 of the 50,000 British soldiers suffered cold injuries. These NFC injuries were attributed to the poor physical status of the troops and to boots that were "defective and quite unsuitable."[11] Although the etiologic importance of a wet and cold environment was not universally appreciated for more than 70 years, precautionary measures to improve foot care reduced the number of British soldiers with NFC injuries to 474 the following winter. As is so often true for medical lessons learned during wars, the knowledge was lost, and during the first December of World War I, the British suffered 4823 NFC injuries.[12] Unfortunately, there have been few clinical or experimental reports on NFC injury since World War II.

A variety of nonfreezing cold injuries are recognized. Chilblain (pernio) is an infrequently used term to describe dermatological changes in skin chronically exposed to wet, nonfreezing cold. "Trench foot" got its name during World War I when the soldiers spent so much time in wet, cold trenches.[13] Survivors of shipwrecks tended to develop a similar problem referred to as "immersion foot."[14] In the Vietnam conflict, "paddy foot" was used to describe a warm water variant with similar tissue changes.[15]

Etiology

AXIOM Nonfreezing cold (NFC) injury is caused by tissue chilling and reduced perfusion of tissues resulting from cold-induced vasoconstriction.[1]

Histologic studies of tissues with NFC injury demonstrate a characteristic pattern of acute inflammatory response with neural and muscular injury and subsequent fibrosis. Factors contributing to NFC injury are: immobility, impaired circulation, venous stasis, debilitation, constrictive footwear or clothing, and dehydration.[1] NFC injury gen-

erally requires moisture because water, which is an excellent conductor of heat, is needed for tissue to lose heat. In very cold and wet conditions, NFC injury can develop in hours, but in less extreme conditions, it may require days of exposure. Reduced perfusion can also speed up tissue changes.

AXIOM Cold injury is much more apt to occur in areas of the body that are not kept dry.

Specific Problems

CHILBLAIN

Chilblain refers to the swelling and reddish or violaceous plaques that may develop on fingers, toes, or ears after repeated or chronic exposure to dampness at temperatures just above freezing.[12] Burning, itching, and tingling are prominent symptoms when the involved part warms. In some instances, erythema and edema may develop into vesiculation and ulceration. Any underlying metabolic or vascular disorder may contribute to this problem.

Local treatment is nonspecific and consists of careful rewarming of the involved part and protection from further cold or trauma.[12] Correction of any underlying problem such as anemia, malnutrition, or hypothyroidism may accelerate healing and reduce the likelihood of injury if further exposure cannot be avoided.

IMMERSION FOOT

The clinical syndrome of immersion foot has been recognized for centuries.[16] It occurs in the setting of prolonged exposure to a wet environment. Immersion foot has accounted for large numbers of casualties in many wars and conflicts of this century. Pseudonyms for the disorder include trench foot, swamp foot, tropical jungle foot, paddy foot, jungle rot, sea boot foot, bridge foot, and foxhole foot.

AXIOM Immersion foot refers to virtually any foot injuries caused by prolonged exposure to cold and wet.

Although many terms have been applied to this syndrome, immersion foot can be used for all such nonfreezing injuries.[17] When the more severe effects of cold but nonfreezing water (less than 15° C) are present, it should be subcategorized as "cold-water immersion foot." The more benign variant occurring at warmer temperatures should be called "warm-water immersion foot."

Immersion foot is characterized by white, wrinkled, painful involvement of the soles of the feet.[16] With more prolonged exposure, the dorsum of the foot may also be involved. Although recovery is complete and without major long-term sequelae in most circumstances, severe complications such as nerve and muscle injury, as well as gangrene, may occasionally be seen.[16]

The pathologic hallmark of immersion foot is waterlogging of the thick stratum corneum of the soles of the feet.[15,16] Natural creases are exaggerated and new creases are produced causing wrinkling.[16] Evidence of absorption of 1 to 2 gm of water per hour by the foot (as much as 47 ml in 24 hours) has been reported.[17] The amount absorbed depends on the salinity of the medium, with fresh water re-

TABLE 37B–2 *Heat Production During Various Activities*[8]

Activity	kcal/hr
Basal	70
Football	102
Light assembly work	108
Exposure to hot sun	150
Walking (4 mph)	340
5-mile run	360
Swimming	660

sulting in much greater absorption. Much of what is absorbed will pass into the circulation, but some is retained in the stratum corneum.

Biopsy specimens of the skin of affected individuals have shown swelling, thickening, and fragmentation of the stratum corneum with variable amounts of edema of the upper dermis.[15] In some cases, the capillaries of the upper dermis may be constricted by edema and/or a lymphocytic vasculitis.[18]

The best treatment of immersion foot is prevention. Adequate foot care, including drying of the feet, is necessary. The military has suggested that it is optimal to air dry feet for at least 8 hours out of every day.[11,12] Boots are apparently better at preventing the syndrome than tennis shoes because of their greater impenetrability to water and grit. Thermal insulation may actually make the situation worse.

AXIOM   Nonfreezing cold injuries to the feet frequently result from inadequate or improperly fitting footwear.

When homelessness is identified, not only the patient's feet but also their footwear should be examined. Referral for social service consultation to replace or repair inadequate footwear is indicated. Instruction in foot care is also of benefit and should be a routine in shelters for the homeless.[16] Some physicians prefer to treat immersion foot by warming the feet in water heated to 100-105° F and then carefully drying them.[1] Others prefer passive rewarming at room temperature because active local rewarming may increase the edema, reactive hyperemia, and pain. Analgesics are often necessary during rewarming, but are usually not needed later because anesthesia of the involved tissues often accompanies the development of hyperemia.

AXIOM   The treatment of immersion foot includes careful protection of the involved tissue as long as hyperemia, anhidrosis, and paresthesias persist.

Gangrene may be present at the time of presentation or may develop during treatment of immersion foot. Supportive treatment with the avoidance of further injury and infection is similar to that described for frostbite. Tetanus prophylaxis is administered if there is breakdown of the skin or any gangrene. Antibiotics are usually unnecessary unless indicated for other injuries. The beneficial effects of sympathectomy, vasodilators, dextran, or anticoagulants are unproven.[1]

AXIOM   Careful atraumatic physical therapy is useful to minimize the formation of contractures in patients with immersion foot.

FROSTBITE

The term frostbite refers to the damage caused by crystallization of water in the skin or subcutaneous tissue by exposure to temperatures at or below freezing.[12]

Etiology

Frostbite generally occurs as a result of exposure to extremely cold temperatures.[19] The majority of soldiers who have developed frostbite were exposed to temperatures below $-12°$ C (10° F) for more than 7 hours.[12] In many instances, the individual exposed to excessive cold may not even be aware that he is in danger of suffering frostbite. Failure to provide adequate protection to the face, ears, and extremities is a common factor in the development of frostbite. The windchill factor may be entirely ignored, and the individual, aware that the outside temperature is only a few degrees below the freezing point, may fail to consider the fact that a 30-mph

wind can reduce the effective temperature to well below zero.[12] Engaging in military actions or some variety of winter sports may be a distracting influence and further reduce awareness of impending frostbite.

AXIOM   Frostbite injury is much less apt to occur in individuals carefully watching each other for early signs of its development.

To clarify the mechanisms of cold temperature on vibration-induced white finger (VWF), Chen et al[20] studied three groups of forestry chain saw operators. Groups I and II worked in a cold, high-altitude area, and group III worked in a warm, low-mountain climate. Group I workers had evidence of VWF (VWF [+]), but groups II and III did not (VWF [−]). Fingernail fold microcirculation before and after cold exposure, finger skin sympathetic alpha receptor response, and sympathetic skin response were measured. The results showed that there was no significantly different neuropathy in any of the groups. However, vibration-induced microcirculatory disturbances, including blood stasis and red blood cell aggregation, were more prominent in the VWF (+) group, whereas both of the VWF (−) groups (groups II and III) had no significant microcirculatory disturbances. This suggests that the severity of the microcirculatory disturbances in VWF were dose-dependent and were aggravated by cold.

Pathophysiologic Changes

The pathophysiological changes of frostbite are extremely complex but usually involve at least two factors: (a) direct tissue damage caused by the cold and (b) tissue injury resulting from vasoconstriction and then later vasodilatation with resultant edema, red cell sludging, and thrombosis of vessels (Fig. 37B–1). Both of these factors play a role, and the resultant decreased blood flow to the surface makes these tissues much more susceptible to direct cold injury.

Experimental studies have shown that rapid freezing and rapid thawing can maintain viable tissue; however, rapid freezing is rarely encountered clinically, and people cannot be thawed rapidly.[1] The

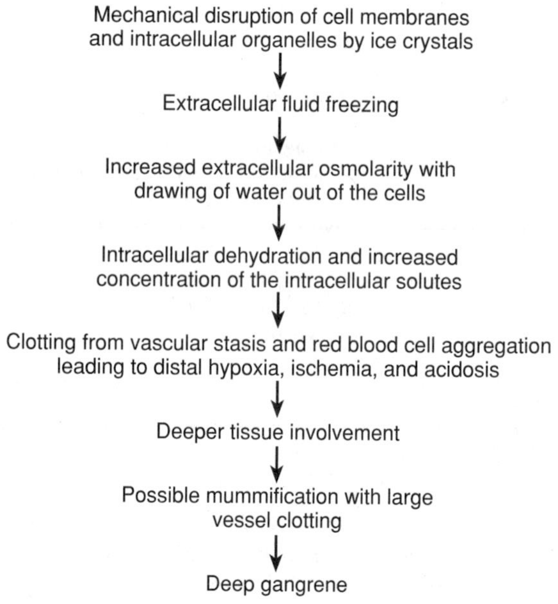

Mechanical disruption of cell membranes
and intracellular organelles by ice crystals
↓
Extracellular fluid freezing
↓
Increased extracellular osmolarity with
drawing of water out of the cells
↓
Intracellular dehydration and increased
concentration of the intracellular solutes
↓
Clotting from vascular stasis and red blood cell aggregation
leading to distal hypoxia, ischemia, and acidosis
↓
Deeper tissue involvement
↓
Possible mummification with large
vessel clotting
↓
Deep gangrene

FIGURE 37B–1   Sequence of events of frostbite. (From Fritz RL. Clin Sports Med 1989;8:111.)

frostbite encountered clinically is a "slow" freezing process characterized by sheets of extracellular ice crystals surrounding dehydrated, collapsed, but unfrozen cells.

Cutaneous vasoconstriction in response to cold results in arteriovenous shunting.[1] This cutaneous arteriovenous shunting is relieved intermittently (every 5 to 7 minutes) by "cold-induced" vasodilatation, the so-called "hunting reaction."[21] The hunting reaction prevents rapid freezing of the skin, but the price paid for this protective vasodilatation is an inappropriate increase in the loss of body heat. Intense or prolonged cold inactivates the hunting reaction, and freezing of tissue then ensues.

Once extracellular freezing begins, unbound intracellular water shifts to the extracellular spaces in response to the hypertonic osmotic gradient surrounding the ice crystals.[1] In clinical frostbite, the temperatures in deep tissues are seldom more than a few degrees below freezing because ice crystallization is an exothermic process, and if the environmental exposure is severe enough to lower tissue temperatures, the resultant total-body hypothermia tends to kill the patient.

Cellular death from freezing is not a simple matter of rupture of cell membranes from osmotic gradients created by tissue freezing.[1] It appears to be a complex process involving damage from ice crystals and osmotic gradients, alterations in intracellular composition (particularly of enzyme systems), changes in membrane permeability, pH alterations, vasoconstriction, capillary injury, increased blood viscosity, and the metabolic status of the tissues during cooling. Additional damage resulting from circulatory stasis, thromboses, and tissue swelling often occurs after thawing.[1]

Diagnosis

SIGNS AND SYMPTOMS
Freezing begins at the skin and progresses toward the core of the body.[1] As with nonfreezing cold injuries, the most distal portions of the involved limb are most severely injured. Sudden blanching or an unusual whiteness of the skin with a pale, glassy appearance may be the first indication of cold injury.[12] There is generally also an uncomfortable sensation of coldness followed by numbness. There is usually a distinct boundary between the frozen and unfrozen areas. Initially, the depth of frostbite cannot be determined accurately, as all the frozen areas are cold, cadaveric in appearance, and without sensation.[1] The severity of the frostbite may not be clear until several days after thawing. As rewarming occurs, there may be increasing tingling, stinging, burning, and/or aching.[12]

CLASSIFYING FROSTBITE (TABLE 37B–3)
The severity of frostbite may be divided into degrees: first-degree (frost nip), characterized by hyperemia and edema after thawing; second-degree, characterized by hyperemia and blisters; third-degree, with necrosis of the skin and subcutaneous tissue; and fourth-degree, involving necrosis of underlying fascia and muscle.[12]

First-degree Frostbite (Frost Nip)
In first-degree frostbite, the skin, after rewarming, becomes mottled blue or purple and then red and swollen.[12] Edema may persist for a week or longer and is followed by skin peeling, which may persist for many weeks or months.

Second-degree Frostbite
With second-degree frostbite, first-degree changes are followed by formation of multiple tiny vesicles or a single large vesicle within 12 to 24 hours of rewarming.[12] The blisters dry and form black eschars in 1 to 3 weeks. These gradually peel away revealing underlying intact skin that is easily injured. Initially the area may be anesthetic, but with rewarming, tingling and burning are followed within 1 to 5 days by throbbing and aching that may be quite severe.

Third-degree Frostbite
Third-degree frostbite involves the full thickness of the skin.[12] There may be severe edema of the entire involved hand or foot, and blisters

TABLE 37B–3 Classification of Frostbite

Signs	Symptoms
First-degree: Partial skin freezing	
Erythema, edema, hyperemia	Transient stinging and burning
No blisters	May have hyperhidrosis
Occasional later desquamation	
Second-degree: Full-thickness skin freezing	
Erythema, edema	Numbness; vasomotor disturbances in severe cases
Vesicles with clear fluid	
Blisters that desquamate and form blackened eschar	
Third-degree: Subcutaneous tissue	
Violaceous/hemorrhagic blisters	Initially no sensation
Skin necrosis	Involved tissue feels like wood
Blue-gray discoloration	Later burning, throbbing, aching
Fourth-degree: Full-thickness freezing down to bone	
Little edema	
Initially mottled, deep red, or cyanotic	
Eventually dry, black, mummified	

Adapted from Britt LD, Dascombe WH, Rodriguez A. New horizon in management of hypothermia and frostbite injuries. SCNA 1991;71:345.

may be proximal to the damaged tissue. In addition to the white, waxy appearance, the areas become firm and there is no "give" to the underlying tissues with compression. The thick, black eschar that subsequently develops separates slowly over the next several weeks and usually reveals underlying granulating tissue that slowly epithelializes. Severe aching or throbbing in the frostbitten tissues may persist for several weeks.

AXIOM Even with what appears to be severe frostbite with black eschar, a great deal of spontaneous healing eventually occurs.

Fourth-degree Frostbite
The destruction of tissue with fourth-degree frostbite extends down to involve bone.[12] The damaged tissue gradually develops the appearance of dry gangrene. Severe paresthesias may be present at the line of demarcation that develops between the gangrenous tissue and that which will survive. This demarcation may not be apparent for at least several weeks.[12]

AXIOM One should not perform early amputations for frostbite unless the patient develops a severe infection that is unresponsive to appropriate antibiotics.

Prevention of Frostbite (Table 37B–4)

Frostbite is best prevented by avoiding extremely cold environments; however, if there is no way to avoid exposure, one should prepare for the worst possible scenario. Loose, dry, layered clothing over as much of the body as possible is extremely helpful. Avoidance of drugs and alcohol is also important. It is helpful to have a companion who can watch for early evidence of frostbite because the initial stages are frequently unrecognized by the involved individual.

Treatment

FROST NIP
The damage resulting from frost nip is usually minor and prompt rewarming and subsequent protection from further exposure generally

TABLE 37B–4   Prevention of Frostbite

1. Suspect the possibility if exposed to cold air in conjunction with wind.
2. Wear adequate, layered, loose-fitting clothing, especially over the hands, feet, nose, and ears.
3. Keep clothing dry.
4. Do not touch bare metal with bare skin.
5. Cover all metal with cloth, tape, or leather.
6. Do not maintain one position for prolonged periods.
7. Avoid cramped quarters.
8. Keep wriggling cold toes and fingers.
9. Keep contracting your facial muscles.
10. Turn your back to the wind whenever possible.
11. Protect localized skin numbness whenever possible from further exposure.
12. Watch companion's exposed skin.
13. Rewarm cold and numb fingers in the crotch or axillae or against companion's stomach.
14. Find immediate shelter from the elements and build a fire if fingers or toes become cold, numb, and begin not to wriggle.

Modified from Fritz RL, Perrin DH. Cold exposure injuries: prevention and treatment. Clin Sports Med 1989;8:111.

TABLE 37B–5   Field Treatment of Frostbite

1. Prevent the victim from further heat loss by avoiding the wind, protecting the frostbitten area, and drying all gear, especially gloves, socks, and boot liners.
2. Protect the victim from further freezing by making emergency camp and leaving for help only after a fire is started and ample firewood obtained.
3. Stay with the victim if there is any chance of a rescue search party.
4. If rapid rewarming by water immersion is possible, remember that this can be painful and that shock and compartment syndrome are a possibility.
5. Once thawed, the frozen part should not be used.
6. Any wrapping should anticipate that thawed tissue swells rapidly.
7. If immediate evacuation is not possible, it is preferable to leave a foot frozen.
8. A frozen body part is unlikely to be further damaged by use.
9. A thawed body part is susceptible to further injury.
10. Once evacuated, all frostbite injuries should be examined in a medical facility or hospital.

Modified from Fritz RL, Perrin DH. Cold exposure injuries: prevention and treatment. Clin Sports Med 1989;8:111.

completely reverses the process.[12] If artificial heat is not available, the area should be warmed by covering it with hands or by breathing on it.

> **AXIOM**   An area of cold injury should never be rubbed, especially with snow or cold water.

SUPERFICIAL FROSTBITE

Prehospital Care (Table 37B–5)

Because frostbite injury is cumulative, the duration of cold exposure should be minimized; however, the frozen tissue should not be thawed if refreezing or physical trauma is likely to occur during evacuation. Patients whose frostbite has thawed are generally incapacitated by pain, while those with unthawed frostbite are better able to cooperate with rescuers because they have little or no pain. If refreezing is likely, the best course is to maintain the local temperature just below freezing and immobilize the involved extremities because motion at the frozen-nonfrozen tissue interfaces is likely to increase the amount of subsequent tissue loss.[1]

Thawing (Table 37B–6)

Once the patient is in a protected environment where the involved tissues will not be traumatized or cooled again, the frozen tissues should be rapidly rewarmed. The frozen area should not be massaged or rubbed.[1] Analgesics are often required during thawing because it can be extremely painful. Rapid thawing by submerging the frozen areas in water preheated to 38-40° C (100.4-104° F) is the method of choice for deep frostbite. Thawing with heat in excess of 40° C (104° F) can increase the loss of tissue. Rewarming is continued until all of the involved tissues are warm and hyperemic. If systemic hypothermia below 32° C (90° F) accompanies the frostbite, rapid, internal rewarming is the treatment of choice.[1]

> **AXIOM**   A patient with a cold injury should not smoke cigarettes or be given any drug that can cause vasoconstriction.

Smoking can cause severe vasoconstriction in the skin, causing a slower rewarming and additional tissue damage.[12]

After Thawing

The goals of treatment after rewarming are to avoid infection and to minimize loss of tissue.[1] Prophylactic antibiotics are not used unless indicated for other injuries. After several days, non-narcotic analgesics should be adequate for controlling pain. The frostbitten areas are

treated in an open fashion on sterile padding and under cradles covered by sterile sheets to avoid secondary injury from pressure. Although some surgeons open bullae and then apply a topical antibiotic, most surgeons allow the vesicles and bullae to resolve spontaneously.

> **AXIOM**   Debridement of frostbitten tissues should be extremely conservative; with time, most of the damage will heal by itself.

Necrotic tissue is debrided by immersion therapy twice a day in whirlpool baths containing a mild soap or detergent. If the tissue becomes infected, the area should be debrided as needed to control the local infection and to prevent systemic sepsis. The injured areas are thoroughly air-dried after the whirlpool treatments, and sterile cotton is placed between the digits to prevent maceration.

The use of topical antibacterial agents between whirlpool treatments is favored by some; however, others claim they delay separation of the eschar.[1] Early careful physical therapy minimizes the loss of motion.

DEEP FROSTBITE

After rewarming, third-degree frostbite tissue remains blanched, and the patient may benefit from the use of intravenous heparin.[12] Little or no pain is experienced except at the margins of viable and nonviable tissue. The presence of pain, purplish mottling, or vesiculation in the frostbitten area suggests that there may be some patchy survival of tissues.

The eschar that forms should be managed like a third-degree burn. If there is no evidence of viability, the eschar and involved subcutaneous tissues may be mechanically debrided after 36 to 48 hours and

TABLE 37B–6   Frostbite Treatment Protocol

Patients with frostbite injuries are admitted to the hospital
On admission, the affected areas are rewarmed rapidly in circulating warm water (104° F) for 15 to 30 minutes
After rewarming
    Topical treatment with aloe vera every 6 hours
    The affected parts are elevated and splinted as needed
    Tetanus prophylaxis
    Analgesia, IV or IM morphine or meperidine, as indicated
    Ibuprofen 12 mg/kg orally per day
    Daily hydrotherapy

Modified from Britt LD, Dascombe WH, Rodriguez A. New horizon in management of hypothermia and frostbite injuries. SCNA 1991;71:345.

split-thickness skin grafts applied.[12] If blistering has occurred, even sparsely, the area may be treated as a deep second-degree burn, from which re-epithelialization may occur from remnants of hair follicles and sweat glands.

The residual damage from severe frostbite may result in extensive areas of gangrene or loss of various body parts, including fingers or toes and parts of the ears or nose.[12] Additionally, severe persisting paresthesias or causalgia may develop which, in some instances, may be benefited by chemical or surgical sympathectomy.

AXIOM   The depth of tissue necrosis in frostbite is usually much less than expected.

Inexperienced observers often incorrectly assume that the black skin of frostbite when the patient is first seen indicates a full-thickness injury and that the necrotic skin means that the underlying deep tissue is also dead. This assumption has led to some unnecessary and inappropriately high early amputations for frostbite.

AXIOM   Surgical debridement or amputations for frostbite should not be performed until the level of mummification or tissue death is clearly demarcated, and this usually takes at least 1 to 3 months.

Early digital escharotomies may be indicated if the eschar restricts motion and limits physical therapy.[1] Prompt fasciotomy is mandatory if compartment syndrome occurs after reperfusion. In suspicious or questionable cases, the diagnosis of compartment syndrome should be confirmed by measuring compartment pressures.

Much of the controversy concerning the management of severe cold injuries has focused on the various methods used to reduce: (a) the vasospastic response to tissue cooling, (b) the vascular injury induced by freezing, and (c) the anoxia secondary to the swelling that accompanies rewarming.[1] The value of low-molecular-weight dextran, anticoagulants, adrenergic blocking agents, sympatholytic drugs, thrombolytic agents, and therapy with hyperbaric oxygen is unproven. Although early sympathectomy decreases the pain and edema of deep frostbite, it is controversial whether it decreases the amount of tissue loss. Indeed, the use of sympathectomy or vasodilators in an attempt to improve peripheral circulation may actually induce compartment syndromes and cause higher levels of amputation.[1]

Borovikov[21] has noted that digitless hands from frostbite injury are typically seen in young men as a result of an episode of intoxication. Such deformities occur bilaterally in 80% of cases and often lead to total loss of prehensile capability. Because of a high degree of motivation in these patients, toe-to-hand transfer in 25 digitless patients had an excellent prognosis. Microanastomoses in these frostbitten hands was as reliable as in mechanically injured hands, provided the ulnar artery and its branches were intact and there was a satisfactory thumb post. Because the amputations tended to occur at the level of the metacarpal heads, the preferred transplant was a second and third toe composite. Well-planned sharing of available toes is necessary for establishing optimum bilateral hand function, especially in the face of simultaneous toe frostbite.

Sequelae of Cold Injury

Supportive therapy usually results in complete recovery from mild cold injuries.[1] Over a period of days or weeks, the blebs, edema, hyperemia, anhidrosis, and paresthesias disappear, and the circulation appears to return to normal. In third- or fourth-degree frostbite, however, recovery without serious sequelae is unlikely[1] (Table 37B–7). In addition to tissue losses, these patients are often incapacitated by limitations of motion, pain on walking, hyperhidrosis, hyperesthesias, cold intolerance, and severe vasospastic attacks to even mild cold. Years after suffering deep frostbite, more than two-thirds of the patients may complain of cold feet, hyperhidrosis, pain, and numbness, particularly during winter months.

TABLE 37B–7   Possible Frostbite Sequelae

Cold sensitivity	Vasospastic attacks
Hyperhidrosis	Hyperesthesias
Intrinsic muscle atrophy	Chronic pain
Color changes in integument	Pinnae calcification (uncommon)
Arthritis	Squamous-cell carcinoma (rare)
Growth plate abnormalities (children)	
Tissue loss	

Britt LD, Dascombe WH, Rodriguez A. New horizon in management of hypothermia and frostbite injuries. SCNA 1991;71:345.

Arthritis is a common sequela in patients with deep frostbite and, in addition, many develop impaired joint mobility. Children may also suffer retardation of bone growth secondary to injury to their epiphyseal plates. Sympathectomy appears to reduce the chronic pain, hyperhidrosis, and vasospastic sequelae of cold injuries to some degree; however, cold intolerance often persists in spite of this procedure.[1]

AXIOM   Patients who have suffered severe cold injury should avoid any repeat cold exposure because they are at increased risk to suffer severe tissue damage and/or pain.

One interesting sequela incurred by patients with superficial frostbite is the lesion referred to as chilblains or pernio.[1] Chilblains are characterized by recurrent localized itching, swelling, and painful erythema. One report suggests that the symptoms and cutaneous lesions of chilblains resolve with the administration of nifedipine, a calcium channel blocker that has been found useful in the treatment of Raynaud's phenomenon.[22]

TOTAL BODY HYPOTHERMIA

Hypothermia is generally defined as a body core temperature of less than 35° C (95° F).[23,24] Unfortunately, most clinical thermometers do not record temperatures at this level.

Incidence

ACCIDENTAL HYPOTHERMIA

The incidence of exposure-induced (accidental) hypothermia has not been accurately determined in the United States.[2] Although accidental hypothermia is a major public health problem, it is frequently unrecognized, especially in the elderly. From 1970 to 1979 the Public Health Service recorded 4826 deaths from hypothermia in the United States.[25] Exposure-induced hypothermia is not unusual during wilderness adventures,[26] but the majority of cases occur in urban areas.

AXIOM   Hypothermia can occur at virtually any temperature below 80° F.

Hypothermia is not that uncommon in southern states, and it also occurs among patients without outdoor exposure.[27] Hypothermia cases have been reported as far south as Texas and Florida, even under relatively mild climatic conditions.[6] Not only is hypothermia relatively common, but it can be extremely dangerous. The experience with exposure hypothermia at Bellevue Hospital was that 13% of the patients died. Of these deaths, 71% occurred while the patient was still hypothermic, and failure to achieve euthermia within 12 hours was uniformly fatal.[28]

AXIOM   Hypothermia can increase the mortality rates with virtually any injury.

There were 68 deaths from hypothermia in the District of Columbia between 1972 and 1982.[25] Among this population, the highest death rate was among black men with a median age of 50. Half of the patients had high ethanol levels, half had inadequate housing, and a third were malnourished. Urban poverty can have a great effect on incidence of hypothermia seen at inner-city medical centers. The growing elderly population is particularly prone to develop this problem.

Although hypothermia may afford some protection against anoxia that might otherwise prove fatal,[29] it is often an ominous sign.[30] Children are at extraordinary risk from accidents that cause hypothermia, especially drowning.[31] This paradox has given rise to the realization that hypothermic protection from hypoxia or ischemia is unusual, and even optimal management may not produce a good outcome.[32]

POST-TRAUMATIC HYPOTHERMIA

The frequency of post-traumatic hypothermia is unclear, but severely injured patients are at great risk for developing post-traumatic hypothermia. In a group of critically injured adults with head injuries, 40% were or became hypothermic during resuscitation.[1] The incidence of hypothermia in patients who are in shock and require massive transfusions is even higher.[31,33,34]

> **AXIOM** One should monitor core temperatures closely in trauma patients, especially those who are in shock, receive massive transfusions, or have prolonged abdominal surgery.

Etiology (Table 37B–8)

ACCIDENTAL HYPOTHERMIA

Exposure hypothermia results from heat loss in excess of heat production. The rate of heat loss is directly proportional to the temperature difference between the body and cooler adjacent structures.[4,35] In the United States, clinically significant hypothermia is most commonly seen in alcoholic patients.[36] In addition to causing CNS changes that result in individuals not seeking appropriate shelter and protection from the environment, alcohol causes cutaneous vasodilation which accelerates heat loss.[3]

MASSIVE BLOOD TRANSFUSIONS

Hypothermia that develops in the hospital in injured patients is often closely related to the amount of cold fluid and blood administered. In one study, hypothermic patients received an average of 8.7 units of blood versus 3.3 units in patients who did not develop hypothermia (P < 0.01).[1] A survey published by Werweth et al[37] in 1984 revealed that only one-third of emergency departments had fluid warming devices.

It should not be surprising that massive transfusions of cold blood cause hypothermia. Collins noted that approximately 300 kcal, which is equal to 2 hours of normal resting caloric expenditure, are needed to warm 10 liters of blood from 4° C (39° F) to core temperature. He also noted that this requirement often comes "precisely at the worst time, when the oxygen supply and energy are being severely stressed."[38]

TABLE 37B–8 Factors Predisposing to Cold Injury Trauma

1. Inadequate insulation from the cold and wind
2. Arterial disease or heart failure
3. Tight footwear or clothing
4. Poor nutrition
5. Mental impairment
6. Hypothyroidism and/or hypoadrenalism
7. Atonic metabolic disease
8. Fatigue
9. Use of alcohol or tobacco
10. Very young or very old

Modified from Fritz RL, Perrin DH. Cold exposure injuries: prevention and treatment. Clin Sports Med 1989;8:111.

TABLE 37B–9 Mechanisms of Heat Transfer

Radiation: energy emissions to a colder object
Conduction: direct contact with a colder or warmer object
Convection: movement of air or water adjacent to the skin
Evaporation: loss of body heat by the conversion of water to gas

Modified from Fritz RL, Perrin DH. Cold exposure injuries: prevention and treatment. Clin Sports Med 1989;8:111.

> **AXIOM** Endogenous warming after hypothermia has developed can put a tremendous metabolic and cardiovascular strain on the patient.

Mechanisms of Heat Loss

The mechanisms of heat transfer are generally considered to involve radiation, conduction, convection, and evaporation (Table 37B–9). Radiation, which is the movement of infrared heat rays from the skin at the speed of light, usually accounts for about 50-60% of the body's heat loss in a warm room.[16] In a cold environment, the radiant heat loss may be much greater. Human skin, especially on the head, is an excellent radiator of heat. In a clothed individual, 75% of the heat loss at −15° C (5° F) can occur from an uncovered head.

At room temperature, heat conduction accounts for about 20% of the heat loss (15% to the air and 5% to adjacent objects). In water, however, heat conduction is 24 times faster than in air.[16,39] Indeed, hypothermia can occur with just 1 or 2 hours of immersion in water as warm as 16° C (65° F). Wet clothing loses most of its insulating ability because of conduction. Cold ground, snow, and metal (such as an airplane fuselage or metal stretcher) are also excellent heat sinks.

Convection occurs as warm air next to the skin is replaced by cool air.[16] If there is no wind, convection carries off only about 25% of lost body heat. Although heat loss by convection currents is increased 14 fold in a 35-mph wind, wind velocity is seldom critical in exposure hypothermia. Once the wind velocity is more than a few miles per hour, heat loss by convection exceeds the body's heat loss by conduction.[4]

Evaporation from the skin accounts for only about 7% of heat loss at rest, but under ideal conditions it can carry off an amount of heat equivalent to six times the body's basal metabolic rate.[16] Pulmonary heat losses account for approximately 14% of heat loss at rest. This loss increases with exertion or at higher altitudes, especially in cold, dry air. Thus, the total heat loss by evaporation from the skin and airways may account for 20% or more of the body's heat loss.

Classification

The three stages of hypothermia have been described as the responsive, slowing, and poikilothermic phases[40] (Table 37B–10). Hypothermia may also be considered as either mild, moderate, or severe, and such classifications may help define the duration and aggressiveness of therapy required, as well as the prospect for a successful outcome.[2]

The responsive or mild hypothermia phase (core temperature 32°-35° C) is characterized by an attempt on the part of the patient to maintain a normal body temperature.[1] Blood pressure, heart rate, and respiratory rate are initially increased, but later decline as the hypothermia becomes more severe.[2] Muscle tone is increased and is frequently accompanied by active shivering. The level of consciousness may also be depressed and is typically manifest as stupor or confusion. Peripheral vasoconstriction is evidenced by diminished pulses, pallor or acrocyanosis, and coolness of the extremities to touch. The increase in central blood volume induced by peripheral vasoconstriction can produce a diuresis (so-called "cold diuresis") that can cause clinically significant hypovolemia. Cardiac output progressively falls

TABLE 37B–10 *Physiologic Changes in Hypothermia*

Stage	Core Temperature	Potential Effects
Mild	32-34.9° C 89.6-94.9° F	Tachypnea Tachycardia Ataxia Dysarthria Shivering Usually conscious Sometimes confused Normal blood pressure
Moderate	28-31.9° C 82.4-89.5° F	Loss of shivering Dysrhythmias Osborne (J) waves Decreased consciousness Semiconscious Combative Muscle rigidity Dilated pupils Decreased breathing rate
Severe	<28° C <82.4° F	Loss of reflexes Coma Hypotension Acidemia VFib/asystole Increasing flaccidity Apnea

Modified from Jolly BT, Ghezzi KT. Accidental hypothermia. Emerg Med Clin N Am 1992;10;3:11.

as the heart cools and myocardial contractility decreases, even if the blood volume is maintained at normal levels.

AXIOM The patient has little or no defense against hypothermia during a general anesthetic or when the core temperature is less than 32° C.

During the slowing phase (core temperature 23-32° C), enzyme kinetics slow, and shivering may be manifest only as a fine tremor. The skin vessels becomes vasodilated and heart rate, respiratory rate, and blood pressure progressively fall. The slowing phase can be subdivided into a superficial slowing phase (28-32° C) and a deep slowing phase (23-28° C).

Below 28° C, the patient is usually comatose. In most clinical settings, a core temperature of less than 28° C is considered severe hypothermia, and some physicians believe that poikilothermia sets in at this temperature. Patients in the poikilothermic phase (core temperature less than 23° C) have no effective way of preventing heat loss.[1]

Pathophysiology (Table 37B–11)

Because cooling retards the velocity of cellular enzymatic reactions, various organ systems begin to fail.[41] Ion pumps become inefficient, cell membranes become inappropriately permeable, and ionic gradients are lost.[42] There is no question that post-traumatic hypothermia is associated with increased mortality rates.[33,34] Despite some experimental data that suggest that moderate hypothermia may promote survival from hemorrhagic shock in rats,[43] the clinical consensus is that euthermic injured patients have a much better chance for survival.[1]

OXYGEN CONSUMPTION

Hypothermia produces a decrease in basal metabolic rate of approximately 6-7% per degree C, so the metabolic rate is 51% of normal at a core temperature of 28° C, and it is 20% of normal at 26.7° C (80° F).[43,44] This decrease in metabolic rate is associated with a con-

comitant decrease in oxygen consumption and a lesser decrease in CO_2 production, so the respiratory quotient falls from 0.82 at 37° C to 0.65 at 30° C.

CARDIAC OUTPUT AND BLOOD PRESSURE

Initially, as the core temperature falls from 37° C toward 32° C, cardiac output stays the same or increases slightly and blood pressure rises primarily because of increasing peripheral vasoconstriction. At lower temperatures, however, both of these values begin to decrease.[1] Cardiac output also progressively decreases because of hypovolemia, bradycardia, and decreased tissue O_2 requirements.

Blood viscosity increases with decreased core temperature as a result of an increase in plasma viscosity and a rising hematocrit.[2,45] Below 32° C, all vital signs tend to be subnormal. Compensatory mechanisms such as shivering tend to disappear below 28° C, but the muscles tend to be quite rigid because of increased muscle tone.[2]

ELECTROCARDIOGRAM

The electrocardiogram (ECG) can be of great importance in hypothermic patients because the greatest immediate danger is death from cardiac dysrhythmias.[46-49] As the core temperature falls to 28° C, there is progressive slowing of myocardial depolarization. This causes widening of QRS complexes, prolongation of the P-R interval, T wave inversion, J waves, arrhythmias (especially atrial fibrillation), and progressive bradycardia.

AXIOM So-called Osborne (J) waves on an ECG may be the first clue that hypothermia is present, especially in anesthetized patients.

TABLE 37B–11 *Characteristics of Hypothermia*

Core Temperature	Characteristics
35.0° C(95.0° F)	Maximum shivering and thermogenesis
34.0° C(93.2° F)	Amnesia, dysarthria, and increasingly poor judgment; normal blood pressure; maximum respiratory stimulation
33.0° C(91.4° F)	Ataxia and apathy
32.0° C(89.6° F)	Stupor; 25% decrease in oxygen consumption
31.0° C(87.8° F)	Shivering and thermogenesis cease
30.0° C(86.0° F)	Atrial fibrillation and other arrhythmias develop; pulse and cardiac output two-thirds of normal; insulin ineffective
29.0° C(84.2° F)	Decreased pulse, reduced consciousness and respiratory rates; pupils dilated
28.0° C(82.4° F)	Decreased fib threshold; 50% decrease in V0$_2$ and pulse rates
27.0° C(80.6° F)	Loss of reflexes and voluntary motion
26.0° C(78.8° F)	Major acid-base disturbances; no reflexes or response to pain
25.0° C(77.0° F)	Cerebral blood flow one-third of normal; cardiac output 45% of normal; pulmonary edema may develop
24.0° C(75.2° F)	Significant hypotension
23.0° C(73.4° F)	No corneal or oculocephalic reflexes
22.0° C(71.6° F)	Maximum risk of ventricular fibrillation; 75% decrease in oxygen consumption
20.0° C(68.0° F)	Pulse rate 20% of normal
19.0° C(66.2° F)	Flat EEG
18.0° C(64.4° F)	Asystole
16.0° C(60.8° F)	Lowest adult accidental hypothermia survival
15.2° C(59.4° F)	Lowest infant accidental hypothermia survival
10.0° C(50.0° F)	92% decrease in oxygen consumption
9.0° C(48.2° F)	Lowest therapeutic hypothermia survival

Modified from Danzl DF, Pozos RS, Hamlet MP. Accidental hypothermia. In: Auerbach PS, Geehr EC, eds. Management of wilderness and environment emergencies. 2nd ed. St. Louis: CV Mosby Co., 1989; 35.

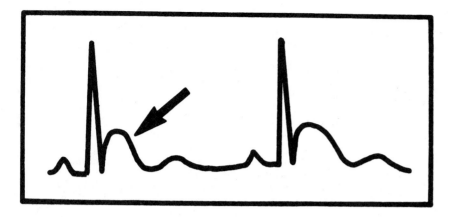

FIGURE 37B–2 Osborne (J) wave (arrow) after QRS complex, pathognomonic of hypothermia. These are often seen best in the lateral precordial leads. (From Farmer JC. Temperature-related injuries. In: Civetta JM, Taylor RW, Kirby RR, eds. Critical care. Philadelphia: JB Lippincott, 1988; 693-700.)

Osborne (J) waves are slow positive deflections in the latter part of the QRS complex. This abnormality is seen most prominently in aVL, aVF, and in the left chest leads (Fig. 37B–2). This deflection enlarges with worsening hypothermia and reverses readily with rewarming.[50] These waves may be in such close proximity to the S wave that it may be difficult to distinguish them from QRS complexes. This ECG change is pathognomonic of hypothermia, but its presence varies a great deal. Indeed, Osborne waves have been reported in 11 to 80% of cases.[51]

Ventricular and supraventricular ectopy are common in severe hypothermia. In addition, the threshold for ventricular fibrillation is decreased and may be precipitated by rough handling, movement of the patient, or insertion of a PA catheter.[32]

KIDNEYS

The "cold diuresis" seen with hypothermia occurs because peripheral vasoconstriction increases the central blood volume and renal perfusion. In addition, there is decreased reabsorption of water and sodium as a result of depressed tubular oxidative activity.[52–54] Renal tubular glucosuria may also result.[52,54] At lower temperatures, a combination of hypovolemia and low cardiac output may induce acute tubular necrosis.

AXIOM The diuresis occurring with hypothermia can cause hypovolemia, and this can cause severe hypotension during rewarming.

PULMONARY FUNCTION AND BLOOD GASES

Respiratory rate and minute ventilation may increase with the metabolic rate initially, but at core temperatures below 32° C, the respiratory rate progressively falls. Below 28° C, the respiratory rate may be less than 4 breaths/min.[3] At such temperatures, there is also often an alveolar pattern on x-ray resembling pulmonary edema.

Pulmonary secretions can be greatly increased during hypothermia, especially during rewarming. Additionally, hypothermia decreases the cough reflex and reduces vital capacity.[54] All of these processes can predispose to severe atelectasis and post-hypothermia pneumonitis.[44]

AXIOM Severely hypothermic patients are particularly apt to develop pneumonia after rewarming.

The oxyhemoglobin dissociation curve shifts to the left as a direct effect of lowered temperatures.[2] The PO_2 and PCO_2 decrease about 5% for each 1° C decrease in temperature (Table 37B–12). Although temperature correction of blood gas values has historically been advocated,[44,55-57] more recent work seems to indicate that these corrections are unnecessary.[58] Maintenance of reasonably normal values as measured by the blood gas analyzer at 37° C appears to indicate adequate gas exchange.

BLOOD CHEMISTRIES

Electrolyte changes with hypothermia include progressive hyponatremia and either hyperkalemia or hypokalemia.[1,2] Platelets and leukocytes may be sequestered in the spleen or liver, resulting in thrombocytopenia and leukopenia.[59] Cold-induced granulocytopenia has been thought to be an indicator of the severity of hypothermia, but it is an inconstant finding.[2]

Hyperglycemia during hypothermia may result from (a) decreased insulin release from the pancreas,[44,59-61] (b) inhibition of peripheral glucose utilization,[59,61] and (c) altered hepatic carbohydrate metabolism.[62] Nevertheless, hypoglycemia is not uncommon in near-drowning victims who present with or without hypothermia.[63] Acute alcohol intoxication, exhaustion from struggling, and/or a prolonged stay in the water may contribute to its development. These patients should be treated with glucose, but hyperglycemia should be avoided because it may impair neurologic function.[64]

COAGULATION

The function of coagulation factors and platelets becomes progressively impaired as the temperature falls below 34-35° C. Below 28-32° C, a clinical picture of DIC may develop.

AXIOM One of the best ways to prevent coagulopathies in trauma patients is to prevent or rapidly correct hypothermia.

BLOOD VISCOSITY

With increasing hypothermia, there is a progressive increase in the viscosity of blood with its filterability decreasing about 2.2% per degree centigrade fall in temperature.[65] Erythrocyte deformability also decreases, especially as the temperature falls from 37° C to 34° C temperature range, averaging a 5.1% decrease per degree. Below 34.0° C, red cell deformability decreases only 1.8% per degree. The greatest increase in plasma viscosity occurs in the lower temperature range (34-30° C).

TABLE 37B–12   Blood Gas Changes with Hypothermia

Temp (° C)	pH	PCO_2 (mm Hg)	PO_2 (mm Hg)
37	7.40	40	80
36	7.42	38	74
35	7.43	37	69
34	7.45	35	64
33	7.46	33	59
32	7.48	32	55
31	7.49	31	51
30	7.51	29	47
29	7.52	28	44
28	7.54	27	41

The viscosity of whole blood normally varies significantly with the shear rate or flow. At low shear or flow rates, cellular aggregation occurs, increasing viscosity. As shear or flow rate increases, erythrocytes disaggregate, resulting in a significant drop in viscosity. This is known as the shear-thinning phenomenon and is a characteristic of the cellular viscosity of whole blood. In the study by Poulos et al,[65] cellular viscosity accounted for 65 to 70% of the total viscosity changes noted throughout the temperature ranges evaluated.

MENTATION AND NEUROLOGICAL FUNCTION

There is approximately a 6-7% decrease in cerebral blood flow for each 1° C decrease in core temperature. At 26.7-31.7° C (80-89° F) there is usually confusion and decreased deep tendon reflexes,[44,66] peripheral nerve conduction, and pain sensitivity.[44,67] Below 26.7° C (80° F), there is usually coma, the pupils are often fixed, and patients are often areflexic. Pupillary dilation is common below 30° C, and the electrocephalogram is generally flat when the core temperature is lower than 20° C.[3] Although core cooling usually lags behind the hypoxic effects of hypothermia, the occurrence of immersion hypothermia before asphyxia may protect the brain from anoxic damage to some degree.

Gooden[68] has noted that the normothermic human brain suffers irreversible damage if subjected to acute asphyxia for longer than 10 minutes. Significant resistance of brain tissue to hypoxia occurs only after its temperature has fallen to 30° C or less. Since body surface cooling depresses core temperature by only one-third of this drop in 10 minutes, an additional factor is required to explain neurological survival from near-drowning. The idea that ingestion and aspiration of large amounts of cold water produce such a temperature drop lacks quantitative evidence.

Although the diving response in marine mammals occurs in humans to a lesser extent, in about 15% of the volunteers tested, a profound diving response was noted. This response, which starts immediately upon submersion, prevents aspiration of water, redistributes oxygen stores to the heart and brain, slows cardiac oxygen use, and initiates a hypometabolic state. Thus, survival from prolonged near-drowning appears to depend upon an interplay between the degree of the diving response, the rapidity of development of the hypothermia, and the resulting speed with which protective hypometabolism develops.

OTHER ORGANS

As core temperatures fall, there is a progressive decrease in gastrointestinal motility, and at temperatures below 32° C there is usually an adynamic ileus.[2,44,59,62] Pancreatic function remains undisturbed until the core temperature drops below 32° C. At temperatures below 28° C, one tends to see stress gastric ulcers and hemorrhagic pancreatitis with increasing serum amylase levels.[2,3] Hepatic function, especially conjugation and detoxification, tends to decrease with worsening hypothermia and serum transaminase levels tend to rise.[44,59,62]

Adrenal cortical activity is decreased at core temperatures below 28° C. Measured cortisol levels may actually rise, however, as a result of decreased hepatic clearance.

Diagnosis

HISTORY

A presumptive diagnosis of environmentally induced hypothermia depends on recognition of the harshness and duration of exposure and of the mental and physical capabilities of the patient during that time.[1] Even if the patient has not suffered prolonged or severe exposure to cold, one should suspect hypothermia if the patient has any one of a number of conditions that predispose patients to hypothermia. These include extremes of age, CNS problems (obtundation or hypothalamic lesions), metabolic abnormalities (malnutrition, hypoglycemia, or depressed thyroid or pituitary function), and the effects of various drugs (alcohol, barbiturates, phenothiazines, and general anesthesia).

> **AXIOM** Seriously injured patients who are hypotensive are at particular risk of developing hypothermia.[69,70]

CLINICAL EXAMINATION

There is generally a fairly standard progression of signs, symptoms, and physiologic changes caused by a progressive decrease in core temperature.[12] As hypothermia develops, there is initially an intense shivering that gradually abates as the individual continues to cool and lapses into an apathetic state. From this point on, cooling is more rapid. Apathy and lethargy deepen until unconsciousness occurs. At this point, there is usually little or no response to external stimuli, and there is a progressive slowing and weakening of the pulse and respirations.

If treatment is begun before the extremities freeze, active warming may permit survival.[12] The problem, however, is frequently complicated by cardiac irregularities, and continuous ECG monitoring is advisable.

LABORATORY TESTS

Laboratory tests should include arterial and venous blood gases, CBC, electrolytes, urinalysis, and coagulation studies (especially platelets, PT, and PTT).[1,2,3] In patients with hypothermia of unknown etiology, one should also perform thyroid function studies, ethanol and illicit drug levels, and blood cultures.

DETERMINING IF THE PATIENT IS DEAD

An oft-quoted dictum in the treatment of hypothermia is that "hypothermic patients are not dead until they are warm and dead." Indeed, all methods of clinical assessment are inaccurate until the patient is adequately rewarmed to at least 32° C, but preferably to 34-35° C.[1,2]

> **AXIOM** Hypothermic patients with recent loss of signs of life should not be pronounced dead until or unless there are still no signs of life after the patient has been warmed to at least 32° C and preferably 35° C.

Prevention of Hypothermia

A great deal of attention has been given to the prevention of hypothermia, particularly during surgery in patients receiving massive blood transfusions.[32,71,72] Traumatized patients can present with a wide variety of anatomic and metabolic problems that impair the body's ability to prevent hypothermia. These aberrations can disrupt feedback loops for temperature control between the skin and CNS. As a result, the patient becomes a passive responder to the ambient temperature.[73]

To prevent or reduce heat loss, the patient can be covered with an aluminum "space blanket" that traps body heat and reflects radiated heat back to the patient.[1] The ED resuscitation area and operating room should be warmed for the comfort of the patient, not the physicians, nurses, and technicians. Most importantly, these patients must receive warmed fluids during resuscitation. Crystalloids and blood should be warmed to 40° C before they are administered to the patient. In the operating room, the patient should be placed on a preheated blanket, and the temperature in the ventilator cascade should be maintained at 48.9° C (120° F). Other measures that may be used include irrigating body cavities, the stomach, and/or the bladder with warmed saline solutions during and/or after the operation.

> **AXIOM** As soon as the major bleeding has been controlled during emergency surgery, the surgeon should irrigate the body cavity being explored with warmed saline until the core temperature is at least 34-35° C.

In some areas, immersion in cold water is the most frequent cause of hypothermia.[32] Even strong swimming skills become useless in icy water, a circumstance in which weakening and incoordination develop rapidly. Children living in areas with ice cold pools and lakes should be taught the heat-escape-lessening position (HELP), in which the arms are held tightly to the anterior axillary line and the knees are flexed to the chest while awaiting rescue.[74]

Prevention of hypothermia is often thought to involve common sense. However, once an individual is exposed to a severely cold environment and stress, thinking may not be as logical as it should be. Consequently, preventive measures (Table 37B–13), including adequate cover, food, and water, should be instituted before exposure occurs. One should also stay dry and avoid alcohol and fatigue.

Treatment of Hypothermia

ADVANCED CARDIOPULMONARY LIFE SUPPORT (FIG. 37B–3)

Prevention of Cardiac Arrest

Patients with severe hypothermia can usually meet their physiologic needs despite significant hypotension, bradycardia, and hypoventilation. Consequently, overly aggressive treatment of hypothermia has been linked with cardiac arrest, usually caused by VF.[32]

AXIOM   As long as the hypothermic patient has a pulse and is breathing, treatment should not be overly aggressive.

Frequent case reports document that many victims of hypothermia, found with signs of life, developed cardiac arrest during resuscitation.[51,75,76] In contrast, other reports describe victims in whom a perfusing cardiac rhythm persisted despite significant hypotension and bradycardia.[72]

TABLE 37B–13   Measures for Prevention of Hypothermia

1. Prepare for the worst possible weather and for the possibility of an unexpected night out.
2. Carry food that contains sugar for a quick-energy source.
3. Eat small amounts often, maintaining a steady flow of body fuel all day.
4. Avoid dehydration by constantly drinking water to a total of at least 3 to 4 quarts of fluid daily.
5. Ingesting snow is inefficient, and it worsens hypothermia.
6. Dress in layers so that clothing may be adjusted for overcooling or overheating.
7. Carry windproof and waterproof outer garments.
8. Stay dry.
9. Do not exhaust yourself; get plenty of rest.
10. Breathe through the nose rather than the mouth to minimize heat and fluid loss.
11. Avoid alcoholic beverages and smoking tobacco.
12. Recognize high-risk individuals and be suspicious of early symptoms.
13. If immersed in cold water and rescue is not immediately accessible, huddle and remain as immobile as possible.

Modified from Fritz RL, Perrin DH. Cold exposure injuries: prevention and treatment. Clin Sports Med 1989;8:111.

One factor that may cause death after rescue is a continued decline in core temperature after the victim is removed from a cold environment.[32] This "afterdrop" was thought to result from the return of cold blood from the periphery to the core; however, experimental

FIGURE 37B–3 Treatment algorithm for accidental hypothermia. (Adapted [with permission] from Zell SC, Kurtz KJ. Severe exposure hypothermia: a resuscitation protocol. Ann Emerg Med 1985;14:339.)

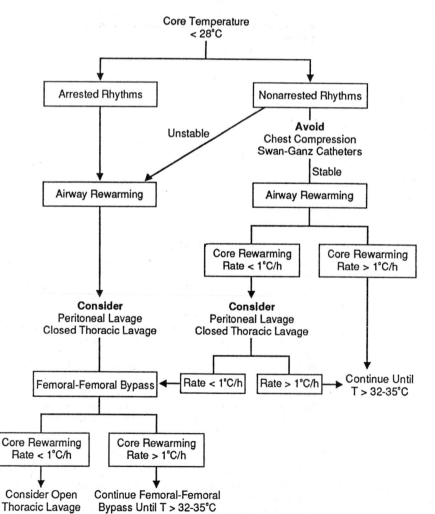

evidence suggests that some of the afterdrop results from ongoing conduction of heat from the warmer core into colder surface layers.[78-80]

> **AXIOM** Blood pressure and cardiac filling pressures must be watched carefully during rewarming when vasodilation causes a strong tendency to hypovolemia and hypotension.

A more important cause of death after rescue may be related to "rewarming shock."[32] Although the patient may be able to maintain adequate perfusion during hypothermia, the additional metabolic burden of rewarming may be too great for the cardiovascular system. Other problems may include vasodilation as the patient is warmed.[81] Rough handling, aggressive manipulation, and/or increased exertion during rescue may also be factors in sudden death.[32]

Several pharmacologic agents have been proposed to prevent ventricular fibrillation in hypothermic patients. Dopamine, which can cause a slight increase in heart rate in hypothermia, has been shown to reduce the threshold of ventricular fibrillation to 12.2° C (54° F).[82] It accomplishes this by blocking both alpha and beta receptors and by competitively inhibiting the epinephrine-induced ventricular fibrillation that may accompany rewarming. Prevention of dysrhythmias during resuscitation also depends on correcting the tendency to metabolic acidosis and associated hyperkalemia. Consequently, frequent determinations of arterial blood gases and electrolytes are important during rewarming.[83]

Ventilation

Most authors believe that if a patient has severe hypothermia, any breathing and any perfusing rhythm are probably adequate, regardless of the rate or depth of respiration or the heart rate or blood pressure. Consequently, many authors would withhold artificial respiration and chest compressions in such patients to avoid the risk of precipitating VF.[84]

If no breathing is present or the respiratory rate is less than 4/min, the patient should have endotracheal intubation. Despite the fact that intubation has precipitated VF in isolated cases, experience with large numbers of patients suggests that intubation in patients with hypothermia is safe; however, hyperventilation with precipitous changes in arterial pH should be avoided.[12]

> **AXIOM** Some ventilation is better than no ventilation, but hyperventilation can precipitate severe arrhythmias or cardiac arrest.

CPR

Knowing when to provide CPR to severely hypothermic individuals can be extremely difficult. If the core temperature is unknown, CPR should be started if there appears to be cardiac arrest.[84] If a patient is known to be severely cold (below 28° C) and an electrocardiographic monitor shows a perfusing rhythm, regardless of the rate, some authors would withhold CPR, even in the absence of a palpable pulse.[85-87] Most physicians, however, would not withhold CPR in a severely hypothermic patient if there were no palpable pulses.[88] In many instances, effective perfusion is restored spontaneously with rewarming, but the process is more effective if some circulation is present.

> **AXIOM** Although CPR may precipitate VF and is not very effective during hypothermia,[89] one should not hesitate to provide CPR if the patient is pulseless after a thorough check.[32]

Prolonged CPR may be tolerated relatively well in hypothermic patients without sequelae. In the past, it was suggested that CPR in hypothermia patients should be performed at half the usual rate; however, until more is known about CPR during hypothermia, normal rates should probably be employed.[32]

> **AXIOM** Electrical cardioversion of the hypothermic heart (below 30-32° C) is difficult, if not impossible.

Attempts to restore a perfusing cardiac rhythm, particularly when ventricular fibrillation is present, are unlikely to succeed until the temperature is raised above 30° C, and generally will not succeed until the core temperature is raised above 34-35° C.[2,90]

Antiarrhythmic Agents

Lidocaine appears safe in hypothermic patients, but its efficacy is uncertain.[32] Bretylium, in some case reports, has been associated with spontaneous defibrillation of hypothermic patients,[91,92] and some investigators believe that bretylium is the drug of choice for raising the fibrillatory threshold. In animal studies, however, bretylium did not appear to provide chemical defibrillation,[93] and it did not significantly protect against the onset of fibrillation.[94] In fact, some dogs developed VF during the infusion of bretylium. Nevertheless, in patients with persistent VF, attempts at chemical defibrillation with bretylium may be warranted.[32]

Electrical defibrillation may be attempted at any temperature, but is usually not successful until the core temperature reaches at least 32-35° C.[32] After cardiopulmonary bypass, many hearts cannot be defibrillated until the core temperature is 34-35° C. Rather than increasing the electrical energy delivered at low temperatures, it may be wiser to suspend attempts at defibrillation until warmer core temperatures are reached.

Correction of Metabolic Acidosis

The indications for the treatment of metabolic acidosis with sodium bicarbonate during cardiac arrest are controversial. The American Heart Association does not recommend empiric sodium bicarbonate during the first 10 minutes of CPR; however it can be given if ABG analysis reveals a severe metabolic acidosis.[95] The Committee on Trauma of the American College of Surgeons recommends sodium bicarbonate treatment to raise the pH of injured patients to 7.20.[96] Physiologically, however, acidosis does not generally interfere with cardiovascular function unless the pH is less than 7.00 to 7.10.

If treatment appears to be indicated for suspected severe metabolic acidosis, most authorities recommend using an initial bolus of 1 mEq $NaHCO_3$/kg of body weight. Further sodium bicarbonate administration should be guided by measurements of the arterial and venous blood gases. Indeed, giving bicarbonate can be extremely hazardous and can increase cellular acidosis if CO_2 is not removed adequately.

> **AXIOM** Bicarbonate should not be used to treat severe metabolic acidosis unless the ventilation is adequate to remove the increased CO_2 that is formed.

MONITORING

Core Temperature

Because the methods used for rewarming are dictated to some extent by the severity of the hypothermia, it is essential that hypothermic patients and those at risk to develop hypothermia have accurate continuous monitoring of their core temperatures.[97] This necessitates the use of a thermistor capable of detecting temperatures below 35° C (95° F).

> **AXIOM** In general, core temperatures are best monitored with an esophageal probe, particularly in the OR.

The ideal site to monitor core temperature clinically is usually the esophagus because it correlates rather closely with the temperature of the heart. Bladder and rectal temperatures tend to lag at least 1-2° C behind the esophageal temperature. Proper rectal temperature monitoring requires that the thermometer be inserted at least 10 cm past the anal verge. If the thermometer tip is not buried in a large collection of feces, such temperatures are helpful, but they are subject to artifact and time lags.[97] Thermistors attached to the bladder end of a Foley catheter are probably more reliable than rectal temperatures. Oral temperatures during hypothermia are unreliable.

Vital Signs

Continuous hemodynamic monitoring of hypothermic patients is extremely important and should include a cardioscope, indwelling arterial and central venous pressure lines, and a Foley catheter for monitoring urine output.[1] Pulmonary artery catheters are generally avoided in severely hypothermic patients because they increase the tendency to dangerous arrhythmias.

Laboratory

Laboratory monitoring in hypothermic patients should include serum glucose and electrolyte levels and arterial blood gases.[39,104] Some authors believe that the blood gas values from the laboratory (measured with the specimen at 37° C) should be corrected to the patient's core temperature. The usual correction is a 0.015 increase in pH, a 4.4% decrease in the PCO_2, and a 7.2% decrease in the PO_2 for each 1° C decrease in temperature below 37° C.[36,98] Thus, if the values obtained in the laboratory at 37° C were pH = 7.40, PCO_2 = 40 mm Hg, PO_2 = 80 mm Hg, the values corrected for a core temperature of 32° C would be pH = 7.48, PCO_2 = 32 mm Hg, and PO_2 = 55 mm Hg. Others believe that the uncorrected values are more meaningful.

AXIOM Uncorrected blood gas values in hypothermic patients may be more meaningful than those that are corrected to 37° C.

Whether or not to correct ABG levels to the patient's core temperature is one of the hottest and longest-lasting controversies in hypothermia. The logic for correcting pH and blood gases to the core temperature of the patient seems intuitively correct, and rational arguments can be offered for such temperature correction.[99]

The most recent school of thought draws on clinical,[100] physicochemical,[71] and even comparative physiologic[101,102] arguments to suggest that, at least for pH and PCO_2, uncorrected values reflect the physiologic status of the patient more accurately and make analysis of the values much easier. Delaney et al[103] explained the implications of both choices and decided against correction of pH and carbon dioxide pressure.

AXIOM ABG values do not have to be corrected to the patient's core temperature.

Patients with hypothermia should probably be given 100% oxygen. Correction of the PO_2 to the patient's core temperature is acceptable but will generally not change the therapy, at least initially.[32] Pulse oximetry and transcutaneous measurement of PO_2 and PCO_2 in severe hypothermia tend to be inaccurate because of the decreased skin perfusion.[32]

WARMING (TABLE 37B–14)

The method of choice for rewarming a hypothermic patient depends on the severity of the hypothermia and the available facilities. The general types of rewarming include: (a) passive warming (warm environment, blankets, etc.), (b) active external warming (immersion in warm water, electric blankets, etc.), and (c) active core warming (irrigation of the stomach or colon or thoracic or peritoneal cavities with warm crystalloids, use of heated ventilatory gases, infusion of warmed intravenous fluids, regional warming with radiowaves, and extracorporeal heat exchangers).[104-106]

Passive External Rewarming

Passive external rewarming consists of adding an insulating layer to the patient (i.e., a blanket) and allowing his or her own heat-generating mechanisms to restore body temperature.[1,2] This raises core temperature approximately 1° C (1.8° F)/hr. Obviously, this

TABLE 37B–14   Treatment Options for Rewarming Patients with Hypothermia

Degree of Hypothermia	Treatment
Mild: Core temperature of 32-34.9° C (89.6-94.9° F)	Passive external rewarming: Shelter from the environment Remove wet or cold clothes Apply layers of clothing or blankets Provide warm fluids
Moderate: Core temperature of 28.0-31.9° C (82.4-89.4° F)	Active external rewarming of truncal areas with: Electric warming blankets Hot-water bottles Heating pads Radiant heat sources Warming beds
Severe: Core temperature <28° C (<82.4° F)	Active core rewarming with: Warm humidified oxygen Nasogastric lavage Peritoneal lavage Open thoracotomy with myocardial/mediastinal irrigation Cardiopulmonary bypass

Modified from Hector MG. Treatment of accidental hypothermia. Amer Family Physic 1992;45:785.

method is generally adequate only in otherwise normal patients with mild hypothermia. Passive external warming is not adequate for treating severe hypothermia, and its use under such circumstances can be associated with a high mortality rate, especially in adults.[107]

Active External Rewarming

Active external warming uses devices that generate their own heat (i.e., hot water bottles, submersion in a tank of warm water, or heating blankets).[2] Hypothermic individuals who have lost the shivering response have no mechanism for increasing their metabolic rate and must be warmed externally or internally. Active external warming is suitable for patients in the upper range of moderate hypothermia who are without dysrhythmias or significant ECG changes.[108] Although there is some controversy as to the best way of warming these patients, direct application of heat in the 100-104° F range appears to be the best therapeutic measure. In neonatal hypothermia, rewarming techniques produce better results if they are rapid.[109]

AXIOM Slow rewarming of patients with moderate-severe hypothermia allows additional ischemic damage to occur.[12]

Unfortunately, active external warming has some hazards. Blankets or warmers more than 45° C can burn the patient's skin. Surface warming also causes cutaneous vasodilation. The resulting shift of blood from the core to peripheral vessels may cause a marginally hypovolemic patient to develop "rewarming shock." This problem, however, is obviated if volume repletion is promptly accomplished and maintained during rewarming.[110]

AXIOM Rapid external rewarming can cause hypotension and use of external devices with temperatures above 45° C can damage the skin.

As a result of external rewarming, the cold, acidotic blood previously trapped in the peripheral circulation of patients with moderate-severe hypothermia can induce core cooling, or afterdrop, as it enters the central circulation.[111] This afterdrop can cause ventricular fibrillation that is unresponsive to pharmacologic or electrical stimuli. Additionally, as the surface temperature rises above that which stimulates shivering, heat production stops even though an acceptable core temperature has not yet been achieved.[1]

> **AXIOM** Despite the shortcomings of active external rewarming, no difference in survival or morbidity has been prospectively demonstrated between this technique and core rewarming.[110,112]

Core Rewarming

The warming methods of choice for patients with moderate-severe hypothermia are those that employ active core warming.[1] With these techniques, the heart and brain are rewarmed first. The heart is quickly brought above the temperature at which spontaneous fibrillation is apt to occur. The central thermal receptors regain their previously cold-inhibited function, and homoeothermic reflexes can now assist rewarming.[1] Passive and active external warming can be used in conjunction with active core warming;[27,113] however, active external warming must be used with some caution.

INHALATION OF HEATED GASES

> **AXIOM** The most effective, easily managed, and readily available method of active core warming is inhalation of heated gases.[1]

Warmed gases for inhalation can be delivered both by heated humidifier and by various portable devices.[113,114] Because stimulation of the oropharynx may induce cardiac arrhythmias, intubation should be accomplished rapidly and efficiently by physicians expert in the technique. The maximal inspired temperature of the heated gases should be 43.3° C (110° F) to prevent thermal injury to the respiratory passages. In awake patients, the gas temperature must be reduced to approximately 40° C (104° F).[111] With this technique, patients have been warmed at a rate of approximately 1.2-1.4° C (2.2-2.5° F)/hr.[1] Because of the high incidence of pneumonia among these patients, the use of prophylactic antibiotics appears to be justified.

WARMED INTRAVENOUS FLUIDS. Parenteral solutions in plastic bags can be heated in a microwave oven.[115] It is important to be sure that the fluids are actually delivering warmth to the patient because the fluid can cool a great deal in the intravenous tubing.[116] Indeed, many of the older commercial blood warmers limit flow rates and, consequently, do not really provide effective heating of the intravenous fluids.[117]

IRRIGATION OF THE GASTROINTESTINAL TRACT. Warmed gastric lavage or enemas can also provide some heat transfer; however, because the surface areas of the stomach and colon are relatively small, these routes are relatively ineffective, and aspiration can occur during gastric lavage.[1,2,35]

> **AXIOM** Warmed gastric lavage for treating hypothermia is quite slow and it increases the risk of aspiration of gastric contents.

PLEURAL AND/OR PERITONEAL LAVAGE. Warmed peritoneal dialysis and closed pleural lavage have the potential to provide large amounts of heat,[118-120] but they are relatively slow and require a large volume of warmed fluid. Hemodialysis with a blood warmer may be especially useful when overdose of certain drugs (e.g., barbiturates) accompanies hypothermia.[32]

CARDIOPULMONARY BYPASS. Extracorporeal circulation with a heart-lung machine has been used successfully in a number of patients with extreme hypothermia.[32] The advantages include extremely rapid rewarming from the core outward, support of circulation, provision of volume replacement and oxygenation, reversal of hemoconcentration, and decreased stress to the myocardium.[121] Core rewarming also shortens the interval during which cardiopulmonary resuscitation is required in patients who had cardiopulmonary arrest, and it decreases

the volume of crystalloid fluids required for repletion of the intravascular volume.[112]

Cardiopulmonary bypass (CPB) circuits generally include a mechanical pump, oxygenator, heat exchanger, and connective tubing.[5] The femoral vessels are cannulated for vascular access with a surgical cutdown[121] or via a percutaneous approach.[122]

> **AXIOM** If rapidly available, partial cardiopulmonary bypass is the most rapid, effective method for correcting severe hypothermia.

Kugelberg et al[123] described the first use of CPB for hypothermia in 1967. Subsequent studies demonstrated that resuscitation from profound hypothermia was possible with CPB after other types of core rewarming were unsuccessful.[124-126] Splittgerber et al[121] showed that CPB rewarms at four times the rate of other types of core rewarming. In 1987, CPB was used to treat multiple victims of severe accidental cold exposure on Mt. Hood, Oregon.[127] Despite having the lowest mean core temperature of any series of patients in the literature (11.5° C), two of these victims survived.

> **AXIOM** CPB is the treatment of choice for resuscitation of patients who have profound hypothermia and cardiac arrest.

Collective data from 11 studies using CPB for profound hypothermia with a cardiac arrest between 1967 and 1987 yielded a 71% overall survival rate.[128] Newer developments such as heparin-bonded circuits, smaller cannulae, and less complicated CPB equipment should increase the future utility of this device in the emergency department.[5]

Vretenar et al[129] reviewed collective data on 68 hypothermic patients resuscitated with cardiopulmonary bypass. The mean initial core temperature was 21° C. Sixty-one patients (90%) were in cardiac arrest. Femorofemoral bypass was used in 72% of the patients. The overall survival was 60%, and 80% of the survivors returned to their previous level of function. Sixty-seven percent of nonsurvivors died because of inability to establish a cardiac rhythm or wean from bypass. There were no survivors among the six patients with a core temperature less than 15° C. Patients in cardiac arrest had a higher mortality than patients who were not (p = 0.02). Climbing and avalanche victims had a higher mortality than other hypothermic patients (p = 0.003).

Although controlled studies comparing the efficacy of cardiopulmonary bypass and alternative warming techniques have not been done, cardiopulmonary bypass has several advantages over other warming methods for profoundly hypothermic patients. Tissue perfusion and oxygenation are maintained while rapid warming occurs. Thus, cardiopulmonary bypass resuscitation is recommended for hypothermic patients in cardiac arrest and for patients with core temperatures lower than 25° C, irrespective of the cardiac rhythm. Patients in stable condition with temperatures between 25-28° C can be treated with cardiopulmonary bypass or conventional warming techniques.

Methods for determining which hypothermic patients to rewarm continue to evolve.[32] It now appears that any patient with any chance of hypothermic protection from cerebral ischemia should have an attempt at rewarming. The lowest core temperature that has been measured in adults who survived accidental hypothermia is approximately 16° C (60.8° F).[130,131] This has led to the frequently quoted adage that "a patient is not dead until he is warm and dead," with "warm" meaning a core temperature of at least 32-35° C (89.6-95.0° F).[90]

> **AXIOM** Hypothermic patients are not dead until they are warm (32-35° C) and dead.

Although severely hypothermic patients can often be resuscitated after they are warmed, there are limits to such resuscitation. Hypothermia does not alter the presence of obviously fatal injuries.[32] In addition, failure to restore a circulating cardiac rhythm within 30 minutes after rewarming to 32-35° C makes further efforts unlikely to be successful. Efforts to develop laboratory markers of "irreversible death" (e.g., severe hyperkalemia above 10 mEq/L or serum ammonia above 250 µmol/L)[76,131] have thus far been based on limited experience and should be viewed as preliminary.[32]

AXIOM Cool-water drowning does not offer the same cerebral protection as drowning by ice-cold water.

Orlowski[132] noted that water colder than 10° C (50° F) accounts for all reported cases of survival after prolonged (15 minutes or longer) submersion, and many cases probably involved water colder than 5° C (41° F). Even in ice-water drowning, hypothermia is no guarantee of survival; such patients still frequently die of anoxia as well as lung injury, multisystem failure, or trauma. Rapid core cooling after only brief immersion suggests a preserved circulation and a better chance of survival; however, slow cooling after a long submersion suggests a grave prognosis.[32]

AXIOM Rapid core cooling after submersion provides a better prognosis than slow cooling.

Fluid Therapy

Hypovolemia induced by cold diuresis[133,134] and concomitant injuries must be corrected early, and volume expansion is an essential component of resuscitation from hypothermia.[110] Various reports indicate that 14 to 35% of the blood volume during cooling falls to temperatures in the range of 20-25° C.[135] In the absence of blood loss, the volume of crystalloid needed to correct hypovolemia can be guided by the degree of hemoconcentration.[40,136]

Lloyd[137] notes that people who die from hypothermia, even if they are alive and uninjured when rescued, probably die from hypovolemia or fluid overload. The traditional explanation that death in these individuals results from ventricular fibrillation from the afterdrop of core temperature was based on inadequate measurement and failure to consider the physiology of cold. The actual mechanism in any individual case depends both on the history of the cooling and the method of rewarming used. Lloyd[137] also notes that some deaths occur as a result of continued cooling of the body or ventricular fibrillation precipitated by rough handling.

As the core temperature rises, vascular capacity increases. A minimum of 500 ml of isotonic fluid is usually needed for each 1° C temperature rise to maintain an adequate blood volume; however, because cardiac depression often accompanies hypothermia, the rate of the volume replacement should be guided by the response of the central venous pressure and cardiac output.[3] Isotonic crystalloid solutions warmed to approximately 40° C can be infused fairly rapidly in doses of 20 ml/kg as often as needed as long as the CVP does not rise abruptly.[32]

AXIOM Some glucose should be present in the fluids used to resuscitate hypothermic patients.

Some glucose should be in the intravenous fluids administered initially to hypothermic patients. Despite the frequent presence of hyperglycemia in these patients, hypoglycemia can develop rapidly.[32]

Drugs

Adrenergic medications, especially dopamine in inotropic dosages, can help support blood pressure during hypothermia.[72,73] Military antishock trousers (MAST), however, are relatively ineffective in hypothermic patients[138] and could theoretically be harmful.[139] Drugs generally not recommended in hypothermic patients include vasoconstrictors, sodium bicarbonate, insulin, corticosteroids, and ethanol.[32,71,140,141]

AXIOM Vasoconstrictors should not be used in patients with hypotension resulting from hypothermia.

Vasoconstrictors can interfere greatly with attempts at rewarming and may cause severe additional tissue damage.[12] As the temperature

rises, myocardial function will usually improve enough to restore the blood pressure to normal if there is adequate preload.

POSTRESUSCITATION THERAPY

Airway Protection

AXIOM Bronchopneumonia is a frequent complication of hypothermia, and it is often made much worse by aspiration.

Hypothermia can cause severe bronchorrhea during rewarming, and aspiration is fairly frequent in patients whose mental status is altered by the hypothermia. Consequently, careful attention should be paid to airway protective mechanisms, such as cough and gag reflexes. If any doubt exists regarding the adequacy of these reflexes, early endotracheal intubation should be performed.[2]

Other Measures

Other measures that may help in the treatment of severely hypothermic patients include vasodilators and correction of severe anemia.[12] Prolonged anticoagulation with Coumadin was thought to help prevent thromboses in tissues with cold injury,[12] but it is now generally avoided.[2]

HEAT-OVERLOAD SYNDROMES

Exposure to hot environments may result in a variety of disorders including heat cramps, heat syncope, heat exhaustion, and heatstroke.[1]

AXIOM Although heat-overload syndromes may be distinguished from each other clinically, their underlying physiologic aberrations differ primarily only with regard to their severity.

Heat-overload syndromes are often associated with dehydration either as a result of hard physical labor or ineffective sweating.[142] Dehydration in a hot, dry environment also predisposes to these disorders. Heat-overload is much more apt to occur in elderly patients with preexisting problems such as alcoholism, heart disease, or obesity[1] (Table 37B–15). Various types of drugs may also predispose to heat-overload syndromes (Table 37B–16).

Although the means by which humans adjust to excessively hot temperatures are not entirely clear, sweating and insensible water evaporation appear to be the main homeostatic mechanisms. As long as sweating continues, humans can withstand remarkably high temperatures provided that the constituents of sweat (water, sodium, chloride, and potassium) are replaced in a timely fashion. Hard labor in a hot environment can put extreme demands on the circulation to de-

TABLE 37B–15 Predisposition to Heat Injury

Behavior	Illness
Injudicious exertion	Congestive heart failure
Inappropriate clothing	Dehydration
Lack of acclimatization	Diabetes mellitus
Poor fluid and salt intake	Neuropathies
Exposure to sun	Skin diseases
Obesity	Scleroderma
Fatigue	Healed major burn
	Hyperthyroidism
	Fever
	Delirium tremens
	Psychosis
	Neonates/elderly
	Prior heatstroke
	Hypokalemia

Modified from Tek D, Olshaker JS. Heat illness. Emerg Med Clin N Am 1992;10:299.

TABLE 37B-16 **Drugs That Increase the Risk of Environmental Heat Injury**

Drug Class	Examples	Mechanism
Diuretics	Furosemide, ethacrynic acid, acetazolamide	Salt depletion and dehydration
Anticholinergics	Atropine, belladonna	Suppression of sweating
Antiparkinsonians	Procyclidine HCl, benztropine mesylate	Suppression of sweating
Phenothiazines	Chlorpromazine, promethazine	Suppression of sweating and (possibly) disturbed hypothalamic temperature regulation
Tricyclics	Tranylcypromine	Increased motor activity and increased heat production
Antihistamines	Diphenyhydramine	Suppression of sweating
Butyrophenones	Haloperidol	(Possibly) disturbed hypothalamic temperature regulation and failure to recognize thirst
Sympathomimetic amines	Dextroamphetamine, phenmetrazine cocaine	Increased psychomotor activity

Knochel JP. Heatstroke and related heat stress disorders. Dis Mon 1989;35:306.

liver nutrients and oxygen to the muscles as well as blood to the skin to facilitate heat transfer. Because blood flow to skeletal muscle takes priority over that to the skin, the cutaneous perfusion may be inadequate to dissipate the heat generated.[1]

> **AXIOM** Decreased sweating, especially while working in a hot environment, can rapidly increase the likelihood of a heat-induced injury.

Heat Cramps

Heat cramps are the most benign type of heat-overload syndrome.[1] Environmental temperatures exceeding body temperature and/or direct exposure to the sun are not necessary. Athletes participating in strenuous activities are particularly susceptible to this problem. These cramps seem to result primarily from electrolyte imbalances, especially hyponatremia, and are characterized by painful spasms of the voluntary muscles. Occasionally, the cramps in abdominal muscles may mimic an acute abdomen.[1] Free water intake, stimulated by thirst, often intensifies the electrolyte imbalance.

> **AXIOM** Heat cramps are usually best corrected by administration of dilute salt solutions after the patient has been placed in a cool environment.

Laboratory studies usually reveal hyponatremia and hypochloremia; however, hemoconcentration may occasionally be observed. The cessation of cramps with the administration of salt (sodium chloride) and water is striking and supports the hypothesis that the pathogenesis of heat cramps is depletion and/or dilution of these essential electrolytes.[1]

> **AXIOM** Because sweat has 5.0 or more mEq of potassium per liter, excessive sweating, corrected only with water and NaCl, can eventually cause hypokalemia.

Heat Syncope

The symptoms of heat syncope can range from lightheadedness to severe fatigue and loss of consciousness.[1] Sweating (in contrast to insensible water loss) is visible, and the body temperature may be quite elevated, especially if the episode is induced by exercise. In spite of the hyperthermia, the patient is often pale as a result of hypotension from peripheral venous pooling. Although cramps may develop in some patients, the skeletal muscles tend to be quite flaccid.

> **AXIOM** Heat syncope is generally self-limiting and often requires no treatment other than removal of the patient from the main heat source and rest in a recumbent position; however, administration of some water and salt will usually speed recovery.

Heat Exhaustion

Heat exhaustion, also called heat prostration, is the most common type of heat-overload syndrome.[1] Heat exhaustion occurs in both physically active and sedentary individuals. Patients typically present with weakness, vertigo, headache, and nausea, all of which may precede physical collapse. The skin is initially cool and clammy, and because prostration usually develops before prolonged exposure to heat, the body temperature is often normal or subnormal.[1]

Although recovery from heat exhaustion is usually spontaneous, intravenous saline can speed up the process. While the underlying defect is not a depletion of salt and water, maintenance of these electrolytes will help prevent the development of heat exhaustion in individuals exposed to persistently high temperatures.[1]

Heatstroke

Heatstroke is a medical emergency, with mortality rates ranging from 10 to 80%.[143] It is characterized by a body temperature equal to or greater than 41.1° C (106° F), or by a body temperature of 40.6° C (105° F) or greater with anhidrosis and/or an altered mental status.[2,8]

ETIOLOGY

Exertional Heatstroke

Heatstroke syndrome may be either exertional or nonexertional (classic heatstroke).[2] Exertional heatstroke is typically seen in healthy young adults who overexert themselves in high ambient temperatures and humidity or in an environment to which they are not acclimatized (Table 37B-17). Their thermoregulatory mechanisms are usually intact initially. Eventually, however, endogenous heat production outstrips the heat-dissipating mechanisms.[2] These patients usually stop sweating before the onset of symptoms, and subsequently they may demonstrate profound homeostatic dysfunction and hyperpyrexia.[1]

> **AXIOM** Heatstroke usually occurs because of severe exertion or because of severe underlying diseases affecting cardiovascular function or heat loss.

Classic Heatstroke

Classic heatstroke is nonexertional and is most common in patients with preexisting diseases, such as congenital absence of sweat glands, scleroderma, atherosclerosis, diabetes mellitus, or alcoholism.[144] Other conditions associated with the development of heatstroke syndrome include congestive heart failure, renal insufficiency, chronic obstructive pulmonary disease, psychoses, cystic fibrosis, and thyrotoxicosis. Although "classic" heatstroke is most commonly a disorder of the elderly during environmental heat waves, all ages are at risk. Infants, for example, may develop heatstroke if wrapped too warmly during a febrile illness or if left in a car in a hot environment. Drugs that may increase the risk of heatstroke include diuret-

TABLE 37B–17   Comparison of Classic and Exertional Heat Stroke*

Feature	Classic	Exertional
Age group	Very young, very old	Men 15-45 years old
Health status	Chronic illness common	Usually healthy
History of febrile illness or immunization	Unusual	Common
Activity	Sedentary	Common in football players, military recruits, competitive runners
Drug use	Sweat depressants, diuretics, haloperidol, phenothiazines	Amphetamines, cocaine
Sweating	Usually absent	Often present
Respiratory alkalosis	Dominant	Mild
Lactic acidosis	Absent or mild	Often marked
Acute renal failure	<5% of patients	30% of patients
Rhabdomyolysis	Seldom severe	Severe
Hyperuricemia	Modest	Severe
Creatinine:BUN† ratio	1:10	Elevated
CPK, aldolase	Mildly elevated	Markedly elevated
Hypocalcemia	Uncommon	Common
DIC†	Mild	Marked
Hypoglycemia	Uncommon	Common

*Some features are common to both types: lack of heat acclimatization, dehydration, salt depletion, hyperthermia (≥106°F), cutaneous flushing and mottling, coma, psychotic behavior, convulsions while cooling, shock, adult respiratory distress syndrome, hypokalemia, hypernatremia, hypophosphatemia or hyperphosphatemia, poikilothermia during recovery.
†BUN = blood urea nitrogen; DIC = disseminated intravascular coagulation.
Knochel JP. Heatstroke and related heat stress disorders. Dis Mon 1989;35:306.

ics, phenothiazines, anticholinergics, beta-blockers, tricyclic antidepressants, and amphetamines.[145,146]

Role of Cytokines

Bouchama et al[147] have noted that endotoxin, tumor necrosis factor alpha (TNF-alpha), interleukin 1 alpha (IL-1 alpha), and other pyrogenic cytokines may be involved in the pathogenesis of heatstroke. In a prospective study, Bouchama et al[147] measured plasma IL-1 beta, IL-6, and interferon gamma (INF-gamma) concentrations in 28 heatstroke patients at the time of hospital admission (precooling) and after complete cooling (postcooling), and in 10 normal control subjects. They also measured C-reactive protein (CRP) as a marker of acute phase response and calculated severity of illness using the simplified acute physiology score. Twenty-five males and 3 females had a mean (+/- SEM) rectal temperature of 41.2+/-0.2° C. IL-6, IL-1 beta, and INF-gamma concentrations were elevated in 100%, 39%, and 50% of the patients, and the CRP values were elevated in 72% of the patients. The IL-6 concentrations correlated with the severity of illness (r = 0.516, p = 0.03) and the two patients with the highest IL-6 concentrations died.

CLINICAL PRESENTATION (TABLE 37B–18)

AXIOM   Multiple organ damage can develop rapidly during severe, untreated heatstroke.

CNS Changes

Heatstroke usually occurs without any prodromal signs or symptoms.[1] As the thermoregulatory mechanisms fail, the body temperature can rapidly rise above 105-106° F, and the patient can quickly lapse into coma or obtundation.[2]

AXIOM   CNS disturbances are characteristically present to some degree in all cases of heatstroke.

During the development of heatstroke, irritability and/or irrationality tend to precede any depression in the level of consciousness, and the majority of patients can quickly become unresponsive to painful stimuli. Seizures and signs of cerebellar dysfunction are common. The pupils are usually pinpoint. In spite of these CNS changes, the cerebrospinal fluid is generally clear, and the opening pressure is usually normal.[1]

Widespread neuronal death can occur rapidly with heatstroke, and the Purkinje cells of the cerebellum are often the most severely affected. Cerebral edema and petechial hemorrhages are also often seen. Survivors of severe heatstroke syndrome often have evidence of cerebral dysfunction, including aphasia, hemiplegia, and ataxia.[148]

Cardiac Changes

The pulse in heatstroke is generally weak and thready. Hypotension is common, but it is not universal. Cardiac muscle damage and occasional frank infarction occur frequently in patients with both exertional and classic heatstroke and are related to the direct cellular toxicity of heat on the myocytes. The cardiac changes may develop more rapidly if there is coronary artery disease and/or hypovolemia.

AXIOM   Patients with severe heatstroke can rapidly develop increasing cardiovascular dysfunction.

Patients with heatstroke typically present with tachycardia and some hypotension. Tachydysrhythmias, particularly those of ventricular origin, may be life-threatening. The circulatory collapse present in such patients is not well understood but probably results from cutaneous vasodilatation and a decreased systemic vascular resistance. Peripheral vasodilatation can lead to a condition of high-output cardiac failure.

TABLE 37B–18   Complications of Heat Stroke

Early	Late
Seizures	Persistent neurologic deficit
Shivering	Liver failure
Hypothermia	Disseminated intravascular coagulation
Rebound hyperthermia	Hyperosmolar coma
Pulmonary edema	Adult respiratory distress syndrome
Rhabdomyolysis	Renal failure
Hypokalmia	Hyperkalemia
Hypernatremia	Hypocalcemia
Electrocardiographic changes	Hyperuricemia
Hypotension	

Tek D, Olshaker JS. Heat illness. Emerg Med Clin N Am 1992;10:299.

Pulmonary Changes

Patients developing heatstroke tend to hyperventilate and may develop severe respiratory alkalosis. Radiographic evidence of pulmonary consolidation frequently occurs, and fatal pulmonary edema can develop rapidly in patients with severe preexisting cardiopulmonary disease.[1]

Skeletal Muscle Changes

Rhabdomyolysis is common in patients with exertional heat stroke and may be severe.[2] In addition to its potential contribution to the development of acute renal failure, the rapid development of hyperkalemia and its potential cardiac effects may be an immediate threat to survival. Severe hypocalcemia may also develop as a result of rhabdomyolysis.[2] Exogenous calcium, however, should not be administered unless serious ventricular ectopy secondary to hyperkalemia develops because hypercalcemia can exacerbate the severity of the rhabdomyolysis.

Renal Dysfunction

Renal damage, to some extent, is seen in almost all patients with heatstroke.[2,149,150] It is commonly manifested initially by mild proteinuria and abnormal urine sediment. Acute renal failure develops five to six times more commonly in patients with exertional heatstroke (30-35%) than in those with the nonexertional type and appears to be related to dehydration, renal hypoperfusion, and the myoglobinuria of rhabdomyolysis.[2]

Uric acid nephropathy may also develop in patients with heatstroke as a result of strenuous muscular activity. Initially, all that may be seen is some increased urine sediment and a mild proteinuria. In the presence of hypotension and myoglobinuria, however, the patient can rapidly progress to complete renal shutdown.

AXIOM The combination of dehydration, hypotension, and rhabdomyolysis can rapidly cause oliguric renal failure in patients with heatstroke.

Hepatic Changes

Some degree of hepatic damage occurs in most patients with heatstroke.[2] During strenuous exercise, the temperature of hepatic venous blood may be more than 3-4° C warmer than the measured core body temperature and may predispose to hepatic cellular injury.[2] Cholestasis and centrilobular necrosis appear responsible for the elevations of both bilirubin and serum transaminase levels.[142] These changes, however, are typically self-limited and without any long-term morbidity.[2] Fulminant hepatic necrosis leading to death is quite rare.

Hassanein et al[151] have noted that, in a minority (less than 10%) of heatstroke victims in whom neurologic injury has not resulted in death within the first 2-3 days, the hepatic injury of heatstroke can result in death that occurs a week or more after the onset of the heat stress, unless the liver is replaced. Two such cases were referred to the University of Pittsburgh for transplantation. On the basis of these two referrals and a review of the literature, Hassanein et al[151] believe that this problem occurs more often than is currently appreciated, principally because of a lack of knowledge about the problem.

Coagulation Changes

Disseminated intravascular coagulation (DIC) in heatstroke may range from an asymptomatic laboratory finding of hypofibrinogenemia and thrombocytopenia to severe clinical bleeding. Assays of coagulation factors, including factors II, V, VII, IX, and X, as well as plasminogen, are normal in most heatstroke patients, including those with prolonged coagulation studies, suggesting that their qualitative function is affected by the heat exposure. Furthermore, heat is known to enhance fibrinolytic activity in blood. Consequently, many patients with heatstroke develop petechiae in the skin and visceral organs.[152] Patients may also develop melena, hematemesis, hematochezia, hemoptysis, or clinical DIC characterized by thrombocytopenia, hypofibrinogenemia, and prolongation of the prothrombin and partial thromboplastin times.

Electrolyte Changes

A number of characteristic laboratory changes have been described in heatstroke. Significant dehydration is frequent in patients with exertional heatstroke and may be reflected by elevated levels of blood urea nitrogen, creatinine, glucose hemoglobin, hematocrit, and white blood cells; however, serum sodium, potassium, phosphate, calcium, and magnesium concentrations are frequently low early in the clinical course.[142,146]

AXIOM Severe electrolyte problems, especially with potassium and calcium, can develop during heatstroke and may be greatly aggravated during fluid resuscitation.

Injudicious rehydration with pure water can cause additional decreases in the serum levels of many electrolytes, and these, in turn, can cause a number of serious problems. Hypokalemia, for example, may decrease the ability of the patient to sweat, decrease skeletal muscle blood flow, and cause a nephrogenic diabetes insipidus with further dehydration.[8] Serum potassium levels, however, are usually normal or high depending on the urine output and the amount of breakdown of tissue, especially muscle.[55]

If significant skeletal muscle damage and cellular lysis occur, severe hyperkalemia can develop.[55] Hypocalcemia is usually seen in patients with significant rhabdomyolysis, and it is primarily a result of calcium salt precipitation in injured skeletal muscle.

TREATMENT

Survival of heatstroke depends on promptly recognizing the syndrome and immediately lowering the core body temperature.[2] Mortality rates appear to be directly related to the severity and duration of the hyperpyrexia.[8,153]

Effective lowering of the core body temperature usually requires only external cooling techniques.[2] Immersion in an ice water bath is frequently used, but it is not as effective as wetting the skin with tepid water (to prevent cutaneous vasoconstriction), followed by the use of fans to facilitate evaporation of the water. Gastric or peritoneal lavage with iced saline is only rarely required in refractory cases or when thermogenesis is ongoing (as in malignant hyperthermia). If an immersion cooling technique is used, vigorous skin massage should be used to prevent the dermal stasis of cooled blood that tends to occur as local cutaneous vasoconstriction occurs. When the falling core temperature approaches 39° C, efforts to cool the patient should be terminated because the body temperature will continue to fall another 1-2° C.

AXIOM Cooling of patients with heatstroke is best done by wetting the patient's skin with tepid water and facilitating its rapid evaporation with fans.

From a practical standpoint, cooling by immersion is unsatisfactory when cardiac monitoring or airway protection is needed.[2] Evaporative techniques are generally more effective and allow the patient to be placed on a bed and treated like the usual intensive care patients. The intravenous administration of chlorpromazine (25 to 50 mg every 6 hours) may help by preventing shivering.

The need for intravascular fluids must be carefully assessed.[2] There may be little or no dehydration in patients with underlying cardiac, renal, or hepatic failure, but dehydration is common in otherwise normal patients with exertional heat injury. Hypotension may result from volume depletion, peripheral vasodilation, and/or myocardial dysfunction.

AXIOM Although insertion of a PA catheter in hypothermic patients can cause severe arrhythmias, it may be essential in the optimal management of severe heatstroke.

Early placement of a pulmonary arterial monitoring catheter is recommended in any circumstance in which uncertainty regarding the patient's volume status or myocardial function exists.[2] Dobutamine may be helpful in patients who have an adequate BP but also have myocardial dysfunction and an inadequate cardiac output.

AXIOM　One should anticipate the possibility of heatstroke in patients developing seizures.

Seizures are commonly seen with heatstroke and should be treated with intravenous diazepam.[2] Airway protection should be established via endotracheal intubation in patients with severe mental status changes and impaired cough or gag reflexes. The role of dehydrating agents, such as mannitol or furosemide, in the management of cerebral edema is unclear. They may, however, be of some benefit in patients who have persistent oliguria in spite of adequate fluid loading and blood pressure.[2]

Acute renal failure, especially in association with rhabdomyolysis, can be a major source of patient morbidity.[2] Measures aimed at its prevention include prompt reestablishment of an adequate intravascular volume, blood pressure, and cardiac output, and correction of any concomitant metabolic abnormalities. Furosemide or mannitol may benefit patients with rhabdomyolysis if oliguria persists in spite of adequate volume loading and hemodynamics.

AXIOM　Serum potassium levels in heatstroke may either be extremely low or high, depending on the urine output and the amount of muscle damage.

Serum potassium levels should be closely monitored in patients with heatstroke. Standard therapy for life-threatening hyperkalemia (including calcium, glucose with insulin, and bicarbonate) should be given to patients with either typical ECG changes or increasing ventricular ectopy. If oliguric renal failure develops, prompt hemodialysis may be required to manage the hyperkalemia.

Coagulation disorders in heatstroke syndrome are relatively common. Some benefit may be achieved with continuous infusions of heparin at 500-800 units/hr in patients who develop laboratory evidence of DIC.[8,16] The use of dextran solutions to maintain an adequate blood pressure is generally discouraged because dextrans may contribute to the development of a clinical bleeding disorder and/or renal failure.

Excess Thermogenesis Syndromes

Malignant hyperthermia (MH) and neuroleptic malignant syndrome (NMS) are disorders of body temperature resulting from excessive endogenous heat production, without the influence of ambient temperature.[2] The hypothalamic regulation of temperature and the physiologic mechanisms to dissipate heat may be impaired, particularly in neuroleptic malignant syndrome. In addition to hyperpyrexia, both of these conditions tend to be associated with profound muscle rigidity.

ETIOLOGY

Although other predisposing conditions have been described, certain drugs appear to be essential for the development of malignant hyperthermia and neuroleptic malignant syndrome.[2] Agents particularly apt to cause malignant hyperthermia in susceptible individuals include halothane and succinylcholine.[154] Agents that tend to be associated with neuroleptic malignant syndrome include phenothiazines, haloperidol, and dopamine-depleting drugs.[155] Sudden withdrawal of dopamine-agonists, such as levodopa, may also cause this syndrome in susceptible individuals.

AXIOM　Core temperature should be watched carefully in all patients with severe trauma, particularly during general anesthesia and/or if the patient has recently taken neuroleptic drugs.

Malignant Hyperthermia

INCIDENCE.　Malignant hyperthermia (MH) is a rare genetic myopathy that was first described as a fatal complication of general anesthesia in 1960.[156] It is estimated to affect approximately 1 in 15,000 pediatric patients and 1 in 40,000 middle-aged patients. It is the most common cause of death as a direct result of general anesthesia.[157] The mode of transmission is genetic. The severest form is autosomal dominant, and the less severe form is autosomal recessive. Thus, both men and women can have MH, although there is a slightly higher incidence in the male pediatric population. Malignant hyperthermia is usually triggered by halogenated anesthetic agents with or without depolarizing muscle relaxants.

CALCIUM CHANGES.　After muscle contraction, calcium is sequestered from the contractile apparatus to allow relaxation of skeletal muscle.[158] Individuals who develop malignant hyperthermia tend to have a genetically inherited predisposition for the administration of certain drugs to cause increased release of stored calcium from the sarcoplasmic reticulum into the myoplasm with decreased subsequent removal of the calcium from the contractile apparatus. This can cause vigorous continued muscle contracture, resulting in rigidity and greatly increased metabolic activity. The resultant surge in thermogenesis can cause the core body temperature to rise 1° C every 5 minutes. Although the hypothalamic regulation of body temperature and the physiologic mechanisms to dissipate heat appear to be intact,[158] they are totally inadequate to deal with this magnitude of heat production.

GENETIC FACTORS.　It increasingly appears that malignant hyperthermia is a heterogeneous disorder that can be caused by a variety of genetic defects, in one of a number of genes.[159] Direct molecular methods will provide a rapid, efficient, noninvasive, and low-cost screening test once the causative genetic mutations have been identified. However, until then, indirect molecular genetic methods can be used to demonstrate the inheritance of an abnormal gene in certain family members at risk. This requires localizing the gene that produces the abnormal phenotype to a subchromosomal segment by linkage analysis and showing the coinheritance of MHS and DNA markers in a number of family members.

McLennan et al[160] have focused their attention on the linkage of MH to defects in the gene (RYR1) encoding the skeletal muscle Ca^{++} release channel. They have cloned and sequenced human RYR1 cDNA and found restriction fragment length polymorphisms (RFLPs) in the human gene. They also localized RYR1 to human chromosome 19q13.1. Studies of the cosegregation of MH with these RFLPs established RYR1/MH linkage on human chromosome 19q13.1. They then sequenced MH and normal porcine RYR1 cDNAs. They found a specific mutation in malignant hyperthermia pigs and a corresponding mutation in 1 of 35 human MH families studied.

The finding of linkage of malignant hyperthermia to markers from chromosome 19q13.1-13.2 and the identification of mutations in a candidate gene have held out hope for the availability of a genetic diagnosis. However, Ball and Johnson[157] have noted that it is likely that only about 50% of families have a mutation of the skeletal muscle calcium release channel gene. With this degree of genetic heterogeneity, presymptomatic testing based on DNA markers can only be offered at present to a limited number of families in whom linkage to markers from 19q13.1-13.2 has been clearly shown.

The combination of halothane and succinylcholine, commonly used for anesthetic induction during pediatric otolaryngologic procedures, is associated with a 1% incidence of masseter spasm, which may be an early sign of malignant hyperthermia. In an 18-month retrospective review of patients undergoing general anesthesia in a pediatric otolaryngology service, Kosko et al[161] found that the incidence of masseter spasm was 2 of 206 (1%) in children who were anesthetized with halothane and received succinylcholine. The agents were not used in patients identified as high risk for developing malignant hyperthermia, and none of those patients developed malignant hyperthermia.

Neuroleptic Malignant Syndrome

The administration of certain neuroleptic drugs can cause a similar, but usually less intense, elevation in core body temperature than that seen with malignant hyperthermia. Caroff et al[158] have suggested that patients with the genetic predisposition for malignant hyperthermia may also be susceptible to developing neuroleptic malignant syndrome. As with malignant hyperthermia, sustained muscle contracture is the major cause of the hyperthermia. In addition, hypothalamic temperature setpoint regulation may be affected by the dopamine receptor blockade caused by these drugs.[162] Thus, mechanisms to dissipate heat may also be impaired.

CLINICAL SYNDROME

> **AXIOM** It may be difficult to detect malignant hyperthermia or neuroleptic malignant syndrome in patients with severe CNS and musculoskeletal injuries.

Severe CNS damage from direct trauma or ischemia can cause severe hyperthermia and can be difficult to differentiate from MH and NMS if anesthesia or neuroleptic drugs are given.

Malignant Hyperthermia

Malignant hyperthermia is characterized by the development of trismus in 50% of patients, followed by total body rigidity and a significant increase in core body temperature.[2] This process may begin at any time during anesthetic induction and can proceed with great rapidity. The metabolic consequences of this syndrome include a combined respiratory and metabolic acidosis, along with elevated serum potassium, sodium, and calcium levels. If significant myonecrosis follows, serum potassium levels may rapidly rise to life-threatening levels, and plasma ionized calcium may fall abruptly as calcium moves into injured muscle.

Early findings that suggest that a malignant hyperthermic crisis may be imminent include excessive masseter muscle contractions or rigidity after succinylcholine administration. Other changes may include cyanosis, hypercarbia, tachycardia, and hypertension. As the syndrome progresses, the rapid severe increase in core body temperature is virtually diagnostic.[2]

> **AXIOM** If the development of malignant hyperthermia is not promptly recognized, patients can rapidly die, especially if they are severely injured.

The classic diagnostic triad consists of skeletal muscle rigidity, metabolic acidosis, and elevated body temperature. The definitive diagnosis is made by exposing intact muscle fibers to caffeine and halothane in varying concentrations.

Neuroleptic Malignant Syndrome

Neuroleptic malignant syndrome should be suspected in patients who are given a neuroleptic drug and subsequently develop signs of muscular rigidity, dystonia, or unexplained catatonic behavior.[2] Diaphoresis, tachycardia, tachypnea, and hypertension or hypotension, are evidence of underlying autonomic instability. Temperature elevation usually follows these findings. Laboratory data are variable; however, serum levels of creatine phosphokinase (CPK) and glutamic-oxaloacetic transaminase (GOT) may rise abruptly in patients who develop rhabdomyolysis.

COMPLICATIONS

> **AXIOM** Failure to recognize excess thermogenesis early can rapidly result in multiple organ failure, especially if the patient is hypovolemic.

The complications that arise with malignant hyperthermia and neuroleptic malignant syndrome are similar to those of heatstroke,[2] but the temperature elevation, rhabdomyolysis, and hepatic necrosis may be much more severe. In addition, DIC is more common with malignant hyperthermia, but it does not appear to correlate with as poor a prognosis as it does in heatstroke.[158] Renal failure is most apt to occur in patients with severe rhabdomyolysis, but primary myocardial damage appears to be less frequent than in heatstroke. The development of ventricular tachydysrhythmias seems to parallel the degree of hypermetabolism and hyperkalemia, but seizures are uncommon. Patients with neuroleptic malignant syndrome have an increased tendency to develop aspiration pneumonia because of dystonia and an impaired ability to handle their secretions.[163]

TREATMENT

Successful treatment of malignant hyperthermia and neuroleptic malignant syndrome depends on early recognition and prompt withdrawal of the suspected inciting agent. In malignant hyperthermia, just discontinuing the inciting agent is often adequate therapy, provided the syndrome is not yet well-established.[158] Recovery from neuroleptic malignant syndrome may similarly occur with discontinuation of the drug; however, the temperature may not return to baseline for 5 to 7 days.

> **AXIOM** The keys to successful treatment of excessive thermogenesis are early diagnosis, discontinuance of the inciting agents, administration of dantrolene, cooling of the patient, and carefully monitored cardiopulmonary and metabolic support.

Dantrolene is the drug of choice in malignant hyperthermia and should be administered to patients in whom hyperpyrexia continues to develop after anesthetic removal. The recommended dose is 2 mg/kg intravenously, repeated every 5 minutes, up to a total of 10 mg/kg. This should be given before instituting any other supportive therapeutic measures. Dantrolene acts by inhibiting calcium release from the sarcoplasmic reticulum, thereby decreasing the amount of calcium available for ongoing excessive muscle contraction; however, respiratory muscle function and airway protection usually remain intact.

The role of dantrolene in neuroleptic malignant syndrome is less well-defined; however, in several case reports it was shown to reduce thermogenesis.[152,164] The doses used are similar to those recommended for malignant hyperthermia. Administration of greater than 10 mg/kg may be associated with hepatic toxicity.

A number of other drugs, such as bromocriptine, amantadine, and levodopa/carbidopa have been used to reduce thermogenesis.[158,163,164] All of these drugs increase central neurologic dopaminergic tone, thereby altering both the hypothalamic and peripheral mechanisms that increase core body temperature.[2]

> **AXIOM** Minute ventilation must usually be much greater than normal in patients with hyperthermia.

Specific emphasis should be placed on assessing airway and ventilatory adequacy in patients with neuroleptic malignant syndrome, but tracheal intubation should not be performed unless needed. All of these patients should be treated in an intensive care unit.[2]

⊘ FREQUENT ERRORS

In the Management of Temperature-related (Nonburn) Injuries

1. *Causing additional injury to frozen tissue by rubbing it or immersing it in excessively hot water in an effort to warm it rapidly.*
2. *Failing to adequately protect frozen tissues from cold or physical trauma after rewarming.*

3. *Inadequate fluid administration during rewarming.*
4. *Allowing a patient with a cold injury to smoke or receive a vasoconstrictor drug.*
5. *Giving inadequate attention to the generalized or systemic effects of cooling while treating frostbite.*
6. *Failing to detect and treat underlying trauma or systemic diseases, such as hypothyroidism or vascular insufficiency.*
7. *Failure to provide adequate salt and potassium to individuals with excessive sweating.*
8. *Failing to adequately correct hypovolemia and failure to look carefully for predisposing conditions in patients with heatstroke.*
9. *Failure to anticipate severe electrolyte abnormalities, especially with potassium and calcium, in patients with heatstroke.*
10. *Failure to anticipate seizures and multiple organ failure in patients with severe heatstroke.*
11. *Failure to adequately monitor core body temperature in patients with severe trauma.*
12. *Delayed diagnosis and treatment of malignant hyperthermia or neuroleptic malignant syndrome.*

▼▼▼▼▼▼▼▼▼▼▼▼▼▼▼▼▼▼▼▼▼▼▼▼▼▼▼▼

SUMMARY POINTS

1. Impairment of mental or cardiovascular function greatly increases the risk of patients developing accidental heat or cold injury.
2. The body's responses to hyperthermia are limited and include cutaneous vasodilation, sweating, and decreased physical activity.
3. Heatstroke syndrome is more likely to occur if there is increased activity and the person is poorly acclimatized.
4. The homeothermic responses to cold are virtually nonexistent at core temperatures below 28° C (83° F).
5. Nonfreezing cold (NFC) injury is caused by tissue chilling and reduced perfusion of tissues resulting from cold-induced vasoconstriction.
6. Cold injury is much more apt to occur in areas of the body that are not kept dry.
7. Immersion foot refers to virtually any foot injuries caused by prolonged exposure to cold and wet.
8. Nonfreezing cold injuries to the feet frequently result from inadequate or improperly fitting footwear.
9. The treatment of immersion foot includes careful protection of the involved tissues as long as hyperemia, anhidrosis, and paresthesias persist.
10. Careful atraumatic physical therapy is useful to minimize the formation of contractures in patients with immersion foot.
11. Frostbite injury is much less apt to occur in individuals carefully watching each other for early signs of its development.
12. Even with what appears to be severe frostbite, a great deal of spontaneous healing eventually occurs.
13. One should not perform early amputations for frostbite unless the patient develops a severe infection that is unresponsive to appropriate antibiotics.
14. An area of cold injury should never be rubbed, especially with snow or cold water.
15. A patient with a cold injury should not smoke cigarettes or be given any drug that can cause vasoconstriction.
16. Debridement of frostbitten tissues should be extremely conservative; with time, most of the frozen tissue will heal by itself.
17. The depth of tissue necrosis in frostbite is usually much less than expected.
18. Surgical debridement or amputations for frostbite should not be performed until the level of mummification or tissue death is clearly demarcated, and this usually takes at least 1 to 3 months.
19. Patients who have suffered severe cold injury should avoid any repeat cold exposure because they are at increased risk to suffer severe tissue damage and/or pain.

20. Hypothermia can occur at virtually any temperature below 80° F.
21. Hypothermia can increase the mortality rates with virtually any injury.
22. One should monitor core temperatures closely in trauma patients, especially those who are in shock, receive massive transfusions, or have prolonged abdominal surgery.
23. Endogenous warming after hypothermia has developed can put a tremendous metabolic and cardiovascular strain on the patient.
24. The patient has little or no defense against hypothermia during a general anesthetic or when the core temperature is less than 32° C.
25. So-called Osborne (J) waves on an ECG may be the first clue that hypothermia is present, especially in anesthetized patients.
26. The diuresis occurring with hypothermia can cause hypovolemia, and this can cause severe hypotension during rewarming.
27. Severely hypothermic patients are particularly apt to develop pneumonia after rewarming.
28. One of the best ways to prevent coagulopathies in trauma patients is to prevent or rapidly correct hypothermia.
29. Seriously injured patients who are hypotensive are at particular risk of developing hypothermia.
30. Hypothermic patients with recent loss of signs of life should not be pronounced dead until or unless there are still no signs of life after the patient has been warmed to at least 32° C or preferably 35° C.
31. As soon as the major bleeding has been controlled during emergency surgery, the surgeon should irrigate the body cavity being explored with warmed saline until the core temperature is at least 34-35° C.
32. As long as the hypothermic patient has a pulse and is breathing, treatment should not be overly aggressive.
33. Blood pressure and cardiac filling pressures must be watched carefully during rewarming when there is a strong tendency to develop hypovolemia and hypotension.
34. Some ventilation is better than no ventilation, but hyperventilation can precipitate severe arrhythmias or cardiac arrest.
35. Although CPR may precipitate VF and is not very effective during hypothermia, one should not hesitate to provide CPR if the patient is pulseless after a thorough check.
36. Electrical cardioversion of the hypothermic heart (below 30-32° C) is difficult, if not impossible.
37. Bicarbonate should not be used to treat severe metabolic acidosis until the ventilation is adequate to remove the increased CO_2 that is formed.
38. In general, core temperatures are best monitored with an esophageal probe, particularly in the OR.
39. Uncorrected blood gas values in hypothermic patients may be more meaningful than those that are corrected to 37° C.
40. ABG values do not have to be corrected to the patient's core temperature.
41. Slow rewarming of patients with moderate-severe hypothermia allows additional ischemic damage to occur.
42. Rapid external rewarming can cause hypotension, and use of external devices with temperatures above 45° C can damage the skin.
43. Despite the shortcomings of active external rewarming, no difference in survival or morbidity has been prospectively demonstrated between this technique and those involved in core rewarming.
44. The most effective, easily managed, and readily available method of active core warming is inhalation of heated gases.
45. Warmed gastric lavage for treating hypothermia is quite slow and it increases the risk of aspiration of gastric contents.
46. If rapidly available, partial cardiopulmonary bypass is the most rapid, effective method for correcting severe hypothermia.
47. CPB is the treatment of choice for resuscitation of patients who have profound hypothermia and cardiac arrest.
48. Hypothermic patients are not dead until they are warm (at least 32-35° C) and dead.

49. Cool-water drowning does not offer the same cerebral protection as drowning by ice-cold water.
50. Rapid core cooling after submersion provides a better prognosis than slow cooling.
51. Some glucose should be present in the fluids used to resuscitate hypothermic patients.
52. Vasoconstrictors should not be used in patients with hypotension resulting from hypothermia.
53. Bronchopneumonia is a frequent complication of hypothermia, and it is often a result of aspiration.
54. Although heat-overload syndromes may be distinguished from each other clinically, their underlying physiologic aberrations differ primarily only with regard to their severity.
55. Decreased sweating, especially while working in a hot environment, can rapidly increase the likelihood of a heat-induced injury.
56. Heat cramps are usually best corrected by administration of dilute salt solutions after the patient has been placed in a cool environment.
57. Because sweat has 5.0 or more mEq of potassium per liter, excessive sweating, corrected only with water and NaCl, can eventually cause hypokalemia.
58. Heat syncope is generally self-limiting and often requires no treatment other than removal of the patient from the main heat source and rest in a recumbent position; however, administration of some water and salt will usually speed recovery.
59. Heatstroke usually occurs because of severe exertion or because of severe underlying diseases affecting cardiovascular function or heat loss.
60. Multiple organ damage can develop rapidly during severe, untreated heatstroke.
61. CNS disturbances are characteristically present to some degree in all cases of heatstroke.
62. Patients with severe heatstroke can rapidly develop increasing cardiovascular dysfunction.
63. Cardiopulmonary failure is apt to occur in patients with heatstroke and preexisting cardiopulmonary disease.
64. The combination of dehydration, hypotension, and rhabdomyolysis can rapidly cause oliguric renal failure in patients with heatstroke.
65. Severe electrolyte problems, especially with potassium and calcium, can develop during heatstroke and may be greatly aggravated during fluid resuscitation.
66. Cooling of patients with heatstroke is best done by wetting the patient's skin with tepid water and facilitating its rapid evaporation with fans.
67. Although insertion of a PA catheter in hypothermic patients can cause severe arrhythmias, it may be essential in the optimal management of severe heatstroke.
68. One should anticipate the possibility of heatstroke in patients developing seizures.
69. Serum potassium levels in heatstroke may either be extremely low or high, depending on the urine output and the amount of muscle damage.
70. Core temperature should be watched carefully in all patients with severe trauma, particularly during general anesthesia and/or if the patient has recently taken neuroleptic drugs.
71. If the development of malignant hyperthermia is not promptly recognized, patients can rapidly die, especially if they are severely injured.
72. It may be difficult to detect malignant hyperthermia or neuroleptic malignant syndrome in patients with severe CNS and musculoskeletal injuries.
73. Failure to recognize excess thermogenesis early can rapidly result in multiple organ failure, especially if the patient is hypovolemic.
74. The keys to successful treatment of excessive thermogenesis are early diagnosis, discontinuance of the inciting agent, administration of dantrolene, cooling of the patient, and carefully monitored cardiopulmonary and metabolic support.

75. Minute ventilation must usually be much greater than normal in patients with hyperthermia.

▲▲▲▲▲▲▲▲▲▲▲▲▲▲▲▲▲▲▲▲▲▲▲▲▲▲▲▲▲▲▲▲

REFERENCES

1. Fisher RP, Souba WW, Ford EG. Temperature-associated injuries and syndromes. In: Moore EE, Mattox KL, Feliciano DV, eds. Trauma. 2nd ed. Norwalk, CT: Appleton & Lange, 1991; 765-776.
2. Farmer JC. Temperature-related injuries. In: Civetta JM, Taylor RW, Kirby RR, eds. Critical care. Philadelphia: JB Lippincott, 1988; 693-700.
3. Bowe EA, Klein EF. Near-drowning. In: Capan LM, Miller SM, Turndorf H, eds. Trauma: anesthesia and intensive care. Philadelphia: JB Lippincott, 1991; 652-653.
4. Guyton AC. Body temperature, temperature regulation and fever. In: Guyton AC, ed. Textbook of medical physiology. 6th ed. Philadelphia: Saunders, 1981; 886.
5. Jolly BT, Ghezzi KT. Accidental hypothermia. Em Med Clin N Am 1992;10:311.
6. Moss JF. Accidental severe hypothermia. Surg Gynecol Obstet 1986; 162:501.
7. Myers RAM, Britten JS, Cowley RA. Hypothermia: quantitative aspects of therapy. JACEP 1979;8:523.
8. Knochel JP. Environmental heat illness. A review. Arch Intern Med 1974;133:841.
9. Moss JF, Haklin M, Southwick HW, et al. A model for the treatment of accidental severe hypothermia. J Trauma 1986;26:68.
10. Knochel JP. Heatstroke and related heat stress disorders. Dis Month 1989;35:306.
11. Francis TJR. Nonfreezing cold injury: a historical review. J R Nav Med Serv 1984;70:134.
12. Vaughn PB. Local cold injury: menace to military operations. Milit Med 1980;145:305.
13. Ramstead KD, Hughes RG, Webb AJ. Recent cases of trench foot. Postgrad Med J 1980;56:879.
14. Ungley CC, Channell GD, Richards RL. The immersion foot syndrome. Br J Surg 1945;33:17.
15. Akers AA. Paddy foot: a warm water immersion foot syndrome variant, part I. The natural disease, epidemiology. Milit Med 1974;139:605.
16. Wrenn K. Immersion foot: a problem of the homeless in the 1990s. Arch Int Med 1991;151:785.
17. Rietschel RL, Allen AM. Immersion feet: a method of studying the effects of protracted water exposure on human skin. Milit Med 1976; 141:778.
18. Willis I. The effects of prolonged water exposure on human skin. J Invest Dermatol 1973;60:166.
19. Bangs CC. Hypothermia and frostbite. Emerg Med Clin North Am 1984; 2:475.
20. Chen GS, Yu HS, Yang SA, et al. Responses of cutaneous microcirculation to cold exposure and neuropathy in vibration-induced white finger. Microvasc Res 1994;47:21.
21. Borovikov A. Toe-to-hand transfers in the rehabilitation of frostbite injury. Ann Plast Surg 1993;31:245.
22. Dowd PM, Rustin MHA, Lanigan S. Nifedipine in the treatment of chilblains. Br Med J 1986;293:923.
23. Miller JW, Danzl DF, Thomas DM. Urban accidental hypothermia: 135 cases. Ann Emerg Med 1980;9:456.
24. Moss J. Accidental severe hypothermia. Surg Gynecol Obstet 1986; 162:501.
25. Rango N. Exposure-related hypothermia mortality in the United States, 1970-79. Am J Public Health 1984;74:1159.
26. Hauty MG, Esrig BC, Hill JG, et al. Prognostic factors in severe accidental hypothermia: experience from the Mt. Hood tragedy. J Trauma 1987;27:1107.
27. Danzl DF, Pozos RS, et al. Multicenter hypothermia survey. Ann Emerg Med 1987;16:1042.
28. White JD. Hypothermia: the Bellevue experience. Ann Emerg Med 1982;11:417.
29. Biggart MJ, Bohn DJ. Effect of hypothermia and cardiac arrest on outcome of near-drowning accidents in children. J Pediatr 1990; 117:170.
30. Jurkovich GJ, Greiser WB, Luterman A, Curreri PW. Hypothermia in trauma victims: an ominous predictor of survival. J Trauma 1987; 17:1019.

31. Orlowski JP. Drowning, near-drowning, and ice-water submersions. Pediatr Clin North Am 1987;34:75.
32. Cornelli HM. Accidental hypothermia. J Pediatrics 1992;120:671.
33. Wilson RF, Mammen E, Walt AJ. Eight years of experience with massive blood transfusions. J Trauma 1971;11:275.
34. Wilson RF. Complications of massive transfusions. Surgical Rounds 1981;4:47.
35. English MJ, Farmer C, Scott WA. Heat loss in exposed volunteers. J Trauma 1990;30:422.
36. Fitzgerald FT. Hypoglycemia and accidental hypothermia in an alcoholic population. West J Med 1980;133:105.
37. Werwath DL, Schwab CW, Scholten JR, et al. Microwave ovens: a safe new method for warming crystalloids. Ann Emerg Med 1984;13:407.
38. Collins JA. Problems associated with the massive transfusion of stored blood. Surgery 1974;75:274.
39. Harries MG. Drowning in man. Crit Care Med 1981;9:407.
40. Willson JT, Miller WR, Eliot TS. Blood studies in the hypothermic dog. Surgery 1958;43:979.
41. Hochachka PW, Somero GN. The adaptation of enzymes to temperature. Comp Biochem Physiol 1968;27:659.
42. Myers RD, Veale WL. Body temperature: possible ionic mechanism in the hypothalamus controlling the set point. Science 1970;170:95.
43. Sori AJ, Et-Assuooty A, Rush BJ, et al. The effect of temperature on survival in hemorrhagic shock. Ann Surg 1987;53:706.
44. Fitzgerald FT, Jessop C. Accidental hypothermia: a report of 22 cases and review of the literature. Adv Intern Med 1982;27:128.
45. Postlethy JC, Dorm J. Hypothermia, thrombosis, and acute pancreatitis. Br Med J 1974;2:446.
46. Paton BC. Accidental hypothermia. Pharmacol Ther 1983;22:331.
47. Towne WD, Geiss WP, Yanes HO, et al. Intractable ventricular fibrillation associated with profound accidental hypothermia: successful treatment with partial cardiopulmonary bypass. N Engl J Med 1972;287:1135.
48. Coniam SW. Accidental hypothermia. Anesthesia 1979;34:250.
49. Carden D, Doan L, Sweeney PJ, et al. Hypothermia. Ann Emerg Med 1982;11:497.
50. Solomon A, Barish RA, Browne B, et al. The electrocardiographic features of hypothermia. J Emerg Med 1989;7:169.
51. O'Keeffe KM, Accidental hypothernia: a review of 62 cases. JACEP (Ann Emerg Med) 1978;6:479.
52. Segar WE, Riley PA, Barila TG. Urinary composition during hypothermia. Am J Physiol 1956;185:528.
53. Kanter GS. Renal clearance of glucose in hypothermic dogs. Am J Physiol 1959;196:366.
54. Hervery GR. Hypothermia: physiologic changes encountered in hypothermia. Proc Roy Soc Med 1973;66:1053.
55. Bradley AF, Stupfel M. Severinghaus JW. Effect of temperature on PCO_2 and PO_2 of blood in vitro. J Appl Physiol 1956;9:201.
56. Kelman GR, Nunn JF. Nomograms for correction of blood PO_2, PCO_2, pH, and base excess for time and temperature. J Appl Physiol 1966; 21:1484.
57. Severinghaus JW. Oxyhemoglobin dissociation curve correction for temperature and pH variation in human blood. J Appl Physiol 1968;12: 485.
58. Ream AK, Reitz BA, Silverberg G. Temperature correction of PCO_2 and pH in estimating acid-base status: an example of the emperor's new clothes? Anesthesiology 1982;56:41.
59. Reuler JB. Hypothermia: pathophysiology, clinical settings and management. Ann Intern Med 1978;89:519.
60. Curry DL, Curry KP. Hypothermia and insulin secretion. Endocrinology 1970;81:750.
61. Maclean D, Murison J, Griffiths PD. Acute pancreatitis and diabetic ketoacidosis in hypothermia. Br Med J 1974;2:58.
62. Brauer RW, Hollway RJ, Krebs JS, et al. The liver in hypothermia. Ann NY Acad Sci 1959;80:395.
63. Boles JM, Mabille S, Scheydecker JL, et al. Hypoglycemia in salt water near-drowning victims. Intens Care Med 1988;14:80.
64. Lanier WL, Stangland KJ, Scheithauer BW, et al. The effects of dextrose infusion and head position on neurologic outcome after complete cerebral ischemia in primates: examination of a model. Anesthesiology 1987;66:39.
65. Poulos ND, Mollitt DL. The nature and reverseability of hypothermia-induced alterations of blood viscosity. J Trauma 1991;31:996.
66. Maclean D, Taig DR, Emslie-Smith D. Achilles tendon reflex in accidental hypothermia and hypothermic myxedema. Br Med J 1973;2:87.
67. Forbes A, Ray LH. Conditions of survival of mammalian nerve trunks. Am J Physiol 1923;64:435.
68. Gooden BA. Why some people do not drown: hypothermia versus the diving responses. Med J Aust 1992;157:629.
69. Luna GK, Maier RV, Pavlin EG, et al. Incidence and effect of hypothermia in seriously injured patients. J Trauma 1987;27:1014.
70. Jurkovich GJ, Greiser WB, Luteman A, et al. Hypothermia in trauma victims: an ominous predictor of survival. J Trauma 1987;27:1019.
71. Swain JA. Hypothermia and blood pH: a review. Arch Intern Med 1988;148:1643.
72. Nicodemus HF, Chaney RD, Herold R. Hemodynamic effects of inotropes during hypothermia and rapid rewarming. Crit Care Med 1981; 9:325.
73. Riishede L, Neilsen KF. Myocardial effects of adrenaline, isoprenaline and dobutamine at hypothermic conditions. Pharmacol Toxicol 1990; 66:354.
74. American Academy of Pediatrics, Committee on Pediatric Aspects of Physical Fitness, Recreation, and Sports. Accidental hypothermia. Pediatrics 1979;63:926.
75. Southwick FS, Dalglish PJ. Recovery after prolonged asystolic cardiac arrest in profound hypothermia: a case report and literature review. JAMA 1980;243:1250.
76. Hauty MG, Esrig BC, Hill JG, Long WB. Prognostic factors in severe accidental hypothermia: experience from the Mt. Hood tragedy. J Trauma 1987;27:1107.
77. Shields CP, Sixsmith DM. Treatment of moderate-to-severe hypothermia in an urban setting. Ann Emerg Med 1984;19:1093.
78. Hayward JS, Eckerson JD, Kemna D. Thermal and cardiovascular changes during three methods of resuscitation from mild hypothermia. Resuscitation 1984;11:102.
79. Webb P. Afterdrop of body temperature during rewarming: an alternative explanation. J Appl Physiol 1986;60:385.
80. Savard GK, Cooper KE, Veale Wl, Malkinson TJ. Peripheral blood flow during rewarming from mild hypothermia in humans. J Appl Physiol 1985;58:4.
81. Lloyd EL. Hypothermia: the cause of death after rescue. Alaska Med 1984;26:74.
82. Nicodemus HF, Chaney RD, Herold R. Hemodynamic effects of inotropes during hypothermia and rapid rewarming. Crit Care Med 1981; 9:325.
83. Zell SC, Kurtz KJ. Hypothermia therapy. Ann Emerg Med 1985;14:1036.
84. Steinman AM. Cardiopulmonary resuscitation and hypothermia. Circulation 1986;74:IV29.
85. Osborne L, Kamal E, Smith JE. Survival after prolonged cardiac arrest and accidental hypothermia. Br Med J (Clin Res Ed) 1984;289:881.
86. Danzl DF, Pozos RS, Auerbach PS, et al. Multicenter hypothermia survey. Ann Emerg Med 1987;16:1042.
87. Robinson M, Seward PN. Environmental hypothermia in children. Pediatr Emerg Care 1986;2:154.
88. Ornato JP. Special resuscitation situations: near drowning, traumatic injury, electric shock, and hypothermia. Circulation 1986;74:IV23.
89. Maningas PA, DeGuzman LR, Hollenbach SJ, et al. Regional blood flow during hypothermic arrest. Ann Emerg Med 1986;15:390.
90. Hector MG. Treatment of accidental hypothermia. Am Fam Physician 1992;45:785.
91. Danzl DF, Sowers MB, Vicario SJ, et al. Chemical ventricular defibrillation in severe accidental hypothermia. Ann Emerg Med 1982;11:698.
92. Kochar G, Kahn SE, Kotler MN. Bretylium tosylate and ventricular fibrillation in hypothermia. Ann Intern Med 1986;105:624.
93. Elenbaas RM, Mattson K, Cole H, et al. Bretylium in hypothermia-induced ventricular fibrillation in dogs. Ann Emerg Med 1984;13:994.
94. Murphy K, Nowak RM, Tomlanovich MC. Use of bretylium tosylate as prophylaxis and treatment in hypothermic ventricular fibrillation in the canine model. Ann Emerg Med 1986;15:1160.
95. Advanced cardiac life support. 2nd ed. Dallas, TX: American Heart Association, 1987.
96. Advanced trauma life support. Committee on Trauma. Chicago: American College of Surgeons, 1989; 66.
97. Nicholson RW, Iserson KV. Core temperature measurement in hypovolemic resuscitation. Ann Emerg Med 1991;20:62.
98. Curry DL, Curry KP. Hypothermia and insulin secretion. Endocrinology 1970;87:750.
99. Myers RA, Britten JS, Cowley RA. Hypothermia: quantitative aspects of therapy. JACEP (Ann Emerg Med) 1979;8:523.
100. Reuler JB. Hypothermia: pathophysiology, clinical settings, and management. Ann Intern Med 1978;89:519.
101. White FN. A comparative physiological approach to hypothermia. J Thorac Cardiovasc Surg 1981;82:821.

102. Ream AK, Reitz BA, Silverberg G. Temperature correction of PCO_2 and pH in estimating acid-base status: an example of the emperor's new clothes? Anesthesiology 1982;56:41.

103. Delaney KA, Howland, MA, Vassallo S, et al. Assessment of acid-base disturbances in hypothermia and their physiologic consequences. Ann Emerg Med 1989;18:72.

104. Marcus P. Laboratory comparison of techniques for rewarming hypothermic casualties. Aviat Space Environ Med 1978;49:692.

105. Hayward JS, Steinman AM. Accidental hypothermia: an experimental study of inhalation rewarming. Aviat Space Environ Med 1976;46:1236.

106. White JD, Bufferfield AB, Greer KA, et al. Comparison of rewarming by radio wave regional hyperthermia and warm humidified inhalation. Aviat Space Environ Med 1984;55:1103.

107. White JD. Hypothermia: the Bellevue experience. Ann Emerg Med 1982;11:417.

108. Wilford DC, Hill EP, Moores WY. Theoretical analysis of oxygen transport and delivery during hypothermia. Physiologist 1982;25:340.

109. Kaplan M, Eidelman AI. Improved prognosis in severely hypothermic newborn infants treated by rapid rewarming. J Pediatr 1984;105:470.

110. Ledingham IM, Mone JC. Treatment of accidental hypothermia. Prospective clinical study. Br Med J 1980;280:1102.

111. Best R, Syverud S, Nowak RM. Trauma and hypothermia. Am J Emerg Med 1985;3:48.

112. Moss JF, Maklin M, Southwick HW, et al. A model for the treatment of accidental severe hypothermia. J Trauma 1986;26:68.

113. Lloyd EL. Accidental hypothermia treated by central rewarming through the airway. Br J Anaesth 1973;45:41.

114. Lloyd EL, Croxton D. Equipment for the provision of airway warming (insulation) in the treatment of accidental hypothermia in patients. Resuscitation 1981;9:61.

115. Leaman PL, Martyak GG. Microwave warming of resuscitation fluids. Ann Emerg Med 1985;14:876-879.

116. Aldrete JA. Preventing hypothermia in trauma patients by microwave warming of I.V. fluids. J Emerg Med 1985;3:435.

117. Flancbaum L, Trooskin SZ, Pedersen H. Evaluation of blood-warming devices with the apparent thermal clearance. Ann Emerg Med 1989;18:355.

118. Jessen K, Hagelsten JO. Peritoneal dialysis in the treatment of profound accidental hypothermia. Aviat Space Environ Med 1978;49:426.

119. Hall KN, Syverud SA. Closed thoracic cavity lavage in the treatment of severe hypothermia in human beings. Ann Emerg Med 1990;19:204.

120. Iversen RJ, Atkin SH, Jaker MA, et al. Successful CPR in a severely hypothermic patient using continuous thoracostomy lavage. Ann Emerg Med 1990;19:1335.

121. Splittgerber FH, Talbert JG, Sweezer WP, Wilson RF. Partial cardiopulmonary bypass for core rewarming in profound accidental hypothermia. Am Surg 1986;52:407.

122. Laub GW, Banaszak D, Kupferschmid J, et al. Percutaneous cardiopulmonary bypass for the treatment of hypothermic circulatory collapse. Ann Thorac Surg 1989;47:608.

123. Kugelberg J, Schuller H, Berg B, et al. Treatment of accidental hypothermia. Scand J Thorac Cardiovasc Surg 1967;1:142.

124. Althaus U, Aerberhard P, Schupbach P, et al. Management of profound accidental hypothermia and cardiorespiratory arrest. Ann Surg 1982;195:492.

125. Towne WD, Geiss WP, Yanes HO, et al. Intractable ventricular fibrillation associated with profound accidental hypothermia: successful treatment with partial cardiopulmonary bypass. N Engl J Med 1972;287:1135.

126. Truscott DG, Firor WB, Clein LJ. Accidental profound hypothermia: successful resuscitation by core rewarming and assisted circulation. Arch Surg 1973;106:216.

127. Hauty MG, Esrig BC, Hill JG, et al. Prognostic factors in severe accidental hypothermia: experience from the Mt. Hood tragedy. J Trauma 1987;27:1107.

128. DaVee TS, Reinberg EJ. Extreme hypothermia and ventricular fibrillation. Ann Emerg Med 1980;9:100.

129. Vretenar DF, Urschel JD, Parrott JC, et al. Cardiopulmonary bypass resuscitation for accidental hypothermia. Ann Thorac Surg 1994;58:895.

130. Nozaki R, Ishibashi K, Adachi N, et al. Accidental profound hypothermia. N Engl J Med 1986;315:1680.

131. Schaller MD, Fisher AP, Perret CH. Hyperkalemia: a prognostic factor during acute severe hypothermia. JAMA 1990;264:1842.

132. Orlowski JP. Drowning, near-drowning, and ice water drowning. JAMA 1988;260:390.

133. Moyer JH, Morris G, DeBakey ME. Hypothermia: effect on renal hemodynamics and on excretion of water and electrolytes in dog and man. Ann Surg 1957;145:26.

134. Segar WE, Riley PA, Barila TG. Urinary composition during hypothermia. Am J Physiol 1956;185:528.

135. Roberts DE, Barr JC, Kerr D, et al. Fluid replacement during hypothermia. Aviat Space Environ Med 1985;56:333.

136. Kanter GS. Hypothermic hemoconcentration. Am J Physiol 1968;214:856.

137. Lloyd EL. The cause of death after rescue. Int J Sports Med 1992;13:S196.

138. Kolodzik PW, Mullin MJ, Krohmer JR, et al. The effects of antishock trouser inflation during hypothermic cardiovacular depression in the canine model. Am J Emerg Med 1988;6:584.

139. Bangs CC. Hypothermia and frostbite. Emerg Med Clin North Am 1984;1:475.

140. Wong KC. Physiology and pharmacology of hypothermia. West J Med 1983;138:227.

141. Fitzgerald FT, Jessop C. Accidental hypothermia: a report of 22 cases and review of the literature. Adv Intern Med 1982;27:127.

142. Clowes GHA, O'Donnell TF. Heatstroke. N Engl J Med 1974;291:564.

143. Khogali M, Hales JRS, eds. Heatstroke and temperature regulation. New York: Academic Press, 1983; 1.

144. Robertshaw D. Contributing factors to heatstroke. In: Khogali M, Hales JRS, eds. Heatstroke and temperature regulation. New York: Academic Press, 1983; 53.

145. Kilbourne EM, Choi K, Jones TS, et al. Risk factors for heatstroke: a case control study. JAMA 1982;247:3332.

146. Curley FJ, Irwin RS. Disorders of temperature control: hyperthermia, part I. J Intensive Care Med 1986;1:5.

147. Bouchama A, al-Sedairy S, Siddiqui S, et al. Elevated pyrogenic cytokines in heatstroke. Chest 1993;104:1498.

148. Beller GA, Boyd AE. Heatstroke: a report of 13 consecutive cases without mortality despite severe hyperpyrexia and neurologic dysfunction. Milit Med 1975;140:464.

149. Knochel JP, Biesel WR, Herndon EG, et al. The renal, cardiovascular, hematologic and serum electrolyte abnormalities of heatstroke. Am J Med 1961;30:299.

150. Gilliland PF, Cirksena WJ, Teschan PE. Renal, metabolic and circulatory responses to heat and exercise. Ann Intern Med 1970;73:213.

151. Hassanein T, Razack A, Gavaler JS, et al. Heatstroke: its clinical and pathological presentation, with particular attention to the liver. Am J Gastroenterol 1992;87:1382.

152. Stefanini M, Spicer DD. Hemostasis breakdown, fibrinolysis, and acquired hemolytic anemia in a patient with fatal heatstroke: pathogenetic mechanisms. Am J Clin Pathol 1971;55:180.

153. Beller GA, Boyd AE. Heatstroke: a report of 13 consecutive cases without mortality despite severe hyperpyrexia and neurologic dysfunction. Milit Med 1975;140:464.

154. Gronert GA. Malignant hyperthermia. Anesthesiology 1980;53:395.

155. Guze GH, Baxter LR. Neuroleptic malignant syndrome. N Engl J Med 1985;313:163.

156. Johnson C, Edleman KJ. Malignant hyperthermia: a review. J Perinatol 1992;12:61.

157. Ball SP, Johnson KJ. The genetics of malignant hyperthermia. J Med Genet 1993;30:89.

158. Caroff S, Rosenburg H, Gerbert JC. Neuroleptic malignant syndrome and malignant hyperthermia. Lancet 1983;1:244.

159. Levitt RC. Prospects for the diagnosis of malignant hyperthermia susceptibility using molecular genetic approaches. Anesthesiology 1992;76:1039.

160. MacLennan DH, Otsu K, Fujii J, et al. The role of the skeletal muscle ryanodine receptor gene in malignant hyperthermia. Symp Soc Exp Biol 1992;46:189.

161. Kosko JR, Brandom BW, Chan KH, et al. Masseter spasm and malignant hyperthermia: a retrospective review of a hospital-based pediatric otolaryngology practice. Int J Pediatr Otorhinolaryngol 1992;23:45.

162. Gronert GA. Malignant hyperthermia. In: Miller RD, ed. Anesthesia. New York: Churchill Livingstone, 1986; 1971-1984.

163. Curley FJ, Irwin RS. Disorders of temperature control: hyperthermia, part II. J Intensive Care Med 1986;1:91.

164. Smego RA, Durack DT. The neuroleptic malignant syndrome. Arch Intern Med 1982;142:1183.

Chapter 38 Metabolic and Nutritional Considerations in Trauma

MICHAEL S. DAHN, M.D., Ph.D.

ROBERT F. WILSON, M.D

INTRODUCTION

Importance of Nutrition

The incidence of malnutrition in hospitalized patients may exceed 25% on admission and 50% during that hospitalization. Such malnutrition is important because it may be associated with a 25% morbidity rate (primarily infections) and a 5% mortality rate.[1]

Although the majority of trauma victims are well nourished prior to hospitalization, the hypermetabolism that is associated with multiple injuries can rapidly lead to severe wasting of lean body mass. Postinjury hypermetabolism leads to malnutrition much more rapidly than simple starvation, and consequently nutritional support is an important part of the management of patients with severe trauma.

History

About 40 years after the discovery of the circulation of blood by William Harvey in 1616, Sir Christopher Wren used a goose quill needle attached to a pig bladder to successfully infuse ale, wine, and opium into the veins of dogs.[2]

In the late 1800s, various forms of intravenous protein administration were attempted, but they often caused severe allergic or febrile reactions.[1] In 1913, Henriques and Anderson claimed they could produce nitrogen balance in dogs by infusing a protein containing nutrient solution intravenously.[3] However, further progress in parenteral alimentation was slow to develop until the mid twentieth century.

Enteral feeding other than by mouth was also very slow in developing. In 1862, Captain H. Bill began rectal installation of wine and beef essence as a standard route of nutrient administration.[4] However, it was not until 1910 that Einhorn introduced "enteral nutrition" via a weighted, rubber duodenal feeding tube. Although they, in 1947, described enteral feeding of protein hydrolysates and glucose via nasogastric and nasojejunal tubes to hypermetabolic postsurgical patients, Reigel et al. failed to achieve nitrogen balance in 67% of their patients.[5]

In the 1930s, Cuthbertson described the hypermetabolic response to injury.[6] In addition to documenting the increased oxygen consumption and protein catabolism following trauma, Cuthbertson also showed that the feeding of injured patients with high-quality protein and adequate calories tended to minimize weight loss, but it did not alter the increased urinary nitrogen excretion associated with major injury.

Elman, in 1937, reported the first true peripheral alimentation of amino acids in humans using hydrolyzed casein.[7] However, intravenous hydrolyzed casein plus glucose could not achieve positive nitrogen balance in severely injured patients.

Finally, in 1951, intravenous fat emulsions became available commercially. These could produce a positive nitrogen balance, but their use was associated with a high incidence of complications including anemia, bleeding, and fat embolism.[8]

The modern era of nutritional support began in 1968 when Dudrick et al. demonstrated that normal growth and development could be accomplished in beagle puppies fed only intravenously using protein hydrolysates and high concentrations (20-25%) of glucose.[9] This led to multiple human trials in which the efficacy of total parenteral nutrition was demonstrated. It was, however, not until 1975 that a safe intravenous lipid preparation (Intralipid) appeared in the United States and balanced intravenous nutrition became possible.

THE METABOLIC RESPONSE TO TRAUMA

Hypermetabolism

AXIOM Clinically, the hypermetabolism of trauma is evidenced by low-grade fever, tachycardia, and tachypnea.

In order to meet the increased tissue demands for oxygen after trauma, the cardiac index is often greater than normal (3.0-3.5 L/min/m^2 in young adult males) and often exceeds 4.5 L/min/m^2. The resultant increases in CO_2 production may require ventilation exceeding 10-15 L/min. (150-250% of normal). Laboratory findings include hyperlactatemia, hyperglycemia, and a urine urea nitrogen (UUN) excretion that may exceed 15 g/day.[1]

The metabolic changes associated with starvation are quite different when compared to severe trauma. Following injury, the increased metabolic energy expenditure (MEE) is reflected by increases in oxygen consumption and CO_2 production; in the starved state, energy expenditure is decreased (Fig. 38–1). In the hypermetabolic state, the respiratory quotient (RQ) ranges 0.80-0.85, reflecting utilization of a mixed fuel source, including carbohydrate, fat, and amino acids (Table 38–1). In the starved state, the RQ tends to approach 0.67-0.70, reflecting the utilization of stored fat as the primary fuel source[1,10] (Table 38–1; Fig. 38–2).

Carbohydrate Metabolism

AXIOM Stress carbohydrate metabolism is characterized by increased glycogenolysis and gluconeogenesis that is poorly suppressed by the exogenous administration of glucose.[1]

Although insulin levels and glucose utilization are increased by stress, the increased glucose production and hyperglycemia seem to be driven largely by an increased glucagon/insulin ratio. Glucose uptake into the cell has variously been found to be depressed (insulin resistance), normal, or increased in the stressed state. Additionally, utilization of glucose by the peripheral tissues tends to be inefficient.[11]

The inefficient use of glucose in trauma may result from a limited capacity of the pyruvate dehydrogenase enzyme complex—which is responsible for the formation of acetyl CoA from pyruvate—and not from a failure of oxidative metabolism (Figure 38–3). This is reflected in the stoichiometric rise in lactate and pyruvate so that the molar ratio of lactate to pyruvate remains < 20:1.[1] The increased lactate is reconverted to glucose via the Cori cycle, with the production of heat and consumption of body energy. In hypovolemic shock, lactate levels rise with relatively little change in pyruvate, producing what Huckabee referred to as "excess lactate."[12]

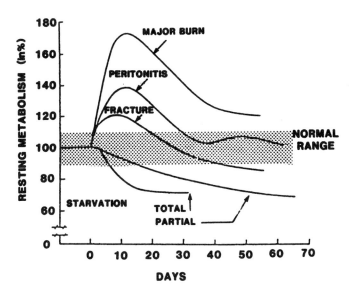

FIGURE 38–1 Percent change from normal of resting metabolism as a function of time in patients with major burns, peritonitis, fractures, and total and partial starvation. (From: Long CL, Schaffel N, Geiger JW, et al. Metabolic response to injury and illness: estimation of energy and protein needs from indirect calorimetry and nitrogen balance. JPEN 1979;3:452.)

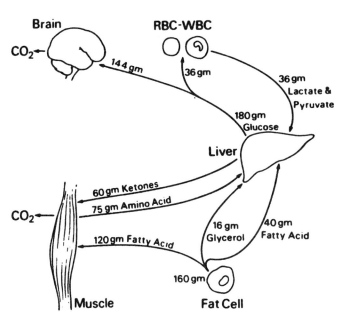

FIGURE 38–2 Substrate distribution in fasting man. (From: Long CL. Carbohydrate metabolic parameters as an assessment of nutritional status. Levenson SM, ed. Nutritional assessment—present status, future directions and prospects. Report of the second Ross Conference on Medical Research. Columbus: Ross Laboratories, 1981; 40).

Hepatic gluconeogenesis normally occurs at a rate of approximately 2.0-2.5 mg/kg/min, but it increases to at least 3.5-5.0 mg/kg/min in the stressed state. This contributes to the requirements of "obligate" glucose-using tissues including brain and, to some degree, kidney, liver, and skeletal muscle. However, the percentage of glucose turnover that is oxidized is relatively constant, ranging 50-55% both in starved and stressed states.

Fat Metabolism

Fat metabolism in both starvation and stress is characterized by increased lipolysis as fat stores are mobilized for energy (Fig. 38–4).

Lipids represent a significant portion of the substrate oxidized for energy in severely injured and septic patients. Serum triglyceride levels rise, and increased activity of "hormone-sensitive lipase" induced by β-adrenergic stimulation causes an accelerated release of free fatty acids (FFA) from fat stores.[13] There is also increased production of very low-density lipoprotein (VLDL) triglycerides by the liver for oxidative metabolism by other tissues.[14] Although hepatic production of ketones may be increased, plasma ketone levels are low.[15]

The turnover of medium- and long-chain fatty acids is also increased. The levels of the various fatty acids in the plasma also change somewhat with oleic acid levels increasing and linoleic and arachidonic acid levels decreasing.[1]

Normally, increased tissue lipoprotein lipase (LPL) activity favors the utilization of triglycerides as oxidative substrates by cardiac and

skeletal muscle.[16] However, during stress, lipid uptake into nonadipose tissue is impaired by tumor necrosis factor-α, interleukin-1-β, and interleukin-2 (factors present during hypermetabolic states) which inhibit the activity of LPL.[16] Clinical studies, however, indicated that the mechanisms resulting in increased availability of fat substrate appear to dominate because fat oxidation is sustained or accelerated in seriously ill patients.[17]

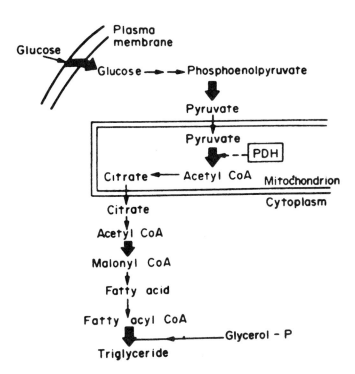

FIGURE 38–3 Outline of nonoxidative metabolism of glucose. (From: Denton RM, Hughes WA. Pyruvate dehydrogenase and the hormonal regulation of fat synthesis in mammalian tissues. Int J Biochem 1978;9:545).

TABLE 38–1 *Respiratory Quotients and Caloric Yield from the Oxidation of Various Substrate Forms*

(1) 1 Glucose + 6 O_2 → 6 CO_2 + 6 H_2O + 673 kcal (RQ = 1.0)
(2) 1 Palmitate + 23 O_2 → 16 CO_2 + 16 H_2O + 2398 kcal (RQ = 0.70)
(3) 1 AA + 5.1 O_2 → 4.1 CO_2 + 0.7 urea + 2.8 H_2O + 475 kcal
  (RQ = 0.80)
(4) 4.5 Glucose + 4.0$_2$ → 1 Palmityl + 11 CO_2 + 11 H_2O + 630 kcal
  (RQ = 2.75)

Flatt J. Energetics of intermediary metabolism. In Assessment of energy metabolism in health and disease. (First Ross Conference of Medical Research). Columbus: Ross Laboratories, 1980.

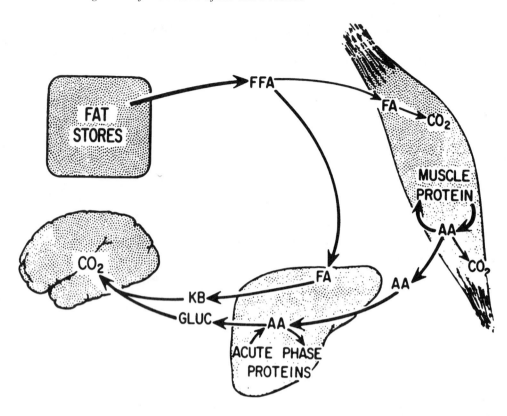

FIGURE 38–4 Metabolic response to injury. The interrelationships of fat, muscle, and liver in meeting energy requirements (FFA = free fatty acids; AA = amino acids; KB = ketone bodies; GLUC = glucose). (From: Blackburn GL, Bistrian BR, Homsy FN. Protein metabolism in the surgical patient. Kirkpatrick JR, ed. Nutrition and metabolism in the surgical patient. Mount Kisco, New York, Futura 1983; 67.)

Nitrogen Metabolism

ACCELERATED NITROGEN LOSS

AXIOM Accelerated hepatic urea formation and urine urea nitrogen (UUN) loss, which may exceed 15 g/day, is a prominent feature of the hypermetabolic response to severe injury and sepsis.

The nitrogen for the increased UUN losses after trauma comes from accelerated total body protein catabolism, particularly of skeletal muscle, connective tissue, and unstimulated gut (Fig. 38–5). Although this catabolism results in increased availability of amino acid substrates for various metabolic processes, there is also marked depletion of lean body mass.

The increased rate of proteolysis appears to be related to the magnitude of trauma. Amino acids coming from this increased proteoly-

sis are liberated primarily from skeletal muscle. They may be utilized for synthesis of new protein or may be degraded by hepatic gluconeogenesis and used for tissue oxidative processes. The use of amino acids as oxidative substrate is particularly increased in skeletal muscle, which prefers utilization of the essential branched-chain amino acids leucine, isoleucine, and valine.

AXIOM UUN losses are usually < 5 g/day in nonstressed starvation but exceed 15 g/day in severe stress.

In contradistinction to starvation, excessive protein catabolism seen after injury is not suppressed by exogenous administration of amino acids or by the administration of other fuel sources, such as fat or glucose.

The increased MEE of trauma usually peaks after 3–5 days and then gradually returns to baseline when convalescence is uncompli-

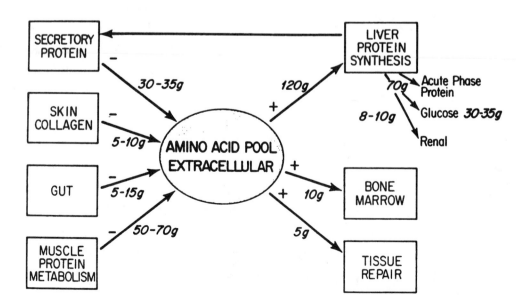

FIGURE 38–5 Functional redistribution of body cell mass after injury provides nitrogen for protein synthesis. Arrows reflect the net release (−) from collagen, gut, and muscle, as well as the uptake (+) of amino acids into tissues whose net anabolism is associated with survival. The conversion of protein to glucose and urea is a trivial source of energy, but is an important role of the liver to produce heat necessary to maintain core temperature. (From: Blackburn GL, Bistrian BR, Homsy FN. Protein metabolism in the surgical patient. Kirkpatrick JR, ed. Nutrition and metabolism in the surgical patient. Mount Kisco, New York, Futura 1983; 60).

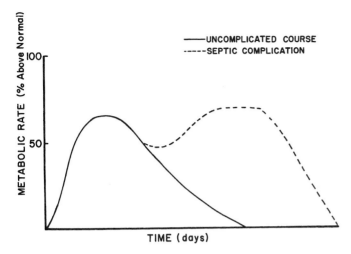

FIGURE 38–6 The metabolic rate typically rises following trauma reaching a peak 3-5 days following the acute event. Thereafter, hypermetabolism gradually subsides when convalescence is uneventful. Persistent or recurrent hypermetabolic episodes develop most commonly when a septic complication occurs.

TABLE 38–2 *Metabolic Changes with Starvation and Stress Hypermetabolism*

	Starvation	*Stress Hypermetabolism*
Resting energy expenditure	–	+ +
Primary fuels	Fat	Mixed
Proteolysis	+	+ + +
Respiratory quotient	Low (0.67)	High (0.85)
Gluconeogenesis	+ +	+ + + +
BCAA	+	+ + +
Urinary nitrogen loss	+	+ + +
Ketone body production	+ + + +	+

cated (Fig. 38–6). The magnitude of this increase in metabolic rate is directly related to the severity of trauma, with the greatest elevations occurring in patients with severe burns. Alterations in urea nitrogen excretion usually tend to parallel changes in MEE.

ACCELERATED PROTEIN TURNOVER

One of the major effects of trauma and sepsis is the stimulation of whole-body protein turnover[18] (Table 38–2). Skeletal muscle proteolysis occurs and significant amounts of the liberated branched-chain amino acids (leucine, isoleucine, and valine) are oxidized as a fuel source (Fig. 38–7). Alanine and glutamine production are increased, and they serve as substrate for accelerated glucose production during stress. Although protein synthesis (anabolism) is also stimulated, it does not keep pace with the rate of protein breakdown (catabolism). As a result, progressively negative nitrogen balance occurs as the severity of stress increases (Fig. 38–8).

One benefit of the increased protein turnover is a greater amino acid availability for hepatic synthesis of acute-phase proteins.[19] This appears to be crucial for host survival during severe stress and sepsis. These liver-derived acute phase proteins include fibrinogen, haptoglobin, ceruloplasmin, C-reactive protein, α-1 acid glycoprotein, and some complement components. These substances plus other opsonic factors and antiproteases serve a vital role by: (a) stimulating reticuloendothelial function, (b) preventing an unimpeded inflammatory response, and (c) providing other incompletely defined survival mechanisms for the body. Because skeletal muscle proteolysis results in tissue protein depletion at the same time that it permits proper evolution of the acute phase response, increased posttraumatic protein turnover may be viewed as a double-edged sword.

AXIOM Although protein breakdown in stress increases the availability of amino acids for visceral protein synthesis, the associated excess nitrogen loss is detrimental.

Wound Healing

Meyer et al. noted that wound healing involves a series of complex physicochemical interactions that require specific micronutrients at every step.[20] Consequently, in critically ill or severely injured patients, wound healing is frequently impaired by the associated protein-catabolic, hypermetabolic response to stress. The hypothalamus responds to cytokine stimulation by increasing the thermoregulatory set-point and by augmenting elaboration of stress hormones (catecholamines, cortisol, and glucagon). In turn, the stress hormones induce futile thermogenic substrate cycling, lipolysis, and proteolysis. This results in increased skeletal muscle degradation to produce amino acid substrates for hepatic gluconeogenesis.

FACTORS RESPONSIBLE FOR METABOLIC CHANGES IN TRAUMA AND SEPSIS

The major identifiable factors that appear to orchestrate hypercatabolic events following trauma include: (a) metabolic demands in the traumatic wound, (b) the interplay between various counterregulatory hormones (especially catecholamines, glucagon, and cortisol), and (c) the effect of cytokines (Fig. 38–9).

Metabolic Demands of the Traumatic Wound

Trauma wounds, especially large burns, can directly increase total body metabolic by stimulating regional blood flow and the rate of glucose consumption.[21] Healing tissue exhibits an apparent preference for glycolytic metabolic activity. This can contribute significantly to the total body glucose turnover, especially since glycolysis is a much less efficient energy source than complete glucose oxidation. Additionally, lactate, which is the major end-product of glycolytic metabolism, requires disposal, and this is done primarily through its reconversion to glucose in the liver. The resulting accelerated lactate recycling also increases energy requirements.[22]

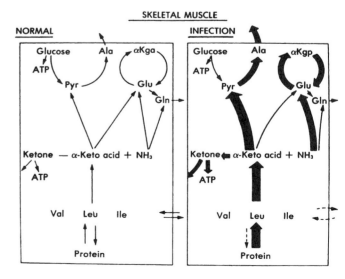

FIGURE 38–7 The role of BCAAs in response to infection. Increased formation of alanine, glutamate, and α-ketoglutarate occurs. (From: Bonau RA, Daly JM. Surgical nutrition. Miller TA, Rowlands BJ, eds. Physiologic basis of modern surgical care. St. Louis: CV Mosby Company, 1988; 66).

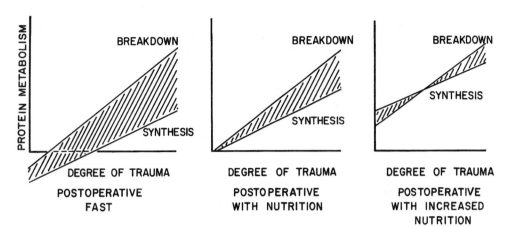

FIGURE 38–8 Net protein metabolism (shaded area) may be schematically represented by the relative balance between whole-body protein synthesis and degradation under deprivational and fed states. Both synthesis and degradation tend to rise in relation to the degree of injury. Under fasting conditions, protein breakdown exceeds synthesis resulting in a negative nitrogen balance. Nutrient administration can overcome this unfavorable state primarily by driving protein synthesis to higher levels. (From: Clague MB, Keir MJ, Wright PD, et al. The effects of nutrition and trauma on whole-body protein metabolism in man. Clin Sci 1983;65:165).

Stress Endocrine Response

> **AXIOM** Following trauma, increased activity of the hypothalamus and sympathetic nervous system result in increased release of ACTH, catecholamines, and glucagon.

Following trauma, multiple stimuli, including changes in arterial and venous pressure and volume, osmolality, pH, arterial oxygen content, pain, anxiety, and toxic mediators from tissue injury reach the hypothalamus. These stimuli are integrated and relayed to the sympathetic nervous system and adrenal medulla. Simultaneously, the pituitary initiates the hormonal response characteristic of the metabolic response to injury. ACTH is released from the anterior pituitary into the systemic circulation in response to corticotropin-releasing factor (CRF), and stimulates the production of cortisol by the adrenal cortex. Vasopressin from the posterior pituitary acts directly on the renal tubule to promote free-water retention. Aldosterone, released from the adrenal cortex, promotes sodium resorption in the renal tubule. The net effect of these "primary stress hormones" is to mobilize energy reserves and to promote the retention of salt and water to support the intravascular volume and central circulation.

Energy availability to the tissues can be viewed in terms of the balance between the effects of insulin, the major storage or anabolic hormone, and the effects of "counter regulatory hormones," glucagon, cortisol, and catecholamines. Insulin lowers blood glucose levels primarily by its effects on the membrane transport and intracellular metabolism of glucose in the peripheral tissues, such as skeletal muscle and fat.[1] Additionally, insulin plays a central regulatory role in tending to cause increased protein synthesis and formation of fat and control of lipogenesis, the net effect being to promote the storage of ingested fuels.

The counter regulatory hormones oppose the effects of insulin.[23] They mobilize energy reserves and elevate blood glucose levels, but at the expense of accelerated body catabolism. Glucagon is released from the α-2 cells of the islets of Langerhans in response to hypoglycemia and to β-adrenergic stimulation. It acts primarily in the liver to promote gluconeogenesis and to enhance hepatic amino acid extraction. Glucagon also acts in concert with cortisol to increase protein catabolism to increase available gluconeogenic substrate or for direct oxidative utilization. Cortisol, by promoting hepatic gluconeogenesis, contributes in large part to the hyperglycemia and apparent "insulin resistance" observed in patients with critical illness.[19] Catecholamines elevate blood glucose levels by stimulating gluconeogenesis and glycogenolysis. Epinephrine, probably through its β-adrenergic agonist properties, also accounts for some of the reduced peripheral tissue responsiveness to insulin after trauma.[24]

Epinephrine, glucagon, and growth hormone may also be involved with accelerated lipolysis associated with stress.[25,26] This occurs despite the presence of hyperinsulinemia (which normally inhibits fat mobilization and oxidation) during intravenous glucose infusion. The triglycerides from mobilized fat are rapidly broken down to glycerol and free fatty acids, which serve as primary fuel sources.

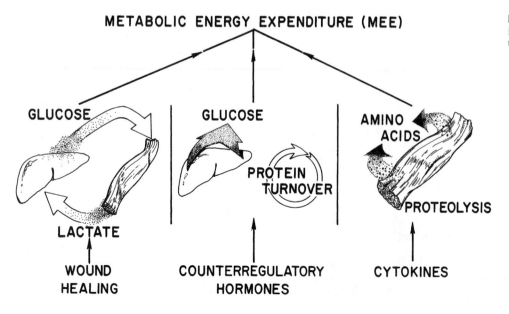

FIGURE 38–9 Factors that contribute to increased metabolic demand following trauma.

TABLE 38–3 Triple Hormone (Cortisol, Glucagon, Epinephrine) Effects on Normal Volunteers

Clinical Data	
Temp	↑
HR	↑
Systolic BP	↑
Laboratory Data	
Glucose levels	↑
Insulin levels	↑
Indirect Calorimetry	
Min vent	↑
VO$_2$	↑
VCO$_2$	↑
MEE	↑
RQ	NC↓
Urine	
Urea N$_2$	↑
N$_2$ bal	↓

One of the most interesting early observations concerning the stress-related actions of the three counterregulatory hormones is their collective effects on hepatic glucose production (Table 38–3). Individually, these three hormones induce only mild- and short-lived elevations in blood glucose levels and hepatic glucose production; however, the simultaneous infusion of epinephrine, glucagon, and cortisol effects a sustained synergistic response which is two- to fourfold greater than the sum of their individual effects.[27] Furthermore, studies showed that numerous other characteristics of the injury response (including increased energy expenditure, ureogenesis, and whole-body protein turnover) can be stimulated in normal volunteers by this triple hormone infusion.[23] This hormone combination also increases total hepatic protein synthesis in experimental models in a manner very similar to that seen following clinical trauma and sepsis. These experimental observations are consistent with clinical findings of accelerated visceral amino acid clearance following injury and sepsis.[28]

AXIOM The increased secretion of counter-regulatory hormones is an important cause of posttraumatic hypermetabolism.

Despite the compelling findings on the role of the counterregulatory hormones in stress, this concept has not gone without some challenges. Although the increased metabolic rate of trauma and sepsis occurs coincident with the protein catabolic response, the counterregulatory hormone elevation occurs out of phase with these changes.[29] The concentrations of stress hormones are highest within 36 hours of injury, and they may be only mildly elevated during the peak metabolic response which may occur several days later. Additionally, the elevation in metabolic rate, which results from the administration of these catabolic hormones, to normal volunteers is generally small (only 10-20% above basal levels) and cannot achieve the markedly elevated levels observed in many critically ill patients. Finally, triple-hormone infusions cannot fully reproduce the metabolic response to injury and sepsis, which includes leukocytosis, fever, and increased hepatic synthesis of acute-phase proteins.[30,31] Because of these concerns, numerous studies have focused increasing attention upon the contribution that cytokines may play in the overall stress response.

AXIOM It is generally believed that the postinjury and septic catabolic response is due largely to the combined influences of stress hormones and cytokines.

Cytokines

The cytokines are a group of proteins secreted primarily by cells of the immune system (i.e., lymphocytes, macrophages, and reticuloen-

dothelial cells). They are believed to serve a local cell-to-cell (paracrine) and perhaps even cell-to-same-cell (autocrine) signaling function within various tissues. However, the cytokines may also exert systemic effects by escaping their local environment into the systemic circulation or by altering organ function enough to cause a whole body effect. These mediator responses are believed to act in conjunction with an altered nutrient intake to determine the metabolic response of the host. Additionally, some of the numerous cytokines released can also cause changes in metabolism by influencing blood levels of insulin, glucagon, and corticosteroids.[32]

Of the numerous cytokines that are produced in increased quantities under stress conditions, interleukin-1 (IL-1), tumor necrosis factor-α (TNFα), and interleukin-6 (IL-6) are considered to be the most important modulators of intermediary metabolism and metabolic rate[32] (Table 38–4). The role of these protein mediators is considered to be greatest during inflammatory or infectious conditions. However, because the inflammatory response may be present to varying degrees, even in the absence of bacteria,[33] these factors should also play a major role in trauma. Furthermore, as may be expected in any new scientific field, some of the early work done with "purified" monokine preparations has been contradicted by the effects of newer recombinant forms of IL-1 and TNFα, and the literature remains somewhat clouded as to the specific metabolic functions of these monokines.

INTERLEUKIN-1

The mobilization of amino acids from skeletal muscle to support increased visceral protein production during stress has been attributed to transmissible plasma factors with IL-1-like activity in the blood.[34] It has been concluded that either IL-1 or an active fragment of IL-1, derived from macrophages activated by sepsis or trauma, can cause skeletal muscle proteolysis by stimulating prostaglandin E$_2$ production. This sequence of events results in increased amino acid loss by peripheral tissues[35] and can account for at least part of the increased liver protein production on the basis of: (a) increased amino acid substrate delivery to the liver, and (b) direct IL-1 stimulation of acute-phase protein gene transcription.[36,37]

Recombinant IL-1 appears to have a synergistic effect with TNF to induce skeletal muscle proteolysis which may be further modu-

TABLE 38–4 Overlapping Roles of Leukocytic Cytokines in the Regulation of Metabolism

Parameter	Response	Cytokines Responsible
General		
Voluntary food intake	↓	IL-1, TNFα
Resting energy expenditure	↑	IL-1, TNFα
Body temperature	↑	IL-1, TNFα, IFN
Glucose metabolism		
Glucose oxidation	↑	IL-1, TNFα
Gluconeogenesis	↑	IL-1
Lipid metabolism		
Lipoprotein lipase activity	↓	IL-1, TNFα, IFN
Adipocyte fatty acid synthesis	↑	TNFα, TNFβ, IFN
Lipolysis in adipocytes	↑	IL-1, TNFα
Protein metabolism		
Hepatic synthesis of acute phase proteins	↑	IL-1, TNFα, IL-6
Skeletal muscle protein degradation	↑	IL-1
Hormone release		
Corticosteroid	↑	IL-1, IL-6
Thyroxin	↓	IL-1
Glucagon	↑	IL-1, TNFα
Insulin	↑	IL-1

Abbreviations: IL-1: interleukin-1, TNFα: tumor necrosis factor, IL-6: interleukin-6, IFN: interferon

lated due to the ability of IL-1β to increase both insulin and glucagon levels; however, *in vitro* recombinant IL-1 by itself does not appear to produce the muscle proteolysis that occurred with earlier preparations of "purified" IL-1. This has suggested that the latter studies may reflect impure preparations or in vivo recruitment of additional endogenous factors which may affect proteolysis.[38]

IL-1 also appears to play a significant role in stress carbohydrate metabolism. In addition to increasing plasma insulin and glucagon levels, it also appears to elevate plasma glucocorticoids via stimulation of pituitary ACTH release, thus creating a hormonal milieu favoring gluconeogenesis.[39]

Less is known about the effect of monokines on stress lipid metabolism; however, TNFα,[40] IL-1β,[41] and IL-2[37] appear to inhibit the activity of lipoprotein lipase. IL-2 appears to activate lipolysis by decreasing the α-adrenergic inhibition of hormone-sensitive lipase.[42]

TUMOR NECROSIS FACTOR

A number of experimental studies have shown that the typical endocrine and metabolic response patterns seen in injury and sepsis can be reproduced by parenteral administration of IL-1 or TNFα (Table 38–4). The temporal evolution of the ensuing stress response is identical to the response seen with endotoxin,[37,43,44] indicating that these cytokines may be primary mediators of the septic/inflammatory response. Additionally, some of the metabolic responses to bacterial endotoxin and TNF, such as stress hormone elevation and increased total body oxygen consumption, can be attenuated by pharmacologic levels of cyclooxygenase inhibitors, reaffirming the possible role of prostaglandins.[45,46]

These findings strongly indicate that the cytokines, TNF in particular, may be important mediators of the hypermetabolic response of stress. It remains unclear, however, whether these factors are the direct regulators of these processes for several reasons: (a) plasma levels of these cytokines are frequently very low or undetectable in sustained clinical sepsis, even when the patients are hypermetabolic, (b) *in vitro* studies show that purified recombinant preparations of IL-1 and TNF have minimal direct effects on skeletal muscle protein turnover, hepatocellular carbohydrate metabolism, and hepatic secretory protein synthesis.[47]

In a recently reported study by Bagby et al., rats were pretreated with a neutralizing goat anti-TNF IgG antibody prior to intravenous lipopolysaccharide (LPS) or subcutaneous live Escherichia coli administration.[48] Pretreatment with anti-TNF attenuated the increase in plasma lactate and glucagon levels, but failed to ameliorate the LPS-induced hyperglycemia. The LPS-stimulated increase of *in vivo* glucose metabolic rate was not altered by anti-TNF. The rats treated with anti-TNF prior to induction of hypermetabolic infection also exhibited the usual increases in whole-body glucose appearance rate and metabolism. These results indicate that the alterations in glucose metabolism that occur in response to LPS are largely independent of endogenous TNF. However, this study does not eliminate the possibility that TNF is at least partially responsible for the increased glucose utilization in selected cells during infectionlike states.

It increasingly appears that additional cytokines may be produced at the same time as IL-1 and TNF during inflammation and that these as yet unidentified factors may be responsible for some of the observed metabolic effects.[49] Nevertheless, despite this confusing array of experimental findings, IL-1 and TNF are currently viewed as important contributors to inflammatory processes, possibly as early initiators of a cascade of secondary mediators.

INTERLEUKIN-6

Interleukin-6, in conjunction with IL-1 and the corticosteroids, appears to function somewhat differently than IL-1 and TNF. It clearly exhibits a direct stimulatory effect upon hepatocyte secretory protein synthesis. It has also been shown the combination of these three mediators (i.e., IL-6, IL-1, corticosterone) reproducibly stimulate vigorous hepatic acute-phase protein production.[50]

IL-6 is induced by TNF and peaks after the TNF maximal response. TNF is frequently difficult to detect in acute illness but IL-6

tends to be sustained and has been suggested as a prognostic indicator.[51] Although some reports indicate that high levels are associated with complicated clinical courses and increased likelihood of mortality, its prognostic utility is not accepted completely.[52]

AXIOM Although some metabolic effects attributable to cytokines may require additional factors, the acute-phase protein response appears to be largely due to the direct effects of IL-6 (formerly known as hepatocyte stimulating factor).

OTHER INTERLEUKINS

Host-derived cytokines (IL-1, TNF) and endogenous chemotactic factors (e.g., leukotriene B_4) can elicit the formation of IL-8 at a local injury site by mononuclear leukocytes, noninflammatory cells, and neutrophils. IL-8 is a chemotactic cytokine or chemokine that can sustain or amplify an inflammatory response through continued neutrophil recruitment and activation. Conversely, IL-4 and IL-10, which are expressed by lymphocytes, appear to regulate these cytokine interactions by exerting suppressive efforts on IL-6, IL-8, TNF, and IL-1. Thus, both positive and negative interactions are found in the cytokine network.[53]

INTERRUPTING THE CYTOKINE CASCADE

Experimental studies indicate that both IL-1 and TNF exert beneficial influences on host immune function when present in limited quantities. However, when produced in excess they are associated with physiologic responses that may be detrimental to the host. As mentioned earlier, exogenous administration of TNF may reproduce many of the physiologic and metabolic responses associated with septic shock. As a result, strategies for altering the cytokine cascade have been developed in order to minimize the noxious effects of these cytokines.

The overall approach can be arbitrarily divided into two modalities. First, because septic shock most commonly is precipitated by gram-negative infections with an associated endotoxin or lipopolysaccharide stimulation of cytokine production, neutralization of lipopolysaccharide would theoretically abrogate this process. Experimental studies utilizing monospecific antibody directed against lipopolysaccharide (or its active component Lipid A) successfully protected the host against lethal endotoxemia. Unfortunately, clinical studies utilizing monoclonal antibodies directed against endotoxin have not yielded similar results.[54] An alternate approach, which is currently under investigation, utilizes bactericidal/permeability increasing protein (BPI), which is a naturally occurring plasma protein with potent antimicrobial activity when directed against gram-negative bacteria *in vitro*.[55] BPI has the capacity to neutralize endotoxin by virtue of a high-affinity binding domain for endotoxin that antagonizes the association between LPS and another naturally occurring plasma protein, lipopolysaccharide binding protein (LBP). LBP-associated endotoxin (i.e., LPS) can stimulate the formation of endogenous TNF to a much greater extent than unbound lipopolysaccharide. Displacement of LBP by BPI attenuates the ability of LPS to stimulate cytokine formation dramatically. Thus, the parenteral administration of recombinant bactericidal permeability increasing protein may serve as an effective mechanism to attenuate the cytokine response during gram-negative sepsis.

A second approach that has undergone extensive investigation is the utilization of anticytokine therapy. The major advantage of this approach is that it is independent of the initiating factor (gram-negative or gram-positive infection) because cytokines are elaborated under a variety of clinical circumstances. Antiinterleukin-1 therapy involves the administration of pharmacologic levels of a naturally occurring protein, interleukin-1 receptor antagonist (IL-1ra) which interferes with ligand (IL-1) binding. Although experimental studies using this agent have shown improved physiologic responses following endotoxin challenges (improvement in blood pressure, decreased mortality) clinical trials have yielded only marginal benefit.[56] Anti-TNF strategies used monoclonal antibody directed against tumor necrosis factor resulting in its neutralization. A second more novel approach takes advantage of the observation that TNF receptors are shed from cellular surfaces during the course of sepsis/inflammation. When these receptors are administered in increased quantities they also have the capacity to neutralize endogenous TNF. This latter approach has not reached clinical trials at this stage. Monoclonal antibody directed against TNF has undergone extensive clinical evaluation; however, no substantial increase in survival in critically ill septic patients has been documented.[56]

The clinical results associated with anticytokine therapies have been disappointing and the reasons for their less-than-expected results remain unclear. Nevertheless, it is likely that studies in this area will continue and will include efforts at earlier administration of these agents, as well as use of combination preparations directed against multiple cytokines simultaneously.

Growth Factors

Research at the cellular and molecular levels has identified and characterized several families of growth factors including colony-stimulating factors (CSF), platelet-derived growth factors (PDGF), epidermal growth factors (EGF), insulinlike growth factors (IGF; e.g., somatomedin-C), heparin binding growth factor (HB-GF), and transforming growth factors (TGF). These factors regulate cell growth and division and are involved in the metabolic and cellular response to injury.[57-59]

GENERAL MANAGEMENT CONSIDERATIONS TO IMPROVE METABOLISM IN CRITICALLY ILL PATIENTS

The current basis for the prevention and treatment of multiple organ failure following trauma includes source control, restoration of oxygen transport, and adequate nutritional support.[1]

Source Control

Tissue directed procedures include measures to surgically control infected wounds, reduce and fixate fractures, and close large, open wounds.

AXIOM Evidence of persistent hypermetabolism or acute organ failure should stimulate a diligent search for an uncontrolled focus of infection or inflamed or necrotic tissue.

It is increasingly clear that large, open wounds or septic foci may serve as ongoing stimuli of the systemic inflammatory response.[59]

This, in turn, is usually accompanied by a hypermetabolic response pattern with increased oxygen consumption and hyperdynamic circulation. After major surgery, this is a normal, appropriate response pattern and usually is self-limited. However, persistence of this response may be a forerunner to increasing organ dysfunction. The likelihood of this progression would be minimized if necrotic or septic foci were controlled by early, appropriate debridement and antibiotic therapy.

Oxygen Transport

The generalized response to shock and major injury is directed at support of the central circulation. Unfortunately, this acute response occurs at the expense of perfusion in the "less vital" vascular beds, such as those in the skin, skeletal muscle, and splanchnic circulation; however, these organs are a major source of toxic inflammatory mediators responsible for stress hypermetabolism. Additionally, hypoperfusion of the gut may play a major role in translocation of bacteria and bacterial products into the blood stream or lymphatics.

AXIOM Following major trauma, tissue perfusion and oxygen transport should probably be maintained at levels 25–50% greater than normal.

It is now clear that tissue hypoxia can dramatically magnify the hypermetabolic response to injury. Experimental studies showed that a localized inflammatory focus, which would normally be self-limited, can be converted to a systemic process and organ failure when superimposed transient hypoxia occurs.[33] Additionally, altered body metabolism due to hypoxic or ischemic organs[59,60] can have a tremendous impact upon the host because metabolites that are normally modified or eliminated by those organs may now accumulate.

The body has little or no capacity to store oxygen; therefore, oxygen consumption is believed to reflect oxygen demand as long as the oxygen supply is adequate. This assumption has resulted in the concept of flow-dependent oxygen consumption (Figure 38–10), which has been described in a number of clinical situations, including sepsis and septic shock.[61] At lower levels of oxygen delivery, oxygen consumption appears to be flow dependent; in other words, oxygen consumption increases as oxygen delivery increases. At some higher level of oxygen delivery, however, oxygen consumption no longer increases with increased delivery and is therefore considered to be flow independent. It is only at that point that oxygen transport can be assumed to be adequate.

FIGURE 38–10 Oxygen consumption as a function of oxygen delivery for normal (solid line) and hypermetabolic (dotted line) patients. Note that oxygen delivery must be increased considerably before flow-independent oxygen consumption is attained in hypermetabolic patients. (Adapted from: Dahn MS. Visceral organ resuscitation, perspective in critical care, 1991;4:1-41.)

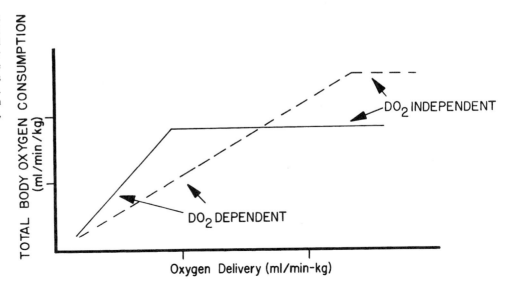

AXIOM Assuring the adequacy of tissue oxygen delivery is an important early part of the overall metabolic support of critically ill or injured patients.

Oxygen delivery (DO_2) is defined as the product of cardiac output (Q) and arterial oxygen content (CaO_2).

$$DO_2 = Q(L/min) \times CaO_2 \ (mL/dL) \times 10$$

Oxygen consumption (VO_2) is defined as the product of cardiac output and arterial-venous O_2 content difference [$C(a-v)O_2$].

$$VO_2 = Q(L/min) \times [C(a-v) \ O_2] \times 10$$

Maintaining an optimal oxygen delivery may require maintaining a cardiac output up to 50% greater than normal, hematocrit of at least 30-35%, and arterial oxygen saturation above 90%. The adequacy of oxygen delivery can be determined to some extent by serial observations of mixed venous oxygen saturation, plasma lactate levels, and acetoacetate/β-hydroxybutyrate ratios. However, the response to increased oxygen delivery may be most important. When raising DO_2 causes no further increase in VO_2, the VO_2 is said to be transport-independent, and the VO_2 is assumed to be at an optimal level.

When transport-dependent oxygen consumption is seen, it implies that the total body oxygen consumption may be suboptimal and that occult areas of anaerobic tissue metabolism may exist. Transport dependence also suggests that such tissue regions may be converted from lactate producers to optimally functioning oxygen-consuming areas only when higher levels of oxygen delivery are provided. Recently, the issue of transport dependency has become controversial for at least two reasons. First, the demonstration of an increase in oxygen consumption following augmentation of oxygen transport may occasionally be accounted for by the algebraic relationship between VO_2 and DO_2. Because these variables share the cardiac output term in their expressions, an artifactual "coupling" may arise suggesting a transport dependency when none exists. This problem may be avoided if oxygen consumption is determined by an independent technique, such as indirect calorimetry. Second, evidence exists that efforts to augment systemic oxygen delivery may fail to improve outcome in critically ill patients.[62] Nevertheless, in view of the seriousness of hypoxia-induced exacerbation of the hypermetabolic syndrome, it would seem wise to avoid oxygen-transport-dependent states.

AXIOM The simplest method for detecting and correcting transport-dependent oxygen consumption is by progressively increasing oxygen transport until total body oxygen consumption (preferably determined by indirect calorimetry) no longer rises.

A correlate of oxygen consumption is lactate production, which has an inverse relationship to cardiac output. Lactate production is considered to be flow independent only when further increases in cardiac output do not produce a decrease in plasma lactate.[1] When using lactate as a measure of the adequacy of the oxygen delivery, it should be remembered that obesity, sepsis, and hepatic insufficiency can cause small elevations in lactate (range: 2.0-3.0 mmol/L) which may be physiologic. When oxygen delivery is inadequate, lactate rises disproportionately to pyruvate. In patients with hemodynamically-compensated sepsis or underlying liver disease, lactate may be elevated, but the lactate/pyruvate ratio is still < 20. This implies that the pyruvate dehydrogenase enzyme complex, rather than insufficient oxygen for aerobic metabolism, is the limiting step in the oxidation of substrate.[1]

Some authors have espoused the use of supernormal hemodynamic criteria as appropriate endpoints for the resuscitation of critically ill patients.[63,64] Although it is clear that survivors of critical illness often require increased levels of oxygen delivery and consumption, serial determinations, rather that fixed goals, may be more appropriate.

Energy Requirements

STRESS STRATIFICATION

The key to successful nutritional support for critically ill or injured patients is an understanding of the altered metabolism characteristic of stress states. Because of the extreme variability of the response between patients, and the dynamic nature of the metabolic response over time within a given patient, it can be helpful to develop a system for categorizing the degree of metabolic changes present.

The severity of the hypermetabolic response is not well predicted from the clinical setting or from various injury severity scores. The use of objective variables that more directly reflect the metabolic response to injury and critical illness include oxygen consumption, urinary nitrogen excretion, blood glucose, and plasma lactate.[1] It is essential to recognize the variability and continuum of metabolic response to stress so that various nutritional formulas can be appropriately modified for the condition of the patient, particularly in relation to nonprotein calories, quantity of protein or amino acids, and nonprotein-calorie-to-nitrogen ratio.

IMPORTANCE OF DETERMINING CALORIC NEEDS

AXIOM The increased caloric energy expenditure occurring after trauma must be provided from external sources in order to minimize the use of endogenous structural and functional protein for cellular fuel.

Because endogenous amino acids can be easily oxidized to serve as an energy source, the goal of nutrient therapy should be to offset this wasteful process by providing sufficient nonprotein calories to keep endogenous protein breakdown to a minimum. Thus, considerable effort has been expended toward the determination or prediction of energy expenditure (EE) in critically ill and injured patients.

The need to determine energy requirements is greatest in patients who are expected to have a protracted recovery from trauma. The previously well-nourished patient who has a brief, uncomplicated acute illness can tolerate short periods of limited nutrient intake with little difficulty. However, patients with severe burns, patients who develop postoperative infections, and patients who are persistently hypermetabolic all require increased caloric and other nutrient support for a prolonged period to avoid rapid loss of body cell mass.

Jeevanandam et al. noted the increasing recognition of the metabolic consequences of excessive nutritional support.[65] They also observed that time-dependent optimal nutritional support is desired for an early and uncomplicated recovery after severe injury or illness. To help provide data for these concepts, the metabolic effects of adding balanced amino acids to glucose infusions during total parenteral nutrition were investigated in 18 patients after major trauma (injury severity score: 35 ± 2). Two studies were conducted on each subject, one about 40-60 hours postinjury in the basal state without any dietary intake and then after four to six days of intravenous nutrition provided solely as glucose (24 ± 2 kcal/kg/day, 80% resting energy expenditure, n = 8) or isocaloric glucose (28 ± 2 kcal/kg/day) with amino acids (275 ± 28 mg of nitrogen/kg/day, n = 10). Whole-body fuel substrate kinetics were studied for energy metabolism (indirect calorimetry), protein kinetics, and lipid mobilization.

Their data indicated that injury-induced hypoaminoacidemia was equally modulated whether the glucose-based nutrition had amino acids or not, and the negative nitrogen balance was reduced similarly in both groups.[65] The protein breakdown rate was significantly (P = .025) decreased in both groups, but it was greater (30% vs 18%) in the patients receiving total parenteral nutrition. Thus, intravenous nutrition did not stimulate protein synthesis. Whole-body lipolysis rate and net fat oxidation rate were suppressed more when glucose alone was given; this also resulted in less reesterification. Thus, provision of intravenous glucose alone, not to exceed the resting energy expenditure, seemed to be superior to isocaloric glucose with amino acids during this early catabolic flow phase of injury because the injured body could not assimilate the exogenous amino acid.

METHODS FOR DETERMINING ENERGY EXPENDITURE

Determination or prediction of resting energy expenditure (REE) has generally been accomplished by one of three approaches:

1. Harris-Benedict or similar equations
2. Estimates based upon patterns reported in clinical studies, and
3. Indirect calorimetry

Harris-Benedict Equations

The Harris-Benedict equations[66] are regression relationships that predict REE in kilocalories per day based upon height, weight, and age:

$$REE \text{ (males)} = 66.47 + 13.75 \text{ (weight)} + 5.0 \text{ (height)} - 6.76 \text{ (age)}$$

$$REE \text{ (females)} = 655.10 + 9.56 \text{ (weight)} + 1.85 \text{ (height)} - 4.68 \text{ (age)}$$

where weight is expressed in kg, height in cm, and age in years. The advantages of REE derived from the Harris-Benedict equations are the ease of use, lack of requirement of expensive equipment and technical support, and rapidity of calculation. However, these relationships were established in normal, unstressed subjects and it has been recognized that the Harris-Benedict equations underestimate energy needs during acute illness. It is believed that when they are applied to ill patients, these equations correctly predict energy requirements in < 50% of patients.[67]

In order to factor in the increases in metabolic rate often associated with trauma, several scaling parameters have been applied to the estimates derived from these equations. For example, to account for the increase in REE due to physical activity, the calculated energy expenditure can be multiplied by a factor of 1.1 to 1.2. Additionally, a stress factor that causes further increases in energy expenditures can also be used. This latter factor may vary from 1.0 for clinically insignificant injury up to 2.1 for a 50-60% (or greater) total body burn.[68] Long et al., using stress factors ranging from 1.2 for patients undergoing minor surgery to 2.1 in patients with extensive burns, found that energy expenditure predicted from the Harris-Benedict equations were within 5% of those measured by indirect calorimetry.[69] Unfortunately, no unequivocal guidelines allowed the clinician to reliably predict this factor for a particular patient, resulting in some uncertainty in the final energy expenditure prediction.

Estimates from Population Studies

Based upon population studies, the maintenance caloric requirements in fasting unstressed subjects is about 25 kcal/kg/day. In injured and septic patients, MEE ranges 35-50 kcal/kg/day.[70,71] This is similar to the estimates derived by multiplying the Harris-Benedict equation by 1.2×1.6. Unfortunately, this wide range leaves considerable room for error.

Some recent reports have indicated that the caloric requirements of seriously ill patients tend to be overestimated by protocols using population estimates and correction factors.[67,72] Apparently, the extent of this discrepancy cannot be determined without indirect calorimetry.

> **AXIOM** When indirect calorimetry is not available, it is probably wise to provide about 35 kcal/kg/day in severely hypercatabolic patients because the needs of up to 90% of such patients can be met by this level of caloric support.

Indirect Calorimetry

Indirect calorimetry involves the measurement of carbon dioxide production and oxygen consumption rates which, based upon the known stoichiometry of glucose and fat oxidation in the body, can be converted to energy expenditure.[73,74] Additionally, the ratio of carbon dioxide produced to oxygen consumed (VCO_2/VO_2), termed the respiratory quotient (RQ), provides an estimate of the relative amounts of glucose and fat that are oxidized.

Starvation, a state in which fat oxidation is dominant, is characterized by an RQ of 0.7, whereas a glucose-based dietary intake is associated with an RQ of 1.0. RQ values > 1.0 are believed to reflect endogenous fat synthesis as a result of excess calories, usually from carbohydrates.

Portable metabolic carts can provide this objective assessment of nutrient metabolism in spontaneously breathing, as well as intubated, mechanically ventilated patients, thereby providing a direct measurement of caloric needs.[75] This approach probably provides the best estimate of caloric needs because it does not require the use of estimated correction factors and can be obtained on demand.

Two studies using indirect calorimetry data have suggested that the MEE of injured septic patients are increased over BEE by only 13% and 14%.[77] More recently, it has been found, that by using indirect calorimetry, that the mean MEE averaged 30% higher than the BEE calculated from the Harris-Benedict equations (P < 0.001) and averaged 11% less than the calculated energy expenditure (CEE) derived by using an estimated stress factor (P < 0.01).[78]

Evidence is accumulating that hypermetabolically injured and septic patients do not require the 4000-6000 kcal/day that was occasionally recommended in the past. Current recommendations for caloric support range from 25 to 35 kcal/kg/day. Caloric intakes exceeding 40 kcal/kg/day have not been shown to further enhance nitrogen retention.[1]

Despite the apparent advantages of indirect calorimetry, some drawbacks exist. Indirect calorimetry is labor and technology intensive, expensive, and not reliably measured in a number of clinical settings, particularly when inspired oxygen concentrations exceed 50% in mechanically ventilated patients and in spontaneously breathing patients on any gas mixture except room air.[1] In addition, routine ICU care maneuvers (e.g., bronchoscopy, nursing care maneuvers, and respiratory therapy efforts) can increase energy expenditure 20-35% above resting levels for up to 1-2 hours after completion.[74] The overall contribution of these procedures to total energy expenditure is small because they are used relatively infrequently over the course of a day; however, measurements made soon after these events provide falsely high estimates of the total daily caloric needs.

> **AXIOM** Improperly timed indirect calorimetry studies may lead to underfeeding or overfeeding which may have a detrimental effect on survival.[78]

In the opposite extreme, patients who have recently been sedated may exhibit transient reductions of energy expenditure by 6-9%. Because this provides a falsely low estimate of energy requirements, underfeeding may result.[79] Furthermore, day-to-day variations in MEE may be as large as 30% in individual ICU patients. Consequently, repeated or serial determinations are needed to ensure proper caloric assessment.[80] In addition, the costs associated with the hardware and specialized personnel to perform these tests places some fiscal constraints upon this monitoring.

> **PITFALL** ⊘
>
> *Although indirect calorimetry provides the most precise means of assessing energy expenditure, it must be recognized that extrapolation of isolated values to average daily caloric needs may result in significant errors.*

Factors Altering Energy Expenditure

NUTRIENT SUPPORT

It is becoming apparent that nutrient substrates can elicit a rise in metabolic rate. The provision of nutrient support may increase MEE by as much as 10% and 25% in nonseptic and septic conditions, respectively.[81] The cause of this thermogenic effect has not been fully investigated but probably reflects: (a) the specific dynamic action of all foods, especially protein, which uses about 15% of the calories consumed to process nutrients and, (b) stimulated protein synthesis in response to increased availability of amino acids.

Some of the recommended levels of caloric intake for trauma patients already have the thermogenic effect of nutrients included, and this must be considered when these data are applied to clinical practice.

Hormonal Changes

Jeevanandam et al. noted that hormonal responses to major trauma trigger a cascade of metabolic adjustments leading to catabolism and substrate mobilization.[82] They also reported that energy deficit and energy surfeit have profound effects on hormone levels. To characterize the changes in regulatory hormone levels after multiple injury, they measured the plasma levels of eight hormones within 48-60 hours of injury in the fasting state and then daily for 5 days during the administration of total parenteral nutrition in 10 hypermetabolic, highly catabolic, severely injured adult patients.

Acute deficiency in anabolic insulin-like growth factor 1 (IGF-1) and growth hormone levels were seen along with elevated levels of counterregulatory stress hormones and insulin.[82] Provision of nutrition on the first day had no effect on IGF-1 and cortisol levels. However, growth hormone levels were raised to normal and nitrogen balance improved. Over the next four days, no appreciable changes occurred in these parameters. The persistently low levels of IGF-1 were believed to reflect the altered nutritional status of the patients, as characterized by the continued negative nitrogen balance and elevated cortisol levels in the early posttraumatic period. IGF-1 and insulin levels showed a significant negative correlation with the catabolic indicators, 3-methylhistidine and catecholamine excretion. The authors believed that these results suggest that IGF-1 is regulated by nutritional intake independent of growth hormone and may be a better nutrition indicator.

Changes in VO₂ and O₂ Extraction

To show the relationship between VO_2 and substrate utilization, Giovannini et al. performed metabolic and hemodynamic measurements in 72 septic and 40 nonseptic surgical patients undergoing total parenteral nutrition.[83] In the septic patients, oxygen extraction (O_2Ex) was inversely related to cardiac index (CI); however, at any given CI, significant increases in O_2Ex with simultaneous increases in O_2 consumption (VO_2) were related to increasing doses of amino acids. Fat had less effect and glucose had no effect on O_2Ex.

In nonseptic patients, O_2Ex was also inversely related to CI; however, at any given CI, there was no evident substrate-supply dependency of O_2Ex.[83] The increase in VO_2/g of administered amino acids was 817 mL in septic patients and 267 mL in nonseptic patients. These results suggest that the impaired O_2Ex and VO_2 in septic patients may at least partially reflect abnormalities in substrate utilization. Consequently, amino acid support may have a role in modulating these abnormal O_2Ex patterns by providing preferential substrate for oxidative metabolism.

Excretion of Polyamines

Poyhonen et al. noted that excretion of polyamines first increases and then decreases in patients with multiple trauma receiving total parenteral nutrition (TPN).[84] To separate the effects of trauma and TPN on polyamine excretion, they studied 12 patients with multiple trauma and 14 patients after surgery for colorectal malignancy. Patients were randomized to receive either TPN or hypocaloric glucose infusion. Urinary excretion of total and free polyamines, putrescine (PU), spermidine (SPD), and spermine (SP), and their metabolites, N1-acetylspermidine (N1-AcSPD) and N8-acetylspermidine (N8-AcSPD), and energy and nitrogen balance were measured.

Excretion of all polyamines except spermine (SP) markedly increased after trauma and surgery, exceeding the normal values by two- to ten-fold.[84] In addition, in patients receiving TPN, the excretion of total polyamines was 48% higher (P < .01), PU 34% higher (P < .05), SPD 35% higher (P < .05), and SP 350% higher (P < .05) than in patients receiving hypocaloric glucose. Although urinary excretion of SP was only 17% of the control values during hypocaloric glucose infusions (P < .05), it was normal during TPN. The difference in polyamine excretion between nutrition groups was even more pronounced when normalized for nitrogen and energy balance. Patients receiving TPN were more hypermetabolic than patients receiving hypocaloric glucose (1.36 ± 0.06 [SE] vs 1.16 ± 0.04 times predicted values, respectively; P < .025). Thus, energy expenditure could explain the difference in polyamine excretion between the nutrition groups.

SPECIAL METABOLIC PROBLEMS

Prediction of MEE in two conditions, burn injury and obesity, deserve special consideration because the Harris-Benedict equations may be particularly misleading under these circumstances.

Burns

Of the various conditions that may stimulate hypermetabolism, burns tend to cause the highest observed metabolic rates. MEE increases with the extent of burn, reaching a plateau at about 50-60% body surface area burn (BSAB).

Various formulas have been proposed to estimate the caloric needs of burn patients when indirect calorimetry is unavailable.[70,85] Characteristically, these regression equations include a factor for the extent of the burn (BSAB). The Toronto Formula has been suggested as one of the best of these predictive formulas[68,86]:

$$MEE = -4343 + (10.5 \, BSAB) + (0.23 \, CI) + (0.84 \, HBEE) + (114 \, T) - (4.5 \, DPB)$$

where CI is the current caloric intake (thermogenic effect), HBEE is the Harris-Benedict equation energy expenditure, T is the average rectal temperature (°C) over 24 hours, and DPB is the day when postburn measurements are taken. Thus, a 50-year-old 5′8″, 154 lb man with a 50% BSAB, 510 kcal/day intake (3 L of 5% G/W), a Harris-Benedict equation EE of 1554 kal, and an average rectal temp of 38°C on the third postburn day would have:

$$MEE = -4343 + (10.5)(50) + (0.23)(510) + (0.84)(1554) + (114)(38) - (4.5)(3)$$
$$= -4343 + 525 + 117.3 + 1305.36 + 4332 - 13.5$$
$$= 6280 - 4357 = 1923 \, kcal$$

Despite the detail of this equation, significant individual variability still exists. This again emphasizes the need for serial monitoring.

Obesity

Estimates of energy expenditure for obese patients using the Harris-Benedict equations are excessively high (compared to measured EE) when actual body weight is used and too low when ideal body weight is used. Regression equations to predict REE have been developed specifically for obese patients;[87] however, their importance may be questioned, based upon clinical studies supporting the use of hypocaloric, protein-sparing nutritional support as a means to sustain lean body mass in critically ill, obese patients. Restriction of nonnitrogen caloric intake to as low as 50% of measured REE has resulted in satisfactory postoperative recovery of seriously ill obese patients provided protein intake was sufficiently high to maintain a positive nitrogen balance.[88]

AXIOM Nitrogen balance can be achieved by carefully matching nitrogen intake with output, even when caloric intake is low.

Summary

No single approach to the prediction of caloric intake is error free. Nevertheless, it seems reasonable to use one of these methods in conjunction with serial estimates of nutritional progress using various indices, such as nitrogen balance, plasma protein concentrations (e.g., albumin, transferrin), and immune competence indicators (delayed cutaneous hypersensitivity, absolute lymphocyte count) to determine the adequacy of nutritional therapy.

NUTRITIONAL SUPPORT

General Considerations

TIMING OF NUTRITIONAL SUPPORT

The provision of early nutrient support after trauma or surgery can be an essential component of general care and convalescence; however, the question of precisely when to initiate such nutrient support remains a judgment issue. Although little definitive data are available, there are suggestions in the surgical literature that early feeding may moderate the metabolic response to injury and improve outcome.[89,90] However, beginning a feeding modality with its potential technical and metabolic complications must be weighed against the likelihood that a patient will develop a protracted illness.[91]

It has been reported that mortality rates and incidence of organ failure in critically ill patients increase substantially when the cumulative, negative caloric balance exceeds 10,000 kcal[92] which can develop after only four to five days in patients receiving only 5% glucose solutions. This suggests that the latitude for beginning nutritional support is relatively small. Many authors suggested that feeding should be instituted within 36-48 hours following the onset of severe illness,[93] and some centers begin burn patients on enteral feedings within 12 hours of admission.

AXIOM   If the trauma victim was severely malnourished prior to injury, the trauma is apt to cause a hypermetabolic response and nutritional therapy should be begun as soon as the patient is hemodynamically stable.

Young, previously well-nourished patients who have simple fracture repair or a routine, uncomplicated laparotomy and who are expected to eat in four to five days probably will not benefit from nutritional support.

GOALS OF NUTRITIONAL THERAPY

The goals of nutritional support include: (a) the maintenance of organ structure and function, and (b) prevention or treatment of malnutrition particularly in settings where malnutrition may become a significant contributor to morbidity and mortality. Although it is reasonable to strive to achieve these goals, it is probably not reasonable, particularly in the setting of severe posttrauma hypermetabolism, to expect real weight gain or increases in muscle mass.

Nutrients

GLUCOSE

Rationale for Use

Glucose has generally been recommended as the primary energy source for patients receiving intravenous nutritional support. Its beneficial effect has been attributed to its ability to suppress hepatic gluconeogenesis. This allows salvage of glucogenic amino acids and suppression of cellular amino acid oxidation. However, large quantities of glucose do not suppress the protein catabolism of severe stress. Furthermore, the maximum rate of glucose oxidation is only about 5 mg/kg/min.[94] Using only glucose to supply the complete caloric needs of patients TPN can cause a number of complications, including hyperglycemia, hyperosmolar coma, osmotic diuresis, hepatic enzyme elevations, and essential fatty acid deficiency.

Current Recommendations

Current recommendations for the provision of carbohydrate in nutritional support depend on the level of stress present.[95] Nonprotein caloric intake should range from 25 to 35 kcal/kg/day for most patients, and the make-up of this caloric level should vary with the level of stress.

In starved, unstressed patients, the entire caloric load may consist of glucose, except for small amounts of fat to prevent essential fatty acid deficiency. This can be given in a nonprotein calorie-to-nitrogen ratio of about 150 to 1.

In highly stressed patients, glucose should probably constitute 60-70% of nonprotein calories, with the remainder of the calories supplied as fat. Carbohydrate calories in the range of 20 kcal/kg/day are an appropriate starting point.[1] In highly stressed patients, TPN containing 25% dextrose is probably inappropriate and glucose should probably be reduced to 15% concentrations, especially when TPN is begun.

LIPIDS

Use of fat emulsions to provide a portion of the nonprotein calories has been fostered by studies indicating that fat clearance and oxidation[96] proceed normally in seriously ill, septic patients. Fat has also been shown to have a protein-sparing effect that is equivalent to glucose.[97] Several reports have argued that fat is used in preference to glucose as a metabolic fuel in critically ill, septic patients.[26,98,99] Many authorities currently believe that fat and glucose are equivalent as an energy substrate for injured and septic patients. It is only in patients with severe, advanced multiple organ or liver failure that the capacity of the patient to clear lipids from the bloodstream may decline.[100] Although short-term studies (< 3 days) indicated that glucose may be more effective in reducing nitrogen loss than isocaloric infusions in which a portion of glucose calories were substituted with fat,[101] other reports showed that the superiority of a carbohydrate-based system is transient and these two different nutrient combinations become equivalent as the duration of TPN administration increases.[102,103] Collectively, the ability of fat emulsions to decrease the metabolic complications of TPN and to produce equivalent nitrogen sparing has resulted in their increased popularity. Consequently, they now constitute at least a portion of the parenteral nutritional regimen for most patients.

In the starved state, the majority of calories can be supplied as glucose with a small amount of lipid (2-5% of the calories) given to prevent essential fatty acid deficiency. In patients with starvation or low-stress metabolism, one or two bottles of intravenous lipid (500 mL of a 10% solution) per week should be more than adequate to prevent the complications of essential fatty acid deficiency.

The signs of essential fatty acid deficiency include skin scaling, impaired wound healing, increased susceptibility to infection, capillary fragility, thrombocytopenia, fatty infiltration of the liver, and alterations in mental status. Evidence of essential fatty acid deficiency can appear earlier than may be expected for the degree of body fat depletion. This is due in part to the suppression of lipolysis by the high insulin levels that are present because of high rates of gluconeogenesis and exogenous glucose infusion.

Although the use of fat calories is generally increased in the setting of postinjury hypermetabolism, excess lipid can also cause complications, particularly when given parenterally. Some of these problems include hypoxemia,[104] neutrophil dysfunction, and decreased phagocytic function of macrophages leading to further immune dysfunction.[105,106] Additionally, omega-6 fatty acids are precursors of dienoic prostaglandins and leukotrienes, many of which are actively involved in the inflammatory response and may be injurious to the host by a variety of mechanisms.[1]

As a result of these unfavorable characteristics of exogenously supplied fat, current recommendations for lipid nutritional support in the stressed patient are that fat should constitute no more than 15-40% of nonprotein calories; in addition, the maximal fat infusion rate should not exceed 2.5 g/kg/day.[107]

Triglyceride Clearance

When using intravenous fat preparations, careful attention must be paid to the rate of administration and to monitoring of lipid clearance. Lipids are often infused at a rate of 0.5-1.0 g/kg/day over 10-20 hours, usually beginning after the morning laboratory blood samples are drawn. Serum triglycerides usually are monitored two or three times weekly, particularly in the early phases of nutritional support, and the lipid infusion rate is decreased if serum triglycerides rise excessively.

Impaired lipid metabolism in the late stages of hypermetabolism

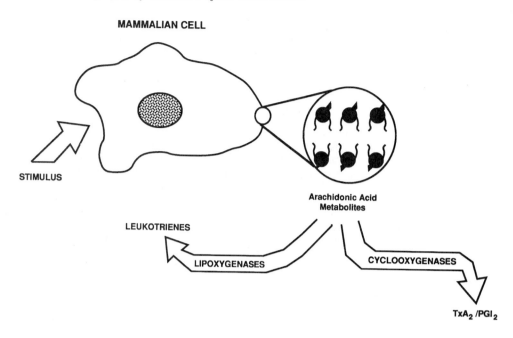

MAMMALIAN CELL

STIMULUS

Arachidonic Acid
Metabolites

LEUKOTRIENES

LIPOXYGENASES

CYCLOOXYGENASES

TxA$_2$ /PGI$_2$

FIGURE 38–11 The accelerated liberation of arachidonic acid from the cell membrane of various tissue cells results in the increased formation of prostaglandins, thromboxane A$_2$, and leukotrienes which exhibit significant metabolic and vasoactive properties. (Tx = thromboxane; PGI$_2$ = prostacyclin).

and organ failure may necessitate discontinuing the lipid infusion. The clearance rate of fat may be assessed by measuring plasma triglyceride levels before and after intravenous fat. Triglyceride concentrations > 300-350 mg/dL six hours after a lipid infusion of 50 g suggests that the use of intravenous fat should be limited. Additionally, when the caloric contribution of fat emulsions (1.1 kcal/mL of a 10% emulsion) exceeds 50-75% of the total caloric intake, problems related to overload of the reticuloendothelial system by lipid particles may arise. This is characterized by hepatosplenomegaly, fatty infiltration of the liver, and increased bacterial trapping in the lung.[108-109] Below this upper range, injured/septic patients appear to adapt well to whatever nutrient mix is administered, indicating that the proportions of fat versus glucose are relatively unimportant in relationship to utilization.

Endstage or preterminal sepsis may be associated with changes to a fixed fuel requirement. Under such circumstances the relative proportions of each substrate oxidized tends to become independent of the amounts administered. Nevertheless, even under these circumstances, relatively similar quantities of glucose and lipid are oxidized.[110] Consequently, in advanced sepsis, most clinical reports recommend a lipid contribution of only 30-50% of the total caloric intake.

Problems with Current Intravenous Lipids

Recently, some deleterious effects of parenteral lipids have been reported, and these appear to be due to the specific lipid formulations currently available. The source of the lipid available in current products is variable, with soybean oil (Intralipid, Travamulsion) and safflower oil (Liposyn) the most commonly used. All currently available lipid products, whether for enteral or parenteral use, consist primarily of omega-6 fatty acids and contain the essential fatty acid linoleic acid. Linoleic acid, which is an omega-6 polyunsaturated essential fatty acid, constitutes 50-75% of the total fatty acid content in fat emulsions made from plant oils. This far exceeds the daily essential fatty acid requirement, which is only 1-4% of the total caloric need.[111] Although the bulk of linoleic acid is oxidized as an energy substrate, some of the excess of this fatty acid is believed to serve as a precursor for the increased production of arachidonic acid metabolites, such as the leukotrienes (LTs), prostaglandins (PGs), and thromboxanes (TXs), many of which are vasoactive and can produce tissue edema (Figure 38–11).

Clinical studies have indicated that intravenous omega-6 intravenous fat emulsions can increase intrapulmonary shunt and pulmonary artery pressures and aggravate states of impaired oxygenation in se-

riously ill patients. Experimental studies have indicated that these effects are at least partially due to increased production of arachidonic acid metabolites derived from polyunsaturated fats which also accumulate in cell membranes (Figure 38–12). These substances can significantly alter ventilation/perfusion matching and reduce pulmonary diffusing capacity.[112] Although the magnitude of this effect is usually relatively small, it may have a significant impact on outcome in some critically ill patients.

Another adverse effect of lipid infusions is an impairment of host immune responses, thereby increasing the susceptibility to infection. Excessive linoleic acid may result in the formation of increased amounts of certain prostaglandins, especially PGE$_2$ and PGI$_2$ which are immunosuppressive agents.[118-120] Prostaglandin E$_2$, in particular, is known to suppress a variety of lymphocyte responses, including T-cell proliferation, antibody and lymphokine production, and macrophage function. To offset these unfavorable characteristics of current lipid emulsions, some authorities have suggested a reduction in the amount of administered lipid to 5-15% of the total nonprotein calories.[113,114]

PITFALL ⊘

Administration of > 30% of the total nonnitrogen caloric intake as lipids can interfere with pulmonary and immune function.

Fish Oils

Several approaches are under study to avoid the noxious effects of currently available lipid emulsions. One strategy to minimize the immunosuppressive effects of currently used lipids is to replace them with marine lipids (fish oils) which contain omega-3 fatty acids, such as eicosapentaenoic acid (EPA; Figure 38–12). Experimental studies have indicated that the presence of omega-3 fatty acids and their metabolites (e.g., PGE$_3$, TxA$_3$, LTB$_5$) have competitive and inhibitory effects on the metabolism of linoleic acid to arachidonic acid and its prostaglandin products. In addition, omega-3-derived metabolites themselves have properties opposing those of the omega-6 metabolites. For example, PGE$_3$ is not immunosuppressive while PGE$_2$ is. Also, excessive quantities of leukotriene B$_4$ (LTB$_4$) which arises from arachidonic acid and contributes to leukocyte chemotaxis can cause adverse pulmonary changes in the lungs. However, EPA from omega-3 lipids inhibits LTB$_4$ production and increases the output of the analogue LTB$_5$ which has markedly attenuated chemotactic properties.[109] Furthermore, macrophage production of proinflammatory

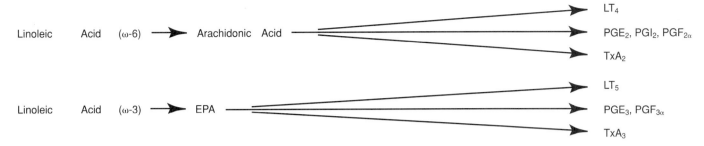

FIGURE 38–12 Polyunsaturated fatty acids may be metabolized to a variety of other products, such as the leukotrienes (LTs), prostaglandins (PGs) and thromboxanes (TXs) which exhibit vasoactive and immunologic effects. (EPA = eicosapentaenoic acid).

cytokines, such as IL-1 and TNF, is reduced with a fish-oil-based lipid intake.[114]

In a recent report of a multicenter, prospective, randomized clinical trial by Bower et al., studying the effects of early enteral administration of a formula (IMPACT) that has arginine, nucleotide, and fish oil, patients who received at least 821 mL/day of the experimental formula had their hospital median length of stay reduced by 8 days (P < .05).[115] In patients stratified as septic, the median length of hospital stay was reduced by 10 days (P < .05). There was also a major reduction in the frequency of acquired infections (P < .01) in patients who received the experimental formula. In the septic subgroup fed at least 821 mL/day of the experimental formula, the median length of stay was reduced by 11.5 days. A major reduction also occurred in acquired infections (both P < .05). In support of this work, another recent report demonstrated improved immunologic responses in postoperative patients using an omega-3 fatty acid and arginine supplemental diet.[116]

Medium-chain Triglycerides

Another approach toward minimizing the adverse effects of the omega-6 polyunsaturated fatty acids is the use of medium-chain fatty acid (MCFA) triglycerides (MCT), which are composed of fatty acids with carbon chain lengths of 6-12. Conventional lipid products usually contain fatty acids of the long-chain fatty acid (LCFA) variety which have more than 12 carbons. Compared to long-chain fats, the MCFA and MCT exhibit some metabolic properties that are desirable for critically ill patients. These include: (a) more rapid clearance from the bloodstream, and (b) ability to enter mitochondria for oxidation without the cofactor carnitine. In critical illness with organ failure, carnitine may be deficient; consequently, LCFA will be slow to enter mitochondria, whereas MCFA may be oxidized much more readily. Finally, the nitrogen sparing potential of MCT appears to be at least equivalent to LCT.[117]

Because MCT cannot supply essential fatty acid requirements, emulsions have been developed known as structured lipids, which contain both MCFA and LCFA esterified onto the same glycerol backbone. It is hoped that this will provide the benefits of both lipid classes. Because neither fish oil nor MCT products are currently approved for parenteral administration in the United States, their use is limited to enteral products.

Combinations of Fat and Glucose

The nutrient support regimens used most frequently now are a mixed substrate formulation of both fat and glucose in order to minimize the adverse effects of each of these individual nutrients. High-glucose loads increase CO_2 levels and the tendency to respiratory failure and also tend to cause liver function test abnormalities associated with fatty infiltration of the liver (hepatic steatosis). Both of these conditions may be managed by replacing some of the carbohydrate with fat.

Singer et al. investigated the effects of glycerol as a fuel source in 22 hypermetabolic trauma patients who were randomly assigned to either glucose or glycerol as the carbohydrate source (220 g glycerol or 320 g dextrose) in a lipid-based system of parenteral nutrition.[118] In the glycerol group, plasma glucose concentrations were significantly lower, whereas glycerol levels increased nearly twenty fold. Insulin levels were greater in the glucose group, and glucagon increased in both groups to a similar degree. Nitrogen balance was restored to equilibrium in the glycerol group, but remained negative in the glucose group. No abnormalities in liver function or differences in serum albumin levels were noted in either group. A 12% thermic effect was noted in the glucose group, but not in the glycerol group.

PROTEIN

Nitrogen Balance in Stress Situations

As already noted, the metabolic response to trauma and sepsis is characterized by increased proteolysis, particularly in skeletal muscle, increased ureagenesis, increased hepatic synthesis of acute-phase reactant proteins, and increased urinary nitrogen losses. The response is incompletely suppressed by adequate nonprotein calories, whether supplied as fat or glucose. Total protein synthesis is increased as a result of wound healing, increased formation of immune and inflammatory cells, and synthesis of acute-phase proteins; however, the protein synthetic rate is exceeded by the rate of protein catabolism in skeletal muscle, gut, and connective tissue with a resultant net negative nitrogen balance (Figure 38–8).

Obtaining a Positive Nitrogen Balance

Survival is generally believed to be best served by the attainment of a positive nitrogen balance. It was formerly believed that this required slightly exceeding the estimated daily energy expenditure with nonprotein calories. However, in severe stress the accelerated protein catabolism is not sensitive to exogenously administered calories or amino acids.[119] Conversely, when enough amino acids are given to compensate for the increased demand in stress, the protein synthetic rate can be increased by exogenously supplied amino acids; as a result, nitrogen balance can be achieved even if the patient's energy expenditures are underestimated.[119,120]

AXIOM An underestimation of energy requirement may be offset by a greatly increased nitrogen intake.

The beneficial effects of achieving nitrogen balance by way of supporting increased protein synthesis would appear to include maintaining proper immune and reparative function until the source of the neuroendocrine and mediator activation can be eliminated. The dose of exogenous amino acids or protein should be increased until nitrogen equilibrium is achieved. Further increases in the amino acid load appear only to enhance ureagenesis and azotemia, but do not improve nitrogen balance.[1]

Current recommendations for amino acid/protein administration depend on the degree of metabolic stress (Table 38–5). In low-stress settings, nitrogen balance can be achieved with protein doses as low

TABLE 38–5 Nutritional Goals

	Uncomplicated Starvation	Mild Stress	Moderate Stress	Severe Stress
Nonprotein calorie nitrogen ratio (kcal/g N)	150/1	150/1	100/1	80/1
Amino acids (g/kg/day)	0.5-1.0	1.0-1.4	1.4-1.9	2.0-2.9
Total nonprotein calories (kcal/kg/day)	20-25	20-25	25-30	30-35

as 0.5-1.0 g/kg/day, as long as the intake of calories, vitamins, and minerals is adequate.[1] Nonprotein-calorie-to-nitrogen ratios approximating 150:1 are appropriate in this setting. With severe stress, protein intake of 1.5-2.5 g/kg/day, is more appropriate.[70,121] These estimates of elevated protein requirements come from reports indicating that the optimal nonprotein-calorie-to-nitrogen ratio of nutritional formulations for normal or unstressed states (150:1) is shifted to lower levels (80-100:1) in critically ill, hypermetabolic patients.[122]

Using Intravenous Albumin to Prevent or Correct Ileus

Studies from the 1930s demonstrated that dogs rendered hypoalbuminemic from plasmapheresis developed progressive gastric and intestinal hypomotility to the point of complete gastric stasis.[123,124] When the plasma proteins were reinfused, motility returned to normal. Barden's group believed that tissue edema was the chief cause of decreased small bowel motility.[123]

Moss noted that following extensive surgery, the decreased ability to absorb fluid from the small bowel is partially due to hypoalbuminemia.[125] He also demonstrated that induced hypoalbuminemia in rabbits caused impaired intestinal absorption of tritiated water and NaI[131] and increased intraluminal fluid and bowel weight.

A strong negative correlation between plasma protein concentration and fluid transport across mucosa was demonstrated by Duffy et al.[126] They found that below a total plasma protein concentration of 4.1 g/100 cc, mucosal fluid flow is from the interstitium to the lumen and absorption from the intestinal lumen is impaired. Pietsch also demonstrated a strong negative correlation between serum protein levels and the ability of the small bowel to absorb water.[127]

Durr et al. found that hypoalbuminemic patients had intolerance to enteral feedings and suggested that a reduced colloid osmotic pressure played an important role.[128] They also noted that the number of days that a patient tolerated enteral feedings was positively correlated (P < 0.01) with the mean serum albumin for each patient.

Ford et al. noted that patients with serum albumin < 3.0 g/dL (18 of 46 patients) were able to take in significantly fewer calories and had more feeding intolerance than patients with serum albumin > 3.0 g/dL.[129] In a second phase of the study, 20 patients with serum albumin < 3.0 g/dL underwent albumin replacement over 2-3 days. Only 2 of these 20 patients had feeding intolerance after albumin replacement, and they attained a caloric level equal to patients who started with higher albumin levels.

Other studies, however, failed to document benefits from albumin replacement. Foley et al., in a prospective, randomized trial of critically ill patients, found no benefit from albumin replacement on a variety of outcome variables, including complication rates, mortality, hospital stay, ventilatory dependence, or tolerance to enteral feedings.[130] Their study, however, had several problems, one of which was that none of their patients attained a plasma albumin level > 3.0 g/dL at any time during the study.

In a recent prospective, randomized study of 69 hypoalbuminemic patients following aortoiliac or iliofemoral bypass, Woods and Kelley gave 37 patients enough intravenous albumin to achieve plasma albumin levels of > 3.5 gm/dl.[131] These albumin-treated patients, when compared to a group of 32 patients not receiving albumin, showed no significant differences in postoperative day of flatus (4.1 vs 4.2

days), day of oral intake (4.0 vs 3.8), day when regular diet was begun (6.1 vs 5.5), or postoperative hospital days (9.2 vs 8.4). Nevertheless, they believed that albumin replacement may still play a role in improving bowel function in chronically hypoalbuminemic patients.

Use of High Concentrations of BCAA

Although it is highly controversial, Barton and Cerra[1] and a few other investigators continue to favor the use of amino acid preparations enriched in branched-chain amino acids (BCAA) in settings of high metabolic stress. During severe stress, the amino acids oxidized for fuel, particularly by skeletal muscle, include a significant portion of the BCAAs. Because of an accelerated oxidative consumption of BCAAs in traumatic stress, provision of additional amounts of these amino acids has been postulated to offset tissue leucine deficits.[91] When standard amino acid preparations are given in dosages sufficient to meet this oxidative rate, the result is an excess of gluconeogenic and aromatic amino acids and a tendency to aggravate the already existing hyperglycemia.

Currently available high-BCAA formulations contain 45-50% BCAAs, with concomitantly decreased amounts of glucogenic and aromatic amino acids; standard amino acid formulations contain only 15-33% BCAAs. High-BCAA formulations have been shown to be more efficient than standard formulations at promoting nitrogen retention, supporting hepatic protein synthesis, and minimizing urea production.[132,133] Some investigators believe that although more expensive on a per gram basis, the high-branched-chain formulations are less expensive than standard amino acids when compared in terms of nitrogen retained.[134] However, the benefits of BCAA have largely been inferred from the *in vitro* ability of leucine to promote protein synthesis and inhibit protein breakdown in skeletal muscle.

In 1990, von Meyerfeldt et al reported on a prospective, randomized, double-blind trial investigating the effects of BCAA enrichment of a TPN regimen on nitrogen balance, 3-methylhistidine excretion, and morbidity (as evidenced by disturbances in organ function, severity of sepsis, and mortality).[135] The study enrolled 101 patients with 52 receiving a standard TPN solution and 49 a BCAA-enriched solution. Both groups received 30 kcal kg^{-1} body-weight, 15% fat calories, and 0.17 g nitrogen kg^{-1} body-weight. In the BCAA-enriched group, patients received 0.56 g BCAA kg^{-1} body-weight. The other group of patients received 0.18 g BCAA kg^{-1} body-weight. Nitrogen balances and 3-methylhistidine excretion were not significantly different between the groups. Mortality (early or late), sepsis or stress-related, also did not differ significantly between the groups. Thus, the authors were not able to confirm the reported beneficial effects of BCAA-enriched TPN in septic and traumatized patients.

Because of the expense and because clinical reports have failed to show that an increased intake of BCAA confers any advantage in outcome over standard amino acid preparations in critically ill patients, their use has declined markedly.[136,137]

Fluid and Electrolyte Management

The typical fluid and electrolyte response to injury is retention of salt and water and loss of intracellular potassium, magnesium, and phosphorus. Malnutrition can cause similar abnormalities and can greatly magnify those caused by injury. Small increases in plasma levels of intracellular ions can reflect large decreases in quantities of these ions in the cellular compartment. Repletion of lean body mass via nutritional support also requires replacement of these intracellular ions.[1]

In a classic study by Rudman et al., malnourished adult patients were treated with intravenous hyperalimentation that the authors made deficient in various nutritional elements.[138] Formulations deficient in phosphorus led to hypophosphatemia, fatigue and restlessness, and negative balances of nitrogen, potassium, and calcium. Formulas deficient in potassium led to hypokalemia, malaise, and negative balances in nitrogen and phosphorus. Although both hypokalemia and hypophosphatemia prevented nitrogen retention, weight gain continued, though at a reduced rate, apparently reflecting expansion of the extracellular space with sodium and water and continued expansion of adipose tissue. Glucose infusion in the absence of intracellular ions led to increased adipose tissue, despite a persistent, negative nitrogen balance. This work demonstrated that the attainment of positive nitrogen balance and increase in lean body mass requires repletion of protoplasm which, in turn, requires not only substrate for protein synthesis, but also provision of adequate amounts of intracellular electrolytes.

AXIOM Obtaining a positive N_2 balance with TPN requires administration of adequate calories, amino acids, and other intracellular components.

The importance of monitoring and maintaining appropriate plasma levels of sodium, potassium, and chloride are usually related to the effects of abnormalities of these electrolytes on neuromuscular and cardiac function and on acid-base status. In patients requiring nutritional support, serum concentrations of magnesium and phosphorus should also be carefully monitored and corrected as indicated.

Fluid requirements may vary considerably, depending on the state of resuscitation, gastrointestinal losses, evaporation from wounds, and renal function. Two commonly used methods of estimating maintenance fluid requirements are body weight and body surface area. On a weight basis, maintenance fluid requirements can be met by providing 100 mL/kg per day for the first 10 kg of body weight, 50 mL/kg per day for the next 10 kg of body weight, and 20 mL/kg per day for any additional body weight. Thus, a 70 kg adult male is given 100

(10) + 50(10) + 20(50) = 2500 mL of fluid per day to cover urine and insensible water loss. When maintenance fluid support is based on body surface area, 1500 mL/m^2 is usually given.

Even when the initial resuscitation is complete, extra fluid must be supplied to replete evaporative losses in ungrafted burns and other open wounds. Additional fluid and electrolytes must also be provided to replace excessive gastrointestinal losses (Table 38–6). The adequacy of fluid support is usually best assessed in terms of urine output. In an adult patient, urinary output of 0.5-1.0 mL/kg/hr is generally accepted as adequate, although in the setting of critical illness, an output in the range of 1.0-1.5 mL/kg/hr is often preferred.

Electrolyte requirements also vary considerably depending on the clinical situation. For the patient deprived of normal food intake for relatively short periods, only sodium, potassium, and chloride must be supplied. The minimum daily requirements of sodium in patients with normal renal function is about 20 mEq/day to compensate for losses due to sweating and skin desquamation.[1] However, 1-2 mEq/kg/day are usually provided to replace obligate losses and to suppress aldosterone secretion sufficiently to prevent potassium wasting (Table 38–7).

Obligate urinary potassium excretion is about 30-40 mEq/day; however, in the setting of normal renal function, at least 40-60 mEq/day are usually needed. Additional potassium must be supplied to patients with excess gastrointestinal losses or polyuria due to diuretics or mobilization of excess resuscitation fluid.

Chloride is often given in quantities equal to that of sodium; however, the relationship of chloride to bicarbonate and acid-base status can be important. Sodium and potassium can be given either as the chloride for patients with a tendency toward metabolic alkalosis, or as the acetate salt for those with a tendency toward metabolic acidosis.

When nutritional support is provided, adequate amounts of the intracellular ions (potassium, magnesium, and phosphorus) must also be supplied. The concentrations of intracellular ions should be monitored at least twice weekly initially.

Judgment should be used when planning nutritional formulations in settings where large doses of insulin or electrolytes, such as potassium, are to be incorporated into the formula. Although it may be convenient to incorporate the patient's entire daily electrolyte and insulin requirement into the TPN, TPN is expensive and wasting a bottle because it contains too much potassium or insulin is extremely careless. Potassium boluses and insulin drips are generally preferred when

TABLE 38–6 *Electrolyte Concentrations of Various Body Fluids*

		Electrolyte Concentration			
	Daily Volume	*Na*	*K*	*Cl*	*HCO₃*
Saliva	1000-1500	(50) 20-80	(15) 10-20	(30) 20-40	(40) 20-60
Stomach (low acid)	1500-2500	(100) 90-100	(10) 5-15	(110) 100-115	30
Stomach (high acid)	1500-2500	(55) 45-60	(15) 10-30	(115) 90-120	(10) 0-25
Bile	1000-1500	(145) 134-156	(5.2) 3.9-6.3	(90) 60-110	35
Pancreas	500-1500	(141) 113-153	(4.6) 2.6-7.4	(77) 54-95	90
Jejunum	1500-2500	(120) 100-140	(5.0) 3.0-7.5	(100) 90-115	
Ileum	1000-2000	(117) 91-140	(5.0) 3.0-7.5	(106) 82-125	25
Ileostomy	1500-3500	(125) 120-130	(16.2) 15-25	(110) 105-115	30
Cecostomy	1000-3000	80	21	48	45
Diarrhea		50-70	30	30-45	45
Urine	1000-1500	40-60	30-50	50-90	
Sweat	0-500	35-50	5	40-55	

Numbers in parentheses = average value

TABLE 38-7 Typical TPN Constituents at DRH for Acute Trauma Patients

Volume	
2,000-3,000 mL/day	
Nutrients	
Amino acids	4.25-8.0%
Dextrose	15-25%
Fat emulsion	500 mL 10-20% BIW-TIW
MVI	10 mL/day
Electrolytes (per liter)	
Sodium	35 mEq
Potassium	30 mEq
Chloride	35 mEq
Acetate	71 mEq
Phosphate	15 mmol
Calcium	4.7 mEq
Magnesium	5.0 mEq
Trace Elements (3 ml)	
Zinc	3 mg
Copper	1.3 mg
Manganese	0.3 mg
Chromium	12 mcg

BIW = 2 times a week
TID = 3 times a week

"excessive quantities of these substances are required, at least until the patient's daily requirements appear to be stable.

Vitamins and Trace Elements

The requirements for vitamins and trace elements in the stressed, hypermetabolic patient are unknown.[1] The dose of each vitamin is at least the recommended daily allowance (RDA); however, increased amounts of various vitamins, especially vitamin C, may be of some benefit. One should also supply at least the RDA for trace elements (Table 38-8), and more is appropriate when deficiencies are present. In oliguric renal failure, trace-element administration can usually be decreased to once or twice weekly.

It is important to prevent vitamin- and trace-element deficiency in critically ill or injured patients. A number of commercially available preparations with vitamins and trace minerals are available, but vitamin K generally has to be administered separately at least once a week. Consequently, one should be familiar with the functions and clinical signs of deficiency for selected vitamins as well as the guidelines for daily intravenous intake (Table 38-9).

Of the various trace-element deficiencies that may occur (Table 38-10), those involving zinc, copper, and selenium deserve some mention. Zinc and copper deficiencies may develop because of excessive gastrointestinal losses[139,140] and both may be excreted in increased quantities in the urine of hypermetabolic trauma patients.[141] Zinc is particularly important in wound healing, and copper is important for proper red cell formation. Selenium deficiency has also been reported in burn patients, although it is unclear whether this deficiency represents increased losses or inadequate intake.[142]

ENTERAL AND PARENTERAL NUTRITION

Although nitrogen balance can be achieved when adequate nutrition is provided by either the parenteral or the enteral route, each has advantages and disadvantages that may be pertinent in individual patients.

Enteral versus Parenteral Nutrition

ADVANTAGES OF PARENTERAL NUTRITION

AXIOM The primary advantage of total parenteral nutrition is that its use does not depend on a functional gastrointestinal tract and it is reliable in the sense that whatever is given will appear in the bloodstream.

Enteral nutrition requires a functioning small intestine and may be somewhat unreliable because the patient may not receive what is ordered or it may not be absorbed. It also often takes several days for enteral nutrition to be advanced to the intended maintenance strength and volume. In addition, enteral feedings often have to be stopped for radiologic diagnostic tests, return trips to the operating room, or because of plugged or dislodged feeding tubes. Abdominal distension and/or excessive diarrhea may also make one discontinue or alter enteral nutrition.

DISADVANTAGES OF ENTERAL NUTRITION

Difficulties in Placing Feeding Tubes

One of the more frequent disadvantages of enteral nutrition is the technical difficulties that may be involved in the placement of feeding tubes. Placement of a jejunostomy feeding tube at surgery is a reasonable alternative to nasojejunal feeding; however, performing a laparotomy only to insert a jejunostomy tube is not without some risk.

Diarrhea

Diarrhea is a problem in at least 20% of enterally fed patients; however, its incidence and severity can be minimized by starting with dilute formulas (usually ¼ strength) initially and by increasing concentration and volume slowly. We generally start with quarter-strength and quarter-volume feedings. Volume is gradually increased as tolerated over 2-4 days for a total of 80-125 mL/hr. The concentration is then increased as tolerated over 2-4 days to full-strength feedings.

Persistent diarrhea can usually be controlled by adding dietary fiber, reducing fat content, and/or using antidiarrheal agents, such as paregoric, diaphenoxylate, or imodium. However, one should check that a Clostridium difficile enterocolitis is not present because of prior or concomitant antibiotic therapy. Antidiarrheal agents are contraindicated in Clostridium difficile enteritis because the systemic symptoms and bowel damage caused by the toxin can be made much worse. H_2 receptor blocking agents may be helpful in controlling diarrhea in the setting of massive small bowel resection.[1]

Risk of Aspiration

Aspiration of enteral feedings into the lungs can be a significant problem in patients with gastric feedings tubes, and it may occur in as many as 40% of such patients. Because of the high incidence of gastric atony and the resultant risk of aspiration, we tend to avoid gastric feeding in critically ill patients, especially those without a good gag reflex.

TABLE 38-8 Suggested Intravenous Requirements for Trace Elements

Element	Plasma Content (μg/L)	Pediatric Patients (kg/day)	Adult Patients
Chromium	27-180	0.14-02 μg	10-20 μg
Copper	980-1200	10-20 μg	0.3-1.5 μg
Fluoride	140-190	1 μg	1-2 mg
Iodine	38-60	3-5 μg	1-2 μg/kg
Iron	580-2100	1 mg	0.5-2.0 mg
Manganese	1.8-3.1	5-20 μg	0.15-1.2 mg
Molybdenum	?	?	0.1-0.2 mg
Selenium	20-220*	?	0.1-0.2 mg
Zinc	1.3-3.0 mg	300[a] 100[b]	2-10 mg[c]

*Whole blood content.
[a]Premature infants up to 3 kg of body weight.
[b]Term infants and children up to five years old. Thereafter, the recommendation for adults applies, up to a maximum dosage of 4 mg/day.
[c]2-3 times this dosage may be required in the first days in patients with clinical signs of zinc deficiency.

TABLE 38–9 *Suggested Formulations for Children Ages 11 Years and Above, and Adults* (Results Do Not Include Requirements for Pregnancy or Lactation)*

Vitamins	RDA Adult Range	Multivitamin Formulation for IV Use	Water-soluble Vitamin Formulation for IM Use
Vitamin A (IU)	4000-5000**	3300	
Vitamin D (IU)	400	200	
Vitamin E (IU)	12-15	10.0	
Ascorbic acid (mg)	45	100.0	100.0
Folacin (μg)	400	400.0	400.0
Niacin (mg)	12-20	40.0	40.0
Riboflavin (mg)	1.1-1.8	3.6	3.6
Thiamine (mg)	1.0-1.5	3.0	3.0
B_6 Pyridoxine (mg)	1.6-2.0	4.0	4.0
B_{12} Cyanocobalamin (μg)	3	5.0	5.0
Pantothenic acid (mg)	5-10	15.0	15.0
Biotin (μg)	150-300	60.0	60.0

*Adapted from guidelines for Multivitamin Preparation for Parenteral Use, AMA, 1975.
**Assumes 50% intake as carotene, which is less available than vitamin A.

Inconsistent or Unreliable Intake

In many patients who have had abdominal surgery or trauma, some difficulty occurs in providing adequate enteral calories in the early postoperative period. Poor gastric emptying, ileus, and diarrhea may all be problems initially, and not infrequently enteral feedings must be discontinued, at least transiently, for certain diagnostic studies, such as CT scans of the abdomen. In 1989, Abernathy et al. reported that the intake of their patients fed via nasoenteric tubes was only 61% of the caloric goals.[143] These findings are similar to those of Rapp et al.[144] and Norton et al.[145] In a more recent report of 22 mechanically-ventilated postoperative patients, Kemper et al. found that eight patients who received only enteral nutrition received only 68% of their caloric requirements, and the day-to-day variation in nutrient intake in the enteral group was 40 ± 56% versus 12 ± 24% in the parenteral group (P < 0.001).[146]

ADVANTAGES OF ENTERAL NUTRITION

Preservation of Gut Barrier Function

AXIOM TPN lacks the ability of enteral nutrition to improve gut trophic factors and gastrointestinal barrier function.

One of the biggest advantages of enteral nutrition is its ability to stimulate gut mucosal development and preservation of gut barrier function. Gut mucosal atrophy occurs during starvation,[147] after long periods of TPN,[148] and in defunctionalized intestinal segments.[149] Animals fed intravenously have decreased gut weights, mucosal thickness, protein, DNA, brush border enzyme activity, and epithelial cell proliferation compared with animals fed enterally.[148,150] In animals having massive small bowel resections, only animals receiving enteral nutrition demonstrated mucosal growth and functional adaptation.[151,152] Some evidence has also suggested that early enteral nutrition may ablate the hypermetabolic response in burned guinea pigs.[90]

The maintenance of gut structure and function has been attributed primarily to intraluminal amino acids, particularly glutamine, which are used by the small bowel as a preferential fuel source.[153] Hopefully this would decrease any tendency to translocation of bacteria and bacterial products which might otherwise cause a systemic inflammatory response and increased sensitivity of the host to bacteremia or endotoxemia.[154]

The mechanisms proposed for increased bacterial translocation during TPN are multifactorial. These include atrophy of the gut barrier, as well as associated lymphoid tissue due to the absence of luminal nutrients and trophic factors.[154] Also, TPN predisposes to the overgrowth of certain gut bacterial species, especially gram-negative aerobes, while simultaneously depressing intraluminal defense mechanisms, which include anaerobic bacteria and secretory IgA.[155] Enteral feeding is also a prime stimulus for IgA secretion in bile.

Bacterial translocation can contribute to the systemic inflammatory response and hypermetabolism of injury and sepsis, and increasing data suggests that the gut is a contributor to hypermetabolism-organ-failure syndromes. Approximately 25% of the circulating blood volume is contained within splanchnic capacitance vessels. In hemorrhage and shock, this blood is redistributed to the central circulation at the expense of gut perfusion. The result is varying degrees of ischemic mucosal injury, which predisposes the patient to translocation of intestinal bacteria or bacterial products into the portal circulation or into the mesenteric lymph nodes and spleen. Although intestinal bacterial translocation does occur in the setting of multiple systemic insults, its true clinical significance is still unclear.

Reduced Stress Hormones and Cytokines

Production of counterregulatory hormones, splanchnic cytokines, especially TNF, and acute-phase proteins are much greater in endotoxin-challenged patients treated with TPN versus enterally fed controls.[156]

TABLE 38–10 *Evidence of Trace Element Deficiencies*

Trace Element	Function	Signs of Deficiency
Chromium	Glucose tolerance; maintenance of normal serum levels	Insulin-resistant glucose intolerance; elevated serum lipids
Copper	Component of ceruloplasmin; connective tissue metabolism; melanin formation	Anemia, leukopenia, depigmentation of skin
Iron	Constituent of hemoglobin, myoglobin, and the cytochrome enzymes	Microcytic hypochromic anemia, fatigue, weakness
Zinc	Lipid, protein, carbohydrate, and nucleic acid metabolism; cell replication and connective tissue synthesis	Dermatitis; impaired wound healing; depressed cell-mediated immunity; alopecia; depressed visceral protein status
Cobalt	—	Pernicious anemia
Manganese	Oxidative phosphorylation; fatty acid metabolism; protein and mucopolysaccharide synthesis	Growth retardation; CNS dysfunction

Reduced Morbidity and Mortality

Although clinical studies have indicated that parenteral and enteral nutrition are essentially equivalent modes of nutritional support in postoperative patients,[157] other reports have noted that enteral nutrition actually reduces mortality compared to TPN in models of hemorrhagic shock[158] and peritonitis.[159] Recently, this survival advantage was related to the influence that enteral nutrition may have on maintenance of gut structure and function.

In 1985, Moore and Jones reported the results of a prospective, randomized study of 75 trauma patients with an ATI > 15.[160] The control group received no nutritional support for 5 days and then, if intolerant to oral intake, they were given high-nitrogen TPN. The treatment group received a high-nitrogen elemental diet, delivered early after surgery, by needle catheter jejunostomy. The authors noted that the TEN group maintained better total lymphocyte counts and had significantly fewer major septic complications (4% versus 26%).

Kudsk et al. reported on constitutive and acute-phase protein levels measured on days 1, 4, 7, and 10 in 68 severely injured patients randomized to enteral or parenteral feedings.[161] Significantly higher levels of constitutive proteins and lower levels of acute-phase proteins were found in the patients randomized to enteral feeding. Although some hepatic protein reprioritization appeared to be caused by the nutrient route, this was only apparent in the less severely-injured patients. A more important factor in increasing visceral protein levels with enteral feeding was the reduction in septic morbidity. The incidence of septic complications was 15% (5 of 33) with enteral feeding and 41% (14 of 34) with the parenteral route (P < 0.03).

Mainous et al. noted that enteral nutrition improves resistance to experimentally-induced infections, blunts the hypermetabolic response to injury, and maintains intestinal structure and function better than parenteral nutrition.[162] They also believed that a policy of early enteral feeding in critically ill patients should be strongly favored. They demonstrated the safety and efficacy of immediate enteral feeding in patients with major burns and in a wide variety of other critically ill patients who had not been believed to be candidates for enteral nutrition due to the presence of ileus or fresh gastrointestinal anastomoses.

In a report by Moore et al., a two-part meta-analysis combined data from eight prospective, randomized trials that were designed to compare the nutritional efficacy of early enteral (TEN) and parenteral (TPN) nutrition in high-risk surgical patients.[163] The combined data gave sufficient patient numbers (TEN = 118; TPN = 112) to adequately address whether the route of substrate delivery affected the incidence of septic complications. The phase I (dropouts excluded) meta-analysis showed that significantly fewer TEN patients experienced septic complications (TEN: 17%, TPN: 44%; P = 0.0001). The phase II meta-analysis, which was an "intent-to-treat" analysis (dropouts included), also showed that fewer TEN patients developed septic complications. Further breakdown by patient type showed that the blunt trauma subgroup had the most significant reduction in septic complications when fed enterally.

Not all studies, however, have shown a clear advantage to enteral nutrition. In a recent report, Borzotta et al. evaluated measured REE and UUN in patients with severe head injury randomized to early parenteral (TPN = 21) or jejunal (ENT = 27) feeding with identical formulations.[164] REE increased to 2400 ± 531 kcal/day in both groups and remained at 135% ± 26% to 146% ± 42% of predicted energy expenditure over 4 weeks. Nitrogen excretion peaked during the second week at 33.4 ± 10 (TPN) and 31.2 ± 7.5 (ENT) g N/day. Both routes were equally effective at meeting the specified nutritional goals (1.2 × REE, 2.5 g protein/kg/day intake, stabilized albumin and transferrin levels). Infections were equally frequent: 1.86 episodes/TPN patient versus 1.89 episodes/ENT patient.

Although patients' charges were much greater for the TPN, hospital costs were similar for TPN and ENT support regimens.[164] In this study, the patients with head injuries were hypermetabolic for weeks, and only 27% were capable of meeting their nutritional requirements by oral intake by the time of discharge. Most importantly, TPN and ENT support were equally effective when pre-scribed according to individual measurements of REE and nitrogen excretion.

Eyer et al. also found that early enteral feeding after blunt trauma did not attenuate the stress response and did not alter the patient's outcome.[165] In a prospective, randomized clinical trial in patients with blunt trauma, 52 patients were randomized to receive early feedings (24 hours) or late feedings (72 hours). Feedings were given via nasoduodenal feeding tubes. The feedings were rapidly advanced to achieve full volume and strength within 24 hours to reach a goal of 1.5 g protein/kg/day. There were 38 patients who underwent at least 5 days of therapy and were considered to have completed the study. Although the patients were similar in age, gender, injury severity score, and mean PaO_2/FiO_2 ratio, the early group had more patients with a $PaO_2/FiO_2 > 150$. After feeding began, the amount fed per day was the same in both groups. There were no significant differences in metabolic responses as measured by plasma lactate and urinary total nitrogen, catecholamines, and cortisol. Both groups achieved nitrogen retention. In addition, no significant differences were recorded in ICU days, ventilator days, organ system failure, specific types of infection, or mortality, although the early feeding group had a greater total number of infections.

DISADVANTAGES OF PARENTERAL NUTRITION

Costs

Several disadvantages to intravenous feeding exist. First, it costs at least three times as much as enteral feeding. Second, the administration of TPN requires the placement of a central venous catheter, and this procedure is associated with a small (usually < 5%), but definite incidence of technical complications, such as pneumothorax, hemothorax, arterial injury, hydrothorax, and catheter embolus. Third, catheter infections can also be a significant problem.

Increased Suppression of Lipolysis

Intravenous administration of high-glucose loads can lead to greater hyperinsulinemia than that which occurs in enterally fed patients. Hyperinsulinemia leads to suppression of lipolysis so that the patient's fat stores cannot be mobilized for energy and serum free fatty acids may decrease to very low levels.[166]

SUMMARY

Enteral nutrition should be the preferred method for feeding injured patients for several reasons: (a) enteral nutrition costs less than one-third of comparable parenteral feeding, (b) it can satisfy most nutrient requirements better than parenteral nutrition, and (c) it exerts beneficial effects upon intestinal mucosa which may influence the incidence and severity of bacterial translocation.

Enteral Nutrition

TIMING

Reversal of intestinal structural and functional atrophy after a period of starvation or TPN is probably much more difficult to accomplish than preventing its occurrence. This point may be very relevant because nutrient support may be withheld for up to one week in some postoperative patients even if they initially do well.

AXIOM The earlier enteral nutrition is begun after trauma, the more likely it is to be of benefit.

Previously, physicians tended to limit the use of enteral nutrition in critically ill or injured patients because of the presence of intestinal ileus. Although return of gastric and colonic motility is rather slow after trauma, the small intestine may begin to function normally within 24-48 hours of abdominal surgery. Thus, provision of feedings through a jejunostomy or nasojejunal tube permits earlier feedings than would otherwise be tolerated by mouth or through a gastric tube. The etiology of diarrhea with enteral feedings varies and must be managed based upon a consideration of the probable causal factors for each patient (Table 38–11).[154,167]

TECHNIQUES

Early feeding via a 16 or 18F nasogastric tube can be very effective because any gastric residual can be easily checked, reducing the risk of aspiration of gastric contents. However, some risk of aspiration still remains, and feeding into the stomach may also enhance colonization of gram-negative bacilli. A risk of developing sinusitis also exists, especially when the other nostril has a nasotracheal tube.

Small, weighted feeding tubes are less irritating to the nose and pharynx, but the gastric residual cannot be easily checked, and a risk of aspiration of gastric contents still remains. Longer feeding tubes passed into the jejunum are thought to be less likely to cause aspiration.

Percutaneous endoscopic gastrostomy (PEG) catheters avoid nasal and pharyngeal irritation and are less likely to clog than small feeding tubes. However, a risk of gastric contents being regurgitated and aspirated exists. Percutaneous endoscopic jejunostomy (PEJ) catheters in which a catheter inserted through a PEG is advanced into the jejunum are also available, but many of these catheters come back into the stomach and have to be repositioned.

Montecalvo et al. compared the nutritional outcomes and pneumonia rate in patients fed either into the stomach via a 12-Fr, 43-inch, radiopaque polyurethane feeding tube or into the jejunum via a similar 12-Fr 60-inch feeding tube advanced past the ligament of Treitz endoscopically.[168] Of 19 patients initially randomized to jejunal feeding, five were placed in the gastric feeding group because the jejunal tube became displaced and could not be replaced. In the final comparison of 24 gastric-fed patients and 14 jejunal-fed patients, the jejunal group received a significantly higher percentage of their daily goal caloric intake (P = .05). They also had greater increases in serum prealbumin concentrations (P = .05) than the patients with gastric tube feeding. Although the jejunal tube group had more days of diarrhea (3.3 ± 6.6 vs 1.8 ± 2.9), this difference was not statistically significant. Nosocomial pneumonia was diagnosed clinically in two (10.5%) patients in the gastric tube group and in no patients in the jejunal tube group.

At Detroit Receiving Hospital, we insert jejunostomy feeding tubes into patients with severe head injuries within five days of admission because of the impression that this reduced the likelihood of aspiration of gastric contents. The use of jejunostomy feeding rather than gastric feeding was partly stimulated by the findings of Saxe et al. who showed that patients with severe head injuries have impaired esophageal function, increasing the likelihood of aspiration of gastric contents.[169] There were, however, a number of jejunostomy complications, resulting in the more frequent use of PEGs.

ENTERAL DIETS

The composition of the enteral formula may be an important determinant of its nutritional effect and may ultimately determine the patient's metabolic response to illness and outcome. One of the impor-

tant factors is the amount of nitrogen (protein) present. The increased nitrogen requirements of critically ill patients must be met whether the patient is receiving enteral feedings or TPN. Although a nonprotein-calorie-to-nitrogen ratio of 150:1 is adequate for nonstressed patients, a ratio of 80-100:1 tends to be associated with better nitrogen retention and higher plasma protein levels in critically ill patients.[132]

The types of protein or amino acids given can also be important. Diets containing nitrogen in the form of intact or partially hydrolyzed protein appear to improve nitrogen retention and liver function and lower mortality rates more than free-amino-acid-based diets.[170,171] Peptide-based diets are reported to exhibit significant advantages in critically ill patients.[172] This conclusion has been supported by data showing that experimental protein hydrolysates high in dipeptides and tripeptides are assimilated more efficiently than equivalent free amino acid mixtures.[160] However, this increased efficiency does not extend to peptides larger than tripeptides. Furthermore, difficulty occurs with extrapolation of experimental data to commercial peptide diets that contain primarily medium-chain peptides which require further intraluminal hydrolysis prior to absorption.

NUTRITIONAL MONITORING

One of the major complications of nutritional support is the failure to achieve the desired goals. Several methods for evaluating the patient's nutritional status and for monitoring the response to therapy are available.

AXIOM Most parameters for monitoring nutrition are only estimates, and trends tend to be much more useful than absolute numbers.

History and Physical Examination

The history and physical examination remain the mainstay of nutritional assessment. Pertinent historic information includes a history of any gastrointestinal symptoms or diseases, weight changes, and exercise status. When appropriate, signs and symptoms of specific nutrient deficiencies should be obtained (Tables 38–7, 38–8).

Anthropometric Measurements

Commonly used anthropometric measurements, such as midarm circumference (MAC), skin fold thickness (SFT), and arm muscle area (AMA), reflect skeletal mass and the amount of fat present. In the absence of edema or ascites, gradual weight changes can be an important indicator of altered lean body mass. An absolute weight loss exceeding 10 pounds has been associated with increased mortality in surgical patients.[1] Because of the increased extracellular water accumulated by critically ill patients, a large variance in their anthropometric characteristics occurs, making these measurements of little use.

Chemical Studies

Chemistry studies reflecting lean body mass primarily involve measurements of nitrogen balance and 3-methylhistidine.

NITROGEN BALANCE

Serial every-other-day or twice weekly nitrogen balance determinations are probably the most reliable, readily available, short-term method for ascertaining the adequacy of nutritional support. Nitrogen balance is calculated as nitrogen intake minus nitrogen output from all sources. Nitrogen intake is relatively easy to calculate with enteral or intravenous feeding. Approximately 1 g of nitrogen is provided by every 6.25 g of protein or amino acids given. Nitrogen output includes stool losses (1-2 g/day in the absence of gastrointestinal disease), skin losses (0.1-0.4 g/m² per day), and urinary losses. Urinary nitrogen consists of several components, including urea, uric

TABLE 38–11 *Causes and Treatment Options to Consider When Patients Develop Diarrhea After Receiving Enteral Products*

Cause	Recommendations
Intestinal mucosal atrophy	Prevent with early enteral feeding; use low-fat, hypotonic diets with partially hydrolyzed protein and oligosaccharides
Excess tonicity of feedings	Avoid elemental diets; reduce the rate of diet progression
Antibiotic-induced colitis	Discontinue antibiotics; Flagyl® for C. difficile, cholestyramine, or Kaopectate®
Lactase deficiency	Avoid lactose in feedings

acid, ammonia, amino acids, and creatinine. Urea usually accounts for 80-90% of urinary nitrogen, but may account for as little as 65-70% in patients with severe stress. In such patients, direct measurements of total urinary nitrogen (TUN) may provide a much more accurate estimate of urinary nitrogen losses than the UUN plus a standard correction factor.

Nitrogen excretion in the absence of abnormal skin or stool losses can be calculated by

$$N_{out} = TUN + 2$$

or

$$N_{out} = UUN (1.2) + 2$$

or

$$N_{out} = UUN + 4$$

In most patients, the total unmeasured nonurea nitrogen losses from the urine, skin, and feces add up to about 4.0 g/day. Unfortunately, this calculation may lead to significant errors in highly catabolic patients because the nonurea N_2 losses in the urine will be increased.[173]

Corrections must be made for increases in the BUN. Because urea diffuses readily in and out of cells, total body content changes are calculated in terms of the total body water, which is assumed to be 60% of the body weight. Thus, a 10 mg/dL rise in the BUN in a 70 kg mass is equivalent to a $(70)(0.6)(10)(10) = 4200$ mg (4.2 g) loss of N_2 from the lean body mass.

Measurements of urinary nitrogen require complete sample collection, ideally over 24 hours. The adequacy of the sample collection can partially be confirmed by the simultaneous measurement of urinary creatinine. Total urine creatinine excretion per day should be about 1500 mg in a normal adult male and 1000-1200 mg in a normal adult female. However, in severe sepsis, it may decrease to 300-600 mg per day.

Assessing nitrogen excretion can be very difficult in the patients with excessive gastrointestinal losses. Burn patients are particularly susceptible to errors in the estimation of nitrogen losses because of unmeasured protein losses through the open burn wound. However, one can collect stool and/or dressings for nitrogen measurements. These losses appear to be greatest in the first week after injury and have been estimated as follows:

Burn Surface Protein Loss (24 hr) = 1.2 × BSA × % BSAB where the protein loss is expressed in grams, body surface area (BSA) is in square meters, and the body surface area burn (BSAB) is in percent.[174] Thus, a patient with a BSA of 1.8 m^2 and a 50% burn would have 108 g of protein loss per day from the burn wound. This would be equivalent to 17.3 g of N_2 per day. Balance studies are also less accurate in renal failure. However, as noted above, changes in total body urea nitrogen can be calculated from changes in the BUN and estimated total body water.

3-METHYLHISTIDINE

3-Methylhistidine is an amino acid that comes only from skeletal muscle. It is excreted unchanged in the urine and therefore reflects the rate of muscle proteolysis. Excretion tends to be increased in patients with larger lean body mass, greater stress, and poor nutritional intake. However, renal failure can inhibit the rate of 3-methylhistidine excretion.[1]

CHEMICAL ANALYSES ASSESSING HEPATIC PROTEIN SYNTHESIS

Chemical analyses used to assess hepatic protein synthesis include serum albumin, transferrin, thyroxine binding prealbumin, and retinol-binding protein. These studies can be reasonably reliable as nutritional indices; however, they are affected to some extent by the state of hydration and by abnormal gastrointestinal or urinary losses.

Albumin

Albumin is a plasma protein containing 575 amino acids with a molecular weight of about 65,000 daltons. It is highly water soluble and has a strong negative charge (19 at pH 7.4). Its negative charge is largely responsible for the Donnan effect, causing colloid oncotic pressure (COP) of the plasma to be about 50% greater than that caused by plasma protein alone. Serum proteins—of which albumin accounts for at least 62%—are responsible for 28 mm Hg in COP, with 19 mm Hg contributed by proteins and 9 mm Hg contributed by cations held in the plasma by the Donnan effect.

Albumin is contained in a large body pool (4-5 g/kg). In stress, plasma levels may decrease precipitously, but the total body content is often unchanged. Serum albumin levels are also decreased in nephrosis, enteropathies, hepatic failure, dialysis, uremia, burn wounds, and acute blood volume expansion. They may be increased by dehydration and by increased cortisol or anabolic hormones, such as growth hormone, insulin, and estrogens.

Because of its long half-life (20-21 days), its plasma levels respond slowly to therapy. When given intravenously, equilibration of the albumin with the interstitial fluid space may occur within the first several minutes. Subsequent loss from the vascular compartment is slow, with complete distribution between the intraplasma and extraplasma compartments normally occurring within 7-10 days. Proteins, including albumin, are the only dissolved substances in the plasma and interstitial fluid that normally do not diffuse easily through the capillary membrane. When they do diffuse through the capillary membrane, proteins are returned to the vascular space via the lymphatic system.

We have noted for many years that critically or injured patients who were able to maintain higher hemoglobin and albumin levels tended to do better than those with lower values, even with comparable degrees of injury. Higher albumin levels may be particularly important in patients with cirrhosis. Burr et al. studied 200 patients admitted within one year of onset of a spinal cord lesion.[175] The main determinant of length of stay was the level of the spinal cord lesion and whether it was complete or incomplete. Within these categories, the length of stay was increased in patients in whom anemia or hypoalbuminemia occurred. Although the causes of the anemia and hypoalbuminemia were not always evident, sepsis and malnutrition were probably factors, and efforts at recognizing and treating the cause of anemia or hypoalbuminemia may be expected to shorten the time required for rehabilitation.

Transferrin

Transferrin is present in smaller quantities (250-300 mg/dl) than albumin and it has a shorter half-life (8-10 days); therefore, it is a more sensitive indicator of the patient's nutritional status. However, transferrin is also adversely affected as a nutritional indicator by the same variables as albumin. In addition, iron deficiency can lead to elevations in transferrin levels.

Prealbumin

Thyroxine-binding prealbumin levels are normally 22 ± 7 mg/dl and it has a short half-life (2 days). Therefore, it is a sensitive indicator of nutritional status. However, it is also affected by the state of hydration. In addition, low levels are seen in hyperthyroidism, cystic fibrosis, chronic illness, and acute stress.

Retinol-binding Protein

Retinol-binding protein is a specific carrier involved in vitamin A transport, and it is linked with thyroxine-binding prealbumin in a constant molar ratio. It has a very short half-life (12 hours) and is very sensitive to synthesis and utilization changes. Normal serum levels are 5.1 ± 2.5 mg/dl and these levels rise in patients with renal disease and excess vitamin A administration. Blood levels are reduced in liver disease, cystic fibrosis, hyperthyroidism, and vitamin A deficiency.

Tests of Immune Competence

A number of tests of immune competence have been described as nutritional indices. However, all of them can be affected by a variety of conditions other than nutritional status and interpretation of results can be difficult.

SKIN TEST ANTIGENS

AXIOM Anergy to recall skin test antigens can be caused by radiation, malignancy, infection, steroids, chemotherapy, collagen vascular diseases, and recent surgery or trauma.

At least four antigens should be used simultaneously to perform skin testing for standard recall antigens; a positive test (i.e., not anergic) is 5 mm of induration at 48-72 hours. Commonly used skin test antigens are PPD, Candida, mumps, and trichophyton. Failure to respond positively to any of the four antigens is referred to as "anergy."

When anergy is found more than 3-4 days after acute surgery or trauma, the patient is either septic or very likely to become septic. In a report by Meakins et al., over 50% of anergic patients became septic and a high percentage died.[176] Responding positively to only one of four antigens is referred to as "relative anergy" and is almost as bad as anergy. A positive response to two or more antigens usually indicates normal immune competence.

Protein-sparing nutrition can improve the postoperative host resistance seen in many patients.[177] Valuable information can be obtained by checking these skin tests weekly in patients with marginal nutrition or possible sepsis.

ABSOLUTE LYMPHOCYTE COUNT

Absolute lymphocyte count (ALC) is probably more reliable than skin testing as an indicator of nutritional status. Normally, the ALC is > 2000-2500/mm^3. An ALC < 1500/mm^3 is believed to reflect moderate malnutrition, whereas an ALC < 800/mm^3 can reflect anergy and/or severe malnutrition. The ALC is also adversely affected by sepsis, steroids, neoplasia, and transplant immunosuppression.

Monitoring Nutritional Therapy

Serum electrolytes (Na$^+$, K$^+$, Cl$^-$, HCO$_3^-$) are measured daily for the first week of nutritional support and less often during long-term therapy in stable patients. Magnesium and phosphorus should be checked twice weekly initially and less often during long-term therapy.

Glucose is checked every 6 hours initially and after increases or decreases in the rate of TPN or enteral formulas. Patients with poorly controlled diabetes may warrant glucose levels two to four times daily; however, when glucose tolerance is not a problem, glucose levels can be obtained at the same intervals as electrolytes.

Liver function tests (bilirubin, alkaline phosphatase, SGOT, and SGPT) and serum albumin should be obtained once or twice weekly. Monthly checks are probably adequate in the setting of long-term nutritional support.

In the acute setting, 24-hour urine collections for nitrogen balance should be obtained twice weekly until positive nitrogen balance is obtained.

Indirect calorimetry should be done at least once or twice weekly until the appropriate nutritional prescription is determined. In hypermetabolic surgical patients, an RQ of 0.80-0.85 suggests utilization of an appropriate mixed fuel source. An RQ of 0.6-0.7 suggests an erroneous measurement or an inadequate caloric intake and the utilization of endogenous fat. An RQ of 1.0 or greater suggests overfeeding, particularly with carbohydrates.

Prothrombin time (PT) should be obtained weekly in the acute setting to monitor the adequacy of vitamin K administration.

Serum triglycerides are checked before and 6 hours after a test dose of triglycerides (usually 500 mL of 10% intralipid) and then weekly unless increased doses of fat, increased sepsis, or abnormal liver function test suggests a need for more frequent monitoring.

ORGAN-SPECIFIC NUTRIENT SUPPORT

Pulmonary Failure

Excess calories, and particularly carbohydrate calories, are associated with an increase in CO$_2$ production that may be clinically significant in patients with compromised pulmonary function. This excess CO$_2$ production can be decreased by providing up to 50% of the nonprotein calories as fat. The oxidation of fat produces much more energy per molecule of CO$_2$ produced than does carbohydrate. To minimize CO$_2$ production, excess carbohydrate calories, as indicated by an RQ exceeding 1.0, should be avoided.

At the opposite extreme, excess intake of currently available fat preparations, particularly when given intravenously, has been associated with a number of potentially detrimental effects with regard to immune and pulmonary function. Excess serum chylomicrons are believed to be cleared by macrophages, and lipid-laden macrophages appear to have decreased phagocytic function, potentially limiting the capacity of pulmonary and other macrophages to clear bacteria and inflammatory debris.

Excessive doses of intravenous fat have also been associated with a number of abnormalities of in vitro tests of immune function, suggesting that they may predispose the host to infection and further pulmonary compromise.[105,106,178,179] It has been found that the omega-6 fatty acids in our current plant oil fat emulsions for intravenous use are substrates for the formation of inflammatory mediators. These mediators, especially prostaglandins and leukotrienes, may contribute significantly to systemic inflammatory response characteristic of severe stress. In addition to a systemic inflammatory response, prostaglandins and leukotrienes may contribute to aberrations in blood flow within the lung, thereby increasing ventilation/perfusion mismatching.[101]

Hepatic Failure

The utility of specific nutritional formulations in patients with hepatic failure, particularly those with hepatic encephalopathy, is controversial. Levels of ammonia, presumably formed from excess dietary protein and/or blood in the intestinal tract, frequently do not correlate with the degree of hepatic encephalopathy.

Encephalopathy in cirrhosis may be partially accounted for by accumulation of methionine and aromatic amino acids (tyrosine, phenylalanine) in the plasma and central nervous system (CNS). Because the liver is the major organ system responsible for clearing these amino acids, an increase in the plasma concentration due to hepatic insufficiency encourages transport across the blood-brain barrier. It has been hypothesized that the resultant excess of aromatic amino acids in the CNS may then serve as precursors for the formation of false neurotransmitters, such as octopamine, which can induce encephalopathy.[180]

Although this amino acid pattern has not consistently been shown to correlate with the degree of encephalopathy, abrupt increases in the levels of aromatic amino acids occur during the terminal phases of hepatic failure. Administration of BCAA may overcome this process by competing for transport systems common to both aromatic and branched-chain amino acids. Another benefit of BCAA may be a concomitant stimulation of hepatic protein synthesis. This would be expected to improve production of host defense proteins and presumably also improve outcome.

The association of excessive dietary protein intake with hepatic encephalopathy leads to attempts to alter hepatic encephalopathy with dietary manipulation. In addition to attempts at gut decontamination with lactulose or nonabsorbable antibiotics, therapy in the past frequently included protein restriction. However, a multicenter, prospective, double-blind, randomized trial demonstrated that the provision of adequate glucose and amino acids enriched with BCAAs and deficient in methionine and aromatic amino acids is superior to a diet containing adequate glucose calories alone in improving hepatic encephalopathy.[181] Although this study confirmed the need for adequate nutrition, including protein, in patients with hepatic encephalopathy, it is less clear whether a specific hepatic nutritional formulation is better than standard nutritional formulation in the treatment or prevention of hepatic encephalopathy.

In a more recent study comparing a formula similar to the one described above (high-branched-chain, low-aromatic amino acids) to an isocaloric, isonitrogenous nutritional formulation containing standard amino acids, there was no difference in terms of subjective or objective measures of encephalopathy, despite the expected reduction in plasma aromatic amino acids and increase in BCAAs in the experimental group.[182] In another controlled, double-blind cross-over study, the effects of oral BCAA supplementation on latent or subclinical hepatic encephalopathy demonstrated significant improvement in psychometric tests as compared to patients receiving isonitrogenous casein supplements.[183]

Adequate nutrition, including amino acids, is needed in patients with hepatic insufficiency. It is less clear whether specialized formulas enriched with BCAAs and deficient in aromatic amino acids are more beneficial than those with standard amino acids. To many physicians, use of the specialized formulations, such as Hepatamine® or Hepatic-Aid®, in patients with hepatic insufficiency and the characteristic plasma amino acid profile may be appropriate. However, no clinical data demonstrate that BCAA preparations offer any significant advantages over standard amino acid preparations for this problem.

Renal Failure

Isolated renal failure is typically treated with protein restriction. However, the catabolic nature of severe trauma and sepsis usually demands an increased protein intake in order to avoid acute protein malnutrition. Furthermore, the occurrence of oliguric renal failure imposes marked constraints on the use of conventional feeding approaches because of fluid volume and electrolyte restrictions.

Traditional management of acute oliguric renal failure consists of infusing highly concentrated (35-50%) dextrose solutions with a high-calorie-to-nitrogen ratio (350/1) in order to limit fluid intake and reduce the rate of BUN accumulation.[25] The caloric intake goal is determined by the estimated or measured MEE. Protein intake can be gradually increased up to 1.0-1.5 g/kg/day when BUN can be maintained < 80 mg/dl.

The use of essential amino acids as a means to control the rate of BUN rise has been reported to be advantageous;[134] however, this approach remains controversial. In a 1980 report, a selected group of patients with renal failure were treated with dextrose and a mixture of essential and nonessential amino acids. These findings were compared to two groups of patients who had been treated either with essential amino acids and dextrose or with dextrose alone 5 years previously.[184,185] Mortality was 91% in the group receiving mixed amino acids and 35% in patients receiving the essential amino acid formula. However, several animal and human studies since then failed to show a benefit of essential amino acids.[186,187] In another controlled study published in 1981, no survival benefit was identified either with TPN containing essential and nonessential amino acids or with TPN containing essential amino acids alone.[188]

> **AXIOM** Although providing adequate protein is important in the nutritional support of surgical patients with acute oliguric renal failure, there is no obvious benefit to providing only essential amino acids.

In spite of the essential amino acid controversy, aggressive nutritional support is indicated to support protein synthesis and maintain nitrogen balance in patients with renal failure. It should also be remembered that in most situations, nutritional support of the hyper-

metabolic patient in renal failure should not be curtailed in an effort to reduce the need for dialysis.

> **AXIOM** Dialysis should be performed as often as needed to allow optimal nutritional support.

Hemodialysis, which can add significant physiologic stress, such as hypotension, is often required in patients with severe, acute oliguric renal failure. However, nutritional efforts in patients on hemodialysis often does not provide the target protein intake required for critically ill patients.

The use of another technique, known as continuous arteriovenous hemofiltration (CAVH), has been shown to be a useful method for managing the metabolic and nutritional difficulties associated with renal failure.[189] Standard substrate concentrations and volumes of TPN may be infused into patients undergoing CAVH because excess extracellular fluid, urea nitrogen, and electrolytes are continuously removed by ultrafiltration. Significantly, the desired protein intake for critically ill patients can usually be attained using this technique.

SPECIALIZED NUTRIENTS

Over the last decade, numerous, specialized nutrient supplements have been recommended in an effort to address specific disease processes or to influence host immune function. These supplements include specific amino acids, nucleic acids, and omega-3 fatty acids.

Glutamine

Glutamine is a nonessential amino acid that has received much attention because it is believed to serve a critical role in sustaining intestinal architecture and mucosal barrier function. Because bacterial translocation is currently viewed as an important mechanism contributing to multiple organ dysfunction in critically ill patients, agents that may inhibit this process are viewed as potentially therapeutic. Glutamine is believed to be the principal energy source for the gut and an important nutrient for enterocyte replication. Because the total body glutamine pool declines following injury and sepsis, it has been postulated that this nutrient may become "conditionally essential" and provision of additional quantities of the amino acid may be beneficial.[190] Glutamine-supplemented TPN solutions have been shown to inhibit intestinal mucosal and functional atrophy and to reduce the bacterial translocation that occurs when standard TPN (which is glutamine-free) is used in animal models.[191,192]

Glutamine also can have beneficial effects upon nonintestinal tissues. Experimental studies showed that it can inhibit skeletal muscle proteolysis and stimulate protein synthesis. Glutamine is also essential for proper lymphocyte proliferation in vitro.[193] Because of its apparent wide-ranging importance, some enteral products are supplemented with free glutamine. Intravenous nutrient solutions are currently glutamine-free because of its instability in solution. Studies are now underway to circumvent this problem by supplementing TPN solutions with glutamine-containing dipeptides that are stable in aqueous media.[194,195]

Arginine

The amino acid arginine has been shown experimentally to improve protein synthesis, wound healing, and immune function when it is provided as a nutritional supplement.[196] Arginine is normally considered to be a nonessential amino acid in mature mammals. However, under conditions of immaturity or severe stress, arginine becomes necessary for adequate nitrogen balance. Arginine supplements to postoperative feeding programs improve nitrogen balance compared to isonitrogenous nonarginine-containing diets.[197] Arginine also improves host immunity in the postoperative state as evidenced by: (a) less severe depression and earlier return to normal of peripheral T lymphocyte mitogen stimulation responses after trauma, and (b) greater expression of the T helper cell phenotype.[197] Arginine has also enhanced collagen synthesis and has increased wound strength in human studies.[196-198]

Animal studies have demonstrated similar positive effects. Arginine attenuates the involution of the rodent thymus gland which usually occurs following trauma. This effect is associated with preservation of the lymphocyte content and function within the gland.[199] Animals treated with arginine are better able to withstand septic and traumatic (burn) injuries compared to untreated controls.[200,201]

Human studies exploring the metabolic benefits of arginine have required doses in the range of 500 mg/kg/day, and these are much greater than those apt to be seen clinically.[196] This has suggested that the effects of arginine do not simply reflect replenishment of a relative amino acid deficiency. Some studies showed that arginine stimulates secretion of pituitary growth hormone, prolactin, insulinlike growth factor 1 (IGF-1), insulin, and glucagon.[197] Increased growth hormone, insulin, and IGF-1 could account for the anabolic responses to arginine administration, and the increased secretion of prolactin—which has immune regulatory properties—could account for some of the immunostimulating actions of arginine. Additional arginine effects include stimulation of polyamine and cyclic guanosine monophosphate synthesis.[196]

Nucleic Acids

Nucleic acids are another group of nutrients that may exert favorable immunomodulating effects upon the host.[202,203] The specific elements that appear to be responsible for these effects include purine and pyrimidine bases of ribonucleic (RNA) and deoxyribonucleic acid (DNA). Although these bases are normally not essential for growth, dietary supplementation may be of benefit when host immunity is depressed.

Experimental studies have indicated that dietary nucleotide deprivation enhances survival of cardiac allografts in rodents, especially when pharmacologic immunosuppression is superimposed.[202] In addition, animal models of infection exhibited a lowered resistance to bacterial and fungal infections when their diets were nucleotide-free. Correspondingly, indices of delayed hypersensitivity, macrophage function, and mortality are improved when supplemental RNA or uracil is provided.[203] This dependence upon exogenous nucleotides for proper immune function appears to be most characteristic of tissues, such as lymphocytes and intestinal cells, that are metabolically hyperactive or exhibit rapid turnover.[203] These findings suggested that supplemental nucleic acids in enteral diets may improve host-defense responses in critically ill patients.

Omega-3 Fatty Acids

Experimental studies have shown that diets supplemented with omega-3 fatty acids improve a variety of nutritional indices and immune responses. Following burn injury, diets containing fish oil appear to preserve weight and transferrin levels better, result in lower metabolic rates, and provide better cell-mediated immune responses than those containing omega-6 fatty acids from plant oils. Dietary restriction of linoleic acid and supplementation with fish oil also attenuates the increases in thromboxane A_2 and prostacyclin usually seen after experimental sepsis, thereby attenuating potentially noxious inflammatory mediator responses[204,205] (Figure 38–12). Clinical studies evaluating omega-3 fatty acids alone, however, are extremely limited. Because these lipids have been combined with several other immune-modulating supplements in commercially available diets, it is difficult to discern the specific roles of individual agents.

Combinations

The clinical and experimental studies demonstrating benefits derived from various nutrient supplements have culminated in the development of enteral preparations containing these specific substrates.

Preliminary studies indicate that Impact®, an enteral preparation containing added arginine, nucleic acids, and omega-3 fatty acids, can improve immune responses and reduce infectious and wound complications compared to unsupplemented, standard enteral formulation.[206]

In 1992, Bower et al. reported the effects of an enteral formula fortified with arginine, RNA, and omega-3 fatty acids (Impact®) on LOS in ICU patients compared to a control formula (Osmolite HN®).[207] This prospective, randomized, double-blind multi-site study included 326 adult ICU patients with APACHE II $\geq$ 10 and/or TISS $\geq$ 20 who were entered within 48 hours of injury or septic event and required 7 days of enteral nutrition. Both groups tolerated administration of their diets well. No significant difference occurred in mortality between the groups, but a trend did exist toward a shorter LOS in the Impact group. Of the patients who met the requirements for study completion, the LOS of the Impact group (25.3 days) was 29% less than for Osmolite HN® (35.6 days; P = 0.038). The incidence of most infectious complications was lower in the Impact group, but this difference was significant only for urinary tract infections (P = 0.005). However, the subgroup of patients who were fed 7 or more days with Impact and had complications had a decreased LOS from the onset of the infectious complication to discharge. This difference (23 versus 34 days) was significant for those who had pneumonia (P = 0.02). Thus, although it did not reduce the incidence of all complications, Impact did reduce the LOS from the onset of pneumonia to discharge.

In a recent study, Brown et al. compared selected nutritional and immunologic markers and infection in trauma patients receiving a specialized enteral formula with those receiving standard enteral therapy.[208] Nineteen patients fed the specialized enteral formula received supplemental arginine, linolenic acid, betacarotene, and hydrolyzed protein for up to 10 days. Eighteen control patients received standard enteral nutrition. The patients who received the specialized formula had fewer infections (3 of 19 vs 10 of 18; P < 0.05), better nitrogen balance, higher C-reactive protein levels, and greater increases in the CD4:CD8 ratio.

Xylitol

Schricker et al. noted that xylitol may help to achieve the two major goals of TPN after trauma and during sepsis: (a) reduced protein catabolism, (b) avoidance of hyperglycemia, and (c) decreased hepatic gluconeogenesis.[209] The authors had previously noted that, after trauma and during sepsis, whole-body glucose metabolism is reduced while the utilization of xylitol is more than doubled. In order to investigate whether these differences were associated with beneficial effects on hepatic glucose production and protein sparing, two animal and two clinical studies were conducted.

In burned rats, Schricker et al. demonstrated that hypocaloric xylitol, in contrast to glucose, significantly reduced hepatic glucose production and gluconeogenesis from three-carbon molecules.[209] In septic rats, exchange of glucose calories with xylitol in a proportion of 1:1 was associated with a significantly reduced nitrogen and 3-methyl-histidine excretion. In studies of surgical ICU patients, the authors were able to confirm these nitrogen-sparing properties of xylitol. Hepatic glucose production and urea synthesis rates were significantly reduced during xylitol infusion after trauma, whereas equicaloric glucose had no effects. In septic patients, xylitol led to significantly lower lactate concentrations and gluconeogenesis rates than did isocaloric glucose.

Thus, Schricker et al. showed that, in animal and human studies, hypocaloric xylitol and a 1:1 mixture of glucose/xylitol were more efficient in preserving body protein than glucose alone.[209] Hepatic gluconeogenesis was significantly reduced by xylitol when compared to isocaloric glucose. Therefore, they recommended, during the acute phase of trauma, carbohydrate supplementation with 3 g/kg BW/d of xylitol. During long-term TPN, they recommended a glucose/xylitol mixture (1:1) of 6 g/kg/d together with amino acids and, if necessary, lipids.

COMPLICATIONS OF NUTRITIONAL SUPPORT

Failure to Set and/or Achieve Therapeutic Endpoints

AXIOM The most important complication of nutritional support is failure to set and/or achieve therapeutic endpoints.

Nutritional support is expensive and not without risk; to provide this therapy in a haphazard fashion, without appropriate goals or monitoring to ensure successful therapy, is not appropriate. The general goals of nutritional support are to support the lean body mass and the function of individual organs. However, more specific goals may include the establishment of a slightly positive (2-3 g/day) nitrogen balance with an RQ of about 0.83. Nitrogen balance requires administration of adequate quantities of amino acids and nonprotein calories. The appropriateness of the caloric intake can be assessed by indirect calorimetry.

Mechanical and Technical Complications

INTRAVENOUS FEEDING

For parenteral nutrition, acute complications relate to the placement of central venous catheters and include arterial injury, pneumothorax, hemothorax, and hydrothorax. In addition, catheters can erode through vessel walls, causing hydrothorax or hydropericardium. In experienced hands, the incidence of these complications ranges 2% or less. The major long-term complication of central venous catheterization is infection, and strict attention must be paid to sterile technique at insertion and during routine catheter care and dressing changes. When possible, blood should not be drawn through these catheters.

Thrombosis of the catheter after several days is not unusual, but can be prevented or retarded by flushing with heparin or by adding some heparin to intravenous solutions. If a symptomatic thrombosis of a subclavian or innominate vein occurs, local thrombolytic therapy may be effective.

ENTERAL NUTRITION

Mechanical complications of enteral nutritional support are primarily related to placement and long-term maintenance of feeding tubes and aspiration of gastric contents into the lungs. Tubes placed nasally can be associated with excess pulmonary secretions, pharyngeal irritation, sinusitis, otitis media, and pressure ulcers of the nasal ala. These problems are most common with stiffer polyethylene nasogastric tubes, but occasionally warrant the removal of even soft feeding catheters. Improper placement of feeding tubes, particularly into the lungs, can lead to catastrophic problems.

AXIOM The placement of feeding tubes should be confirmed radiographically before feeding is initiated.

The incidence of aspiration may be as high as 40% with gastric feedings. This can be minimized by elevating the head of the bed at least 30° at all times and by frequently checking for gastric distention and high gastric residuals. Many of these complications can be avoided by operatively placed jejunostomy feeding tubes, although intraperitoneal leaks around such a tube may be catastrophic.

AXIOM Aspiration of gastric contents and enteral feedings, especially in neurologically impaired patients, can be greatly reduced by keeping the patient's head elevated and feeding through jejunostomy catheters.

One of the most troublesome problems seen in small-caliber nasojejunal or needle-catheter jejunostomy tubes is clogging of the lumen. Crushed medications can be a major cause of occluded tubes. A number of remedies for clogged tubes have been proposed, including flushing with solutions of meat tenderizer, streptokinase, or carbonated soft drinks; however, the best treatment is prevention.

Substrate Intolerance

Substrate intolerance with intravenous feeding may include chills, fever, sweating, cyanosis, dizziness, and headache. These are more likely to occur with intravenous fat administration.

The development of gastrointestinal symptoms, such as bloating, cramping, or diarrhea as a result of enteral nutrition, are usually related primarily to the osmolarity of the formula or to inappropriate rates of administration (Table 38–10). Diarrhea may complicate nutritional therapy in over 25% of patients on enteral feedings. The problem can often be avoided by gradual increases in formula concentration and infusion rates. Excess fat, hyperosmolar feeding formulas, and lactose intolerance can also predispose to diarrhea and cramping. Chronic malnutrition with gut mucosal atrophy, short gut syndromes, and pancreatic insufficiency may also contribute to the problem.

Lactose intolerance or difficulties with osmolarity can often be corrected with a change in formula. Pancreatic insufficiency may respond to commercially available pancreatic enzymes given four times daily.

PITFALL ⊘

Assuming that all diarrhea developing when enteral feeding is begun is due to the enteral feeding rather than more serious problems.

In critically ill patients with diarrhea, infectious causes, especially pseudomembranous enterocolitis due to overgrowth of Clostridium difficile, should be ruled out, particularly in patients who have received broad-spectrum antibiotics. Stool analyses should be performed in these patients. The presence of fecal leukocytes suggests an infectious etiology and warrants evaluation, which should include stool cultures for pathogens, such as Clostridium difficile, Campylobacter, and Yersenia. Serologic tests should also be done for C. difficile toxin. Sigmoidoscopy to identify pseudomembranous colitis may also be warranted.

Bacterial contamination of the feeding formula is a potential cause of diarrhea, but it is rarely a problem when manufacturers' recommendations are observed.

When all correctable causes of diarrhea have been ruled out or treated, antidiarrheal therapy is appropriate. Lomotil® or Imodium® can be quite effective, but such drugs are contraindicated with C. difficile enterocolitis. Bulk-forming agents, such as Metamucil®, may decrease stool liquidity, but they do not alter fluid and electrolyte losses. When antidiarrheals are used, they should be given on a regular basis to prevent diarrhea rather than merely to treat it.

Metabolic Complications

WATER BALANCE

Disturbances in water balance due to intravenous feedings are most commonly due to excess free-water, as reflected by hyponatremia, hypoproteinemia, and anemia. The etiology is related not only to fluid in the form of nutrition, but also to fluids given with medications and "keep-open" IVs. Lipid infusions may also contribute to water excess when 10% solutions are used instead of 20% solutions.[206]

Problems with fluid overload are encountered less frequently in enterally fed patients. Enteral feeding is more apt to cause volume depletion, as reflected by hypernatremia, prerenal azotemia, and hemoconcentration. These are most commonly seen in patients who also have abnormal fluid losses, such as in burns, large open wounds, or gastrointestinal problems.

ELECTROLYTE ABNORMALITIES

Electrolyte abnormalities occur during nutritional support, but they tend to be less frequent and less severe when nutrition is managed by special teams. In one report, electrolyte imbalance occurred in 36% and pH disturbances in 19% of 164 patients given TPN by a variety of physicians, whereas similar complications occurred in only 3% of 211 patients managed by a nutrition support service.[210]

Sodium

Hyponatremia in spite of an excess of total body sodium (as reflected by edema, ascites, and fluid overload) occurs frequently in critically ill patients as the result of the initial resuscitation and the hormonal changes associated with trauma and sepsis. This hyponatremia is usually dilutional, and may be due to a number of factors which include: prolonged administration of hypotonic fluids; cardiac, renal, or liver disease; or the syndrome of inappropriate antidiuretic hormone secretion (SIADH). Hypernatremia is most common in infants and comatose individuals who cannot respond to normal thirst by drinking. However, water depletion may be precipitated by diabetes insipidus, diuretics, and inadequate water in nutritional formulations.

Potassium

Potassium needs are increased during TPN, particularly when glucose is the primary caloric source. Increased potassium is also needed during protein synthesis.[138] Diuretics and high urinary outputs can cause severe potassium losses, usually with at least 30-40 mEq of potassium in each liter of urine. Hyperkalemia may be precipitated by renal failure or by acidosis, whereas alkalosis tends to be associated with hypokalemia.

Phosphate

Hypophosphatemia is one of the more common electrolyte abnormalities associated with intravenous feeding, and it occurs in up to 30% of patients.[211,212] Adequate phosphorus is required for the attainment of nitrogen balance; without adequate phosphate supplementation, hypophosphatemia can develop within 48 hours of institution of TPN.[213]

Hyperphosphatemia is most commonly associated with renal failure, but it may also be associated with the use of 10% solutions of intravenous fat as a result of the phosphorous content of the solution.[206]

Magnesium

Magnesium deficiency can be precipitated by excess gastrointestinal losses, alcoholism, diuretic use, and rapid protein anabolism. Symptoms of hypomagnesemia are similar to those of hypocalcemia and include perioral tingling, positive Trousseau's sign, and tetany. Unfortunately, a discrepancy often occurs between serum magnesium levels and total body content.[214] Hypomagnesemia is often not seen until a moderate-to-severe total body magnesium deficiency is present.

AXIOM Total body magnesium may be quite low and serum levels can still be normal.

Hypermagnesemia occurs most often in the setting of renal failure and may lead to weakness, nausea and vomiting, and cardiac arrhythmias.

Calcium

Abnormalities of serum calcium are unusual as a complication of nutritional support alone. Total calcium levels are frequently low in critically ill patients because of hypoalbuminemia. However, ionic hypocalcemia is uncommon unless the patient is septic or hypotensive.[215] Bone stores of calcium are extremely large and serum ionized calcium levels tend to be maintained at the expense of bone decalcification.

PROBLEMS RELATED TO GLUCOSE

Hyperglycemia

Hyperglycemia in stressed patients is one of the most common complications of TPN administration, occurring in at least 25% of non-diabetic patients. Hyperglycemia can occur with both parenteral and enteral nutritional support, but complications of hyperglycemia, such as hyperosmolar states, are much more common with TPN.[211,213]

Hyperglycemic complications with intravenous glucose for TPN are particularly common in patients who are septic because the hepatic gluconeogenesis appears to be relatively nonsuppressible. In fasting nonstressed humans, hepatic gluconeogenesis can be readily suppressed by moderate doses (4 mg/kg/min) of exogenous glucose. In contrast, septic patients exhibit only partial inhibition of liver glucose output during such infusions.[98] Consequently, blood glucose levels are usually higher in septic patients due to the continued influx of endogenous glucose into the total body glucose pool.[98,99]

Liver Dysfunction

TPN-induced liver dysfunction has been attributed primarily to deposition of fat in hepatocytes resulting from high-glucose loads. At infusion rates of 4-8 mg/kg/min, only 50% of the glucose given is actually oxidized, and much of the remainder is converted into fat, a portion of which is deposited in the liver.[99] As glucose administration rates approach and exceed 5 mg/kg/min in injured patients, an increasing proportion of patients will have RQs > 1.0, indicating that the administered glucose is being directed into fat production rather than being used as a metabolic fuel.[99,216]

Increased CO_2 Production

AXIOM RQ values > 1.0 usually indicate an excessive carbohydrate intake.

The additional carbon dioxide derived from increased fat synthesis during high rates of glucose infusion may contribute to increased minute ventilation to maintain a normal blood CO_2 level. Consequently, a further increase in total body oxygen consumption occurs due to the increased effort of breathing. The potential for inducing respiratory failure also exists in patients with marginal pulmonary function. Although the relative contribution of this mechanism to respiratory insufficiency in critically ill patients is probably minimal, it may be significant in the patients with severe COPD or ARDS. In such patients, intravenous fat emulsions are increasingly used to provide a portion of the nonnitrogen caloric support.

PITFALL ⊘

A purely glucose-based nutritional support program may increase oxygen consumption (VO_2) and arterial PCO_2, increasing ventilatory demands and retarding weaning of patients from assisted mechanical ventilation.

LIPIDS

Complications related to lipid administration can result from both inadequate fat intake and excessive fat intake. When no lipids or lipids lacking long-chain fatty acids are given, essential fatty acid deficiency may develop in 4 weeks in starving patients.[1] In stressed patients receiving large amounts of glucose, hyperinsulinemia tends to suppress lipolysis. This can prevent mobilization of endogenous essential fatty acids, leading to clinical essential fatty acid deficiency in as little 10 days. Medium-change triglycerides, which can only be given enterally, can also cause essential fatty acid deficiencies.

Signs of essential fatty acid deficiency include malabsorption, diarrhea, dry skin, coarse hair, brittle nails, impaired wound healing, thrombocytopenia, hemolytic anemia, and increased capillary permeability.[213] Prevention of the problem involves administering lipids on a twice weekly basis. Toxic and/or allergic reactions have on rare occasions been associated with intravenous lipid infusions and include headache, dizziness, flushing, sweating, and cyanosis. These symptoms can be minimized with slower lipid infusion rates.

AMINO ACIDS

Problems resulting from protein or amino acid administration are primarily related to production of excess nitrogenous wastes. In critically ill patients, prerenal azotemia resulting from amino acid administration, increased muscle catabolism, and volume depletion from other causes is not unusual and may lead to osmotic diuresis, dehydration, and death. Prevention includes adequate hydration and limiting amino acid infusions to the amount required for attaining nitrogen balance.

Hepatobiliary Complications

The most common hepatic complication of short-term parenteral nutritional support is hepatic steatosis (fatty infiltration of the liver). Etiologic factors include infusion of carbohydrate as the sole source of calories, infusion of excess calories, essential fatty acid deficiency, and carnitine deficiency. High rates of glucose infusion appear to stimulate hyperinsulinemia, which stimulates lipogenesis and inhibits lipid mobilization from fat stores. Essential fatty acid deficiency promotes fat accumulation in the liver as a result of decreased synthesis of phospholipids which are required for lipid transport. Carnitine deficiency, although unusual, may also lead to impaired transport and reduced mitochondrial oxidation of lipids.

Fatty infiltration of the liver can occur within the first 1-3 weeks of intravenous feeding. Liver biopsies show periportal infiltration in mild cases, but panlobular or centrilobular infiltration may be seen in the more severe cases. In mild cases, blood chemistry changes may only be evident with moderate elevations in the aminotransferases and alkaline phosphatase; however, in severe cases, clinical changes (hepatic enlargement and right upper quadrant pain) as well as marked elevations in both hepatocellular and canalicular enzymes are manifest. Enzymatic changes often improve with time even when TPN is continued. Fatty infiltration by itself seldom causes progressive hepatic injury; however, in the presence of sepsis, it may accelerate hepatic failure.

Intrahepatic cholestasis tends to occur later than fatty infiltration, usually only appearing in liver biopsies taken after 3-4 weeks of TPN. Histologically, the lesion presents as pericentral or periportal canalicular bile plugging, bile staining of surrounding hepatocytes, and some degree of triaditis with a predominantly lymphocytic infiltrate. Triaditis may persist for several months after discontinuation of TPN.[217] Clinically, cholestasis presents with an elevated alkaline phosphatase developing after three or more weeks of TPN. This is followed by elevations in bilirubin, and jaundice is usually the only symptom.

Extrahepatic cholestasis and cholelithiasis can also occur with long-term TPN. Gallbladder sludge is common after 4 weeks of TPN and is almost universal after 6 weeks of TPN.[218] The development of biliary sludge is aggravated by gallbladder stasis resulting from a lack of enteral feedings and the resultant lack of neural and hormonal stimulation for gallbladder contraction.[219,220] Other causes of cholestasis include increased production of the hepatotoxic bile acid lithocholate by intestinal bacteria,[221] excess calories, and toxic amino acid metabolites.[222]

Nonspecific triaditis, although associated with cholestasis, can occur independent of cholestasis, particularly in patients with inflammatory bowel disease receiving TPN. Nonspecific triaditis may represent an early form of the lesion that presents as cholestasis.[222] Clinically, triaditis appears early in the course of TPN, with elevations of bilirubin and alkaline phosphatase and high amino transferase levels.

Hepatobiliary complications of nutritional support are usually diagnosed because of blood chemistry changes. Elevation in amino transferase is suggestive of hepatocellular injury and usually reflects fatty infiltration or triaditis, whereas hyperbilirubinemia and elevation of alkaline phosphatase are more suggestive of cholestasis.

AXIOM Mild alterations in hepatic function that resolve with dietary maneuvers usually reflect a relatively benign cholestatic process. Progressive liver dysfunction in spite of dietary changes probably reflects toxic manifestations of other disease processes, such as sepsis or drug toxicity.

In the deteriorating patient, liver biopsy may be required to prove a diagnosis of fatty infiltration, whereas cholangiography may be required to confirm the ultrasound diagnosis of biliary sludge or obstruction. Other more serious causes of hepatic dysfunction, such as

ischemic or infectious hepatitis, cholecystitis, and mechanical biliary obstruction, should also be considered before attributing abnormal hepatobiliary enzymes to nutritional support. Management of hepatobiliary complications of nutritional support are primarily aimed at prevention. Excess calories should be avoided and 15-30% of the nonprotein calories should be provided as fat to include essential long-chain fatty acids. Cyclic TPN, to allow mobilization of fat between periods of hyperinsulinemia, may minimize the tendency toward steatosis. Enteral nutrition, even when only partial, tends to minimize biliary stasis.

EXPERIMENTAL DRUGS

Meyer et al. recently reported that protein catabolism cannot be reversed by providing increased amino acids alone, due at least partially to defects in amino acid transport.[20] These defects can be reversed to some extent by anabolic agents, such as growth hormone and insulinlike growth factor-1 (IGF-1).

Growth Hormone

Growth hormone treatment dramatically improves wound healing in severely burned children, and supplementation with protein and vitamins, especially arginine and vitamins A, B, and C, provides optimum nutrient support of the healing wound.

The administration of parenteral human growth hormone (hGH) reduces nitrogen excretion under a variety of clinical conditions.[223-225] Early studies suggested that hGH exhibited anabolic actions primarily during the convalescent phase after injury; however, a complete nutrient intake was required for this to occur. Although the increment of protein retention induced by hGH is greatest under those conditions, it has become clear that it can reduce body protein losses, even during hypocaloric intravenous feeding[223] in the acute phase of critical illness.[224,225]

Following hGH administration, whole-body protein synthesis rises while protein degradation remains relatively stable. Part of the anabolic effect of hGH may depend upon its ability to stimulate endogenous IGF-1, which is a potent anabolic peptide and can itself induce protein retention. This may be important because IGF-1 production following hGH intake is inhibited in some critically ill, septic patients.[226] Despite this process, the nutritional benefits of hGH in the care of most surgical patients are potentially great. Because it can be produced in large quantities through genetic technology, it also appears likely that hGH will eventually play a significant adjunctive role in the nutritional care of trauma patients.

Recently, Jeevanandam and Peterson investigated the basic lipid kinetics of trauma and its modification after 7 days of TPN with or without daily rhGH in 20 severely injured, highly catabolic, hypermetabolic adult multiple-trauma victims.[227] Compared to the control group, the treatment group showed significantly ($P = 0.006$) enhanced rates of lipolysis and free fatty acid resterification. A trend toward increased net glucose oxidation and decreased fat and protein oxidation rates was also found. The simultaneously increased lipolytic and reesterification processes seen with rhGH may allow the adipocyte to respond rapidly to changes in peripheral metabolic fuel requirements in injury.

Insulinlike Growth Factor

Cioffi et al. recently reported on the effect of IGF-1 on energy expenditure and protein and glucose metabolism in patients with thermal injury.[228] Because accelerated protein catabolism is an important part of the hypermetabolic response to thermal injury, and because IGF-1 minimizes protein catabolism and normalizes energy expenditure in animal models of thermal injury, the authors studied the effects of IGF-1 on resting energy expenditure and whole-body protein kinetics in burn patients before and after 3-day infusions of IGF-1 (20 mcg/kg/hr). REE was not altered by IGF-1 (40.3 + 2.2 vs 39.1 + 0.021 kcal/kg/day; $P < 0.05$). However, glucose uptake was promoted and protein oxidation was decreased significantly (0.118 ± 0.029 vs 0.087 ± 0.021 g/kg/day; $P < 0.05$) by IGF-1. In addition, insulin secretion, in response to glucose challenge, was blunted. Thus, IGF-1 appears to have a beneficial effect in preserving lean body mass during severe stress conditions by minimizing the oxidation of amino acids.

⊘ FREQUENT ERRORS

In Nutritional Therapy in Trauma Patients

1. *Failure to optimize oxygen delivery and oxygen consumption to eliminate oxygen debt as soon as possible in critically injured patients.*
2. *Under- or overestimating the metabolic requirements in severely injured patients.*
3. *Delaying nutritional therapy in poorly nourished and/or hypermetabolic trauma patients.*
4. *Inadequate monitoring of nutritional parameters in severely injured or malnourished trauma patients.*
5. *Allowing continued stress in trauma patients with major metabolic problems.*
6. *Inadequate attention to organ function, thereby delaying recognition of organ failure.*
7. *Failure to promptly reverse the causes of increasing organ dysfunction or failure.*
8. *Relying on clinical estimates of nutritional needs in severely injured or malnourished patients.*
9. *Administration of too many calories and not enough protein or amino acids to severely injured or malnourished patients.*
10. *Allowing patients with head injuries to have blood glucose levels > 200 mg/dl.*
11. *Failing to begin enteral nutrition as soon as possible.*
12. *Assuming that diarrhea in patients on enteral nutrition is due only to nutritional therapy.*
13. *Failing to keep the stomach decompressed in patients who are unable to protect their airways.*
14. *Giving intravenous lipids without adequately monitoring triglyceride clearance.*
15. *Failing to look for and/or diagnose hepatic steatosis due to intravenous nutrition in its earlier phases.*

▼▼▼▼▼▼▼▼▼▼▼▼▼▼▼▼▼▼▼▼▼▼▼▼▼▼▼▼▼▼▼▼

SUMMARY POINTS

1. Clinically, the hypermetabolism of trauma is evidenced by low-grade fever, tachycardia, and tachypnea.
2. Stress carbohydrate metabolism is characterized by increased glycogenolysis and gluconeogenesis that is poorly suppressed by the exogenous administration of glucose.
3. Accelerated hepatic urea formation and UUN loss, which may exceed 15 g/day, are prominent features of the metabolic response to severe injury and sepsis.
4. UUN losses are usually < 5 g/day in nonstressed starvation, but > 15 g/day in severe stress.
5. Although protein breakdown in stress increases the availability of amino acids for visceral protein synthesis, the associated excess nitrogen loss is detrimental.
6. Following trauma, increased activity of the hypothalamus and sympathetic nervous system occurs, resulting in increased release of ACTH, catecholamines, and glucagon.
7. The increased secretion of counterregulatory hormones is an important cause of posttraumatic hypermetabolism.
8. It is increasingly believed that the postinjury and septic hypercatabolic response is due largely to the combined influences of stress hormones and cytokines.
9. Although some metabolic effects attributable to cytokines may require additional factors, the acute-phase protein response appears

to be largely due to the direct effects of IL-6 (formerly know as hepatocyte stimulating factor).
10. Evidence of persistent hypermetabolism or acute organ failure should stimulate a diligent search for an uncontrolled focus of infection or inflamed or necrotic tissue.
11. Following major trauma, tissue perfusion and oxygen transport should probably be maintained at levels 25-50% greater than normal.
12. Assuring the adequacy of tissue oxygen delivery is an important early part of the overall metabolic support of critically ill or injured patients.
13. The simplest method for detecting and correcting transport-dependent oxygen consumption is by progressively increasing oxygen transport until total body oxygen consumption no longer rises.
14. The increased caloric energy expenditure occurring after trauma must be provided from external sources in order to minimize the use of endogenous structural and functional protein for cellular fuel.
15. When indirect calorimetry is not available, it is probably wise to provide about 35 kcal/kg/day in severely hypercatabolic patients because the needs of up to 90% of such patients can be met by this level of caloric support.
16. Improperly timed indirect calorimetry studies may lead to underfeeding or overfeeding which may have a detrimental effect on survival.
17. Although indirect calorimetry provides the most precise means of assessing energy expenditure, it must be recognized that extrapolation of isolated values to average daily caloric needs may result in significant errors.
18. Nitrogen balance can be achieved by carefully matching nitrogen intake with output even when the caloric intake is low.
19. If the trauma victim was severely malnourished prior to the injury, the trauma is apt to cause a hypermetabolic response and nutritional therapy should be begun as soon as the patient is hemodynamically stable.
20. Administration of more than 30% of the total nonnitrogen caloric intake as lipids can interfere with pulmonary and immune function.
21. An underestimation of energy requirement may be offset by a greatly increased nitrogen intake.
22. Obtaining a positive N_2 balance with TPN requires administration of adequate calories, amino acids, and other intracellular components.
23. The primary advantage of TPN is that its use does not depend on a functional gastrointestinal tract and it is reliable in the sense that whatever is given will appear in the bloodstream.
24. TPN lacks the ability of enteral nutrition to improve gut trophic factors and gastrointestinal barrier function.
25. The earlier enteral nutrition is begun after trauma, the more likely it is to be of benefit.
26. Most parameters for monitoring nutrition are only estimates, and trends tend to be much more useful than absolute numbers.
27. Anergy to recall skin test antigens can be caused by radiation, malignancy, infection, steroids, chemotherapy, collagen vascular diseases, and recent surgery or trauma.
28. Although providing adequate protein is important in the nutritional support of surgical patients with acute oliguric renal failure, there is no obvious benefit to providing only essential amino acids.
29. Dialysis should be performed as often as needed to allow optimal nutritional support.
30. The most important complication of nutritional support is failure to set and/or achieve therapeutic endpoints.
31. The placement of feeding tubes should be confirmed radiographically before feeding is initiated.
32. Aspiration of gastric contents and enteral feedings, especially in neurologically impaired patients, can be greatly reduced by keeping the patient's head up and feeding through jejunostomy catheters.
33. One should not assume that all diarrhea developing when enteral feeding is begun is due to the enteral feeding rather than more serious problems.

34. Total body magnesium may be quite low and serum levels can still be normal.

35. RQ values > 1.0 usually indicate an excessive carbohydrate intake.

36. A purely glucose-based nutritional support program may increase oxygen consumption (VO_2) and the arterial PCO_2, increasing ventilatory demands and retarding weaning of patients from assisted mechanical ventilation.

37. Mild alterations in hepatic function that resolve with dietary maneuvers usually reflect a relatively benign cholestatic process. Progressive liver dysfunction in spite of dietary changes probably reflects toxic manifestations of other disease processes, such as sepsis or drug toxicity.

▲▲▲▲▲▲▲▲▲▲▲▲▲▲▲▲▲▲▲▲▲▲▲▲▲▲▲▲▲▲▲▲▲▲▲▲▲▲

REFERENCES

1. Barton RG, Cerra FB. Metabolic and nutritional support. Moore EE, Feliciano DV, Mattox KL, eds. Trauma, 2nd ed. Appleton and Lange. 1991; 965.
2. Philosophical Transactions of the Royal Society of London (1656). London: Royal Soc London, 1809; 45.
3. Henriques V, Anderson AC. Ueber parenterale ernahrung durch intravenose injecktion. Z Physiol Chem 1913;88:357.
4. Bill H. Notes on arrow wounds. Boston Med Surg J 1862;88:378.
5. Riegel C, Koop CE, Drew J, et al. The nutritional requirements for nitrogen balance in surgical patients during the early postoperative period. J Clin Invest 1947;26:18.
6. Cuthbertson DP. Further observations on the disturbance of metabolism caused by injury, with particular reference to the dietary requirements of fracture cases. Br J Surg 1935;23:505.
7. Elman R. Amino acid content of the blood following intravenous injection of hydrolyzed casein. Proc Soc Exp Biol Med 1937;37:437.
8. Fischer JE. Metabolism in surgical patients: protein, carbohydrate, and fat utilization by oral and parenteral routes. Sabiston DL, ed. Textbook of surgery: the biological basis of modern surgical practice. Philadelphia: WB Saunders, 1986.
9. Dudrick S, et al. Long-term parenteral nutrition with growth, development and positive nitrogen balance. Surgery 1968;64:134.
10. McClave SA, Snider HL. Use of indirect calorimetry in clinical nutrition. Nutr Clin Pract 1992;7:207-221.
11. Dahn MS, Jacobs LA, Smith S, Hans B, Lange MP, Mitchell RA. The relationship of insulin production to glucose metabolism in severe sepsis. Arch Surg 1985;120:166-172.
12. Huckabee WE. Abnormal resting blood lactate: I. The significance of hyperlacticemia in hospitalized patient. Am J Med 1961;30:833.
13. Wolfe RR, Shaw JHF. Glucose and FFA in kinetics in sepsis: role of glucagon and sympathetic nervous system activity. Am J Physiol 1985; 248:E236.
14. Spitzer JJ, Bagby CJ, Meszaros K. Alterations in lipid and carbohydrate metabolism in sepsis. JPEN 1988;12:53S.
15. Dahn MS, Kirkpatrick JR, Blasier R. Alterations in the metabolism of exogenous lipid associated with sepsis. JPEN 1984;8:169.
16. Bagby GJ, Spitzer JA. Lipoprotein lipase activity in rat heart and adipose tissue during endotoxin shock. Am J Physiol 1980;238:H325.
17. Askanazi J, Carpentier YA, Elwyn DH, et al. Influence of total parenteral nutrition on fuel utilization in injury and sepsis. Ann Surg 1980; 191:40.
18. Clague MB, Keir MJ, Wright PD, et al. Protein flux, nutrition and injury. Clin Sci 1983;65:165.
19. Hasselgren PO, Pederson P, Sax HC, et al. Current concepts of protein turnover and amino acid transport in liver and skeletal muscle during sepsis. Arch Surg 1988;123:992.
20. Meyer NA, Mueller MJ, Herndon DN. Nutrient support of the healing wound. New Horiz 1994;2:202.
21. Aulick LH, Baze WB, McLeod VC, et al. Control of blood flow in a large surface wound. Ann Surg 1980;191:249.
22. Wolfe RR, Herndon DN, Jahoor F, et al. Effect of severe burn injury on substrate cycling by glucose and fatty acids. N Engl J Med 1987;317:403.
23. Bessey PQ, Watters JM, Aoki TT, et al. Combined hormonal infusion simulates the metabolic responses to injury. Ann Surg 1984;200:264.
24. Bessey PQ, Brooks DC, Black PR, et al. Epinephrine acutely mediates skeletal muscle insulin resistance. Surgery 1983;94:172.
25. Bynoe RP, Kudsk KA, Fabian TC, et al. Nutrition support in trauma patients. Nutr Clin Pract 1988;3:137.
26. Askanazi J, Carpentier YA, Elwyn DH, et al. Influence of total parenteral nutrition on fuel utilization in injury and sepsis. Ann Surg 1980; 191:40.
27. Eigler N, Sacca L, Sherwin RS. Synergistic interactions of physiologic increments of glucagon, epinephrine and cortisol in the dog. J Clin Invest 1979;63:114.
28. Rosenblatt S, Clowes GHA, George BC, et al. Exchange of amino acids by muscle and liver in sepsis: comparative studies in vivo and in vitro. Arch Surg 1983;118:167.
29. Frayn KN. Hormonal control of metabolism in trauma and sepsis. Clin Endocrinol 1986;24:577.
30. Pederson P, Hasselgren PO, Angeras U, et al. Protein synthesis in liver following infusion of the catabolic hormones corticosterone, epinephrine, and glucagen in rats. Metabolism 1989;38:927.
31. Watters JM, Bessey PQ, Dinarello CA, et al. Both inflammatory and endocrine mediators stimulate host responses to sepsis. Arch Surg 1986; 121:179.
32. Klasing KC. Nutritional aspects of leukocytic cytokines. J Nutr 1988; 118:1436.
33. Nuytinck JRS, Goris RJA, Weerts JG, et al. Acute generalized microvascular injury by activated complement and hypoxia: the basis of the adult respiratory distress syndrome and multiple organ failure? Br J Exp Pathol 1986;67:537.
34. Clowes GHA, George BC, Villei CA, et al. Muscle proteolysis induced by a circulating peptide in patients with sepsis or trauma. N Engl J Med 1983;308:545.
35. Baracos V, Rodemann P, Dinarello CA, et al. Stimulation of muscle protein degradation and prostaglandin E2 release by leukocytic pyrogen (interleukin-1). N Engl J Med 1983;308:553.
36. Loda M, Clowes GHA, Dinarello CA, et al. Induction of hepatic protein synthesis by a peptide in blood plasma of patients with sepsis and trauma. Surgery 1984;96:204.
37. Flores E, Bistrian BR, Blackburn GL, et al. Acute phase response to human recombinant mediators. Surg Forum 1987;30:28.
38. Pomposelli JJ, Flores EA, Bistrian BR. Role of biochemical mediators in clinical nutrition and surgical metabolism. JPEN 1988;12:212.
39. Bebedovsky H, Del Rey A, Sorkin E, et al. Immunoregulatory feedback between interleukin-1 and glucocorticoid hormones. Science 1986; 233:652.
40. Bagby GJ, Corll CB, Thompson JJ, et al. Lipoprotein lipase-suppressing mediator in serum of endotoxin-treated rats. Am J Physiol 1986;251:E470.
41. Beulter BA, Cerami A. Recombinant interleukin-1 suppresses lipoprotein lipase activity in 3T3-L1 cells. J Immunol 1985;135:3969.
42. Gagner M, Shizgal HM, Forse RA. The effect of interleukin-1 and interleukin-2 on the adrenergic control of hormone-sensitive lipase in the human adipocyte. Surgery 1986;100:298.
43. Tracey KJ, Lowery SF, Fahey TJ, et al. Cachectin/tumor necrosis factor induces lethal shock and stress hormone response in the dog. Surg Gynecol Obstet 1987;164:415.
44. Michie HR, Spriggs DR, Manogue KR, et al. Tumor necrosis factor and endotoxin induce similar metabolic responses in human beings. Surgery 1988;104:280.
45. Evans DA, Jacobs DO, Revhaug A, et al. The effects of tumor necrosis factor and their selective inhibition by ibuprofen. Ann Surg 1989; 209:312.
46. Revhaug A, Michie HR, Manson JM, et al. Inhibition of cyclooxygenase attenuates the metabolic response to endotoxin in humans. Arch Surg 1988;123:162.
47. Moldawer LL, Svaninger G, Gelein J, et al. Interleukin-1 and tumor necrosis factor do not regulate protein balance in skeletal muscle. Am J Physiol 1987;253:C766.
48. Bagby GJ, Lang CH, Skrepnik N, et al. Regulation of glucose metabolism after endotoxin and during infection is largely independent of endogenous tumor necrosis factor. Circ Shock 1993;39:211.
49. Goldberg AL, Kettehut IC, Furono V. Activation of protein breakdown and prostaglandin E2 production in rat skeletal muscle in fever is signaled by a macrophage product distinct from interleukin-1 or other known monokines. J Clin Invest 1988;81:1378.
50. Marinkovic S, Jahreis GP, Wong GG, et al. IL-6 modulates the synthesis of a specific set of acute phase plasma proteins. J Immunol 1989; 142:808.
51. Damas P, Ledonx D, Nys M, et al. Cytokine serum level during severe sepsis in human IL-6 as a marker of severity. Ann Surg 1992;215:356-362.

52. Calandra T, Gerain J, Heumann D, et al. High circulating levels of interleukin-6 in patients with septic shock: evolution during sepsis, prognostic value, and interplay with other cytokines. Am J Med 1991;91:23-29.

53. Kunkel SL, Lukacs NW, Strieter RM. The role of interleukin-8 in the infectious process. Ann N Y Acad Sci 1994;730:134-143.

54. Bone RC, Balk RA, Fein A, et al. A second large controlled clinical study of E5, a monoclonal antibody to endotoxin: results of a prospective, multicenter, randomized, controlled trial. Crit Care Med 1995;23:994-1005.

55. Fisher CJ, Marra MN, Palardy JE, et al. Human neutrophil bactericidal/permeability increasing protein reduces mortality rate from endotoxin challenge: a placebo-controlled study. Crit Care Med 1994;22:553-558.

56. Moldawer LL. Biology of proinflammatory cytokines and their antagonists. Crit Care Med 1994;22:S3-S7.

57. Lynch SE, Colvin RB, Antoniades HN. Growth factors in wound healing. J Clin Invest 1989;84:640.

58. Rifkin DB, Moscatelli D. Recent developments in the cell biology of basic fibroblast growth factor. J Cell Biol 1989;109:1.

59. Dahn MS, Wilson RF, Lange MP, et al. Hepatic parenchymal oxygen tension following injury and sepsis. Arch Surg 1990;125:441.

60. Dahn MS, Lange P, Lobdell K, et al. Splanchnic and total body oxygen consumption differences in septic and injured patients. Surgery 1989; 101:69.

61. Astiz ME, Rackow EC, Falk JL, et al. Oxygen delivery and consumption in patients with hyperdynamic septic shock. Crit Care Med 1987; 15:26.

62. Hayes MA, Timmins AC, Yau EHS, et al. Elevation of systemic oxygen delivery in the treatment of critically ill patients. N Engl J Med 1994; 330:1717.

63. Shoemaker WC, Appel PL, Kram HB, et al. Prospective trial of supranormal values of survivors as therapeutic goals in high-risk surgical patients. Chest 1988;94:1176.

64. Edwards JD, Brown CS, Nightingale P, et al. Use of survivors' cardiorespiratory values as therapeutic goals of septic shock. Crit Care Med 1989;17:1098.

65. Jeevanadam M, Shamos RF, Petersen SR. Substrate efficacy in early nutrition support of critically ill multiple trauma victims. JPEN 1992; 16:511.

66. Harris JA, Benedict FG. A biometric study of basal metabolism in man. Washington, DC: Carnegie Institute, 1919.

67. Makk LJK, McClave SA, Creech PW, et al. Clinical applications of the metabolic cart to the delivery of total parenteral nutrition. Crit Care Med 1990;18:1320.

68. Cunningham JJ. Factors contributing to increased energy expenditure in thermal injury: a review of studies employing indirect calorimetry. JPEN 1990;14:649.

69. Long CL, Schaffel N, Geiger JW, et al. Metabolic response to injury and illness: estimation of energy and protein needs from indirect calorimetry and nitrogen balance. JPEN 1979;3:452.

70. Shigzal HM, Martin MF. Caloric requirements of the critically ill septic patient. Crit Care Med 1988;16:312.

71. Jeevanandam M, Young DH, Schiller WR. Influence of parenteral nutrition on rates of net substrate oxidation in severe trauma patients. Crit Care Med 1990;18:467.

72. Swinamer DL, Phang PT, Jones RC, et al. Twenty-four hour energy expenditure in critically ill patients. Crit Care Med 1987;15:637.

73. Weir JB de V. New methods for calculating metabolic rate with special reference to protein metabolism. J Physiol 1949;109:1.

74. Kleiber M. Energy. The fire of life. New York: John Wiley, 1961; 105.

75. Nelson LD, Anderson HB, Garcia H. Clinical validation of a new metabolic monitor suitable for use in critically ill patients. Crit Care Med 1987;15:951.

76. Askanazi J, Carpentier Ya, Elwyn DH, et al. A controlled trial of the effect of parenteral nutritional support on patients with respiratory failure and sepsis. Clin Nutr 1983;2:97.

77. Roulet M, Detsky AS, Marliss EB, et al. A controlled trial of the effect of parenteral nutritional support on patients with respiratory failure and sepsis. Clin Nutr 1983;2:97.

78. Alexander JW, Gonce SJ, Miskell PW, et al. A new model for studying nutrition in peritonitis. The adverse effect of overfeeding. Ann Surg 1989;209:334.

79. Swinamer DL, Phang PT, Jones RC, et al. Effect of routine administration of analgesia on energy expenditure in critically ill patients. Chest 1988;92:4.

80. Veramelj CG, Feenstra BWA, Van Lanschot JJB, et al. Day-to-day variability of energy expenditure in critically ill surgical patients. Crit Care Med 1989;17:623.

81. Giovannini I, Chiarla C, Boldrini G, et al. Calorimetric response to amino acid infusion in sepsis and critical illness. Crit Care Med 1988;16:667.

82. Jeevanandam M, Holaday NJ, Petersen SR. Post traumatic hormonal environment during total parenteral nutrition. Nutrition 1993;9:333.

83. Giovannini I, Chiarla C, Boldrini G, et al. Substrate supply as determinant of O₂ extraction in sepsis and nonseptic trauma. Nutrition 1993; 9:33.

84. Poyhonen MJ, Takala JA, Pitkanen O, et al. Urinary excretion of polyamines in patients with surgical and accidental trauma: affect of total parenteral nutrition. Metabolism 1993;42:44.

85. Ireton-Jones CS, Turner WW, Baxter CR. The effect of burn wound excision on measured energy expenditure and urinary nitrogen excretion. J Trauma 1987;27:217.

86. Allard JP, Pichard C, Hoshino E, et al. Validation of a new formula for calculating the energy requirements of burn patients. JPEN 1990;14:115.

87. Pavlou KN, Hoefer MA, Blackburn GL. Resting energy expenditure in moderate obesity. Ann Surg 1986;203:136.

88. Dickerson RN, Rosato EF, Mullen JL. Net protein anabolism with hypocaloric parenteral nutrition in obese stressed patients. Am J Clin Nutr 1986;44:747.

89. Moore EE, Jones TN. Benefits of immediate jejunostomy feeding after major abdominal trauma: a randomized prospective study. J Trauma 1986;26:874.

90. Mochizuki H, Trocki O, Dominion L, et al. Mechanism of prevention of post burn hypermetabolism and catabolism by early enteral feeding. Ann Surg 1984;200:297.

91. Freund HR, Rinon B. Sepsis during total parenteral nutrition. JPEN 1990;14:39.

92. Bartlett RH, Dechert RE, Mault JR, et al. Measurement of metabolism in multiple organ failure. Surgery 1982;92:771.

93. Cerra FB, McPherson JP, Konstantinides KN, et al. Enteral nutrition does not prevent multiple organ failure syndrome (MOFS) after sepsis. Surgery 1988;104:727.

94. Long CL. Fuel preferences in the septic patient: glucose or lipid? JPEN 1987;11:333.

95. Cerra FB, Hirsch J, Mullen K, et al. The effect of stress level, amino acid formula, and nitrogen dose on nitrogen retention in traumatic and septic stress. Ann Surg 1987;205:282.

96. Nordenstrom J, Carpentier YA, Askanazi J, et al. Metabolic utilization of intravenous fat emulsion during total parenteral nutrition. Ann Surg 1982;196:221.

97. Nordenstrom J, Askanazi J, Elwyn D, et al. Nitrogen balance during total parenteral nutrition: glucose vs fat. Ann Surg 1983;197:27.

98. Shaw JH, Klein S, Wolfe RR. Assessment of alanine, urea and glucose interrelationships in normal subjects and in patients with sepsis with stable isotopic tracers. Surgery 1985;97:557.

99. Shaw JHF, Wolfe RR. Response to glucose and lipid infusions in sepsis: a kinetic analysis. Metabolism 1985;34:442.

100. Lindholm M, Rossner S. Rate of elimination of the intralipid fat emulsion from the circulation in ICU patients. Crit Care Med 1982;10:740.

101. Long JM, Wilmore DW, Mason AD, et al. Effect of carbohydrate and fat intake on nitrogen excretion during total intravenous feeding. Ann Surg 1977;185:417.

102. Tracey KJ, Legaspi A, Albert JD, et al. Protein and substrate metabolism during starvation and parenteral refeeding. Clin Sci 1988;74:123-132.

103. Meguid MM, Schimmel E, Johnson WC, et al. Reduced metabolic complications in total parenteral nutrition: pilot study using fat to replace one-third of glucose calories. JPEN 1982;6:304.

104. Hunt CE, Gora P, Inwood RJ. Pulmonary effects of intralipid: the role of intralipid as a prostaglandin precursor. Prog Lipid Res 1981;20:199.

105. Wiernik A, Jarstrand C, Julander I. The effect of intralipid on mononuclear and polymorphonuclear phagocytes. Am J Clin Nutr 1983; 37:256.

106. Nugent KM. Intralipid effects on reticulo-endothelial function. J Leukoc Biol 1984;36:123.

107. Pelham LD. Rational use of intravenous fat emulsions. Am J Hosp Pharm 1981;38:198.

108. Sobrado J, Moldawer LL, Pomposelli JJ. Lipid emulsions and reticuloendothelial system function in healthy and burned guinea pigs. Am J Clin Nutr 1985;42:855.

109. Wan JMF, Teo TC, Babayan VK, Blackburn GL. Invited comment: lipids and the development of immune dysfunction and infection. JPEN 1988;2:435.

110. Fried RC, Bailey PM, Mullen JL, et al. Alterations in exogenous substrate metabolism in sepsis. Arch Surg 1986;121:173.

111. Roesner M, Grant JP. Intravenous lipid emulsions. Nutr Clin Pract 1987;2:96.
112. Skeie B, Askanazi J, Rothkopf MM, et al. Intravenous fat emulsions and lung function: a review. Crit Care Med 1988;6:193.
113. Trochi O, Heyd TJ, Waynack JP, et al. Effects of fish oil on postburn metabolism and immunity. JPEN 1987;11:521.
114. Billiar TR, Bankey PE, Svingen BA, et al. Fatty acid intake and Kupffer cell function: fish oil alters eicosanoid and monokine production to endotoxin stimulation. Surgery 1988;104:343.
115. Bower RH, Cerra FB, Bershadsky B, et al. Early enteral administration of formula (IMPACT®) supplemented with arginine, nucleotides, and fish oil in intensive care unit patients: results of a multicenter, prospective, randomized, clinical trial. Crit Care Med 1995;23:436.
116. Kemen M, Senkal M, Homann HH, et al. Early postoperative enteral nutrition with arginine-W-3 fatty acids and ribonucleic acid-supplemented diet versus placebo in cancer patients: an immunologic evaluation of impact. Crit Care Med 1995;23:652.
117. Bach AC, Storck D, Meraiki Z. Medium-chain triglyceride-based fat emulsions: an alternative energy supply in stress and sepsis. JPEN 1988;12:825.
118. Singer P, Bursztein S, Kirvela O, et al. Hypercaloric glycerol in injured patients. Surgery 1992;112:509.
119. Shaw JHF, Wildbore M, Wolfe RR. Whole body protein kinetics in severely septic patients. Ann Surg 1987;205:288.
120. Echenique MM, Bistrian BR, Blackburn GL. Theory and techniques of nutritional support in the ICU. Crit Care Med 1982;10:46.
121. Wolfe RR, Goodenough RD, Burke JF, et al. Response of protein and urea kinetics in burn patients to different levels of protein intake. Ann Surg 1983;197:163.
122. Cerra FB, Shronts EP, Raup S, et al. Enteral nutrition in hypermetabolic surgical patients. Crit Care Med 1989;17:619.
123. Barden RP, Thompson WD, Ravdin IS, et al. The influence of the serum protein on the motility of the small intestine. Surg Gynecol Obstet 1938;66:819.
124. McCray PM, Barden RP, Ravdin. Nutritional edema: its effects upon the gastric emptying time before and after gastric operations. Surgery 1937;1:53.
125. Moss G. Postoperative metabolism: the role of plasma albumin in the enteral absorption of water and electrolytes. Pac Med Surg 1967;75:355.
126. Duffy PA, Granger DN, Taylor AE. Intestinal secretion induced by volume expansion in the dog. Gastroenterology 1978;75:413.
127. Pietsch JB. Effects of hypoproteinemia on intestinal absorption. Surg Forum 1985;153:153.
128. Durr ED, Hunt DR, Roughneen PT, et al. Hypoalbuminemia and gastrointestinal intolerance to enteral feeding in head injured patients. Gastroenterology 1986;90:1401.
129. Ford EG, Jennings LM, Andrassy RJ. Serum albumin (oncotic pressure) correlates with enteral feeding tolerance in the pediatric surgical patient. J Pediatr Surg 1987;22:597.
130. Foley EF, Borlase BC, Dzik WH, et al. Albumin supplementation in the critically ill. A prospective, randomized trial. Arch Surg 1990;125:739.
131. Woods MS, Kelley H. Oncotic pressure, albumin and ileus: the effect of albumin replacement on postoperative ileus. Am Surg 1993;59:75.
132. Yu Y, Wagner DA, Walesreswski JC, et al. A kinetic study of leucine metabolism in severely burned patients. Ann Surg 1988;207:421.
133. Bower RH, Muggin-Sullam M, Fisher J. Branched chain amino acid-enriched solutions in the septic patient. Ann Surg 1986;203:13.
134. Cerra FB, Blackburn B, Hirsch J, et al. The effect of stress level, amino acid formula, and nitrogen dose on nitrogen retention in traumatic and septic stress. Ann Surg 1987;205:282.
135. von Meyenfeldt MF, Soeters PB, Vente JP, et al. Effect of branched chain amino acid enrichment of total parenteral nutrition on nitrogen sparing and clinical outcome of sepsis and trauma: a prospective randomized double blind trial. Br J Surg 1990;77:924.
136. Brennan MF, Cerra F, Daly JM, et al. Report of a research workshop: branched-chain amino acids in stress and injury. JPEN 1986;10:446.
137. Brown RO, Buonpane EA, Vehe KL, et al. Comparison of modified amino acids and standard amino acids in parenteral nutrition support of thermally injured patients. Crit Care Med 1990;18:1096.
138. Rudman D, Millikan WJ, Richardson TJ, et al. Elemental balances during intravenous hyperalimentation of underweight adult subjects. J Clin Invest 1975;55:94.
139. Wolman SL, Anderson GH, Marliss EB, et al. Zinc in total parenteral nutrition: requirements and metabolic effects. Gastroenterology 1979;76:458.
140. Bozetti F, Inglese MG, Terno G, et al. Hypocupremia in patients receiving total parenteral nutrition. JPEN 1983;7:563.
141. Askari A, Long CL, Blakemore WS. Urinary zinc, copper, nitrogen and potassium losses in response to trauma. JPEN 1979;3:151.
142. Triplett WC. Clinical aspects of zinc, copper, manganese, chromium and selenium metabolism. Nutr Int 1985;1:60.
143. Abernathy GB, Heizer WD, Holcombe BJ, et al. Efficacy of tube feeding in supplying energy requirements of hospitalized patients. JPEN 1989;13:387.
144. Rapp RP, Young B, Taryman D, et al. The favorable effect of early parenteral feeding on survival in head-injured patients. J Neurosurg 1983;58:906.
145. Norton JA, Ott LG, McClain C, et al. Intolerance of enteral feeding in the brain injured patient. J Neurosurg 1988;68:62.
146. Kemper M, Weissman C, Hyman AI. Caloric requirements and supply in critically ill surgical patients. Crit Care Med 1992;20:344.
147. Wilmore DW, Smith RJ, O'Dwyer ST, et al. The gut: a central organ after surgical stress. Surgery 1988;104:917.
148. Levine GM, Deren JJ, Steiger E, et al. Role of oral intake in maintenance of gut mass and disaccharide activity. Gastroenterology 1974;67:975.
149. Gleeson MH, Dowling RH, Peters TJ. Biochemical changes in intestinal mucosa after experimental small bowel by-pass in the rat. Clin Sci 1972;43:743.
150. Eastwood GL. Small bowel morphology and epithelial proliferation in intravenously alimented rabbits. Surgery 1977;82:613.
151. Feldman EJ, Dowling RH, McNaughton J, et al. Effect of oral versus intravenous nutrition on intestinal adaptation after small bowel resection in the dog. Gastroenterology 1976;70:712.
152. Ford WDA, Boelhauwer RU, King WWK, et al. Total parenteral nutrition inhibits intestinal adaptive hyperplasia in young rats: reversal by feeding. Surgery 1984;96:527.
153. Lo CW, Walker WA. Changes in the gastrointestinal tract during enteral or parenteral feeding. Nutr Rev 1989;47:193.
154. Rolandelli RH, Rombeau JL. Enteral nutrition in critically ill patients. Perspect Crit Care 1989;2:1.
155. Alverdy JC, Avys E, Moss GS. Total parenteral nutrition promotes bacterial translocation from gut. Surgery 1988;104:185.
156. Fong Y, Marano MA, Barber A, et al. Total parenteral nutrition and bowel rest modify the metabolic response to endotoxin in humans. Ann Surg 1989;210:449.
157. Bower RH, Talamini MA, Sax HC, et al. Postoperative enteral vs parenteral nutrition. Arch Surg 1986;121:1040.
158. Zaloga GP, Knowles R, Black KW, et al. Total parenteral nutrition increases mortality after hemorrhage. Crit Care Med 1991;19:54.
159. Kudsk KA, Stone JM, Carpenter G, et al. Enteral and parenteral feeding influences mortality after hemoglobin—E. coli peritonitis in normal rats. J Trauma 1983;23:606.
160. Moore EE, Jones TN. Benefits of immediate jejunostomy feeding after major abdominal trauma: a prospective randomized study. J Trauma 1986;26:874.
161. Kudsk KA, Minard G, Wojtysiak SL, et al. Visceral protein response to enteral versus parenteral nutrition and sepsis in patients with trauma. Surgery 1994;116:516.
162. Mainous MR, Block EF, Deitch EA. Nutritional support of the gut: how and why. New Horiz 1994;2:193.
163. Moore FA, Feliciano DV, Andrassy RJ, et al. Early enteral feeding, compared with parenteral, reduces postoperative septic complications. Ann Surg 1992;216:172.
164. Borzotta AP, Pennings J, Papasadero B, et al. Enteral versus parenteral nutrition after severe closed head injury. J Trauma 1994;37:459.
165. Eyer SD, Micon LT, Konstatinides FN. Early enteral feeding does not attenuate metabolic responses after blunt trauma. J Trauma 1993;34:639.
166. McArdle AH, Palmason C, Morency I. A rationale for enteral feeding as the preferable route for hyperalimentation. Surgery 1981;90:616.
167. Gottschlich MM, Warden GD, Michel M, et al. Diarrhea in tube-fed burn patients: incidence, etiology, nutritional impact and prevention. JPEN 1989;12:338.
168. Montecalvo MA, Steger KA, Farber HW, et al. Nutritional outcome and pneumonia in critical care patients randomized to gastric versus jejunal tube feedings. Crit Care Med 1992;20:1377.
169. Saxe JM, Ledgerwood AM, Lucas CE, et al. Lower esophageal sphincter dysfunction precludes safe gastric feeding after head injury. J Trauma 1993;35:170.
170. Zaloga GP. Physiologic effects of peptide-based enteral formulas. Nutr Clin Pract 1990;5:231.
171. Jones BJM, Lees R, Andrews J, et al. Comparison of an elemental and polymeric enteral diet in patients with normal gastrointestinal function. Gut 1983;24:78.

172. Grimble GK, Rees RG, Keohone PP, et al. Effect of peptide chain length on absorption of egg protein hydrolysates in the normal jejunum. Gastroenterology 1987;92:136.

173. Konstantinides FN, Cerra FB. Can urinary urea nitrogen be substituted for total urinary nitrogen when calculating nitrogen balance in clinical nutrition. JPEN 1988;11:18S.

174. Waxman K, Rebello T, Pinderski L, et al. Protein loss across burn wounds. J Trauma 1987;27:136.

175. Burr RG, Clift-Peace L, Nuseibeh I. Hemoglobin and albumin as predictors of length of stay of spinal injured patients in a rehabilitation center. Paraplegia 1993;31:473.

176. Meakins JL, Pietch JB, Burenick O, et al. Delayed hypersensitivity: indicator of acquired failure of host defenses in sepsis and trauma. Ann Surg 1977;186:241.

177. Christou NV, Superina R, Broadhead M, et al. Postoperative depression of host resistance: determinants and effect of peripheral protein-sparing therapy. Surgery 1982;92:786.

178. Jarstrand C, Berghem L, Lahnborg G. Human granulocyte and reticuloendothelial system function during intralipid infusion. JPEN 1978;2:663.

179. Nordenstrom J, Jarstrand C, Wiernik A. Decreased chemotactic and random migration of leukocytes during intralipid infusion. Am J Clin Nutr 1979;32:2416.

180. Fischer JE. Branched-chain enriched amino acid solutions in patients with liver failure: an early example of nutritional pharmacology. JPEN 1990;14:249S.

181. Cerra FB, Cheung NK, Fischer JE, et al. Disease-specific amino acid infusion (FO80) in hepatic encephalopathy: a prospective, randomized, double-blind, controlled trial. JPEN 1985;93:288.

182. Kanematsu T, Koyanagi N, Matsumata T, et al. Lack of preventive effect of branched-chain amino acid solution on postoperative hepatic encephalopathy in patients with cirrhosis: a randomized, prospective trial. Surgery 1988;104:482.

183. Egberts EH, Schomerus H, Hamster W, et al. Branched chain amino acids in the treatment of latent portosystemic encephalopathy: a double-blind placebo-controlled crossover study. Gastroenterology 1985;88:887.

184. Abel RM, Beck CH, Abbott WM, et al. Improved survival from acute renal failure after treatment with intravenous essential L-amino acids and glucose: results of a prospective double blind study. N Engl J Med 1973;288:695.

185. Freund H, Atamina S, Fischer JE. Comparative study of parenteral nutrition in renal failure using essential and nonessential amino acid containing solutions. Surg Gynecol Obstet 1980;151:652.

186. Leonard CD, Luke RG, Siegel RR. Parenteral essential amino acids in acute renal failure. Urology 1975;6:154.

187. Oken DE, Sprinkel FM, Landwehr DM, et al. Ineffectiveness of amino acid infusions in the treatment of rats with acute renal failure. J Am Soc Nephrol 1978;11:96A.

188. Feinstein EI, Blumenkrantz MJ, Healy M, et al. Clinical and metabolic responses to parenteral nutrition in acute renal failure. A controlled double-blind study. Medicine 1981;60:124-137.

189. Barlett RH, Mault JR, Dechert RE, et al. Continuous arteriovenous hemofiltration: improved survival in surgical acute renal failure. Surgery 1986;100:400.

190. Smith RJ, Wilmore DW. Glutamine nutrition and requirements. JPEN 1990;14:945.

191. Grant JP, Snyder PJ. Use of glutamine in total parenteral nutrition. J Surg Res 1988;44:506.

192. Burke DJ, Alverdy JC, Aoys E, et al. Glutamine-supplemented total parenteral nutrition improves gut immune function. Arch Surg 1989;124:1396.

193. Souba WW, Herskowitz K, Austgen TR, et al. Glutamine nutrition: theoretical considerations and therapeutic impact. JPEN 1990;14:237S.

194. Adibi S. Experimental basis for use of peptides as substrates for parenteral nutrition: a review. Metabolism 1987;36:1001.

195. Karner J, Roth E, Ollenschlager G, et al. Glutamine-containing dipeptides as infusion substrates in the septic state. Surgery 1989;106:893.

196. Kirk SJ, Barbul A. Role of arginine in trauma, sepsis and immunity. JPEN 1990;14:226S.

197. Daly JM, Reynolds J, Thom A, et al. Immune and metabolic effects of arginine in the surgical patient. Ann Surg 1988;208:512.

198. Barbul A, Lazarou SA, Efron DT, et al. Arginine enhances wound healing and lymphocyte immune responses in humans. Surgery 1990;108:331.

199. Barbul A, Wassenkrug HL, Seifter E, et al. Immunostimulatory effects of arginine in normal and injured rats. J Surg Res 1980;29:228.

200. Madden HP, Breslin RJ, Wassenkrug HL, et al. Stimulation of T cell immunity enhances survival in peritonitis. J Surg Res 1988;44:658.

201. Saito H, Trocki O, Wang S, et al. Metabolic and immune effects of dietary arginine supplementation after burns. Arch Surg 1987;122:784.

202. Van Buren CT, Kulkarni AD, Rudolph F. Synergistic effect of a nucleotide-free diet and cyclosporine on allograft survival. Transplant Proc Suppl 1983;1:2967.

203. Rudolph FB, Kulkarni AD, Fanslow WC, et al. Role of RNA as a dietary source of pyrimidines and purines in immune function. Nutrition 1990;61:45.

204. Muakkassa FF, Koruda MJ, Ramadan FM, et al. Effect of dietary fish oil on plasma thromboxane B_2 and 6-keto-prostaglandin $F_{1\alpha}$ levels in septic rats. Arch Surg 1991;126:179.

205. Meydani SN, Dinarello CA. Influence of dietary fatty acids on cytokine production and its clinical implications. Nutr Clin Pract 1993;8:65.

206. Cerra FB, Lehman S, Konstantinides N, et al. Effect of enteral nutrients on in vitro tests of immune function in ICU patients: a preliminary report. Nutrition 1990;6:84.

207. Bower RH, Lavin PT, LiCari JJ, et al. A modified enteral formula reduces hospital length of stay (LOS) in patients in intensive care units (ICU). Clin Nutr, Special Supplement, Vol. 11, 1992.

208. Brown RO, Hunt H, Mowatt-Larssen CA, et al. Comparison of specialized and standard enteral formulas in trauma patients. Pharmacotherapy 1994;14:314.

209. Schricker T, Kugler B, Trager, et al. Effects of xylitol on carbohydrate and protein metabolism after trauma and during sepsis. Nutr Hosp 1993;8:471.

210. Nehme AE. Nutritional support of the hospitalized patient. JAMA 1980;243:1906.

211. Vanlingingham S, Simpson S, Daniel P, et al. Metabolic abnormalities in patients supported with enteral tube feeding. JPEN 1982;6:503.

212. Weinsier RL, Bacon J, Butterworth CE Jr. Central venous alimentation: a prospective study of the frequency of metabolic abnormalities among medical and surgical patients. JPEN 1982;6:421.

213. Giner M, Curtas S. Adverse metabolic consequences of nutritional support: macronutrients. Surg Clin North Am 1986;66:1025.

214. Chernow B, Smith S, Rainet TG, et al. Hypomagnesemia: implications for critical care specialists. Crit Care Med 1983;10:193.

215. Wilson RF, Soullier G, Antonenko D. Ionized calcium levels in critically ill surgical patients. Am Surg 1979;45:485.

216. Goodenough RD, Wolfe RR. Effect of total parenteral nutrition on free fatty acid metabolism in burned patients. JPEN 1984;8:357.

217. Sheldon GF, Petersen SR, Sanders R. Hepatic dysfunction during hyperalimentation. Arch Surg 1978;113:504.

218. Messing B, Bories C, Kunstlinger F, et al. Does total parenteral nutrition induce gallbladder sludge formation and lithiasis? Gastroenterology 1983;84:1012.

219. Pitt HA, King W III, Mann LL, et al. Increased risk of cholelithiasis with prolonged total parenteral nutrition. Am J Surg 1983;145:106.

220. Roslyn JJ, Pitt HA, Mann LL, et al. Gallbladder disease in patients on long-term parenteral nutrition. Gastroenterology 1983;84:148.

221. Popper H. Cholestasis. Annu Rev Med 1968;19:39.

222. Baker AL, Rosenberg IH. Hepatic complications of total parenteral nutrition. Am J Med 1987;82:489.

223. Manson JM, Wilmore DW. Positive nitrogen balance with human growth hormone and hypocaloric intravenous feeding. Surgery 1986;100:88.

224. Ziegler TR, Young LS, Ferrari-Baliviera E, et al. Use of human growth hormone combined with nutritional support in a critical care unit. JPEN 1990;14:574.

225. Ponting GA, Ward HC, Halliday D, Sim AJW. Protein and energy metabolism with biosynthetic human growth hormone in patients on full intravenous nutritional support. JPEN 1990;14:437.

226. Dahn MS, Lange P, Jacobs LA. Insulin-like growth factor-1 production is inhibited in human sepsis. Arch Surg 1988;123:1409.

227. Jeevanandam M, Petersen SR. Altered lipid kinetics in adjuvant recombinant human growth hormone-treated multiple-trauma patients. Am J Physiol 1994;267:E560.

228. Cioffi WG, Gore DC, Rue LW 3rd, et al. Insulin-like growth factor-1 lowers protein oxidation in patients with thermal injury. Ann Surg 1994;220:310.

Chapter **39** Sepsis in Trauma

ROBERT F. WILSON, M.D.

JAMES G. TYBURSKI, M.D.

STEPHEN W. JANNING, Pharm. D.

"There is at bottom only one genuinely scientific treatment for all diseases, and that is to stimulate the phagocytes. Drugs are a delusion." —"The Doctors Dilemma," George Bernard Shaw

INTRODUCTION

Incidence

As surgeons have become increasingly successful in their resuscitation of severely injured patients, the incidence of infections and related complications has also risen.[1,2] In patients with major trauma, the incidence of infection is at least 15-20%,[3,4] and the incidence of bacteremia is at least 10%.[5] Approximately 5% of patients with penetrating injuries and 8% of patients with blunt injuries who die, do so because of sepsis.[6]

AXIOM In patients surviving for at least 48 hours, sepsis is the single most frequent cause of later morbidity and mortality.

Up to 80% of late, nonneurologic deaths following trauma are due to infection and resultant multiple organ failure (MOF).[7,8] In one study of patients surviving at least 48 hours after major abdominal vascular trauma, almost half developed serious infections causing death or at least 14 days of hospitalization.[9] In another survey, 10% of all deaths following motor vehicle accidents were due to infections.[7] Of those who lived at least 48 hours, 54% died from infectious complications. In another study, 24% of patients admitted to a shock trauma unit developed nosocomial infections, and infection was a direct cause of death in a third of their mortalities.

Of trauma patients who required 5 or more days of intensive care unit (ICU) treatment, nosocomial infection developed in 60%.[10] In another series, 81 (24%) of 338 consecutive patients treated surgically for penetrating abdominal trauma developed postoperative infections and nine of 10 deaths were caused by infection.[4] Of 111 posttraumatic infections in that series, 53 (48%) were directly related to trauma (wound infection, peritonitis, abdominal abscess) and 58 (52%) were classified as nosocomial (pneumonia or urinary tract infection).

Several factors can directly predispose patients to infections after trauma.[1] These include the mechanism of wounding, the numbers and types of organ injury, the presence of shock, and blood transfusions. Stab wounds of the abdomen are usually associated with a 1-2% incidence of abdominal infection, whereas gunshot wounds tend to have an incidence of abdominal infection that is about 5-10 times higher.[11] Colon injuries are associated with abdominal infection rates of 12-20%, and the amount and duration of fecal contamination is important. Mild contamination produces infection rates of approximately 5%, while major contamination produces infection rates of 30-40%.[12]

Penetrating wounds of the stomach are associated with an infection rate almost as high as with colon injuries in some series,[13] probably because the stomach in injured patients is often filled with partially digested food which neutralizes the gastric acid and allows bacterial colonization.

Stratification systems, including the Abdominal Trauma Index (ATI) and Injury Severity Score (ISS), also correlate with and are predictive of sepsis.[11,14] An ATI > 25 was associated with a 27% incidence of abdominal infection, while an ISS of $\geq$ 16

is associated with a 10% incidence of infection in patients requiring laparotomy.

An increasing number of critically ill patients with advanced age and preexisting medical problems are being kept alive following major trauma because of sophisticated intensive care. Unfortunately, many of these patients have greatly impaired host defenses and, consequently, are very likely to develop sepsis. In a sense, these patients may suffer a double jeopardy; not only are they more apt to become septic, but their impaired host defenses, by reducing the tendency for fever, leukocytosis, and signs of local inflammation, also make the early diagnosis and localization of infection much more difficult. Consequently, it is not surprising that the mortality rate of invasive infection in these critically ill patients may exceed 60-70%.[15]

Definitions

Infection is defined as invasion of pathogenic microorganisms into body tissues.[1] Bacteremia is the presence of bacteria in the bloodstream documented by positive blood cultures. Sepsis is the host response to infection, and it is characterized by (a) hypothermia (temperature < 95° F) or hyperthermia (temperature > 101° F), (b) tachycardia (heart rate > 90), (c) tachypnea (respiratory rate > 20 while spontaneously breathing), and (d) clinical evidence of infection. The "sepsis syndrome" includes all of the criteria for sepsis, along with evidence of abnormal end-organ function, such as altered cerebral function, oliguria (urine output < 30 mL/hour or < 0.5 mL/kg/hour for at least 1 hour), hypoxemia (PaO_2/FiO_2 ratio < 300) in the absence of other pulmonary or cardiovascular disease), or elevated lactate levels.[16] Septic shock has all of the criteria for the sepsis syndrome, in addition to hypotension (systolic BP < 90 mm Hg or a 40 mm Hg decrease from baseline for > 1 hour despite adequate volume resuscitation).

FACTORS INCREASING THE RISK OF INFECTION

Some sepsis following trauma may be prevented by careful attention to wound care, avoiding blood transfusions, and maintaining increased oxygen delivery to tissues, particularly during the first 12-24 hours after injury. The balance between bacterial factors, host defenses, and various preventative or therapeutic maneuvers determine whether an infection becomes established and how it responds to treatment.

Bacterial Factors

AXIOM The ability of microorganisms to cause infection is a function of their virulence, numbers present, presence of other bacteria, the patient's host defenses, and the appropriateness of the antimicrobial agents used.

VIRULENCE

Toxins

The virulence or ability of bacteria to invade and cause infection varies tremendously. Some of the best-studied virulence factors are the various toxins or enzymes that these organisms can release. These substances may either directly or indirectly damage the host or they may counteract host defense mechanisms. Clostridium tetani organisms produce a powerful exotoxin which can damage neurologic tissue remote from the area of infection, and C. welchii produces several powerful exotoxins which can cause severe tissue damage and necrosis (gas gangrene) in and around the area of infection.

The lipopolysaccharides in the outer membrane of the cell wall of gram-negative bacteria can cause a wide variety of systemic changes, including fever, tachycardia, hyperventilation, hypotension, intravascular coagulation, and death.

The endotoxins of so-called "smooth" bacteria (bacteria that appear to form smooth colonies when cultured in the laboratory) are macromolecules composed of three main regions: an inner layer of lipid A, an intermediate layer of core polysaccharides, and an outer layer of "O" antigens. The "O" antigens are made up of repeating oligosaccharide units, which usually contain three to five sugars each. The arrangement of these sugars generally determines the specific antigenicity of that organism. Absence of "O" antigens makes bacterial colonies appear to be "rough" on culture media.

Antibodies to either "O" or "core" lipopolysaccharide antigens can prevent the toxicity of endotoxin. The protection provided by "O" antibody, however, is much more specific and is limited to the species or subspecies from which it was derived. In contrast, "core" antibody provides broad protection against endotoxin from a wide variety of gram-negative bacteria with unrelated "O" antigens. Large multicenter trials studying the effectiveness of monoclonal antibodies to endotoxin have thus far failed to consistently reduce mortality rates. Lack of an early indicator of gram-negative sepsis appears to be a major limiting factor.

Capsules

Bacterial capsules can greatly increase virulence. These loose, gelatinous coverings of mixed polysaccharides can impede or completely block phagocytosis. Some Gram-negative bacilli, such as certain Klebsiella species, have extremely thick capsules.

NUMBER OF ORGANISMS

PITFALL ⃠

> *Assuming that a wound is almost "sterile" just because it looks clean.*

The incidence and degree of infection developing in any wound correlates directly with the number of contaminating organisms. The number of bacteria necessary to cause infection is often referred to as the critical inoculum, and this varies considerably with the local environment.

AXIOM Foreign bodies, blood, and dead space in a wound can reduce the critical inoculum of bacteria needed to cause infection from 10^6 for many wounds to 10^2, (i.e., factor of 1:10,000).[17]

COMBINATIONS OF ORGANISMS

Another important bacterial factor is the number and types of other bacteria in the area. These other bacteria may be antagonistic and reduce the chance of infection by competing for nutrients; however, in many clinical situations they are synergistic and increase the likelihood of infection. For example, aerobic bacteria in a wound may consume the oxygen that is present, thereby improving the environment for the growth and multiplication of anaerobic bacteria. Anaerobic bacteria may help the aerobic bacteria by elaborating various toxins that reduce the ability of phagocytes to remove the aerobes.

ANTIBIOTIC RESISTANCE

A bacterial population may become resistant to an antimicrobial agent either by spontaneous mutation or by transfer of genetic material from resistant bacteria to sensitive bacteria. The organisms most frequently causing sepsis at present are not the classic high-virulence organisms, such as β-hemolytic streptococci, but rather organisms, such as Pseudomonas, which, although they are usually of relatively low virulence, have great genetic versatility.

Most bacteria that can cause infection in humans can replicate by binary fission every 20 minutes. Therefore, when the proper nutrients and temperature are available, one organism can produce over 10 billion (10^9) other organisms within 10 hours. With such large numbers of bacteria, the mutation rate, which is usually about 1×10^7 or 1 in 10 million is more than adequate for mutant organisms to be seen regularly.

In some situations, mutant bacteria are given an advantage over the other bacteria present, and they proliferate. One way to "select out" such organisms is to administer antibiotics to which the mutant strain is resistant but the others are sensitive. When the mutant is the only organism capable of replicating in the presence of the antibiotics, it can replace the current microbial population with descendants of the antibiotic-resistant mutants within 24-48 hours.

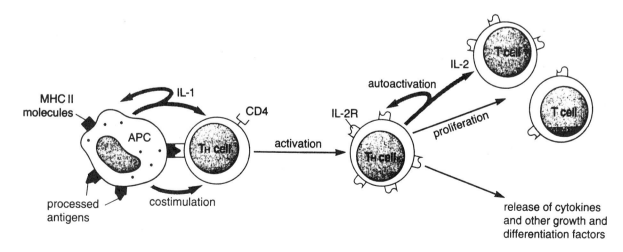

FIGURE 39–1 TH cell activation. The APC presents an antigen in the context of a class II MHC to the TH cell and also provides a constimulatory signal. The two signals lead to activation of the TH cell. The APC also releases IL-1, which acts on both the APC and the TH cell to promote activation. Activation leads to IL-2 receptor expression and IL-2 secretion by the TH cell, resulting in autocrine growth stimulation (From: Goodman JW. The immune response. Stites DP, Terr AI, Parslow TG, eds. Basic & clinical immunology, 8th ed. Norwalk: Appleton & Lange, 1994; 45).

A great deal of evidence has accumulated to show that bacteria can directly transmit antibiotic resistance to other bacteria.[18] The genetic information controlling antibiotic resistance is frequently contained in extrachromosomal deoxyribonucleic acid (DNA) molecules called plasmids. These special DNA molecules, which are also called resistance (R) factors, are self-replicating and may be passed on to or exchanged with adjacent bacteria. This material does not diffuse from one organism to another; actual physical contact (which may be considered almost "sexual") is required.

Host Defenses

Probably the most important activities of our host defenses involve the reticuloendothelial system (RES). The cells in the RES can act against invading microorganisms by: (a) elaborating substances (lymphokines or monokines) which stimulate the inflammatory response and tend to enhance the body's defense mechanisms, (b) phagocytosing the microorganisms, or (c) forming antibodies that react with them or their toxins to destroy them, inactivate them, or enhance their removal by phagocytes.

Hypovolemic animals tend to have impaired host defenses and have an increased likelihood of developing infections.[19,20] It has also been shown clinically that the most significant factor predictive of postoperative infections is the number of blood transfusions during the first 24 hours.[3,4,9,21]

IMMUNE FUNCTION

The immune system may be arbitrarily divided into nonspecific and specific response systems. Nonspecific systems include anatomical and physiologic barriers, the inflammatory response, the complement cascade, and nonspecific cellular responses by macrophages and neutrophils. The specific response system includes the humoral (antibody) response of B-lymphocytes and the cell-mediated response of T-lymphocytes.

Nonspecific Immune Response System

EPITHELIAL DEFENSES

The usual first line of defense against external pathogens is provided by epithelial cells and tissue macrophages lining the body's surfaces, such as the skin or linings of the gastrointestinal and genitourinary tracts. Anything that disrupts this integrity is associated with an increased risk of infection. These epithelial surfaces can be damaged directly by trauma or by attempts to treat the patient, such as inserting intravenous lines. Hypoxia and hypoperfusion due to trauma can also indirectly damage epithelial surfaces, including the gastrointestinal tract, which may cause loss of mucosal integrity, thereby allowing bacteria or their toxins to enter intestinal lymphatics, portal venous blood, or peritoneal cavity.

A number of reports have shown the importance of the degree of wound contamination[22,23] and the condition of the wound at the time of closure[22] in the subsequent development of infection. In a similar manner, in traumatic wounds associated with fractures, the risk of infection is directly related to the severity of local soft-tissue injury.[2]

Open fractures are graded depending on the degree of associated soft-tissue injury.[2] Grade 1 open fractures which have a skin wound < 1 cm in length and are without any significant soft-tissue damage have a reported wound infection rate of 0-9%. Grade 2 open fractures, which have larger wounds or more underlying tissue damage have a reported infection rate of 1-12%. Grade 3 open fractures, which include segmental fractures, and fractures with extensive soft-tissue damage, flaps, or avulsions, or associated neurologic or vascular injuries requiring repair have a reported infection rate of 9-55%.[24-26] When Grade 3 open fractures are further subdivided, fractures with associated vascular injuries have an infection rate three times higher than those in which the vessels are intact.[26]

The importance of translocation of bacteria in patients with nonthermal injuries is unknown.[2] Prolonged lack of enteral feeding and sepsis can reduce intestinal mucosal thickness and blood flow. Intestinal mucosa that has become thin and/or ischemic may allow increasing amounts of bacteria and bacterial products to translocate from the intestinal lumen into the portal venous system or peritoneal cavity.

Trauma patients may have hypoperfusion of the gut for a variety of reasons, including direct tissue injury, hemorrhage, and various inflammatory mediators.[27] In a study by Rush et al. of hypotensive trauma patients, 56% had positive blood cultures within three hours of injury.[28] However, a study by Moore et al., in which portal venous blood and peripheral blood were sampled for five days after injury, found that bacteremia was uncommon following major torso trauma.[29] This may be partially explained by studies which revealed that bacteria from the intestine may preferentially enter the bloodstream via the thoracic duct.[30] Peitzman et al. noted that of 25 critically ill trauma patients, none had positive mesenteric lymph node culture, even at second operations three to five days after the original injury.[27]

INTRAVENOUS CATHETERS

Intravenous catheters left in place longer than two to three days can be an important cause of thrombophlebitis and sepsis in critically ill patients. About 20-40% of intravenous catheters eventually become colonized with bacteria or fungi and ultimately contribute to bacteremia and septicemia in about 2-8% of patients.[31,32] Catheters inserted via a cutdown are more apt to become infected.

AXIOM Fever developing two to three days after surgery or trauma is often due to infected intravenous catheters.

Intravenous catheters placed in the emergency department are often inserted with less than ideal sterile technique and should be replaced within 12-24 hours. When any catheter that may be infected is being removed, a blood culture should be drawn through it; the catheter tip and intracutaneous portion should also be cultured.

AXIOM Any patient who becomes septic without another obvious cause should be considered to have an infected intravenous line until proved otherwise.

To reduce the risk of infection with intravenous plastic catheters, there appears to be some value in having increased distance between the puncture site or incision in the skin and the point at which the catheter enters the vein. When permanent Hickman or other types of catheters are inserted, the subcutaneous tunnel between the skin incision and vein should generally be at least 2-3 inches long.

URETHRAL CATHETERS

Urethral catheters and/or instrumentation in patients with infected urine is a frequent source of serious infection, particularly by gram-negative rods, such as Escherichia coli.[33] When a Foley catheter is in place for more than five days, bacterial counts in the urine often exceed 100,000 (10^5) per mL urine. Most physicians consider this to be evidence of a urinary tract infection; however, others believe that increased polymorphonuclear leukocytes (PMNs) in the urine help to differentiate between colonization and actual infection. In some series, urinary tract infections account for up to 40% of hospital-acquired infections, and most of these infections are associated with indwelling urethral catheters.

Although some bacteria may move up into the bladder along side the urethral catheter, most bacteria probably enter the bladder by movement up through the urine in the lumen of the drainage tubing. Consequently, maintenance of a closed-drainage system is extremely important. A high rate of urine flow may also help to decrease the number of organisms ascending the tubing. Careful cleansing of the catheter at the urethral meatus once or twice daily is also important.

ENDOTRACHEAL TUBE

> **AXIOM** The longer that ventilatory assistance is required, the more likely it is that the patient will develop pneumonia.

Freedland et al. reported that when a ventilator was required on trauma patients for more than seven days, at least 50% of them developed pneumonia.[34] In patients with flail chest, need for ventilatory assistance for seven days or more was associated with the development of pneumonia in 100% of patients.

If an endotracheal tube is required for more than 7-10 days, an early tracheostomy should be considered. Rodriguez et al. showed that, when long-term ventilatory support is required, performing a tracheostomy by the fourth or fifth day results in a shortened hospital stay.[35] However, even if the physician believes that an endotracheal tube is preferable to a tracheostomy for patients who require prolonged intubation, tracheostomy probably should be performed within the first 5-10 days when: (a) the patient tolerates the endotracheal tube poorly, (b) pulmonary secretions cannot be removed adequately through the endotracheal tube, or (c) the endotracheal tube appears to be damaging the vocal cords, nasal septum, or paranasal sinuses.

GASTRIC pH

A low gastric pH is a physiologic barrier to microorganisms that enter the upper gastrointestinal tract. It has been demonstrated that decreased acidity in the stomach allows a greatly increased number of bacteria to survive and multiply there. This has been believed to cause both higher pneumonia rates and increased translocation of bacteria in the distal bowel. Consequently, the routine use of H_2 blockers for the prevention of stress gastritis has been challenged, and cytoprotective agents, such as sucralfate, have been recommended to lower infection rates. The literature is controversial on this point with series showing both increases and no differences in infection rates with the use of sucralfate versus H_2 blockers.[36-38]

Inflammatory Response

RESPONSE TO INFECTION

Inflammation is the tissue response to injury or infection. Several processes are involved, including vasodilation, increased capillary permeability, and chemotaxis (i.e., attraction of various cells, especially neutrophils and macrophages to an inflamed area).[39,40] Vasodilatation results in an increased supply of blood, bringing more PMNs, macrophages, and antibodies to the involved area. Chemotaxis is first manifested as margination, which refers to adherence of PMNs to the walls of the capillaries of involved tissue. This occurs in response to chemicals liberated in that area from bacteria, involved tissue cells, or complement.

The increased local capillary permeability allows the PMNs and macrophages plus large quantities of fluid and protein to leak into the involved tissues. Antibodies and complement that enter the tissue can attach to microorganisms there to assist in their destruction and removal by phagocytes. Fibrinogen that also enters may coagulate and thereby help to isolate the noxious agent or bacteria from the rest of the body.

The tissue response to infection appears to be mediated largely by substances released during complement activation and by kinins. Kinins involved in inflammation are a group of polypeptides, usually 9-11 amino acids in length, which can produce profound hemodynamic effects, including increased capillary and small-vein permeability.[41]

Bradykinin, the best known of the kinins, is an extremely potent vasodilator. Even in nanogram (10^{-9}) quantities, bradykinin can cause profound vasodilation and increased permeability of capillaries and small veins. Much of the flushing seen with sepsis, alcoholism, and pancreatitis appears to be due to bradykinin.

The other kinin of particular interest in sepsis is myocardial depressant factor (MDF). MDF is believed to be liberated from isch-

emic pancreatic cells, and it depresses myocardial function and causes splanchnic vasoconstriction.[42]

Excess activation of these vasoactive substances can cause inappropriate vasoconstriction (resulting in local ischemia) or vasodilation (with increased capillary permeability causing increased loss of fluid into tissues). A vicious, downward cycle of increased release of vasoactive substances, hypovolemia, and progressively impaired cardiovascular activity may then develop.

> **AXIOM** Early eradication of all underlying infection is the best way to stop the downward spiral of organ dysfunction in sepsis.

Complement

NORMAL FUNCTION. Complement refers to a group of at least 11 proteins in serum which can be activated in a proteolytic cascade fashion to destroy or assist in the destruction of bacteria, abnormal cells, or particulate matter.[43] The complement cascade can be initiated by the classic pathway via C_1 activation by antigen-antibody reactions or via the alternative pathway by activation of C_3 by endotoxin, natural antibody, or several other substances.

Complement acts to enhance standard antigen-antibody immune reactions by: (a) promoting chemotaxis, immune adherence, and phagocytosis, and (b) by liberating anaphylotoxins, especially C_{3a} and C_{5a}.[43] These two substances, which are released during the complement cascade, appear to be extremely important in the development of the adult respiratory distress syndrome (ARDS) in septic patients. They stimulate PMN chemotaxis and cause them to stick to pulmonary capillary endothelium. Liberation of lysosomal enzymes and superoxides from these PMNs is generally the major cause of ARDS.

COMPLEMENT DEFICIENCIES. Isolated deficiencies of individual components of the complement system have been associated with an increased risk of recurrent or serious infections.[43] A wide variety of bacterial pathogens have been recovered from patients with deficiencies of the early components of the classic or alternative complement pathways. C_{3b} appears to have a critical role in the opsonization of most bacterial species, and C_{5a} is important in normal leukocyte chemotaxis.

In addition to genetically determined generalized serum complement deficiencies, some studies have suggested that local deficiencies of complement at various body sites, such as the peritoneal cavity, may be a risk factor in the development of spontaneous peritonitis in patients with alcoholic cirrhosis.[43] Patients maintained on chronic peritoneal dialysis commonly have low peritoneal fluid complement and immunoglobulin levels, and a local opsonic deficiency also may play a role in the pathogenesis of peritonitis in these patients.

Asplenia

The spleen is a major site of antibody and complement production and is the major filter for removing microorganisms from the bloodstream.[44,45] Thus, asplenic individuals can have greatly impaired host defenses, particularly for removing encapsulated organisms entering the body through the respiratory tract. They also have decreased levels of IgM, properdin, and tuftsin and have decreased activation of the complement system.

Fibronectin

NORMAL FUNCTION. Fibronectin is a high-molecular weight (440,000-450,000) glycoprotein that occurs in two forms.[46] The soluble form functions in blood and tissue fluids as an opsonin. The insoluble form is located near the basement membrane of small vessels and is important in vascular integrity. The general terms "plasma fibronectin" and "tissue fibronectin" have also been used to refer to the soluble and insoluble forms, respectively.

The importance of plasma fibronectin to phagocytic function gained much attention when it was discovered that plasma fibronectin is identical to opsonic glycoprotein, which has been known to modulate macrophage uptake of various collagen-coated nonbacterial test particles.[46] MOF in septic patients may be partially related to excess macrophage activation or dysfunction mediated by plasma opsonic fibronectin deficiency which may be reversed in some patients by intravenous infusion of fibronectin-rich plasma cryoprecipitate.[46]

FIBRONECTIN DEFICIENCIES. Plasma fibronectin deficiencies following trauma and/or major surgery may be a contributing factor to altered RES function and to organ dysfunction in septic patients. Consequently, fibronectin deficiency may increase susceptibility to a wide variety of stresses. Cryoprecipitate contains 8-12 times as much fibronectin as plasma. Infusion of cryoprecipitate into septic trauma and burn patients who have low immunoreactive and biosayable fibronectin levels has reversed opsonic deficiency in some patients.[46] This has resulted in a decline in the febrile and septic states of patients, as well as a transient improvement in pulmonary function.

In septic, injured patients, an abnormality of fluid balance related to increased vascular permeability often exists. Abnormalities in the amount or distribution of tissue fibronectin may be related to altered endothelial cell adherence to the subendothelium, as well as altered cell-to-cell binding of endothelial cells.

Macrophages

AXIOM   In addition to providing cell-mediated immunity (CMI) and activating antibody production, macrophages secrete multiple cytokines that influence immune response.

Macrophages play a remarkably diverse role in host defense. The fixed (tissue) phagocytes (macrophages) are believed to be derived from monocytes formed in bone marrow. They include (a) special sessile cells lining capillaries or sinusoids in various organs (such as Kupffer cells in the hepatic sinusoids) and (b) reticular cells, such as those found in the spleen (particularly in the red pulp) and in lymph nodes (in the medullary sinuses).

Macrophage activation is a complex process, and cytokines produced by tissue macrophages, circulating monocytes, or T (thymus-derived) lymphocytes are generally believed to be the principal mediators of CMI. Once activated by the proper cytokine, macrophages exhibit increased phagocytosis, enhanced oxidative metabolism with generation of microbicidal oxygen radicals, increased production of hydrolytic enzymes, and augmented killing of a wide variety of intracellular organisms.

Whenever bacteria invade the body, macrophages are activated. These, in turn, stimulate specific lymphocytes by processing and presenting antigens to them. Activation of T-lymphocytes produces the cellular immune response, and the activation of B-lymphocytes causes them to produce specific antibodies against invading microorganisms.

Polymorphonuclear Leukocytes

Once an epithelial barrier has been breached, PMNs assume a critical role in checking the spread of invasive organisms.[47] For PMNs to perform, they must be capable of carrying out a number of activities including margination on the vascular endothelium, migration through the capillary wall, directed movement toward a stimulus (chemotaxis) in the tissue, phagocytosis (ingestion), and intracellular killing.

AXIOM   Tissue oxygen tension is an important variable influencing the risk of infection because PMNs require oxygen to kill bacteria.[2]

It has been shown that hypoxic animals are more susceptible to bacterial infection and, when hyperoxic, these animals are more resistant to infection.[48] This effect is most marked immediately following bacterial contamination.

Defective PMN chemotaxis may be the result of inadequate generation of the signals that normally attract them, abnormalities of PMN receptors for chemoattractants, or disorders of the complex "machinery" involved in cell locomotion. Staphylococcus aureus is the most important pathogen in patients with abnormal PMN chemotaxis, and recurrent cutaneous or deep-seated abscesses are the most common manifestation of this disorder.[49] Patients with the hyperimmunoglobulin recurrent infection syndrome (Job's syndrome) have been evaluated most extensively, and recent studies have incriminated a monocyte-derived chemotactic inhibitory factor.[50]

Specific Immune Response Functions

AXIOM   Specific immune responses are divided into two broad categories: cell-mediated and humoral. The cell-mediated response is primarily directed against intracellular pathogens, such as viruses, while the humoral response (antibody-producing) is primarily against extracellular pathogens, such as bacteria.

In the specific immune response (Fig. 39–1),[50] an antigen presenting cell (APC), often a macrophage, presents antigen to T-helper lymphocytes (which are identified by a surface protein designated as CD-4). The T-helper cells become activated when the antigen is presented along with various co-stimulatory factors, including interleukin-1 (IL-1), which is produced by activated macrophages. Only T-helper cells with the specific receptor for the presented antigen is activated. This prevents simultaneous activation of all T-helper cells to one antigen. The T-helper cells then activate the cell-mediated or humoral (or both) arms of the immune system. Which specific arm is turned on depends on the mixture of cytokines presented and produced. The end result is production of either (a) cytotoxic (CD-8) lymphocytes capable of killing diseased cells (Fig. 39–2), or (b) plasma cells which produce soluble antibody against the antigen (Fig. 39–3).

HUMORAL IMMUNITY

Antibodies are specific proteins that develop in response to a particular antigen, which may be an invading microorganism or any foreign substance.[43] These antibodies have a wide variety of functions, but basically they attempt to destroy or inactivate the antigen and/or enhance its phagocytosis and subsequent removal from the body. Almost all antibodies are formed in plasma cells, which are found primarily in lymph nodes, spleen, and bone marrow.

The macrophage plays a critical role in initiating this process for many antigens, and helper (CD-4) cells are also involved. When stimulated by activated CD-4 cells or their cytokines, B (bursa-derived) lymphocytes mature into plasma cells, which are activated to secrete specific antibodies.[43]

Receptors on the surface of each of the cell types participating in antibody production have been partially characterized.[43] T-cells recognize antigens only in the context of "self," in relationship to molecules that are coded for major histocompatibility complex (MHC) genes on the surface of macrophages and B-lymphocytes. These gene loci are found on chromosome 6 in human cells, and they are termed the human leukocyte A (HLA) system.

The ability of macrophages to present antigens to T-cells is restricted to subpopulations of cells expressing HLA-DR (class II) molecules on their surfaces. The genetic basis of decreased responsiveness to certain antigens or increased susceptibility to certain types of infection may ultimately be linked to defects in this HLA system.

Severe dysfunction of antibody production has been described in patients after trauma. Changes in both absolute production and in antibody repertoires have been shown in hemorrhagic shock models.[51,52] Reductions in certain T-helper cell lymphokines and increases in suppressor lymphokines have been postulated as causes for these defects.

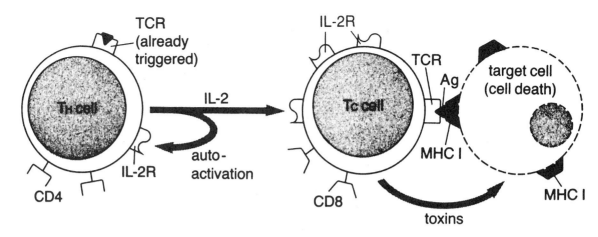

FIGURE 39–2 Tc cell activation requires contact with specific antigen in the context of a class 1 MHC molecule on the surface of a target cell. It also requires IL-2 from a nearby activated TH cell. The activated Tc cell kills the target cell either by secreting cytotoxins (as shown) or by inducing it to commit suicide. (From: Goodman JW. The immune response. Stites DP, Terr AI, Parslow TG, eds. Basic & clinical immunology, 8th ed. Norwalk: Appleton & Lange, 1994; 46).

AXIOM One of the major immune defects after severe trauma is reduced antigen-presenting capability.

A central figure in the specific immune response system is the APC, which is prototypically, the macrophage. Several studies have shown reduced antigen presentation in the form of decreased cell surface activity markers following trauma.[53-55] This has led to clinical trials in which attempts were made to increase macrophage activity by administering interferon-γ[56] or PPG-glucan[57] in high-risk surgical patients. The results of these small studies were mixed, and larger studies are pending.

CMI involves the production of cytotoxic T-lymphocytes (CTLs), which have receptors for CD-8. CTLs seek out and destroy cells that have specific altered proteins on their surfaces. These CTLs are produced when a T-helper cell presents an antigen to a resting CTL with the specific receptor for the presenting antigen. The antigen presented must be MHC consistent. The costimulating signal is IL-2 which is produced by activated T-helper cells.

Changes in CMI have been described following trauma and during sepsis.[53,58] Delayed type hypersensitivity reactions have been found to be depressed following injury, and patients with persistent anergy have a high incidence of subsequent sepsis and death.[59] In vitro lymphocyte proliferative capability and IL-2 production, its receptor expression[60] and lymphocyte production of interferon-α,[61] are altered following trauma.[60] Indeed, cells from trauma patients can suppress allogeneic responses in mixed lymphocyte cultures.[62] These phenomena may be a reflection of an increase in suppressor T-cell activity,[63] which may also explain an observed reduction in the production of antibody by B cells.[64] However, the increase in suppressor T-cell activity by itself may be a secondary phenomenon due to increased prostaglandin E$_2$ release from macrophages.[65]

The pattern of lymphocyte subpopulation responses following major trauma remains poorly defined, with conflicting reports about the significance of changes in T-helper and suppressor populations or ratios.[66,67] Some evidence has suggested that lymphocytes taken from peripheral blood may function much differently than lymphocytes taken from the spleen or mesenteric lymph nodes.[68] In a recent report on patients admitted to three trauma centers with injury severity scores of 20 or more, Cheadle et al. were able to characterize different lymphocyte phenotypic subsets throughout their hospital courses.[58]

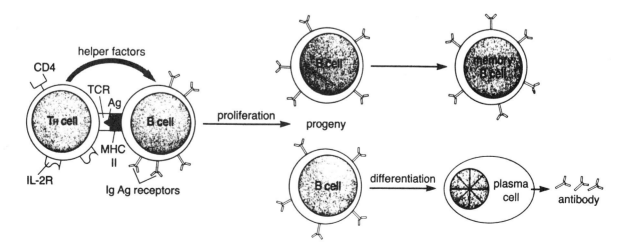

FIGURE 39–3 B cell activation. Antigen-binding to surface immunoglobulins, coupled with soluble or contact-mediated helper factors from an activated TH cell, leads to proliferation and differentiation. Cytokines involved in TH cell stimulation include IL-2, IL-4, and IL-6. (From: Goodman JW. The immune response. Stites DP, Terr AI, Parslow TG, eds. Basic & clinical immunology, 8th ed. Norwalk: Appleton & Lange, 1994; 45).

Cytokines and Other Chemical Responses

AXIOM The main substances involved in the host response to trauma and infection include tumor necrosis factor (TNF), various ILs (especially IL-1), platelet-activating factor, and various arachidonic acid metabolites.

TUMOR NECROSIS FACTOR. TNF, also known as cachectin, is produced by macrophages and multiple other cells (Table 39–1). It has been demonstrated in mice and humans that infusion of endotoxin stimulates the release of TNF[69] which can cause virtually every symptom and sign of infection.[70] Nevertheless, minimal-to-moderate levels of TNF may be beneficial and can prevent death in experimental animals receiving inoculations of live bacteria that would otherwise be lethal.

TNF is a pyrogen, as well as a stimulant for release of IL-1, IL-6, and IL-8, platelet-activating factor, leukotrienes, thromboxane A_2, and prostaglandins. It induces expression of adhesion molecules which promote the adhesion of neutrophils to endothelial cells. It also activates complement and the coagulation cascade.

INTERLEUKINS. IL-1 is identical to endogenous pyrogen, the messenger molecule frequently involved in fever production. IL-1 is also capable of enhancing T-cell responsiveness to almost any activating stimulus. Together with IL-2, a lymphokine produced by T-helper cells, IL-1 participates in the activation of T-lymphocytes. IL-2 also activates neutrophils and T- and B-lymphocytes and promotes muscle wasting. Activated T-cells, in turn, can produce cytokines that activate macrophages to kill intracellular organisms.

IL-2 production can be stimulated by gram-positive organisms. It causes decreases in systemic vascular resistance and a tendency for cardiac output to increase even though the cardiac ejection fraction tends to decrease.[70] It stimulates the release of TNF and causes endothelial cell damage by lymphocytes. IL-2 can also stimulate blast transformation of cytotoxic T-cells that have the capacity to kill certain viruses.

IL-6 is similar to IL-1 in that it stimulates acute-phase protein production by the liver and is also a pyrogen. Its release can be stimulated by endotoxin, TNF, and IL-1. It augments activation of neutrophils and T- and B-lymphocytes.

PLATELET-ACTIVATING FACTOR. Platelet-activating factor (PAF) is an important phospholipid mediator of the sepsis cascade.[1] It is released by many cells including endothelial cells, neutrophils, pneumocytes, and platelets. Release is stimulated by a number of compounds including TNF, leukotrienes, and histamine. Low concentrations of PAF

TABLE 39-1. *Inflammatory Mediators in Sepsis*

Inflammatory Mediator	Alternate Designations	Cell(s) of Origin	Actions
Interleukin-1	Lymphocyte-activating factor B-cell activating factor IL-1	Monocytes	Promotes T-cell production of IL-2 Stimulates T-cell expression of IL-2 receptors Supports B-cell proliferation and antibody production Proteolytic effects Stimulates hepatic synthesis of acute phase proteins Pyrogenic
Interleukin-2	T-cell growth factor IL-2	T-cells	Promotes T-cell activation and replication Stimulates B-cell maturation and activation Promotes expression of IL-2 receptors Stimulates production of mature PMNs Promotes limited self renewal of some multipotential stem cells
Interleukin-4	B-cell growth factor I (BSF-1)	T-cells	Stimulates IgG and IgE synthesis by activated B-cells Sustains autocrine growth of T-cell clones
Interleukin-6	B-cell stimulating factor-2 (BSF-2) Hepatocyte stimulating factor IL-6	Monocytes Kupffer cells	Autocrine stimulation of monocytes Stimulates B-cells Stimulates hepatocytes
Interleukin-8	IL-8	Monocytes Fibroblast Keratinocytes	Activates and attracts neutrophils Chemotactic for T-cells
Interleukin-10	Cytokine synthesis inhibitory factor IL-10	Activated TH2, CD8 T, and B-lymphocytes, macrophages	Inhibition of cytokine production by TH1 cells, NK cells, and APCs Promotion of B-cell proliferation and antibody responses Suppression of cellular immunity Mast cell growth
Prostaglandins	PGE_1 PGE_2 PGI_2 $PGF_{2\alpha}$	Macrophages Endothelial cells	Vasodilation (PGI_2, PGE_2) Suppression of monocytes, T-helper cell and B-cell function (PGE_2) Increases intracellular cyclic AMP (PGE_2
Thromboxanes	TxA_2, TxB_2	Endothelial cells Leukocytes	Vasoconstriction (TxA_2) Platelet aggregation Increases vascular permeability
Interferon	IFN_γ IFN_α IFN_β	T-cells (γ) Macrophages (α and β)	Promotes expression of IL-2 receptors Activates macrophage Mediates an antiviral effect by binding with responsive cells Mediates antitumor effects
Tumor necrosis factor	Cachectin TNF	Monocytes Kupffer cells	Direct cell killing Enhancement of antiviral INF effects

prime inflammatory cells, while higher concentrations stimulate neutrophils to adhere to endothelial cells, causing them to degranulate and produce toxic oxygen radicals. PAF has been shown to produce hypotension and increase vascular permeability, particularly in the lung, and has been implicated as a causative agent of ARDS.[1] It decreases peripheral vascular resistance along with cardiac output and causes coronary vasoconstriction. It is also believed to be involved in the gastrointestinal ulceration and neurotoxicity seen with sepsis.

ARACHIDONIC ACID METABOLITES. Metabolism of arachidonic acid produces increased amounts of thromboxane A_2, leukotrienes, and prostaglandins.[1] Thromboxane A_2 is a potent vasoconstrictor and bronchoconstrictor. It increases vascular permeability and increases platelet aggregation. Various leukotrienes can cause vasoconstriction, bronchoconstriction, and/or increased vascular permeability.

A particularly important prostaglandin in sepsis is prostacyclin (PGI_2). It causes vasodilation, decreases platelet aggregation, and may contribute to the low systemic vascular resistance seen in septic shock.

Prostaglandin E_2 (PGE_2) causes vasodilatation and may have a protective effect on the microvasculature. It has a direct pyrogen effect on the hypothalamus, and depending on the dose, it may either stimulate or inhibit TNF release. It may also be immunosuppressive, with particular effects on monocyte function.[71]

OPSONINS

> **AXIOM** Opsonins refer to a group of substances in serum that attach themselves to the surface of antigens (usually microorganisms or particulate matter) and thereby enhance the ability of phagocytes to recognize and engulf the antigens.

The three main types of opsonins are antibodies, complement, and fibronectin. IgG and IgM antibodies to specific microorganisms are the most common immunoglobulins that can function as opsonins. Complement and fibronectin are relatively nonspecific opsonins that can react immediately to invading microorganisms or foreign substances.

Other Factors Affecting Host Defenses

Other factors that may impinge on the host's ability to defend itself against microorganisms include various drugs that may be administered, extremes of age, and severe metabolic problems.

IMMUNOSUPPRESSIVE DRUGS

Immunosuppressive drugs (to prevent transplant rejection) and cytotoxic drugs (for treating malignancies) can profoundly depress bone marrow and the RES. This may be particularly important in patients who, because of advanced malignancy, already have a reduction in phagocyte- and antibody-forming tissues. In addition, cytotoxic drugs tend to injure rapidly growing cells, such as intestinal mucosa, thereby creating additional portals of entry for various microorganisms.

ANTIBIOTICS

Antibiotic therapy can profoundly alter the host microflora and may thereby determine which microorganisms are likely to cause infection. Almost all antibiotics in therapeutic doses cause changes in gastrointestinal, oropharyngeal, and skin flora, replacing these microorganisms with other organisms that are more antibiotic-resistant. Antimicrobial agents can also reduce host resistance by inducing certain vitamin deficiencies.

CORTICOSTEROIDS

> **AXIOM** Corticosteroid therapy is frequently associated with an increased incidence of infection by opportunistic bacteria, viruses, fungi, and parasites.

Glucocorticoids depress the inflammatory response and can induce lysis of mononuclear cells.[72] Corticosteroids also redistribute T cells from the circulation, thereby impairing their access to inflammatory sites.[73] Although corticosteroids appear to affect PMN function in vitro, in vivo prednisone has no discernible effect on PMN function except at pharmacologic doses.[74]

AGE

Host resistance is most apt to be impaired in individuals who are younger than three months of age or older than 70 years.[75,76] In addition to impaired host defenses, aged patients are more apt to have cardiovascular, pulmonary, and other organ dysfunction. Infections in older patients are also particularly apt to be caused by gram-negative bacilli.

METABOLIC ABNORMALITIES

Diabetes Mellitus

Patients with uncontrolled diabetes mellitus have an incidence of infections up to several times higher than nondiabetics.[77,78] Increased blood glucose levels apparently play only a minor role; however, ketoacidosis can cause defective inflammatory responses with sluggish polymorphonuclear migration, ineffective phagocytosis, and decreased killing and fibroblast proliferation.[79] In addition, the small blood vessel changes that often complicate diabetes mellitus may interfere with local tissue blood flow, reduce absorption of drugs given intramuscularly or subcutaneously, and cause renal and cardiovascular dysfunction.

Uremia

Uremic acidosis has a number of effects on host defense which include: (a) impaired early phases of the acute inflammatory response, (b) reduced immune responses to antigenic stimuli, (c) impaired delayed cellular hypersensitivity, (d) altered production of all types of immunoglobulins, and (e) defective cell division.[80]

Cirrhosis

Patients with severe cirrhosis have a greatly reduced resistance to infection, and these patients can develop fatal septic shock from relatively mild infections. In addition to the impaired liver metabolism and reduced hepatic RES function seen in cirrhosis, there is shunting of portal venous blood, which may contain enteric bacilli or endotoxin, around the hepatic RES, directly into the systemic circulation.

Malnutrition

Severe malnutrition tends to increase the risk and severity of infection.[81] Although most trauma victims have increased nutritional demands after trauma,[82] their gastrointestinal tracts often do not function for several days. A patient's nutritional status is not usually an important early risk factor for trauma-related infection, but it may be a significant factor in the patient's eventual ability to survive infection.[2]

> **PITFALL** ⊘
>
> *Patients with major trauma who receive no nutrition for four to five days can develop cumulative caloric and protein deficits that can result in greatly increased complication rates.*

Severe, acute protein or calorie malnutrition can be associated with impairment of CMI functions.[81] Both the number and functional capability of T-lymphocytes are markedly reduced, as is the delayed hypersensitivity response to antigens and sensitizing chemicals. Severe nutritional deficiencies also interfere with lymphokine production by T-lymphocytes and may increase the number of suppressor cells. The efficacy of vaccines is also impaired in severely malnourished patients.

Resistance to infection may be returned to normal in some of these patients by early, adequate enteral feedings. Enteral feeding, which should be used whenever possible, appears to be more effective than intravenous hyperalimentation at maintaining or restoring host defenses.[83] Many trauma patients, however, require some TPN initially while enteral nutrition is progressively titrated to adequate levels.

Lack of Enteral Nutrition

Prolonged TPN is believed to reduce intestinal mucosal thickness and increase the tendency to bacterial translocation. This may be partially due to lack of free glutamine in commercially available parenteral preparations. An increased tendency also exists for patients on TPN to develop acalculous cholecystitis.

Some of the factors that may cause acute acalculous cholecystitis include decreased mucosal blood flow, increased intraluminal pressure, viscous bile, bacterial colonization, and edema or spasm of the ampulla of Vater.[84] In a review of 21 cases, Petersen and Sheldon in 1979 emphasized that intravenous hyperalimentation caused gallbladder distention with bile stasis and inspissation and played an important role in the etiology of acalculous cholecystitis.[85] Glenn and Becker noted severe focal necrosis of the blood vessels in the muscularis and serosa of the gallbladder in patients with this problem, and in six (40%) of their 15 patients, the gallbladder was completely gangrenous.[86] Intravenous cholecystokinin, however, by causing the gallbladder to contract and empty may help to prevent this complication.[87]

CARDIOVASCULAR FUNCTION

Any impairment of tissue perfusion increases the likelihood that otherwise harmless endogenous bacteria may cause infection. Patients with shock have an increased tendency to develop infection, especially if shock persists for > 30 minutes and the patient received massive transfusions.[9]

PULMONARY DISEASES

Physical Defense Mechanisms

The first line of host defense for the lungs is the upper airway with various physical mechanisms to reduce access of particulate matter to the lungs. Nearly all particles with a diameter > 10 microns are deposited within the nose and nasopharynx and only particles smaller than 1-2 microns tend to reach the alveoli.[88] This is important because droplets carrying infectious microorganisms are often smaller than 2 microns in diameter, particularly when they are produced by sneezing or coughing.

The respiratory tract is normally sterile below the glottis. This sterility is mechanically maintained by alveolar macrophages and the mucociliary clearance apparatus. In smokers and patients with chronic obstructive lung disease, the mucociliary clearance mechanisms are impaired.[89] These patients often have infected bronchial secretions and have an increased risk of developing severe pneumonitis following trauma.

If a ventilator has been required on our trauma patients for more than seven days, at least 50% of them have developed pneumonia. In our patients with a flail chest, need for ventilatory assistance for seven days or more was associated with the development of pneumonia in 100% of patients.[34]

If an endotracheal tube is required for more than 7-10 days, a tracheostomy is often performed by the fourth or fifth day. However, even if the physician believes that an endotracheal tube is preferable to a tracheostomy for patients who require prolonged intubation, a tracheostomy probably should be performed within the first five to 10 days if: (a) the patient tolerates the endotracheal tube poorly, (b) the pulmonary secretions cannot be removed adequately through the endotracheal tube, or (c) the endotracheal tube appears to be damaging the vocal cords, nasal septum, or paranasal sinuses.

Cellular Defense Mechanisms

In spite of the physical defense mechanisms of the airways, a substantial quantity of fine particulate and soluble material is deposited

in alveoli where they are dealt with by alveolar macrophages.[89,90] If the immediate phagocytic responses of the alveolar macrophages are inadequate, immunologically-specific mechanisms will be initiated by local lymphocytes. Interaction of these lymphocytes with alveolar macrophages appears necessary for the initiation, modulation, and expression of pulmonary immune reactivity.

DIAGNOSIS OF INFECTION

Diagnosis involves not only determining that an infection is present but also finding its source and determining the organisms involved. Although the diagnosis of many surgical infections is usually "relatively easy," some intraabdominal abscesses may be extremely difficult to identify.

AXIOM   Severe infections may sometimes develop without pain, fever, or leukocytosis, especially in patients who have impaired host defenses.

In anergic patients, large abscesses may be present with little or no fever, tenderness, or leukocytosis. In overwhelming infections developing in spite of antibiotic therapy, particularly in debilitated patients, the only evidence of infection may be a shift in the differential white blood cell (WBC) count to the left (i.e., more band or immature forms) with little or no change in the total WBC count.

History

Medical histories may be helpful in some patients, particularly when they reveal infections that tend to recur or illnesses that can reduce the patient's host defenses. The most frequent symptoms of infection include chills and fever, pain, cough, dysuria, and night sweats. Pain and discomfort may also help to localize the probable site of infection.

CHILLS AND FEVER

Although fever is one of the classic signs or symptoms of infection, significant sepsis can occur without fever; some of the worst infections, especially those caused by gram-negative organisms, may be associated with hypothermia.[91] Fevers > 105° F-106° F often indicate a neurologic or metabolic problem, which may be complicating sepsis. Musher et al., however, reported that fever patterns often lack clinical significance.[91]

The great majority of fevers that occur in the first 48 hours after surgery or trauma are noninfectious in origin.[92,93] In a series of 329 patients undergoing operation for penetrating abdominal injuries, the overwhelming majority demonstrated elevated temperatures on one or more of the first five postoperative days.[94] Only when fever persisted beyond the fourth postinjury day did it begin to become useful in distinguishing infected from uninfected patients.[94] Nevertheless, some highly lethal infections should be considered when a high fever occurs during this period.[95] One possibility is an undetected intestinal injury or a leaking anastomosis causing worsening peritonitis. This can cause an early dramatic fever that can be accompanied by striking cardiovascular disturbances.[2]

Certain invasive, soft-tissue infections caused either by β-hemolytic streptococci or by Clostridium species, especially C. perfringens, can also cause striking systemic signs of sepsis within the first 24-48 hours after injury. Diagnosis of these infections is made by inspection of the wound and Gram stain of any exudate.

Streptococcal infections usually have surrounding erythema, and Gram stain of the fluid from the wound reveals large numbers of gram-positive cocci and PMNs. A clostridial infection displays little or no erythema, but marked swelling and edema are usually present. Fluid from the wound typically has gram-positive rods (without spores) on Gram stain and does not usually contain any WBCs. The wound should be reinspected within 24 hours regardless of the findings at diagnosis and/or surgical debridement.[96,97]

Initially, many infections, particularly when the patient is receiving antibiotics, may cause only mild, temporary temperature elevations which may be missed unless the temperature is taken every four hours. When the patient has any fever, it is most apt to occur in the late afternoon and early evening, and special efforts should be made to take the temperature during that time. In patients who are stuporous or mouth breathers, the temperature should be taken rectally.

PAIN

Pain is usually well localized to the site of infection when somatic nerves are involved. Pain sensation from intraabdominal infections, however, often is carried by splanchnic nerves, which tend to produce only vague, poorly localized discomfort that may be referred to another area. Tenderness from intraabdominal collections of pus is usually better localized than pain and may be of great diagnostic value.

COUGH

A new or increased cough in a septic patient generally indicates a tracheobronchial or pulmonary infection of some type, particularly when copious or purulent sputum is produced. It may also indicate that aspiration has occurred. Copious amounts of foul sputum are typically associated with anaerobic involvement in lung abscesses or bronchiectasis. Sharp chest pain with cough or deep breaths generally indicates pleuritic inflammation.

DYSURIA

Acute cystitis is characterized by frequency of urination, dysuria, and urgency. Such symptoms are not uncommon in injured patients who have had a urinary catheter for more than two or three days even if the urine is sterile.

Physical Examination

The classic signs of inflammation are pain, redness, heat, and swelling. If, in addition, the involved area is indurated and there is fluctuation in its center, this would be strongly indicative of an abscess. Swelling of the lower leg, especially at the calf, may indicate thrombophlebitis or phlebothrombosis. Rales in the lung may be associated with pneumonia, atelectasis, or congestion. Flank tenderness may indicate infection in the kidney or subphrenic space. A pelvic abscess is often first noted as lower abdominal tenderness and severe cervical motion tenderness on vaginal examination.

The value of physical examination of the abdomen is extremely variable. A report by Gibson et al. demonstrated that only 19 (33%) of abdominal abscesses were diagnosed on clinical grounds.[98] The experience of Gibson et al. parallels our own relative lack of success with physical examination in patients with postoperative intraabdominal infections.

General Signs of Sepsis

A wide variation may be seen in the physical appearance of septic patients. However, five fairly characteristic types of clinical presentation may be noted, including: (a) failure to thrive, (b) typical sepsis (without shock or organ failure), (c) progressive MOF, (d) hyperdynamic (warm) septic shock, and (e) hypodynamic (cold) septic shock.

FAILURE TO THRIVE

In older patients, particularly those with severe trauma or malnutrition, recovery from surgery is often extremely slow, probably because of preexisting organ dysfunction. However, this failure to recuperate properly, (i.e., "failure to thrive") may also be due to unsuspected sepsis. Host defenses in these patients are often so impaired that, even with severe sepsis, few objective signs of infection may be evident, except for increasing confusion.

The patient with failure to thrive tends to be lethargic. Although blood gases may be relatively good, the patient is often too weak to be extubated. Although the BUN and serum creatinine are usually normal, measured creatinine clearance is often < 40-50 mL/minute. Gastrointestinal function is slow to return. Bowel sounds are present, but the abdomen tends to be somewhat distended, and the patient may not pass gas per rectum for many days. Liver function tests are usually only slightly abnormal initially.

TYPICAL SEPSIS

Although fever is seen in most typical cases of sepsis without shock or organ failure, up to 13% of septic patients may have temperatures < 36.4° C (96.6° F). Another 5-20% are afebrile.[91]

Careful observation of septic patients has shown that hyperventilation is often an early clinical finding. A sudden onset of tachypnea is an indication for drawing blood and for arterial blood gas analysis and blood cultures. The respiratory rate in typical sepsis is often more than double normal and the tidal volume is usually only slightly reduced, producing a minute ventilation which is often at least 1.5-2.0 times normal. Even without pulmonary infection or fluid overload, rales are often present at the bases.

Not infrequently, increasing confusion or restlessness is the first sign that a patient is becoming septic. In some instances, the increasing confusion and restlessness may be difficult to differentiate from delirium tremens. However, some patients with gram-negative sepsis are remarkably awake and alert until just prior to death.

As long as an adequate blood volume is maintained, pulse pressures tend to widen as the severity of sepsis increases. Tachycardia is also common, and tachyarrhythmias may be the first clinical sign of sepsis.[99] The pulse, although fast, is usually full and almost bounding in septic patients.

The abdomen is often somewhat distended. Septic patients tend to develop an ileus early, even without an abdominal focus of infection. If abdominal or renal sepsis is present, the ileus can rapidly become much more severe.

The skin in early sepsis is typically warm and dry with a flushed or pink color. Occasionally, acrocyanosis may develop due to intravascular clotting. A characteristic skin lesion, ecthyma gangrenosum, occurs in up to 25% of patients with Pseudomonas bacteremia, but may occasionally be due to E. coli.[100] Findings obtained from Gram stains of exudate can often help to provide an initial microbiologic diagnosis.

MULTIPLE ORGAN FAILURE SYNDROME

It has been increasingly recognized that MOF can be important evidence of sepsis. In one of the first reports on the subject, Eiseman et al. in 1977 described 42 postoperative patients with MOF.[101] Sepsis was judged to be the etiology in 69%. Nevertheless, the presence of sepsis in critically ill patients is frequently not clear. Up to 50% of patients with MOF or shock have repeated negative blood cultures, even though evidence of advanced sepsis can be found eventually in up to 90% of patients.[101,102]

Polk and Shields reported that organ failure, especially if it involves the lungs and kidneys, may indicate the presence of occult intraabdominal infection in postoperative trauma victims.[103] They believed that support of organ function without definitive correction of the underlying infection is only palliative. Fry et al., in a study of 38 patients with MOF who had a mortality rate of 74%, found that: (a) the incidence of MOF was about 7% after emergency surgery, (b) MOF was primarily due to infection, (c) the temporal sequence of MOF was usually lung, liver, gastric, and kidney, and (d) MOF is the most common fatal expression of uncontrolled infection.[104]

Pulmonary Failure

The need for ventilator assistance for more than three to four days is often defined as pulmonary failure, and this is often the earliest finding in MOF. ARDS is characterized by increasing hyperventilation and progressive hypoxemia. The lungs have increasing rales, decreasing compliance, and increasing physiologic shunting.[105] Once the shunt (Q_s/Q_t) exceeds 20-25%, increasing ventilatory assistance, usually with at least 5-10 cm H_2O positive end-expiratory pressure (PEEP), is required.

Pulmonary artery pressure and pulmonary vascular resistance (PVR) tend to increase with sepsis; if pulmonary hypertension develops, it is usually associated with an increased mortality rate. An indirect indication of increased PVR is an increased pulmonary artery diastolic pressure (PADP)—pulmonary artery wedge pressure (PAWP) gradient. Of 37 septic patients studied by Sibbald et al., 12 had a PADP-PAWP gradient > 5 mm Hg, and 10 (83%) of these patients died within 48 hours.[106] Of 25 patients with a more normal PADP-PAWP gradient, only 6 (24%) died. An increase in CVP in patients with pulmonary hypertension may be incorrectly interpreted as evidence of fluid overload or right heart failure. As a consequence, the CVP response to a fluid challenge provides much more accurate information than isolated CVP levels.[107]

Hepatic Failure

Hepatic failure in MOF is often defined as a serum bilirubin > 2.0-3.0 mg/dL with SGOT, LDH, and/or alkaline phosphatase levels at least double normal.[108-110] An early increase in serum bilirubin levels after trauma may be due to ischemic liver damage or hemolysis, but jaundice developing after 8-10 days is usually due to sepsis.

AXIOM   Patients with jaundice developing eight or more days after trauma should be assumed to be septic until proved otherwise.

Several theories exist to explain the factors causing hepatic dysfunction in sepsis. It has been postulated that sepsis causes decreased effective hepatic blood flow which, in turn, causes hepatic and ischemic dysfunction.[111] However, animal studies have demonstrated no change in indocyanine green clearance after direct hepatic ischemia.[112] In addition, Dahn et al., using direct hepatic vein catheterization, showed that hepatic/splanchnic blood flow is increased in patients with sepsis.[113] Although it has not yet been demonstrated, hepatic dysfunction may be a result of cytokine production in the gut or from peripheral tissues.[1]

Renal Failure

In the context of MOF, renal failure is often defined as a 0.5-1.0 mg/dL increase in serum creatinine or a serum creatinine > 2.0 mg/dL. With increasing sepsis, usually a progressive tendency exists for oliguria to develop unless large quantities of fluid are given. However, even if the urine output is well maintained at over 1.0 mL/kg/hour, creatinine clearance (Cl_{Cr}) will often decrease rapidly to < 50 mL/minute.[114] If the patient is receiving an aminoglycoside, it is particularly important to follow the Cl_{Cr} level.

Occasionally, because of a concentrating defect in the kidneys, an "inappropriate polyuria" develops in septic patients. It is called inappropriate because the polyuria may persist even when the plasma volume becomes extremely low and the urine sodium concentration decreases to < 10 mEq/L. At times it may be difficult to differentiate inappropriate polyuria from the fluid mobilization that typically occurs as a patient begins to improve following major surgery or trauma.

Cardiovascular Failure

Cardiovascular changes of early sepsis typically include vasodilation and an increased cardiac output and vascular permeability. Vasodilation and increasing capillary permeability result in the patient often requiring intravenous fluids > 200-300 mL/hour above measured losses to maintain an adequate BP and urine output. The volume status of septic patients may be very confusing because these patients are often edematous, and an increasing PVR tends to increase CVP; however, PAWP is usually normal or only slightly elevated.

As early as 1965 it was reported that, with increasing sepsis, cardiac output usually increases and systemic vascular resistance decreases.[115] If the cardiac index decreases below 2.5 L/min/m² in septic patients, the mortality rate may exceed 75%, even if hypotension is not present. Calvin et al. also noted that survivors tended to demonstrate greater increases in CI and left ventricular stroke work index (LVSWI) as PAWP increased than did nonsurvivors.[116] Other studies using cardioscintography to measure left-ventricular end-diastolic volumes (LVEDV) and ejection fractions (LVEF) seem to indicate that myocardial contractility is usually not depressed in early sepsis.[117]

Oxygen consumption (VO_2) is one of the most important measurements in septic patients.[118] In early sepsis it is usually greater than the normal of 130-160 mL/minute/m². However, if the AV oxygen difference is > 5.0 vol%, oxygen delivery (DO_2) tends to be lower than needed. If VO_2 falls to < 50 mL/minute/m², or if the VO_2 stays < 100 mL/min/m², most patients die.[118]

AXIOM   Generally, the higher the VO_2 is maintained in critically injured patients, especially during the first 12-24 hours, the better the patient's prognosis will be.

Neurologic Failure

Signs of increasing neurologic failure in sepsis include progressive lethargy, alternating with restlessness and confusion, evolving to semi-coma, and finally deep coma. These signs may be extremely variable from time-to-time and day-to-day, but usually a progressive decline occurs as long as sepsis continues.

Gastrointestinal Failure

One of the most frequent signs of gastrointestinal failure in sepsis is a progressive ileus. Consequently, a well-functioning nasogastric tube is essential to prevent excessive abdominal distension. The presence of sepsis also predisposes patients to stress-related gastric mucosal damage, which is believed to be due to decreased mucosal perfusion. Prophylaxis with acid-reducing therapy or sucralfate decreases the incidence of clinically significant bleeding. Sucralfate is preferred by some because it preserves gastric acidity, thereby decreasing bacterial colonization and (presumably) subsequent pneumonia, but this is controversial. When gastric pH stays < 3.0 in spite of acid suppression therapy and hourly antacids, abdominal sepsis is often present.

PITFALL ⊘

Although upper gastrointestinal feeding may reduce stress-related gastric mucosal damage, jejunostomy feedings are not as effective.

Metabolic Failure

Even with adequate calories (25-35 cal/kg/day) and protein (1.3-2.0 g/kg/day), nitrogen balance in septic patients tends to be negative.[119] Albumin and transferrin levels tend to become progressively lower, and urine creatinine, which is normally about 1500 mg/day in adult males,[114] may decrease to < 600 mg/day. A greatly reduced daily creatinine excretion combined with high urinary nitrogen loss may be an indication of increased catabolism of vital organs rather than muscle.

Intolerance to administered glucose is an excellent sign of increased stress, usually due to sepsis.[120,121] Inhibition of pyruvate dehydrogenase (PDH) by long-chain fatty acyl coenzyme A (CoA) results in accumulation of pyruvate, lactate, and other gluconeogenic precursors. Conversion of pyruvate to acetyl CoA is also inhibited in sepsis. Elevated plasma triglyceride levels seen in sepsis result in increased fatty acyl CoA concentrations, and these inhibit PDH.[122] If the patient is receiving parenteral nutrition, glucose intolerance will usually be obvious much earlier. In terminal sepsis, the patient may also become intolerant to intravenous lipids.[119]

Immunologic Failure

Impaired host-defense may be characterized by anergy with a complete lack of response to standard, delayed hypersensitivity skin test antigens, such as candida, mumps, PPD, histoplasmin, and trichophyton. An absolute lymphocyte count (ALC) < 800-1500/mm^3 may also be an indication of anergy.[123]

Endocrine Failure

Up to 15% of critically ill patients with sepsis may have at least transient adrenal insufficiency as evidenced by cortisol levels that are normal or only slightly elevated and little or no response to ACTH.[124] All patients with adrenal insufficiency and sepsis die unless they are given corticosteroids. If shock develops, these patients tend to have good responses to massive doses of corticosteroids.

Relative parathormone insufficiency may occur in sepsis; however, ionized calcium levels usually decrease in advanced sepsis,[125] and tend to remain low in spite of increased parathormone activity as reflected by increased nephrogenous production of cyclic AMP.[126]

HYPERDYNAMIC (WARM) SEPTIC SHOCK

AXIOM Characteristically, patients in early septic shock are vasodilated, have a normal or increased cardiac output, and have warm, dry, pink, or flushed skin.

It may be difficult at times to determine precisely when severe sepsis with a slightly low BP becomes hyperdynamic septic shock. However, shock is generally considered to be present if: (a) the systolic BP decreases to < 90 mm Hg, the mean BP decreases to < 65 mm Hg, or either pressure decreases by > 25%, (b) urine output decreases to < 0.4 mL/kg/hour, (c) metabolic acidosis develops, or (d) the VO$_2$ is < 100 mL/minute/m^2.

Even with a normal oxygen delivery (DO$_2$), oxygen extraction in sepsis may be ≤ 15%. We found that a low or decreasing VO$_2$ often indicates that shock is developing before there is a significant decrease in BP. Furthermore, failure of the VO$_2$ to increase to normal or higher levels with treatment is a grave prognostic sign.

Even if hypotension becomes severe, the cardiac index in early sepsis tends to be normal (2.5-4.0 L/minute/m^2) or high, particularly if the blood volume is adequately maintained or increased.[127] Anemia or cirrhosis tends to increase cardiac output even more. The increased stroke volume and pulse pressure tend to make arterial pulses in early sepsis easily palpable.

HYPODYNAMIC (COLD) SEPTIC SHOCK

Low-cardiac output is characteristic of late septic shock. It is usually unrelated to the types of bacteria involved.[128] Oxygen delivery is generally reduced and oxygen consumption is often less than half of normal. With increasing vasoconstriction, the skin becomes cold, clammy, mottled, or cyanotic, and severe oliguria tends to develop.

AXIOM Hypodynamic (cold) septic shock usually occurs late in sepsis and indicates that cardiac failure and some element of hypovolemia are present.

The main causes of the low-cardiac output of late-septic shock are cardiac failure and hypovolemia. In a study of 48 septic shock patients, Parker et al. reported that right and left ventricular ejection fractions tended to decrease, while left and right ventricular end-diastolic volumes tended to increase.[128] These changes, which are characteristic of a failing heart, can occur within the first 24 hours of septic shock and persist for at least one week.[129] These changes are believed to be due to a myocardial depressant factor.[1] In several different animal models, myocyte depression has been elicited by addition of serum from septic patients, TNF, gram-negative bacteria, gram-positive bacteria, and endotoxin.[130,131] Similar results have been obtained when TNF, IL-2, or endotoxin are given to humans.[130,132]

As sepsis progresses, capillaries and small veins throughout the body, particularly in infected tissues, develop greatly increased permeability, and increasing amounts of fluid become sequestered in the interstitial spaces. In a period of 12-24 hours, ≥ 10 L of extra fluid may be required to replace this loss.

Water, sodium, and calcium tend to move into cells whose metabolism is impaired. Consequently, even though the total body water may be much greater than normal and the patient appears to be overhydrated, an increasing tendency exists for the development of absolute or relative hypovolemia.

Laboratory Studies

WHITE BLOOD CELL COUNT

In most septic patients, the WBC count is elevated to 15,000/mm^3 or more, usually with a "shift to the left" (i.e., > 5% immature [band] forms). In some patients, the total WBC may be normal, and the only evidence of sepsis may be a shift to the left. In severe, advanced sepsis, particularly due to gram-negative bacilli, the WBC count occasionally may be low (< 4,000/mm^3), and this is often an ominous prognostic sign.

In a study of patients with penetrating abdominal injuries, the WBC count during the first five posttrauma days averaged 15,500/mm^3 for patients without infection and 19,800/mm^3 for patients with infections.[2] In uninfected patients, 90% had at least one WBC count above 10,000/mm^3.

AXIOM Although a leukocytosis after trauma raises the suspicion of infection, specific additional evidence for infection should be sought before antibiotics are begun.[2]

The absolute lymphocyte count (ALC), which is normally 2,500/mm^3 or more, may provide some indication of the type of infection present and the status of the patient's host defenses. If the absolute lymphocyte count is < 1500/mm^3, one should suspect the presence of impaired host defenses. If the absolute lymphocyte count is < 800/mm^3, host defenses are generally impaired, and the patient will usually be nonreactive to standard, delayed hypersensitivity skin tests.[123]

BLOOD CHEMISTRIES

Glucose Levels

Blood glucose levels tend to be elevated in sepsis, particularly if TPN is started. The response to insulin is also often impaired.[133]

Ionized Calcium Levels

In septic patients, plasma ionized calcium levels can rapidly decrease to values less than the normal of 2.1-2.4 mEq/L (1.05-1.20 mmol/L). Because the ECF-ionized calcium is about 10^{-3} molar and the intracellular ionized calcium levels may be as low as 10^{-7}, the gradient across many cell membranes is about 10,000 to 1.[134] When cell metabolism becomes impaired, increased amounts of ionized calcium move into the cytoplasm, and the plasma ionized calcium can rapidly decrease to levels of < 0.9 mmol/L. In general, when ionized calcium levels decrease to < 0.7 mmol/L, cardiovascular performance is often impaired and prognosis can be severely reduced.

AXIOM A progressive decrease in plasma-ionized calcium levels should make one look for sepsis, impaired tissue perfusion, or some other cause of altered cell metabolism.

COAGULATION STUDIES

In sepsis, increasing activation of platelets occurs, and stimulation of the coagulation cascade results in a progressive reduction in the platelet count and the concentrations of most clotting factors.[135,136] Neame et al., using sensitive tests for detecting thrombin and plasmin activation, found evidence of disseminated intravascular coagulation (DIC) in almost all patients with bacteremia who had platelet counts of $< 50,000/mm^3$.[137]

Wilson et al. attempted to predict or diagnose early sepsis by measuring plasma antithrombin III levels in patients at risk for developing infection.[138] Antithrombin (AT) accounts for 80% of the body's defense against intravascular coagulation. As each molecule of thrombin is formed, a molecule of antithrombin binds with it irreversibly. Thus, any stimulation of the clotting system, which occurs early in sepsis, can rapidly reduce antithrombin levels below the normal of 75% to 120% of control.

AXIOM Low antithrombin levels in the absence of extensive clotting or severe liver disease generally indicate that infection is present or will develop.

AT levels $< 60\%$, especially if progressively decreasing, in the absence of liver disease, bleeding, deep venous thrombosis, or recent, massive transfusions are strong predictors of sepsis.[138] If AT levels have not risen to 70% by four days after trauma, a 70-80% chance exists that the patient is infected or will become infected.

BLOOD GASES

Sepsis is a powerful stimulus to ventilation. Initial blood gas analyses in patients developing septic shock generally reveal a $PaCO_2 < 30\text{-}35$ mm Hg, normal bicarbonate levels (21-26 mEq/L), and pH > 7.45.[139,140] Early hyperventilation so frequently accompanies sepsis that, if a patient with other evidence of infection is not hyperventilating, one should suspect that the patient has metabolic alkalosis or is developing respiratory failure.

The initial respiratory alkalosis in sepsis is generally a nonspecific response and not compensatory for hypoxemia or metabolic acidosis. However, if shock were to develop and/or oxygen consumption were to decrease, lactic acid levels would tend to increase, causing the patient to hyperventilate even more as a compensatory response.

As shock becomes more severe, anaerobic metabolism increases, eventually producing lactic acidemia. Baker et al. demonstrated a significant difference in initial lactate levels between survivors and non-survivors (5.1 vs 8.2 mEq/L).[141] On recovery of shock or just prior to death, nonsurvivors' lactate levels were 7.7 compared with 2.6 in the survivor group. In addition, many septic patients had an increased anion gap metabolic acidosis that could not be explained by lactic acid alone.[142]

Metabolic alkalosis has been noted in an increasing number of clinically ill and injured patients, particularly when severe sepsis is present.[143] The etiology of the increased bicarbonate levels, often developing in spite of concurrent respiratory alkalosis, is not always clear. Some of the most frequently recognized possible causes of this metabolic alkalosis include bicarbonate administration, instillation of antacids into the stomach to reduce gastric acidity, removal of large quantities of acidic gastric secretions, hypokalemia due to excessive diuresis and/or the use of corticosteroids, and increased metabolism of citrate (from blood transfusions) or lactate (from Ringer's lactate) to bicarbonate.

BACTERIOLOGIC STUDIES

Smears

PITFALL ⊘

When smears are not obtained before antibiotic therapy is begun, bacteriologic diagnosis may be delayed or inaccurate.

Whenever possible, pus or exudate from any infected or contaminated areas should be smeared and Gram stained prior to beginning antibiotic therapy. Often this simple approach of obtaining and reading a Gram-stained smear of pus or exudate is ignored, thereby losing potentially valuable information regarding the etiologic agent. Not infrequently, various factors or technical errors may cause either no organisms or the wrong organisms to grow on culture. Under such circumstances, the information obtained from examination of the initial smear may be especially valuable.

Quantification of the number of PMNs and bacteria on sputum smears may help to differentiate between positive sputum cultures due to colonization, tracheobronchitis, and pneumonitis. With colonization, few, if any, PMNs are manifest and only a small number of organisms (10^1-10^2/mL) are present. Tracheobronchitis is characterized by sputum with more bacteria (10^3-10^4/mL) and moderate numbers of PMNs. In pneumonitis, generally many bacteria ($\geq 10^5$/mL) and many PMNs are seen.

AXIOM Bronchial secretions obtained during bronchoscopy by bronchoalveolar lavage or protected brush specimens are generally more reliable than induced sputum or tracheal aspirates.

For a smear to be accurate, it must be a good representative sample of the material available. Obtaining proper samples of tracheobronchial secretions, except by protected brush specimens or bronchoalveolar lavage during bronchoscopy, may be difficult, but they can be very helpful.[144,145] Many sputum samples consist largely of mouth and pharyngeal secretions. When alveolar macrophages (dust cells) can be recognized in the specimen, a relatively good sample of lower respiratory tract material has probably been obtained.

AXIOM Occasionally, pleural fluid can be obtained by thoracentesis in patients with pneumonia, and the organisms found there usually are the same as those in the underlying lung infection.

Obtaining a good urine specimen can be a problem in some patients with suspected urinary tract infection. Some believe that if the patient is catheterized, the specimen should be obtained by aspirating the Foley catheter tubing with a needle rather than by disconnecting the tube and breaking the closed drainage system. If the patient is not catheterized, a clean, midstream catch in a man is usually a fairly accurate specimen. In women, suprapubic aspiration of the bladder provides the greatest accuracy.

AXIOM Even when urine contains more than 10^5 microorganisms/mL, pyuria should also be present to warrant diagnosis and treatment of a urinary tract infection.

Culture and Sensitivity Studies

As with smears, the accuracy of culture studies depends primarily on how representative the material submitted is of the involved fluid or organ. It also depends on how rapidly and carefully the specimen is handled. At Detroit Receiving Hospital (DRH), specimens of pus taken from a variety of abscesses will show "no growth" in about 50% of cases if it takes more than two hours for the specimen to reach the lab. If the specimen is taken directly to the laboratory and is plated almost immediately, bacteria grow out in almost 100% of cases.

AXIOM Exudate or pus that is not cultured rapidly in the microbiology laboratory often yields inconclusive or deceptive results, particularly if mixed infections are present.

Great care must also be taken to avoid skin contaminants when taking blood cultures or culturing exudate from wound infections. Cultures taken with swabs should be taken from the edges of abscesses and not the center. Material from the center of abscesses is more likely to contain only necrotic material and dead PMNs.

AXIOM The ideal specimen for detecting the microorganisms responsible for an abscess is a tissue biopsy from the edge of the abscess.

Whenever possible, both aerobic and anaerobic cultures should be made of all infected or contaminated material recovered from tissue abscesses. Anaerobic cultures must be taken with the same precautions as arterial blood gases and then placed immediately into tubes containing carbon dioxide and no oxygen. The material should then be placed into appropriate media and incubated as soon as possible.

AXIOM False-negative anaerobic cultures are common, and this should be considered when choosing antibiotic therapy based on laboratory studies.

When rapid information on aerobic bacteria is desired, a direct smear of infected material onto blood agar plates may yield characteristic colonies within a few hours. When this is done with antibiotic discs already on the agar plate, helpful information on sensitivities may also be available within 24 hours.

Blood Cultures

In patients with bacteremias, at least two blood cultures should be obtained at intervals of at least 20-30 minutes because one or more of these blood cultures are often negative, and a single positive blood culture may be due to a contaminant. Diurnal variations in temperature are probably related primarily to cortisol production by the body rather than to the presence of organisms in blood. Ideally, blood cultures should be drawn just before a patient spikes a fever.

For suspected, acute, untreated bacterial pneumonia, meningitis, or acute bacterial endocarditis, two sets of samples (20 mL/set for adults) should be obtained from separate sites (left and right arms) before empiric antibiotics are started. For patients with fever of unknown origin or suspected subacute bacterial endocarditis, three sets of blood samples should be obtained on the first day with the samples drawn at least 60 minutes apart. If the culture results are negative after 24 hours, three more samples should be drawn. If six blood-culture results are negative, special culture techniques may be needed.

When the patient has received antibiotics, inoculation of at least one hypertonic blood culture bottle or one resin-containing bottle should be done to remove the antibiotics. Although previous antimicrobial therapy may delay the growth of organisms, drawing more than six blood cultures does not usually increase the yield of positive results.

Getting positive blood cultures can be a special problem in patients with gram-negative bacteremia because these are often relatively low-grade infections, and the bacteremia may be transient. Observation of the cultures for as long as two weeks and blind subculturing often increases the yield.

AXIOM The "rule of threes" for blood cultures states that three blood cultures per day for three days will generally detect gram-negative bacteremia in untreated patients.

Cultures of Intravenous Catheters

If an intravenous catheter infection is suspected, blood cultures should be drawn through that catheter and directly from another vein. In addition, the tip and intracutaneous portion of the catheter should be cultured. Intravenous catheter tips must be cultured carefully because of the high incidence of contamination as the catheter is removed.

Invasive Burn Wound Infection

Quantitative cultures of potentially infected tissue can be extremely useful. It is now clear that colony counts that are $\geq 10^5/g$ of burned tissue generally indicate invasive infection. Furthermore, skin ulcers or wounds containing more than this concentration of organisms usually cannot be skin-grafted successfully. With β-hemolytic streptococci, however, as few as 10 organisms/g of tissue in an open wound can prevent successful skin grafting.

Problems with Culture Results

Often the most rapidly growing organisms, rather than the ones responsible for infection, are grown out on culture. When the culture result correlates with what is found on the Gram stain, the results usually are reliable. When the results do not correlate, one must use clinical judgment and/or obtain further cultures and smears.

AXIOM Smears and cultures should be obtained, whenever possible, before antibiotic therapy is begun.

Once they are started, antibiotics can stop growth of all or some bacteria unless specific steps are taken to inhibit or dilute the antibiotic. When the patient has been receiving antibiotics but continues to have evidence of sepsis and the cultures keep showing "no growth" or "normal flora," a special effort should be made to culture anaerobic organisms and fungi, especially candida.

AXIOM The location and extent of an infection and the bacteria involved may be masked while the patient receives antibiotics.

In some instances, antibiotics do not control infection, but they mask its signs, can make it extremely difficult to locate, and prevent the responsible organisms from growing in culture. If the infection is not controlled after one or more changes of antibiotics or if the location of the infection causing the sepsis cannot be determined, it may be advisable to stop all antibiotics for 24-48 hours. After that time, cultures are more apt to be positive and the abscess or site of infection is more likely to be identified. The decision to stop antibiotics in critically ill or injured patients must be individualized because the patient's infection may get considerably worse while the antibiotics are discontinued.

In some instances, a relatively high, spiking fever disappears after antibiotics have been discontinued. When the fever does not reappear in 48-72 hours, it can generally be assumed that the patient had antibiotic (drug) fever.

Opportunistic Infections

An increasing number of opportunistic infections of the lungs occurs, especially in patients with granulocytopenia or AIDS. Although giving a multitude of drugs designed to treat the organisms most likely to cause these infections is frequently successful, bronchoalveolar lavage or protected brush specimens may be required to make a definitive diagnosis and provide effective treatment.

If the diagnosis is still in doubt, thoracotomy with open-lung biopsy may be required. In many instances, open-lung biopsy is of value because it shows that the infiltrate is not due to microorganisms, and this allows several potentially toxic antimicrobial agents to be discontinued. However, the risk of open-lung biopsy in such patients can be high and, even with appropriate therapy, the mortality rate often exceeds 60-70%.

Skin Testing

Failure of the patient to react to skin testing of four or more skin-recall antigens, including mumps, candida, trichophyton, histoplasmin, and/or purified protein derivative (PPD), indicates severe impairment of host defenses and is referred to as anergy.[59] Most of our patients with severe trauma and/or massive transfusions are anergic for two to three days. If anergy persists beyond the fourth day, the patients generally develop one or more infections. Over 95% of our ICU patients with serum albumin levels below 2.2 g/dL and absolute lymphocyte counts (ALC) < 800/mm³ have been anergic.

AXIOM When skin testing shows a patient to be persistently anergic, one should look carefully for an infection and make sure that nutritional intake is adequate.

Radiologic Procedures

PLAIN RADIOGRAPHIC AND CONTRAST STUDIES

Plain radiographs are usually of relatively little help in diagnosing sepsis, especially in the abdomen. However, air-fluid levels outside the bowel, such as between the liver and diaphragm, are highly suggestive of a subphrenic abscess. Displacement of bowel loops or other abdominal organs may also be evidence of an abscess. In a study of the reliability of various tests for diagnosing abdominal abscesses, Glick et al. found that KUB radiographs had a sensitivity of 33% and accuracy of 20%.[146] Contrast enemas had a sensitivity of 43% and an accuracy of 40%.

RADIOIOSOTOPIC SCANS

The main isotopes used to diagnose and localize infections in the abdomen have been gallium and indium. HIDA and PIPIDA scans have been used to diagnose acute cholecystitis.

Gallium Scans

Gallium scanning is seldom used for investigating possible intra-abdominal infections. The gallium scanner is not portable, and the cost is significantly higher than for ultrasonography. Furthermore, the results of ultrasonography are available immediately, while it requires 48 hours for an adequate gallium scan assessment.[147] Significant numbers of false-positive diagnoses occur with gallium scanning, due, in part, to its normal excretion into the bowel and kidneys.[147] In some patients, it is impossible to differentiate an abscess from normal bowel excretion. The gallium scan will also be positive in areas of recent trauma or surgery. Some physicians believe that the accuracy of gallium scanning for diagnosing abdominal abscess is about 50% (i.e., it is no better than flipping a coin).

Indium Scans

Indium-111-labeled leukocytes can be of particular value as an adjunct to ultrasonography and CT scans, which can detect fluid collections, but cannot identify the contents.[148] Unfortunately, indium-111-labeled leukocyte uptake is nonspecific. Accumulation of indium may occur in the colon after multiple enemas and in bowel with vasculitis or ischemia. Uptake in a wide variety of tissues with nonspecific inflammatory changes, tumors, and even hematomas has also been described.[148]

AXIOM Gallium and/or indium scans are of little value for detecting acute infections in trauma patients.

HIDA-PIPIDA Scans

Acalculous cholecystitis is an increasingly recognized complication in critically ill patients and now comprises about 5-10% of all acute cholecystitis.[86] Gallstones are absent in up to 62% of patients in whom acute cholecystitis develops after an unrelated surgical procedure.[149] Gallstones may also be absent in 87% of patients with acute cholecystitis after major trauma.[150]

AXIOM The preferred test for evaluating the biliary tract is ultrasonography with or without HIDA or PIPIDA hepatobiliary scanning.[151,152]

When ultrasonography shows dilatation of the gallbladder or thickening of its wall in a patient who may have acute cholecystitis, a PIPIDA scan should be done.[152] If this shows excretion of the isotope into the small bowel but no visualization of the gallbladder, the diagnosis of acute cholecystitis is fairly accurate. Unfortunately, PIPIDA scanning requires movement of the patient to the radiologic suite for imaging for up to two hours. Furthermore, it is poor in diagnosing chronic cholecystitis and cholelithiasis unless the cystic duct is occluded.

AXIOM Patients who have been on TPN for five to seven days may not have their gallbladders visualized on a PIPIDA scan even when the cystic duct is patent and the gallbladder is normal.

ULTRASONOGRAPHY

Ultrasonographic examination of the abdomen can be performed quickly, is relatively inexpensive, and can be done in the emergency department, OR, or ICU. However, special problems with drains and ostomies exist, and the accuracy of the study is technician-dependent. Even under ideal circumstances, it is usually only 50-60% accurate.[152]

Ultrasonography can be particularly helpful in screening for acute acalculous cholecystitis by demonstrating progressive gallbladder dilatation, increasing wall edema, and sludge in the lumen. However, dilatation of the gallbladder and sludge formation on ultrasonography are also common findings in normal gallbladders after prolonged fasting.[85]

Ultrasonography has been recommended for some time for guiding percutaneous drainage of abdominal abscesses or loculated fluid collections in the chest. Visualization of abdominal organs with ultrasound is better than with fluoroscopy, and the pathway for the drainage catheter can be adequately planned in most cases. However, the actual placement of the needle, guide wire, and catheter cannot be observed; thus, the danger of injury to uninvolved abdominal organs still exists.

CT SCANS

CT scan is now generally considered the most accurate, noninvasive technique for diagnosing abscesses or other fluid collections in the abdomen or chest. In some reports it has had 98% sensitivity and 95% specificity.[153] However, it is expensive, and the patient must be moved to the CT scan suite. Furthermore, it may be difficult to differentiate pus from other fluid, tumors, thick cysts, or cellulitis (phlegmon). It is useful for directing the insertion of percutaneously-placed catheters to drain intraabdominal or intrathoracic fluid collections.

AXIOM CT scans are the ideal tests for detecting intraabdominal abscesses, but they are relatively unreliable during the first five days after trauma.

Clinical Characteristics of Infections Caused by Various Microorganisms

The signs, symptoms, and clinical courses of the most frequent infections following trauma are often characteristic and, in some instances, may be virtually diagnostic.

STAPHYLOCOCCAL INFECTIONS

The typical lesion produced by (coagulase-positive) Staphylococcus aureus is usually well localized and consists of an indurated area that undergoes central necrosis and abscess formation with the development of a thick, creamy, odorless pus. Fever and leukocytosis are usually present, especially if the infection is uncontrolled, spreading, or causing septicemia. Bacteremia or septicemia can be dangerous because of the high frequency with which metastatic abscesses can develop.

Occasionally, S. aureus can produce a relatively mild wound infection with severe systemic signs and symptoms due to a specific toxin (toxic-shock Staphylococcal toxin) which can cause hypotension, red rash, and MOF.[154,155]

Coagulase-negative Staphylococci are being recognized increasingly in intravenous catheter infections and following operations on the cardiovascular system. In some centers, it is the most frequent cause of infection following cardiac surgery. Because of the concern that a positive blood culture with S. epidermidis may be a contaminant, at least two separate positive cultures are often required for diagnosis.

STREPTOCOCCAL INFECTIONS

A wide variety of streptococcal infections may be seen following trauma; however, because most of the infections caused by these organisms respond so well to penicillin, they are rarely a problem once recognized. Most of these infections are caused by Streptococcus pyogenes (group A, β-hemolytic); however, other streptococci, such as Streptococcus viridans, may also be encountered.

Streptococcus Pyogenes

The lesions cause by S. pyogenes are characterized by a rapid progression of cellulitis, lymphangitis, lymphadenitis, and extension of the inflammation along fascial planes. Thin, watery pus may develop, but frank abscess formation rarely occurs. Erysipelas, which classically appears as a superficial spreading cellulitis with indurated, raised, and irregular margins, is most often caused by Streptococcus hemolyticus. Bacteremia occurs frequently and may result in septic shock within 24 hours of infection. It is characterized by chills, high fever, a rapid thready pulse, and general signs of toxemia.

AXIOM   Septic shock developing within 24-48 hours of trauma is usually due to Streptococcus pyogenes or Clostridium welchii.

Streptococcal Gangrene

Streptococcal gangrene, usually caused by anaerobic streptococci, is a rapidly spreading, invasive, fascial, and subcutaneous infection that may be associated with thrombosis of nutrient vessels resulting in necrosis and slough of the overlying skin. Occasionally, the patient may also develop clear, bullous lesions which may coalesce and become filled with hemorrhagic fluid. These infections usually occur in wounds of the lower extremities or abdomen.

Enterococci

Infections containing enterococcus organisms typically develop relatively late (seven or more days after trauma) and usually only in combination with gram-negative aerobes or anaerobes in debilitated individuals who had been receiving broad-spectrum antibiotics.

INFECTIONS CAUSED BY GRAM-NEGATIVE BACILLI

Gram-negative bacilli are involved in most infections associated with injury to the gastrointestinal or genitourinary tracts. These infections are usually polymicrobial and typically involve both anaerobic and aerobic organisms. Wound infections caused by gram-negative aerobes generally have a longer incubation period than those caused by staphylococci or streptococci, and often cause less systemic toxicity, at least initially.

After several days or weeks of treatment with broad-spectrum antibiotics, the likelihood of antibiotic-resistant gram-negative aerobes being cultured from many parts of the body increases, particularly in the tracheobronchial tree.

MIXED INFECTIONS

AXIOM   Mixed soft-tissue infections after trauma usually occur in wounds contaminated by soil, bites, gastrointestinal contents, or infected urine.[155]

Soft-tissue infections caused by mixed gram-positive and gram-negative organisms are characterized by necrosis of subcutaneous and fascial tissues with progressive gangrene in the skin from thrombosis of local nutrient vessels (Table 39-2). A wide variety of etiologic agents have been associated with this condition, including Bacteroides, anaerobic streptococci, and various coliforms. Crepitation in the wound because of local gas formation may be caused by many different bacteria, including Clostridium welchii, the etiologic agent for most cases of gas gangrene.

INFECTIONS CAUSED BY ANAEROBES

With improved culturing techniques, anaerobic organisms are recognized increasingly as a cause of infections following trauma or surgery. Anaerobic bacteria are divided into five main groups: (a) gram-negative nonsporulating rods, such as Bacteroides and Fusobacteria, (b) gram-positive nonsporulating rods, including the Eubacterium and Bifidobacterium, (c) large gram-positive sporulating rods, such as clostridial organisms, (d) gram-positive cocci, such as the Peptostreptococci, and (e) gram-negative cocci, such as the Veillonella.[156] The most frequently encountered anaerobes in surgical infections, particularly after colon injuries, are Bacteroides species, followed by Peptostreptococci and clostridial organisms.

Bacteroides Infections

Various bacteroides species are, by far, the most frequent organisms in the colon. Because these organisms may cause only minimal local inflammatory changes, at least initially, infections by these organisms may be difficult to identify or localize. Although Bacteroides fragilis subspecies fragilis organisms are the only Bacteroides organisms with a capsule and although they make up only 7% of the Bacteroides organisms found in normal colons, its capsule increases its virulence so much that they are cultured in over 40% of infections where Bacteroides species are found. The nonfragilis species of Bacteroides are more common than the fragilis types in some series and are more resistant to certain antibiotics, such as cefotetan.

Peptostreptococcus

Peptostreptococcus is the most important anaerobic gram-positive coccus. It is often associated with anaerobic myositis, joint infection, breast abscess, septic abortion, liver abscesses, and empyema. It has often been associated with Bacteroides in a variety of mixed infections.[156] With the exception of Peptococcus niger, all pathogenic species formerly in the genus Peptococcus have been transferred to the genus Peptostreptococcus. Both Peptococcus and Peptostreptococcus can produce a foul odor and gas. Peptostreptococcus organisms are normally present in the vagina, mouth, and feces.

TABLE 39-2   Clinical Clues to Possible Polymicrobial Infection

---

I. Clinical setting suggestive of infection due to colonization by bacteria normally resident on mucosal or skin surfaces
 A. Soft-tissue infection due to acute or chronic skin breaks, especially in the perineum region and/or on the feet
 B. Intra-abdominal infection due to a torn hollow viscus
 C. Gynecologic infections after instrumentation or operation
 D. Soft-tissue infections of head and neck due to mucosal trauma or disease
 E. Infection after human or animal bites
II. Infection associated with malignancy or other process resulting in tissue destruction
III. Necrotic tissue, gangrene, or pseudomembrane formation
IV. Gas in tissues or wound drainage
V. Foul-smelling discharge

From: Ahrenholz and Simmons, 1988.[155]

Clostridial Infections

The clostridial infections most apt to occur in injured patients include clostridial cellulitis, clostridial myositis, and tetanus. Surgeons faced with a patient who has any infected gangrenous tissue must try to categorize the lesion accurately because the extent and urgency of the treatment required may differ markedly (Table 39–3).[155]

AXIOM Most gangrenous infections with gas in the tissues are not gas gangrene, but these lesions should be treated as such until proven otherwise.

Gangrene, even when associated with gas in the tissue, is often due to nonclostridial organisms, and even if clostridial organisms are present, they are not all of the same seriousness. For example, although clostridial cellulitis may be extremely painful and have an ominous appearance, it is seldom fatal unless the patient is debilitated and the treatment is inadequate. Clostridial myositis, conversely, can cause sudden, severe prostration of the patient and may be rapidly fatal. In some instances, this organism can cause septic shock, or even death, within 24 hours of the onset of infection.

CLOSTRIDIAL CELLULITIS. Clostridial cellulitis can be caused by several Clostridia species, but Clostridium welchii is the most frequent.[157] This infection of the skin, subcutaneous, and connective tissues is a crepitant cellulitis which spreads rapidly along fascial planes and typically produces a gray or reddish-brown discharge. Eventually, necrosis and sloughing of the involved superficial fascia, subcutaneous tissue, and skin may occur as a result of thrombosis or local blood vessels. Pain in and around the wound is severe.

CLOSTRIDIAL MYOSITIS. Gas gangrene, which is also known as clostridial myositis, is usually caused by Clostridium welchii; however, C. novyi, C. septicum, and C. sordellii may also cause this problem.[157] This dreaded complication should be anticipated in any wound in which extensive destruction of muscle has occurred combined with severe contamination of tissues, particularly when any delay in therapy or an associated vascular injury was present.

This infection is characterized by rapidly spreading gangrene of muscle and a profound toxemia. Swelling and pain occur early, often within the first 24 hours after injury. Gas formation with crepitation within the muscle and along fascial planes is usually found, but may be absent in some patients. The infected muscle quickly becomes soft, swollen, and dark red, and frequently a foul-smelling, brown, watery exudate is evident.

AXIOM Because of a clostridial leukocidin, relatively few white blood cells are present in the exudate from gas gangrene.

The prostration of the patient with gas gangrene is often far out of proportion to the fever. Early diagnosis is facilitated by examination of the wound discharge which may contain many large gram-positive rods, usually without spores.

TETANUS. Tetanus, caused by Clostridium tetani, is an extremely serious anaerobic infection. It is much less common in the United States now than in past decades because most citizens have had at least partial immunization. Nevertheless, many patients have failed to obtain subsequent booster doses at the prescribed intervals.

Tetanus is a unique infection in that virtually all the symptoms are caused by a powerful exotoxin released by growing bacteria.[158] Although this infection is most apt to occur with deep and dirty wounds, it is occasionally seen in patients with relatively small, innocuous-appearing lacerations.

After an incubation period of about 4-12 days, the patient typically begins to experience restlessness, headache, stiffness of the jaw muscles, and intermittent tetanic muscle contractions near the wound. Tachycardia, excessive sweating, and salivation are also often present. Generalized tonic contractions may follow within 12-24 hours, producing a classic facial distortion (risus sardonicus), opisthotonos, and rigidity. Clonic muscle contractions may result from even the slightest stimulation.

FUNGAL INFECTIONS

Within the past few years, the incidence of fungal infections, particularly by Candida species, has risen sharply, especially in patients receiving intravenous hyperalimentation and those with diminished host resistance from severe debilitation or prolonged therapy with steroids or antineoplastic agents.[159] Candida superinfection is always a threat in severely injured patients who have been receiving broad-spectrum antibiotics for two weeks or longer.

TABLE 39-3 *Differential Diagnosis of Crepitant Soft-Tissue Wounds*

Parameter	Clostridial Cellulitis	Nonclostridial Anaerobic Cellulitis	Gas Gangrene	Streptococcal Myositis	Necrotizing Fasciitis	Infected Vascular Gangrene
Predisposing conditions	Local trauma or surgery	Diabetes mellitus; preexisting localized infection	Local trauma or surgery; colon cancer	Local trauma	Diabetes mellitus, abd. surg. perineal inf. drug addiction	Peripheral arterial insuff.
Skin appearance	Minimal discoloration	Minimal discoloration	Yellow-bronze; dark bullae; green-black necrosis[a]	Erthema	Erythematous cellulitis	Discolored or black
Exudate	Thin, dark	Dark pus	Serosanguineous	Abundant seropurulent	Seropurulent	0
Gas	++++	++++	++	±	++ to ++++	0 to +++
Odor	Sometimes foul	Foul	Variable; slightly foul or peculiarly sweet	Slight; sour	Foul	0 to foul
Systemic toxicity	Minimal	Moderate	Marked	Only late in course	Moderate or marked	Minimal
Muscle involvement	0	0	++++	+++	0	Variable

0 = none; ± = mild; ++ = moderate; +++ = severe; ++++ = very severe
[a]Early changes are minimal; these are late findings.
From: Ahrenholz and Simmons, 1988.[155]

Failure to consider candidiasis when bacterial cultures are repeatedly negative in a septic patient who has been on broad-spectrum antibiotics.

Most fungal infections cause relatively few systemic symptoms.[159] Their presence is often not suspected until the organisms are identified in pulmonary secretions or wound drainage. Systemic Candida infections, however, may closely resemble gram-negative septicemia. These infections should be suspected when cultures from patients with this clinical picture are repeatedly negative for aerobic and anaerobic bacteria. Even when they cannot be cultured from the blood, the presence of Candida organisms should be suspected when they are found in large quantities in the mouth, urine, and/or feces.

Monitoring

AXIOM Increasing data suggest that great efforts should be made in patients with severe trauma to increase their oxygen delivery index (DO_2I) to 600 mL/minute/m^2 or more and their oxygen consumption index (VO_2I) to 150-170 mL/minute/m^2 or more as soon as possible after injury.

Shoemaker et al. showed that a $DO_2I > 600$ mL/minute/m^2 and a $VO_2I \geq 170$ mL/minute/m^2 in a variety of high-risk surgical patients reduced organ failure rates and mortality rates.[160] Moore et al. showed that patients in whom a VO_2I of ≥ 150 mL/minute/m^2 was achieved within 12 hours of trauma had a decreased incidence of later MOF ($17\% = 4/24$ vs $80\% = 12/15$).[161]

Fleming et al. prospectively tested the effect of the early postinjury attainment of supranormal values of oxygen delivery (≥ 670 mL/minute/m^2), and oxygen consumption (≥ 166 mL/minute/m^2) on outcome in traumatized patients who had an estimated blood loss of ≥ 2000 mL.[162] The goals in control patients were to attain normal values for all hemodynamic measurements. During a six-month period, 33 protocol patients and 34 control patients with similar vital signs, estimated blood losses, and severity of injuries were enrolled in the study. Eight (24%) protocol patients died, while 15 (44%) control patients died. The protocol patients had fewer mean ($\pm$ SEM) organ failures per patient (0.76 ± 1.21 vs 1.59 ± 1.60), shorter stays in the ICU (5 ± 3 vs 12 ± 12 days), and fewer mean days requiring ventilation (4 ± 3 vs 11 ± 10) than did the control patients ($P < .05$ for each).

PREVENTING INFECTION

Controlling Bleeding

Bleeding should also be controlled as soon as possible. This not only reduces the loss of cells and proteins that are important in host defense, but also reduces the number of needed blood transfusions. If 15 units or more blood transfusions are required, the incidence of serious infections after major trauma can exceed 85%.[9]

Maintaining Tissue Perfusion

Shock must be corrected rapidly. Hypotension should not be allowed to persist for > 15-30 minutes. Maintaining normal or increased blood flow to an injured area is particularly important.

AXIOM Many wound infections following trauma can be prevented by good surgical technique, early, thorough debridement of all contamination or necrotic tissue, and complete drainage of any collections of blood or other fluid.

Although much attention has been given to antibiotics, strict adherence to the surgical principles of good wound care and mainte-

nance of optimal tissue perfusion are by far the most effective means for preventing infection following trauma. Tscherne et al. showed that the infection rate following open fractures was reduced by 75% in patients who had sterile dressings in place from the scene of the accident to the operating room when compared with those who did not.[163]

Quantitative wound cultures reveal an increasing frequency of significant bacterial contamination and risk of wound infection as the duration from injury to wound closure increases.[164] Edlich et al. showed that a wound closed soon after injury is subject to fewer and less severe infections than wounds closed at 12-24 hours.[165]

Careful debridement of contaminated wounds is necessary to reduce bacterial contamination and remove blood and nonviable tissue that can promote bacterial growth.[166] When the wound cannot be completely debrided, irrigation of the wound may help.[167] The appropriate irrigation force may be obtained from commercial irrigation devices or a 50 mL syringe with a 19-gauge needle. Rubber bulb syringe irrigation or irrigation by gravity from intravenous bags is generally ineffective.[168] High-pressure irrigation should be used on dirty or contaminated wounds that cannot be adequately debrided by lesser procedures.[169] Various antiseptic solutions used as wound irrigants have been found to be ineffective for killing bacteria in contaminated wounds. In addition, antiseptics can directly damage the host-defense mechanisms in wounds.[170]

"Wet" wounds with increased amounts of blood and/or serum are at greater risk for infection than dry wounds,[22] and a subcutaneous hematoma with its iron and protein can greatly increase the incidence and severity of infection.[171] Fluid in the dead space of a wound is low in antibody and complement, and provides an environment within which bacteria can grow and WBCs do not function effectively.[172] Nevertheless, the placement of additional sutures, which can function as foreign bodies and increase tension in the wound in an attempt to eliminate dead space, may have the paradoxical effect of increasing infection.[173] Leaving drains, especially of the open (Penrose) type, also increases the risk of infection.[174,175]

Tissues must be handled as gently as possible so as to keep tissue injury to a minimum. The finest sutures capable of repairing the wound should be used. Monofilament, nonabsorbable wire or plastic sutures, such as nylon, cause less tissue reaction than those that are braided and/or absorbable.

In heavily contaminated wounds or where all foreign material or devitalized tissue cannot be satisfactorily removed, the wound should be left open.[165] After the wound edges are granulating well and the risk of infection is past, usually by three to five days, and the quantitative bacteriologic count is $< 10^5$/g of tissue, the wound can be closed safely.[176]

Prophylactic Antibiotics

INDICATIONS

Antibiotics given at the time the trauma victim is first seen are usually not "prophylactic" because some degree of local contamination is present if any mucosal or skin barrier has been damaged. Antibiotics are most apt to be effective when given with two hours of injury.

AXIOM Antibiotic therapy should not be delayed when its use is clinically indicated.

Antibiotics are now generally recommended for: (a) all contaminated or dirty wounds, including dog bites, (b) all surgical procedures or wounds involving bowel, lungs, or urinary tract, (c) clean wounds where infection would be particularly dangerous, including neurosurgical and cardiovascular procedures, especially when prosthetic materials are implanted, and (d) immunosuppressed patients. Old age, massive transfusions, and prolonged surgery may also be indications for prophylactic antibiotics.

Abdominal Trauma

> **AXIOM** Antibiotics effective against anaerobic GI bacteria and gram-negative aerobes should be administered as soon as possible to patients with abdominal trauma involving the distal small bowel or colon.

It is now clear from a large number of prospective double-blind studies[177-184] that proper use of appropriate prophylactic antibiotics can reduce infection rates in patients with abdominal trauma.[1,2] In injured patients, particularly those with intraabdominal wounds, the amount of contamination present may not be apparent clinically for at least several hours. Nevertheless, the sooner antibiotics are started, the more effective they are likely to be.[185] When evidence of bowel injury exists, continued contamination of the peritoneal cavity should be controlled surgically, and the area irrigated, as soon as possible, until it is clean.

Pulmonary Contusions

Some clinicians have recommended the administration of antibiotics to patients with pulmonary contusions because the damaged lung parenchyma is more susceptible to bacterial infection. The risk is increased a great deal if the patient requires endotracheal intubation and mechanical ventilation. The futility of trying to prevent pneumonia in high-risk patients by the use of antibiotics, however, has been known for many years. Furthermore, if an infection were to develop, it often would be caused by resistant organisms. The most effective means of preventing these infections include optimal resuscitation of the patient, strict aseptic management of the endotracheal tube or tracheostomy, aggressive pulmonary toilet, and the earliest possible safe extubation of the patient.[2]

Chest Tubes

Because of the urgent circumstances under which chest tubes are often inserted in an emergency department after trauma, an increased rate of subsequent pleural infection may occur. The use of antibiotics for the treatment of traumatic hemothorax and/or pneumothorax in patients with chest tubes is controversial. Several prospective studies have been published, the majority of which suggest that antibiotics are helpful (Table 39–4).[186-192] Overall, the incidence of lung infection or empyema was reduced by antibiotics from 16.2% (47 of 290) to 2.3% (7 of 301) (P < 0.001). The only

questions still being debated are (a) the best antibiotics to be used and (b) the duration required. It now appears that for most types of trauma, a preoperative dose and one to two additional doses is probably adequate.[193]

> **AXIOM** Although controversial, data from five of seven prospective double-blind studies support using prophylactic antibiotics when chest tubes are inserted for traumatic pneumothorax or hemothorax.

Basilar Skull Fractures

The use of prophylactic antibiotics in basilar skull fractures has been quite controversial.[194] In 1970, Hand and Sanford reported several patients with meningitis following basilar skull fractures.[195] The route of infection appeared to involve a communication between the sinuses or the middle ear and the subarachnoid space. Leech and Paterson believed that preventive antibiotics, when compared with historic or literature controls, showed efficacy for prophylactic antibiotics when a CSF leak was present.[196] Klastersky et al., however, showed acceptably low rates of infection without prophylactic antibiotics.[197] Furthermore, when infections developed in patients on antibiotics, the organisms were more likely to be antibiotic-resistant.

> **AXIOM** Prophylactic antibiotics for uncomplicated traumatic CSF leaks do not reduce the incidence of infection but do increase the likelihood of infection by an antibiotic-resistant organism.

On theoretical grounds, basilar skull fracture with a CSF leak is a setting in which it is preferable not use preventive antibiotics because the risk of infection continues over several days.[2] Every circumstance in which prophylactic antibiotics have been effective in preventing infection has involved a limited time during which contamination may occur.

> **AXIOM** In settings where the risk of infection continues over an extended period of time, preventive antibiotics have uniformly failed to prevent subsequent infection; furthermore, the bacteria involved are more apt to become antibiotic-resistant.[2]

TABLE 39-4 *Summary of Studies Comparing Prophylactic Antibiotics with Placebo for Traumatic Hemopneumothorax in Patients with Chest Tubes*

Reference	Regimen	Incidence of Postoperative Infections					
		Antibiotic Therapy			Placebo		
		Lung[a]	Empyema	Total	Lung[a]	Empyema	Total
Grover et al,[(186)]	Clindamycin 300 mg/IV q 6 h	4/38	1/38	4/38	13/37	6/37	13/37[b]
Stone et al,[(187)]	Cefamandole 1 q 6 h	0/60	1/60	1/60	5/60	3/60	8/60[b]
Mandal et al,[(188)]	Doxycycline 200 mg (1 dose), then 100 mg q 12 hr	0/40	0/40	0/40	0/40	1/40	1/40
LeBlanc and Tucker, 1985[(189)]	Cephapirin 1 q IV q 6 h	1/26	0/26	1/26	1/23	1/23	2/23
LoCurto et al,[(190)]	Cefoxitin 1 g q 6 h	0/30	0/30	0/30	4/28	5/28	8/28[b]
Brunner et al,[(191)]	Cefazolin 1 g IV q 6 h	1/44	0/44	1/44	3/46	6/46	9/46[b]
Nichols et al,[(192)]	Cefonicid 1 g IV daily	0/63	0/63	0/63	3/56	4/56	6/56
TOTAL		6/301 (2.0%)	2/301 (0.7%)	7/301 (2.3%)	29/290 (10.0%)	26/290 (9.0%)	47/290[c] (16.2%)

[a]Pneumonia or lung abscess.
[b]P < 0.5.
[c]P < 0.001 versus antibiotic therapy total.
From: Wilson RF, Janning SW. Handbook of antibiotic therapy for surgery—related infections, 3rd ed. Springfield: Scientific Therapeutics, Inc., 1995; 43.

TIMING OF ANTIBIOTICS

Several investigations have shown that maximum protection from infection in wounds is achieved when antibiotics are administered within two to three hours of bacterial tissue contamination.[2,17,198,199,200]

The optimal duration of prophylactic antibiotics is still unclear. Some clinical trials have relied on a three-dose, 12-hour regimen[22,199]; however, successful prophylactic antibiotic use has ranged from one dose to 14 days.[2] Nevertheless, in virtually all studies, the shorter durations of therapy have consistently been as effective as those given for several more days.[201-203]

In patients with abdominal trauma and suspicion of bowel injury, Fullen et al.[185] and others reported that the early administration of antibiotics with activity against aerobic and anaerobic bowel flora is warranted during resuscitation.[2] If no bowel injury is demonstrated at surgery, the antibiotics can be discontinued after a single dose. When bowel injury is documented, several articles have reported success if the antibiotics are given for 48 hours or less.[13,201-204] Although giving antibiotics for only a short time after trauma may be effective, adequate dosing is extremely important, especially in patients requiring large quantities of fluid.[205]

ANTIBIOTIC CHOICES FOR PARTICULAR INJURIES

Organisms Most Likely to be Involved

The main organisms likely to cause wound infections are staphylococci and streptococci. The staphylococci are generally sensitive to penicillinase-resistant penicillins (such as nafcillin and oxacillin) or first-generation cephalosporins, such as cefazolin (Ancef). β-Hemolytic streptococci are usually sensitive to penicillin.

For Particular Injuries

OPEN SKULL FRACTURES. Open skull fractures or missile penetration of the cranial vault can lead to meningitis or brain abscess. The most common infecting organism in brain abscesses is S. aureus, but Enterobacteriaceae may occasionally be involved. A penicillinase-resistant penicillin with or without a third-generation cephalosporin is usually appropriate.[206] With early cranial or spinal meningitis after trauma, S. pneumoniae is the most common pathogen. When meningitis develops later, it is usually a mixed infection, and the organisms present are influenced by antecedent antibiotic therapy.

If preventive antibiotics are used for an open basilar skull fracture, they should be able to penetrate the blood-brain barrier well; however, after the meninges are inflamed, most antibiotics penetrate the blood-brain barrier adequately.

FACIAL TRAUMA. Severe trauma to the face can cause fractures of the skull, jaws, and other facial bones. In general, antibiotics, such as penicillinase-resistant penicillin, are effective.[206] Prophylaxis for major surgical procedures involving an injury or incision through oral or pharyngeal mucosa calls for more broad-spectrum coverage, to include the oral anaerobes.

THORACIC-PULMONARY TRAUMA. The most common pathogens causing pulmonary infections after thoracic trauma include S. aureus, coagulase-negative staphylococci, S. pneumoniae, Group A streptococci, and Enterobacteriaceae. Late infections are typically caused by Pseudomonas species. Cefazolin is adequate for the gram-positive organisms apt to be involved.[206] For more severe injuries that also involve the digestive tract or for injuries that involve the lungs of patients with chronic bronchitis, broader coverage is indicated.

ABDOMINAL TRAUMA

Parenteral Antibiotics. The incidence of postoperative infections after abdominal trauma varies with the type and number of organs injured, the severity and duration of hypotension, and the number of blood transfusions required.[3,9,207] Organisms in the colon and distal ileum are predominately anaerobic bacteria, such as bacteroides, clostridia, and peptostreptococci. Many gram-negative aerobes, such as E. coli, are also present (Table 39–5). The coliform organisms generally respond well to aminoglycosides or second- or third-generation cephlosporins. Anaerobes usually respond well to clindamycin or metronidazole.

Antibiotic trials in which a variety of expanded-spectrum single agents have been compared with aminoglycoside-based combinations (usually including gentamicin and clindamycin) show similar efficacy.[3,180,208] In addition, short-duration prophylaxis (12 hours) appears to be as effective as prolonged coverage.[201,209]

Antibiotic Irrigation. The use of antibiotic irrigation at laparotomy for gastrointestinal perforation is controversial.[210] Some authors have reported clinical benefits with antibiotic irrigation,[211-213] whereas others have demonstrated no benefit over that obtained with systemic antibiotics plus irrigation with plain saline.[214]

AXIOM Although extremely controversial, antibiotic irrigation of heavily contaminated areas of the peritoneal cavity may be of some value in selected patients.

In an important study in rabbits in which peritonitis was produced with intraperitoneal instillation of human feces, and a two-hour delay before treatment occurred, cefotetan intramuscularly BID and irrigation with plain saline resulted in an 80% mortality (11 of 14).[215] Cefotetan intramuscularly BID plus cefotetan 1.0 mg/mL in the saline washout reduced mortality to 21% (3 of 14; P = 0.003) and markedly reduced the number of intraperitoneal abscesses.

ORTHOPEDIC TRAUMA. Early, complete, operative debridement and drainage are of paramount importance in preventing infection in open fractures. Single agents, such as cefazolin, with activity against S. aureus have been used with success to help prevent infections in such wounds (Table 39–6).[216-218] The addition of an aminoglycoside has been recommended in larger, more complex wounds and in those that may be contaminated with gram-negative aerobes.[219] Late infections associated with open fractures are often caused by hospital-acquired bacteria.[218]

DEEP, SOFT-TISSUE LACERATIONS. Antibiotic administration following deep, soft-tissue lacerations should include agents active against gram-positive organisms and anaerobes.[206,220,221] If the status of tetanus vaccination is unknown, tetanus toxoid should be administered.

TABLE 39-5 *Presumptive Antimicrobial Therapy after Abdominal Trauma*

Infection or circumstance	Abdominal trauma involving gastrointestinal tract, but especially colon or distal small bowel
Common pathogens	Polymicrobial: E. coli, other Enterobacteriaceae, Enterococci, B. fragilis, other anaerobes, S. aureus, coagulase-negative staphylococci
Recommendation(s)	Single agents: ticarcillin/clavulanate, ampicillin/sulbactam, pipercillin/ tazobactum, cephamycin Third generation cephalosporin with clindamycin Aminoglycoside with clindamycin
Alternatives	Mezlocillin, pipercillin, ciprofloxacin with clindamycin Ceftizoxime

From Wilson RF, Janning SW. Handbook of antibiotic therapy for surgery-related infections, 3rd ed. Springfield, NJ: Scientific Therapeutics, Inc. 1995; 33.

TABLE 39-6 **Presumptive Antimicrobial Therapy after Orthopedic Trauma**

Infection or Circumstance	Common Pathogens	Recommendation(s)	Alternatives
Open fractures, low-to-moderate risk	S. aureus	Cefazolin	Penicillinase-resistant penicillins MRS: vancomycin alone or with rifampin and/or aminoglycoside
Open fractures, high-risk (extensive soft-tissue damage, neurologic or vascular injury)	S. aureus Pseudomonas, Enterococci, Enterobacteriaceae	Pencillinase-resistant penicillin, cefazolin Ticarcillin/clavulante, extended-spectrum penicillin, or third generation cephalosporin (ceftazidime for Pseudomonas)	Consider addition of aminoglycoside for gram-negative coverage

MRS = methicillin-resistant staphylococci
From: Wilson RF, Janning SW. Handbook of antibiotic therapy for surgery-related infections, 3rd ed. Springfield, NJ: Scientific Therapeutics, Inc., 1995; 36.

In patients with tetanus-prone wounds, early extensive debridement and irrigation should be provided along with tetanus toxoid, tetanus immune globulin (250 units), and appropriate antibiotics.

HUMAN AND ANIMAL BITES

AXIOM One should assume that all human bites are contaminated with a large number of virulent mouth aerobes and anaerobes.

Penicillin G is often recommended for human and animal bites because it covers most of the aerobic and anaerobic organisms contaminating such injuries; however, it is ineffective against S. aureus, which is isolated in approximately 35% of hand infections. In addition, an increasing number of other microorganisms in the oral flora of humans and animals have become β-lactamase-resistant. Consequently, for serious injuries where the risk of infection is high, a parenteral combination of a penicillin and a β-lactamase inhibitor (e.g., ticarcillin/clavulanate, ampicillin/sulbactam), may be more effective (Table 39–7).[222,223] For individuals taking oral antibiotics at home, amoxicillin/clavulanate or a combination of penicillin and dicloxacillin may be appropriate.

PROBLEMS WITH ANTIBIOTICS

PITFALL ⊘

Too much reliance on prophylactic antibiotics to prevent infection may produce the opposite result.

Although they are frequently of benefit in injured patients, prophylactic antibiotics have great potential for harm when given for prolonged periods, particularly in otherwise healthy patients in whom the risk of infection is small and the consequences of infection are not grave.

It is increasingly recognized that early administration of a short course of antibiotics, combined with early, effective resuscitation, and early operation result in a low rate of postoperative infection following penetrating abdominal trauma.[2,4,201] Additional benefits achieved with a short course of antibiotics include a reduction in adverse effects and suprainfections, less development of antibiotic-resistant organisms, and decreased costs.[224-226]

A nosocomial infection seen almost exclusively in patients receiving antibiotics for another cause is antibiotic-associated colitis caused by overgrowth of Clostridium difficile.[227] This infection should be suspected in any patient who has recently received antibiotics and then develops diarrhea.[2] These patients may have abdominal tenderness, fever, and leukocytosis. Treatment consists of adequate intravenous fluids, cessation of all antibiotic therapy if possible, administration of oral metronidazole if possible (otherwise intravenous), and avoidance of antidiarrheal preparations, such as opiates.[2]

Vaccines and Antitoxins

Vaccines (for active immunization) and antitoxins (for passive immunization) have an important place in the prevention of tetanus and rabies. Their role in gas gangrene is controversial.

SDD/SPEAR Prophylaxis

In recent years, a number of reports have explored the use of antibiotic prophylaxis programs called selective decontamination of the digestive tract (SDD)[228] or selective parenteral and enteral antisepsis regimen (SPEAR).[229] These programs use an oral application of an ointment containing polymyxin E, tobramycin, and amphotericin. The same drugs are also given in an enteral suspension via a nasogastric tube throughout the patient's stay in the ICU. Intravenous cefotaxime is given for five days.

AXIOM SDD and SPEAR prophylaxis are expensive and work-intensive, and are not likely to improve outcome for the great majority of ICU trauma patients.

TABLE 39-7 **Presumptive Antimicrobial Therapy for Human and Animal Bites**

Infection or Circumstance	Common Pathogens	Recommendation(s)	Alternatives
Human bites	β-Hemolytic streptococci S. aureus, anaerobes, anaerobes, E. corrodens	Amoxicillin/clavulanate, clindamycin Parenteral: ticarcillin/clavulanate, ampicillin/sulbactam, piperacillin/tazobactam	Cephamycin, erthromycin
Animal bites[a]	α-Hemolytic streptococci, S. aureus, P. multocida Corynebacterium species peptostreptococci, Bacteroides species	Penicillin V potassium with dicloxacillin, amoxicillin/clavulanate Parenteral: ticarcillin/clavulanate, ampicillin/sulbactam, pipercillin/tazobactam	Erythromycin Parenteral: cephamycin, imipenem/cilastatin

[a]Rabies prophylaxis may be necessary.
From: Wilson RF, Janning SW. Handbook of antibiotic therapy for surgery-related infections, 3rd ed. Springfield: Scientific Therapeutics, Inc., 1995; 37.

The proponents of these programs believe that they reduce gram-negative colonization of the gastrointestinal tract while preserving the normal anaerobic gastrointestinal flora, thereby significantly reducing nosocomial infections in patients in the ICU. However, almost all of the studies used historic rather than concurrent controls and had rather subjective and poorly defined definitions of infection so that their validity is difficult to judge.[2] Furthermore, only one of the studies showed a difference in mortality in patients admitted for trauma;[229] because these patients constituted < 15% of the entire group, this subgroup analysis has been considered suspect.[2]

In a report by Cerra et al. in 1992, 46 patients were randomized to receive either selective gut decontamination as norfloxacin (500 mg suspension every 8 hours) together with nystatin (1 million units every 6 hours) or matching placebo solutions administered through a nasogastric tube within 48 hours of surgical ICU admission.[230] The selective gut decontamination group had a lower number of nosocomial infections (22 infections in 25 patients vs 42 infections in 21 patients; P < 0.0002) and reduced hospital stays (33 ± 5 vs 50 ± 8; P < 0.07). However, no decrease in the incidence of progressive MOF syndrome (6 of 25 vs 5 of 21), ARDS (7 of 25 vs 8 of 21), or mortality (13 of 25 vs 10 of 21) occurred.

TREATMENT OF INFECTIONS

> **AXIOM**   Early, adequate drainage and debridement is the most important treatment of localized infections.

Surgical Drainage

Following hollow viscus injury, 80% of major infections are abdominal or retroperitoneal abscesses, with the remaining 20% being necrotizing fasciitis or diffuse suppurative peritonitis.[13] Surgical control of the primary or underlying infectious process in the abdomen is usually far more important than are the antimicrobial agents used. Most failures of antimicrobial therapy are due to inadequate or delayed removal, drainage, or debridement of infected secretions, fluid, or tissue. Most large collections of pus can cause severe toxicity and do not resolve unless drained.

DRAINING ABDOMINAL ABSCESSES

Laparotomy

Drainage of abdominal abscesses should be as complete as possible without spreading the infected material into uninvolved areas. Postoperative catheter drainage should be dependent, when possible. In situations in which drainage of the abdomen can only be accomplished anteriorly, soft sump tubes should be used. With posterior drains, the nurse must exercise judgement in determining the best balance between position changes to prevent pulmonary complications and those promoting optimal drainage. Anterior abdominal drainage in children who can be mobile is facilitated when they are encouraged to play on their hands and knees with toys that can be pushed along the floor.

> **AXIOM**   Continued leakage of intestinal contents, particularly from the colon or distal small bowel, into the peritoneal cavity is tolerated poorly.

With any gastrointestinal leak, the involved bowel should be excised or exteriorized, as soon as possible. Nasogastric suction alone is usually not adequate to prevent continued leakage from injured bowel.

> **AXIOM**   An abscess cavity, which continues to drain large quantities of pus or fluid for several days after surgical drainage, is usually inadequately drained or is associated with a fistula.

When the amount of drainage from an abdominal abscess exceeds 100-200 mL/day for several days, it can usually be assumed that either the abscess is inadequately drained or that a fistula from the gastrointestinal or urinary tract is present. When the drainage fluid continues to be malodorous, a strong possibility exists that anaerobic organisms are present, and the incision and drainage procedure was inadequate.

Percutaneous Drainage

Increasing reports described percutaneous catheter drainage of abdominal abscesses using ultrasonography or CT radiologic guidance. Although this technique can be safe and effective, it is now fairly clear that percutaneous drainage should probably not be done when:[231-233] (a) three or more abscesses are present, (b) one would have to traverse bowel or pleura to provide drainage, (c) the source of the infection has not been controlled (i.e., a bowel leak is present), or (d) fungal abscess is present (i.e., pus is too thick and peel must be removed surgically).

Thus, a single hepatic abscess is ideal for percutaneous drainage, particularly if the patient is a poor risk for surgery. However, irrigation of the catheter should be performed with small quantities (5-20 mL) sterile saline, preferably with a high concentration of appropriate antibiotics, every 8-12 hours.

Although cure rates of 86% (61 of 71),[231] 84% (49 of 581),[232] and 82% (28 of 33)[233] have been reported with percutaneous drainage of abdominal abscesses, major complication rates have been as high as 15-24%.[234] Furthermore, surgeons reported failure rates with this technique to be as high as 9 of 17 (56%)[235] and 12 of 21 (57%).[234]

Blind Laparotomy

In a study of 77 patients with intraabdominal infections by Pitcher and Musher in 1982, a clear preoperative diagnosis was possible in only about half the patients.[236] Because the overall mortality was 64% with peritonitis and 63% with intraperitoneal abscess, the authors believed that, in the absence of a clear diagnosis, failure to respond to four to five days of antibiotic therapy may be an indication for exploratory laparotomy. Polk and Shields also believed that MOF may be an indication for abdominal exploration.[103]

When a surgical patient becomes increasingly septic after surgery or trauma involving the abdomen and no other obvious infected site can be found, the abdomen is often the source. Consequently, if such a patient is deteriorating in spite of all other therapy, it may be wise to perform a "blind laparotomy" (i.e., without objective evidence of peritonitis or abscess).

> **AXIOM**   In patients who are, in spite of all other therapy, progressively deteriorating with sepsis after abdominal trauma, exploratory laparotomy should be considered even if all diagnostic tests for abscess or peritonitis are negative.

Since CT scanning has become available, blind laparotomies are needed much less often. Sinanen et al. found that their laparotomies for suspected intraabdominal sepsis were most likely to be positive when objective evidence of intraabdominal focus existed by:[237] (a) physical examination, ultrasonography, or CT, or (b) septic shock with positive blood cultures.

In a study by LeGall et al., intraabdominal sepsis was found in 66 of 100 febrile postlaparotomy patients.[238] Six factors that were associated with a significantly increased chance that the infection was intraabdominal included: (a) lack of positive blood cultures, (b) white blood cell count > 12,000/mm^3, (c) ileus, (d) mental disturbances, (e) contaminated first laparotomy, and (f) abdominal tenderness. In our own experience, an infectious process requiring surgical drainage is found in about 50% of blind laparotomies. Unfortunately, many patients with MOF who have abdominal abscesses drained will not survive because their general condition has already deteriorated too far.

Although the operative mortality for reoperation for intraabdominal infections after trauma has been quoted at 30%,[1] only the most seriously ill patients are usually considered for reoperation.[239] Furthermore, the mortality of patients with intraabdominal infections that are not controlled is nearly 100%. Hinsdale and Jaffe demonstrated a 91% positive laparotomy rate when a group of general surgery patients were explored on the basis of physical findings, positive radiographs, or MOF.[240] These patients had an overall mortality of 43%. Similar findings were reported by Machiedo et al.[241] Their mortality rate for reexploration of trauma patients was only 11%, which was significantly different from nontraumatic, emergency patients. Although no control group was randomized to nonoperative therapy, it was assumed that all of those patients would have died without surgery.

Leaving the Abdomen Open

When severe, generalized peritonitis is found, it may be wise to leave the abdomen open and reexplore it on a daily basis. Most of these severe infections have two to three anaerobic and one to two aerobic bacterial species present. On an extremity, one can easily see the advantage of debriding a severe, mixed infection daily, but it is more difficult for the average surgeon to perform daily debridements within the abdomen. Continued postoperative irrigation through catheters to treat residual peritoneal contamination is usually ineffective.[242]

If the abdomen is to be left open, the peritoneal cavity should be cleaned and irrigated thoroughly with 10-20 L of saline upon completion of the procedure. Fibrin that is firmly adherent is left undisturbed. A final rinse with an antibiotic solution (either 1.0 g of cefazolin or a combination of 500 mg neomycin and 500,000 units of polymyxin/L) can be used, but the irrigant should then be removed as completely as possible. The bowel loops are then covered with rayon or nylon dressing (to prevent adhesions to the abdominal wall) followed by moist fluff gauzes. Two binders are then applied to the abdomen.

Postoperatively, the patient is sedated, kept on a ventilator in the ICU, and brought to the OR daily. The packs are removed and any fluid collections or debris accumulating in the previous 24 hours is cultured and removed. For two to three days, most of these patients have pockets of infected, cloudy fluid from which organisms can often be cultured. When the peritoneal cavity looks clean, often by the fifth day, the abdominal fascia can generally be closed safely. If the fascia cannot be approximated without too much tension, prosthetic mesh can be used to close the abdomen. The skin and subcutaneous tissue should be left open.

AXIOM   Even when a surgeon does not believe in leaving the abdomen open in patients with severe, diffuse peritonitis, initial improvement followed by later deterioration should be an indication for early reexploration.

BRONCHOSCOPY

Bronchoscopy can be helpful in the treatment of lobar atelectasis and some pulmonary infections. The incidence of arrhythmias, which are the most frequent complication of therapeutic bronchoscopies, can be reduced by ensuring adequate ventilation and oxygenation during the procedure. This is best accomplished by performing bronchoscopy through a T-piece on an endotracheal tube while the patient is ventilated with 100% O_2.

AXIOM   Repeated bronchoscopies for toilet should be strongly considered in patients with severe atelectasis or pneumonia not responding promptly to other therapy.

REMOVAL OF INTRAVENOUS CATHETERS

Intravenous catheters are a frequent source of bacteremia. Fever beginning two to three days after surgery is particularly apt to be due to infection of an intravenous catheter. When even a vague possibility exists that an intravenous catheter is infected and other veins are available, the intravenous catheter site(s) should be changed and the catheter tip(s) cultured. The benefits of replacing intravenous cath-

eters prophylactically in the same site over wires every 48-72 hours are controversial. However, such a technique may be useful in patients who have no other venous access.

REMOVAL OF URINARY CATHETERS

Catheterization of the urinary tract should be avoided whenever possible. However, if the urine is infected and the urinary tract is even partially obstructed, infection usually would be impossible to correct without adequate drainage.

Antimicrobial Agents

AXIOM   No antibiotic, or combination of antibiotics, "covers everything."

GENERAL CONSIDERATIONS

Choosing Appropriate Antibiotics

Whenever possible, only one or, at the most, two antibiotics should be used at a time. In addition, the antibiotic(s) should not have a spectrum extending beyond that necessary to control the organisms involved. "Shotgun" therapy with three or more broad-spectrum antibiotics should be discouraged, except in the presence of life-threatening infections in which the involved microorganisms and their sensitivities are unknown. Although it takes at least 48-72 hours to grow-out and identify most aerobes and seven to nine days to grow-out and identify most anaerobes, these results are helpful when the patient does not respond to the initial antibiotics. Furthermore, once antibiotics have been given, the accuracy of the later cultures is greatly reduced.

Some of the factors that may help in deciding on the proper choice of antibiotics include: location of infection, culture and sensitivity reports, severity of infection, status of organ systems that may be damaged by antibiotics, and toxicity and side effects of available antibiotics.

Route of Administration

In critically ill patients, absorption of drugs by the oral route is erratic and often inadequate. In addition, even if the gastrointestinal tract is working well, gram-negative organisms often require much higher antibiotic doses than could be achieved or tolerated by oral administration.

For certain drugs, the intramuscular route should not be used because of: (a) poor absorption and a tendency to form sterile abscesses (tetracycline, chloramphenicol, erythromycin), (b) excessive pain at the injection site (cephalothin, methicillin, aqueous penicillin), or (c) inability to achieve adequate blood levels (carbenicillin). The intramuscular route is also inappropriate in shock and in patients with severe vascular disease because of impaired circulation. Conversely, the amount of penicillin or cephalosporin given intravenously must be higher than the intramuscular dose because of rapid urinary excretion of these drugs.

Organ Failure

It is necessary to know which drugs require either dosage change or complete avoidance with various types of organ failure. This is particularly true of aminoglycosides and vancomycin in patients with severe renal dysfunction. When such agents must be used, peak and trough blood levels of these agents must be followed closely.

Peak and Trough Levels

With aminoglycosides and vancomycin, it is essential to get frequent peak and trough levels to determine whether the levels are high enough to adequately treat the infection and low enough to prevent toxic side effects. In general, the incidence of nephrotoxicity and/or ototoxicity with aminoglycosides averages about 11-16% in most studies, with the ototoxicity often being irreversible.[243] Nevertheless, doses that are 50-100% higher than normal are often needed to achieve adequate peak levels in patients with severe trauma and much third-spacing of fluid. Under such circumstances, the interdose interval must be increased to reduce the incidence and severity of toxic side effects.

AXIOM The only way to ensure maximum effectiveness and safety with aminoglycosides in critically ill patients is to serially monitor peak and trough levels at least every two to four days.

Alternatively, in the absence of preexisting renal insufficiency, a single daily dose (SDD) regimen may be prescribed for aminoglycosides. Targeted peak concentrations are twice as high as traditional regimens in order to take advantage of the concentration-dependent bactericidal activity of these agents. The long interdose interval takes advantage of the postantibiotic effect and also minimizes exposure to toxic effects. To date, no increase in the ototoxicity with SDD regimens has been documented. Data showing increased efficiency and decreased nephrotoxicity with SDD aminoglycosides are still evolving.

Evaluating Response

AXIOM Once treatment of an infection is begun with a carefully selected antibiotic, it should be continued for at least 48-72 hours before empirically adding or changing to another agent.

If a patient continues to have fever and/or leukocytosis after 48-72 hours of antibiotic therapy, one should suspect that a continuing or recurrent infection is still present.[244] One should look for both trauma-related and nosocomial infections. One should also review the possible causes of antibiotic treatment failure (Table 39–8).

When multiple cultures and diagnostic studies are unrevealing, one should consider discontinuing the antibiotic(s) and looking for noninfectious causes of fever (Table 39–9). When a patient who has had a recent laparotomy becomes increasingly septic without any other obvious source, "blind" exploration of the abdomen should be considered, even when an abscess cannot be demonstrated clinically or radiologically.

AXIOM An infection in an abdominal incision that drains increased fluid or exhibits signs of fascial necrosis may be evidence of an underlying intraabdominal infection and/or anastomotic leak.

In one study of 65 patients treated for intraabdominal infections, no recurrent infections developed in 30 patients who became afebrile

TABLE 39-8 Possible Causes of Antibiotic Treatment Failure

Inappropriate antibiotic
  Erroneous initial diagnosis
  Failure of drug to reach site of infection
  Organism not susceptible to antibiotic at concentrations achievable at
    site of infection
  Inactivation of antibiotic by bacterial enzymes
  Unrelated infection elsewhere in body
  Superinfection
Appropriate antibiotic but insufficient treatment
  Drug administered by inappropriate route
  Dose too small, too infrequent
  Inadequate dosing in patients with expanded volume of distribution
  Massive blood or other fluid loss during therapy
  Course of therapy too short
Appropriate antibiotic but other problems or other therapy required
  Impaired host defenses
  Failure to institute appropriate surgical measures in addition to antibiotics

TABLE 39-9 Noninfectious Causes of Fever in Trauma Patients

Hematomas, seromas
Necrotic or inflamed tissues
Transfusion reactions
Thrombophlebitis, pulmonary emboli
Pancreatitis
Drug-induced (amphotericin B, vancomycin, sulfonamides, penicillins,
  phenytoin, quinidine)
Adrenocortical insufficiency

and had white blood cell counts that became normal.[245] However, of 14 patients with persistent fever, 11 (79%) developed recurrent infections. Of 15 patients who had postoperative intraabdominal infections, only 4 responded to appropriate antibiotic treatment without surgery.

ANTIBIOTIC CHOICES FOR VARIOUS SITES OF INFECTION

Wound Infections

Infections can occur in any incision or traumatic wound. In a study of over 1000 trauma patients, abdominal incisions with less than a six-hour delay in operation after trauma and without any associated intraabdominal injuries were called "clean" and had an infection rate of almost 3%.[246] Abdominal wounds with colon injuries or with more than a six-hour delay (and penetrating extremity wounds with more than a six-hour delay) were called "contaminated" and had an infection rate of 24%. All other abdominal incisions, (and penetrating extremity wounds treated within six hours, and blunt extremity wounds treated after six hours) were called "clean-contaminated" and had an infection rate of 11%.

Wound infections are usually diagnosed more than 5 days after operation or injury.[2] Local pain, swelling, erythema, and drainage are the most common signs. Most wound infections are adequately treated by opening the wound. Some wounds may also require debridement and irrigation.

Many wound infections developing outside the hospital in patients who have no involvement of the GI or female genitourinary tracts are caused by penicillin-sensitive staphylococci and streptococci which can be treated well by a first-generation cephalosporin.[206,247] The staphylococci causing wound infections in the hospital, however, are generally coagulase-positive organisms which are resistant to penicillin, but some are responsive to β-lactamase-resistant penicillins, such as methicillin or first-generation cephalosporins. Methicillin-resistant staphylococcus aureus (MRSA) requiring antibiotic therapy must be treated with vancomycin.

PITFALL ⊘

Overzealous use of vancomycin has led to the development of vancomycin-resistant enterococci; consequently, empiric use of this agent should be discouraged.

If the patient is allergic to penicillin, drugs such as erythromycin or clindamycin, which are relatively nontoxic, may be used effectively. The drug-of-choice for life-threatening staphylococcal infection in the patient with anaphylactic penicillin allergy is vancomycin.[10]

AXIOM Wound infections developing in patients who have had intraabdominal injury or have been receiving broad-spectrum antibiotics are often caused by gram-negative bacilli.

Pulmonary Infections

The generally accepted clinical criteria for making a diagnosis of pneumonia include a new or changing infiltrate on chest radiography, in addition to fever (> 101.5°F), purulent sputum (> 25 white blood cells/low-power field), many bacteria on Gram stain, one or more positive sputum cultures, and a white blood cell count > 15,000/mm^3 or with more than 10% immature forms.[1] A wide variety of organisms may cause pulmonary infections after trauma, and a Gram stain of the sputum is essential. Although protected brush specimens and bronchoalveolar lavage probably improve diagnostic accuracy, data are not conclusive.[2]

> **AXIOM**   Although about a third of positive sputum cultures in ICU patients are due to colonization, one should consider treating for that organism—especially Pseudomonas—if the patient is severely immunodepressed.

When the patient has a community-acquired pneumonia, S. pneumoniae or H. influenzae is apt to be the causative agent, and erythromycin with or without cefuroxine is recommended (Table 39-10).[248-251] Smears of sputum can be helpful for determining which antibiotics to use. Gram-positive cocci in chains (streptococci) are usually sensitive to penicillin. Gram-positive cocci in clusters (staphylococci) are often responsive to cephalosporins or penicillinase-resistant penicillins.

> **AXIOM**   Before treating pneumonia with antibiotics, great efforts should be made to perform Gram stain and culture and sensitivity testing on a good sputum or bronchoscopic specimen.

Mild-to-moderate pulmonary infections caused by Gram-negative bacilli may be treated with extended-spectrum penicillins, cephalosporins, a fluoroquinolone, or a β-lactamase inhibitor combination. Severe gram-negative pulmonary infections developing after several days of antibiotic therapy are often caused by Pseudomonas, which should generally be treated with an aminoglycoside plus an extended-spectrum penicillin, such as piperacillin. This combination is preferred because it has synergistic bactericidal effects against pseudomonas and other gram-negative aerobes, and it decreases emergence of resistance during treatment.

Aspiration pneumonitis can be a severe problem in trauma patients, especially those who are unconscious or have facial injuries.[252,253] Even though fairly large amounts of food, pharyngeal or gastric secretions may be aspirated into the tracheobronchial tree, leukocytosis and abnormal chest radiography may not be evident for another 12-24 hours or longer. Pulmonary changes in the first few hours following aspiration usually represent chemical injury rather than infection. No well-documented treatment plan exists for such patients. It is common practice to start antibiotics to treat the expected aspiration pneumonia, but the efficacy of this is unproved.[2]

Emergency bronchoscopy is performed as soon as possible after suspected aspiration to ensure that no foreign material, such as food or dental work, remains in the tracheobronchial tree.[2] With removal of the foreign material, the problem is one of bacterial contamination combined with chemical and/or physical injury to the trachea and bronchi. A logical choice of antibiotics for aspiration occurring in the first few hours of hospitalization is the immediate administration of cefazolin followed by two more doses at six-hour intervals.[2] This covers most oral and gastric flora as well as most Staphylococcus aureus. When brief contamination has occurred, infection may be aborted. When infection develops, culture and sensitivity testing on the pulmonary secretions is essential.

> **AXIOM**   The best ways to prevent pulmonary infection are to prevent aspiration, to relieve pain enough to facilitate optimal coughing, to perform timely tracheostomy when indicated, and to promptly and completely drain any hemopneumothorax that may develop.

Pulmonary abscesses due to aspiration are generally caused initially by aerobic gram-positive cocci and mouth anaerobes, including the fusospirochetes. A growing number of these organisms are resistant to penicillin, and clindamycin is increasingly the initial drug of choice for pulmonary infections that may be caused by aspiration.

Empyema of the pleural space can occur after pneumonia, and it is a not uncommon cause of infection after thoracic trauma.[254] Empyema should be particularly suspected in a patient who has systemic signs of infection plus an increasing pleural effusion after chest trauma. The risk of empyema following trauma is greatly increased when the treating physician does not succeed in completely evacuating a traumatic hemothorax from the pleural space.[255] Diagnosis is made by Gram stain and culture of the pleural fluid. If the insertion of a thoracostomy tube and specific antibiotic therapy does not resolve the clinical evidence of sepsis within a reasonable period (48-72 hours), thoracotomy for decortication of the lung should be considered.[256]

TABLE 39-10   **Empiric Antimicrobial Therapy of Pneumonia**

Infection or Circumstance	Common Pathogens	Recommendations (s)	Alternatives
Community-acquired pneumonia	S. pneumoniae,[a] H. influenzae	Erythromycin with or without cefuroxime or other second generation cephalosporin	Ampicillin/sulbactam amoxicillin/clavulanate
Nosocomial pneumonia	Enterobacteriaceae, P. aeruginosa, K. pneumoniae, S. pneumoniae, S. aureus	Extended-spectrum penicillin or antipseudomonal third-generation cephalosporin with aminoglycoside	Third-generation cephalosporin or ciprofloxacin with clindamycin Ticarcillin/clavulanate, imipenem/cilastatin, ampicillin/sulbactam,[b] piperacillin/tazobactam[b]
Nosocomial pneumonia in aspiration-prone patients	As above and Bacteroides, other oral anaerobes	Penicillinase-resistant penicillin with aminoglycoside and clindamycin	Third-generation cephalosporin with clindamycin Ticarcillin/clavulanate, ampicillin/sulbactam,[b] piperacillin/tazobactam,[b] imipenem/cilastatin

[a]In some areas, up to 10-20% of S. pneumoniae are penicillin-resistant.
[b]Does not provide Pseudomonas coverage.
Abramowicz, 1994[248]; Brittain et al, 1985[249]; Musher, 1991[250]; Rodriguez et al, 1991[35] Wisinger, 1993[251]
From: Wilson RF, Janning SW. Handbook of antibiotic therapy for surgery-related infections, 3rd ed. Springfield, NJ: Scientific Therapeutics, Inc., 1995; 59.

Peritonitis

AXIOM The most important method for diagnosing posttraumatic peritonitis early is repetitive examinations by a physician who is familiar with the patient's injuries and treatment. This may be supplemented with chest radiography, abdominal ultrasonography, and CT as needed.

Intraabdominal infection is one of the most serious infections to follow trauma, and it has a mortality rate of 10-30%.[4,21] The organisms most likely to cause intraperitoneal infections are of the family Enterobacteriaceae (including Escherichia, Klebsiella, Enterobacter, and Proteus species). Other organisms also likely to be present are streptococci, enterococci, and various anaerobic organisms, particularly Bacteroides species. Although Bacteroides species are involved in most infections following trauma to the colon, this may not be reflected in the culture reports because these anaerobic organisms can be difficult to culture and often grow out slowly.

For mild-to-moderate peritoneal contamination, one can use a wide variety of agents that are effective against gram-negative aerobes and the intestinal anaerobes. The best-studied and documented antibiotic regimen for intraabdominal infection is an aminoglycoside combined with either clindamycin or metronidazole.[2] Alternatives to aminoglycoside include third-generation cephalosporins, ciprofloxacin, or aztreonam. Aztreonam should only be combined with clindamycin because neither metronidazole nor aztreonam has significant activity against gram-positive aerobes.

Two single-agent regimens with appropriate activity for empiric treatment of intraabdominal infection are imipenem/cilastatin and ticarcillin/clavulanic acid. For severe peritoneal contamination, especially by colon or distal small-bowel injuries, triple antibiotics can be used, including ampicillin, aminoglycoside, and either clindamycin or metronidazole.

The clinician should be prepared to reoperate and to change antibiotics depending on the patient's clinical course and the results of sensitivity testing. In several combined series of patients with serious intraabdominal infections, up to 25% of patients required a second operation to resolve infection. In two series, half of the patients required either a change in antibiotics, reoperation, or both.[257,258]

Urinary Tract Infections

Although they are the most frequently used drugs for treating mild-to-moderate urinary tract infections in ambulatory patients, sulfa preparations are seldom used in patients with severe infections. Ampicillin may be effective against the gram-negative organisms that are usually involved, but gentamicin is the antibiotic of choice for most severe kidney infections. Ampicillin plus gentamicin is often indicated in severe cases because this combination is also the regimen of choice against enterococci.

Bacterial cystitis may often be prevented by irrigating the bladder with dilute neosporin solutions containing 40 mg of neomycin and 20 mg of polymyxin B per liter of fluid at an infusion rate of 40 mL/hour. Some physicians, however, believe that irrigation with antibiotic solutions should be avoided and that a closed urinary drainage system is the only effective method for preventing catheter cystitis. When fungal infection develops in the bladder, 20-50 mg of amphotericin B added to a liter of sterile water may be an effective irrigating solution; routine treatment of positive urine fungal cultures in the absence of actual infection is controversial.

Infected Vascular Prostheses

Infections of vascular prosthetic grafts are uncommon, but they can be a severe threat to life and limb. They are most likely to occur in the groin,[259] and contamination is believed to occur at the time the graft is sutured into place; however, infection may take months to become clinically apparent. Prosthetic grafts become infected more often than saphenous vein grafts. Prostheses that allow more tissue ingrowth are more resistant to late infection.

AXIOM Any abnormality in the groin following femoral vascular surgery, even months later, should be considered evidence of an infected vascular prosthesis until proven otherwise.

A variety of microorganisms has been isolated from infections of vascular grafts. The most frequent isolates are coagulase-negative staphylococci, S. aureus, and E. coli. Klebsiella, Proteus, and Pseudomonas strains are encountered less frequently.[259] Mucin-producing strains of S. epidermidis show increased adherence to prosthetic vascular grafts.[260] Early infections are caused more often by S. aureus, while late infections tend to be caused by coagulase-negative staphylococci.

Infections around patent vascular prostheses can sometimes be managed with drainage, debridement, and intensive antibiotic therapy, but infected, occluded grafts require resection of the graft. If a limb is threatened, an extraanatomic vascular bypass will also be needed. Parenteral antibiotics are administered for at least two to four weeks after resection of an infected graft. If a superficially infected graft is left in place, parenteral and then oral antibiotics should be continued for three to six months or longer. The selection of antibiotics is based on the organisms cultured from the infection.

Septic Phlebitis

Septic phlebitis has become much more common since the introduction of plastic intravenous cannulas.[259] The rate of infection is approximately 40 times higher than with steel cannulas. Infection is particularly common when cutdowns are performed and after emergency placement of intravenous lines. Multiple lumen lines and prolonged cannulation (> 48-72 hours) are also associated with an increased rate of infection.

AXIOM Intravenous catheter infection with a positive S. aureus culture requires at least 10-14 days of intravenous antibiotics and should be considered due to septic phlebitis until proven otherwise.

Removal of the catheter is usually enough to resolve the infection, but intravenous antibiotics are needed for at least 10-14 days when S. aureus bacteremia occurs or fever persists.[259] Suppurative thrombophlebitis is uncommon, but when gross pus can be demonstrated in the vein radiologically, by aspiration, or during incision and drainage, treatment generally requires surgical excision of the involved portion of the vein in addition to antibiotic therapy. Suppurative thrombophlebitis is most commonly caused by S. aureus and may persist after the catheter is removed.[261]

Treatment of Specific Infections

STAPHYLOCOCCUS

Treatment of S. aureus infections of soft tissue is primarily complete surgical drainage. Antibiotics are not an important part of the treatment of such infections, but if S. aureus bacteremia were to manifest, it should generally be treated aggressively with appropriate intravenous antibiotics for at least 10-14 days.

Community-acquired S. aureus usually responds well to nafcillin, oxacillin, or first-generation cephalosporins[262] (Table 39–11). However, an increasing number of MRSA are being found, especially in intravenous drug abusers. At Detroit Receiving Hospital, over 70% of the S. aureus cultured from the blood of intravenous drug abusers are MRSA. In such patients, vancomycin is usually effective. Although S. epidermidis is usually sensitive to first-generation cephalosporins or antistaphylococcal penicillins, an increasing number are becoming resistant to such agents and require vancomycin for effective therapy.

TABLE 39-11 **Drugs of Choice in Serious Infections Caused by Gram-Positive Organisms**

Organism	Drug of Choice	Alternative Drugs

Aerobes
S. aureus or
  S. epidermidis
  penicillin-sensitive
	Penicillin G	First-generation cephalosporin, vancomycin, or clindamycin[a]

Penicillinase-producing	Oxacillin or nafcillin	First-generation cephalosporin, vancomycin, ticarcillin/clavulanate, ampicillin/sulbactam, piperacillin/tazobactam, or clindamycin[a]
Methicillin-resistant[b]	Vancomycin	Trimethoprim/sulfamethoxazole
Nonenterococcal streptococci	Penicillin G	First-generation cephalosporin, vancomycin, or clindamycin[a]
Enterococci	Penicillin or ampicillin with aminoglycoside	Vancomycin with aminoglycoside
Pneumococcus	Penicillin G[c]	First-generation cephalosporin, vancomycin, erythromycin
Anaerobes: C. difficile	Metronidazole	Vancomycin, tetracycline, chloramphenicol, clindamycin, metronidazole, tetracycline
C. tetani	Penicillin G[d]	
C. perfringens	Penicillin G[e]	

[a]First-generation cephalosporins are most active. When endocarditis is suspected, do not use clindamycin; some authorities recommend the addition of aminoglycoside for endocarditis caused by nonenterococcal streptococci or moderately resistant staphylococci.
[b]Methicillin-resistant staphylococci should be assumed resistant to all cephalosporins even if disk testing were to suggest sensitivity.
[c]An increasing number of pneumococci are penicillin-resistant.
[d]As an adjunct to passive and active immunization.
[e]As an adjunct to debridement of infected tissue.
From: Crawford GE. An approach to use of antimicrobial agents. Civetta JM, Taylor RW, Kirby RR, ed. Critical care. Philadelphia: JB Lippincott Co., 1988; 769-783.

STREPTOCOCCI

Most streptococci are sensitive to penicillin; however, necrotizing infections caused by streptococci also require radical incision or excision and drainage. The enterococci, which used to be considered with the genus Streptococcus, have now been reclassified as the genus Enterococcus. They are resistant to many antibiotics, but generally respond well to a combination of ampicillin or vancomycin plus aminoglycoside. In a five-year study by Garrison et al., 123 episodes of enterococcal bacteremia were studied.[263] No primary source of bacteremia was identified in 42% of the patients, and the infection was polymicrobial in 35%. The overall mortality was 54% and was increased in patients with intraabdominal sepsis and in patients in whom no primary source of infection could be identified.

GRAM-NEGATIVE AEROBES

Gram-negative aerobic bacilli, such as E. coli and Klebsiella, generally respond well to aminoglycosides (Table 39–12); however, these bacilli typically become increasingly resistant to whatever antibiotics are being used most frequently in each hospital.

PITFALL ⊘

If the sensitivities of bacteria found within hospitals are not checked on a regular basis, the initial empiric antibiotic choices made by physicians are likely to be increasingly incorrect.

Treatment of Pseudomonas pulmonary infections may be extremely difficult. Flexible bronchoscopy may be helpful, especially if there is concomitant atelectasis of a segment or a lobe. Rotating beds to improve drainage of various pulmonary segments can also be helpful. For the most severe Pseudomonas infections, combinations of aminoglycosides plus an extended-spectrum penicillin, such as piperacillin, are often required. Alternatives include third-generation cephalosporins, such as ceftazidime, or the fluoroquinolones.

TETANUS

Although tetanus could be almost eliminated by universal active immunization during childhood, approximately 100 patients with clinical tetanus are reported in the United States each year.[158,264] Approximately one million cases occur worldwide annually, and it has been estimated that at least 250-300 cases occur annually in the United States.[265]

Immunization

Proper immunization is the best method for preventing tetanus from developing. Although Arthus reactions have been reported from over administration of tetanus toxoid, judicious use of immunization is safe (Table 39–13).[264] Any patient with suspected tetanus should be immunized in addition to being given tetanus immunoglobulin. Instances of repeated tetanus infections have been reported when the initial infection did not present enough of an immunologic challenge to cause permanent immunity.[1] Once the diagnosis of tetanus is suspected, tetanus immunoglobulin is given in repeated doses of 500-1000 mg. If not already administered, tetanus toxoid is given 0.5 mL at another site.

Surgical Debridement

AXIOM Any finding suggesting the presence of anaerobic infection is an indication for early, aggressive exploration, incision, and debridement.

All necrotic and potentially infected tissue should be excised with wide incision of adjacent tissue so that the wound is well exposed to air. Careful reexamination of the wound every 12-24 hours is essential and often reveals additional tissue that must be incised or debrided. Frequent irrigations with hydrogen peroxide or zinc peroxide may also be beneficial. Oxygen should be added to the inhaled gas mixtures to keep the arterial Po_2 at $\geq$ 100 mm Hg.

Sedation and Antiepileptic Drugs

AXIOM Death due to tetanus is most likely to result from respiratory arrest occurring during generalized convulsion.

Adequate sedation is important in patients with tetanus and may require continuous intravenous drip of 0.1% Thiopental. Lorazepam, 1-2 mg intramuscularly or intravenously every four to six hours, may also be helpful. The patient should be placed in a dark room and protected from as much auditory, visual, and other stimuli as possible. Maintenance of adequate fluid and calories is essential, preferably through a feeding catheter with its tip in the distal duodenum or jejunum to help prevent vomiting and aspiration.

Antibiotics

Antibiotics have no effect on tetanus toxin already released, but they should be given to prevent further multiplication of Cl. tetani organisms and to control or prevent secondary infections of the wound or

TABLE 39-12 **Drugs of Choice in Serious Infections Caused by Gram-Negative Organisms**

Organism	Drug of Choice	Alternative Drugs
Enteric aerobes:		
Mixed Enterobacteriaceae	Aminoglycoside, second- or third-generation cephalosporin	Piperacillin, mezlocillin, imipenem/cilastatin, ticarcillin/clavulanate, ampicillin/sulbactam, piperacillin/tazobactam, ciprofloxacin
E. coli	Aminoglycoside, first-generation cephalosporin	Imipenem/cilastatin, ticarcillin/clavulanate, ampicillin/sulbactam, pipercillin/tazobactam, TMP/SMX, piperacillin, mezlocillin, other cephalosporins, ciprofloxacin
Klebsiella	Aminoglycoside, first-generation cephalosporin	Imipenem/cilastatin, ticarcillin/clavulanate, ampicillin/sulbactam, piperacillin/tazobactam, piperacillin, mezlocillin, other cephalosporins, ciprofloxacin
Proteus		
P. mirabilis	Ampicillin	Aminoglycoside, first-generation cephalosporin, piperacillin, mezlocillin, ticarcillin/clavulanate, ampicillin/sulbactam, piperacillin/tazobactam, ciprofloxacin
Other Proteus species	First-generation cephalosporin, gentamicin	Same as above, imipenem/cilastatin[a]
Serratia	Gentamicin	Piperacillin, mezlocillin, ticarcillin/clavulanate, TMP/SMX, ciprofloxacin, imipenem/cilastatin, piperacillin/tazobactam
Other aerobes:		
Acinetobacter[b]	Aminoglycoside	Imipenem/cilastatin piperacillin, mezlocillin, ticarcillin/clavulanate, ampicillin/sulbactam, piperacillin/tazobactam, tetracycline, ciprofloxacin
H. influenzae	TMP/SMX	First-generation cephalosporin, amoxicillin/clavulanate, ciprofloxacin
P. multocida	Amoxicillin/clavulanate	Tetracycline, first-generation cephalosporin, ciprofloxacin
P. aeruginosa	Extended spectrum penicillin with an aminoglycoside	Ceftazidime or cefoperazone with an aminoglycoside
P. cepacia	TMP/SMX	Chloramphenicol
X maltophilia	TMP/SMX	Ticarcillin/clavulanate, third-generation cephalosporin
Anaerobes:		
Bacteroides		
Oral flora	Clindamycin	Cephamycin,[c] metronidazole
GI strains	Clindamycin or metronidazole	Cephamycin,[c] imipenem/cilastatin, ticarcillin/clavulanate, ampicillin/sulbactam, piperacillin/tazobactam, ceftizoxime

TMP/SMX = trimethoprim/sulfamethoxazole
GI = gastrointestinal
[a]Not recommended for indole-positive Proteus
[b]Resistant Acinetobacter may require imipenem/cilastatin or ticarcillin/clavulanate, ampicillin/sulbactam, or piperacillin/tazobactam plus amikacin
[c]Cefoxitin, cefotetan, or cefmetazole
From: Crawford GE: An approach to use of antimicrobial agents. Civetta JM, Taylor RW, Kirby RR, ed. Critical Care. Philadelphia, JB Lippincott Co., 1988, 769-783.

respiratory tract. The antibiotics used are similar to those used for gas gangrene.

Hyperbaric Oxygen

PITFALL ⊘

Excessive reliance on hyperbaric oxygenation to control anaerobic infections may reduce the efforts of the surgeon to provide optimal incision and drainage.

Hyperbaric oxygenation can be extremely helpful in controlling severe infections caused by anaerobic organisms, particularly Clostridia. The clinical results, however, have often been inconclusive and, unless hyperbaric oxygen facilities are readily available, the risks of moving critically ill patients often outweigh the potential benefits. Furthermore, a tendency may exist to be less vigorous with debridement and surgical drainage when use of hyperbaric oxygenation is contemplated. Finally, hyperbaric oxygen itself has certain risks and may be dangerous in the hands of personnel who are not thoroughly trained and experienced in its use.

CLOSTRIDIAL CELLULITIS AND MYOSITIS

Surgical treatment of clostridial cellulitis or myositis (gas gangrene) must be prompt with extensive decompression and thorough debridement of all involved tissue. If the infection continues to advance up an extremity in spite of adequate surgical incision and drainage plus antibiotics, early amputation may be the only hope of cure. Speed is extremely important in the management of these patients because the

infection may progress to shock and death within 24-48 hours. High doses of intravenous antibiotics, particularly penicillin, with or without concomitant cephalosporins, chloramphenicol, or clindamycin, should also be started immediately (Table 39–14). In patients not responding to antibiotics and surgical debridement and drainage, hyperbaric oxygen should also be used when available.

TABLE 39-13 **Tetanus Prophylaxis**

Tetanus immunization history	Clean wound	"Tetanus-prone" wound[a]
Fully immunized; last booster injection:		
< 5 years	None	None
5-10 years	None	Toxoid booster
> 10 years	Toxoid booster	Toxoid booster + TIG-H
Incompletely immunized or uncertain history	Toxoid + completion of immunization	Toxoid + TIG-H + completion of immunization

TIG-H = tetanus immune globulin-human
[a]Such as, but not limited to, wounds contaminated with dirt or feces, puncture wounds, deep avulsions, and wounds resulting from missiles or crushing.
From: Brand DA, et al: Adequacy of antitetanus prophylaxis in six hospital emergency rooms. N Engl J Med 1983; 309:636.

TABLE 39-14   *Empiric Antimicrobial Therapy of Necrotizing Infections*

Infection or Circumstance	Common Pathogens	Recommendation (s)	Alternatives
Necrotizing fasciitis, infected vascular gangrene	Mixed aerobic-anaerobic, clostridia (gangrene)	Ampicillin with aminoglycoside and clindamycin or metronidazole	Ticarcillin/clavulanate, imipenem/cilastatin, ampicillin/sulbactam, piperacillin/tazobactam, cephamycin
Streptococcal myositis	Group A streptococci	Penicillin G	First-generation cephalosporin, vancomycin
Gas gangrene, clostridial cellulitis	C. perfringens, C. novyi, C. septicum	Penicillin G (high dose)	Clindamycin, imipenem/cilastatin, erythromycin
Nonclostridial anaerobic cellulitis	Anaerobic streptococci, other mixed anaerobes, S. aureus, Group A streptococci	Penicillinase-resistant penicillin, cephamycin ticarcillin/clavulanate, ampicillin/sulbactam, piperacillin/tazobactam	Clindamycin

From: Simmons and Ahrenholz, 1988.[157]

Gas gangrene antitoxin is rarely used because it is of little or no benefit and has a high incidence of allergic reactions.[266] The best prophylaxis for gas gangrene is early, aggressive debridement and drainage of contaminated wounds plus appropriate antibiotics in high dosage. Hyperbaric oxygen in selected patients may also be of benefit.

HUMAN BITE INFECTIONS

Infections after human bites are usually excellent examples of bacterial infections caused by mixed aerobic and anaerobic organisms. Lacerations over a knuckle of a clenched fist tend to close off when the hand is opened. These infections are characterized by rapid development of marked swelling and tenderness, a thick, foul-smelling purulent exudate, and necrosis of adjacent tissues. Such wounds should be promptly explored and debrided in the OR. Antibiotics effective against mouth bacteria should be continued until the wound is well-healed. In the past, penicillin was adequate, but increasingly, newer antibiotics, such as beta-lactamase inhibitor combinations (ticarcillin/clavulanate, ampicillin/sulbactam, or piperacillin/tazobactam), are being used.

NECROTIZING FASCIITIS

Necrotizing fascitis requires prompt opening of the involved area, excision of all involved tissues, and adequate drainage. Reinspection and debridement of the wound should be performed again within 24-48 hours.[97] Antibiotic coverage should be effective against aerobic gram-positive cocci, aerobic gram-negative rods, and anaerobes.

SINUSITIS

Acute sinusitis is not infrequent in trauma patients, and it can cause serious morbidity.[1] It is most common in patients with nasogastric and nasotracheal tubes in place and in patients who have sustained facial fractures.[267,268] At Detroit Receiving Hospital, CT scans of the head and/or face show fluid in the maxillary sinuses in about a third of the patients who have a nasogastric tube and a nasotracheal tube in place for a week or more. Of those with fluid in a maxillary sinus, drainage of the sinus results in recovery of significant numbers of PMNs and bacteria in about a third of patients.

Some patients complain of headache and/or pain over the involved sinuses. Plain radiography can be helpful, but CT scans are more sensitive. The definitive diagnosis is made by sinus puncture, which obtains material for Gram stain, culture, and sensitivity testing. The ideal treatment is complete drainage of the involved sinuses, removal of all nasal tubes, and administration of nasal decongestants and antibiotics.

CANDIDA INFECTIONS

AXIOM   Fungal infection should be suspected in septic ICU patients who have received broad-spectrum antibiotics for > 10-14 days and have no obvious sites of infection, particularly if multiple cultures of all possible infected foci are negative for bacteria.

In patients with persisting fever of unknown etiology after 10-14 days of broad-spectrum antimicrobial therapy, use of antifungal therapy should be considered. Amphotericin B or fluconazole should also be given to patients with two or more sites (e.g., mouth, sputum, urine, drain sites) positive for C. albicans.[269] One should not wait for positive blood cultures to begin therapy. Short-term, limited dosing with amphotericin B (total dose: 6-8 mg/kg) appears to be adequate for many patients.[270]

In some instances, a swish and swallow administration of nystatin (1,000,000 units every four hours) may help to reduce the tendency for Candida overgrowth in the gastrointestinal tract of patients receiving prolonged, broad-spectrum antibiotics.

RABIES

All dog or other animal bites should be irrigated vigorously with saline and all nonviable or excessively contaminated tissue should be debrided thoroughly. Tetanus toxoid should be given in virtually all patients. Antibiotics should be given for deep wounds and wounds caused by wild animals. When any reasonable chance exists that the animal had rabies, the patient should be started on a course of human rabies immune globulin (HRIG) along with a rabies vaccine.[271]

The dose of HRIG is 20 IU/kg. If HRIG is not available, equine antirabies serum may be used after proper allergy testing. A human diploid-cell-strain (HDCS) rabies vaccine has been 100% protective. HDCS is given in 5 mL doses intramuscularly on days 0, 3, 7, 14, and 28. Because of possible severe allergic reactions, duck embryo vaccine should be used to start therapy only if HDCS is not immediately available.

Improving Host Defenses

ERADICATION OF NEGATIVE FACTORS

Removal of Foreign Bodies

Foreign bodies greatly increase the likelihood of infection. Infected foreign bodies that are not essential to the life or function of the patient should be removed as soon as possible.

Diabetic Control

Control of diabetes mellitus during sepsis is often extremely difficult. Diabetic ketoacidosis reduces resistance to infection, and sepsis tends to make the diabetic ketoacidosis worse, creating a vicious, downward cycle. Aggressive eradication of the infection and careful monitoring of blood glucose and acetone levels are essential.

AXIOM If hyperglycemia cannot be controlled with insulin and reduced carbohydrate intake, one should suspect an uncontrolled infection.

Improving Renal Function

Renal function is generally best improved by providing enough fluid to maintain a high urine output without loop diuretics. Reduction of nitrogenous waste products in the blood by early, complete debridement of necrotic tissue may also be important. Hypercatabolic renal failure, characterized by an increase in BUN of > 25 mL/dL/day, has a poor prognosis and is much easier to prevent than to treat. Early administration of proper nutritional support may also help to reduce mortality rates in patients with impaired renal function.

AXIOM Proper monitoring of renal function requires serial creatinine clearance studies. Serum creatinine changes are relatively insensitive in patients with sepsis.

Improving Hepatic Function

Hepatic failure is best prevented or corrected by providing optimal blood flow, oxygenation, and glucose, and by reducing the amount of ammonia reaching the liver from the intestinal tract. Reduction of blood ammonia levels is best achieved by cleaning the bowel with cathartics or enemas, administration of nonabsorbable antibiotics to reduce the number of bacteria in the bowel, and lactulose. Administration of nutrients with high levels of branched-chain amino acids (BCAAs) and low concentrations of aromatic amino acids may also help to treat hepatic encephalopathy.

IMPROVED NUTRITION

Hyperalimentation of severely malnourished individuals can help to restore phagocytosis toward normal levels. This is particularly important if the patient has albumin levels < 2.2 g/dL and an ALC < 800/mm^3. These patients may require more than 35 nonprotein calories and 1.5-2.5 g of protein per kg body weight daily to restore immunologic competence. The negative nitrogen balance of sepsis, however, usually cannot be reversed by exogenous nutritional support until all infections are controlled.

During septic hypermetabolism, energy production seems to be primarily protein-based, and the most that can often be achieved with hyperalimentation is some degree of protein sparing. This seems to be best achieved by providing high amino acid loads (2-3 g/kg every 24 hours), with approximately 80-90 glucose calories per gram of administered nitrogen (e.g., 5% amino acids in 20% glucose), together with multivitamins and adequate trace elements. Early enteral nutritional support may be very helpful for reducing the risk of infection in trauma patients.[83,272,273]

Some septic patients have hyperglycemia that is resistant to insulin. Exogenous insulin administration (except in patients with diabetes mellitus) may potentiate the tendency for hepatic steatosis. Increased use of fats, to provide up to 40% of nonprotein calories, can be helpful in patients who do not tolerate high-glucose loads. Serum triglycerides levels, however, must be monitored closely.

In 1984 Cerra et al. reported great interest in the use of BCAAs in septic patients.[274] They postulated that the septic process, in some unknown way (possibly via a defect in mitochondrial oxidative processes), triggered progressive sequential fuel failure in which BCAAs were preferentially utilized as a fuel source in skeletal muscle due to septic-induced abnormalities in the utilization of glucose, fat, and ke-

tone bodies. As a result, the body autocannibalized its skeletal muscle protein in order to obtain adequate amounts of BCAA fuel substrate.

Cerra et al. demonstrated that the nitrogen-retaining effect of the BCAAs was proportional to the BCAA load, that the effect started at 0.5 g of BCAA/kg/day in the setting of balanced nutritional support, and that the effect was consistent with a BCAA influence on protein synthesis.[274] Furthermore, a 1983 study of patients with septic stress documented a return of skin test reactivity and an increase in total lymphocyte count in patients receiving high-dose BCAAs when compared with patients receiving standard amino acid solutions.[275] Efforts to duplicate these results in other surgical patients, however, have generally been unsuccessful.

In the patient who is recovering from severe sepsis, a program of physical therapy and exercise seems to be advisable during convalescence. Deposition and incorporation of amino acids into skeletal protein is facilitated by active muscular activity. Ill patients usually have marked limitations of activity and require planned exercise programs to maintain active and functional skeletal mass.

AXIOM Physical therapy is an important part of any successful nutritional program.

In a recent report of a multicenter, prospective, randomized clinical trial by Bower et al., studying the effects of early enteral administration of a formula (Impact®) which has arginine, nucleotides, and fish oil, patients who received at least 821 mL/day of the experimental formula had a median hospital stay reduced by 8 days (P < .05).[276] In a subset of patients stratified as septic, the median hospital stay was reduced by 10 days (P < .05). A major reduction also occurred in the frequency of acquired infections in the same subset of patients receiving the experimental formula (P < .01).

AXIOM Early enteral nutrition, particularly with immunostimulatory nutrients, should be considered in injured patients who have a high probability of developing infection.

FRESH-FROZEN PLASMA

Administration of fresh-frozen plasma may help to restore host defenses, particularly complement, in patients with prolonged infections or severe malnutrition. Unfortunately, relatively large amounts of plasma may be required to restore immunoglobulin and complement levels to normal, and this is considered a poor use of a precious resource. In addition, a 0.1-0.5% risk of hepatitis exists with each unit of blood product infused.

CRYOPRECIPITATE

Saba et al. showed that effective phagocytosis of circulating nonmicrobial particulate matter by the RES requires opsonization by circulating fibronectin (also known as α_2 surface-binding glycoprotein).[2] Fibronectin appears to be the major opsonin for clearance of wound and tissue debris, collagen fragments, and macroaggregates of fibrin by tissue macrophages. Although it binds weakly to S. aureus and may promote phagocytosis of the organism, fibronectin does not bind to most gram-negative organisms, and it is not believed to be a significant bacterial opsonin.[277]

In trauma and burn patients, depressed fibronectin levels may correlate with the extent of injury. Fibronectin-rich cryoprecipitate has been administered to trauma patients in an attempt to reverse MOF. Although resolution of sepsis and clinical improvement were reported in some ad hoc trials, the observations have not been confirmed in controlled trials.[277]

IMMUNOTHERAPY

Because 50-75% of posttraumatic infections are due to gram-negative organisms, much attention has been directed toward therapy against endotoxin, particularly the lipid-A component of lipopolysaccharide which is the most highly conserved area between species and probably the most toxic.[1] Initially, rabbit antibodies were generated against the J-5 mutant of E. coli, which lacks the ability to attach side chains to core polysaccharide. When these antibodies were injected into rabbits infected with E. coli, Klebsiella, or Pseudomonas, enhanced survival was demonstrated.[278]

In a randomized, prospective, double-blind trial, a similar vaccine made by injecting boiled J-5 cells into healthy humans was administered to 304 patients believed to have gram-negative sepsis. Mortality was significantly decreased from 39% to 22%.[279] A similar study in 1985 reported the results of administering antiserum to E. coli J-5 to surgical patients at high-risk of gram-negative bacteremia.[280] Although the incidence of gram-negative infections was not reduced, the risk of developing gram-negative septic shock was decreased in the treatment group.

Over the next several years, monoclonal antibody (HA-1A), which was an IgM antibody to the lipid-A moiety, was developed. In a randomized, double-blind trial of 543 patients with presumed gram-negative sepsis, no significant effect was demonstrated on mortality overall.[281] However, in the subgroup of 200 patients that had gram-negative bacteremia, a significant decrease in mortality from 49% in the control group to 30% in the treatment group occurred. This was even more marked in the patients with shock, in whom the mortality was reduced from 57% to 33%.

Although these initial results were extremely encouraging, confirmatory follow-up studies have not been forthcoming. In a study of 600 patients, no evidence of increased survival was noted in patients with gram-negative bacteremia; however, some increases in mortality were noted in patients who did not have gram-negative bacteremia.[282]

Because TNF appears to be the main initiator of the sepsis cascade, immunization against this protein has important therapeutic potential. Some degree of protection was demonstrated in mice injected with TNF antiserum from rabbits prior to receiving endotoxin.[283] Mortality was not affected when the antiserum was given at the same time or three or six hours after lipopolysaccharide administration.

OTHER RESEARCH WORK

Work has been performed on cyclooxygenase inhibitors, such as ibuprofen and pentoxifylline, a methylxanthine. Pentoxifylline was shown to increase survival in mice when given up to four hours after a lipopolysaccharide challenge.[284] Pretreatment with the platelet-factor-activating antagonist BN-52021 was shown to attenuate the hypotension caused by lipopolysaccharide infusion in rats. Survival increased from 20% to 85%.[285]

In another study, high-dose methylprednisolone was administered in a double-blind, randomized trial to septic patients and compared with placebo. No difference in 14-day mortality could be shown.[286] Naloxone was similarly evaluated in a prospective, randomized, double-blind trial in patients with a clinical diagnosis of septic shock. Mortality at seven days was 62% in the placebo-treated patients as opposed to 67% in the naloxone-treated patients. Currently, neither drug is recommended in the therapy of sepsis; however, a role does exist for administration of corticosteroids in adrenal insufficiency.[1]

Correction of Pathophysiologic Changes

If MOF is allowed to develop, the patient will probably die even if the infectious process that initiated the MOF is finally controlled.

PULMONARY SYSTEM

In critically ill or injured patients, the first priority of treatment is generally to ensure adequate ventilation, not only for proper oxygen and carbon dioxide exchange, but also to prevent atelectasis and other pulmonary complications. If the $Paco_2$ is > 45-50 mm Hg in patients who do not have metabolic alkalosis, or if the Pao_2 is < 50 mm Hg in spite of oxygen administration, ventilatory assistance is needed.

> **AXIOM** Maintaining early, optimal perfusion of vital organs with well-oxygenated blood is one of the best ways to prevent infection and later MOF after trauma.

Maintenance of optimal pulmonary function may require adding PEEP. Because it tends to reduce venous return and cardiac output, particularly in hypovolemic patients, PEEP should not be added until or unless the blood volume is normal or greater than normal. If > 10 cm H_2O PEEP is used, cardiac output and oxygen transport (cardiac output multiplied by arterial oxygen content) should also be monitored.

CARDIOVASCULAR FUNCTION

Fluid Therapy

In sepsis, it is extremely important to maintain a cardiac index that is normal (2.5-3.75 L/min/m^2) or preferably higher. However, septic patients tend to become hypovolemic because of increased permeability of capillaries and venules. Consequently, early aggressive fluid administration is extremely important. It is important to insert two, and preferably three, large intravenous catheters and any hypovolemia should be corrected rapidly. Generally, septic patients require at least 200-300 mL of fluid per hour over and above measured losses.

The relative amounts of crystalloid, colloid, and blood that should be given to septic patients is controversial. Albumin levels are often low in septic patients, and some investigators believe that albumin administration can be helpful;[287,288] however, continued administration of large amounts of albumin may cause more harm than good.[289] Some investigators believe that, in sepsis, exogenous albumin moves rapidly into the interstitial space, particularly in the lungs, drawing water with it, thereby increasing the tendency for respiratory failure. In addition, it has been shown that albumin infusions can reduce the production of coagulation factors and immunoglobulins.[290] Albumin is also expensive and frequently in short supply.

Optimal Oxygen Delivery

Several methods exist for trying to ascertain whether oxygen delivery is optimal. One method is to progressively increase oxygen delivery (DO_2) until no further increase in oxygen consumption occurs (VO_2). Another method for optimizing DO_2 is to increase it until lactate levels and/or base deficit are normal.[291-294] Some studies have shown that if lactate levels are normal, further increases in DO_2 will generally not increase the VO_2.[291]

Another technique optimizing DO_2 is to try to achieve a set of optimal goals, such as a cardiac index > 4.5 L/min/m^2, $DO_2I > 600$ mL/min/m^2, and $VO_2I > 17$ mL/min/m^2. Using these "optimal" values as a goal, Shoemaker et al. were able to reduce the mortality rate in high-risk surgical ICU patients from 35% (using normal values as the goal) to 4%.[160]

In our experience, each unit of packed red blood cells increases O_2 content by about 8-10% and increases O_2 delivery by about 5-7%. We have also noted that septic patients who have a VO_2 which is persistently < 100 mL/min/m^2 have a mortality rate approaching 100%. However, increasing DO_2 above normal (500-600 mL/min/m^2) does not always increase VO_2 above a normal of 130-160 mL/min/m^2. Haupt et al., for example, found that as oxygen delivery (DO_2) increases, VO_2 can usually only be driven beyond normal in patients who have lactic acidosis in spite of a normal VO_2.[291]

SUMMARY

In many series, sepsis is the most frequent, single cause of death after trauma, especially in the patients who survive at least 48 hours. Development of sepsis should be anticipated in elderly patients or in those with trauma causing intestinal injury, particularly if the patient had massive transfusions or shock.

The diagnosis of infection may be extremely difficult, particularly if the infection is intraperitoneal. Furthermore, patients with impaired host defenses may show only a failure to thrive and then progressive MOF. Physical examination is usually not helpful. Gallium and indium scans and ultrasonography are only about 50-60% accurate. Ultrasound followed by HIDA/PIPIDA scans may be helpful in diagnosing acute acalculous cholecystitis which appears to be an increasingly frequent problem in these patients. CT scans are at least 80-90% accurate in diagnosing intraabdominal abscesses, but the diagnosis of peritonitis is still largely clinical.

Even without clear evidence of infection, the patient with increasing sepsis after abdominal trauma, in spite of all other treatment efforts, should probably be explored (i.e., have a "blind laparotomy"). If generalized peritonitis is found, it may be wise to leave the abdomen open and reexplore and debride it daily until it is clean. Percutaneous drainage of abdominal abscesses is being performed increasingly and is of particular value in the 30-50% of patients with single bacterial abscesses where the drainage tract does not cross bowel or peritoneum and no underlying intestinal leak is present.

Antibiotics are only a second line of defense against infection, and their use should be directed by smear and culture results whenever possible. For abdominal infections, coverage for gram-negative anaerobes and Bacteroides fragilis is essential. When infection persists for more than one to two weeks, infection by enterococci and fungi must be considered.

When shock develops, maintaining an oxygen consumption of at least 150-170 mL/min/m^2 is a particularly important part of resuscitation. Although controversial, increasing hematocrit to 40% or higher in critically ill, septic patients may also be of value. Enteral nutrition should be started as soon as possible.

⊘ FREQUENT ERRORS

In the Prevention and Management of Infections After Trauma

1. *Depending on prophylactic antibiotics instead of sound surgical principles.*
2. *Excessively long courses of prophylactic antibiotics.*
3. *Masking the presence of all fever with antipyretics.*
4. *Beginning antibiotics without appropriate cultures and smears.*
5. *Improper collecting and handling of material for cultures, particularly for anaerobes.*
6. *Administering an agent with broad-spectrum coverage when specific therapy is possible.*
7. *Selecting antibiotic doses that are inappropriate for the clinical status of the patient and/or preexisting organ system failure.*
8. *Failing to check antibiotic sensitivities in the hospital at frequent intervals.*
9. *Discontinuing antibiotics before the infecting organisms have been adequately controlled.*
10. *Assuming that the cause of persistent fever is an antibiotic-resistant organism.*
11. *Failing to search for hidden abscesses.*
12. *Mistaking colonization for superinfection.*
13. *Failing to consider unusual organisms when cultures are repeatedly negative.*

▼▼▼▼▼▼▼▼▼▼▼▼▼▼▼▼▼▼▼▼▼▼▼▼▼▼▼▼▼▼▼▼

SUMMARY POINTS

1. In patients surviving for at least 48 hours, sepsis is the single, most frequent cause of later morbidity and mortality.
2. The ability of microorganisms to cause infection is a function of their virulence, numbers present, presence of other bacteria, the patient's host defenses, and the appropriateness of the antimicrobial agents used.
3. One should not assume that a wound is almost "sterile" just because it looks clean.
4. Foreign bodies, blood, and dead space in a wound can reduce the critical inoculum of bacteria needed to cause an infection from 10^6 for many wounds to 10^2, (i.e., by a factor of 10,000).
5. Fever developing two to three days after surgery or trauma is often due to an infected intravenous catheter.
6. Any patient who becomes septic without another obvious cause should be considered to have an infected intravenous line until proved otherwise.
7. The longer ventilatory assistance is required, the more likely it is that the patient will develop pneumonia.
8. Early eradication of all underlying infection is the best way to stop the downward spiral of organ dysfunction in sepsis.
9. In addition to providing cell-mediated immunity and activating antibody production, macrophages secrete multiple cytokines that influence immune response.
10. Tissue-oxygen tension is an important variable influencing the risk of infection because PMNs require oxygen to kill bacteria.
11. Specific immune responses are divided into two broad categories, cell-mediated and humoral. The cell-mediated response is primarily directed against intracellular pathogens, such as viruses, while the humoral response (antibody-producing) is primarily against extracellular pathogens, such as bacteria.
12. One of the major immune defects after severe trauma is reduced antigen-presenting capability.
13. The main substances involved in the host response to trauma and infection include TNF, the ILs (especially IL-1), platelet-activating factor, and various arachidonic acid metabolites.
14. Opsonins refer to a group of substances in serum which attach themselves to the surface of antigens (usually microorganisms or particulate matter) and thereby enhance the ability of phagocytes to recognize and engulf them.
15. Corticosteroid therapy is frequently associated with an increased incidence of infection by opportunistic bacteria, viruses, fungi, and parasites.
16. Patients with major trauma who receive no nutrition for 4-5 days can develop cumulative caloric and protein deficits that can result in greatly increased complication rates.
17. Severe infections may sometimes develop without pain, fever, or leukocytosis, especially in patients who have impaired host defenses.
18. In trauma patients who may develop infections, temperatures should be taken at least every four hours, particularly in the early evening.
19. When daily rectal examinations are not performed on patients who may develop pelvic abscesses, severe systemic toxicity may develop before the diagnosis is made.
20. Septic patients tend to be restless, anxious, and/or confused.
21. Once MOF syndrome has developed, the process becomes self-perpetuating, and the patient's prognosis is poor, even if the initiating factors are then controlled.
22. Patients with jaundice developing eight or more days after trauma should be assumed to be septic until proven otherwise.
23. Generally, the higher the VO$_2$ is maintained in critically injured patients, especially during the first 12-24 hours, the better the patient's prognosis will be.
24. Although upper gastrointestinal feeding may reduce stress-related gastric mucosal damage, jejunostomy feedings are not as effective.
25. Characteristically, patients in early septic shock are vasodilated, have normal or increased cardiac output, and have warm, dry, pink, or flushed skin.
26. Hypodynamic (cold) septic shock usually occurs late in sepsis and indicates that cardiac failure and some element of hypovolemia are present.
27. Although leukocytosis after trauma raises the suspicion of infection, specific additional evidence for infection should be sought before antibiotics are begun.

28. A progressive decrease in plasma-ionized calcium levels should make one look for sepsis, impaired tissue perfusion, or some other cause of altered cell metabolism.

29. Low antithrombin levels in the absence of extensive clotting or severe liver disease generally indicate that infection is present or will develop.

30. When smears are not obtained before antibiotic therapy is begun, bacteriologic diagnosis may be delayed or inaccurate.

31. Bronchial secretions obtained during bronchoscopy by bronchoalveolar lavage or protected brush specimens are more reliable than induced sputum or tracheal aspirates.

32. Occasionally, pleural fluid can be obtained by thoracentesis in patients with pneumonia, and the organisms found there will usually be the same as those in the underlying lung infection.

33. Even when urine contains $> 10^5$ microorganisms/mL, pyuria should also be present to warrant diagnosis and treatment of a urinary tract infection.

34. Exudate or pus, which is not cultured rapidly in the microbiology laboratory, often yields inconclusive or deceptive results, particularly if mixed infections are present.

35. The ideal specimen for detecting the microorganisms responsible for an abscess is a tissue biopsy from the edge of the abscess.

36. False-negative anaerobic cultures are common and should be considered when choosing antibiotic therapy based on laboratory studies.

37. The "rule of threes" for blood cultures states that three blood cultures taken on three consecutive days will usually document a gram-negative bacteremia in untreated patients.

38. Smears and cultures should be obtained, whenever possible, before antibiotic therapy is begun.

39. The location and extent of an infection and the bacteria involved may be masked while the patient is receiving antibiotics.

40. When skin testing shows a patient to be persistently anergic, one should look carefully for an infection and make sure that nutritional support is adequate.

41. Gallium and/or indium scans are of little value for detecting acute infections in trauma patients.

42. The preferred test for evaluating the biliary tract is ultrasonography with or without HIDA or PIPIDA hepatobiliary scanning.

43. Patients who have been on TPN for five to seven days may not have their gallbladders visualized on a HIDA or PIPIDA scan, even when the cystic duct is patent and the gallbladder is normal.

44. CT scans are the ideal test for detecting intraabdominal abscesses, but they are relatively unreliable during the first five days after trauma.

45. Septic shock developing within 24-48 hours of trauma is usually due to Streptococcus pyogenes or Clostridium welchii.

46. Mixed soft-tissue infections after trauma usually occur in wounds contaminated by gastrointestinal or infected genitourinary contents.

47. Most gangrenous infections with gas in the tissues are not gas gangrene, but the infections should be approached as if they may be.

48. Because of clostridial leukocidin, relatively few white blood cells are found in the exudate from gas gangrene.

49. One should consider the possible presence of candidiasis if bacterial cultures are repeatedly negative in a septic patient who has been on broad-spectrum antibiotics.

50. Increasing data suggest that great efforts should be made in patients with severe trauma to increase their oxygen delivery index (DO_2I) to 600 mL/minute/m^2 or more and their oxygen consumption index (VO_2I) to 150-170 mL/min/m^2 or more as soon as possible after injury.

51. Many wound infections following trauma can be prevented by good surgical technique, early thorough debridement of all contaminated or necrotic tissue, and complete drainage of any collections of blood or other fluid.

52. Antibiotic therapy should not be delayed when its use is clinically indicated.

53. Antibiotics effective against anaerobic GI bacteria and gram-negative aerobes should be administered as soon as possible to patients with abdominal trauma that may involve the distal small bowel or colon.

54. Although controversial, data from five of seven prospective double-blind studies support using prophylactic antibiotics when chest tubes are inserted for traumatic pneumothorax or hemothorax.

55. Prophylactic antibiotics for uncomplicated traumatic CSF leaks do not reduce the incidence of infection but do increase the likelihood of infection by an antibiotic-resistant organism.

56. In settings where the risk of infection continues over an extended period of time, preventive antibiotics have uniformly failed to prevent subsequent infection; furthermore, the bacteria eventually involved are more apt to be antibiotic-resistant.

57. Although extremely controversial, antibiotic irrigation of heavily contaminated areas of the peritoneal cavity may be of some value in selected patients.

58. One should assume that all human bites are contaminated with a large number of virulent mouth aerobes and anaerobes.

59. SDD and SPEAR prophylaxis are expensive and work-intensive, and they are not likely to improve outcome for the great majority of ICU trauma patients.

60. Early, adequate drainage and debridement is the most important treatment of localized infections.

61. Continued leakage of intestinal contents, particularly from the colon or distal small bowel, into the peritoneal cavity is tolerated poorly.

62. An abscess cavity, which continues to drain large quantities of pus or fluid for several days after surgical drainage, is usually inadequately drained or is associated with a fistula.

63. In patients who are, in spite of all other therapy, progressively deteriorating with sepsis after abdominal trauma, an exploratory laparotomy should be considered even if all diagnostic tests for abscess or peritonitis are negative.

64. Even when a surgeon does not believe in leaving the abdomen open in patients with severe, diffuse peritonitis, initial improvement followed by later deterioration should be an indication for early re-exploration.

65. Repeated bronchoscopies for toilet should be strongly considered in patients with severe atelectasis or pneumonia not responding promptly to other therapy.

66. No antibiotic, or combination of antibiotics, "covers everything."

67. The only way to ensure maximum effectiveness and safety with aminoglycosides in critically ill patients is to serially monitor peak and trough levels at least every two to four days.

68. Once treatment of an infection is begun with a carefully selected antibiotic, it should be continued for at least 48-72 hours before empirically adding or changing to another agent.

69. An infected abdominal incision that drains increased fluid or exhibits signs of fascial necrosis may be evidence of an underlying intraabdominal infection and/or anastomotic leak.

70. Overzealous use of vancomycin has led to the development of vancomycin-resistant enterococci; consequently, empiric use of this agent should be kept to a minimum.

71. Wound infections developing in patients who have had intraabdominal injury or have been receiving broad-spectrum antibiotics are often caused by gram-negative bacilli.

72. Although about a third of positive sputum cultures in ICU patients are due to colonization, one should consider treating for that organism, especially if it is Pseudomonas, and the patient is severely immunodepressed.

73. Before treating pneumonia with an antibiotic, great efforts should be made to perform Gram stain and culture and sensitivity testing on a good sputum or bronchoscopic specimen.

74. The best ways to prevent pulmonary infection are to prevent aspiration, to relieve pain enough to facilitate optimal coughing, to perform a timely tracheostomy when indicated, and to promptly and completely drain any hemopneumothorax that may develop.

75. The most important method for diagnosing posttraumatic peritonitis early is repetitive examinations by a physician who is familiar with the patient's injuries and treatment. This may be supplemented with chest radiography, abdominal ultrasonography, and CT as needed.

76. Any abnormality in the groin following femoral vascular surgery, even months later, should be considered evidence of an infected vascular prosthesis until proved otherwise.

77. Intravenous catheter infection with a positive S. aureus culture requires at least 10-14 days of intravenous antibiotics and should be considered due to a septic phlebitis until proven otherwise.

78. Any finding suggesting the presence of an anaerobic infection is an indication for early, aggressive exploration, incision, and debridement.

79. Death due to tetanus is most likely to result from respiratory arrest occurring during a generalized convulsion.

80. If the sensitivities of the bacteria found within hospitals are not checked on a regular basis, the initial empiric antibiotic choices are likely to be increasingly incorrect.

81. Fungal infection should be suspected in septic ICU patients who have received broad-spectrum antibiotics for > 10-14 days and have no obvious sites of infection, particularly if multiple cultures of all possible infected foci are negative for bacteria.

82. When hyperglycemia cannot be controlled with insulin and reduced carbohydrate intake, one should suspect the presence of uncontrolled infection.

83. Proper monitoring of renal function in septic patients requires serial creatinine clearance studies; serum creatinine changes are relatively insensitive.

84. Physical therapy is an important part of any successful nutritional program.

85. Early enteral nutrition, particularly with immunostimulatory nutrients, should be considered in injured patients with a high probability of developing infection.

86. Maintaining early optimal perfusion of vital organs with well-oxygenated blood is one of the best ways to prevent infection and later MOF after trauma.

▲▲▲▲▲▲▲▲▲▲▲▲▲▲▲▲▲▲▲▲▲▲▲▲▲▲▲▲▲▲▲▲▲

REFERENCES

1. Fabian TC, Minard G. Sepsis. Mattox KL, ed. Complications of trauma. New York: Churchill Livingstone, 1994; 61-79.
2. Dellinger EP. Prevention and management of infections. Moore EE, Mattox KL, Feliciano DV, eds. Trauma, 2nd ed. Norwalk: Appleton & Lange, 1991; 231-244.
3. Nichols RL, Smith JW, Klein DB, et al. Risk of infection after penetrating abdominal trauma. N Engl J Med 1984;311:1065.
4. Dellinger EP, Oreskovich MR, Wertz MJ, et al. Risk of infection following laparotomy for penetrating abdominal injury. Arch Surg 1984;119:20.
5. Stillwell M, Caplan ES. The septic multiple-trauma patient. Crit Care Clin 1988;4:345.
6. Carmona R, Catalona R, Trunkey DO. Septic shock. Shires GT, ed. Shock and related problems. New York:, Churchill Livingstone, 1984; 156.
7. Baker CC, Oppenheimer L, Stephens B, et al. Epidemiology of trauma deaths. Am J Surg 1980;140:144.
8. Goris RJA, Draaisma J. Causes of death after blunt trauma. J Trauma 1982;22:141.
9. Wilson RF, Wiencek R, Balog M. Predicting and preventing infection after abdominal vascular injuries. J Trauma 1989;29:1371.
10. Schimpff SC, Miller RM, Polakavetz S, Hornick RB. Infection in the severely traumatized patient. Ann Surg 1974;179:352.
11. Croce MA, Fabian TC, Stewart RM, et al. Correlation of abdominal trauma index and injury severity score with abdominal septic complications in penetrating and blunt trauma. J Trauma 1991;32:380.
12. George SM, Fabian TC, Voeller GR, et al. Primary repair of colon wounds: a prospective trial in nonselected patients. Ann Surg 1989;209:728.
13. Fabian TC, Croce MA, Payne LW, et al. Duration of antibiotic therapy for penetrating abdominal trauma: a prospective trial. Surgery 1992;112:788.
14. Moore EE, Dunn EL, Moore JB, et al. Penetrating abdominal trauma index. J Trauma 1981;21:439.
15. Weisel RD, Vito L, Dennis RC, et al. Myocardial depression during sepsis. Am J Surg 1977;133:612.
16. Bone RC. The pathogenesis of sepsis. Ann Intern Med 1991;115:457.
17. Miles AA, Miles EM, Burke J. The value and duration of defense reactions of the skin to the primary lodgement of bacteria. Br J Exp Pathol 1957;38:79.
18. Sanders CC, Sanders WE Jr. Emergence of resistance during therapy with the newer beta-lactam antibiotics: role of inducible beta-lactamases and implications for the future. Rev Infect Dis 1983;5:639.
19. Esrig BC, Frazee L, Stephenson SFS, et al. The predisposition to infection following hemorrhagic shock. Surg Gynecol Obstet 1977;144:915.
20. Livingston DH, Malangoni MA. An experimental study of susceptibility to infection after hemorrhagic shock. Surg Gynecol Obstet 1988;168:138.
21. Dawes LG, Aprahamian C, Condon RE, Malangoni MA. The risk of infection after colon injury. Surgery 1986;100:796.
22. Polk HC Jr, Lopez-Mayor JF. Postoperative wound infection: a prospective study of determinant factors and prevention. Surgery 1969;66:97.
23. Robson MC, Krizek TJ, Heggers JP. Biology of surgical infection. Curr Prob Surg 1973;3:2.
24. Gustilo RB, Anderson JT. Prevention of infection in the treatment of one thousand and twenty-five open fractures of long bones. J Bone Joint Surgery 1974;56A:532.
25. Chapman MW, Mahoney M. The role of early internal fixation in the management of open fractures. Clin Orthop 1979;138:120.
26. Dellinger EP, Miller SD, Wertz MJ, et al. Risk of infection after open fracture of the arm or leg. Arch Surg 1988;123:1320.
27. Peitzman AB, Udekwu AO, Ochoa J, Smith S. Bacterial translocation in trauma patients. J Trauma 1991;31:1083.
28. Rush BF Jr, Sori AJ, Murphy MS, et al. Endotoxemia and bacteremia during hemorrhagic shock. Ann Surg 1988;207:549.
29. Moore FA, Moore EE, Poggetti R, et al. Gut bacterial translocation via the portal vein: a clinical perspective trial in patients with major torso trauma. J Trauma 1991;31:629.
30. Redan JA, Rush BF, McCullough JN, et al. Organ distribution of radiolabeled enteric Escherichia coli during and after hemorrhagic shock. Ann Surg 1990;211:663.
31. Pinill JC, Ross DF, Martin T, et al. Study of the incidence of intravascular catheter infection and associated septicemia in critically ill patients. Crit Care Med 1983;11:21.
32. Collignon P, Suni N, Pearson I, et al. Sepsis associated with central venous catheters in critically ill patients. Intensive Care Med 1988;14:227.
33. Jarvis WR, White JW, Munn VP, et al. Nosocomial infection surveillance 1983. MMWR 1984;33:9SS.
34. Freedland M, Wilson RF, Bender JS, Levison MA. The management of flail chest injury: factors affecting outcome. J Trauma 1990;30:1460.
35. Rodriguez JL, Gibbons KJ, Bitzer LG. Pneumonia: incidence, risk factors, and outcome in injured patients. J Trauma 1991;31:907.
36. Driks MR, Craven DE, Celli BR, et al. Nosocomial pneumonia in intubated patients randomized to sucralfate versus antacids and/or histamine type 2 blockers: the role of gastric colonization. N Engl J Med 1987;317:1376.
37. Tryba M. Sucralfate versus antacids or H2 antagonists in stress ulcer prophylaxis: a meta-analysis on efficacy and pneumonia rate. Crit Care Med 1991;19:942.
38. Fabian TC, Boucher BA, Croce MA, et al. Pneumonia and stress ulceration in severely injured patients. Arch Surg 1993;128:11.
39. Baue AE. Mediators of injury and inflammation. Deitch EP, ed. Multiple organ failure—patient care and prevention. St. Louis: Mosby–Year Book, 1990; 29-66.
40. Stevenson TR, Mathes SJ. Wound healing. Miller TA, Rowlands BJ, eds. Physiologic basis of modern surgical care. St. Louis: CV Mosby Co, 1988; 1010-1011.
41. Aasen AO, Smith-Erichsen N, Amundson E. Plasma kallikrein-kinin system in septicemia. Arch Surg 1983;118:343.
42. Lefer AM. Role of a myocardial depressant factor in the pathogenesis of circulatory shock. Fed Proc 1970;29:1836.
43. Root RK, Ryan JL. Humoral immunity and complement. Mandell JL, Douglas RG, Bennett JE, eds. Principles and practice of infectious disease, 2nd ed. New York: John Wiley & Sons, 1985; 31-57.
44. Downey EC, Shackford SR, Fridlund PH, et al. Long-term depressed immune function in patients splenectomized for trauma. J Trauma 1987;27:661.
45. Sullivan JL, Ochs HD, Schiff G. Immune responses after splenectomy. Lancet 1987;1:181.

46. Saba TM, Blumestock FA, Scovill WA, Bernard H. Cryoprecipitate reversal of opsonic glycoprotein deficiency in septic surgical and trauma patients. Ann Surg 1981;195:177.

47. Meakins JL, Hohn DC, Simmons RL, et al. Host defenses. Howard RJ, Simmons RL, eds. Surgical infectious diseases, 2nd ed. Norwalk: Appleton & Lange, 1988; 152.

48. Knighton DR, Fiegelvo, Halverson T, et al. Oxygen as an antibiotic. The effect of oxygen on bacterial clearance. Arch Surg 1990;125:97.

49. Hohn DC. The phagocytes. Howard RJ, Simmons RL, eds. Surgical infectious diseases, 2nd ed. Norwalk: Appleton & Lange, 1988; 158-166.

50. Goodman JW. The immune response. Stites DP, Terr AI, Parslow TG, eds. Basic & clinical immunology. Norwalk: Appelton & Lange, 1994; 45-46.

51. McRitchie DI, Girotti MJ, Rotstein OD, Teodorczyk-Injeyan JA. Impaired antibody production in blunt trauma—possible role for T-cell dysfunction. Arch Surg 1990;125:91.

52. Schneider RP, Christou NV, Meakins JL, Nohr C. Humoral immunity in surgical patients with and without trauma. Arch Surg 1991;126:143.

53. Faist E, Kupper T, Baker CC, et al. Depression of cellular immunity after major burn injury: its association with posttraumatic complications and its reversal with immunomodulation. Arch Surg 1986;121:1000.

54. Hershman MJ, Cheadle WG, Wellhausen SR, et al. Monocyte HLA-DR antigen expression characterizes clinical outcome in the trauma patient. Br J Surg 1990;77:204.

55. Ertel W, Meldrum DR, Morrison MH, et al. Immunoprotective effect of a calcium channel blocker on macrophage antigen presentation function, major histocompatibility class II antigen expression, and interleukin-1 synthesis after hemorrhage. Surgery 1990;108:154.

56. Polk HC Jr, Cheadle WG, Livingston DH, et al. A randomized prospective clinical trial to determine the efficacy of interferon-gamma in severely injured patients. Am J Surg 1992;163:191.

57. Babineau TJ, Marcello P, Swails W, et al. Randomized phase I/II trial of a macrophage-specific immunomodulator (PGG-Glucan) in high risk surgical patients. Ann Surg 1994;220:601.

58. Cheadle WG, Pemberton RM, Robinson D, et al. Lymphocyte subset responses to trauma and sepsis. J Trauma 1993;35:844.

59. Christou NV. Host-defense mechanisms in surgical patients: a correlative study of the delayed hypersensitivity skin-test response, granulocyte function and sepsis. Can J Surg 1985;28:39.

60. Rodrick ML, Wood JJ, O'Mahoney JB, et al. Mechanisms of immunosuppression associated with severe nonthermal traumatic injuries in man: production of IL-1 and -2. J Clin Immunol 1986;6:310.

61. Livingston DH, Appel SH, Wellhausen SR, et al. Depressed interferon-gamma production and monocyte HLA after severe injury. Arch Surg 1988;123:1309.

62. O'Mahony JB, Palder SB, Wood JJ. Depression of cellular immunity after multiple trauma in the absence of sepsis. J Trauma 1984;24:869.

63. Keane RM, Munster AM, Birmingham W, et al. Suppressor cell activity after major injury: direct and indirect functional assays. J Trauma 1982;22:770.

64. McRitchie DI, Girotti MJ, Rotstein OD, et al. Impaired antibody production in blunt trauma. Arch Surg 1990;125:91.

65. Faist E, Mewer A, Baker C, et al. Prostaglandin E2 dependent suppression of interleukin-2 production in patients with major trauma. J Trauma 1987;27:837.

66. Fosse E, Trumpy JH, Skulberg A. Alterations in T-helper and T-suppressor lymphocyte populations after multiple injuries. Injury 1987;18:199.

67. Baker CC, Faist E. Immunologic response. Moore EE, Mattox KL, Feliciano DV, eds. Trauma, 2nd ed. Norwalk: Appleton & Lange, 1991; 887-888.

68. Tyburski JG, Diebel LN, Pieroni M, et al. Regional differences in lymphocyte function following resuscitated hemorrhagic shock. J Trauma 1994;37:469.

69. Beutler B, Cerami A. Cachectin: more than a tumor necrosis factor. N Engl J Med 1987;316:379.

70. Ognibene FP, Rosenberg SA, Lotze M, et al. Interleukin-2 administration causes reversible hemodynamic changes and left ventricular dysfunction similar to those seen in septic shock. Chest 1988;94:750.

71. Miller-Graziano CL, Fink M, Wu JY, et al. Mechanisms of altered monocyte prostaglandin E2 production in severely injured patients. Arch Surg 1988;123:293.

72. Ilfeld DN, Krakauser RS, Blease RM. Suppression of autologous mixed lymphocyte reaction by physiologic concentration of hydrocortisone. J Immunol 1977;119:428.

73. Fauci AS, Dale DC, Balow JE. Glucocorticoid therapy: mechanisms of action and clinical considerations. Ann Intern Med 1976;84:304.

74. Losito A, Williams DG, Cooke G, et al. The effects on polymorphonuclear leukocyte function of prednisolone and azathioprine in vivo and prednisolone, azathioprine, and 6 mercaptopurine in vitro. Clin Exp Immunol 1978;32:423.

75. Cruse PJE. Wound infections: epidemiology and clinical characteristics. Howard RJ, Simmons RL, eds. Surgical infectious diseases, 2nd ed. Norwalk: Appleton & Lange, 1988; 319-329.

76. Gardner IO. The effect of aging on susceptibility to infection. Rev Infect Dis 1980;2:801.

77. Robertson HD, Polk HC Jr. The mechanism of infection in patients with diabetes mellitus: a review of leukocyte malfunction. Surgery 1974;75:123.

78. Kune GA. Life-threatening surgical infection: its development and prediction. Ann R Coll Surg Engl 1978;60:92.

79. Allen JC. The diabetic as a compromised host. Allen JC, ed. Infection and the compromised host. Clinical correlations and therapeutic approaches, 2nd ed. Baltimore: Williams & Wilkins, 1981; 229.

80. Goldbaum SE, Reed WP. Host defenses and immunologic alterations associated with chronic hemodialysis. Ann Intern Med 1980;93:597.

81. Alexander JW. Nutrition and infection—new perspectives for an old problem. Arch Surg 1986;121:966.

82. Barton RG, Cerra FB. Metabolic and nutritional support. Moore EE, Mattox KL, Feliciano DV, eds. Trauma, 2nd ed. Norwalk: Appleton & Lange, 1991; 965-993.

83. Moore FA, Feliciano DV, Andrassy RJ, et al. Early enteral feeding, compared with parenteral, reduces postoperative septic complications. Ann Surg 1992;216:172.

84. Orlando R III, Gleason E, Drezner AD. Acute acalculous cholecystitis in the critically ill patient. Am J Surg 1983;145:472.

85. Petersen SR, Sheldon GF. Acute acalculous cholecystitis: a complication of hyperalimentation. Am J Surg 1979;138:814.

86. Glenn F, Becker CG. Acute acalculous cholecystitis. Ann Surg 1982;195:131.

87. Sitzmann JV, Pitt HA, Steinborn PA, et al. Cholecystokinin prevents parenteral nutrition induced biliary sludge in humans. Surg Gynecol Obstet 1990;170:25.

88. Proctor DF, Andersen I, Lundquist G. Clearance of inhaled particles from the human nose. Arch Intern Med 1973;131:132.

89. Newhouse M, Sanchis J, Bienenstock J. Lung defense mechanisms-I. N Engl J Med 1976;295:990.

90. Newhouse M, Sanchis J, Bienenstock J. Lung defense mechanisms-II. N Engl J Med 1976;295:1045.

91. Musher DM, Fainstein V, Young EJ, et al. Fever patterns, their lack of clinical significance. Arch Intern Med 1979;139:1225.

92. Dykes MHM. Unexplained postoperative fever. Its value as a sign of halothane sensitization. JAMA 1971;216:641.

93. Garibaldi RA, Brodine S, Matsumiya S, et al. Evidence for the noninfectious etiology of early post-operative fever. Infect Control 1985;6:273.

94. Dellinger EP, Wertz MJ, Oreskovich MR, et al. Specificity of fever and leukocytosis after laparotomy for penetrating abdominal trauma. J Trauma 1983;26:633.

95. Dellinger EP. Approach to the patient with postoperative fever. Gorbach SL, Bartlett JG, Blacklow NR, eds. Infectious diseases. Philadelphia: WB Saunders, 1992; 753-758.

96. Dellinger EP. Severe necrotizing soft-tissue infections. JAMA 1981;246:1717.

97. Dellinger EP. Crepitus and gangrene. Kass EH, Platt R, eds. Current therapy in infectious disease-3. Toronto: BC Decker, 1990; 232.

98. Gibson DM, Feliciano DV, Mattox KL, et al. Intra-abdominal abscess after penetrating abdominal trauma. Am J Surg 1981;142:699.

99. Kirkpatrick JR, Wilson RF. The significance of cardiac arrhythmias in the septic patient. Mich Med 1975;74:645.

100. Rajan RK. Spontaneous bacterial peritonitis with ecthyma gangrenosum due to Escherichia coli. J Clin Gastroenterol 1982;4:145.

101. Eiseman B, Beart R, Norton L. Multiple organ failure. Surg Gynecol Obstet 1977;144:323.

102. Fry DE, Pearlstein L, Fulton RL, Polk HC Jr. Multiple system organ failure. Arch Surg 1980;115:136.

103. Polk HC Jr, Shields CL. Remote organ failure: a valid sign of occult intra-abdominal infection. Surgery 1977;81:310.

104. Fry DE, Garrison N, Heitsch RC, et al. Determinants of death in patients with intra-abdominal abscess. Surgery 1980;88:517.

105. Wilson RF, Larned PA, Corr JJ, et al. Physiologic shunting in the lung in critically ill or injured patients. J Surg Res 1970;12:571.

106. Sibbald WJ, Paterson NAM, Holliday RL, et al. Pulmonary hypertension in sepsis. Chest 1978;73:583.

107. Wilson RF, Sarver E, Birks R. Central venous pressure and blood volume determinations in clinical shock. Surg Gynecol Obstet 1971;132:631.

108. Sarfeh IJ, Balint JA. The clinical significance of hyperbilirubinemia following trauma. J Trauma 1978;18:58.

109. Cerra FB, Seigel JH, Border JR, et al. The hepatic failure of sepsis: cellular versus substrate. Surgery 1979;86:409.

110. Fath JJ, St. Cyr JA, Konstantinides FN, et al. Alterations in amino acid clearance during ischemia predict hepatocellular ATP changes. Surgery 1985;98:396.

111. Macheido GW, Hurd T, Rush BF, et al. Temporal relationship of hepatocellular dysfunction and ischemia in sepsis. Arch Surg 1988;123:424.

112. Minard G, Fabian TC, Croce MA, et al. Effect of isolated hepatic ischemia on organic anion clearance and oxidative metabolism. J Trauma 1992;32:514.

113. Dahn MS, Lange MP, Lobdell K, et al. Splanchnic and total body oxygen consumption differences in septic and injured patients. Surgery 1987;101:69.

114. Wilson RF, Soullier G, Antonenko D. Creatinine clearance in critically ill surgical patients. Arch Surg 1979;114:461.

115. Wilson RF, Thal AP, Kindling PH, et al. Hemodynamic measurements in septic shock. Arch Surg 1965;91:121.

116. Calvin JE, Driedger AA, Sibbald WJ. An assessment of myocardial function in human sepsis utilizing ECG gated cardiac scintigraphy. Chest 1981;80:579.

117. Parker MM, Shelhammer JH, Bacharach SL. Severe reversible myocardial depression in septic shock. Crit Care Med 1983;11:229.

118. Wilson RF, Christensen C, Ali M, et al. Oxygen consumption in critically ill surgical patients. Ann Surg 1972;176:801.

119. Cerra FB, Siegel JH, Coleman B, et al. Septic autocannibalism: a failure of exogenous nutrient support. Ann Surg 1980;192:570.

120. Dahn M, Bouwnard D, Kirkpatrick JR. The sepsis-glucose intolerance riddle: a hormonal explanation. Surgery 1979;86:423.

121. Vary TC, Siegel JH, Nakatani T, et al. Regulation of glucose metabolism by altered pyruvate dehydrogenase activity in sepsis. JPEN 1986;10:351.

122. Kispert P, Caldwell MD. Metabolic changes in sepsis and multiple organ failure. Deitch EA, ed. Multiple organ failure. New York: Thieme Medical Publishers, Inc., 1990; 104-125.

123. Meakins JL, Pietsch JB, Bubenick O, et al. Delayed hypersensitivity: indicator of acquired failure of host defenses in sepsis and trauma. Ann Surg 1977;186:241.

124. Sibbald WJ, Short A, Cohen MP, Wilson RF. Variations in adrenocortical responsiveness during severe bacterial infections. Ann Surg 1977;186:29.

125. Wilson RF, Soullier G, Antonenko D. Ionized calcium levels in critically ill surgical patients. Am Surg 1979;45:485.

126. Sibbald WJ, Sardesai V, Wilson RF. Hypocalcemia and nephrogenous cyclic AMP production in critically ill and injured patients. J Trauma 1977;17:677.

127. Wilson RF, Sarver EJ, LeBlanc LP. Factors affecting hemodynamics in clinical shock with sepsis. Ann Surg 1971;174:939.

128. Parker MM, Shelhamer JH, Natanson C, et al. Serial cardiovascular variables in survivors and nonsurvivors of human septic shock: heart rate as an early predictor of prognosis. Crit Care Med 1987;15:923.

129. Parker MM, McCarthy KE, Ognibene FP, et al. Right ventricular dysfunction and dilatation, similar to left ventricular changes, characterize the cardiac depression of septic shock in humans. Chest 1990;97:126.

130. Parrillo JE, Burch C, Shelhamer JH, et al. A circulating myocardial depressant substance in humans with septic shock. J Clin Invest 1985;76:1539.

131. Natanson C, Danner RL, Elin RJ, et al. Role of endotoxemia in cardiovascular dysfunction and mortality. J Clin Invest 1989;83:243.

132. Suffredini AF, Fromm RE, Parker MM, et al. The cardiovascular response of normal humans to the administration of endotoxin. N Engl J Med 1989;321:280.

133. Gump FE, Long CL, Killian P, Kinney JM. Studies of glucose intolerance in septic injured patients. J Trauma 1974;14:378.

134. White BC, Winegar CD, Wilson RF, Trombley JH. The possible role of calcium blockers in cerebral resuscitation: a review of the literature and synthesis for future studies. Crit Care Med 1983;11:202.

135. Corrigan JJ Jr. Vitamin K-dependent coagulation factors in gram-negative septicemia. Am J Dis Child 1984;138:240.

136. Mammen EF, Miyakawa T, Phillips TF, et al. Human antithrombin concentrates and experimental disseminated intravascular coagulation. Semin Thromb Hemost 1985;11:373.

137. Neame PB, Kelton JG, Walker IR, et al. Thrombocytopenia in septicemia: the role of DIC. Blood 1980;56:88.

138. Wilson RF, Farag A, Mammen EF, Fujii Y. Sepsis and antithrombin III, prekallikrein and fibronectin levels in surgical patients. Am Surg 1989;55:450.

139. Wilson RF. The diagnosis and treatment of acute respiratory failure in sepsis. Heart Lung 1976;5:614.

140. Wilson RF, Sibbald WJ. Adrenal corticosteroids for the acutely ill or injured. Compr Ther 1976;2:61.

141. Baker J, Coffernils M, Leon M, et al. Blood lactate levels are superior to oxygen-derived variables in predicting outcome in human septic shock. Chest 1991;99:956.

142. Rackow EC, Mecher C, Astiz ME, et al. Unmeasured anion during severe sepsis with metabolic acidosis. Circ Shock 1990;30:107.

143. Wilson RF, Gibson DB, Percinel AK, et al. Severe alkalosis in critically ill patients. Arch Surg 1972;105:197.

144. Marquene CH, Herengt F, Mathieu, et al. Diagnosis of pneumonia in mechanically ventilated patients: repeatability of the protected specimen brush. Am Rev Respir Dis 1993;147:211.

145. Cook DJ, Brun-Buisson C, Guyatt GH, Sibbald WJ, et al. Evaluation of new diagnostic technologies: bronchoalveolar lavage and the diagnosis of ventilator-associated pneumonia. Crit Care Med 1994;22:1314.

146. Glick PL, Pellegrini CA, Stein S, Way LW. Abdominal abscess. A surgical strategy. Arch Surg 1983;118:646.

147. Moir C, Robins RE. Role of ultrasonography, gallium scanning and computed tomography in the diagnosis of intra-abdominal abscess. Am J Surg 1982;143:582.

148. Wing VW, Van Sonnenberg E, Kipper S, Bieberstein MP. Indium-III-labelled leukocyte localization in hematomas: a pitfall in abscess detection. Radiology 1984;152:173.

149. Gatley JF, Thomas EJ. Acute cholecystitis occurring as a complication of other diseases. Arch Surg 1983;118:1137.

150. Dupriest RW Jr, Khaneja SC, Cowley RA. Acute cholecystitis complicating trauma. Ann Surg 1979;189:84.

151. Suarez CA, Balock F, Bernstein D, et al. The role of HIDA/PIPIDA scanning in diagnosing cystic duct obstruction. Ann Surg 1980;191:391.

152. Matolo NM, Stadalnik RC, McGahan JP. Comparison of ultrasonography, computerized tomography, and radionuclide imaging in the diagnosis of acute and chronic cholecystitis. Am J Surg 1982;144:676.

153. Aeder MI, Wellman JL, Haaga JR, Hau T. Role of surgical and percutaneous drainage in the treatment of abdominal abscess. Arch Surg 1983;118:273.

154. Chesney PJ, Bergdoll MS, Davis JP, et al. The disease spectrum, epidemiology and etiology of toxic shock syndrome. Ann Rev Microbiol 1984;38:315.

155. Ahrenholz DH, Simmons RL. Mixed and synergistic infections. Howard RJ, Simmons RL, eds. Surgical infectious diseases, 2nd ed. Norwalk: Appleton & Lange, 1988; 87-99.

156. Finegold SM. Anaerobic bacteria. Howard RJ, Simmons RL, eds. Surgical infectious diseases, 2nd ed. Norwalk: Appleton & Lang, 1988; 49-62.

157. Simmons RL, Ahrenholz DH. Infections of the skin and soft tissues. Howard RJ, Simmons RL, eds. Surgical infectious diseases, 2nd ed. Norwalk: Appleton & Lang, 1988; 377-441.

158. Furste W, Aguirre A, Lutter K. Tetanus. Howard RJ, Simmons RL, eds. Surgical infectious diseases, 2nd ed. Norwalk: Appleton & Lang, 1988; 837-847.

159. Davies SF, Sarosi GA. Fungi of surgical significance. Howard RJ, Simmons RL, eds. Surgical infectious diseases, 2nd ed. Norwalk: Appleton & Lang, 1988; 101-114.

160. Shoemaker WC, Appel PL, Kram HB, et al. Prospective trial of supranormal values of survivors as therapeutic goals in high-risk surgical patients. Chest 1988;94:1176.

161. Moore FA, Haenel JB, Moore EE, Whitehill TA. Incommensurate oxygen consumption in response to maximal oxygen availability predicts postinjury multiple organ failure. J Trauma 1992;33:58.

162. Fleming A, Bishop M, Shoemaker W, et al. Prospective trial of supranormal values as goals of resuscitation in severe trauma. Arch Surg 1992;127:1175.

163. Tscherne H, Oestern HJ, Sturm J. Osteosynthesis of major fractures in polytrauma. World J Surg 1983;7:80.

164. Robson MC, Duke WF, Krizek TJ. Rapid bacterial screening in the treatment of civilian wounds. J Surg Res 1973;14:426.

165. Edlich RF, Rogers W, Kaspar G, et al. Studies in the management of

contaminated open wounds. II. Comparison of resistance to infection of open and closed wounds during healing. Am J Surg 1969;117:323.

166. Dhingra U, Schauerhamer RR, Wangensteen OH. Peripheral dissemination of bacteria in contaminated wounds: role of devitalized tissue: evaluation of therapeutic measures. Surgery 1976;80:535.

167. Rodeheaver GT, Pettry D, Thacker JG, et al. Wound cleansing by high pressure irrigation. Surg Gynecol Obstet 1975;141:357.

168. Brown LL, Shelton HT, Bornside GH, Cohn I Jr. Evaluation of wound irrigation by pulsatile jet and conventional methods. Ann Surg 1978;187:170.

169. Wheeler CB, Rodeheaver, Thacker JG, et al. Side effects of high pressure irrigation. Surg Gynecol Obstet 1976;143:775.

170. Rodeheaver G, Bellamy W, Kody M, et al. Bactericidal activity and toxicity of iodine-containing solutions in wounds. Arch Surg 1982;117:181.

171. Krizek TJ, Davis JH. The role of the red cell in subcutaneous infection. J Trauma 1965;5:85.

172. Alexander JW, Koerlitz J, Alexander NS. Prevention of wound infection: a case for closed suction drainage to remove wound fluids deficient in opsonic proteins. Am J Surg 1976;132:59.

173. deHoll D, Rodeheaver G, Edgerton MT, Edlich RF. Potentiation of infection by suture closure of dead space. Am J Surg 1974;127:716.

174. Magee C, Rodeheaver GT, Golden GT, et al. Potentiation of wound infection by surgical drains. Am J Surg 1976;131:547.

175. Cerise EJ, Pierce WA, Diamond DL. Abdominal drains: their role as a source of infection following splenectomy. Ann Surg 1970;171:764.

176. Gottrup F, Fogdestam I, Hunt TK. Delayed primary closure: an experimental and clinical review. J Clin Surg 1982;1:113.

177. Nichols RL. Prevention of infection in high risk gastrointestinal surgery. Am J Med 1984;76:111.

178. Heseltine PNR, Berne TV, Yellin AE, et al. The efficacy of cefoxitin vs clindamycin/gentamicin in surgically treated stab wounds of the bowel. J Trauma 1986;26:241.

179. Rowlands BJ, Ericsson CD, Fischer RP. Penetrating abdominal trauma: the use of operative findings to determine length of antibiotic therapy. J Trauma 1987;27:250.

180. Moore FA, Moore EE, Ammons LA, McCroskey BL. Presumptive antibiotics for penetrating abdominal wounds. Surg Gynecol Obstet 1989;169:99.

181. Sims EH, Lou MA, Williams SW, et al. Piperacillin monotherapy compared with metronidazole and gentamicin combination in penetrating abdominal trauma. J Trauma 1993;34:205.

182. Nichols RL, Smith JW, Robertson GD, et al. Prospective alterations in therapy for penetrating abdominal trauma. Arch Surg 1993;128:55.

183. Griswold JA, Muakkassa FF, Betcher E, Poole GV. Injury severity dictates individualized antibiotic therapy in penetrating abdominal trauma. Am Surg 1993;59:34.

184. Fabian TC, Hess MM, Croce MA, et al. Superiority of aztreonam/clindamycin compared with gentamicin/clindamycin in patients with penetrating abdominal trauma. Am J Surg 1994;167:291.

185. Fullen WD, Hunt J, Altemeier WA. Prophylactic antibiotics in penetrating wounds of the abdomen. J Trauma 1972;12:282.

186. Grover FL, Richardson JD, Fewel JG, et al. Prophylactic antibiotics in the treatment of penetrating chest wounds: a prospective double blind study. J Thorac Cardiovasc Surg 1977;74:528.

187. Stone HH, Symbas PN, Hooper CA. Cefamandole for prophylaxis against infection in closed tube thoracostomy. J Trauma 1981;21:975.

188. Mandal AK, Montano J, Thadepalli H. Prophylactic antibiotics and no antibiotics compared in penetrating chest trauma. J Trauma 1985;25:639.

189. LeBlanc KA, Tucker WY. Prophylactic antibiotics and closed tube thoracostomy. Surg Gynecol Obstet 1985;160:259.

190. Locurto JJ Jr, Tischler CD, Swan KG, et al. Tube thoracostomy and trauma: antibiotics or not? J Trauma 1986;26:1067.

191. Brunner RG, Vinsant GO, Alexander RH, et al. The role of antibiotic therapy in the prevention of empyema in patients with an isolated chest injury (ISS 9-10): a prospective study. J Trauma 1990;30:1148.

192. Nichols RL, Smith JW, Muzik AC, et al. Preventive antibiotic usage in traumatic thoracic injuries requiring closed tube thoracostomy. Chest 1994;106:1493.

193. Demetriades D, Breckon V, Breckon C, et al. Antibiotic prophylaxis in penetrating injuries of the chest. Ann R Coll Surg Engl 1991;73:348.

194. Petersdorf RG, Curtin JA, Hoeprich PD, et al. A study of antibiotic prophylaxis in unconscious patients. N Engl J Med 1957;257:1001.

195. Hand WL, Sanford JP. Posttraumatic bacterial meningitis. Ann Intern Med 1970;72:869.

196. Leech PJ, Paterson A. Conservative and operative management of cerebrospinal-fluid leakage after closed head injury. Lancet 1973;1:1013.

197. Klastersky J, Sadeghi M, Brihaye J. Antimicrobial prophylaxis in patients with rhinorrhea or otorrhea: a double-blind study. Surg Neurol 1976;6:111.

198. Burke JF. The effective period of preventive antibiotic action in experimental incisions and dermal lesions. Surgery 1961;50:161.

199. Bernard HR, Cole WR. The prophylaxis of surgical infection. The effect of prophylactic antimicrobial drugs on the incidence of infection following potentially contaminated operations. Surgery 1964;56:151.

200. Classen DC, Evans RS, Pestotnik SL, et al. The timing of prophylactic administration of antibiotics and the risk of surgical-wound infection. N Engl J Med 1992;326:281-286.

201. Dellinger EP, Wertz MJ, Lennard ES, et al. Efficacy of short-course antibiotic prophylaxis after penetrating intestinal injury: a prospective randomized trial. Arch Surg 1986;121:23.

202. DiPiro JT, Cheung RPF, Bowden TA Jr. Single dose systemic antibiotic prophylaxis of surgical wound infections. Am J Surg 1986;152:552.

203. Hofstetter SR, Pachter HL, Bailey AA, et al. A prospective comparison of two regimens of prophylactic antibiotics in abdominal trauma: cefoxitin vs triple drug. J Trauma 1984;24:307.

204. Feliciano DV, Gentry LO, Bitondo CG. Single agent cephalosporin prophylaxis for penetrating abdominal trauma. Am J Surg 1986;152:674.

205. Ericsson C, Fischer R, Rowlands B, et al. Prophylactic antibiotics in trauma: the hazards of underdosing. J Trauma 1989;29:1356.

206. Kaiser AB. Antimicrobial prophylaxis in surgery. N Engl J Med 1986;315:1129.

207. Page CP, Bohnen JMA, Fletcher R, et al. Antimicrobial prophylaxis for surgical wounds—guidelines for clinical care. Arch Surg 1993;128:79.

208. Nelson RM, Benitez PR, Newell MA, Wilson RF. Single-antibiotic use for penetrating abdominal trauma. Arch Surg 1986;121:153.

209. Demetriades D, Lakhoo M, Pezikis A, Charalambides D. Short-course antibiotic prophylaxis in penetrating abdominal injuries: ceftriaxone versus cefoxitin. Injury 1991;22:20.

210. Ablan CJ, Olen RN, Dobrin PB, et al. Efficacy of intraperitoneal antibiotics in the treatment of severe fecal peritonitis. Am J Surg 1991;162:453.

211. Lord JW Jr, LaRaja RD, Daliana M, Gordon MT. Prophylactic antibiotic wound irrigation in gastric, biliary, and colonic surgery. Am J Surg 1983;145:209.

212. Nomikos IN, Katsouyanni K, Papaioannous AN. Washing with or without chloramphenicol in the treatment of peritonitis: a prospective, clinical trial. Surgery 1986;99:20.

213. Silverman SH, Ambrose NS, Youngs DJ, et al. The effect of peritoneal lavage with tetracycline solution on postoperative infection. A prospective, randomized clinical trial. Dis Colon Rectum 1986;29:165.

214. Sauven P, Playforth MJ, Smith GM, et al. Single dose antibiotic prophylaxis of abdominal surgical wound infection: a trial of preoperative latamoxef against preoperative tetracycline lavage. J R Soc Med 1986;79:137.

215. Rappaport WD, Holcomb M, Valente J, Chvapil M. Antibiotic irrigation and the formation of intra-abdominal adhesions. Am J Surg 1989;158:435.

216. Johnson KD, Bone LB, Scheinberg R. Severe open tibial fractures: a study protocol. J Orthop Trauma 1988;2:175.

217. Patzakis MJ, Wilkins J. Factors influencing infection rate in open fracture wounds. Clin Orthop 1989;243:36.

218. Roth AI, Fry DE, Polk HC Jr. Infectious morbidity in extremity fractures. J Trauma 1986;26:757.

219. Dellinger EP. Antibiotic prophylaxis in trauma: penetrating abdominal injuries and open fractures. Rev Infect Dis 1991;13(suppl 10):S847.

220. Bohnen JMA, Solomkin JS, Dellinger EP, et al. Guidelines for clinical care: anti-infective agents for intra-abdominal infection. A Surgical Infection Society policy statement. Arch Surg 1992;127:83.

221. Sacks T. Prophylactic antibiotics in traumatic wounds. J Hosp Infect 1988;11(suppl A):251.

222. Brown DM, Young VL. Hand infections. South Med J 1993;86:56.

223. Edlich RF, Rodeheaver GT, Thacker JG. Wounds, bites, and stings. Mattox KL, Moore EE, Feliciano DV, eds. Trauma. Norwalk: Appleton & Lange, 1988; 697.

224. Weinstein L, Musher DM. Antibiotic-induced suprainfection. J Infect Dis 1969;119:663.

225. Maki DG, Schuna AA. A study of antimicrobial misuse in a university hospital. Am J Med Sci 1978;275:271.

226. Stone HH, Haney BB, Kolb LD, et al. Prophylactic and preventive antibiotic therapy. Timing, duration and economics. Ann Surg 1979;189:691.

227. Bartlett JG, Willey SH, Chang TW, Lowe B. Cephalosporin-associated

pseudomembranous colitis due to Clostridium difficile. JAMA 1979;242:2683.

228. Stoutenbeek CP, vanSaene HK, Miranda DR, et al. The effect of oropharyngeal decontamination using topical nonabsorbable antibiotics on the incidence of nosocomial respiratory tract infections in multiple trauma patients. J Trauma 1987;27:357.

229. Ledingham IMcA, Alcock SR, Eastaway AT, et al. Triple regimen of selective decontamination of the digestive tract, systemic cefotaxime, and microbiological surveillance for prevention of acquired infection in intensive care. Lancet 1988;1:785.

230. Cerra FB, Maddaus MA, Dunn DL, et al. Selective gut contamination reduces nosocomial infections and length of stay but not mortality or organ failure in surgical intensive care unit patients. Arch Surg 1992;127:163.

231. Gerzof SG, Robbins AH, Johnson WC, et al. Percutaneous catheter drainage of abdominal abscess. J Med 1981;305:653.

232. Von Sonnenberg E, Ferrve JT, Mueller PR, et al. Percutaneous drainage of abscesses and fluid collections: technique, results and applications. Radiology 1982;142:1.

233. Haaga JR, Weinstein AJ. CT-guided percutaneous aspiration and drainage of abscesses. AJR 1980;135:1187.

234. Sunshine J, McConnell DB, Weinstein CJ, et al. Percutaneous abdominal abscess drainage. Am J Surg 1983;145:615.

235. Glass CA, Cohn I Jr. Drainage of intra-abdominal abscess. Am J Surg 1984;147:315.

236. Pitcher WD, Musher DM. Critical importance of early diagnosis and treatment of intra-abdominal infection. Arch Surg 1982;117:328.

237. Sinanan M, Maier RV, Carrico J. Laparotomy for intra-abdominal sepsis in patients in an intensive care unit. Arch Surg 1984;119:652.

238. LeGall JR, Fagniez PL, Meakins J, et al. Diagnostic features of early high post-laparotomy fever: a prospective study of 100 patients. Br J Surg 1982;69:451.

239. Halpern NA, McElhinney AJ, Greenstein RJ. Postoperative sepsis: reexplore or observe? Accurate indication from diagnostic abdominal paracentesis. Crit Care Med 1991;19:882.

240. Hinsdale JG, Jaffe BM. Re-operation for intra-abdominal sepsis. Indications and results in modern critical care setting. Ann Surg 1984;199:31.

241. Machiedo GW, Tikellis J, Suval W, et al. Reoperation for sepsis. Am Surg 1985;51:149.

242. Hunt MG. Generalized peritonitis. Arch Surg 1982;117:209.

243. Moore RD, Smith CR, Lietman PS. Risk factors for the development of auditory toxicity in patients receiving aminoglycosides. J Infect Dis 1984;149:23.

244. Sabath LD, Simmons RL, Howard RJ. Antimicrobial agents. Howard RJ, Simmons RL, eds. Surgical infectious diseases, 2nd ed. Norwalk: Appleton & Lange, 1988; 259-306.

245. Lennard ES, Dellinger EP, Wertz MJ, Minshew BH. Implications of leukocytosis and fever at conclusion of antibiotic therapy for intra-abdominal sepsis. Ann Surg 1982;195:19.

246. Weigelt JA. Risk of wound infections in trauma patients. Am J Surg 1985;150:782.

247. Barie PS, Christou NV, Dellinger EP, et al. Pathogenicity of the Enterococcus in surgical infections. Ann Surg 1990;212:155.

248. Abramowicz M. A reminder: piperacillin/tazobactram is not for pseudomonas. Med Lett 1994;36:110.

249. Brittain DC, Scully BE, Neu HC. Ticarcillin plus clavulanic acid in the treatment of pneumonia and other serious infections. Am J Med 1985;79(suppl 5B):81.

250. Musher DM. Pneumococcal pneumonia including diagnosis and therapy of infection caused by penicillin-resistant strains. Infect Dis Clin North Am 1991;5:509.

251. Wisinger D. Bacterial pneumonia: S. pneumoniae and H. influenzae are the villains. Postgrad Med 1993;93:43,49,52.

252. Tinstman TC, Dines DE, Arms RA. Postoperative aspiration pneumonia. Surg Clin North Am 1973;53:859.

253. Aldrete JA, Liem ST, Carrow DJ. Pulmonary aerobic bacterial flora after aspiration pneumonitis. J Trauma 1975;15:1014.

254. Caplan ES, Hoyt NJ, Rodriguez A, Cowley RA. Empyema occurring in the multiply traumatized patient. J Trauma 1984;24:785.

255. Eddy AC, Luna GK, Copass M. Empyema thoracis in patients undergoing emergent closed tube thoracostomy for thoracic trauma journal Am J Surg 1989;157:494.

256. Coon JL, Shuck JM. Failure of tube thoracostomy for post-traumatic empyema: an indication for early decortication. J Trauma 1975;15:588.

257. Dellinger EP, Wertz MJ, Meakins L, et al. Surgical infection stratification system for intra-abdominal infection. Arch Surg 1985;120:21.

258. Lennard ES, Minshew BH, Dellinger EP, et al. Stratified outcome comparison of clindamycin-gentamicin vs chloramphenicol-gentamicin for treatment of intra-abdominal sepsis. Arch Surg 1985;120:889.

259. Wilson RF, Janning SW, eds. Handbook of antibiotic therapy for surgery-related infections, 3rd ed. Springfield: 1995.

260. Schmitt DD, Brandyk DF, Pequet AJ, et al. Mucin production by Staphylococcus epidermidis: a virulence factor promoting adherence to vascular grafts. Arch Surg 1986;121:89.

261. Fry DE, Fry RV, Borzotta AP. Nosocomial blood-borne infection secondary to intravascular devices. Am J Surg 1994;167:268.

262. Crawford GE. An approach to use of antimicrobial agents. Civetta JM, Taylor RW, Kirby RR, eds. Critical care. Philadelphia: JB Lippincott Co., 1988; 769-783.

263. Garrison RN, Fry DE, Berberich S, Polk HC Jr. Enterococcal bacteremia: clinical implications and determinants of death. Ann Surg 1982;196:43.

264. Brand DA, Acampora D, Gottlieb LD, et al. Adequacy of antitetanus prophylaxis in six hospital emergency rooms. N Engl J Med 1983;309:636.

265. Sutter RW, Cochi SL, Brink EW, et al. Assessment of vital statistics and surveillance data for monitoring tetanus mortality, United States, 1979-1984. Am J Epidemiol 1990;131:32.

266. Alexander JW, Babcock GF, Waymack JP. Immunotherapeutic approaches to the prevention and treatment of infection in the surgical patient. Howard RJ, Simmons RL, eds. Surgical infectious diseases. Norwalk: Appleton & Lange, 1988; 307-317.

267. Deutschman CS, Wilton P, Sinow J, et al. Paranasal sinusitis associated with nasotracheal intubation: a frequently unrecognized and treatable source of sepsis. Crit Care Med 1986;14:111.

268. Grindlinger GA, Niehoff J, Hughes SL, et al. Acute paranasal sinusitis related to nasotracheal intubation of head-injured patients. Crit Care Med 1987;15:214.

269. Slotman GJ, Shapiro E, Moffa SM. Fungal sepsis: multisite colonization versus fungemia. Am Surg 1994;60:107.

270. Solomkin JS, Simmons RL. Candida infections in surgical patients. World J Surg 1980;4:381.

271. Howard RJ. Rabies. Howard RJ, Simmons RL, eds. Surgical infectious diseases, 2nd ed. Norwalk: Appleton & Lange, 1988; 126-127.

272. Adams S, Dellinger EP, Wertz MJ, et al. Enteral versus parenteral nutritional support following laparotomy for trauma: a randomized prospective trial. J Trauma 1986;26:882.

273. Kudsk KA, Croce MA, Fabian TC, et al. Enteral versus parenteral feeding: effects on septic morbidity after blunt and penetrating abdominal trauma. Ann Surg 1992;215:503.

274. Cerra FB, Mazuski JE, Chute E, et al. Branched chain metabolic support. A prospective, randomized, double-blind trial in surgical stress. Ann Surg 1984;199:286.

275. Nuwer N, Cerra FB, Shronts EP, et al. Does modified amino acid total parenteral nutrition alter immune-response in high level surgical stress. JPEN 1983;7:521.

276. Bower RH, Cerra FB, Bershadsky B, et al. Early enteral administration of a formula (Impact®) supplemented with arginine, nucleotides, and fish oil in intensive care unit patients: results of a multicenter, prospective, randomized, clinical trial. Crit Care Med 1995;23:436.

277. Hesselvic JF. Plasma fibronectin levels in sepsis: influencing factors. Crit Care Med 1987;15:1092.

278. Ziegler EJ, McCutchan JA, Douglas H, et al. Prevention of lethal Pseudomonas bacteremia with epimerase-deficient mutant. J Immunol 1973;111:433.

279. Ziegler EJ, McCutchan JA, Fierer J, et al. Treatment of gram-negative bacteremia and shock with human antiserum to a mutant Escherichia coli. N Engl J Med 1982;307:1225.

280. Baumgartner JD, Glauster MP, McCutchan JA, et al. Prevention of gram-negative shock and death in surgical patients by antibody to endotoxin core glycolipid. Lancet 1985;2:59.

281. Ziegler EJ, Fisher CJ, Spring CL, et al. Treatment of gram-negative bacteremia and septic shock with HA-1A human monoclonal antibody against endotoxin. N Engl J Med 1991;324:429.

282. The National Committee for the Evaluation of Centoxin. The French national registry of HA-1A (Centoxin) in septic shock. Arch Intern Med 1994;154:2484.

283. Beutler B, Milsark IW, Cerami AC. Passive immunization against cachectin/tumor necrosis factor protects mice from lethal effect of endotoxin. Science 1985;229:869.

284. Schade UF. Pentoxifyllin increases survival in murine endotoxin shock and decreases formation of tumor necrosis factor. Circ Shock 1990;31:171.

285. Fletcher JR, DiSimone AG, Earnest MA. Platelet activating factor receptor antagonist improves survival and attenuates eicosanoid release in severe endotoxemia. Ann Surg 1990;211:312.

286. Hinshaw L, Peduzzi P, Young E, et al. Effect of high-dose glucocorticoid therapy on mortality in patients with clinical sign of systemic sepsis. N Engl J Med 1987;317:659.

287. Hauser CJ, Shoemaker WC, Turpin I, et al. Oxygen transport responses to colloids and crystalloids in critically ill surgical patients. Surg Gynecol Obstet 1980;150:811.

288. Poole GV, Meredity JW, Pernell T, et al. Comparison of colloids and crystalloids in resuscitation from hemorrhagic shock. Surg Gynecol Obstet 1982;15:577.

289. Kovalik SG, Ledgerwood AM, Lucas CE. The cardiac effect of altered calcium hemostasis after albumin resuscitation. J Trauma 1981;21:275.

290. Johnson D, Lucas CE, Gerrick SJ. Altered coagulation after albumin supplements for treatment of oligemic shock. Ann Surg 1979;114:379.

291. Haupt MT, Gilbert EM, Carlson RW. Fluid loading increases oxygen consumption in septic patients with lactic acidosis. Am Rev Respir Med 1985;131:912.

292. Kruse JA, Haupt MT, Puri VK, Carlson RW. Lactate levels as predictors of the relationship between oxygen delivery and consumption in ARDS. Chest 1990;98:959.

293. Rutherford EJ, Morris JA, Reed GW, et al. Base deficit stratifies mortality and determines therapy. J Trauma 1992;33:417.

294. Hayes MA, Yau EHS, Timmins AC, et al. Response of critically ill patients to treatment aimed at achieving supranormal oxygen delivery and consumption. Chest 1993;103:886.

Chapter **40** Posttraumatic Pulmonary Insufficiency

ROBERT F. WILSON, M.D.

"And the Lord God formed man of the dust of the ground and breathed into his nostrils the breath of life." —Genesis 2:7

INTRODUCTION

Pulmonary Insufficiency

"Pulmonary insufficiency" has been defined as a clinical state in which the gas exchange in the lungs is inadequate to maintain body function without mechanical support.[1,2,3] This term also refers to pathophysiologic changes that cause a patient to have $PO_2 < 60$ mm Hg on room air and/or a PCO_2 of ≥ 46 mm Hg with a normal or low pH.[4]

Spectrum of Acute Lung Injury

Critically ill patients commonly manifest diffuse cellular malfunction of lung parenchyma as a result of severe systemic insults, such as sepsis,[5] hypoperfusion,[6] or multiple trauma[7] (Table 40–1). This pathologic condition, which has become known as adult respiratory distress syndrome (ARDS),[8] is now recognized to be part of a pathologic spectrum known as acute lung injury (ALI).[9] It has been suggested that the term "acute" replace "adult" in the ARDS acronym[10] to more appropriately reflect the severe manifestations of ALI. Although evidence exists that appropriate application of conventional ventilator management techniques improves survival in patients with mild-to-moderate ARDS,[11-13] these techniques have not changed outcome in patients with severe ARDS.[10,11,14,15]

Prevailing knowledge of ALI supports the concept of a spectrum of disease processes.[9,10] Mild ALI, often referred to as noncardiogenic pulmonary edema, is characterized by vascular endothelial cell damage.[15] The increased capillary permeability results in movement of water into the interstitium which, in turn, causes diminished lung volume and decreased compliance.

Moderate ALI, often referred to as early ARDS, is characterized by a significant decrease in lung compliance due to increasing interstitial edema, sloughing of type 1 alveolar epithelial cells, insufficient or abnormal production of surfactant, and increasing alveolar fluid.[16] Because the interstitial and alveolar edema of ARDS tends to accumulate in gravity-dependent areas, the alveoli in those areas tend to collapse fairly readily.[17] These atelectatic alveoli, however, are potentially recruitable with appropriate CPAP/PEEP therapy.[15]

Severe ALI, often referred to as late ARDS, involves an extensive atelectasis and consolidation at least partially attributable to dysfunctional type 2 epithelial cells.[17] The consolidated lung is not recruitable and results in a significantly diminished number of alveoli that can be ventilated. This has been described as "baby lung syndrome" because the adult patient has no more lung tissue available for ventilation than a small baby.[17] Metabolic endothelial dysfunction also tends to occur in late ALI and this may partially account for its association with multiple organ failure (MOF).[18]

ARDS

Between 150,000 and 200,000 cases of ARDS occur in the United States each year.[1] The mortality rate of approximately 40-50%, however, has not changed in most centers during the last 20 years despite other advances in medical care.[19,20]

AXIOM ARDS, which develops in some patients after severe trauma and in many with severe sepsis, is a nonspecific response of the lungs to a wide variety of insults.

ARDS is a clinical syndrome of diverse etiology characterized by diffuse lung injury and dysfunction.[1] Although published incidence rates and mortality figures show a great deal of variation, a consistent finding in most studies is the higher incidence of ARDS in patients with multiple risk factors.[21,22] In addition, a definite relationship exists between the severity of injury or sepsis and the likelihood of the subsequent development of ARDS.[22]

Posttraumatic Pulmonary Insufficiency

As the management of severe trauma has improved, increasing numbers of patients have survived the initial period of shock only to die later with severe, progressive MOF which usually begins as pulmonary insufficiency.[4,23] In an analysis of 3289 trauma patients, Hoyt et al. found that 368 (11.2%) developed pulmonary complications.[24] The most frequent pulmonary complications and their incidence were pneumonia (7.5%), atelectasis (3.4%), respiratory failure/distress (1.6%), aspiration (1.5%), ARDS (1.2%), and pulmonary embolus (0.7%). The most important predictors of pulmonary complications included: ISS ≥ 16, blunt trauma, shock on admission, trauma score < 13, chest surgery, pedestrian-MVA, head injury (AIS ≥ 3), and age > 55 years.

HISTORICAL PERSPECTIVE

In 1936, Moon observed pulmonary edema in patients dying late after shock and ascribed it to direct injury to pulmonary capillary endothelium with resultant plasma extravasation.[25] In 1945, Burford and Burbank used the term "traumatic wet lung" to describe the vicious cycle of increased pulmonary exudation, secretions, and atelectasis seen in many of their patients with chest trauma or with isolated abdominal or head injuries.[26]

In 1950, Mallory described similar pathologic changes in the lungs in late deaths following trauma.[27] In 1950, Jenkins et al., on the basis of their study of eight such patients, believed that many of the changes were due to excessive administration of intravenous fluids.[28] The term, "congestive atelectasis" was used to distinguish these lung changes from "obstructive atelectasis."[2] In 1963, Burke referred to the reduced oxygen extraction in spite of an increased minute ventilation and increased work of breathing in patients with trauma and peritonitis as characteristic of "high-output respiratory failure."[29]

These characteristic pulmonary changes are associated with a large number of clinical problems and have been referred to by a wide variety of names (Table 40–2).[30] In 1967, Ashbaugh et al. coined the term, "adult respiratory distress syndrome" for these changes because of their similarity to those seen in the infant respiratory distress syndrome (IRDS).[31] One major difference between these two entities, however, is that in IRDS primary surfactant deficiency exists,[32] whereas in the adult syndrome, the surfactant deficiency is a secondary phenomenon.[33]

TABLE 40–1   Interpretation of PaO₂/FiO₂ Ratio

PaO_2	FiO_2	Ratio	Q_s/Q_t (%)	Abnormality
240	0.4	600	5	None
120	0.4	300	10	Minimal
100	0.4	250	15	Mild
80	0.4	200	20	Moderate
60	0.4	150	30	Severe
40	0.4	100	40	Very severe

AXIOM   Although it develops in relatively few trauma patients, severe pulmonary dysfunction continues to have a high mortality rate.

Of 6196 trauma patients admitted to San Francisco General Hospital over a 4-year period, Lewis et al. found that only 390 (6.3%) required intubation and mechanical ventilatory support.[34] The mortality in this group, however, was 38% (148 of 390), versus 3.1% (180 of 5806) in the other patients.

CLINICAL ETIOLOGIC FACTORS

Shock

Inadequate blood flow to the lungs can cause a decrease in mucociliary clearance and surfactant production.[35,36] Surfactant, a phospholipid produced in the lungs by type II alveolar cells, lowers surface tension in alveoli and thereby helps to prevent atelectasis.[36] Henry found that lung tissue from animals in shock had decreased oxygen uptake and reduced capacity to convert inorganic 32P to phosphoprotein.[35] Surfactant activity may also be reduced by various proteins and fluid leaking into the alveoli through damaged or abnormal alveolar lining cells.

AXIOM   Hemorrhagic hypotension by itself seldom produces ARDS; significant tissue damage or inflammation must usually also be present.

Fluid Overload

Any increase in pulmonary capillary pressure can greatly increase the rate at which fluid leaves "leaky" pulmonary capillaries and enters the pulmonary interstitial spaces. Most patients who die following severe, prolonged shock or sepsis have extremely heavy, wet lungs at autopsy. This is often believed to be evidence that the physician overloaded the patient with fluid; however, the lungs in these patients can become loaded with fluid even when cardiac filling pressures are kept low.[37]

Although examination of intake and output records of these patients often reveals that a great deal of fluid has been given to pa-

TABLE 40–2   Hemoglobin Levels, Oxygen Consumption, and Mortality Rates

No. of Patients	Hemoglobin (gm/dl)	VO_2 (ml/min/m²)	Mortality Rate (%)
13	> 15	186	23
31	12.5-15.0	138	42
80	10.0-12.4	114	64
58	7.5-9.9	99	72
18	< 7.5	97	72

tients with ARDS, unpublished studies on isolated, perfused dog lung showed that lungs quickly developed congestive atelectasis and pulmonary edema after exposure to E. coli endotoxin, even if mean pulmonary venous pressure were kept at zero. However, if pulmonary venous pressure was allowed to increase, the rate of development of pulmonary edema was greatly accelerated.

AXIOM   Giving excess fluid to a patient developing ARDS greatly accelerates the pulmonary dysfunction.

Massive Blood Transfusions

Patients who receive massive blood transfusions (> 10 units in 24 hours) have an increased risk of death, infections, and pulmonary complications.[38,39] ARDS following multiple blood transfusions has been believed to be due to microemboli of clumps of various cells and particulate matter. Micropore filtration of blood, however, failed to reduce the incidence of these problems.[40] Another possibility is capillary flow reduction because of increased blood viscosity as well as tissue hypoxia from the low P_{50} of the transfused red blood cells.[37,41] Passive transfer of immune factors may also play a role.[42]

AXIOM   Patients who receive massive blood transfusions have an increased chance of developing ARDS, primarily because of the increased risk of becoming septic.

Although massive blood transfusions can cause transient abnormalities of pulmonary function, the evidence that it leads to ARDS is controversial.[41] In one study, patients without other predisposing factors did not have an increased incidence of ARDS unless > 22 units of blood were given within a 12-hour period.[20]

Pulmonary Contusion

Pulmonary contusion is usually diagnosed on the basis of infiltrates seen on radiography within six hours of chest trauma. The contusions generally worsen for the next 24-48 hours and then begin to clear, but the changes in the lung that are seen during thoracotomy at that time are usually much more extensive than is suggested by chest radiography.[43] In patients with flail chest injuries, the hypoxemia is believed to be due to the underlying pulmonary contusion. Furthermore, severe contusions seem to increase the likelihood of patients with a flail chest developing pneumonia and requiring prolonged ventilatory support.[43]

Fat Emboli

AXIOM   One should assume that all patients with long bone fractures will have some degree of fat embolism, which is most easily quantified by the decrease in platelet count and the increased alveolar-arterial oxygen difference.

"Fat embolism" is the name given to a clinical syndrome characterized by cerebral and respiratory dysfunction following long bone fractures. A relatively asymptomatic interval of 12-48 hours occurs after injury, following which the patient begins to demonstrate increasing tachypnea, restlessness, and confusion.[44] If this progresses to the full-blown syndrome of severe hypoxemia and coma, the mortality rate may exceed 10-20%.

Fat emboli come primarily from the marrow of fractured bones[45] but some fat emboli may also develop in blood because of increased lipolysis.[46,47] Platelets adhere to these particles so that, characteristically, the platelet count decreases and petechiae may appear transiently on the chest and conjunctivae or in the axillas. An increase in the $P(A-a)O_2$ and a decrease in the platelet count occur in virtually all patients with major fractures.[48-50]

AXIOM Relatively mild nonthoracic trauma may cause significant blood gas and platelet abnormalities, and these changes may be due to subclinical fat emboli.

One of the major reasons for early operative fixation of fractures is to reduce the incidence and severity of fat emboli.[51] Continued motion at fracture sites can increase the incidence and severity of pulmonary failure following trauma. In addition, early fixation of lower-extremity fractures allows patients to be mobilized out of bed sooner, thereby reducing the incidence of pneumonia and DVT.

Central Nervous System Injuries

Patients with central nervous system (CNS) injuries have a greatly increased risk of developing pulmonary complications because of aspiration, atelectasis, and prolonged ventilatory support. In addition, neurogenic pulmonary edema may be a factor.

Neurogenic pulmonary edema is a poorly defined syndrome which is seen most frequently in patients who die soon after massive head or spinal cord injury.[52] Increased pulmonary venous tone resulting from massive sympathetic discharge raises pulmonary capillary hydrostatic pressure and may dilate intercellular clefts, causing noncardiogenic pulmonary edema.[53,54] Transient cardiac depression may also be present.

Pneumonitis

AXIOM Making an accurate diagnosis of pneumonia in ICU patients can be extremely difficult; however, any trauma patient on a ventilator for > 7-14 days probably has some pneumonitis and/or atelectasis.

It can be extremely difficult to make an accurate diagnosis of pneumonia in the presence of ARDS.[55] The major distinguishing features of pneumonia are said to be fever (≥ 101°F), leukocytosis (> 12,000/mm^3), new pulmonary infiltrate, and sputum with increased numbers of PMNs and bacteria on Gram stain and culture. To confirm which organisms are responsible for pneumonia, organisms should be shown on blood culture, in a pleural effusion, or from a protected brush (bronchoscopic) or bronchoalveolar lavage (BAL) specimens. Infection of the lung directly causing ARDS is believed to be unusual, but the incidence of pulmonary sepsis does tend to increase after ARDS has become established.[55]

Pneumonia following surgery or accidental trauma can be thought of as having three main causes: (a) atelectasis, (b) prolonged ventilatory support, and/or (c) aspiration of gastric or oral contents.

PNEUMONIA DUE TO ATELECTASIS

AXIOM Atelectasis is the most common complication of trauma to the chest or abdomen.

Abdominal or chest-wall pain, which prevents the patient from taking deep breaths or coughing properly, can greatly impair the patient's ability to clear secretions from the tracheobronchial tree. Excessive sedation or injuries which keep the patient in bed also increase the tendency for atelectasis. Occasionally, blood gas changes of postoperative or posttraumatic atelectasis can be confused with ARDS; however, ARDS does not usually cause significant hypoxemia during the first 24-48 hours.

VENTILATOR-INDUCED PNEUMONIA

Prolonged (> 5-10 days) ventilatory support is associated with an increased tendency to develop pneumonia. In patients with chest trauma, the incidence of pneumonia after one week of mechanical ventilation is at least 30-40%, and after three weeks of ventilatory

support, most patients will have developed pneumonia.[1] In one flail chest study, ventilatory support for more than seven days resulted in a 100% incidence of pneumonia.[43]

ASPIRATION PNEUMONITIS

Aspiration of gastric contents is particularly apt to occur in individuals with head trauma or drug or alcohol intoxication, and aspiration of food and/or acid can cause severe damage to the lungs.[3,20,21] Aspiration is most apt to occur either at trauma or during the induction of or emergence from anesthesia. It is good practice, therefore, to insert a nasogastric tube when a patient with severe trauma is first seen to remove as much gas or fluid from the stomach as possible.

PITFALL ⊘

Failure to carefully monitor nasogastric tube suction of the stomach increases the risk of aspiration of gastric contents into the lung.

If aspiration of gastric contents occurs, food particles and any remaining acid or bile should be removed promptly with a bronchoscope. Oral contents in patients with severe gum or dental disease may have bacterial counts exceeding 10^{10}-10^{12} organisms/mL and aspiration of these combined aerobes and anaerobes into the lungs can rapidly cause severe necrotizing pneumonia.

The anatomical portions of the lung involved can be helpful in diagnosing aspiration. For example, aspiration of gastric or oral contents into the lung while the patient is supine tends to involve the superior segments of the lower lobes and/or the posterior segments of the upper lobes.

AXIOM Severe acidity is not needed in aspirated material to cause severe lung injury.

Although acid can be extremely damaging to the lungs, gastric aspirates with a pH > 2.5 are also capable of causing ARDS,[56] especially when large volumes of fluid and particulate matter are aspirated.

Sepsis

AXIOM The best known major predisposing factor for ARDS is sepsis.[19,21,57]

In one study, 18% of all patients admitted to the hospital with positive blood cultures developed ARDS.[58] In another study, 23% of patients with gram-negative sepsis developed ARDS, and the combination resulted in a 90% mortality.[59]

The clinical picture of sepsis without positive blood cultures is more likely to occur in trauma patients than in any other group, possibly because of prophylactic antibiotic coverage.[60] Sepsis can also be caused by necrotic or inflamed tissue or by endotoxemia rather than by viable bacteria in the bloodstream.[61]

Pulmonary Embolism

INCIDENCE

Pulmonary embolism (PE) is a relatively frequent complication of severe trauma. Coon found a 14.3% incidence of PE during autopsies of 224 patients who died after accidental trauma.[62] In another series, approximately 5% of trauma deaths that occurred > 1 week after blunt trauma were caused by PE.[63]

SOURCE

In at least 85-90% of patients who develop PE, the sources of the emboli are the deep veins of the pelvis and thighs, particularly the femoral and iliac veins. In the remainder, the right heart and upper limb veins are the sources.[64]

AXIOM About 10-20% of calf vein thrombi propagate into iliofemoral veins and 10-20% of these cause pulmonary emboli with an overall mortality rate of approximately 10-20%.

PATHOPHYSIOLOGIC CHANGES

The ventilation-perfusion (V/Q) mismatch seen with pulmonary emboli is the main cause of hypoxemia.[65] Decreased mixed venous oxygen saturation, such as may occur with low-cardiac output, makes arterial hypoxemia even worse, particularly when the shunt (Q_{sp}/Q_t) is > 20%.

DIAGNOSIS

The majority (70-80%) of patients with documented PE do not have clinical evidence of lower extremity DVT. Arterial hypoxemia occurs in 80-90% of patients.[66] However, even when PaO_2 is normal because of hyperventilation, the alveolar-arterial oxygen gradient is generally increased.

AXIOM Many more pulmonary emboli occur than are suspected or proven antemortem.

The common clinical symptoms and signs of PE, which include dyspnea, tachypnea, tachycardia, and chest pain, are nonspecific. The sudden appearance of hypotension plus hypoxemia, however, is strongly suggestive of PE.[65]

With a pulmonary embolus, the $PaCO_2$ is usually decreased because of hyperventilation, even though a widened arterial-end tidal Pco_2 gradient is often present because of increased dead-space ventilation.[67] Normally, the $P(A-a)co_2$ is only 2-3 mm Hg, but a PE, by increasing pulmonary dead space, can increase this markedly.

AXIOM Any sudden decrease in the $PETCO_2$ or increase in the $P(a-ET)co_2$ difference should make one suspect a pulmonary embolus.

Perfusion lung scanning with technetium-labeled albumin microspheres is a sensitive test, and a normal result is deemed by many to virtually exclude PE.[68] Chronic obstructive pulmonary disease and pneumonia, however, can also cause perfusion defects.

AXIOM A normal lung scan is accurate for ruling out a significant pulmonary embolus.

The accuracy of a perfusion scan of the lung is greatly enhanced when a simultaneous ventilation scan using ^{133}Xenon is also performed and the resultant V/Q scan shows perfusion defects involving two or more areas as big as segments with normal ventilation. Such a finding is considered a high-probability scan and in a high-risk individual allows a PE to be diagnosed with 85-90% accuracy.[69] Nevertheless, some patients with PE may have low-probability scans with matching defects (i.e., defects on both the ventilation and perfusion scans). When a strong clinical suspicion of PE exists, but the lung scan is not helpful, pulmonary angiography should be obtained.

AXIOM Pulmonary arteriography is the gold standard for diagnosing pulmonary emboli.

Smoke Inhalation

Clinical manifestations of chemical tracheobronchitis and pneumonitis of an inhalation injury during the first 36 hours may include: bronchospasm, tracheobronchitis, atelectasis, coughing episodes, and upper airway edema.[1] The clinical manifestations in the second stage of inhalation injury are due to pulmonary edema, which usually occurs to some degree two to six days after injury.[2,70] During the next

one to two weeks, the patient may expectorate mucus casts formed in the tracheobronchial tree and develop bronchopneumonia.[1]

Ventilator-induced Lung Injury (Volutrauma)

As gas volume increases toward the alveolar limit of distensibility, the elastic forces diminish and the contiguous epithelial, interstitial, and endothelial structures are subject to mechanical distortions that may cause lung injury.[17,71] Ventilator-induced lung injury can be produced in mice with normal lungs if they are persistently ventilated at tidal volumes that cause alveolar pressures > 35 cm H_2O.[72] However, if the same high-inflation pressures are applied to alveoli which cannot be overdistended because of an artificial restriction to chest-wall expansion, lung injury usually does not occur.[73] Furthermore, in animal models of moderate ALI, tidal volumes that can cause lung injury no longer do so when lung compliance is improved by appropriate levels of CPAP/PEEP.[74] Such data suggest that alveolar hyperdistention, rather than high-alveolar pressure, is the cause of ventilator-induced lung injury;[10,71] hence, the term, volutrauma, rather than barotrauma, is increasingly used to describe ventilator-induced lung injury.[15]

AXIOM Ventilator-induced lung injury appears to be due to overdistension of alveoli (i.e., volutrauma) rather than just exposure of the alveoli to high pressures (i.e., barotrauma).

PATHOPHYSIOLOGY

Pathologic Stages

ARDS usually follows a rather predictable course characterized by overlapping phases which include: an acute or exudative phase (0-6 days), a proliferative phase (4-10 days), and a chronic or fibrotic phase (after 8-14 days)[76] (Fig. 40–1).

EXUDATIVE PHASE

The initial or "exudative" phase (0-4 days) is characterized by altered pulmonary capillary endothelial integrity and increased numbers of inflammatory cells in the interstitium.[2] Once it enters the interstitial space, fluid tends to move centrally along the peribronchial and perivascular spaces. Because interstitial pressure in peribronchial tissue is negative relative to that in the alveolar interstitial spaces, it can drain fluid from the alveolar interstitium readily, at least initially.[77] As a result of the large amount of interstitial fluid that can be taken up without affecting the alveoli, total lung water may increase by 70-100% before changes in arterial blood gases are detectable.

Any increase in central venous pressure, as in right heart failure, tends to decrease pulmonary lymphatic flow and increase edema formation. In addition, an increase in the size of the effective filtration surface of pulmonary capillaries due to increased cardiac filling increases the movement of fluid from capillaries into the interstitium.[78]

Several studies have shown that in ARDS, in contrast to cardiogenic pulmonary edema, no correlation exists between the amount of lung water and the degree of hypoxia or shunt.[78,79] In ARDS, however, there is also evidence of a significant release of humoral mediators.

AXIOM Once alveolar flooding begins, lung mechanics can change abruptly.

Edema fluid in alveoli in ARDS is generally rich in protein, inflammatory cells, and mediators of lung injury, and increased alveolar fluid tends to decrease the quantity and effectiveness of surfactant in the alveoli.[80] The chemical composition of surfactant in ARDS patients is abnormal and has been found to have a reduced ability to reduce surface tension.[81]

As ARDS continues, a wide range of inflammatory cells, including lymphocytes and other mononuclear cells, move into the intersti-

FIGURE 40–1 A schematic representation of the time course of the evolution of ARDS. During the early or exudative phase, the lesion is characterized by a pulmonary capillary leak with edema. Within a few days, a proliferative phase may appear, with marked interstitial inflammation, followed by increasing fibrosis. (From: Hall JB, Schmidt GA, Wood LDH, eds. Principles of critical care. New York: McGraw-Hill, Inc., 1992; 1638)

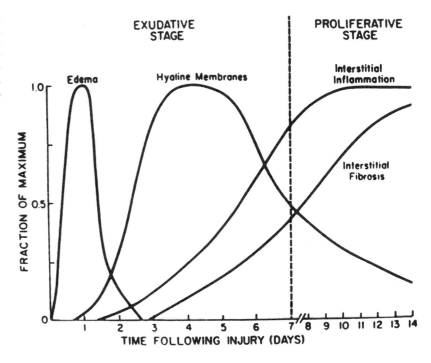

tium and alveoli. Early destruction of type I alveolar cells occurs, leaving a denuded basement membrane. Eosinophilic hyaline membranes consisting of proteinaceous fluid, cellular fragments, fibrin strands, and remnants of surfactant also increase in the alveoli along their walls, especially along the alveolar ducts.[82]

The original concept that ARDS was a homogeneous pathologic process has been refuted by CT studies showing a heterogeneous, but essentially gravitational distribution of pathologic changes.[18,83] The heterogeneous distribution of the pathologic changes is supported by multiple inert gas studies showing a mixture of high, low, and normal ventilation-to-perfusion matching.[15]

PROLIFERATIVE PHASE

The proliferative stage of ARDS typically occurs after four to ten days and is characterized by increasing fibrosis and alveolitis.[2] Capillary endothelial cells begin to show more damage and focal swelling. The inflammatory cells that infiltrate the lung tissue during this stage are primarily mononuclear cells, especially lymphocytes, macrophages, and plasma cells. These cells are accompanied by proliferating fibroblasts and increasing deposition of collagen around the air spaces. The interstitium remains edematous, and there is proliferation of the cuboidal type II pneumocytes to line the alveoli.[1]

CHRONIC PHASE

In the final or chronic stage of ARDS (11-20 days) there is evidence of increasing lung tissue destruction and emphysema, with progressive fibrosis of the interstitium and intraalveolar spaces. In some areas of the lung, complete obliteration of the alveolar structures may occur.[1,2]

Pulmonary Vasculature

AXIOM The pulmonary vasculature in ARDS is characterized by increasing capillary permeability and vasoconstriction.

Full-blown ARDS typically is associated with moderate-to-severe pulmonary hypertension due initially to humoral mediators, such as thromboxane A_2, leukotrienes, and serotonin. Perivascular "cuffing" by edema fluid in the interstitium can also reduce vascular compliance and increase right ventricular afterload, thereby reducing cardiac output and the delivery of oxygen to peripheral tissues.[84] Ob-

struction of the pulmonary microvasculature with particulate microemboli, such as neutrophils or platelets, probably also plays a later role.

As ARDS progresses, much of the pulmonary vascular bed may be disrupted or obliterated, and the remaining patent vessels respond to increased blood flow with initial dilation and then reactive edema. Later in the process, extension of vascular smooth muscle may occur into the smaller, normally nonmuscular pulmonary arterioles.[85] This remodeling appears to be essential to the development of persistent pulmonary hypertension. Hypoxia and vascular thrombosis probably also contribute to this effect.

As pulmonary hypertension progresses, loss of the hypoxic vasoconstriction response occurs. This loss of normal pulmonary autoregulation results in increased shunting of blood through atelectatic areas of the lung.

AXIOM Loss of pulmonary autoregulation contributes to the hypoxemia of late ARDS.

Etiologic Factors

Some of the earliest observations regarding posttraumatic pulmonary insufficiency concluded that, because interstitial and alveolar edema can develop without elevated pulmonary capillary pressures, pulmonary capillary permeability must be increased.[86] Using the Staub pulmonary lymph fistula studies in sheep, it was found that infusion of many substances, including endotoxin, histamine, fibrin degradation products, thrombin, and microemboli can cause alterations in microvascular permeability similar to those seen in ARDS.[87]

Mediators of Acute Lung Injury

Many inflammatory mediators have been implicated in the pathogenesis of acute lung injury (Table 40–3).[1-3] It seems clear that when the areas of trauma or infection are remote from lung, various inflammatory mediators causing pulmonary dysfunction are released from injured tissue into venous blood which then perfuses the lungs. Resident macrophages in pulmonary capillaries and alveolae can also elaborate potent monokines that can further increase acute lung injury.[1,2]

TABLE 40–3 *Clinical Conditions Associated with Various Mixed Venous Oxygen Saturations*

S_vO_2	Cardiac Output $(L/min/m^2)$	Situations to Consider
80% or more	> 4.0 +	Sepsis, cirrhosis, L to R shunts; wedge PA catheter
70-75%	3.0-3.5	Normal
50-65%	2.5-3.0	Slight cardiac decompensation or increased VO_2
50-60%	2.0-2.5	Moderate cardiac decompensation; lactic acidosis
32-50%	1.5-2.0	Increasing shock, coma

From: Wilson RF: Critical care system and monitoring. In Moore EE, Mattox KL, Feliciano DV, eds. Trauma (2nd ed). Norwalk, Appleton & Lange 1991, p 867.

VASOACTIVE SUBSTANCES

A number of vasoactive substances, including catecholamines, serotonin, histamine, and polypeptides is released during shock, sepsis, and trauma. Sukhnandan and Thal showed that these agents may have profound effects on pulmonary perfusion in experimental animals.[88] Our later unpublished studies on isolated perfused dog lungs demonstrated that these substances greatly accelerated the development of congestive atelectasis and pulmonary edema.

LEUKOCYTE ACTIVATION

Sections from the lungs of patients dying with "shock lung" typically show large numbers of PMNs in pulmonary capillaries and in the pulmonary interstitium.[89] Most experimental evidence suggests that the lung injury of ARDS is caused by activation of these leukocytes and their subsequent release of toxic products. In addition to the role of complement, especially C_{5a}, causing PMNs to stick to pulmonary capillary endothelium, alveolar macrophages can also release chemotaxins that cause increased numbers of neutrophils to adhere to pulmonary capillary endothelium.[1]

AXIOM Neutrophils can cause or contribute to the development of pulmonary edema by increasing pulmonary capillary permeability.

In a recent study, Law et al. showed that serum levels of endothelial intracellular adhesion molecules for neutrophils (ICAM-1) for 13 trauma patients at end-resuscitation correlated well (r = 0.95) (P < 0.05) with their MOF scores.[90] They also showed that six pa-

tients who developed MOF had a mean ICAM-1 level that was significantly higher than that found in those who did not develop MOF.

The mechanism of leukocyte activation in ARDS seems to involve stimulation of a ligand-receptor complex which enhances the activity of membrane-bound guanine nucleotide regulatory protein (GNRP). This, in turn, increases phospholipase C (PLC) activity and can result in production of three types of substances that may injure the lung: (a) toxic free radicals, (b) neutral proteases, especially elastase, and (c) arachidonic acid metabolites.[91]

Toxic Oxygen Metabolites

AXIOM Toxic oxygen radicals released from neutrophils attached to pulmonary capillary endothelium are probably the most important cause of the early changes in ARDS.

Reperfusion of ischemic tissue can result in formation of a variety of toxic oxygen species (Fig. 40–2). Activated PMNs can also release highly reactive free-radical species, including superoxide anion (O_2^-), hydrogen peroxide (H_2O_2), hydroxyl radicals (HO·), and peroxide radicals (ROO·).[91] Because they have an unpaired electron in their outer orbits, free radicals are unstable. They can give up the electron and act as a reducing agent, or they can accept another electron and act as an oxidizing agent.[1] Superoxide anion (O_2^-) is moderately unstable and, with the addition of an electron and two H^+ ions, it can be converted to H_2O_2, which is freely diffusible across capillary and cell membranes (Fig. 40–3). In the presence of Fe^{2+}, superoxide anions produce the extremely unstable HO· radical, which can induce damage only when it is close to its target. H_2O_2, in the presence of Cl^- ion and the lysosomal enzyme myeloperoxidase, may be converted to hypochlorous acid (HOCl), another powerful oxidant, which is important for killing bacteria in phagolysosomes.[91]

Large amounts of superoxide anions are generated during the respiratory burst that accompanies phagocytosis.[91] Normally, these reactive oxygen intermediaries cause little problem because they are neutralized rapidly by endogenous defense systems that protect the integrity of cells and tissues.[92] Endogenous free-radical scavengers include superoxide dismutase, (for oxygen free radicals), catalases (to convert hydrogen peroxide to H_2O and O_2), glutathione peroxidase and glutathione reductase, which alter cellular susceptibility to oxidants, and a variety of other scavengers that can absorb free electrons. When free radicals are released in massive amounts, however, intracellular defenses may be overcome, and the toxic radicals may enter the extracellular space, where defenses are weaker, and cause extensive tissue damage.[93]

Oxygen radicals usually cause damage to biologic membranes by lipid peroxidation with resultant alteration of the physical properties

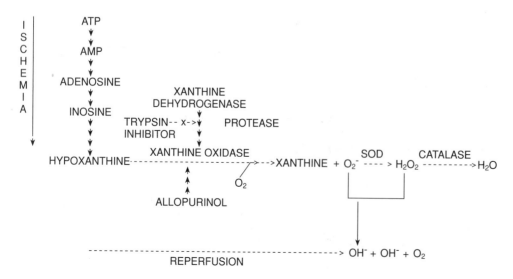

FIGURE 40–2 Mechanism of oxygen radical production during reperfusion of ischemic tissue. (ATP = adenosine triphosphate, AMP = adenosine monophosphate, SOD = superoxide dismutase, DMSO = dimethyl sulfoxide.) (From: RJ Korthius, DN Granger. Ischemia-reperfusion injury: role of oxygen-derived free radicals. Taylor AE, Matalon S, Ward P, eds. Physiology of oxygen radicals. Bethesda: American Physiological Society, 1986; 213.)

$$(1) \quad O_2 + A^{2+} - - - - - -> O_2^- + A^{3+}$$

$$(2) \quad O_2 + H_2A - - - - -> H_2O_2 + A$$

$$(3) \quad O_2 + H_2O_2 \xrightarrow{\quad Fe^{3+} \quad} OH\cdot + OH^- + O_2$$

FIGURE 40–3 Mechanisms for generating toxic oxygen species. (1) Superoxide anion (O_2^-) is generated by one-electron reduction of molecular oxygen (O_2) through a variety of electron donors (A^{2+}). (2) Hydrogen peroxide (H_2O_2) is generated by the two-electron reduction of molecular oxygen, usually via enzymatic catalysis. (3) The interaction of superoxide and hydrogen peroxide in the presence of metals can generate hydroxyl radical. (From: Fisher AB. Molecular mechanisms of oxygen toxicity. Appl Cardiopulmonary Pathophysiol 1989;3:121).

of membrane phospholipids.[94] As a consequence, important membrane-bound enzymes (such as Na-K ATPase, adenylate cyclase, and cytochrome oxidase) may be inactivated. Membrane fluidity is also decreased, thereby increasing entrapment of platelets and leukocytes on endothelial surfaces. Lipid peroxidation also increases the production of reactive fatty acid hydroperoxides that are also toxic to plasma membranes.

Hydrogen peroxide, in concentrations believed to be similar to those normally found around stimulated PMNs, is capable of causing lysis of a variety of cells.[2] Such cell lysis is accompanied by activation of (ADP-ribose) polymerase and depletion of intracellular nicotinamide adenine dinucleotide (NAD).[94] This polymerase is activated in the nucleus in response to DNA strand breaks and various chemical changes that include a reduction in available NAD, depletion of adenosine triphosphate, influx of intracellular Ca^{++}, and actin polymerization.[95]

Additional studies performed in vitro have demonstrated that reactive oxygen-derived metabolites can damage endothelial cells, lung parenchymal cells,[96] and fibroblasts.[97] Although they did not detect lysis of human endothelial cells exposed to stimulated PMNs, Harlan et al. were able to demonstrate endothelial cell detachment, probably due to PMN release of lysosomal neutral proteinases.[98]

AXIOM Early use of free-radical scavengers may be one of the best ways to reduce the pathophysiologic changes in ARDS.

In a recent study by Marzi et al., administration of recombinant human superoxide dismutase (rhSOD) after polytrauma caused attenuation of MOF, particularly in respect to cardiovascular and pulmonary function.[99] The authors also speculated that, because the rhSOD had been started relatively late (about the end of the first day after trauma), earlier administration of rhSOD (such as at the onset of resuscitation) may provide even better results.

Neutrophil Proteases

Acute inflammatory lung injury has been shown to be associated with the release of various proteases from granules in the lysosomes of neutrophils. These proteases (such as elastase, β-glucuronidase, cathepsin G, and collagenase) can destroy various components of the vascular basement membrane.[100] Some of these enzymes, particularly elastase, have been found in bronchoalveolar lavage fluid from patients with ARDS.[101] These proteases may not only directly destroy interstitial architecture, but may also amplify lung injury by activating other agents that can cause further leukocyte aggregation and tissue infiltration.[102]

AXIOM Proteases from neutrophils attached to pulmonary capillary endothelium may be a major cause of later pathophysiologic changes in ARDS.

In order for protease activities and tissue injury to occur, antiproteases, which are normally present, must be consumed or inactivated. Evidence for this was provided by Cochrane et al., who found oxidative inactivation of α1-proteinase inhibitor in patients with ARDS.[103] The reactions responsible for reducing the effectiveness of protease inhibitors may also be derived from toxic oxygen free-radical species, such as hydrogen peroxide.

Arachidonic Acid Metabolites

Arachidonate bound to phospholipids is a normal component of cell membranes. When any injury to the cell membrane occurs, such as by free radicals or lysosomal enzymes, an increase in intracellular calcium is manifest which activates phospholipase. This results in the release of free arachidonic acid from the cell membrane.[1] Once released, arachidonic acid can be metabolized by cyclooxygenase and lipooxygenase (Fig. 40–4).

CYCLOOXYGENASE DERIVATIVES. The cyclooxygenase pathway leads to the production of prostaglandins PGE_2, prostacyclin (PGI_2), $PGF_{2\alpha}$, and thromboxane (T_xA_2). PGI_2 is a vasodilator and inhibitor of platelet aggregation; however, PGF_2 and T_xA_2 (thromboxane) are vasoconstrictors and enhance platelet aggregation. In sheep challenged with endotoxin, thromboxane A_2 predominates in the early phase of lung injury and appears to be responsible for much of the associated pulmonary hypertension.[104]

PGI_2 is produced in the lung following endotoxin infusion, and metabolites of prostacyclin appear in the efferent lymph of mediastinal lymph nodes draining the lungs of animals infused with endotoxin.[105] Prostacyclin and other prostaglandins may also increase PMN influx into the lung.[106]

AXIOM The ratio of PGI_2 to T_xA_2 production determines the ultimate effects of cyclooxygenase metabolism on the lungs and other organs.

LIPOXYGENASE DERIVATIVES. The lipoxygenase pathway leads to production of several leukotrienes. In this pathway hydroperoxyeicosatetraenoic acid (HPETE) is rapidly converted to hydroxyeicosatetraenoic acid (HETE) and leukotriene A4 (LTA4). HETE is chemotactic,

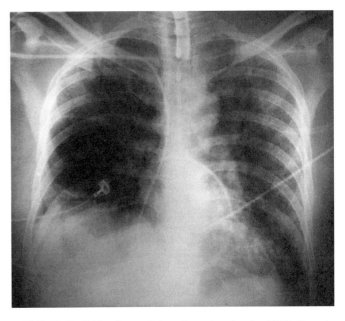

FIGURE 40–4 Fairly characteristic radiographs of early ARDS. In early ARDS, usually some reduction in lung volume occurs, accompanied by blurring of the bronchovascular margins and subtle perihilar ground-glass infiltrates.

and LTB4 aggregates white cells and stimulates them to release lysosomal products. The leukotrienes constrict smooth muscle, increase vascular permeability, and can contribute to the edema associated with lung injury.[107-111]

Studies in Neutropenic Patients

Recently, some doubt has been cast on the role of neutrophils in the development of ARDS, because it has been found in neutropenic patients.[112,113] Once the pulmonary endothelium has been damaged by neutrophil-independent mechanisms, however, the reappearance of circulating neutrophils in neutropenic patients coincides with worsening of the syndrome.[114,115]

AXIOM   ARDS can occur in animals and patients with neutropenia and complement deficiencies, but the presence of complement and activated PMNs can greatly accelerate and intensify the process.

Complement Activation

When complement-activated plasma is infused into rabbits, neutropenia and hypoxemia rapidly occur.[116] With sheep, complement activation causes similar results in addition to provoking an increase in pulmonary artery pressure and an increased flow of lung lymph.[117] Severe neutropenia has also been observed early in the course of ARDS, suggesting that complement products cause PMN sequestration in the lungs.[118]

C_{5a} des arginine, a low-molecular weight cleavage product of complement, appears to be particularly important for pulmonary vascular leukosequestration.[2] It can then initiate the respiratory burst in PMNs that results in production of superoxide anion and selective release of lysosomal contents.[119] Studies with primates have demonstrated that anti-$C5a_{des\ Arg}$ antibodies can reduce the hypoxia, extravascular lung water, pulmonary hypotension, and mortality rates following infusion of live E. coli.[115]

Many investigators now agree that, although elevated levels of $C5a_{des\ Arg}$ and $C3a_{des\ Arg}$ reflect the degree of complement activation, such alterations fail to consistently predict the presence or severity of acute lung injury.[21,110,120] Major lung inflammation seems to require additional stress, such as hypoxia or prostaglandin E_2 infusion. In addition, severe lung injury has been demonstrated in C_5-depleted animals, and leukocyte aggregation in the lungs can occur via other mechanisms.[1]

AXIOM   Although it may be necessary to start the processes that result in ARDS, complement activation does not appear to be a necessary condition in all patients.[121]

PLATELETS

A wide variety of physiologic process can cause extensive platelet aggregation and embolization to the lungs with resultant pulmonary changes.[122] When pulmonary reticuloendothelial and fibrinolytic activities are normal, large amounts of platelets, procoagulants, products of coagulation, and other substances may be cleared from the microcirculation with minimal morbidity. When reticuloendothelial function has been overwhelmed by intravascular coagulation or microvascular debris because of shock, sepsis, or trauma, the stage may be set for progressive pulmonary thromboembolic obstruction.[3]

PITFALL ⊘

> *Failure to use adequate in-line microfilters when giving massive blood transfusions may contribute to more rapid development of pulmonary insufficiency.*

The ability of endotoxin or thrombin to increase airway resistance, pulmonary vascular resistance, and microvascular permeability in thrombocytopenic sheep is not altered if platelet numbers are decreased.[123] Although platelet aggregation provoked by infusion of ADP can cause hypoxemia in sheep, pulmonary vascular resistance

is not increased.[124] In contrast, collagen infusion into cats can cause platelet aggregation, pulmonary vasoconstriction, and decreased lung compliance.[125]

AXIOM   Human lung tissue obtained from septic patients shows platelet sequestration, but it is not certain what role they play in the pathophysiology of lung injury.[126]

PLATELET-ACTIVATING FACTOR

AXIOM   PAF can cause many of the changes seen with ARDS, but its role in the process is unclear.

Platelet-activating factor (PAF) is a phospholipid mediator of inflammation that is produced by platelets, PMNs, monocytes, and alveolar macrophages.[2] It exerts at least some of its effects through stimulation of prostaglandin and leukotriene synthesis. It can cause protein-rich pulmonary edema, increased pulmonary vascular resistance, and decreased compliance when infused into experimental animals.[127] When it is infused into rabbits, PAF causes vesiculation of pulmonary endothelial cells.[128] Nevertheless, PAF has not been recovered from the lungs of injured animals, possibly because of its short half-life and the insensitivity of currently available assays.[2]

CYTOKINE AMPLIFICATION

AXIOM   Of the various cytokines released by inflammatory processes, tumor necrosis factor, interleukin-1, and interleukin-8 appear most likely to have a role in ARDS.

Tumor Necrosis Factor

Tumor necrosis factor (TNF) is produced by monocytes following various types of stimulation, including bacterial endotoxins.[2] When it is injected into experimental animals, TNF can produce acute injury in the lungs and other tissues similar to that produced by infusion of endotoxin.[129] Although endotoxin and TNF cause pulmonary margination of PMNs, TNF also directly increases pulmonary capillary permeability.[130] Antibodies against TNF can prevent shock and increase survival when animals are pretreated before exposure to endotoxin.[131]

Interleukin-1

Interleukin-1 (IL-1), which is derived from several different cells, including macrophages and endothelial cells, amplifies the inflammatory response to a wide variety of stimuli, including TNF.[2] The biological activities of IL-1 and TNF overlap considerably and include activation of acute-phase protein synthesis by the liver, activation of fibroblast collagen production, and augmentation of endothelial cell production of a leukocyte-adherence-promoting glycoprotein.[132]

Interleukin-8

Interleukin-8 (IL-8), which is a potent neutrophil chemoattractant, and which can induce neutrophil superoxide anion production, also appears to be important in the development of ARDS.[133] Kunkel et al. believed that alveolar macrophages generate TNF and IL-1, which are potent stimulants for the production of IL-8 by lung fibroblasts and by type II pneumocytes.[134] Rodriguez et al. found that 70% of 151 patients undergoing mechanical ventilation had bronchial secretions that tested positive for IL-8 within 36 hours of admission.[133] The presence of IL-8 in the lungs was significantly associated with multiple injuries, pulmonary dysfunction, and need for more prolonged ventilatory support.

PULMONARY CAPILLARY ENDOTHELIUM

The pulmonary capillary endothelial surface provides about one-fourth of the total capillary surface area of the body and accounts for 40% of the cells in the lungs.[2] Instead of displaying a fenestrated surface like other capillary endothelium, pulmonary capillaries have vesicles that are lined by enzymatic proteins, such as ATPase and 5-nucleotidase, which may be important for transport of certain plasma compounds into the interstitium.[135]

Tight gap junctions (0-5 nm) are normally found between pulmonary endothelial cells, and these restrict the passage of water-soluble macromolecules into the interstitial space.[136] When the lung is injured by endotoxin, the gap junctions become wider and allow increased extravasation of fluid and protein into the interstitium.[2]

LUNG METABOLISM

Pulmonary endothelial cells can alter the biological activity of a number of substances.[2] For example, pulmonary capillary endothelium has angiotensin-converting enzyme (ACE), which cleaves one amino acid from angiotensin I to produce angiotensin II, which is a potent vasoconstrictor. ACE is also important for the metabolism of bradykinin which is an extremely potent vasodilator and which greatly increases permeability of capillaries and their related venules. Serum ACE activity is markedly reduced in primates following induction of sepsis.[137] Pulmonary capillaries are also capable of inactivating other biologically active substances, such as serotonin, prostaglandins, and anaphylatoxins.[138]

> **AXIOM** Pneumonocytes and pulmonary capillary endothelial cells can produce and/or inactivate many substances involved in inflammatory changes in the body.

Lung cells can produce a large number of compounds, including histamine, complement, arachidonic acid metabolites, platelet-activating factor, fibronectin, and Factor VIII antigen.[2] Certain proteases released by alveolar macrophages are part of the protection against transbronchial influx of bacteria or foreign matter.

ALVEOLAR EPITHELIUM

In addition to its role in reducing the tendency for alveolae to collapse, surfactant has antibacterial properties, especially to several gram-positive species.[139] Type II cells also play a role in the clearance of fluid from the alveoli through an active Na transport mechanism.[140] When type II epithelial cells are injured, however, the biochemical components of surfactant are altered and are less effective.[81]

VASCULAR OCCLUSION

In addition to capillary endothelial lesions, ARDS is characterized by occlusion of capillaries and other small pulmonary vessels. The importance of vascular occlusion was first recognized by Blaisdell et al. in 1966[141] and has since been observed in pathologic specimens by numerous investigators.[2] PMNs, platelets, and fibrin may contribute to occlusion of pulmonary capillaries, via the action of inflammatory mediators that cause them to adhere to endothelium.

OTHER FACTORS

Other factors that may play a role in the development of ARDS include fibrin degradation products, and elevated levels of Factor VIII,[142] Factor XIII,[115] and fragment D.[143] Whether these are modulators or markers of an ongoing process remains unclear. In experimental ARDS, platelets may also have an important role.[144]

> **AXIOM** Excess activation of the coagulation and fibrinolytic cascades appears to contribute to the development of ARDS.

PATHOLOGY

The pathologic changes that occur in the lungs during the development of respiratory failure following trauma and/or sepsis tend to follow a sequence of: (a) adherence of PMNs to pulmonary capillaries, (b) disruption of pulmonary capillary endothelium, (c) interstitial edema, (d) congestive atelectasis, (e) alveolar edema, (f) hyaline membrane formation, and (g) varying amounts of pneumonitis.

> **AXIOM** By the time ARDS becomes apparent clinically, an advanced degree of congestive atelectasis is usually present.

PMN Adherence

Soon after shock or trauma, increasing numbers of PMNs begins to adhere to pulmonary capillaries.[145] On electron photomicrography, it can be seen that the limiting membrane of these PMNs becomes tightly opposed to the plasmalemma of the endothelium especially in capillaries and venules.

Pulmonary Capillary Damage

As the lysosomes in these attached PMNs break down, the powerful toxic radicals and hydrolytic enzymes that are released can cause severe damage to the capillary endothelium and adjacent tissue. Progressively enlarging spaces between endothelial cells develop and allow increasing quantities of fluid and protein, and eventually even red blood cells, to enter the interstitial spaces.[3]

Interstitial Edema

Increasing interstitial edema causes the lungs to stiffen, reduces alveolar space for gas exchange, and interferes with the movement of oxygen from alveoli into capillaries.[145] The development of this interstitial edema is accelerated if increased crystalloids are administered at this time.

> **AXIOM** Regardless of the cause of ARDS, anything that increases PAWP tends to accelerate the pathologic process.

Congestive Atelectasis

> **AXIOM** Pathologically, ARDS is characterized by congestive atelectasis, which is usually worse in the dependent portions of the lungs.

As the process continues, a progressive, congestive atelectasis develops, especially in dependent areas. It is this increasing, diffuse, congestive atelectasis that is so characteristic of posttraumatic pulmonary insufficiency.

Alveolar Edema

If the inciting process is not corrected, increasing quantities of fluid eventually move into the alveoli.[4] This alveolar fluid is relatively high in protein which, not only interferes with ventilation and gas exchange, but also inactivates surfactant.

Pneumonitis

Eventually most patients with persistent ARDS develop a superimposed pneumonitis.[3] This pneumonitis further compounds the pulmonary problem by increasing the amount of secretions and atelectasis. Sudden development of large areas of pneumonitis, particularly in dependent portions of the lung, may be due to aspiration of gastric or oral contents.

PATHOPHYSIOLOGIC CHANGES

The three main pathophysiologic changes seen with ARDS include: (a) gas exchange abnormalities, (b) pulmonary hypertension, and (c) decreased pulmonary compliance.[1,2]

TABLE 40–4 Weaning Criteria

Test	Minimal	Optimal
Q_s/Q_t	< 20%	< 10-15%
PaO_2/FiO_2	> 200	> 300
$P(A-a)O_2$ on FiO_2 1.0 (mm Hg)	< 350	< 250
PCO_2 with pH $\leq$ 7.40	< 45	35-40
V_d/V_t	< 0.6	< 0.45
Vital capacity	> 10 cc/kg	$\geq$ 15 cc/kg
Negative inspiratory force	−25 cm/H_2O	−30 cm H_2O
V_t (spontaneous)	$\geq$ 5 cc/kg	$\geq$ 6 cc/kg
Minimum ventilation (V_E)	< 12 L	< 10 L
Respiratory rate	< 30/min	< 20/min

From: Wilson RF: Critical care systems and monitoring. In Moore EE, Mattox KL, Feliciano DV, eds. Trauma (2nd ed). Norwalk, Appleton & Lange, 1991, p 862.

Gas Exchange Abnormalities

HYPOXEMIA

Etiology

AXIOM The most prominent laboratory abnormality in ARDS is hypoxemia which responds poorly to increases in FiO_2.

The unique structure of alveolar-capillary junctions provides a "thin-side" and "thick-side" at various points where they are in contact.[2] In areas with thin alveolar-capillary junctions, almost no interposed interstitial tissue exists and gas exchange is efficient. Because the thick side of the alveolar-capillary complex is the first area to widen with pulmonary edema or other infiltrative processes, oxygen exchange is relatively unaffected by pulmonary edema in its initial phases.[2]

AXIOM Ventilation-perfusion (V/Q) inequalities are believed to be the major cause of hypoxemia in ARDS.

V/Q abnormalities in ARDS are believed to be due principally to atelectasis and alveolar flooding.[146] This, in turn, results in shunting of venous blood through the lungs into the arterial circulation without being completely oxygenated. Once alveolar edema is apparent clinically, arterial hypoxemia tends to increase rapidly.[147]

The later stages of ARDS are characterized by progressive alveolar flooding, atelectasis, decreased functional residual capacity, and pulmonary hypertension.[148] At this point, greatly increased intrapulmonary shunting of blood and lack of response to increased oxygen are evident.[23,24]

Quantitation of Hypoxemia

The quantitation of hypoxemia in patients breathing oxygen-enriched gases is best done with the PaO_2/FiO_2 ratio or the amount of physiologic shunting in the lungs (Q_{sp}/Q_t).

AXIOM A PaO_2/FiO_2 ratio (PFR) falling below 200 or a physiologic shunt in the lungs (Q_{sp}/Q_t) exceeding 20% developing more than two to three days after trauma usually indicates ARDS.

PaO_2/FiO_2 RATIO. Because arterial oxygen tension (PaO_2) varies directly with the fraction of inspired oxygen (FiO_2), it is convenient to express oxygenation as the ratio of PaO_2 to FiO_2 (PaO_2/FiO_2 ratio). Normal values are about 600, which is equivalent to a shunt (Q_{sp}/Q_t) of about 3-5% (Table 40–4). If the ratio were to decrease acutely to 200 in a patient with previously normal lungs, the Q_{sp}/Q_t usually would be about 20%, and the patient generally would need mechanical ventilatory assistance.

PHYSIOLOGIC SHUNTING IN THE LUNG (Q_{sp}/Q_t)

Interpreting the Q_{sp}/Q_t

AXIOM Physiologic shunting in the lung is usually the most sensitive test for diagnosing impending or early respiratory failure.

Normally, the amount of blood that is shunted through the lungs without being completely oxygenated is about 3-5% of the cardiac output. Mild-to-moderate ARDS may increase the shunt to 15-20%, at which point one should strongly consider providing ventilatory assistance and PEEP to the patient. When the pulmonary shunt exceeds 25%, however, patients with severe trauma or sepsis are apt to develop increasing respiratory failure unless the primary inciting process can be eradicated.

AXIOM Trends are much more important than absolute numbers when evaluating blood gases or pulmonary function tests.

Calculating Q_{sp}/Q_t

All that is needed to calculate physiologic shunting in the lung (Qsp/Qt) is an airtight system for providing a specific FiO_2 and apparatus for accurately measuring oxyhemoglobin saturation and Po_2. After the patient receives a certain FiO_2 for 15 or preferably 30 minutes, arterial and mixed venous samples are drawn. Using the differences between the maximum possible (theoretical) pulmonary capillary oxygen content (C_cO_2), the actual arterial oxygen content (C_aO_2), and the actual mixed venous oxygen content (C_vO_2), the percentage of physiologic shunting may be determined from a modified Berggren's formula:[24]

$$\% \text{ Physiologic shunting} = Q_{sp}/Q_t$$
$$= \frac{C_cO_2 - C_aO_2}{C_cO_2 - C_vO_2} \times 100\%$$

C_cO_2 = Oxygen content of pulmonary capillary blood
C_aO_2 = Oxygen content of arterial blood
C_vO_2 = Oxygen content of mixed venous blood

Thus, when the theoretical oxygen content of pulmonary venous blood is 20 vol %, the arterial content is 19 vol %, and the mixed venous oxygen content is 15 vol %, the shunt is:

$$Q_{sp}/Q_t = \frac{20 - 19}{20 - 15} = \frac{1}{5} = 20\%$$

The formula for calculating oxygen content (ml/dl):

$$\frac{[Hb \times O_2 \text{ satn} \times 1.34]}{100} + [(PaO_2) \times 0.003]$$

Thus, when the Hb is 10.0 g/100 mL, the oxygen saturation is 90% and the Po_2 is 60 mm Hg, the oxygen content is $[(10.0) \times (0.9) \times (1.34)] + [(60) \times (0.003)] = 12.24$ mL/100 mL. If a Swan-Ganz catheter were in place, the venous blood from the pulmonary artery would be ideal for these calculations. When pulmonary artery or right ventricular blood is not available, blood drawn from the superior vena cava through a CVP line has an oxygen content that is normally relatively close to that of mixed venous blood. The C_cO_2 on 100% O_2 is calculated as $(Hb)(1.34) + (2)(FiO_2)$. With an Hb of 10.0 gm/dl on 60% O_2, $C_cO_2 = (10)(1.34) + (2)(0.4) = 14.2$.

Effect of Cardiac Output

AXIOM Any maneuver that increases cardiac output tends to increase the amount of physiologic shunting in the lungs.

The relationship between respiratory and hemodynamic function in ARDS can be extremely complex.[149,150] When reduced cardiac output is manifest, pulmonary blood flow tends to go to the better oxygenated areas of the lung. When pulmonary blood flow increases, the additional blood flow must go to less well-oxygenated portions of the lung. Thus, an increase in cardiac output tends to increase the amount of shunting in the lungs.[23,24]

The reverse of this observation is also true. Because vessels in the more severely affected areas of the lung are more apt to have hypoxic vasoconstriction, any reduction in perfusion pressure or cardiac output tends to cause these vessels to collapse completely, forcing the blood to go through better oxygenated areas of the lung. However, with a low cardiac output, the mixed venous PO_2 will tend to be low, and this will also tend to make the arterial PO_2 low.

AXIOM A low arterial PO_2 in a patient with a low-cardiac output tends to indicate more pulmonary dysfunction than the same PaO_2 in a patient with high-cardiac output.

To factor in the effect of the cardiac output on the Q_{sp}/Q_t, the "shunt index" (% Q_{sp}/Q_t divided by the cardiac index) was used to follow the changes in pulmonary function.[151] For example, at a normal cardiac index of 3.5 liters·min^{-1}·m^{-2} and a normal shunt of 5.0%, the SI is 5.0/3.5 = 1.4. If a patient were to have a shunt of 20%, with a cardiac index of 2.5 liters·min^{-1}·m^{-2}, the SI would be 8.0. Patients with an SI above 5.0 usually require ventilatory support.

CARBON DIOXIDE LEVELS
Although most physicians believe that it is relatively normal until late in ARDS, CO_2 exchange in the lungs is frequently altered almost as early as oxygen exchange.

AXIOM The need for increased minute ventilation to maintain normal levels of $PaCO_2$ in ARDS is primarily due to increased dead space (V_d/V_t).

When the dead space fraction is normal (i.e., about 30%), minute ventilation (V_e) in an adult male is generally 5-6 L/min. When the dead space fraction increases to 60-70% due to large numbers of non-perfused alveoli, the minute ventilation (V_e) must increase to 12-15 L/min or more to maintain an eucapnic state.

One can estimate the dead space/tidal volume ratio (V_d/V_t) by the following formula:

$$V_d/V_t = \frac{(V_e)\,(Paco_2)}{800}$$

Thus, with a normal minute ventilation (V_e) of 6 L/min and a normal $PaCO_2$ of 40 mm Hg,

$$V_d/V_t = \frac{(6)(40)}{800} = \frac{240}{800} = 0.3$$

If the V_e is 15 L/min and $Paco_2$ is 30 mm Hg:

$$V_d/V_t = \frac{(15)(35)}{800} = \frac{525}{800} = 0.66$$

AXIOM V_d/V_t exceeding 0.60-0.65 usually indicates a severe degree of ventilation-perfusion mismatch.

CAPNOGRAPHY
Capnography, by providing a real-time estimate of $PaCO_2$, can be a useful means of assessing ventilatory adequacy, respiratory gas exchange, carbon dioxide production, and cardiovascular status. Sudden decreases in the end-tidal Pco_2 ($PETCO_2$) suggest mechanical problems in the airway, hypoventilation, or a sudden decrease in pulmonary blood flow. In a recent study of $PETCO_2$ changes during emergency surgery in 100 critically ill or injured patients, Domsky et

al. found that the $PETCO_2$ and the arterial end-tidal Pco_2 difference [P(a-ET)CO_2], could provide important prognostic information.[152] $PETCO_2$ was usually 28 mm Hg or more in the patients who survived. The patients who survived usually also had a P(a-ET)CO_2 difference of less than 8 mm Hg.

AXIOM A $PETCO_2$ persistently < 28 mm Hg and an arterial-$ETCO_2$ difference greater than 8 mm Hg following resuscitation are associated with a poor prognosis.

Pulmonary Hypertension

In young, previously healthy adults, the pulmonary artery (PA) pressure averages about 12/5 with a mean PA pressure (mPAP) of about 8 mm Hg. If the PAWP is 4.0 mm Hg and the cardiac output is 5.0 L/min, pulmonary vascular resistance (PVR) would be:

$$\frac{mPAP - PAWP}{CO} \times 80 = \frac{8-4}{5} \times 80 = 64 \text{ dyne·sec·cm}^{-5}$$

In older individuals, PA pressure may normally be as high as 25/10 with an mPAP of 15 mm Hg. If the PAWP is 5.0 mm Hg and CO is 5 L/min, the PVR would be:

$$\frac{15-5}{5} \times 80 = \frac{10}{5} \times 80 = 160 \text{ dyne·sec·cm}^{-5}$$

A normal PVR is considered to be 40-160 dyne·sec·cm^{-5}.

AXIOM Increasing pulmonary hypertension is probably the most frequent and consistent hemodynamic evidence of a poor prognosis following trauma.

In the early stages of ARDS, pulmonary hypertension is primarily the result of neurohumoral activity, including increased thromboxane A_2, leukotrienes, and serotonin. In the later stages of ARDS, various types of microemboli and interstitial edema are probably more important. Visconi et al., in determining the cause of pulmonary hypertension in ARDS, found pulmonary microthrombosis in 80% of polytrauma patients, but in only 25% of septic patients.[153]

Decreased Pulmonary Compliance

The increased stiffness of the lung in ARDS, which is due primarily to interstitial and alveolar edema, makes it more difficult to inflate the lung, reduces lung volumes, and increases the work of breathing.[2]

AXIOM Tachypnea is usually the first indication of increased lung stiffness in ARDS.

The overall work of breathing is needed to: (a) overcome airway resistance and gas inertia, and (b) provide the mechanical force necessary to expand the lung parenchyma and chest wall. For patients with a constant minute ventilation, a reduced rate of breathing (i.e., using slow, deep breaths) decreases the work of breathing due to airway resistance but increases parenchymal work.[2] Conversely, an increase in the rate of breathing (rapid, shallow breaths) increases airway work and decreases parenchymal work. In ARDS, airway resistance is increased relatively little compared to the parenchymal resistance; consequently, it is more efficient for the patient to breathe rapidly and shallowly.

AXIOM When a low and decreasing static and dynamic pulmonary compliance cannot be corrected, the prognosis with ARDS is poor.

The compliance of the lung and chest wall can be quantitated relatively easily when the patient is intubated (Fig. 40-6). Dynamic com

TABLE 40–5 **Clinical Indicators Suggestive of a Failed Weaning Attempt**

Parameters	Value*
Respiratory rate	Increase > 10 breaths/min
Pulse	Increase > 20 beats/min
Blood pressure	Increase or decrease > 20 mm Hg systolic
PaO_2	Decrease to < 60 mm Hg with supplemental O_2
$PaCO_2$	Increase > 10 mm Hg
pH	Decrease > 0.10 unit

* value indicating that the weaning attempt is likely to fail
From: Hyzy RC, Popovich J Jr: Mechanical ventilation and weaning (Chap. 84). In Carlson RW, Geheb MA, eds. Principles and Practice of Medical Intensive Care. Philadelphia, WB Saunders Co., 1993, p 924.

pliance (C_D) is obtained by dividing the tidal volume by the peak inspiratory pressure (PIP) minus PEEP during inspiration. Static compliance (C_S) is equal to the tidal volume divided by the inspiratory plateau pressure (IPP) (obtained during a 0.5 second respiratory hold) minus the PEEP. Thus, when the PIP is 40 cm H_2O, the IPP is 30 cm H_2O, the PEEP is 10 cm H_2O, and the V_t 1000 mL:

$$C_D = \frac{Vt}{PIP-PEEP} = \frac{1000}{40-10} = 33 \text{ mL/cm } H_2O$$

$$C_S = \frac{Vt}{IPP-PEEP} = \frac{1000}{30-10} = 50 \text{ mL/cm } H_2O$$

Normal values are 60-100 mL/cm H_2O for C_D and 100-200 mL/cm H_2O for C_S. With ARDS, C_S values < 50 mL/cm H_2O are commonly seen; in severe cases, they may be < 30 mL/cm H_2O.

AXIOM In general, tidal volumes and PEEP should be adjusted, as needed, to provide the best static compliance for ventilated patients.

Clinical Progression

The clinical progression of ARDS can be described as occurring in four stages[2] (Table 40–5). In the first stage, some dyspnea and tachypnea can be noted, but generally no changes are manifest on chest radiography. In the second stage, the patient begins to develop some hypoxemia and respiratory distress. A decrease in the functional residual capacity, an increase in the dead-space ventilation, and an increase in pulmonary vascular resistance are usually present. These changes can occur within hours and often precede the appearance of infiltrates on chest radiography.

AXIOM The presence of ARDS is often not detected clinically until its third stage.

The third stage of ARDS is marked by a progressive clinical pulmonary insufficiency that requires aggressive ventilatory support. At this stage, patients often require an FiO_2 in excess of 0.6 and a V_E of 12 L/min or more. This stage is often also recognizable by the appearance of diffuse, pulmonary infiltrates on chest radiography.

In the fourth stage, patients become increasing refractory to ventilatory support and PEEP, and terminally, the hypoxemia is accompanied by hypercapnia. Severe alterations in compliance make ventilation increasingly difficult. A complete white-out of the lungs may develop on chest radiography. These patients eventually develop right ventricular failure with low ejection fractions, and tissue oxygenation may become so poor that hypercapnia and increasingly severe lactic acidosis may also develop. Patients reaching this stage of ARDS often develop MOF and die.

DIAGNOSIS

Criteria

The criteria for diagnosis of ARDS vary somewhat from author to author, but generally include: (a) an inciting problem, such as sepsis, trauma, or an inflammatory process, (b) normal PAWP (< 12 mm Hg), (c) hypoxemia with a PaO_2/FiO_2 ratio (PFR) of < 200, (d) presence of diffuse, patchy infiltrates on chest radiography, and (e) absence of any other conditions that could cause these changes.

AXIOM Generally, a PFR < 300 following trauma in a previously healthy individual indicates acute lung injury, a PFR < 200 indicates ARDS and a PFR < 120 indicates severe ARDS.

Prediction of ARDS

Pepe et al. were able to predict the onset of ARDS in 50% of their patients with an 80% accuracy.[19] The four major risk factors that were identified included: a high injury severity score (> 25), multiple transfusions, sepsis syndrome, and initial PaO_2/FiO_2 ratio of < 200 in patients on mechanical ventilation. The major goal of predicting ARDS is to stimulate aggressive therapy to try to improve oxygen delivery to tissues to try to prevent the development of MOF.

AXIOM Ventilatory assistance in critically injured patients should not be delayed until there is clinical evidence of severe respiratory failure.

Clinical Criteria for Diagnosis
HISTORY

Timing
ARDS usually develops within two to three days of an initiating event, especially when multiple risk factors are present. Mortality more than 72 hours after major trauma is most commonly secondary to the sepsis syndrome; in one study, six times as many ARDS patients had sepsis syndrome as patients with similar risk factors who did not develop ARDS.[19]

Clinical Situations
Some clinical situations that are frequent precursors for acute respiratory failure following trauma, especially with a flail chest, include shock, three or more organ injuries or large bone fractures, sepsis, flail chest, coma, previous pulmonary disease, and age greater than 65 years.[154] Although much individual variation exists, the greater the number of these situations or factors that are present, the greater the chance that ARDS will develop.

AXIOM Virtually all patients with shock and persistent sepsis, especially from severe peritonitis, develop some degree of respiratory failure.

Sepsis is the most frequent cause of ARDS, but evidence in trauma patients suggests that increased pulmonary capillary permeability may precede the development of clinically apparent sepsis.[155]

PHYSICAL EXAMINATION
Increasing tachypnea is often the first sign of posttraumatic pulmonary insufficiency, but it is a nonspecific sign. Examination of the lungs at this time usually reveals nothing more than some basilar rales and a decrease in breath sounds.[1]

Although the clinical response to a low PaO_2 is undoubtedly responsible for some of the signs of ARDS, most ARDS patients continue to hyperventilate even after administration of enough oxygen to correct the hypoxemia.[1] A possible mechanism for this may be stimulation of J-receptors in the pulmonary interstitium because of disturbance of normal length-tension relationships so that decreased lung expansion occurs for a given amount of change in pleural pressure.[86,156]

One can estimate the relative increased work of breathing (WOB) in many patients by the following formula:

$$WOB = \frac{RR}{10} \times EF$$

where RR is the respiratory rate and EF is the effort factor. EF is 1.0 with normal, quiet breathing, but it is 2.0 when even mild evidence of increased effort exists, and 3.0 or more when the patient is obviously laboring.

Thus, when a patient has an RR of 30/minute and is working fairly hard at breathing, the WOB is $\frac{30}{10} \times 3 = 9$ times normal. In general, a patient who is not a trained athlete cannot maintain a WOB exceeding six to eight for more than a few hours without developing so much fatigue that efforts at breathing may cease entirely.

AXIOM Restlessness should be considered as due to hypoxia until proved otherwise.

If restlessness is due to hypoxia, the patients' movements tend to be purposeless, abrupt, and irregular, whereas the actions of a patient who is restless because of pain, but is adequately oxygenated are generally directed to reducing a particular irritant and are slower and more repetitive. When in doubt, it is best to assume that a restless patient is hypoxic until proved otherwise.

AXIOM If narcotics or sedatives are given to a patient with restlessness due to pulmonary problems, ventilation will be further reduced.

Cyanosis is a late sign of respiratory failure and generally does not develop in patients with hemoglobin levels < 10.0 g/dL until or unless severe impairment of blood flow to the skin or mucous membranes occurs. It usually takes a minimum of 5.0 g of reduced hemoglobin in the capillaries of the skin or lips before a patient appears cyanotic.

PITFALL ⊘

One should not assume that a patient's oxygenation is adequate because no cyanosis is present, especially when the Hb ≤ 10 g/dL.

Laboratory Studies

MARKERS FOR SEPSIS AND/OR INFLAMMATORY CHANGES

The most important laboratory studies for following the progress of posttraumatic pulmonary insufficiency are arterial blood gas analyses. Tests demonstrating the presence of sepsis and/or other organ failure, however, are also important. With fat embolism syndrome, it can be helpful to track platelet counts and $P(A-a)O_2$ levels.

AXIOM In patients who have had minimal bleeding and little or no shock, fat embolism is the most frequent cause for a decrease in the platelet count below normal in the first 24-48 hours after trauma.

Maunder suggested a number of cellular and biochemical markers that can be used to help identify patients who are developing ARDS.[21] Some of the proposed markers include increased neutrophil activity,[115] increased levels of elastase in alveolar lavage fluid,[157] and increased serum complement levels.[110,120]

BLOOD GASES AND DERIVED VALUES

AXIOM With blood gases, one should follow not only the PaO_2 and $PaCO_2$, but also the PaO_2/FiO_2 ratio, the $P(A-a)O_2$, PvO_2, SvO_2, and Q_{sp}/Q_t.

PaCO₂

With adequate alveolar ventilation, the $PaCO_2$ should correlate closely with the pH_a. Generally, the $PaCO_2$ in mm Hg should be ≤ 8.0 + 1.5 times the HCO_3. Thus, if the HCO_3 is 24 mEq/L, the $PaCO_2$ should be ≤ 44 mm Hg. If the HCO_3 is 16 mEq/L, the $PaCO_2$ should be [8 + (1.5)(16)] = 32 mm Hg or less.

AXIOM A low $PaCO_2$ does not necessarily indicate that the patient's ventilation is adequate, especially when hypocarbia is mild in the face of moderate-to-severe metabolic acidosis.

In an effort to reduce excessive alveolar distension with resultant "volutrama" to the lungs, low-tidal volumes with resulting "permissive hypercarbia" are being increasingly used.[15] Most clinicians agree that a gradual rise in the $PaCO_2$ to 60 mm Hg is not life-threatening provided that the $pH_a \geq 7.30$. A $pH_a \geq 7.25$ is usually well tolerated by patients free of preexisting cardiac disease.[15] However, although permissive hypercapnia has been safely applied in limited studies,[158] it is premature to assume that this practice is completely without risk.[15]

PaO₂

Ideally, PaO_2 in patients with ARDS should be kept < 80 mm Hg (SaO_2 = 95%) to reduce the chances of damage to the lung by hyperoxia. An arterial $PO_2 \geq 60$ mm Hg (SaO_2 = 90%) is traditionally considered acceptable in critically ill patients on ventilators. If severe lung disease is present, an arterial PO_2 as low as 50 mm Hg may be justified to avoid use of potentially deleterious high FiO_2 levels or large amounts of PEEP.[159]

PaO₂/FiO₂ Ratio

When the PaO_2/FiO_2 ratio is decreasing, one must be suspicious that ARDS or some other pulmonary problem is developing. When the PaO_2/FiO_2 ratio decreases to < 200 (such as with a PaO_2 < 80 mm Hg on an $FiO_2 \geq 0.4$), this generally indicates moderate-to-severe pulmonary changes requiring ventilatory support.

Physiologic Shunting in the Lung (Q_{sp}/Q_t)

In general, the Q_{sp}/Q_t is a more accurate and sensitive index of pulmonary function than the PaO_2 or the PaO_2/FiO_2 ratio. In patients with a large Q_{sp}/Q_t, a low PvO_2 tends to also keep the PaO_2 low. A low PvO_2 or SvO_2 usually results from reduced O_2 delivery (DO_2) relative to oxygen consumption (VO_2).

AXIOM A decrease in PaO_2 may be caused by poor pulmonary function, but in ARDS it may also be caused by high-oxygen consumption and/or low-oxygen delivery.[160]

OXYGEN CONSUMPTION

Although oxygen consumption (VO_2) may be expected to decrease when a patient develops pulmonary insufficiency with a reduced DO_2, VO_2 often remains relatively normal until late, even with advanced pulmonary insufficiency.[161] Measurements of oxygen consumption, therefore, may be deceptive when attempting to diagnose early respiratory failure.

AXIOM Peripheral defects in oxygen utilization can become increasingly apparent as ARDS becomes more severe.

In several studies,[162] it has been shown that a decreased oxygen supply to peripheral tissues during ARDS is often not accompanied by an increased percent of extraction.[1] Below a critical threshold of DO_2, a decrease in oxygen uptake or utilization without a shift to anaerobic metabolism can occur until relatively low VO_2 levels are found.

AXIOM In patients who are apt to develop ARDS, one should maintain an optimal VO_2 or at least a VO_2 that is not flow-dependent.

Lung Compliance

Most of the increase in inflation pressure needed as acute respiratory failure develops is due to increased lung water. For example, if it were to take 40 cm H_2O to inflate the lungs with a tidal volume of 1000 mL, it probably would take about 30 cm H_2O of that pressure to inflate the lungs themselves. Thus, the stiffness of the lungs in such an individual would probably be about three to six times greater than normal and, as a corollary, lung compliance would only one-third or one-sixth of normal.

AXIOM   Decreasing static lung compliance in a patient after trauma, in the absence of hemopneumothorax or abdominal distension, is usually due to increased lung water and may indicate developing ARDS.

Although a gradual increase in lung resistance or stiffness is characteristic of ARDS, a sudden increase in airway pressure should make one suspect pneumothorax or major airway obstruction.

AXIOM   If the inflation pressures on a ventilator were to increase suddenly, pneumothorax or major airway obstruction should be suspected.

Lung Water

Measuring lung water, such as with the thermal dye dilution technique, has severe limitations for diagnosing ARDS and has not been useful clinically.[163] The pulmonary lymphatics are able to compensate for a severe degree of increased capillary permeability, and studies showed a marked increase in lung lymph flow before extravascular lung water (EVLW) increases. In ARDS, a pulmonary weight increase of as much as 50% may be required before PaO_2 decreases.

Radiologic Studies

Lung infiltrates seen immediately after trauma are usually due to pulmonary contusion. Localized infiltrates appearing after 24-48 hours are often due to aspiration, and diffuse infiltrates at that time are often due to fat emboli. Diffuse infiltrates appearing after 48-72 hours tend to be due to ARDS from continuing tissue necrosis, inflammation, or infection.

AXIOM   It cannot be assumed that pulmonary function is satisfactory when the lungs appear relatively normal on chest radiography.

The earliest changes noted on chest radiography in ARDS usually include: (a) scattered areas of mild platelike atelectasis, particularly at the lung bases posteriorly, and (b) signs of vascular congestion with increased prominence of perihilar vascular markings (Fig. 40–4). Many of these patients then develop scattered, fluffy, irregular areas of increased density, similar to those seen with interstitial pneumonitis. These pulmonary infiltrates may then enlarge and coalesce (Fig. 40–5). Eventually both lung fields may be completely "whited out" on chest radiography.

AXIOM   The amount of lung damage initially seen on plain chest radiography usually greatly underestimates the severity and extent of the ARDS.

CT scans of the chest, particularly in the early phases, generally reveal the extent of the parenchymal involvement in ARDS much better than chest radiographs (Fig. 40–6). The typical appearance of ARDS on CT scans includes ground-glass opacities with air bronchograms, followed by increasingly dense areas of consolidation in the dependent portions of the lungs. The high frequency of involvement of the lower, more dependent lung parenchyma, with less involvement of the non-dependent areas is seen better on CT. CT can

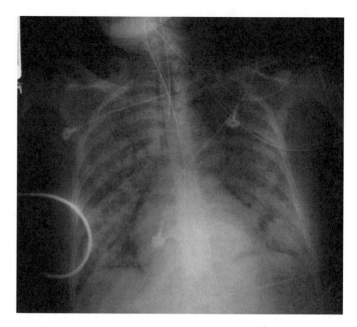

FIGURE 40–5   As ARDS progresses, the chest films tend to show increasingly dense, patchy infiltrates and then increasing consolidation throughout both lungs. In some instances, small tension pneumothoraces may develop in both chests, particularly when high-peak inflation pressures are used.

also identify pleural fluid collections much earlier and more accurately than plain radiographs.

PAWP Monitoring

PAWP monitoring is often necessary to differentiate the increased lung water of ARDS from cardiogenic pulmonary edema. Furthermore, one should make efforts to ensure that patients developing ARDS are not overloaded with fluid.

Typically, ARDS is characterized by a PAWP < 12 mm Hg; however, an increased level of PEEP, especially > 10 cm H_2O may artificially increase PAWP. When a large amount of PEEP is being used, a "corrected PAWP" (i.e., PAWP at zero PEEP) can be estimated by subtracting one-third of the PEEP from the PAWP. In other words, when 20 cm H_2O (14.7 mm Hg) PEEP is used and the measured PAWP is 15.0 mm Hg, the "corrected PAWP" is probably about 10.1 mm Hg.

AXIOM   When large amounts of PEEP are used, one should follow changes in the PAWP rather than absolute levels to obtain a more accurate impression of cardiac-filling.

Taking the patient off high levels of PEEP to determine the "true PAWP" is not warranted and can allow increased pulmonary edema to develop rapidly. Furthermore, one should be following *changes* in the level of PAWP and not relying on absolute *levels* to determine therapy. If PAWP is not available, one could follow changes in the CVP or pulmonary artery diastolic pressure.[164]

THERAPEUTIC GOALS

Infection

AXIOM   If ARDS is developing or getting worse, it usually implies that an inadequately treated infection is present.

One of the primary goals in the treatment of ARDS is to control the underlying etiologic factors.[1] Although it frequently does not correlate well with the degree of the shunt or amount of extravascular lung water, the mortality for ARDS does correlate with the severity

FIGURE 40–6 CT scan of the lungs in ARDS tends to reveal much more extensive parenchymal changes than does corresponding chest radiography.

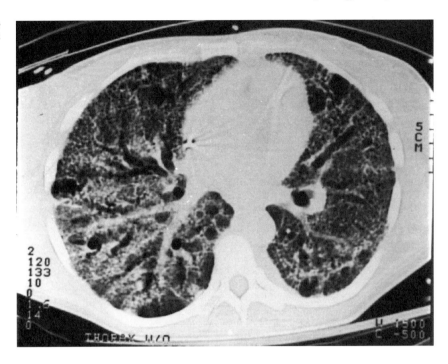

and duration of uncontrolled sepsis and the number of other organ failures.[165,166]

> **AXIOM** Early and complete eradication of pus and/or necrotic tissue is extremely important in patients with ARDS.

Despite aggressive diagnostic efforts, it is often extremely difficult to find the source of sepsis in patients with ARDS. It has been hypothesized that a systemic inflammatory response syndrome (SIRS) in patients without apparent infection may be due to bacterial translocation from the gastrointestinal tract. Although it has been well documented in experimental animals, the frequency and importance of bacterial translocation in the gut in humans is controversial. Moore et al. were unable to document the presence of bacteria in portal venous blood of injured patients with a wide variety of injuries.[167]

If infection develops, the antibiotic(s) chosen should be tailored to the specific organism(s) likely to be present. With pulmonary infections this can often be determined initially by a Gram stain of sputum or, preferably, a protected brush specimen, prior to the culture and sensitivity reports. The duration of treatment is determined by the patient's response, but in general, shorter rather than longer courses are recommended to reduce the risk of superinfections by resistant organisms or fungi.[168]

> **AXIOM** Persistent fever, leukocytosis, and pulmonary dysfunction in critically injured patients after 7-10 days of antibiotic therapy may be due to fungal infection, and it may be prudent to begin antifungal therapy in such individuals.

Improving Pulmonary Function

The prevention and treatment of respiratory failure may be divided into the following categories: nursing care, general supportive measures, fluid management, drug therapy, inhalation therapy, correction of airway problems, and ventilatory support.

NURSING CARE

Encouraging the patient to cough and take deep breaths, frequent position changes, elevation of the head and chest, and chest physiotherapy should be routine in any nursing unit caring for critically ill or injured patients.

GENERAL SUPPORTIVE MEASURES

Reduction of Abdominal Distension

Distended bowel and increased ascitic fluid may elevate the diaphragm markedly, thereby reducing tidal volume and increasing the work of breathing. This should be prevented or corrected with early nasogastric suction or paracentesis as needed.

> **AXIOM** Patients who may develop pulmonary problems and require prolonged gastrointestinal intubation may benefit from having such tubes passed through a gastrostomy or jejunostomy rather than through the nose or mouth.

Reduction of Pain

One of the greatest deterrents to effective breathing and coughing following trauma is pain from an injury or surgical incision involving the chest or upper abdomen. Such pain can be controlled with multiple small doses of intravenous morphine, but these narcotics can also depress the cough reflex and ventilation markedly. In such patients, epidural analgesia may produce dramatic benefit.

> **AXIOM** Controlling pain so that the patient can take deep breaths and cough effectively is probably the single best way to prevent atelectasis and/or pneumonia following truncal trauma or surgery.

Reduction of Oxygen Demand

When the patient has a high fever or is agitated, oxygen requirements may be greatly increased. To reduce increased VO_2, one should reduce the patient's temperature with drugs, sponging, or induced hypothermia. When the patient is in pain, this is generally best corrected by epidural analgesia or local anesthetic block. Sedatives and/or muscle relaxants may also be used, but with caution, especially when the patient is not on a ventilator.

> **AXIOM** When restlessness is due to pain, analgesics may be indicated; however, when restlessness is due to hypoxia, such agents may be lethal.

Chest Tubes

A restricted tidal volume, especially in patients with chest trauma or peritonitis, may be due to increased pleural fluid in one or both sides of the chest. Although > 500-1000 mL of pleural fluid may not be detected on a supine chest radiograph, such fluid should be suspected in patients with marginal pulmonary function, especially when peak inspiratory pressures on a ventilator exceed 50 cm H_2O. In patients with severe ARDS, each pleural cavity usually has at least 100-200 mL of fluid. Removal of such fluid often causes the peak ventilator pressure to decrease by at least 5-10 cm H_2O.

> **AXIOM** A gradual increase in PIP in ARDS may be at least partially due to pleural effusions, but a sudden increase is due to an obstructed airway or pneumothorax until proved otherwise.

FLUID THERAPY

"Keep the Patient Dry"

Although rapid restoration of the blood volume after bleeding has been controlled and maintenance of a high-oxygen delivery to tissues is important to survival, the continued administration of fluid must be done carefully, with close attention to vital signs, CVP, PAWP, urine output, and tissue perfusion.[169] Frequent auscultation of the lungs is also important.

Right Ventricular End-diastolic Volume

A modification of the pulmonary artery catheter with a rapid thermistor has allowed thermodilution studies to determine the right ventricular end-diastolic volume index (RVEDVI) at the bedside.[170] In a study of 32 trauma patients,[171] cardiac index correlated much better with RVEDVI, than with PAWP. Of 83 studies in which the PAWP was > 18 mm Hg, additional fluid could be given in 71 (86%) because the RVEDVI was low (< 90 mL/m^2) or mid-range (90-140 mL/m^2). At the other PAWP extreme, of 50 studies in which PAWP was < 12 mm Hg, RVEDVI was > 140 mL/m^2 in 12 (24%). Thus, 25 (78%) of these trauma patients had PAWPs at some time that may have encouraged a clinician to increase or decrease preload when the RVEDVI would have indicated the opposite.

> **AXIOM** In attempting to find the ideal cardiac filling volume, one should use the RVEDVI or the hemodynamic response to fluid challenges rather than isolated PAWP or CVP levels.

Prevent Severe Reductions in Colloid Osmotic Pressure

Although the use of colloids to resuscitate trauma patients has been extremely controversial, some value may exist in maintaining a colloid osmotic pressure (COP) of at least ½-⅔ of the normal value of 22-28 mm Hg.[172-174] Administration of albumin to maintain an adequate COP, however, may also cause problems.[175-177] For example, in patients with increased capillary permeability due to severe sepsis or shock, albumin may rapidly enter the interstitial space of the lungs and draw fluid with it, thereby increasing interstitial edema. Consequently, albumin or other colloids must be given carefully, noting how well the cardiovascular and pulmonary systems respond. Changes in the DO_2I, VO_2I, and Q_{sp}/Q_t are particularly important.

> **AXIOM** Although the role of colloids in the prevention or treatment of ARDS is controversial, low COP tends to increase the water content of the lungs.

In order to determine whether a high-molecular-weight colloid may help to reduce EVLW, Oppenheimer and Landolfo used macromolecular hetastarch (HES), with an average molecular weight of 450,000, to try to maintain the plasma COP gradient.[178] In 13 isolated, perfused canine left lower lobes with ARDS produced by oleic acid (to simulate the respiratory dysfunction seen with fat embolism syndrome), addition of HES to the perfusate increased COP from 11.9 ± 4.5 mm Hg to 13.4 ± 3.2 mm Hg. Although the control lung

continued to form edema at a rate of 0.94 ± 0.31 mL/minute/100 g tissue, the lungs with HES perfusate reduced their water content at a rate of 0.25 ± 0.12 mL/minute/100 g. Thus, an increased COP due to a high MW colloid helped to reduce edema fluid in experimental ARDS due to fat embolism.

Maintain Adequate Hemoglobin Levels

Hemodilution to a hemoglobin < 10.0 g/dL in critically injured patients not infrequently causes some reduction in DO_2 and VO_2. Although the optimal hemoglobin in critically injured patients is debated and is believed by many physicians to be about 10 g/dL with a hematocrit of about 30%, Wilson and Gibson noted that critically ill or injured patients with higher hemoglobin levels tended to have better survival rates.[179]

Shoemaker and Appel also noted that survivors tended to have higher hemoglobin levels.[180] In a study by Fenwick et al., patients with ARDS and lactic acidosis were transfused from a hemoglobin of 9.7 to 12.3 g/dL; this increased DO_2 from 452 to 585 mL/minute/m^2 and VO_2 from 117 to 131 mL/minute/m^2.[181] Similar increases in VO_2 were achieved by transfusion in a report by Gilbert et al.[182] However, when DO_2 and VO_2 are already at supranormal (optimal) levels and the patient does not have lactic acidosis, increasing the Hb further is not apt to significantly increase VO_2.

> **AXIOM** Although extremely controversial, patients with severe ARDS or other severe cardiopulmonary dysfunction tend to have a better prognosis when the Hb level is 12.0 g/dL or more.

We noted significant improvements in physiologic shunting in the lung in our own patients with severe ARDS when the Hg was > 12.0 g/100 mL. Even when the initial hematocrit was 30%, each unit of packed red blood cells increased oxygen content 7-10% and increased DO_2 4-6%. Increased oxygen-carrying capacity of the blood can be particularly important in patients who have cardiac or respiratory failure and in those who have had multiple blood transfusions.

OPTIMAL DO₂ AND VO₂

Numerous studies have shown the benefit of "optimal" (supranormal) levels of DO_2 and VO_2 in preventing organ failure after surgery or trauma. Shoemaker et al. showed that increasing the DO_2 to > 600 mL/minute/m^2 and the VO_2 to ≥ 170 mL/minute/m^2 reduced the incidence of pulmonary complications in high-risk surgical patients from 27% (16 of 60) to 4% (1 of 28).[183] Likewise, Cryer et al. found that a high DO_2 and a low $P(A-a)O_2$ on the third day after the diagnosis of ARDS were the two most important correlates predicting survival.[184]

> **AXIOM** Achieving optimal (supranormal) DO_2 and VO_2 levels soon after trauma or surgery in high-risk patients seems to reduce the incidence and severity of organ failure and death.

Fleming et al., in a prospective study of resuscitation in 67 patients with severe trauma (mean ISS = 27), found that early postinjury attainment of supranormal cardiac index (≥ 4.5 L/minute/m^2), DO_2 (≥ 670 mL/minute/m^2), and VO_2 (≥ 166 mL/minute/m^2) resulted in fewer deaths (14% vs 44%) and a lower incidence of respiratory failure (39% vs 68%).[185]

NUTRITIONAL SUPPORT

> **AXIOM** Early, aggressive enteral nutrition appears to reduce complications after trauma.

Moore and Moore showed that early, aggressive enteral feeding of trauma patients is feasible despite major intraabdominal injuries and is preferable to parenteral nutrition because of the reduced incidence of septic complications.[186] In a review of immunonutrition as an emerging strategy in the ICU, Alexander reported the potential value of arginine, dietary nucleotides (RNA), and lipids from fish oil (ω-3-fatty acids).[187] Glutamine may also be helpful by improving N_2 balance, improving enterocyte metabolism, and reducing the loss of skeletal muscle.

PREVENTION OF STRESS GASTRITIS

A great deal of controversy exists concerning the best method for preventing stress gastritis in trauma patients because increasing gastric pH may allow bacterial overgrowth in the stomach. This could increase the tendency for bacterial pneumonia secondary to subclinical aspiration of gastric contents.

AXIOM Although preventing stress gastritis seems to be a worthwhile goal in high-risk patients, allowing bacterial overgrowth in a highly alkaline stomach may increase the risk of pulmonary complications.

Two recent meta-analyses provided conflicting conclusions as to whether sucralfate or increasing gastric pH is superior.[188,189] This discrepancy may have occurred because the patient groups varied greatly, the controls were poorly matched, and many different regimens were analyzed.[190] In a recently well-controlled, randomized, prospective trial comparing sucralfate with either bolus or continuous cimetidine administration in nonburned trauma patients, Fabian et al. found no difference in the incidence of nosocomial pneumonia.[191]

In another recent study, however, Cioffi et al. performed a randomized study of 96 burn patients using either sucralfate (1 g/20 mL water q 5 hours; n = 48) or cimetidine (300 mg q 6 hours) plus antacids as needed every two hours to keep gastric pH $\geq$ 4.5 (n = 48).[190] They found that the intubated patients treated with sucralfate had a higher incidence of pneumonia (43%) versus the antacid-cimetidine group (18%; P < 0.05).

DRUGS

Bronchodilators

AXIOM Although it is not usually a prominent feature in respiratory failure following trauma, bronchospasm or wheezing should be treated aggressively when it occurs.

Inhaled β-adrenergic agonists are increasingly considered to be the therapy of choice for the treatment of acute bronchospasm, particularly in critically ill patients.[192] Other indications for their usage include prophylaxis of chronic and exercise-induced asthma. In hospitalized patients, isoetharine and metaproterenol are the most commonly used inhalation agents for administration by nebulization.[192]

Inotropic Agents

One of the digitalis preparations should be given when atrial fibrillation is present, particularly when evidence of cardiac failure exists, but it is a relatively weak inotrope and has many side effects. Dopamine and/or dobutamine are generally the inotropes of choice in the ICU. Dopamine is probably the ideal agent when one wishes to increase both BP and cardiac output. If the preload and BP are adequate, dobutamine is probably the inotrope of choice.[193]

AXIOM Inotropic agents may be helpful for increasing DO_2 and VO_2 to optimal levels. The resulting tachycardia and increased shunting in the lung, however, can be a problem.

Diuretics

Intravenous diuretics may be required to prevent or to help correct pulmonary insufficiency in patients with heart failure or evidence of fluid overloading. Great care must be taken, however, to prevent hypovolemia as a result of excessive diuresis, particularly during the obligatory fluid sequestration phase after trauma. This phase, which

is present from the completion of the initial fluid resuscitation and surgery for about 48 hours, is often characterized by reduced blood volume because of increased movement of fluid from the intravascular to the interstitial fluid space.

AXIOM It is extremely dangerous to give diuretics when oliguria is due to a deficit in the functional ECF.

In patients with severe abdominal trauma and postoperative oliguria, one should look for abdominal compartment syndrome in spite of good BPs and cardiac outputs.[194] When it is clear that the oliguria is present in spite of a more than adequate preload, dopamine in doses of 1-3 μmcg/kg/minute can often help to promote diuresis. Occasionally, mannitol (12.5-25.0 g bolus and 6.25-12.5 g/hour) and/or furosemide (5-20 mg by intermittent intravenous injection) may also be needed.

If the patient still were to have excessive fluid, continuous AV hemofiltration (CAVH) can be helpful. Garzia et al. used this in 14 nonoliguric patients who had severe ARDS.[195] Three grossly unstable patients died early, but the other 11 patients improved markedly.

INHALATION THERAPY

Oxygen

Unless FiO_2 exceeding 0.6 is required, the arterial PO_2 should be kept > 60 mm Hg and preferably at 70-80 mm Hg in patients who have recently had severe trauma. The initial efforts to increase arterial Po_2 should be directed toward improving the patient's ventilation. Although the data concerning the relationships between FiO_2 and oxygen toxicity are relatively poor,[196] it is generally believed that inhaled oxygen concentrations of $\leq$ 40% are relatively safe, but prolonged use of inhaled oxygen concentrations > 50%, may be associated with increased atelectasis and shunting in the lungs.

AXIOM Concern about oxygen toxicity should not prevent the administration of a high FiO_2 (fraction of inspired oxygen) if this is the only way to maintain PaO_2 of at least 50 mm Hg in patients with severe ARDS.

Aerosolization and Nebulization

Aerosolization and nebulization refers to the introduction of droplets of fluid, mechanically mixed with air or oxygen, into the respiratory tract with or without medications. Humidification may be of benefit by: (a) decreasing the viscosity of mucoid secretions in the respiratory tract, thereby permitting the cilia to function more efficiently, and (b) counteracting the drying effects of various gases introduced by the ventilator.

An important consideration in aerosolization or nebulization is the particle size. Widely differing estimates of the site of the ultimate deposition of particles of various sizes while breathing through the mouth have been reported; however, particles of 1-5 micron diameter may be most effective.

Ultrasonic nebulizers can provide large quantities of fluid particles of small size (0.5-3.0 microns), and these can rapidly cause fluid overload, especially in infants. Mucolytic agents can cause severe bronchospasm, and they should never be given without a bronchodilator.

MAINTENANCE OF AN OPEN AIRWAY

Nasotracheal Suction

In patients who are not already intubated and who do not cough adequately to remove tracheobronchial secretions, properly performed nasotracheal suction may not only directly remove such secretions, but it may also cause the patient to cough much more forcefully.

Bronchoscopy

When excess secretions collect in the tracheobronchial tree that cannot be removed by coughing or tracheal aspiration, bronchoscopy is indicated. During bronchoscopy, the patient should be constantly monitored to prevent unsuspected hypoxemia or hypotension from developing. Bronchoscopy on these patients can be performed through an existing tracheostomy tube or an endotracheal tube. If a tube is not already in place, one can usually be inserted under topical anesthesia to make sure that ventilation and oxygenation are adequate during the bronchoscopy.

VENTILATORY SUPPORT

Indications for Using Ventilators

A ventilator should be used in trauma patients whenever the clinical situation or laboratory studies suggest that the patient has inadequate ventilation or is likely to develop respiratory failure.

PITFALL ⊘

If ventilatory assistance is delayed in injured patients until definite clinical evidence of respiratory failure exists, the lung changes can be very difficult to reverse.[11-13]

Some of the more frequent clinical indications for early ventilatory assistance in injured patients include:

1. Flail chest, particularly when it involves seven or more ribs or is bilateral.
2. Severe pulmonary contusion with hypoxemia.
3. Severe CNS depression due to trauma, drugs, or infection.
4. Injury to three or more major organs requiring surgery.
5. Previous severe pulmonary disease.
6. Severe, prolonged shock.
7. Massive smoke inhalation or aspiration of vomitus.

Some of the laboratory values that may indicate a need for ventilatory assistance in injured patients include:

1. Arterial $PO_2 < 60$ mm Hg on room air, and/or $PaO_2 < 80$ mm Hg on $\geq 40\%$ oxygen.
2. Arterial PCO2 > 50 mm Hg (in the absence of metabolic alkalosis).
3. Alveolar-arterial oxygen difference > 55 mm Hg on room air or > 350-400 mm Hg on 100% O_2.
4. Physiologic shunting in the lung of $\geq 20\%$.
5. PaO_2/FiO_2 ratio of < 200.

On clinical grounds, subjective respiratory distress, labored breathing, or tachypnea at rates in excess of 35/minute may be indications for ventilatory support.[1] These findings may be accompanied by worsening of the chest radiographs.

TRACHEAL INTUBATION

Endotracheal Intubation

AXIOM   When any question exists about the adequacy of the upper airway or minute ventilation in a trauma victim, the patient should probably have early ventilatory support.

Endotracheal intubation can be accomplished either orally or nasally. When it must be accomplished rapidly because of respiratory distress, the oral route is preferred. For long-term support over several days, however, the nasal route is usually more stable and comfortable.

Orotracheal tubes have a larger lumen and can generally be inserted more rapidly and accurately. Nasotracheal tubes have a narrower lumen and are 5 cm longer, thereby increasing the resistance to ventilation and the passage of suction catheters. Trauma to the turbinates during passage of nasotracheal tubes can also produce significant hemorrhage which may occasionally require nasal packing and blood transfusions. In addition, prolonged use of a nasotracheal tube, particularly when a nasogastric tube is present in the other nostril, increases the tendency for the patient to develop sinusitis.

Tracheal cartilage necrosis that can be caused by high pressures in the balloon of endotracheal or tracheostomy tubes can eventually cause tracheal stenosis, tracheoesophageal fistula, or tracheoinnominate artery fistula.[197] The incidence of these tracheal complications has been reduced by using soft, compliant cuffs. Another way to reduce the pressure against the tracheal cartilages is to inflate the balloon only partially, and allow a slight leak around it during the inspiratory phase. One can also use an external pressure control device to keep cuff pressures < 20-25 mm Hg.

TRACHEOSTOMY

Although it had generally been believed that the complications of tracheostomy exceeded those of prolonged endotracheal intubation, many surgeons now perform earlier tracheostomies on patients who will require long-term ventilatory support. Rodriquez et al. presented data that performing a tracheostomy before five days in patients requiring prolonged ventilatory support results in significantly less time on the ventilator and in the ICU.[198]

AXIOM   If a patient requires long-term ventilation or protection of the upper airway, early tracheostomy may be indicated.

Ordering Ventilatory Care

Orders for ventilatory assistance should include:

1. The type of ventilatory support to be used.
2. The gases to be delivered.
3. The tidal volume.
4. The ventilatory pressure range.
5. The ventilatory rate.
6. PEEP.
7. The frequency of sighing.
8. Nebulization and humidification.

TYPE OF VENTILATORY SUPPORT

Types of Ventilatory Assistance

PRESSURE-CYCLED VENTILATORS.   The Bird MK VIII is an example of a pressure-cycled ventilator that delivers gas until the pressure limit selected is reached, at which point the exhalation valve opens. Delivery of a specific volume of gas with each breath may be difficult; however, by assessing the airway resistance encountered and the dynamic compliance of the patient's lungs, the flow rates and pressure limits can usually be adjusted to provide adequate tidal volumes.

AXIOM   Pressure-cycled ventilators are generally easier to use, but when ARDS develops, volume-cycled ventilators are often preferable.

Pressure-cycled ventilation can be used when the patient has only minimal pulmonary difficulty, is alert and cooperative, has a stable chest wall, and has relatively normal lung compliance. It is generally much easier for patients to synchronize with pressure-limited ventilators, but this limits the tidal volume that can be delivered to patients with stiff lungs.

TIME-CYCLED VENTILATORS.   The Bourns BP-200 is a time-cycled ventilator. The length of the inspiratory phase is controlled by a master timer that integrates several mechanical functions. Flow is continuous across the patient's airway, and as the number of mandatory ventilations from the ventilator is reduced during weaning, the patient can supplement the minute ventilation by breathing spontaneously from passing fresh gas flow.

FIGURE 40–7   Modes of gas transport during HFV and a sketch of their zones of dominance. These modes of transport are not mutually exclusive and may interact extensively, depending on HFV settings and the effects of disease on lung mechanics. (HFO = high-frequency oscillator) (From: Chang HK. Mechanisms of gas transport during ventilation by high-frequency oscillation. J Appl Physiol Respirat Environ Exercise Physiol 1984;56:553).

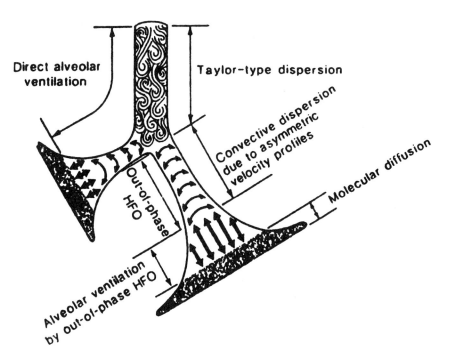

VOLUME-CYCLED VENTILATORS.   Volume-cycled ventilators, in which inspiration is terminated by delivery of a preset volume, are often far more suitable than pressure-cycled machines for patients with "stiff" lungs due to ARDS or other problems because it delivers a preset volume regardless of the pressure required.

AXIOM   Most patients with ARDS require volume-cycled ventilators to ensure adequate gas exchange.

Volume-cycled ventilators have a pressure-limit control that can be adjusted, as needed, to a level slightly higher than the peak airway pressure generated by delivery of the preset tidal volume; however, one may have to lower inspiratory-flow rates and prolong the time for inspiration if the inspiratory pressure gets too high.

HIGH-FREQUENCY VENTILATORS.   High-frequency ventilation (HFV) involves several different methods by which the lung is ventilated at a frequency exceeding 60 cycles/minute (cpm). The modes of gas transport during HFV involve several different types of gas dispersion (Fig. 40–7). Compared to conventional ventilatory modes, HFV has several potential advantages. It reduces both mean airway pressure (P_{aw}) and PIP. This results in less impairment of venous return, reduced right ventricular afterload, and decreased likelihood of pulmonary barotrauma. Unfortunately, the tracheal mucosa can be seriously damaged by the low humidity of the gases often used.

AXIOM   HFV use after trauma is generally limited to upper airway surgery or management of bronchopulmonary fistulas.

HFV has proved suitable for bronchoscopy, laryngoscopy, and laryngeal or tracheal surgery.[199] It also appears to be helpful in treating large bronchopleural fistulas and controlling increased intracranial pressure.

In a prospective clinical trial of 35 patients suffering from severe posttraumatic and/or septic ARDS who were refractory to conventional controlled mechanical ventilatory (CMV) support, Borg et al. found that combined high-frequency ventilation (CHFV) resulted in a 23% survival of patients who were clinically and physiologically indistinguishable from those in the ARDS nonsurvivor group who were treated by CMV alone.[200]

CHFV utilizes two different breath rates. These include a base rate of six breaths/min and a superimposed HFV rate of 50 Hz. The superimposed HFV pulses are believed to improve gas distribution through enhanced convection, while the basal breath provides sufficient pressure to open and stabilize the airways. However, the base rate of six breaths/min combined with HFV tends to increase the effective end-expiratory pressure and mean airway pressures to unacceptable levels in some patients with noncompliant lungs.

Levels of Ventilatory Support

Various levels of ventilator support (full, partial, and total) have been defined.[15,201]

FULL VENTILATORY SUPPORT.   With full ventilatory support all of the work of breathing required to maintain eucapnia is provided by the ventilator.[15] This may be provided by controlled ventilation or with assist-control ventilation. With most patients, it is prudent to initiate full ventilator support and then consider either partial or total support when the patient is stabilized and the patient's cardiopulmonary status is more clearly defined.

Controlled Ventilation.   The control mode of ventilation is utilized when one wants the patient's breathing rate to be completely determined by the ventilator.[2] In this mode, the patient is not able to trigger inspiration independently, but receives breaths at a predetermined rate. To utilize this mode, one must slightly "overbreathe" the patient to lower arterial PCO_2 to remove the patient's ventilatory drive. The other alternative is to paralyze or heavily sedate the patient.

Assist-control Ventilation.   The assist-control mode of ventilatory support allows patients to initiate inspiration as directed by respiratory drive. In this mode, the machine is triggered to deliver a breath by inspiratory effort of the patient, which is sensed at the ventilator as slight negative pressure. A preset tidal volume is then delivered in the same way that it would have if the machine had been triggered by itself. If the patient breathes too rapidly, expiratory time (T_e) may be reduced to the point that air may be trapped in the alveoli producing auto-PEEP (Fig. 40–8). When the patient does not initiate any breaths, the ventilator is set to deliver tidal volumes at a rate to provide reasonable blood gases.

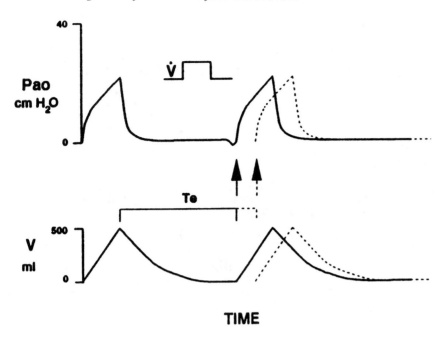

FIGURE 40–8 Airway opening pressure (Pao) and lung volume (V) during assist-control ventilation of a patient who is triggering the ventilator. The second breath was set to be delivered at the time marked by the dotted arrow; however, the patient triggered the ventilator at the time marked by the solid arrow, thereby decreasing the expiratory time (T_e) (From: Schmidt GA, Hall JB, Wood LDH. Management of the ventilated patient. Murray JF, Nadel JA, eds. Textbook of respiratory medicine, vol 2. Philadelphia: WB Saunders, 1994; 2645).

Unfortunately, many patients, particularly those with sepsis, delirium tremens, or severe brain damage, are tachypneic regardless of their minute ventilation and blood gases and can develop severe respiratory alkalosis. In some of these patients, intravenous sedatives or morphine can be used successfully to correct the excessive tachypnea. Occasionally, however, severe tachypnea cannot be controlled until or unless the patient is paralyzed pharmacologically.

PARTIAL VENTILATORY SUPPORT.   With partial ventilatory support, the patient provides an essential portion of the required work of breathing.[15] Ventilators designed to provide partial support permit the patient to breathe spontaneously to whatever extent is desirable without physiologic detriment, while the ventilator supplies the remaining work of breathing. In comparison with full ventilatory support, partial ventilatory support techniques have been shown to enhance cardiac output in patients with normal left ventricular function,[202] cause less hemodynamic compromise in conjunction with CPAP/PEEP therapy,[203] and allow for significantly greater urine output and renal blood flow.[204]

Patients who are not usually candidates for partial ventilator support include those with severe ventilatory muscle fatigue or severe chronic obstructive pulmonary disease.[205] Patients with cardiogenic shock and poor left ventricular reserve also tend to maintain better left ventricular function when all of the work of breathing is supplied by the ventilator.[206]

Intermittent Mandatory Ventilation.   Intermittent mandatory ventilation (IMV) has been proposed as a technique to help wean adults from mechanical-ventilatory support.[207] IMV consists basically of two independent circuits connected to the patient. In one circuit, patients can breath spontaneously from a reservoir bag, at whatever rate and depth they desire. The other circuit is connected to the ventilator, which delivers mandatory inspirations of a preset volume at a set rate. This allows the patient to breathe spontaneously as much as desired with mechanical inflations supplied at regular preset intervals that cannot be influenced by the patient.

One of the main physiologic advantages of IMV is the lower inspiratory intrapleural pressures during spontaneous breathing. This results in increased right-ventricular filling and cardiac output. Thus, IMV allows higher PEEP with fewer deleterious effects on venous return and cardiac output. Spontaneous breathing with IMV also promotes more normal matching of ventilation to perfusion.

AXIOM   Physiologic advantages to IMV include increased venous return and better V/Q relationships during spontaneous breathing. IMV also improves weaning from the ventilator in some patients.

Synchronized Intermittent Mandatory Ventilation.   Synchronized intermittent mandatory ventilation (SIMV) allows spontaneous breathing between mechanically-delivered ventilator breaths, but the mandatory ventilator breaths are synchronized to begin with the patient's next spontaneous inspiratory effort (Fig. 40–9). This technique was introduced because of concern that a mechanical breath may be introduced along with a spontaneous breath, causing great increases in peak inspiratory airway and intrapleural pressures.

Pressure-support Ventilation.   Pressure-support ventilation (PSV) is a form of mechanical ventilation in which the patient's spontaneous inspiratory efforts are augmented with a previously selected level of positive pressure so that airway pressure is held constant at an increased level throughout the inspiratory period.[208] The inspiratory pressure support in PSV is usually in the range of 5-15 cm H_2O. This pressure is held constant through servocontrol of the delivered flow and is terminated when the patient's inspiratory flow demand decreases to a preselected percentage of the initial peak mechanical inspiratory flow. Following this, passive exhalation occurs. PSV is different from conventional volume-cycled ventilation in that, with PSV, the clinician selects only the inspiratory pressure; the patient controls the ventilatory timing and interacts with the delivered pressure to determine the inspiratory flow and tidal volume (Fig. 40–10).

The patient's spontaneous work of breathing with PSV is less than with CPAP at the same pressure, and the technique is entirely different. In the PSV mode, the ventilator is triggered by the patient and continues to supply gas at a preselected positive-pressure limit throughout inspiration.[208] As long as the patient's inspiratory effort is maintained, the preselected airway pressure stays constant, with a variable flow of gas from the ventilator. The airway pressure, flow, and lung volume changes during PSV are more akin to assisted-mechanical ventilation than to spontaneous breathing with CPAP.

When 3-8 cm H_2O-pressure support is incorporated with SIMV or CPAP, the work of breathing imposed by the endotracheal tube, ventilator circuit, and demand valve system is reduced to that of a continuous flow system.[209] With levels > 10 cm H_2O, pressure sup-

FIGURE 40–9 Airway opening pressure (Pao), flow (V̇), and lung volume (V) during synchronized, intermittent, mandatory ventilation. Breath 1 (a mandatory breath) is not triggered by the patient. The rectangle near-breath 2 denotes the interval during which the ventilator is programmed to synchronize with an inspiratory effort by the patient, thereby delivering the mandatory breath slightly ahead of schedule. In breath 2, the patient triggers a breath within the window, receiving the same volume and flow as during a mandatory breath. Breath 3 is initiated before the synchronization interval and, therefore, it is not assisted. Flow and tidal volume (V_T) are totally determined by the patient's effort. When the patient fails to trigger another breath within the next synchronization window, a mandatory breath (4) is delivered (From: Schmidt GA, Hall JB, Wood LDH. Management of the ventilated patient. Murray JF, Nadel JA, eds. Textbook of respiratory medicine, vol 2. Philadelphia: WB Saunders, 1994; 2646).

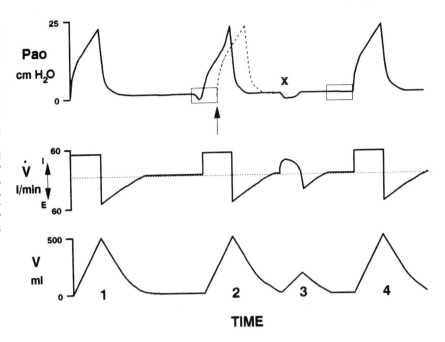

port may be considered an independent mode of ventilation. Most patients exhibit increases in tidal volume when pressure-support levels exceed 10 cm H_2O and decreases in respiratory rates at PSV levels of 20 cm H_2O.[210]

Pressure support is alleged to be superior to IMV or SIMV as a partial support mode because the work of breathing is assisted with every breath and many patients are more comfortable;[211] however, data confirming this assumption are not available.[15] In addition, when the patient initiates more than 20 cycles/minute, a higher incidence of auto-PEEP occurs.[212]

AXIOM Although the medical literature has not shown improved weaning from the ventilator with PSV, it seems to be extremely helpful.

The principle advantages of PSV are decreased patient work of breathing and improved subjective comfort. Wong et al. also noted that PSV can lower airway pressure (P_{aw}) compared to conventional positive-pressure or volume ventilation.[213] PSV can also enhance spontaneous tidal volume (V_T), thereby decreasing the need for mechanical breaths. Reducing the required number of mechanical breaths also decreases P_{aw}. Therefore, PSV may be helpful in ventilating some patients with bronchopleural fistulas.

Mandatory Minute Volume. Hewlett et al. described a technique called mandatory minute volume (MMV) in which the patient is guaranteed a preselected minute ventilation.[214] If the entire amount were breathed spontaneously, no augmentation by the ventilator would occur. When the spontaneous minute ventilation does not reach the pre-

FIGURE 40–10 Pressure-support ventilation. When a breath is triggered, airway opening pressure (Pao) increases to the set level (Pinsp). The flow and tidal volume (V_T) delivered depend on the Pinsp, respiratory system mechanics, and the patient effort. The first breath shown represents a patient who triggered the ventilator, then remains fully passive. During the middle breath, the patient makes a small but prolonged inspiratory effort. The Pao remains at the set inspiratory level as long as patient effort maintains some air flow, and a much longer inspiratory time (T_I) and a larger V_T result. In the final breath, a more powerful but briefer inspiratory effort is made, shortening the T_I but generating a larger V_T than during the passive breath. (I = inspiratory flow; E = expiratory flow.) (From: Schmidt GA, Hall JB, Wood LDH. Management of the ventilated patient. Murray JF, Nadel JA, eds. Textbook of respiratory medicine, vol 2. Philadelphia: WB Saunders, 1994; 2647).

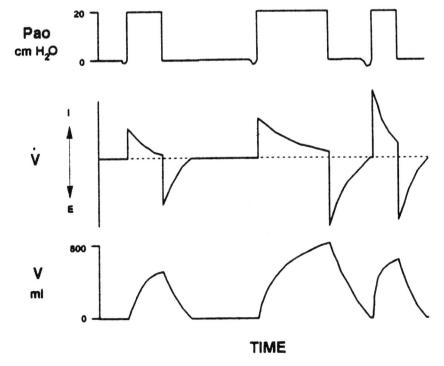

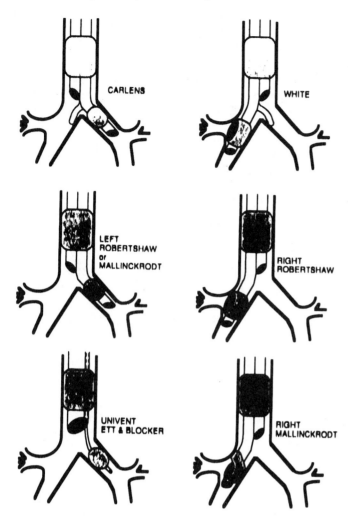

FIGURE 40–11 Schematic drawings of some common double-lumen tubes that can be used for synchronous, independent lung ventilation. (From: Tuxen D. Independent lung ventilation. Tobin MJ, ed. Principles and practice of mechanical ventilation. New York: McGraw-Hill, Inc., 1994; 572).

selected level, the portion that has not been breathed spontaneously is collected by the ventilator and delivered automatically. This is done by having the ventilator automatically add PS in 1-2 cm H_2O increments until the desired minute ventilation is reached.

Synchronous Independent Lung Ventilation. Significant unilateral lung injury is not infrequently encountered during the management of patients with severe multiple-organ system trauma. In many of these patients, the standard forms of mechanical ventilation can make the ventilation-perfusion abnormality worse by overexpanding the more normal lung. In such instances, use of an appropriately sized, double-lumen endobronchial catheter (Fig. 40–11) and synchronous independent lung ventilation can be much more effective.[215]

TOTAL VENTILATORY SUPPORT. With total ventilator support, pressure preset modes are applied to maintain a constant inspiratory pressure below a certain level for the purpose of avoiding volutrauma. Shapiro and Peruzzi believed that the term "total ventilatory support" is appropriate because neuromuscular blockade is imperative to optimize ventilation and oxygenation.[15]

No data justify the application of total ventilatory support techniques to patients without severe, acute lung disease.[15] Total ventilator support has three major liabilities that must be considered: (a) hemodynamic instability is commonly encountered when the technique

is initiated, (b) neuromuscular blockade must be initiated and maintained, and (c) eucapnic ventilation may not be obtained.[15]

Pressure-controlled Ventilation. With pressure-controlled ventilation (PCV), inspiratory gas flow is provided in the same manner as the pressure-support mode, but the cycle is both initiated and ended by preset time factors[15] (Figs. 40–12, 40–13). Both pressure-control and pressure-release modes begin inspiration at preset time intervals, rapidly achieve the preset circuit pressure, maintain the preset inspiratory pressure while inspiratory flow varies, and end the inspiratory cycle at a preset time interval. Assuming an adequate inspiratory time, the delivered tidal volume is determined by the preset airway pressure and pulmonary compliance.

Hickling et al. managed 50 patients with severe ARDS by limitation of the peak inspiratory pressure, disregarding the resultant hypercapnia.[216] Tidal volumes were reduced to as low as 5 mL/kg. The mean maximum $PaCO_2$ was 62 torr and the highest $PaCO_2$ was 129 torr. No specific treatment was given for the respiratory acidosis that developed, and no statistical difference was found in the maximum

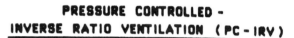

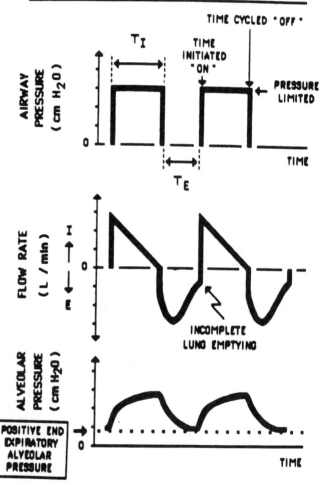

FIGURE 40–12 In this example of PC-IRV, the inhalation time (T_I) is approximately twice as long as the exhalation time (T_E). The mechanical inhalation phase is time-initiated "ON," pressure-limited, time-cycled "OFF," and a decelerating inspiratory flow waveform is generated. Because the decreased exhalation time prevents full exhalation, incomplete lung emptying occurs, resulting in intrinsic or auto-PEEP. (From: Banner MJ, Lampotang S, Blanch PB, Kirby RR. Mechanical ventilation. Civetta JM, Taylor RW, Kirby RF, eds. Critical care, 2nd ed. Philadelphia: JB Lippincott Co, 1992; 1403).

FIGURE 40–13 Pressure-control ventilation. The left-hand tracing shows a pressure-control breath with normal resistance, during which inspiratory pressure (Pao) equilibrates with alveolar pressure (Palv) before the inspiratory cycle is terminated. Tidal volume (V_T) can be predicted from the Pinsp and static respiratory system compliance. In the right-hand tracing, inspiratory resistance is elevated. At the same Pao, inspiratory flow is reduced, and the V_T (solid line) falls below what is predicted by the Cstat and Pinsp (dotted line) (From: Schmidt GA, Hall JB, Wood LDH. Management of the ventilated patient. Murray JF, Nadel JA, eds. Textbook of respiratory medicine, vol 2. Philadelphia: WB Saunders, 1994; 2646).

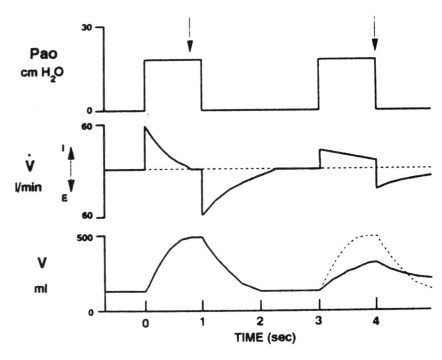

$PaCO_2$ of survivors and nonsurvivors. The group mortality rate of 16% was significantly lower than what was predicted by the Acute Physiology and Chronic Health Evaluation II (APACHE II) scoring system (40%), and only a single death was attributed to respiratory failure.

AXIOM Use of PCV should be considered in virtually all patients who require peak inspiratory pressures > 50 cm H_2O.

Volume Support Ventilation. Volume support ventilation (VSV), a mode of ventilation used in some patients with severe respiratory failure, involves a combination of pressure-regulated volume control and pressure support.[217] With VSV, when the patient triggers the ventilator, a controlled tidal volume is delivered in a pressure-limited way with decelerating flow using the lowest possible pressure. Each inspiration is terminated when the inspiratory flow has decreased to

20% of peak flow or after 80% of the set cycle time has elapsed. In this way, patients can determine their own frequency and inspiration times; ventilation is adapted to changes in the each patient's compliance, breath by breath.[217]

Inverse Ratio Ventilation. Normally, the ratio of inspiratory time (I) to expiratory time (E) is 1:2, 1:3, or 1:4. Positive-pressure ventilation with the inspiratory time (I) equal to or less than the expiratory time (E) is referred to as inverse ratio ventilation (IRV). IRV can be provided with PCV or volume control ventilation (VCV) (Fig. 40–14) and has been used successfully to treat a number of infants and adults with severe respiratory failure not responding to other types of ventilatory support.[218,219] IRV improves gas exchange by a progressive alveolar recruitment, but it may take several hours for such recruitment to be fully accomplished. In a study of 18 adults with acute respiratory failure, Ravizza et al. found that compared to IPPV, 6

FIGURE 40–14 Inverse ratio ventilation (IRV). The first panel shows pressure-controlled IRV (PC-IRV) in which airway opening pressure (Pao) during inspiration is held constant and expiratory time (T_E) is shortened to invert the inspiratory to expiratory (I:E) time ratio. With the short T_E, interruption of expiratory flow occurs at end-expiration (i.e., intrinsic PEEP is present). The second panel shows volume controlled IRV (VC-IRV) with a square-wave-flow pattern in which an end-inspiratory pause is used to invert the I:E ratio. The peak pressure is higher than during equivalent PC-IRV because flow remains high at end-inspiration (when elastic recoil is maximal). Auto-PEEP is also present. In the third panel, IRV is created by using a decelerating flow profile. The peak airway pressure is midway between the other two modes because a small end-inspiratory flow is present. In all three cases, the mean lung volume and mean alveolar pressure are increased compared to ventilator modes having normal I:E ratios (From: Schmidt GA, Hall JB, Wood LDH. Management of the ventilated patient. Murray JF, Nadel JA, eds. Textbook of respiratory medicine, vol 2. Philadelphia: WB Saunders, 1994; 2649).

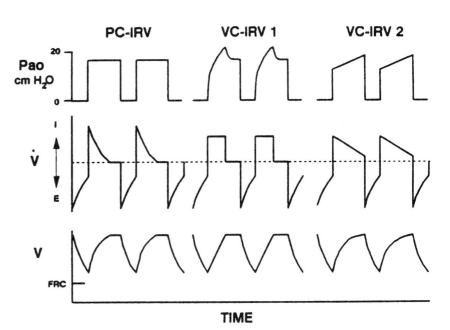

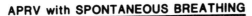

APRV with SPONTANEOUS BREATHING

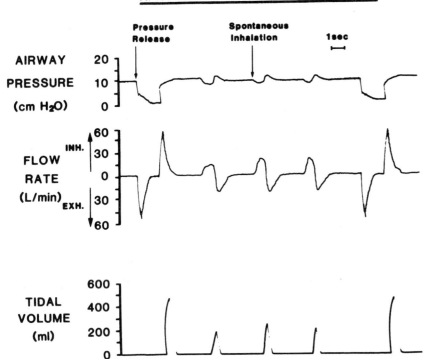

FIGURE 40–15 Airway pressure, flow rate, and tidal volume waveforms of a spontaneously breathing patient receiving airway pressure release ventilation (APRV). With APRV, the patient is allowed to breathe spontaneously, as desired, on continuous positive airway pressure. At regular, preselected intervals, a release valve opens, allowing pressure and volume from the lungs to be released. After a preselected release time has elapsed, the release valve closes and the level of CPAP is restored, gas flow fills the lungs, and a tidal volume is applied (From: Banner MJ, Lampotang S, Blanch PB, Kirby RR. Mechanical ventilation. Civetta JM, Taylor RW, Kirby RF, eds. Critical care, 2nd ed. Philadelphia: JB Lippincott Co, 1992; 1411).

hours of IRV significantly improved PaO_2/FiO_2 ratios and static compliance.[220] A decrease also occurred in the PIP.

In a study of 11 trauma patients with severe ARDS, Samuels et al., found that within 24 hours, IRV-PC significantly increased the mean PaO_2/FiO_2 ratio from 70 to 149 mm Hg with little change in DO_2 (996 versus 1053 mL/minute) or VO_2 (336 versus 357 mL/minute).[221] In a similar study of 16 trauma patients, Simon et al. found that IRV significantly reduced PIP in all patients, and in 13 of 16 patients an increase in PaO_2/FiO_2 ratio also occurred.[222] Oxygen delivery decreased (774 to 721 mL/min²) as did cardiac output (9.8 to 8.9 L/minute), but these values were still above normal. In spite of these data, no general agreement exists about the advantages of IRV over conventional I:E ratios with sufficient PEEP to obtain the same increase in lung volume.[223]

Airway Pressure Release Ventilation. Airway pressure release ventilation (APRV) increases alveolar ventilation by intermittently releasing continuous positive pressure generated by the ventilator (Fig. 40–15). In passive patients, APRV is identical to PC-IRV; however, the patient's ability to breathe spontaneously during APRV creates a markedly different intrapleural pressure waveform.[224]

Two types of APRV can be used: APRV during which the pressure release time is preset,[225] and intermittent mandatory pressure release ventilation (IMPRV). Both are specifically designed for assisting spontaneously breathing patients.[224] When compared with CMV plus PEEP in patients with acute respiratory failure, APRV has been shown to produce similar hemodynamic effects at similar mean airway pressures.[226] However, it is not intended for patients with severe airflow obstruction; if the patient's respiratory rate were to increase above 30/minute, auto-PEEP would become a limiting factor and IMPRV would no longer be an efficient method of ventilatory support.

GASES TO BE DELIVERED

The gases most frequently used in mechanical ventilation are oxygen and compressed air. Whenever possible, the oxygen concentration is limited to the minimum required to provide reasonable oxygenation of the blood (i.e., arterial oxygen saturation of at least 90%), particularly when an $FiO_2 > 0.5$ is required to do that. When high ventila-

tory pressures are required, one may have to be satisfied with a PaO_2 of 50-59 mm Hg.

AXIOM In most situations where a ventilator is used, the injured patient needs mechanical assistance, and providing additional oxygen is only a secondary consideration.

When initially ventilating the patient, it may be wise to use 100% oxygen ($FiO_2 = 1.0$) for at least 20 minutes, and then obtain a set of blood gases. This allows one to determine what FiO_2 is probably needed to maintain PaO_2 of about 60-80 mm Hg.

TIDAL VOLUME

AXIOM Efforts to keep $PaCO_2$ normal or low with high-tidal volumes or minute ventilation may damage the lungs.

Tidal volume is generally started at about 10-12 mL/kg. Using a ventilatory rate of 10-18/min, V_t is usually adjusted to provide a $PaCO_2$ of 35-40 mm Hg. An increasing tendency, however, exists to use low-tidal volumes as low as 5-7 mL/kg to prevent volutrauma (overdistension of alveoli). This hypoventilation results in "permissive hypercapnia" which appears to be well-tolerated as long as the $PaCO_2$ is allowed to increase slowly so that plasma bicarbonate levels can increase and prevent severe decreases in arterial pH.

AIRWAY PRESSURE

AXIOM Efforts should be made to keep the PIP from exceeding 50 cm H_2O.

The airway pressure required to inflate the lungs properly varies greatly from patient to patient and is largely dependent on the tidal volume used, the inspiratory flow rate, and the resistance of the airway, lungs, and chest wall. In general, plateau pressures (during an inspiratory hold) < 40 cm H_2O in a paralyzed patient or 50 cm H_2O in patient without paralysis are relatively safe, but alveolar inflation pressures > 50-60 cm H_2O increase the risk of trauma to the lungs.[207]

When a certain tidal volume seems to be needed, but the ventilatory pressures are too high, one can often reduce these pressures by decreasing the inspiratory flow rate, prolonging the inspiratory time, or using PCV. Patients with high ventilatory pressures may also have increased pleural fluid that may not be detected clinically.

VENTILATORY RATE

Normally, a ventilatory rate of 8-18/minute with an inspiration-to-expiratory-time ratio (I/E) of 1:2 is used. In patients with either acute or chronic restrictive lung disease, ventilatory rates exceeding 20/minute may be necessary, depending on the desired V_E and targeted $PaCO_2$.

POSITIVE END-EXPIRATORY PRESSURE

PEEP is probably the most effective supportive therapy in ARDS.[228] The major pulmonary effects of CPAP/PEEP therapy are redistribution of extravascular lung water from the less compliant interstitial spaces (between the alveolar epithelium and capillary endothelium where gas exchange occurs) to the more compliant interstitial spaces (toward the peribronchial and hilar areas). Recruitment of collapsed alveoli also occurs.[228] The redistribution of extravascular lung water also results in improved oxygen diffusion and improved lung compliance when pulmonary edema is present.[229]

The use of PEEP was shown by Ashbaugh and Petty in 1973 to improve oxygenation markedly and thereby reduce the need for high-inspired concentrations of oxygen in hypoxemic patients.[230] PEEP can be used for any mode of ventilation, even for patients breathing spontaneously.

Actions of PEEP

AXIOM The main functions of PEEP are to keep alveoli expanded during expiration and increase the patient's functional residual capacity back toward normal.

PEEP reduces intrapulmonary shunting and can usually correct hypoxemia that is unresponsive to a high FiO_2 by recruiting (reopening) previously collapsed alveoli.[1] Reopening alveoli often cannot be accomplished by simply ventilating the lungs with large tidal volumes because many collapsed alveoli are on a relatively flat compliance curve,[231] and their reexpansion requires not only elevated airway pressure but also prolonged maintenance of those pressures.

The second role of PEEP is to "splint" the lung in an inflated state by keeping unstable alveoli open at end-expiration.[232] The third role of PEEP is to improve lung compliance and thereby facilitate ventilation. Because less effort must be spent to open alveoli on the flat portion of the compliance curve, the amount of lung expansion per unit of alveolar-distending-pressure increases. Finally, PEEP acting on alveoli that contain fluid tends to "spread the fluid out" over a larger area so that the distance for oxygen to diffuse from alveoli into capillaries is reduced.

In a study of the effects of high levels of PEEP ($>$ 15 cm H_2O) in 59 trauma patients with ARDS, Miller et al. increased PEEP until the Q_{sp}/Q_t was $\leq$ 20% and the FiO_2 was $\leq$ 0.50.[233] This therapy increased the PaO_2/FiO_2 ratio from 138 $\pm$ 89 to 243 $\pm$ 87 mm Hg, decreased the Q_{sp}/Q_t from 39 $\pm$ 18% to 22 $\pm$ 12%, and increased the DO_2I from 396 $\pm$ 132 to 476 $\pm$ 136 mL/min/m^2 (P $<$ 0.05).

Limitations of PEEP

AXIOM Although PEEP appears to be an important part of the treatment of ARDS, in many studies, it does not prevent ARDS, reduce its incidence, or alter its course or outcome.[234]

Little or no need appears to exist for instituting more than "physiologic" levels of PEEP (3-5 cm H_2O), unless increasing hypoxemia is present with ventilated patients. Increasing lung volume and airway pressure by the use of PEEP can block pulmonary lymphatics.[235] Finally, PEEP may compress the capillaries of compliant alveoli,

shifting blood from these vessels to those perfusing noncompliant, poorly ventilated alveoli.[1] Thus, when PEEP is initially added, it may paradoxically increase intrapulmonary shunt and decrease PaO_2.

Problems with PEEP

AXIOM The major problems with PEEP are related to its tendency to reduce venous return and cardiac output, especially with levels $>$ 10-15 cm H_2O.

The relationship between PEEP and cardiac output is determined by several mechanisms.[236] PEEP increases intrathoracic pressure which, in turn, decreases venous return to the heart. To some extent, this effect can be offset by increasing intravascular volume. PEEP also increases pulmonary vascular resistance and right ventricular afterload. PEEP can also cause sufficient right ventricular dilation to impinge on the left ventricle and decrease its filling;[237] however, the extent of these changes is controversial.

Applying PEEP

PEEP is usually applied in 2.5-5.0 cm H_2O increments. PEEP can be changed fairly rapidly, but it takes at least 20-30 minutes for it to exert its full effect on oxygenation. If the improvement in PaO_2 were not adequate, PEEP can be increased by another increment.[1] Simultaneous monitoring of SaO_2 by pulse oximeter and of SvO_2 by continuous, mixed venous oximetry catheter may expedite estimation of intrapulmonary shunt (Q_{sp}/Q_t), oxygen utilization, and oxygen extraction.[238] These indices may be estimated as follows:

$$Q_{sp}/Q_t = 1\text{-}SaO_2 \: / \: 1\text{-}SvO_2$$
$$O_2 \text{ extraction} = SaO_2\text{-}SvO_2/SaO_2$$

In other words, if the SaO_2 is 90% and the SvO_2 is 70%, the Q_s/Q_t would be (1.0-0.90)/(1.0-0.70) = .10/.30 = 33%. The O_2 extraction would be 20/90 = 22%.

It is also important to monitor cardiac output, oxygen delivery (DO_2), and oxygen consumption (VO_2), particularly when PEEP is increased $>$ 10 cm H_2O. PEEP tends to reduce venous return, cardiac output, and oxygen delivery unless increased fluids or blood and/or inotropes are given as the PEEP is increased.

AXIOM When optimizing the level of PEEP in a patient, it is essential to also maintain optimal DO_2 and VO_2 by giving fluids, blood, or inotropes as needed.

End-points for PEEP

Although PEEP has been used for almost 20 years since it was first described by Ashbaugh and Petty,[230] the "optimal" level of PEEP is still controversial. Initially, optimal PEEP was believed to be the level that provided the best overall lung compliance[239] (Fig. 40–11). Later, "best PEEP" was believed to be the level of PEEP that achieved the lowest Q_{sp}/Q_t without a physiologically significant decrease in cardiac output.[240] The term, "rational PEEP" has been used by some to indicate the level of PEEP that maintains an adequate DO_2 but allows FiO_2 to be reduced to $\leq$ 0.5. Many physicians increase PEEP until the PaO_2 is at least 60 mm Hg on an FiO_2 of $\leq$ 0.5.

Other goals that have been emphasized as therapeutic end-points for PEEP include: (a) pulmonary shunt of $<$ 15-20% (even if "super-PEEP" [greater than 30 cm H_2O] must be used),[241] (b) decreased dead space determined by monitoring arterial to end-tidal CO_2 gradients,[242] (c) PaO_2/FiO_2 ratio $>$ 200,[234] and/or (d) the "least PEEP" possible so as to minimize complications.[235]

Auto-PEEP

Patients with airflow limitation or high-minute ventilation may have end-expiratory lung volumes exceeding normal FRC because the rate of lung emptying is slowed and expiration is interrupted by the next inspiratory effort.[243,244] This abnormally increased end-expiratory

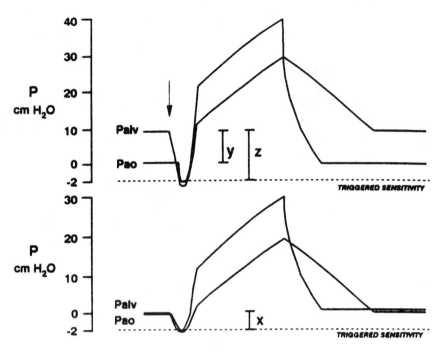

FIGURE 40–16 Effects of intrinsic PEEP on triggering. The lower tracings of airway opening pressure (PaO) and alveolar pressure (Palv) represent a patient who is triggering volume-cycled ventilator breaths and who does not have intrinsic PEEP. The upper tracing shows a patient similarly ventilated, but who has about 10.0 cm H_2O auto-PEEP. The patient without PEEP has to lower the Palv by only 2 cm H_2O to trigger a breath. In contrast, the patient with auto-PEEP must lower the Palv by about 10 cm H_2O before having any impact on Pao, then the Palv must be reduced a further 2 cm H_2O negative pressure to trigger the ventilator (From: Schmidt GA, Hall JB, Wood LDH. Management of the ventilated patient. Murray JF, Nadel JA, eds. Textbook of respiratory medicine, vol 2. Philadelphia: WB Saunders, 1994; 2648).

lung volume is termed dynamic hyperinflation, auto-PEEP, or intrinsic PEEP.

Although PEEP may be helpful in managing patients with severe pulmonary dysfunction, excessive auto-PEEP should be avoided. Adverse effects of auto-PEEP include: (a) the respiratory muscles operate at an unfavorable position on their length-tension curve, (b) an increased elastic load exists, and (c) breathing takes place at a higher, less compliant portion of the pressure-volume curve of the lung. A much greater reduction in alveolar pressure may also be required to trigger the ventilator (Fig. 40–16).

AXIOM If further increases in tidal volume and/or ventilatory rate in a patient with a high-minute ventilation cause an increase in the PaCO$_2$, one should suspect that significant auto-PEEP is present.

When the expiratory port of the ventilator circuit is occluded immediately before the onset of the next breath, the pressure in the lungs and ventilator circuit will equilibrate, and the level of auto-PEEP will be displayed on the ventilator manometer. The level of auto-PEEP can also be estimated from continuous recordings of airway pressure and flow during mechanical ventilation. Auto-PEEP has also been determined by monitoring changes in end-expiratory volume using inductive plethysmography.[245]

AXIOM When the patient's ventilatory flow rate tracing indicates that the next inspiration interrupts an expiratory effort, auto-PEEP is present.

Therapeutic measures to reduce the level of auto-PEEP include bronchodilators, a larger diameter endotracheal tube, decreased minute ventilation by controlling fever and pain, and decreased inspiratory time/expiratory time (I:E) ratio by increasing the inspiratory flow rate and/or using nondistensible tubing in the ventilator circuit.

CPAP and sPEEP

Continuous positive airway pressure (CPAP) and spontaneous positive end-expiratory pressure (sPEEP) are positive-pressure modes used during spontaneous breathing[246] (Fig. 40–17). With CPAP, both the inspiratory and expiratory pressures are positive, although the inspiratory level may be less. With sPEEP, airway pressure is zero or negative (subambient) during inspiration, but it is increased at the end of expiration to a predetermined positive pressure. The level of CPAP

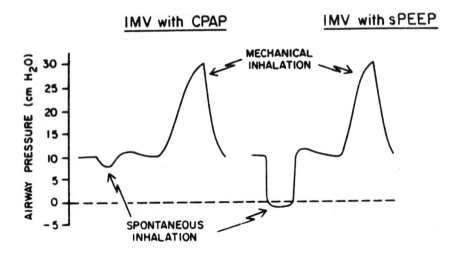

FIGURE 40–17 Intermittent, mandatory ventilation combined with CPAP and sPEEP. Less work of breathing is required with CPAP (From: Banner MJ, Lampotang S, Blanch PB, Kirby RR. Mechanical ventilation. Civetta JM, Taylor RW, Kirby RF, eds. Critical care, 2nd ed. Philadelphia: JB Lippincott Co, 1992; 1403).

or sPEEP used is designed to increase expiratory transpulmonary pressure and functional residual capacity.

FREQUENCY OF SIGHING

AXIOM Intermittent sighing is an important method for preventing atelectasis in patients taking frequent, small, spontaneous or ventilator breaths.

Under normal circumstances, individuals spontaneously take at least four to six deep breaths (sighs) each hour. This inflates many of the alveoli that are not expanded with the usual tidal volumes. When a patient is put on a ventilator, especially of the volume-limited type, the resultant fixed tidal volume, when provided for prolonged periods, allows atelectasis to develop in areas that are poorly ventilated. To prevent this from occurring, it is important to hyperinflate the lungs at least two to three times each hour with a tidal volume $1\frac{1}{2}$ to 2 times greater than normal, providing that the inflation pressures do not exceed 50-60 cm H_2O. The optimal frequency of sighing varies from patient to patient, but 6 times per hour appears to be satisfactory for most patients.

NEBULIZATION AND HUMIDIFICATION

In general, one should provide the maximum humidity possible to patients on a ventilator because of the drying effect that most ventilators have on the tracheobronchial tree. In small patients, however, particularly those with heart disease, some of the newer machines can provide so much moisture that the quantity of fluid absorbed through the alveoli and bronchial mucosa may overload the circulation and cause congestive heart failure.

Monitoring Ventilatory Support

MONITORING THE VENTILATOR

Ventilatory parameters requiring frequent monitoring are tidal volume, respiratory rate, PIP, plateau pressure (during an inspiratory hold), PEEP, FiO_2, and minute ventilation. The patient and the ventilatory equipment should be monitored at least every one to two hours. This includes auscultation of the chest for bilateral air entry and the location of rales and rhonchi.

PITFALL ⊘

Failure to follow PIP levels in ventilated patients can result in delayed diagnosis of tension pneumothorax or worsening of pulmonary function.

A rapid increase in PIP may be the result of a mucous plug, pneumothorax, kinking of the endotracheal tube, or slipping into a mainstem bronchus. A slow increase in airway pressure is usually an indication of increasing lung stiffness and deteriorating pulmonary function. A rapid decrease in pressure usually indicates a ventilator or circuit disconnection or an endotracheal cuff leak. A slow decrease in airway pressure may indicate improvement in lung compliance, decrease in airway resistance, or slow air leak.

MONITORING THE PATIENT

AXIOM The patient who is awake, alert, comfortable, and cooperative, and has normal vital signs on a ventilator is generally doing well, even if arterial blood gases are not optimal.

When the patient appears to be anxious or fighting the ventilator, something is usually wrong with the airway, the ventilatory, or its settings, and should be corrected as soon as possible. In comatose patients, it can be difficult to judge how well the patient is tolerating ventilatory support.

BLOOD GASES

AXIOM In critically injured patients in the ICU, obtaining venous blood gases at the same time as arterial blood gases provides a great deal more physiologic information.

Arterial and Venous Samples

Arterial blood gases (ABG) and mixed venous blood gases (VBG) should be analyzed at least once a day for every patient on a ventilator. In addition, ABG and VBG should be drawn with any clinical cardiopulmonary change or with any change in therapy.

Arterial Po_2 should be kept > 60 mm Hg, and preferably at 70-80 mm Hg, unless one would have to increase the $FiO_2 > 0.5$ or use high-ventilatory pressures. Although $PaCO_2$ has traditionally been kept at about 35-40 mm Hg in most trauma patients on a ventilator, an increasing tendency exists to allow some hypercapnea to reduce high-inflation pressures. In a recent study by Simon et al. of 10 trauma patients, hypercarbia to a mean PCO_2 of 54 mm Hg (range = 45-96) was permitted for 6 ± 3 days.[247] Mean HCO_3 increased to 30.9 ± 3.9 mEq/L. Cardiovascular function remained supranormal with a mean cardiac output of 11.3 ± 2.6 L/minute and mean DO_2 of 878 ± 252 mL/minute/m². Neurologic status was also unchanged.

The oxygen delivery index (DO_2I), oxygen consumption index (VO_2I), and pulmonary shunting (Q_{sp}/Q_t) should also be followed. Efforts should be made to increase DO_2I until: (a) VO_2I is at least 160 mL/minute/m² or (b) VO_2I does not increase any further when DO_2 is increased. There should also be no lactic acidosis.

Pulmonary Artery Saturation

A number of pulmonary artery catheters has been developed to continuously monitor mixed venous oxygen saturation (SvO_2). Normal SvO_2 is about 70-75%. When decreases occur in cardiac output, arterial oxygen content, or oxygen delivery, or oxygen consumption increases, mixed venous oxygen saturation tends to decrease. Thus, changes in the SvO_2 can provide early warning of problems with the lungs or cardiovascular system.

When SvO_2 increases to $\geq 80\%$, the catheter tip may have wedged into a small pulmonary artery so that pulmonary capillary (oxygenated) blood is being analyzed. Other possibilities include an increase in cardiac output (as from sepsis or use of vasodilator) or a decrease in oxygen consumption (as with excess sedation or hypothermia). Development of a left-to-right shunt or severe hyperoxia ($PaO_2 > 200$-300 mm Hg) may also make SvO_2 increase.

A decrease in $SvO_2 < 50$-60% is usually due to a significant decrease in cardiac output or lung function so that oxygen delivery to the tissues is reduced. It could also be due to an increase in oxygen consumption.[248] Although a sudden decrease in SvO_2 often indicates important physiologic changes, the patient's condition can deteriorate seriously sometimes without any change in SvO_2.

PITFALL ⊘

Assuming that a patient's cardiovascular and pulmonary systems are stable because the SvO_2 hasn't changed.

Intraarterial Probes

Intravascular probes using fiberoptic light channels and specific fluorescent compounds to continuously measure pH, PaO_2, and $PaCO_2$ have been developed.[249] One of these probes is so small that it will pass through a 20-gauge catheter, leaving sufficient clearance for pressure measurements and for blood sampling. Although clinical experience with them is limited, these intravascular fiberoptic "blood gas machines" should find wide acceptance as the technology is perfected.

Pulse Oximetry

AXIOM The main value of pulse oximetry is its ability to provide early warning of potentially dangerous trends in pulmonary or cardiovascular function.

Continuous monitoring of oxygen saturation and pulse amplitude in the fingers, toes, or ears with pulse oximetry can provide early warning of pulmonary or cardiovascular deterioration before it becomes clinically apparent.[250] This technique employs a microprocessor that continuously measures pulse rate and oxyhemoglobin saturation. When compared with ABGs, pulse oximeter is accurate ± 2-3%.

Pulse oximetry has many advantages that make it ideal for use in the ICU.[251] However, impaired local perfusion, abnormal hemoglobin, and high PO_2 can limit its accuracy and usefulness. Carboxyhemoglobin and fetal hemoglobin falsely increase oximeter-saturation readings, whereas methemoglobin decreases them.[251]

Capnography

Capnography, by monitoring the PCO_2 in expired gases, can provide a real-time estimate of $PaCO_2$. This can assess ventilatory adequacy, respiratory gas exchange, carbon dioxide production, and the cardiovascular status of the patient.[252] Although the measurement of end-tidal carbon dioxide ($ETCO_2$) underestimates $PaCO_2$ by 2-6 mm Hg in patients on a ventilator, the difference is constant for a given patient provided the dead space/tidal volume ratio (V_d/V_t) and airway resistance do not change.

AXIOM An increase in $P(a-ET)CO_2$ may reflect increased dead space on the lungs, and this should make one suspect pulmonary embolus, a drastic reduction in cardiac output, and/or increased ventilation-perfusion mismatching in the lung.

Because carbon dioxide production is directly dependent on metabolic rate, many conditions can decrease $ETCO_2$. However, sudden decreases in $ETCO_2$ suggest mechanical problems in the airway or hypoventilation. A gradual decrease in $ETCO_2$ is usually due to increased dead space or to reduced pulmonary blood flow. Increases in $ETCO_2$ are generally due to hypermetabolic states.[252] If a simultaneous $PaCO_2$ were available, one could calculate the arterial-end tidal PCO_2 difference [$P(a-ET)CO_2$].

AXIOM Whenever possible, tissue perfusion should be increased and tidal volume adjusted to keep $P_{ET}CO_2$ at ≥ 29 mm Hg and the $P(a-ET)CO_2$ ≤ 7 mm Hg.[152]

In a recent study of 100 critically ill or injured patients during general anesthesia, patients with $P_{ET}CO_2$ values of 29 mm Hg or more and $P(a-ET)CO_2$ of 8 mm Hg or less had a much better prognosis than patients who did not.[152] Even when other parameters suggested that the patient was doing well, a $P_{ET}CO_2$ ≤ 28 mm Hg or a $P(a-ET)CO_2$ ≥ 9 mm Hg indicated that resuscitation and/or ventilation of the patient were not optimal.

Transcutaneous Monitoring

Transcutaneous oxygen and carbon dioxide tensions ($PTC-O_2$ and $PTC-CO_2$) can be used to provide early warning of disturbed pulmonary function or systemic circulation, as well as for the evaluation of local tissue perfusion. Comparative studies have indicated that $PTC-O_2$ and $PTC-CO_2$ are often more sensitive indicators of circulatory changes than are arterial pressure, heart rate, CVP, ECG, and urine output.[253] If tissue perfusion is severely reduced, $PTC-O_2$ and $PTC-CO_2$ values deviate from their relationship with arterial partial pressures and become flow-dependent.

Conjunctival O_2 and CO_2 Measurements

If cardiac output is adequate, conjunctival PO_2 ($PCJ-O_2$) would reflect PaO_2. However, during hemorrhagic shock, $PCJ-O_2$ reflects car-

diac output rather than PaO_2. If the PaO_2 is adequate, the $PCJ-O_2$, like the $PTC-CO_2$, would reflect local tissue perfusion.[254] Because the conjunctivae are supplied by the ophthalmic branch of the internal carotid artery, the $PCJ-O_2$ may also reflect carotid arterial oxygen transport.[255]

Criteria for Ventilatory Weaning

GENERAL CONDITION OF THE PATIENT

One should not attempt to wean patients from a ventilator when they are hemodynamically unstable or when the problem that initially necessitated the mechanical support has not been corrected. The patient to be weaned should not be septic, and chest radiography should be improving or at least "stable."

PHYSICAL EXAMINATION

AXIOM Rapid, shallow breathing, respiratory alternans, or abdominal paradox during attempts at spontaneous breathing generally indicate that the patient is not ready to be weaned from the ventilator.

Three physical findings that can be seen during spontaneous ventilation that generally predict weaning failure include: (a) rapid shallow breathing, (b) respiratory alternans (i.e., alternating between abdominal and rib cage breathing), and (c) abdominal paradox (inward movement of the abdominal wall during inspiration). All of these tend to indicate that the patient's ventilatory muscles are weak and/or will fatigue easily.

WEANING PARAMETERS

Tests to help determine whether a patient is ready for withdrawal from ventilatory support can be separated into three areas of assessment: ability to oxygenate, resting ventilatory needs, and ventilatory mechanical capability. Young, cooperative, otherwise healthy patients can often be successfully weaned even though they do not meet these criteria.

AXIOM In elderly and uncooperative individuals, particularly those with other organ system dysfunction, even the presence of optimal criteria does not guarantee successful weaning.

Oxygenation

In general, the lower the FiO_2 needed to maintain a PaO_2 of at least 60 and preferably 70-80 mm Hg, the more likely the weaning process is to be successful. Ear or finger oximetry measurements may occasionally be substituted for PaO_2 values when the patient is on ≤ 30% oxygen. The venous admixture or shunting in the lungs (Q_{sp}/Q_t), which is normally 3-5%, should also be < 15-20% before one attempts to wean the patient from ventilatory support.

Ventilatory Performance at Rest

pH-PCO_2. Arterial PCO_2 is largely dependent on alveolar ventilation and metabolic rate of the patient. Increased carbon dioxide production or increased dead space must be matched with an increased minute ventilation to maintain a steady $PaCO_2$. Fever, sepsis, shivering, and/or high-glucose loads during TPN increase carbon dioxide production and ventilatory demands. A PCO_2 higher than one would expect from the pH generally indicates that one should not attempt weaning, unless the patient has COPD with chronic hypercarbia.

V_D/V_T. The normal dead space/tidal volume ratio (V_d/V_t) is about 0.3. If it exceeds 0.6, the patient cannot usually be weaned from ventilatory support. Small increases in V_d/V_t > 0.6 generally require large increases in minute ventilation (V_E) in order to maintain a given $PaCO_2$ level.

MINUTE VENTILATION. Normal minute ventilation (V_E) in a typical adult male is about 6 L/minute or about 3.5 L/minute/m². It should usually be < 10-12 L/minute (5.8-7.0 L/minute/m²) before the patient can be weaned from the ventilator. The maximal voluntary ventilation that a patient can maintain for prolonged periods is usually only about double the resting minute ventilation.[256]

RESPIRATORY RATE. The respiratory rate (machine breaths plus spontaneous breaths) ideally should be < 20/minute, and preferably < 30/minute, before attempting weaning. During a minute of spontaneous breathing, it has been found that when the respiratory rate (RR) increases to > 37/minute, the weaning failure rate was 80% (12/15).[256] In contrast, if RR was ≤ 25/minute, the failure rate was only 13% (2/15).

RESPIRATORY RATE/TIDAL VOLUME RATIO. Yang and Tobin, in a retrospective study of indices predicting the outcome of trials of weaning from mechanical ventilation, found that rapid, shallow breathing, as reflected by RR/tidal volume ratio (RR/V_t) during one minute of spontaneous breathing, was the most accurate predictor of weaning failure.[257] If the RR/V_t ratio were ≥ 100 breaths/minute/L (i.e., RR ≥ 30 with a V_t ≤ 0.3 L), 95% (19/20) of the patients failed the weaning attempt. At an RR/V_t ratio of 80-100 breaths/minute/L, the failure rate was 50% (6/12), and with an RR/V_t ratio ≤ 80, the weaning failure rate was 9% (3/32).

OXYGEN COST OF BREATHING. The oxygen cost of breathing (OCOB) is calculated from the difference in oxygen consumption between spontaneous breathing and total mechanical ventilation. Shikora et al. studied 28 patients, five of whom could be successfully extubated;[258] the OCOB was 1 ± 9% in those who were weaned successfully and 22 ± 19% in those who could not be weaned (P < 0.02).

MECHANICAL CAPABILITY. The two mechanical ventilatory parameters that have been used most frequently to evaluate a patient's ability to be weaned are forced vital capacity (FVC) and maximum negative inspiratory force (NIF).[256]

AXIOM   An FVC < 10 mL/kg or NIF < 25 cm H₂O usually indicates that the patient is not ready for weaning.

FVC. FVC depends on muscular strength, motivation, and respiratory system compliance. A normal vital capacity in young adults is about 65-70 mL/kg, and patients usually need an FVC of at least 10 mL/kg, and preferably 15 mL/kg, before they are ready to be taken off the ventilator.

NIF. Normal individuals can develop an NIF > 100-150 cm H₂O. It is generally believed that a patient should be able to develop at least 25-30 cm H₂O negative inspiratory force to be weaned successfully. Sahn et al. reported that an NIF of 30 cm H₂O invariably resulted in successful weaning and an NIF < 20 cm H₂O invariably resulted in weaning failure.[256]

Techniques of Weaning

The three most frequent methods used for weaning patients from mechanical ventilatory support are the traditional (trial-and-error) T-piece trials, IMV, and PSV.[259]

T-PIECE TRIALS

With T-piece weaning, one can either use an abrupt "sink-or-swim" trial or gradually increase the periods of spontaneous ventilation on the T-piece. If the duration of the intubation was brief in a relatively healthy individual, one can usually force the patient to assume the work of breathing fairly abruptly. The trial period can extend from a few minutes to several hours prior to extubation. If the trial fails, one

can try again 12-24 hours later, or one can switch to a gradual withdrawal technique.

In patients who have been on a ventilator for more than a few days or who have severe muscle weakness, gradually prolonged trial periods of spontaneous ventilation are generally used. During these periods, the patient breathes a humidified gas mixture with enough O₂ to maintain an SaO₂ of at least 90%.

AXIOM   Patients on T-piece weaning trials tend to have fixed, low-tidal volumes and should be encouraged to sigh (take deep breaths or be bagged) at least four to six times per hour.

When the patient becomes anxious or restless, or becomes tachycardic and/or tachypneic, the trial period is ended.[110] One can then start a series of gradually increasing periods of spontaneous ventilation ("stress") with adequate periods of ventilatory support ("rest") in between. Increasing the ventilatory support at night may be helpful to make sure that the patient is getting adequate rest.[249]

AXIOM   In weaning patients from prolonged ventilatory support, it is essential to provide adequate rest between periods of stress.

IMV TECHNIQUE

With the IMV technique of weaning, the patient is allowed to progressively assume the work of breathing by gradually reducing the number of ventilator breaths between the patient's spontaneous efforts. The number of ventilator breaths can generally be reduced as long as: (a) pH is ≥ 7.35, (b) PCO₂ is ≤ 45 mm Hg, and (c) ventilator rate plus spontaneous breaths is ≤ 30/minute. When any question exists about the patient's blood gases, they should be checked after each ventilator adjustment. A pulse oximeter can greatly reduce the number of ABG determinations required.

When the patient remains clinically stable at an IMV rate of two to four breaths/minute, one can usually discontinue mechanical ventilation successfully. If the patient is unable to progress beyond an IMV of two to four per minute, further weaning on 5-10 cm H₂O CPAP or PSV could be tried.

PSV TECHNIQUE

PSV is increasingly used to gradually decrease the level of ventilator support.[208] The level of PSV is gradually decreased to whatever low level compensates for the resistance of the ET tube and ventilatory circuit. The patient can often then be extubated at that level of PSV.[260]

Improving the Chance of Weaning

When failure to wean occurs, in spite of all of these efforts to improve ventilation, one should consider doing the following:

1. Improve nutrition, especially protein, but reduce the carbohydrate load.
2. Correct any potassium, calcium, phosphorus, or thyroid deficiencies.
3. Discontinue all sedatives.
4. Consider epidural analgesia for continued chest or abdominal pain.
5. Try theophylline in therapeutic doses to improve diaphragm strength.[261]
6. Consider the use of progesterone as a respiratory center stimulant (20 mg Provera TID for 7-10 days).[262]
7. Search for organic neuromuscular disease.
8. Consider reversing drug-induced neuromuscular dysfunction with Tensilon.[263]
9. Consider methylprednisolone in COPD patients or in those with evidence of pulmonary fibrosis (0.5 mg/kg daily and then gradually withdrawn over 1-2 weeks).
10. Vitamin B₁₂ 1000 mcg intramuscularly to improve muscle strength.

OTHER THERAPY

Nutritional Support

Supplying early enteral nutrition in severely traumatized patients can be helpful, and increasing malnutrition may exacerbate the immune depression documented in many patients with trauma, sepsis, and ARDS.

> **AXIOM** Early enteral nutrition can reduce the incidence and severity of infections after trauma.[264]

Drugs

ANTIINFLAMMATORY AGENTS

Corticosteroids

> **AXIOM** If the patient is not making progress in weaning from the ventilator after two to three weeks of intensive therapy, one may consider using corticosteroids to retard the development of pulmonary fibrosis.

In patients who have ARDS but cannot be weaned from the ventilator after two to three weeks in an ICU, in spite of eradication of all infection, methylprednisolone has been of some help in selected patients with evidence of increasing pulmonary fibrosis. The dose of methylprednisolone used by Ashbaugh and Maier under such circumstances was 125 mg intravenously every six hours (plus antacids and H_2-blockers) until evidence of improvement occurred.[265] The dose was then gradually tapered. They used this regimen successfully in eight of 10 selected surgical patients. Previously, similar patients of theirs had a mortality rate exceeding 85%.

Nonsteroidal Antiinflammatory Drugs

Animal studies showed that some of the effects of endotoxin administration are reduced when inhibitors of arachidonic acid metabolism are administered prior to the endotoxin.[61] Indomethacin (1 mg/kg), presumably by inhibiting the cyclooxygenase pathway, has improved PaO_2 in patients with severe bacterial pneumonia.[266] Byrne et al. showed that ibuprofen prevents deterioration in static transpulmonary compliance and transalveolar protein flux in septic pigs; however, supporting clinical data are still lacking.[267]

Prostaglandins

Prostacyclin (PGI_2) is a vasodilator that inhibits platelet and leukocyte adhesion and stabilizes cell membranes.[268] Infusions of this agent have been used in ARDS, but it is not recommended for clinical use.[268]

Prostaglandin E_1 (PGE_1) in high doses blocks coagulation and the inflammatory response by inhibiting platelet aggregation, macrophage activation, neutrophil chemotaxis, and neutrophil release of oxygen radicals and lysosomal enzymes. It dilates pulmonary and systemic vessels, but has minimal effects on pulmonary hypoxic vasoconstriction.[269] Although PGE_1 was shown in one study to improve survival in patients with ARDS,[269] a multicenter, randomized trial failed to show significant benefit.[270]

ANTIPROTEOLYTIC AGENTS

Aprotinin (Trasylol®), a proteinase inhibitor, was believed to be of some value in experimental ARDS; however, a randomized trial on 78 polytrauma patients did not produce increased survival or decreased duration or severity of ARDS.[271]

SURFACTANT

In neonates with the respiratory distress syndrome, aerosolized surfactant repletion via the endotracheal tube has had some success.[272] It is unknown whether this type of therapy is applicable in adults in whom surfactant depletion is a secondary phenomenon.

NITRIC OXIDE

In 1987, nitric oxide was reported to be an important endothelium-derived relaxing factor.[359] Although inhaling high concentrations of nitric oxide can be lethal because it causes severe, acute pulmonary edema and methemoglobinemia, little evidence of toxicity is present when the concentration is < 50 parts per million (ppm).

Rossaint et al. reported on nine patients with severe ARDS who inhaled two different concentrations of nitric oxide for 40 minutes each.[274] They also treated seven patients with continuous inhalation of nitric oxide in concentrations of 5-20 ppm for 3-53 days. The nitric oxide reduced the mean (± SE) pulmonary-artery pressure from 37 ± 3 mm Hg to 30 ± 2 mm Hg (P = 0.008), decreased the shunting from 36 ± 5% to 31 ± 5% (P = 0.028), and increased the PaO_2/FiO_2 ratio from 152 ± 15 mm Hg to 199 ± 23 mm Hg (P = 0.008). Ogura et al. noted that nitric oxide inhalation may also be helpful in smoke inhalation injuries.[275]

In a recent position paper, Zapol et al. indicated that several clinical studies have firmly established inhaled nitric oxide as a selective pulmonary vasodilator.[276] Freeman, in an accompanying article, however, noted that the toxicity of inhaled nitric oxide is poorly and incompletely described, and there is limited mechanistic understanding of how nitric oxide affects various pathologic pulmonary conditions.[277]

TRI-IODOTHYRONINE

The "sick euthyroid syndrome" is frequently seen in critically ill or injured patients, and it is associated with an acute decrease in circulating levels of free tri-iodothyronine (T_3).[278] Noting that lung cellular function, growth, and repair are dependent on thyroid hormonal stimulation, Dulchavsky and Bailey experimentally demonstrated improved lung compliance, histologic integrity, and surfactant availability with T_3 administration during sepsis-induced hypothyroidism.[279] They also showed that administration of T_3 to septic animals helps to restore pulmonary vascular permeability and compliance to normal without affecting cellular metabolic rates.[280]

> **AXIOM** In patients not progressing well on ventilator therapy, one may wish to consider measuring and possibly administering T_3.

ANTIOXIDANTS

Antioxidant agents, such as glutathione reductase and superoxide dismutase, have been used to protect the lung against toxic oxygen radicals, but experience with these agents in humans is limited. Likewise, fibronectin repletion by administering cryoprecipitate has been investigated as a possible therapeutic modality for ARDS.[281] We have had some success using large amounts (8-12 units) of cryoprecipitate in occasional, selected patients who had low antithrombin levels.

N-acetylcysteine has been shown to attenuate the severity of ARDS in a porcine model of ARDS.[282] This mucolytic agent increases intracellular levels of glutathione, which is an excellent endogenous free-radical scavenger, and it has attenuated the severity of ARDS in porcine ARDS. No prospective, double-blind, randomized clinical studies, however, have shown improvement in PaO_2/FiO_2 ratios.

MONOCLONAL ANTIBODIES

Advances in cytokine biology led to the development of immunologic approaches to the treatment of ARDS, directed at three levels of the inflammatory cascade: (a) inciting event (e.g., endotoxin), (b) mediators (e.g., TNF), and (c) effector cells (e.g., PMNs).[283]

Murine monoclonal antibodies that cross-react with endotoxin can protect experimental animals from the deleterious effects of live gram-negative bacteria.[284] However, no conclusive benefits were found in two large multicenter clinical trials in which antiendotoxin monoclonal antibodies (HA-1A and E5) were used in patients with gram-negative bacteremia or septic shock.[285,286]

The strongest evidence supporting the role of TNF in septic shock and ARDS came from studies showing a significant reduction in the development of ARDS, MOF, and death when anti-TNF antibodies were given one hour before a lethal dose of E. coli in primates.[287] In a study by Exley et al. of 14 patients with septic shock, monoclonal antibody to TNF significantly increased BP without any apparent adverse effects.[288]

Attention has also been focused on a recombinant IL-1 receptor antagonist (IL-I_{ra}) which blocks the in vivo and in vitro effects of IL-1 but possesses no agonist activity.[289] IL-I_{ra} significantly reduces PMN infiltration into the lungs and decreases mortality rates seen with experimental endotoxin or live E. coli infusions.[290] Even more importantly, in a recent clinical trial in septic patients, IL-I_{ra} treatment was associated with a dose-dependent, 28-day survival benefit (P < 0.05.)[291]

In a preliminary study in primates, pretreatment with infusions of anti-C5a des arginine antibody protected animals against subsequently infused E. coli.[115] Arterial BP decreased slightly with the infusion of E. coli, but no evidence suggested respiratory failure despite the development of profound and sustained neutropenia.

EXTRACORPOREAL MEMBRANE OXYGENATOR

Standard Extracorporeal Membrane Oxygenator

Extracorporeal membrane oxygenation (ECMO) is the term used to describe prolonged cardiopulmonary bypass using a membrane lung to exchange oxygen and carbon dioxide. A multicenter, prospective, randomized study of ECMO in 90 adults with acute, severe respiratory failure was reported in 1979.[292] The survival rate in patients receiving continued conventional ventilatory treatment was 8.3%, and with ECMO the survival rate was 9.5%.

In spite of these dismal results, the benefits seen with ECMO in newborns with severe congenital cardiac and pulmonary problems stimulated continued research into its use in various types of acquired respiratory failure. In 1993, Moler et al. reported a survival rate of 46% in 220 pediatric patients, ages 1 month to 18 years, who received extracorporeal life support (ECLS) for 247 ± 164 hours for severe pulmonary failure.[293] Such results with ECMO have now also begun to be seen in adults. Anderson et al. reported on the use of ECLS for severe ARDS in 17 multiply injured patients who were considered moribund despite conventional mechanical ventilation.[294] Eleven patients recovered lung function and were successfully weaned off ECLS. Nine patients were discharged from the hospital (53% survival).

Extracorporeal Carbon Dioxide Removal

Extracorporeal carbon dioxide removal (ECCO$_2$R) is a venovenous technique introduced in 1980 to provide carbon dioxide removal in adults.[295] This technique may decrease mortality rate in adults with severe, acute respiratory failure by allowing adequate carbon dioxide removal with significantly reduced tidal volumes and thereby reduced airway pressures.[296] Although ECCO$_2$R requires fewer resources than ECMO, current ECCO$_2$R techniques still demand facilities and personnel beyond the capabilities of the average ICU.[15]

In some centers in Europe, ECCO$_2$R has become standard therapy for severe ARDS, especially for patients who do not respond to PEEP.[293] In a report by Brunet et al. from Paris in 1993, 23 adults with severe respiratory failure meeting the ECMO criteria were treated with ECCO$_2$R and low-frequency, positive-pressure ventilation with a 52% survival rate.[297]

Comparison with Recent Ventilator Studies

In a recent report by Morris et al., a randomized, controlled, clinical trial compared a combination of ECCO$_2$R and pressure-controlled (IPC)-IRV with conventional ventilator therapy in patients who met ECMO entry criteria.[298] No survival advantage was demonstrated for the ECCO$_2$R-PCIRV patients (33%: 7 of 21; vs 42%: 8 of 19). These data are supported by a report by Suchyta et al. in 1991 in which they noted that, using current therapy on 51 patients who met ECMO blood gas criteria, 23 (45%) survived.[299] Thus, great caution must be

used when comparing survival with ECMO in nonrandomized trials with historical controls.

INTRAVASCULAR OXYGENATOR

The intravascular oxygenator (IVOX) is a temporary, implantable, intravascular membrane oxygenator that is designed to transfer gas intravenously.[300] It is made up of several hundred, gas-permeable, hollow fibers that are inserted into the vena cava by femoral venous cutdown. Flow of gas through each fiber adds O$_2$ and removes CO$_2$ from the bloodstream. Unlike ECMO, which can be used as a total lung replacement, IVOX is only an assist device.[301]

Gentilello et al. used the IVOX in 10 patients with ARDS, and the IVOX increased PaO$_2$ and reduced PaCO$_2$, but the quantity of gas transfer was not sufficient to allow a reduction in PEEP, FiO$_2$, or minute ventilation.[300] Insertion of the IVOX also decreased cardiac index and systemic oxygen delivery despite maximum fluid and inotropic support, and the mortality was 80%.

OUTCOME

Early Survival

The overwhelming majority of deaths associated with ARDS take place within two weeks of onset and are usually caused by MOF.[1]

> **AXIOM** Few patients actually die from ARDS; they usually die of MOF, often with uncontrolled sepsis.[55,60]

In one large series of patients with sepsis-induced ARDS, the cause of death in the first three days after the onset of ARDS was respiratory failure in < 10% of patients. After three days, the cumulative death rate due to respiratory failure was 18%; most of these patients also had pneumonia.[302]

> **AXIOM** Deaths in ARDS patients can often be linked to concomitant infections; with this combination, the mortality rate often exceeds 70%.[303]

MOF is the usual cause of death in patients with ARDS.[304] Death is usually due to an inability to control an underlying inflammatory process, such as untreated or untreatable infection, an abscess needing drainage, or persistent necrotic tissue.[304]

Late Sequelae

Hypoxemia with exercise, reduced lung volumes, and lowered carbon dioxide diffusing capacity can be detected in 40% of survivors of ARDS for up to six months following apparent clinical recovery.[2] However, by the end of the first year, activities in most of these patients are not restricted. The patients who had the most prolonged need for oxygen concentrations exceeding 60% were more apt to develop permanent restrictive changes and pulmonary hypertension.[2]

SUMMARY-CONCLUSIONS

ARDS is one of the most frequent and serious complications of major trauma. Sepsis is a particularly important cause; if the underlying infection is not eliminated, ARDS will not resolve and MOF will develop. Once MOF develops, the prognosis for patients with ARDS is extremely poor.[165,166,304]

The best results with posttraumatic pulmonary insufficiency seem to be obtained by preventing it, by keeping hypotension and blood transfusions to a minimum, and by achieving supranormal VO$_2$ as early as possible. Efforts to: (a) fixate fractures and get patients out of bed promptly, (b) provide early, adequate enteral nutrition, and (c) eradicate sepsis and other inflammatory foci as early as possible also appear to be important.

⊘ FREQUENT ERRORS

In the Management of Posttraumatic Respiratory Failure

1. *Forgetting that even relatively mild nonthoracic trauma may be associated with significant pulmonary changes.*
2. *Failing to use adequate in-line filters when giving massive transfusions to patients in shock.*
3. *Delaying ventilatory assistance until obvious clinical evidence of severe pulmonary insufficiency exists.*
4. *Assuming that a patient's lungs are functioning well when the patient is not in distress, has "good color," and has relatively normal chest radiographs.*
5. *Failing to realize that when severely injured or septic patients are not hyperventilating, they are likely to have damage to brain, airway, lungs, or chest wall or cerebral depression from drugs or alcohol.*
6. *Failing to realize that an injured patient with only a mild reduction in arterial PO_2 but a large reduction in PCO_2 may actually have severe alveolar-arterial O_2 differences associated with significant pulmonary changes.*
7. *Relying on absolute values rather than on trends in the patient's ventilation and blood gases.*
8. *Relying on an $FiO_2 > 0.4$-0.5 rather than on improved ventilation to increase reduced arterial Po_2.*
9. *Delaying or performing inadequate or excessive, rapid dehydration of patients with respiratory failure.*
10. *Failure to adequately monitor DO_2 and VO_2 when increasing PEEP to > 10 cm H_2O.*

▼▼▼▼▼▼▼▼▼▼▼▼▼▼▼▼▼▼▼▼▼▼▼▼▼▼▼▼▼▼▼▼

SUMMARY POINTS

1. ARDS, which develops in some patients after very severe trauma, is a nonspecific response of the lungs to a wide variety of insults.
2. Although it develops in relatively few trauma patients, severe pulmonary dysfunction continues to have a high mortality rate.
3. Hemorrhagic hypotension by itself seldom produces ARDS; significant tissue damage or inflammation must usually also be present.
4. Giving excess fluids to a patient developing ARDS greatly accelerates the pulmonary dysfunction.
5. Patients who receive massive blood transfusions have an increased chance of developing ARDS, primarily because of the increased chance of becoming septic.
6. One should assume that all patients with large bone fractures will have some degree of fat embolism, which is most easily quantified by the decrease in platelet count and increased alveolar-arterial oxygen difference.
7. Relatively mild nonthoracic trauma may cause significant blood gas and platelet abnormalities, and these changes may be due to subclinical fat emboli.
8. Making an accurate diagnosis of pneumonia in ICU patients can be extremely difficult; however, any trauma patient on a ventilator for more than 7-14 days probably has some pneumonitis and/or atelectasis.
9. Atelectasis is the most common complication of trauma to the chest or abdomen.
10. One should carefully monitor nasogastric tube suction of the stomach so as to prevent aspiration of gastric contents into the lung.
11. Severe acidity is not needed in aspirated material to cause severe lung injury.
12. The best known major predisposing factor for ARDS is sepsis.
13. About 10-20% of calf vein thrombi propagate into iliofemoral veins and 10-20% of these cause pulmonary emboli with an overall mortality rate of approximately 10-20%.
14. Many more pulmonary emboli occur than are suspected or proved antemortem.
15. Any sudden increase in the $P(a\text{-}ET)CO_2$ difference should make one suspect pulmonary embolus.
16. A normal lung scan is extremely accurate for eliminating significant pulmonary embolus.
17. Pulmonary arteriography is the gold standard for diagnosing pulmonary emboli.
18. Ventilator-induced lung injury appears to be due to overdistension of alveoli (i.e., volutrauma), rather than just exposure of the alveoli to high pressures (i.e., barotrauma).
19. Once alveolar flooding begins, lung mechanics can change abruptly.
20. The pulmonary vasculature in ARDS is characterized by increasing capillary permeability and vasoconstriction.
21. Loss of pulmonary autoregulation contributes to hypoxemia in late ARDS.
22. Neutrophils can cause or contribute to the development of pulmonary edema by increasing pulmonary capillary permeability.
23. Toxic oxygen radicals released from neutrophils attached to pulmonary capillary endothelium are probably the most important cause of early changes in ARDS.
24. Early use of free-radical scavengers may be one of the best ways to reduce the pathophysiologic changes in ARDS.
25. Proteases from neutrophils attached to pulmonary capillary endothelium may be a major cause of later pathophysiologic changes in ARDS.
26. The ratio of PGI_2 to TxA_2 production determines the ultimate effects of cyclooxygenase metabolism on the lungs and other organs.
27. ARDS can occur in animals and patients with neutropenia and complement deficiencies, but the presence of complement and activated PMNs can greatly accelerate and intensify the process.
28. Although complement activation usually starts the processes resulting in lung injury in ARDS, it does not appear to be a necessary condition in all patients.
29. Failure to use adequate in-line microfilters when giving massive blood transfusions may contribute to more rapid development of pulmonary insufficiency.
30. Human lung tissue obtained from septic patients shows platelet sequestration, but it is not certain what role they play in the pathophysiology of lung injury.
31. PAF can cause many of the changes seen with ARDS, but its role in the process is unclear.
32. Of the various cytokines released by inflammatory processes, TNF, IL-1, and IL-8 appear most likely to have a role in ARDS.
33. Pneumonocytes and pulmonary capillary endothelial cells can produce and/or inactivate many substances involved in inflammatory changes in the body.
34. Excess activation of coagulation and fibrinolytic cascades appears to contribute to the development of ARDS.
35. By the time that ARDS becomes apparent clinically, a rather advanced degree of congestive atelectasis is usually present.
36. Regardless of the cause of ARDS, anything that increases PAWP tends to accelerate the pathologic process.
37. Pathologically, ARDS is characterized by congestive atelectasis which is usually worse in the dependent portion of the lungs.
38. The most prominent laboratory abnormality in ARDS is hypoxemia which responds poorly to increases in FiO_2.
39. Ventilation-perfusion (V/Q) inequalities are believed to be the major cause of hypoxemia in ARDS.
40. A PaO_2/FiO_2 ratio < 200 or a physiologic shunt in the lungs $(Q_{sp}/Q_t) > 20\%$ developing more than two to three days after trauma usually indicates that ARDS is developing.
41. Physiologic shunting in the lung is usually the most sensitive test for diagnosing impending or early respiratory failure.
42. Trends are much more important than absolute numbers when evaluating blood gases or pulmonary function tests.
43. Any maneuver that increases cardiac output tends to increase the amount of physiologic shunting in the lungs.

44. Low-arterial PO_2 in a patient with a low-cardiac output tends to indicate more pulmonary dysfunction than the same PaO_2 finding in a patient with a high-cardiac output.

45. The need for an increased minute ventilation to maintain normal levels of $PaCO_2$ in ARDS is primarily due to increased dead space (V_d/V_t).

46. V_d/V_t exceeding 0.60-0.65 usually indicates a severe degree of ventilation-perfusion mismatch.

47. A $PETCO_2$ persistently < 28 mm Hg and an arterial-$ETCO_2$ difference greater than 8 mm Hg following resuscitation is associated with a poor prognosis.

48. Increasing pulmonary hypertension is probably the most frequent and consistent hemodynamic evidence of poor prognosis following trauma.

49. Tachypnea is usually the first indication of increased lung stiffness in ARDS.

50. When a low and decreasing static and dynamic pulmonary compliance cannot be corrected, the prognosis with ARDS is poor.

51. In general, tidal volumes and PEEP should be adjusted, as needed, to provide the best static compliance for ventilated patients.

52. The presence of ARDS is often not detected clinically until its third stage.

53. Generally, a PFR < 300 following trauma in a previously healthy individual indicates acute lung injury; a PFR < 200 indicates ARDS; and a PFR < 120 indicates severe ARDS.

54. Ventilatory assistance in critically injured patients should not be delayed until there is clinical evidence of severe respiratory failure.

55. Virtually all patients with shock and persistent sepsis will develop severe ARDS.

56. Ventilatory assistance in critically injured patients should not be delayed until clinical evidence suggests severe respiratory failure.

57. Virtually all patients with shock and persistent sepsis, especially from severe peritonitis, develop some degree of respiratory failure.

58. Restlessness should be considered as due to hypoxia until proved otherwise.

59. When narcotics or sedatives are given to a patient with restlessness due to pulmonary problems, ventilation is further reduced.

60. One should not assume that a patient's oxygenation is adequate because he or she is not cyanotic, especially when the Hb is $\leq$ 10 g/dL.

61. In patients who have had minimal bleeding and little or no shock, fat embolism is the most frequent cause for a decrease in the platelet count below normal in the first 24-48 hours after trauma.

62. With blood gases, one should document not only the PaO_2 and $PaCO_2$, but also the PaO_2/FiO_2 ratio, $P(A-a)O_2$, PvO_2, SvO_2, and Q_{sp}/Q_t.

63. Low $PaCO_2$ does not necessarily indicate that the patient's ventilation is adequate, especially when hypocarbia is only mild in the face of moderate-to-severe metabolic acidosis.

64. A decrease in PaO_2 may be caused by poor pulmonary function, but in ARDS it may also be caused by high-oxygen consumption and/or low-oxygen delivery.

65. A peripheral defect in oxygen utilization can become increasingly apparent as ARDS becomes more severe.

66. In patients who are apt to develop ARDS, one should maintain an optimal VO_2 or at least a VO_2 that is not flow-dependent.

67. Decreasing static lung compliance in a patient after trauma, in the absence of hemopneumothorax or abdominal distension, is usually due to increased lung water and may indicate developing ARDS.

68. When inflation pressures on a ventilator suddenly increase, pneumothorax or major airway obstruction should be suspected.

69. It cannot be assumed that pulmonary function is satisfactory when the lungs appear to be relatively normal on chest radiography.

70. The amount of lung damage seen initially on plain chest radiography usually greatly underestimates the severity and extent of ARDS.

71. When large amounts of PEEP are used, one should follow changes in PAWP rather than absolute levels to obtain a more accurate impression of cardiac filling.

72. If ARDS is developing or getting worse, it usually implies that an inadequately treated infection is present.

73. Early and complete eradication of pus and/or necrotic tissue is extremely important in patients with ARDS.

74. Persistent fever, leukocytosis, and pulmonary dysfunction in critically injured patients after 7-10 days of antibiotic therapy may be due to fungal infection, and it may be prudent to begin antifungal therapy in such individuals.

75. Patients who may develop pulmonary problems and require prolonged gastrointestinal intubation may benefit from having such tubes passed through a gastrostomy or jejunostomy rather than through the nose or mouth.

76. Controlling pain so that the patient can take deep breaths and cough effectively is probably the single best way to prevent atelectasis and/or pneumonia following truncal trauma or surgery.

77. When restlessness is due to pain, analgesics may be indicated; however, when restlessness is due to hypoxia, such agents may be lethal.

78. A gradual increase in PIP in ARDS may be at least partially due to pleural effusions, but a sudden increase is due to an obstructed airway or pneumothorax until proved otherwise.

79. In attempting to find the ideal cardiac-filling volume, one should use the RVEDVI or hemodynamic response to fluid challenges rather than isolated PAWP or CVP levels.

80. Although the role of colloids in the prevention or treatment of ARDS is controversial, low COP tends to increase the water content of the lungs.

81. Although controversial, patients with severe ARDS or other cardiopulmonary dysfunction tend to have a better prognosis when the hemoglobin level is 12.0 g/dL or more.

82. Achieving optimal (supernormal) DO_2 and VO_2 levels soon after trauma or surgery in high-risk patients seems to reduce the incidence and severity of organ failure and death.

83. Early, aggressive enteral nutrition appears to reduce complications after trauma.

84. Although preventing stress gastritis seems to be a worthwhile goal in high-risk patients, allowing bacterial overgrowth in a highly alkaline stomach may increase the risk of pulmonary complications.

85. Although it is not usually a prominent feature in respiratory failure following trauma, bronchospasm or wheezing should be treated aggressively when found.

86. Inotropic agents may be helpful for increasing DO_2 and VO_2 to optimal levels. The resulting tachycardia and increased shunting in the lung, however, can be a problem.

87. It is extremely dangerous to give diuretics if oliguria is due to a persistent deficit in the functional ECF.

88. Concern about oxygen toxicity should not prevent the administration of high FiO_2 (fraction of inspired oxygen) if this is the only way to maintain PaO_2 of at least 50 mm Hg in patients with severe ARDS.

89. If ventilatory assistance is delayed in injured patients until there is definite clinical evidence of respiratory failure, the lung changes can be very difficult to reverse.

90. When any question exists about the adequacy of the upper airway or minute ventilation in a trauma victim, the patient should probably have early ventilatory support.

91. When a patient requires long-term ventilation or protection of the upper airway, early tracheostomy may be indicated.

92. Pressure-cycled ventilators are generally easier to use, but when ARDS is developing, volume-cycled ventilators are often preferable.

93. Most patients with ARDS require volume-cycled ventilators to ensure adequate gas exchange.

94. HFV use after trauma is generally limited to upper airway surgery or management of bronchopulmonary fistulas.

95. Physiologic advantages of IMV include increased venous return and better V/Q relationships during spontaneous breaths. IMV also improves weaning from the ventilator in some patients.

96. Although the medical literature has not shown improved weaning from the ventilator with PSV, it seems to be extremely helpful in many patients.

97. Use of pressure-controlled ventilation should be considered in virtually all patients who require peak inspiratory pressures > 50 cm H_2O.

98. In most situations where a ventilator is used, the injured patient needs mechanical assistance, and providing additional oxygen is only a secondary consideration.

99. Efforts to keep $PaCO_2$ normal or low with high-tidal volumes or minute ventilation may damage the lungs.

100. Efforts should be made to keep PIP from exceeding 50 cm H_2O.

101. The main functions of PEEP are to keep alveoli expanded during expiration and increase the patient's functional residual capacity back towards normal.

102. Although it appears to be an important part of the treatment of ARDS, in many studies, PEEP does not prevent ARDS, reduce its incidence, or alter its course or outcome.

103. The major problems with PEEP are related to its tendency to reduce venous return and cardiac output, especially when levels > 10-15 cm H_2O are used.

104. When optimizing the level of PEEP in a patient, it is essential to also maintain optimal DO_2 and VO_2 by giving fluids, blood, or inotropes as needed.

105. If further increases in tidal volume and/or ventilatory rate in a patient with high minute ventilation cause an increase in $PaCO_2$, one should suspect that significant auto-PEEP is present.

106. When the patient's ventilatory flow rate tracing indicates that the next inspiration interrupts an expiratory effort, auto-PEEP is probably present.

107. Intermittent sighing is an important method for preventing atelectasis in patients taking frequent, small, spontaneous, or ventilator breaths.

108. Failure to follow PIP levels in ventilated patients can result in delayed diagnosis of a tension pneumothorax or worsening of pulmonary function.

109. The patient who is awake, alert, comfortable, and cooperative, and has normal vital signs on a ventilator is generally doing well, even if ABGs are not optimal.

110. In critically injured patients in the ICU, obtaining VBGs at the same time as ABGs can provide a great deal more physiologic information.

111. One should not assume that a patient's cardiovascular and pulmonary systems are stable because the SvO_2 hasn't changed.

112. The main value of pulse oximetry is its ability to provide early warning of potentially dangerous trends in pulmonary or cardiovascular function.

113. An increase in $P(a-ET)CO_2$ may reflect increased dead space on the lungs; this should make one suspect pulmonary embolus, drastic reduction in cardiac output, and/or increased ventilation perfusion mismatching in the lung.

114. Whenever possible, tissue perfusion should be increased and tidal volume adjusted to keep $PETCO_2 \geq 29$ mm Hg and $P(a-ET)CO_2 \leq 7$ mm Hg.

115. Rapid, shallow breathing, respiratory alternans, or abdominal paradox during attempts at spontaneous breathing generally indicate that the patient is not ready to be weaned from the ventilator.

116. In elderly and uncooperative individuals, particularly those with other organ system dysfunction, even the presence of the optimal weaning criteria do not guarantee successful weaning.

117. An FVC < 10 mL/kg or NIF < 25 cm H_2O usually indicates that the patient is not ready for weaning.

118. Patients on T-piece weaning trials tend to have fixed, low-tidal volumes and should be encouraged to sigh at least four to six times per hour.

119. In weaning patients from prolonged ventilatory support, it is essential to provide adequate rest between periods of stress.

120. Early enteral nutrition can reduce the incidence and severity of infections after trauma.

121. If the patient is not making progress in weaning from the ventilator after two to three weeks of intensive therapy, one may consider corticosteroids to retard the development of pulmonary fibrosis.

122. In patients not progressing as well as expected on ventilator therapy, one may wish to consider measuring and/or administering T_3.

123. Few patients actually die from ARDS; they usually die of MOF, often with uncontrolled sepsis.

124. Deaths in ARDS patients can often be linked to concomitant infections; with this combination, the mortality rate often exceeds 70%.

▲▲▲▲▲▲▲▲▲▲▲▲▲▲▲▲▲▲▲▲▲▲▲▲▲▲▲▲▲▲▲▲▲▲▲

REFERENCES

1. Nacht A, Kahn RC, Miller SM. Adult respiratory distress syndrome and its management. Capan LM, Miller SM, Turndorf H, eds. Trauma: anesthesia and intensive care. Philadelphia: JB Lippincott, 1991; 725-753.
2. Horn JK, Lewis FR Jr. Respiratory insufficiency. Moore EE, Mattox KL, Feliciano CV, eds. Trauma, 2nd ed. Norwalk: Appleton & Lange, 1992; 909-926.
3. Wilson RF, Norton ML. Respiratory failure in trauma. Walt AJ, Wilson RF, eds. The management of trauma: pitfalls and practice. Philadelphia: Lea & Febiger, 1975; 501-531.
4. Wilson RF, Kafi A, Asuncion Z, et al. Clinical respiratory failure after shock or trauma: prognosis and methods of diagnosis. Arch Surg 1969;98:538.
5. Anderson RR, Holliday RL, Driedger AA, et al. Documentation of pulmonary capillary permeability in the adult respiratory distress syndrome accompanying human sepsis. Am Rev Respir Dis 1979;119:869.
6. Anderson RW, DeVries WC. Transvascular fluid and protein dynamics in the lung following hemorrhagic shock. J Surg Res 1976;20:281.
7. Webb WR. Pulmonary complications in non-thoracic trauma: summary of the National Research Council conference. J Trauma 1959;9:700.
8. Ashbaugh JDG, Petty T. Acute respiratory distress in adults. Lancet 1967;2:319.
9. Shapiro BA, Cane RD. Metabolic malfunction of lung: noncardiogenic edema and adult respiratory distress syndrome. Surg Annu 1981;13:271.
10. Bernard GR, Artigas A, Brigham KL, et al. The American European Consensus Conference on ARDS: definitions, mechanisms, relevant outcome, and clinical trial coordination. Am J Respir Crit Care Med 1994;149:818.
11. Slutsky SS. Mechanical ventilation ACCP Consensus Conference. Chest 1993;104:1833.
12. Suchyta MR, Clemmer TP, Orme JF, et al. Increased survival of ARDS patients with severe hypoxemia: ECMO criteria. Chest 1991;99:951.
13. Montgomery AB, Stager MA, Carrico CJ, et al. Causes of mortality in patients with adult respiratory distress syndrome. Am Rev Respir Dis 1985;132:485.
14. Morris AH, Wallace CJ, Clemmer TP, et al. Extracorporeal CO_2 removal therapy for adult respiratory distress syndrome patients. Respir Care 1990;35:224.
15. Shapiro BA, Peruzzi WT. Changing practices in ventilator management: a review of the literature and suggested clinical correlations. Surgery 1995;117:121.
16. Demling RH. Adult respiratory distress syndrome: current concepts. New Horizons 1993;1:388.
17. Gattinoni L, Pesenti A, Avalli L, et al. Pressure-volume curve of the total respiratory system in acute respiratory failure: a computed tomographic scan study. Am Rev Respir Dis 1987;136:730.
18. Bone RC, Balk R, Slotman G, et al. Adult respiratory distress syndrome: sequence and importance of development of multiple organ failure. Chest 1992;101:320.
19. Pepe PE, Potkin RT, Reus DH, et al. Clinical predictors of the adult respiratory distress syndrome. Am J Surg 1982;144:124.
20. Fowler AA, Hamman RF, Good JT, et al. Adult respiratory distress syndrome: risk with common predispositions. Ann Intern Med 1983;98:593.
21. Maunder RJ. Clinical prediction of the adult respiratory distress syndrome. Clin Chest Med 1985;6:413.
22. Weigelt J, Mitchell RA, Snyder WHO. Early identification of patients prone to develop the respiratory distress syndrome. Am J Surg 1981;142:687.
23. Wilson RF, Sibbald WJ. Acute respiratory failure. Crit Care Med 1976;4:79.

24. Hoyt DB, Simons RK, Winchell RJ, et al. A risk analysis of pulmonary complications following major trauma. J Trauma 1993;35:524.

25. Moon VH. Pathological features following shock with delayed death. Am J Pathol 1936;12:788.

26. Burford TH, Burbank B. Traumatic wet lung: observations on certain physiologic fundamentals in thoracic trauma. J Thoracic Cardiac Surg 1954;14:415.

27. Mallory TB. The general pathology of traumatic shock. Surgery 1950;27:629.

28. Jenkins MT, Jones RF, Wilson B, et al. Congestive atelectasis—a complication of the intravenous infusion of fluids. Ann Surg 1950;132:327.

29. Burke JF. High output respiratory failure. Ann Surg 1963;158:4.

30. Petty TL. Adult respiratory distress syndrome: historical perspective and definition. Semin Respir Med 1981;2:99.

31. Ashbaugh DG, Bigelow OB, Petty TL, et al. Acute respiratory distress in adults. Lancet 1967;2:319.

32. Pfenninger J, Gerber A, Tschappeler H, et al. Adult respiratory distress syndrome in children. J Pediatr 1982;101:352.

33. Petty TL, Fowler AA. Another look at ARDS. Chest 1982;82:98.

34. Lewis FR, Blaisdell FW, Scholbohm RM. Incidence and outcome of post-traumatic respiratory failure. Arch Surg 1977;112:436.

35. Henry JN. The effect of experimental hemorrhagic shock on pulmonary alveolar surfactant. J Trauma 1967;5:691.

36. Levin SE, et al. Surface active alveolar lining material and pulmonary disease. Surg Gynecol Obstet 1966;123:53.

37. Shoemaker WC, Appel P, Czer LSC, et al. Pathogenesis of respiratory failure (ARDS) after hemorrhage and trauma. Crit Care Med 1980;8:504.

38. Wilson RF, Mammen E, Walt AJ. Eight years of experience with massive blood transfusions. J Trauma 1971;11:275.

39. Wilson RF, Dulchavsky SA, Soullier G, et al. Problems with 20 or more blood transfusions in 24 hours. Am Surg 1987;53:410.

40. Durtschi MB, Haisch CE, Reynolds L, et al. Effect of micropore filtration on pulmonary functions after massive transfusion. Am J Surg 1979;138:8.

41. Rutledge R, Sheldon GF, Collins ML. Massive transfusion. Crit Care Clin 1986;2:791.

42. Popovsky MA, Abel MD, Moore SB. Transfusion related acute lung injury associated with passive transfer of antileukocyte antibodies. Am Rev Respir Dis 1983;128:689.

43. Freedland M, Wilson RF, Bender JS, et al. The management of flail chest injury: factors affecting outcome. J Trauma 1990;30:1460.

44. Shier MR, Wilson RF. Fat embolism syndromes: traumatic coagulopathy with respiratory distress. Surg Ann 1980;12:139.

45. Gauss H. The pathology of fat embolism. Arch Surg 1924;9:593.

46. Lehman EP, Moore RM. Fat embolism. Arch Surg 1927;14:621.

47. LeQuire VA. A study of the pathogenesis of fat embolism based on human necropsy material and animal experiments. Am J Pathol 1959;35:999.

48. Wilson RF, McCarthy B, LeBlanc LP, et al. Respiratory and coagulation changes after uncomplicated fractures. Arch Surg 1973;106:395.

49. Shier MR, James RE, Riddle J, et al. Fat embolism prophylaxis: a study of four treatment modalities. J Trauma 1977;17:621.

50. Bergentz SE. Studies on the genesis of post-traumatic fat embolism. Acta Chir Scand 1961;282(Suppl):1.

51. Riska EB, Myllynen P. Fat embolism in patients with multiple injuries. J Trauma 1982;22:891.

52. Milak AB. Pulmonary vascular response to increase in intracranial pressure. Role of sympathetic mechanisms. J Appl Physiol 1977;42:335.

53. Wray NP, Nicotra MB. Pathogenesis of neurogenic pulmonary edema. Am Rev Respir Dis 1978;118:783.

54. Colice GL. Neurogenic pulmonary edema. Clin Chest Med 1985;6:473.

55. Campbell GD, Coalson JJ, Johanson WG. The effect of bacterial superinfection on lung function after diffuse alveolar damage. Am Rev Respir Dis 1984;129:974.

56. Schwartz DJ, Wynn JW, Gibbs CP, et al. The pulmonary consequences of aspiration of gastric contents at pH values greater than 2.5. Am Rev Respir Dis 1980;121:119.

57. Vito L, Dennis RC, Weisel RD. Sepsis presenting as acute respiratory insufficiency. Surg Gynecol Obstet 1974;138:896.

58. Fein AM, Lippmann H, Holtzman H, et al. The risk factors, incidence, and prognosis of ARDS following septicemia. Chest 1983;83:40.

59. Kaplan RL, Sahn SA, Petty TL. Incidence and outcome of the respiratory distress syndrome in Gram-negative sepsis. Arch Intern Med 1979;139:867.

60. Hudson LD. Causes of the adult respiratory distress syndrome—clinical recognition. Clin Chest Med 1982;3:195.

61. Newman JH. Sepsis and pulmonary edema. Clin Chest Med 1985;6:371.

62. Coon WW. Risk factors of pulmonary embolism. Surg Gynecol Obstet 1976;143:385.

63. Goris RJA, Draaisma J. Causes of death after blunt trauma. J Trauma 1982;22:141.

64. Bell WR, Simon TL. Current status of pulmonary thromboembolic disease: pathophysiology, diagnosis, prevention, and treatment. Am Heart J 1982;103:239.

65. Kaufman B. Deep vein thrombosis and pulmonary embolism in the injured patients. Capan LM, Turndorf H, eds. Trauma: anesthesia and intensive care. Philadelphia: JB Lippincott, 1991; 821.

66. Dantzker DR, Bower JS. Alterations in gas exchange following pulmonary thromboembolism. Chest 1982;81:495.

67. Hatle L, Rokseth R. The arterial to end-expiratory carbon dioxide tension gradient in acute pulmonary embolism and other cardiopulmonary diseases. Chest 1974;66:352.

68. Menzoian JO, Williams LF. Is pulmonary angiography essential for the diagnosis of acute pulmonary embolism? Am J Surg 1979;137:543.

69. Hull RD, Hirsh J, Carter CJ, et al. Diagnostic value of ventilation-perfusion lung scanning in patients with suspected pulmonary embolism. Chest 1985;88:819.

70. Thorning DR, Howard ML, Hudson LD, et al. Pulmonary responses to smoke inhalation. Human Pathol 1982;13:255.

71. Parker JC, Hernandez LA, Peevy KJ. Mechanics of ventilator-induced lung injury. Crit Care Med 1993;21:131.

72. Tsuno K, Miura K, Takeya M, et al. Histopathologic pulmonary changes from mechanical ventilation at high peak airway pressure. Am Rev Respir Dis 1991;143:1115.

73. Hernandez LA, Peevy KJ, Moise AA, et al. Chest wall restriction limits high airway pressure-induced lung injury in young rabbits. J Appl Physiol 1989;66:2364.

74. Corbridge TC, Wood LDH, Crawford GP, et al. Adverse effects of large tidal volume and low PEEP in canine acid aspiration. Am Rev Respir Dis 1990;142:311.

75. Katz JA, Aberman A, Frand V, et al. Heroin pulmonary edema: evidence for increased pulmonary capillary permeability. Am Rev Respir Dis 1972;106:472.

76. Meyrick BO. Pathology of the adult respiratory distress syndrome. Crit Care Clin 1986;2:405.

77. Matthay MA. Pathophysiology of pulmonary edema. Clin Chest Med 1985;6:301.

78. Brigham KL, Kariman K, Harris T, et al. Lung water and vascular permeability surface areas in humans during respiratory failure. Am Rev Respir Dis 1980;121:426.

79. Lava J, Rice C, Moss G, et al. Pulmonary dysfunction in sepsis. Is pulmonary edema the culprit? J Trauma 1982;22:280.

80. Snapper JR, Hutchison AA, Olgetree ML, et al. Lung mechanics in pulmonary edema. Clin Chest Med 1985;6:393.

81. Hallman M, Spragg R, Harrell JH, et al. Evidence of lung surfactant abnormality in respiratory distress syndrome. Crit Care Med 1984;12:14.

82. Pietra GG, Ruttner JR, Wust W, et al. The lung after trauma and shock: fine structure of the alveolar capillary barrier in 23 autopsies. J Trauma 1981;21:454.

83. Maunder RJ, Shuman WP, McHugh JW, et al. Preservation of normal lung regions in the adult respiratory distress syndrome. J Clin Invest 1982;69:543.

84. Bachofen M, Weibel ER. Structural alterations of lung parenchyma in the adult respiratory distress syndrome. Clin Chest Med 1982;3:35.

85. Snow RL, Davis P, Pontoppidan H, et al. Pulmonary vascular remodeling in adult respiratory distress syndrome. Am Rev Respir Dis 1982;126:887.

86. Bernard GR, Brigham KL. Pulmonary edema: pathophysiologic mechanisms and new approaches to therapy. Chest 1986;89:594.

87. Staub NC. Pathophysiology of pulmonary edema. Staub NC, Taylor AE, eds. Edema. New York: Raven Press, 1984; 719.

88. Sukhnandan R, Thal AP. Effect of endotoxin and vasoactive agents on dibenzyline pretreated lungs. Surgery 1965;58:185.

89. Tate RM, Repine JE. Neutrophils and the adult respiratory distress syndrome. Am Rev Respir Dis 1983;128:552.

90. Law MM, Cryer HG, Abraham E. Elevated levels of soluble ICAM-1 correlated with the development of multiple organ failure in severely injured trauma patients. J Trauma 1994;37:100.

91. Fantone JC, Feltner DE, Brieland JK, et al. Phagocytic cell-derived inflammatory mediators and lung disease. Chest 1987;91:428.

92. Bertrand Y. Oxygen-free radicals and lipid peroxidation in adult respiratory distress syndrome. Intensive Care Med 1985;11:56.

93. Ward PA, Till GO, Hatherill JR, et al. Systemic complement activation, lung injury and products of lipid peroxidation. J Clin Invest 1986; 76:517.

94. Schraufstatter IU, Hyslop PA, Hinshaw DB, et al. Hydrogen peroxide-induced injury of cell and its prevention by inhibitors of poly (ADP-ripose) polymerese. Proc Natl Acad Sci USA 1986;83:4908.

95. Schraufstatter IU, Hinshaw DB, Hyslop PA, et al. Oxidant injury of cells. DNA strand-breaks activate polyadenosine diphosphate-ribose polymerase and lead to depletion of nicotinamide adenine dinuclotide. J Clin Invest 1986;77:1312.

96. Martin JW, Gadek JE, Hunninghake GW, et al. Oxidant injury of lung parenchymal cells. J Clin Invest 1981;68:1277.

97. Simon RH, Scoggin CH, Patterson D. Hydrogen peroxide causes the fatal injury to human fibroblasts exposed to oxygen radicals. J Biol Chem 1981;256:7181.

98. Harlan JM, Killen PD, Harker LA, et al. Neutrophil-mediated endothelial injury in vitro. Mechanisms of cell detachment. J Clin Invest 1981;68:1394.

99. Marzi I, Buhren V, Schuttler A, et al. Value of superoxide dismutase for prevention of multiple organ failure after multiple trauma. J Trauma 1993;35:110.

100. Westaby S. Mechanism of membrane damage and surfactant depletion in acute lung injury. Intensive Care Med 1986;12:2.

101. Lee CT, Fein AM, Lippman M, et al. Elastolytic activity in pulmonary lavage fluid from patients with the adult respiratory distress syndrome. N Engl J Med 1981;304:192.

102. Rinaldo JE, Rogers RM. Adult respiratory distress syndrome: changing concepts of lung injury and repair. N Engl J Med 1982;306:900.

103. Cochrane CG, Spragg R, Revak SD. Pathogenesis of the adult respiratory distress syndrome. Evidence of oxidant activity in bronchoalveolar lavage fluid. J Clin Invest 1983;71:754.

104. Perkowski SZ, Havill AM, Flynn JT, et al. Role of intrapulmonary release of eicosanoids and superoxide anion as mediators of pulmonary dysfunction and endothelial injury in sheep with intermittent complement activation. Circ Res 1983;53:574.

105. Johnston MG, Hay JB, Movat HZ. Kinetics of prostaglandin production in various inflammatory lesions measured in draining lymph. Am J Pathol 1979;95:225.

106. Issekutz AC, Movat HZ. The effect of vasodilator prostaglandin on polymorphonuclear leukocyte infiltration and vascular injury. Am J Pathol 1982;107:300.

107. Garcia JGN, Noonan TC, Jubiz W, et al. Leukotrienes and the pulmonary microcirculation. Am Rev Respir Dis 1987;136:161.

108. Gadaleta D, Davis JM. Pulmonary failure and the production of leukotrienes. J Am Coll Surg 1994;178:309.

109. Malik AB, Perlman MB, Cooper JA, et al. Pulmonary microvascular effects of arachidonic acid metabolites and their role in lung vascular injury. Fed Proc 1985;44:36.

110. Weinberg P, Matthay MA, Webster RO, et al. Biologically active products of complement and acute lung injury in patients with sepsis syndrome. Am Rev Respir Dis 1984;130:791.

111. Cramer EB, Migliorisi G, Pologe L, et al. Effect of leukotrienes on endothelium and the transendothelial migration of neutrophils. J Allergy Clin Immunol 1984;74:386.

112. Maunder RJ, Hackman RC, Riff E, et al. Occurrence of the adult respiratory distress syndrome in neutropenic patients. Am Rev Respir Dis 1986;133:313.

113. Ognibene FP, Martin SE, Parker MM, et al. Adult respiratory distress syndrome in patients with severe neutropenia. N Engl J Med 1986;315:547.

114. Rinaldo JE, Rogers RM. Adult respiratory distress syndrome. N Engl J Med 1986;315:578.

115. Tate RM, Repine JE. Neutrophils and the adult respiratory distress syndrome. Am Rev Respir Dis 1983;128:552.

116. Hohn DC, Meyers AJ, Gherini ST, et al. Production of acute pulmonary injury by leukocytes and activated complement. Surgery 1980;88:48.

117. Horn JK, Flick MR, Hoeffel JH, et al. Pulmonary responses to intravascular complement activation in sheep. Clin Res 1985;33:466A.

118. Thommasen HV, Russell JA, Boyko WJ, et al. Transient leucopenia associated with adult respiratory distress syndrome. Lancet 1984;8:809.

119. Goldstein IM, Perez HD. Biologically active peptides derived from the fifth component of complement. Prog Hemost Thromb 1980;5:41.

120. Duchateau J, Haas M, Schreyen H, et al. Complement activation in patients at risk of developing the adult respiratory distress syndrome. Am Rev Respir Dis 1984;130:1058.

121. Tennenberg SD, Jacobs MP, Solomkin JS. Complement-mediated neutrophil activation in sepsis and trauma related adult respiratory distress syndrome. Arch Surg 1987;122:26.

122. Stallone RJ, Lim RC Jr, Blaisdell FW. Pathogenesis of the pulmonary changes following ischemia of the lower extremities. Ann Thorac Surg 1969;7:539.

123. Snapper JR, Hinson JM Jr, Ledfferts P, et al. Effect of antiplatelet antibody (APA) on the awake sheep and platelet depletion on the sheep's response to endotoxin. Fed Proc 1983;42:477A.

124. Minnear FL, Moon DG, Kaplan JE, et al. Effect of ADP-induced platelet aggregation on lung fluid balance in sheep. Am J Physiol 1982;242:H645.

125. Bo G, Hognestad J. Effects on the pulmonary circulation of suddenly induced intravascular aggregation of platelets. Acta Physiol Scand 1972;85:523.

126. Schneider RC, Zapol WM, Carvalho AC. Platelet consumption and sequestration in severe acute respiratory failure. Am Rev Respir Dis 1980;122:445.

127. Mojarad M. Hamasaki Y, Said SI. Platelet-activating factor increases pulmonary microvascular permeability and induces pulmonary edema: a preliminary report. Clin Respir Physiol 1983;19:253.

128. Lewis JC, O'Flaherty JT, McCall CE, et al. Platelet-activating factor effects on pulmonary ultrastructure in rabbits. Exp Mol Pathol 1983;38:100.

129. Tracey KJ, Beutler B, Lowry SF, et al. Shock and tissue injury induced by recombinant human cachectin. Science 1986;234:470.

130. Horvath CJ, Ferro TJ, Jesmok G, et al. Recombinant tumor necrosis factor increases pulmonary vascular permeability independent of neutrophils. Proc Natl Acad Sci USA 1988;85:9219.

131. Beutler B, Milsark IW, Cerami A. Passive immunization against cachectin/tumor necrosis factor protects mice from the lethal effect of endotoxin. Science 1985;229:869.

132. Okusawa Gelfand JA, Ikejima T, et al. Interleukin-1 induces a shock-like state in rabbits: synergism with tumor necrosis factor and the effect of cyclooxygenase inhibition. J Clin Invest 1988;81:1162.

133. Rodriguez JL, Miller CG, DeForge LE, et al. Local production of interleukin-8 is associated with nosocomial pneumonia. J Trauma 1992;33:74.

134. Kunkel SL, Standiford T, Kasahara K, et al. Interleukin-8: the major neutrophil chemotactic factor in the lung. Exp Lung Res 1991;17:17.

135. Ryan JW, Smith U. Metabolism of adenosine 5′-monophosphate during circulation through the lungs. Trans Assoc Am Physicians 1971;84:297.

136. Schneeberger EE. Barrier function of intercellular junctions in adult and fetal lungs. Fishman AP, Renkin EM, eds. Pulmonary edema. Bethesda: American Physiological Society, 1979.

137. Rice CL, Kohler JP, Casey L, et al. Angiotensin-converting enzyme (ACE) in sepsis. Circ Shock 1983;11:59.

138. Ferriera SH, Vane JR. Half-lives of peptides and amines in the circulation. Nature 1976;215:1237.

139. Smith FB, Kikkawa Y. The type II epithelial cells of the lung. V. Synthesis of phosphatidyl glycerol in isolated type II cells and pulmonary alveolar macrophages. Lab Invest 1979;40:172.

140. Matthay MA, Berthiaume Y, Staub NC. Long-term clearance of liquid and proteins from the lungs of unanesthetized sheep. J Appl Physiol 1985;59:928.

141. Blaisdell FW, et al. Pulmonary microembolism: a cause of morbidity and death after major vascular surgery. Arch Surg 1966;93:776.

142. Carvalho A, Bellman SM, Saullo V, et al. Altered factor VIII in acute respiratory failure. N Engl J Med 1982;307:1113.

143. Manwaring D, Curreri PW. Platelet and neutrophil sequestration after fragment D-induced respiratory distress. Circ Shock 1982;9:75.

144. Heffner JE, Sahn SA, Repine JE. The role of platelets in adult respiratory distress syndrome. Am Rev Respir Dis 1987;135:482.

145. Wilson JW, Ratliff NR, Harkel DB. The lung in hemorrhagic shock. In vivo observations of pulmonary microcirculation in cats. Am J Pathol 1970;58:337.

146. Dantzker DR, Brook CJ, Dehart P, et al. Ventilation-perfusion distribution in the adult respiratory distress syndrome. Am Rev Respir Dis 1979;120:1039.

147. Bongard FS, Matthay M, Mackersie RC, et al. Morphologic and physiologic correlates of increased extravascular lung water. Surgery 1984;96:395.

148. Zapol WM, Snider MT. Pulmonary hypertension in severe acute respiratory failure. N Engl J Med 1977;296:476.

149. Jardin F, Gurdjian F, Desfonds P, et al. Effect of dopamine on intrapulmonary shunt fraction and oxygen transport in severe sepsis with circulatory and respiratory failure. Crit Care Med 1981;7:273.

150. Cheney F, Colley PS. The effect of cardiac output on arterial blood oxygenation. Anesthesiology 1980;52:496.

151. Wilson RF. Blood gases: pathophysiology and interpretation. Wilson RF, ed. Critical care manual applied physiology and principles of therapy, 2nd ed. Philadelphia: FA Davis Publishing Company, 1992; 411.

152. Domsky M, Wilson RF, Hines J. Intraoperative end-tidal carbon dioxide values and derived calculations correlated with outcome: prognosis and capnography. Crit Care Med 1995;23:1497.

153. Visconi S, Rossi GP, Pesenti A, et al. Pulmonary microthrombosis in severe adult respiratory distress syndrome. Crit Care Med 1988;16,111:1.

154. Sankaran S, Wilson RF. Factors affecting prognosis in patients with flail chest. J Thorac Cardiovasc Surg 1970;60:402.

155. Sturm JA, Wisner DH, Oestern HJ, et al. Increased lung capillary permeability after trauma. A prospective clinical study. J Trauma 1986;26:409.

156. Newman JH. ARDS, new insights and unresolved problems. Intensive Care Med 1983;9:303.

157. Nuytinck J, Goris R, Redl H, et al. Post-traumatic complications and inflammatory mediators. Arch Surg 1986;121:886.

158. Hickling KG. Low volume ventilation with permissive hypercapnia in the adult respiratory distress syndrome. Clin Intensive Care 1992;3:67.

159. Shapiro BA. A historical perspective on ventilator management. New Horizons 1994;2:8.

160. Schuster DP, Trulock EP. Correlation of changes in oxygenation, lung water and hemodynamics after oleic acid-induced acute lung injury in dogs. Crit Care Med 1984;12:1044.

161. Wilson RF, Christensen C, Ali M, et al. Oxygen consumption in critically ill surgical patients. Ann Surg 1972;176:801.

162. Pepe PE, Culver BH. Independently measured oxygen consumption during reduction of oxygen delivery by positive end-expiratory pressure. Am Rev Respir Dis 1985;132:788.

163. Cutillo AG. The clinical assessment of lung water. Chest 1987;92:319.

164. Wilson RF, Beckman B, Tyburski JG, et al. Pulmonary artery diastolic and wedge pressure relationships in critically ill and injured patients. Arch Surg 1988;123:933.

165. Fry DE, Pearlstein L, Fultin RL, et al. Multiple system organ failure. The role of uncontrolled infection. Arch Surg 1980;115:136.

166. Knaus WA, Draper EA, Wagner DP, et al. Prognosis in acute organ-system failure. Ann Surg 1985;202:685.

167. Moore FA, Moore EE, Poggetti, et al. Gut bacterial translocation via the portal vein: a clinical perspective with major torso trauma. J Trauma 1991;31:626.

168. Dellinger EP, Wertz, MJ, Lennard ES, et al. Efficacy of short-course antibiotic prophylaxis after penetrating intestinal injury: a prospective randomized trial. Arch Surg 1986;121:23.

169. Prewitt RM, McCarthy J, Wood LDH. Treatment of acute low pressure edema in dogs: relative effects of hydrostatic and oncotic pressure, nitroprusside and positive end-expiratory pressure. J Clin Invest 1981;67:409.

170. Diebel LN, Wilson RF, Tagett MG, et al. End-diastolic volume: a better indicator of preload in the critically ill. Arch Surg 1992;127:817.

171. Diebel L, Wilson RF, Heins J, et al. End-diastolic volume versus PAWP in evaluating preload in ICU trauma patients. J Trauma 1993;35:988.

172. Skillman JJ, Restall DS, Salzman EW. Randomized trial of albumin vs electrolyte solutions during abdominal aortic operations. Surgery 1995;78:291.

173. Hauser CJ, Shoemaker WC, Turpin I. Oxygen transport responses to colloids and crystalloids in critically ill surgical patients. Surg Gynecol Obstet 1980;150:811.

174. Appel PL, Shoemaker WC. Evaluation of fluid therapy in adult respiratory failure. Crit Care Med 1981;9:862.

175. Ledgerwood AM, Lucas CE. Post-resuscitation hypertension, etiology, morbidity and treatment. Arch Surg 1974;108:531.

176. Lucas CE, Ledgerwood AM, Mammen EF. Altered coagulation protein content after albumin resuscitation. Ann Surg 1982;196:198.

177. Clift DR, Ledgerwood AM, Lucas CE, et al. The effect of albumin resuscitation for shock on the immune response to tetanus toxoid. J Surg Res 1982;32:449.

178. Oppenheimer L, Landolfo KP. Treatment of permeability pulmonary edema with macromolecular solutions. J Trauma 1991;31:1036.

179. Wilson RF, Gibson DB. The use of arterio-central venous oxygen differences to calculate cardiac output and oxygen consumption in critically ill surgical patients. Surgery 1978;84:362.

180. Shoemaker WC, Appel PL. Use of physiological monitoring to predict outcome and to assist in clinical decisions in critically ill postoperative patients. Am J surg 1983;146:43.

181. Fenwick J, Russell JA, Phang T, et al. Blood transfusion identifies delivery dependent oxygen consumption in patients with adult respiratory distress syndrome and lactic acidosis. Chest 1988;94:74S.

182. Gilbert EM, Haupt MT, Mandanas RY, et al. The effect of fluid loading, blood transfusion, and catecholamine infusion on oxygen delivery and consumption in patients with sepsis. Am Rev Respir Dis 1986;134:873.

183. Shoemaker WC, Appel PL, Kram HB, et al. Prospective trial of supranormal values as therapeutic goals in high-risk surgical patients. Chest 1988;94:1176.

184. Cryer HG, Richardson JD, Longmire-Cook S, et al. Oxygen delivery in patients with adult respiratory distress syndrome who undergo surgery. Arch Surg 1989;124:378.

185. Fleming A, Bishop M, Shoemaker W, et al. Prospective trial of supranormal values as goals of resuscitation in severe trauma. Arch Surg 1992;127:1175.

186. Moore EE, Moore FA. Aggressive enteral feeding reduces sepsis and multiple organ failure? A review of recent studies. J Crit Care Nutr 1993;1:5.

187. Alexander JW. Immunonutrition: an emerging strategy in the ICU. J Crit Care Nutr 1993;1:21.

188. Cook DJ, Laine LA, Guyatt GH, et al. Nosocomial pneumonia and the role of gastric pH: a meta-analysis. Chest 1991;100:7.

189. Tryba M. Sucralfate versus antacids or H_2-antagonists for stress ulcer prophylaxis: a meta-analysis of efficacy and pneumonia rate. Crit Care Med 1991;19:942.

190. Cioffi WG, McManus AT, Rue LW, et al. Comparison of acid neutralizing and non-acid neutralizing stress ulcer prophylaxis in thermally injured patients. J Trauma 1994;36:541.

191. Fabian TC, Boucher BA, Croce MA, et al. Pneumonia and stress ulceration in severely injured patients. Arch Surg 1993;128:195.

192. Seligman M. Bronchodilators. Chernow B, ed. The pharmacologic approach to the critically ill patient, 2nd ed. Baltimore: Williams & Wilkins, 1988; 446.

193. Shoemaker WC, Appel PL, Kram HB. Hemodynamic and oxygen transport effects of dobutamine in critically ill surgical patients. Crit Care Med 1986;14:1032.

194. Diebel LN, Dulchavsky SA, Wilson RF. Effect of increased intra-abdominal pressure on hepatic arterial, portal venous, and hepatic microcirculatory blood flow. J Trauma 1992;33:289.

195. Garzia F, Todor R, Scalea T. Continuous arteriovenous hemofiltration countercurrent dialysis (CAVH-D) in acute respiratory failure (ARDS). J Trauma 1991;21:1277.

196. Jackson RM. Oxygen therapy and toxicity. Ayres SM, Grenvik A, Holbrook PR, Shoemaker WC, eds. Textbook of critical care, 3rd ed. WB Saunders Company, 1995; 784-789.

197. Pearson FG, Andrews MJ. Detection and management of tracheal stenosis following cuffed tube tracheostomy. Ann Thorac Surg 1971;12:371.

198. Rodriguez JL, Steinberg SM, Luchetti FA, et al. Early tracheostomy for primary airway management in the surgical critical care setting. Surgery 1990;108:655.

199. Dreyfuss D, Jackson RS, Coffin LH, et al. High frequency ventilation in the management of tracheal trauma. J Trauma 1986;26:287.

200. Borg UR, Stoklosa JC, Siegel JH, et al. Prospective evaluation of combined high frequency ventilation in post-traumatic patients with adult respiratory distress syndrome refractory to optimized conventional ventilatory management. Crit Care Med 1989;17:1129.

201. Marini JJ, Kelsen SG. Re-targeting ventilatory objectives in adult respiratory distress syndrome. New treatment prospects; persistent questions. Am Rev Respir Dis 1992;146:2.

202. Mathru M, Rao TL, El-Etr AA, et al. Hemodynamic response to changes in ventilatory patterns in patients with normal and poor left ventricular reserve. Crit Care Med 1982;10:423.

203. Shah DH, Newell JAC, Dutton RE, et al. Continuous positive airway pressure versus positive end-expiratory pressure in response distress syndrome. J Thorac Cardiovasc Surg 1977;75:577.

204. Steinhoff HH, Hohlhoff RJ, Falke KJ. Facilitation of renal function by intermittent mandatory ventilation. Intensive Care Med 1984;10:59.

205. Roussos C, Maklem PT. Diaphragmatic fatigue in man. J Appl Physiol 1977;43:198.

206. Tokioka H, Saito S, Kasaka F. Effects of pressure support ventilation on breathing patterns and respiratory work. Intensive Care Med 1989;15:491.

207. Downs JB. New modes of ventilatory assistance. Chest 1986;90:626.

208. MacIntyre NR. Respiratory function during pressure support ventilation. Chest 1986;89:677.

209. Katz JA, Kraemer RW, Gjerde GE. Inspiratory work and airway pres-

sure with continuous positive airway pressure delivery systems. Chest 1985;88:519.

210. MacIntyre NR, Leatherman NE. Ventilatory muscle loads and the frequency-tidal volume pattern during inspiratory pressure assisted (pressure supported) ventilation. Am Rev Respir Dis 1990;141:327.

211. MacIntyre N, Nishimura M, Usada Y, et al. The Nagoya Conference on system design and patient-ventilator interactions during pressure support ventilation. Chest 1990;97:1463.

212. MacIntyre NR. Pressure support ventilation. Respir Care 1986;31:189.

213. Wong DH, Stemmer EA, Gordon I. Acute massive air leak and pressure support ventilation. Crit Care Med 1990;18:114.

214. Hewlett AM, Platt AS, Terry VG. Mandatory minute volume. A new concept in weaning from mechanical ventilators. Anaesthesia 1977;32:163.

215. Shapiro BA, Cane RD, Harrison RA. Positive end-expiratory pressure in adults with special reference to acute lung injury. A review of the literature and suggested clinical corrections. Crit Care Med 1984;12:127.

216. Hickling KG, Henderson SJ, Jackson R. Low mortality associated with low volume pressure limited ventilation with permissive hypercapnia in severe adult respiratory distress syndrome. Intensive Care Med 1990;16:372.

217. Hazelzet JA, Pwetru R, Den Ouden C, et al. New modes of mechanical ventilation for severe respiratory failure. Crit Care Med 1993;21:S366.

218. Greaves TH, Cramolini GM, Waler DH, et al. Inverse ratio ventilation in a 6 year old with severe post-traumatic adult respiratory distress syndrome. Crit Care Med 1989;17:588.

219. Wilson RF, Christensen C, Ali M, et al. Oxygen consumption in critically ill surgical patients. Ann Surg 1972;176:801.

220. Ravizza AG, Carugo D, Cerchairi EL, et al. Inverse ratio and conventional ventilations: comparison of the respiratory effect. Anesthesiology 1989;59:A523.

221. Samuels JB, Rochon B, Stanford GC, et al. Pressure controlled inverse ratio ventilation in severe ARDS. J Trauma 1992;33:162.

222. Simon R, Ivatury R, Hayard V. Failure of standard ventilatory parameters to predict IRV success. J Trauma 1993;34:183.

223. Hyzy RC, Popovic J. Mechanical ventilation and weaning. Carlson RW, Geheb MA, eds. Principles and practice of medical intensive care. Philadelphia: WB Saunders, 1993; 937.

224. Rouby JJ, Ben Ameur M, Jawish D, et al. Continuous positive airway pressure (CPAP) vs intermittent mandatory pressure release ventilation (IMPRV) in patients with acute respiratory failure. Intensive Care Med 1992;18:69.

225. Stock MC, Downs JB, Frolieher DA. Airway pressure release ventilation. Crit Care Med 1987;15:462.

226. Rasanen J, Downs JB, Stock MC. Cardiovascular effects of conventional positive pressure ventilation and airway pressure release ventilation. Chest 1988;93:911.

227. Lawler PGP, Nunn JF. A reassessment of the validity of the isoshunt graph. Br J Anaesth 1984;56:1325.

228. Shapiro BA, Cane RD, Harrison RA. Positive end-expiratory pressure therapy in adults with special reference to acute lung injury. Crit Care Med 1984;12:127.

229. Miller WC, Rice DL, Unger KM, et al. Effect of PEEP on lung water content in experimental noncardiogenic pulmonary edema. Crit Care Med 1981;9:7.

230. Ashbaugh DG, Petty TL. PEEP: physiology indications and contraindications. J Thorac Cardiovasc Surg 1973;65:195.

231. Norwood SH, Civetta JM. Ventilatory support in patients with ARDS. Surg Clin North Am 1985;65:895.

232. Katz JA, Marks JD. Inspiratory work with and without continuous positive airway pressure in patients with acute respiratory failure. Anesthesiology 1985;63:598.

233. Miller RS, Nelson LD, DiRusso S, et al. High level positive end-expiratory pressure (PEEP) management in trauma associated with adult respiratory distress syndrome (ARDS). J Trauma 1991;31:1719.

234. Pepe PE, Hudson LD, Carrico CJ. Early application of positive end-expiratory pressure in patients at risk for the adult respiratory distress syndrome. N Engl J Med 1984;311:281.

235. Albert RK. Least PEEP: primum non nocere. Chest 1985;87:2.

236. Sibbald WJ, Driedger AA, Cunningham DG, et al. Right and left ventricular performance in acute hypoxemic respiratory failure. Crit Care Med 1986;14:852.

237. Broaddus VC, Berthiaume Y, Biondi JW, et al. Hemodynamic management of the adult respiratory distress syndrome. J Intensive Care Med 1987;2:190.

238. Rasanen J, Downs JB, DeHaven B. Titration of continuous positive airway pressure by real-time dual oximetry. Chest 1987;92:853.

239. Suter PM, Fairley HB, Isenberg MD. Optimum end-expiratory airway pressure in patients with acute pulmonary failure. N Engl J Med 1975;292:284.

240. Shapiro B. General principles of airway pressure therapy. Shoemaker WC, Ayres S, Grenvik A, et al., eds. Textbook of critical care. Philadelphia: WB Saunders, 1989; 505.

241. Kirby RR, Downs JB, Civetta JM, et al. High level positive end-expiratory pressure (PEEP) in acute respiratory insufficiency. Chest 1975;67:156.

242. Murray IP, Modell JH, Gallagher TJ, et al. Titration of PEEP by the arterial minus end-tidal carbon dioxide gradient. Chest 1984;85:100.

243. Bolin RW, Pierson DJ. Ventilatory management in acute lung injury. Crit Care Clin 1986;2:585.

244. Tobin MJ, Lodato RF. PEEP, auto-PEEP and water falls. Editorial. Chest 1989;96:449.

245. Hoffman RA, Ershowsky P, Krieger BP. Determination of auto-PEEP during spontaneous and controlled ventilation by monitoring changes in end-expiratory thoracic gas volume. Chest 1989;96:613.

246. Banner MJ, Smith RA. Mechanical ventilation. Civetta JM, Taylor RK, Kirby RR, eds. Critical care. Philadelphia: JB Lippincott, 1988; 1168.

247. Simon R, Mawilmada S, Ivatury R. Hypercapnia—is there a cause for concern. J Trauma 1993;35:171.

248. Gilbert EM, Haupt MT, Mandanas RY, et al. The effect of fluid loading, blood transfusion, and catecholamine infusion on oxygen delivery and consumption in patients with sepsis. Am Rev Respir Dis 1986;134:873.

249. Shapiro BA, Cane RD, Chomka CM, et al. Preliminary evaluation of an intra-arterial blood gas system in dogs and humans. Crit Care Med 1989;17:455.

250. Taylor MB, Whitman JG. The current status of pulse oximetry. Anesthesia 1986;41:943.

251. Stasic AF. Continuous evaluation of oxygenation and ventilation. Civetta JM, Taylor RW, Kirby RR, eds. Critical Care. Philadelphia: JB Lippincott, 1988; 317.

252. Triner L, Sherman J. Potential value of expiratory carbon dioxide measurement in patients considered to be susceptible to malignant hyperthermia. Anesthesiology 1981;55:482.

253. Nolan LS, Shoemaker WC. Transcutaneous O_2 and CO_2 monitoring of high risk surgical patients during the perioperative period. Crit Care Med 1982;10:762.

254. Kram HB, Shoemaker WC. Transcutaneous, conjunctival, and organ P_{O_2} and P_{CO_2} monitoring in the adult. Shoemaker WC, Ayres S, Grenvik A, et al., eds. Textbook of critical care. Philadelphia: WB Saunders, 1989; 283.

255. Kram HB, Shoemaker WC, Bratanow N, et al. Noninvasive conjunctival oxygen monitoring during carotid endarterectomy. Arch Surg 1986;121:914.

256. Sahn SA, Laushminarayan, Petty TL. Weaning from mechanical ventilation. JAMA 1976;232:2208.

257. Yank KL, Tobin MJ. A prospective study of indices predicting the outcome of trials of weaning from mechanical ventilation. N Engl J Med 1991;324:445.

258. Shikora SA, Benotti PN, Johannigman JA. The oxygen cost of breathing may predict weaning from mechanical ventilation better than the respiratory rate to tidal volume ratio. Arch Surg 1984;129:269.

259. Slatsky AS. ACEP Consensus Conference: mechanical ventilation. Chest 1993;104:1833.

260. Kaemerek RM. Inspiratory pressure support: does it make a difference? Intensive Care Med 1989;15:337.

261. Irwin RS, Demers RR. Mechanical ventilation. Rippe JM, Irwin RS, Alpert IS, Dalen JE, eds. Intensive care medicine. Boston: Little, Brown, 1985; 462.

262. Goldman AL, Morrison D, Foster LJ. Oral progesterone therapy: oxygen in a pill. Arch intern Med 1981;141:574.

263. Argov Z, Mastaglia FL. Disorders of neuromuscular transmission caused by drugs. N Engl J Med 1979;301:409.

264. Moore FA, Moore EE, Jones TN, et al. TEN versus TPN following major abdominal trauma—reduced septic morbidity. J Trauma 1989;29:916.

265. Ashbaugh DG, Maier RV. Idiopathic pulmonary fibrosis in adult respiratory distress syndrome. Diagnosis and treatment. Arch Surg 1985;120:530.

266. Hanly PJ, Dobson K, Roberts D, et al. Effect of indomethacin on arterial oxygenation in critically ill patients with severe bacterial pneumonia. Lancet 1987;1:351.

267. Byrne K, Carey PC, Sielaff TD, et al. Ibuprofen prevents deterioration in static transpulmonary compliance and transalveolar protein flux in septic porcine acute lung injury. J Trauma 1991;31:155.

268. Bone RC, Jacobs ER. Advances in pharmacologic treatment of acute lung injury and septic shock. Adv Anesth 1987;4:327.

269. Holcroft JW, Vassar MJ, Weber CJ. Prostaglandin E$_1$ and survival in patients with the adult respiratory distress syndrome. Ann Surg 1986;203:371.

270. Bone RC, Slotman G, Maunder R, et al. Randomized double-blind, multicenter study of prostaglandin E$_1$ in patients with the adult respiratory distress syndrome. Prostaglandin E$_1$ Study Group. Chest 1989;96:114.

271. Tuxen DV, Case JF. Effect of aprotinin in adult respiratory distress syndrome. Anaesth Intensive Care 1986;14:390.

272. Svenningsen N, Robertson B, Andreason B, et al. Endotracheal administration of surfactant in very low birth weight infants with respiratory distress syndrome. Crit Care Med 1987;15:918.

273. Palmer RMJ, Ferrige AG, Moncada S. Nitric oxide release accounts for the biological activity of endothelium-derived relaxing factor. Nature 1987;327:524.

274. Rossaint R, Falke KJ, Lopez F, et al. Inhaled nitric oxide for the adult respiratory distress syndrome. N Engl J Med 1993;328:399.

275. Ogura H, Cioffi WG, Jordan BS, et al. The effect of inhaled nitric oxide on smoke inhalation injury in an ovine model. J Trauma 1993;35:167.

276. Zapol WM, Falke KJ, Hurford WE, et al. Inhaling nitric oxide: a selective pulmonary vasodilator and bronchodilator. Chest 1994;105:875.

277. Freeman B. Free radical chemistry of nitric oxide: looking at the dark side. Chest 1994;105:795.

278. Burman KD. Thyroid hormones. Chernow B, ed. The pharmacologic approach to the critically ill patient. Baltimore: Williams & Wilkins, 1994; 752-755.

279. Dulchavsky SA, Bailey J. T$_3$ maintains surfactant synthesis in sepsis. Surgery 1992;112:475.

280. Dulchavsky SA, Hendrick HR, Dutta S. Pulmonary biophysical effects of triiodothyronine augmentation during sepsis-induced hypothyroidism. Crit Care Med 1993;35:104.

281. Downs JB. New modes of ventilatory assistance. Chest 1993;90:626.

282. MacIntyre NR. Respiratory function during pressure support ventilation. Chest 1986;89:677.

283. St. John RC, Dorinsky PM.: Immunologic therapy for ARDS, septic shock, and multiple organ failure. Chest 1993;103:932.

284. Silva AT, Appelmelk BJ, Buurman WA, et al. Monoclonal antibody to endotoxin core protects mice from Escherichia coli sepsis by a mechanism independent of tumor necrosis factor and interleukin-6. J Infect Dis 1990;162:454.

285. Ziegler EJ, Fisher CJ Jr, Sprung CL, et al. Treatment of Gram-negative bacteremia and septic shock with Ha-1A human monoclonal antibody against endotoxin: a randomized, double-blind, placebo-controlled trial. N Engl J Med 1991;324:429.

286. Greenman RL, Schein RM, Martin MA, et al. A controlled clinical trial of E5 murine monoclonal IgM antibody to endotoxin in the treatment of Gram-negative sepsis. JAMA 1991;266:1097.

287. Tracey KJ, Lowrey SF, Cerami A, et al. Anti-cachectin/TNF monoclonal antibodies prevent septic shock during lethal bacteremia. Nature 1987;330:662.

288. Exley AR, Cohen J, Buurman W, et al. Monoclonal antibody to TNF in severe septic shock. Lancet 1990;335:1275.

289. Dripps DJ, Brandhuber BJ, Thompson RC, et al. Interleukin-1 (IL-1) receptor antagonist binds to the 90-kDa IL-1 receptor but does not initiate IL-1 signal transduction. J Biol Chem 1991;226:1033.

290. Ulich TR, Yin S, Guo K, et al. The intratracheal administration of endotoxin and cytokines: III. The interleukin-1 (IL-1) receptor antagonist inhibits endotoxin- and IL-1-induced acute inflammation. Am J Pathol 1991;138:521.

291. Fisher CJ Jr, Slotman GJ, Opal SM, et al. Initial evaluation of human recombinant interleukin-1 receptor antagonist in the treatment of sepsis syndrome. A randomized, open-label, placebo-controlled multicenter trial. Crit Care Med 1994;22:3.

292. Zapol WM, Snider MT, Hill JD. Extracorporeal membrane oxygenation in severe acute respiratory failure. A randomized prospective study. JAMA 1979;242:2193.

293. Moler FW, Palmisano J, Custer JR. Extracorporeal life support for pediatric respiratory failure: predictors of survival from 220 patients. Crit Care Med 1993;21:1604.

294. Anderson HL, Shapiro MB, Steimle CN, et al. Extracorporeal life support for respiratory failure due to trauma—a viable alternative. J Trauma 1993;35:158.

295. Gattinoni L, Agnostomi A, Pesenti A, et al. Treatment of acute respiratory failure with low frequency positive pressure ventilation and extracorporeal CO$_2$ removal. Lancet 1980;2:292.

296. Morris AH, Wallace J, Menlove RL, et al. Final report: a computerized protocol controlled randomized clinical trial of new therapy that includes LFPPV-ECCO$_2$R. Am Rev Respir Dis 1992;145.A184.

297. Brunet F, Belghith M, Mira JP, et al. Extracorporeal carbon dioxide removal and low-frequency positive-pressure ventilation: improvement in arterial oxygenation with reduction of risk of pulmonary barotrauma in patients with adult respiratory distress syndrome. Chest 1993;104:889.

298. Morris AH, Wallace J, Menlove RL, et al. Randomized clinical trial of pressure-controlled inverse ratio ventilation and extracorporeal CO$_2$ removal for adult respiratory distress syndrome. Am J Respir 1994;149:295.

299. Suchyta MR, Clemmer TP, Orme JF, et al. Increased survival of ARDS patients with severe hypoxemia (ECMO criteria). Chest 1991;99:951.

300. Gentilello LM, Jurkovich GJ, Gubler KD, et al. The intravascular oxygenator (IVOX): preliminary results of a new means of performing extrapulmonary gas exchange. J Trauma 1993;35:399.

301. Mortensen JD. Conceptual and design features of a practical, clinically effective, intravenous, mechanical blood oxygen/carbon dioxide exchange device (IVOX). Int J Artif Organs 1989;12:384.

302. Montgomery AB, Stager MA, Carrico CJ, et al. Causes of mortality in patients with the adult respiratory distress syndrome. Am Rev Respir Dis 1985;132:485.

303. Seidenfeld JJ, Pohl DF, Bell RC, et al. Incidence, site, and outcome of infections in patients with the adult respiratory distress syndrome. Am Rev Respir Dis 1986;134:12.

304. Bell RC, Coalson J, Smith JD, et al. Multiple organ system failure and infection in adult respiratory distress syndrome. Ann Intern Med 1983;99:293.

305. Bitterman PB, Polunovsky VA, Ingbar DH. Repair after acute lung injury. Chest 1994;105:118S.

Chapter **41** Cardiovascular Failure Following Trauma

ROBERT F. WILSON, M.D.

INTRODUCTION

Cardiac failure is an increasingly important cause of death or major complications in injured patients.[1] This is true partly because of the increasing number of elderly patients who are injured and partly because of our improving ability to resuscitate individuals with prolonged hypotension or cardiovascular injuries.

Although some heart failure seen after trauma is due to prolonged, severe hypotension, much of it is related to preexisting cardiac disease. It is estimated that 2.4 million Americans suffer from heart failure, and approximately 400,000 new cases are added each year.[2] The prevalence rate is about 1-2% at age 50, while at 80 years and above, about 10-15% have heart failure. A diagnosis of heart failure carries a grim prognosis, with up to 35-50% of patients dying within the next two years.[4]

Within six years of the initial diagnosis of heart failure in the Framingham study, 63% of women and 70% of men had experienced one or more recurrences. In addition, these patients had a fourfold greater risk of stroke and a 2.5-5 times greater probability of myocardial infarction than did the general population.[5]

In most previously healthy patients who develop cardiac failure, the process develops rather suddenly because of cardiac arrest or severe, prolonged shock, aggravated by rapid, severe fluid overloading.[1] In some, it develops insidiously over several days because of myocardial depression caused by sepsis and/or increasing demands placed on the cardiovascular system by other organ failure.

CARDIOVASCULAR PHYSIOLOGY

Functional Anatomy of the Heart

The heart is composed primarily of interlacing fibers of specialized muscle. It weighs about 300 g in the average adult male and 250 g in the average adult female, or about 2 g for each pound of ideal body weight.

ATRIA

The atria act as reservoirs and booster pumps for filling the ventricles. During the early phase of ventricular diastole, blood flows passively from the atria into the ventricles, but during the last phase, the atria contract, pumping in about 20-30% of the end-diastolic volume of the ventricles (Fig. 41–1). Loss of atrial systole in a normal heart has only minimal effect, but with any impediment to left ventricular (LV) filling, such as with mitral stenosis, left atrial systole may account for more than 50% of LV filling.

VENTRICLES

The walls of the left ventricle are much thicker (8-12 mm) than those of the right ventricle (3-4 mm) to pump against a systemic vascular resistance which is normally at least six times greater than that present in the pulmonary circuit (Table 41–1).

Although the normal upper limit of systolic pressure in the right ventricle in older individuals is 25 mm Hg, in young adults this limit is normally only 12-15 mm Hg. The right ventricle often cannot achieve a systolic pressure > 40 mm Hg unless preexisting right ven-

tricular hypertrophy occurs. The normal left ventricle often cannot achieve aortic pressure > 180 mm Hg without dilating and developing some dysfunction.

AXIOM When aortic systolic pressure exceeds 160-180 mm Hg, the LV end-diastolic pressure (LVEDP), even in a normal heart, often doubles and the left ventricle may dilate and go into failure.

CONDUCTING SYSTEM

The conducting system of the heart has the capability of rhythmic electrical impulse formation and can conduct electrical impulses much more rapidly than typical cardiac muscle. Electrical impulses in the heart normally begin in the sinoatrial (SA) node. The impulse then spreads over the atria to stimulate atrial contraction along special upper, middle, and lower internodal tracts to the atrioventricular (AV) node.

AXIOM In infants, the elderly, and patients with diseased hearts, stroke volume may be relatively fixed. Consequently, bradycardia after trauma may be extremely dangerous.

Impulses picked up or generated by the AV node are transmitted along the AV bundle of His to the Purkinje fibers and then to the ventricular myocardium.[6] The Purkinje fibers not only act as the terminal portion of the conduction system, but they can also function as a backup pacemaker for the heart. However, their discharge rate is only 20-40 beats per minute. Thus, they seldom initiate a heartbeat except when there is a complete AV block and complete absence of AV nodal impulses.

AXIOM Unusual ventricular complexes in a patient with a very slow heart rate may represent escape beats (not premature ventricular contractions) and should not be suppressed.

CORONARY ARTERIES

Coronary blood flow in an adult male at rest averages about 250-300 mL/min which is about 1.0 mL/g of heart muscle, or 4-5% of the total cardiac output.[6] During systole, blood flow through the LV myocardium decreases to very low levels. Coronary sinus blood has the lowest P_{O_2} (18-20 mm Hg) and lowest saturation (30-35%) of any venous blood in the body. Thus, even in the normal resting state, 65-70% of the oxygen present in coronary artery blood is removed as blood passes through the heart. Therefore, there is no so-called "oxygen reserve" in coronary blood.

AXIOM When increased oxygen is required by the heart, it can only be provided by increasing coronary blood flow.

The heart is one of the few organs that can utilize lactate for fuel; therefore, coronary venous lactate levels normally are lower than those in the arteries.

FIGURE 41-1 The phases of the cardiac cycle correlated with the occurrence of heart sounds and changes in aortic, LV, and left atrial pressures (From: Shatz IJ, Wilson RF. Cardiovascular failure. Walt AJ, Wilson RF, eds. Management of trauma: pitfalls and practice. Philadelphia: Lea & Febiger, 1975; 537).

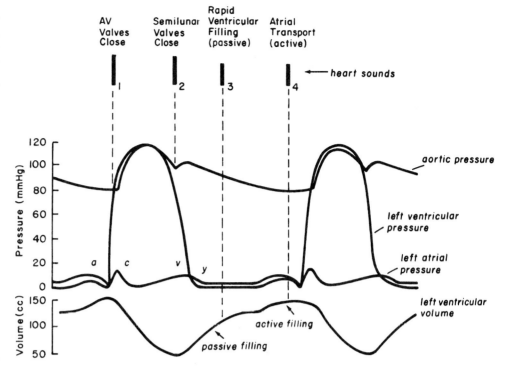

AXIOM Increased coronary sinus lactate usually indicates myocardial ischemia.

Basic Physiology of Muscle Contraction

All striated muscle, including skeletal and cardiac muscle, consists of numerous muscle fibers about 10-100 microns in diameter which, in turn, consist of several hundred to several thousand myofibrils.[6] Myocardial cells are separated from each other by sarcolemma and intercalated disks. Each cell contains: (a) an energy generation system (the mitochondria), (b) intracellular transportation and storage system for calcium and other ions (the transverse tubular system and sarcoplasmic reticulum), and (c) an electromechanical apparatus (the myofibrils) that converts chemical energy into mechanical work. Each myofibril contains about 1500 myosin and about 3000 actin filaments which lay parallel to each other. These large, polymerized protein molecules, which are responsible for muscle contraction, are sus-

pended within the sarcoplasm. Depolarization is initiated by a short-duration increase in the permeability of the cell membrane to Na^+ and Ca^{2+}.

Factors Affecting Cardiac Function

The main factors that affect cardiac function and cardiac output include preload (filling of the heart during diastole), afterload (resistance against which the heart must pump), contractility of the heart, the coordinated pattern of the contractions, and heart rate.[6]

PRELOAD

Preload refers to the tension on a muscle fiber as it begins to contract. In the heart, this is determined by the quantity of blood in the ventricle at the end of diastole.[6] As early as 1884, Howell and Donaldson[7] presented evidence that the heart has intrinsic mechanisms by which its output is adjusted to its venous input. In 1895, Frank published his classic studies on "the dynamics of heart muscle." He showed that the reactions of cardiac muscle to its precontractile tension were similar to the response of skeletal muscle to its initial length of tension. Frank also showed that, within limits, stepwise increases in the end-diastolic volume in the frog heart determine the magnitude of the next cardiac contraction.

In 1914, Wiggers demonstrated that the reactions established by Frank for the frog's ventricle were also applicable to the naturally beating right ventricle of dogs.[9] In that same year, Straub[10] and Patterson and Starling[11,12] independently reported their studies of the effect of changes in initial tension and length on the response of isolated hearts.[9] Starling, on the basis of highly suggestive, but not quite conclusive, studies on heart-lung preparations, concluded that "the mechanical energy set free on passage from the resting to the constricted state depends on the area of chemically active surfaces; i.e., on the length of the muscle fibers."[13] Starling, because of his clear descriptions of these inclusions in his Linacre lecture in 1918[13] received most of the recognition, and this principle is often referred to as "Starling's law of the heart."

Wiggers[14] reported that although there is a general impression that the "law" presented so eloquently by Starling was based on data from his own experiments, the careful reader will discover that the pub-

TABLE 41-1 Pressure and Oxygen Saturation in Various Chambers of the Heart

	Pressure (mm Hg)	O_2 Saturation (%)
Superior vena cava	0-5	70-75
Inferior vena cava	0-5	75-80
Coronary sinus	—	30-40
Right atrium	0-5	70-75
Right ventricle	12-25/0-5	70-75
Pulmonary artery	12-25/5-10 (8-15)*	70-75
Pulmonary capillaries	6-12	98-100
Left atrium	5-10	95-98
Left ventricle	120/0-5	95-98
Aorta	120/80 (92)	95-97

*Parentheses refer to mean pressure
From: Wilson RF. Cardiovascular physiology. Wilson RF, ed. Critical care manual: applied physiology and principles of therapy, 2nd ed. Philadelphia: FA Davis Company, 1992; 6.

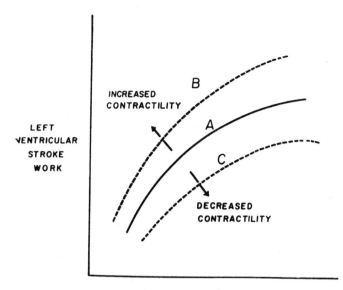

FIGURE 41–2 Relationship between LV end-diastolic fiber length and LV stroke work. Curve A represents normal function; Curve B illustrates a "shift to the left" associated with increased contractility, such as may result from infusion of epinephrine or norepinephrine. Curve C represents a "shift to the right" associated with decreased contractility, such as may result from ventricular failure from ischemia or myocardial depressant drugs (From: Schlant RC. Normal anatomy and function of the cardiovascular system. Hurst JW, Logue RB, eds. The heart. New York: McGraw-Hill Book Company, 1966; 29).

lished curves were acknowledged to be reproductions of graphs previously published by Blix and Frank.[8]

Sarnoff and Berglund[15] and Sarnoff[16] demonstrated that a "family of curves" correlating end ventricular diastolic volume and pressure exists for each ventricle. They also noted that many factors, such as humoral agents, neural influences, and the metabolic condition of the myocardium determine which particular "curve" the ventricle is operating on at a given moment (Fig. 41–2). This form of intrinsic autoregulation of the heart (in which the size of the ventricular chamber determines its contractility) has been referred to as heterometric autoregulation. In contrast, hemometric autoregulation refers to changes in ventricular activity due to alterations in heart rate (Bowditch effect) or aortic pressure (Anrep effect) without any change in diastolic ventricular fiber length.

AXIOM Increased filling of the heart, increased pulse rate, and increased aortic pressure all tend to increase myocardial contractility.

All of these effects are interrelated. For example, increased filling of the heart increases the resting heart rate (Bainbridge reflex) at the same time that it increases pumping effectiveness. The Bainbridge reflex appears to be initiated primarily by receptors in the walls of the right atrium or venae cavae that transmit impulses to the vasomotor center by way of vagal afferent fibers.

Increased blood volume, by increasing atrial distention, also causes increased secretion of atrial natriuretic peptide (ANP), primarily by the left atrium.[17] ANP is a potent natriuretic diuretic and vasodilating substance. The resultant loss of salt and water in the urine and dilatation of vessels act to reduce cardiac filling. Patients with increased cardiac filling pressure and congestive heart failure usually have significantly elevated plasma levels of immunoreactive ANP.

AXIOM Use of positive end-expiratory pressure (PEEP) reduces the net distending pressure of the atria, thereby reducing ANP secretion; therefore, PEEP can reduce urine output by decreasing venous return and by decreasing ANP production.

AFTERLOAD

Afterload for a ventricle is defined as its wall tension during ejection. It may also be defined as the "load" the cardiac muscle must overcome when it contracts.[18] The two principal determinants of this tension, according to LaPlace's formula, are the systolic pressure and the radius of the ventricle.[16] LV radius is related to its end-diastolic volume, and its systolic pressure is related to the impedance to blood flow in the aorta.[18] The impedance to LV ejection is determined by the total systemic vascular resistance (SVR).

The formula for calculating SVR is:

$$SVR = \frac{MAP - CVP}{CO} \times 80$$

where MAP = mean arterial pressure, CVP = central venous pressure, CO = cardiac output, and normal SVR = 900-1400 dyne·sec·cm^{-5}.

As ventricular radius increases, wall tension also increases. If afterload were to increase but preload and contractility were to remain constant, decreased muscle shortening during contraction and prolonged presystolic ejection time would occur.[19] Increasing the duration of the isovolemic contraction phase markedly increases myocardial oxygen consumption, and this can be detrimental to trauma patients with coronary artery disease.

AXIOM Increased afterload decreases stroke volume and increases myocardial oxygen consumption.

An increase in systemic vascular resistance (SVR) increases intrinsic ventricular contractility, but stroke volume and cardiac output tend to decrease. In the failing heart, an increased SVR tends to cause a much greater decline in cardiac output (Fig. 41–3). A decline in cardiac output is often seen when vasopressors are used to correct hypotension; however, if the systemic BP is below the critical closing pressure of diseased coronary arteries, the increase in BP may improve coronary blood flow and myocardial performance much more than it increases myocardial oxygen consumption (MVO$_2$).[20]

PITFALL ⊘

Failing to recognize that drugs that increase blood pressure also tend to reduce cardiac output, tissue perfusion, and oxygen delivery (DO$_2$), but will increase MVO$_2$.

CARDIAC CONTRACTILITY

The rate of generation of cross linkings between actin and myosin determines the state of myocardial contractility which, in turn, con-

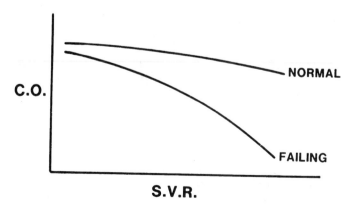

FIGURE 41–3 Qualitative relationship of cardiac output (CO) and systemic vascular resistance (SVR). A normal heart can tolerate elevations of SVR or afterload because pump function is adequate. The failing heart has poor ability to maintain cardiac output in the face of increasing SVR (From: Grande CM, Tissot M, Bhatt V, et al. Preexisting compromising conditions. Capan LM, Miller SM, Turndorf H, eds. Philadelphia: JB Lippincott, 1991; 249).

FIGURE 41–4 During excitation-contraction coupling, depolarization of the sarcolemma is accompanied by opening of calcium channels, allowing movement of calcium ions by passive influx down an electrochemical gradient from a region of high activity outside the cell to a region of low Ca^{++} activity inside the cell. Influx of small amounts of Ca^{++} across the sarcolemma triggers much larger Ca^{++} release from the sarcoplasmic reticulum, providing the large amounts of Ca^{++} needed for binding to contractile proteins and initiation of contraction. Relaxation occurs when the ATP-dependent Ca^{++} pump in the sarcoplasmic reticulum drives Ca^{++} back into the intracellular membrane system (From: Majid PA, Roberts R. Heart failure. Civetta JM, Taylor RW, Kirby RR, eds. Critical care. New York: JB Lippincott, 1988; 947).

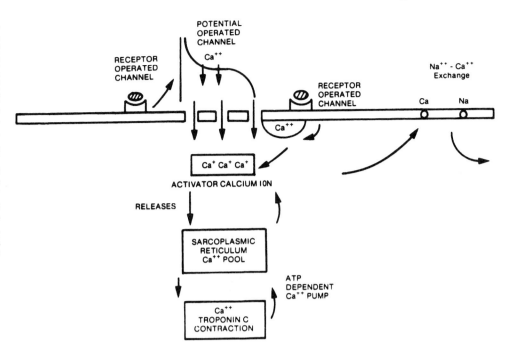

trols stroke volume when preload and afterload are constant. Until recently, there was no readily available way to quantify cardiac contractility. With special pulmonary artery (RIF) catheters, one can now determine right ventricular ejection fraction (RVEF).[21] One can also look at cardiac output and oxygen delivery at various preloads and afterloads.

Some of the mechanical and biochemical abnormalities seen with decreased myocardial contractility include decreases in: (a) velocity of muscle shortening at a given set of loading conditions, (b) maximum rate of force development, and (c) the force developed.[20] From a biochemical standpoint, mechanisms regulating the strength of myocardial contraction include actomyosin adenosine triphosphatase (ATPase) activity and the amount of activator calcium that is made available for binding to troponin C and to calmodulin during each systole (Fig. 41–4).[21] Actomyosin ATPase activity is uniformly decreased in the failing myocardium.[22] Although this results in a slower velocity of shortening, the associated reduction in oxygen consumption helps to conserve the limited supply of ATP and creatine phosphate.

Calcium fluxes across the sarcoplasmic reticulum are also impaired in the failing myocardium.[20] At the onset of depolarization, calcium crosses the muscle cell membrane during the plateau phase of the action potential. This triggers the release of internal calcium stores which, in turn, activates the contractile process by binding to troponin C and to calmodulin. The strength of the myocardial contraction is directly related to the amount of calcium released.[20]

A heart that is hypertrophied or is strongly stimulated by sympathetic impulses is capable of pumping greater quantities of blood than normal against a standard amount of resistance and may be considered to have increased myocardial contractility.

COORDINATED CONTRACTIONS
Even when all individual muscle units in the heart are functioning properly, failure of these units to beat in a coordinated fashion can greatly impair cardiac function.[6] Some of the more frequent causes of uncoordinated myocardial contraction include: (a) bundle-branch blocks due to ischemia or trauma, (b) ischemia or trauma to portions of the myocardium causing slower and/or weaker contraction than normal, (c) arrhythmias, and (d) excessive dilation of the ventricle.

HEART RATE
When stroke volume remains constant, an increased heart rate up to about 150 beats/min will tend to increase cardiac output.[18] The heart rate is determined primarily by a balance between stimulation of the parasympathetic nervous system's cholinergic receptors in the sinoatrial node—producing a decreased rate—and the sympathetic nervous system's stimulation of β-adrenergic receptors—producing an increased rate.[23,24] Cardiac output in very young and very old individuals with a relatively fixed stroke volume is rate-dependent; however, in patients with coronary artery disease, the benefits of improving cardiac output by increasing heart rate must be weighed against the detrimental increase in myocardial oxygen consumption that occurs with tachycardia.[26]

If the pulse rate is < 50 or > 150 per minute, cardiac output often decreases and the tendency to arrhythmias increases. However, in well-trained athletes, it is not unusual for the resting pulse rate to be < 50 at rest and greater that 180 during maximal exertion.

HEART RATE VARIABILITY
Tunin-inga et al. showed that heart rate variability is a relatively accurate, noninvasive technique for evaluating LV function and prognosis.[25] In patients with acute myocardial infarction, reduced variability in heart rate tends to correlate with poor prognosis.[26,27] In one study, 44% of patients with low HR variability (SD of RR intervals < 50 ms) had signs of heart failure, compared with only 8% of patients with high HR variability. In patients with chronic heart failure, Saul et al.[28] and Casolo et al.[29] reported that patients with advanced heart failure had considerably reduced HR variability, due apparently to abnormal sympathetic and parasympathetic control.[30]

OTHER FACTORS
Other factors that may influence cardiac function include hypoxia, anemia, and concentrations of various cations.

Hypoxia
Mild hypoxia tends to cause a moderate increase in sympathetic stimulation which, in turn, increases cardiac contractility. However, severe hypoxia impairs myocardial function.[9]

Anemia
Anemia decreases the viscosity of blood which, in turn, decreases the afterload for the heart and the resistance to blood flow in tissues. In addition, severe anemia may cause tissue hypoxia with resultant di-

lation of peripheral vessels further decreasing afterload.[9] As a result, cardiac output tends to increase in an almost linear fusion as hematocrit decreases; however, with hematocrit levels < 15-20%, blood flow may be too fast to unload O_2 in the capillaries adequately and cardiac output may have to increase geometrically to keep the tissues supplied with O_2 properly.

Effects of Various Cations

With hyperkalemia or hypocalcemia, contraction of the heart becomes progressively weaker and slower.[9] In contrast, a decrease in plasma potassium or an increase in ionized calcium concentrations tends to increase myocardial contractility. Shock and sepsis increase the movement of ionized calcium into cells. The reduced transcellular calcium gradient reduces myocardial contractility.

Myocardial Oxygen Consumption

KINETIC AND POTENTIAL ENERGY

Ordinarily, 96-98% of the work output of the left ventricle is in the form of pressure (potential energy).[9] Only 2-4% of the work output of the heart is used to create the kinetic energy associated with blood flow out of the heart. However, in certain conditions (such as aortic stenosis), as much as 50% of the total work output may be required to create blood flow.

HEAT PRODUCTION

During cardiac contraction, most of the chemical energy used is converted into heat and only a small portion into work.[9] The ratio of cardiac work output to the energy expenditure is called the efficiency of cardiac contraction. The efficiency of the heart under normal circumstances is only about 5-10%. However, during maximum work output, it may increase to 15-20%.

SYSTOLIC TENSION-TIME INDEX

Multiple studies have attempted to correlate MVO_2 with various measurements of cardiac activity. From Sarnoff's studies on isolated hearts, it is now generally agreed that MVO_2 correlates well with the calculated systolic tension-time index (STTI).[24] STTI is equal to the average tension developed by the left ventricle during systole multiplied by the duration of systole per minute. Because the tension developed in the ventricular wall during systole is a function of systolic pressure and ventricular volume, the greater the systolic pressure and the volume (radius) of the ventricle, the greater the MVO_2. As the pulse rate increases, the amount of time that the heart is in systole each minute also increases and causes the MVO_2 to increase. Conversely, when a vasodilator is given, stroke volume increases, but mean ventricular pressure is decreased. Thus, if the pulse rate were to remain constant, a vasodilator could cause cardiac output to increase without increasing MVO_2.

PULSE-PRESSURE PRODUCT

Changes in the pulse-pressure product (PPP), which is equal to the systolic BP multiplied by the heart rate, can be used to estimate changes in MVO_2. For example, if the BP is 120/80 and the pulse rate is 70/minute, the PPP is 120×70 or 8400. If the BP were to rise to 140/90 and the pulse rate to 120/minute, the new PPP would be 16,800 and the MVO_2 would also double. Efforts to reduce PPP after aortic surgery with calcium-channel blockers may reduce the incidence of myocardial ischemia.[31]

> **AXIOM** Increases in heart rate and systolic BP cause a geometric increase in myocardial oxygen demands.

Increases in heart rate and contractility can improve cardiac output somewhat but they can also greatly increase MVO_2.[28] In contrast, increases in preload will increase cardiac output with only a small increase in MVO_2.[28] Ideally, decreases in afterload can increase cardiac output while decreasing MVO_2.

> **AXIOM** The best relationship between cardiac output and MVO_2 is achieved by increasing preload and decreasing afterload rather than by inotropic or chronotropic stimulation.

No direct mechanism to measure myocardial work clinically exists, but it can be indirectly calculated. LV stroke work index (LVSWI) is the work preformed by the left ventricle. It is equal to the stroke volume index (SV divided by body surface area) times the mean arterial pressure. Thus, a vasodilator can appear to be improving myocardial contractility because the patient can have an increased stroke volume at a lower CVP and pulmonary artery wedge pressures (PAWP). However, the LV stroke work index (LVSWI) will usually not be increased because the BP tends to decrease more than the SV increases.

DEFINING HEART FAILURE

> **AXIOM** Cardiac failure is often defined as an inability of the heart to pump enough blood to meet the metabolic demands of the body; however, it is usually diagnosed clinically from evidence of pulmonary or systemic venous overload.

Clinical vs Physiologic Definitions

The term "cardiac failure" tends to have different meanings to clinicians and physiologists. To many clinicians, it refers to signs and symptoms related to venous hypertension, pulmonary congestion, and/or reduced cardiac output. However, cardiac output is not reduced in all instances of heart failure. In some patients with heart failure, cardiac output is normal or even elevated, provided the venous return is high enough to offset any decrease in cardiac contractility.

> **AXIOM** From the physiologist's viewpoint, cardiac failure is often defined as a diminished work output of the heart in relation to its filling pressure or volume.[32]

The pumping ability or contractility of the heart may be defined by cardiac function curves that correlate the stroke work of the heart (mean blood pressure multiplied by stroke volume) with the filling pressure or diastolic volume of the heart. Under these circumstances, left heart failure is considered to be present when low LVSWI occurs with a high PAWP (Fig. 41–1). Right heart failure would be reflected by a low RVSWI and a high CVP.

Right and Left Heart Failure

The terms, right heart failure and left heart failure are sometimes used clinically to describe the two major types of signs and symptoms seen with cardiac failure.[9,20] With "right" heart failure, the main signs and symptoms are pedal edema, hepatomegaly, and distended neck veins. With "left" heart failure, the usual problems are pulmonary congestion and dyspnea, often with weakness or fatigue and light-headedness.

Because the left and right sides of the heart are two separate pumping systems, it is possible for one of the ventricles to fail independently of the other, at least transiently. The most frequent causes of heart failure, such as myocardial infarction, hypertension, or valvular heart disease, often affect only the left ventricle initially.

> **AXIOM** Right heart failure is usually due to left heart failure and right heart failure can impair LV filling.

Isolated right heart failure due to chronic obstructive lung disease, acute pulmonary embolus, or right ventricular infarction is much less common than biventricular failure. When one side of the heart becomes weakened or fails, a sequence of events begins that eventually

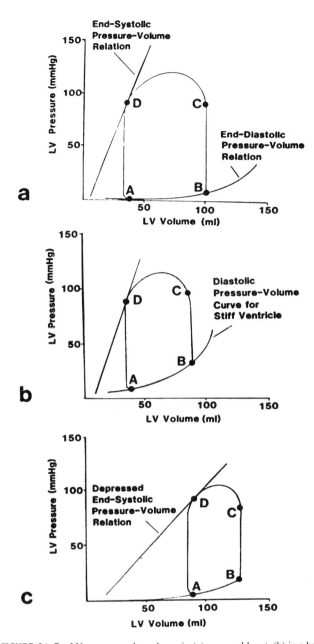

FIGURE 41–5 LV pressure-volume loops in (a) a normal heart, (b) in a heart with diastolic dysfunction, and (c) in a heart with systolic dysfunction. The pressure-volume loop in diastolic dysfunction differs from the normal curve in that end-diastolic pressure is elevated (point B) without a concomitant increase in end-diastolic volume. In systolic dysfunction, there is a depressed end-systolic pressure-volume relationship resulting in a decreased ejection fraction (EF) (From: Grande CM, Tissot M, Bhatt V, et al. Preexisting compromising conditions. Capan LM, Miller SM, Turndorf H, eds. Philadelphia: JB Lippincott, 1991; 249).

causes the opposite side to also fail. Thus, in most patients with heart failure, both chambers are eventually involved.

Systolic and Diastolic Dysfunction

Heart failure can mechanistically also be considered as diastolic dysfunction and/or systolic dysfunction.[33] Each of these occurs by different mechanisms and can best be appreciated by examining ventricular pressure-volume loops (Fig. 41–5).

Heart failure due to diastolic dysfunction is characterized by high-filling pressures at normal or lower diastolic volumes. It may be caused by severe LV hypertrophy due to hypertension, aortic steno-

sis, or hypertrophic cardiomyopathy.[20,34,35] Myocardial hypertrophy increases ventricular stiffness and can lead to delayed and reduced filling. Filling may also be impaired, in part, by abnormal relaxation of myocardial fibers due to ischemia.[36] Because calcium transport back into the sarcoplasmic reticulum at the end of contraction requires ATP, even a modest decrease in cellular ATP may slow relaxation.

Heart failure due to systolic dysfunction is characterized by a reduced ejection fraction. This typically occurs when ventricular contractility diminishes because of myocardial ischemia, infarction, or degeneration (myocarditis or cardiomyopathy).

AXIOM Systolic cardiac dysfunction is characterized by a reduced ejection fraction and need for higher end-diastolic volumes; diastolic dysfunction is characterized by a poorly relaxing heart requiring high-filling pressures.

Systolic dysfunction is much more common than diastolic dysfunction.[33] One can increase the cardiac output of a heart with systolic dysfunction by increasing preload, but the increase in cardiac output will be less than with a normal ventricle; however, the failing ventricle cannot tolerate the stress of an increased afterload, and cardiac output may decrease markedly as SVR increases.[36] Thus, in acute trauma, the reflex increase in SVR caused by hypovolemia or pain can place a major strain on a failing heart and can cause a substantial decrease in cardiac output.

Rate of Onset

Some degree of cardiac failure is present in many critically ill patients. It may develop acutely (after a myocardial infarction, cardiac surgery, or cardiac arrest) or it may develop somewhat more slowly over a period of hours or days in patients with sepsis.

ETIOLOGY OF HEART FAILURE

When a broad definition of cardiovascular failure is used (i.e., inadequate blood flow to meet the body's metabolic demands), three principal causes can be identified. These include primary myocardial failure, inadequate venous return, and circulatory overload (Table 41–2).

Primary Myocardial Failure

The primary or direct causes of inadequate cardiac function can be categorized into myocardial insufficiency, interference with diastolic filling, arrhythmias, and electrolyte and acid-base abnormalities.

ACUTE MYOCARDIAL INFARCTION

AXIOM The most frequent cause of inadequate cardiac function is myocardial infarction.

TABLE 41–2 Causes of Cardiovascular Failure

A. Primary
  1. Cardiac changes
     Myocardial infarction, valve disorders, etc.
     Cardiomyopathy (alcoholic)
     Hypothyroidism
  2. Interference with diastolic filling (tamponade), constrictive pericarditis)
  3. Arrhythmias
  4. Electrolyte and acid-base abnormalities
B. Inadequate venous return (e.g., hypovolemia, vasodilators, anesthesia)
C. Circulatory overload
  1. Increased blood volume
  2. Increased venous return (e.g., high output failure, A-V fistulas)

Myocardial Loss

It is reasonable to assume that most trauma victims over 50 years of age have some degree of coronary artery disease (CAD) and may develop myocardial ischemia or even infarction under the stress of trauma and surgery, especially with severe, prolonged hypotension. This may cause a reduced cardiac output which, in turn, can further compromise organ perfusion.[33]

With reduced cardiac output, tissues of the body are forced to extract more oxygen from the blood. This "oxygen reserve" is important in most vital organs, but it is less useful to the myocardium, which normally extracts all available oxygen coming to it.[37] If the available oxygen is still inadequate, tissues are forced to resort to anaerobic metabolism which, if persistent, will eventually cause progressive cellular death and dysfunction of the heart and other vital tissues.

A linear correlation exists between the extent of LV damage after an acute myocardial infarction and the amount of systolic dysfunction.[20] Clinical heart failure generally develops when 20-35% of the ventricular myocardium shows contractile abnormalities (hypokinesis, akinesis, or dyskinesis).[38] Loss of more than 40% of the ventricular myocardium results in cardiogenic shock, and loss of function of more than 60-70% of the left ventricle is usually rapidly fatal.[39]

In the early stages of myocardial infarction, compliance of the infarcted myocardium may be normal or even increased, so that passive bulging during systole may develop.[40] Paradoxical systolic expansion of a ventricular segment decreases stroke volume. Within 6-24 hours, however, edema and cellular infiltration in the infarct leads to decreased ventricular compliance, which improves systolic function somewhat by preventing paradoxical expansion of the ventricular chamber during systole.[41]

When diminished stroke output in myocardial infarction causes a decrease in blood pressure, this leads to a reflex increase in heart rate and systemic vascular resistance, as well as stimulation of increased sympathetic nervous system activity. The increased adrenergic activity not only increases heart rate and peripheral vascular tone but also increases the contractility of the noninfarcted muscle. All of these changes increase MVO_2, and this increase in MVO_2 in the face of reduced coronary blood flow can cause more myocardial ischemia or even death.[20]

In some patients who became hypotensive following acute myocardial infarction, cardiac output is normal or only slightly reduced, and hypotension in such individuals is related primarily to inadequate peripheral arteriolar vasoconstriction.[42]

Acute Mitral Regurgitation

Up to 25% of patients develop a mild-to-moderate mitral regurgitation within one week following an acute myocardial infarction.[43] In two-thirds of these patients, the acute mitral regurgitation is associated with inferior wall infarction and involves the posteromedial papillary muscle. If mitral regurgitation is due to rupture of a papillary muscle, the onset of severe heart failure usually will be almost immediate. If the failure is accompanied by shock, 90% of these patients will die within two weeks if the condition is not promptly corrected surgically.[44]

Mitral regurgitation may also be due to annular dilatation associated with progressive LV failure in patients with extensive myocardial infarction. This type of regurgitation rarely needs surgical correction.[45]

Ventricular Septal Defect

Rupture of the ventricular septum is seen in approximately 2% of hospitalized patients with an acute myocardial infarction, and it accounts for 5% of postinfarction deaths.[20] In 50% of patients with ventricular septal rupture, sudden hemodynamic deterioration and cardiac shock occur.[46] As many as one-third of these patients also have some degree of mitral regurgitation. Over 90% of these patients die within the first year if the defect is not corrected surgically.

LV Aneurysm

Some LV aneurysmal dilatation develops in up to 38% of patients who have a myocardial infarction.[47] The functional abnormalities produced by the aneurysm depend on its size, location, and compliance characteristics. When more than one-fourth of the LV wall area is involved in the aneurysm and a compensatory increase in the contractility of the residual myocardium fails to maintain an adequate cardiac output, clinical heart failure may ensue.[48]

Patients with severe hemodynamic impairment from an LV aneurysm can benefit considerably from surgical reconstruction of the left ventricle.[49] However, LV ejection fraction values of < 35% tend to predict a poor functional result.[50]

Right Ventricular Infarction

AXIOM Acute right ventricular infarction can closely resemble pericardial tamponade.

Right ventricular involvement in patients with inferoposterior wall infarction can cause a positive Kussmaul sign (i.e., inspiratory rise in jugular venous pressure), elevation of jugular venous pressure, right ventricular gallop, and pulsus paradoxus (i.e., decrease of > 10-15 mm Hg in systemic systolic pressure during inspiration).[20] Hemodynamic measurements usually demonstrate elevated right atrial pressures, reduced systolic and elevated diastolic pressures in the right ventricle, an early dip in the RV diastolic pressure followed by a plateau (square-root sign), normal or near normal pulmonary artery wedge pressures (PAWP), reduced systemic pressures, and depressed cardiac output. Chest radiography usually shows clear lung fields. Radionuclide angiography reveals a markedly reduced right ventricular ejection fraction. The differential diagnosis includes pulmonary embolism and pericardial tamponade.

Volume expansion and judicious use of inotropes, such as dobutamine, can greatly improve prognosis, with a 60% survival rate reported in some series.[51] Nitrates and diuretics, which reduce preload, should be avoided.[20]

CARDIOMYOPATHIES

Cardiomyopathy is a frequent cause of heart failure in the United States.[20] The most popular classification recognizes three types of cardiomyopathy: congestive (dilated), restrictive (nondilated), and hypertrophic (Fig. 41-6; Table 41-3).

Dilated Cardiomyopathy

The most common forms of congestive (dilated) cardiomyopathy are: idiopathic (the most frequent type), alcoholic, ischemic, diabetic, and viral; congestive cardiomyopathy may also be seen following adriamycin therapy.[20]

Whether alcohol is a primary causal factor or just a risk factor in the development of cardiomyopathy is controversial.[52] Evidence suggests that there are direct toxic effects of alcohol on the myocardium because ventricular performance is decreased even when healthy subjects ingest alcohol in moderate quantities; however, typical alcoholic cardiomyopathy is usually seen in individuals who have been drinking heavily for more than a decade.[52] Interestingly, patients with alcoholic cardiomyopathy rarely have liver disease.[53]

Although most dilated cardiomyopathies are idiopathic, it is increasingly suggested that autoantibodies against cardiac tissue are important.[54,55] Other molecular markers of impairment of cardiac performance in dilated cardiomyopathy include structural and functional alterations in the myosin heavy and light chains and other myofibrillar proteins,[56] abnormalities in intracellular calcium handling, decreased density and responsiveness of myocardial β adrenoceptors,[57] and alterations in the levels of the stimulatory and inhibitory subpopulations of regulatory guanine nucleotide-binding proteins.[58]

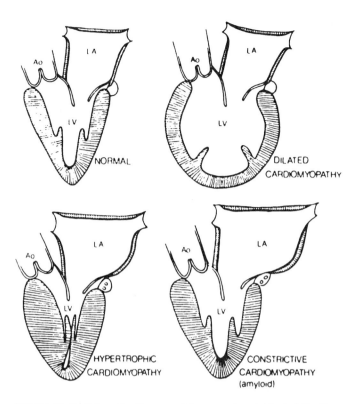

FIGURE 41–6 Schematic diagrams of the normal ventricle and the three types of cardiomyopathies (From: Kavinsky CJ, Parrillo JE. Severe heart failure in cardiomyopathy: pathogenesis and treatment. Ayres SM, Grenvik A, Holbrook PR, Shoemaker WC, eds. Textbook of critical care. Philadelphia: WB Saunders Co, 1995; 584).

Hypertrophic Cardiomyopathy

Hypertrophic cardiomyopathy includes severe LV hypertrophy without identifiable cause, which is associated with microscopic myocardial fiber disarray in 90% of patients.[59] Hypertrophy is asymmetric and affects the septum in 90% of patients. The atria also tend to be hypertrophied and dilated, indicating either increased resistance to filling of the ventricle and/or increased atrioventricular valve regurgitation. Mitral valve leaflets are usually thickened. Hypertrophic cardiomyopathy is familial in about one-third of patients, with autosomal-dominant inheritance. A history of sudden death is common in such families.[59]

Restrictive Cardiomyopathy

The characteristic feature of restrictive cardiomyopathy is impaired ventricular distensibility during diastole in the presence of relatively normal systolic function.[60] The functional abnormalities closely resemble those of constrictive pericarditis, and differentiating the two can be difficult. Restrictive cardiomyopathy is usually secondary to specific diseases, such as amyloidosis, sarcoidosis, hemochromatosis, glycogen storage disease, and endomyocardial fibrosis.[60]

SEVERE SHOCK OR CARDIAC ARREST

AXIOM   The most frequent cause of severe cardiovascular failure after trauma in young, previously healthy patients is severe, prolonged shock or cardiac arrest.

Severe, prolonged ischemia due to cardiac arrest or shock can cause either myocardial dysfunction or death. The low-flow state reduces cellular oxygenation and allows membrane integrity to be breached. Sodium, calcium, and water enter the cell and potassium leaves it. Adenosine triphosphate (ATP) is consumed and lactate production increases. Cyclic adenosine monophosphate (cAMP) concentrations decrease and calcium regulation is compromised. Histologically, these "sick cells" begin to swell. Eventually, their lysosomes leak and progressive cellular disruption develops.

In patients with severe continued shock from intraabdominal bleeding, prelaparotomy thoracotomy to cross-clamp the descending thoracic aorta can help to restore myocardial perfusion and reduce bleeding.[61] However, when systolic BP does not increase to 90 mm Hg within five minutes of aortic cross-clamping and continued aggressive fluid resuscitation, the patient is in irreversible cardiac failure; in a report by Wiencek and Wilson, all patients in whom this occurred died during surgery, regardless of additional cardiovascular support.[61]

Although severe shock after trauma is usually due to continued bleeding and hypovolemia, it may also be due to interference with diastolic filling because of pericardial tamponade or tension pneumothorax.

Cardiac failure in patients with pulmonary injuries may also be due to systemic air emboli involving the coronary arteries. This occurs most frequently in individuals with hemoptysis who are mechanically ventilated.[62] Clamping the descending thoracic aorta and allowing proximal aortic pressures to increase above 160-180 mm Hg can also cause acute LV dilatation and pulmonary edema.[63,64]

ARRHYTHMIAS

Arrhythmias are not uncommon in trauma victims.[35] In some instances they were the cause of the trauma, but trauma to the heart,

TABLE 41–3 Classification of the Cardiomyopathies

	Dilated	Restrictive	Hypertropic	
			Non-obstructive	*Obstructive*
Left ventricular end-diastolic pressure	↑↑	↑↑	↑↑	↑↑
Left ventricular end-diastolic volume	↑↑	nl or ↓	nl or ↓	nl or ↓
Diastolic compliance	↑	↓↓	↓↓	↓↓
Left ventricular ejection fraction	↓↓	nl or ↑	nl or ↑	nl, ↓, ↑
Echocardiography	↑↑ LV dimension ↓↓ Ventr. systolic function AV valve regur.	nl or ↓ LV dimension nl Ventr. systolic function ↑ LV wall thickness and mass	nl or ↓ dimension nl or ↑ systolic function Localized ↑ LV wall thickness (septum)	LV outflow tract obst. Systolic ant. motion of mitral valve Mitral regur.

Abbreviations: AV = atrioventricular; nl = normal; LV = left ventricle; ↑ = slightly increased; ↓ slightly decreased; ↑↑ = greatly increased; ↓↓ = greatly decreased.
From: Kavinsky CJ, Parrillo JE. Severe heart failure in cardiomyopathy: pathogenesis and treatment. Ayres SM, Grenvik A, Holbrook PR, Shoemaker WC, eds. Textbook of critical care. Philadelphia: WB Saunders, 1995; 584.

spinal cord,[65] or head[66] can cause a variety of arrhythmias. Although most postoperative arrhythmias are not associated with acute myocardial infarction, one should look for an underlying myocardial ischemia.[28]

Bradycardia is usually due to increased vagal tone. Because stroke volume is relatively fixed in most patients with heart failure, an increased heart rate is important for increasing cardiac output in times of stress. Consequently, bradycardia can have severe detrimental effects in patients with heart failure.

Sinus tachycardia secondary to physiologic stress is common, but it can also occur with inadequate resuscitation. Consequently, persistent tachycardia suggests that the resuscitation is not complete.

AXIOM Although tachycardia up to 160-180/minute can improve cardiac output in young individuals, it can also severely limit myocardial blood flow when CAD is present.

Severe tachyarrhythmias reduce the time available for diastolic ventricular filling and coronary blood flow. Consequently, tachycardia in the presence of significant CAD can cause myocardial ischemia.

AXIOM Atrial fibrillation should generally be prevented or rapidly corrected, especially in patients with severe mitral stenosis.

Atrial fibrillation or flutter may indicate an ischemic myocardial event, pulmonary embolus, or congestive heart failure. In most instances, atrial arrhythmias do not cause clinical heart failure unless a significant reduction of ventricular function is already present.[67]

Even when the ventricular response rate is controlled by digitalis, atrial fibrillation decreases cardiac output and increases any tendency for congestive failure, presumably by causing loss of the normal "booster-pump" function of the atrium.[9] Atrial fibrillation in patients with LV hypertrophy and/or diastolic dysfunction can cause pulmonary edema.

Ventricular premature beats (VPBs) that are frequent, are multifocal, or occur during T-waves can be precursors of life-threatening ventricular tachycardia and ventricular fibrillation, especially following acute myocardial infarction.[9] Ventricular dysrhythmias are frequent in patients with dilated cardiomyopathy, and they can cause further impairment of ventricular function.

MYOCARDIAL CONTUSION

Significant myocardial damage can be caused by the impact of the heart against the decelerating chest wall or by crushing the chest. Blunt injuries to the heart can range from a mild contusion to ventricular rupture.[68] Cardiac trauma has been implicated as the cause of death in at least 5% of fatal motor vehicle accidents. Nonfatal cardiac contusions can usually be differentiated from myocardial infarction at autopsy because the contusion: (a) has an abrupt transition zone between the injured and normal myocardium, (b) is patchy, and (c) is often confined to specific bundles.[68]

The diagnosis and management of myocardial contusion remain very controversial. Changes on electrocardiography (ECG) are usually nonspecific. The most common arrhythmia is sinus tachycardia, which occurred in 72% of such patients studied by Cane and Shamroth[69]; however, this finding can be caused by shock, pain, anxiety, hypoxemia, or hypocapnia. Premature atrial or ventricular beats are the second most frequent abnormalities seen in many series.[68]

S-T segment or T-wave abnormalities are considered more specific for myocardial contusion. Kron and Cox reported that 26 of 50 patients with myocardial contusions had ECG abnormalities, and 22 of these 26 patients had changes in their ST-T segments.[70] Nineteen of the ST-T segment changes were transient while three were persistent. Consequently, many patients with abnormalities of myocardial wall motion immediately after trauma do not have elevated CPK-MB levels.[71]

Some investigators believe that the most reliable criterion for the diagnosis of myocardial contusion is increased levels of CPK-MB isoenzymes.[68] The CPK-MB isoenzyme is released from damaged myocardial cells and can be detected by either electrophoresis or immunoassay. It is usually expressed as a percentage of the total serum CPK concentration, and a CPK-MB concentration > 5% of the total CPK is believed to be sensitive and specific for the diagnosis of myocardial injury.[68] However, the half-life of the CPK-MB isoenzyme is short, and frequent sampling is necessary to detect any elevation, which is usually maximal at about 18 hours. Fabian et al. found an increased CPK-MB concentration in 53 of 56 (85%) patients with myocardial contusions by using a sampling interval of 6 hours.[72] Unfortunately, the CPK-MB fraction in the myocardium of young, healthy people may be < 1%.

AXIOM Patients with myocardial contusion do not require ICU monitoring unless they have arrhythmias, heart failure, other severe injuries, or preexisting cardiac disease.

Echocardiography is a noninvasive and relatively inexpensive means of evaluating patients with a possible myocardial contusion.[68] The application of this technique to blunt cardiac trauma was proposed by Coleman et al. in 1976,[73] and the Mayo Clinic group developed an extensive experience with this technology.[74] The most common finding is abnormal wall motion, such as hypokinesis or dyskinesis. It also can detect acute valvular injury, pericardial effusions, or intracavitary clots.

Radionuclide angiography can also be used to detect wall-motion abnormalities, decreased ejection fractions, and depressed Starling function curves.[68,73]

AXIOM Patients with wall-motion abnormalities from myocardial contusion have an increased risk of shock or arrhythmias during general anesthesia until up to one month later.[74]

Surgery is not absolutely contraindicated in patients with myocardial contusion; however, when a wall-motion abnormality exists, the incidence of intraoperative arrhythmias and hypotension is increased.[74] Consequently, if the surgery is very important, these patients should have careful monitoring of preload (PAWP or RVEDVI) and cardiac output. If a patient with myocardial contusion develops intraoperative cardiogenic shock that does not respond to fluids and inotropes, intraaortic balloon pumping may be helpful.[75]

ELECTROLYTE AND ACID BASE ABNORMALITIES

Hypokalemia

Hypokalemia hyperpolarizes the cell membrane and prolongs the cardiac action potential.[76] These changes are associated with characteristic ECG abnormalities which include ST segment depression, depressed T waves, and appearance of U waves. However, these changes are nonspecific.

Hypokalemia is also associated with an increased incidence of arrhythmias and conduction defects, and it increases the cardiac toxicity of digitalis glycosides.[77] In individuals hospitalized with acute myocardial infarction, hypokalemia increases the incidence of ventricular tachycardia and fibrillation.[78] Hypokalemia in these patients usually results from diuretics but may be aggravated by increased cellular uptake of potassium due to high circulating catecholamine levels.

AXIOM Patients with hypokalemia often also have hypomagnesemia.

Severe Hypocalcemia

CHF may occur in patients with hypocalcemia and may improve only with correction.[79] Some of the more frequent causes of hypocalcemic myocardial dysfunction include hypoparathyroidism, hypocalcemia associated with end-stage renal disease, and hypocalcemia attrib-

TABLE 41–4 Cardiac Effects of Hypomagnesemia

Electrocardiogram
  Prolonged PR interval
  Prolonged QT interval
  Flattening of T wave
Supraventricular tachycardias
Ventricular arrhythmias
  Premature contractions
  Ventricular tachycardia
  Torsades de pointes

From: Oster JR, Preston RA, Materson BJ. Fluid and electrolyte disorders in congestive heart failure. Semin Nephrol 1994;14:485.

uted to rapid transfusion of citrated blood.[80,81] The well-described electrophysiologic effects of hypocalcemia include prolongation of the ST segment and prolongation of the QT interval.

Magnesium Depletion

Causes of magnesium depletion in patients with CHF include diuretics, liver disease, and poor intake.[79,82] Magnesium deficiencies should be suspected in any patient with an arrhythmia; however, serum magnesium levels may be normal in individuals with moderate-to-severe tissue magnesium depletion (Table 41–4).

AXIOM Serum magnesium levels may be normal in patients with moderate-to-severe tissue magnesium deficiencies.

Gottlieb et al. found that patients with serum magnesium levels < 1.6 mEq/L had more frequent ventricular arrhythmias than did patients with higher levels.[83] Even more interesting was the observation that patients with low serum magnesium levels seemed to have a significantly worse one-year survival rate (45% vs 71%). This may be related to worsening of cardiac contractility as well as an increase in the incidence of severe ventricular arrhythmias.

AXIOM Serum magnesium levels may be a prognostic indicator in patients with established CHF.

Severe Phosphorous Depletion

Normal phosphorous metabolism is required for adequate utilization of high-energy compounds. Moderate hypophosphatemia, defined as a serum phosphorous level of 1.0-2.5 mg/dL, is a relatively common finding in hospitalized patients, but it is not usually associated with significant symptoms. Severe hypophosphatemia (< 1.0 mg/dL), however, may be associated with a constellation of clinical findings, including reversible ventricular dysfunction.[79]

Acidosis

AXIOM Acidosis tends to depress cardiac contractility, but the increased catecholamine release it stimulates tends to override the depression unless the pH is < 7.10.

Mild acidosis may improve cardiac action, but severe acidosis (pH < 7.10) tends to reduce ejection fraction and cardiac output. Many patients with metabolic acidosis have compensatory respiratory alkalosis, and $Paco_2$ levels of < 20 mm Hg can also interfere with myocardial contractility and coronary blood flow.

Mechanisms that have been suggested to explain the effect of acidosis on myocardial contractility include: inhibition of slow Ca^{2+} current, decreased Ca^{2+} pool and Ca^{2+} release, altered binding and uptake of intracellular Ca^{2+}, and decreased tension generated by myofibrils in response to Ca^{2+}.[84]

The decrease in cardiac contractility associated with respiratory acidosis is often greater than that seen from metabolic acidosis.[85] Carbon dioxide rapidly enters cells, reducing intracellular pH, whereas both hydrogen and bicarbonate ions enter and exit myocytes relatively slowly, causing a smaller reduction in intracellular pH.[85,86]

Patients with chronic CHF have high levels of circulating catecholamines[87] and reduced myocardial norepinephrine receptor concentrations.[88] In this population of patients, systemic acidosis may produce a more profound negative inotropic effect and may be seen with a lesser degree of acidosis because compensatory sympathoadrenal mechanisms may be blunted. Patients on β-adrenergic blockers also tend to have more deleterious effects from systemic acidosis.[89]

PULMONARY HYPERTENSION

AXIOM The hemodynamic change most significantly associated with an increased mortality rate more than 48 hours after trauma is pulmonary hypertension.

Increased pulmonary vascular resistance after trauma is associated with an increased mortality rate in many series.[90-92] Strum et al. found that nonsurvivors of multiple trauma had an increased pulmonary vascular resistance and right ventricular stroke work index when compared to survivors.[90] Eddy et al. used a special pulmonary artery catheter to measure right ventricular ejection fractions (RVEFs) in multiple-trauma patients.[91] He found an early decrease in RVEF following trauma that improved over the subsequent 8-12 hours in survivors but did not improve in the nonsurvivors. LV function was similar in survivors and nonsurvivors.

Thus, instead of being a simple conduit, the right ventricle may be important for maintaining pulmonary blood flow after trauma.[28] Because excess fluid administration can cause RV dilation which, in turn, can impair LV filling, inotropes and pulmonary vasodilators may be the preferred therapy for posttraumatic pulmonary hypertension.[93,94]

CIRCULATORY OVERLOAD

In healthy individuals, the difference in blood volume between hypovolemic shock and heart failure may exceed 3-4 L. However, patients with preexisting cardiac disease or myocardial dysfunction due to prolonged shock may progress from hypovolemic hypotension to pulmonary edema with fluid infusions of as little as 1,000 mL.

Although fluid overloading may occur during the initial resuscitation from shock or trauma, it is more likely to occur during the fluid mobilization phase, which usually begins 48-72 hours after acute injury or surgery. When large volumes of fluid are given during the fluid mobilization phase, or when urine output cannot keep pace with the shift of fluid from the interstitial space into the vascular space, hypertension and/or heart failure may result. Patients with renal or hepatic failure are particularly apt to accumulate extracellular fluid and have an increased tendency to develop heart failure.

When cardiac filling is increased by > 30-50%, cardiac muscle fibers may be stretched beyond their normal physiologic limits. This can decrease the effectiveness of the heart as a pump and start a vicious cycle of increasing fluid retention and cardiac failure.

AXIOM Cardiac failure from fluid overload is rare in patients without preexisting cardiac disease, cardiac trauma, or severe, persistent shock.

SEPSIS

Later in the hospital course after trauma, cardiovascular failure may be caused by severe sepsis. This cardiovascular failure may occur because of unrecognized hypovolemia and/or the presence of myocardial depression factors.

Hypovolemia

AXIOM Patients with sepsis often require greatly increased intravenous fluids.

TABLE 41–5 *Clinical Manifestations of Heart Failure*

Reduced cardiac output	Fatigue Tiredness Dizziness Syncope	Cold, blue extremities Malar flush Muscle wasting Cachexia
Pulmonary venous congestion	Dyspnea Orthopnea Paroxysmal nocturnal dyspnea	Tachypnea Shallow breathing Pulsus alterans Gallop rhythm Pulmonary basal rales Bronchospasm (rare)
Systemic venous congestion	Right hypochondrial pain and tenderness (hepatic congestion) Ankle swelling Abdominal swelling	Hepatojugular reflux Jugular venous distension Hepatomegaly Ankle/sacral edema

*COPD = chronic obstructive pulmonary disease.
From: Majid PA, Roberts R. Heart failure. Civetta JM, Taylor RW, Kirby RR, eds. Critical care. New York: JB Lippincott, 1988; 946.

It may be extremely difficult to maintain an adequate intravascular fluid volume in patients with severe sepsis. The vasodilation and greatly increased capillary permeability associated with severe infection often increase fluid needs by more than 200-500 mL/hr over and above measured losses. Because of the increased capillary permeability, the lungs may also become quite edematous, even when the patient is hypovolemic.

AXIOM Patients with sepsis may develop pulmonary edema in spite of reduced cardiac filling pressures.

Myocardial Depressant Factors

Myocardial depressant factors (MDF) have been detected in hemorrhagic, endotoxin, cardiogenic, ischemic, traumatic, hypovolemic, and burn shock from various species.[92] Most of these agents are small peptides with molecular weights of 250-1000 daltons.[95] They usually arise from splanchnic organs, especially the pancreas, and exert a negative inotropic effect.

In a study of MDF by Demeules, rabbit papillary muscle was exposed to septic shock serum obtained from dogs.[96] Action potential amplitude, action potential duration, and resting membrane potential were all depressed. Hyperkalemia blocked these effects, suggesting that the myocardial defects in septic shock may be mediated through abnormalities in fast sodium channel activity.[90,92]

Many pharmacologic agents can decrease the activity of MDF in hemorrhagic and traumatic shock, but the improvement seen may only be secondary to better perfusion of the splanchnic bed.[92] It has also been found that leukotriene antagonists,[97] prostaglandin E₁,[98] iloprost,[99] and platelet-activating factor antagonists[100] decrease MDF activity in trauma shock. Reilly et al. found a significant correlation between serum MDF activity in septic patients and a reversible decrease in LV ejection fraction.[101]

HIGH-OUTPUT CARDIAC FAILURE

Although cardiac output may be high in patients with severe anemia, cirrhosis, arteriovenous fistulas, or thyrotoxicosis, the heart may actually have difficulty keeping up with the increased venous return. As a consequence, filling pressures and volumes may be much higher than normal, so that ejection fractions are low, producing a condition that may be referred to as high-output cardiac failure.

AXIOM Cardiac indices exceeding 5.0-6.0 L/min/m² may not only be detrimental to the heart, but may also reduce oxygen transfer peripherally and in the lungs because of inadequate time spent by red cells in the capillaries.

COMPENSATORY CHANGES IN HEART FAILURE

Three principal compensatory mechanisms occur over time in patients with heart failure: (a) (acutely) increased release of catecholamines that increase heart rate and contractility, (b) (subacutely) retention of salt and water to increase preload, and (c) (chronically) myocardial hypertrophy.

Acute Cardiovascular Changes

AXIOM Acute cardiovascular responses to reduced BP or cardiac output are primarily due to increased sympathetic nervous system activity.[102]

BARORECEPTOR REFLEXES

Whenever cardiac output or blood pressure decreases, a number of acute circulatory reflexes attempt to restore blood pressure and flow to normal.[102] The best known of the acute circulatory reflexes involved in heart failure is the baroreceptor reflex. This is activated by reduction in arterial blood pressure, thereby reducing stimulation of the baroreceptors in the carotid sinus. Normally the carotid sinus is stimulated by an increase in BP which then inhibits the vasomotor center and causes a lowering of BP to more normal levels. With hypotension, the normal inhibition of the vasomotor center by the carotid sinus is removed.

If systolic pressure decreases to very low levels (below 60 mm Hg), the central nervous system (CNS) ischemic reflex is activated, causing a powerful simulation of the sympathetic nervous system. At the same time, the parasympathetic system is reciprocally inhibited.

In chronic heart failure (CHF), the ability of cardiac and arterial baroreceptors to suppress sympathetic activity and reduce the release of vasopressin and catecholamines is impaired.[103] Left atrial receptors are no longer appropriately activated by the increase in atrial pressure that follows volume expansion. The cause of this abnormal baroreceptor sensitivity may be related to changes in cardiac and arterial compliance as well as to disruption and fragmentation of receptor endings. This baroreflex dysfunction greatly impairs the ability of the circulation to limit the release of vasoconstrictor neurohormones, even after the threat of cerebral perfusion has subsided.[104]

AXIOM Most patients with heart failure demonstrate an increased activation of the sympathetic nervous system with elevated plasma norepinephrine levels, even at rest.

CARDIAC EFFECTS

Sympathetic stimulation of adrenergic receptors in the heart during heart failure can cause a profound increase in the rate and force of myocardial contraction.[105] If a portion of the myocardium is damaged but not dead, sympathetic stimulation will usually strengthen the contraction of abnormal myocardium. If < 40% of the ventricular myocardium is nonfunctional due to infarction, normal muscle can often compensate for the nonfunctional portion.

The chronic failing heart often lacks adequate stores of norepinephrine because of defective local catecholamine synthesis and storage.[106] Consequently, the chronically failing heart may have to depend on epinephrine and norepinephrine released from the adrenal medulla and peripheral nerve endings for much of its adrenergic stimulation.[107]

Despite high circulating levels of catecholamines, the heart rate may not be greatly increased in patients with CHF. Such observations suggest that some adaptation to prolonged sympathetic stimulation occurs. This reduced responsiveness to catecholamines is not related to a defect in myocardial contractile elements because the failing myocardium usually responds normally to digitalis and calcium. The problem appears to be related to a specific intracellular deficiency of cyclic AMP in the failing heart.

AXIOM Continuing heart failure is characterized by down-regulation of β-adrenergic receptors.

The cause of intracellular myocardial deficiency of cyclic AMP in CHF is most likely related to defects in β-adrenergic receptors. The failing myocardium also becomes depleted of catecholamines because of defects in the synthesis and uptake of norepinephrine.[108] In addition, the density of β-adrenergic receptors is markedly decreased, and this receptor loss is accompanied by a proportional decrease in the activity of adenylate cyclase and agonist-stimulated muscle contraction.[109]

Prolonged, excessive catecholamine stimulation may damage the myocardium directly, leading to an increase in transsarcolemmal calcium influx and an intracellular calcium overload. Generation of free radicals by catecholamine metabolites, such as adrenochrome, may also contribute to myocardial damage.[110]

AXIOM High levels of catecholamines and an increase in peripheral vascular tone may contribute not only to functional circulatory impairment but also to progression of myocardial dysfunction.

VASCULAR EFFECTS

Sympathetic stimulation of α-adrenergic receptors causes increased arteriolar vasoconstriction, and this tends to raise the blood pressure and shift blood flow to vital organs, especially the heart and brain.[111] The associated increase in venous tone reduces vascular capacity, thereby increasing venous return which, in turn, can help return cardiac output to nearly normal levels.

INCREASED OXYGEN EXTRACTION

With increasing heart failure and decreased perfusion, tissues are forced to extract more oxygen from the blood. Under normal circumstances, the body extracts about 25% of the oxygen available in the blood. However, when blood flow is greatly reduced, systemic tissues may extract more than 40-50% of the oxygen present. If the tissues are still not getting enough oxygen, the tissues will be forced into anaerobic metabolism with development of progressive lactic acidosis.

Subacute Compensatory Changes

The main change in subacute heart failure is increased salt and water retention.

RETENTION OF SODIUM AND WATER

The subacute compensatory changes in heart failure result in an increase in extracellular fluid due to retention of salt and water by the kidneys. This fluid retention is caused by shifts of blood flow in the kidneys and by elevated levels of vasopressin[112] and aldosterone.[113]

The reduced cardiac output seen in heart failure causes renal vasoconstriction which further reduces renal blood flow. Renal blood flow is also diverted from the outer renal cortex to the inner (juxtamedullary) renal cortex where there are less glomeruli, but the tubules have long loops of Henle; consequently, absorption of water and sodium is increased. Thus, in heart failure, urine tends to become more concentrated (particularly with urea), but it usually has a low ($<$ 10-20 mEq/L) sodium concentration.

Increased sympathetic tone, decreased renal arterial perfusion, and decreased sodium concentrations in the distal tubule fluid all can activate the juxtaglomerular apparatus (JGA) to release renin. Renin cleaves angiotensin I from an α_2-globulin, and angiotensin-converting enzyme (ACE) converts angiotensin I to angiotensin II. Angiotensin II is a potent vasoconstrictor, especially on the renal afferent arterioles, and it stimulates the adrenal cortex to release aldosterone. Aldosterone causes even more sodium and water retention.

When blood flow to brain or filling of the atria is reduced, increased amounts of ADH are released from the posterior pituitary.[114] ADH causes increased absorption of water in the distal and collecting tubules, further expanding the ECF and reducing urinary output.

The fluid retention in moderate cardiac failure may increase blood volume by 15% or more, and the resultant increased diastolic filling of the heart may restore cardiac output to relatively normal levels. In severe cardiac failure, however, salt and water retention may increase blood volume and venous return by 30-50% or more and stretch the myocardial muscle fibers beyond their normal physiologic limits, causing a further decrease in cardiac output.

Aldosterone, by promoting salt and water retention, causes interstitial edema and, possibly, increased sodium content of vascular walls.[20,115] Increased sodium concentration in the vascular wall causes increased stiffness of the blood vessel which, together with extrinsic compression from interstitial edema, may further increase vascular tone.[116] Other hormones, including arginine vasopressin, also tend to increase systemic vascular resistance in heart failure.[20]

INCREASED ERYTHROPOIESIS

Another cause of increased blood volume in patients with cardiac failure is increased production of red blood cells.[20] Whenever oxygen delivery to the tissues is reduced, the bone marrow is stimulated to increase its erythropoietic activity, resulting in an increase in red blood cell volume. However, as the hematocrit rises, particularly above 55%, the increased viscosity can increase cardiac work and decrease cardiac output, thereby aggravating the tendency to heart failure.

Chronic Compensatory Changes

In chronic heart failure, cardiac hypertrophy and various changes try to improve local organ blood flow and to reduce excessive accumulation of salt and water.

MYOCARDIAL HYPERTROPHY

Physiologic Effects

The principal chronic hemodynamic adjustment to heart failure is hypertrophy of the LV myocardium.[102] The rapidity and extent to which the myocardium will hypertrophy varies with the acuteness of the problem and the type of overload with which the heart must contend. Acute overload—as may develop with acute mitral insufficiency secondary to a rupture of a papillary muscle—is usually tolerated very poorly. However, when the same degree of mitral insufficiency develops slowly over a period of months or years, the changes may be tolerated well for quite some time.

AXIOM Volume overloads (such as those resulting from aortic insufficiency) are tolerated better than pressure overloads (as may occur with aortic stenosis).

Gradually increasing pressure overloads tend to cause hypertrophy. Cardiac dilatation usually does not occur until relatively late, after severe failure has developed.

Although it may be an important compensatory mechanism, myocardial hypertrophy makes the heart more susceptible to ischemia. Blood flow to the endocardium through long, narrow transmyocardial arterioles in thickened heart muscle can decrease very rapidly when diastolic aortic pressures decrease and LV diastolic pressures increase.

Types of Hypertrophy

MYOCYTE HYPERTROPHY. The most complex etiologic factor in cardiac enlargement in patients with heart failure is that of myocyte cell hypertrophy to allow the left ventricle to maintain wall stress in the presence of a rising afterload and preload.[117] Katz, in a recent review, reported that cells of the hypertrophied, failing heart are not normal.[118] The synthesis of myosin heavy chains, which determine myosin ATPase activity and muscle-shortening velocity, is altered by chronic heart failure. This increases the tendency for arrhythmias, slowed relaxation, and desensitization to sympathetic neurotransmitters. The decreased response to adrenergic stimulation is due to decreased numbers of β-adrenergic-receptor molecules and altered guanine nucleotide-binding proteins (also known as G-proteins).

Although cardiac hypertrophy and dilation is an adaptive process, there is concern that the heart can "overadjust" to its reduction in performance.[119] In many patients, the increase in size and change in the shape of the heart contribute to the poor prognosis.[120]

COLLAGEN CHANGES. Normal myocytes are held together by a complex network of collagen struts.[121] As the heart enlarges, dissolution of these collagen struts occurs, allowing for "slippage" of individual myocytes or whole bundles of myocytes. This increases the tendency of the heart to dilate in the presence of increasing end-diastolic volume.

It remains unclear as to how dissolution of the collagen scaffold actually occurs. One possibility is that acute myocardial injury activates collagenase enzymes which, in turn, dissolve the complex network of collagen that normally binds the myocardial cells together.

Ultimately, synthesis of new collagen occurs, and a number of hypotheses exist as to how this may occur. One possibility is that fibroblasts express membrane-bound angiotensin II receptors,[120] and that angiotensin II may expedite the synthesis of new collagen as a nonspecific response to injury. The hormone aldosterone may also help cause excess or abnormal distribution of myocardial collagen, leading to ischemic and dilated cardiomyopathy.

Experimental evidence now suggests that ACE inhibitors are capable of reducing the amount of myocardial collagen synthesis that occurs in the setting of acute myocardial injury.[122] Moreover, drugs designed to inhibit aldosterone, such as spironolactone, may also be beneficial in this regard.[123]

Drugs Affecting Cardiac Hypertrophy

Drugs designed to inhibit or attenuate LV hypertrophy in heart failure may have an increasing role. In the SAVE trial, not only did the early use of captopril after myocardial infarction improve survival in patients with LV ejection fraction of ≤ 40%, but substantial attenuation of subsequent LV remodeling also occurred.[124] Inhibition of LV dilation was also observed in the SOLVD trial,[125] where enalapril tended to reduce LV mass and ventricular sphericity.

INCREASED ATRIAL NATRIURETIC FACTOR

Atrial natriuretic factor (ANF) promotes sodium excretion by the kidneys and may be thought of as an endogenous natriuretic released in response to CHF.[126] Some of the other effects of ANF include: (a) direct vasodilator actions by its ability to increase intracellular cyclic GMP and thereby antagonize the actions of most endogenous vasoconstrictors, (b) enhanced baroreceptor sensitivity, thereby reducing central activation of the sympathetic nervous system, (c) suppressed formation of renin, (d) inhibition of the actions of angiotensin II, including its vasoconstrictor actions and its ability to stimulate thirst and aldosterone secretion, and (e) inhibition of the release of vasopressin and its vasoconstrictor effects on systemic vessels and its antidiuretic effects on the collecting ducts.

Thus, ANF is a neurohormonal antagonist to many of the physiologic changes occurring in heart failure. This antagonism may not only reduce cardiac distension but may also decrease the adverse effects of endogenous vasoconstrictors on the kidneys. This may explain why renal function is less impaired in patients with cardiac failure than in those with hypovolemia, even when the cardiac output is reduced to the same degree.[126]

Unfortunately, many ANF studies were performed with doses far greater than those likely to be used in clinical conditions.[127] Roach et al., for example, reported that physiologic levels of ANF do not alter reflex sympathetic control in the vascular system.[128]

AXIOM PEEP, which decreases the distension of the atria, can significantly reduce ANF production, thereby reducing urine output and causing more fluid retention in heart failure.

INCREASED PROSTAGLANDIN PRODUCTION

In the final phases of heart failure, ANF may no longer be able to exert its renal effects, and prostaglandins may increasingly assume the role of antagonizing the intrarenal effects of systemic vasoconstrictor hormones.[129,130] Unlike ANF, however, prostaglandins can also increase the release of renin from juxtaglomerular cells and thereby lead to further activation of endogenous vasoconstrictors. The critical reduction in renal blood flow seen in the final phases of CHF may explain why hyponatremia—an important clinical indicator of severe renal hypoperfusion—has prognostic significance.

AXIOM Decreasing serum sodium levels is a bad prognostic sign in patients with CHF.

With severe heart failure and hyponatremia, indomethacin (a prostaglandin synthesis inhibitor) can cause significant decreases in cardiac index and increases in PAWP; however, patients with normal serum sodium levels usually have no significant hemodynamic change after indomethacin.[129] Thus, the vasodilator effects of prostaglandins may be an important compensatory mechanism in severe heart failure complicated by hyponatremia.

PITFALL ⊘

Use of prostaglandin synthesis inhibitors in patients with severe CHF increases the tendency for renal failure.

Organ Changes in Heart Failure

HEART

AXIOM Myocardial oxygen consumption increases in heart failure, but coronary blood flow tends to decrease.

In ventricular failure, end-diastolic volume and fiber length tend to increase. As the ventricle dilates and radius (R) increases, each fiber must develop more tension (T) at a given intraventricular pressure (P) to eject blood from the heart. This can result in a substantial increase in myocardial oxygen requirements. However, the reduced cardiac output, tachycardia, and high LV diastolic pressures reduce coronary blood flow. In addition, the increased tension required to develop a given intraventricular pressure results in a decreased rate of myocardial fiber shortening, and consequently the preejection phase of systole is prolonged, further increasing MVO$_2$. Excessive dilation also tends to make contraction of the ventricles less coordinated and less effective.

LUNGS

AXIOM One of the most sensitive indicators of increasing cardiac failure is a decrease in arterial Po$_2$.

In cardiac failure, the vital capacity and functional residual capacity in the lungs are decreased because of increased blood in the pulmonary vessels and increased fluid in the pulmonary interstitial space. This increases the work of breathing and the tendency towards atelectasis. When fluid accumulates in the alveoli, oxygen diffusion can be impaired; any protein present in alveolae can inactivate surfactant, increasing the tendency to atelectasis. When pleural effusions develop, even greater impairment of ventilation occurs.

The forces involved in the translocation of water into the lungs and other tissues in heart failure were defined by Starling in 1896.[131] These have been described by the formula:

$$Qf = K_tA [(P_c - P_i) - \sigma (\pi_c - \pi_i)]$$

Q_f is the net flow of water across a capillary, K_t is the filtration coefficient that defines the fluid conductance across capillary membranes, A is the cross-sectional area of the involved capillaries, and sigma (σ) is the Staverman reflection coefficient that defines the effectiveness of the membrane in preventing protein leakage through the capillary membrane.

When no protein can move across the capillary membrane, the reflection coefficient is 1.0. If capillary permeability is greatly increased, as in sepsis, so that no capillary barrier to protein exists, the value of the reflection coefficient approaches zero. P_c and P_i are the hydrostatic pressures in the capillary and interstitial spaces, respectively, and π_c and π_i are the osmotic pressures in the capillaries and interstitial water. In the lungs, only two of these forces, P_c and π_c, can be readily measured as the PAWP and plasma colloid osmotic pressure (COP).

Assuming a normal plasma COP of 22-25 mm Hg and a normal PAWP of 6-15 mm Hg, the COP-PAWP gradient ranges 7-19 mm Hg (average: 16 mm Hg). This favors fluid remaining inside the pulmonary capillaries. When the COP-PAWP is reduced by either elevation of PAWP or reduction of COP, increased fluid flux into the pulmonary extravascular space may occur.

Some studies indicate that critically ill patients with heart failure and a COP-PAWP gradient of $<$ +4 mm Hg tend to develop pulmonary edema as determined by chest radiographic changes.[132] However, most investigators have found a poor correlation between the COP-PAWP gradient and either the amount of extravascular lung water (EVLW) or the amount of shunting (Q_{sp}/Q_t) in the lungs.

LIVER, SPLEEN, AND INTESTINES

The increased right atrial pressure present in heart failure tends to reduce venous return from the splanchnic circulation and to produce increasing congestion in the liver, spleen, and intestines. Occasionally, the pain and tenderness of an acutely congested liver produces pain and tenderness in the right upper quadrant of the abdomen, suggesting a diagnosis of acute cholecystitis.

If cardiac failure is severe and persistent, the reduction in liver blood flow caused by severe congestion may impair liver function. Eventually, the liver may become fibrotic, developing what has been referred to as cardiac cirrhosis.

KIDNEYS

Severe cardiac failure decreases glomerular filtration and urinary output predominantly via increased angiotensin II activity and can produce a prerenal azotemia with an elevated BUN.[79] If NSAIDs are given, thereby reducing the renal vasodilation caused by prostaglandins, oliguric renal failure may develop rapidly.

ENDOCRINE ORGANS

The secretion of renin, ADH, and norepinephrine tends to increase during acute heart failure, but the secretion of these substances is often relatively normal in patients with stable CHF. After trauma or during sepsis or shock, these substances are usually present in much greater concentrations, and an increased tendency for heart failure exists when the myocardium has been damaged in any way.

DIAGNOSIS OF CARDIAC FAILURE

Clinical

HISTORY

The history should try to determine whether any direct injury to the heart, prolonged shock, cross-clamping of the thoracic aorta, or cardiac arrest occurred.

Past History

When a past history can be obtained, especially in older individuals, one should inquire about preexisting evidence of LV dysfunction, such as easy fatigability, dyspnea at rest or with minimal exertion, orthopnea, and paroxysmal nocturnal dyspnea.

Current Symptoms

DYSPNEA. Patients with left-sided heart failure classically complain of feeling "short of breath" (due to congestion of the lungs) and/or weakness and fatigue (due to inadequate cardiac output). Dyspnea with mild exertion is often the first symptom of heart failure and is usually associated with an increased respiratory rate (tachypnea).

The precise cause of dyspnea is unknown, but it appears to be related to increased interstitial edema and pulmonary congestion which decrease lung compliance, increase the work of breathing, and tend to cause hypoxemia. In addition, interstitial edema in the vicinity of the pulmonary capillaries may stimulate juxtacapillary receptors ("J-receptors") thereby reflexly causing rapidly shallow breathing. A disproportion between the increased work required by ventilatory muscles and reduced blood flow to ventilatory muscles may also cause some sensation of breathlessness.

COUGH. In some patients, coughing with excitement or physical efforts may be the first symptom of heart failure and may erroneously lead to the assumption that a pulmonary, rather than a cardiac, problem is present. In some instances, sputum may appear bloody or rusty because of the presence of hemosiderin-laden alveolar macrophages, further increasing the suspicion of a pulmonary lesion.

PITFALL ⊘

Assuming that an increasing cough or hemoptysis can only be due to a pulmonary problem.

ORTHOPNEA AND PND. Orthopnea and paroxysmal nocturnal dyspnea (PND) are particularly interesting symptoms of left heart failure.[20] When the patient with moderate-to-severe heart failure is in the upright position, blood tends to pool in the most dependent portions of the body. Because of increased systemic capillary pressure in dependent areas, as much as 15% of the intravascular water can leak into the tissue spaces of the legs, producing dependent pedal edema. When the patient lies down, however, the blood that was pooled in the legs can now return to the heart, causing increased congestion in the lungs. When shortness of breath occurs as soon as the patient lies down, the patient is said to have orthopnea. Conversely, patients who are relatively comfortable when they first lie down but awaken suddenly with severe dyspnea several hours later are said to have PND.[20] The mechanism causing PND is probably related not only to the gradual uptake of fluid from areas of peripheral edema but also to a reduction in cardiac output because of increased vagal tone during sleep.

OTHER SYMPTOMS. Breathlessness, orthopnea, and PND are often the cardinal symptoms of LV failure in "younger" patients. However, in elderly patients, confusion, restlessness, and fatigue are more common. Other symptoms that may develop (because of severe congestion of the intestines) include anorexia, nausea, vomiting, and abdominal distention. Weakness and fatigue, which are most often considered symptoms of left heart failure, may also be prominent in isolated right heart failure.

AXIOM Nausea, vomiting, and abdominal pain and distension in patients with heart failure can sometimes simulate an acute surgical abdomen.

PHYSICAL EXAMINATION

Chest Wall

Physical examination may reveal chest wall bruises, or rib tenderness that should make one suspect underlying myocardial or pulmonary injuries. A sternal fracture should make one particularly concerned about the possibility of myocardial contusion.

Heart

TACHYCARDIA AND CARDIAC ENLARGEMENT. Sinus tachycardia, although a very nonspecific sign, is almost invariably present with cardiovascular failure. Pulsus alternans in which only every other heart beat produces a palpable peripheral pulse, although uncommon, is a reliable sign of severe LV failure. Palpation may reveal a hyperactive precordium with or without cardiac enlargement. Cardiac dilatation may occur rapidly, but muscle hypertrophy usually requires at least several weeks or months to develop; it is seldom found in acutely injured patients without preexisting cardiac disease.

GALLOP RHYTHM

AXIOM A gallop rhythm should be considered a sign of LV failure until proven otherwise.

A third heart sound during diastole is an important sign of LV failure, but it is easily overlooked. The cadence produced by the fixed sequence of two normal heart sounds followed by an abnormal third heart sound can, especially when the heart is beating rapidly, produce a sound very much like that of a galloping horse.

PITFALL ⊘

Failure to listen closely for a third heart sound in all patients with cardiac or pulmonary symptoms.

In children and young adults, a third heart sound is often a normal finding. With advancing age, however, the significance of these auscultatory findings is altered. Over the age of 50, the detection of a fourth heart sound is less specific because it can also be found in some relatively healthy individuals.[20] In contrast, a third heart sound in older patients usually indicates ventricular dysfunction.

MURMURS. Dilatation of the left ventricle may cause enlargement of the mitral valve annulus resulting in the systolic murmur of mitral insufficiency radiating towards the axilla.

BLOOD PRESSURE CHANGES

PITFALL ⊘

Failure to appreciate that a decrease in pulse pressure may be an important sign of increasing cardiac failure.

Unless heart failure is severe, systemic blood pressure tends to be elevated or at high-normal levels. The return towards normal of an elevated blood pressure is often considered a good clinical sign, but sometimes it indicates increasing cardiovascular failure. A low-pulse pressure, in particular, tends to suggest the presence of hypovolemia, aortic stenosis, tamponade, or severe cardiac failure.

Lungs

RALES. In early LV failure, rales may be present only at the lung bases; however, as heart failure worsens, rales become higher and more generalized. At times, rales of congestion may be difficult to differentiate from those of atelectasis, particularly in patients with trauma or severe sepsis who may not be able to clear their bronchial secretions properly.

WHEEZES

AXIOM All that wheezes is not asthma.

Wheezing is usually considered to be due to bronchial asthma. However, it may also occur with cardiac failure (in the absence of pulmonary disease) because of swelling and congestion of the mucosa in smaller bronchioles.

PLEURAL EFFUSIONS. Pleural effusions resulting from heart failure empirically occur slightly more frequently on the right, whereas a left hydrothorax may be slightly more suggestive of a pulmonary embolus.

PULMONARY EDEMA. Occasionally, acute, severe LV failure may develop rather suddenly, while the right ventricle is still functioning relatively well. The abrupt rise in pulmonary venous and capillary pressures can cause fluid to accumulate rapidly in pulmonary interstitial spaces and alveoli producing clinical pulmonary edema. Frothy pink-tinged sputum may begin to advance up the bronchioles into the trachea, greatly impairing ventilation as well as gas exchange.

Neck Veins

One of the most obvious signs of heart failure is distention of the deep jugular veins to at least 3.0 cm above the sternal notch when the patient is sitting up at a 45° angle.[6] This may be a helpful sign, but it is much less accurate than direct readings of the CVP or PAWP. Severe, acute heart failure may also cause annular dilatation of the tricuspid valve with enough tricuspid regurgitation to cause pulsations of the dilated neck veins.

Liver

Enlargement of the liver and a positive hepatojugular reflux (pushing on the liver producing increased neck-vein distention) are important corroborative signs of congestive heart failure. When severe cardiac failure causes tricuspid insufficiency, the liver may pulsate.

Pedal or Sacral Edema

Swelling of the feet and ankles is frequently caused by chronically increased venous pressure in the legs resulting from right heart failure. Such patients also often develop incompetence of the valves in the leg veins due to chronic distention. In the bedridden patient with heart failure, the sacral area, rather than the feet and legs, is the dependent portion of the body. Consequently, this is the area that should be examined for edema.

PITFALL ⊘

Failing to examine the presacral area for edema in bedridden patients.

Laboratory Studies

With acute heart failure, usually some hemodilution occurs because of increased plasma water. With chronic heart failure, increased bone marrow production of red blood cells, as a compensatory response to chronic hypoxemia, may cause Hb and Hct values to rise above normal, thereby increasing blood viscosity and afterload. In addition, increasing renal ischemia may cause a progressively increasing BUN. Later, with further reduction in arterial inflow and increased venous congestion, progressive renal and hepatic dysfunction may cause rising plasma creatinine and bilirubin levels. Chronic use of diuretics and a low-salt diet tend to cause hyponatremia and hypokalemia and these, in turn, can also increase the tendency for renal dysfunction.

AXIOM In patients with heart failure, a decreasing arterial P_{O_2} is generally a sensitive indicator that the process is getting worse.

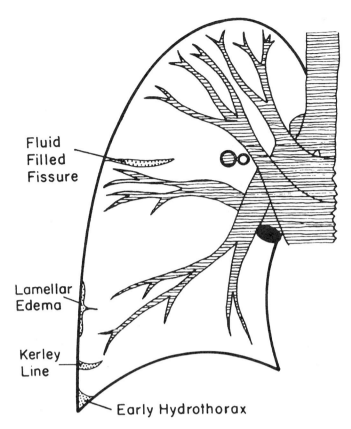

Fluid
Filled
Fissure

Lamellar
Edema

Kerley
Line

Early Hydrothorax

FIGURE 41–7 The radiographic features of CHF include edema, Kerley lines, and pleural effusion. (From: Shatz IJ, Wilson RF. Cardiovascular failure. Walt AJ, Wilson RF, eds. Management of trauma: pitfalls and practice. Philadelphia: Lea & Febiger, 1975; 538).

A decreasing Pao$_2$ usually indicates that heart failure is increasing, whereas an increasing Pao$_2$ is generally a sign of improvement. When LV function appears to be good, but the arterial Po$_2$ is decreasing, one must be concerned about the possibility of recurrent pulmonary emboli, especially in older or bed-ridden individuals.

AXIOM A relatively sudden decrease in arterial Po$_2$ in a patient with heart failure should make one look carefully for pulmonary emboli.

Serial evaluation of CPK-MB and LDH isoenzymes may also help to detect myocardial contusion or myocardial infarction.

Radiologic Studies

PLAIN RADIOGRAPHY

Lungs
On upright chest radiography, fine, transverse lines of increased density, particularly near the hilum (Kerley's A lines) or near the costophrenic angles in the lung bases (Kerley's B lines), are often the first radiographic signs of increased lung water[20] (Fig. 41–7). Increased prominence and dilatation of central lung markings are usually detected somewhat later. Accumulation of fluid in the interlobar fissures and blunting of the costophrenic angles by free pleural fluid are usually relatively late signs, but care should be taken to look for them, especially on the right.

Heart
An enlarged heart suggests a chronic, underlying cardiac problem. When the cardiac silhouette enlarges rapidly, chronic heart failure

with a superimposed, severe, acute process is usually present. Patients with pure mitral stenosis usually maintain a relatively normal cardiac size until right heart failure begins to develop. The patient with chronic, obstructive lung disease tends to have a relatively small cardiac silhouette because the diaphragm tends to flatten and move lower in the chest, giving the heart a more vertical position.

AXIOM An enlarged cardiac silhouette in spite of moderate-to-severe COPD is usually evidence of advanced heart failure.

PULMONARY ARTERIOGRAPHY
Pulmonary arteriography is used most frequently to detect pulmonary emboli, and pulmonary emboli should be considered when heart failure develops without obvious cause more than 1-2 weeks after trauma.

RADIONUCLIDE ANGIOGRAPHY
First-pass, gated radionuclide angiography can be used to evaluate RV and LV ejection fractions, regional wall motion, and end-diastolic volumes.[133,134] Heart failure due to systolic dysfunction is usually clinically evident when the left ventricle ejection fraction is reduced to < 40%. The ejection fraction (ratio of stroke volume to ventricular end-diastolic volume) is normally about 0.55-0.70 for the left ventricle and 0.45-0.60 for the right ventricle.

AXIOM Changes in end-systolic and end-diastolic volumes provide much more accurate estimates of the functional capabilities of the right and left heart than do the CVP and PAWP.

Electrocardiographic Findings

ECG findings do not indicate the presence or absence of CHF. However, RV or LV hypertrophy tends to indicate a chronic strain, usually due to increased afterload. Evidence of ischemia, infarction, conduction disturbances, tachyarrhythmias, or bradyarrhythmias may also provide important clues to the etiology of heart failure. When symptoms are intermittent, 24-hour Holter (ECG) monitoring may be helpful.

AXIOM Although continuous Holter monitoring picks up many more ECG changes in acutely injured patients, the significance of these changes is not clear.

The detection of myocardial ischemia by ECG or other means is of great importance in patients with evidence of heart failure after trauma.[33] Although optimal electrode placement may be limited by prior surgical procedures, ECG monitoring with at least two simultaneous leads will permit detection of myocardial ischemia in most instances. Lead II provides good P-wave morphology and monitors ischemic events in the inferior wall, and the V$_5$ lead detects such changes in the anterolateral wall. Whenever possible, use of three simultaneous leads, particularly II, V$_4$, and V$_5$, appears to be superior to two-lead monitoring.[135]

Hemodynamic Monitoring

For uncomplicated trauma patients, sophisticated monitoring is not required, and one can manage fluids by balancing outputs with intake and following blood pressure, heart rate, and urine output. When the hemodynamic picture becomes confusing, and particularly when perfusion is inadequate in spite of apparently adequate fluid loading, it becomes necessary to monitor cardiac function more closely, and a central venous pressure or pulmonary artery catheter should be inserted.

CENTRAL VENOUS PRESSURE

CVP monitoring can provide helpful data for appropriate fluid management in most young patients with normal cardiac function.[136] At least five variables control CVP: (a) blood volume, (b) the distensibility of the right heart, (c) systemic venous constriction, (d) pulmonary vasoconstriction, and (e) intrathoracic pressure. The measured CVP is the result of all of these factors and does not necessarily reflect the adequacy of the circulating blood volume or the competence of right or LV function.

A CVP of 4-8 cm H_2O is usually considered normal. Although a CVP of 0-4 cm H_2O is considered normal by some, a CVP < 4-6 cm H_2O in critically injured patients usually indicates hypovolemia. In contrast, CVP exceeding 16 cm H_2O often indicates an adequate or increased blood volume; however, positive-pressure ventilation, increased pulmonary vascular resistance, pneumothorax, and abdominal distension can all cause high CVP values in spite of hypovolemia.

AXIOM	Trends and the response of CVP or PAWP to fluid challenges are much more important than absolute values.[136]

In patients who may have cardiac or pulmonary problems, the rate of fluid infusion should be gauged by the response of CVP or PAWP. A minimal response to rapid infusions of fluid is characteristic of hypovolemia. In contrast, a rapid rise in CVP or PAWP with a fluid challenge suggests that the rate of fluid infusion should be reduced or stopped.

When blood volumes, fluid administration, and CVP were measured serially in 124 critically ill and injured patients at Detroit General Hospital, no correlation between these values was found.[136] The CVP response to the administration of fluid was much more reliable than isolated CVP readings in evaluating the amount of fluid needed; however, none of the single parameters studied (blood volume, central venous pressure, or clinical impression) correlated consistently with the amount of fluid required to restore normal tissue perfusion.

AXIOM	Although CVP is usually elevated to at least 12-16 cm H_2O in patients with heart failure, it may be normal (4-8 cm H_2O), at least temporarily, if the decompensation is primarily left sided.

An occasional patient with acute LV failure following a cardiac arrest or an acute myocardial infarction develops acute, severe pulmonary edema in spite of a CVP < 5.0 cm H_2O.[136]

PULMONARY ARTERY CATHETERS

Indications

Because of the poor correlation between CVP and filling pressures in the left heart in patients with sepsis, respiratory failure, or myocardial ischemia, clinicians have become increasingly interested in monitoring pulmonary artery wedge pressures (PAWP).[137]

Quinn and Quebbeman used pulmonary artery catheterization for unknown fluid status in 43 patients, for hypotension in 28 patients, and for sepsis in 13 patients.[138] Therapy was altered because of pulmonary artery wedge pressure and cardiac output measurements in only 30% of the patients. Eight patients were believed clinically to have heart failure but actually required additional fluid. In addition, seven patients believed to be hypovolemic clinically, actually had fluid overload.

Insertion

PA catheters are usually inserted through an internal jugular or subclavian vein.[92,138] Once the catheter is in its proper position, the balloon should be inflated and the catheter pulled back until a slight resistance is met. This tends to remove excess catheter from the right ventricle and helps prevent excessive distal migration.

If there is difficulty in placing the catheter, it is preferable to allow the catheter to be too far peripheral and to withdraw it after confirmation by chest radiography than to advance the catheter after the sterile field has been broken.[92] The catheter tip on chest radiography should not extend more than half the distance to the chest wall. If a persistent wedge pattern is seen, the catheter should be withdrawn until a good pulmonary artery tracing is seen. During measurement of the PAWP, the balloon should be inflated with as little air as possible, certainly < 0.75-1.0 cc of air to reduce the chances of pulmonary artery rupture.

AXIOM	Chest radiography should be obtained after attempts to insert a central catheter, regardless of success or failure.

Arrhythmias During Insertion

Premature ventricular beats occur during at least 10-17% of pulmonary artery catheter insertions.[139] These are not related to technique but are primarily due to catheter irritation of the endocardium.[92] Lidocaine can be used prophylactically, but most of the rhythm abnormalities resolve after catheter manipulation ceases. Arrhythmias during insertion are more frequent when the patient is hypothermic, acidotic, or hypoxic.[92] These conditions should be corrected, if possible, before attempting catheter placement.

AXIOM	When a left-bundle branch block is present, an external pacemaker should be present while inserting a PA catheter.

One must be particularly careful when the patient has a left-bundle branch block (LBBB) prior to insertion. If a right-bundle branch block (RBBB) develops during insertion in such an individual, the resultant complete heart block could be disastrous unless an external pacer is immediately available.

Monitoring with a PA Catheter

AXIOM	When a pulmonary catheter is inserted to monitor a critically injured patient, it should be used to determine the "optimal" hemodynamic values and then maintain them for at least 24-48 hours.

Sequential measurements of PAWP and cardiac output in order to construct ventricular function curves can be helpful in patients with cardiac or pulmonary dysfunction. A patient with an elevated PAWP that increases abruptly with a standard fluid challenge (3.0 mL/kg of a balanced electrolyte in 10 minutes) without an increase in cardiac output or LV stroke work index, is said to have a flat ventricular function curve; this indicates that one should not push further intravenous fluids at that time.

Patients with severe pulmonary dysfunction may have an elevated CVP and pulmonary artery pressures, but a normal or low PAWP. A fluid challenge in such patients often results in an increased cardiac output and LV stroke work without a significant increase in CVP or pulmonary arterial wedge pressures, indicating that further fluid administration may be beneficial.

Left heart failure is usually associated with a PAWP exceeding 18-22 mm Hg. Our studies with right ventricular end-diastolic volume indices (RVEDVI), however, indicate that many of these patients with "high" PAWPs can still respond favorably to fluid loading.[21]

Mixed Venous Oxygen Saturation

The pulmonary artery catheter permits mixed venous blood sampling through the distal pulmonary artery port; when the cardiac output, hemoglobin, and Pao_2 are also known, one can calculate oxygen consumption.[140] The normal mixed venous blood saturation is 70-75% with a Pao_2 of approximately 40 mm Hg. The mixed venous oxygen tension is an indirect assessment of oxygen utilization for the entire body. It depends on many hemodynamic factors, including tissue perfusion, variations in different organ oxygen requirements by various organs, and the affinity of hemoglobin for oxygen.

One can also use a sensor on the PA catheter tip to continuously monitor mixed venous (pulmonary artery) oxygen saturation (Svo_2). Svo_2 of 60-65% often indicates decreased oxygen delivery (DO_2) relative to the oxygen consumption (VO_2), and an $Svo_2 < 60\%$ is often indicative of frank or impending shock.

> **AXIOM** Mixed venous oxygen saturation can provide early warning of cardiopulmonary dysfunction, but one cannot rely on a stable Svo_2 to exclude such problems.

A decrease in Svo_2 often occurs before other clinical signs of cardiovascular dysfunction develop, and the Svo_2 can be very useful as an "early warning" for these problems.[141]

CARDIAC OUTPUT

Techniques and Accuracy

The most frequently used method for measuring cardiac output at the bedside is the thermodilution technique, which measures the change in temperature caused by an ice cold solution injected into the right atrium 30 cm from the end of the catheter in the pulmonary artery.[92] The end of the catheter contains a thermistor that determines the temperature changes in the surrounding blood. The temperature change from the right atrium to the pulmonary artery is inversely proportional to the cardiac output.[142]

The accuracy of the thermodilution determination depends on the technique used. The volume of injectate must be uniform because even small increases in injectate volume can cause falsely low determinations. As a corollary, decreases in the volume of the injectate gives falsely high cardiac outputs.[143]

Either iced or room-temperature solutions may be used, but the temperature at the injection port in the right atrium is most important. When using iced solutions, the chance for a temperature increase from the ice container to the right atrium is greater than with room-temperature solutions. However, use of iced saline increases the signal-to-noise ratio over that of room-temperature solutions and tends to minimize errors.[144]

> **AXIOM** One should not assume that thermodilution cardiac output determinations are always accurate, especially if the cardiac outputs are very high or very low.

Ideally, each thermodilution cardiac output curve should be visually inspected because a smooth, uninterrupted curve is necessary for accurate results.[145] The injectate should be delivered in < 4 seconds with only a single peak on the curve. Three determinations should be made at end expiration and the average taken as the true cardiac output. Although we have tried to have the determinations be within 5% of each other, variation among the three determinations of < 15% according to Stetz[146] is not statistically significant and does not need to be repeated.

Estimating Cardiac Contractility

Although less than ideal, contractility can be assessed by the relationship between cardiac filling pressures and ventricular work indices. LVSWI in g-m/m^2/beat is calculated by mBP × SVI × .0136. Normal values for LVSWI at a PAWP of 15-18 mm Hg are about 65-70 g-m/m^2/beat. Ideally, a curve is constructed with LVSWI plotted against three different PAWPs.

Optimizing Cardiac Output and Oxygen Delivery

> **AXIOM** If a patient is sick enough to require PA catheter monitoring, the catheter should be used to optimize cardiac output and oxygen delivery (DO_2).

To optimize hemodynamic function, preload is increased with boluses of fluid until the CO does not increase appreciably but the PAWP increases substantially. If the cardiac index (CI) is still < 4.0-4.5 L/min/m^2, inotropes can be used to raise it to that level. DO_2 is then

also increased by increasing hemoglobin levels and then SaO_2 until oxygen consumption (VO_2) no longer increases or is at least 160 mL/min/m^2. This should be done as soon after the initial trauma as possible.

END-DIASTOLIC VOLUMES

PAWP vs LVEDP and LVEDV

It is generally believed that a a fairly good correlation exists between PAWP, left atrial pressure, and LVEDP. However, because of variations in LV compliance, LVEDP does not always provide an adequate indication of the LV end diastolic volume (LVEDV).[92,117]

> **AXIOM** A high PAWP does not necessarily indicate that end-diastolic volumes are also increased, especially in patients with cardiac disease.

Measuring Right Ventricular End-diastolic Volume Index

> **AXIOM** End-diastolic volumes are a more accurate guide for fluid resuscitation of critically ill patients than are PAWP levels.

Within the past several years, bedside measurements of RV ejection fraction (RVEF) by a thermodilution technique using a specially modified pulmonary artery catheter have become available. Reuse et al. reported the results of measuring RV volumes before and after fluid challenges with 300 mL of 4.5% albumin in 41 ICU patients.[148] In patients with a right ventricular end-diastolic volume index (RVEDVI) < 140 mL/m^2, fluid tended to raise cardiac output. However, in 20% (8 of 4l) of patients with a RVEDVI > 140 mL/m^2, the fluid challenge tended to decrease cardiac output.

Diebel et al., studied the relative value of PAWP and RVEDVI in reflecting preload status of 29 critically ill patients.[21] Regression analysis of 136 hemodynamic studies demonstrated that CI correlated better with RVEDVI (r = 0.61) than it did with PAWP (r = 0.42). Comparisons of PAWP and RVEDVI showed that possible misleading information concerning filling volume was provided by the PAWP at some time in 15 (52%) of these patients. Of 15 patients given 22 fluid challenges, seven patients with high PAWPs (≥ 18 mm Hg) but a RVEDVI < 139 mL/m^2 "responded" with a rise in CI. All fluid challenges in patients with a RVEDVI < 90 mL/m^2 responded with a rise in CI.

> **AXIOM** RVEDVI more accurately predicts preload recruitable increases in cardiac output than do PAWP levels.

ECHOCARDIOGRAPHY

Right ventricular imaging by two-dimensional echocardiography (2-D echo) is increasing in popularity and utility and can be used to identify a failing right ventricle. Starling et al. studying patients with chronic obstructive lung disease showed good correlation between right ventricular variables determined by 2-D echo and radionuclide techniques.[150]

Using M-mode and two-dimensional echocardiography, the majority of cardiac structural abnormalities can be recognized and the severity of stenotic valve lesions can be estimated by measurement of the cross-sectional area. With the additional use of Doppler ultrasound, the direction and velocity of blood flow can be determined, permitting quantitative assessment of valve gradients. Echocardiographic studies can also be used to determine the mean velocity of circumferential fiber shortening and the ejection fraction.[151]

> **AXIOM** Echocardiography, especially transesophageally, is an excellent technique for evaluating the heart, pericardium, and mediastinum after trauma.

Transesophageal echocardiography is increasingly being used to evaluate the aorta after trauma. It has already been used extensively to detect intraoperative myocardial ischemia and infarction[152] and to assess mitral regurgitation,[153] chorda tendinea rupture,[154] and aortic stenosis.[155]

CARDIAC CATHETERIZATION

When the patient has progressive heart failure that is of unknown etiology and is not responding to standard treatment, cardiac catheterization may provide extremely useful diagnostic information, particularly when pressures and oxygen contents are studied in each chamber. Cardiac catheterization can also be used to detect lesions that may be corrected surgically. When surgical management of CAD is contemplated, coronary angiography is also performed.

TRANSVENOUS ENDOMYOCRADIAL BIOPSY

Since Kono and Sakakibara introduced the percutaneous, transvenous technique for obtaining endomyocardial biopsies in 1962, physicians have used it for diagnosing a wide variety of cardiac problems.[156] Serial histologic evaluation of heart transplant recipients as a means of monitoring rejection and immunosuppressive therapy is the most frequent indication for transvenous endomyocardial biopsy (TEB).[54] Endomyocardial biopsy is also useful for monitoring the cardiotoxic effects of anthracycline chemotherapeutic agents and for diagnosing myocarditis, particularly in patients with a recent onset of heart failure.

PREVENTION AND TREATMENT OF CARDIAC FAILURE

Other than preventing cardiac failure by removing precipitating events, the therapeutic approaches to heart failure are based on improving the four main determinants of cardiac performance: preload, afterload, contractility, and heart rate.

Prevention of Cardiac Failure

PROMPT CORRECTION OF SHOCK AND HYPOXEMIA

AXIOM   The best way to prevent cardiac dysfunction after trauma is to keep hypotension and hypoxemia to a minimum and to prevent cardiac fluid and pressure overloads.

Prevention of heart failure in trauma patients primarily involves rapid treatment of shock to keep myocardial ischemia to a minimum. This involves aggressive resuscitation with fluids and blood and rapid control of bleeding sites. Pericardial tamponade, tension pneumothorax, and any other causes of hypotension should also be corrected promptly.

Care must be taken not to overload the heart with fluids or cause an excessive afterload on the left or right ventricle. For the left ventricle this involves keeping the use of vasoconstrictor agents and/or aortic clamping to a minimum. For the right ventricle this involves avoiding high pulmonary inflation pressures and preventing ARDS and pulmonary emboli.

PREVENTION AND CORRECTION OF HYPOTHERMIA

AXIOM   The hypothermic heart does not function well and it is difficult to resuscitate.

Core temperatures < 32-33°C tend to impair cardiovascular function. Consequently, core temperatures should be monitored carefully, and hypothermia prevented by a variety of techniques, including giving warmed blood and fluids. Shock must also be corrected as rapidly as possible. Keeping room temperatures elevated, keeping patient exposure to a minimum, and instituting active rewarming as soon as possible are also important.

PROMPT CORRECTION OF ACID-BASE ELECTROLYTE ABNORMALITIES

Severe acidosis with arterial pH < 7.00-7.10 should be corrected to a pH of at least 7.20 as soon as possible, preferably by improving tissue perfusion. When bicarbonate is given, one must be certain that the minute ventilation and lung function are adequate to keep both the arterial and venous P_{CO_2} within proper limits [$(1.5 \times HCO_3) + 8$]; otherwise the bicarbonate can cause a "paradoxical" cellular acidosis because the liberated CO_2 from the HCO_3 can rapidly enter cells, but the HCO_3 cannot.

Severely abnormal magnesium, potassium, calcium, or phosphate levels can cause arrhythmias and/or impair cardiovascular function. Such abnormalities are particularly apt to occur during massive blood transfusions to hypothermic individuals in severe shock. Prolonged aortic clamping can cause a severe washout acidosis after the clamp is released.

AXIOM   Severe phosphate deficiencies (< 1.0 mg/dL) can interfere with cellular metabolism and should be corrected promptly.[157]

Removing Precipitating Factors

REDUCING METABOLIC DEMANDS

Increased afterload and tachycardia should be controlled as soon as possible to prevent myocardial ischemia. Stress and pain also place a burden on the failing heart.

AXIOM   The increased catecholamine release associated with stress, pain, and anxiety can cause heart failure to progress in spite of all other therapy.

DISCONTINUING CARDIODEPRESSIVE MEDICATIONS

The physician should be alert to the possibility that patients with heart failure may be taking medications, such as β-adrenergic blockers or calcium-channel blockers, that have negative inotropic effects.

THIAMINE

Chronic alcoholics occasionally develop severe myocardiopathy which, like beriberi heart disease, may respond to large doses of thiamine (100 mg BID or TID).

GLUCOSE-INSULIN-POTASSIUM SOLUTIONS

Glucose-insulin-potassium (GIK) solutions can support ischemic myocardium and improve myocardial performance.[158] The ingredients in GIK solutions vary, but usually contain (per liter) 100-200 g of glucose, 20-40 units of regular insulin, and 40-80 mEq of potassium chloride. The infusion is usually given at 100-250 mL/hr as long as the patient is not overloaded with fluid.

GIK solutions, in both animals and humans, often increase RV and LV contractility independent of preload and may reduce the tendency for arrhythmias. In one study, a GIK solution produced a 40% higher cardiac index than an equivalent amount of mannitol, and the effect lasted for at least 45 minutes.[158] An increase in oxygen consumption usually occurs after a GIK solution is started secondary to an increased cardiac output and oxygen delivery.[159] Use of a GIK solution may be particularly helpful in patients who do not have an adequate cardiac output in spite of maximal inotropic therapy.

Optimization of Preload

CORRECTING HYPOVOLEMIA

AXIOM   Continuing hypotension in trauma patients is usually due to inadequate volume replacement.

Volume expansion generally has little detrimental effect on myocardial oxygen consumption, but it can cause a dramatic improvement in BP and cardiac output.[23] In addition, the detrimental effects of increased intrathoracic pressure because of ventilatory support can almost always be overcome by adequate fluid infusions.

AXIOM The usual first step to improving cardiac output in trauma patients is increasing preload to adequate levels.

Patients with underlying heart failure tolerate the stress of trauma poorly; however, identifying preexisting LV dysfunction can be extremely difficult in acutely injured patients. Nevertheless, the initial management of major trauma patients with massive hemorrhage is rapid control of bleeding and then aggressive resuscitation, regardless of what preexisting conditions may be present.

AXIOM In patients with heart failure, more precise monitoring during resuscitation may be required because of the small blood volume difference that may exist between hypovolemia and fluid overload.

The fluids that are administered to acutely injured patients can be either balanced salt solutions, colloid, or blood, and considerable debate has occurred over the effects of these on pulmonary function. The use of colloids or balanced salt solutions does not seem to make any difference in lung function, as long as they are given to equivalent intravascular filling end-points.

OPTIMAL HEMATOCRIT

Hemoglobin and hematocrit concentrations in blood have been measured for over 100 years and the optimal hematocrit is still debated.[160] It is generally believed that a hemoglobin level of 10.0 g/dL, which corresponds to a hematocrit of about 30%, is adequate for most injured patients; however, this author prefers higher levels (12.0 g/dL or more) in patients with cardiopulmonary dysfunction. In respiratory failure, a hematocrit of 40% has been correlated with increased survival,[161] and in trauma and septic shock patients, hematocrits of 38% or more have been associated with increased survival.[162]

FILLING PRESSURES

Generally, the preload in acutely injured patients should be adjusted to a CVP of 10-15 cm H_2O and/or a PAWP of 12-15 mm Hg.[92] Following trauma, fluid requirements are frequently underestimated, and much higher filling pressures may be required.

AXIOM When the fluid status of a patient is in doubt, one should carefully evaluate the response to a standard fluid challenge, such as 3.0 mL/kg of a balanced electrolyte solution given over 10 minutes.

USING VENTRICULAR RESPONSE CURVES

Under optimal conditions, a ventricular response curve can be generated by watching the change in cardiac output or LVSWI as the preload is increased. The point at which the cardiac output or LVSWI no longer increases and/or the filling pressures (CVP and/or PAWP) begin to increase abruptly with an additional increment of fluid is usually the ideal filling pressure.

OPTIMIZING OXYGEN DELIVERY AND OXYGEN CONSUMPTION

AXIOM The best way to reduce morbidity and mortality in critically injured patients is to promptly optimize oxygen delivery and oxygen consumption.

Oxygen consumption is independent of oxygen delivery as long as oxygen delivery is maintained above a certain critical value, which has been called the "critical oxygen delivery."[161] Below this value, oxygen delivery is inadequate to meet the tissue demands, and at least some cells must utilize anaerobic metabolism to maintain cellular function.[92] If tissue hypoxemia is severe enough, lactic acidosis will develop eventually.

TABLE 41-6 Methods of Preload Reduction

Salt restriction
Diuretic therapy
   Thiazides
   Loop diuretics (furosemide, bumetamide, ethacrynic acid)
   Potassium-sparing agents (spironolactone, amiloride, triameterene)
Fluid removal by phlebotomy, hemodialysis, or ultrafiltration
Parenteral vasodilators
   Nitroglycerine
   Nitroprusside
Oral vasodilators
   Nitrates (also effective in ointment or sublingual forms)
   Prazosin
   Captopril and enalapril
Mechanical
   Surgical correction of regurgitant valvular lesions and shunts

---

Shoemaker showed that increasing the cardiac index to 4.5 L/min/m^2, DO_2 to 700 mL/min/m^2, and VO_2 to 170 mL/min/m^2 reduced morbidity rate and time in the ICU for high-risk postoperative surgical patients.[162] Moore et al. also showed that patients who achieved a VO_2 of at least 150 mL/min/m^2 within 12 hours of injury had the best outcome.[163]

REDUCING EXCESSIVE PRELOAD (TABLE 41-6)

Decreased Salt and Water Intake

When blood volume is excessively high relative to the ability of the cardiovascular system to handle it, efforts must be made to: (a) reduce the intake of salt and water, (b) increase the excretion of salt and water, and/or (c) increase venous capacitance. Restriction of water and salt intake can be a vital, nonpharmacologic means of reducing excessive preload; however, this may be difficult to manage in patients with acute, severe trauma. Later in the hospital course, such efforts may be more practical.

Fluid restriction after the obligatory fluid sequestration phase may help to correct the hyponatremia often observed in patients with CHF; however, because fluid restriction is poorly tolerated by many trauma patients, treatment of hyponatremia with a variety of drugs, particularly captopril and furosemide, is often necessary.[79]

Diuretics

THIAZIDES

AXIOM Diuretics can cause severe problems if given to patients who are hypovolemic.

Hydrochlorothiazide and thiazidelike diuretics increase the delivery of sodium to the distal nephron by blocking its reabsorption in the cortical diluting segment of the nephron.[79] These diuretics are often recommended for the initial treatment of mild-to-moderate cardiac failure in nonstress situations. However, thiazides have a greater tendency to impair glucose tolerance and have been reported to occasionally cause severe hyponatremia. They are ineffective when the glomerular filtration rate is < 25 mL/min, and they may adversely affect renal function by causing vasoconstriction of afferent renal arterioles.

LOOP DIURETICS. Loop diuretics (ethacrynic acid, furosemide, and bumetanide) act by inhibiting active reabsorption of chloride, sodium, potassium, calcium, and magnesium across the thick, ascending limb of the loop of Henle.[164] They can be specially useful in correcting the refractory edema of moderate-to-severe acute cardiac failure. They are often able to induce diuresis even when renal blood flow is markedly reduced. They are also able to reverse the shunting of blood from cortical to juxtamedullary nephrons that occurs commonly in heart failure or trauma.[92]

In situations with obvious fluid overload, the initial intravenous dose of furosemide is generally 40-80 mg; however, in patients with recent trauma, it is probably safer to start with doses of 10-20 mg and then double the dose every 15-30 minutes until a satisfactory urinary output is obtained. Interestingly, the very rapid relief of pulmonary edema that can be seen with furosemide appears to be due to its ability to cause venodilation and thereby reduce venous return to the heart.[165]

The margin of safety between fluid overload and hypovolemia in critically ill or injured patients may be very small, and many chronically hypertensive patients are actually hypovolemic. If diuresis is excessive, patients with poorly functioning hearts can easily be made severely hypovolemic; however, the "braking phenomenon" helps to prevent continued action of diuretics at the renal level when plasma volume is severely depleted.[166] Loop diuretics are also less effective in patients with severe respiratory acidosis and hypoxemia.[167]

Severe electrolyte problems, such as hypokalemia, hypomagnesemia, hypochloremia, and metabolic alkalosis, may develop during diuresis. These abnormalities may alter the cardiac response to digitalis and can precipitate dangerous arrhythmias. Hypomagnesemia may be a particularly important problem in debilitated patients (especially those who abuse ethanol or are uremic).

POTASSIUM-SPARING DIURETICS. Spironolactone is a steroid that competes for cytosolic receptor sites with aldosterone, which tends to have high levels in CHF. Spironolactone not only increases urinary sodium excretion, but it also decreases potassium, magnesium, and hydrogen ion loss in the urine.

Triamterene and amiloride act on the distal tubular epithelium to markedly reduce the transmembrane electrochemical gradient. This reduces the loss of potassium and hydrogen ions as well, but it has no effect on magnesium or calcium excretion.[79]

AXIOM Potassium-sparing diuretics and ACE-inhibitors should generally not be given at the same time.

Hyperkalemia can occur relatively easily if the use of potassium-sparing agents is not carefully monitored, and potassium supplements can cause gastrointestinal side effects. It is also important to avoid potassium-sparing diuretics when ACE inhibitors are being given.

AXIOM The most frequent electrolyte cause of arrhythmias is hypokalemia due to excessive diuresis.

Many elderly patients with cardiac failure have underlying ischemic heart disease, and a dietary deficiency of protein and potassium is not unusual in such individuals. With additional potassium loss due to loop diuretics, hypokalemia may become severe, greatly increasing the risk of arrhythmias.

Vasodilators
Vasodilators, such as nitroglycerin, which mainly affect capacitance veins, can dramatically reduce venous return and cardiac filling pressures. One must be certain, however, that vasodilators are not given to patients who may be hypovolemic. In addition, cardiac filling pressures should be monitored closely.

Positive-pressure Ventilation
Positive-pressure ventilation, especially with some PEEP, can dramatically reduce venous return to the heart. In patients with acute pulmonary edema, this may be the most rapid and effective way to restore the arterial Po_2 to normal levels.

Tourniquet/Phlebotomy
In desperate situations, such as acute pulmonary edema, venous return can be reduced rapidly be elevating the head and chest and ap-

plying rotating tourniquets to the extremities. Phlebotomy is rarely used now; however, in desperate situations, removal of 50-100 mL of blood at five to ten minute intervals up to a total 250-400 mL may help in the urgent management of acute pulmonary edema until previously administered drugs become effective.

Inotropic Support

AXIOM Once preload is optimized, the next step in improving hemodynamic function and oxygen delivery generally includes inotropes and/or vasodilators.

After the optimal preload has been determined, one can proceed to either inotropic support and/or afterload reduction to optimize cardiac output. When heart failure is predominantly due to systolic dysfunction (with a reduced ejection fraction), inotropic agents may be appropriate. However, when diastolic dysfunction disturbs adequate cardiac diastolic filling to require the use of high end-diastolic pressures, arterial vasodilators may be indicated. One may also have to avoid inotropes, especially digitalis, that can adversely affect ventricular relaxation.[168]

AXIOM The great majority of patients with heart failure after trauma will have systolic dysfunction.

DIGITALIS GLYCOSIDES

Indications
Digitalis glycosides have both negative chronotropic and positive inotropic effects. They improve contractile function, augment LV ejection fraction, and reduce symptoms due to heart failure.[169] In patients with heart failure and atrial fibrillation with a rapid ventricular response, digoxin is extremely effective for slowing the ventricular heart rate, improving diastolic filling, and augmenting ventricular systolic function. Digitalis compounds can also be useful in the conversion of ectopic rhythms, especially atrial and nodal tachycardias. An excellent response to digitalis can also be expected in many patients with heart failure due to aortic valvular disease or mitral regurgitation.

A less satisfactory response or no response to digitalis preparations can be expected in patients with mitral stenosis and sinus rhythm, diffuse myocardial disease, chronic cor pulmonale, constrictive pericarditis, or CHF associated with thyroxicosis, anemia, or peripheral arteriovenous fistulae.[1] Evidence also exists that chronic pulmonary disease predisposes patients to digoxin toxicity at relatively low serum levels.

AXIOM Unless chronic pulmonary disease is accompanied by atrial fibrillation or LV failure, digoxin should be avoided.[184]

Mechanisms of Action
Digitalis glycosides increase the force and velocity of cardiac contraction in normal, as well as diseased, myocardium by inhibition of sodium-potassium ATPase (Na^+-K^+-ATPase) activity.[20,170] This results in a net increased sodium influx into cells, and increased calcium accumulation in exchange for sodium through sodium-calcium exchange systems. This enhances contractility of the failing myocardium and can lead to a significant increase in cardiac output and LV stroke work.[20]

Digitalis also acts on cardiac conduction tissue to prolong its refractory period and reduce its conduction velocity. However, in myocardium the reverse occurs with shortening of the refractory period. Digitalis in therapeutic doses augments vagal tone, and this also retards atrioventricular conduction. At doses in the toxic range, sympathetic nerve activity is enhanced, and may increase the tendency for ventricular dysrhythmias.[20]

Administration

AXIOM The optimal digitalizing dose is extremely variable from patient to patient.

For rapid digitalization of a patient (as in patients with atrial fibrillation with fast ventricular responses), digoxin 0.75-1.0 mg can be given by slow intravenous injection.[20] Additional doses of 0.125-0.25 mg may be needed in the next four to six hours. Alternatively, 0.75-1.50 mg of digoxin can be given in 250 mL of 5% dextrose by intravenous infusion over a period of two hours.

AXIOM Digoxin levels should not be checked sooner than six hours after the last dose.

Normal digoxin levels are 1-2 mcg/mL, determined 6 hours after the last dose.[20] Values > 2-3 mcg/mL are frequently associated with signs and symptoms of toxicity; however, toxicity can occur at much lower levels in the presence of hypokalemia or hypercalcemia. Regardless of the serum digoxin levels, digoxin should be discontinued temporarily if potassium levels are < 3.0 mEq/L or if calcium levels are high.

AXIOM Little or no correlation exists between serum digoxin levels and therapeutic responses to the drug.

The beneficial hemodynamic effects of digitalis can be obtained without any ECG changes. If ECG changes occur, some element of toxicity is usually present.

Side Effects

Because the increased contractility produced by digitalis usually also increases myocardial oxygen requirements, it should be used with caution in patients with severe CAD.[102] However, when cardiac dilatation due to heart failure is present, digitalis may decrease heart size enough to decrease myocardial oxygen consumption.

AXIOM Any arrhythmia that develops in a patient receiving digitalis should be considered due to the digitalis until proven otherwise.

One of the main drawbacks to digitalis preparations is that it can precipitate severe arrhythmias.[102] Paroxysmal atrial tachycardia (PAT) with varying AV block is particularly apt to be due to digitalis toxicity. Consequently, before digitalis is given to a patient in heart failure, it is important to determine whether the patient is hypokalemic or hypercalcemic and whether any digitalis preparation has been given within the past 7-14 days. Furthermore, because it is largely excreted by the kidneys, the maintenance dose of digoxin should be reduced if renal function is impaired.

AXIOM Because it tends to slow the conduction of impulses through the AV node and the Bundle of His, digitalis should generally be avoided in patients with AV block.

Severe digitalis intoxication is increasingly treated with digoxin-specific antibody fragments which are developed in sheep and then isolated, purified, and fragmented.[171]

DOPAMINE

AXIOM Dopamine is probably the best inotrope to give to patients who continue to have a low BP and cardiac output in spite of optimal fluid loading.

Dopamine is probably the inotropic agent used most frequently to increase blood pressure and cardiac output in patients who have already been adequately fluid-loaded. It is a naturally-occurring compound and is the immediate precursor of norepinephrine in the biosynthesis of catecholamines.[92]

Like all catecholamines, the effects of dopamine are dose-dependent with different receptor populations stimulated at different concentrations. With increasing doses, dopamine sequentially stimulates dopaminergic, β-adrenergic, and then α-adrenergic receptors.[92] Vasoconstriction occurring at higher doses probably also involves serotonin- and tryptamine-sensitive receptors.[172]

Dopamine receptors are located in the coronary, mesenteric, and renal vascular beds, and these splanchnic receptors are stimulated at doses of 1-3 mcg/kg/min. However, dopaminergic receptors are relatively weak, and their effects are easily negated by simultaneous stimulation of β- or α-adrenergic receptors.

Stimulation of dopaminergic receptors causes relaxation of renal vessels, whereas high doses stimulate α-receptors to cause vasoconstriction of renal vessels. Most critical illnesses are associated with high endogenous catecholamine levels which result in α-receptor stimulation. This may explain why dopamine frequently fails to improve renal blood flow and renal function in critically ill patients.[28]

AXIOM Administration of low-dose dopamine to patients with high endogenous catecholamine levels usually does not cause dilation of renal or mesenteric vessels.

As dopamine doses are raised to 5-10 mcg/kg/min, they increase myocardial contractility by acting directly on β-adrenergic receptors in the myocardium. This increase in contractility is often accompanied by some increase in heart rate and myocardial oxygen consumption.[92] Filling pressures may remain unchanged or may increase. The increase in preload is apparently due to α-adrenergic stimulation of venous receptors. This can be seen at doses as low as 2 mcg/kg/min and can be blocked by α-receptor antagonists. Usually, the increase in preload does not have any adverse hemodynamic effects, but it does limit the usefulness of dopamine in patients with failure secondary to excessive volume overload.

AXIOM Dopamine is not the ideal inotropic agent when excessive volume overload occurs.

With doses of dopamine above 20-30 mc/kg/min, α-adrenergic stimulation can predominate, and this can decrease renal and mesenteric blood flow. When afterload increases significantly, the beneficial effects of dopamine on cardiac contractility are offset by the increased impedance to ventricular ejection, and this causes cardiac output to decrease.

AXIOM In conditions associated with a decreased systemic vascular resistance, such as sepsis, dopamine can often be used in rather high doses without causing excessive vasoconstriction.[189]

Dopamine is a relatively safe drug, except for tachyarrhythmias when the dose is increased too rapidly, or when it is given to a patient who already is tachycardic. Because part of the effect of dopamine is due to release of endogenous myocardial catecholamines, it is less likely to be of benefit in CHF when the myocardium tends to have depleted catecholamine stores.[173] Dopamine may also precipitate angina pectoris in patients with CAD.[173] In patients with preexisting peripheral vascular disease, the intense vasoconstriction caused by high doses of dopamine may occasionally cause gangrene of digits.[174]

DOBUTAMINE

Dobutamine is a synthetic catecholamine with minimal α-adrenergic effects. At doses of 5-10 mcg/kg/min, it selectively stimulates β-₁ receptors producing an increase in cardiac contractility with relatively minor increases in heart rate.[175] At higher doses, increasing β-₂ adrenergic activity results in increasing tachycardia and peripheral and often pulmonary vasodilatation.[175,176] Dobutamine lowers central venous pressure, pulmonary artery pressure, and PAWP through its effect on contractility. Although it causes a redistribution of blood flow from mesenteric and renal vascular beds to coronary and skeletal muscle beds, urine output is frequently increased because of increased cardiac output.[63,175]

Dobutamine is most useful in circumstances where a selective inotropic agent is indicated and the blood pressure is high-normal or increased. The infusion should be started at 2-5 mcg/kg/min and titrated to the maximal effect on cardiac output. In patients with high systemic vascular resistance, the dobutamine dose can be increased relatively rapidly in order to provide β_2-mediated arterial vasodilation. Tachycardia is usually the main factor limiting its dose.

Relatively few problems occur with dobutamine. However, it can occasionally cause hypotension in patients with unrecognized hypovolemia, and it occasionally causes tachyarrhythmias.[22] Tolerance to dobutamine can also develop within 72 hours, especially when larger doses are used.

DOPAMINE PLUS DOBUTAMINE

One of our favorite inotropic combinations in critically ill elderly patients is dopamine at 5 mcg/kg/min and dobutamine at 5-10 mcg/kg/min. We have used this combination so frequently in older patients with low-cardiac outputs that we often refer to it as "vitamin D".

Richard et al. reported eight mechanically-ventilated patients in cardiogenic shock treated with dopamine and dobutamine.[177] Each patient received three infusions in a randomly assigned order: (a) dopamine at 15 mcg/kg/min; (b) dobutamine at 15 mcg/kg/min combined with dopamine at 7.5 mcg/kg/min, and (c) dobutamine at 7.5 mcg/kg/min. Stroke volume-index increased similarly with all infusions, but dopamine by itself increased oxygen consumption (P < .05) and tended to increase hypoxemia. The dopamine-dobutamine combination increased mean arterial pressure, maintained PAWP within normal limits, and prevented the worsening of hypoxemia induced by dopamine alone. It also produced increases in renal blood flow, glomerular filtration rate, urine flow, and sodium excretion. This may be of particular importance in patients with severe heart failure, particularly if they are on a ventilator, which tends to reduce glomerular filtration and increase sodium retention.

DOPEXAMINE

Dopexamine is a newer synthetic catecholamine that is structurally and functionally related to dopamine[92]; however, it is only one-third as active as dopamine at DA-1 sites and one-fifth as active at DA-2 sites. It has no α-adrenergic activity, and it is a potent β_2-agonist. Dopexamine acts as an inotrope by an initial baroreceptor-mediated stimulation of the release of norepinephrine in the myocardium followed by an inhibition of neuronal reuptake of norepinephrine, probably mediated through DA-2 receptors. This combined effect results in a potentiation of endogenous and exogenous catecholamines.[178] Dopexamine also increases cardiac output through vasodilator effects mediated predominantly through β_2-receptor stimulation.[92]

Dopexamine decreases renal vascular resistance but to a lesser extent than dopamine.[92] It also reduces hepatic-splanchnic vascular resistance leading to augmented splanchnic blood flow.[179] As the dose of dopexamine is increased, the augmentation of splanchnic and renal blood flow is reduced.

Doses above 4 mcg/kg/min increase heart rate with a resultant increase in myocardial oxygen consumption. When compared to dobutamine in patients with chronic CHF, dopexamine caused greater increases in cardiac output and greater reductions in central filling pressures and pulmonary vascular resistance.[180]

ISOPROTERENOL

AXIOM	Isoproterenol should probably only be used in patients who have a slow, weak heart.

In patients with bradycardia and a low cardiac output, such as may occur after valvular cardiac surgery, isoproterenol in doses of 1.0-2.0 mcg/min (0.015-0.030 mcg/kg/min) may improve cardiac output without an excess increase in heart rate. It may be particularly helpful for the patient who also has increased pulmonary vascular resistance. However, when the pulse rate is > 120/min, isoproterenol tends to reduce diastolic aortic pressure and coronary blood flow while it increases myocardial oxygen consumption. This may be particularly detrimental in patients with acute myocardial infarction or pulmonary embolism.

EPINEPHRINE

Epinephrine in doses of 1-2 mcg/min (0.015-0.030 mcg/kg/min) may dramatically increase blood pressure and cardiac output in patients who are unresponsive to dopamine and/or dobutamine. The lower doses have a relatively greater inotropic effect, while large doses are more vasoconstrictive. Large doses also increase the tendency for severe tachycardia and ventricular arrhythmias. Tachyphylaxis can develop fairly rapidly.

AMRINONE

AXIOM	Amrinone is an excellent inotrope for improving cardiac function in patients with pulmonary hypertension, but its long half-life can be a major problem if an undesirable response occurs.

Amrinone is a potent inotrope and vasodilator.[92] It is believed to act through inhibition of cardiac phosphodiesterase which cleaves cyclic AMP. This inhibition results in an increase in intracellular cyclic AMP which then increases intracellular calcium concentrations. Amrinone may also act by inhibiting calcium uptake by the sarcoplasmic reticulum and by sensitizing the contractile proteins to calcium so that contraction is initiated and maintained at lower concentrations of intracellular calcium.

Because increases in intracellular cAMP cause vascular smooth muscle to relax, phosphodiesterase inhibitors are potent vasodilators. Although amrinone and milrinone decrease systemic, pulmonary, and coronary vascular resistance, heart rate and blood pressure usually do not change.[181]

Indications for amrinone include: (a) severe CHF refractory to conventional treatment with digoxin, diuretics, and vasodilators; and (b) acute heart failure associated with myocardial infarction (to reduce pulmonary vascular resistance and to improve cardiac output).

Amrinone requires a loading dose and then a maintenance infusion. A 0.75 mg/kg bolus is administered over 2-3 minutes, and then a maintenance infusion of 5-10 mcg/kg/min is begun. Another bolus of 0.75 mcg/kg may be given in 30 minutes as needed. An alternative approach is to give it at 40 mcg/kg/min for 1 hour, followed by 10 mcg/kg/min as a maintenance infusion. Either way, the maximum dose should not exceed 18 mg/kg in 24 hours.

Adverse effects of amrinone include nausea and vomiting (0.5%-2.0%), thrombocytopenia (2.4%), and increased ventricular dysrhythmogenicity.[92] Although hypotension is believed to be rare, these agents can cause a sudden, severe decrease in BP in patients who are hypovolemic.

CALCIUM

Ionized calcium levels < two-thirds of normal (which is 1.05-1.2 mmol/L) can impair cardiac contractility. Hypocalcemia can develop rapidly in patients with shock or congestive failure, particularly when they are getting massive blood transfusions at a rate faster than one unit every five minutes.[182-184]

AXIOM	Calcium should not be given to improve cardiac function, except possibly in patients with shock or heart failure after multiple blood transfusions, after calcium-blockers, or in patients with severe hyperkalemia.

Calcium should not be administered indiscriminately to all patients in shock because it can interfere with resuscitation, especially if an adequate cardiac output is not established soon after its administra-

TABLE 41–7 *Vasodilators for Use during Intraoperative and Early Recovery Phases*

Drug	Dosage	Action	Comments
Nitroprusside	0.25-10 µg/kg/min	Arterial and venous dilatation Direct action on vessels	May cause reflex tachycardia Tachyphylaxis may occur Cyanide toxicity may occur May impair thyroid uptake of iodine May cause coronary steal
Nitroglycerine	0.25-10 µg/kg/min	Mainly venodilator Some arteriolar dilatation Direct effect	Reflex tachycardia may occur Does not cause coronary steal
Hydralazine	2.5-20 mg IV every 4-6 hrs 20-40 mg IM every 4-6 hrs	Direct vasodilator More prominent dilator effect on arterioles than on veins	May cause reflex tachycardia Increases cerebral, coronary, renal, and splanchnic blood flows
Trimethaphan	1-4 mg/min	Vasodilatation through ganglionic blockade	Histamine release Tachyphylaxis may occur Potentiates effects of succinylcholine
Phentolamine	2-5 mg IV	Alpha blockade Mainly arterial dilator	Reflex tachycardia Hypoglycemia

From: Grande CM, Tissot M, Bhatt V, et al. Preexisting compromising conditions. Capan LM, Miller SM, Turndorf H, eds. Philadelphia: JB Lippincott, 1991; 250.

tion.[185,186] Hypocalcemia can also blunt the effects of catecholamines[187] and glucagon.[188] Calcium tends to move into cells that have impaired metabolism. This lowers plasma calcium levels and causes an intracellular calcium excess which stimulates phospholipase A_2 and can also precipitate organic anions and phosphates.[92,185,186]

AXIOM Calcium administration except to counteract excess citrate or potassium may impair resuscitative efforts.

GLUCAGON

Glucagon is a polypeptide hormone produced by the alpha cells of the pancreatic islets. It helps to maintain plasma glucose levels during fasting and stress, primarily by increasing hepatic glycogenolysis. Glucagon has also been shown to have inotropic and some chronotropic cardiac effects that are independent of the β-adrenergic receptors.[188]

Glucagon's inotropic action is not affected by norepinephrine depletion or by α- or β-adrenergic receptor blockade. Glucagon is also effective in restoring stable cardiovascular states in some patients with β-blocker or calcium-channel-blocker overdoses.[188-190] Glucagon operates through adenyl cyclase to increase cyclic AMP formation and thereby increases transcellular calcium flux. Glucagon has been reported to be a particularly effective inotropic agent because of antiarrhythmic properties, additive effects with digitalis glycosides, and secondary coronary vasodilation.

AXIOM Glucagon can be helpful in patients with a poor cardiac output due to beta blockers or calcium blockers.

The dosage of glucagon used is extremely variable. Boluses of 1-5 mg intravenously every 30-60 minutes may be effective. An infusion of 10 mg/hr may also be effective in some patients. Disturbing side effects may include severe hyperglycemia and nausea and vomiting, especially with large doses.

Vasodilators (Table 41–7)

AXIOM Vasodilators should not be given to patients who are hypovolemic or hypotensive.

Vasodilators may be used to reduce afterload and/or preload. Afterload reduction is particularly important when cardiac output remains low because of elevated systemic vascular resistance.

Widespread use of vasodilators in the treatment of heart failure has highlighted the importance of systemic vascular resistance in regulating the performance of a diseased left ventricle.[20,191] When myocardial function is normal, cardiac output is dependent on venous return. In the presence of systolic dysfunction, however, cardiac output is extremely sensitive to changes in the systemic vascular resistance, and increased venous return has little effect because the left ventricle is already operating at or near the top of a depressed cardiac function curve.[20]

A wide variety of vasodilators are currently available for treating heart failure. These include nitrites and nitrates, α-adrenergic blockers, calcium blockers, ganglionic blockers, and other agents.[20] The hemodynamic effects of vasodilator drugs in severe LV failure vary somewhat according to whether their predominant activity is on the arterial or venous circulation. Agents that are venoselective tend to reduce cardiac filling pressure (preload) more than vascular resistance (afterload).

AXIOM Preload should be optimized before using afterload-reducing agents.

Vasodilators can cause sudden, severe hypotension in patients with unrecognized hypovolemia, especially in younger patients, if an adequate BP is being maintained primarily by high catecholamine levels.[18] Even with an adequate preload, vasodilators tend to cause some decrease in BP; however, it is essential to not let the BP decrease too far. In a review of 13 studies, Farnett et al. found that diastolic BP levels reduced to < 85 mm Hg were associated with a significantly increased risk of adverse cardiac events.[192]

NITRATES

Nitrates are potent, direct dilators of smooth muscle in veins and arteries.[20] Veins appear to have a greater affinity for nitrates, with venodilation occurring at much lower plasma concentrations than arteriolar vasodilation. Nitrates are most effective in patients with high-filling pressures and a low-cardiac output. The resultant decrease in ventricular wall tension is associated with a more favorable myocardial blood supply: demand ratio, and the decreased central filling pressure helps alleviate pulmonary congestion. Cardiac output tends to increase in patients who maintain an adequate preload.

Nitrates can be particularly useful in patients with predominant diastolic dysfunction, especially when it is due to ischemia. Correction of dyspnea by nitrates often increases exercise tolerance, even when cardiac output is not substantially improved.[20]

Nitroprusside

Sodium nitroprusside is an extremely potent, short-acting vasodilator that relaxes vascular smooth muscle in both arteries and veins.[193] Because of its potency, rapid onset, short duration of action, and remarkably linear dose-response relationships, sodium nitroprusside is frequently used to manage acute, severe heart failure. It is also the drug of choice for many hypertensive crises. However, with dissecting aneurysms, the increased dp/dt and reflex tachycardia that it causes may be a problem; consequently, simultaneous use of a beta-blocker is required.

Sodium nitroprusside is considered a "balanced" vasodilator because it dilates both venous capacitance and arterial resistance vessels, thereby causing a decrease in both preload and afterload.[193] In patients with a normal blood volume, the venous pooling may cause relative hypovolemia and this, combined with a decreased afterload, can cause BP and cardiac output to decrease abruptly.[194] In contrast, when preload is very high, venous return will still be adequate following nitroprusside, and the decrease in afterload caused by nitroprusside usually causes an increase in cardiac output. Myocardial ischemia may also be caused by nitroprusside because of its ability to dilate normal coronary vessels in nonischemic areas, thereby stealing blood from ischemic areas that have diseased, nonresponsive vessels.[195] Pulmonary vascular resistance also decreases during nitroprusside infusions, probably due to a direct effect on the pulmonary vascular bed.

The dose of sodium nitroprusside required to produce a satisfactory reduction of afterload in cardiac failure varies from 15 to 400 mcg/minute (0.2-6.0 mcg/kg/min), averaging approximately 50 mcg/minute (0.7 mcg/kg/min).

Other than hypotension, the major side effects of nitroprusside include thiocyanate/cyanide toxicity and mild reductions in arterial oxygen tension due to nitroprusside-induced inhibition of the pulmonary vasoconstrictor response. Thiocyanate toxicity, which usually only occurs in patients with renal failure, is manifested by confusion, hyperreflexia, and convulsions. Cyanide toxicity is usually first manifested by metabolic acidosis due to cyanide combining with cytochromes and inhibiting aerobic cellular metabolism. Thiocyanate or cyanide toxicity occurs almost exclusively in patients receiving high doses of nitroprusside for a prolonged period. Infusion rates of < 3 mcg/kg/min for < 72 hours are generally not associated with toxicity.

AXIOM Nitroprusside should not be used in high doses (> 3.0 mg/kg/min) for more than 72 hours.

Some deaths during prolonged infusions of high doses of nitroprusside have been ascribed to cyanide toxicity. If metabolic acidosis and confusion do not improve rapidly after discontinuation of nitroprusside, one should consider using thiosulfate, sodium nitrate, or hydroxocobalamin (vitamin B_{12a}) to facilitate conversion of cyanide to thiocyanate. Monitoring blood thiocyanate levels can be used to follow toxicity in patients requiring infusions for longer than two to three days.

Rapid discontinuation of nitroprusside infusion can cause a rebound decrease in cardiac output and increase in SVR, BP, and PAWP.

Nitroglycerin

In addition to its ability to dilate coronary arteries and relieve ischemic myocardial pain, nitroglycerin also dilates systemic vessels, usually with a greater reduction in venous return than arterial resistance.[196] Nitroglycerin also dilates ureteral, uterine, and gastrointestinal smooth muscle.

If nitroglycerin is administered to patients with only mild heart

failure, cardiac output may decrease. However, in severe heart failure with a more than adequate preload, the mild arterial dilating effect of nitroglycerin is usually enough to produce an increase in cardiac output. Nitroglycerin also tends to reduce pulmonary arterial pressure, and this may be helpful in patients with COPD or severe ARDS.

AXIOM Intravenous nitroglycerin by slow infusion may be the vasodilator of choice in patients with heart failure when high preload is the main problem and/or the patient has moderate-to-severe ischemic heart disease.[197]

Intravenous nitroglycerin can be started in doses of 0.3 mcg/kg/min and gradually increased to about 3.0 mcg/kg/min. One of the main drawbacks to continued intravenous nitroglycerin therapy is the rapid development of tolerance and the occasional development of methemoglobinemia.[198] It has been found that oral administration of N-acetylcysteine (Mucomyst) in doses of 200 mg/kg can at least partially reverse the tolerance that develops during continuous intravenous nitroglycerin therapy.

Sublingual nitroglycerin is used primarily to relieve angina; however, the responses can be quite variable. It has been postulated that sustained levels of nitrates tend to be less effective than the peaks associated with intermittent administration due to interactions with membrane receptors.[199]

α-ADRENERGIC BLOCKERS

Phentolamine

Phentolamine is considered one of the classic α-adrenergic blocking agents, and it causes blockade at both postsynaptic (α_1) and presynaptic (α_2) receptors.[200] Phentolamine can relax arteriolar and, to a lesser extent, venous smooth muscle and thus can increase cardiac output and reduce pulmonary and systemic venous pressure in patients with moderate-to-severe heart failure of all etiologies.[200] The increased cardiac output and less-than-expected decreases in venous tone may be caused by a secondary increase in the release of norepinephrine, which increases cardiac contractility and causes venous vasoconstriction. Although phentolamine is generally well tolerated in nonischemic cardiac failure, the tachycardia and norepinephrine release that it causes can increase ischemia in patients with CAD.

Phentolamine is usually given as an intravenous infusion starting at 0.1 mg/min which can be increased slowly up to 2.0 mg/min as needed. Because of the tachycardia that it can cause and its high cost, phentolamine is rarely used now to treat heart failure. Other major side effects of phentolamine include vomiting, crampy abdominal pain, and diarrhea.

Prazosin

Prazosin is a selective, α_1 (postsynaptic) adrenergic receptor antagonist that causes arteriolar and venous vasodilation by its receptor-blocking effects.[201] In patients with heart failure, prazosin has balanced hemodynamic actions similar to those of nitroprusside, producing reductions in both systemic and pulmonary venous pressures. Cardiac output tends to increase when adequate preload is maintained; however, this drug is of limited use in acute trauma patients because it is only given orally.

CALCIUM-CHANNEL BLOCKERS

Calcium-channel blocking agents interfere with muscular excitation-contraction coupling by reducing the movement of calcium into cells via the so-called "slow channels." This results in peripheral and coronary artery vasodilation and a negative inotropic effect. However, decreased contractility may be offset by decreased LV afterload, resulting in a favorable net effect on LV function.[202]

Nifedipine

Nifedipine has been widely used in the treatment of angina pectoris, and it may be of benefit in selected patients with heart failure. In patients with severe LV failure, nifedipine tends to cause an increase in cardiac output and a decrease in systemic vascular resistance.[203] Nevertheless, many clinicians are reluctant to use calcium-channel blockers in heart failure because of their direct depressant effect on the myocardium. However, with nifedipine, the decrease in afterload is often more profound than the myocardial depressant effect, resulting in overall enhanced hemodynamics.[204]

Verapamil

Verapamil has vasodilator properties, but its direct myocardial depressant effect is more profound, and this may seriously aggravate myocardial dysfunction in patients with severe heart failure. It may, however, be of value in treating tachyarrhythmias which may be contributing to the severity of the heart failure.

ARTERIAL VASODILATORS

Hydralazine

Hydralazine is a potent, direct dilator of vascular smooth muscle, especially in arterioles. Consequently, it primarily affects afterload. In patients with severe heart failure and very high SVR, hydralazine can produce impressive increases in stroke volume.[205] It has only a modest tendency to lower systemic and pulmonary venous pressures. For a given change in blood pressure, hydralazine increases cardiac output more than nitroprusside or nitrates.[45] Hydralazine can also increase renal blood flow, thereby promoting diuresis.

When hydralazine is used in critically ill patients, intravenous administration is the most reliable route, but it must be given slowly and with constant hemodynamic monitoring to avoid sudden, severe hypotension. Administration is usually started by giving 5-10 mg by a slow intravenous drip over at least 20-30 minutes. The maximal effect occurs 25-45 minutes after injection and the effect may last 4-24 hours. Subsequent doses of up to 20 mg can be administered intravenously every six hours.

After hydralazine administration, some patients with heart failure develop severe tachycardia which can exacerbate angina pectoris in patients with ischemic heart disease.

Minoxidil

Minoxidil is a potent, direct-acting, vascular smooth muscle relaxant that acts primarily on the arterial bed.[206] Because it is only given orally, minoxidil has limited use in the ICU, but it can be very helpful later.

ACE INHIBITORS

Captopril

Activation of the renin-angiotensin-aldosterone axis in CHF can cause excessive vasoconstriction and salt and water retention. Interruption of this system with ACE inhibitors, such as captopril, has several potentially beneficial hemodynamic effects.[207,208] The primary mechanism of action is to reduce production of angiotensin II by competitive inhibition of the enzyme that converts angiotensin I into angiotensin II. Reduced levels of angiotensin II, in turn, promote vasodilation and lower aldosterone production. Captopril interferes not only with the action of angiotensin at peripheral vascular receptor sites but also at central brain receptor sites, thereby decreasing sympathetic outflow and reducing thirst.[209] Furthermore, it may retard the breakdown of bradykinin and prostaglandins,[210] resulting in an increased tendency for vasodilation and increased levels of prostaglandins.

Multiple clinical trials of the oral forms of ACE inhibitors showed both acute and chronic improvements in cardiac output, stroke work index, and functional status along with lowered systemic and pulmonary vascular resistance and reduced ventricular-filling pressures. This agent may work even in individuals who have become refractory to digoxin, diuretics, and other vasodilators.[211]

Captopril is only available in an oral preparation. Therapy is started with 25 mg every six hours and increased to a maximum daily dosage of 450 mg. Maximal drug effectiveness is frequently obtained when an ACE inhibitor is used in combination with a diuretic, such as furosemide.[212]

AXIOM   Captopril should not be used in patients who are or may become hyperkalemic.

Side effects with captopril include rash, hypotension, deterioration of renal function, and hyperkalemia. By lowering plasma aldosterone and thereby reducing urinary potassium excretion, ACE inhibitors may elevate serum potassium.

When internal potassium homeostasis is perturbed (e.g., by noncardio-selective beta-blockers), or when external potassium homeostasis is impaired (e.g., by potassium supplementation, renal insufficiency, hypoaldosteronism, or potassium-sparing diuretics), the patient receiving catopril is at high risk for developing hyperkalemia.[79] Theoretically, older patients may also be at a higher risk. Development of sepsis while the patient receives an ACE inhibitor may result in extremely high rates of capillary leakage because ACE is also important in inactivating bradykinin.

Enalapril

A Consensus Trial concluded that the addition of enalapril, a newer ACE inhibitor, to other conventional therapy (including vasodilators) significantly improves signs and symptoms and reduces mortality in patients with New York Heart Association class IV heart failure and a relatively well-preserved BP.[213] It has a long half-life and is clinically effective on a once-daily dose.[214]

GANGLIONIC BLOCKERS

Trimethaphan (Arfonad) is a short-acting ganglionic blocking agent which, in the past, was used primarily for treatment of hypertensive crises. The inhibition of reflex sympathetic discharge by ganglionic blockade usually prevents an undesirable reflex tachycardia. However, the variability of response to the drug and the occasional occurrence of severe orthostatic hypotension make its use somewhat difficult.

OXYGEN

AXIOM   Oxygen can be a very effective pulmonary vasodilator.

Because hypoxia can cause pulmonary artery vasoconstriction, giving oxygen to a hypoxic individual can significantly reduce the afterload on the right ventricle. Severe hypoxia may also cause myocardial and peripheral tissue damage. Consequently, patients with CHF often benefit from the administration of sufficient oxygen to maintain an arterial P_{O_2} of at least 80 mm Hg.

β-ADRENERGIC BLOCKERS

Historically, the negative inotropic properties of β-adrenergic receptor antagonists were believed to preclude their use in patients with CHF. However, it is now clear that a chronic excess of circulating catecholamines may have direct toxic effects on the myocardium and may increase myocardial oxygen demands by increasing afterload, heart rate, and contractility.

In 1975, Waagstein et al. reported beneficial effects of β-adrenergic blocking agents in patients with dilated cardiomyopathy, presumably by decreasing resting symptomatic tone and reversing the down-regulation of β-receptors caused by chronically elevated norepinephrine levels.[215] Randomized trials in patients with idiopathic dilated cardiomyopathy demonstrated that cautious β-adrenergic blocker therapy can decrease filling pressures and improve cardiac function and exercise tolerance.[216]

DRUG COMBINATIONS

AXIOM   Drug combinations, if monitored properly, tend to produce better results and fewer side-effects than single agents.

Nitrates Plus Inotropes

The combination of vasodilators (such as nitroprusside or nitroglycerin) with inotropic agents (such as dopamine or dobutamine) may increase cardiac output much more than either type of agent alone.[216,217] The PAWP and pulse rate may also be lower than they would be with an inotropic agent alone.

Miller et al. used dopamine at an average dose of 2.6 ± 0.7 mcg/kg/min with sodium nitroprusside at an average dose of 0.5 ± 0.2 mcg/kg/min in patients who had recently undergone cardiopulmonary bypass and were being treated for LV dysfunction.[218] The average systemic vascular resistance was 3520 dyne-sec/cm.[5] Combination therapy increased cardiac index by 45% and reduced systemic vascular resistance by 41%. Similarly, with adequate preload, the combination of a vasodilator with furosemide can produce better excretion of water and sodium than either agent alone.[219]

Miller et al. also used the term "preload reserve" to indicate the shift in Starling's curve resulting from the administration of low-dose dopamine and nitroprusside to patients with marked vasoconstriction[218]; however, without adequate preload, two-drug therapy can cause hypotension and a decrease in cardiac output.[92]

Hydralazine and Nitrates

The addition of hydralazine and isosorbide dinitrate to a long-term therapeutic regimen of digoxin and diuretics can have a very favorable effect on LV function and mortality.[220] One study demonstrated a mortality reduction of 36% at three years in heart failure patients treated with hydralazine and isosorbide dinitrate compared with the results in similar patients taking only prazosin or a placebo.

Norepinephrine Plus Phentolamine

Another combination of drugs that can be used to treat heart failure and/or hypotension is the infusion of an α- and β-stimulator (norepinephrine) with an α-blocking agent (phentolamine).[221] Norepinephrine has about 15% β-adrenergic effects and 85% α-adrenergic effects. With phentolamine blocking excessive α-adrenergic effects, the β-adrenergic effects are unmasked and cardiac output may increase markedly.

Gray et al. used various norepinephrine doses with phentolamine, at a ratio of 2.5 mg of phentolamine to each 1 mg of norepinephrine in patients with a low-cardiac output after open heart surgery.[222] This combination consistently increased systemic arterial pressure without causing tachycardia or ventricular irritability. Phentolamine also prevents the severe decreases in renal blood flow found when levarterenol is given alone.[223]

Amrinone Combinations

A combination of dobutamine and amrinone can be extremely beneficial. Sympathomimetic amines stimulate synthesis of cyclic AMP and amrinone prevents degradation of cyclic AMP. The resultant greatly increased cAMP concentrations increase the availability of calcium to the contractile elements.[224] The vasodilation seen with these two drugs may be complementary by increasing cardiac output without compromising flow to any peripheral vascular beds.[181]

Treatment of Arrhythmias

NEED FOR TREATMENT

AXIOM   When an arrhythmia is asymptomatic and may be chronic, one should think twice and/or obtain cardiology consultation before treating it.

A failing heart may attempt to maintain an adequate cardiac output by increasing its rate; thus, tachycardia in trauma patients with CHF may continue despite an adequate resuscitation. Consequently, efforts to lower heart rate by giving more fluid than needed could lead to pulmonary edema.

Pain, anxiety, hypovolemia, anemia, acidosis, and hypoxia are major causes of tachycardia in acute trauma victims and should be treated aggressively. However, when severe tachycardia persists in spite of all other therapy in a patient with heart failure but an adequate cardiac output and BP, a short-acting β-adrenergic agent may be given cautiously.[33]

AXIOM   Magnesium depletion can be an important cause of arrhythmias in CHF.

Serum magnesium concentration is normally 1.4-2.1 mEq/L. Because the relative amount of Mg contained in the plasma compartment is small compared with the skeletal muscle pool of exchangeable Mg, serum Mg levels may be normal in spite of moderate-severe Mg depletion in tissues.[79]

AXIOM   Serum Mg levels may be normal in spite of serious Mg tissue depletion.

CLASSIFICATION OF ANTIARRHYTHMIC DRUGS

Antiarrhythmic drugs can be classified into five categories based on their mechanism of action.[92]

Group I Drugs

Group I drugs, such as quinidine and procainamide, act by depressing sodium conductance.[225] This results in: (a) decreased conduction velocity, (b) increased refractoriness of myocardial muscle, (c) decreased automaticity of the myocardium, and (d) direct suppression of conduction in the AV node, His bundle, and ventricular muscle. They are most effective in supraventricular and ventricular arrhythmias that are due to either an automatic focus or reentry. These agents can cause prolongation of the PR interval and QRS complex. Toxic levels of group I agents may result in complete heart block.

Group II Drugs

Group II drugs, such as phenytoin and lidocaine, have little effect on the conduction velocity of normal tissue, but they selectively decrease conduction velocity through ischemic myocardium.[225] These agents are frequently used to treat reentry ventricular arrhythmias. Phenytoin (Dilantin®) may be of particular benefit in patients with tachyarrhythmias due to digitalis toxicity.

Group III Drugs

Group III drugs have β-adrenergic blocking capability and some group I and group II effects.[225] They are commonly used to treat supraventricular and ventricular arrhythmias, but in high doses they can cause AV nodal block and suppress lower pacemaker function, which may result in asystole. They can also be used to treat excessive sinus tachycardia.

Increased heart rate not only increases myocardial oxygen consumption but may also decrease presystolic ejection time to the point that stroke volume may be reduced. Therefore, one should try to reduce tachycardias to 100-120 beats/min to decrease these detrimental side effects.

AXIOM   β-Adrenergic blocking agents are generally contraindicated in cardiac failure and low-output states unless problems are due to a tachyarrhythmia that is unresponsive to other therapy.

Group IV Drugs

Group IV drugs, such as bretylium, are quaternary ammonium compounds whose major action is to reduce the disparity in duration of action potential between normal and ischemic myocardium.[225] Bretylium is as effective as lidocaine in controlling ventricular fibrillation, but it can cause severe hypertension initially and then severe hypotension.

Group V Drugs

Group V drugs, such as verapamil, act by blocking or reducing calcium influx into myocardial cells.[225] They depress activity in the sinoatrial node, AV node, and in diseased myocardial fibers which have slow channel-dependent properties. They have a mild, negative inotropic effect, but can often provide excellent control of supraventricular tachycardias that are resistant to group I, II and IV agents. A verapamil dose of 5-10 mg intravenously is used in patients with supraventricular tachycardia (SVT); however, if atrial fibrillation or flutter is due to an accessory conduction pathway (e.g., WPW), agents such as verapamil, beta blockers, or lidocaine may cause a ventricular fibrillation which is very difficult to reverse. With atrial fibrillation or flutter that may be due to an accessory pathway, procaineamide is the drug of choice.

Group VI Drugs

A sixth group of antiarrthymic drugs may be considered for the therapy of bradycardia. Patients with symptomatic bradycardia, particularly when associated with a second- or third-degree heart block, may respond dramatically to atropine, isoproterenol, or a pacemaker.

SPECIFIC ARRHYTHMIAS

Arrhythmias can be grouped into five categories: tachyarrhythmias, bradyarrhythmias, conduction defects, ectopic beats, and electromechanical dissociation.[33]

Tachyarrhythmias

SINUS TACHYCARDIA

AXIOM The most frequent cause of persistent sinus tachycardia in trauma patients is inadequate volume resuscitation.

Treatment of sinus tachycardia is directed at correction of the underlying cause.[226,227] In elderly patients with possible CAD, invasive monitoring should be considered, and one should try to reduce the heart rate to < 100-120/minute.

When the underlying etiology of severe sinus tachycardia cannot be determined and control of the heart rate is necessary, a β-adrenergic blocker may be administered cautiously. If hypotension develops, the BP should be promptly raised with an $α_1$-adrenergic agonist.[33]

AXIOM If a beta blocker is used to treat severe, persistent tachycardia in a patient with heart failure, a short drug half-life can be very helpful.

Esmolol is an excellent choice for treating severe sinus tachycardia in trauma patients because it has a half-life of only nine minutes; therefore, if hypotension were to develop, it would be of short duration.[33] The patient is given a slow initial intravenous dose of 0.5 mg/kg. This dose is repeated every 4-5 minutes until adequate control of heart rate is obtained. For continuing control after the pulse has been reduced, esmolol infusion can be administered at 25-300 mcg/kg/min.

ATRIAL FLUTTER AND FIBRILLATION. The choice of treatment for atrial flutter or fibrillation depends on the patient's hemodynamic stability and the acuteness of the onset of the arrhythmia. A hemodynamically unstable patient with an acute onset of atrial fibrillation or flutter should have synchronous cardioversion. If the patient's hemodynamic instability is secondary to blood loss, fluid resuscitation should be performed prior to cardioversion.

When an adequate history cannot be obtained, a persistent, excessively rapid ventricular rate should be controlled with digoxin, a beta-blocker, or verapamil.[33] Cardioversion should not be attempted in patients with chronic atrial fibrillation because of the possibility of embolization from an atrial thrombus. Verapamil or beta-blockers must be given cautiously to patients with CHF. However, simultaneous or prior administration of calcium may reduce the negative inotropic effects of verapamil, without significantly affecting its ability to slow the ventricular response.

Once the ventricular rate has been controlled, quinidine or procainamide can be used to convert the arrhythmia to a normal sinus rhythm, but quinidine increases the risk of digoxin toxicity.[228]

PAROXYSMAL SUPRAVENTRICULAR TACHYCARDIA. Important causes of SVT include underlying heart disease and chronic lung disease.[33] When SVT is associated with an AV block, digitalis toxicity must be strongly suspected. Vagal stimulation often terminates SVT.[33] If digitalis toxicity is responsible for arrhythmia, digoxin is withheld and phenytoin is given in repeated doses of 50-100 mg intravenously every 5 minutes until a therapeutic effect is obtained or up to 15 mg/kg have been given. Verapamil (2.5-10 mg intravenously) is the drug of choice in treatment of SVT, but beta blockers and digoxin are also effective in slowing conduction through the AV node.

Quinidine and nifedipine block conduction in the retrograde pathway, and are the drugs of choice in the treatment of SVT resulting from reentry or automatic atrial tachycardia as long as the ventricular response is first controlled.[33] Procainamide may also be used (100 mg intravenous doses over 5 minutes) and repeated until a therapeutic effect is obtained or a total dose of 1 g has been given. Administration of procaineamide should be discontinued if hypotension develops or if the QT interval is prolonged by 50% or more.

AXIOM If SVT causes hemodynamic instability, the patient should be electrically cardioverted.

WOLFF-PARKINSON-WHITE SYNDROME. WPW is present in about 0.15% of the general population.[229] The characteristic QRS complex is wider than 0.12 second because of a delta wave that results from early depolarization of the ventricles via an accessory bundle (Fig. 41–8).

Reentry accounts for 80% of the tachycardias associated with WPW; atrial fibrillation and flutter account for the remaining 20%.[229] The tachycardia is often initiated by a premature atrial contraction or by a rapid sinus rate. Therefore, a trauma patient with sinus tachycardia and an anomalous pathway may develop an extremely rapid tachycardia. When the ventricular rate is above 200 and hemodynamic compromise is present, cardioversion is the treatment of choice.

AXIOM Verapamil should not be used to treat atrial fibrillation or flutter in a patient with WPW syndrome.

Verapamil, beta blockers, and lidocaine may all be used in the treatment of WPW. However, they are contraindicated when associated with atrial flutter or fibrillation. All of these drugs decrease the refractory period of the accessory pathway, increase the ventricular response, and may precipitate ventricular fibrillation.[230] In this setting, procainamide is the treatment of choice.

VENTRICULAR TACHYCARDIA. The most common cause of ventricular tachycardia is ischemic heart disease. Other etiologies include valvular heart disease, myocardial contusion, myocarditis, cardiomyopathies, hypoxia, hypercapnia, hypokalemia, and hypomagnesemia. The underlying cause obviously should be corrected whenever possible.

In hemodynamically stable patients, lidocaine is the treatment of choice. Intravenous procainamide or bretylium can be used if lidocaine is unsuccessful. In hemodynamically unstable patients, cardioversion is attempted.

TORSADES DE POINTES. Torsades de pointes presents as a ventricular tachycardia with QRS complexes of varying amplitude and axis (Fig. 41–8). It is an unstable arrhythmia, spontaneously converting to sinus rhythm or degenerating to ventricular fibrillation. It is often associated with the quinidine or procainamide therapy, mitral value prolapse, myocarditis, hypomagnesemia, hypokalemia, or hypocalcemia.[226]

Treatment involves discontinuing quinidine or procainamide, use

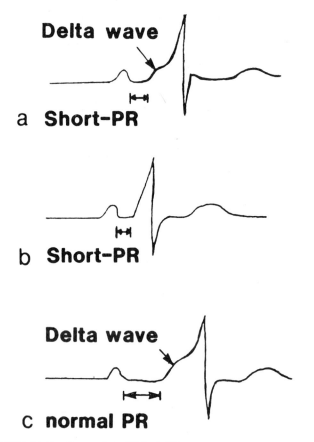

FIGURE 41–8 Characteristic ECG of WPW syndrome utilizing (a) Kent bundle, (b) James fiber, or (c) Mahaim pathway (From: Grande CM, Tissot M, Bhatt V, et al. Preexisting compromising conditions. Capan LM, Miller SM, Turndorf H, eds. Philadelphia: JB Lippincott, 1991; 249).

of overdrive pacing, and administration of intravenous Mg. When the rhythm degenerates into ventricular fibrillation, cardioversion must be performed.

Bradyarrhythmias

Bradyarrhythmias may be caused by direct trauma to the heart, head, spinal cord, neck, or eyes. Increased intracranial pressure (ICP) may result in sinus bradycardia associated with hypertension (Cushing's reflex).[231] Acute compression of the spinal cord may also result in bradyarrhythmias and even sinus arrest.

Severe hemorrhage immediately after trauma may also produce a paradoxical bradycardia instead of tachycardia. These patients usually remain conscious but hypotensive.[232]

SINUS BRADYCARDIA. If a slow heart rate is not associated with hypotension or impaired perfusion, no treatment is required. When hypotension may be secondary to blood loss, fluid should be given rapidly.

AXIOM Administration of atropine in the presence of hypovolemic bradycardia can cause ventricular fibrillation.[232]

When bradycardia results from causes other than severe hemorrhage, atropine (0.5-1.0 mg) is the drug of choice. Occasionally, atropine causes more severe bradycardia unless 1.0 mg is given. Isoproterenol or epinephrine (1-2 mcg/min intravenously) may be tried if atropine fails; however, if the patient is hypovolemic, isoproterenol could cause severe hypotension. If the heart rate fails to respond to these measures, external pacing or insertion of a temporary transvenous pacemaker is indicated.

JUNCTIONAL BRADYCARDIA. Junctional bradycardia results from suppression of the SA node with a resulting escape rhythm.[33] The resulting P-waves may be inverted or lost in the QRS complex or may follow it. When CVP monitoring is in place, diagnostic cannon A waves, resulting from contraction of the atrium against a closed AV valve, may be noted. Although junctional bradycardia is occasionally due to contusion of the SA node, this rhythm is usually caused by inhalation anesthetic agents. Treatment, when required for hypotension, includes decreasing the anesthetic concentration and/or giving atropine. If hypotension and bradycardia persist despite treatment, pacing may be required.

Conduction Defects

AXIOM Conduction defects can be caused by trauma to the head, eyes, spine, or heart.

Conduction defects in young trauma victims are more likely to be caused by trauma than by preexisting cardiac disease.[33] They are most apt to be seen after myocardial contusion or penetrating injuries to coronary arteries. Autonomic dysfunction after closed-head injury may also result in acute myocardial changes that can cause conduction defects or ventricular arrhythmias.[231]

FIRST-DEGREE HEART BLOCK. First-degree heart block is characterized by a PR interval larger than 0.2 second. It can be caused by ischemic heart disease, chronic degenerative changes of the conduction system, myocarditis, increased vagal tone associated with neck, eye, or head injuries, digoxin toxicity, and anesthetic agents. It is usually asymptomatic and requires no treatment. If treatment is needed, atropine is the drug of choice.

SECOND-DEGREE HEART BLOCK. Second-degree AV block is most likely to be encountered in elderly trauma victims with chronic degenerative changes in the AV node or the His-Purkinje conduction system; however, it is occasionally caused by myocardial injury.[32]

Second-degree heart block can be divided into Mobitz I (Wenckebach) and Mobitz II blocks (Fig. 41–9). A Mobitz I block is characterized by a progressive prolongation of the PR interval until a P-wave occurs without a QRS complex. This is caused by delayed conduction through the AV node. No treatment is required because it is a stable arrhythmia and is unlikely to progress to complete heart block. Pacing is indicated only if the patient is symptomatic.

A Mobitz type II, second-degree AV block is caused by changes in the His-Purkinje conduction system and is a precursor of third-degree heart block. This type of second-degree heart block requires placement of a pacemaker.

BIFASCICULAR BLOCKS. A bifascicular conduction block is defined either as a left bundle branch block or as a right bundle branch block associated with a block of either the anterior or posterior fascicle of the left bundle branch.[33] Right bundle branch block associated with a left anterior hemiblock is the most common bifascicular block, and it occurs in about 1% of the adult population.

Patients with a bifascicular block do not require prophylactic pacemaker insertion unless the conduction defect is associated with a history of syncope. However, pacing capability in the form of an external pacemaker, transvenous pacemaker, or a pacing pulmonary artery catheter should be available when the patient has: (a) chronic bifascicular block plus a first-degree heart block, (b) evidence of trifascicular disease, or (c) trauma-induced acute bifascicular block.

A right bundle branch block develops in up to 8% of patients during pulmonary artery catheterization.[196] The incidence of complete heart block during passage of a pulmonary artery catheter in patients with preexisting left bundle branch block varies from 0 to 1%.[170,173,176,193] Thus, complete heart block during this procedure is rare, but its consequences are grave. A reasonable approach to take with patients who have LBBB and need a PA catheter is to have an external pacemaker at the bedside in order to immediately initiate pac-

FIGURE 41–9 (a) An example of second-degree AV block of the Wenckebach type. The rhythm strip reveals progressive lengthening of the PR interval until the P wave is completely blocked, (b) An example of Mobitz type II block in which the P wave is intermittently completely blocked without lengthening of the prior PR interval (From: Grande CM, Tissot M, Bhatt V, et al. Preexisting compromising conditions. Capan LM, Miller SM, Turndorf H, eds. Philadelphia: JB Lippincott, 1991; 244).

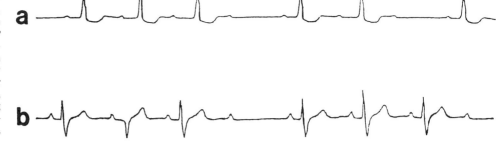

ing if a complete heart block develops. Occasionally, emergency insertion of a transvenous pacemaker may be required.

COMPLETE HEART BLOCK. Complete heart block is an absolute indication for pacemaker insertion. If the AV node is blocked, the QRS complexes are narrow and heart rate is 45-55 beats/minute. If the block occurs below the AV node, the QRS complexes are wide, and the heart rate is 30-40 beats/minute.

Causes of complete heart block include chronic degenerative changes of the conduction system, coronary heart disease, cardiomyopathies, myocarditis, increased vagal tone, digitalis toxicity, beta-blockers, and hyperkalemia. Acute complete heart block can occur following trauma as a result of myocardial contusion, increased vagal tone, or hyperkalemia during massive blood transfusion to hypovolemic and hypothermic patients. Lidocaine should not be used to treat the wide QRS complexes of a complete heart block because it will slow the rate further.

Ectopic Beats

Ectopic beats are of three types: premature atrial contractions, premature junctional contractions, and premature ventricular contractions.[33] Premature atrial contractions are usually of no significance and do not require treatment. Premature junctional contractions usually do not require treatment unless the patient is hemodynamically unstable and requires a faster heart rate to maintain a reasonable cardiac output.

Premature ventricular contractions (PVCs) arise from an ectopic focus below the AV node. The QRS complex is wide and often bizarre in appearance. PVCs in trauma patients are usually associated with hypokalemia, CAD, hypoxia, hypercapnia, or cardiac contusion.[33] Treatment should be started if the PVCs are multifocal in origin, if more than five/minute occur, or if they occur on the ascending limb of the prior T-wave. Lidocaine is the drug of choice.

AXIOM If the patient has PVCs and a slow heart rate, the "PVCs" are probably escape beats and should not be suppressed.

Electrical-mechanical Dissociation

Electrical-mechanical dissociation (EMD) is characterized by normal cardiac electrical activity but no mechanically effective heart beat.[33] This problem may be caused by trauma, massive bleeding, hypocalcemia, tension pneumothorax, acute pericardial tamponade, or inhalation anesthetic overdose. Insertion of an arterial catheter may reveal some mechanical cardiac function that is not apparent clinically.

AXIOM When EMD appears to be present, one should look carefully for pericardial tamponade, pneumothorax, or hypovolemia.

Treatment of any underlying cause plus aggressive volume repletion and ventilation with 100% oxygen may restore cardiac output and be lifesaving.

Other Treatment

ANTICOAGULATION

Deep venous thrombosis and pulmonary emboli are common in patients with CHF and may, in themselves, precipitate or aggravate cardiac failure.

AXIOM The diagnosis of pulmonary emboli should be strongly considered in patients with recurrent heart failure of unknown etiology.

Although anticoagulant therapy probably has little or no effect on the incidence or severity of coronary artery thrombosis itself, it may significantly reduce venous thrombosis, pulmonary emboli, and systemic emboli from left atrial or LV thrombi.

In patients with an active thromboembolic process, 5,000 units of heparin should be given rapidly intravenously as a loading dose, followed by 600-1500 units/hour (18 units/kg/hr) by constant intravenous infusion, to maintain thrombin times or partial thromboplastin times (PTT) at 1½-2 times normal. Convincing evidence exists, some dating back more than 40 years, to indicate that heparin and related agents are also aldosterone-suppressing and/or natriuretic.[79] The entity of heparin-induced hyperkalemia, however, is not widely appreciated.

AXIOM Heparin can aggravate a tendency to hyperkalemia.

After the acute thrombotic or embolic episode has subsided, coumadin is started and the heparin is discontinued after the coumadin has become effective. The coumadin should then generally be continued for at least three to six months. Coumadin may also be used prophylactically in patients who are at high risk for suffering an acute thromboembolic process.

Chronic anticoagulation is also now widely advocated in dilated cardiomyopathy and is based on several retrospective studies suggesting an increased incidence of thromboembolic events in nonanticoagulated patients. The data are conflicting, however, and definitive resolution of this issue awaits a prospective, randomized trial.[233] Chronic warfarin administration in dilated cardiomyopathy is best prescribed for patients with severe atrial or ventricular dilatation, especially in the setting of atrial fibrillation.

CORTICOSTEROIDS

The use of pharmacologic doses of corticosteriods in septic or other shock states has largely been abandoned; however, if there is any clinical evidence that adrenal insufficiency may be present, as has been seen in up to 15% of ICU patients,[234] hydrocortisone in doses of 100 mg intravenously every 8 hours may be lifesaving.

OPIATE ANTAGONISTS

Endogenous opioid peptides are released along with ACTH in response to all types of stress, including shock.[33] The effects of these endogenous neurotransmitters can be blocked with opiate antagonists, such as naloxone. Naloxone increases blood pressure, cardiac output, and survival in almost all types of experimental shock. Clinically, however, naloxone increases BP but does not improve survival.[235]

Treatment of Acute Pulmonary Edema

The emergency treatment of acute pulmonary edema should proceed in rapid, previously determined manner.

AXIOM The most rapid and effective method for treating severe acute pulmonary edema is positive-pressure ventilation with increased oxygen.

---

1. When pulmonary edema is mild, oxygen may be given by nasal catheter, mask, or intermittent positive-pressure breathing. Positive-pressure ventilation with an endotracheal tube is indicated in the most severe cases and may help to retard the development of pulmonary edema fluid by increasing intraalveolar pressure and reducing venous return.
2. Elevation of the patient's head and chest to an upright sitting position can improve ventilation and reduce venous return.
3. Morphine sulfate, 5-15 mg, may be given intramuscularly or slowly intravenously, depending on the patient's blood pressure, with careful observation for respiratory depression or hypotension. However, morphine may be contraindicated in patients with pulmonary edema when the following are present: (a) increased intracranial pressure, (b) severe pulmonary disease, or (c) severe lethargy or semicoma.
4. Furosemide, 40-80 mg intravenously, is given and repeated as needed to obtain at least 200-500 ml of urine in the next 1-2 hours.
5. Tourniquets can be applied to three extremities and rotated every 15 minutes to decrease venous return. Vasodilators and/or phlebotomy may also be used in particularly severe cases to reduce venous return. Vasodilators should not be used in hypotensive patients.
6. In undigitalized patients, 0.5-1.0 mg digoxin may be given intravenously followed by additional increments of 0.25 mg every 4-6 hours for 3-4 doses as indicated. The dose must be lowered if renal function is impaired or if the patient is hypokalemic or hypercalcemic.
7. Cardioversion should be used if the patient has a supraventricular or ventricular tachycardia that does not respond rapidly to the usual antiarrhythmic drugs. It is generally preferable to try cardioversion before a patient is given digitalis.

AXIOM When a patient has been digitalized, attempts at cardioversion may precipitate severe ventricular arrhythmias.

Mechanical Support of Cardiac Function

Over the past decade, considerable advances have been made in developing devices to support the heart during cardiogenic shock and/or severe heart failure. Sometimes these devices are used to support the heart until a donor heart is available for cardiac transplantation.

Criteria for considering use of mechanical support for a failing heart include hypotension (mean BP < 60 mm Hg), and/or a low cardiac index (< 1.5-2.0 L/min/m^2) which persists in spite of a more than adequate preload (determined by CVP and or PAWP responses to fluid challenges) and maximal drug therapy.[236]

INTRAAORTIC BALLOON PUMPING

Although relatively few exclusion criteria exist for intraaortic balloon pump (IABP) support for acute cardiac failure or cardiogenic shock, especially after cardiac surgery, long-term mechanical support is generally not advocated if the patient has irreversible renal hepatic or pulmonary failure, severe peripheral vascular disease, symptomatic cerebrovascular disease, incurable cancer, coagulopathies, blood dyscrasias, or severe persisting infection.[236]

AXIOM IABP should be considered in patients with cardiogenic shock or acute, severe left heart failure persisting in spite of all other therapy.

Inserting an IABP involves passage of a catheter-balloon system through one of the femoral arteries and positioning it in the descending aorta just distal to the left subclavian artery.[75,237] The balloon is connected to an external pneumatic pump that inflates and deflates the intraaortic balloon in time with the patient's ECG or arterial pressure waves. Rapid inflation of the balloon as soon as the aortic valve closes (usually during the T-wave) increases aortic diastolic pressure and augments coronary perfusion.[238] Sudden deflation of the balloon at the beginning of systole (just following the QRS complex) reduces resistance to LV emptying, thereby increasing cardiac output and reducing systolic time, LV pressures, and end-systolic volume. The resultant decrease in systolic tension time index reduces myocardial oxygen consumption.[239] At the same time, increased aortic diastolic pressure, increased diastolic time, and decreased end-diastolic RA and LV pressure, all improve coronary artery blood flow.

The major use of IABP support has been in cardiac surgery patients unable to come off cardiopulmonary bypass. It has also been used extensively in patients with acute LV failure or cardiogenic shock due to acute myocardial infarction.[240] Use of IABP support to treat cardiogenic shock allows the use of vasodilators and inotropic agents to aid in improving hemodynamic status. The technique also permits relatively safe performance of cardiac catheterization and angiography so that patients can be evaluated for possible emergency surgical intervention.

Contraindications to IABP include aortic regurgitation, aortic aneurysm, and severe peripheral vascular disease.[20] Tachydysrhythmias or irregular heart rhythms are also relative contraindications. Complications of IABP support are relatively infrequent.[20] These include damage or perforation of the aortic wall, ischemia distal to the catheter insertion site in the femoral artery, peripheral arterial embolization, thrombocytopenia, and hemolysis.

ECMO

An extracorporeal membrane oxygenator (ECMO) system consists of a membrane lung, centrifugal pump, and heat exchanger, all connected to a gas source through a mixer that allows appropriate changes in gas flow.[241] Blood flows through the membrane lung while oxygen and carbon dioxide diffuse through the membrane.

ECMO systems have generally proved ineffective for periods of support longer than 48 hours, but they do allow for rapid resuscitation and further patient evaluation.[241] ECMO systems should not be used for bridging patients to transplantation because of a potentially long wait for a suitable donor. Also, these systems require continuous heparin for anticoagulation and provide incomplete biventricular support.

EXTERNAL CENTRIFUGAL PUMPS

External centrifugal pumps utilizing rotating cones for impellers to circulate blood are used primarily for postcardiotomy support, although they have been used successfully to bridge patients to transplantation.[242] They are attached to cannulas that may be placed in any cardiac chamber (except the right ventricle) to provide univentricular or biventricular support. Although they are easily inserted, and capable of providing cardiac outputs of 2-6 L/min, and are well-suited for short durations of support (< 7 days), these pumps have several disadvantages. These include limited mobility of the patient, a need for continuous intravenous anticoagulation with heparin, and a high incidence of hemolysis and thrombus formation.

EXTERNAL LVAD

External pulsatile LV assist devices (LVAD) have been used successfully as a bridge to transplantation and in postcardiotomy and acute myocardial infarction cardiogenic shock applications.[243] These sac-type or dual-chamber pumps are powered by compressed air and positioned paracorporeally allowing the patient some mobility. Cannulae attach directly to the patient's heart, exiting through the chest wall and connecting to pumps and an external console. A sternotomy and cardiopulmonary bypass are required to insert the device. A major advantage is that right, left, or biventricular support can be provided.

IMPLANTABLE LVAD

Implantable LVADs are electrically or pneumatically actuated pumps that are implanted in the abdominal wall or peritoneal cavity.[244] An external power cable or pneumatic line transverses the skin, allowing for excellent patient mobility. The pulsatile LVADs are designed for LV cannulation and should only be used in patients with isolated LV failure.

If a patient also develops refractory right ventricular failure, another device (i.e., an external centrifugal pump) could be used for right ventricular support. Cardiopulmonary bypass and a midline incision are required for insertion. Implantable LVADs are primarily used to bridge patients to transplantation and have been successfully used for long-term support. These temporary devices may be a prototype for a permanent nontethered system that will provide an alternative for patients with end-stage heart disease who are not suitable candidates for heart transplantation.

DYNAMIC CARDIOMYOPLASTY

Over the past ten years, skeletal muscle-cardiac assist has been increasingly proposed as a biomechanical means to augment the systolic function of a failing heart using the patient's endogenous skeletal muscle (usually latissimus dorsi). Unlike cardiac transplantation, concerns such as graft rejection, complications from chronic immunosuppression, and accelerated CAD are avoided with skeletal muscle-cardiac assist.[245]

In general, the patient's latissimus dorsi muscle is detached and wrapped around a portion of the heart, usually the right ventricle.[245] The latissimus dorsi muscle may also be used to provide counterpulsation by being wrapped around the aorta and stimulated to pump during diastole. It may also be attached to the aorta as an extraaortic counterpulsator.

There appears to be general agreement that dynamic cardiomyoplasty can be considered for otherwise healthy patients with NYHA functional class III or IV heart failure.[245] It is not offered to patients who stand a reasonably good chance of receiving cardiac transplantation, but if the cardiomyoplasty fails, cardiac transplantation could continue to be a therapeutic option.

Most clinical reports based on patient follow-up are still in the early stages of investigation. Abry and Carpentier in Paris have the oldest and largest series.[246] Of their 20 patients having the procedure by June, 1989, nine died. However, the mortality rate was only 30% in a more recent group of 10 patients. In Doppler studies on nine survivors more than six months postoperatively, the group by Abry and Carpentier reported an increase, ranging from 12-42%, in LV ejection fraction in six patients.

TABLE 41-8 Indications for Cardiac Transplantation

Accepted Indications
   Maximal VO$_2$ < 10 mL/kg/min with achievement of anaerobic
     metabolism
   Severe ischemia consistently limiting routine activity not amenable to
     bypass surgery or angioplasty
   Recurrent, symptomatic ventricular arrhythmias refractory to all accepted
     therapeutic modalities
Probable Indications
   Maximal VO$_2$ < 14 mL/kg/min and major limitation of the patient's
     daily activities
   Recurrent, unstable ischemia not amenable to bypass surgery or
     angioplasty
   Instability of fluid balance and renal function not due to patient
     noncompliance
Inadequate Indications
   Ejection fraction < 20%
   History of functional class III or IV symptoms of heart failure
   Previous ventricular arrhythmias
   Maximal VO$_2$ > 15 mL/kg/min without other indications

From: Mudge GH, Goldstein S, Addonzio IJ, et al. Bethesda Conference Task Force 3: cardiac transplantation recipient guidelines/priortization. J Am Coll Cardiol 1993;22:21.

TABLE 41-9 Tailored Therapy for Heart Failure before Transplantation

1. Measurement of baseline hemodynamics
2. Intravenous nitroprusside and diuretics tailored to hemodynamic goals:
   • Pulmonary capillary wedge pressure ≤15 mm Hg
   • Systemic vascular resistance ≤1200 dyne·s/cm^5·m^2
   • Right atrial pressure 8 mm Hg
   • Systolic blood pressure 80 mm Hg
3. Definition of optimal hemodynamics by 24-48 hours
4. Titration of high-dose vasodilators as nitroprusside is weaned:
   • Captopril, hydralazine, isosorbide dinitrate
5. Monitored ambulation and diuretic adjustment for 24-48 hours
6. Maintain digoxin levels at 0.9-2.0 ng/dL if no contraindication
7. Detailed patient education
8. Flexible outpatient diuretic regimen including intermittent metolazone
9. Progressive walking program
10. Vigilant follow-up

From: Kavinsky CJ, Parrillo JE. Severe heart failure in cardiomyopathy: pathogenesis and treatment. Ayres SM, Grenvik A, Holbrook PR, Shoemaker WC, eds. Textbook of critical care. Philadelphia: WB Saunders Co, 1995; 594.

The data from the study by Magovern et al. indicated that LV ejection fraction in three patients increased from 28% to 48%, 30% to 44%, and 25% to 33% at approximately 1 year postoperatively.[248] However, a follow-up report showed a great deal of variation in the results in these patients.

Cardiac Transplantation

In a 1993 report from the International Society for Heart and Lung Transplantation, it was noted that cardiac transplantation was performed in over 26,000 recipients worldwide since 1967. The total actuarial 1-year survival was 79%.[249] For 1990 to 1991, the report from the Transplant Cardiology Research Data Base, which includes first heart transplants in 911 patients from 25 major United States institutions showed a one-year survival of 84%.[250] The most common indication for transplantation was dilated heart failure, with CAD accounting for 51% of these recipients.[250]

Cardiac transplantation provides the only effective therapy for meaningful long-term survival in patients who have ejection fractions < 15-25% and who are in severely decompensated heart failure despite maximal medical therapy, in patients with refractory ventricular dysrhythmias, and in patients dependent on intravenous inotropic agents or mechanical circulatory support devices (Table 41-8).[54] However, current indications for transplantation now focus on peak oxygen uptake and specific clinical features, rather than the previous, more general guidelines that included ejection fraction and the New York Heart Association classification.[251]

Contraindications to cardiac transplantation have been changing. Patients with previous malignancy may now be accepted before the general 3- to 5-year tumor-free interval frequently advocated in the past. Patients with refractory endocarditis have also undergone transplantation without postoperative infection.[252] The impact of older recipient age on survival is still controversial. Patients over age 65 have a 3-year survival of 70%, compared with 77% for younger patients.[249]

Most institutions reject patients with transpulmonary gradients above 15 mm Hg or pulmonary vascular resistance above 4 Wood units after optimization of left-sided filling pressures and therapy with intravenous vasodilators. Although a remote history of alcohol or drug use is no longer a criterion for exclusion in most programs, extended abstinence must be convincingly demonstrated.[253]

Optimal medical therapy for heart failure prior to transplantation has continued to evolve (Table 41-9).[254] Guidelines from the Bethesda Conference on Cardiac Transplantation suggest that therapy should be adjusted until clinical congestion has been resolved or until further therapy has been repeatedly limited by severe hypotension or marked azotemia.[251] Decompensation should not be considered refractory until "therapy with vasodilators has been pursued using continuous hemodynamic monitoring to approach hemodynamic goals." Such therapy should include ACE inhibitors in combination with oral nitrates.[254]

SUMMARY

The best method for preventing cardiovascular failure in trauma patients is to keep hypotension and hypoxemia as brief as possible, especially in patients with preexisting cardiovascular disease. Rapid resuscitation to optimal (supranormal) levels of DO_2 and VO_2 appear to be helpful.

If cardiovascular failure develops, an etiologic diagnosis should be established whenever possible; diastolic dysfunction with preserved systolic function should be identified because a different therapeutic approach is needed. Complications, such as pulmonary emboli, should be anticipated.

For patients with NYHA class I or II heart failure who are in sinus rhythm but have decreased LV function, treatment with an ACE inhibitor may improve both symptoms and life expectancy. The routine use of digitalis is not recommended unless concomitant atrial fibrillation is present.

Patients with NYHA class III or IV heart failure are candidates for treatment with digitalis, along with diuretics and an ACE inhibitor. When optimal results are not obtained with this regimen, one should consider adding nitrates and/or hydralazine. The management of patients who do not respond to optimal medical therapy should include a careful search for anemia, infection, pulmonary emboli, or hyper- or hypothyroidism.

The outcome of cardiovascular failure after trauma is related to its etiology and the severity of any pre-existing disease.[92] Cardiac failure as a single cause of mortality in the postinjury period is unusual. Cardiac failure developing more than 48 hours after injury is usually a part of the multiple organ failure syndrome.

Pulmonary dysfunction in the postresuscitative phase can cause pulmonary hypertension and right ventricular failure.[256] These changes are usually transient when proper support is given to the cardiopulmonary systems, including accurate fluid replacement, pharmacologic support of the heart, and early mechanical ventilation.[92] Mechanical assistance and/or transplantation should also be considered in patients not responding to maximal medical therapy.

⊘ FREQUENT ERRORS

1. *Delayed or inadequate correction of hypovolemia in a trauma patient because of a fear of overloading the patient with fluid.*
2. *Failure to consider hypovolemia a probable cause of continued severe tachycardia in older trauma patients with a history of heart failure.*
3. *Any delay in detecting or treating K, Mg, or Ca abnormalities in a patient with heart failure.*
4. *Failing to provide an adequate preload in a patient with diastolic cardiac dysfunction because CVP and/or PAWP is high.*
5. *Assuming that bronchospasm or coughing in an elderly patient is due to a pulmonary problem.*
6. *Attempting to increase BP with vasoconstrictor drugs in a patient with cardiac systolic dysfunction.*
7. *Not trying diligently to keep pulse rate and systolic BP at normal levels, especially when CAD is present.*
8. *Using a vasodilator without ensuring a continuing adequate preload and without monitoring PAWP and BP closely.*
9. *Reducing BP without considering the aortic BP-LVEDP gradient to the subendocardial myocardium.*
10. *Delay in providing ventilatory support and oxygen to patients with pulmonary edema.*
11. *Using a digitalis preparation when it is not definitely indicated.*

▼▼▼▼▼▼▼▼▼▼▼▼▼▼▼▼▼▼▼▼▼▼▼▼▼▼▼▼

SUMMARY POINTS

1. When aortic systolic pressure exceeds 160-180 mm Hg, the LVEDP, even in a normal heart, often doubles, and the left ventricle may dilate and go into failure.
2. In infants, the elderly, and patients with diseased hearts, stroke volume may be relatively fixed. Consequently, bradycardia after trauma may be extremely dangerous.
3. Unusual ventricular complexes in a patient with a very slow heart rate may represent escape beats (not premature ventricular contractions) and should not be suppressed.
4. When increased oxygen is required by the heart, it can only be provided by increasing coronary blood flow.
5. Increased coronary sinus lactate usually indicates myocardial ischemia.
6. Increased filling of the heart, increased pulse rate, and increased aortic pressure all tend to increase myocardial contractility.
7. Use of positive end-expiratory pressure (PEEP) reduces the net distending pressure of the atria, thereby reducing ANP secretion; therefore, PEEP can reduce urine output by reducing venous return and by decreasing ANP production.
8. Increased afterload decreases stroke volume and increases myocardial oxygen consumption.
9. Drugs that increase BP increase MVO_2 but they also tend to reduce cardiac output, tissue perfusion, and oxygen delivery (DO_2).
10. Increases in heart rate and systolic BP cause a geometric rise in myocardial oxygen demands.
11. The best relationships between cardiac output and MVO_2 are achieved by increasing preload and decreasing afterload rather than by inotropic or chronotropic stimulation.
12. Cardiac failure is often defined as an inability of the heart to pump enough blood to meet the metabolic demands of the body; however, it is usually diagnosed clinically from evidence of pulmonary or systemic venous overload.
13. From the physiologist's viewpoint, cardiac failure is often defined as a diminished work output of the heart in relation to its filling pressure or volume.
14. Right heart failure is usually due to left heart failure and right heart failure can impair LV filling.
15. Systolic cardiac dysfunction is characterized by reduced ejection fraction and need for higher end-diastolic volumes. Diastolic dysfunction is characterized by a poorly relaxing heart requiring high-filling pressures.
16. The most frequent cause of inadequate cardiac function is myocardial infarction.
17. Acute right ventricular infarction can closely resemble pericardial tamponade.
18. The most frequent cause of severe cardiovascular failure after trauma in young previously healthy patients is severe prolonged shock or cardiac arrest.
19. Although tachycardia up to 160-180/minute can improve cardiac output in young individuals, it also limits myocardial blood flow when CAD is present.
20. Atrial fibrillation should generally be prevented or rapidly corrected, especially in patients with severe mitral stenosis.
21. Patients with myocardial contusion do not require ICU monitoring unless they have arrhythmias, heart failure, other severe injuries or preexisting cardiac disease.
22. Patients with wall-motion abnormalities from myocardial contusion have an increased risk of shock or arrhythmias during general anesthesia until up to one month later.
23. Patients with hypokalemia often also have hypomagnesemia.
24. Serum Mg levels may be normal in patients with moderate-to-severe tissue Mg deficiency.
25. Serum Mg levels may be a prognostic indicator in patients with established CHF.
26. Acidosis tends to depress cardiac contractility, but the increased

catecholamine release it stimulates tends to override the depression unless the pH is < 7.10.

27. The hemodynamic change most significantly associated with an increased mortality rate more than 48 hours after trauma is pulmonary hypertension.

28. Cardiac failure from fluid overload is rare in patients who do not have preexisting cardiac disease, cardiac trauma, or severe, persistent shock.

29. Patients with sepsis often require greatly increased intravenous fluids.

30. Patients with sepsis may develop pulmonary edema in spite of reduced cardiac-filling pressures.

31. Cardiac indices exceeding 5.0-6.0 L/min/m^2 may not only be detrimental to the heart, but may also reduce oxygen transfer peripherally and in the lungs because of inadequate time spent by red cells in the capillaries.

32. Acute cardiovascular responses to reduced BP or cardiac output are primarily due to increased sympathetic nervous system activity.

33. Most patients with heart failure demonstrate increased activation of the sympathetic nervous system with elevated plasma norepinephrine levels, even at rest.

34. Continuing heart failure is characterized by down-regulation of β-adrenergic receptors.

35. High levels of catecholamines and an increase in peripheral vascular tone may contribute not only to functional circulatory impairment, but also to progression of any myocardial dysfunction.

36. Volume overloads (such as those resulting from aortic insufficiency) are tolerated better than pressure overloads (as may occur with aortic stenosis).

37. PEEP, which decreases distension of the atria, can significantly reduce ANF production, thereby reducing urine output and causing more fluid retention in heart failure.

38. Decreasing serum sodium levels is a bad prognostic sign in patients with CHF.

39. Use of prostaglandin synthesis inhibitors in patients with severe CHF increases the tendency for renal failure.

40. Myocardial oxygen consumption increases in heart failure, but coronary blood flow tends to decrease.

41. One of the most sensitive indicators of increasing cardiac failure is a decrease in arterial Po$_2$.

42. Assuming that an increasing cough or hemoptysis can only be due to a pulmonary problem.

43. Nausea, vomiting, abdominal pain, and distension due to intestinal vascular congestion in patients with heart failure can sometimes simulate acute surgical abdomen.

44. A gallop rhythm should be considered a sign of LV failure until proven otherwise.

45. All that wheezes is not asthma.

46. In patients with heart failure, a decreasing arterial Po$_2$ is generally a sensitive indicator that the process is getting worse.

47. A relatively sudden decrease in arterial Po$_2$ in a patient with heart failure should make one look carefully for pulmonary emboli.

48. An enlarged cardiac silhouette in spite of moderate-to-severe COPD is usually evidence of advanced heart failure.

49. Changes in end-systolic and end-diastolic volumes provide much more accurate estimates of the functional capabilities of the right and left heart than do the CVP and PAWP.

50. Although continuous Holter monitoring can document many more ECG changes than a standard ECG in acutely injured patients, the significance of these changes is not clear.

51. Trends and the response of CVP or PAWP to fluid challenges are much more important than absolute values.

52. The CVP may be normal, at least temporarily, if the heart failure is primarily left-sided.

53. Chest radiography should be obtained after attempts to insert a central catheter, regardless of success or failure.

54. If an LBBB is present, an external pacemaker should be available while inserting a PA catheter.

55. If a pulmonary catheter is inserted to monitor a critically injured patient, it should be used to determine and then maintain "optimal" hemodynamic values.

56. Mixed venous oxygen saturation can provide early warning of cardiopulmonary dysfunction, but one cannot rely on a stable SvO$_2$ to exclude such problems.

57. One should not assume that thermodilution cardiac output determinations are always accurate, especially when the values are very high or very low.

58. If a patient is sick enough to need PA catheter monitoring, the catheter should be used to optimize cardiac output and oxygen delivery (DO$_2$).

59. A high PAWP does not necessarily indicate that end-diastolic volumes are also increased, especially in patients with cardiac disease.

60. End-diastolic volumes are a more accurate guide for fluid resuscitation of critically ill patients than are PAWP levels.

61. RVEDVI more accurately predicts preload recruitable increases in cardiac output than does the PAWP level.

62. Echocardiography, especially if done transesophageally, is an excellent technique for evaluating the heart, pericardium, and mediastinum after trauma.

63. The best way to prevent cardiac dysfunction after trauma is to keep hypotension and hypoxemia to a minimum and to prevent fluid and pressure overloads.

64. The hypothermic heart does not function well, and it is difficult to resuscitate.

65. Severe phosphate deficiencies (< 1.0 mg/dL) can interfere with cellular metabolism and should be corrected promptly.

66. Increased catecholamine release associated with stress, pain, and anxiety can cause heart failure to progress in spite of all other therapy.

67. Continuing hypotension in trauma patients is usually due to inadequate volume replacement.

68. The usual first step to improving cardiac output in trauma patients is increasing preload to adequate levels.

69. In patients with heart failure, more precise monitoring during resuscitation may be required because of the small blood volume difference that may exist between hypovolemia and fluid overload.

70. When the fluid status of a patient is in doubt, one should carefully evaluate the response to a standard fluid challenge, such as 3.0 mL/kg of a balanced electrolyte solution, given over 10 minutes.

71. The best way to reduce morbidity and mortality in critically injured patients is to promptly optimize oxygen delivery and oxygen consumption.

72. Diuretics can cause severe problems if given to patients who are hypovolemic.

73. Potassium-sparing diuretics and ACE-inhibitors should generally not be given at the same time.

74. The most frequent electrolyte cause of arrhythmias is hypokalemia due to excessive diuresis.

75. Once preload is optimized, the next step in improving hemodynamic function and oxygen delivery generally includes inotropes and/or vasodilators.

76. The great majority of patients with heart failure after trauma will have systolic dysfunction.

77. Unless chronic pulmonary disease is accompanied by atrial fibrillation or LV failure, digoxin should be avoided.

78. The optimal digitalizing dose is extremely variable from patient to patient.

79. Digoxin levels should not be checked sooner than six hours after the last dose.

80. Little or no correlation exists between serum digoxin levels and therapeutic responses to the drug.

81. Any arrhythmia that develops in a patient receiving a digitalis preparation should be considered due to that drug until proven otherwise.

82. Because it tends to slow the conduction of impulses through the AV node and the bundle of His, digitalis should generally be avoided in patients with AV block.

83. Dopamine is probably the best inotrope to give to patients who continue to have a low BP and cardiac output in spite of optimal fluid loading.

84. Administration of dopamine to patients with high endogenous catecholamine levels will usually not cause dilation of renal or mesenteric vessels.

85. Dopamine is not the ideal inotropic agent when excessive volume overload occurs.

86. In conditions associated with decreased systemic vascular resistance, such as sepsis, dopamine can often be used in rather high doses without causing excessive vasoconstriction.

87. Isoproterenol should probably only be used in patients who have a slow, weak heart.

88. Amrinone is an excellent inotrope for improving cardiac function in patients with pulmonary hypertension, but its long half-life can be a major problem if undesirable responses occur.

89. Calcium should not be given to improve cardiac function except perhaps in patients with shock or heart failure after multiple, rapid blood transfusions, after calcium-blockers, or in patients with severe hyperkalemia.

90. Calcium administration except to counteract excess citrate or potassium may impair resuscitative efforts.

91. Glucagon can be helpful in patients with a poor cardiac output due to beta blockers or calcium blockers.

92. Vasodilators should not be given to patients who are hypovolemic or hypotensive.

93. Preload should be optimized before using afterload reducing agents.

94. Nitroprusside should not be used in high doses (> 0 mg/kg/min) for more than 72 hours.

95. Intravenous nitroglycerin by slow infusion may be the vasodilator of choice in patients with heart failure when a high preload is the main problem and/or the patient has moderate-to-severe ischemic heart disease.

96. Captopril should not be used in patients who are hyperkalemic or apt to become hyperkalemic.

97. Oxygen can be a very effective pulmonary vasodilator.

98. Drug combinations, when monitored properly, tend to produce better results and fewer side-effects than single agents.

99. If an arrhythmia is asymptomatic and may be chronic, one should think twice and/or obtain cardiology consultation before treating it.

100. Mg depletion can be an important cause of arrhythmias in CHF.

101. Serum Mg levels may be normal in spite of moderate-severe Mg depletion in tissues.

102. β-Adrenergic blocking agents are generally contraindicated in cardiac failure and low-output states unless the problems are due to tachyrhythmias that are unresponsive to other therapy.

103. The most frequent cause of persistent sinus tachycardia in trauma patients is inadequate volume resuscitation.

104. If a beta blocker is used to treat severe, persistent tachycardia in a patient with heart failure, a short drug half-life can be very helpful.

105. When SVT results in hemodynamic instability, the patient should be electrically cardioverted.

106. Verapamil should not be used to treat atrial fibrillation or flutter in a patient with WPW syndrome.

107. Administration of atropine in the presence of hypovolemic bradycardia can cause ventricular fibrillation.

108. Conduction defects can be caused by trauma to the head, eyes, spine, or heart.

109. When the patient has PVCs and a slow heart rate, the "PVCs" are probably escape beats and should not be suppressed.

110. When EMD appears to be present, one should look carefully for pericardial tamponade, pneumothorax, or hypovolemia.

111. The diagnosis of pulmonary emboli should be strongly considered in patients with recurrent heart failure of unknown etiology.

112. Heparin can aggravate a tendency to hyperkalemia.

113. The most rapid and effective method for treating severe acute pulmonary edema is positive-pressure ventilation with increased oxygen.

114. When a patient has been digitalized, attempts at cardioversion may precipitate severe ventricular arrhythmias.

115. IABP should be considered in patients with cardiogenic shock or acute severe left heart failure persisting in spite of other therapy.

▲▲▲▲▲▲▲▲▲▲▲▲▲▲▲▲▲▲▲▲▲▲▲▲▲▲▲▲▲▲▲▲

REFERENCES

1. Schatz IJ, Wilson, RF. Cardiovascular failure following trauma. Walt AJ, Wilson RF, eds. The management of trauma: practice and pitfalls. Philadelphia: Lea & Febiger, 1975; 532-544.
2. Furburg CD, Yusuf S, Thom TJ. Potential for altering the natural history of congestive heart failure: need for large clinical trials. Am J Cardiol 1985;55:45A.
3. Eriksson H. Heart failure: a growing public health problem. J Int Med 1995;237:135.
4. Smith WM. Epidemiology of congestive heart failure. Am J Cardiol 1985;55:3A.
5. Kannel WB. Epidemiological aspects of heart failure. Cardiol Clin 1989;7:1.
6. Schlant RC. Normal anatomy and function of the cardiovascular system. Hurst JW, Logue RB, eds. The heart. New York: McGraw Hill, 1966; 28-30.
7. Howell WH, Donaldson FJ. Experiments upon the heart in the dog with reference to the maximum volume of blood sent out by left ventricle in a single beat. London: Philosphical Tr, Part 1 1894; 154.
8. Frank O. Die grundfform des arteriellen pulses. Z Biol 1898;37:483.
9. Wiggers CJ. Some factors controlling the shape of the pressure curve in the right ventricle. Am J Physiol 1914;33:383.
10. Straub H. Dynamik des saugetierherzens. I Deutsche Arch klin. Med 1914;115:531. II Ibid, 1914;116:409.
11. Patterson SW, Starling EH. On the mechanical factors which determine the output of the ventricles. J Physiol 1914;48:357.
12. Patterson SW, Piper H, Starling EH. The regulation of the heart beat. J Physiol 1914;48:465.
13. Starling EH. "The Linacre lecture on the law of the heart." London: Longmans, Green, and Co., Ltd., 1918.
14. Wiggers CJ. Determinants of cardiac performance. Circulation 1951;4:485.
15. Sarnoff SJ, Berglund E. Ventricular function. I. Starling's laws of the heart studied by means of simultaneous right and left ventricular function curves in the dog. Circulation 1954;9:706.
16. Sarnoff SJ. Myocardial contractility as described by ventricular function curves: observations on Starling's law of the heart. Physiol Rev 1955;35:107.
17. Goy JJ, Waeber B, Nussberger J, et al. Infusion of atrial natriuretic peptide to patients with congestive heart failure. J Cardiovasc Pharmacol 1988;12:562.
18. Norwood SH, Civetta CM. ICU management of the trauma patient. Kreis DJ Jr, Gomez GA, eds. Trauma management. Boston: Little, Brown & Co, 1989; 431-452.
19. Cohn JN. Blood pressure and cardiac performance. Am J Med 1973;55:351.
20. Majid PA, Roberts R. Heart failure. Civetta JM, Taylor RW, Kirby RR, eds. Critical care. Philadelphia: JB Lippincott, 1988; 945-974.
21. Diebel LN, Wilson RF, Taggett MG, et al. End-diastolic volume: a better indicator of preload in the critically ill. Arch Surg 1992;127:817.
22. Span JF, Buccino RA, Sonnenblick EH, et al. Contractile state of cardiac muscle obtained from cats with experimentally produced ventricular hypertrophy and heart failure. Circ Res 1967;21:341.
23. Sibbald WJ, Calvin JE, Holliday RL, et al. Concepts in the pharmacologic and nonpharmacologic support of cardiovascular function in critically ill surgical patients. Surg Clin North Am 1983;63:455.
24. Sarnoff SJ. Hemodynamic determinants of oxygen consumption of the heart with special reference to the tension-time index. Am J Physiol 1958;192:148.
25. Tuninga YS, van Veldhuisen DJ, Brouwer J, et al. Heart rate variability in left ventricular dysfunction and heart failure: effects and implications of drug treatment. Br Heart J 1994;72:509.
26. Pipilis A, Flather M, Ormerod O, Sleight P. Heart rate variability in acute myocardial infarction and its association with infarct size and clinical course. Am J Cardiol 1991;67:1137.

27. Farrell TG, Bashir Y, Cripps T, et al. Risk stratification for arrhythmic events in postinfarction patients based on heart rate variability, ambulatory electrocardiographic variables and the signal-averaged electrocardiogram. J Am Coll Cardiol 1991;18:687.

28. Saul JP, Aria Y, Berger RD, et al. Assessment of autonomic regulation in chronic congestive heart failure by heart rate spectral analysis. Am J Cardiol 1988;61:1292.

29. Casolo G, Balli E, Taddei T, et al. Decreased spontaneous heart rate variability in congestive heart failure. Am J Cardiol 1989;64:1162.

30. Binkley PF, Nunziata E, Haas GJ, et al. Parasympathetic withdrawal is an integral component of autonomic imbalance in congestive heart failure: demonstration in human subjects with verification in a paced canine model of ventricular failure. J Am Coll Cardiol 1991;18:464.

31. Dahn MS, Wilson RF, Lange MP, et al. Hemodynamic benefits of verapamil after aortic reconstruction. J Vasc Surg 1989;9:806.

32. Braunwald E. Pathophysiology of heart failure. In Heart disease, a textbook of cardiovascular medicine. Philadelphia: WB Saunders, 1980; 453.

33. Grande CM, Tissot M, Bhatt VP, et al. Preexisting compromising conditions. Capan LM, Miller SM, Turndorf H, eds. Trauma: anesthesia and intensive care. Philadelphia: JB Lippincott, 1991; 240-251.

34. Peterson KL, Tsuji J, Johnson A, et al. Diastolic left ventricular pressure-volume and stress-strain relations in patients with valvular aortic stenosis and left ventricular hypertrophy. Circulation 1978;58:77.

35. Gaasch WH, Bing OHL, Mirsky I. Chamber compliance and myocardial stiffness in left ventricular hypertrophy. Eur Heart J 1982;3:139.

36. Mason DT, Awan NA, Joyce JA, et al. Treatment of acute and chronic congestive heart failure by vasodilator-afterload reduction. Arch Intern Med 1980;140:1577.

37. Messer JV, Neill WA. The oxygen supply of the human heart. Am J Cardiol 1962;9:384.

38. Rackley CE, Russell RO Jr, Mantle JA, et al. Modern approach to the patient with acute myocardial infarction. Curr Probl Cardiol 1977;1:49.

39. Page DL, Caulfield JB, Kastor JA, et al. Myocardial changes associated with cardiogenic shock. N Engl J Med 1971;285:133.

40. Forrester JS, Diamond G, Parmeley WW, et al. Early increase in left ventricular compliance after myocardial infarction. J Clin Invest 1972;51:598.

41. Smith M, Ratshin RA, Harrel FE, et al. Early sequential changes in left ventricular dimensions and filling pressures in patients after myocardial infarction. Am J Cardiol 1974;33:363.

42. Hughes JL, et al. Abnormal peripheral vascular dynamics in patients with acute myocardial infarction: diminished reflex arteriolar vasoconstriction. Clin Res 1971;19:321.

43. Debusk RE, Harrison DC. The clinical spectrum of papillary muscle disease. N Engl J Med 1969;281:1458.

44. Mundeth ED, Buckley MJ, Daggett WM, et al. Surgery for complications of myocardial infarction. Circulation 1972;45:1279.

45. Gahl K, Sutton R, Pearson M, et al. Surgical treatment of papillary muscle rupture complicating myocardial infarction. N Engl J Med 1968;278:1137.

46. Radford MJ, Johnson RA, Buckly MJ, et al. Ventricular septal rupture: a review of clinical and physiological features and analysis of survival. Circulation 1979;60(suppl):39.

47. Majid PA, Warden R, Defeyter PJF, et al. Left ventricular aneurysm. Pre- and postoperative hemodynamic studies at rest and during exercise. Eur J Cardiol 1980;12:215.

48. Cheng TO. Incidence of ventricular aneurysm in coronary artery disease, an angiographic appraisal. Am J Med 1971;50:340.

49. Bjork VO, Henze A, Jonasson R, et al. Survival and cardiac performance after left ventricular aneurysmectomy. Scand J Thorac Cardiovasc Surg 1978;12:37.

50. Stephens DJ, Dymond DS, Stone DL, et al. Left ventricular aneurysm and congestive heart failure: value of exercise and isosorbide dinitrate in predicting the hemodynamic results of aneurysmectomy. Am J Cardiol 1980;45:932.

51. Lorrell B, Leinbach RC, Pohost GM, et al. Right ventricular infarction. Am J Cardiol 1979;43:465.

52. Friedman HS, Lieber CS. Cardiotoxicity of alcohol. Cardiovasc Med 1977;2:111.

53. Regan TJ, Haider B. Ethanol abuse and heart disease. Circulation 1981;64(suppl 3):111.

54. Kavinsky CJ, Parrillo JE. Severe heart failure in cardiomyopathy: pathogenesis and treatment. Ayres SM, Grenvik A, Holbrook RR, Shoemaker WC, eds. Textbook of critical care, 3rd ed. Philadelphia: WB Saunders, 1995; 583-595.

55. Caforio ALP, Bonifacio E, Stewart JT, et al. Novel organ-specific circulating cardiac autoantibodies in dilated cardiomyopathy. J Am Coll Cardiol 1990;15:1527.

56. Margossian SS, White HD, Caulfield JB, et al. Light chain 2 profile and activity of human ventricular myosin during dilated cardiomyopathy. Identification of a causal agent for impaired myocardial function. Circulation 1992;85:1720.

57. Ungerer M, Bohm M, Elce JS, et al. Altered expression of beta-adrenergic receptor kinase and beta-adrenergic receptors in the failing human heart. Circulation 1993;87:454.

58. Morgan HE. Cellular aspects of cardial failure. Circulation 1993;87 (Suppl IV):IV-4.

59. Wigle ED, Sasson Z, Henderson MA. Hypertrophic cardiomyopathy: the importance of the site and the extent of the hypertrophy. A reveiw. Prog Cardiovasc Dis 1985;28:1.

60. Shabatai R. Restrictive cardiac disease. Heart Failure 1985;1:231.

61. Wiencek RG, Wilson RF. Injuries to the abdominal vascular system: how much does aggressive resuscitation and prelaparotomy thoracotomy really help? Surgery 1987;102:731.

62. Wiencek RG, Wilson RF. Central lung injuries. A need for early vascular control. J Trauma 1988;28:1418.

63. Wilson RF. Thoracic vascular trauma. Bongard FS, Wilson SE, Perry MO, eds. Vascular injuries in surgical practice. Norwalk: Appleton & Lange, 1991; 107-130.

64. Wilson RF. Injury to the heart and great vessels. Henning RJ, Grenvik A, eds. Critical care cardiology. New York: Churchill, Livingstone, 1989; 111.

65. Evans DE, Kobrine AJ, Rizzoli HV. Cardiac arrhythmias accompanying acute compression of the spinal cord. J Neurosurg 1980;2:52.

66. Weilder DJ. Myocardial damage and cardiac arrhythmias after intracranial hemorrhage: a critical review. Stroke 1974;5:759.

67. Brill IC, et al. Congestive failure due to auricular fibrillation in an otherwise normal heart. JAMA 1960;173:784.

68. Tenzer ML. The spectrum of myocardial contusion: a review. J Trauma 1985;25:620.

69. Cane RD, Schamroth L. Prolongation of the Q-T interval with myocardial contusion. Heart Lung 1978;7:652.

70. Kron IL, Cox PM. Cardiac injury after chest trauma. Crit Care Med 1983;11:524.

71. Roberts R. Where, oh where, has the MB gone. N Engl J Med 1985;313:1081.

72. Fabian TL, Mangiante EC, Patterson CR, et al. Myocardial contusion in blunt trauma: clinical characteristics, means of diagnosis, and implications for patient management. J Trauma 1988;28:50.

73. Coleman J, Gonzalez A, Harlaftis N, Symbas P. Myocardial contusion: diagnosis value of cardiac scanning and echocardiography. Surg Forum 1976;32:293.

74. Frazee RD, Mucha P, Farnell MB, et al. Objective evaluation of blunt cardiac trauma. J Trauma 1986;26:510.

75. Snow N, Lucas AE, Richardson JD. Intra-aortic balloon counterpulsation for cardiogenic shock from cardiac contusion. J Trauma 1982;22:426.

76. Geheb MA, Desai TK. Clinical disorders of calcium and magnesium metabolism in critically ill patients. Carlson RW, Geheb MA, eds. Principles and practice of medical intensive care. Philadelphia: WB Saunders, 1993; 1196-1212.

77. Steiness E. Diuretics, digitalis and arrhythmias. Acta Med Scand Suppl 1981;75:647.

78. Nordrehaug JE, Von Der Lippe G. Hypokalemia and ventricular fibrillation in acute myocardial infarction. Br Heart J 1983;50:525.

79. Oster JR, Preston RA, Materson BJ. Fluid and electrolyte disorders in congestive heart failure. Semin Nephrol 1994;14:485.

80. Wilson RF, Mammen E, Walt AJ. Eight years of experience with massive blood transfusions. J Trauma 1971;11:275.

81. Wilson RF, Dulchavsky SA, Soullier G, Beckman B. Problems with 20 or more blood transfusions in 24 hours. Am Surg 1987;53:410.

82. Smith TW, Braunwald E, Kelly RA. The management of heart failure. Braunwald E, ed. Heart disease. Philadelphia: WB Saunders, 1990; 631-645.

83. Gottlieb SS, Baruch L, Kukin ML, et al. Prognostic importance of the serum magnesium concentration in patients with congestive heart failure. J Am Coll Cardiol 1990;16:827.

84. Mehta PM, Kloner RA. Metabolic and toxic effects on the cardiovascular system. Carlson RW, Geheb MA, eds. Principles and practice of medical intensive care. Philadelphia: WB Saunders, 1993; 1038-1049.

85. Cingolani HE, Mattiazi AR, Blesa ES, et al. Contractility in isolated mammalian heart muscle after acid base changes. Circ Res 1970;26:269.

86. Cingolani HE, Blesa ES, Gonzales NC, et al. Extracellular vs intracellular pH as a determinant of myocardial contractility. Life Sci 1969;8:775.

87. Thomas JA, Marks BH. Plasma norepinephrine in congestive heart failure. Am J Cardiol 1978;41:233.

88. Bristow MR, Ginsburg R, Minobe W, et al. Decreased catecholamine sensitivity and beta-adrenergic receptor density in failing human hearts. N Engl J Med 1982;307:205.

89. Steinhart CR, Purmutt S, Gurtner GH, et al. Beta-adrenergic activity and cardiovascular response to severe respiratory acidosis. Am J Physiol 1983;244:H46.

90. Sturm JA, Lewis FR, Trentz O, et al. Cardiopulmonary parameters and prognosis after severe multiple trauma. J Trauma 1979;19:305.

91. Eddy AC, Rice CL, Anardi DM. Right ventricular dysfunction in multiple trauma victims. Am J Surg 1988;155:712.

92. Weigelt JA, Stanford GG. Cardiovascular failure. Moore EE, Mattox KL, Feliciano DV, eds. Trauma, 2nd ed. Norwalk: Appleton & Lange, 1991; 941-964.

93. Weber KT, Janicki JS, Shroff S, et al. Contractile mechanics and interaction of the right and left ventricles. Am J Cardiol 1981;47:685.

94. Weber KT, Janicki JS, Shroff SG, et al. The right ventricle: physiologic and pathophysiologic considerations. Crit Care Med 1983;11:323.

95. Lefer AM. Properties of cardioinhibitory factors produced in shock. Fed Proc 1987;27:2734.

96. Demeules JE. A physiologic explanation for cardiac deterioration in septic shock. J Surg Res 1984;36:553.

97. Levitt MA, Lefer AM. Efficacy of two leukotriene antagonists in rat traumatic shock. Methods Find Exp Clin Pharmacol 1987;9:269.

98. Levitt MA, Lefer AM. Beneficial effects of prostaglandin E₁ infusion in experimental traumatic shock. Crit Care Med 1987;15:769.

99. Levitt MA, Lefer AM. Anti-shock properties of the prostacyclin analog, iloprost, in traumatic shock. Prostaglandins Leukot Med 1986;25:175.

100. Terashita Z, Stahl GL, Lefer AM. Protective effects of a platelet activating factor (PAF) antagonist and its combined treatment with prostaglandin (PG) E₁ in traumatic shock. J Cardiovasc Pharmacol 1988; 12:505.

101. Reilly JM, Cunnion RE, Burch-Whitman C, et al. A circulating myocardial depressant substance is associated with cardiac dysfunction and peripheral hypoperfusion (lactic acidemia) in patients with septic shock. Chest 1989;95:1072.

102. Wilson RF. Heart failure. Wilson RF, ed. Critical care manual: applied physiology and principles of therapy, 2nd ed. Philadelphia: FA Davis, 1992; 187-223.

103. Harris P. Congestive cardiac failure: central role of the arterial blood pressure. Br Heart J 1987;58:190.

104. Langer SZ. Presynaptic regulation of the release of catecholamines. Pharmacol Rev 1980;32:337.

105. Sole MJ. Alterations in sympathetic and parasympathetic hemotransmitter activity in congestive heart failure. Braunwald E, Mock MB, Watson JT, eds. Congestive heart failure. Orlando: Grune & Stratton, 1982; 101.

106. Cohn JN, Levilne TB, Francis GS, et al. Neurohumoral control mechanisms in congestive heart failure. Am Heart J 1981;102:509.

107. Packer M. Neurohormonal interactions and adaptations in congestive heart failure. Circulation 1988;77:721.

108. Chidsey CA, Braunwald E. Sympathetic activity and neurotransmitter depletion in congestive heart failure. Pharmacol Rev 1966;15:685.

109. Bristow MR, Ginsberg R, Minobe W, et al. Decreased catecholamine sensitivity and beta-adrenergic receptor density in failing human hearts. N Engl J Med 1982;307:205.

110. Singal PK, Yater JC, Beamish RE, et al. Influence of reducing agents over adrenochrome-induced changes in the heart. Arch Pathol Lab Med 1981;105:664.

111. Leithe ME, Margorien RD, Hermiller JB, et al. Relationship between central hemodynamics and regional blood flow in normal subjects and in patients with congestive heart failure. Circulation 1984;69:57.

112. Goldsmith SR, Francis GS, Cowley AW, et al. Increased plasma arginine vasopressin in patients with congestive heart failure. J Am Coll Cardiol 1983;1:1385.

113. Klockowski P, Levy G. Kinetics of drug action of disease states: effect of experimental hypovolemia on the pharmacodynamics and pharmacokinetics of desmethyl diazepam. J Pharmacol Exp Ther 1988;245:508.

114. Rieger GAJ, Liebau G, Kochsiek K. Antidiuretic hormone in congestive heart failure. Am J Med 1982;72:49.

115. Zelis R, Delea CS, Coleman HN, et al. Arterial sodium content in experimental congestive heart failure. Circulation 1970;41:213.

116. Magrini F, Niarchos AP. Ineffectiveness of sublingual nitroglycerin in acute left ventricular failure in presence of massive peripheral edema. Am J Cardiol 1980;45:841.

117. Katz AM. Cardiomyopathy of overload: a major determinant of prognosis in congestive heart failure. N Engl J Med 1990;322:l00.

118. Francis GS, McDonald K, Chu C, et al. Pathophysiologic aspects of end-stage heart failure. Am J Cardiol 1995;75:11A.

119. Weber KT, Brilla CG. Pathological hypertrophy and cardiac interstitium: fibrosis and renin-angiotensin-aldosterone system. Circulation 1991; 83:1849.

120. Villarreal FJ, Kim NN, Ungab GD, Printz MP, Dillmann WH. Identification of functional angiotensin II receptors on rat cardiac fibroblasts. Circulation 1993;88:2849.

121. van Krimpen C, Smits JFM, Cleutjens JPM, et al. DNA synthesis in the non-infarcted cardiac interstitium after left coronary artery ligation in the rat: effects of captopril. J Mol Cell Cardiol 1991;23:1245.

122. Anversa P, Sonnenblick EH. Ischemic cardiomyopathy: pathophysiologic mechanisms. Progr Cardiovasc Dis 1990;33:49.

123. Katz AM. Is heart failure an abnormality of myocardial cell growth? Cardiology 1990;77:346.

124. Sutton JSJ, Pfeffer MA, Plappert T, et al. Quantitative two-dimensional echocardiographic measurements are major predictors of adverse cardiovascular events after acute myocardial infarction. The protective effects of captopril. Circulation 1994;89:68.

125. Konstam MA, Kronenberg MW, Rousseau, et al. Effects of the angiotensin converting enzyme inhibitor enalapril on the long-term progression of left ventricular dilatation in patients with asymptomatic systolic dysfunction. Circulation 1993;88:2277.

126. Giles TD. Defining the role of atrial natriuretic factor in health and disease. J Am Coll Cardiol 1990;15:1331.

127. Cody RJ, Atlas SA, Laragh JH, et al. Atrial natriuretic factor in normal subjects and heart failure patients: plasma levels and renal, hormonal, and hemodynamic responses to peptide infusion. J Clin Invest 1986;78:1362.

128. Roach PJ, Sanders JS, Berg WJ, et al. Pathophysiologic levels of atrial natriuretic factor do not alter reflex sympathetic control: direct evidence from microneurographic studies in humans. J Am Coll Cardiol 1990;15:1318.

129. Dzau VJ, Packer M, Lilly LS, et al. Prostaglandins in severe congestive heart failure. N Engl J Med 1984;310:347.

130. Oliver JA, Sciacca R, Pinto J, et al. Participation of the prostaglandins in the control of renal blood flow during acute reduction of cardiac output in the dog. J Clin Invest 1981;67:229.

131. Starling EH. On the absorption of fluids from the connective tissue spaces. J Physiol 1896;18:312.

132. Rackow EC, Fein A, Siegel J. The relationship of the colloid osmotic-pulmonary artery wedge pressure gradient to pulmonary edema and mortality in critically ill patients. Chest 1982;4:433.

133. Berger HJ, Zaret BL. Nuclear cardiology. N Engl J Med 1981;305:855.

134. Matthay RA, Berger HJ. Noninvasive assessment of right and left ventricular function in acute and chronic respiratory failure. Crit Care Med 1983;11:329.

135. London MJ, Hollenberg M, Wong MG, et al. Intraoperative myocardial ischemia: localization by continuous 12-lead electrocardiography. Anesthesiology 1988;69:232.

136. Wilson RF, Sarver E, Birks R. Central venous pressure and blood volume determinations in clinical shock. Surg Gynecol Obstet 1971; 132:631.

137. Swan HJC, et al. Catheterization of the heart in man with use of a flow-directed balloon-tipped catheter. N Engl J Med 1970;283:447.

138. Quinn K, Quebbeman EJ. Pulmonary artery pressure monitoring in the surgical intensive care unit. Arch Surg 1981;116:872.

139. Boyd KD, Thomas SJ, Gold J, Boyd AD. A prospective study of complications of pulmonary artery catheterizations in 500 consecutive patients. Chest 1983;84:245.

140. Kasnitz P, Druger GL, Yorra F, Simmons DH. Mixed venous oxygen tension and hyperlactatemia. JAMA 1976;236:570.

141. Nelson LD. Continuous venous oximetry in surgical patients. Ann Surg 1986;203:329.

142. Branthwaite MD, Bradley RB. Measurement of cardiac output by thermal dilution in man. J Appl Physiol 1968;24:434.

143. Keefer JR, Borash PG. Pulmonary artery catheterization. Blitt CD, ed. Monitoring in anesthesia and critical care medicine. New York: Churchill Livingstone, 1985; 180.

144. Elkayam U, Berkley R, Azen S, et al. Cardiac output by thermodilution techniques: effect of injectate volume and temperature on accuracy and reproducibility in the critically ill patient. Chest 1968;84:418.

145. Norris SL, King EG, Grace M, et al. Thermodilution cardiac output. An in vitro model of low flow states. Crit Care Med 1986;14:57.
146. Stetz CW, Muller RG, Kelly GE, et al. Reliability of the thermodilution method in the determination of cardiac output in clinical pratice. Am Rev Respir Dis 1982;126:1001.
147. Raper R, Sibbald WJ. Misled by the wedge? The Swan-Ganz catheter and left ventricular preload. Chest 1986;89:427.
148. Reuse C, Vincent JL, Pinsky MR. Measurements of right ventricular volumes during fluid challenge. Chest 1990;98:l450.
149. King RM, Mucha P, Seward JB, et al. Cardiac contusion: a new diagnostic approach utilizing two-dimensional echocardiography. J Trauma 1983;23:610.
150. Starling MR, Crawford MH, Sorenson SG, et al. Two dimensional echocardiographic technique evaluating right ventricular size and performance in patients with obstructive lung disease. Circulation 1982;66:612.
151. Peterson KL, Skloven D, Ludbrook P, et al. Comparison of isovolemic and ejection phase indices of myocardial performance in man. Circulation 1974;49:1088.
152. Smith JS, Cahalan MK, Benefiel DJ, et al. Intraoperative detection of myocardial ischemia in high-risk patients: electrocardiography versus two dimensional transesophageal echocardiography. Circulation 1985;72:1015.
153. Shively B, Cahalan M, Benefiel D, Schiller N. Intraoperative Doppler echocardiography: intraoperative assessment of mitral valve regurgitation by transesophageal Doppler echocardiography. J Am Coll Cardiol 1986;7:228A.
154. Schluter M, Kremer P, Hanrath P. Transesophageal 2-D echocardiographic features of flail mitral leaflet due to ruptured chordae tendinae. Am Heart J 1984;108:609.
155. Hofmann T, Kasper W, Meinertz T, et al. Determination of aortic valve orifice area in aortic stenosis with two-dimensional transesophageal echocardiography. Am J Cardiol 1987;59:330.
156. Mason JW, O'Connell JB. Clinical merit of endomyocardial biopsy. Circulation 1989;79:971.
157. O'Conner LR, Wheeler WS, Bethune JE. Effect of hypophosphatemia on myocardial performance in man. N Engl J Med 1977;297:901.
158. Dennis RD, Harlow C, Egdahl RH, Hechtman HB. Enhancement of myocardial function with glucose, insulin and potassium. Surg Gynecol Obstet 1980;151:185.
159. Tuynman HARE, Thijs LG, Straub JP, et al. Effects of glucose-insulin-potassium (GIK) on the position of the oxyhemoglobin dissociation curve. 2,3-diphosphoglycerate, and oxygen consumption in canine endotoxin shock. J Surg Res 1983;34:246.
160. Czer LSC, Shoemaker WC. Optimal hematocrit value in critically ill postoperative patients. Surg Gynecol Obstet 1978;147:363.
161. Hill EP, Willford DC, Moores WY, et al. Oxygen transport and oxygen consumption vs. cardiac output at different haematocrits. Perfusion 1987;2:39.
162. Wilson RF, Walt AJ. Blood replacement. In Management of trauma: practices and pitfalls. Philadelphia: Lea, and Febiger, 1975; 136.
163. Moore FA, Haenel JB, Moore EE, Whitehill TA. Incommensurate oxygen consumption in response to maximal oxygen availability predicts postinjury multiple organ failure. J Trauma 1992;33:58.
164. Dikshit K, Vyden JK, Forrester JS, et al. Renal and extra-renal hemodynamic effects of furosemide in congestive heart failure after myocardial infarction. N Engl J Med 1973;288:1087.
165. Babini R, du Souich P. Furosemide pharmacodynamics: effects of respiratory and acid base disturbances. J Pharmacol Exp Ther 1986;237:623.
166. Chonko A, Grantham JJ. Treatment of edema states. Maxwell MH, Kleeman CR, Narins RG, eds. Disorders of sodium content and concentration. New York: McGraw-Hill, 1987; 429.
167. Materson BJ. Insights into intrarenal sites and mechanisms of action of diuretic agents. Am Heart J 1983106:188.
168. Naylor WG, Williams A. Relaxation in heart muscle: some morphological and biochemical considerations. Eur J Cardiol 7 1978;(Suppl):35.
169. Gheorghiade M, Zarowitz BJ. Review of randomized trials of digoxin therapy in patients with chronic heart failure. Am J Cardiol 1992;69:48G.
170. Smith TW, Haber E. Digitalis (Parts 1-4). N Engl J Med 1973;289:945,1010,1063,1125.
171. Martiny SS, Phelps SJ, Massey KL. Treatment of severe digitalis intoxication with digoxin-specific antibody fragments: a clinical review. Crit Care Med 1988;16:629.
172. Gilbert JC, Goldbert LI. Characterization by cyproheptadine of the dopamine-induced contraction in canine isolated arteries. J Pharmacol Exp Ther 1975;193:435.
173. Goldberg LI. Cardiovascular and renal actions of dopamine: potential clinical application. Pharmacol Rev 1972;24:1.
174. Alexander CS, Sako Y, Mikulic E. Pedal gangrene associated with use of dopamine. N Engl J Med 1975;293:591.
175. Sonnenblick EH, Frishman WH, Lejemtel TH. Dobutamine: a new synthetic cardioactive sympathetic amine. N Engl J Med 1979;300:17.
176. Leier CV, Unverferth DV, Kates RE. The relationship between plasma dobutamine concentrations and cardiovascular responses in cardiac failure. Am J Med 1979;66:238.
177. Richard C, Ricome JL, Rimailho A, et al. Combined hemodynamic effects of dopamine and dobutamine in cardiogenic shock. Circulation 1983;67:620.
178. Bass AS, Murphy MB, Kohli JD, Goldberg LI. Potentiation by dopexamine of the cardiac responses to circulating and neuronally released norephinephrine: a possible mechanism for the therapeutic effects of the drug. J Cardiovasc Pharmacol 1989;13:667.
179. Leier CV. Regional blood flow responses to vasodilators and inotropes in congestive heart failure. Am J Cardiol 1988;62:86E.
180. Baumann G, Gutting M, Pfafferot C, et al. Comparison of acute haemodynamic effects of dopexamine hydrochloride, dobutamine and sodium nitroprusside in chronic heart failure. Eur Heart J 1988;9:503.
181. Mancini D, Lejemtel T, Sonnenblick E. Intravenous use of amrinone for the treatment of the failing heart. Am J Cardiol 1984;56:8B.
182. Wilson RF, Soullier G, Antonenko D. Ionized calcium levels in critically ill surgical patients. Am Surg 1979;45:485.
183. Wilson RF, Dulchavsky SA, Soullier G, Beckman B. Problems with 20 or more blood transfusions in 24 hours. Am Surg 1987;53:410.
184. Wilson RF, Binkley LE, Sabo FM, et al. Electrolyte and acid base changes with massive blood transfusions. Am Surg 1992;58:535.
185. White BC, Winegar CD, Wilson RF, Hoehner PJ. Calcium blockers in cerebral resuscitation. J Trauma 1983;23:788.
186. White BC, Winegar CD, Wilson RF, Trombley JH. The possible role of calcium blockers in cerebral resuscitation: a review of the literature and synthesis for future studies. Crit Care Med 1983;11:202.
187. Zaloga GP, Willey S, Malcolm D, et al. Hypercalcemia attenuates blood pressure reponse to epinephrine. J Pharmacol Exp Ther 1988;247:949.
188. Chernow B, Zaloga GP, Malcolm D, et al. Glucagon's chronotropic action is calcium dependent. J Pharmacol Exp Ther 1987;241:833.
189. Hall-Boyer K, Zaloga GP, Chernow B. Glucagon: hormone or therapeutic agent? Crit Care Med 1984;12:584.
190. Zaritsky AL, Horowitz M, Chernow B. Glucagon antagonism of calcium channel blocker-induced myocardial dysfunction. Crit Care Med 1988;246-251.
191. Chatterjee K, Parmley WW. The role of vasodilator therapy in heart failure. Prog Cardiovasc Dis 1977;19:301.
192. Farnett L, Mulrow CD, Linn WD, et al. The J-curve phenomenon and the treatment of hypertension. JAMA 1991;265:489.
193. Miller RR, Awan NA, Mason DT. Pharmacologic mechanisms for left ventricular unloading in clinical congestive heart failure. Circ Res 1976;39:127.
194. Chiariello M, Gold HK, Leinback RC, et al. Comparison between effects of nitroprusside and nitroglycerin in ischemic injury during acute myocardial infarction. Circulation 1976;54:766.
195. Gold HK, Chiariello M, Leinbach RC, et al. Deleterious effects of nitroprusside on myocardial injury during acute myocardial infarction. N Engl J Med 1975;293:1003.
196. Ogilvie RI. Effects of nitroglycerin in peripheral blood flow distribution and venous return. J Pharmacol Exp Ther 1978;207:362.
197. Miller RR, Vismara L, Williams DO, et al. Pharmacologic mechanisms for left ventricular unloading in clinical congestive heart failure: differential effects of nitroprusside, phentolamine and nitroglycerin on cardiac function and peripheral circulation. Circ Res 1976;39:127.
198. Bojar RM, Rastegar H, Payne DD. Methemoglobinemia from intravenous nitroglycerin: a word of caution. Ann Thorac Surg 1987;43:332.
199. Packer M, Lee WH, Kessler PD, et al. Prevention and reversal of nitrate tolerance in patients with congestive heart failure. N Engl J Med 1987;317:799.
200. Majid PA, Sharma B, Taylor SH. Phentolamine for vasodilator treatment of severe heart failure. Lancet 1971;2:719.
201. Miller RR, Awan NA, Maxwell KS, et al. Effect of prazosin on cardiac impedance and preload in congestive heart failure. N Engl J Med 1977;297:303.
202. Braunwald E. Mechanism of action of calcium-channel blocking agents. N Engl J Med 1982;307:1618.
203. Lundbrook PA, Tiefenbrunn AJ, Reed FR, et al. Acute hemodynamic responses to sublingual nifedipine: dependence on left ventricular function. Circulation 1982;65:489.
204. Elkayam U, Weber L, Behrooz T, et al. Acute hemodynamic effect of

oral nifedipine in severe chronic congestive heart failure. Am J Cardiol 1983;52:1041.

205. Moulds RFW, Jauernig JA, Shaw JA. A comparison of the effects of hydralazine, diazoxide, sodium nitrite and sodium nitroprusside on human isolated arteries and veins. Br J Clin Pharmacol 1981;1:57.

206. Markham RV, Gilmore A, Pettinger, et al. Central and regional hemodynamic effects and nonhumoral consequences of minoxidil in severe congestive heart failure and comparison to hydralazine and nitroprusside. Am J Cardiol 1983;52:774.

207. Colluci WS, Wynne J, Holman BL, et al. Long-term therapy of heart failure with captopril: an oral inhibitor of angiotensin converting enzyme. N Engl J Med 1979;301:117.

208. Galvao M. Role of angiotensin-converting enzyme inhibitors in congestive heart failure. Heart Lung 1990;19:505.

209. Johnson AK, Mann JFE, Rascher W, et al. Plasma angiotensin II concentrations and experimentally induced thirst. Am J Physiol 1981;240:R229.

210. Davis R, Ribner HS, Keung E, et al. Treatment of chronic congestive heart failure with captopril: an oral inhibitor of angiotensin converting enzyme. N Engl J Med 1979;301:117.

211. The Captopril Multicenter Research Group. A placebo-controlled trial of captopril in refractory chronic congestive heart failure. J Am Coll Cardiol 1983;2:775.

212. Cleland JGF, Gillen G, Dargie HJ. The effects of furosemide and angiotensin-converting enzyme inhibitors and their combination on cardiac and renal hemodynamics in heart failure. Eur Heart J 1988;9:132.

213. The Consensus Trial Study Group. Effects of enalapril on mortality in severe congestive heart failure: results of the cooperative North Scandinavian Enalapril Survival Study (Consensus). N Engl J Med 1987;316:1429.

214. Sharpe N, Murphy J, Coxon R. Enalapril in chronic heart failure: a double-blind placebo-controlled trial. J Am Coll Cardiol 1984;3:4761.

215. Waagstein F, Bristow MR, Swedberg K, et al. Beneficial effects of metoprolol in idiopathic dilated cardiomyopathy. Lancet 1993;342:1441.

216. Loeb HS, Rahimtoola SH, Gunnar RM. The failing myocardium: I. Drug management. Med Clin North Am 1973;57:167.

217. Miller RR, Awan NA, Joye JA, et al. Combined dopamine and nitroprusside therapy in congestive heart failure. Circulation 1977;55:881.

218. Miller DC, Stinson EB, Oyer PE, et al. Postoperative enhancement of left ventricular performance by combined inotropic-vasodilator therapy with preload control. Surgery 1980;88:108.

219. Nelson GIC, Silke B, Forsyth DR, et al. Hemodynamic comparison of primary venous or arteriolar dilation and the subsequent effect of furosemide in left ventricular failure after acute myocardial infarction. Am J Cardiol 1983;52:1035.

220. Pierpont GL, Cohn JN, Franciosa JA. Combined oral hydralazine-nitrate therapy in left ventricular failure, hemodynamic equivalency to sodium nitroprusside. Chest 1978;73:8.

221. Wilson RF, Sarver EJ, Rizzo J. Hemodynamic changes, treatment and prognosis in clinical shock. Arch Surg 1971;102:21.

222. Gray R, Shah PK, Singh B, et al. Low cardiac output states after open heart surgery. Chest 1981;80:16.

223. Cimmino VM, Bove El, Argenta LC, et al. The effect of simultaneous administration of levarterenol and phentolamine on renal blood flow. Ann Thorac Surg 1976;21:158.

224. Gage J, Strom J, Jordan A, et al. Synergistic effects of dobutamine and amrinone on cardiac performance and contractility in chronic heart failure. Clin Res 1985;33:187.

225. Federman J, Vleitstra RE. Antiarrhythmic drug therapy. Mayo Clin Proc 1979;54:531.

226. Zaidan JR, Curling PE. Cardiac dysrhythmias: recognition and management. Stoelting RK, Barash PG, Gallagher TJ, eds. Advances in anesthesia. Chicago: Year Book, 1985; 207.

227. Walsh KA, Ezri MD, Denes P. Emergency treatment of tachyarrhythmias. Med Clin North Am 1986;70:791.

228. Leahey EB, Reiffel JA, Drusin RE, et al. Interaction between quinidine and digoxin. JAMA 1978;240:565.

229. Sazama KJ. The syndrome known as WPW: a review. JAMA 1976;31:56.

230. Madrid AH, Moro C, Marin Huerta EM, et al. Atrial fibrillation in Wolff-Parkinson-White syndrome: reversal of isoproterenol effects by sotalol. PACE 1992;15:2111.

231. Jackuck SJ, Ramani PS, Clark F, et al. Electrocardiographic abnormalities associated with raised intracranial pressure. Br Med J 1975;1242.

232. Barriot P, Riou B. Hemorrhagic shock with paradoxical bradycardia. Intensive Care Med 1987;13:203.

233. Dunkman WB, Johnson GR, Carson PE, et al. Incidence of thromboembolic events in congestive heart failure. Circulation 1993;87(Suppl VI):VI-94.

234. Benton EW. Naloxone and TRH in the treatment of shock and trauma: what future roles? Ann Emerg Med 1985;14:729.

235. Safani M, Blair J, Ross D, et al. Prospective, controlled, randomized trial of naloxone infusion in early hyperdynamic septic shock. Crit Care Med 1989;17:1004.

236. Pennington DG, Joyce LD, Pae WE, Burkholder JA. Patient selection. Ann Thorac Surg 1989;47:77.

237. Orlando R, Drezner AD. Intra-aortic balloon counterpulsation in blunt cardiac injury. J Trauma 1983;23:424.

238. Carleton RA, Hauser RG. The failing myocardium: II. Assisted circulation. Med Clin North Am 1973;57:187.

239. Cohn L. Intra-aortic balloon counterpulsation in low cardiac output states. Surg Clin North Am 1975;55:545.

240. Hagneijer F, Laird JD, Haalebros MMP. Effectiveness of intraaortic balloon pumping without cardiac surgery for patients with severe heart failure secondary to recent myocardial infarction. Am J Cardiol 1977;40:951.

241. Mooney MR, Arom KV, Joyce LD, et al. Emergency cardiopulmonary bypass support in patients with cardiac arrest. J Thorac Cardiovasc Surg 1991;101:450.

242. Killen DA, Prehler JM, Borkon AM, Reed WA. Bio-medicus ventricular assist device for salvage of cardiac surgical patients. Ann Thorac Surg 1991;52:230.

243. Champsaur G, Ninet J, Vigneron M, Cochet P, et al. Use of the Abiomed BVS System 5000 as a bridge to cardiac transplantation. J Thorac Cardiovasc Surg 1990;100:122.

244. Frazier OH, Rose EA, Macmanus Q, et al. Multicenter clinical evaluation of the HeartMate 1000 IP left ventricular assist device. Ann Thorac Surg 1992;53:1080.

245. Lee KF, Wechsler AS. Dynamic cardiomyoplasty. Adv Cardiac Surg 1993;4:207.

246. Abry B, Carpentier A. Hospital Broussais clinical experience II. Preassist period. Carpentier A, Chachques JC, Grandjean P, eds. Cardiomyoplasty. Mount Krisco: Futura Publishing Co, 1991; 149-153.

247. Mihaileanu S, Chachques JC. Hospital Broussais III. Postassist period. Carpentier A, Chachques JC, Grandjean P, eds. Cardiomyoplasty. Mount Krisco: Futura Publishing Co, 1991; 154-157.

248. Magovern GJ, Heckler FR, Park SB, et al. Paced skeletal muscle for dynamic cardiomyoplasty. Ann Thorac Surg 1991;45:614.

249. Kaye MP. The registry of the International Society for Heart and Lung Transplantation: tenth official report, 1993. J Heart Lung Transplant 1993;12:541.

250. Bourge RC, Naftel DC, Constanzo-Nordin MR, et al. Pretransplantation risk factors for death after heart transplantation: a multiinstitutional study. J Heart Lung Transplant 1993;12:549.

251. Mudge GH, Goldstein S, Addonzio IJ, et al. Bethesda Conference Task Force 3: cardiac transplantation recipient guidelines/prioritization. J Am Coll Cardiol 1993;22:21.

252. DiSosa VJ, Slose IJ, Cohn IH. Cardiac transplantation for intractable prosthetic valve endocarditis. J Heart Lung Transplant 1990;9:142.

253. Rovelli M, Palmeri D, Vossler E, et al. Noncompliance in organ transplant recipients. Transplant Proc 1989;21:833.

254. Stevenson LW. Selection and management of patients for cardiac transplantation. Curr Opin Cardiol 1994;9:315.

255. Fodarow GC, Chelimsky-Fallick C, Stevenson LW, et al. Effect of direct vasodilation vs angiotensin converting-enzyme inhibition on mortality in advanced heart failure: the Hy-C trial. J Am Coll Cardiol 1992;19:842.

256. Sibbald WJ, Driedger AA. Right ventricular function in acute disease states: pathophysiologic considerations. Crit Care Med 1983;11:339.

Chapter 42 Renal Response to Severe Injury and Hypovolemic Shock

CHARLES E. LUCAS, M.D.

ANNA M. LEDGERWOOD, M.D.

INTRODUCTION

The kidneys play a critical role in the homeostatic responses to injury and hemorrhagic shock. Knowledge of these responses helps one make the best decisions for optimizing fluid therapy after severe injury. The kidneys, working through complicated physiologic pathways distributed throughout the nephron, provide the key linkage between the cardiovascular system and the interstitial fluid space.

An average patient is composed of 60% water with its contained solutes. The maintenance of life in health and in disease states revolves around a fine balance of the fluxes between the various body compartments. Many of these fluid and electrolyte shifts are controlled or influenced by the kidneys which help regulate the fluid balance between the extracellular and intracellular fluid spaces. They also help to maintain total body fluid and electrolyte balance, modulate acid-base homeostasis, excrete undesirable metabolites, and help to maintain perfusion of core organs during hemorrhage.

NORMAL STATE

Renal Blood Flow (Table 42-1)

Both kidneys weigh about 300 g and receive 20-25% of the cardiac output so that renal blood flow (RBF) averages about 1250-1500 mL/minute in adults. This is equivalent to a mean renal plasma flow (RPF) averaging about 625-650 mL/minute. During severe shock, RBF may decrease to about 100 mL/minute.

RBF sequentially passes through the interlobar, arcuate, and intralobar arteries. About 85% of the RBF perfuses the outer cortical (component I) glomeruli and the remaining 15% of the RBF enters the juxtamedullary glomeruli located in the inner cortex and outer medulla (component II).

Glomerular Filtration

The normal glomeruli permit about 20% of the plasma to be filtered as a cell-free and protein-free filtrate. Thus, the normal glomerular filtration rate (GFR) averages about 125 mL/minute or about 180 L/day. GFR can be determined by calculating the renal clearance (urine/plasma concentration times urine volume) of exogenously administered inulin or endogenous creatinine. Inulin is completely filtered and is neither secreted nor reabsorbed by the tubules. When inulin is used to monitor GFR, extracellular fluid space (ECF) can also be calculated.

Creatinine is almost completely filtered and relatively little is secreted by the tubules except in severe renal disease so that its clearance can be used to estimate the GFR. The work of GFR is performed by the heart, and the volume of protein-free filtrate reflects perfusion pressure and various osmolar and oncotic factors.

Proximal Convoluted Tubule

Protein-free glomerular filtrate traverses the proximal convoluted tubules where 80% of the sodium and water are reabsorbed. The nonfiltered plasma, now rich in protein, perfuses the efferent arteriole and the peritubular vessels which are involved in active tubular reabsorption and secretion. The volume of effective RPF (ERPF) through these vessels may be monitored by paraamino hippurate clearance (C_{PAH}) which is filtered and secreted but not reabsorbed. ERPF averages about 650 mL/minute and correlates directly with renal work and renal oxygen consumption (Table 42-1). The distribution of RBF may be monitored by radioactive xenon-133 (Xe-133). Most of the RBF perfuses the outer cortical segment (C_I) with a smaller fraction entering the inner cortex/outer medulla (C_{II}) and only a tiny fraction entering the inner medulla (C_{III}).[1] The juxtamedullary (C_{II}) nephrons are unique in that they possess a loop of Henle which descends into the inner medulla (C_{III}) and then ascends back to the inner cortex (Fig. 42-1).

Loops of Henle

The loops of Henle are the site for active sodium reabsorption against a gradient. This active sodium reabsorption causes the inner medullary interstitium to become hypertonic and this hypertonicity facilitates the subsequent concentration of filtrate with preservation of salt and water. This hypertonicity is further regulated by the peritubular vessels passing close to the loops of Henle, thus modulating the fine osmolar and oncotic balances between the plasma in these vessels and the medullary interstitial fluid space (IFS).

When hemorrhagic shock causes a decrease in C_I flow and a redistribution of RBF to C_{III}, the rapid flow through these peritubular vessels may "wash out" the ions and osmoles causing a transient "paralysis" of the renal concentrating mechanisms. Low ERPF during hypovolemic shock may cause ischemia to these tubular cells, thereby impeding sodium reabsorption and disrupting the maintenance of medullary hypertonicity.

AXIOM Prolonged shock can interfere with the kidney's ability to preserve water and sodium after renal perfusion is reestablished.

Distal Convoluted Tubule

Twenty percent of the glomerular filtrate (25 mL/minute or 36 L/day) not reabsorbed in the proximal convoluted tubules enters the distal convoluting tubules where additional salt and water are reabsorbed under the influence of aldosterone and antidiuretic hormone (ADH). The distal tubules also exchange sodium for potassium or hydrogen depending upon pH and potassium delivery. Each distal tubule passes near its glomerulus at the afferent arteriole at a special site where the macula densa and Polkissen body combine to form the juxtaglomerular apparatus (JGA), which functions as a feedback loop affecting sodium and water balance.

TABLE 42-1   *Normal Cardiovascular and Renal Hemodynamics*

System	Flow (L/min)	Work (g/m/m²)	Pressures (mm Hg)	Resistance (d · sec/cm⁵)	Renal Clearance (mL/min)
Systemic	5	50	120/80 (MAP = 93)	1000-1500	Na ± = 1−3
Pulmonary	5	10	25/10 (PAWP = 5)	75-125	mOsm = 2−4
Renal	1.3	0.5	120/80	4500-5000	Urine = 1.0

Renin is released from the JGA in response to renal sympathetic nerve stimulation, renal catecholamine perfusion, afferent arteriolar perfusion changes, and reduced tubular sodium delivery. Once secreted, renin cleaves an α-2 globulin to produce angiotensin I, a decapeptide, which is a weak vasoconstrictor. This is converted to its highly active form, angiotensin II, which is an octapeptide. Renin may also be released and consumed within the kidney as part of the process known as autoregulation which plays an important role after injury. In addition to the renal effects, angiotensin II also stimulates adrenal secretion of aldosterone, which augments sodium reabsorption in the distal convoluting tubules.

Collecting Ducts

After exiting the distal tubules, the remaining hypotonic filtrate (15 mL/minute or 20 L/day) enters the collecting ducts where water reabsorption occurs as the filtrate passes though the hypertonic inner medulla. Water reabsorption is regulated by ADH which, in turn, is released from the posterior pituitary in response to baroreceptor (hypotension) and osmolar (increased tonicity) stimuli. Antidiuretic hormone promotes increased water reabsorption from the distal tubule and collecting ducts depending on the osmolar gradient between these sites and the inner medullary interstitium (Figure 42-1).

In response to shock, blood flow to the kidneys may decrease from a normal of 1250 mL/min to < 100 mL/min. Despite the severity of this vasoconstriction, the kidneys still would be able to respond to replacement therapy with restoration of function if ischemia were not too severe or too prolonged. Thus, the final urine concentration and volume varies with a number of factors, including plasma volume (PV), serum osmolality (S_{osm}), ADH and aldosterone secretion, colloid oncotic pressure (COP), and other factors.

Urine concentration normally ranges from isosmolar (275-295) to 1400 milliosmoles/L. The cumulative effects of these activities lead to an average urine output of 1 mL/minute with a sodium and osmolar clearance of 1-3% of the GFR. Free water clearance (C_{H2O}) is normally negative reflecting the excretion of a concentrated urine.

RENAL RESPONSE TO HEMORRHAGIC SHOCK

Following trauma and blood loss, the renal response correlates directly with the severity of the injury and degree of hypovolemia.[2-5]

Pathophysiology

High RBF allows the kidneys to preserve plasma volume and maintain renal function during mild-to-moderate (class I) hemorrhage.[6] Experimental and clinical studies indicated that autoregulation allows GFR to be rather well maintained even when RBF is decreased to 70% of normal. To accomplish this, the filtration fraction (GFR/ERPF) is increased from a normal of about 20% to over 30%. This autoregulation, a process influenced largely by intrinsic renin activity, results from selective postglomerular or efferent arteriolar vasoconstriction in the absence of preglomerular vasoconstriction.

Class II hemorrhage exceeds the autoregulatory capacity of the kidney, and there is vasoconstriction at both the pre- and postglomerular arterioles causing renal vascular resistance (RVR) to increase.[6] This causes a reduction in RBF to about 30% of normal and, in spite of a further increase in the filtration fraction, GRF decreases to about 50-60% of normal. This allows the reduced cardiac output to be selectively redirected to vital organs while the most critical renal functions are maintained. During a class III hemorrhage with a systolic blood pressure < 70 mm Hg, RBF decreases to about 10% of normal and GFR to < 20% of normal. Excretion of urine is < 0.1 mL/min.

Class IV hemorrhage is characterized by impending cardiac arrest with very low systemic pressure, tachycardia, and anuria, reflecting extreme renal vasoconstriction with absence of measurable perfusion or filtration.[6]

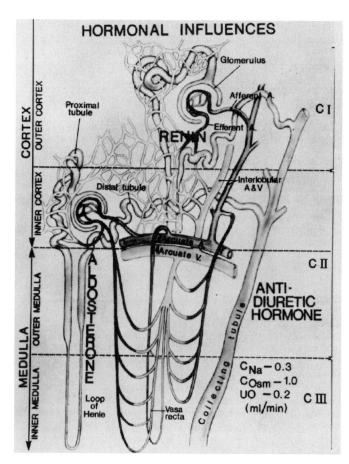

FIGURE 42-1   Component I (C_I) is outer cortex with greatest blood flow. Component II (C_{II}) is inner cortex/outer medulla which contains the juxtamedullary glomeruli which have, within their nephrons, loops of Henle which extend into component III (C_{III}), the inner medulla which helps to regulate the countercurrent mechanism.

AXIOM During hypovolemia, the combination of increased RVR, decreased RBF, and decreased GFR results in salt and water conservation which augments the total homeostatic response to the hemorrhagic insult.

After adequate resuscitation has restored the plasma volume and cardiac output, renal vasoconstriction subsides, but relatively slowly, first in the afferent arterioles and later in the efferent arterioles. Once the process of renal vasoconstriction has been established, it may persist for several hours or even days following volume restoration, depending upon the severity of the renal insult (Table 42-2).

Other humeral factors involved in the intricate balance of renal function include the prostaglandins and kinins. The prostaglandins, which are unsaturated fatty acids synthesized ubiquitously from arachidonic acid, are intimately involved with renal humoral control and serve as the modulators of the renal response to critical insults. The prostaglandins, PGE_2, PGD_2, and PGI_2 are vasodilators which increase RBF and redistribute RBF toward the outer cortex.[7] Kallikrein is a protease that cleaves bradykininogen to form bradykinin which then increases capillary permeability and is a vasodilator. Kallikrein, however, also causes smooth muscle contraction and cleavage of prorenin with renin release. These substances increase RBF to C_{II} and C_{III}. As studies on these complex humeral interactions continue, more knowledge will be forthcoming about the responses to critical illness and the potential for beneficial manipulation of these responses.

Treatment

AXIOM Oliguria and reduced sodium excretion immediately following trauma are generally due to hypovolemia and should not be treated by diuretics.

The treatment of oliguria after trauma should be directed toward rapid replenishment of the circulatory volume and cardiac output. When the volume deficit results from hemorrhagic shock, volume restoration should be provided in the form of both blood and balanced electrolyte solution (BES). We currently recommend that the volume of BES replacement be 3 L for every 1 L of estimated blood loss. This high ratio of crystalloid solution replacement to blood loss is designed to correct the ongoing reduction in the IFS during the period of severe hemorrhage and shock. Consequently, a patient with an acute 2.5 L hemorrhagic insult will present with severe hypotension and require about 7.5 L of BES plus restoration of the red cell mass. The crystalloid solution helps to correct the IFS deficit and also

augments the soon-to-be-expanded intracellular fluid space. Osmotic and loop diuretics in this setting are usually contraindicated.

PITFALL ⊘

Mannitol used to treat increased intracranial pressure (ICP) from head trauma may have adverse renal effects when the patient has been hypovolemic.

INTRAOPERATIVE RENAL RESPONSE AFTER INJURY

When a severely injured patient undergoes surgery for control of hemorrhage, the renal autoregulatory response to the PV deficit is affected by the altered systemic cardiovascular status, general anesthesia, and intraoperative surgical manipulation. The sudden reduction in the protective preoperative renal and systemic vasoconstriction due to the anesthetic agents combined with continued bleeding from injured organs can precipitate a marked reduction in cardiac output and blood pressure, increased RVR, decreased RBF, and anuria. This response may occur even though the preoperative blood pressure had been restored to low-normal levels.

AXIOM Protection of the kidney during emergency surgery after acute trauma is best provided by administering enough fluid before and during surgery to achieve a urine output of 2 mL/minute without diuretics.

Emphasis should be placed preoperatively on generous volume replacement to increase urine output to 2 mL/minute when the patient's problems permit this extra time to be spent on resuscitation. If hypovolemia were to develop following the induction of anesthesia, efforts must be directed toward rapid restoration of circulatory volume.

AXIOM Intraoperative protection of kidney function is best achieved by improving the cardiovascular status by the administration of BES, blood, plasma, and, when appropriate, inotropic agents.

Following severe injury, persistent hypotension and anuria is best treated by additional BES replacement with the expectation that both blood pressure and then urine flow will be restored. An initial increase in CVP with fluids should not deter such needed fluid administration. Both clinical and laboratory studies showed that a transient delay occurs in the reestablishment of urine flow after hypotension has been corrected and the mean arterial pressure (MAP) has been restored to normal or higher levels by fluid and blood therapy. This

TABLE 42-2 *Renal Clearances and Renal Vasoconstriction After Major Trauma*

Parameters Measured	Acute		Convalescent
	RVR*=<10,000 d-s/cm⁵(25 pts)	RVR*=>10,000 d-s/cm⁵(23 pts)	RVR*=4000-8000 d-s/cm⁵(26 pts)
GFR (mL/min)	112 ± 16	87 ± 21 (P < 0.10)	116 ± 11
ERPF (mL/min)	456 ± 46 (P < 0.05)	323 ± 41 (P < 0.05)	680 ± 112
C_{osm} (mL/min)	4.5 ± 1.6 (P < 0.05)	4.7 ± 2.1 (P < 0.10)	3.4 ± 0.4
C_{osm}/GFR (%)	4.1 ± 0.8 (P < 0.05)	5.1 ± 1.0 (P < 0.05)	3.3 ± 0.4
C_{Na} (mL/min)	3.2 ± 0.7 (P < 0.05)	3.4 ± 0.9 (P < 0.05)	1.82 ± 0.2
C_{H20} ±0.7	−0.48 ± 0.2 (P < 0.05)	−0.43 ± 0.3 (P < 0.05)	1.37 ± 0.7 1.37

GFR = Glomerular filtration rate, ERPF = Effective renal plasma flow.
All values expressed as mean ± S.D.; both groups studied acutely are statistically compared to the convalescent studies using the Student t test. The patients received an average of 11 blood transfusions during resuscitation.

continued oliguria results from persistent renal vasoconstriction and continued movement of fluid from the PV into the IFS which had become markedly depleted during the period of hypotension and hypovolemia. Because a blood-volume deficit of as much as 2 L and an interstitial fluid deficit of up to 4 L may still exist when the MAP has just been restored to normal during surgery, aggressive replacement of 1-2 L of BES over the next 15-45 minutes usually provides enough circulatory volume to reverse intraoperative oliguria and to circumvent the need for intraoperative diuresis. Most patients respond well to this intraoperative regimen which is usually followed by good postoperative renal function.

POSTOPERATIVE RENAL FUNCTION AFTER INJURY

Transient Postoperative Polyuria

AXIOM Postoperative polyuria after hemorrhagic shock may mimic fluid overload and lead to hypovolemia when fluids are restricted.

A potentially hazardous renal response to severe hemorrhagic shock is a transient period of polyuria that may occur immediately after resuscitation and surgical intervention.[8] This increased urine output usually is not excessive, and it seldom exceeds 250 mL for 30 minutes or lasts for more than 3 hours after conclusion of surgery to control bleeding.

The mechanism for this early postoperative polyuria is not clear. Several postulates have been presented. One purported mechanism involves a "wash out" of osmoles from the inner medullary interstitium during the period of hypovolemic shock when the RBF is moved from the outer cortex to the inner medulla. Because the juxtamedullary nephrons are the only nephrons that have loops of Henle that descend into the inner medulla, this can lead to an inner medullary wash-out of sodium and other osmoles; this, in turn, can temporarily paralyze the countercurrent concentrating mechanism.[9,10]

Another possible mechanism for postresuscitative or postoperative polyuria involves possible ischemia to the juxtamedullary nephrons during hypovolemic insult. Such ischemia could cause transient disruption of tubular cell function, thereby inhibiting sodium reabsorption and preventing maintenance of inner medullary hypertonicity. This reason for the transient postoperative polyuria seems unlikely because the polyuric phenomenon only lasts for a short period following surgery.

AXIOM Glucose should not be present in resuscitation fluids because of severe hyperglycemia and osmotic diuresis that can result.

A third possible mechanism for transient postoperative polyuria is an osmotic diuresis resulting not only from release of glucose and other osmoles from endogenous stores but also from osmoles in the resuscitation fluids, particularly when they contain glucose. Marked hyperglycemia exceeding 1000 mg/dL with consequently increased osmotic diuresis has been seen in patients resuscitated with BESs containing 5% dextrose. The use of resuscitation fluids containing 5% dextrose should be avoided in order to circumvent this hazard.

AXIOM Polyuria immediately following surgery in a patient who had preoperative or intraoperative hypotension is usually due to renal changes during hypotension and not fluid overload.

Regardless of the mechanism(s) leading to early postoperative polyuria in patients following resuscitation from hemorrhagic shock, the surgeon should recognize that the polyuria does not necessarily reflect an excess circulatory volume. High-urine volume should be ignored while addressing the resuscitation needs of the patient according to changes in blood pressure, pulse, pulse pressure, and the function of other organs. Fortunately, this polyuric phase is of short du-

TABLE 42-3 *Altered Renal Concentration After Resuscitation From Shock*

Study Time	GFR	U/O	C_{Na}	C_{osm}	C_{H2O}
Operation	35	8.5	5.9	8.1	0.4
5 hr postop	90	3.9	4.3	6.0	−2.0
15 hr postop	110	1.6	1.8	3.1	−1.5
Day 2	115	3.1	2.6	4.0	−0.9
Day 4	113	1.6	2.1	4.0	−2.3

All data are expressed in mL/minute as mean ± S.D.
GFR = Glomerular filtration rate.

ration, after which the surgeon will be able to use the volume of urine as one of the critical monitors of ongoing resuscitation (Table 42-3).

Postoperative Obligatory Extravascular Fluid Sequestration

AXIOM Following shock and resuscitation, a period of obligatory extravascular fluid sequestration occurs.

The most challenging therapeutic tasks after severe hemorrhagic shock occur in the postoperative period when the patients enter a period of obligatory extravascular fluid sequestration, sometimes referred to as phase II.[11] The hallmarks of this postoperative fluid uptake phase, which lasts 12-36 hours after severe hemorrhagic shock, include tachycardia, decreased MAP, reduced pulse pressure, oliguria, weight gain, increased central-filling pressures, and some degree of respiratory insufficiency. The patient usually has extensive extravascular fluid sequestration in both the interstitial and intracellular spaces. Fluid administration is often restricted or diuretics are given at this time because it is mistakenly believed that the patient is overloaded with fluid. As the consequence of such changes in therapy, the plasma-volume deficit worsens and the likelihood of acute renal failure (ARF) and death increases. This obligatory expansion of both interstitial and intracellular fluid spaces is comparable to that seen in severely burned patients with the prime differences being the mechanism of tissue injury and the sites of fluid sequestration.

The volume of this obligatory fluid expansion is directly related to the severity and duration of the hemorrhagic shock insult. Maintenance of optimal cardiovascular function during this phase is facilitated by keeping hemoglobin levels above 10.0 g/dL and correcting the PV deficit with BESs. Once the PV has been reestablished, the kidneys usually respond with an increase in GFR and urine flow even though the RBF may still be low because renal vasoconstriction may persist 2-4 days following severe hemorrhagic hypotension.

AXIOM Even with adequate fluid resuscitation, urine flow may be somewhat reduced following severe shock because of persistent renal vasoconstriction.

Severe hemorrhagic shock insult also affects other organs, such as the lungs, causing an increase in central filling pressure with impaired oxygenation postoperatively. Because extravascular fluid sequestration occurs at the expense of plasma volume, the combination of increased total body water, deranged oxygenation, hyperventilation, marginal perfusion pressures, and oliguria suggests a diagnosis of combined failure of the kidneys, heart, and lungs. The high central filling pressures and impaired oxygenation are often misdiagnosed as "fluid overload." This term has unfortunate therapeutic implications because fluid restriction and/or diuresis at this time could rapidly lead to renal shutdown, and oliguric renal failure developing during the obligatory extravascular fluid sequestration phase almost always results in death. The question then arises: Should therapy be directed toward inadequate circulatory volume, as reflected by low blood pressure and oliguria, or should it be directed at the so-called vascular overload, as reflected by edema, weight gain, increased filling pressures, and decreased oxygenation?

AXIOM Restriction of fluids during the first 24-48 hours after traumatic shock can greatly increase morbidity and mortality.

The use of diuretics during the fluid sequestration phase often leads to profound diuresis and can cause a severe reduction in plasma volume.[12] This postdiuretic decrease in plasma volume can further reduce perfusion pressures and RPF which, in turn, may result in treatment with vasopressors. Although the reduction in cardiac work after diuretic therapy would be beneficial if patients experienced heart failure, myocardial decompensation in this setting is very uncommon.[12,13] Because precise definition of the cause of oliguria is often difficult, therapy should be adjusted according to organ response to careful administration of fluids and/or inotropic agents.

Fluid Mobilization Phase

Following the period of extravascular fluid sequestration, the patient enters a period of fluid mobilization and diuresis, which is sometimes referred to as phase III.[11] Fluid mobilization from the interstitial and intracellular fluid spaces into the vascular space may begin within 24-48 hours after adequate fluid resuscitation and operation. During the fluid mobilization phase, systolic and diastolic BPs may increase above 150/100 torr producing what has been referred to as "postresuscitation hypertension."[13] Despite the combination of hypertension, expanded PV, increased total body water, and elevated cardiac index, RVR remains elevated and RBF tends to remain depressed (Table 42-4).

The humoral and physiologic events that allow the coexistence of hypertension, increased BP, and decreased RBF are complex and not fully understood. This "postresuscitative hypertension" does not appear to be only due to acute hypervolemia due to previously sequestered extravascular fluid rapidly reentering the plasma space.[11] Thus, treatment by fluid restriction and aggressive diuresis in carefully monitored patients may successfully reduce BP to < 150/100 torr, but it also tends to cause increased tachycardia, a narrowed pulse pressure, increased renin release, reduced GFR, and progressive oliguria, which occasionally is fatal. This sequence of clinical findings suggests that a relative hypovolemic state has been induced by the fluid restriction and diuresis even though BP is above the normal range for that particular patient.

AXIOM Current therapeutic guidelines for postresuscitative hypertension include fluid restriction and avoidance of colloids but no longer include aggressive diuresis.

During the period of postresuscitative hypertension, the patient usually exhibits spontaneous diuresis which allows BP to return to normal levels within 24-48 hours by which time PV, GFR, RBF, and renal excretory function have also usually returned to normal. When concomitant central filling pressures are excessive or when spontaneous diuresis appears to be slow in onset, gentle exogenous diuresis with 5-10 mg of intravenous furosemide may help to initiate the fluid mobilization phase. When gentle diuresis seems to be beneficial, one must be careful not to give larger doses of furosemide to reduce BP < 150/100 torr because it may have adverse effects on the kidneys.

Vasoactive drugs may be useful in maintaining cardiac support and urine output. The use of low-dose dopamine (1-3 μg/kg/min) and/or dobutamine infusion (5-10 μg/kg/min) may help to increase peripheral perfusion pressure, cardiac output, and oxygen delivery even when the fluid infusion rate is reduced. Although infusion of a vasoactive drug has theoretic appeal in injured patients with cardiac insufficiency, overuse of this regimen may lead to drug tachyphylaxis and subsequent death.

A low-dose infusion of dopamine may augment cardiac output without increasing peripheral vascular resistance or reducing flow to vital organs. The increase in blood flow also increases urine output. Although this diuretic effect has been attributed to renal vasodilation, our own studies (unpublished data) indicated that RPF and distribution of RBF remained constant or else fluctuated in proportion to the change in cardiac output after low-dosage dopamine infusion. These findings were corroborated by Hilberman et al. who suggested that diuresis and natriuresis caused by dopamine may occur independently of any effects on RBF.[14] It is possible that dopamine directly inhibits tubular solute reabsorption and thus causes diuresis[14] or that it causes a decrease in ADH release. Ultimately, the place for infusion of vasoactive drugs to reduce fluid needs in the critically ill patient will be determined by careful monitoring of cardiopulmonary function.

AXIOM Hypotension due to diuresis and fluid restriction is usually much more dangerous than mild-to-moderate degrees of postresuscitation hypertension.

If antihypertensive agents were used during the fluid mobilization phase to control elevated BP, cardiovascular function should be monitored carefully to avoid hypotension. Incremental intravenous doses of labetalol (5-20 mg; total: 60-80 mg) can often provide adequate BP and HR control without causing hypotension. In some patients, a total labetalol dose up to 220 mg may be required to control hypertension.[15]

Renal Response to Colloids After Hemorrhagic Shock

The extravascular fluid sequestration state after resuscitation from hemorrhagic shock is associated with decreased intravascular proteins and low intravascular COP. Some surgeons believed that low serum albumin (SA) levels seen at this time cause or contribute to extravascular sequestration. Consequently, addition of human serum albumin (HSA) to the resuscitation regimen for hemorrhagic shock has been proposed by several physicians as a means to increase intravascular COP.[16-18] Hopefully, this would reduce extravascular water sequestration, and the increased fluid returned to the vascular space could be excreted by the kidneys. Unfortunately, HSA does not prevent fluid sequestration and it does not increase renal excretion of fluid. Based

TABLE 42-4 *Renal Response to Fluid Mobilization and Postresuscitative Hypertension*

Parameter Measured	Hypertensive (12 pts)	Nonhypertensive (14 pts)
GFR (mL/min)	90 ± 13 (P < 0.10)	118 ± 12
ERPF (mL/min)	346 ± 34 (P < 0.05)	601 ± 68
TRBF (mL/min)	838 ± 51 (P < 0.05)	1153 ± 163
C_{osm} (mL/min)	6.5 ± 1.6	4.9 ± 0.4
C_{osm}/GFR (%)	6.6 ± 1.2 (P < 0.10)	4.4 ± 0.5
C_{Na} (mL/min)	3.3 ± 1.0	3.0 ± 0.4
U/Na (mEq/L)	51 ± 8.6 (P < 0.05)	85 ± 14
MAP (mm Hg)	114 ± 4 (P < 0.05)	98 ± 3
CVP (cm H_2O)	10 ± 2 (P < 0.05)	4 ± 0.6
C.I. (L/mm)	3.6 ± 0.5	3.9 ± 0.4
TPR (d-s cm^5)	1340 ± 126	1210 ± 110
RVR (d-s cm^5)	16,290 ± 1430 (P < 0.05)	5780 ± 1065

BP > 150/100 mm Hg for 6 or more hours. Patients received an average of 15.2 blood transfusions. Values expressed as mean ± SE.

upon extensive controlled studies in severely injured patients, the renal effects of HSA have been elucidated. When given in a random fashion as a supplement to blood and fluid resuscitation for hemorrhagic shock, HSA produces an increase in serum albumin levels, PV, and RBF. However, despite the increase in PV and RBF, a decrease in GFR, osmolal clearance (C_{Osm}), osmolal clearance (C_{Na}), and urinary output occurs.[10] In many patients, the decrease in urinary output after HSA supplementation has led to an increased need for loop diureses and an increased incidence of ARF.

AXIOM   Colloids may increase plasma volume more than crystalloids but they reduce GFR and urine output, thereby increasing the incidence of renal failure.

The mechanism for the decreased GFR and urine output after albumin administration appears to be related to an increase in COP and osmolality within the glomerular tuft, thereby maintaining salt and H_2O in the PV. Furthermore, HSA increases COP in the peritubular vessels of the inner medulla and this increases sodium and water reabsorption in response to aldosterone and ADH. The resultant increased water and salt retention during the extravascular fluid sequestration phase causes the patient to gain even more weight. This increased fluid retention also impairs pulmonary function as reflected by reduced oxygenation and prolonged need for ventilation support.

AXIOM   Based upon the renal response to colloid resuscitation, HSA should not be used during the fluid sequestration phase.

Effects of Artificial Ventilation on Fluid Therapy

Patients with severe hemorrhage may later develop varying degrees of pulmonary insufficiency requiring ventilatory support.[6] Controlled mechanical ventilation (CMV), even with zero end-expiratory pressure (ZEEP), has been shown to produce significant changes in renal function.[19,20] With the addition of positive end-expiratory pressure (PEEP), alteration of renal function is even more pronounced.[21-23] In one study in head-injured patients, addition of 10 cm H_2O of PEEP to CMV reduced urine output by 34%, GFR by 19%, RBF by 32%, and sodium by 33%.[24] Decreased water and sodium excretion results in water retention, weight gain, tissue edema, and decreased hematocrit, plasma osmolality, and plasma sodium concentrations.[25] Thus, ventilatory adjustments designed to improve arterial oxygen content may significantly alter fluid therapy.

AXIOM   Positive-pressure ventilation, especially with PEEP, can greatly reduce urine output and sodium excretion.

Respirator-induced changes of renal function have been attributed to several mechanisms.[26] Experimentally, it has been suggested that increases in inferior vena cava (IVC), hepatic, and renal vein pressures, which accompany administration of PEEP, may reduce RBF and thereby contribute to the altered renal function.[27,28] However, reduction of hepatic congestion by means of a vena cava to jugular venous shunt during PEEP does not improve renal function.[29] In addition, despite significant increases in IVC pressure during PEEP, deterioration of renal function has been shown to occur only in hypovolemic and normovolemic animals but not in those that are hypervolemic.[30] Thus, renal congestion secondary to increased IVC pressure by PEEP appears to contribute little to altered renal function. It has been suggested that redistribution of RBF from cortical to juxtamedullary nephrons could cause impairment of renal function[31]; however, a more recent study by the same group using radioactive microspheres failed to demonstrate any blood flow redistribution in the kidneys when PEEP was added.[32]

At present, available evidence suggests that the decreased cardiac output induced by PEEP, and to a lesser extent by CMV, is the primary cause of the renal effects. Both high tidal volumes and PEEP reduce venous return and cardiac output,[33,34] probably as a result of diminished left ventricular end-diastolic volume caused by elevated intrathoracic pressure, autonomic reflex alterations, and decreased venous return.[35,36] Increased pulmonary vascular resistance[35,36] and altered ventricular geometry with cardiac septal or lateral free-wall shifting[37,38] caused by PEEP may also reduce cardiac output.

AXIOM   CMV with PEEP can improve oxygenation but can also reduce cardiac output with a resultant decrease in tissue oxygen delivery.[39]

The frequently associated decrease in arterial BP with PEEP inhibits baroreceptor discharge which, in turn, enhances sympathetic tone, catecholamine secretion, and renin-angiotensin-aldosterone activity.[40] These acute compensations maintain circulatory homeostasis and minimize further decreases in BP but can also produce severe hemodynamic changes in the kidney.

The extent and severity of renal and cardiovascular changes caused by PEEP are dependent on the pulmonary, cardiac, and intravascular volume status of the patient, the amount of PEEP applied, and the types of anesthetic and sedative drugs used.[25] For instance, in patients with decreased lung compliance, the elevated airway pressures may not be transmitted to the intrapleural space, and thus the elevation of intrathoracic pressure may be relatively small.[25,41,42] This, of course, results in less reduction in venous return, BP, and renal function. Likewise, patients who have increased intravascular volume are not affected much by the otherwise deleterious renal and hemodynamic effects of PEEP.[29,30,43]

AXIOM   CMV and PEEP are much less apt to have deleterious cardiac and renal effects when the patient is hypervolemic.

Although elevated plasma ADH levels have been demonstrated during the initial phases of PEEP therapy, resultant decreases in free-water clearance have been observed only infrequently.[25] This suggests that, under these circumstances, ADH acts as a vasoconstrictor rather than as an antidiuretic. Furthermore, a small number of patients demonstrated that ADH was not involved in the antidiuretic effect of PEEP.[40]

Several mechanisms may be responsible for increased ADH levels during ventilation with PEEP. These may include stimulation of low-pressure (atrial) and high-pressure (arterial) baroreceptors by decreased central blood volume,[44,45] angiotensin release,[24] and increased plasma osmolality.

Recently, atrial natriuretic factor (ANF) has been shown to contribute to the development of PEEP-induced antidiuresis.[46,47] ANF is secreted from the atrial wall in response to increased atrial transmural pressure. The sites of action of ANF are the kidneys, the adrenals, vascular smooth muscle, and possibly the central nervous system. ANF levels increase in congestive failure and volume overload to induce diuresis; however, during ventilation with PEEP the increase in intrathoracic pressure tends to decrease transmural pressures within the heart and results in decreased ANF secretion which, in turn, results in antidiuresis.

AXIOM   CMV and PEEP tend to reduce the formation of ANF.

After a period of mechanical ventilation, retained water and exogenously administered fluids can cause a significant increase in intravascular and total body water. When the ventilator is removed, the increased intravascular volume improves cardiac filling pressures and cardiac output.[48] The resultant decrease in sympathetic tone and ADH and renin-angiotensin activity, together with increased ANF secretion, can greatly increase cardiac output, RBF, urine output, and sodium excretion.

ACID-BASE BALANCE AFTER HEMORRHAGIC SHOCK

Hemorrhagic shock tends to cause a continuous decline in arterial pH until vascular volume and tissue perfusion are reestablished. However, even after intravascular volume is repleted, metabolic acidosis may persist for several hours due to slow metabolism of the acids formed during cellular ischemia.

AXIOM Arterial metabolic acidosis may persist to some degree for several hours after shock has been corrected by adequate fluid resuscitation.

Interestingly, the homeostatic response to shock permits the interstitial pH to be maintained at relatively normal levels despite severe hemorrhagic insults which may reduce arterial pH values to < 7.0. Presumably, this homeostasis is designed to protect cellular integrity and thereby maintain vital cellular functions. The mechanism of this protection is unclear and is currently under investigation.

When acid production exceeds acid elimination, the resultant intravascular acidosis is managed by buffering the hydrogen ions and by elimination of acid through the lungs and kidneys. Pulmonary elimination of acid through carbon dioxide excretion is limited by the inability of severely injured, hypovolemic patients to maintain a greatly increased minute ventilation for prolonged periods. In addition, the plasma bicarbonate system may become depleted, and intracellular buffering mechanisms may become impaired by cellular damage.

The renal mechanisms of acid excretion include tubular reabsorption of sodium bicarbonate and the excretion of acid with phosphate and ammonia (Table 42-5). The latter two processes enable adults to normally excrete 70-80 mEq of acid per day through the kidneys. Even though acid excretion may be greatly increased by the kidneys in the presence of severe metabolic acidosis, these three mechanisms require a reasonably normal GFR and RBF and intact renal tubules. The renal changes associated with hemorrhagic shock disrupt these processes. Consequently, the acid load generated from hypoxic tissues may overwhelm the excretory capacity of the lungs and kidneys.

Treatment of acid-base abnormalities during hemorrhagic shock is best accomplished by rapid restoration of PV and tissue perfusion to reduce the need to generate lactic acid because of tissue hypoxia. BES is preferred for resuscitation because of its ready availability and its ability to correct volume deficits in the vascular and interstital fluid spaces. Normal saline resuscitation without supplemental sodium bicarbonate may cause a further decrease in blood pH. Ringer's lactate also helps to buffer acidosis as the lactate within Ringer's lactate is metabolized to bicarbonate.

AXIOM No resuscitation fluid returns pH to normal in patients with severe hemorrhagic shock until fluid resuscitation and oxygen delivery are adequate.

Correction of metabolic acidosis in severe shock may require therapy with bicarbonate. A patient with persistent hypotension, acidosis, and severe hypocarbia (arterial PCO_2 < 15-20 mm Hg) generally has a total extracellular fluid deficit of at least 4 L and a bicarbonate deficit > 200 mEq. Consequently, the rapid infusion of 4 L of Ringer's lactate (which contains 28 mEq of lactate/L) plus one am-

TABLE 42-5 *Renal Control of Fluid and Acid Base Balance*

Mechanism	Capacity (mEq/day)
Bicarbonate production	40-80
Titratable acid generation	10-30
Ammonia excretion	30-50

ARF with impaired renal plasma flow precludes tubular generation of ammonia and reduces renal bicarbonate production. Consequent acidosis requires parenteral correction.

pule of sodium bicarbonate (44.3 mEq) per liter should correct both the volume deficit and metabolic acidosis. Once the intravascular volume is restored, renal perfusion and filtration will improve and the renal mechanisms for acid excretion will again become operative. When the shock insult leads to acute oliguric renal failure, the renal component of acid-base balance must be accomplished with dialysis or hemofiltration.

RENAL RESPONSE TO SEPSIS

Sepsis is one of the feared complications following severe injury, and it is particularly likely to develop when hollow viscus injury leads to extensive peritoneal soilage in a patient with severe hypotension. When infection develops, the byproducts of cellular and microbial damage must be cleared from the infected area for elimination by the kidneys. When the quantity of circulatory byproducts exceeds excretory capacity, the typical peripheral organ changes of sepsis evolve. Thus, the renal response to sepsis reflects the total changes within the cardiovascular system.

Hyperdynamic Sepsis

SYSTEMIC HEMODYNAMIC CHANGES

Prior to 1965, sepsis was generally characterized as a hypodynamic state with decreased cardiac output and increased systemic vascular resistance (SVR). With this characterization, the kidneys were also believed to respond to sepsis with increased RVR and decreased RBF. More recently, treatment of septic patients with aggressive fluid replacement has resulted in significant improvements in cardiac output and renal blood. Many septic patients develop a hyperdynamic state associated with increased cardiac output, decreased systemic vascular resistance, expanded extracellular fluid volume, and increased urine output.

POLYURIA OF SEPSIS

Prospective studies demonstrated that polyuria tends to occur in severely septic patients when aggressive fluid resuscitation is initiated soon after the septic insult begins and prior to the development of renal ischemia and severe oliguria. The syndrome of "inappropriate polyuria" may persist for some time despite fluid restriction and the development of hypovolemia, and this can cause a sudden decrease in systolic BP < 90 mm Hg.

AXIOM The polyuria of sepsis can cause abrupt, severe hypovolemia when fluid intake is restricted because of an impression that the patient is overloaded with fluid.

Mechanisms for Polyuria in Sepsis

HYPEROSMOLEMIA. The mechanisms for "inappropriate polyuria" in septic patients with a hyperdynamic cardiovascular state remain controversial. Some have postulated that polyuria is due to osmotic diuresis. Hyperosmolemia occurs in septic patients and can be determined either by direct measurement or by calculation from the serum sodium, blood urea nitrogen (BUN), and serum glucose concentrations:

$$Osm_{calc} = 2[Na^+] + \frac{BUN}{2.8} + \frac{Glucose}{18}$$

The severity of sepsis correlates closely with the difference between calculated and measured serum osmolality. However, measured osmolar clearances in septic patients usually range 2-3% of the GFR, and this is at the upper end of normal. Thus, the hyperosmolemia of sepsis may contribute to inappropriate polyuria but it does not appear to be the primary problem.

RENAL VASODILATION. Another possible mechanism for inappropriate polyuria involves the tendency for sepsis or its associated hyperosmolemia to be a potent vasodilator in many vascular beds, including the kidney. Thus, hyperosmolemia may facilitate diuresis by means of renal vasodilation and through the effects of increased RPF on the concentrating mechanism.

MEDULLARY WASHOUT. The polyuria of sepsis may also be caused by a juxtamedullary "wash out" due to increased RBF to the inner cortex and medulla. Studies in severely septic patients with polyuria indicated that the total RBF is elevated even though effective RBF, as monitored by PAH clearance, is reduced. This paradoxical finding can only be explained on the basis of intrarenal shunting of an increased blood flow to the renal medulla, and this which could produce an osmolar washout. Similar increases in RBF were reproduced in an experimental model of hind limb sepsis.

| AXIOM | When a patient with a severe infection has been appropriately resuscitated, the kidneys share in the hyperdynamic state of sepsis. |

Inadequate ADH Secretion

Another mechanism by which the inappropriate polyuric syndrome is produced has been proposed by Hermreck and Thal as a result of studies in dogs with septic hind limbs.[49] Inappropriate polyuria seen with the septic hind limb model was initially believed to result from decreased release of ADH from the posterior pituitary gland. Experimental studies suggested that when ADH is given to septic animals with polyuria, it will counter the polyuric state. Clinical studies, however, demonstrated that the polyuric state generally persists in septic patients despite the administration of physiologic doses of ADH (1-2 mcg/kg/hour).

BLOCKADE OF ALDOSTERONE RECEPTORS. The polyuria of sepsis has also been attributed to a distal tubular blockade of aldosterone receptor sites. The calculated aldosteronelike effect of the renal tubules ($C_{PAH}/C_{H2O} + C_{Na}$) in septic patients with positive free-water clearance, however, shows no impairment of aldosteronelike activity. In contrast, most septic patients can reabsorb sodium with great efficiency even up to the point of developing acute oliguric renal failure.

SUMMARY. The polyuria of sepsis may be due to a variety of factors, including a septic or toxic insult to the juxtamedullary tubules leading to decreased medullary hypertonicity with reduced reabsorption of water from the collecting ducts. In a sense, the polyuria of sepsis is the renal response to the early release of the byproducts of the ongoing conflict between bacteria and white blood cells.

Treatment of Polyuria of Sepsis

| AXIOM | "Normal" urine output of 0.5 mL/kg/hour is often inadequate in septic patients. |

The therapeutic implications of the polyuric syndrome are clear. Physicians must recognize that a "good urine output" of 35-50 mL/hour may not be adequate in the early septic period. Polyuria, together with large, insensible water losses, extracellular fluid space expansion, and increase in nasogastric secretions over a period of days may lead to rather severe hypovolemia which may go unrecognized prior to a "sudden" cardiovascular collapse.

Careful monitoring of ongoing intake and output, vital signs, and urine sodium concentrations can help prevent this sudden catastrophe. When urine sodium concentration decreases below 20 mEq/L, one must look carefully for a perfusion deficit. If urine sodium decreases below 10 mEq/L, sudden, severe hypovolemia and impending prerenal failure may be imminent.

| AXIOM | High urine output with a urine sodium concentration < 10 meq/L may indicate that the polyuria of sepsis is present in spite of significant hypovolemia. |

Hypodynamic Sepsis

At least 35% of patients with severe sepsis subsequent to injury and hypovolemic shock develop a hypodynamic state with decreased cardiac output and increased systemic vascular resistance despite aggressive fluid replacement. These patients also tend to have a hypodynamic response to sepsis in the kidneys as evidenced by increased RVR and decreased RBF and GFR. These changes are associated with a decrease in RBF to the outer renal cortex. When these hemodynamic changes occur in the presence of normal concentrating function, the renal response leads to oliguria with reduced sodium and osmolar clearances. Various antibiotics, particularly aminoglycosides, may add to the potential for renal injury.

| AXIOM | Hypodynamic sepsis with oliguria is best treated with aggressive fluid resuscitation. |

Therapy in the hypodynamic septic patient with oliguria must be directed toward reestablishing urine flow by providing an effective PV to support compromised myocardium and peripheral perfusion. Persistent oliguria in fully resuscitated patients may require exogenous diuresis with mannitol or furosemide in order to improve the preload to the heart. Fortunately, the combination of hypodynamic sepsis and oliguria after trauma is not common.

| AXIOM | If oliguria were to persist in spite of adequate fluid resuscitation, BP, and cardiac output, cautious loop diuretic therapy might be helpful. |

When a patient has appropriate PV and cardiac output but oliguria persists, septic-induced ARF is imminent. Some patients in this state respond to aggressive diuresis with furosemide. This can be administered by giving 40 mg and then doubling this dose every 30 minutes until diuresis is obtained or until a total cumulative dose of 500 mg of furosemide has been given. If a diuretic response were not to occur with this regimen, the patient usually would have established acute oliguric renal failure.

ACUTE RENAL FAILURE

Incidence and Implications

Posttraumatic renal failure was first recognized as a special entity in casualties during World War II.[50] The incidence of ARF among those who were severely injured was 42% and the resultant mortality was 90%.[51] The incidence of ARF declined to 35% during the Korean War and to less than 1% during the latter years of the Vietnam war. This improvement was probably due to rapid evacuation and early, aggressive resuscitation with crystalloids.

| AXIOM | Acute oliguric renal failure in sepsis or after trauma requiring hemodialysis is almost invariably fatal. |

ARF in the trauma patient is a formidable complication. The mortality of ARF in the posttrauma patient is reportedly as high as 50-60%.[52] Oliguric renal failure after major trauma carries a mortality of 90%.[53] In contrast, nonoliguric ARF is associated with a mortality of slightly less than 20%.[54] Only about one-third of patients suffer ARF during the initial trauma and surgical treatment phase (phase I), whereas the remaining two-thirds develop renal failure later in phases II or III as a result of postoperative complications or therapy.

Etiology

RENAL ISCHEMIA

The most common causes of renal dysfunction within the first few days after trauma are prerenal azotemia, ATN, and renal vascular injury. Renal dysfunction that develops 1-2 weeks after trauma is usually caused by: (a) ATN secondary to drug or radiocontrast dye-induced ischemia, (b) drug-induced acute tubular interstitial nephritis

(ATIN), (c) postinfectious glomerulonephritis, or (d) prerenal azotemia.

A number of conditions are associated with an increased risk of an injured patient developing ATN,[55-59] including cardiac arrest, prolonged systemic hypotension or aortic cross-clamping, extensive muscle damage with myoglobinuria, major blood transfusion reactions, severe burns, and gram-negative sepsis.[55,56]

Other important conditions increasing the risk of developing ATN include advanced age, preexisting renal vascular disease, previous hypertension, aminoglycoside therapy,[60] and radiocontrast dye studies.[61,62]

NONISCHEMIC CAUSES OF ACUTE TUBULAR NECROSIS

Acute Tubular Necrosis Associated with Sepsis

As mentioned previously, early sepsis in normovolemic patients is often accompanied by a hyperdynamic circulatory state, with an increase in cardiac output and a decrease in total peripheral resistance. Increased urine volume during the early phases of sepsis combined with plasma leakage into the extravascular compartment leads to reduced effective circulatory volume and decreased RBF. The resultant severe reduction in GFR can rapidly progress to ATN.

Pigment-induced Acute Tubular Necrosis

Severe myoglobinuria from muscle necrosis or red blood cell destruction from hemolytic transfusion reactions may cause ATN in trauma patients.[63-65] High urine output (> 200-300 mL/hr) helps to prevent this type of renal failure.

RHABDOMYOLOSIS AND MYOGLOBINURIA. Each kilogram of skeletal muscle contains approximately 110 mEq of potassium, 500-750 mL of H_2O, 0.75 mmol (2.25 g) of phosphate, and 4 g of myoglobin.[64-65] Crush injury causes hyperkalemia, hyperphosphatemia, azotemia, hypocalcemia, disseminated intravascular coagulation, systemic hypotension, and myoglobinuria. Skeletal muscle injury raises creatine phosphokinase (CPK), aldolase, glutamic-oxaloacetic transaminase, and lactic dehydrogenase.

Myoglobin concentrations exceeding 100-150 mg/dL discolors the plasma and urine.[64] Because myoglobin is not bound to serum proteins, it is freely excreted in the urine which becomes reddish-brown, but the plasma remains clear. Myoglobin or hemoglobin nephrotoxicity is due to ferrihemate, is dose dependent, and is unlikely to occur in the absence of hypovolemia or acidotic urine.

> **AXIOM** ARF due to hemoglobinuria or myoglobinuria is unlikely unless the patient is hypotensive and has an acid urine.[65]

Another problem seen with crush injuries is the so-called "second-wave phenomenon".[63] CPK released from damaged muscles reaches its maximal plasma concentration 24-36 hours after injury. Persistent elevations of CPK at this time often indicate residual muscle necrosis. An inadequately treated compartment syndrome at this time leads to gangrene and ARF. This second-wave phenomenon occurs after fluid resuscitation, and purportedly results from the decomposition of muscle into smaller proteins and amino acids which raises tissue oncotic pressure and promotes fluid expansion of the involved compartment.

ARF caused by rhabdomyolysis and myoglobinuria is treated with fluids, loop diuresis, and mannitol, as needed, to maintain a urine output of at least 200 mL/hour and with sodium bicarbonate to keep urine pH above 6.5.[66]

During the oliguric phase of rhabdomyolysis-induced ARF, moderate-to-severe hypocalcemia may develop from several mechanisms, including: (a) movement of calcium into damaged or ischemic cells, (b) decreased synthesis of 1,25-$(OH)_2$ vit D, and (c) hyperphosphatemia.[67] During the polyuric recovery phase of rhabdomyolysis-induced ARF, hypercalcemia occurs. The overall mortality rate of rhabdomyolysis-induced ARF is about 15%.[68]

HEMOGLOBIN-INDUCED ACUTE RENAL FAILURE. Release of free hemoglobin from hemolyzed red blood cells can cause ARF, especially when hypotension and ischemia coexist.[69,70] Incompatible blood transfusions and thermal injury are the most common causes of hemoglobinuria in the trauma patient.[70] Advances in blood banking techniques decreased the frequency of primary hemolytic transfusion reactions. Delayed transfusion reactions that occur 4-14 days after transfusion also may cause hemoglobinuric ARF.[70]

The initial symptoms of hemoglobinuric ARF include fever and urticaria. Hemoglobinuria, oliguria, and hemolytic anemia can occur rapidly. Administration of mannitol and increased fluids immediately after detection of hemoglobinuria helps to prevent ARF. The likelihood of recovery from transfusion-reaction-induced ARF, especially when it occurs 1-3 weeks after the transfusion, is good.[71]

Drug-induced Acute Renal Failure

The pathogenesis of ARF secondary to drugs varies with the specific agent.[59] The major mechanisms involved in drug-induced ARF include (a) acute tubular necrosis, (b) immunologic reactions, (c) obstructive nephropathy, and (d) excessive vasoconstriction.

The most widely publicized type of direct tubular toxicity is that produced by aminoglycosides. Renal failure in patients receiving these drugs can occur even when peak and trough antibiotic levels have been meticulously measured. Predisposing nephrotoxicity factors for these antibiotics include (a) preexisting renal disease, (b) advanced patient age, (c) volume depletion, and (d) prolonged therapy.[72] Cephalosporins and clindamycin potentiate aminoglycoside nephrotoxicity in humans.[73]

Azotemia, with serum creatinine levels increasing to more than 1.3 mg/dL, occurs in 8-11% of all hospitalized patients receiving aminoglycoside therapy.[74] Clinically significant ARF (i.e., serum creatinine > 2.0 mg/dL) occurs in only 3-5% of patients.[74] The nephrotoxicity of aminoglycosides is increased in elderly patients and when they are used concurrently with diuretics, radiographic contrast media, or antifungal agents. Generally, the nephrotoxic potential of aminoglycosides is increased when (a) trough serum levels are > 2 mcg/mL, (b) peak serum levels are > 12-15 mcg/mL, and (c) the drug is used for longer than 2 weeks.[54]

> **AXIOM** Renal function, especially creatinine clearance, should be monitored closely in patients receiving prolonged courses and/or high doses of aminoglycosides.

The major lesion in aminoglycoside-induced ARF is proximal tubular necrosis with relative sparing of the glomeruli and blood vessels.[75] Aminoglycosides also inhibit phospholipase activity in the Na^+–K^+ pump of the inner mitochondrial membrane.[76] Aminoglycoside nephrotoxicity usually presents as nonoliguric ARF that may be delayed for several days.[77] The first functional defect is often a decrease in urine concentrating ability, resulting in polyuria. Before the onset of azotemia, increases in urinary microglobulins, muramidase, β-glucuronidase, and N-acetyl hexosaminidase occur. However, finding these tubular proteins in urine is not pathognomonic of ARF. The appearance of mild proteinuria and granular casts precedes the development of azotemia. After the discontinuation of aminoglycosides, resolution of ARF may take several weeks.[78] Other antimicrobials that are more likely to produce ATN include amphotericin B, polymyxin B, and polymyxin E.[59] The penicillin class of antibiotics, in particular methicillin, can cause a hypersensitivity reaction resulting in acute interstitial nephritis which is usually rapidly reversible when the offending drug has been removed.[79] Furosemide, thiazide, and allopurinol have also produced this type of allergic interstitial nephritis.

Intratubular precipitation of oxalate, resulting in obstructive nephropathy, is the major mechanism associated with irreversible nephrotoxicity secondary to methoxyflurane.[80]

> **AXIOM** Nonsteroidal antiinflammatory drugs should not be used in patients who may have renal impairment because of hypotension or other drugs.

A reversible decline in GFR has been reported after the administration of nonsteroidal antiinflammatory agents, such as aspirin and indomethacin, that inhibit prostaglandin synthesis.[59] These agents appear to have no deleterious effect on renal function in healthy persons, but they may have adverse effects on activation of the renin-angiotensin or catecholamine systems in patients with hypovolemia, preexisting hepatic or renal disease, or advanced CHF. Gentamicin, amphotericin, and heavy metals can also cause renal vasoconstriction.

Radiocontrast-induced Nephropathy

FACTORS CAUSING ATN. Trauma patients are often exposed to radiographic contrast studies, and such tests are the ones most likely to cause ARF.[61] The incidence of ARF after administration of radiocontrast agents varies 1-13%.[61,62] Two medical centers reported that 9-11% of all ARF is caused by radiocontrast media.[4,81] Most investigators showed that preexisting renal insufficiency and intravascular volume depletion are important predisposing factors.

The most commonly used contrast agents are 2, 4, 6-triiodinated benzoic acid derivatives, which are markedly hyperosmolar and contain 26-37% iodine by weight.[61,62] They are excreted entirely by the kidney, and their serum half-lives are normally 30-60 minutes. They increase urinary excretion of uric acid and oxalate and also stimulate ADH production.

The pathogenesis of ATN secondary to radiocontrast dye appears to be multifactorial.[61] Possible mechanisms include direct tubular toxicity, renal ischemia, intratubular obstruction, and immunologic abnormalities.[2] Changes in red blood cell morphology and function have also been implicated. Important risk factors for contrast-medium-induced ARF are preexisting renal impairment, peripheral vascular disease, dehydration, multiple myeloma, hypertension, and age over 60 years.

Contrast-medium-induced nephropathy is characterized by serum creatinine levels beginning to increase about 24 hours after dye injection, peaking between the third and fifth day, and returning to baseline within 10 days. Urine specific gravity is often high initially (> 1.025) due to the high osmolarity of the contrast medium. Urine sodium levels and 24-hour urine sodium excretion may be low. Renal function usually returns to normal unless the patient was allowed to become oliguric. Acute hemodialysis is seldom needed.[82,83]

AXIOM   High urine output should be maintained in patients who are at risk for developing contrast-medium-induced nephrotoxicity.

PREVENTION. Anto et al. advocated prevention of contrast-medium-induced renal failure by intravenous infusion of 250 mL of 20% mannitol over 1 hour after administration of intravenous contrast, followed by infusion of 0.45% saline in 5% dextrose at a rate equivalent to the urine output.[84] Berksett and Kjellstrand proposed that all patients with precontrast serum creatinine levels > 2.0 mg/dL receive 500 mL of 20% mannitol.[85] The infusion starts 1 hour before the contrast media and continues for 6 hours thereafter. Furosemide, in a dose of 100 mg for each 1.0 mg/dL elevation of serum creatinine, is added.

Terminology

ACUTE RENAL FAILURE
ARF is a sudden, severe deterioration in renal function occurring from any cause.[59] Renal insufficiency is generally characterized by an increase in BUN and serum creatinine; these can occur without changes in urine volume. The term, acute tubular necrosis (ATN) refers to a specific form of ARF occurring after shock or certain nephrotoxic agents; a more appropriate term is vasomotor nephropathy.

OLIGURIA AND ANURIA
Oliguria is defined as a urine output < 400 mL/day. This represents the minimal amount of urine in which the normal daily solute load of 500 mOsm can be excreted when the urine is maximally concentrated to 1200 mOsm/kg of H_2O.[59] A lower urine output results in azotemia even if the kidney can concentrate.

Anuria is a urine volume < 50 mL/day. Mechanical blockage of the bladder drainage system is the most common cause of sudden anuria. Other causes include bilateral renal cortical necrosis, vascular occlusion, or obstructive uropathy.

Nonoliguric renal failure is defined as progressive azotemia in patients voiding over 400 mL/day.[59] High-output renal failure is defined as acute renal insufficiency in patients with daily urine volumes > 4000 mL/day.

Classification of Acute Renal Failure

From an etiologic standpoint, acute renal failure or dysfunction is often divided into prerenal, postrenal, and renal causes.

PRERENAL AZOTEMIA

AXIOM   The most common cause of oliguria after injury is decreased renal perfusion due to inadequate or delayed fluid resuscitation.

Because the morbidity and mortality of established acute oliguric renal failure are so great, prerenal oliguria must not be allowed to progress to intrinsic acute oliguric renal failure because of inadequate fluids or inappropriate use of loop diuretics.

Prerenal azotemia develops only after renal responses to decreased glomerular blood flow fail to maintain normal kidney perfusion, filtration, and reabsorption.[5] Azotemia per se usually occurs as a result of increased tubular reabsorption of urea due to slowing of the tubular fluid flow rate. The compensatory mechanisms utilized by the healthy kidney include autoregulatory dilation of the afferent arterioles, tubuloglomerular feedback, modulation of the actions of systemic vasoconstrictors by intrarenal vasodilator prostaglandins, constriction of the efferent arterioles, and the fluid-retaining ability of the kidney.[86]

Autoregulatory vasodilation occurs primarily at the level of the afferent arterioles.[59] Perfusion pressure below the limits of autoregulation results in maximally dilated afferent arterioles.

As glomerular perfusion pressure decreases below the autoregulatory range (mean arterial pressure: 80-120 mm Hg), the glomerular filtration rate declines, resulting in a reduced volume of glomerular filtrate entering the tubules.[59] Aldosterone and antidiuretic hormone (ADH), which are both secreted in response to hypovolemia and/or hypotension, alter the amount and composition of the urine by conserving sodium and water. The result is a small volume of urine with a high specific gravity and a low-sodium content.

Prerenal azotemia becomes irreversible when RBF has been reduced so severely that oxygen and substrate delivery to the renal tubular cells is inadequate to keep them alive.[59] Prevention of these irreversible changes requires prompt recognition of hypovolemia and hypotension.

Another problem that can cause prerenal azotemia is increased intraabdominal pressure. This may occur in the trauma patient after the application of MAST or from abdominal distension secondary to ileus, bowel obstruction, or postoperative hemorrhage.[59] Decreases in RBF and glomerular filtration rate occurred as a result of this increased intraabdominal pressure.[87] Recent studies showed that the impairment in renal function occurring because of increased intraabdominal pressure is a local phenomenon due to direct renal compression and markedly increased renal vascular resistance.[87]

POSTRENAL AZOTEMIA
Anuria is rare in the absence of bilateral ureteral or lower urinary tract obstruction.[59] Obstruction of the urinary tract of the trauma pa-

tient may occur acutely secondary to pelvic fractures because of (a) bilateral ureteral compression from a large retroperitoneal hematoma, (b) rupture of the bladder, or (c) complete transection of the urethra.[88] Intraoperative injury to one or both ureters may occur in trauma patients requiring emergency surgical procedures for retroperitoneal injuries. Obstruction of urine flow may also occur because of prostatic hypertrophy or because of Foley catheter obstruction. When the possibility of obstructive uropathy cannot be excluded, renal ultrasound imaging should be performed. B-mode scanning provides the most reliable confirmatory test with an accuracy > 90%,[89] but real-time ultrasonography is equally sensitive and can shorten the examination time considerably.[90] Chronic obstruction of the lower urinary tract eventually results in anatomical and functional abnormalities in the kidneys. Increased back pressure reduces glomerular filtration rate and causes a resultant increase in urea reabsorption.[59] Prolonged obstruction to urine flow also causes renal vasoconstriction with further reduction in RBF which may be severe enough to cause ischemic injury.

> **AXIOM** Prompt recognition and therapy of urinary tract obstruction are necessary to prevent renal parenchymal damage.

ACUTE INTRINSIC RENAL FAILURE

Persistent prerenal or postrenal causes of azotemia may eventually lead to ATN.[59] In the majority of patients, however, the morphologic changes of ATN are due to tubular toxins or profound ischemia.[91] With toxic injury, both functional and morphologic changes occur in all segments of the nephron. In contrast, renal ischemic damage tends to be characterized by extensive, patchy cortical necrosis of any or all parts of the renal tubule along with disruption of the basement membrane.[92]

ACUTE TUBULAR INTERSTITIAL NEPHRITIS

ATIN usually presents as oliguric ARF without a history suggesting acute glomerulonephritis or ATN.[5] In trauma patients, it is almost invariably drug-induced. The drugs that most commonly cause this entity are (a) antibiotics (especially penicillins, sulfadiazines, and cephalosporins), (b) nonsteroidal antiinflammatory agents (with the possible exception of Sulindac), (c) diuretics, and (d) others, including cimetidine, allopurinol, and diphenylhydantoin. Many systemic infections may also cause ATIN.

Only a minority of patients with ATIN have the classic features of rash, arthralgias, and fever in association with ARF. Peripheral blood eosinophilia and elevated serum IgE levels help to confirm the diagnosis of ATIN, but their absence does not exclude this disorder. Eosinophiliuria is the most useful indicator of ATIN.[93] Improvement in urine output and renal function within several days of removing the offending drug or agent is also suggestive of the diagnosis. The renal uptake of gallium citrate, as quantitated by scanning, is markedly increased in ATIN but not in ATN, vasculitis, or pyelonephritis (Table 42-1).[94,95] This test offers a promising, noninvasive method of confirming the diagnosis of ATIN. The diagnosis of ATIN can also be made by renal biopsy, if necessary. Although most patients make good recoveries from ATIN after withdrawal of the offending agents, some patients may deteriorate and develop advanced renal failure requiring dialysis.

Pathophysiology of Acute Renal Failure

Some of the pathophysiologic changes believed to occur in kidneys developing ARF include (a) tubular obstruction, (b) passive backflow of glomerular filtrate, (c) preglomerular arterial vasoconstriction with subsequent decrease in glomerular plasma flow,[59] and (d) ultrastructural changes induced in the glomerular capillary bed resulting in decreased glomerular permeability.

RENAL TUBULAR OBSTRUCTION

Many investigators postulated that tubular obstruction, possibly associated with back diffusion, is the principal pathologic factor in ARF.[96,97] This is based on frequent histologic findings of interstitial edema, tubular casts, and regenerating tubular cells.[98] Most data supporting this mechanism were derived from micropuncture studies following temporary renal ischemia in the rat.[99,100] However, morphologic studies in patients with ATN did not support the theory of tubular obstruction by casts.[101]

PASSIVE BACKFLOW

An alternative theory for ATN is the passive backflow hypothesis in which glomerular filtrate is reabsorbed from the damaged tubule into the renal interstitium and then into the circulation, resulting in oliguria or anuria.[102-104] Although it may occur in many types of ARF, the precise significance of this hypothesis is not clear.

ARTERIOLAR VASOCONSTRICTION

Several investigators suggested that renal vasomotor abnormalities are the cause of oliguria in ATN due to toxins and ischemia and suggested the name, "acute vasomotor nephropathy," to describe the pathophysiologic changes in this process.[105,106] Renal hemodynamic studies using dye dilution techniques and radioactive microspheres showed a pattern of preferential cortical ischemia in patients with ARF of a magnitude great enough to depress glomerular filtration.[107,108]

Many reports support the hypothesis that the local production of renin by JGA is responsible for preglomerular vasoconstriction.[63,109] Increased sodium delivery to the macula densa, because of tubular damage and decreased ability to reabsorb sodium, results in increased release of renin and production of angiotensin followed by constriction of afferent arterioles.

> **AXIOM** The pathogenesis of ATN is multifaceted, with decreased glomerular capillary pressure and permeability, changes in RBF, and tubular obstruction all interrelated and contributing to the problem.[59]

Clinical Pathophysiology

The most prominent effects of renal failure include retention of metabolic endproducts, primarily creatinine, urea, and uric acid.[59]

> **AXIOM** Characteristic electrolyte and acid-base changes in ARF include hyponatremia, hyperkalemia, metabolic acidosis, hyperphosphatemia, hypermagnesemia, and hypocalcemia.

CREATININE

The increase in serum creatinine in ARF is a direct result of decreasing rates of glomerular filtration. In the patient with near cessation of glomerular filtration, serum creatinine can be expected to increase at a rate of about 1.0-1.5 mg/dL/day.[53]

UREA

BUN levels increase as GFRs decrease. In contrast to creatinine, however, urea is partially reabsorbed in the tubules. In hypercatabolic states associated with dehydration, the increases in urea may exceed 25 mg/day.[59]

URIC ACID

Serious increases in plasma uric acid are infrequent in ARF unless it is secondary to rhabdomyolysis.[59] Retention of uric acid is an additional threat to renal function because it may crystallize and obstruct the tubular lumen.

HYPONATREMIA

> **AXIOM** Hyponatremia in oliguric renal failure is largely due to excessive intake of salt-free fluids.

Some degree of hyponatremia is present in the majority of patients with ARF due to excessive intake of salt-poor fluids and to an increased production of endogenous water.[59] If serum sodium concentrations were to decrease rapidly below 125 mEq/L, the signs and symptoms of water intoxication may appear. Urinary sodium concentrations in ARF usually exceed 40 mEq/L and reflect diminished reabsorption of sodium by the acutely damaged tubular epithelium.

Endogenous water of oxidation formed from the catabolism of body fat and protein is normally about 300 mL/day.[59] In oliguric renal failure patients, catabolism of both fat and protein and, therefore, the production of endogenous water may be much greater than in a healthy person. If there is also an increased intake of salt and water, rapid expansion of both the intracellular and extracellular fluid spaces may occur.

HYPERKALEMIA

The marked reduction of urinary potassium excretion in ARF results from decreased GFR and disruption of tubular secretion of potassium into the tubular fluid.[59] In the presence of continuing breakdown of muscle protein, potassium levels in the extracellular fluid can increase quickly in oliguric patients.

> **AXIOM**   Hyperkalemia can rapidly become a life-threatening problem in hypercatabolic patients who are oliguric, particularly when they are also acidotic.

METABOLIC ACIDOSIS

Accelerated protein catabolism because of trauma combined with the declining ability of the kidney to excrete an acid load result in the rapid accumulation of sulfuric, phosphoric, and organic acids.[59] Lactic acidosis may also contribute to this metabolic acidosis, which can become severe enough to require dialysis.

PHOSPHORUS, CALCIUM, AND MAGNESIUM

Plasma phosphorus and magnesium levels increase and calcium levels decrease in acute oliguric renal failure. Hypocalcemia or hypermagnesemia rarely causes symptoms.[59]

Differential Diagnosis of Acute Azotemia and Oliguria

ARF after trauma often occurs in a background of multiorgan damage. The primary goal in the initial evaluation of such patients is to exclude disorders for which prompt specific therapy can be curative.[9,10,59]

URINARY TRACT OBSTRUCTION (POSTRENAL AZOTEMIA)

> **AXIOM**   Obstruction of the urinary tract, particularly in men with prostatic hyperplasia, is the most common cause of sudden cessation of urine output.[59]

The incidence of acute urinary tract obstruction may be increased after trauma because of anticholinergic agents given during anesthesia or urethral swelling occurring secondary to instrumentation.[53] Therefore, anuric or severely oliguric patients should be examined promptly for bladder distention. In a patient without an indwelling catheter, the bladder should be catheterized. Ultrasonography may be used to evaluate upper urinary tract obstruction. If this study were equivocal, CT, radionuclide scanning, or retrograde pyelography may be employed.[110,111]

HYPOVOLEMIA (PRERENAL OLIGURIA)

> **AXIOM**   Early differentiation of prerenal oliguria from intrinsic failure is crucial to reduce the morbidity and mortality associated with ARF.

BUN and Serum Creatinine Levels

Normal kidneys respond to diminished RBF by conserving water and Na^+. In ARF, the GFR is severely decreased and the ability of the kidneys to concentrate urine and conserve Na^+ is impaired.[112] The most prominent effect of filtration failure on blood chemistry is retention of urea and creatinine.

The kidneys excrete creatinine mainly by glomerular filtration. Normally, creatinine is not reabsorbed from the tubules, and only a minute amount is secreted by the distal renal tubular cells. Low GFR in ARF causes decreased creatinine excretion, and the usual daily plasma creatinine increase is 0.5-1.0 mg/dL.[5] After severe trauma, creatinine may increase 2.0-2.5 mg/dL/day.[53,113] The relative daily rate of plasma urea increase exceeds that seen with creatinine.

BUN: Serum Creatinine Ratio

Normally, the BUN-to-plasma-creatinine ratio is 10-15. With accelerated tissue catabolism, this ratio increases. Conversely, with rhabdomyolysis, the ratio tends to decrease because muscle creatine is converted to creatinine.[5]

Creatinine Clearance

> **AXIOM**   Serum creatinine levels may not reflect severe decreases in creatinine clearance or GFR for some time after renal dysfunction has developed.

At very low glomerular filtration rates, some tubular excretion of creatinine by the acutely damaged tubular epithelium also occurs.[114,115] Consequently, creatinine clearance in these instances may overestimate GFR by 100%.[114] For instance, when the actual (inulin) GFR is 15 mL/minute, creatinine clearance may be 30 mL/minute, a value that is still below the normal range.

Creatinine clearance is calculated using the equation:

$$C_{cr} = U_{cr} \times V/P_{cr}$$

where C_{cr} is the creatinine clearance, U_{cr} is the urinary creatinine concentration in mg/dL, V is the urinary flow in mL/minute, and P_{cr} is the plasma creatinine concentration. A 1- or 2-hour creatinine clearance is reasonably accurate when hydration is adequate, urine flow is normal, and serum proteins are normal. Added value accrues when sequential tests are compared with each other.[116] Weinrauch et al. used this assay in traumatized patients and demonstrated that a C_{cr} below 25 mL/minute within 6 hours after trauma often led to renal failure.[58]

U/P Urea and U/P Creatinine Ratios

The ratios of urinary to plasma creatinine (U_{cr}/P_{cr}) and urea (U_{urea}/P_{urea}) concentrations may help to differentiate between prerenal and renal azotemia.[112] Normal U/P creatinine ratio is > 20-30, and normal U/P urea ratio is > 5-10.[53] In prerenal azotemia, the kidney is capable of excreting the maximum amount of creatinine and urea; therefore, both U/P creatinine and urea ratios increase. However, the U/P creatinine ratio is a more reliable index than the U/P urea ratio because part of the filtered urea is reabsorbed by the renal tubules. In ARF, the U/P creatinine and urea ratios usually decrease below 20 and 4, respectively. A U/P urea ratio 8-10 may be observed in patients who are developing renal dysfunction. An infusion of 500-1000 mL crystalloid solution usually results in normalization of the U/P urea ratio in patients who do not have renal impairment.

> **AXIOM**   The U/P urea ratio is low and remains unaltered or decreases when a fluid challenge is given to patients who have already developed ARF.

Urine Sodium Levels

Urinary sodium concentration (U_{Na}) is elevated in ARF because the renal tubules are unable to reabsorb sodium. U_{Na} in excess of 40 mEq/L is common in patients with established ARF. In contrast, in prerenal azotemia, sodium is conserved by the kidney, and the U_{Na} is usually < 10-20 mEq/L.

Renal Failure Index

Simultaneous determination of U_{Na} and U_{cr}/P_{cr} may provide a more accurate differential diagnosis between prerenal azotemia and ARF than either test alone. Handa and Morrin described the "renal failure index" in which the urinary sodium concentration is divided by the U_{cr}/P_{cr} ratio.[122] A value > 1 suggests ATN, whereas a value < 1 usually indicates prerenal azotemia (Table 42-3).

Fractional Excretion of Sodium

The fractional excretion of sodium (FE_{Na}) is an index of tubular Na^+ reabsorption and glomerular filtration. It represents the fraction of the total filtered Na^+ load that is excreted in the urine. This index is calculated according to the following equation:

$$FE_{Na} (\%) = [(U_{Na}/P_{Na}) / (U_{cr}/P_{cr})] \times 100\%$$

An FE_{Na} value $< 1\%$ is consistent with prerenal azotemia, whereas values exceeding 2-3% suggest renal parenchymal damage (Table 42-3). This test requires only simultaneously collected "spot urine" and blood samples. Espinel and Gregory made an accurate diagnosis of renal failure in 86 of 87 patients solely on the basis of FE_{Na} values.[117] Occasionally, FE_{Na} is $< 1\%$ in patients with ARF, especially after burn injury.[118,119] FE_{Na} does not always detect renal dysfunction in nonoliguric patients.[120,121]

Osmolar and Free-water Clearance

The injured kidney is defective in handling water. Impairment of water reabsorption by the tubular epithelium results in isosthenuric urine (specific gravity < 1.010). The amount of plasma containing the solutes excreted in the urine per minute is referred to as osmolar clearance (C_{osm}); urine volume (V) $- C_{osm}$ is the free-water clearance ($C_{H_2O} = V - C_{osm}$). Simultaneous measurement of urinary and plasma osmolality is used to determine osmolar clearance, which may be calculated as:

$$C_{osm} = U_{osm} \times V/P_{osm}$$

where U_{osm} is the urinary osmolality, V is the urinary flow in mL/min, and P_{osm} is the plasma osmolality. C_{H_2O} has a negative value when the urine is hypertonic, and a positive value when the urine is hypotonic. In a normally functioning kidney the value of C_{osm} is greater than that of urinary volume (V). Thus, the normal C_{H_2O} is -15 to -50 mL/hour. In ARF, C_{osm} decreases, and the C_{H_2O} moves toward a positive value. Monitoring of C_{H_2O} and C_{osm} in the traumatized patient during the early postoperative period may predict the development of ARF. By using this test, Baek et al. were able to predict ARF in 93% of their patients 48 hours before establishment of the diagnosis by other criteria.[123] C_{H_2O} in ARF usually ranges -15 to $+15$ mL/hour; however, a markedly positive C_{H_2O} value ($> +60$ mL/hour) may be observed immediately after reversal of shock. Therefore, under such circumstances, it is not predictive of ARF.

> **AXIOM** Changes in free-water clearance can be used to help predict the onset of ARF but are much more accurate when used in conjunction with creatinine clearance.

The observation that free-water clearance can be used to predict the onset of ARF before the development of oliguria has been supported by several studies.[4,124,125] However, Shin et al. demonstrated in severely injured patients that the C_{cr} during the first 6 hours after surgery was a more sensitive index than the C_{H_2O}.[121] Simultaneous measurement of C_{cr} and C_{H_2O} has been suggested to reinforce the reliability of C_{H_2O} as an early predictor of ARF.[124]

Urinalysis

Considerable differences exist between urinary indices in oliguric and nonoliguric ARF. A high urinary specific gravity (> 1.025) is generally inconsistent with acute tubular necrosis or obstructive uropathy and suggests a diagnosis of prerenal azotemia.[59] However, elevated urinary specific gravity may occur in patients with ATN when increased glucose, protein, contrast dye, or mannitol is present in urine.

Heavy proteinuria is suggestive of primary glomerular disease.[59] Prerenal azotemia or extrarenal urinary obstruction is not characterized by significant proteinuria. With acute allergic interstitial nephritis, sterile pyuria is frequently present and the demonstration of eosinophils in the urinary sediment is almost diagnostic. Urine in prerenal azotemia and obstructive uropathy is usually unremarkable except for hyaline casts.

In patients with ATN, it is common for urine to contain granular casts, white blood cells, tubular cells, and trace protein, especially when oliguria is present.[59] Gross hematuria is unusual in ATN and suggests bilateral renal arterial occlusion or obstruction. A positive dipstick for heme or red-brown pigmentation of the urine in the absence of red blood cells suggests renal failure secondary to hemoglobin or myoglobin.

Summary and Cautions

> **AXIOM** Single laboratory determinations of blood and urinary indices may be misleading when attempting to perform a differential diagnosis of the cause of oliguria.

Urine and renal function tests should be performed at 2-4-hour intervals to ensure accurate diagnosis of ATN.[121,124] Measurements of serum creatinine or BUN taken immediately after an abrupt decrease in GFR, such as after hemorrhagic shock, can be misleading. BUN and plasma creatinine increase slowly after a sudden decline in GFR, and it usually takes several hours for these indices to reflect the new steady-state GFR.

> **AXIOM** Before making a diagnosis of ARF, a fluid bolus should be given to eliminate hypovolemia.

If renal failure is developing and the patient is not already overloaded with fluid, an intravenous fluid challenge of 500-1000 mL of normal saline should be administered over 15-30 minutes. If urine output were to fail to increase, a Swan-Ganz catheter should be inserted to monitor additional fluid challenges.

TREATMENT OF ACUTE RENAL FAILURE

General Management

The importance of rapidly correcting hypovolemia and removing aggravating factors has already been stressed; however, when a reasonable urine output can be obtained, prognosis is improved and management is greatly simplified.

DIURETICS

> **AXIOM** Indiscriminate use of diuretics in trauma patients with oliguria may precipitate the development of ATN. When hypovolemia has been eliminated, diuretics may have both a diagnostic and therapeutic value in early oliguric renal failure.

When hypovolema has been eliminated, diuretics given within the first day or two of oliguria may favorably alter the course of ARF.[129] The other theoretical advantage is that successful diuresis may convert oliguric renal failure to the nonoliguric variety that has a much better prognosis.

Mannitol

Mannitol is an osmotic diuretic that decreases proximal tubular sodium reabsorption.[59] Purported beneficial effects include an increase in GFR, a decrease in renin secretion, and a washout of any tubular casts.[130] More likely, mannitol functions solely as an osmotic diuretic.

Mannitol administration (25 g intravenous bolus) may be beneficial when given during the onset of oliguric renal failure after circulatory insufficiency has been eliminated. Mannitol facilitates intratubular hydration in patients with muscle injury, mismatched transfusion, intravascular hemolysis, and acute hyperuricemia.[131]

Furosemide

Furosemide is a loop diuretic that acts primarily by inhibiting active sodium and chloride transport in the medullary, thick ascending limb of Henle.[59] One must correct hypovolemia before giving furosemide. Failure to do so may precipitate ATN in a patient with otherwise reversible prerenal oliguria. Although it is reported to increase RBF and modulate renin secretion by the macula densa, furosemide probably functions only as a loop diuretic.[132,133] Furosemide is given as a bolus followed by doubling the dose every 15 minutes if no diuresis results. The recommended maximum total dose to reverse impending oliguric renal failure is 2 g.

Dopamine

Dopamine, when infused intravenously at a dose of 1-3 mcg/kg/min, is reported to increase total RBF and shift blood flow from the renal medulla to the cortex.[134] More likely, diuresis and natriuresis seen after low-dose dopamine infusion are due to the effects of dopamine on ADH.

Fluid and Electrolyte Balance

SODIUM AND WATER

AXIOM   Fluid restriction is an important part of the treatment of established acute oliguric renal failure but this must be placed in perspective according to other organ function and total body needs.

The daily fluid requirement for a patient with established acute oliguric renal failure is equivalent to measured losses from the gastrointestinal (GI) tract and kidneys plus either two-thirds of the estimated insensible water loss or 600 mL/day, whichever is less.[59] Provision of water in excess of this amount can rapidly lead to volume expansion and hyponatremia. Accurate daily weights and measurement of intake and output are essential. Sodium intake in patients with ARF should be limited to measured losses. However, even when the total body content of sodium increases, serum sodium levels may be decreased because of dilution.[136,137] Maximum water and sodium retention usually occurs during the first two days following acute posttraumatic oliguric renal failure and persists 4-7 days[138]; however, it may not be possible or practical to restrict fluid in catabolic trauma patients because of their high caloric and protein needs.

A mild degree of fluid overload may usually be treated with fluid restriction. However, serum sodium levels < 125 mEq/L may require therapy with hypertonic (3%) saline and diuretics or dialysis. With more severe fluid overload in patients who still have some urine output, large doses of loop diuretics may be used to prevent pulmonary edema. A less frequently used therapy to remove excess water is oral sorbitol 70% (2 mL/kg) or rectal sorbitol 20% (10 mL/kg) provided that no trauma to the gastrointestinal tract exists. When the above treatments are not effective, emergency dialysis or continuous arteriovenous hemofiltration (CAVH) may be necessary.

METABOLIC ACIDOSIS

In normal adults who consume an average diet, approximately 1 mEq/kg of nonvolatile acid is produced daily by metabolism. Hypercatabolic patients with trauma may generate larger acid loads so that serum HCO_3 levels decline more rapidly. The specific cations released during catabolism include sulfate and a number of organic acids, including lactic acid. The accumulation of these ions in the body results in the development of an anion gap acidosis. Bicarbonate administration can help to correct this acidosis, but the amount of bicarbonate that can be given is limited by the concomitant sodium load.

AXIOM   Severe metabolic acidosis of established acute oliguric renal failure is best treated with dialysis, not sodium bicarbonate.

Reversal of severe metabolic acidosis is preferably accomplished by dialysis. Abrupt correction of this acidosis in patients with hypocalcemia can precipitate tetany. Therefore, acidosis should be corrected gradually and supplemental calcium should be administered as needed.

HYPERKALEMIA

AXIOM   Hyperkalemia is the most rapidly fatal complication of acute oliguric renal failure.

Etiology

Hyperkalemia is a frequent cause of death in patients with ARF.[138] Even when potassium intake is restricted, hyperkalemia is a hazard, especially when tissue breakdown and metabolic acidosis coexist. Blood transfusions add to this hazard. Renal tubular acidosis accentuates hyperkalemia. With each 0.1 unit decrease in pH, an increase of about 0.5 in serum K^+ levels occurs.

AXIOM   Metabolic acidosis can cause hyperkalemia even when respiratory compensation restores pH to normal.

Hyperkalemia may accompany hyperosmolemia. Thus, hyperkalemia may occur in oliguric patients with acute head injury treated with mannitol. Other factors that may cause hyperkalemia include β-adrenergic receptor blockers, blood transfusions, salt substitutes, captopril, and nonsteroidal antiinflammatory drugs.

Diagnosis

Hyperkalemia is defined as a serum potassium level > 5.5 mEq/L. Hyperkalemia causes peaked T waves and prolongation of PR and QRS intervals. Early ECG changes of hyperkalemia require prompt therapy.

AXIOM   Hyponatremia, hypocalcemia, and acidosis increase the cardiotoxic effects of hyperkalemia. These should be corrected promptly.

Treatment

AXIOM   The treatment of hyperkalemia is directed at antagonizing the effect of K^+ on the cardiac conduction system, shifting K^+ intracellularly, and removing K^+ from the body.

CALCIUM.   A calcium infusion moderates the effects of K^+ on myocardial membrane potentials, myocardial threshold, and cardiac conduction without lowering serum K^+ levels. Such therapy with intravenous $CaCl_2$ transiently raises serum Ca^{++} levels.[139]

BICARBONATE.   Potassium can be shifted into cells by administration of alkali ($NaHCO_3$ 8.4%, 50-100 mL) which raises pH.

GLUCOSE AND INSULIN.   The hypokalemic effect of glucose and insulin is concentration-dependent[140]; therefore, intermittent bolus insulin injections (plus glucose) every few hours is more effective than a continuous infusion. Serum K^+ can also be reduced by inducing respiratory alkalosis; for each 0.1 unit increase in pH, serum potassium levels decrease about 0.5 mEq/L.

KAYEXALATE.   Kayexalate (50 g) given orally or rectally every 2-3 hours decreases the total body potassium pool.[5] Because resin releases sodium in exchange for potassium, one must monitor the effects of sodium on central volume.

AXIOM   Kayexelate must be used carefully in hypervolemic patients.

DIALYSIS. Hemodialysis can extract 100-200 mEq/L of K^+ in 4 hours. This maintains appropriate K^+ levels in most patients. Hypercatabolic and acidotic patients may require more frequent dialysis.

CALCIUM ABNORMALITIES IN ARF

Shortly after the onset of ARF, plasma phosphate levels start to increase and Ca^{++} levels start to decline[5]; calcitonin and parathyroid hormone concentrations also increase.[141] Tetany rarely occurs in ARF patients with hypocalcemia unless total serum calcium levels decrease below 6.0 mg/dl. Metabolic acidosis increases the concentration of ionized calcium and thus offers some protection against tetany.

Medication Adjustments in Renal Failure

Loss of renal function requires dosage adjustment of all drugs that are excreted by the kidneys. Therapeutic concentrations also vary with hemodialysis and to a lesser degree with peritoneal dialysis.

> **AXIOM** Throughout the period of renal failure and during the subsequent recovery phase, drugs given must be selected and doses administered with great care to provide maximum benefit without aggravating renal dysfunction.

Complications

GASTROINTESTINAL COMPLICATIONS

Stress gastric ulcers develop in up to 20% of ARF patients and contribute to the mortality from this disease.[142] They may result from a number of factors, including elevated gastrin levels.[143] Aluminum hydroxide antacids not only decrease gastric acidity and the risk of peptic ulcer disease but can also help to control hyperphosphatemia, which is a common finding in ARF. Constipation caused by aluminum-containing antacids may be minimized by administering them with sorbitol.

Magnesium-containing antacids should not be given because of their potential for causing magnesium toxicity. Cimetidine can also prevent stress ulceration; however, it can cause mental confusion and encephalopathy, especially in elderly patients with ARF.[144]

ANEMIA

Anemia develops in severe oliguric ARF because of reduced serum erythropoietin levels.[5] Other factors, such as gastrointestinal bleeding and hemolysis, may contribute to anemia. Consequently, hematocrit should be measured frequently and anemia corrected with packed red blood cell transfusions as needed. With the recent introduction of erythropoietin as therapy for the anemia of chronic renal failure, the need for blood transfusions in these patients should decrease.

PLATELET DYSFUNCTION

> **AXIOM** Even when the platelet count is normal, bleeding time should be measured before any invasive or surgical procedure is undertaken in a patient with renal failure.

Bleeding secondary to platelet dysfunction is common in ARF patients. Dialysis may ameliorate this problem.[145] Prolonged bleeding time is improved with cryoprecipitate[20] or 1-deamino-8-D-arginine vasopressin (DDAVP) given as a 0.3 mcg/kg bolus in 50 mL normal saline for 30 minutes before a procedure.[146] Some success has also been reported with the use of intravenous conjugated estrogens which have a longer half-life than DDAVP.

Trauma victims often receive massive transfusions that cause dilution thrombocytopenia.[147,148] Injured ARF patients frequently have both a qualitative and quantitative platelet defect. Transfusion of platelet concentrates may reverse this defect.

INFECTIONS

Sepsis and associated multiple organ failure account for most trauma deaths after 48 hours.[149] Unfortunately, the diagnosis of sepsis may be difficult because severe trauma, burns, and ARF impair host defenses. The usual signs of infection, such as fever, leukocytosis, and local inflammation, may be minimal or absent.

> **AXIOM** The only indication of sepsis in patients with ARF may be progressive multiorgan failure.

Urinary tract or pulmonary infections are common in ARF patients. Consequently, indwelling bladder catheters should be removed at the earliest opportunity. Likewise, good pulmonary physiotherapy is helpful. Another major source of infection is phlebitis, especially from central venous cannulas.

PERICARDITIS AND PERICARDIAL OR PLEURAL EFFUSION

Pericarditis, with or without pleuritis or pleural effusion, also occurs in patients with ARF.[150] The clinical picture of acute pericarditis secondary to ARF has a wide spectrum. Pericardial friction rub is the most common clinical finding; this usually disappears as the effusion increases in size. Chest pain is seldom a dominant feature. Fever with or without leukocytosis is likely.

> **AXIOM** If cardiac failure or hypotension were to develop in a patient with chronic renal failure, one should suspect pericardial effusion with tamponade.

Pericardial tamponade is a well recognized complication of ARF.[151] Uremic pericardial tamponade can cause signs of acute right-sided heart failure with elevated jugular venous pressure, hepatic enlargement, generalized edema, and pulsus paradoxus. Systemic hypotension occasionally occurs and may cause cerebral ischemia.

Treatment of uremic pericarditis is directed toward treating the uremia with dialysis. Hypovolemia after dialysis or ultrafiltration, however, is a potential hazard. If cardiac tamponade were to occur, a pericardial window and/or pericardiectomy may be required.

Nutritional Support

Nutrition is important in patients with ARF. Nutritional support may be complicated by high-energy requirements, insulin resistance, and negligible free-water and urea clearance. Supplemental carbohydrate is provided to minimize protein breakdown. Fluid overload is prevented by infusing a 35%-glucose solution. Essential amino acids are infused to maintain nitrogen needs. These hypertonic solutions often have a caloric-nitrogen ratio exceeding 450 to 1 with a high proportion of essential amino acids.

Nutritional support is best when administered orally in a volume compatible with the cardiovascular system. Unless the patient had nutritional problems before the onset of ARF, hyperalimentation can be delayed for several days. Each 6.25 g of protein contains 1 g of nitrogen. Thus, patients with severe ARF receiving hyperalimentation may rapidly accumulate significant amounts of nitrogenous waste products. Amino acid loss during hemodialysis averages 10-15 g per run. CAVH mobilizes about 6 g every 12-24 hours. Because they are lost into the dialysate outflow, water-soluble vitamins must be replaced after dialysis.

> **AXIOM** When nutritional protein causes BUN to increase rapidly, dialysis or CAVH helps control BUN while adequate nutrition is provided.

Large volumes of hyperalimentation solutions may be required to maintain adequate nutrition in severely hypercatabolic patients. Intralipid infusions may be added 2-3 times per week.[152] To maintain fluid balance in such patients, daily hemodialysis or CAVH may be necessary. The injured patient with ARF also may develop phosphate, potassium, and magnesium depletion requiring dietary supplementation.

Renal Support

BEDSIDE ULTRAFILTRATION

AXIOM When injured patients develop oliguria and impaired renal function, fluid and electrolyte abnormalities can often be treated by bedside continuous arteriovenous hemofiltration.

CAVH, using small hollow-fiber hemofilters without pumps, is an alternative to conventional acute dialysis methods.[154] Arterial blood, usually from the radial artery, passes through an ultrafiltration apparatus by the force of the patient's BP and then returns to the patient usually via a cephalic or brachial vein line.

AXIOM CAVH provides a slow, continuous removal of fluid and unwanted solutes and avoids fluid and electrolyte shifts that are poorly tolerated in unstable trauma patients.

CAVH causes little or no hemodynamic change and is useful in ARF patients who develop hypotension during standard hemodialysis. Another important advantage of this method is that filtrate removal of up to 500-800 mL/hour permits administration of large volumes of parenteral nutrition solutions needed by hypercatabolic oliguric patients without the risk of volume overload. Thus, CAVH can produce space for intravenous medications and more aggressive use of intravenous or enteral nutrition.

AXIOM Continuous arteriovenous hemofiltration is *not* a substitute for hemodialysis in trauma patients with ARF and uremia.

CAVH requires continuous heparinization and constant supervision. A Scribner shunt (radial artery to vein or femoral artery to vein) facilitates CAVH, but this shunt uses an important artery that makes subsequent use for long-term dialysis problematic. Vascular access can be obtained by venovenous shunts with a double-lumen catheter via either a subclavian or femoral vein. Femoral catheters can be placed for at least one week and subclavian catheters for as long as three weeks. Complications are minimal, but include bleeding, hypovolemia, hypotension, and infection.

HEMOPERFUSION

Charcoal hemoperfusion is used infrequently in the treatment of ARF. However, impressive results have been obtained in patients with fulminant hepatic failure (hepatorenal syndrome) using this technique. Prostacyclin can be used to prevent platelet activation during hemoperfusion.[155]

HEMODIALYSIS

Hemodialysis, the mainstay of therapy for ARF, is urgently needed in patients who have (a) refractory pulmonary edema, (b) hyperkalemic crises, (c) uremic encephalopathy, (d) uremic complications, such as pericarditis, or (e) symptomatic derangements of azotemia and acidosis.[156]

The beneficial role of hemodialysis in ARF has been confirmed by epidemiologic studies showing a mortality rate of 25% in fully dialyzed patients versus 73% in sporadically dialyzed patients and 90% in nondialyzed patients.[157] Prophylactic dialysis may further reduce mortality.[158]

AXIOM Hemodialysis, done prophylactically, is beneficial in the hemodynamically stable patient, with severe ARF.

Hemodialysis rapidly corrects uremia, fluid and electrolyte disturbances, and acidosis. Routine "prophylactic" dialysis simplifies management by liberalizing water and electrolyte restriction and enhances the well-being of the patient by keeping the levels of urea and other nitrogenous substances at more normal levels.[59] Perhaps the greatest benefit of aggressive or prophylactic hemodialysis is the provision of adequate calories and nutrition to minimize catabolism and promote wound healing.

Severe hypoxemia may develop during hemodialysis. This is largely due to complement activation and an increased adherence of platelets and polymorphonuclear leukocytes to pulmonary capillary endothelium. Thus, hypoxia and thrombocytopenia may appear during the first hour of dialysis.[159] These values usually return to baseline within 2 hours after treatment.

Other complications of hemodialysis include hypotension, hypoxemia, hemorrhage, arrhythmias, and problems related to technical errors (e.g., air embolism, dialysate contamination). "Disequilibrium syndrome," manifest by headache, nausea, vomiting, disorientation, tremors, and increased CSF pressure, may also appear with hemodialysis. These symptoms are probably caused by cerebral edema due to sudden changes in the osmotic gradient between brain and blood during hemodialysis.[30] Paradoxical acidosis may also develop in the CSF during hemodialysis and cause similar symptoms.[160] Elevation of ICP has been described in head-injured patients during dialysis.[161] Thus, ICP monitoring may be necessary in these patients.

AXIOM Hemodialysis must be performed with extreme caution in patients with increased ICP.

Hypotension, which is common during hemodialysis, can result from excessive fluid removal, sudden osmolar changes, plasticizer infusion, blood-membrane incompatibility, or acetate toxicity.[5,162]

AXIOM Even mild hypovolemia can cause severe hypotension when hemodialysis is started.

Bleeding from heparin anticoagulation during hemodialysis can be reduced by using a constant low-dose heparin infusion to maintain activated clotting time or PTT twice normal. Occasionally, it may be necessary to use protamine in the venous return channel of the dialysis system. Other dangers with hemodialysis include infected or thrombosed arteriovenous shunts or grafts. Careful attention to detail regarding these frustrating problems increases the likelihood of a successful outcome.

PERITONEAL DIALYSIS

AXIOM Peritoneal dialysis, although slower than hemodialysis, has the advantages of widespread availability, technical simplicity, and a low incidence of complications.

Peritoneal dialysis is the treatment of choice in ARF involving children, GI bleeding, shock, acute myocardial infarction, and acute pancreatitis. Contraindications include abdominal sepsis or recent laparotomy for abdominal trauma. Hypercatabolic patients cannot be adequately dialyzed by this technique.[164] Complications of peritoneal dialysis include peritonitis and compromised pulmonary function.

Diuretic Phase of Oliguric ATN

Most patients who survive acute oliguric ARF can expect return of adequate renal function in three weeks.[156] Once the oliguric phase has passed and the patient enters the diuretic phase, the likelihood for survival is greatly increased, but one must still be careful to prevent recurrent hypotension, hypokalemia, or hyponatremia due to persistent impaired tubular reabsorption of free water and electrolytes. When polyuria manifests, serum and urinary electrolytes and body weight must be measured at least daily. In most patients, diuresis and natriuresis appear to be secondary to excretion of edema fluid; however, diuresis can also reduce the effective intravascular volume. Large urinary potassium losses may require supplementation during the polyuric phase.

The duration of dialysis for ARF does not appear to correlate with the degree of functional recovery, but the patient's age does. Older patients progress to chronic renal failure much more often and rarely make a complete recovery.[138] Of the 50% of patients who survive acute oliguric renal failure, 15% recover completely, 25% have incomplete but stable recovery of renal function for the rest of their lives, 5% have renal recovery but progress gradually to endstage renal disease, and 5% have no renal recovery and must be treated for endstage renal disease.

Nonoliguric Acute Renal Failure

The incidence of nonoliguric ATN is increasing.[166,167] This increase is probably related to (a) earlier and more aggressive fluid resuscitation and (b) an increased incidence of nephrotoxin-induced ATN. With more frequent monitoring of blood levels of nephrotoxic substances, milder forms of nonoliguric ARF are diagnosed with greater accuracy. The use of diuretics may also convert some cases of early oliguric ATN to a nonoliguric form.

Generally, management of nonoliguric patients is easier than of those with oliguric ARF because they have fewer fluid, electrolyte, and acid-base abnormalities.[113] Few of these patients require dialysis and nonoliguric ATN has a lower mortality rate.[168,169]

Prognosis of Acute Renal Failure Following Trauma

Mortality rates in trauma patients developing ARF still exceed 50-60%; sepsis is the most frequent contributor to death.[135,138] The development of sepsis-induced ARF after trauma is particularly lethal and carries a reported mortality of 90%.[170] Other factors include CHF, hyperkalemia, respiratory failure, and GI hemorrhage. Ominous prognostic factors include shock, respiratory failure, GI hemorrhage, CHF, ascites, myocardial infarction, and peritonitis.[171]

Although ARF after trauma is usually self-limited, many survivors have long-term impaired renal function.[54,138,172] The best recovery of renal function is found in younger patients with shorter periods of oliguria.[131]

SUMMARY

The renal changes with trauma, hypovolemia, and sepsis are complex. Many factors act together to cause extravascular sequestration of fluid following trauma, thereby reducing intravascular volume and decreasing RBF. Aggressively correcting hypovolemia and restoring renal perfusion along with prevention or avoidance drugs or tests associated with an increased incidence of ARF are essential.[173]

The overall mortality in ARF is high, although early corrective therapy is beneficial. Trauma patients may develop ARF not only because of the initial hypovolemic insult but also from later drug- or contrast-medium-induced nephrotoxicity.

Improved hyperalimentation, antibiotic therapy, and meticulous attention to drug therapy offer the best chances for survival.

Any additional insult to the kidneys during the course of ARF carries a poor prognosis. Careful preoperative evaluation and preparation, use of regional anesthetic methods whenever possible, adequate perioperative monitoring, elimination of potential risk factors, and appropriate use of anesthetic and adjunct drugs are some of the important principles of management for these patients.

In the future, synthetic or recombinant proteolytic inhibitors may be of some benefit in injured patients with ARF.[174] Continuing research on endothelin,[175,176] endothelium-derived relaxing factor, and calcium entry blockers[177,178] may also have an impact on future treatment.

⊘ FREQUENT ERRORS

Made in the Prevention, Diagnosis, and Treatment of Acute Renal Failure after Trauma

1. *Assuming that oliguria occurs on the basis of renal failure without adequately eliminating hypovolemia and mechanical obstruction.*
2. *Assuming that elevated central venous pressure indicates adequate blood volume.*
3. *Failing to appreciate that a large volume of urine does not necessarily mean volume overload.*
4. *Failing to recognize that polyuria without adequate fluid replacement may result in severe plasma volume deficit and acute oliguric vasomotor nephropathy.*
5. *Restricting sodium in patients who were already volume- or sodium-depleted prior to injury or operation.*
6. *Administering loop diuretics when not necessary and without being careful to maintain an adequate circulating volume.*
7. *Failing to maintain high-volume urine flow during extensive operative manipulations.*
8. *Failing to be aggressive in the control of sepsis by early drainage, debridement, and appropriate antibiotics.*
9. *Administering potassium-containing fluids before ascertaining that renal function is adequate.*
10. *Restricting fluids in the hopes of preventing pulmonary insufficiency in an oliguric patient.*
11. *Failing to carefully monitor fluid and electrolyte balance during the recovery (diuretic) phase of acute vasomotor nephropathy.*

▼▼▼▼▼▼▼▼▼▼▼▼▼▼▼▼▼▼▼▼▼▼▼▼▼▼▼▼▼

SUMMARY POINTS

1. Prolonged shock can interfere with the kidney's ability to preserve water and sodium for at least several hours after renal perfusion is reestablished.
2. During hypovolemia, the combination of increased RVR, decreased RBF, and decreased GFR results in salt and water conservation which augments the total homeostatic response to the hemorrhagic insult.
3. Oliguria and reduced sodium excretion immediately following trauma are generally due to hypovolemia and should not be treated by diuretics.
4. Mannitol used to treat head trauma may cause renal failure if the patient is hypovolemic and oliguric.
5. Protection of the kidney during emergency surgery after acute trauma is best provided by administering enough fluid preoperatively to achieve a urine output of at least 2 mL/minute without diuretics.
6. Intraoperative protection of renal function is best achieved by improving the cardiovascular status by the early administration of BES and blood as needed.
7. Polyuria immediately following surgery on a patient who had been hypotensive before or during surgery is usually due to renal changes during hypotension and not fluid overload.
8. Following shock and its resuscitation, a period of obligatory extravascular fluid sequestration occurs that can cause hypovolemia if inadequate fluids are given.
9. Even with adequate fluid resuscitation, urine flow may be somewhat reduced postoperatively because of persistent renal vasoconstriction.
10. Current therapeutic guidelines for postresuscitative hypertension include fluid restriction with avoidance of all colloids but no longer include aggressive diuresis to reduce BP to normal levels.

11. Any hypotension developing during the obligatory extravascular sequestration fluid mobilization phases can be extremely detrimental to the kidneys.

12. Based upon the renal response to colloid resuscitation, HSA should no longer be used during the fluid sequestration phase.

13. CMV and PEEP are much less apt to have deleterious cardiac and renal effects when the patient is hypervolemic.

14. PEEP tends to reduce the formation of ANF, causing even further reductions in urine output.

15. Arterial metabolic acidosis tends to persist to some degree for several hours after shock has been corrected by adequate fluid resuscitation.

16. No resuscitation solution returns pH to normal in patients with severe hemorrhagic shock until fluid resuscitation and oxygen delivery are adequate.

17. The polyuria of sepsis can cause abrupt, severe hypovolemia when the fluid intake is restricted because of an impression that the patient is overloaded with fluid.

18. When a patient with a severe infection has been appropriately resuscitated, the kidneys share in the hyperdynamic state of sepsis.

19. A "normal" urine output of 0.5 mL/kg/hour may not be adequate in septic patients.

20. High-urine output with a urine sodium concentration < 10 mEq/L may indicate the polyuria of sepsis is present in spite of significant hypovolemia.

21. ARF due to hemoglobinuria or myoglobinuria is unlikely unless the patient is hypotensive and has acidic urine.

22. Renal function, especially creatinine clearance, should be monitored closely in patients receiving prolonged courses or high doses of aminoglycosides.

23. High-urine output should be maintained in patients who are at risk for developing contrast-medium-induced nephrotoxicity.

24. The most common cause of oliguria after injury is decreased renal perfusion due to inadequate or delayed fluid resuscitation.

25. Prompt recognition and therapy of urinary tract obstruction are necessary to prevent renal parenchymal damage.

26. Early differentiation of prerenal oliguria from intrinsic renal failure is crucial to reduce morbidity and mortality following trauma.

27. The U/P urea ratio is low and remains unaltered or decreases in patients with established ARF when a fluid challenge is given.

28. Before making a diagnosis of ARF, a fluid bolus should be given to be absolutely certain that hypovolemia is not present.

29. Indiscriminate use of diuretics in trauma patients with oliguria may actually precipitate ATN in the patient with prerenal azotemia. However, when hypovolemia is eliminated, such agents may have both diagnostic and therapeutic value.

30. The treatment of acute oliguric renal failure centers around fluid restriction, but this must be placed in perspective according to other organ function and total body needs.

31. Hyperkalemia is the most rapidly fatal complication of ARF.

32. Metabolic acidosis can still cause hyperkalemia even though respiratory compensation corrects the pH to normal.

33. Throughout the period of ARF and during the subsequent recovery phase, antibiotics and other drugs must be selected with great care to provide maximum benefit without aggravating the renal status.

34. When injured patients develop oliguria and impaired renal function, fluid and electrolyte abnormalities can often be treated by bedside continuous hemofiltration.

35. CAVH can provide a slow, continuous removal of fluid and may avoid fluid and electrolyte shifts that are poorly tolerated in unstable trauma patients.

36. CAVH is not a substitute for hemodialysis in trauma patients with ARF and uremia.

37. Hemodialysis must be performed with caution in patients who may have increased ICP or who may be hypovolemic.

▲▲▲▲▲▲▲▲▲▲▲▲▲▲▲▲▲▲▲▲▲▲▲▲▲▲▲▲▲▲▲

REFERENCES

1. Hope A, Clausen G, Aukland K. Intrarenal distribution of blood flow in rats determined by 125I-iodoantipyrine uptake. Circ Res 1976;39: 362-370.
2. Barsoum RS, Payne JL, Inagaki M. Halothane-induced renal vasodilation. Anesthesiology 1981;50:609.
3. Ghoneheim MM, Pandya H. Plasma protein binding of thiopental in patients with impaired renal or hepatic function. Anesthesiology 1975;42:545.
4. Landes RG, Lillehei RC, Lindsay WG, et al. Free-water clearance and the early recognition of acute renal insufficiency after cardiopulmonary bypass. Ann Thorac Surg 1976;22:41.
5. McGoldrick MD, Capan LM. Acute renal failure in the injured. Capan LM, Miller SM, Turndorf H, eds. Anesthesia and intensive care. Philadelphia: JB Lippincott Co, 1991; 755-785.
6. Lucas CE, Ledgerwood AM. Hemodynamic management of the injured. Capan LM, Miller SM, Turndorf H, eds. Anesthesia and intensive care. Philadelphia: JB Lippincott Co, 1991; 83-113.
7. Dunn MJ, Hood VL. Prostaglandins and the kidney. Am J Physiol 1977;233:F169-F184.
8. Hayes DF, Werner MH, Rosenberg IK, Lucas CE, Westreich M, Bradley V. Effects of traumatic hypovolemic shock on renal function. J Surg Res 1974;16:490-497.
9. Lucas CE. The renal response to acute injury and sepsis. Surg Clin North Am 1976;56:953.
10. Lucas CE. Renal considerations in the injured patient. Surg Clin North Am 1982;62:133.
11. Lucas CE. Resuscitation of the injured patient: The three phases of treatment. Surg Clin North Am 1977;57:3.
12. Lynam DP, Cronnelly R, Castagnoli KP, et al. The pharmacodynamics and pharmacokinetics of vecuronium in patients anesthetized with isoflurane with normal renal function or with renal failure. Anesthesiology 1988;69:227.
13. Maguire WC, Anderson RJ. Continuous arteriovenous hemofiltration in the intensive care unit. J Crit Care 1986;1:54.
14. Glassock RJ, Conen AJ, Bennett CM, et al. Primary glomerular diseases. Brenner BM, Rector FC, eds. The kidney, 2nd ed. Philadelphia: WB Saunders Publishing, 1981; 1351.
15. Miller ED, Kistner JR, Epstein RM. Whole-body distribution of radioactively labelled microspheres in the rat during anesthesia with halothane, enflurane, or ketamine. Anesthesiology 1980;52:296.
16. Donohoe JF. Acute bilateral cortical necrosis. Brenner BM, Lazarus MS, eds. Acute renal failure. Philadelphia: WB Saunders Publishing, 1983; 252.
17. Sladen RN, Endo E, Harrison T. Two-hour versus 22-hour creatinine clearance in critically ill patients. Anesthesiology 1987;67:103.
18. Handa SP. Acute renal failure in association with hyperurecemia: its recovery with ethacynic acid. South Med J 1971;64:676.
19. Hobika GH, Evers JL, Mostert JW, et al. Comparison of hemodynamic effects of glucagon and ketamine in patients with chronic renal failure. Anesthesiology 1972;37:654.
20. Janson PA, Jubeliker SJ, Weinstein MJ, et al. Treatment of the bleeding tendency in uremia with cryoprecipitate. N Engl J Med 1980;303:1318.
21. Berry AJ, Geer RT, Marshall C, et al. The effect of long term controlled mechanical ventilation with positive end expiratory pressure on renal function in dogs. Anesthesiology 1984;61:406.
22. Marquez JM, Douglas ME, Downs JB, et al. Renal function and cardiovascular responses during positive airway pressure. Anesthesiology 1979;50:393.
23. Priebe HJ, Heiman JC, Headley-Whyte J. Mechanisms of renal dysfunction during positive end-expiratory pressure ventilation. J Appl Physiol 1981;50:643.
24. Adams AP. Enflurane in clinical practice. Br J Anaesth 1981;53:27S.
25. Annest SJ, Scovill WA, Blumenstock PA, et al. Increased creatinine clearance following cryoprecipitate infusion in trauma and surgical patients with decreased renal function. J Trauma 1980;20:276.
26. Cousins MJ, Skowronski G, Plummer JL. Anaesthesia and the kidney. Anaesth Intens Care 1983;11:292.
27. Mazze RI. Fluorinated anaesthetic nephrotoxicity: an update. Can Anaesth Soc J 1984;31:S16.
28. Shafi T, Chou S, Porush JG, et al. Infusion intravenous pyelography and renal function. Arch Intern Med 1978;138:1218.
29. Philbin DM, Coggins CH. Plasma antidiuretic hormone levels in cardiac surgical patients during morphine and halothane anesthesia. Anesthesiology 1978;49:95.

30. Walkin KG. The pathophysiology of the dialysis disequilibrium syndrome. Mayo Clin Proc 1969;44:406.

31. Fish K, Sievenpiper T, Rice SA, et al. Renal function in Fischer 344 rats with chronic renal impairment after administration of enflurane and gentamicin. Anesthesiology 1980;53:481.

32. Powell DR, Miller RD. The effects of repeated doses of succinylcholine on serum potassium in patients with renal failure. Anesth Analg 1975;54:746.

33. Eknoyan G, Wacksman SJ, Glueck HI, et al. Platelet function in renal failure. N Engl J Med 1969;280:677.

34. Fraley DS, Adler S. Isohydric regulation of plasma potassium by bicarbonate in the rat. Kidney Int 1976;9:333.

35. Cattell WR, Fry IK. Urography in acute renal failure. Am Heart J 1975;90:124.

36. Quebbeman EJ, Maierhofer WJ, Piering WF. Mechanisms producing hypoxemia during hemodialysis. Crit Care Med 1984;12:359.

37. Halpern M, Bear R, Goldstein MB, et al. Interpretation of the serum potassium concentration in metabolic acidosis. Clin Invest Med 1979;2:55.

38. Miller RD, Matteo RS, Benet LZ, et al. The pharmocokinetics of d-tubocurarine in man with and without renal failure. J Pharmacol Exp Ther 1977;202:1.

39. Martin R, Beauregard L, Tetrault JP. Brachial plexus blockade and chronic renal failure. Anesthesiology 1988;69:405.

40. Myers BD, Moran SM. Hemodynamically mediated acute renal failure. N Engl J Med 1986;314:97.

41. Tobimatsu M, Ueda Y, Saito S, et al. Effects of a stable prostacyclin analog on experimental ischemic-acute renal failure. Ann Surg 1988;208:65.

42. Ward S, Boheimer N, Weatherley BC, et al. Pharmacokinetics of atracurium and its metabolites in patients with normal renal function, and in patients in renal failure. Br J Anesth 1987;59:697.

43. Wacker W, Merrill JP. Uremic pericarditis in acute renal failure. JAMA 1954;156:764.

44. Mazze RI, Escue HM, Houston JB. Hyperkalemia and cardiovascular collapse following administration of succinylcholine to traumatized patients. Anesthesiology 1969;31:540.

45. Schimpff SC, Caplan FS. Role of the host in aminoglycoside nephrotoxicity. Curr Opinions: Aminoglycoside Nephrotoxicity 1984;1:16.

46. Hou SH, Bushinsky DA, Wish JB, et al. Hospital acquired renal insufficiency: a prospective study. Am J Med 1983;74:243.

47. Kono K, Philbin DM, Coggins CH, et al. Renal function and stress response during halothane and fentanyl anesthesia. Anesth Analg 1981;60:552.

48. Anto HR, Chou SY, Porush JG, et al. Mannitol prevention of acute renal failure associated with infusion intravenous pyelography. Clin Res 1979;27:407A.

49. Hermreck AS, Thal AP. Mechanisms for the high circulatory requirements in sepsis and shock. Ann Surg 170:677-694.

50. Abel RM, Beck CH, Abbott WM, et al. Improved survival from acute renal failure after treatment with intravenous essential L-amino acids and glucose. N Engl J Med 1973;288:695.

51. Aitkenhead AR, Vater M, Achola K, et al. Pharmacokinetics of single dose I.V. morphine in normal volunteers and patients with end-stage renal failure. Br J Anaesth 1984;56:813.

52. Barsoum RS, Rihan ZEB, Baligh OK, et al. Acute renal failure in the 1973 Middle East war—experience of a specialized base hospital: effect of the site of injury. J Trauma 1980;20:303.

53. Etheredge EE, Hruska KA. Acute renal failure in the surgical patient. Zuidema GD, Rutherford RB, Ballinger WF, eds. The management of trauma, 4 ed. Philadelphia: WB Saunders, 1985; 169.

54. Whelton A. Post-traumatic acute renal failure. Bull NY Acad Med 1979;2:150.

55. Gotta AW, Murray D, Sullivan CA, et al. Postoperative renal failure caused by disseminated intravascular coagulation. Can Anaesth Soc J 1975;22:149.

56. Fischer RP, Polk HC. Changing etiologic patterns of renal insufficiency in surgical patients. Surg Gynecol Obstet 1975;140:85.

57. Rasmussen HH, Ibels LS. Acute renal failure. Multivariate analysis of causes and risk factors. Am J Med 1982;73:211.

58. Weinrauch LA, Healy RW, Leland OS, et al. Coronary angiography and acute renal failure in diabetic azotemic nephropathy. Ann Intern Med 1977;86:56.

59. Sirinek KR, Hura CE. Renal failure. Moore EE, Mattox KL, Feliciano DV, eds. Trauma, 2nd ed. Norwalk: Appleton & Lange, 1991; 927-939.

60. Byrd L, Sherman RL. Radiocontrast-induced acute renal failure: a clinical and pathophysiologic review. Medicine 1979;58:270.

61. Goormaghtigh N. Vascular and circulatory changes in renal cortex in the anuric crush-syndrome. Proc Soc Exp Biol Med 1945;59:303.

62. Heneghan M. Contrast-induced acute renal failure. AJR 1978;131:1113.

63. Knochel JP. Rhabdomyolysis and myoglobinuria. Semin Nephrol 1981;1:75.

64. Koskelo P, Kekki M, Wager O. Kinetic behavior of 1-labelled myoglobin in human beings. Clin Chim Acta 1967;17:339.

65. Eneas JF, Schoenfeld PY, Humphreys MH. The effect of infusion of mannitol-sodium bicarbonate on the clinical course of myoglobinuria. Arch Intern Med 1979;139:801.

66. Llach F, Felsenfeld AJ, Haussler MR. The pathophysiology of altered calcium metabolism in rhabdomyolysis-induced acute renal failure. Interactions of parathyroid hormone, 25-hydroxycholecalciferol, and 1, 25 dihydroxychole-calciferol. N Engl J Med 1981;305:117.

67. Cocoran AC, Page IH. Renal damage from ferroheme pigments in myoglobin, hemoglobin, hematin. Tex Rep Biol Med 1945;3:528.

68. Itagneyik K, Gordon E, Linus L, et al. Glycerol induced hemodialysis with hemoglobinuria and acute renal failure. Lancet 1974;1:75.

69. Holland PV, Schmidt PJ. Pathogenesis of acute renal failure associated with incompatible transfusion. Lancet 1967;2:1169.

70. Horowitz HI, Stein IM, Cohen BD. Further studies on the platelet inhibitor effect of guanidinosuccinic acid and its role in uremic bleeding. Am J Med 1970;49:336.

71. Meltz D, Berties J, David D, et al. Delayed hemolytic transfusion reaction with renal failure. Lancet 1971;1:1348.

72. Kahlmcter G, Hallberg T, Kamme C. Gentamicin and tobramycin in patients with various infections-nephrotoxicity. J Antimicrob Chemother 1978;4(Suppl A):47.

73. Butkus DE, deTorrente A, Terman DS. Renal failure following gentamicin in combination with clindamycin. Nephron 1976;17:307.

74. Bennett WM. Aminoglycoside nephrotoxicity. Nephron 1983;35:73.

75. Zaske DE. Pharmacokinetics and host factors on dosage requirements and nephrotoxicity. Curr Opinions: Aminoglycoside Nephrotoxicity 16, 1984.

76. Cronin RE. Acute renal failure in the experimental animal. Semin Nephrol 1981;1:5.

77. Cronin RE. Aminoglycoside nephrotoxicity: pathogenesis and prevention. Clin Nephrol 1979;2:251.

78. Appel GB, Neu HC. Gentamicin, 1979. Ann Intern Med 1978;89:528.

79. Ditlove J, Weidmann P, Bernstine M, et al. Methicillin nephritis. Medicine 1977;56:483.

80. Frascino JA, Vanamee P, Rosen PP. Renal oxalosis and azotemia after methoxyflurane anesthesia. N Engl J Med 1970;283:676.

81. McGoldrick MD. Diagnosis and management of acute renal failure: Part I. Cardiovasc Rev Rep 1984;5:1031.

82. Parfrey PS, Griffiths SM, Barrett BJ, et al. Contrast material-induced renal failure in patients with diabetes mellitus, renal insufficiency, or both. A prospective controlled study. N Engl J Med 1989;320:143.

83. Schwab SJ, Hlatky MA, Pieper KS, et al. Contrast nephrotoxicity: a randomized controlled trial of a nonionic and an ionic radiographic contrast agent. N Engl J Med 1989;320:149.

84. Anto HR, Chou SY, Porush JG, et al. Infusion intravenous pyelography and renal function: effects of hypertonic mannitol in patients with chronic renal failure. Arch Intern Med 1981;141:1652.

85. Berksett RD, Kjellstrand C. Radiological contrast-induced nephropathy. Med Clin North Am 1984;68:351.

86. Badr KF, Ichikawa I. Prerenal failure: a deleterious shift from renal compensation to decompensation. N Engl J Med 1988;319:623.

87. Harman PK, Kron IL, McLachlan HD, et al. Elevated intra-abdominal pressure and renal function. Ann Surg 1982;196:594.

88. Jacques T, Lee R. Improvement of renal function after relief of raised intra-abdominal pressure due to traumatic retroperitoneal haematoma. Anaesth Intensive Care 1988;16:478.

89. Talner LB, Scheible W, Ellenbogen PH, et al. How accurate is ultrasonography in detecting hydronephrosis in axotemic patients? Urol Radiol 1981;3:1.

90. Lee JKT, Baron RL, Meison GL, et al. Can real-time ultrasonography replace static b-scanning in the diagnosis of renal obstruction? Radiology 1981;139:161.

91. Griffith GL, Maull KI, Coleman K, et al. Acute reversible intrinsic renal failure. Surg Gynecol Obstet 1978;146:631.

92. Heptinstall RH. Pathology of the kidney. Boston: Little, Brown, 1974; 781.

93. Martinez-Maldonado M, Benabe JE, Lopez-Novoa JM. Acute renal failure associated with tubulo-interstitial disease including papillary necrosis. Brenner BM, Lazarus JM, eds. Acute renal failure. Philadelphia: WB Saunders, 1983; 434.

94. Linton AL, Clark WF, Driedger AA, et al. Acute interstitial nephritis due to drugs. Ann Intern Med 1980;93:735.

95. Van Ypersele de Strihou C. Acute oliguric interstitial nephritis. Kidney Int 1979;16:751.

96. Arendshorst WJ, Finn WF, Gottschalk CW. Pathogenesis of acute renal insufficiency after temporary renal ischemia in the rat. Am Soc Nephrol 1973;6:4.

97. Eisenbach GM, Steinhausen M. Micropuncture studies after temporary ischemia in the rat. Pflugers Arch Ges Physiol 1973;343:11.

98. Bywaters EGL, Stead JK. The production of renal failure following injection of solutions containing myohaemoglobin. Q J Exp Physiol 1944;33:53.

99. Finn WF, Arendshorst WJ, Gottschalk CW. Pathogenesis of oliguria in acute renal failure. Circ Res 1975;36:675.

100. Tanner GA, Sloan KL, Sophasan S. Effects of renal artery occlusion on kidney function in the rat. Kidney Int 1973;4:377.

101. Bohle A, Jahnecke J, Meyer D, et al. Morphology of acute renal failure: Comparative data from biopsy and autopsy. Kidney Int 1976;10:S9.

102. Cox JW, Baehler RW, Sharma H, et al. Studies on the mechanism of oliguria in a model of unilateral acute renal failure. J Clin Invest 1974;53:1546.

103. Oliver J, MacDowell M, Tracy A. The pathogenesis of acute renal failure associated with traumatic and toxic injury: renal ischemia, nephrotoxic damage, and the ischemic episode. J Clin Invest 1951;30:1307.

104. Stein JH, Gottschalk J, Osgood RW, et al. Pathophysiology of a nephrotoxic model of acute renal failure. Kidney Int 1975;8:27.

105. Edwards JG. The renal tubule (nephron) as affected by mercury. Am J Pathol 1942;18:1011.

106. Steinhausen M, Eisenbach GM, Helmstadter V. Concentration of lissamine green in proximal tubules of antidiuretic and mercury poisoned rats and the permeability of these tubules. Pflugers Arch Ges Physiol 1969;311:1.

107. Hollenberg NK, Epstein M, Rosen SM, et al. Acute oliguric renal failure in man: evidence for preferential renal cortical ischemia. Medicine 1968;47:455.

108. Reubi FC, Gurtlea R, Gossweiler NA. A dye dilution method of measuring renal blood flow in man with special reference to the anuric subject. Proc Soc Exp Biol Med 1962;111:760.

109. Flamenbaum W. Pathophysiology of acute renal failure. Arch Intern Med 1973;131:911.

110. Orecklin JR, Brosman SA. Current concepts in the diagnosis of acute renal failure. J Urol 1972;107:892.

111. Sherwood T, Doyle FH, Boulton-Jones, et al. The intravenous urogram in acute renal failure. Br J Radiol 1974;47:368.

112. Okem DE. On the differential diagnosis of acute renal failure. Am J Med 1981;71:916.

113. Anderson RJ, Schrier RW. Acute renal failure. Petersdorf RG, Adams RD, Braunwald E, Isselbacher KJ, Martin JB, Wilson JD, eds. Harrison's principles of internal medicine, 10th ed. New York: McGraw-Hill, 1983; 606.

114. Kim KE, Onesti G, Osvaldo R, et al. Creatinine clearance in renal disease: a reappraisal. Br Med J 1969;4:11.

115. Myers BD, Hiberman M, Spencer RJ, et al. Glomerular and tubular function in non-oliguric acute renal failure. Am J Med 1982;72:642.

116. Wilson RF, Soullier G. The validity of two-hour creatinine clearance studies in critically ill patients. Crit Care Med 1980;8:281.

117. Espinel CH, Gregory AW. Differential diagnosis of acute renal failure. Clin Nephrol 1980;13:73.

118. Diamond JR, Yoburn DC. Nonoliguric acute renal failure associated with a low fractional excretion of sodium. Ann Intern Med 1982;96:597.

119. Kirschbaum BB. Low FE_{Na} acute renal failure. J Trauma 1982;22:511.

120. Miller TR, Anderson RJ, Linas SL, et al. Urinary diagnostic indices in acute renal failure: a prospective study. Ann Intern Med 1978;89:47.

121. Shin B, MacKenzie CF, Helrich M. Creatinine clearance for early detection of post-traumatic renal dysfunction. Anesthesiology 1986;64:605.

122. Handa SP, Morrin PAF. Diagnostic indices in acute renal failure. Can Med Assoc J 1967;96:78.

123. Baek SM, Makaball GG, Brown RS, et al. Free-water clearance patterns as predictor and therapeutic guides in acute renal failure. Surgery 1975;77:632.

124. Brown R, Babcock R, Talbert J, et al. Renal function in critically ill postoperative patients: sequential assessment of creatinine, osmolar and free-water clearance. Crit Care Med 1980;8:68.

125. Kosinski JP, Lucas CE, Ledgerwood AM. Meaning and value of free water clearance in injured patients. J Surg Res 1982;33:184.

126. Schrier RW. Acute renal failure. Kidney Int 1979;15:205.

127. De Torrente A. Acute renal failure. Int Anesthesiol Clin 1984;22:83.

128. Lucas CE, Zito JG, Carter KM, et al. Questionable value of furosemide in preventing renal failure. Surgery 1977;82:315.

129. Luke RG, Briggs JD, Allison MEM, et al. Factors determining response to mannitol in acute renal failure. Am J Med Sci 1970;259:168.

130. Franklin SS, Maxwell MH. Acute renal failure. Mazwell MH, Kleeman CR, eds. Clinical disorders of fluid and electrolyte metabolism, 3rd ed. New York: McGraw-Hill, p 745.

131. Levinsky NG, Alexander EA. Acute renal failure. Brenner BM, Rector FC, eds. The kidney. Philadelphia: WB Saunders, 1976; 806.

132. Birch AG, Zakheim RM, Jones LG, et al. Redistribution of renal blood flow produced by furosemide and ethacrynic acid. Circ Res 1967;21:869.

133. Wright FS, Schnermann J. Interference with feedback control of glomerular filtration rate by furosemide, triflorin, and cyanide. J Clin Invest 1974;53:1965.

134. Golberg LI. The pharmacologic basis of the use of dopamine. Proc R Soc Med 1977;70(Suppl 2):7.

135. Lindner A, Sherrad DJ, Shan T, et al. Dopamine plus furosemide diuresis in furosemide resistant oliguric acute renal failure. Tel Aviv Satellite Symposium on Acute Renal Failure, 1981; 126.

136. Shoemaker WC. Fluids and electrolytes in the acutely ill adult. Shoemaker WC, Thompson WL, Holbrook PR, eds. Textbook of critical care. Philadelphia: WB Saunders, 1984; 614.

137. Verney EB. Some aspects of water and electrolyte excretion. Surg Gynecol Obstet 1958;106:441.

138. Finn W. Recovery from acute renal failure. Brenner BM, Lazarus MJ, eds. Acute renal failure. Philadelphia: WB Saunders, 1983; 753.

139. Eriksen C, Sorensen MB, Bille-Brahe NE, et al. Hemodynamic effects of calcium chloride administered intravenously to patients with and without cardiac disease during neuroleptanesthesia. Acta Anaesth Scand 1983;27:13.

140. Guerra SMO, Kitabchi AE. Comparison of the effectiveness of various routes on insulin injection: insulin levels and glucose response in normal subjects. J Clin Endocrinol Metab 1976;42:869.

141. Ardaillou R, Beaufils M, Nevez MP, et al. Increased plasma calcitonin in early acute renal failure. Clin Sci Mol Med 1975;49:301.

142. Kleinknecht D, Jungers P, Chanard J, et al. Uremic and nonuremic complications in acute renal failure: evaluation of early and frequent dialysis on prognosis. Kidney Int 1972;1:190.

143. Skillman JJ, Silen W. Stress ulceration in the acutely ill. Annu Rev Med 1976;27:9.

144. Weddington WW, Muelling AE, Moosa HH, et al. Cimetidine toxic reactions masquerading as delirium tremens. JAMA 1981;245:1058.

145. Remuzzi G, Livio M, Marchiaro G, et al. Bleeding in renal failure: altered platelet function in chronic uraemia only partially corrected by haemodialysis. Nephron 1978;22:347.

146. Mannucci PM, Remuzzi G, Pusineri F, et al. Deamino-8-D arginine vasopressin shortens the bleeding time in uremia. N Engl J Med 1983;308:8.

147. Counts RB, Haisch C, Simon TL, et al. Hemostasis in massively transfused trauma patients. Ann Surg 1979;190:91.

148. Reed RL, Ciavarella D, Heimbach DM, et al. Prophylactic platelet administration during massive transfusion. A prospective, randomized, double blind clinical study. Ann Surg 1986;203:40.

149. Fry DE. Infection in the trauma patient: the major deterrent to good recovery. Heart Lung 1978;7:257.

150. Thompson ME, Rault RM, Reddy PS. Uremic pericarditis. Cardiovasc Rev Rep 1981;2:755.

151. Beauary C, Nakamoto S, Kolff WJ. Uremic pericarditis and cardiac tamponade in chronic renal failure. Ann Intern Med 1966;64:990.

152. Wesson DE, Witch WE, Wilmore DW. Nutritional considerations in the treatment of acute renal failure. Brenner BM, Lazarus MJ, eds. Acute renal failure. Philadelphia: WB Saunders, 1983; 609.

153. Abel RM, Shih VE, Abbott WM, et al. Amino acid metabolism in acute renal failure: influence of intravenous essential L-amino acid hyperalimentation therapy. Ann Surg 1974;180:350.

154. Kaplan AA, Longnecker RE, Folkert VW. Continuous arteriovenous hemofiltration. Ann Intern Med 1984;100:358.

155. Gimson AES, Langley PG, Hughes RD, et al. Prostacyclin to prevent platelet activation during charcoal hemoperfusion in fulminant hepatic failure. Lancet 1980;1:173.

156. Hakim R, Lazarus M. Hemodialysis in acute renal failure. Brenner BM, Lazarus MJ, eds. Acute renal failure. Philadelphia: WB Saunders, 1983; 643.

157. Eliahou HE, Boichis H, Bott-Kranner G, et al. An epidemiologic study of renal failure II. Acute renal failure. Am J Epidemiol 1975;101:281.

158. Teschan PE, Baxter CR, O'Brein TF, et al. Prophylactic hemodialysis in the treatment of acute renal failure. Ann Intern Med 1960;53:992.

159. Craddock P, Fehr J, Bringham K, et al. Complement and leukocyte-mediated pulmonary dysfunction in hemodialysis. N Engl J Med 1977;296:769.

160. Arieff AI, Gusado R, Massry SG, Lazarowitz VC. Central nervous system pH in uremia and the effects of hemodialysis. J Clin Invest 1976;58:306.

161. Betrand YM, Hermant A, Mahieu P, et al. Intracranial pressure changes in patients with head trauma during hemodialysis. Intensive Care Med 1983;9:321.

162. Aizawa Y, Ohmori J, Imai K, et al. Depressant action of acetate upon the human cardiovascular system. Clin Nephrol 1977;8:477.

163. Zusman RM, Rubin RH, Cato AE, et al. Hemodialysis using prostacyclin instead of heparin as the sole antithrombotic agent. N Engl J Med 1981;204:934.

164. Bolger PM, Eisner GM, Ramwell PW, et al. Renal actions of prostacyclin. Nature 1978;271:467.

165. Lindseth RE, Hamburger RJ, Szwed JJ, et al. Acute renal failure following trauma. J Bone Joint Surg 1975;57A:830.

166. London RE, Burton JR. Post-traumatic renal failure in military personnel in Southeast Asia. Am J Med 1972;53:137.

167. Shin B, MacKenzie CF, McAslan TC, et al. Postoperative renal failure in trauma patients. Anesthesiology 1979;51:218.

168. Anderson RJ, Schrier RW. Clinical spectrum of oliguric and non-oliguric acute renal failure. Brenner BM, Stern JH, eds. Acute renal failure. New York: Churchill Livingstone, 1980; 1.

169. Anderson RJ, Linas SL, Berns AS, et al. Non-oliguric acute renal failure. N Engl J Med 1977;296:1134.

170. Baek SM, Makabali GG, Shoemaker WC. Clinical determinants of survival from postoperative renal failure. Surg Gynecol Obstet 1975;140:685.

171. Wish JB, Cohen JJ. Renal disease and hypertension. Molitch ME, ed. Management of medical problems in surgical patients. Philadelphia: FA Davis, 1982; 543.

172. Hall JW, Johnson WJ, Maher FT, et al. Immediate and long-term prognosis in acute renal failure. Ann Intern Med 1970;73:515.

173. Bullock M, Umen A, Findelstein M, et al. The assessment of risk factors in 462 patients with acute renal failure. Am J Kidney Dis 1985;5:2.

174. Coleman RW. The role of plasma proteases in septic shock. N Engl J Med 1989;320:1207.

175. Firth JD, Ratcliff PJ, et al. Endothelin: an important factor in acute renal failure. Lancet 1988;2:1179.

176. Yanagisawa M, Kurihara H, et al. A novel potent vasoconstrictor peptide produced by vascular endothelial cells. Nature 1988;332:411.

177. Russell JD, Churchill DN. Calcium antagonist and acute renal failure. Am J Med 1989;87:306.

178. Schrier RW. Cellular mechanism in ischemic acute renal failure: role of calcium entry blockers. Kidney Int 1987;32:313.

Chapter 43 Gastrointestinal Complications Following Trauma

INTRODUCTION

A large number of gastrointestinal complications can occur after major trauma. Of these, some of the more important problems are related to antibiotics, gastric or duodenal ulcerations, gastrointestinal fistulas or obstruction, wound disruptions, and acalculous cholecystitis. Complications associated with individual organ injuries are discussed in more detail in the chapters dealing specifically with those organs.

COMPLICATIONS OF ANTIBIOTICS

Thrush

The incidence of moniliasis of the oral cavity (thrush) is increased in patients who are given broad-spectrum antibiotics on a long-term basis. The diagnosis is usually readily apparent by the multiple adherent, raised white patches scattered over the oropharyngeal mucosa.

> **AXIOM** One should look carefully for Candida infections in trauma patients who are not doing well after 7-14 days of broad-spectrum antibiotics.

Monilial esophagitis is rare except in debilitated patients and in those with AIDS or diabetes mellitus. Proximal dysphagia is a frequent symptom, but its onset may be insidious. The diagnosis is best made by endoscopy. Typically, multiple, whitish plaques overlay friable mucosa, which mimics reflux and herpetic esophagitis. The presence of Candida on esophageal washing is not necessarily diagnostic because the fungus is a commensual organism. Thus, demonstration of fungal mycelia on smear and/or in tissue biopsies are generally considered essential. Stricture, perforation, fistula, and invasive candidiasis are complications of untreated monilial esophagitis.[1] Most patients respond to a polyene antibiotic, such as oral nystatin, but in severe, unresponsive patients, parenteral amphotericin-B or fluconazole may be required.

Candida is not an infrequent colonizer in the trachea or bronchi, but it seldom causes pneumonia except in patients who are severely immunosuppressed.

Candida peritonitis usually occurs after bowel perforations and is especially apt to develop in individuals who have persistent secondary peritonitis and have been on multiple broad-spectrum antibiotics for more than 10-14 days.

Monilial vaginitis can also complicate antibiotic treatment in women and is more common than thrush or esophagitis. Vaginal discharge and itching are frequent symptoms. A white, watery discharge and vaginal erythema suggest the diagnosis, which is confirmed by the presence of mycelia on a fresh preparation of vaginal discharge. Treatment consists of intravaginal nystatin suppositories.

Pseudomembranous Colitis

Pseudomembranous or antibiotic-associated colitis is an acute exudative infection of the large intestine caused by Clostridium difficile. This organism is an anaerobic, spore-forming, Gram-positive bacillus that produces at least four toxins: toxin A (or enterotoxin, which is the most active one), toxin B (or cytotoxin), a heat labile toxin, and a motility-altering factor.[2] Colitis has been reported to follow commonly used antibiotics. It is believed that antibiotic treatment reduces native resistance to colonization by C. difficile.

> **AXIOM** Diarrhea in a patient who has been on broad-spectrum antibiotics should be considered as due to pseudomembranous colitis until proved otherwise.

Colitis following antibiotic use also is referred to as pseudomembranous colitis because in the advanced form, necrotic membranes adhere to the mucosal surface. The distribution and pattern of grossly affected mucosa is variable. The clinical presentation also is variable, ranging from mild, self-limited diarrhea to toxic megacolon.

> **AXIOM** The presentation and distribution of pseudomembranous colitis are extremely variable, but this problem should be suspected in anyone who has received antibiotics and has diarrhea.

The time of onset of symptoms from pseudomembranous colitis is extremely variable. They may begin in two to three days or develop as late as three to four weeks after the antibiotics are started. Multiple liquid bowel movements are common, but bloody diarrhea and/or colonic perforation are quite rare. The responsible organism (C. difficile) and its toxin are found in feces of affected patients. Diagnosis is readily made by examining feces for toxin. Fiberoptic sigmoidoscopy will obviously miss lesions that are restricted to the right colon.

> **PITFALL** ⊘
>
> *Using antidiarrheal drugs to control diarrhea in a patient who may have a proximal partial bowel obstruction or pseudomembranous colitis.*

The treatment of choice for pseudomembranous colitis at present is either oral vancomycin or metronidazole. When the patient cannot take oral medication, intravenous metronidazole or vancomycin may control the problem. Antidiarrheal medications, such as Lomotil®, are contraindicated because they may cause increased bowel damage or toxicity by having C. difficile toxin in contact with the bowel for a longer period of time. Clinical improvement is usually apparent within 48 hours of starting the metronidazole or vancomycin. Treatment failures and/or recurrences are more likely with parenteral administration of these agents.

Cholestryramine can be used to bind the toxin, but it does not appear to significantly influence the clinical course of colitis. When continued treatment with the inducing antibiotic is required, concomitant treatment with vancomycin may be successful, but data are sparse. Relapse can occur after appropriate antibiotic treatment. Repeat treatment with an inducing antibiotic is not contraindicated at a later time for a patient who has recovered from pseudomembranous colitis.

In rare circumstances, appropriate antibiotic treatment does not cause improvement of severe forms of the disease, and subtotal colectomy with temporary ileostomy may be necessary.

UPPER GASTROINTESTINAL ULCERATION

Stress Ulcerations

PATHOPHYSIOLOGY

Stress ulcers are superficial and occur on a background of erosive mucosal inflammation. Stress ulcer, unlike peptic ulcer, is not a primary disease of the upper gastrointestinal tract but rather a manifestation of severe underlying illness. Predisposing conditions include trauma, shock, hemorrhage, sepsis, and burns.

> **AXIOM** All patients with prolonged stress, particularly when due to severe sepsis, will develop some degree of stress gastritis.

The endoscopic appearance of stress ulcers can be similar to the superficial gastric and duodenal ulcerations associated with intracranial disease or erosive gastritis induced by commonly ingested drugs, such as aspirin, nonsteroidal antiinflammatory agents, and alcohol. Although their pathogenesis differs, the distribution of stress ulcers in the stomach does not necessarily differ. Although acute recurrence of chronic peptic ulcer disease may develop during the course of a stressful illness, the pathogenesis and histology of peptic ulcer differs from true stress ulcers, which tend to be acute and relatively superficial ulcerations not associated with scar tissue.

Interspersed foci of pallor and hyperemia of gastric mucosa are often noted within hours of the insult. Punctate or linear hemorrhagic foci of variable number may appear. Areas of superficial mucosal necrosis, referred to as erosions, often appear within 24-48 hours. When they extend to and beyond the muscularis mucosa, these erosions are referred to as ulcers; this may occur by 48-96 hours. These changes usually develop in the midst of diffuse, superficial erosions, and various stages of the disease process are often seen simultaneously.

> **AXIOM** Stress ulcerations are usually greatest in the body of the stomach, and the antrum is usually either spared or only minimally involved.

The process generally begins in the proximal portion of the stomach, and spreads distally. The body of the stomach is usually involved much more severely than the antrum.

Stress ulcers of the duodenum evolve on a background of duodenitis which may also occur within hours of insult or injury. Unlike gastric ulcerations, those of the duodenum generally are not observed within 72 hours of injury. Lesions of the antrum and duodenum are infrequent in the absence of severe disease in the fundus.

ETIOLOGY

> **AXIOM** Stress ulcerations are not a primary disease; they are a manifestation of severe underlying illness.

A large amount of data in experimental animals suggest that shock or any other process that decreases gastric mucosal blood flow, when combined with gastric acid and possibly duodenal contents, can cause acute ulcerations similar to stress ulcers in humans.[3,4] Acid in the gastric lumen is essential for the development of lesions, and as protons back-diffuse into the mucosa, the development of the gastritis and ulcerations is related to the balance between the amount of diffusing acid and the ability of the mucosa to neutralize acid.

Neutralization of acid diffusing into the mucosa is accomplished with bicarbonate from the blood, mucosal secretion of bicarbonate into the lumen, and/or ion exchange processes that permit mucosa cells to rid themselves of intracellular hydrogen ion.[5,6] The concentration of acid in the gastric lumen and the amount of acid diffusing into the gastric mucosa can be quite low at times and still cause injury if the tissue is ischemic.

> **AXIOM** Although patients with stress gastritis do not hypersecrete acid, some acid is necessary to cause the luminal pH to decrease to < 3.5 to cause the lesions.

The role of pepsin in the etiology of stress gastritis is less clear and may be more applicable to mucosa that is already injured by acid. The presence of duodenal contents (particularly bile salts) is not essential, but it can aggravate lesions that are already present.

A decrease in mucosal blood flow is important in the initial development of experimentally-induced gastric ulcerations. Once damage occurs, however, mucosal blood flow increases, probably because of increased local release of endogenous histamine and prostaglandin. The initial decrease in blood flow not only results in cellular and systemic acidosis, but also causes a decrease in tissue bicarbonate. Reperfusion, after the period of ischemia, can cause increased production of hydroxyl and other injurious free radicals. A differential energy deficit also occurs.

> **AXIOM** Although factors other than acid may aggravate tissue damage, stress gastric mucosal lesions are not apt to occur in the absence of luminal acid.

Experimental studies showed that the stomach is able to repair itself rapidly by restitution.[7] This is a process whereby cells in the region of the neck of the gastric glands creep over an intact basal lamina and cover the superficial defects. If the mucosal injury were deeper than the basal lamina, cell replication would be necessary to cover the defect.

> **AXIOM** Both restitution and replication of gastric mucosal cells are inhibited by luminal acid.

Stress ulcers are painless unless perforation occurs; because the lesions are generally superficial, this complication is rare. Upper gastrointestinal hemorrhage is the major manifestation of stress ulcer disease. Although some bleeding may be encountered within hours of injury, it generally takes four to five days for significant bleeding to occur, and this is more apt to occur with sepsis.

Gastric fundic lesions occur in 100% of patients with severe shock or trauma[8] and in 85% of patients with burns of > 35% body surface area.[9] Gastric mucosal disease also occurs in nearly all patients who are septic and have positive blood cultures, but it is present in less than half of nonseptic, critically ill patients.[10]

> **AXIOM** As long as severe sepsis persists, stress gastritis also tends to progress, regardless of treatment.

DIAGNOSIS

The clinical diagnosis of stress gastritis is generally made after blood begins to appear in the nasogastric aspirate of an ICU patient; however, a hazard exists in assuming that such blood is due to stress ulcer and not some other condition, such as a bleeding peptic ulcer, recent suture line, or missed injury. Upper gastrointestinal radiographs may demonstrate peptic ulcers, but they will not demonstrate most stress ulcerations because the lesions are too superficial. Definitive diagnosis is established by esophagogastroduodenoscopy (EGD).

> **AXIOM** Gastrointestinal bleeding in a stressed patient is not necessarily due to stress ulcerations.

A few patients (1% or less) have significant bleeding from an upper gastrointestinal suture line within 24 hours of surgery even in the face of normal coagulation parameters. Anastomotic bleeding rarely requires reoperation because it usually stops spontaneously, even if two to four blood transfusions are required. Anastomotic bleeding may also be noted on about the seventh postoperative day. This rarely requires transfusion and is probably related to some tissue necrosis and slough at the suture line. Anastomotic hemorrhage can easily be confused with stress ulcer bleeding, and the surest way to differentiate between the two is by EGD.

Erosions due to stress gastritis must also be distinguished from those due to mucosal trauma caused by suction applied to a nasogastric tube. The latter generally are not accompanied by fundal gastritis.

> **AXIOM** Antacids or H$_2$-receptor antagonists usually prevent severe stress gastritis as long as severe shock or sepsis is controlled and gastric luminal pH is kept above 3.5.

Prospective trials showed that either antacid or cimetidine significantly reduce the risk of upper gastrointestinal bleeding in critically ill patients, but antacids appear to be somewhat more effective.[11] This may be related to experimental data indicating that inhibited gastric mucosa is more susceptible to ulceration than stimulated mucosa in the presence of luminal acid[12]; however, H$_2$-receptor antagonists may not cause enough inhibition of acid secretion in every patient, particularly in those with severe sepsis, to prevent mucosal damage.

An effective prophylactic regimen for most patients with stress gastritis involves instillation of 30 mL of antacid into the stomach via a nasogastric tube which is then clamped. The tube is aspirated at the end of one hour, and the pH of the aspirate is measured using pH paper. When pH is $\geq$ 3.5, 30 mL of antacid are reinstalled again for one hour; however, when pH is $<$ 3.5, 60 mL of antacid are given. This sequence is repeated hourly. When regurgitation occurs, the tube is suctioned for 30 minutes before pH is measured again. This method is quite nurse-intensive, and diarrhea can be a problem.

H$_2$-receptor antagonists may be almost as good as antacids and require much less work by nurses; however, if bleeding occurs while using these agents, adding an antacid and/or carafate often causes the bleeding to cease.[13]

Uncontrolled bleeding from stress ulcers rarely occurs, providing that rapid resuscitation from shock, control of sepsis, and proper metabolic care to maintain gastric pH $>$ 3.5 are ensured. Upper gastrointestinal bleeding has been almost eliminated in burn patients in whom gastric luminal pH is carefully controlled.[14]

Once stress gastric bleeding begins, the stomach should be irrigated with warm (not cold) saline. Iced saline has a detrimental effect on the gastric mucosa,[15] and experimental studies showed no advantage of using iced saline to stop stress hemorrhage. Saline irrigation alone may be associated with cessation of bleeding in about 80% of patients. Irrigation with antacids may be equally or even more effective.

A number of methods have been proposed to deal with uncontrollable bleeding from stress ulcers. Except for the use of antacids or cimetidine (and presumably other H$_2$-receptor antagonists), however, these methods are difficult to evaluate because of the great variation in the rates of hemorrhage, and the severity of the underlying risk factors causing stress gastritis. The situation is further complicated by the fact that the mortality rate is high no matter what is done when there is no correction of the underlying condition that led to the stress bleeding.

Infusion of vasopressin—which can cause severe vasoconstriction of gastrointestinal vessels—is anecdotally successful, providing the gastric luminal contents remain continuously neutralized with antacid; however, the effectiveness of vasoconstriction by itself is controversial. The adverse effects of pitressin (e.g., hypertension, coronary artery constriction, cardiac arrhythmia, congestive heart failure, water retention) are not avoided by selective perfusion into the left gastric artery. The dose of pitressin is 0.1-0.4 units/minute intravenously, and the patient should be on a cardiac monitor because arrhythmias can occur frequently.

Most bleeding from stress ulcers tends to occur within the distribution of the left gastric artery.[16] When this is confirmed by arteriography, the left gastric artery can be occluded by the injection of autologous clot, and this has been successful in some patients.

> **AXIOM** Surgical intervention is rarely necessary for stress gastritis but obviously it may be indicated when nonsurgical methods fail to control bleeding.

The operative procedure of choice for severe stress gastric bleeding is controversial because of the high incidence of rebleeding after vagotomy and pyloroplasty, vagotomy and antrectomy, or subtotal gastrectomy. The operative mortality also is high, ranging 17-34% in some series.[17] Although it is a major procedure in these critically ill patients, total gastrectomy is probably the procedure of choice when bleeding persists despite rigorous control of gastric pH. Alternatively, the stomach can be devascularized by ligating both gastroepiploic and both gastric arteries, leaving only the short gastric vessels intact.[18]

In all operative procedures for bleeding stress gastritis, with the exception of total gastrectomy, the major mucosal bleeding points should be suture-ligated; however, this may be impractical in diffusely affected mucosa. When total gastrectomy is not done, the operative management of bleeding stress ulcerations must be accompanied by continued control of the gastric pH, and every effort must be made to correct the underlying illness which led to the stress ulcers.

In the rare instance in which perforation of a stress ulcer occurs, the perforation is repaired by simple closure. More extensive surgery is unnecessary; however, control of gastric pH and underlying illnesses is required.

Cushing's Ulcer

In 1933, Harvey Cushing described several patients with isolated, deep gastric, duodenal, and/or esophageal ulcers that appeared to be related to head trauma or surgery. Gastric mucosal changes due to stress ulcer in the majority of patients are identical to those associated with intracranial trauma; however, patients with typical Cushing's ulcers due to head injuries tend to have high gastrin levels and secrete more acid.[19]

> **AXIOM** Cushing's ulcers (versus common stress ulcers) tend to be associated with greater gastrin and acid secretion and are usually deeper and more apt to perforate.

Classic Cushing's ulcers related to intracranial trauma or surgery tend to be much deeper and involve full thickness areas of dissolution of the wall of the esophagus, stomach, or duodenum. Consequently, perforation is much more common with Cushing's ulcers. Furthermore, shock and sepsis are not necessary for the development and progression of Cushing's ulcers.

Confusion between stress and Cushing's ulcers can arise if central nervous system trauma is associated with sepsis or hypotension due to other injuries. Although a crossover effect may occur between stress and Cushing's ulcers in such patients, classic Cushing's ulcers are rarely seen today because of the effectiveness of treatment available for preventing hypersecretion of acid. In the rare event that an operation for continuing hemorrhage is required for a Cushing's ulcer, suture ligation of individual bleeding points and vagotomy are anecdotally effective.

Curling's Ulcer

Acute duodenal ulcerations associated with burns were reported in 1923 by a London surgeon, Joseph Swan, and termed Curling's ulcers after the 1843 report by Thomas Blizard Curling (1811-1888). Gastric ulcers occurring in the setting of thermal trauma are often erroneously referred to as Curling's ulcers. Curling's original description involved burn patients with acute duodenal, not gastric, ulceration, a situation that occurs rarely today.

> **AXIOM** Patients with severe burns should have their gastric luminal pH monitored while a nasogastric tube is present, and antacids and/or H$_2$ blockers should be given until the patient's burns are completely healed.

ENTERIC FISTULAS

Enterocutaneous Fistulas

ETIOLOGY

Although the majority of them are the result of an operative injury to the intestine or an anastomotic disruption, a few enterocutaneous fistulas developing after trauma are due to an incomplete abdominal exploration, resulting in a missed bowel injury or inadequate debridement of the initial injury.[20] Small perforations can easily be missed at operation unless there is a careful, direct inspection of all possibly injured bowel. This is particularly true for posterior penetrating injuries that may involve retroperitoneal colon, especially near the splenic flexure. Serosal tears made by the initial trauma or at surgery can also progress to form enterocutaneous fistulas. Forcing distended bowel into the peritoneal cavity without decompressing the lumen can also cause delayed iatrogenic leak. Direct erosion of bowel may also be caused by the bowstring effect of fascial sutures used to close a large abdominal wall defect under tension.

PATHOPHYSIOLOGY

Fistulas involving any part of the small intestine have a higher mortality than those of the stomach or colon. Mortality ranges 6.5-21%, but the overall mortality today is about 10%.[21] It is difficult to get precise figures for the mortality of a fistula in a trauma population because of the large number of confounding variables.

The size of an intestinal fistula, usually expressed as volume of output, also plays a role, but the dividing line between high and low output is somewhat arbitrary. The definition of a high-output fistula ranges from an effluent > 200 mL/day[22] to one > 1,000 mL during the first 48 hours[23]; however, it is generally accepted that the mortality rate is higher when the fistula output exceeds 1 L/day. For example, the mortality in one series for fistulas draining < 1 L/day was only 6%, but fistulas draining > 1 L/day had a mortality rate more than five times greater.[23]

> **AXIOM** The greater mortality of high-output fistulas is due to the increased risk of developing intraabdominal infection and the significantly lower rate of spontaneous closure.

Several other important variables affect the outcome of a patient with an enterocutaneous fistula. Obstruction of distal bowel is the most frequent reason for an intestinal fistula to persist. Other causes of a persistent intestinal fistula include foreign bodies (such as sutures), carcinoma, Crohn's disease, prior radiation therapy, short tract between the bowel and skin, adjacent infection, or large abdominal wall defect.

> **AXIOM** Although many factors tend to make an intestinal fistula persist, the most important is distal obstruction.

The essential principles in managing most intestinal fistulas include: (a) control of the fistula, (b) control of any associated sepsis, and (c) nutritional support.[22] Control of the fistula means that the effluent is well drained from the peritoneal cavity, the skin or surface wound is protected from enzymatic digestion, and fluid and electrolyte balance is maintained. In some instances, surgery may be required to achieve control of the fistula output. If an intestinal fistula were recognized early in its development and the surrounding inflammatory reaction were not excessive, the fistula could be converted to a tube enterostomy, thereby effecting control. Unfortunately, by the time the presence of a fistula is recognized, the inflammatory reaction is usually so advanced that it is difficult to mobilize the involved intestine or precisely visualize the site of origin. Thus, the drainage can often only be established at a point near the origin of the fistula.

Although they can generally provide effective drainage, sump tubes or closed-drainage systems are easily plugged by debris. Thus, if an operation were required to place sump tubes near a fistula, it may be advisable to place additional drains in the area in case the sump tubes should fail. This is important because it can be extremely difficult to replace an intraperitoneal sump tube through its original tract. Once an intestinal tube dislodges, the abdominal wall opening can rapidly close down because of edema and/or muscle spasm. Another problem with sump tubes or closed-drainage systems is their occasional erosion into adjacent bowel creating another fistula. Although soft latex and even silastic tubes are not immune from this complication, such occurrences appear to be more prevalent with stiff plastic tubes.

Once a satisfactory tract between the fistula and skin has developed, it may be preferable to avoid continued use of the sump tube because it can act as a foreign body and perpetuate the fistula. When the fistula tract is long, however, a sump tube whose tip is just below the level of the abdominal wall and at least 2 cm away from the bowel opening can be useful.

A sump tube may protect the skin, but additional measures, such as the use of karaya powder or protective skin wafers and ointments, are often necessary. If the fistula opening on the skin were far enough away from the incision and bony prominences, such as ribs or the iliac crest, application of a disposable ileostomy appliance usually would be possible. The bag should be attached to suction in order to minimize puddling of intestinal juice within the fistulous tract. Some surgeons have placed great emphasis on keeping the tract dry, but this can be extraordinarily difficult, and usually the best one can hope to accomplish is to prevent puddling.

> **AXIOM** Metabolic support with adequate calories and protein plus accurate replacement of the fistula output of water and electrolytes are essential for maintaining optimal healing and host-defense systems in the patient.

Electrolyte measurements of the fistula output are helpful. Fluid loss from a fistula should be replaced on an electrolyte-for-electrolyte and volume-for-volume basis. The previous 24-hour fistula output is a useful guide for planning the subsequent 24-hour fluid intake.

> **AXIOM** Prolonged nasogastric tube drainage is probably of little benefit for successfully treating well-established intestinal fistulas.

Once the tract of an upper gastrointestinal fistula is well-formed, it is not clear that the use of a nasogastric or longer tube adds to the management. An H_2-receptor antagonist may significantly reduce fistula output, and it is preferable to a nasogastric tube, not only in terms of comfort, but also in reducing fluid and electrolyte losses. Somatostatin or one of its analogues can also reduce gastrointestinal secretions, but the influence of such agents on healing is not known.

Antidiarrheal agents, such as opiates or Kaopectate®, may be helpful adjuncts in the control of lower gastrointestinal fistulas.[24] A "drain me/feed me" arrangement can be made with a proximal and distal tube in the lumen, thereby conserving fluid and electrolyte losses. However, this approach requires frequent surveillance to work properly.

> **AXIOM** Intestinal fistulas generally do not heal unless local and systemic sepsis have been controlled.

Sepsis is the most frequent complication associated with intestinal fistulas. Culture of fistula drainage nearly always grows organisms, but this is not an indication for antibiotics. Although they should be used when evidence of sepsis exists,[25] antibiotics are of little value unless the fistula contents are well-drained. Furthermore, antibiotics are not a substitute for drainage of intraabdominal abscesses, which must be monitored aggressively and continuously. When the patient is septic and no other source is evident, exploration of the abdominal cavity is indicated, even when abscesses cannot be localized preoperatively.

> **AXIOM** Definitive surgical treatment of a gastrointestinal fistula should not be attempted at the same time that an abscess is drained.

Although simultaneous drainage of an abscess and surgical closure of an intestinal fistula are occasionally successful, such efforts often result in larger fistulas with even greater spread of infection. Nevertheless, control of a fistula causing an abscess that is being drained may require a bypass procedure or a proximal stoma with a distal mucous fistula.

Once control of the fistula and any associated sepsis is achieved, radiography with contrast may be helpful for determining the site of origin of the fistula, the continuity of the proximal and distal bowel, and the presence or absence of a distal obstruction. This information is useful for planning the next phase of management, which involves provision of adequate enteral nutrition when possible; however, attempts to provide adequate nutrition are of little value when sepsis persists.

AXIOM   Enteral feeding is preferred over parenteral nutrition whenever possible.

Enteral nutrition is usually much more effective and much less expensive than TPN and it also provides a convenient portal for refeeding proximal fistula effluent. In some instances, a feeding tube can be passed beyond a proximal fistula or a feeding jejunostomy can be constructed distal to the fistula. It is generally unnecessary to resort to parenteral nutrition for small, well-drained distal ileal or colonic fistulas, which are no different in principle from ileostomy or colostomy. Because the volume of refed fistula drainage may restrict the total amount of calories that can be simultaneously administered enterally, some larger volume fistulas are best treated by a combination of enteral and parenteral nutrition.

Once adequate nutrition is provided, definitive surgical closure of the fistula should not be rushed. Distal obstruction, lack of bowel continuity, origin in a segment involved with inflammatory bowel disease, continued massive fluid loss, a stoma at skin level, and/or the presence of a foreign body generally requires surgical correction; however, several weeks or months may be required to obtain adequate nutritional repletion. Further wound healing during that interval may also help to provide better soft tissue for closing the abdominal wall at definitive repair.

Bleeding (other than from stress ulcers or reactivation of peptic ulcers) associated with a fistula is usually due to acute erosion of a drainage tube into the bowel or into granulation tissue lining an inflammatory cavity. Bleeding from the wall of inflammatory cavities can be massive at times, and complete excision of the granulation tissue may occasionally be necessary for control.

AXIOM   Spontaneous closure of a fistula should not be expected to occur until adequate control of the fistula, eradication of the sepsis, and nutritional repletion occur.

Spontaneous closure of intestinal fistulas cannot be expected until all of the factors tending to keep the fistula open are removed; furthermore, if spontaneous closure of an intestinal fistula were to occur, it would usually be within two to three months.[21,24] Of the intestinal fistulas that close spontaneously, about 90% do so within one month of the eradication of infection.

The overall figures for spontaneous closure vary 30-70%, but select series reported even higher rates. Longer fistula tracts are more apt to heal. Only 17% of fistulas with tracts <2 cm in length close spontaneously.[21] If the fistula output were to continue to decrease after one month of nonoperative treatment, such therapy should be continued as long as there appears to be a reasonable hope of spontaneous healing.

AXIOM   When an intestinal fistula has not closed spontaneously within one month of proper control of infection and provision of adequate nutrition, definitive surgical correction is generally required.

Patients with large abdominal wall defects may require a period of nonoperative treatment in order for enough healing of the abdominal wall to occur to facilitate operative repair. Intestinal fistulas associated with large abdominal wall defects rarely close spontaneously.[24] Consequently, it is advisable at definitive operative treatment to provide soft-tissue coverage of the abdominal cavity. Reconstruction of the abdominal wall with polypropylene mesh would be inadvisable if omentum could not be placed between the bowel and the mesh. If the bowel and mesh were in direct contact, the mesh would eventually become incorporated into the bowel wall; this in itself could cause a formation of new enterocutaneous fistulas.[26] An additional problem in using prosthetic mesh is that it can become contaminated and a nidus for later persistent infection because of the presence of a fistula.

Persistence of a deep enterocutaneous fistula in the absence of sepsis and in the presence of adequate nutrition frequently is attributed to epithelialization of the tract; however, this rarely occurs. Persistence of an intestinal fistula originating from otherwise normal bowel is usually due to eversion of the mucosa creating, in effect, a subcutaneous or subperitoneal stoma. This also applies to fistulas whose openings are at the level of the skin.

AXIOM   The most successful operative approach for an enterocutaneous fistula is resection of the involved segment of bowel with reanastomosis of normal tissue.

Attempts at simple direct closure of fistulas are associated with a high rate of recurrence.[21,24] When resection is not anatomically feasible, a bypass procedure may be necessary. The most effective bypass is one of total exclusion where the involved segment is no longer in continuity with the remaining intestine.[24]

Lateral Duodenal Fistulas

Controversy continues to exist about the treatment of lateral duodenal fistulas. Perhaps the number of variables involved can be best appreciated by the wide differences in incidence of spontaneous closure, with two separate series reporting healing rates of 27% and over 90%.[21,27]

Many authors advocate a Billroth II gastrectomy or "diverticularization" of the duodenum with closure of the pylorus and construction of a gastrojejunostomy. This converts the fistula to an "end-fistula" rather than a "side-fistula", and some believe that end-fistulas are more likely to close. However, the only clearly documented advantage of performing gastrojejunostomy, with or without antrectomy, is the ability to more easily institute enteral feeding. Exclusion of the gastric contents from the duodenum as treatment for a duodenal side fistula, especially in patients with pharmacologically induced inhibition of acid secretion by H_2-receptor antagonists, has not been objectively shown to be beneficial.

A more moderate approach to side duodenal fistulas is to perform gastrojejunostomy only in those patients who have distal duodenal obstruction as a result of an inflammatory reaction related to the fistula.[27] Other measures helpful in the control of a lateral duodenal fistula include a feeding jejunostomy and insertion of a tube into the fistula itself, which results in more rapid formation of an established tract.

The principle of resection and reanastomosis is difficult to apply to a persistent duodenal fistula. In this circumstance, at least two options exist. One is to use an onlay jejunal patch graft. The use of ileum is inadvisable because, if an enteroenteric fistula were to develop subsequently at the site of the patch, much of the functional small intestine would have been bypassed and/or ileal bacteria would enter the upper gastrointestinal tract causing significant malabsorption. Although poorly documented in the literature, there is a general feeling that onlay patches to treat an established fistula are prone to leak. Perhaps a more preferable approach is to drain the duodenal fistula with a Roux-en-Y jejunal limb, a principle that is generally applicable to all well-established upper gastrointestinal fistulas.[28]

Enteroenteric Fistulas

Most enteroenteric fistulas occurring in the absence of Crohn's disease follow an operation involving colonic anastomosis or resection. Most of these fistulas occur as a result of a bowel leak causing an abscess which then erodes into an adjacent segment of bowel. Such fistulas usually are diagnosed several days after the initial surgery or trauma.

A fistula between the small intestine and colon frequently presents with diarrhea, which is usually due to reflux of colonic organisms into the small bowel causing malabsorption. In some instances, diarrhea is incapacitating and difficult to treat without surgery; however, definitive repair may be inadvisable for some time due to debility of the patient and/or the local inflammatory reaction. In these circumstances, a colostomy proximal to the fistula is often a simple, effective procedure because the bacterial reflux into the small intestine will be greatly reduced.

Enteroenteric fistulas rarely heal spontaneously but definitive repair is undertaken only when they are symptomatic and the patient is in optimal condition for operation. Enteroenteric fistulas that are not symptomatic usually do not require further treatment; however, occasionally bowel obstruction may be caused by the surrounding scar tissue.

Anastomotic Disruptions

About half of the disruptions of bowel anastomoses are manifest on the second through the fourth postoperative days, and most of the remainder are recognized on the fifth through seventh postoperative days. Early diagnosis may be difficult because early free leakage from a gastric or small intestinal suture line can be easily confused with the onset of acute pancreatitis. Satisfactory radiographic demonstration of all suture lines is essential when suspicion of an anastomotic disruption exists. Water-soluble contrast media should be used instead of barium because barium can be irritating to the peritoneal cavity and can act as an adjuvant to increase the seriousness of intraperitoneal infections.

AXIOM Suspected intestinal anastomotic disruptions should be treated surgically as soon as possible. If the diagnosis were uncertain, radiographic studies should be performed promptly, preferably with a water-soluble contrast agent.

By the time the diagnosis of an anastomotic disruption is made, the involved bowel is often edematous and inflamed. This generally precludes simple placement of additional sutures to close the defect. Tension on the sutures resulting from local inflammatory edema permits them to cut through the tissue easily. Recurrent anastomotic disruptions may also be due to contamination or infection of the tissues at repair. Thus, the safest approach is to exteriorize the anastomotic disruption either as a loop stoma or as a proximal stoma and distal mucous fistula. Although an intestinal stoma, particularly in proximal small intestine, can pose additional morbidity for the patient, it should generally only be taken down again after the patient has regained a normal state of health.

AXIOM Patients with persistent fever plus ileus or delayed gastric emptying following small bowel repairs should be considered to have an anastomotic disruption until proved otherwise.

A suture line disruption with contained leakage usually presents with persistent fever—often attributed to another cause, such as atelectasis—and delayed gastric emptying or ileus. These symptoms are nonspecific and may even be confused with such diverse problems as mild esophageal reflux. Serum amylase levels may also be elevated making clinical differentiation from acute pancreatitis difficult.

AXIOM Anastomotic leak can sometimes be confused clinically with persistent posttraumatic pancreatitis.

An intestinal leak that is contained and is not causing sepsis need not be drained, providing it has good communication with the lumen. Under these circumstances, antibiotic treatment is usually adequate therapy.

INTESTINAL OBSTRUCTION

Complete Bowel Obstruction

ETIOLOGY

Adhesions

Adhesions are the commonest cause of small intestinal obstruction, particularly following surgery or trauma. The majority of these adhesions appear to be related to foreign body reactions, and the most frequent foreign materials are glove powder, lint or threads off sponges, and sutures.[29,30] Peritoneum has high plasminogen activity which can prevent some of those adhesions, but this protection is lost when the bowel has been ischemic. Ischemic tissue can actively inhibit fibrinolysis, and fibrinous exudate that may normally be lysed can then become organized into a fibrin and then a collagenous adhesion. Another mechanism involves serosal injury from trauma, operative manipulation, or drying during operative exposure.[30]

AXIOM Although they cannot be completely prevented, peritoneal adhesions can often be reduced by careful surgical technique.

Unnecessary adhesion formation can be reduced by meticulous surgical technique which includes prevention of granuloma formation as a response to foreign materials, such as glove powder, redundant ends of nonabsorbable sutures, tissue crushed by rough handling, or excessive amounts of tissue left distal to a ligature. Use of moist laparotomy pads or sponges decreases the amount of lint that may stick to mesothelial surfaces. Thorough irrigation of the peritoneal cavity in order to clean it of any intestinal contents immediately after any spill and prior to closure of the abdomen is also beneficial; however, irrigation with saline at temperatures exceeding 37° C can also cause some tissue damage with subsequent adhesion formation.[31]

The incidence of clinically significant reactions in the peritoneal cavity to glove powder is comparatively rare today and is probably due to changes in the technique for sterilizing powder.[32] Starch peritonitis, manifested by obstruction, ascites, and fever, may be due to an immunologic response and may respond dramatically to corticosteroid treatment.[33] The diagnosis can be made by observing microscopic crystals in a specimen of peritoneal fluid, but most often the diagnosis is made at reoperation when one sees the peritoneum studded with raised, white plaques about 2 mm in diameter. Such granulomas can sometimes be confused with peritoneal tuberculosis.

Other Causes

Small bowel obstruction occurring in the immediate postoperative period may be due to intraperitoneal infection, with or without anastomotic leak, and occasionally is the first sign of a dehiscence of the abdominal fascia. Entrapment of a loop of bowel by an abdominal wall suture, usually of the retention type, is a rare, but avoidable, cause of postoperative obstruction. Internal hernias can also occur, and these are usually due to failure to adequately close a surgically created space in the mesentery or between an ostomy and the lateral abdominal wall. Small intestinal obstruction also can occur in patients with disruption of the anterior longitudinal ligaments or with an extensively distorted pelvic fracture.[34] Bowel that becomes entrapped by a grossly displaced fracture can easily become obstructed and/or leak.[35]

DIAGNOSIS

Simple Obstruction

The majority of patients with bowel obstruction have cramping, intermittent abdominal pain, distention, and absence of flatus or stool.[36,37] A distinction should be made between the crampy lower abdominal pain that patients frequently experience prior to first passing flatus and the periumbilical cramping pain characteristic of small bowel obstruction which tends to get progressively worse. Making the diagnosis early is more difficult if flatus or stool were initially passed before the bowel obstruction became complete.

> **AXIOM** Abdominal distention developing after the fourth postoperative day should be considered a result of bowel obstruction until proved otherwise.[37]

The patient who has undergone recent operation for extensive trauma may be particularly difficult to evaluate. This circumstance emphasizes the importance of a "high index of suspicion."

> **AXIOM** A high index of suspicion and frequent careful examinations are particularly important for diagnosing early bowel obstruction after extensive abdominal trauma.

When the small bowel is obstructed, bacterial count in the bowel becomes increasingly high, and anaerobic bacteria may increase rapidly. Once the number of anaerobes exceeds 10^8/g of feces, the intestinal contents begin to look and smell increasingly like large bowel contents.

> **AXIOM** A feculent odor or appearance of nasogastric aspirate or vomitus is often a sign of complete small bowel obstruction.

An early and sensitive indication of a developing small bowel obstruction is large or increasing amounts of drainage from a nasogastric tube postoperatively. In the absence of a nasogastric tube, development of increased belching or symptoms consistent with esophageal reflux may precede the clinical diagnosis of obstruction by several days.

> **AXIOM** High-volume gastric aspirates after abdominal trauma should make one suspicious of a bowel obstruction or peritonitis.

Abdominal distension and failure to pass stool or flatus in the immediate postoperative period are often initially attributed to continuing "adynamic" ileus. Although the presence of high-pitched tinkling bowel sounds coincident with crampy abdominal pain is characteristic of a mechanical small bowel obstruction, the presence or absence of bowel sounds or the type of bowel sounds heard are frequently of little help in differentiating between ileus and mechanical obstruction.

> **AXIOM** Although cramping abdominal pain is not characteristic of adynamic ileus, the absence of such pain does not exclude mechanical obstruction.

Evidence of continuing third space fluid loss for more than 72 hours after operation is a sensitive indicator of a postoperative complication, such as peritonitis or obstruction. Such fluid retention, however, may not be readily apparent unless accurate intake and output records are kept and correlated with changes in daily weight.

> **AXIOM** A tendency for the patient to require increased intravenous fluids after the third day postoperatively should make one suspect complications, such as bowel obstruction or infection.

With small bowel obstructions, plain radiography of the abdomen typically shows dilated small bowel loops with differential air-fluid levels on upright abdominal radiography and a paucity of gas in the colon. Serial radiography frequently is of value in helping to distinguish between complete and partial small bowel obstruction when such differentiation is not clinically apparent or when uncertainty exists.

Contrast studies can often help clarify confusing situations; however, a distal obstruction may not be evident with water-soluble contrast material because it becomes too diluted when it reaches that area. Nevertheless, diarrhea due to the hyperosmotic effect of water-soluble contrast medium may occur if only a partial obstruction were present. Barium can outline distal bowel fairly well, even when it is diluted; delayed radiography with this material may be helpful in distinguishing between partial and complete obstruction.

Contrast material instilled through the rectum is a rapid means for differentiating between a dilated transverse colon and a massively distended loop of small intestine. This distinction is not always easy on plain radiography.

> **AXIOM** When it is not clear whether a loop of bowel is dilated small bowel or colon, contrast enema should be performed.

Strangulation

When possible, bowel obstruction should be diagnosed before strangulation occurs; however, this can be extremely difficult to do at times. After placement of a functioning nasogastric tube and restitution of plasma volume losses, the patient may feel somewhat better even if strangulated bowel were present. The observation that the patient has had a bowel movement or passed flatus can also be deceptive because the stool and gas may have been present in the colon at the time that the more proximal obstruction developed.

The onset of vague but constant abdominal pain localized to one abdominal quadrant without a history of nausea or vomiting may also be an early sign of bowel strangulation. Peritoneal signs are typically present when the bowel is strangulated, but not infrequently they are mild or subtle.

> **AXIOM** Bowel obstruction associated with constant abdominal pain out of proportion to the physical findings in the appropriate clinical setting is a fairly reliable indication of strangulation of bowel.

Unfortunately, the classic picture of strangulation is absent in many patients with this problem. In addition, the presence of pancreatitis or biliary or renal calculi should be excluded. Other so-called classic signs of strangulation obstruction, such as fever, leukocytosis, tachycardia, abdominal tenderness, and presence of a mass are also relatively unreliable for differentiating between strangulation and simple mechanical obstruction.[38]

A diagnosis of strangulation on plain abdominal radiography can be made when gas is seen in the portal vein or the wall of the involved intestine, but these are infrequent and late radiographic signs that are usually not seen until other grave clinical signs are present. Radiographs with contrast are usually of little help in differentiating between strangulation and simple, complete mechanical obstruction.

Strangulating bowel obstruction can easily be confused with acute pancreatitis because both may present with elevated serum amylase. However, normal serum amylase does not exclude strangulation and elevated amylase may occur with simple mechanical obstruction. When the differential diagnosis between strangulation and pancreatitis is unclear, it is safer to operate. CT scan or ultrasound showing clear evidence of pancreatic swelling or a pseudocyst can be helpful, but overreliance on such studies can be dangerous.

TREATMENT

Prevention

Numerous methods have been used to prevent adhesions, but it is sometimes forgotten that adhesions can be beneficial. They can help to seal an anastomosis, prevent or contain a leak, or serve as a lattice work for vessels bridging to an ischemic area. Most experimental attempts to prevent adhesion formation have been chemical in nature and do not offer significant benefit.

Indications for Operation

Complete obstruction occurring in the immediate postoperative period should be treated like any other complete bowel obstruction, and up to a third of these obstructions may require immediate surgical attention. The biggest hazard of delaying surgery is development of a strangulating obstruction. Pain out of proportion to the physical findings, especially occurring a few days after operation, or associated with increased fluid requirements, should be viewed with concern.

AXIOM Severe abdominal pain out of proportion to the physical findings should be considered an indication for urgent surgical intervention until proved otherwise.

A major problem in differentiating between the expected postoperative abdominal pain and unusual pain suggesting an underlying problem occurs in patients who recently received surgery for extensive abdominal trauma, particularly when they are elderly. In such patients, the ileus may last much longer than it would if the same operation had been performed electively. The diagnosis of an obstruction, however, is still suggested by the observation that the patient's progress lags behind that which is expected.

Fortunately, strangulating obstruction is rare shortly after a celiotomy for trauma, but therein lies its danger. Given the high incidence of septic complications following major abdominal trauma, the diagnosis of bowel obstruction may not be correct even though it is suggested by the clinical situation. Thus, even though the signs and symptoms may be due to another complication, the indications for an operation are still present.

The dilemma presented by a patient with possible small bowel obstruction due to adhesions is that, short of frank peritonitis or septic shock, no definite clinical criteria exist to distinguish between simple mechanical and early strangulating obstructions. With prompt treatment, the mortality rate for a strangulating bowel obstruction should be < 5%; however, higher rates usually occur because of delayed or improper treatment. The mortality rate for promptly treated strangulating bowel obstruction should not be significantly different from that for simple mechanical obstruction.[39]

AXIOM One of the main reasons to operate early on what is probably a simple intestinal obstruction is the difficulty in excluding the presence of strangulation.

An emergent operation should be done on most patients who present with a picture suggestive of a complete bowel obstruction, particularly when: (a) vital signs are getting worse, (b) subtle but increasing signs of peritoneal irritation appear, (c) progression of the initial abdominal findings occurs, or (d) third space fluid losses continue or increase beyond anticipated limits. A less aggressive approach is hazardous not only because of the morbidity and mortality associated with necrotic intestine in a trauma patient who is already prone to infection, but also because there is no way of knowing the extent or condition of the involved intestine before operation.

With the possible exception of a Richter's hernia, partially obstructed bowel is not strangulated; however, a partial obstruction may only briefly precede the development of strangulation or herald the development of an intraabdominal abscess.

AXIOM When the patient continues to have flatus, indicating that a suspected bowel obstruction is probably only partial, little risk of strangulated bowel is present.

One study indicated that if one of four signs (pulse > 96/minute, oral temperature more than 37°C, abdominal tenderness, or white blood cell count > 10,000/mm³) were present, a 7% incidence of strangulation would be present.[39] If two or three of those findings were present, the incidence of gangrenous bowel increased to 24% and if all four findings were present, the incidence reached 67%. Although these data may be different at other centers, they offer a practical set of guidelines for following and managing these patients.

Problems at Surgery

DETERMINING BOWEL VIABILITY. Following reduction of a strangulating obstruction, it can be difficult, sometimes, to determine whether the bowel is viable. Criteria, such as mesenteric pulsations, color of the bowel wall, bleeding from a superficial incision in the bowel, and presence of peristalsis, are not always reliable indicators of intestinal viability. Other methods that have been proposed for determining bowel viability include isotopic techniques, fluorescent dyes, electromyography, temperature gradients, and Doppler ultrasound. Another problem with intraoperative assessment in borderline cases is that bowel perfusion is directly related to cardiac output, which may not be optimal at the time that the bowel is being examined.

When only a small portion of the small bowel is questionably viable, it is usually safer to resect the area in question rather than to procrastinate. When the viability of a majority of the small intestine is in question, however, it is usually safer to observe it and perform a "second-look" operation within 24 hours. A rare patient may even require a third look to ensure viability.

AXIOM Failure to perform a second-look operation on marginally viable bowel greatly increases the risk of nonviable bowel being left in place and causing fatal peritonitis.

Dissatisfaction with second-look operations is usually more emotional than real; it is usually much safer to perform a second (or even third) operative procedure than to resect most of a patient's intestine unnecessarily or to allow subsequent peritonitis to develop because necrotic bowel was left in place.

LOSS OF DOMAIN. At laparotomy for posttraumatic bowel obstruction, the small intestine can become so edematous or distended that, even though the obstruction is relieved, it will not fit back into the peritoneal cavity. This situation can sometimes be corrected by removing the bowel contents, either by milking them into the colon or aspirating them using a closed technique (e.g., Leonard tube) or open method (e.g., enterotomy or needle aspiration)[40]; however, if one were to allow leakage of the obstructed luminal contents into the peritoneal cavity, a greatly increased risk of peritonitis would occur. In addition, if the skin were closed in such patients, the incidence of wound infection may approach 60%.[38]

AXIOM When any spill of the contents of obstructed bowel occurs, the skin and subcutaneous tissues should not be closed.

The bacterial count of obstructed bowel rises rapidly and any spill of the intraluminal contents of obstructed bowel can rapidly cause severe peritonitis. Aspiration of the liquid luminal contents from bowel which is obstructed distally can also be associated with significant plasma volume losses. Fluid tends to rapidly reaccumulate in the lumen of the previously obstructed bowel because the mucosal blood vessels in that area have a greatly increased permeability.

AXIOM Large ECF deficits can occur rapidly after a distal bowel obstruction has been decompressed.

COMPLICATIONS

All patients undergoing operation for intestinal obstruction should have a nasogastric tube in place to empty the stomach and minimize the risk of aspiration of gastric contents into the lungs. Anesthetic practices to minimize the chances of aspiration vary, but close cooperation between surgeon and anesthesiologist is essential. During the operation, manipulation of the bowel may cause pooling of fluid in the proximal small bowel and stomach. Under such circumstances, a Valsalva maneuver during extubation may be associated with reflux of large quantities of small intestinal contents into the stomach and possibly up the esophagus into the pharynx and larynx. Aspiration of such fluid into the lungs can result in severe necrotizing pneumonia.

This type of pneumonia frequently is accompanied by a rapidly progressive respiratory failure requiring prompt ventilatory support.

AXIOM   One must be careful to not allow powerful Valsalva maneuvers to cause regurgitation of gastrointestinal contents into the lungs at the end of an operation for obstructed bowel.

Partial Obstruction

Partial bowel obstruction that is not due to an abscess or intussusception usually resolves with nonoperative treatment; however, it may take as long as a month before complete resolution occurs, especially if the obstruction were at the site of an anastomosis.

AXIOM   Diarrhea associated with small bowel distention frequently is due to partial obstruction.

DIAGNOSIS

When the patient with a suspected bowel obstruction has continuing passage of flatus or feces, even in relatively small amounts, the likelihood is that the bowel obstruction is incomplete; however, it must be remembered that occasionally some feces and gas can be passed from bowel distal to a complete obstruction for several days.

Serial plain radiography of the abdomen may be helpful in determining whether the obstruction is partial, especially when progression of gas into the colon occurs; however, care must be taken not to overinterpret such radiographs, as it may be difficult at times to distinguish between colon and dilated small intestine.

A small bowel follow-through examination may be of some value in helping to determine whether an intestinal obstruction is complete or incomplete. Several problems, however, occur with the routine use of such studies. For example, water-soluble contrast material is hypertonic and causes a decrease in plasma volume as it pulls fluid into the bowel lumen. This additional variable may confuse the clinical picture. In addition, water-soluble contrast can become so dilute so quickly in the small bowel that it is of little help in determining the completeness of distal small bowel obstructions. However, diarrhea occurring subsequent to ingestion of water-soluble contrast indicates that the obstruction is partial.

Barium can usually demonstrate distal small bowel obstructions relatively well; however, any barium that has reached the colon will remain there and become progressively inspissated for the duration of the postoperative ileus. The patient may then experience considerable difficulty passing the inspissated barium.

An additional hazard with follow-through contrast studies is that it may take considerable time for the contrast to reach the point of obstruction. If the patient were to stay in the radiology department for that time, unattended by a surgeon, a number of complications could occur. In some cases, because of the severity of the patient's condition, important changes in the patient's clinical picture may be missed. Consequently, it may be safer to explore the abdomen to exclude the diagnosis on just clinical grounds.

TREATMENT

When a course of nonoperative treatment for a possible postoperative bowel obstruction is chosen, a number of surgeons believe that use of a long intestinal tube achieves more rapid resolution of the process; however, no substantive clinical data indicated that a long tube is any more effective than a nasogastric tube in such circumstances.

Patients with partial small bowel obstruction due to adhesions should have effective gastric decompression and must be carefully observed because any increased distension may cause incomplete obstruction to become complete. Prolonged, nonoperative treatment of partial bowel obstruction generally requires the use of parenteral nutrition. This, in itself, can cause a number of mechanical, metabolic, or infectious complications.

Intussusception

ETIOLOGY

Twenty-seven percent of intussusceptions occur in the immediate postoperative period, and most of these involve the proximal jejunum.[41] Of these early intussusceptions, 52% occur in intubated bowel, 28% are presumably caused by adhesions, and 20% are related to a suture line. These figures are in contrast to intussusception occurring in adults without prior operation in whom 90% have associated pathologic processes, such as benign or malignant tumors or inflammatory or congenital lesions.

Both prograde and retrograde intussusception can occur after removal of a long intestinal tube, either shortly after removing the tube or even several weeks later; however, it is more common for the intussusception to occur while the tube is in place.[42]

DIAGNOSIS

AXIOM   Intussusception usually presents as a partial small bowel obstruction.

Obstructive symptoms from an intussusception typically develop about five days postoperatively. Because of the partial nature of the obstruction caused by most intussusceptions, patients are often erroneously treated nonoperatively for prolonged periods.

The presence of periumbilical cramping pain and vomiting without distention in a patient with a long intestinal tube in place should raise suspicion of this diagnosis. The diagnosis can also be made sometimes with careful radiographic examination.

AXIOM   Although spontaneous reduction of an intussusception may occur, it is safer to undertake operation in order to prevent irreducibility as a result of edema or necrosis.

Reduction of an intussusception at surgery is accomplished most safely and effectively by gently squeezing the intussuscipiens (i.e., that portion of intestine containing the invaginated bowel) so that the intussusceptum is literally pushed out from the lumen. The temptation to pull the intussusception apart should be resisted because this can tear intestine easily. The reduction should not be forceful, and any portion that cannot be readily reduced should be considered to be ischemic or to contain a lesion. Either consideration is an indication for resection of the unreduced bowel.

AXIOM   Any intussuscepted bowel that cannot be readily reduced at surgery should be resected.

DELAYED DIAGNOSIS OF BOWEL INJURY

Duodenum

HEMATOMA

Duodenal hematomas usually occur in children with severe, blunt injury to the upper abdomen. Intramural hematoma usually involves the second portion of the duodenum and may produce complete obstruction of the lumen; however, it may take several days for the obstruction to become clinically apparent.[43-45]

Upper gastrointestinal radiographs using contrast are usually diagnostic and will typically show a partial or complete obstruction of the second part of the duodenum with a "coiled spring" sign. The diagnosis can also be made with CT of the abdomen using intraluminal and intravenous contrast.

When a duodenal hematoma is found at surgery, it should be evacuated and the serosa then closed and buttressed with omentum or a loop of jejunum. Treatment of patients in whom the diagnosis is not made at surgery involves tube decompression of the stomach and intravenous feeding, usually for at least 7-14 days. Most duodenal obstructions due to intramural hematoma resolve over a one to two week period. If the obstruction were more prolonged, operative treatment with evacuation of the hematoma and closure of the surgical opening in the serosa should be considered.

PERFORATIONS

AXIOM Without a high index of suspicion, blunt duodenal tears may not become clinically apparent until 24-48 hours later.

The diagnosis of blunt duodenal tears is often delayed because: (a) injury was not believed to be a diagnostic possibility, (b) injury was not detected during incomplete abdominal exploration, or (c) some perforations may require hours or days to develop.[43] Reliance on peritoneal lavage for the diagnosis is dangerous because it is not diagnostic in up to 50% of patients with retroperitoneal duodenal injury.[44] The diagnosis, however, should be suspected on plain radiography of the abdomen when retroperitoneal air is found around the right kidney or along the paraspinal muscles. The most accurate nonoperative diagnostic procedure is an upper gastrointestinal radiographic study using gastrografin.

AXIOM When one does not look carefully for retroperitoneal air on flat plates of the abdomen of patients with severe, blunt abdominal trauma, the diagnosis of duodenal tears may be delayed or missed completely.

Debate continues about the best method for repairing duodenal tears. Although some surgeons found that over 80% of penetrating duodenal injuries can be managed by simple debridement and closure,[44] others advocated the use of a serosal patch with or without addition of pyloric exclusion and/or tube decompression of the duodenum. Retrospective analyses make it difficult to compare the efficacy of one method for repair with another.

When a serosal patch is chosen, it is best to use proximal jejunum because an enteroenteric fistula may develop at the site of repair. When the resulting fistula involves distal bowel, the bypass of most of the small bowel could cause malnutrition and overgrowth of bacteria with resultant malabsorption syndrome.

It is claimed that tube decompression of duodenal repair may facilitate healing or at worst provide a controlled fistula; however, evidence that decompression of the duodenum minimizes complications has not been proved. One must also be alert to the possible development of a drain tract infection after the duodenostomy tube is removed.

Advocates of pyloric exclusion believe that it decreases the incidence of duodenal fistula. It is further believed that should a fistula occur, it would be an "end fistula" and, therefore, associated with less loss of gastrointestinal fluid, a lower incidence of complications, and a better chance of closing spontaneously. Pyloric exclusion can be performed by closing the pylorus with a running suture or staples through a gastrotomy incision and then creating a gastrojejunostomy. Unfortunately, the gastrojejunostomy itself can be associated with additional complications, such as bleeding, obstruction, or ulceration. Marginal ulceration occurs in at least 10% of patients who have a pyloric exclusion for duodenal diverticulization, but most of these appear to respond to nonoperative treatment.[45]

With most pyloric exclusions, the pylorus remains occluded for at least two weeks, but patency of the pylorus is spontaneously reestablished within three weeks of the exclusion in 94% of patients.[45] Of the patients with iatrogenic pyloric occlusion persisting for more than two months, 71% had closures done with polypropylene sutures rather than with catgut.[46]

When combined injury of the pancreas and duodenum is manifest, the incidence of duodenal complications appears to be about the same as in isolated duodenal trauma.[47,48] It has also been reported in a retrospective study that the incidence of duodenal fistulas is decreased and intraabdominal abscesses increased when gastrostomy or jejunostomy tubes are used.[48] The reasons for this are not clear and may be due to study biases. A higher incidence of problems also appears to occur when a Roux-en-Y loop of jejunum is anastomosed to the pancreas during the acute phase of injury.

Perforations of the Jejunum or Ileum

Isolated perforation of the jejunum or ileum as a result of blunt trauma is an unusual injury that can be difficult to diagnose early. It is often not apparent or even considered until 10 hours or more after injury.

Three types of jejunal or ileal perforations may occur. Tears near points of attachment, such as the ligament of Treitz, ileocecal valve, or adhesions are due to mobile bowel moving away from an area of fixation. The other type of perforation is presumably due to a blowout injury and can occur anywhere in the small bowel. A third type is due to ischemic necrosis of a badly contused area. Regardless of the mechanism, the perforation is usually discreet, less than 2 cm long, and on the antimesenteric border.[49] Free perforation of the colon due to blunt trauma can also occur on rare occasions.[50]

AXIOM The major factor associated with morbidity and mortality with blunt small bowel injuries is a delay in diagnosis.

Some abdominal pain and tenderness may be present at admission with intraperitoneal small bowel injuries, but it is often minimal. Free intraperitoneal air on radiography also is characteristically absent initially.

Peritoneal lavage can be a valuable diagnostic tool, especially when it shows an excess white blood cell (WBC) count compared to peripheral blood[51]; however, it often takes at least six hours for a significant elevation of WBCs to appear in the peritoneal fluid.[52] Thus, early, negative diagnostic peritoneal lavage does not exclude the diagnosis. Finding alkaline phosphatase > 10 IU/L in the peritoneal lavage effluent has been reported to strongly suggest small or large bowel perforation in an otherwise equivocal lavage fluid analysis.[53]

AXIOM Early, negative diagnostic peritoneal lavage does not exclude intraperitoneal intestinal perforation.

Acute peritoneal signs or a change in abdominal findings eventually develop in almost all patients with small bowel perforation, but severe peritonitis is almost always present if the diagnosis is delayed more than 12-24 hours. Radiography employing water-soluble contrast media may be helpful when perforation has already occurred; however, when perforation occurs later as a result of ischemia, this study may be normal initially. The important point is that any new complaint, especially following blunt trauma, should be taken seriously.[54]

The majority of patients with blunt, small bowel injuries have associated intraabdominal injuries, and thus a diagnosis in those patients is generally made at laparotomy. Mesenteric hematomas associated with transverse tears of the mesentery are not infrequent, and occasionally may cause delayed necrosis of the small bowel.[49]

AXIOM Blunt injuries of small bowel and its mesentery should be suspected with crush injuries of the spine.

Crush injuries of the small bowel and its mesentery are often associated with fractures of the lumbar spine, especially in high-speed accidents in which a seat belt was incorrectly applied to the abdomen rather than across the lap of the patient.[53] When a full-thickness perforation of the bowel becomes sealed by adjacent structures, some patients recover from jejunal injury without operation; however, such patients may present weeks or months later with a stricture at the site of injury.[54]

Posttraumatic Intestinal Strictures

Strictures of the small intestine following blunt trauma are believed to follow direct impact of the bowel against the vertebral column, producing a severe contusion, shearing the bowel from its mesentery, or tearing the mesentery and some of the vessels near its base. These strictures typically involve the mid jejunum or terminal ileum and are usually < 10 cm in length. Patients with posttraumatic intestinal stricture generally present with intermittent episodes of partial intestinal obstruction.

Some of these posttraumatic intestinal stricture patients present atypically. A few present with steatorrhea as a result of bacterial overgrowth above the partial obstruction.[55] The stricture may also mimic Crohn's disease[56,57] or a colonic obstruction, especially on the left side.[58] Mucosal ulcers just proximal to the stricture are frequent, and this is a feature that is not typically associated with chronic, partial small bowel obstruction due to adhesions.

Although injury to the mesentery is often found in blunt abdominal trauma, ischemic stricture is rare and usually occurs in patients who did not undergo operation at the time of the acute injury. Thus, little justification exists to prophylactically resect viable intestine associated with a mesenteric tear or hematoma.

The diagnosis of ischemic stricture may be difficult to establish when a radiographic contrast study of the small intestine is done during a phase when the patient is asymptomatic. Conversely, operation without a contrast study is only justifiable when a clear history of blunt abdominal trauma and a typical presentation of intestinal obstruction exist.

Hemorrhage

Rarely, focal disruption of the mucosa and submucosa without perforation or damage to the adjacent mesentery may present with massive gastrointestinal hemorrhage as late as 16 hours after blunt abdominal trauma.[59] Traumatic false aneurysms communicating with the gastrointestinal tract are another cause of delayed gastrointestinal hemorrhage, and such hemorrhages are apt to be intermittent in nature.[60] When the patient is hemodynamically stable and can safely be moved to the radiology suite, these problems can often be diagnosed and possibly treated angiographically by an interventional radiologist.

Nonocclusive Bowel Infarction

Nonocclusive bowel infarction may occur as a result of severe, persistent hypotension due to blood loss from a nonabdominal source. The diagnosis becomes evident once peritoneal signs develop, and such signs usually develop within 12-18 hours of admission.[61] The nonocclusive ischemic injury generally involves the right colon, but small intestine may also be involved. The distribution of ischemia may also be patchy in nature.

Resection with a proximal stoma and distal mucous fistula or Hartmann pouch is the safest approach. A second-look procedure may be indicated, depending upon the operative findings; however, by the time full thickness necrosis is evident clinically, development of new areas of infarction is unusual.

Improperly Functioning Ileostomy

Creation of an imperfect, albeit temporary, ileostomy can generate inordinate morbidity for a patient. Some of the more common technical errors include improper location of the ostomy so that it is difficult to place an appliance, too short an ileostomy bud, inadequate fascial apertures, tension, stripping of mesentery from the end of the stoma, and failure to close the intraperitoneal space around the bowel leading to the stoma. Although it may be temporary, some months may pass before the stoma is removed. Timing of the ileostomy removal should not be at a fixed, arbitrary interval. It is safest to do electively after all of the patient's wounds have healed, and good nutritional balance and usual state of health has returned.

COMPLICATIONS OF TUBE JEJUNOSTOMY FEEDINGS

Tube jejunostomy feedings are often tolerated relatively well in the immediate postoperative period in patients with major abdominal trauma. In one prospective study, 63% of patients were able to toler-

ate 3000 mL of an elemental diet daily by 72 hours[62]; however, patients with abdominal trauma indexes > 40 were initially less tolerant of such early feedings.

> **AXIOM**   Early enteral feeding can be beneficial in patients with severe trauma, but careful construction of the feeding jejunostomy and monitoring of intestinal acceptance of the diet are extremely important.

Although they can be beneficial to injured patients, early tube jejunostomy feedings can be associated with a number of complications. A dislodged or nonfunctioning jejunostomy tube can cause severe peritonitis or may be a nuisance. No substantive advantage of a needle catheter jejunostomy over slightly larger catheters exists; furthermore, the smaller needle catheters are more likely to occlude and usually could not be replaced if they were dislodged prematurely.[63] A catheter jejunostomy, however, may also have problems. With the Witzel technique, partial small bowel obstruction may occur if too much jejunum were plicated over the catheter. In addition, successful replacement is rare when premature dislodgement occurs.

The Stamm technique may be a more satisfactory method than the Witzel method for inserting feeding jejunostomy catheters. This involves tunneling the catheter straight through the abdominal wall and through a small enterotomy. One or two absorbable purse string sutures can provide a temporary water-tight seal around the catheter at the level of the jejunum. The jejunum immediately surrounding the catheter is then circumferentially attached to the anterior peritoneum with interrupted sutures at the site where the catheter penetrates the abdominal wall. This permits a seal to form between the peritoneum and the jejunal serosa around the catheter site.

A 12 French catheter usually works well as a jejunostomy feeding tube. If it were to become dislodged, it usually could be replaced easily, providing it were done within a short time of the incident. It is essential, however, to confirm successful replacement of the catheter by obtaining a radiograph while flushing water-soluble contrast material through the new catheter. This will avoid instillation of enteral feedings into the free peritoneal cavity if the jejunum has separated from the parietal peritoneum.

> **AXIOM**   The position of the jejunostomy feeding tube within the bowel lumen should be confirmed after any manipulation or replacement prior to beginning or resuming feedings.

Aggressive, early postoperative enteral feedings through a jejunostomy catheter can result in severe pain.[64] It may also cause so much proximal jejunal distention that the bowel can become dusky. This usually occurs soon after the feedings are begun but may also occur weeks later. It is usually manifested clinically by abdominal pain, progressive abdominal distention, and occasional diarrhea. Bacterial translocation[65] and/or necrosis of the jejunum are potential complications of excessive bowel distension. Although such distension may be due to fermentation of carbohydrates and/or hypertonicity of the feeding formula, in many of reported patients, feeding of full-strength enteral formulas at high initial rates (> 50-100 mL/hour) may have been the main factor.

> **AXIOM**   Excessive distension of bowel by enteral feeding should be suspected when the patient has increasing abdominal pain or distension.

A safe, but initially less efficient, nutritional regimen is to instill full-strength formula at 10 mL/hour and increase the infusion by 10 mL/hour every 24 hours. The infusion can be increased at a faster rate once passage of flatus occurs. The majority of patients ultimately tolerate 70-80 mL/hour without difficulty. Poor tolerance to a slowly progressive increase in the infusion rate may indicate the presence of small bowel obstruction. This problem should also be suspected if the jejunostomy catheter were to drain > 200 mL of fluid in 24 hours.

Such catheters (12 French size), placed on gravity drainage, usually drain < 100 mL/24 hours.

A rare, but significant, complication seen with feeding jejunostomies is wrapping of a loop of intestine around the jejunum at the ostomy site, producing a closed-loop intestinal obstruction. This generally is a late complication, but it is one that can rapidly jeopardize a significant length of intestine.

POSTTRAUMATIC COMPLICATIONS INVOLVING LARGE BOWEL

Delayed Perforation

Delayed perforation of the colon may not occur until hours or weeks after the initial trauma. The vast majority of serosal tears and intramural hematomas heal without complication; however, a few of these seemingly innocuous injuries can lead to complications, such as delayed perforation or stricture as a result of: (a) liquefaction of the hematoma within a pseudocapsule and subsequent osmotic expansion of the contained fluid causing compression of the intestinal blood supply, or (b) intramural abscess formation. In addition, omentum or small bowel may initially wall off an acute perforation, only to subsequently break down.

> **AXIOM** Evidence of sepsis or multiple organ failure after abdominal trauma should be considered due to an intraabdominal infection until proved otherwise.

Development of signs of peritonitis obviously prompts immediate operation. In less obvious situations, laparotomy may be indicated for the patient who develops an ileus more than 12 hours after injury or has an initial ileus that fails to resolve after 3-4 days.[66]

Most postoperative septic complications reported after intraperitoneal repair of colonic injuries are not due to suture line disruption; however, confirmation of an intact suture line is essential.

Problems with Exteriorized Colon Repairs

> **AXIOM** Colon repair that is exteriorized without colostomy must be kept moist.

Although petrolatum gauze may be effective for keeping exteriorized colon repair moist, later removal of the gauze can be traumatic. Moist saline gauze coverage is more effective, but such dressings can dry out quickly.

About to 60-75% of exteriorized colon repairs heal properly and can be returned to the peritoneal cavity within 6-8 days. If the suture line were to break down, attempts at suture repair would be almost always fruitless; the failed repair should be accepted as a colostomy. If the repair were to break down early, one would have to be sure that the colon contents were not leaking back into the peritoneal cavity.

Colostomy Complications

The indications for colostomy in blunt pelvic or perineal injuries are not always obvious at admission.[67] Later development of progressive edema, blisters, and necrosis in the perineum is evidence of severe local infection, and a colostomy should be done promptly in order to reduce contamination of injured tissue.

Colostomy performed for perineal or extraperitoneal rectal injuries should be accompanied by washing out of the residual feces in the defunctionalized bowel. If this were not done, retained feces could act as a persistent source of contamination and cause a higher incidence of sepsis and fistula formation.[65]

Colostomy that is brought out to the skin under tension invites disaster because retraction into the subcutaneous tissues can lead to a devastating necrotizing infection of the abdominal wall and/or severe peritonitis. Thus, retraction of the stoma in the early postoperative period is an indication for immediate operative revision. Suturing the colon wall to the abdominal fascia probably does little to prevent such retraction because the bowel pulls away from the fascia when enough tension is present. When such sutures are used, they can pull through the bowel wall as it retracts and cause prestomal fistulas.

> **AXIOM** Suturing colon to abdominal fascia to try to prevent a colostomy from retracting is apt to cause more complications than it prevents.

Stripping mesentery away from the colostomy stoma so that it can come through the hole in the abdominal wall easier is not advised because it increases the risk of necrosis developing in the protruding colon. The abdominal wall aperture should not constrict the colon, and fascial stenosis is best avoided by an adequate cruciate incision. When any change in the color of the exposed bowel occurs, one should assume that the viability of the bowel is threatened. Failure to close the intraperitoneal pericolostomy space invites an internal hernia.

> **AXIOM** Colostomy stoma that becomes progressively more dusky demands immediate revision.

Placement of the colostomy stoma lateral to the rectus sheath increases the likelihood of peristomal hernia; however, placement of a stoma too close to a midline abdominal incision increases the likelihood of a wound infection and/or a poorly fitting appliance.

Some controversy continues about what type of colostomy should be used to treat trauma patients to provide adequate fecal diversion. Proximal end stoma results in complete diversion, but this can make later closure of the colostomy much more difficult. In general, loop colostomy provides effective temporary diversion for the first few postoperative weeks.[66] Incomplete fecal diversion by loop colostomy can be due to several factors, including partial retraction of the colostomy loop into the abdominal wall.

Rectal and Perirectal Complications

With extraperitoneal rectal trauma one should: (a) perform proximal colostomy, (b) remove feces from the distal colon and rectum, and (c) perform presacral drainage up to the site of injury.[69,70] Drains placed within the abdomen and led out through the abdominal wall do not provide adequate drainage, even when sump or other suction catheters are used.[71]

Presacral drains are best inserted with the patient in the lithotomy position. An incision is made posterior to the anus, beyond the external anal sphincter, and lateral to the anococcygeal raphe. A curved clamp is used to dissect upward to the edge of the sacrum, at which point, the levator sling is penetrated. Damage to the rectum can usually be prevented by directing the clamp posteriorly towards the hollow of the sacrum.

Occasionally, even when colostomy and presacral drainage are provided, extraperitoneal rectal injury can cause a necrotizing deep pelvic infection. When adequate debridement cannot be provided from within the abdomen, additional exposure can be obtained by removing the coccyx and lower two sacral segments and then incising the levator sling in the posterior midline. The resulting exposure is greater than one may imagine from anatomic drawings.

HERNIAS AND EVISCERATIONS

Preexisting Inguinal or Femoral Hernias

The necessity for rapid operation in a severely traumatized patient sometimes precludes detection of preexisting inguinal and/or femoral hernias. When such hernias are present, bowel distension in the postoperative period can cause obstruction within the hernia.

> **AXIOM**   One should look carefully for hernias in any patient who develops signs or symptoms of postoperative bowel obstruction.

Internal Hernias

Internal hernias can develop for a variety of reasons following a celiotomy for abdominal trauma. Mesenteric defects may not be closed, particularly when the patient is unstable and efforts are made to complete the operation as rapidly as possible. Such defects are notorious for trapping small bowel and causing later bowel obstruction. Failure to close the space between a colostomy or ileostomy and the lateral peritoneum may also allow an internal hernia to develop. Occasionally, the remaining bowel twists around the bowel leading up to the ostomy site.

Wound Dehiscence

Another form of postoperative hernia is dehiscence or separation of the fascial closure, even when the skin closure remains intact. This situation is sometimes manifest by the discharge of serosanguinous fluid ("red pop") from the incision.

> **AXIOM**   Drainage of serosanguinous fluid from an abdominal incision postoperatively is due to fascial dehiscence until proved otherwise.

Bowel in the subcutaneous tissues may be palpable in thin patients, but can be extremely difficult to detect in obese patients. A cross-table radiograph or CT scan of the abdomen can help to confirm the diagnosis in questionable circumstances.

Necrotizing Fascitis

When the patient appears to develop an infection with necrotic superficial fascia, adequate debridement generally necessitates removal of most, if not all, of the sutures used to close the abdomen. The debridement should continue all around the wound until normal, uninfected fascia is identified. Even though the bowel may appear to be adherent to either the parietal peritoneum or to omentum covering it, the bowel may later eviscerate. This is prevented with suitable packs or by application of a prosthetic material. Use of an abdominal binder and a large occlusive dressing may help to prevent evisceration, but danger still exists that bowel may work its way up between the compressive dressing and the skin and necrose there.

> **AXIOM**   Bowel that appears to be adherent to the peritoneum can still eviscerate out an open abdominal incision and/or develop fistulas unless the bowel is carefully kept below the plane of the peritoneum of the anterior abdominal wall.

Eviscerations

Repair of an evisceration should generally be performed as an emergency procedure in order to minimize the risk of bowel damage and resultant peritonitis. Preparation of the abdominal wall prior to repair must be done with care because soaps or detergents can harm exposed bowel.

Attempting to reclose the abdomen by just resuturing the fascia is prone to failure, and the safest approach is to use full thickness abdominal wall retention sutures. When omentum is not available to cover the underlying bowel, the sutures should be placed through the properitoneal fat so that they will not contact underlying distended intestine. Retention sutures are generally left in place for at least three weeks. Even then, however, a 30% chance of developing a ventral hernia exists.

> **AXIOM**   Eviscerations should generally be closed, at the very least, with full-thickness retention sutures.

POSTTRAUMATIC LIVER COMPLICATIONS

The most frequent complications of liver injury are subcapsular or intrahepatic hematomas, continued or recurrent bleeding, intrahepatic abscesses, intraabdominal abscesses, biliary fistulas, and liver failure.[72] Delayed rupture of a blunt hepatic injury may not become evident until 8 hours to 30 days after injury.[73]

Hematomas

SUBCAPSULAR HEMATOMA
Most subcapsular hematomas of the liver resolve spontaneously, but a few require operation within the next few days when they increase in size and/or cause increasing right upper abdominal pain. This can occur because of clot lysis and movement of fluid into the hyperosmolar hematoma space causing increasing distention of Glisson's capsule. Even though active bleeding is not found after evacuation of the hematoma in the majority of patients, operation is still indicated because one cannot always be certain of the cause of the symptoms. In addition, hepatic injuries are frequently associated with serious injuries to other organs, such as the duodenum or colon, that may have been initially overlooked.

INTRAHEPATIC HEMATOMAS

> **AXIOM**   Intrahepatic hematomas can be associated with fever and leukocytosis even though no infection is present.

Most sterile central hepatic hematomas cause few, if any, signs or symptoms; however, some of these hematomas can cause increasing right upper abdominal pain, fever, leukocytosis, and even an angiographic picture of abscess. Such fever may last for several days or weeks even though no obvious infection is manifest, even on biopsy. When percutaneous or operative aspiration shows no bacteria, hematoma need not be opened or resected.

> **AXIOM**   Intrahepatic hematomas should not be opened surgically unless a complication, such as infection or bleeding, develops.

Closing a deep liver laceration with superficial sutures or placing foreign hemostatic material into the depths of the wound can cause complications in up to one-half of patients.[73] Superficially placed sutures in the presence of a deep injury will not necessarily stop arterial bleeding. Superficial sutures may allow continued intrahepatic bleeding to damage the parenchyma even more and increase the tendency to a later abscess or hemobilia. If the hepatic artery were ligated to achieve hemostasis, even more parenchyma may be rendered ischemic or damaged.

Use of perihepatic packs to control bleeding from the liver is again gaining popularity.[74] The pack is generally removed 24-72 hours after the patient is hemodynamically stable and has normal coagulation parameters. Hazards in the use of such packs include compression of the inferior vena cava and additional injury to ischemic liver tissue. Consequently, extensive debridement of devitalized liver may be required at the time of removal of the pack.

Continued Bleeding or Rebleeding from Injured Liver

Coagulation studies are essential in patients who continue to bleed or rebleed from liver injuries; however, it is hazardous to assume that the bleeding is solely the result of a coagulopathy found on the laboratory tests. Most continued or recurrent postoperative bleeding is from a correctable source, but if such bleeding were allowed to continue, it would eventually result in development of a clotting abnormality.

To adequately access and control sites of delayed bleeding, it is often necessary to completely mobilize the liver if this were not already done at the initial operation. The liver wound is then opened as needed to visualize its depths. Obtaining adequate exposure may require finger fracture of normal hepatic parenchyma.[75] A particularly dangerous area of dissection is along the inferior surface of the liver in the vicinity of the portal structures. Inadequate exposure in this region can easily result in inadvertent ligation of a major hepatic duct. When any question of this exists, operative cholangiography is essential.

After adequate exposure is obtained, any bleeding vessels or lacerated bile ducts can be secured with sutures or clips under direct vision. Adequate debridement of necrotic liver tissue is important, and sometimes requires a lobectomy or segmentectomy. Provision of adequate postoperative drainage, preferably with closed-drainage systems is also preferable.

Hepatic Artery Ligation

When significant arterial bleeding stems from the liver and direct ligation of the bleeding artery is not possible, the appropriate branch of the hepatic artery can be ligated[76]; however, hepatic artery ligation in a setting of compromised collateral flow can lead to central hepatic necrosis and later sepsis or hemorrhage.[73] This may be manifested by the appearance of hypoglycemia and hypoalbuminemia in some patients.[77] If the area of necrosis is very large, it may be necessary to perform extensive hepatic debridement, even to the point of a formal lobectomy.

Hemobilia

Blunt trauma is the commonest cause of bleeding into the bile ducts, and this is called hemobilia or hematobilia. This usually occurs as a result of injury to an intrahepatic artery and an adjacent bile duct. Hemobilia may also occur following a wound that extends through the substance of liver and into the gallbladder lumen.[78] A rather rare cause of late hemobilia is intermittent bleeding of an intrahepatic false aneurysm into the biliary tract.

> **AXIOM** Gastrointestinal bleeding after liver trauma should be considered due to hemobilia until proved otherwise.

Hemobilia classically presents with right upper abdominal pain followed by hematemesis or melena within one to four weeks of the original trauma. The bleeding may give relief of the pain; however, the bleeding can be limited or intermittent and not even be associated with biliary colic. Fever may occur, but it is only rarely due to an associated cholangitis.[79] Hemobilia may also be a manifestation of hepatic abscess with associated cholangitis.

Diagnosis of hemobilia is usually best made on hepatic arteriography. The treatment of hemobilia varies, depending on its severity and etiology. Treatment usually is not necessary when: (a) bleeding was minimal and does not recur, (b) neither sepsis nor aneurysm occurs, and (c) the patient continues to improve. Nevertheless, the bleeding branch of the hepatic artery can usually be embolized successfully by the radiologist at arteriography.

Hepatic Abscesses

> **AXIOM** Sepsis following major liver injury is due to hepatic abscess until proved otherwise.

Hepatic abscesses usually develop within two to three weeks of injury. For early abscesses, operative drainage probably is preferable to the percutaneous approach because debridement of necrotic tissue can also be done. Such debridement must be done carefully because it can cause significant bleeding. Late hepatic abscesses that are well walled off can often be drained successfully percutaneously using ul-

trasound or CT guidance, but controversy continues about the ultimate effectiveness of this approach.

BILIARY TRACT COMPLICATIONS

Biliary Fistulas

> **AXIOM** Extrahepatic biliary tract injuries that are not recognized at surgery usually present as a biliary fistula, bile peritonitis, or progressive jaundice.[80]

ETIOLOGY

Blunt injuries to the extrahepatic biliary tree, especially the common hepatic or right or left hepatic ducts, are uncommon, and the only initial indication of such an injury at surgery may be a hematoma in the porta hepatis with or without bile staining. An even rarer situation involves delayed rupture of the gallbladder due to an initially incomplete transmural tear, intramural hematoma, or breakdown of omental seal at a site of injury. Consequently, evidence of a posttraumatic bile leak, manifested by jaundice, with or without ascites and vomiting, may not occur for days or weeks. Partial avulsion of the gallbladder from its bed while its blood supply and ductal connection are intact can present as a late acute cholecystitis, particularly if the gallbladder were to twist on its pedicle.

DIAGNOSIS

When a bile leak is suspected, HIDA scan can be performed. If the initial images were negative or inconclusive, delayed images should be taken.

Endoscopic retrograde choledochopancreatography (ERCP) can be helpful for detecting bile duct injuries, but there may be an increased risk of causing infection with this technique. If a bile duct injury is demonstrated but continuity between the biliary tract and the duodenum is manifest, an indwelling catheter passed retrograde through an endoscope may act as a stent while the area heals.

Percutaneous transhepatic cholangiography (PTC) can provide good definition of the bile ducts, but it may be difficult to perform successfully in the absence of ductal dilatation.

TREATMENT

> **AXIOM** Premature attempts at operative closure of biliary fistulas are fraught with problems.

Extrahepatic Biliary Fistulas

It is not necessary to rush for operative repair of a noninfected extrahepatic biliary fistula. Early exploration in a patient without sepsis or pain is usually unwise because most of these fistulas eventually heal spontaneously without any problem. The tissue associated with early biliary fistula is frequently inflamed or edematous and the duct may be quite small. Attempts to perform reconstructive surgery on a small duct in the presence of acute inflammatory edema may cause further damage and make subsequent treatment even more difficult. It is far safer in this situation to allow a stricture to develop because this causes proximal dilatation of the bile ducts, making later definitive repair much easier.

The principles to be followed in the treatment of extrahepatic biliary tract fistulas include: (a) adequate drainage, (b) control of infection, and (c) provision of nutrition. Inadequate drainage tends to result in pooling of bile in or near Morrison's pouch, and this is a frequent forerunner of subhepatic abscesses.

The amount of biliary drainage from a torn common hepatic duct or common bile duct over a period of several days can be substantial and can eventually result in significant fluid and electrolyte disorders. When biliary drainage is collected and returned to the stomach, clinically significant bile gastritis can develop; however, refeeding through a jejunostomy tube can usually be done without ill effects.

Bile Peritonitis and Bile Ascites

Bile peritonitis should be distinguished from bile ascites. Bile ascites is the result of sterile bile and reactive ascitic fluid collecting in the peritoneal cavity with only a mild inflammatory response. Bile peritonitis, in contrast, is associated with clinically apparent inflammation of parietal peritoneum. Although infection is generally believed to be present in bile peritonitis, bacteria are not always detectable. Bile ascites is relatively benign but the mortality rate for bile peritonitis may approach 20% and requires urgent control of the fistula. Early definitive repair of bile ascites or bile peritonitis is seldom possible, but insertion of a catheter into the biliary system may greatly reduce the amount of bile leak.

Biliary Strictures

AXIOM   Progressive, unfluctuating jaundice occurring relatively soon after biliary tract trauma usually indicates that a stricture is present.

Bile duct strictures with jaundice should be corrected as soon as possible after the patient has recovered as much as is safely possible from the original trauma. Although definitive repair may not be possible at this time, intubation of the bile duct through the stricture can be extremely beneficial.

If suppurative cholangitis were to develop, biliary drainage should be provided on an emergency basis. When the duct cannot be intubated by ERCP or a transhepatic approach, operative drainage is required. In some late cases, hepatic transplantation has been necessary because of the unreconstructable nature of injured bile ducts.

Intrahepatic Biliary Fistulas

A biliary fistula from a disrupted intrahepatic bile duct may not become evident for several days. After adequate drainage is provided, most of these fistulas heal with little problem. With the recent trend toward nonoperative management of blunt injuries to the liver, one must be alert to the development of a biliary fistula, especially if it were to present as bile peritonitis.[81] Early, profound jaundice may indicate the presence of a biliary-hepatic vein fistula.[82]

It is hazardous to assume that a biliary fistula occurring after a liver resection for trauma is nothing more than leakage from the cut hepatic surface. When the fistula is a result of unrecognized hilar damage or incorrectly placed deep sutures to control bleeding, the bile leak may persist for a prolonged period and can result in cholangitis.

Repair or intubation of injured intrahepatic ducts can be extremely difficult because of the small size of the ducts and the distorted anatomy occurring from local inflammation and any hepatic regeneration that may have occurred. Adequate external drainage may be the best that one can hope for until a fibrous fistula tract is well established.

Acalculous Cholecystitis

ETIOLOGY

Acalculous cholecystitis develops most frequently in severely traumatized patients who become septic and receive prolonged parenteral nutrition with no enteral feedings. Dehydration and poor tissue perfusion may also be predisposing factors.

DIAGNOSIS

The clinical manifestations of acute acalculous cholecystitis are variable but not different from those of acute cholecystitis with stones. What makes the diagnosis of acalculous cholecystitis difficult in critically ill patients are the subtle signs and symptoms that it may produce. The actual time of onset of acalculus cholecystitis after trauma is extremely varied but typically develops after two to three weeks of parenteral nutrition.

AXIOM   Unless one has a high index of suspicion for the development of acalculous cholecystitis in critically ill patients who are on prolonged parenteral nutrition, the diagnosis may be greatly delayed.

Ultrasonography and hepatobiliary scintigraphy have been reported to be helpful, but this is not a uniform experience.[83,84] On ultrasound, acalculus cholecystitis typically reveals nonspecific dilatation of the gallbladder with a thickened wall, some sludge, and surrounding fluid. When air is seen in the wall of the gallbladder, severe infection is generally present. Increased viscosity of bile from prolonged fasting may prevent sufficient isotopic entry into the gallbladder to visualize it. Consequently, the HIDA scan tends to falsely indicate a cystic duct obstruction compatible with acute cholecystitis.

TREATMENT

Administration of oral fat to critically ill patients and those on parenteral nutrition has been suggested as a means of preventing acalculus cholecystitis. Although fat in the duodenum releases cholecystokinin which should cause the gallbladder to contract, the efficacy of such a regimen is not known.

When acute acalculus cholecystitis is diagnosed, the gallbladder should be resected as soon as possible. Although it may be tempting to perform a cholecystostomy in some critically ill patients, multiple scattered areas of gangrene are evident in at least 40% of these gallbladders. If only a cholecystostomy were performed, local areas of gangrene could leak and cause later severe peritonitis.

The mortality rate for acute acalculous cholecystitis can be quite high, ranging in some series 17-66%,[85] with higher death rates generally due to severe underlying problems. Depending upon how early the diagnosis is made, the operative findings may vary from just edema of the gallbladder wall to gangrene with perforation.

PANCREATIC COMPLICATIONS AFTER TRAUMA

A number of complications can develop following injury to the pancreas. Of the complications seen, up to 35% are pancreatic fistulas, 25% acute pancreatitis, 20% pancreatic abscesses and/or necrosis, and up to 10% pseudocysts. Obviously, a patient may develop more than one of these complications.

Pancreatic Fistulas

TREATMENT OF PANCREATIC FISTULAS

Pancreatic fistulas and pseudocysts are more common after unrecognized blunt trauma to the pancreas. Most pancreatic fistulas close spontaneously in one to three months. With larger fistulas, careful monitoring of fluid and electrolyte balance may be necessary during this period. The role of somatostatin in reducing the volume of pancreatic secretions and facilitating spontaneous healing is beneficial in some, but not all patients. Even after spontaneous closure of a fistula, the patient must be carefully followed because occlusion of the fistula may result in the formation of an infected pseudocyst or ductal stricture.

External pancreatic fistulas lasting more than five to six months generally are treated by operation. Outlining the anatomy of the main pancreatic duct by ERCP is helpful in planning the procedure. If a proximal stricture were present, a Puestow procedure (anastomosis of the pancreatic duct in the body of the pancreas to a Roux-en-Y loop of jejunum) may permit preservation of islet cell-bearing tissue. Chronic fistulas often can be simply diverted into a Roux-en-Y jejunal limb without dissecting the pancreatic duct; however, certain patients may require distal pancreatectomy. If this were done, one should try to perform the resection without sacrificing the spleen.

PANCREATIC ASCITES

Pancreatic ascites occurs as a result of injury to a major duct, rupture of an uninfected pseudocyst, or pancreatic necrosis. Other than vague distension and discomfort from the ascites, relatively few symptoms may occur. In pancreatic ascites, amylase concentration in the peritoneal fluid is generally at least three to five times greater than in blood.

If pancreatic ascites were tolerated reasonably well, the patient could be observed for one to three months in the hope that the internal fistula would close spontaneously. Somatostatin may also be of value. This is not unrealistic when ERCP reveals no proximal obstruction of the pancreatic duct. If the patient were to have severe or increasing symptoms, ERCP should be performed; if an injured duct were found, the operative principles would be the same as those for a pancreatic fistula.

Posttraumatic Pancreatitis

ETIOLOGY

Virtually any significant injury to the pancreas can result in a local inflammatory response which may or may not be apparent clinically. The commonest operative injury to the pancreas occurs during splenectomy, particularly when the intimate relationship between the splenic hilum and the tail of the pancreas is not adequately appreciated. Clamping splenic vessels more than about 1 cm from the spleen can easily result in traumatic pancreatitis and occasional formation of a pseudocyst or fistula.

Pancreatic trauma occasionally results in chronic pancreatic ductal obstruction. The traumatic incident may have been relatively minor and a detailed history may be required to have the patient recall the event. The diagnosis of pancreatic ductal obstruction is suggested by recurrent episodes of acute pancreatitis or a late-appearing pseudocyst. Depending upon the anatomical circumstances, ductal obstruction is best managed by either distal pancreatic resection or Roux-en-Y pancreaticojejunostomy.

DIAGNOSIS

Clinical

Traumatic pancreatitis is usually diagnosed on the basis of the clinical findings and elevated serum or urine amylase levels. Elevated serum lipase levels may also be strongly suggestive of the diagnosis. Persistent upper abdominal pain radiating straight through to the back with ileus and nausea and vomiting and increasing intravenous fluid requirements should make one suspicious of the diagnosis. Evidence of pancreatic injury at initial operation obviously also helps to establish the diagnosis.

Amylase and Lipase Levels

Although elevated serum amylase levels are often considered the single most important test in diagnosing acute pancreatitis, many false-positive and false-negative results occur. False-positive results are particularly likely to be seen with associated injury to small bowel or the salivary glands.[86,87] False-negative results most often are a consequence of the test being done too late in the course of the illness. Serum amylase levels can return to normal within 8-12 hours. In addition, severe pancreatitis with extensive necrosis may not even produce an increase in serum amylase levels. This may occur because of: (a) inability of a severely injured gland to release amylase, (b)

pouring of amylase into the retroperitoneum rather than into the blood stream, or (c) enhanced renal amylase clearance; however, urinary or peritoneal fluid amylase levels may be elevated even though serum levels are normal.[88]

Many causes can elevate serum amylase levels apart from pancreatic inflammation. Isoenzyme analysis—which is usually only available in experimental laboratories—permits distinction between pancreatic amylase and amylase of nonpancreatic origin, such as from the salivary glands.[89] Urine amylase clearance ratios are not specific, but can be helpful in the appropriate clinical setting.

Elevated lipase levels in blood and urine may be due to injury to fat or to development of the fat embolism syndrome, and they offer no advantage over amylase measurements.

Radiography

Plain radiography of the abdomen is not helpful in diagnosing posttraumatic pancreatitis, but ultrasonographic and CT scans can be extremely helpful when they clearly demonstrate pancreatic pathology. When chest radiography shows a left pleural effusion, which on thoracentesis contains a very high amylase level, and there is no evidence of an esophageal leak, the diagnosis is almost certain.

TREATMENT

Supportive Therapy

Therapy of acute traumatic pancreatitis is directed primarily at its complications, especially hypovolemia. Fluid losses around the pancreas may be extremely high. Multiple organ system failure may also occur in severe, acute pancreatitis. Manifestations include respiratory and renal failure, jaundice, diabetes, hypocalcemia, metabolic acidosis, coagulopathy, ECG changes, ophthalmologic problems, skeletal disorders, cutaneous fat necrosis, and psychiatric disturbances.

VENTILATORY SUPPORT

Severe lung changes can occur in acute pancreatitis because of: (a) the effect of pancreatic enzymes on complement, (b) the effects of lipase on surfactant, and (c) the development of pleural effusions and reduced diaphragmatic movement. More than half of the patients with severe, acute pancreatitis develop abnormalities in pulmonary function. If the arterial PO_2 were to begin to decrease significantly, prompt intubation and ventilatory support should be provided to maintain arterial PO_2 at levels of at least 60 and preferably 70-80 mm Hg without exceeding an FiO_2 of 0.5.

FLUID RESUSCITATION. One of the major goals of treatment of traumatic pancreatitis is rapid restoration of the extracellular fluid (ECF) volume to normal or higher levels. In experimental acute pancreatitis, this may require relatively rapid infusion of a fluid volume exceeding 80% of the normal ECF. Although earlier studies suggested that albumin-containing solutions were important in the resuscitation of acute pancreatitis, Ringer's lactate appears to be equally effective.

Metabolic acidosis can occur as a result of a blood volume deficit and is best corrected by improving tissue perfusion. Hematocrit should be monitored frequently because any increase indicates the necessity for more aggressive fluid administration.

Renal failure usually can be prevented by prompt restoration of the plasma volume; however, evidence suggests that renal failure associated with acute pancreatitis can occur even in the absence of demonstrable hypotension.

NASOGASTRIC SUCTION.   Controversy exists about the importance of nasogastric suction in treating acute pancreatitis. In the mild forms of the disease, it probably adds little; however, in more serious cases, it may be of some help. The inflammatory process in severe, acute pancreatitis can produce a functional obstruction of the duodenum and/or stomach, which can be symptomatically relieved by nasogastric tube; however, aspiration of gastric acid does not permit the pancreas to "rest".[90]

CALCIUM.   Hypocalcemia is common in severe, acute pancreatitis and was believed to be primarily related to formation of calcium soaps with free fatty acids. It is known that parahormone effects are also suppressed, but it is not clear whether this is related to just suppression of parahormone secretion or whether the tissues are less responsive to circulating parahormones. The low, total-calcium levels seen in severe, acute pancreatitis are also at least partially due to hypoalbuminemia which can be quite marked. Low calcium levels in acute pancreatitis are rarely associated with symptoms of hypocalcemia, and little evidence suggests that empiric treatment of hypocalcemia changes the course of underlying pancreatitis. Nevertheless, administration of albumin in the presence of low, total-serum-calcium levels can occasionally cause tetany, presumably due to increased calcium binding.

AXIOM   Hypocalcemia occurs frequently in severe pancreatitis, but it usually doesn't require treatment unless it is symptomatic.

ANTIBIOTICS.   No substantive data indicate that the prophylactic use of antibiotics is effective in reducing the incidence of septic complications in traumatic pancreatitis.

AXIOM   Routine administration of antibiotics to patients with acute pancreatitis will probably not reduce the rate of infection.

DRUGS.   Some of the drugs that have been used to treat acute pancreatitis include: (a) H_2-receptor antagonists to diminish gastric acid secretion, (b) aprotinin (Trasylol®) to inhibit serum proteases, and (c) anticholinergic drugs or somatostatin to decrease pancreatic secretion. Unfortunately, no substantive data indicate that any benefit exists from using these agents.

NUTRITION.   When a feeding jejunostomy was placed at the initial operation and no small bowel injury distal to the catheter occurred, tube feedings with a low-fat, elemental diet can be started early without fear of aggravating the pancreatic inflammation. When a jejunostomy tube is not in place, total parenteral nutrition should be begun early. When serum triglyceride levels are not elevated, fat can be given relatively freely, but its levels before and after a fat load should be monitored periodically.

SURGERY.   Laparotomy is recommended in patients with traumatic pancreatitis who do not respond to initial treatment or who initially respond but then later relapse: however, no precise guidelines exist as to how soon patients should have adequate responses to nonoperative management, especially with injuries to other organs.

AXIOM   Patients with posttraumatic pancreatitis that continues to worsen for more than 48 hours should generally have exploratory laparotomy.

Several reasons exist for performing surgery in patients with severe, acute pancreatitis that is not improving. For example, several situations require surgical treatment that may mimic acute pancreatitis and sometimes the distinction can only be made by surgical exploration. A missed injury to the duodenum, jejunum, or ileum is especially important and can be confused with acute pancreatitis both clinically and chemically.

Even when the diagnosis of acute pancreatitis is correct and nothing is found at operation that requires repair, repeated large-volume peritoneal lavage has been reported to correct the acute metabolic abnormalities that may be associated with this process.[91] It is unknown whether this is simply a temporizing measure that postpones mortality from other complications, such as sepsis. Certainly, in nontraumatic pancreatitis, lavage does not influence mortality.

PERITONEAL LAVAGE.   Continuing peritoneal lavage postoperatively carries some hazard of introducing intraperitoneal infection, but potential benefits also exist from removing activated enzymes from the peripancreatic spaces. One approach to peritoneal irrigation for acute pancreatitis involves placement of a catheter in the lesser sac and a second one in the right pericolic gutter.[92] One liter of Ringer's lactate or peritoneal dialysate is introduced into the abdominal cavity through these catheters, left for an hour, and then drained via the same catheters. Peritoneal irrigation can be continued on an hourly basis until systemic signs improve. Catheters are left in place for another 12-24 hours so that the lavage could easily be reinstituted if systemic signs or symptoms were to recur.

Splenectomy for Splenic Vein Thrombosis.   Focal portal hypertension as a result of splenic vein thrombosis may occasionally follow severe, acute pancreatitis and produce esophageal or isolated gastric varices.[93] If these varices produce any significant bleeding, the treatment of choice is splenectomy.

Pancreatic Infections

TERMINOLOGY

The prognosis of infection related to pancreatitis differs, depending upon the nature of the infection; thus, precise definition is essential. There is some agreement that pancreatic abscess should refer to a grossly purulent, liquified collection contained within a fibrous capsule. This definition includes infected pseudocysts. The terms, acute necrotizing pancreatitis or pancreatic necrosis, are generally used to refer to either pancreatic or peripancreatic necrosis. Some authors, however, include any purulent liquid collection and/or necrosis in the area of the pancreas in their definition of a pancreatic abscess. The distinction between pancreatic abscess and pancreatic necrosis is important because abscesses are generally diagnosed later than necrosis and have a less fulminant course and lower mortality. Furthermore, patients who also have extrapancreatic fat necrosis tend to be more severely ill. If the extrapancreatic necrotic tissue were to become infected, the morbidity and mortality rates may rise precipitously.

DIAGNOSIS

A diffuse, necrotizing retroperitoneal infection can be difficult to diagnose, but its presence is suggested clinically in patients with severe, acute pancreatitis who remain seriously ill or who are becoming much more septic. Not infrequently, sepsis may appear to be due to pulmonary changes which are often also present. Positive blood culture in a septic patient with pancreatic injury often requires an exploratory laparotomy to confirm the diagnosis of necrotizing peripancreatic infection and treat it. The organisms most frequently involved with these infections are gram-negative aerobes of gastrointestinal origin.

Plain radiography of the abdomen showing "soap bubbles" in and around the pancreas can be diagnostic when this finding can be differentiated from stool mixed with gas in the colon; however, the presence of pancreatic "soap bubbles" is a late finding.

Conventional CT is not a reliable method for establishing the diagnosis of retroperitoneal necrosis. Dynamic CT of the pancreas, which involves pressure injection of a large volume of intravenous contrast so that specific time-density reconstructions of the pancreas and its perfusion can be accomplished, is usually much more accurate. The majority of patients with positive dynamic CT scans have been reported to have infected retroperitoneal necrosis, but as experience is gained with this diagnostic modality, its value is becoming less certain. Although it is not necessarily an indication for operation, positive dynamic CT scan appears to be useful for determining the necessity for other diagnostic procedures, such as percutaneous needle aspiration. When the needle aspiration shows bacteria, urgent operation is generally needed. When no bacteria are found, indications for operation are based primarily on the patient's clinical course. Pragmatically, however, clinical findings lead to exploration in most patients.

Necrotizing peripancreatic infections are best diagnosed at surgery by the presence of diffuse, thick, pastelike necrotic material in and around the pancreas. The full extent of the process usually is not appreciated preoperatively. Necrosis can extend down into both gutters and into the folds of the small and large bowel mesentery. Occasionally, the process can even occlude mesenteric or retroperitoneal vessels.

TREATMENT

AXIOM	Percutaneous drains placed under radiographic control will not adequately drain infected necrotic pancreatic or peripancreatic tissue.

Necrotizing retroperitoneal peripancreatic infections cannot generally be controlled until the infected tissue is adequately debrided.[94] Multiple operations may be necessary to gain control of the infection, and mortality may be as high as 50%. Suction drains left in the areas of debridement may erode into adjacent intestine, but the risk of this complication theoretically may be reduced by interposing omentum between the drains and bowel.

When an infected pseudocyst is present, percutaneous aspiration under radiologic guidance can be attempted for diagnosis and treatment. It is difficult to see, however, how this could provide better control than open surgical drainage.

Posttraumatic Pancreatic Pseudocysts

ETIOLOGY

Pseudocyst of the pancreas can be a complication of acute pancreatitis regardless of its etiology. Pseudocysts are usually due to a tear in a moderate-to-large-sized pancreatic duct allowing pancreatic secretions to drain into a peripancreatic space where it becomes sealed off from the remainder of the peritoneal cavity. A pseudocyst may not become clinically apparent for weeks or months after a relatively innocuous, blunt injury to the abdomen. Such pseudocysts often are associated with a crack in the pancreas over the lumbar spine, but isolated or multiple injuries to the head and tail of the pancreas can also occur as a result of blunt trauma.[95-96] The appearance of a pseudocyst or recurring episodes of acute pancreatitis may indicate the presence of a ductal stricture,[96] which is usually definable by endoscopic retrograde pancreatography.

DIAGNOSIS

Suspicion of a pseudocyst is raised by a variety of symptoms and/or signs that includes presence of an upper abdominal mass, persistent upper abdominal or back pain, or a persistently elevated serum amylase. The diagnosis is confirmed by ultrasonography or CT.

TREATMENT

Nonoperative Management

Controversy continues about the management of small (< 4-5 cm diameter) asymptomatic, stable pseudocysts. Such cysts seldom cause harm, and an increasing tendency to just observe them exists. Even when the cyst is > 5 cm in diameter, progressive clinical improvement without evidence of infection indicates that only observation is necessary.

AXIOM	The sequential evaluation of pseudocysts by ultrasonography permits relatively accurate determination of changing size.

Timing of Surgery

In symptomatic patients, it is usually desirable to provide early nourishment either intravenously or via a jejunostomy catheter, and postpone any operation for four to six weeks to permit enough maturation of the cyst wall to hold sutures.[97] This time line is changing as a result of CT scans showing earlier thickening of the pseudocyst wall. Conversely, when the pseudocyst is expanding and rupture appears to be imminent, more urgent surgical treatment is indicated. When increasing pain or evidence of infection or bleeding occurs, operation becomes an urgent matter.

Techniques of Pseudocyst Drainage

When the pseudocyst wall is too thin to hold sutures well, external drainage is required. When operative drainage is required and the cyst wall is of adequate thickness, internal drainage with a cystgastrostomy, cystduodenostomy, or Roux-en-Y cystjejunostomy are the preferred operative techniques, depending on the location of the pseudocyst. Some believe that internal drainage of an infected pseudocyst is undesirable, but this is not the case when the cyst wall is thick and the purulent contents are removed prior to completing the anastomosis.

COMPLICATIONS

External drainage of pancreatic pseudocysts is complicated by a 25% incidence of pancreatic fistula. Bleeding from the pseudocyst wall as a result of varices from splenic vein occlusion, pseudoaneurysm formation, or erosion into an adjacent vessel can occur following drainage.[98] Occasionally, pseudocyst recurs after apparently adequate drainage. This is usually due to a proximal or ductal obstruction which is usually detectable by ERCP.

Hemorrhage

When one suspects that hemorrhage has occurred into a pseudocyst or into the retroperitoneum, angiography can be effective for diagnosis and treatment by embolizing the involved vessel(s). Successful embolization of an artery that is bleeding into pseudocyst can avoid a potentially hazardous operation; however, angiography is not uniformly successful in identifying the involved vessel.

When bleeding is persistent or severe and/or the involved vessels have been identified angiographically, they can potentially be ligated outside the pseudocyst. Otherwise, the pseudocyst has to be opened and the open bleeding vessels controlled directly with sutures. Unfortunately, such ligatures may cause necrosis and recurrence of bleeding. In the case of bleeding into the pseudocyst from focal varices due to splenic vein thrombosis, splenectomy may be all that is required.

Splenic Rupture

Spontaneous rupture of the spleen is a rare complication of acute pancreatitis with or without pseudocyst formation. This is believed to be due to thrombosis of the splenic vein with residual patency of the splenic artery, leading to continued expansion of the spleen. Splenectomy is the treatment of choice.

⊘ FREQUENT ERRORS

In the Management of Gastrointestinal Complications Following Trauma

1. *Failing to eliminate Clostridium difficile colitis in posttraumatic diarrhea when the patient has been receiving antibiotics.*
2. *Failing to monitor gastric pH and its response to therapy in critically ill posttraumatic patients.*
3. *Providing inadequate attention to nutrition and peritoneal drainage in patients with posttraumatic enterocutaneous fistulas.*
4. *Failing to consider the possibility of mechanical bowel obstruction in patients who have prolonged ileus and/or excessive gastric aspirate.*

5. *Providing inadequate tube decompression of the stomach during induction and maintenance of anesthesia in a patient with small bowel obstruction.*
6. *Having reluctance to perform second-look operations in patients with bowels of questionable viability.*
7. *Assuming that an early (< 3 hr) negative, diagnostic, peritoneal lavage or CT scan effectively eliminates traumatic bowel injury.*
8. *Not working aggressively to detect intraabdominal infection in patients developing multiple-organ failure after abdominal trauma.*
9. *Failing to perform colostomy, clearing of feces from the distal colon and rectum, and presacral drainage in patients with rectal injuries.*
10. *Providing inadequate debridement of devitalized liver tissue after trauma.*
11. *Failing to consider the possibility that hemobilia may be the cause of gastrointestinal bleeding after abdominal trauma.*
12. *Failing to attempt to definitively correct asymptomatic biliary fistula early.*
13. *Failing to consider the possibility of acute acalculus cholecystitis in patients receiving TPN for more than two to three weeks.*
14. *Relying excessively on serum amylase levels to confirm or eliminate posttraumatic pancreatic complications.*
15. *Failing to differentiate between sterile and infected abscesses associated with acute pancreatitis.*

▼▼▼▼▼▼▼▼▼▼▼▼▼▼▼▼▼▼▼▼▼▼▼▼▼▼▼▼

SUMMARY POINTS

1. One should look carefully for Candida infections in trauma patients who are not doing well after 7-14 days of broad-spectrum antibiotics.
2. Diarrhea, in a patient who has been on broad-spectrum antibiotics, should be considered as due to pseudomembranous colitis until proved otherwise.
3. The presentation and distribution of pseudomembranous colitis is extremely variable, but should be suspected in anyone who develops diarrhea after receiving antibiotics.
4. All patients with prolonged stress, particularly when due to severe sepsis, have some degree of stress gastritis.
5. Stress ulcerations are usually greatest in the body of the stomach, and the antrum is usually either spared or only minimally involved.
6. Stress ulcerations are not a primary disease; they are a manifestation of severe underlying illness.
7. Although many patients with stress gastritis do not hypersecrete acid, some acid is necessary to cause the luminal pH to decrease to < 3.5 to cause the lesions.
8. Although factors other than acid may aggravate tissue damage in the stomach, stress gastric mucosal lesions are not apt to occur in the absence of luminal acid.
9. Both restitution and replication of gastric mucosal cells are inhibited by luminal acid.
10. As long as severe sepsis persists, stress gastritis also tends to progress, regardless what treatment is used.
11. Gastrointestinal bleeding in a stressed patient is not necessarily due to stress ulceration.
12. Antacids or H_2-receptor antagonists can usually prevent severe stress gastritis as long as severe shock or sepsis is controlled and the gastric luminal pH is kept > 3.5.
13. Surgical intervention is rarely necessary for stress gastritis, but it may be indicated when nonoperative methods fail to control bleeding.
14. Cushing's ulcers—versus usual stress ulcers—tend to be associated with greater gastrin and acid secretion and are usually deeper and more apt to perforate.

15. Patients with severe burns should have gastric luminal pH monitored while nasogastric tubes are present, and antacids and/or H_2 blockers should be given until the burns are completely healed.
16. The greater mortality from high-output fistulas is due to increased risk of developing intraabdominal infection and the significantly lower rate of spontaneous closure.
17. Although many factors tend to make an intestinal fistula persist, the most important is a distal obstruction.
18. Metabolic support with adequate calories and protein plus accurate replacement of the fistula output of water and electrolytes are essential for maintaining optimal healing and host defense systems in the patient.
19. Prolonged nasogastric tube drainage is probably of little benefit for curing well-established intestinal fistulas.
20. Intestinal fistulas generally do not heal unless local and systemic sepsis have been controlled.
21. Definitive surgical treatment of a gastrointestinal fistula should not be attempted at the same time that an abscess is drained.
22. Spontaneous closure of a fistula should not be expected until adequate control of the fistula, eradication of sepsis, and provision of nutritional repletion occur.
23. When an intestinal fistula has not closed spontaneously within one month of proper control of infection and provision of adequate nutrition, definitive surgical correction is generally required.
24. The most successful operative approach for enterocutaneous fistula is resection of the involved segment of bowel with reanastomosis of normal tissue.
25. Suspected intestinal anastomotic disruptions should be treated surgically as soon as possible. If the diagnosis were uncertain, preoperative radiographic studies should be performed promptly, preferably with a water-soluble contrast agent.
26. Patients with persistent fever plus ileus or delayed gastric emptying following small-bowel repairs should be considered to have an anastomotic disruption until proved otherwise.
27. A contained anastomotic leak can sometimes be confused clinically with persistent posttraumatic pancreatitis.
28. Although they cannot be completely prevented, peritoneal adhesions can often be reduced by careful surgical technique.
29. Abdominal distention developing after the fourth postoperative day should be considered to be due to bowel obstruction until proved otherwise.
30. A high index of suspicion and frequent careful examinations are particularly important for diagnosing early bowel obstruction after extensive abdominal trauma.
31. A feculent odor or appearance of nasogastric aspirate or vomitus is often a sign of complete small bowel obstruction.
32. Although cramping abdominal pain is not characteristic of adynamic ileus, the absence of such pain does not exclude mechanical obstruction.
33. A tendency for the patient to require increased intravenous fluids after the third day postoperatively should make one suspect complications, such as bowel obstruction or infection.
34. When it is not clear whether a loop of bowel is dilated small bowel or colon, a contrast enema should be performed.
35. Bowel obstruction associated with constant abdominal pain out of proportion to the physical findings in the appropriate clinical setting is a fairly reliable indication of strangulation of bowel.
36. Severe abdominal pain out of proportion to the physical findings should be considered an indication for urgent surgical intervention until proved otherwise.
37. One of the main reasons to operate early on what is probably a simple intestinal obstruction is the difficulty in eliminating the presence of strangulation.
38. When the patient continues to have flatus, indicating that a suspected bowel obstruction is probably only partial, there is less risk that strangulated bowel is present.
39. Failure to perform a second look operation on marginally viable bowel greatly increases the risk of nonviable bowel being left in place and causing fatal peritonitis.

40. When any spill of the contents of obstructed bowel occurs, the skin and subcutaneous tissues should not be closed.
41. Large ECF deficits can occur rapidly when a distal small bowel obstruction is decompressed with a long tube.
42. One must be careful to not allow powerful Valsalva maneuvers to cause regurgitation of gastrointestinal contents into the lungs at the end of an operation on obstructed bowel.
43. Diarrhea associated with small bowel distention frequently is due to partial obstruction.
44. Intussusception usually presents as a partial small bowel obstruction.
45. Although spontaneous reduction of an intussusception may occur, it is safer to undertake operation in order to prevent irreducibility as a result of edema or necrosis.
46. Any intussuscepted bowel that cannot be readily reduced at surgery should be resected.
47. Without a high index of suspicion, blunt duodenal tears may not become clinically apparent until 24-48 hours later.
48. When one does not look carefully for retroperitoneal air on plain radiography of the abdomen of patients with severe blunt abdominal trauma, the diagnosis of duodenal tears may be delayed or missed completely.
49. The major factor associated with morbidity and mortality with blunt small bowel injuries is a delay in diagnosis.
50. A negative diagnostic peritoneal lavage within 2-3 hours of trauma does not exclude intraperitoneal intestinal perforations.
51. Blunt injuries of small bowel and its mesentery should be suspected with crush injuries of the spine.
52. Early enteral feeding can be beneficial in patients with severe trauma, but careful construction of feeding jejunostomy and monitoring of intestinal acceptance of the diet are extremely important.
53. The position of a jejunostomy feeding tube within the bowel lumen should be confirmed after any manipulation or replacement prior to beginning or resuming feedings.
54. Excessive distension of bowel by enteral feeding should be suspected when the patient has increasing abdominal pain or distension.
55. Evidence of sepsis or multiple organ failure after abdominal trauma should be considered due to intraabdominal infection until proved otherwise.
56. Colon repair that is exteriorized without colostomy must be kept moist.
57. Suturing colon to abdominal fascia to try to prevent a colostomy from retracting is apt to cause more complications than it prevents.
58. A colostomy stoma that becomes progressively more dusky demands immediate revision.
59. One should look carefully for hernias in any patient who develops signs or symptoms suggestive of postoperative bowel obstruction.
60. Drainage of serosanguinous fluid from an abdominal incision postoperatively is due to a fascial dehiscence until proved otherwise.
61. Bowel that appears to be adherent to the peritoneum can still eviscerate out an open abdominal incision and/or develop fistulas unless the bowel is carefully kept below the plane of the peritoneum of the anterior abdominal wall.
62. Eviscerations should generally be closed with full-thickness retention sutures.
63. Intrahepatic hematomas can be associated with fever and leukocytosis even though no infection is present.
64. Intrahepatic hematomas should not be opened surgically unless a complication, such as infection or bleeding, develops.
65. Gastrointestinal bleeding after liver trauma should be considered due to hemobilia until proved otherwise.
66. Sepsis following a major liver injury is due to hepatic abscess until proved otherwise.
67. Extrahepatic biliary tract injuries that are not recognized at operation usually present as a biliary fistula, bile peritonitis, or progressive jaundice.

68. Premature attempts at operative closure of biliary fistulas are fraught with problems.
69. Progressive, unfluctuating jaundice occurring relatively soon after biliary tract trauma usually indicates that a stricture is present.
70. Unless one has a high index of suspicion for the development of acalculous cholecystitis in critically ill patients who are on prolonged parenteral nutrition, the diagnosis may be greatly delayed.
71. Asymptomatic pancreatic fistulas or pancreatic ascites can be treated nonoperatively in many instances.
72. One should assume that all patients with pancreatic injuries will develop some degree of pancreatitis and treat them accordingly.
73. The main problem in using hyperamylasemia to diagnose pancreatic disease or injury is its lack of specificity.
74. Patients with severe, acute pancreatitis tend to develop some degree of respiratory dysfunction.
75. Hypocalcemia occurs frequently in pancreatitis, but it usually doesn't require treatment unless it is symptomatic.
76. Routine administration of antibiotics to patients with acute pancreatitis probably does not reduce the rate of infection; however, if infection were to develop, it would more likely be due to antibiotic-resistant organisms.
77. Patients with posttraumatic pancreatitis that continues to worsen for more than 48 hours should generally have exploratory laparotomy.
78. Percutaneous drains placed under radiographic control usually do not drain infected necrotic pancreatic or peripancreatic tissue adequately.
79. The sequential evaluation of pseudocysts by ultrasonography permits relatively accurate determination of changing size.

▲▲▲▲▲▲▲▲▲▲▲▲▲▲▲▲▲▲▲▲▲▲▲▲▲▲▲▲▲▲▲▲▲▲▲▲

REFERENCES

1. Mathieson R, Dutta SK. Candida esophagitis. Digest Dis Sci 1983;28:365.
2. Guandalini S, Fasano A, Migliavacca M, et al. Pathogenesis of postantibiotic diarrhea caused by Clostridium difficile: an in vitro study in the rabbit intestine. Gut 1988;29:598.
3. Fromm D. Gastric mucosal "barrier." Johnson LR, ed. Physiology of the digestive tract, vol I. New York: Raven Press, 1981; 733.
4. Silen W. Experimental models of gastric ulceration and injury. Am J Physiol 1988;255:G395.
5. Olender EJ, Fromm D, Furukawa T, Kolis M. H^+ disposal by rabbit gastric mucosal surface cells. Gastroenterology 1984;86:698.
6. Furukawa T, Olender E, Fromm D, Kolis M. The effects of cyclic AMP and prostaglandins on Na^+ and HCO_3-induced dissipation of a proton gradient in isolated gastric mucosal surface cells of rabbits. Gastroenterology 1985;89:500.
7. Svanes K, Ito S, Takeuchi K, et al. Restitution of the surface epithelium of the in vitro frog gastric mucosa after damage with hyperosmolar NaCl. Gastroenterology 1982;82:1409.
8. Lucas CE, Sugawa C, Riddle J, et al. Natural history and surgical dilemma of "stress" gastric bleeding. Arch Surg 1971;102:266.
9. Czaja AJ, McAlhany JC, Pruitt BA Jr. Acute gastroduodenal disease after thermal injury: an endoscopic evaluation of incidence and natural history. N Engl J Med 1974;291:925.
10. LeGall JR, Mignon F, Bader JP, et al. Injury of gastric mucosa in sepsis. N Engl J Med 1975;292:1242.
11. Shuman RB, Schuster DP, Zuckerman GR. Prophylactic therapy for stress ulcer bleeding: a reappraisal. Ann Intern Med 1987;106:562.
12. Smith P, O'Brien P, Fromm D, et al. Secretory state of the gastric mucosa and resistance to injury by exogenous acid. Am J Surg 1976;184:429.
13. Priebe HJ, Skillman JJ, Bushnell LS, et al. Antacid versus cimetidine in preventing acute gastrointestinal bleeding. N Engl J Med 1980;302:426.
14. Counce JS, Cone JB, McAlister L, et al. Surgical complications of thermal injury. Am J Surg 1988;156:556.
15. Menguy R, Masters YF. Influence of cold on stress ulceration and on gastric mucosal blood flow and energy metabolism. Ann Surg 1981;194:29.
16. Kelemouridis V, Athanasoulis CA, Waltman AC. Gastric bleeding sites: an angiographic study. Radiology 1983;149:643.
17. Wilson WS, Gadacz AT, Olcott C III. Superficial gastric erosions. Am J Surg 1973;126:133.
18. Richardson JD, Aust JB. Gastric devascularization. Ann Surg 1977;185:649.

19. Norton L, Greer J, Eiseman B. Gastric secretory response to head injury. Arch Surg 1970;101:200.

20. Gates JD. Delayed hemorrhage with free rupture complicating the nonsurgical management of blunt hepatic trauma. J Trauma 1994; 36:572.

21. Reber HA, Roberts C, Way LW, et al. Management of external gastrointestinal fistulas. Ann Surg 1978;188:460.

22. Chapman R, Foran R, Dunphy JE. Management of intestinal fistulas. Am J Surg 1964;108:157.

23. Sitges-Serra A, Jaurrieta E, Sitges-Creus A. Management of postoperative enterocutaneous fistulas: the roles of parenteral nutrition and surgery. Br J Surg 1982;69:147.

24. Edmunds LH Jr, Williams GM, Welch CE. External fistulas arising from the gastrointestinal tract. Ann Surg 1960;152:445.

25. Abascal J, Diaz-Rojas F, Jorge J, et al. Free perforation of the small bowel in Crohn's disease. World J Surg 1982;6:216.

26. Voyles CR, Richardson JD, Bland KI, et al. Emergency abdominal wall reconstruction with polypropylene mesh. Ann Surg 1981;194:219.

27. Sandler JT, Deitel M. Management of duodenal fistulas. Can J Surg 1981;24:124.

28. Ujiki GT, Shields TW. Roux-en-Y operation in the management of postoperative fistula. Arch Surg 1981;116:614.

29. Myllarniemi H. Foreign material in adhesion formation after abdominal surgery. Acta Chir Scand 1967;133(Suppl):377.

30. Weibel MA, Majno G. Peritoneal adhesions and their relation to abdominal surgery. Am J Surg 1973;126:345.

31. Kappas AM, Fatouros M, Papadimitriou K, et al. Effect of intraperitoneal saline irrigation at different temperatures on adhesion formation. Br J Surg 1988;75:854.

32. Ellis H. The causes and prevention of intestinal adhesions. Br J Surg 1982;69:241.

33. Grant JBF, Davies JD, Espiner HJ, et al. Diagnosis of granulomatous starch peritonitis by delayed hypersensitivity skin reaction. Br J Surg 1982;69:197.

34. Eldridge TJ, McFall TM, Peoples JB. Traumatic incarceration of the small bowel. J Trauma 1993;35:960.

35. Ashai F, Mam MK, Iqbal S. Ileal entrapment as a complication of fractured pelvis. J Trauma 1988;28:551.

36. Quatromoni JC, Rosoff L Sr, Halls JM, et al. Early postoperative small bowel obstruction. Ann Surg 1980;191:72.

37. Sykes PA, Schofield PF. Early postoperative small bowel obstruction. Br J Surg 1974;61:594.

38. Silen W, Hein MF, Goldman L. Strangulating obstruction of the small intestine. Arch Surg 1962;85:121.

39. Stewardson RH, Bombeck CT, Nyhus LM. Critical operative management of small bowel obstruction. Ann Surg 1978;187:189.

40. Fromm D. Small intestine. Fromm D, ed. Gastrointestinal surgery. New York: Churchill Livingstone, 1985; 376.

41. Sarr MG, Nagorney DM, McIlrath DC. Postoperative intussusception in the adult. Arch Surg 1981;116:144.

42. Shub HA, Rubin RJ, Salvati EP. Intussusception complicating intestinal intubation with a long Cantor tube. Dis Colon Rectum 1978;21:130.

43. Stevens A, Little JM. Duodenal trauma. Aust N Z J Surg 1987;57:709.

44. Levison MA, Petersen SR, Sheldon GF, et al. Duodenal trauma: experience of a trauma center. J Trauma 1984;24:475.

45. Freeark RJ, Moss GS, Sheldon G, et al. A.A.S.T. panel: controversies in management of duodenal injuries. J Trauma 1984;24:481.

46. Martin TD, Feliciano DV, Mattox KL, et al. Severe duodenal injuries. Treatment with pyloric exclusion and gastrojejunostomy. Arch Surg 1983;118:631.

47. Snyder WH, Weigetti JS, Watkins WL, et al. The surgical management of duodenal trauma. Arch Surg 1980;115:422.

48. Stone HH, Fabian TC. Management of duodenal wounds. J Trauma 1979;19:334.

49. Schenk WG, Lonchyna V, Moylan J. Perforation of the jejunum from blunt abdominal trauma. J Trauma 1983;23:56.

50. Winton TL, Girotti MJ, Manley PN, et al. Delayed intestinal perforation after nonpenetrating abdominal trauma. Can J Surg 1985;29:437.

51. Harris CR. Blunt abdominal trauma causing jejunal rupture. Ann Emerg Med 1985;14:916.

52. Burney RE, Mueller GL, Coon WW, Thomas EJ, Mackenzie JR. Diagnosis of isolated small bowel injury following blunt abdominal trauma. Ann Emerg Med 1983;12:71.

53. Jaffin JH, Ochsuer MG, Cole FJ, et al. Alkaline phosphatase levels in diagnostic peritoneal lavage fluid as a predictor of hollow visceral injury. J Trauma 1993;34:829.

54. Enderson BL, Beath DB, Meadors J, et al. The tertiary trauma survey: a prospective study of missed injury. J Trauma 1990;30:666.

55. Lien G, Mori M, Enjoji M. delayed posttraumatic ischemic stricture of the small intestine. Acta Pathol Jpn 1987;37:1367.

56. Taylor D, Magee F, Stordy SN, et al. Small bowel injury simulating Crohn's disease after blunt abdominal trauma. J Clin Gastroenterol 1987;9:99.

57. Brownstein EG. Blunt abdominal trauma simulating Crohn's disease of the terminal ileum. Aust N Z J Surg 1984;54:287.

58. Davidson BR, Everson NW. Colonic stricture secondary to blunt abdominal trauma—report of a case and review of the aetiology. Postgrad Med J 1987;63:911.

59. McBoyle MF, Schiller WR, Hurt AV. Massive gastrointestinal bleeding following blunt abdominal trauma: an unusual case presentation. J Trauma 1984;24:1057.

60. Taylor DW, Babchuk WI, Walz DJ, et al. Gastrointestinal hemorrhage from fistula between traumatic pseudoaneurysm of the right hepatic artery and the duodenum. Clin Nucl Med 1988;13:337.

61. Byrd RL, Cunningham MW, Goldman LI. Nonocclusive ischemic colitis secondary to hemorrhagic shock. Dis Colon Rectum 1987;30:116.

62. Moore EE, Jones TN. Benefits of immediate jejunostomy feeding after major abdominal trauma—a prospective, randomized study. J Trauma 1986;26:874.

63. Sillin L. Methods of enteral nutrition. Fromm D, ed. Gastrointestinal surgery. New York: Churchill Livingstone, 1985; 470.

64. Bruining HA, Schattenkerk ME, Obertop H, et al. Acute abdominal pain due to early postoperative elemental feeding by needle jejunostomy. Surg Gynecol Obstet 1983;157:40.

65. Deitch EA. Simple intestinal obstruction causes bacterial translocation in man. Arch Surg 1989;124:699.

66. Stahl KD, Geiss AC, Bordan DL, et al. Blunt trauma and delayed colon injury. Curr Surg 1985;42:4.

67. Nallathambi MN, Ivatury RR, Shah PM, et al. Penetrating right colon trauma. The ever diminishing role for colostomy. Am Surg 1987; 53:209.

68. Fontes B, Fontes W, Utiyama EM, et al. The efficacy of loop colostomy for complete fecal diversion. Dis Colon Rectum 1988;31:298.

69. Kusminsky RE, Shbeeb I, Makos G, et al. Blunt pelviperineal injuries. An expanded role for the diverting colostomy. Dis Colon Rectum 1982;25:787.

70. Shannon FL, Moore EE, Moore FA, et al. Value of distal colon washout in civilian rectal trauma-reducing gut bacterial translocation. J Trauma 1988;28:989.

71. Schaupp WC. Drainage of low anterior anastomoses. Am J Surg 1969;118:627.

72. Lim RC Jr, Lau G, Steele M. Prevention of complications after liver trauma. Am J Surg 1976;132:156.

73. Olsen WR. Late complications of central liver injuries. Surgery 1982;92:733.

74. Feliciano DV, Mattox KL, Jordan GL Jr, et al. Management of 1000 consecutive cases of hepatic trauma (1979-1984). Ann Surg 1986; 204:438.

75. Pachter HL, Spencer FC, Hofstetter SR, et al. Experience with the finger fracture technique to achieve intra-hepatic hemostasis in 75 patients with severe injuries of the liver. Ann Surg 1983;197:771.

76. Mays ET. The hazards of suturing certain wounds of the liver. Surg Gynecol Obstet 1976;143:201.

77. Mays ET, Conti S, Fallahzadeh H, et al. Hepatic artery ligation. Surgery 1979;86:536.

78. Saad SA, Rush BF Jr, Devanesan JD, et al. Traumatic hematocele of the gallbladder with hemobilia. J Trauma 1979;19:67.

79. McGehee RN, Townsend CM Jr, Thompson JC et al. Traumatic hemobilia. Ann Surg 1974;179:311.

80. Blumgart LH. Bile duct strictures. Fromm D, ed. Gastrointestinal surgery. New York: Churchill Livingstone, 1985; 771.

81. Barker S, Fromm D. Bile peritonitis following expectant management of liver fracture. NY State J Med 1987;87:565.

82. Visner SL, Helling TS, Watkins M. Early profound jaundice following blunt hepatic trauma. J Trauma 1994;36:576.

83. Fox MS, Wilk PJ, Weissmann HS, et al. Acute acalculous cholecystitis. Surg Gynecol Obstet 1984;159:13.

84. Lee AW, Proudfoot WH, Griffen WO Jr. Acalculous cholecystitis. Surg Gynecol Obstet 1984;159:33.

85. Flancbaum L, Majerus TC, Cox EF. Acute posttraumatic acalculous cholecystitis. Am J Surg 1985;150:252.
86. Arvanitakis C, Cooke AR, Greenberger NJ. Laboratory aids in the diagnosis of pancreatitis. Med Clin North Am 1973;62:107.
87. Adams JT, Libertino JA, Schwartz SI. Significance of an elevated serum amylase. Surgery 1968;63:877.
88. Doubilet H, Mulholland JH. Eight-year study of pancreatitis and sphincterotomy. JAMA 1956;160:521.
89. Warshaw AL, Lee KH. Aging changes of pancreatic isoamylases and the appearance of old amylase in the serum of patients with pancreatic pseudocyst. Gastroenterology 1980;79:1246.
90. Levant JA, Secrist DM, Resin H, et al. Nasogastric suction in the treatment of alcoholic pancreatitis. JAMA 1974;229:51.
91. Carey LC. Extraabdominal manifestations of acute pancreatitis. Surgery 1979;86:337.
92. Carey LC, Ellison C. Pancreas. Fromm D, ed. Gastrointestinal surgery. New York: Churchill Livingstone, 1985; 871.
93. Yale CE, Cruming AB. Splenic vein thrombosis and bleeding esophageal varices. JAMA 1971;217:317.
94. Frey CF, Lindenauer SM, Metler TA. Pancreatic abscess. Surg Gynecol Obstet 1979;149:722.
95. Lewis G, Krige JEJ, Bornman PC, et al. Traumatic pancreatic pseudocysts. Br J Surg 1993;80:89.
96. Carr ND, Carins SJ, Lees WR, et al. Late complications of pancreatic trauma. Br J Surg 1989;76:1244.
97. Cooperman A, Ellison EC, Carey LC. Pancreatic pseudocyst. Dent TL, et al, eds. Pancreatic disease. New York: Grune and Stratton, 1981; 247.
98. Stanley JC, Frey CF, Miller TA, et al. Major arterial hemorrhage: a complication of pancreatic pseudocyst and chronic pancreatitis. Arch Surg 1976;111:435.

Chapter **44** Liver Failure After Trauma

ROBERT F. WILSON, M.D.

INTRODUCTION

Throughout history, the liver has been regarded as an important organ. The word "liver" originates from the old English word "lifer" reflecting its vital nature. During the Assyro-Babylonian era (3000-2000 B.C.),[1] sheep liver was frequently used to portend the future. Hepatoscopy or the art of "reading" the liver of sacrificial animals reached its pinnacle among the Babylonians and was a part of haruspicy, which is "reading" the entrails of animals.

Some ancient writers must have had an inkling that the liver can regenerate itself to some degree. In Greek mythology, the titan Prometheus stole fire from the gods to benefit mankind. Zeus, in his anger, had Prometheus chained to a mountain in the Caucasus. Every day an eagle ate a portion of his liver, and during the night it would regenerate.

ANATOMY

The liver is the largest organ in the body, weighing about 1200 g in adult women and 1500 g in adult men.[2,3] The liver parenchymal cells or hepatocytes are arranged in plates that are distributed in the form of lobules. Between the lobules are the portal triads, which contain branches of the portal vein, hepatic artery, and bile ducts. The branches of the portal vein and hepatic artery divide and subdivide, and then empty directly into dilated hepatic capillaries or sinusoids.

The hepatic sinusoids are lined by endothelium which is much more permeable to large molecules than are systemic capillaries. This allows large nutrient particles to get to the liver cells. Within each lobule is a central vein that drains into sublobular veins, which drain finally into the major hepatic veins entering the inferior vena cava.

The bile canaliculi drain into small cholangioles known as the canals of Hering which empty into intralobular ductules. These, in turn, empty into larger and larger ducts, which finally unite to form segmental ducts and then the right and left hepatic bile ducts.

PHYSIOLOGY

The liver is vital to life, and despite significant advances in medicine, an individual can seldom survive for more than a few hours without a liver because of its multiple metabolic, detoxification, reticuloendothelial, and bile secretory functions.[3-6] It is also the only vital organ that can regenerate itself to any significant degree.

Metabolic Functions

The liver has multiple metabolic functions, including the uptake, synthesis, conversion, and storage of various carbohydrates, proteins, fat molecules, vitamins, and coagulation factors.

CARBOHYDRATE METABOLISM

AXIOM Inadequate glycogen stores in the liver can greatly reduce the ability of the patient to tolerate severe trauma.

Glucose absorbed from the intestine is converted by the liver into glycogen, the main storage form for carbohydrates. Other simple sugars, such as fructose, are first converted to glucose and then to glycogen. The liver has the largest readily available supply of glycogen (about 150 g) for rapid glucose production during acute stress; however, the amount of liver glycogen present in patients who have severe diabetes mellitus or cirrhosis may be greatly reduced.

The liver converts glucose into pentoses (via the hexosemonophosphate shunt) for energy and for synthesis of adenosine to make ATP and nucleic acids. With inadequate delivery of oxygen, the liver must metabolize the glucose anaerobically into pyruvate with the net release of only 2 moles of ATP from each mole of glucose. Pyruvate can then be converted into acetyl coenzyme A (CoA) to enter the tricarboxylic acid (Krebs) cycle. This three-carbon molecule can then be broken down into carbon dioxide and hydrogen ions in the Krebs cycle if adequate oxygen is available to oxidize the released hydrogen ions via the cytochrome oxidase system.

The complete metabolism of glucose aerobically can release a total of 34 moles of ATP for each mole of glucose. This, plus the 2 moles of ATP released from the conversion of glucose to pyruvate, can provide a total of 36 moles of ATP produced by aerobic metabolism from each mole of glucose. When inadequate oxygen is available, the Kreb's cycle stops and pyruvate is converted into lactate and only 2 moles of ATP are released per mole of glucose.

PROTEIN METABOLISM

Large quantities of nitrogenous compounds are synthesized, changed, or broken down in the liver daily. The liver is the body's major source of plasma proteins. It produces all of the albumin and α-globulins and some of the β-globulins found in the blood.

AXIOM Bilirubin excretion is impaired relatively early in multiple systemic organ failure (MOF), but protein synthesis is preserved until relatively late.[7]

Chemical tests used to assess hepatic protein synthesis include serum or plasma levels of albumin, transferrin, thyroxine-binding prealbumin, and retinol-binding protein.[1] These tests can be reasonably reliable as nutritional indices, but they are affected by a number of variables other than nutritional status, such as hydration, sepsis, and abnormal gastrointestinal or urinary losses.

AXIOM Decreasing levels of albumin usually imply the presence of sepsis and/or malnutrition.

Albumin is contained in a large body pool (4-5 g/kg), and it has a long half-life (20-22 days).[7] As a result, it is relatively insensitive to acute changes and responds slowly to therapy. Plasma levels are decreased by sepsis, malnutrition, hepatic failure, dialysis, uremia, and acute volume expansion. Plasma albumin levels may be increased in patients who are dehydrated and those who have increased levels of cortisol, growth hormone, insulin, or estrogen.

AXIOM Albumin, because of its long half-life and because its plasma levels are affected by so many factors, is generally not a good guide to the adequacy of nutritional support.

Transferrin is contained in a smaller body pool than albumin. It has a shorter half-life (8-10 days) and much lower normal serum levels (250-300 mg/dl).[8] Therefore, it is a more sensitive indicator of the patient's current nutritional status; however, it is adversely affected as a nutritional indicator by the same variables as albumin. It is also affected by serum iron in that iron deficiency leads to elevations in transferrin, and iron overload depresses transferrin levels.

Thyroxin-binding prealbumin is involved in the transport of thyroid hormone and is a carrier for retinol-binding protein.[8] Its normal serum content is 22 ± 7 mg/dl, and it has a short half-life (2 days). It can be a sensitive indicator of nutritional status, but it is affected by the same variables that affect albumin and transferrin. In addition, low levels are seen in hyperthyroidism, cystic fibrosis, chronic illness, and acute stress.

Retinol-binding protein is a specific carrier involved in vitamin A transport, and it is linked with thyroid-binding prealbumin in a constant molar ratio.[7] Normal serum levels are 5.1 ± 2.5 mg/dl. It has a very short half-life (12 hours) and is very sensitive to synthesis and utilization changes. Levels rise in the setting of renal disease and excess vitamin A administration, but are reduced in liver disease, cystic fibrosis, hyperthyroidism, and vitamin A deficiency.

The liver can also deaminate various amino acids to form simple sugars or fatty acids, and it can form amino acids by transaminating various nonnitrogenous compounds. The ammonia formed from the breakdown of protein and amino acids is largely converted into urea by the liver. In severe liver disease, blood urea nitrogen (BUN) levels may decrease below 5 mg/dl. These low BUN levels tend to indicate severe liver impairment and are apt to be associated with increasing levels of ammonia and aromatic amino acids.

AXIOM   If the bun is below 5.0 mg/dL, one should suspect severe hepatic disease or hepatic failure.

Following trauma or during sepsis, the liver reorients protein synthesis to favor the production of acute phase reactants, such as α_1-antitrypsin, lactoferrin, C-reactive protein, fibrinogen, and ceruloplasmin.[8] Simultaneously, proteolysis of skeletal muscle increases, and the resulting amino acids are transported to the liver to be used for energy production (alanine) or new protein synthesis (i.e., tyrosine, phenylalanine, leucine, isoleucine). Increasing evidence indicates that proteolysis is stimulated by IL-1, and protein synthesis by hepatocytes is stimulated by IL-6 and by other mediators produced by Kupffer cells.

The role of cytokines on hepatic acute-phase protein production has been demonstrated both in vitro and in vivo.[9,10] Although such responses were previously attributed to tumor necrosis factor (TNF) and IL-1,[11,12] more recent in vitro studies with human hepatocytes suggest that IL-6 is primarily responsible for regulation of acute-phase hepatic protein synthesis,[13] with the maximal response requiring concomitant glucocorticoid administration.[13]

Apparently, a glucocorticoid response to injury is necessary to achieve an optimal IL-6 influence on acute-phase protein synthesis. However, glucocorticoids tend to reduce production, probably by attenuating TNF and IL-1 activity.[14]

FAT METABOLISM

The liver can synthesize fatty acids and triglycerides or it can break them down into glycerol and smaller fatty acids. Glycerol is usually then converted to acetyl CoA. Fatty acids are converted to either acetyl CoA or ketone bodies. The liver is also the major source of cholesterol, cholesterol esters, and phospholipids. The ability of the liver to metabolize triglycerides and fatty acids is one of the last metabolic liver functions to fail in hepatic dysfunction.

AXIOM   Rising serum triglyceride levels in patients with sepsis are often a sign of terminal liver failure.

PRODUCTION OF COAGULATION FACTORS

Most coagulation factors are made in the liver. These include Factor I (fibrinogen), Factor II (prothrombin), Factor V (proaccelerin), Factor VII (Proconvertin), Factor IX (plasma thromboplastin component), Factor XI (plasma thromboplastin antecedent), and Factor XII (Hageman Factor). Some Factor VIII (antihemophilic globulin) is also made in the liver, but it is formed principally by endothelial cells outside the liver.

VITAMIN METABOLISM

All vitamins, particularly, A, D, E, K, and B_{12} are stored in the liver and either used there or released as needed by other parts of the body.

Detoxification

A large variety of endogenous and exogenous chemicals are rendered harmless by the liver and then released into the blood (for excretion in the urine) or into the bile (for excretion through the bowel). The detoxification process may involve a large number of chemical reactions, including oxidation, reduction, methylation, acetylation, esterification, and conjugation.

Hepatic function tends to progressively deteriorate with increasing age even when the clinical examination and routine laboratory tests are normal. The most sensitive indicator of altered hepatic function in the elderly is the gradual increase in bromosulfophthalein (BSP) retention that occurs in these individuals.[15] This test is considered abnormal when more than 10% of BSP is retained in the serum 30 minutes after injection.

With decreasing hepatic function, the capacity of the liver to conjugate lipid-soluble drugs is impaired. Consequently, such drugs tend to have a prolonged increase in concentration and reduced dose requirement in the elderly. Thiopental dosage, for instance, is decreased in patients over the age of 60 years.[16] A five-fold increase in the plasma concentration of propranolol, which is eliminated almost entirely on the first pass through the liver, may be seen in patients over 65-70 years of age, even when they have no clinical evidence of hepatic, renal, or cardiac disease.[16] Diazepam elimination is also prolonged in the elderly because of altered hepatic biodegradation.[16]

Reticuloendothelial Functions

The liver is the initial filter for whatever bacteria and bacterial products are absorbed from the intestine into the portal venous system.[2-6] It is not surprising that the liver is one of the most important parts of the reticuloendothelial system (RES) and over 60% of the cells of the RES are present in the liver.

AXIOM   In severe hepatic failure, increased quantities of bacteria and bacterial products from the gut can traverse the liver and get into the systemic circulation.

Bile Formation and Secretion

The hepatocytes of the normal adult male process most of the nutrients ingested, and they secrete about 1000 mL of bile per day.[2-6] This is an active process that depends upon functioning hepatocytes and bile ducts and an adequate hepatic blood flow (HBF) and oxygen supply.

STIMULATION OF BILE SECRETION

Bile secretion is responsive to neurogenic, humoral, and chemical controls. Vagal stimulation increases bile secretion and flow, whereas stimulation of the splanchnic (sympathetic) nervous system decreases bile flow and causes stasis of bile in the gallbladder. The main hormonal stimulus for bile formation and secretion is secretin. Peptides and fatty acids also increase bile flow. Bile salts are particularly effective choleretics and greatly increase the rate of bile formation and secretion by the liver.

BILE CONSTITUENTS

AXIOM   High serum levels of unconjugated bilirubin in adults during the first four to five days after trauma are often due to hemolysis of red cells in hematomas and/or transfused blood.

The most important compounds in bile are bilirubin, bile salts, cholesterol, phospholipids (especially lecithin), mucin, water, and various electrolytes.

Bilirubin

Bilirubin is formed in the RES as the end product of the breakdown of hemoglobin from destroyed red blood cells. Under normal circumstances, approximately 6-35 g of hemoglobin are broken down daily and 30-300 mg of bilirubin are formed. The initial step involves release of biliverdin from hemoglobin. Biliverdin is reduced to unconjugated bilirubin in the extrahepatic RES, then bound to albumin and transported to the liver. In the liver, unconjugated (indirect) bilirubin is conjugated by the enzyme UDP glucuronyl transferase to form bilirubin diglucuronide (direct bilirubin), which is excreted in the bile and gives bile its pale green color. In the bowel, bacteria convert conjugated bilirubin into urobilinogen, about 40% of which is reabsorbed and excreted again in the bile as bilirubin or urobilinogen. The urobilinogen that escapes from the liver is excreted in the urine.

Bile Salts and Bile Acids

Bile salts are essential for fat digestion because they can emulsify triglycerides and thereby lower the surface tension of oil droplets. Phospholipids in the bile greatly increase the ability of bile salts to also form micelles which are necessary for effective absorption of lipids.

In individuals on a normal diet, the liver secretes an average of 24 (16-72) g of bile acids per day. These combine with cations, particularly sodium, to form bile salts. Although only about 3-6 g of bile acids are present in the body at any one time, this bile-acid pool is circulated about eight (3-14) times per day. Over 95% of the bile acids secreted in bile are normally reabsorbed in the intestine. Reabsorption occurs primarily in the distal ileum, which actively absorbs bile acids, particularly those conjugated with taurine or glycine. The enterohepatic circulation refers to the circulation of bile acids from the liver through the bile ducts to the intestine, reabsorption from the terminal ileum into the portal vein, and then back to the liver.

AXIOM Resection or severe disease of the distal ileum can rapidly cause severe bile acid deficiencies.

Two major types of bile acids are recognized. The primary bile acids are those synthesized by the liver; they include cholic acid (with three hydroxyl groups) and chenodeoxycholic acid (with two hydroxyl groups). Within the bowel, these primary bile acids may be converted by bacteria to the secondary bile acids, deoxycholic acid, and lithocholic acid. When they are absorbed and returned to the liver in the portal blood, the secondary bile acids are secreted into bile along with primary bile acids.

After absorption by the intestine, bile acids are transported to the liver. Normally, about 50 mg of bile acids are lost in the feces and replaced by the liver daily. Although the liver can temporarily increase its synthesis of new bile acids to about 3 g/day, any factor that interferes with their absorption in the distal ileum can eventually deplete the bile acid pool.

When bile salt malabsorption occurs, the resulting high concentration of bile salts in the colon may interfere with the absorption of sodium and water, and a severe watery diarrhea may develop. The ZE syndrome or any excess production of gastric acid may also cause diarrhea because excess acid reaching the small intestine interferes with bile salt absorption.

Cholesterol

Cholesterol is generally present in bile in concentrations similar to those found in plasma. Although much attention has been directed to the tendency for high-fat diets to raise blood cholesterol levels, most cholesterol in the blood is actually formed in the liver.

Much attention has been directed to the solubility of cholesterol in bile because cholesterol crystals appear to be the nidus of many gallstones. Both bile salts and lecithin are polar molecules that absorb lipids at one end and water-soluble substances at the other end. In a micelle, their fat-insoluble portions from a hydrophilic shell. Cholesterol, which is almost totally insoluble in water, dissolves in the hydrophobic core of the micelle. Low ratios of bile salts and lecithin to cholesterol or increased concentrations of cholesterol in the bile seem to increase the likelihood of cholesterol crystals forming, and this predisposes to the formation of gallstones.

AXIOM Although there is much concern about high plasma cholesterol levels in the development of atherosclerosis, very low levels (< 100 mg/dL) usually indicate a dangerous degree of malnutrition.

Phospholipids

Lecithin, formed in the liver, is the principal phospholipid in the bile. Low levels of lecithin increase the tendency to gallstone formation.

Fluid and Electrolytes

The pH of hepatic bile is usually near 7.0. It is isosmotic with respect to plasma. The sodium concentration is somewhat higher than in plasma, but the calcium concentration is slightly lower.

Hepatic Hemodynamics

BLOOD FLOW

The liver receives about 25-30% of the cardiac output or about 1500 mL/min.[2-6] The hepatic artery carries fully oxygenated blood and provides approximately 25% of the HBF and about 30-50% of its oxygen. The portal vein drains the splanchnic circulation, has an oxygen saturation of about 80%, and provides the remaining 75% of the HBF. A reciprocal relationship exists between hepatic artery and portal vein flow. If, for some reason the flow through one is reduced, the flow in the other tends to increase.

AXIOM Patients with cirrhosis or any other intrahepatic obstruction to portal venous blood flow are particularly sensitive to any reduction in cardiac output and/or hepatic artery blood flow.

PRESSURES

The pressure in the portal vein is normally 7-10 mm Hg (100-140 mm H_2O). A portal vein pressure exceeding 15 mm Hg (200 mm H_2O) is considered to be portal hypertension. In the hepatic sinusoids, where blood from the hepatic artery and portal veins joins, the pressure is about 2-6 mm Hg. Hepatic venous pressure is normally 1-5 mm Hg.

BLOOD RESERVOIR

About 25-30% (400-500 mL) of the liver volume is blood. If the patient becomes hypovolemic, up to half of hepatic blood can be expelled into the systemic circulation.

CAUSES OF JAUNDICE

Jaundice (icterus) is a yellow discoloration of tissue due to staining with bilirubin. It is best observed in tissues containing elastic tissue, such as the sclerae and the skin of the face and neck. Jaundice can usually be detected when the concentration of conjugated bilirubin is > 2-3 mg/dL or the concentration of unconjugated bilirubin is > 3-4 mg/dL. If bilirubin levels increase, plasma levels may exceed 4-5 mg/dL without the patient appearing jaundiced because it takes at least several hours for the tissue to pick up adequate levels of bilirubin to be visible. The reverse is true as bilirubin levels decrease. Consequently, someone with resolving bile duct obstruction may seem jaundiced in spite of normal bilirubin levels.

AXIOM To facilitate diagnosis, the causes of jaundice are often divided into prehepatic, hepatic, and posthepatic (bile-duct) disorders.[4,17,18]

Prehepatic Disorders

The most important prehepatic cause of jaundice is excessive hemolysis of red blood cells. In trauma, large hematomas are often associated with elevations of bilirubin. Various immune or transfusion reactions, infections, and chemicals can cause so much hemolysis that bilirubin is produced faster than the liver can excrete it. Increased hemolysis may also occur after massive blood transfusions.

It is estimated that about 10% of the erythrocytes in transfused blood that is 14 days old undergo hemolysis daily during the first few days.[19] Thus, one unit of blood (with a hemoglobin concentration of 15 g/100 mL) would liberate about 7.5 g of hemoglobin per day for several days. This amount of hemoglobin (7.5 g) results in the formation of about 250 mg of bilirubin following phagocytosis by the reticuloendothelial system. This equals the usual daily physiologic bilirubin load of 250 mg resulting from the breakdown of senescent red cells, which approximates 1% of the circulating red cell mass.[20] Similarly, resolving hematomas liberate a pigment load in direct relation to the amount of sequestered hemoglobin and serve as an additional source of bilirubin. A large hematoma combined with multiple transfusions can lead to fairly severe hyperbilirubinemia, especially if impaired hepatocellular function exists because of other factors, especially a significant period of hypotension.[19]

Damaged muscle (releasing myoglobin and cytochromes) and hematomas are also causes of increased pigment loads to be handled by the liver. Flint estimated that the heme pigment load with a closed femur fracture may exceed 1000 mg, whereas a major pelvic fracture with hemorrhage may result in an excess pigment load of 7500 mg to be converted to bilirubin.[21]

In younger individuals, congenital disorders (such as spherocytosis, sickle-cell anemia, and thalassemia) should also be considered in the differential diagnosis of jaundice.

Prehepatic jaundice is usually associated with a high fraction of indirect (unconjugated bilirubin) and relatively normal liver enzymes (serum-glutamic oxaloacetic transaminase: SGOT and alkaline phosphatase). Anemia and increased reticulocytes in the peripheral blood smear should also make one suspect hemolysis and prehepatic jaundice.

Hepatic Disorders

The most common medical hepatic problems causing jaundice are the various types of hepatitis, cirrhosis, and congenital hepatic disorders. Following accidental trauma, the most frequent causes of hepatocyte damage or dysfunction include shock with ischemic injury of the liver, severe respiratory insufficiency, drugs, sepsis, infectious hepatitis, and halothane anesthesia.[19] Halothane hepatitis, which rarely (1 of 10,000 general anesthetics) causes severe hepatic necrosis, usually occurs after repeated exposure and prior sensitization to halothane.[22] This problem can be ruled out if no prior halothane anesthesia was given and/or no characteristic recent or resolving centrilobular necrosis is noted microscopically.

Shock not only reduces cardiac output, but also increases resistance to blood flow across the liver,[23] and it can rapidly cause ischemic injury to the liver.[24] Hepatic hypoperfusion in turn results in hepatic excretory impairment. Animal studies showed that, following trauma, there is a marked reduction of hepatic energy-dependent excretory function.[25,26] Furthermore, this energy impairment persists for some time after hypotension in animals has been corrected.

Typical morphologic changes of shock seen on biopsy or autopsy include centrilobular congestion and necrosis plus bile stasis.[23] Bile stasis implies failure of the bile secretory apparatus. Patients who have the greatest degree of hepatic dysfunction also usually have had the most prolonged hypotension and have required the most intensive resuscitative and supportive measures.[27]

Jaundice resulting from shock usually becomes apparent by the third to fourth postoperative day and is generally associated with mild elevations in alkaline phosphatase and SGOT. This syndrome is also commonly associated with other vital organ dysfunction, such as acute renal and respiratory failure.

Sepsis resulting in impaired hepatocellular function has been recognized for some time as the most common cause of persistent jaundice developing a week or more after major abdominal operations. The pathophysiologic process is not clear, but a histologic picture of cholestasis with relatively little inflammation or hepatocellular necrosis is often observed.

Three major intraoperative hepatic procedures may also contribute to liver failure.[21] Right hepatic lobectomy is regularly followed by an early increase in bilirubin to > 5 mg/dL, but usually for only a few days. Similar findings of jaundice and elevation of hepatic enzymes are common when hepatic artery ligation or portal vein ligation is used to achieve hemostasis in patients with liver injury. Packing a liver after ligation of a major hepatic artery branch may cause very severe hepatic lobar necrosis.

DEFICIENT HEPATIC UPTAKE OF BILIRUBIN

Deficient hepatic uptake of bilirubin is seen in most types of acquired liver disease. However, this may also be seen in Gilbert's disease, which is a congenital disorder characterized by normal liver biopsy and intermittent low-grade hyperbilirubinemia (< 5 mg/dL) consisting mainly of unconjugated bilirubin.

DEFICIENT CONJUGATION OF BILIRUBIN

Some degree of deficient conjugation of bilirubin is seen with virtually all types of acquired liver disease. It is also seen, but much less frequently, with: (a) inadequate glucuronyl transferase, as in physiologic jaundice of the newborn and in Crigler-Najjar syndrome, (b) inhibition of glucuronyl transferase by large doses of vitamin K analogs (in premature infants) or by increased blood levels of pregnanediol or novobiocin, and (c) competitive inhibition of glucuronyl transferase by drugs that are detoxified as glucuronides.

DEFICIENT SECRETION OF BILIRUBIN

Deficient liver-cell (hepatocyte) secretion of bilirubin in the adult is usually due to acquired liver disease. In infants and children, it may be due to immaturity of the liver, Dubin-Johnson syndrome, or Rotor syndrome. Dubin-Johnson syndrome characteristically produces a slate-gray or black liver (due to excess bilirubin pigment), which can be seen at surgery and on liver biopsy. The Rotor syndrome is similar physiologically, but does not result in pigment deposition in the liver.

INTRAHEPATIC BILE DUCT OBSTRUCTION

Bile duct obstructions are characterized by elevated levels of conjugated bilirubin and alkaline phosphatase and may occur at the level of the canaliculi, in the large intrahepatic bile ducts, or in the extrahepatic bile ducts. Many acquired liver disorders, particularly viral hepatitis and sepsis, produce canalicular and/or intrahepatic bile duct obstruction which may be difficult at times to differentiate from extrahepatic (posthepatic) obstruction.

Posthepatic Disorders

AXIOM In patients with increasing jaundice after trauma, one should make a special effort to rule out extrahepatic biliary obstruction.

The most frequent posthepatic cause of jaundice is mechanical occlusion of the common hepatic duct or common bile duct by a calculus. Posthepatic jaundice, however, can also be caused by strictures, carcinomas, or pancreatitis.

Percutaneous transhepatic catheterization is used occasionally to diagnose and/or relieve obstruction jaundice. In many patients, one can advance the catheter beyond the obstruction into the duodenum. The catheter can be used to obtain cholangiography, decompress the biliary tract prior to surgery, and/or provide permanent decompression for some tumors. Initially it was believed that reducing bilirubin levels to < 10 mg/dL prior to definitive major surgery reduced operative morbidity and mortality. However, in many studies in which PTC reduced bilirubin levels by over 50%, the mortality rate was higher than that seen with immediate surgery.[28-31]

AXIOM Preoperative transhepatic catheter decompression of an obstructed biliary tract may cause more harm than good.

Despite the diagnostic accuracy and therapeutic potential of PTC with biliary drainage (PTBD), several clinicians have cautioned against its routine use.[28-31] These authors contended that complications of PTBD, especially cholangitis, offset whatever therapeutic benefit the decreased serum bilirubin levels could provide. In a randomized, controlled, prospective study, McPherson et al. showed a higher postoperative mortality rate (32% vs 19%) in patients who had preoperative biliary decompression compared with patients who went directly to surgery.[30]

More recently, Sirinek and Levine, in a nonrandomized study of 221 patients with biliary tract obstruction, found that preoperative biliary decompression, although technically (95%) and physiologically (82%) successful in the majority of patients, had no therapeutic benefit when compared to patients who did not have alleviation of jaundice prior to surgical intervention.[32]

ACUTE HEPATOCELLULAR DISEASES

Of acute hepatic diseases, the one most frequently seen is viral hepatitis.[33] Less frequent causes of acute liver diseases or failure include toxic (drug-induced) hepatitis, alcoholic hepatitis, "septic jaundice," and postanoxic (shock) changes.

Viral Hepatitis

Viral hepatitis is an acute disease affecting all parts of the body, but the predominant clinical and pathologic manifestations are those related to acute hepatocellular necrosis. Epidemiologic studies have demonstrated five relatively distinct types of viral hepatitis: A, B, C, D, and E.[34]

TYPES OF CONTAGIOUS HEPATITIS

Infectious Hepatitis

Infectious or type A hepatitis (IH) is primarily an enteric disease. It is usually transmitted by the fecal-oral route, but it can also be transmitted parenterally. It has a relatively short incubation period (15-40 days). During the prodromal and early icteric phase, the IH virus is present in both blood and feces. A little later in the preicteric stage, fever may be present and symptoms of liver tenderness may develop. The virus usually disappears from blood and feces within a week after the onset of jaundice. About 2-5% of patients with IH die either rapidly from the acute process or later from complications of postnecrotic cirrhosis. IH neither has a propensity for chronicity nor is believed to predispose one to hepatic carcinoma.[35]

Serum Hepatitis

Serum hepatitis (SH) is usually transmitted via contaminated needles or blood. Hepatitis B (and probably hepatitis C) can also be acquired sexually. The incidence of SH in narcotic addicts is extremely high. The incubation period for SH is much longer (60-90 days) than for IH. The virus is found in the serum, but has not been demonstrated in feces. The severity and mortality rate of SH is usually somewhat higher than for IH. It should be considered highly infectious via blood or bloody secretions until high levels of antibodies are found in the blood.

AXIOM One should make an effort to keep the use of blood or blood products in trauma patients to a minimum so as to reduce the chances of transmitting blood-borne diseases, especially hepatitis and AIDS.

Non-A Non-B Hepatitis (Hepatitis C)

Relatively little is known about hepatitis C, but its incidence is becoming increasingly recognized. It now appears to be the most common cause of viral hepatitis following blood transfusions. Less than 10% of cases of posttransfusion hepatitis (PTH) are caused by hepatitis B surface antigen.

AXIOM Non-A, non-B hepatitis is the most frequent type of hepatitis transmitted by infusion of blood or blood products.

The use of so-called surrogate screening tests to eliminate donors at increased risk of transmitting non-A, non-B hepatitis have reduced the risk of transmission to as low as 1-2%. Recent isolation of a hepatitis C virus and the characterization of hepatitis C virus antibody in both blood donors and recipients may further decrease the likelihood of this complication.[36]

Acute symptoms from hepatitis C may be noted 1-3 months after transfusions. They are characteristically mild and easily mistaken for a nondescript viral syndrome. Jaundice is unusual and severe illness from overwhelming hepatic necrosis is uncommon. Thus, unless one carefully screens transfusion recipients with serial liver function tests, the majority of non-A, non-B hepatitis cases will be missed. This is probably the main reason that many physicians underestimate the incidence of hepatitis following blood transfusions.

AXIOM Most patients with posttransfusion hepatitis will be missed unless serial liver function tests are performed weekly or biweekly for three months following transfusion of blood products.

Although few transfusion recipients die acutely from PTH, up to one-half of patients in some series fail to recover completely and subsequently develop chronic liver disease.[37] The prognosis of chronic hepatitis caused by the non-A, non-B virus is not known with certainty, but liver biopsies reveal changes, such as chronic aggressive hepatitis with bridging necrosis or cirrhosis, in a significant percentage of these patients.[38]

Hepatitis D

Hepatitis D is prevalent in the Mediterranean area and deserves consideration when severe hepatitis develops in a patient with serologic evidence of concomitant hepatitis B infection.

AXIOM Hepatitis D will probably not be diagnosed unless one tests serially for hepatitis B after blood transfusions.

Hepatitis delta virus (HDV) is a small RNA virus which replicates and causes hepatitis only in patients who are concurrently infected with the hepatitis B virus (HBV).[39] Delta hepatitis is marked by the presence of HDV in both the liver and serum and by antibody to HDV (anti-HD) in serum. Delta hepatitis infection is endemic in some geographic areas of the world, in particular, countries in the Mediterranean basin.[40] In the United States and most other parts of the world, HDV infection has occurred mainly in intravenous drug abusers and in patients, such as hemophiliacs, who receive multiple blood transfusions.[41,42]

HDV can be either transmitted simultaneously with HBV (coinfection) or infect a subject who is already an HBV carrier (superinfection). It is important to distinguish between these two types of infection because superinfection is much more likely to result in chronic HDV infection and because of the difference in serologic changes that may occur.[39] Patients with acute HDV infection are likely to develop severe acute or fulminant hepatitis,[43,44] and those with chronic delta infection often subsequently develop cirrhosis and endstage liver disease.[45]

The diagnosis of delta hepatitis may be difficult for several reasons. First, HDV infection is associated with a poor and variable antibody response, so that in acute delta hepatitis, only low levels of anti-HD may appear, even after several weeks. Second, the use of commercially available assays to measure delta antigen and antibody in serum is not yet widespread, particularly in the United States. Finally, many of the most sensitive assays are technically difficult to perform, and their use is still restricted to research laboratories.

Hepatitis E

Hepatitis E is transmitted via contaminated food or water and is a common cause of sporadic and epidemic hepatitis in underdeveloped areas of the world.[34] It is found endemically in Central and South America and in Africa and should be considered in the traveler who presents with features of acute hepatitis and negative hepatitis A, B, and C serologies. Like hepatitis A, chronicity of infection is not a common consequence of this disease.

DIAGNOSIS

Most patients with hepatitis have severe anorexia, often with a strong intolerance of fatty foods. They also are lethargic and tire easily. The severe anorexia often improves as jaundice develops.

Viral hepatitis is generally characterized by extremely high SGOT levels (often exceeding 1000 units) and varying, but usually elevated, levels of bilirubin and alkaline phosphatase. Serial viral hepatitis antigen and antibody studies are important to determine the diagnosis and prognosis. Patients with serum hepatitis often have a positive (Australian) antigen in their blood for several days, weeks, or even months.

MANAGEMENT

The management of viral hepatitis consists primarily of providing adequate physical rest and nutrition. In severe cases, steroids may be of some help, particularly if the patient appears to be developing acute hepatic necrosis; although steroids usually make the patients feel better, they probably have little effect on eventual mortality. In some of the most severe cases, exchange transfusions have been used to reduce the toxicity secondary to the severe chemical abnormalities that may develop.

Toxic Hepatitis

Many environmental and therapeutic agents when inhaled, ingested, or administered parenterally can produce hepatic injury; however, many of these substances that damage the liver are not true hepatotoxins, but cause injury indirectly by sensitization reactions (Table 44–1).

Alcoholic Hepatitis

Acute alcoholic hepatitis is caused by excessive alcohol ingestion in a patient who usually already has a fatty or cirrhotic liver. Enzyme changes, especially SGOT, are usually not as severe as those in viral hepatitis; however, alkaline phosphatase may be somewhat higher. The stigmata of cirrhosis (ascites, spider nevi, and bleeding problems) may develop rapidly in patients with alcoholic hepatitis.

Hepatic Dysfunction After Shock and Trauma

Clinicopathologic studies in patients following shock and trauma have correlated light and electron microscopic changes in the liver with clinical and biochemical evidence of several phases of hepatic dysfunction.[46] Patients developing evidence of acute liver dysfunction after trauma increased the risk of dying at least nine-fold.[47,48]

TABLE 44–1   Drugs That Should Be Used with Caution or Not at All in Liver Disease Patients

Group I:	Drugs capable of causing hepatic damage
	Acetaminophen
	Acetylsalicylic acid
	Chlorpromazine
	Erythromycin estolate
	Methotrexate
	Methyldopa
Group II:	Drugs that can compromise liver function
	Anabolic and contraceptive steroids
	Prednisone
	Tetracycline
Group III:	Drugs that may make complications of liver disease worse
	Cyclooxygenase inhibitors (indomethacin)
	Diuretics
	Meperidine and other CNS depressants
	Morphine
	Pentazocine
	Phenylbutazone

(From: Kubisty CA, Arns PA, Wedlund PJ, et al. Adjustment of medications in liver failure. Chernow B, ed. The pharmacologic approach to the critically ill patient, 3rd ed. Baltimore: Williams & Wilkins, 1994; 98.)

PHASES

Phase I (During Shock)

With mild ischemia, electron microscopy (EM) may reveal minimal changes, except for the absence of intramitochondrial granules.[46] With moderate ischemia, EM changes include small hypoxic vacuoles and slight dilatation of the rough and smooth endoplasmic reticulum. During sublethal hepatic ischemia, there is a consistent increase in lipids in the hepatocytes with varying numbers of acute inflammatory cells in the central and midzonal areas of the hepatic lobule.[46] Irreversible damage is indicated by: (a) clumping of chromatic in the nucleus, (b) mitochondrial swelling with flocculent densities, and (c) marked dilatation of the endoplasmic reticulum.

AXIOM   Severe, traumatic shock can cause significant hepatic damage, which is often not clinically apparent.

It has been demonstrated that plasma levels of TNF and IL-6 increase significantly during hemorrhage and remain elevated even after crystalloid resuscitation.[49] The increased levels of circulating TNF, alone or in combination with IL-6, may be responsible for producing the hepatocellular dysfunction observed after trauma and hemorrhagic shock.[49,50] Pentoxifylline treatment during and after hemorrhage in experimental animals can decrease serum levels of TNF and IL-6, restore or improve hepatic blood flow,[51] and increase survival.[52,53]

Phase II (Functional Impairment)

The functional impairment phase of hepatic dysfunction extends from the time of reestablishment of liver perfusion until hepatic function begins to improve.[46] This phase usually only lasts about 4-8 days. Any hepatic failure or jaundice developing or worsening 8-10 days after trauma is usually due to sepsis.

BILIRUBIN.   Patients receiving massive transfusions may have early hemolytic jaundice with bilirubin levels peaking at about 3-4 mg/dL during the first 48 hours. Bilirubin levels tend to decrease until the fifth day. Sarfeh and Balint found that total bilirubin levels on day 4 were an excellent predictor of outcome with higher levels (3.6 ± 0.6 mg/dL) in nonsurvivors than in survivors (1.6 ± 0.3 mg/dL).[27] Nearly 60% of patients with major burns also developed early increases in serum bilirubin levels, presumably from hypovolemia and impaired perfusion of the liver.[54,55] If the bilirubin levels then increase again to over 5 mg/dL by days 8-10, the secondary hyperbilirubinemia is

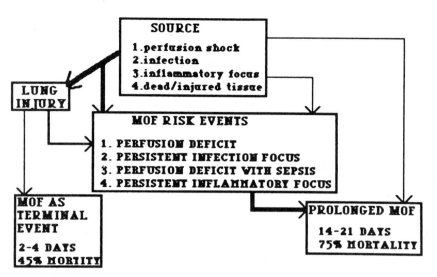

frequently associated with sepsis.[46] Once the sepsis is controlled, the bilirubin levels should gradually decrease back to normal.

AXIOM Jaundice developing 8-10 days after trauma or later is due to sepsis until proven otherwise (Fig. 44–1).

LDH AND SGOT. Lactic dehydrogenase (LDH) and SGOT levels may increase to 400-500 and 100-200 units, respectively, within a few hours of moderate-to-severe anoxic liver damage. Indeed, over 60% of patients with severe burns develop hepatic enzyme elevations, presumably due to ischemia and/or hypoxemia.[54,55] These levels gradually return to normal over the next 3-4 days. With additional hepatic insults, such as the development of sepsis, a secondary rise in LDH and SGOT often precedes the secondary rises in bilirubin by 3-5 days.[48]

Liver enzymes may remain elevated even after the patient is doing well clinically and is discharged from the hospital. A sudden increase in serum levels of alanine and aspartate transferase after discharge may be caused by transfusion-related non-A non-B hepatitis.[48] The late mortality rates in patients who develop liver dysfunction are nine times those of patients who have no evidence of hepatic failure.[47,48]

ALKALINE PHOSPHATASE AND GAMMA GLUTAMYL TRANSPEPTIDASE. The blood levels of alkaline phosphatase and gamma glutamyl transpeptidase (GGTP) tend to increase in patients with obstructive or cholestatic patterns of hepatic dysfunction.[46] These enzymes gradually increase and peak about 2-5 days after the bilirubin peak and then slowly decrease unless other problems develop.

AXIOM Increasing jaundice with high alkaline phosphatase levels soon after trauma should be considered due to extrahepatic biliary tract obstruction until proven otherwise.

METABOLISM OF DRUGS. The duration of action of a number of drugs, including diazepam, may be prolonged in patients with severe burns because biotransformation in the liver is depressed.[56,57] For example, both diazepam and chlordiazepoxide are metabolized in the liver by cytochrome p450 oxidases (phase I reaction), which are depressed in patients with severe burn injuries. Lorazepam, conversely, is metabolized by hepatic glucuronidation (phase II reaction), which is less apt to be impaired by severe burns.[47,56,57]

Phase III: Recovery of Hepatic Function
During recovery of hepatic function, bilirubin, LDH, and SGOT gradually fall to normal. Alkaline phosphatase and GGTP levels be-

gin to decrease several days later.[46] Bile plugs, bile duct proliferation, and acute and chronic inflammatory changes may persist for some time. EM examination tends to show may autophagic vacuoles and residual bodies. Focal necrotic cells may also be present.

THERAPY
Therapy for post-ischemic hepatic dysfunction is directed primarily at correcting any other medical problems and supplying adequate blood flow, oxygen, and glucose to the liver. Eradication of necrotic tissue or areas of inflammation, especially in the abdomen, is also essential.

MULTIPLE ORGAN FAILURE AND SEPSIS

Incidence

The incidence of hepatic dysfunction following trauma is only occasionally reported. Fry noted the development of liver failure in 50 (9%) of 553 patients requiring emergency operations, 61 (18%) of 337 with splenic trauma, 42 (43%) of 98 patients with Bacteroides bacteremia, and 66 (46%) of 143 patients with intraabdominal abscesses (Table 44–2).[58]

Etiology

Risk factors for developing liver failure after trauma or during sepsis include perfusion deficits, dead or injured tissue, uncontrolled infection and pre-existing liver disease.[7]

INADEQUATE PERFUSION

Physiologic Studies
The liver has a double blood supply through the hepatic artery and portal vein, and ligation of either the hepatic artery or the portal vein does not usually result in fatal liver necrosis. However, pathologists occasionally encounter massive hepatic necrosis as a result of disturbances of the hepatic microcirculation in patients with MOF or disseminated intravascular coagulation (DIC).[59] In 1946, Bywaters reported 42 patients who died within 9 days of injury.[60] Although only two (5%) developed jaundice, 12 (31%) had evidence of hepatic necrosis on light microscopy.

In a clinicopathologic study of 15 patients with massive hepatic necrosis after shock, three were diagnosed clinically as having fulminant hepatitis and 12 were diagnosed as having DIC and/or MOF.[59] The areas of liver necrosis were clearly demarcated from the surrounding liver parenchyma, producing an appearance of a so-called "map-like necrosis." Microscopically, the lesions showed a pattern of centrilobular necrosis.

TABLE 44–2 *Frequency of Clinical Failure of Each of Four Organ Systems in 1200 Patients with Different Fundamental Disease Processes*

	Frequency of Organ Failure			
	Lung Failure	Liver Failure	Stress Bleeding	Kidney Failure
Emergency Operations (N = 553)	8%	0%	3%	7%
Intra-abdominal Abscess (N = 143)	32%	46%	12%	27%
Bacteroides Bacteremia (N = 98)	23%	43%	11%	38%
Splenic Trauma (N = 337)	18%	18%	5%	7%

(From: Fry DE, Pearlstein L, Fulton RL, et al. Multiple system organ failure: the role of uncontrolled infection. Arch Surg 1980;115:136.)

In another study of hepatic dysfunction following shock, Champion et al. found that light microscopy of the liver 2-24 hours after shock showed a consistent increase in intracellular lipid and, in some patients, moderate numbers of acute inflammatory cells.[46] Focal necrosis only occurred in patients later exhibiting severe hepatic dysfunction. Bile plugs and cellular swelling were less frequently observed.

On EM, mild-to-moderate hepatic changes following shock were characterized predominantly by swollen mitochondria and dilated endoplasmic reticulum.[46] More severe ischemic damage resulted in greater numbers of cells with irreversible changes, such as flocculent densities in the mitochondria. In the patients with the most severe ischemia, such changes were more widespread (Fig. 44–2).

The liver necrosis was believed to result from severe systemic or intrahepatic circulatory disturbances due to Shwartzman-type reactions and/or repeated shock insults. Fibrin thrombi were found in liver capillaries in 13 (87%) of 15 patients and appeared to impair tissue perfusion. However, these thrombi can lyse rapidly and are not usually seen at autopsy unless the autopsy is performed soon after the initiating event.

Experimental Studies

Fath et al. showed that 60 minutes of complete hepatic ischemia in dogs is associated with a decrease in the hepatic clearance of amino acids.[61] Becker et al. later reported that this decrease in blood flow could be directly correlated with a decrease in hepatocellular, high-energy phosphate stores.[62]

Early studies by Schumer et al. (1970)[63] and Mela et al. (1971)[64] suggested that hepatic mitochondrial injury during endotoxemia may explain the oxygen extraction defects which appear to be responsible for the hepatic dysfunction.[58] Data from studies of rat peritonitis[55] have demonstrated increased uncoupling of oxidative phosphorylation in liver mitochondria along with reduced liver surface oxygen tension. These data were confirmed in studies with E. coli bacteremia, which seemed to indicate that microcirculatory injury resulted in defective hepatic oxidative metabolism and hepatocellular damage.[65]

Some experimental studies have indicated that the effective HBF declines after septic insult and this impaired perfusion precedes alterations in vital metabolic processes.[66-68] Studies of experimental peritonitis,[69] endotoxemia,[70] and bacteremia[71] using indocyanine green (ICG) clearance at doses consistent with first-order clearance kinetics have shown reduced effective hepatic nutrient blood flow prior to development of arterial hypotension.

Studies of effective (nutrient) HBF by Chaudry et al. using galactose elimination kinetics in rat peritonitis due to cecal ligation and puncture technique indicated that effective HBF was 84% of control at 5 hours, 75% of control at 10 hours, and 68% of control at 20 hours.[72]

The mechanism of the microcirculatory injury has been extensively studied. The increased systemic activation of complement appears to inversely correlate with the reduction in effective HBF.[73] The blood flow defect of nonspecific complement activation can be prevented by systemic pretreatment with a combination of superoxide dismutase and catalase,[74] but not with allopurinol.[75] These observations have suggested that the microcirculatory injury may be caused by oxygen radicals derived from neutrophils and not from reperfusion injuries associated with xanthine oxidase activity. Finally, imidazole treatment of rats with peritonitis significantly improved survival and also prevented the flow defect in the hepatic microcirculation.[76]

Clinical Studies

Gottlieb et al. measured splanchnic oxygen consumption and effective HBF in patients without sepsis who had episodes of systolic

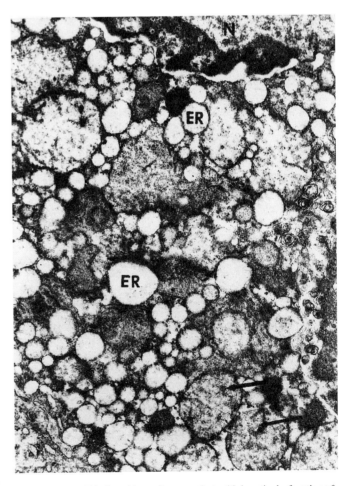

FIGURE 44–2 This liver biopsy from a patient with hepatic dysfunction after shock shows irreversible changes that include clumping of chromatin in the nucleus (N), mitochondrial swelling with flocculent densities (arrows), and marked dilatation of endoplasmic reticulum (ER) (From: Champion HR, Jones RT, Trump BJ, et al. A clinicopathologic study of hepatic dysfunction following shock. Surg Gynecol Obstet 1976;142:657).

BP < 90 mm Hg after severe trauma.[77] They found a significant elevation in splanchnic oxygen consumption. This occurred in spite of a 50% decrease in effective HBF by 12 hours postinjury despite a normal or elevated systemic BP. This decrease in effective hepatic perfusion persisted for about four to five days after injury. Evaluation of hepatocellular function with indocyanine green also showed a decrease in the hepatic clearance of the dye, which was worst about day four and resolved by day seven.[78]

In an effort to more accurately characterize the clinical hemodynamic response of the liver to sepsis, Dahn et al. measured HBF in 10 controls and nine patients with sepsis.[79] HBF was determined using two different indicators and three methods of analysis, including ICG dye clearance (HBF_{ICG}), galactose clearance (GC), and GC with splanchnic galactose gradient measurements (HBF_{GG}). For the 10 controls, HBF determined by the three analytic methods were essentially identical and averaged 0.75 ± 0.15 L/min/m^2. With hepatic venous sampling, the HBF in patients with sepsis was significantly higher than normal, both with ICG clearance (HBF_{ICG}) = 1.28 ± 0.50 and with splanchnic galactose gradient studies (HBF_{GG}) = 1.17 ± 0.52 L/min/m^2 (P < 0.025); however, effective HBF by the GC technique (0.89 ± 0.41 L/min/m^2), which uses peripheral venous sampling, was not significantly increased because of reduced splanchnic galactose extraction which appears to be characteristic of sepsis. Thus, estimates based on peripheral venous sampling showed a decreased effective HBF in sepsis, even though total splanchnic blood flow is increased. As sepsis worsened, the total HBF tended to increase, but effective HBF (galactose extraction) tended to decrease. Gottlieb et al. found that a decreased ICG clearance was a much earlier indication of hepatic failure after injury than was hyperbilirubinemia.[77]

In another study, Dahn et al. estimated mean blood and tissue oxygen tensions in the liver using Krogh-Erlang analysis.[80] This analysis considers each hepatic sinusoid to be a tissue cylinder with the blood capillary at its center. Oxygen tension at any point in the cylinder is determined by the passive radial diffusion characteristics of oxygen in the tissue and the local rates of oxygen utilization. Additionally, when it represents the lowest oxygen tension along the length of a capillary bed, venous oxygen tension may be used to estimate the lowest oxygen tension at which aerobic metabolism would be possible (critical oxygen tension) in this tissue cylinder.

AXIOM The total hepatic blood flow (HBF) in hypermetabolic sepsis is generally increased, even though peripheral extraction studies usually indicate that *effective* HBF is reduced.

Data from 10 septic patients revealed an HBF of 1.24 ± 0.32 L/min/m^2, a splanchnic oxygen consumption of 69.6 mL/min/m^2, and a hepatic venous oxygen tension of 28.8 ± 5.2 mm Hg.[80] Application of these data to the Krogh-Erlang tissue model indicated that despite an increase in oxygen delivery to the splanchnic bed during sepsis, the liver is more likely to have hypoxic events compared with normal patients and patients with trauma. This is indicated by reduced centrilobular oxygen tension and increased critical oxygen tension. The major factor responsible for this is the regional hypermetabolism present in sepsis. This analysis emphasized the critical importance of maintaining high-oxygen deliveries in critically ill patients with sepsis.[80]

AXIOM A higher than normal cardiac index and oxygen delivery is required to maintain adequate hepatic oxygenation after trauma and during sepsis.

Uncontrolled Focus of Infection

The mechanisms by which a persistent focus of infection causes MOF appears to be related to uncontrolled activation of the neuroendocrine system, complement, and cytokines.[7] This is largely due to the toxic effects of endotoxin (lipopolysaccharide); however, injection of Staphylococcus aureus or lipoteichoic acid (a staphylococcal cell-wall

constituent) into rabbits also impairs liver function.[81] Endotoxin causes its damage by activating mononuclear cells which, in turn, alter tissue cellular function causing a hypermetabolic and hyperdynamic state.[7,82,83,84]

Marshall et al. found that sepsis in patients with MOF could come from a wide variety of sources, but the organisms recovered from the blood of these patients most commonly were also cultured from the upper gastrointestinal tract.[85] The mechanisms by which these organisms enter the bloodstream is still debated. Splanchnic blood flow restriction and loss of mucosal integrity due to inadequate enteral nutrition have been suggested as mechanisms promoting bacterial translocation.[82,86] O'Dwyer et al. showed that a single intravenous dose of lipopolysaccharide could increase human intestinal permeability to many previously excluded substances.[87]

Persistent Focus of Dead or Injured Tissue[7]

To determine whether debridement of injured tissue has any effect on liver function, Schirmer et al. compared three groups of animals: those with a closed femur fracture, those with open fractures with tissue debridement, and those with a sham operation.[88] In both the closed- and open-fracture groups, HBF was decreased at 24 hours, but in the closed-fracture group, the decrease in HBF persisted for 48 hours. These results are consistent with the observations of Seibel et al. who reported that immediate treatment of orthopedic patients with open reduction and internal fixation rarely led to hepatic dysfunction, whereas liver failure was more common in patients treated by traction alone.[89] They also noted that bilirubin levels correlated positively with the duration of femur traction. The studies of Amaral et al[90] and Morris et al[91] also indicate that the local wound may release products that influence hepatic metabolism.

Preexisting Fibrotic Liver Disease

Fibrotic liver disease (cirrhosis) predisposes patients to the development of hepatic dysfunction and MOF.[7] These patients already have some hepatocellular dysfunction, and a perfusion deficit or septic insult causes further damage.[92] Because they are often malnourished and immunocompromised, these patients are also more likely to develop systemic infections. One study found that 92% of the "healthy" cirrhotics evaluated had chronic low-grade endotoxemia that was not seen in noncirrhotic individuals.[93] This chronic endotoxic state may explain why cirrhotic patients often have systemic oxygen consumptions well above those of normal unstressed noncirrhotic patients.

Inflammatory Response

COMPLEMENT ACTIVATION. From experimental observations, it appears that the liver dysfunction seen after trauma and with sepsis is at least partially due to excess complement activation by bacteria and bacterial cell products via the alternative pathway.[58] This releases the complement cleavage products C3a and C5a which stimulate neutrophil margination within the visceral microcirculation. The margination of activated neutrophils results in local free-radical-mediated injury which, in turn, causes local fibrin deposition and platelet aggregation. Platelet aggregation may then cause local release of thromboxane. The net effect of this process is that a biomechanical "plug" combined with microcirculatory vasoconstriction causes reduced nutrient flow. The resulting tissue ischemia or hypoxia causes an additional inflammatory response. Tissue reaction may become a self-energizing process such that correction of the underlying septic process may not change the course of events within the microcirculation.[58] This may explain some of the cynicism that has been expressed concerning attempts at aggressive surgical management of intraabdominal infection in patients who already have MOF.[94,95]

Another response of some significance is the concept of bacterial translocation.[96-98] Ischemic microcirculatory injury within the intestinal microcirculation may adversely affect gastrointestinal barrier function so that bacteria from the gut can enter the blood stream and become an additional factor to "fuel the engine" of MOF.[58]

ACTIVATION OF KUPFFER CELLS. Kupffer cells make up about 60-70% of the body's tissue macrophages and comprise up to 80% of the non-parenchymal cells isolated from the liver.[7] Kupffer cells are located along the hepatic sinusoids and lay in direct contact with hepatic parenchymal cells. These cells have immune and phagocytic functions and are the primary hepatic source of IL-1, TNF, and eicosanoids.

The number of Kupffer cells can increase severalfold in sepsis. Bouwens et al. found that about 75% of the Kupffer cell increase in rat livers during sepsis was due to proliferation of local Kupffer cells, and the remainder of the increase was due to the stimulation of peripheral macrophage precursors.[99]

Recently, increasing attention has been given to the effects of bacteria and endotoxin on liver cells, particularly in the presence of hypoxemia and reduced perfusion. The gut is perceived as a major source of the bacteria and bacterial toxins damaging the liver after trauma or burns.[100] Liver dysfunction under such circumstances may be largely due to the effects of activated Kupffer cells on liver cell metabolism.[101-106] The precise nature of the substances responsible for the liver changes are not yet completely characterized, but interleukin-1 (IL-1), interleukin-2 (IL-2), tumor necrosis (TNF), and prostaglandin E_2 (PGE$_2$) appear to be involved. Dietary polyunsaturated fatty acids may also affect mediator release by Kupffer cells.[107]

Mazuski et al. found that cultured Kupffer cells released significant quantities of IL-1, TNF, and PGE$_2$ into the surrounding media when stimulated with endotoxin.[108] Production of IL-1 after lipopolysaccharide stimulation is enhanced by the addition of IL-2.[109] IL-2 production is also augmented by incubation of Kupffer cells with hepatocytes or in media in which hepatocytes have been grown.[110] Endotoxin-induced TNF production by Kupffer cells can also be increased by platelet-activating factor (PAF), a substance that leads to platelet aggregation and increased platelet adhesion to endothelial surfaces.[7]

> **AXIOM**   Increased bacterial translocation of gut bacteria or endotoxin because of gut ischemia, prolonged absence of enteral feeding, or alterations of gut flora may cause excessive activation of Kupffer cells with resulting changes in hepatocyte function.

Coccia et al. have shown that pentoxifylline treatment after hemorrhage significantly improves tissue oxygenation and survival rates.[111] In their study, infusion of pentoxifylline during and after crystalloid resuscitation restored the hemorrhage-induced depression of hepatocellular function back toward normal and decreased elevated plasma levels of TNF and IL-6.

Several studies clearly have demonstrated that pentoxifylline can block TNF mRNA production by macrophages after endotoxin administration.[112-114] As a methylxanthine derivative, pentoxifylline exerts its pharmacologic effects by inhibiting intracellular phosphodiesterase, thus increasing the intracellular concentrations of cyclic AMP[115] which, in turn, suppresses TNF gene transcription.[115] Although it blocks TNF mRNA production, pentoxifylline has no effect on the efficiency of reported mRNA translation.[113]

MEDIATORS. Many mediators are believed to be involved in the changes in the physiologic parameters seen in MOF. Key roles are played by IL-1, IL-2, TNF, and eicosanoids.[7]

Interleukin-1. IL-1 is a protein secreted by many cells, including endothelial cells and cells of the monocyte-macrophage line.[7] Mononuclear cells can be stimulated to produce IL-1 by activated T-cells, immune complexes, C5a, and endotoxin. In myelohematopoetic tissues, the presence of IL-1 is important for optimal cellular activation and proliferation to occur. Other extrahepatic functions of IL-1 include induction of fever, prostaglandin production, fibroblast release of collagenase, and induction of proteolysis in skeletal muscle.[116]

Interleukin-2. IL-2 is a protein secreted by T-lymphocytes after stimulation by IL-1 or by antigen in association with accessory cells

(monocytes or B-cells).[7] The functions of IL-2 include stimulation of lymphocyte proliferation, antibody production, and lymphokine-activated killer activity by some classes of lymphoid cells.[117]

Tumor Necrosis Factor. TNF can induce hemorrhagic necrosis of tumors in certain experimental models.[7,118] This factor previously was called, cachectin, because it was capable of producing anorexia and metabolic disorders leading to cachexia. TNF is the initial cytokine released by macrophages in response to endotoxin or infection. It is produced by activated macrophages, and endotoxin has been identified as one of the most potent stimulators of its production.

Receptors for TNF are present on all somatic cells with the exception of erythrocytes. TNF causes a wide range of metabolic alterations, which include enhancement of neutrophil phagocytic and cytotoxic activities, induction of endothelial production of IL-1 and procoagulant factors, and augmentation of lymphocyte proliferation in response to IL-2. Infusion of TNF by itself can produce the entire clinical picture of severe sepsis.[118]

Eicosanoids. Eicasanoids are derivatives of arachidonic acid and include the prostaglandins, thromboxanes, and leukotrienes.[7] Miller-Graziano et al. documented an association between immune suppression and high circulating levels of PGE$_2$ in burn patients with multiple serious infections.[119] They also noted that after 12 days, these patients also had increased numbers of T-suppressor cells. These T-suppressor cells stimulated monocyte production of PGE$_2$, as well as a higher than normal proportion of circulating monocytes with receptors for the Fc portion of the antibody heavy chain. These monocytes with Fc-receptors have also been identified as a major source of PGE$_2$.[117] Kupffer cells in some species have also been noted to have a high percentage of cells with Fc receptors.[120]

Pathophysiology

Some of the more important pathophysiologic changes seen with hepatic dysfunction after trauma or with sepsis include altered metabolism of carbohydrates, proteins, and fats.

CARBOHYDRATE METABOLISM

> **AXIOM**   Carbohydrate stress metabolism is characterized by: (a) increased glucagon:insulin ratios, (b) increased insulin resistance, (c) increased glycogenolysis and gluconeogenesis in spite of exogenous glucose, (d) hyperglycemia, and (e) increased lactate production.

Total body energy expenditure following trauma or with sepsis may increase > 1.5-2 times normal, and substrate preferences change so that there is a greater emphasis on protein as an energy source.[7] The hyperglycemia that develops is relatively refractory to exogenous insulin. Consequently, decreased glucose utilization is manifest relative to the degree of hyperglycemia present. Additionally, increased levels of catecholamines cause a progressive increase in the glucagon-to-insulin ratio far out of proportion to that expected from the blood glucose levels.[7]

One of the liver's responses to increased catecholamines and glucagon is increased glycogenolysis. A great increase in gluconeogenesis from lactate, alanine, glutamine, glycine, serine, and glycerol also occurs. Although much of this response is directed by the neuroendocrine axis, it can be altered by sepsis. In rats subjected to an infusion of endotoxin, hepatic gluconeogenesis is initially increased, but at 48 hours, the level of gluconeogenesis is not significantly different from that of the control animals, despite the fact that endotoxemic animals have hyperglycemia and hyperlactacidemia and elevated glucagon and catecholamine levels.[121] In the presence of endotoxin, the hepatic conversion of lactate to glucose is no longer sensitive to stimulation from glucagon or norepinephrine. Therefore, although hepatic conversion of lactate to glucose continues, it may not be capable of coping with the increased lactate production. In the final stages of hepatic failure, serum glucose levels decrease and lactate levels increase.

The increased blood lactate levels seen in MOF may be due to several factors, including: (a) increased substrate flow through glycolytic pathways, (b) down-regulation of the tricarboxylic acid cycle, and (c) inadequate gluconeogenic pathways to handle lactate.[7] The primary tissue sources of lactate are muscle and inflammatory cells. Lactate levels in aerobic glycolysis increase if: (a) increased pyruvate is produced, (b) the amount of fat and amino acids (particularly alanine and glutamine) utilized as a source of two-carbon fragments in the Krebs cycle increases, and (c) pyruvate dehydrogenase activity is reduced.

Because the conversion of pyruvate to lactate is not blocked in sepsis, the ratio of lactate to pyruvate remains normal and is associated stoichiometrically with the release of alanine.[23,122] When the patient has an elevated lactate level in the presence of an increased lactate to pyruvate ratio, it indicates inadequate tissue perfusion, and the patient should be resuscitated with intravenous fluids to increase oxygen delivery. Conversely, increased lactate in the presence of a normal lactate-to-pyruvate ratio suggests aerobic glycolysis and/or reduced hepatic clearance which is often due to sepsis.[7]

PROTEIN METABOLISM

AXIOM   The protein metabolism of stress is characterized by: (a) increased total body catabolism that is refractory to exogenous amino acids, (b) reduced muscle amino acid uptake, (c) increased release of muscle amino acids, (d) increased hepatic amino acid uptake, and (e) increased synthesis of acute-phase proteins.[107]

Peripheral protein autocannibalism is an important characteristic of the hypermetabolic response to sepsis.[7] Amino acids released from protein catabolism, particularly of skeletal muscle, become the primary energy source for the body.[123] The increased protein release from skeletal muscle is mediated by a number of factors, including cortisol, cytokines (especially IL-1), and prostaglandins.[116] Data from Cerra et al. have indicated that increased utilization of branched-chain amino acids (BCAA) occurs in patients with sepsis in the following order of preference: leucine, isoleucine, and valine.[124] In the worst patients, hepatic protein synthesis may gradually decrease, especially in nonsurvivors (Fig. 44–3).

To assess the differential effects of liver dysfunction on plasma amino acid profiles in septic and nonseptic states, Cerra et al. studied patients with preexistent cirrhosis after elective surgery, and compared this profile to the profiles seen in noncirrhotic patients, noncirrhotic patients with sepsis, and cirrhotic patients with sepsis.[92] Patients with cirrhosis had increased levels of aromatic amino acids (phenylalanine, tyrosine, and tryptophan), which are known to be predominantly metabolized by the liver. They also had decreased levels of BCAA.

Cirrhotic and noncirrhotic patients who developed sepsis had similar responses, with elevated aromatic amino acid levels and decreased BCAA levels, as well as altered peripheral energy metabolism. Nonsurvivors with sepsis developed increased BCAA levels as death approached, indicating premorbid collapse of peripheral metabolism.

Pittiruti et al. compared patients with and without sepsis after trauma[125] and found similar results to those of Cerra et al.[92] Increased levels of aromatic amino acids, particularly phenylalanine, were also found to correlate directly with increased degrees of hepatic dysfunction, elevated levels of bilirubin, reduced rates of amino acid clearance, and eventual death.[7,61,62]

FAT METABOLISM

AXIOM   Stress fat metabolism is characterized by: (a) increased adipocyte lipolysis, (b) decreased lipogenesis, (c) increased fatty acid oxidation, (d) increased triglyceride turnover, and (e) decreased ketosis.[107]

Hypermetabolism is accompanied by hypertriglyceridemia despite increased peripheral utilization relative to the starvation state.[7] Although much of this increase is caused by release from adipocytes, increased hepatic lipolysis and lipogenesis also contribute to the hypertriglyceridemia. Feingold and Grunfeld found that TNF helps to increase hepatocyte lipogenesis in rats.[126]

Metabolism of lipids to ketones for energy utilization is increased in hypermetabolism.[7] As liver function deteriorates, the release of β-hydroxybutyrate progressively increases demonstrating a decreasing capability of hepatocyte mitochondria to utilize ketones as an energy source. Simultaneously, the serum level of acetoacetate, which is produced by the liver and extracted by peripheral tissues, may decrease to the point of disappearance.[122] The ratio of acetoacetate to β-hydroxybutyrate has been believed to reflect the hepatic mitochondrial redox potential.[7] Ozawa et al. found that postoperative patients with a ratio of > 0.4 in the arterial blood did well, whereas a level < 0.4 was associated with MOF, and a level of < 0.25 was associated with eventual death.[127]

In hepatic lipogenesis, the respiratory quotient (RQ) tends to exceed 1.0.[107] This can easily occur with overfeeding of carbohydrates. Terminally, in sepsis, triglyceride intolerance may develop so that a reduced ability to clear exogenous triglycerides and long-chain fatty acids also occurs.

AXIOM   When fully developed, the liver failure of sepsis has a bad prognosis and is usually followed or is closely associated with the development of renal failure.[107]

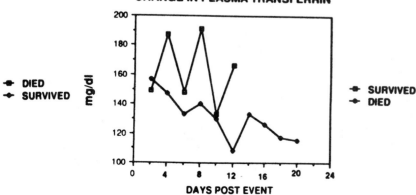

CHANGE IN HEPATIC PROTEIN SYNTHESIS AS CHANGE IN PLASMA TRANSFERRIN

DIED
SURVIVED

SURVIVED
DIED

FIGURE 44–3 In these patients sepsis was the inciting event for hypermetabolism and organ failure. Between days 7-19 postinjury, progressive failure of hepatic protein synthesis occurred, as reflected by decreasing plasma transferrin levels in the patients who died (From: Cerra FB, Mazuski JE, Bankey PE, et al. Role of monokines in altering hepatic metabolism in sepsis. Roth BL, Nielsen TB, McKee AE, eds. Molecular and cellular mechanisms of septic shock. New York: Alan R. Liss, 1989; 267).

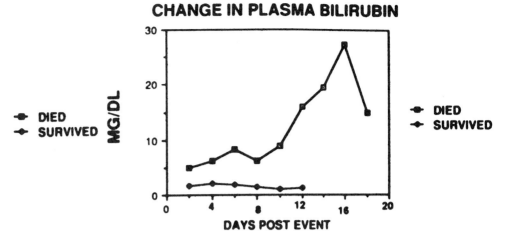

FIGURE 44–4 In patients in whom sepsis was the inciting event for hypermetabolism and organ failure, a progressive increase occurred in bilirubin at days 7-10 postinjury (From: Cerra FB, Mazuski JE, Bankey PE, et al. Role of monokines in altering hepatic metabolism in sepsis. Roth BL, Nielsen TB, McKee AE, eds. Molecular and cellular mechanisms of septic shock. New York: Alan R. Liss, 1989; 267).

Diagnosis

The systemic response to severe trauma is often recognized as a clinical syndrome of tachycardia, tachypnea, altered mentation, leukocytosis, hyperdynamic physiologic state, and hypermetabolism.[107,128] Stimuli, such as severe infection, inflammatory tissue, and perfusion defects, seen in burns and pancreatitis, can also induce the same systemic response.

AXIOM Inadequate control or eradication of infection, inflammation, or necrotic tissue is the most common cause of MOF development.

The usual metabolic response to injury peaks on days 2 and 3 and is usually gone by days 7-10.[107] Severe hypermetabolism persisting for more than 3-4 days is usually associated with some form of persisting injury or impaired perfusion (Fig. 44–4). When the hypermetabolism persists for several more days, serum bilirubin and serum creatinine begin to progressively increase. When severe hypermetabolism persists for more than 2-3 weeks, most patients eventually die.[7]

AXIOM One of the first signs of sepsis and/or increasing hepatic dysfunction is a progressively increasing cardiac output and decreasing systemic vascular resistance.

The increasing organ failure of sepsis is characterized by high-cardiac output, low-systemic-vascular resistance, and increased oxygen consumption (Table 44–3).[107]

AXIOM The two physical findings typically seen with hepatic failure are jaundice and encephalopathy.

Cholestatic jaundice with elevation of serum bilirubin and alkaline phosphatase levels is the most common manifestation of hepatic failure in sepsis.[107] It is particularly apt to be seen with severe, generalized peritonitis involving anaerobic organisms, particularly Bacteroides fragilis.[46] Because hyperbilirubinemia is predominantly of the conjugated form, the problem is primarily impaired excretion rather than impaired hepatocellular uptake.[27]

In some instances, the liver changes due to rapidly progressive sepsis may be difficult to differentiate from other causes of elevated bilirubin, especially within the first five days after trauma; however, with sepsis, alkaline phosphatase levels are often much higher than would be expected for the degree of hyperbilirubinemia, and the hyperbilirubinemia of sepsis is often delayed until 8-10 days after trauma (Figs. 44–4, 44–5).

AXIOM Bilirubin levels > 5 mg/dL in the absence of biliary tract obstruction, transfusion reaction, or resolving hematoma are strongly suggestive of liver dysfunction due to sepsis.[7]

SGOT and SGPT are often elevated in posttraumatic or septic liver failure, but seldom to levels more than two to three times normal. Plasma albumin levels are often very low, but the prothrombin time is usually normal until relatively late. The WBC count is generally elevated, and increased numbers of PMNs are evident, often with a shift to the left (i.e., increased band forms).

AXIOM Early jaundice occurring within five days of trauma should be considered as due to hemolysis or a biliary tract obstruction; jaundice developing after seven days is due to sepsis until proven otherwise.

Sepsis tends to be associated with hyperglycemia which is relatively resistant to insulin. Occasionally, however, when sepsis is overwhelming, the liver either cannot make glucose or mobilize glycogen, resulting in severe hypoglycemia. Septic hypoglycemia generally indicates a poor prognosis and it is usually a preterminal event.[107]

TABLE 44–3 *Metabolic Criteria for Stress Stratification*

Stress Level	Clinical Prototype	Urinary Nitrogen g/day	Oxygen Consumed mL/m²	Blood Glucose mg/dL	Plasma Lactate mM/L	Glucago Insulin Ratio
0	Starvation	< 5	90 ± 10	100 ± 20	1.0 ± 0.5	2.0 ± 0.5
1	Elective surgery	5-10	130 ± 10	150 ± 25	1.5 ± 0.5	2.5 ± 0.8
2	Trauma	10-15	150 ± 20	150 ± 25	2.0 ± 0.5	3.0 ± 0.7
3	Sepsis	> 15	180 ± 20	250 ± 50	> 2.5	8.0 ± 1.5

(From: Cerra FB, Mazuski JE, Bankey PE, et al. Role of monokines in altering hepatic metabolism in sepsis. Roth BL, Nielsen TB, McKee AE, eds. Progress in clinical and biological research. New York: Alan R Liss, 1988; 268.)

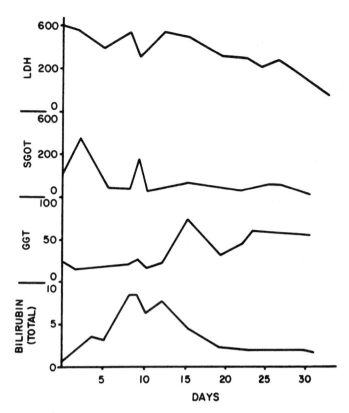

FIGURE 44–5 Serum bilirubin levels in this patient with severe trauma from a motor vehicle accident initially rose because of blood transfusions and retroperitoneal hematoma. A second rise in bilirubin levels began on the fifth day and peaked on day 13 because of hemolytic staphylococcal septicemia (From: Champion HR, Jones RT, Trump BF, et al. Post-traumatic hepatic dysfunction as a major etiology in post-traumatic jaundice. J Trauma 1976;16:650).

AXIOM   When the etiology of persistent jaundice in a patient with major abdominal surgery or trauma cannot be determined in any other manner, exploratory celiotomy should be performed.

As Flint has noted, subjecting a critically ill patient to an operation constitutes a difficult therapeutic decision, but one that is rewarded by positive findings and patient improvement in up to 50% of patients where postoperative or posttraumatic jaundice may be due to peritonitis.[21] Furthermore, exclusion of intraabdominal sepsis allows the clinician to concentrate efforts in other areas. Liver biopsy is less useful as a prognostic measure in septic liver failure than in other conditions, such as hepatitis or cirrhosis.

Pathology

Histologic findings from liver biopsies or autopsies taken from patients with MOFs have consistently revealed: (a) evidence of centrilobular hepatocellular congestion or necrosis, and (b) biliary stasis, with bile noted both intracellularly and inspissated in the canaliculi.[23,27,59] Both of these findings seem to correlate with the degree of elevation of the serum bilirubin.

In 1950, Mallory et al. noted that soldiers who had received lethal, shock-producing injuries and survived < 12 hours had no remarkable hepatic histologic changes at autopsy.[129] In contrast, of the patients surviving 12-96 hours, 87% had fat vacuolation of the liver parenchymal cells in a centrilobular distribution. These pathologic changes were particularly severe in patients with peritonitis.

Treatment

CONTROL OF THE SOURCE

Prevention remains the best mode of treatment of MOF, and control of the source of sepsis is the first principle.[107] Whenever possible, one must stop continued stimulation of the mediator system by areas of inflammation or necrosis as soon as possible. When the primary process can be controlled, the patient's condition and the liver function tests soon begin to improve; however, the WBC count may continue to increase for several days before beginning to fall back toward a normal level.[46]

AXIOM   Correction of hepatic failure in MOF requires debridement of infected or necrotic tissue, drainage of abscesses, and treatment of existing infection with appropriate antibiotics.

Norton et al.[130] and Fry et al.[131] have suggested that exploratory laparotomy is indicated when jaundice develops or recurs in patients at risk for undiagnosed peritonitis or intraperitoneal abscesses. Strawn et al. made similar recommendations in patients who developed septic complications following liver injury.[132] Flint noted that persistent jaundice (i.e., bilirubin > 5 mg/dL lasting longer than three days) was associated with intraperitoneal infection in 75% of patients.[21] Although necrotizing pulmonary and soft-tissue infections causing jaundice are usually easy to diagnose, the presence of occult intraperitoneal sepsis can often only be detected by exploratory laparotomy.

OPTIMAL OXYGEN DELIVERY

AXIOM   Rapid restoration and maintenance of optimal (supranormal) oxygen delivery is extremely important for trying to prevent hepatic failure after trauma.

In many clinical settings in which MOF develops, early optimization of oxygen delivery and consumption may reduce the incidence of MOF and mortality.[107] Following experimental hemorrhagic shock, hepatic and intestinal mucosal blood flow may be only 60-70% of normal after the systolic BP has been restored to normal.[133] It appears that a cardiac output 25-50% greater than normal is required to provide adequate splanchnic blood flow.[133]

Dahn et al. observed that resuscitation of patients was not complete until hyperdynamic splanchnic perfusion could be demonstrated.[134] This may require the use of inotropes and/or vasodilators as well as large quantities of fluid. In addition, it must be remembered that effective HBF may be lower than normal despite a systemic hyperdynamic cardiovascular response. Dopamine in low doses (1-3 mcg/kg/min) may help to improve splanchnic blood flow; however, in large doses (> 20-30 mcg/kg/min), it may decrease hepatic perfusion.

AXIOM   Early optimization of oxygen delivery with fluids, blood, and possibly inotropes should be monitored closely by oxygen consumption, S_vO_2, and serum lactate to ensure a more than adequate splanchnic blood flow.[7]

EARLY ENTERAL NUTRITION

Metabolic support can be an important part of the treatment of hepatic failure.[107] Early enteral nutrition may be particularly important for preserving intestinal mucosa and helping to prevent translocation of bacteria and bacterial products from the gut into intestinal lymphatics and portal venous blood.[100,107]

The source of fat provided for nutrition may also be important. Macrophages from rats fed a diet enriched in omega-3 fats (fish oil) showed a decrease in PGE_2, prostacyclin, and thromboxane A_2 production, as well as a decrease in IL-1 and TNF release in response to endotoxin. Furthermore, the increased PGE_2 production seen with omega-6 fatty acids from intravenous fat may be associated with immunosuppression. After 6 weeks of omega-3 fat therapy, macrophages continued to show a decreased production of IL-1 and TNF. In contrast, in rats fed a diet enriched in omega-6 fats (safflower oil), IL-1 and TNF production in response to endotoxin was increased.[135]

Unfortunately, no good source of omega-3 fatty acids for parenteral nutrition exists. It is increasingly suggested that dietary manipulation of substrate may be a means of improving survival by altering the response of macrophages to certain stimuli. Thus, early enteral nutrition may be extremely important.

AXIOM Early enteral nutrition, which may help decrease bacterial translocation in the gut, may be an important part of reducing hepatic dysfunction in critically ill or injured patients.

EXTRACORPOREAL PERFUSION

With the aim of temporarily assisting the liver whose function rapidly deteriorates after surgery, Matsubara et al. conducted extracorporeal blood purification therapy (EBPT; plasma exchange and/or hemofiltration) in 26 postoperative patients.[136] Initiation of EBPT was instituted when the serum bilirubin exceeded 15 mg/dL or the patient developed grade 2 encephalopathy or coma. Plasma exchange was performed 235 times in 23 patients, and hemofiltration was performed 28 times in seven patients. Plasma exchange was found to control progression of DIC and endotoxemia, and nine patients (35%) were weaned from EBPT. In survivors, the levels of blood ammonia and the number of major complications were significantly lower compared to nonsurvivors. The patients treated only with hemofiltration all died. Among the comorbid factors present, renal failure, respiratory failure, and preexisting cirrhosis were associated with a poor prognosis.

FATTY LIVER

Alcohol

The so-called fatty liver may be an acute or chronic problem. Fat may accumulate in the liver parenchyma as a result of alcohol ingestion, obesity, malnutrition, diabetes mellitus, administration of certain antibiotics (e.g., tetracycline), and exposure to various chemicals (e.g., poisoning by carbon tetrachloride or DDT).

AXIOM Fatty liver is the most frequently noted hepatic abnormality in alcoholics and in patients on TPN.

The precise cause of fat deposition in the liver in alcoholics is unknown; however, factors that appear to be involved include: an increased influx of fatty acids (from fat stores), increased hepatic synthesis of triglycerides (from fatty acids or excess carbohydrates derived from the diet), decreased oxidation of fatty acids, and impaired hepatic synthesis of lipoprotein.

Hepatobiliary Complications of Nutritional Support

A number of hepatobiliary complications of parenteral nutritional support have been reported and include hepatic steatosis, cholestasis, and nonspecific triaditis.[8,137] Progression to chronic liver disease has been reported most frequently in premature infants,[138-140] but it can also occur in adults. When chronic liver dysfunction has occurred during parenteral nutritional support, it has been generally associated with very long-term therapy, and it has presented histologically as steatohepatitis or steatonecrosis with progression to micromodular cirrhosis, similar to lesions seen in alcoholic liver disease.[137-139]

TYPES OF LIVER CHANGES

Hepatic Steatosis

One of the more common complications of relatively short-term (2-3 weeks) parenteral nutrition support is fatty infiltration of the liver, which is also known as hepatic steatosis.[8] A number of factors that seem to be associated with fatty infiltration of the liver include carbohydrate as the sole source of TPN calories, infusion of excess calories, and deficiencies of essential fatty acids or carnitine. The etiology of the fat deposition may also be related to high rates of glucose infusion stimulating hyperinsulinemia which, in turn, stimulates lipogenesis and inhibits lipid mobilization from fat stores. An RQ > 1.0 indicates that carbohydrate nutrients are being converted into fat, and such fat is apt to accumulate in the liver.

AXIOM Indirect calorimetry to monitor RQ may be of great help in optimizing nutritional intake and preventing hepatic steatosis.

Essential fatty acid deficiency can be caused by inadequate intake or by high-insulin levels suppressing the mobilization of endogenous fatty acids. This promotes fat accumulation in the liver as a result of decreased synthesis of phospholipids which are required for lipid transport. Carnitine deficiency, though unusual, may also lead to impaired fat transport and subsequent decreased mitochondrial oxidation of lipids.

Fatty infiltration of the liver may appear within the first one to three weeks of TPN administration.[8] Liver biopsies show that fatty infiltration is confined to periportal areas in mild cases, but in the more severe cases, it is also panlobular or centrilobular.

Extensive fatty infiltration presents clinically with moderate elevations in aminotransferases and mild elevations of alkaline phosphatase. In the most severe cases, hepatic steatosis may present with hepatic enlargement, right upper quadrant pain, and marked elevations in both hepatocellular enzymes and alkaline phosphatase. Fortunately, the lesion does not appear to result in progressive hepatic injury, and enzymatic changes often improve even when TPN is continued.

Intrahepatic Cholestasis

Intrahepatic cholestasis tends to occur later than fatty infiltration and is not usually seen in liver biopsies until after at least three weeks of TPN.[8] Clinically, it presents with an elevated alkaline phosphatase followed by elevations in bilirubin. Jaundice is usually the only symptom. Histologically, the lesion presents as periportal canalicular bile plugging, bile staining of surrounding hepatocytes, and some degree of triaditis with a predominantly lymphocytic infiltration. This triaditis may persist for several months after discontinuation of TPN.[140]

Extrahepatic Cholestasis

Gallbladder sludge is common after four weeks of TPN and is present in almost all patients after six weeks of TPN.[141] Gallstone development has also been associated with long-term TPN.[142-143] The development of biliary sludge appears to be related to gallbladder stasis caused by lack of enteral feedings and the resultant lack of gallbladder contraction.[142,143] Several other mechanisms for TPN-induced cholestasis have been proposed.[8] For example, a deficiency of taurine, which is necessary for bile acid conjugation, has been suggested as a cause of cholestasis in premature infants.[144,145] Increased production of the bile acid lithocholate by intestinal bacteria has also been proposed as a potential cause of cholestasis.[146] Excesses in calories and toxic amino acid metabolites have also been associated with cholestasis.[139]

Nonspecific Triaditis

Although it is often associated with cholestasis, nonspecific triaditis appears to occur independent of this problem, particularly in patients with inflammatory bowel disease receiving TPN.[8] In many patients it is unknown whether the nonspecific triaditis primarily represents a TPN-related condition or is related to the pericholangitis often seen in patients with inflammatory bowel disease not receiving TPN. Nonspecific triaditis may represent a mild or early form of intrahepatic cholestasis.[139] Clinically, triaditis can appear early in the course of TPN, and it is characterized by moderate elevations of hepatocellular enzymes. In patients with high aminotransferase levels, bilirubin and alkaline phosphatase levels may also be elevated.

DIAGNOSIS

The diagnosis of hepatobiliary complications of TPN is usually made on the basis of laboratory findings.[8] Elevations in amino transferase are suggestive of hepatocellular injury and usually reflect fatty infiltration or triaditis, whereas hyperbilirubinemia and elevations of alkaline phosphatase are more suggestive of cholestasis. In a stable patient, laboratory improvements following manipulation of the nutritional formula may be virtually diagnostic.

> **AXIOM**   Patients on TPN should be monitored closely for elevated levels of aminotransferase, bilirubin, and alkaline phosphatase.

In deteriorating patients, liver biopsy may be required to prove a diagnosis of fatty infiltration, and ultrasound or cholangiography may be required to confirm the diagnosis of biliary sludge or obstruction. Other more serious causes of hepatic dysfunction, such as ischemic or infectious hepatitis, biliary calculi, cholecystitis, and/or mechanical biliary obstruction, should also be considered before attributing abnormal hepatobiliary enzymes to nutritional support.[8]

TREATMENT

Management of hepatobiliary complications of TPN are primarily aimed at prevention.[8] Excess calories should be avoided. In most patients, except those with severe malnutrition, and/or hypermetabolism, total nonprotein caloric intake probably should only be about 25 kcal/kg/day.

> **AXIOM**   Using resting energy expenditures and RQs to adjust TPN should help to prevent hepatic complications due to under or overfeeding.

About 20-30% of the nonprotein calories can be given as fat to provide essential long-chain fatty acids. Cyclic TPN, to allow mobilization of fat between periods of hyperinsulinemia, may also minimize the tendency toward steatosis.

Enteral nutrition, even when only partial, should be instituted as soon as possible so as to minimize biliary stasis.[8] In our experience at Detroit Receiving Hospital, 30-60 ml of isosmotic enteral feedings, rather than antacids, can be instilled into the stomach via a nasogastric tube every hour. Clamping the tube for 45-50 minutes and aspirating for 10-15 minutes prevents gastric accumulation of feedings, and about 20-30% of the feedings reach the small bowel.

CIRRHOSIS AND PORTAL HYPERTENSION

Definition

Portal hypertension is usually a complication of liver disease that results in portal vein pressures exceeding 200 mm H_2O (15 mm Hg). Because portal vein pressures are partly dependent on inferior venal cava pressures, one can also consider portal hypertension to exist when the difference between the pressure in the portal vein and inferior vena cava exceeds 150 mm H_2O.

Etiology

INTRAHEPATIC CAUSES

Intrahepatic disease causes about 95% of all portal hypertension. Of these liver diseases, nutritional cirrhosis, posthepatic (postnecrotic) cirrhosis, and biliary cirrhosis are the most common. Other hepatic diseases that can cause portal hypertension include: toxic (drug) hepatitis, metabolic cirrhosis (including hemochromatosis, Wilson's disease, and galactosemia), intestinal bypass, alcoholic hepatitis, neoplasms, and schistosomiasis.

> **AXIOM**   Patients who drink excessive amounts of alcohol are prone to develop nutritional cirrhosis, and this greatly increases the risk of hepatic failure during sepsis or after trauma.

Nutritional Cirrhosis

Nutritional cirrhosis—also referred to as Laennec's, alcoholic, or portal cirrhosis—is the underlying disorder in about two-thirds of patients with portal hypertension. It is usually caused by alcohol abuse and associated malnutrition. Fibrosis and formation of nodules of regenerating liver distort the liver's architecture and impair its function. On gross examination, the liver has uniform, diffuse, small nodules. Microscopically, the nodules consist of proliferating liver cells and fibrosis, particularly around the portal triads.

Postnecrotic Cirrhosis

The cirrhosis that follows severe viral or toxic hepatitis is much less common than nutritional cirrhosis, but it causes about 10-20% of portal hypertension. Postnecrotic cirrhosis may be associated with severe fibrosis in the liver. These patients tend to have a small, shrunken liver with large, irregular nodules. Consequently, the liver in these patients is often called "macronodular" as opposed to the "micronodular" appearance typically seen with nutritional cirrhosis.

Biliary Cirrhosis

Prolonged jaundice eventually causes portal and periportal inflammation and fibrosis. Over a period of months or years, contracture of fibrous tissue eventually produces a macronodular pattern in the liver similar to that seen in postnecrotic cirrhosis. The initial biliary obstruction may be in the small intrahepatic biliary radicles (primary biliary cirrhosis) or in the major extrahepatic ducts (secondary biliary cirrhosis).

> **PITFALL** ⊘
>
> *One should not allow an extrahepatic cause of jaundice to persist any longer than absolutely necessary because of the secondary liver changes it can cause.*

Extrahepatic biliary tract obstruction causing jaundice should be corrected rapidly. No matter how strongly jaundice is believed to be due to intrahepatic disease, if it does not improve after one to two weeks of intensive medical therapy, efforts must be made to rule out extrahepatic biliary duct obstruction.

EXTRAHEPATIC DISEASE

The most frequent extrahepatic problems causing portal hypertension include portal vein obstruction, hepatic vein obstruction, and excessive portal venous blood flow.

Portal Vein Obstruction

Portal vein obstruction is most frequently due to thrombosis which, in children, is usually due to neonatal omphalitis. Cavernous transformation of the portal vein is probably due to recanalization of a previously thrombosed portal vein. These patients tend to develop their portal hypertension in childhood or early adult life and tend to have good liver function. As a consequence, they usually tolerate surgery for portal hypertension well.

> **AXIOM**   Patients with prehepatic portal hypertension can tolerate trauma and surgery much better than patients with other causes of esophageal varices.

Hepatic Vein Obstruction

Extrahepatic obstruction of the hepatic venous outflow system is caused by a group of rare conditions and is often referred to as the Budd-Chiari syndrome. These problems include neoplastic and inflammatory disorders involving the hepatic veins or adjacent inferior vena cava. The most striking clinical findings in the Budd-Chiari syndrome are marked hepatomegaly and ascites.

AV Fistulas

AV fistulas between the hepatic artery and portal vein or between the splenic artery and vein are rare causes of portal hypertension. However, this is a frequent method for producing portal hypertension in experimental animals.

Pathophysiology

Continuing destruction of liver parenchyma can lead to excessive formation of scar tissue and regenerative nodules. This rearranges the hepatic architecture and compresses the vessels inside the liver. Because they have a low pressure and thin walls, the intrahepatic veins are more easily obstructed than other hepatic vessels. This results in an obstruction just distal to the hepatic sinusoids. This postsinusoidal obstruction results in increased portal vein pressure and decreased blood flow to the liver. As portal venous flow decreases, hepatic artery flow increases. As the portal venous pressure increases, increasing amounts of blood from the portal venous system use collateral channels to enter the systemic circulation.

> **AXIOM** The main collaterals between the systemic and portal venous systems include: (a) the coronary (left gastric) vein to the lower esophageal veins and then to the azygous vein, (b) periumbilical veins, and (c) the hemorrhoidal venous system.

In severe portal hypertension, blood may flow retrograde from the liver back into the portal vein and then via collateral veins into the systemic circulation.

Natural History

The prognosis of patients with cirrhosis and portal hypertension is extremely poor.[64] Hepatic cirrhosis is the predominant cause of death in approximately 30,000 patients each year.[147] Not only is cirrhosis the sixth leading cause of death in the United States, but once jaundice, ascites, or esophageal variceal bleeding develop, the one-year survival rate is only 21-35%.[148] Cirrhosis, as a co-morbid factor, also contributes to the demise of many patients.

> **AXIOM** Sepsis or major trauma in cirrhotic patients with jaundice or ascites has an extremely high mortality rate.

The most frequent causes of death in patients with cirrhosis are hemorrhage and hepatic failure. With bleeding esophageal varices due to severe liver disease, the 30-day mortality may be as high as 73%. Child showed that the degree of hepatic decompensation correlated strongly with operative mortality in these patients (Table 44-4).[149]

> **AXIOM** Any surgery requiring laparotomy poses a grave risk to cirrhotic patients.

Schwartz,[150] Cryer et al.,[151] and Arahna et al.[152] reported mortality rates of 27%, 21%, and 24%, respectively, in cirrhotic patients undergoing biliary tract surgery. These rates greatly exceeded the 1.7% reported mortality rate for noncirrhotic patients undergoing similar surgery.[153] Garrison et al. reviewed 100 consecutive patients with biopsy-proved cirrhosis undergoing a variety of intraabdominal operations.[154] The mortality rates for small bowel surgery (60%), colon resection (56%), gastroduodenal surgery (35%), biliary tract surgery (21%), and open liver biopsy (20%), were exceedingly high as compared to the rates in noncirrhotic patients. In 1986, Arahna and Greenlee reviewed their experience with cirrhotic patients undergoing intraabdominal surgery, exclusive of biliary tract or postsystemic shunting, and reported an overall operative mortality rate of 64%.[155]

> **AXIOM** Emergency surgery is tolerated poorly by cirrhotic patients.

When compared to elective procedures, mortality rates with emergency surgery in cirrhotic patients of similar Child's class are up to three times higher than with elective procedures.[154,155] Arahna and Greenlee reported a mortality rate of 86% in patients with advanced cirrhosis who underwent emergency surgery.[155]

In a recent study of 40 cirrhotic patients with trauma, the average mortality rate of 30% was significantly higher than the predicted mortality rate (7%) in relationship to the severity of the specific injuries as reflected by TRISS.[156] Blunt abdominal trauma with hemoperitoneum or visceral injury requiring laparotomy was associated with a mortality rate of 67%.

Bleeding Esophageal Varices

DIAGNOSIS

> **AXIOM** Mild-to-moderate upper GI bleeding in patients with cirrhosis is usually due to gastritis or peptic ulcer disease, not varices.

Bleeding esophageal varices should be suspected in any cirrhotic patient with severe upper GI bleeding, particularly if splenomegaly is present. However, mild-to-moderate upper GI bleeding is more likely to be due to gastritis.

CONTROLLING BLEEDING VARICES

Therapy for bleeding esophageal varices include attempts to: (a) control bleeding, (b) reduce absorption of ammonia and other nitrogenous products from the intestine, and (c) support the failing liver.

Sclerotherapy

> **AXIOM** Sclerotherapy is now generally considered the overall safest and most effective technique for preventing recurrent bleeding from esophageal varices.

Injection of sclerosing agents into and around esophageal varices is the most frequent method for controlling mild-to-moderate variceal bleeding.[157,158]

Pitressin

> **AXIOM** While awaiting sclerotherapy, intravenous pitressin should be started on virtually all patients who appear to be bleeding from esophageal varices.

When the Sengstaken tube does not adequately control variceal bleeding, pitressin, to reduce splanchnic blood flow, can be infused either into a peripheral vein or into the superior mesenteric artery.[159,160] The classic method for infusing pitressin into a peripheral vein consisted of diluting 20 units of vasopressin in 200 mL of fluid which is then given over a period of 20 minutes. This pitressin injection may be repeated every four to six hours as needed or it may be given as a constant infusion of 0.4 units/min. Pitressin has also been administered directly into the superior mesenteric artery as a constant infusion of 0.1-0.4 units/minute; however, this route has been shown to be no more effective or less toxic than the intravenous route.

Unfortunately, the dosage of vasopressin required to reduce portal hypertension is often associated with significant systemic hypertension, increased cardiac afterload, reduced cardiac output, slowing of the heart rate, and arrhythmias. Simultaneous administration of a vasodilator, such as nitroglycerin by constant intravenous infusion or skin patch, can be very helpful under such circumstances.

Esophageal Balloon Tamponade

If properly inflated, the gastric and esophageal balloons of a Sengstaken tube can usually control bleeding from esophageal varices.[159] Because a Sengstaken tube is fairly large, it may be difficult to insert through the nose and down the esophagus. During the process of passing the tube, the patient may aspirate significant quantities of blood or even have a respiratory arrest. Therefore, if the patient is lethargic or comatose and is not be able to protect the airway well, an endotracheal tube should first be inserted to ensure adequate ventilation and to protect the airway while the Sengstaken tube is inserted.

> **AXIOM** When a patient does not have a good cough and gag reflex and is not alert, an endotracheal tube should be inserted prior to inserting a Blakemore-Sengstaken tube to control bleeding esophageal varices.

Because the lumen in the Sengstaken tube used to aspirate material from the stomach is relatively small, an 18F nasogastric tube can be passed down into the stomach alongside the Sengstaken tube.

> **AXIOM** The position of a Sengstaken tube should be checked radiologically whenever possible prior to inflating the gastric balloon to more than 20-30 mm Hg pressure.

Generally, chest radiography is taken after 60-90 mL of air is injected into the gastric balloon to ensure that it is in the stomach and not the esophagus. An alternative technique is to monitor the pressure needed to inflate the gastric balloon. If the pressure remains < 20-30 mm Hg while the gastric balloon is inflated to 150-250 cc, almost no danger of rupturing the esophagus with the gastric balloon exists.

The gastric balloon of the Sengstaken tube must be well-seated just below the gastroesophageal junction, and its position must be maintained by gentle, continuous traction on the tube. Having the patient wear a football helmet so that the tube can be taped to the face guard under mild tension helps to keep the tube in place. If bright-red bleeding continues above a properly inflated and positioned gastric balloon, the diagnosis of bleeding varices is essentially confirmed and the esophageal balloon should be inflated gradually until the bleeding stops or until the pressure in the esophageal balloon reaches 30 mm Hg. The esophageal balloon is usually kept inflated for < 6-12 hours. Using either higher pressures or longer periods of inflation can cause esophageal necrosis. If bleeding recurs when the esophageal balloon is deflated, the balloon can be immediately reinflated.

REDUCING GI ABSORPTION OF NH₃

> **AXIOM** The tendency for GI bleeding in severe cirrhotics to cause encephalopathy can be reduced by decreasing protein intake and giving lactulose, cathartics, and enteral nonabsorbable antibiotics.

Diet

All dietary protein should be stopped temporarily in cirrhotic patients with GI bleeding and/or prehepatic coma.[161] At least 1600 calories should be supplied daily by intravenous infusion or enterally. During recovery, protein can be added to the diet in 20 g increments on alternate days. Any tendency for increased encephalopathy is treated by return to a lower protein intake.

Antibiotics

Oral neomycin is effective for decreasing gastrointestinal ammonia formation[162]; however, impaired hearing or deafness can follow its long-term use. In acute cases, 4-6 g are given daily in divided doses. With such therapy, the EEG usually improves, blood ammonia levels decrease, and fetor hepaticus tends to disappear; however, clinical improvement is difficult to correlate with changes in fecal flora.[162]

Metronidazole (0.2 g orally four times per day) seems to be as effective as neomycin[163]; however, because of a dose-related central nervous system toxicity, it should not be used long-term.

Lactulose

The human intestinal mucosa does not produce an enzyme capable of splitting lactulose, which is a synthetic disaccharide. When given by mouth, lactulose reaches the cecum where it is broken down by bacteria to fatty acids, and causes fecal pH to decrease. The increased colonic acidity favors the growth of lactose-fermenting organisms, and at the same time, organisms which are ammonia formers, such as bacteroides, are suppressed. It may also detoxify the short-chain fatty acids which are produced in the presence of blood and proteins. The colonic fermentative bacteria prefer lactulose to blood when both are present.[164] It may be of particular value in hepatic encephalopathy caused by GI bleeding.

In spite of these findings, the mode of action of lactulose is still uncertain. Fecal acidity should reduce the ionization of ammonia, and hence its absorption; however, fecal ammonia levels are not increased. Nevertheless, lactulose more than doubles the colonic output of bacterial mass and "soluble" nitrogen.[165] This "soluble nitrogen" is no longer available for absorption as ammonia, and a reduced urea production also results.[165]

> **AXIOM** The diarrhea produced by high doses of lactulose can cause severe fluid and electrolyte problems.

The aim of lactulose therapy is to produce acid stools without diarrhea. The initial dose is 10-30 mL three times a day, and this is adjusted to produce two large semisolid stools daily. Side effects include flatulence, diarrhea, and abdominal cramps. The diarrhea can be so profound that serum sodium levels may increase to over 145 mEq/L. At the same time, serum potassium levels may decrease rapidly, and blood volume may decrease enough to impair renal function. These side effects are particularly likely to occur if the daily dose of lactulose exceeds 100 mL.

Lactilol

Lactilol (β-galactoside sorbitol) is a second-generation disaccharide which is not broken down or absorbed in the small intestine, but it is metabolized by colonic bacteria.[166] As a powder, it is more convenient than liquid lactulose and can easily be used as a sweetening agent. It is more palatable and tastes less sugary than lactulose. It is given in a dose of approximately 30 g daily. Lactilol seems to be as effective as lactulose in acute portal systemic encephalopathy,[167] and patients respond considerably more quickly to lactilol and with less diarrhea and flatulence.[168]

Purgation

Constipation can be a precipitating factor for hepatic encephalopathy, and remissions are often associated with improved bowel function. Enemas and purgation with magnesium sulphate may be extremely beneficial in patients with hepatic coma. Lactulose or lactose enemas may also be used, and these are superior to water enemas.[169] All enemas should have a neutral or acidic pH to reduce ammonium absorption. Although magnesium sulphate enemas can occasionally cause dangerous hypermagnesemia, phosphate enemas tend to be safe.

Postoperative Complications in Cirrhotics

SHOCK

> **AXIOM** Prolonged shock in patients with cirrhosis is almost invariably fatal.

Shock for more than 30 minutes in spite of massive transfusions (10 or more units of blood in 24 hours) in cirrhotic patients with bleeding varices is almost invariably fatal.[170] Liver perfusion in these patients depends on hepatic artery flow and any reduction in BP or cardiac output may cause severe hepatic ischemia. Consequently, shock must be prevented or kept to the absolute minimum in patients with cirrhosis. We have also noted that the higher the cardiac index and the lower the total systemic vascular resistance, the poorer the prognosis and the less stress that the cirrhotic patient can tolerate. In addition, if the cardiac output and systemic vascular resistance are normal, the patient is usually hypovolemic.

BLEEDING

AXIOM Cirrhotic patients often have an increased bleeding tendency because they tend to have reduced levels of all coagulation factors (except VIII), thrombocytopenia, and increased fibrinolysis.

Cirrhotic patients may have an increased tendency to bleed for a wide variety of reasons.[171] The cirrhosis itself reduces the production of prothrombin, and factors VII, IX, and X. Fibrinogen is also made by the liver, but its levels are extremely variable in cirrhosis. There may also be increased fibrinolysis because the liver is unable to remove plasminogen activators.

Bleeding may also be a serious problem because of thrombocytopenia due to hypersplenism and because of associated metabolic abnormalities that can interfere with platelet aggregation. Administration of FFP and platelets should be considered in any cirrhotic patient who is bleeding and has abnormal bleeding and coagulation studies. It is generally believed that the prothrombin time should be less than three seconds longer than control before any surgery is performed.

HEPATIC COMA

Etiology

Hepatic encephalopathy usually increases pari passu with hepatic failure. Although the CNS changes often do not correlate well with blood ammonia levels, removal of blood from the GI tract and reducing the number of ammonia-forming organisms in the gut can be of value.[161]

AXIOM Although blood levels of ammonia often do not correlate with the presence or severity of encephalopathy in liver failure, efforts to reduce blood ammonia levels often cause encephalopathy to improve.

Diagnosis

Increasing data suggest that hepatic coma is due to or related to decreased plasma levels of BCAA (leucine, isoleucine and valine) and increased levels of aromatic amino acids (AAA) (phenylalanine and tyrosine) and methionine. A decreased BCAA/AAA ratio in the plasma of patients with encephalopathy may be associated with increased levels of false neurotransmitters, such as octopamine, in brain.[8,172]

Signs of hepatic encephalopathy include changes in personality progressing to confusion, obtundation, and finally coma. Convulsions can occasionally occur. Asterixis or "liver flap" is a characteristic sign of hepatic failure. It consists of a flapping rough tremor of the hands that is best demonstrated when the patient extends the arms, dorsiflexes the wrists, and spreads the fingers. EEG may show paroxysms of bilateral synchronous high-voltage, slow waves.

Therapy

It has been shown in a multicenter, prospective, double-blind, randomized trial of patients with hepatic decompensation that the provision of adequate glucose and amino acids in the form of a mixture enriched with BCAA and deficient in methionine and aromatic amino acids is superior to a diet containing adequate glucose calories alone in terms of improvement of hepatic encephalopathy.[173] Although this study confirmed the need for adequate nutrition, including protein, in patients with hepatic encephalopathy, it is less clear whether a specific hepatic nutritional formulation is better than standard adequate nutrition.[8]

AXIOM Although data are not conclusive, patients developing hepatic failure, especially with encephalopathy, may benefit from diets high in BCAA and low in aromatic amino acids.

TABLE 44–4 *Child's Classification of Patients with Laennec Cirrhosis*

Characteristic	*Child's Class**		
	A	*B*	*C*
Serum albumin (g/dL)	> 3.5	3.0-3.5	< 3.0
Serum bilirubin	> 2.0	2.0-3.0	> 3.0
Ascites	None	Mild, easily correctable	Moderate-to-severe
Muscle wasting	None	Mild	Moderate-to-severe
Encephalopathy	None	None	Present
Mortality risk of elective shunt	2%	10%	50%

*Only one laboratory or clinical characteristic is needed to place a patient in a lower (high risk).

Bromocriptine, a dopamine receptor agonist, has been reported to be of help in chronic hepatic encephalopathy by increasing cerebral blood flow and cerebral oxygen and glucose consumption[174]; however, it is not widely used.

DELIRIUM TREMENS

Delirium tremens (DTs) are not unusual in patients who have been taking large amounts of alcohol just prior to admission. DTs in themselves can have a high mortality rate and may make management of these patients extremely difficult. Some patients require restraints to keep them from harming themselves. Because therapy may require much sedation and restraints, it is important to rule out hypoxemia, sepsis, hypoglycemia, and various electrolyte abnormalities (especially hyponatremia and hypocalcemia) which can cause a DT-like picture.

AXIOM A diagnosis of delirium tremens should not be accepted until sepsis, hypoxemia, and metabolic abnormalities have been ruled out.

Therapy of frank or impending DTs may include large amounts of MgSO$_4$, up to 1-2 g every 4-6 hours the first day and then every 6-8 hours thereafter as needed. If renal failure develops, the amount of MgSO$_4$ may have to be greatly reduced. Deep tendon reflexes should be checked frequently in patients receiving large doses of MgSO$_4$ to avoid excessive hypermagnesemia.

Chlordiazepoxide (Librium®) in doses of 25-50 mg or more may be required every 4-6 hours to keep the patient manageable; however, excessive sedation increases the risk of pneumonia. Large doses of thiamine may also be helpful, and should be given before glucose loads are begun in patients who have not been eating. When large amounts of glucose are given to alcoholic patients without adequate thiamine, they may develop Wernicke's encephalopathy. Alcohol to prevent or treat DTs should probably not be given except in unusual cases.

PULMONARY FAILURE

Pulmonary function may be markedly impaired in cirrhotic patients, especially if severe ascites and muscle wasting occur or if the patient has had prolonged shock, massive transfusions, or sepsis. The Pao$_2$ may be deceptively high in spite of a large pulmonary shunt because of the high P$_V$O$_2$ that tends to be associated with the high-cardiac output present in these patients.

AXIOM ARDS tends to get much worse if the patient develops hepatic failure.

Evidence suggests that severe hepatic dysfunction increases the likelihood of pulmonary dysfunction or ARDS. Matuschak et al. re-

TABLE 44–5 *Acute Vasomotor Nephropathy Versus Hepatorenal Syndrome*

Characteristic	AVN	Hepatorenal Syndrome
Preceding hypotension	Usually present	Often absent
Oliguria	Severe	Mild-to-moderate
Urine osmolarity	Fixed and low	Normal or high
Urine sodium	High	Low
Casts and RBCs in urine	Frequent	Less likely

ported acute respiratory failure manifested by bilateral radiographic pulmonary infiltrates accompanied by progressive hypoxemia requiring mechanical ventilation in 20 of 25 patients with endstage liver failure awaiting hepatic transplantation.[175] Sepsis predisposed to acute respiratory failure in 15 (75%) of these 20 patients. Despite aggressive support, all 20 patients with end-stage liver disease who developed acute respiratory failure died.

RENAL FAILURE

AXIOM One should look carefully for early renal dysfunction in patients with hepatic failure by serially determining creatinine clearance (Cl_{cr}) and the fractional excretion of sodium (Fe_{Na}).

Two types of renal failure may develop in patients with liver failure. These include acute vasomotor nephropathy (AVN) (previously referred to as ATN) and the hepatorenal syndrome. AVN is usually due to prolonged hypotension and renal ischemia, but it may also occur as part of the syndrome of MOF in sepsis. In patients with hepatic failure, little or no evidence of sepsis or renal ischemia may be noted. AVN is usually characterized by oliguria, increasing serum creatinine, a rising BUN (which may be relatively mild if the liver cannot make urea), a low, fixed urine osmolality, relatively high urine sodium levels, and the presence of casts and RBCs in the urinary sediment (Table 44–5).

AXIOM When diuretics are used to reduce ascites due to hepatic failure, one must be careful not to cause prerenal oliguria.

The other type of renal failure which tends to occur coincidentally with hepatic failure (hepatorenal syndrome) is characterized by an increasing creatinine and BUN without striking oliguria.[176] The urine osmolality tends to be normal or high; urine sodium levels are usually very low, and urine sediment tends to be normal. Diuretics may make the hepatorenal syndrome worse.

INFECTION

Impaired RES and malnutrition in cirrhotic patients can contribute greatly to impaired host defenses. Intraperitoneal infections after portosystemic shunts are uncommon, but pulmonary and urinary tract infections are frequent. Antibiotics must be used with some care in these patients because renal excretion and liver detoxification may be severely impaired (Table 44-6).

SEPSIS AND MULTIPLE ORGAN FAILURE

Both the direct immunosuppressive effects of alcohol and the impaired reticuloendothelial and synthetic functions of the liver that accompany cirrhosis and portal hypertension contribute to the higher frequency of MOF in patients with liver disease.[177]

AXIOM Although MOF can occur without sepsis, one should make special efforts to diagnose and eradicate any infectious or inflammatory processes as soon as possible in patients developing this problem.

FLUID AND ELECTROLYTE DISORDERS

Cirrhotic patients tend to have increased total body water, hyponatremia, hypokalemia, and hypomagnesemia. They also have a tendency to develop metabolic alkalosis. Some of this problem may be related to impaired hepatic breakdown of adrenal corticoids. Large quantities of potassium and magnesium may be needed in these patients, but one must be careful not to give sodium except to replace measured losses (as in the nasogastric aspirate). Water is given only to keep up with measured losses plus 800-1000 mL of insensible water loss per day. Any fluid loss from the peritoneal cavity due to ascitic fluid leaking through recent incisions is best replaced with fresh frozen plasma.

AXIOM Although increased protein in the gut may increase the tendency for hepatic encephalopathy, one should make every effort to prevent protein malnutrition.

MALNUTRITION

Most cirrhotic patients who develop liver failure postoperatively are severely malnourished. Serum albumin levels may be < 1.5-2.0 g/dL as a reflection of severe visceral protein deficiencies. Carbohydrates should be given as tolerated by TPN, along with 0.5-1.0 g/kg of protein per day, as soon as the patient is hemodynamically stable. When a tendency for hepatic encephalopathy exists, protein administration may have to be reduced below 0.25-0.50 gm/kg/day. Fat emulsions may be needed, but one should check triglyceride levels closely to be sure they are being cleared properly from the blood.

TABLE 44–6 *Mean (± SD) of Values Obtained at Time of Bilirubin Peak in Jaundiced Patients Following Successful Resuscitation from Severe Shock*

	Surgical Transfusion	Hepatic Dysfunction	Sepsis Septicemia	P
Episodes of jaundice	12	23	15	
Day of bilirubin peak	3.2 (±1.6)	10.2 (±2.0)	19.3 (±89)	≤.0005
Height of bilirubin peak	3.7 (±1.3)	9.5 (±5.5)	18.3 (±9.7)	≤.0005
Bilirubin ratio D/I	2.30 (±3.67)	1.46 (±.54)	1.29 (±.57)	NS
White cell count	9.1 (±2.4)*	10.8 (±2.1)*	20.3 (±4.6)+	≤.005
LDH	252 (±68)	270 (±102)	273 (±92)	NS
GOT	68 (±71)	62 (±71)	113 (±157)	NS
GGT	32 (±30)*	59 (±28)*	174 (±83)+	≤.005
AP	55 (±31)	77 (±50)	126 (±71)	NS

(From: Champion HR, Jones RT, Trump BF, et al. Post-traumatic hepatic dysfunction as a major etiology in post-traumatic jaundice. J Trauma 1976;16:650.)

Ascites

PATHOGENESIS

The primary mechanism for the development of ascites in cirrhotic patients is high pressure in the liver sinusoids with greatly increased movement of fluid into the perisinusoidal space of Disse.[176] Although increased thoracic duct flow can remove much of the excess fluid from the hepatic lymphatics, the remainder moves into the peritoneal cavity through the liver capsule. An increased tendency to fluid overload, hyponatremia, or hypoalbuminemia can contribute to this problem.

THERAPY

Control of the underlying hepatic failure is important. Keeping the patient "on the dry side" and limiting sodium intake may help. Diuretics, especially the antialdosterone types, can also be helpful. If a portosystemic shunt is needed in selected patients, especially those with hepatofugal portal venous blood flow, a side-to-side portacaval shunt is generally preferred over an end-to-side shunt. If there is any possibility of hepatic transplantation later, the shunt should probably be an H-graft away from the portal vein or a TIPS (transcutaneous intrahepatic portosystemic shunt) procedure.

AXIOM End-to-side portacaval shunts may reduce portal venous pressure, but they also tend to make ascites worse and greatly interfere with the later possibility of liver transplantation.

In poor-risk patients with severe, intractable ascites, a peritoneovenous shunt may be helpful. The shunt apparatus, which connects the peritoneal cavity with the superior vena cava via the internal jugular vein, has a special valve that opens when intraperitoneal pressure is 3.0 H_2O higher than central venous pressure. Diuretics are also important following peritoneovenous shunts because one must be careful to not allow the patient to develop CHF because of a sudden influx of ascitic fluid into the circulation.

AXIOM One must make every effort to prevent excessive cardiac filling pressures in patients with peritoneovenous shunts.

Other complications of peritoneovenous shunting include DIC—especially if the ascitic fluid is infected—local infection, systemic sepsis, thrombosis of the vena cava, and air embolism. Not infrequently, these shunts eventually require reoperation because of failure to function properly.

Ⓧ FREQUENT ERRORS

In the Management of Hepatic Failure After Trauma

1. *Failing to optimize cardiac output and oxygen delivery rapidly enough in trauma patients with preexisting liver disease.*
2. *Failing to consider biliary tract obstruction as a cause of increasing bilirubin levels in the first five days after trauma.*
3. *Failing to rule out sepsis as a cause of bilirubin levels rising more than seven days after trauma.*
4. *Administering blood or blood products, with its potential for transmitting hepatitis or AIDS, when it is not necessary.*
5. *Supplying too much carbohydrate so that the RQ is > 1.0, thereby increasing the tendency to hepatic steatosis.*
6. *Allowing efforts to reduce ascites to reduce hepatic perfusion below normal.*
7. *Allowing obstructive jaundice (which itself can cause biliary cirrhosis) to persist longer than absolutely necessary.*
8. *Operating on bleeding esophageal varices only after the patient has had multiple units of blood and prolonged shock.*
9. *Inadequate or delayed removal of blood from the GI tract of a patient who has a tendency to develop hepatic encephalopathy.*
10. *Accepting a diagnosis of DTs in a patient without first ruling out hypoxemia, sepsis, and metabolic problems.*
11. *Not maintaining a good urine output and closely following renal function in patients with hepatic failure.*

▼▼▼▼▼▼▼▼▼▼▼▼▼▼▼▼▼▼▼▼▼▼▼▼▼▼▼▼▼▼

SUMMARY POINTS

1. Inadequate glycogen stores in the liver can greatly reduce the ability of the patient to tolerate severe trauma.
2. Bilirubin excretion is impaired relatively early in MOF, but protein synthesis is preserved until relatively late.
3. Decreasing levels of albumin usually imply the presence of sepsis and/or malnutrition.
4. Albumin, because of its long half-life and because its plasma levels are affected by so many factors, is generally not a good guide to the adequacy of nutritional support.
5. If the BUN is below 5.0 mg/dl, one should suspect severe hepatic disease or hepatic failure.
6. Rising serum triglyceride levels in patients with sepsis are often a sign of terminal liver failure.
7. In severe hepatic failure, increased quantities of bacteria and bacterial products from the gut can traverse the liver and enter the systemic circulation.
8. High serum levels of unconjugated bilirubin in adults during the first four to five days after trauma are often due to hemolysis of red cells in hematomas and/or transfused blood.
9. Resection or severe disease of the distal ileum can rapidly cause severe bile acid deficiencies.
10. Although there is much concern about high plasma cholesterol levels in the development of atherosclerosis, low levels (< 100 mg/dL) usually indicate a dangerous degree of malnutrition.
11. Patients with cirrhosis or any other intrahepatic obstruction to portal venous blood flow are particularly sensitive to any reduction in cardiac output and/or hepatic artery blood flow.
12. To facilitate diagnosis, the causes of jaundice are often divided into prehepatic, hepatic, and posthepatic (bile-duct) disorders.
13. In patients with increasing jaundice after trauma, one should make a special effort to rule out extrahepatic biliary obstruction.
14. Preoperative transhepatic catheter decompression of an obstructed biliary tract may cause more harm than good.
15. One should make an effort to keep the use of blood or blood products in trauma patients to a minimum so as to reduce the chances of transmitting blood-borne diseases, especially hepatitis and AIDS.
16. Non-A, non-B hepatitis is the most frequent type of hepatitis transmitted by infusion of blood or blood products.
17. Most cases of posttransfusion hepatitis will be missed unless serial liver function tests are performed weekly or biweekly for three months following transfusion of blood products.
18. Hepatitis D will probably not be diagnosed unless one tests serially for hepatitis B after blood transfusions.
19. Severe traumatic shock can cause significant hepatic damage, which is often not clinically apparent.
20. Jaundice developing 8–10 days after trauma or later is due to sepsis until proven otherwise.
21. Increasing jaundice with high alkaline phosphatase levels soon after trauma should be considered due to extrahepatic biliary tract obstruction until proven otherwise.
22. The total hepatic blood flow (HBF) in hypermetabolic sepsis is generally increased even though peripheral extraction studies usually indicate that *effective* HBF is reduced.
23. A higher than normal cardiac index and oxygen delivery is required to maintain adequate hepatic oxygenation after trauma and during sepsis.
24. Increased bacterial translocation of gut bacteria or endotoxin because of gut ischemia, prolonged absence of enteral feeding, or alterations of gut flora may cause excessive activation of Kupffer cells with resulting impairment of hepatocyte function.

25. Carbohydrate stress metabolism is characterized by: (a) increased glucagon:insulin ratios, (b) increased insulin resistance, (c) increased glycogenolysis and gluconeogenesis in spite of exogenous glucose, (d) hyperglycemia, and (e) increased lactate production.

26. The protein metabolism of stress is characterized by: (a) increased total body catabolism that is refractory to exogenous amino acids, (b) reduced muscle amino acid uptake, (c) increased release of muscle amino acids, (d) increased hepatic amino acid uptake, and (e) increased synthesis of acute phase proteins.

27. Stress fat metabolism is characterized by: (a) increased adipocyte lipolysis, (b) decreased lipogenesis, (c) increased fatty acid oxidation, (d) increased triglyceride turnover, and (e) decreased ketosis.

28. When fully developed, the liver failure of sepsis has a very bad prognosis and is usually followed or is closely associated with the development of renal failure.

29. Inadequate control or eradication of infection, inflammation, or necrotic tissue is the most common cause for patients to develop MOF.

30. One of the first signs of sepsis and/or increasing hepatic dysfunction is a progressively increasing cardiac output and decreasing systemic vascular resistance.

31. The two physical findings typically seen with hepatic failure include jaundice and encephalopathy.

32. A bilirubin level > 5 mg/dL in the absence of biliary tract obstruction, transfusion reaction, or resolving hematoma is strongly suggestive of liver dysfunction due to sepsis.

33. Early jaundice occurring within five days of trauma should be considered as due to hemolysis or a biliary tract obstruction; jaundice developing after seven days is due to sepsis until proven otherwise.

34. When the etiology of persistent jaundice in a patient with major abdominal surgery or trauma cannot be determined in any other manner, an exploratory celiotomy should be performed.

35. Correction of hepatic failure in MOF requires debridement of infected or necrotic tissue, drainage of abscesses, and treatment of existing infections with appropriate antibiotics.

36. Rapid restoration and maintenance of optimal (supranormal) oxygen delivery is extremely important for trying to prevent hepatic failure after trauma.

37. Early optimization of oxygen delivery with fluids, blood, and possibly inotropes to provide adequate substrate delivery should be monitored closely by oxygen consumption, S_vO_2, and serum lactate to ensure a more than adequate splanchnic blood flow.

38. Early enteral nutrition, which may help to decrease bacterial translocation in the gut, may be an important part of reducing hepatic dysfunction in critically ill or injured patients.

39. Fatty liver is the most frequently noted hepatic abnormality in alcoholics and in patients on TPN.

40. Indirect calorimetry to monitor RQ may be of great help in optimizing nutrition and preventing hepatic steatosis.

41. Patients on TPN should be monitored closely for elevated levels of aminotransferase, bilirubin, and alkaline phosphatase.

42. Using resting energy expenditure and RQ to adjust TPN should help to prevent hepatic complications due to under or overfeeding.

43. Patients who drink excessive amounts of alcohol are prone to develop nutritional cirrhosis, and this greatly increases the risk of hepatic failure during sepsis or after trauma.

44. One should not allow an extrahepatic cause of jaundice to persist longer than absolutely necessary because of the secondary liver changes it can cause.

45. Patients with prehepatic portal hypertension can tolerate trauma and surgery much better than patients with other causes of esophageal varices.

46. The main collaterals between the systemic and portal venous systems include: (a) the coronary (left gastric) vein to lower esophageal veins and then to the azygous vein, (b) periumbilical veins, and (c) the hemorrhoidal venous system.

47. Sepsis or major trauma in cirrhotic patients with jaundice or ascites has an extremely high mortality rate.

48. Any surgery requiring laparotomy poses a grave risk to cirrhotic patients.

49. Emergency surgery is tolerated poorly by cirrhotic patients.

50. Mild-to-moderate upper GI bleeding in patients with cirrhosis is usually due to gastritis or peptic ulcer disease, not varices.

51. Sclerotherapy is now generally considered the overall safest and most effective technique for preventing recurrent bleeding from esophageal varices.

52. While awaiting sclerotherapy, intravenous pitressin should be started on virtually all patients who appear to be bleeding from esophageal varices.

53. When a patient does not have a good cough and gag reflex and is not alert, an endotracheal tube should be inserted prior to inserting a Blakemore-Sengstaken tube to control bleeding esophageal varices.

54. The position of a Sengstaken tube should be checked radiologically whenever possible prior to inflating the gastric balloon to more than 20-30 mm Hg pressure.

55. The tendency for GI bleeding in severe cirrhotic patients to cause encephalopathy can be reduced by decreasing protein intake and giving lactulose, cathartics, and enteral nonabsorbable antibiotics.

56. The diarrhea produced by high doses of lactulose can cause severe fluid and electrolyte problems.

57. Prolonged shock in patients with cirrhosis is almost invariably fatal.

58. Cirrhotic patients often have an increased bleeding tendency because they tend to have reduced levels of all coagulation factors (except VIII), thrombocytopenia, and increased fibrinolysis.

59. Although blood levels of ammonia often do not correlate with the presence or severity of encephalopathy in liver failure, efforts to reduce blood ammonia levels often cause encephalopathy to improve.

60. Although data are not conclusive, patients developing hepatic failure, especially with encephalopathy, may benefit from diets high in BCAA and low in aromatic amino acids.

61. A diagnosis of delirium tremens should not be accepted until sepsis, hypoxemia, and metabolic abnormalities have been ruled out.

62. ARDS tends to get much worse if the patient develops hepatic failure.

63. One should look carefully for early renal dysfunction in patients with hepatic failure by serially determining creatinine clearance (Cl_{cr}) and the fractional excretion of sodium (FE_{Na}).

64. When diuretics are used to reduce ascites due to hepatic failure, one must be careful not to cause prerenal oliguria.

65. Although MOF can occur without sepsis, one should make special efforts to diagnose and eradicate any infectious or inflammatory process as soon as possible in patients developing this problem.

66. Although increased protein in the gut may increase the tendency for hepatic encephalopathy, one should make every effort to prevent protein malnutrition.

67. End-to-end portacaval shunts may reduce portal venous pressure, but they also tend to make ascites worse.

68. One must make every effort to prevent excessive cardiac filling pressures in patients with peritoneovenous shunts.

▲▲▲▲▲▲▲▲▲▲▲▲▲▲▲▲▲▲▲▲▲▲▲▲▲▲▲▲▲▲▲▲▲▲▲▲

REFERENCES

1. Schwartz SI. Historical background. McDermott WV, ed. Surgery of the liver. Boston: Blackwell Scientific Publications, 1988; 1-14.
2. Calne RY. Surgical anatomy of the liver. McDermott WV, ed Surgery of the liver. Boston: Blackwell Scientific Publications, 1988; 15-24.
3. Sherlock S. Anatomy and function. Sherlock S, ed. Diseases of the liver and biliary system, 8th ed. Boston: Blackwell Scientific Publications, 1989; 1-18.
4. Sherlock S. Liver function. McDermott WV, ed. Surgery of the liver. Boston: Blackwell Scientific Publications, 1988; 25-36.
5. Sherlock S. Assessment of liver function. Sherlock S, ed. Diseases of the liver and biliary system, 8th ed. Boston: Blackwell Scientific Publication, 1989; 19-34.

6. Merrell RC. Hepatic physiology. Miller TA, ed. Physiologic basis of modern surgical care. St. Louis: CV Mosby, 1988; 404-416.

7. Walvatne C, Cerra FB. Hepatic dysfunction in multiple organ failure. Deitch EA, ed. Multiple organ failure: pathophysiology and basic concepts of therapy. New York: Thieme Medical Publishers, 1990; 241.

8. Barton RG, Cerra FB. Metabolic and nutritional support. Moore EE, Mattox KL, Feliciano DV, eds. Trauma, 2nd ed. Norwalk: Appelton & Lange, 1991; 965-994.

9. Moshage HJ, Jansen JAM, Franssen JH, et al. Study of the molecular mechanism of decreased liver synthesis of albumin in inflammation. J Clin Invest 1987;79:1634.

10. Moshage HJ, Kleter BEM, van Pelt JF, et al. Fibrinogen and albumin synthesis are regulated at the transcriptional level during the acute phase response. Biochem Biophys Acta 1988;950:450.

11. Ramadori G, Sipe JD, Dinarello CA, et al. Pretranslational modulation of acute phase hepatic protein synthesis by murine recombinant interleukin 1 (IL-1) and purified human IL-1. J Exp Med 1985;162:930.

12. Perlmutter DH, Dinarello CA, Punsal PI, et al. Cachectin/tumor necrosis factor regulates hepatic acute phase gene expression. J Clin Invest 1986;78:1349.

13. Marinokovic S, Jahreis GP, Wong GG, Baumann H. IL-6 modulates the synthesis of a specific set of acute phase plasma proteins in vivo. J Immunol 1989;142:808.

14. Rock CS, Coyle SM, Keogh CV, et al. Influence of hypercortisolemia on the acute-phase protein response to endotoxin in humans. Surgery 1992;112:467.

15. Thompson EN, Williams R. Effect of age on liver function with particular reference to bromosulphalein excretion. Gut 1965;6:266.

16. McLeskey CH. Anesthesia for the geriatric patient. Adv Anesth 1985;2:32.

17. Muller EL, Pitt HA. The jaundiced patient. Miller TA, ed. Physiologic basis of modern surgical care. St. Louis: CV Mosby Co, 1988; 479.

18. Sherlock S. Jaundice. Sherlock S, ed. Diseases of the liver and biliary system, 8th ed. Boston: Blackwell Scientific Publications, 1989; 230.

19. Hermreck AS, Proberts KS, Thomas JH. Severe jaundice after rupture of abdominal aortic aneurysm. Am J Surg 1977;134:745.

20. Kantrowitz PA, Jones WA, Greenberger NJ, et al. Severe postoperative hyperbilirubinemia simulating obstructive jaundice. N Engl J Med 1967;276:591.

21. Flint LM. Liver failure. Surg Clin North Am 1982;62:157.

22. Sherlock S. Halothane hepatitis. Gut 1971;12:324.

23. Shoemaker WC, Szanto PB, Fitch LB, et al. Hepatic physiologic and morphologic alterations in hemorrhagic shock. Surg Gynecol Obstet 1964;118:823.

24. Nunes G, Blaisdell FW, Margaretten W. Mechanism of hepatic dysfunction following shock and trauma. Arch Surg 1970;100:546.

25. Smith LL, Veragut VP. The liver and shock: initiating and perpetuating factors. Prog Surg 1964;4:55.

26. Sarfeh IJ, Balint JA. Hepatic functional and morphological changes following trauma. Gastroenterology 1975;69:862.

27. Sarfeh IJ, Balint JA. The clinical significance of hyperbilirubinemia following trauma. J Trauma 1978;18:58.

28. Joseph PK, Bizer LS, Sprayregen SS, et al. Percutaneous transhepatic biliary drainage: results and complications in 81 patients. JAMA 1986;255:2763.

29. Smith RC, Pooley M, George CR, et al. Preoperative percutaneous transhepatic internal drainage in obstructive jaundice: a randomized, controlled trial examining renal function. Surgery 1985;97:641.

30. McPherson GA, Benjamin IS, Hodgson HJ, et al. Preoperative percutaneous transhepatic biliary drainage: the results of a controlled trial. Br J Surg 1984;71:371.

31. Audisio RA, Bozzetti F, Severini A, et al. The occurrence of cholangitis after percutaneous biliary drainage: evaluation of some risk factors. Surgery 1988;103:507.

32. Sirinek KR, Levine BA. Percutaneous transhepatic cholangiography and biliary decompression. Arch Surg 1989;124:885.

33. Sherlock S. Viral hepatitis. Sherlock S, ed. Diseases of the liver and biliary system, 8th ed. Boston: Blackwell Scientific Publications, 1989; 301.

34. Saxe SE, Gardner P. The returning traveler with fever. Inf Dis Cl N Am 1992;6:427.

35. Alter HJ. The changing epidemiology of hepatitis B in the United States. JAMA 1990;263:1218.

36. Alter HJ. Discovery of the non-A, non-B hepatitis virus: the end of the beginning or the beginning of the end. Trans Med Rev 1989;3:77.

37. Dienstag JL. Non-A, non-B hepatitis: I. recognition, epidemiology, and clinical features. Gastroenterology 1983;85:439.

38. Lashner BA, Jonas KB, Tang HS, et al. Chronic hepatitis: disease factors at diagnosis predictive of mortality. Am J Med 1988;85:609.

39. Hoofnagle JH. Type D (delta) hepatitis. JAMA 1989;261:1321.

40. Rizzetto M, Purcell RH, Gerin JL. Epidemiology of HBV-associated delta agent: geographical distribution of anti-delta and prevalence in polytransfused HGsAg carriers. Lancet 1980;1:1215.

41. Lattau LA, McCarthy JG, Smith MH, et al. Outbreak of severe hepatitis due to delta and hepatitis B viruses in parenteral drug abusers and their contacts. N Engl J Med 1987;317:1256.

42. Rizzetto M, Morello C, Mannucci PM, et al. Delta infection and liver disease in hemophiliac carriers of hepatitis B surface antigen. J Infect Dis 1982;145:18.

43. Govindarajan S, Chin KP, Redeker AG, et al. Fulminant B viral hepatitis: role of delta agent. Gastroenterology 1984;86:1417.

44. DeCock KM, Govindarajan S, Chin KP, et al. Delta hepatitis in the Los Angeles area: a report of 126 cases. Ann Intern Med 1986;105:108.

45. Rizzetto M, Verme G, Recchia S, et al. Chronic HBsAg hepatitis with intrahepatic expression of delta antigen: an active and progressive disease unresponsive to immunosuppressive therapy. Ann Intern Med 1983;98:437.

46. Champion HR, Jones RT, Trump BF, et al. A clinicopathologic study of hepatic dysfunction following shock. Surg Gynecol Obstet 1976;142:657.

47. Welch GW. Care of the patient with thermal injury. Capan LM, Miller SM, Turndorf J, eds. Trauma: anesthesia and intensive care. Philadelphia: JB Lippincott, 1991; 629-648.

48. Chiarelli A, Casadei A, Pornaro E, et al. Alanine and aspartate aminotransferase serum levels in burned patients: a long term study. J Trauma 1987;27:790.

49. Ayala A, Wang P, Ba ZF, et al. Differential alterations in plasma IL-6 and TNF levels following trauma and hemorrhage. Am J Physiol 1991;206:R167.

50. Wang P, Ayala A, Dean RE, et al. Adequate crystalloid resuscitation restores but fails to maintain active hepatocellular function following hemorrhagic shock. J Trauma 1991;31:601.

51. Flynn WJ, Cryer HG, Garrison RN. Pentoxifylline restores intestinal microvascular blood flow during resuscitated hemorrhagic shock. Surgery 1991;110:350.

52. Coccia MT, Waxman K, Soliman MH, et al. Pentoxifylline improves survival following hemorrhagic shock. Crit Care Med 1989;17:36.

53. Barroso AJ, Schmid-Schonbein GW. Pentoxifylline pretreatment decreases the pool of circulating activated neutrophils, reduces in vivo adhesion to endothelium, and improves survival from hemorrhagic shock. Biorheology 1990;27:401.

54. Chiarellia A, Siliprandi L, Casadei A, et al. Aminotransferase changes in burned patients. Intensive Care Med 1987;13:199.

55. Czaja AJ, Rizzo TA, Smith WR, et al. Acute liver disease after cutaneous injury. J Trauma 1975;15:887.

56. Martyn JAJ. Clinical pharmacology and drug therapy in the burned patient. Anesthesiology 1986;65:67.

57. Martyn JAJ, Greenblatt DJ, Quinby WC. Diazepam kinetics in patients with severe burns. Anesth Analg 1983;62:293.

58. Fry DE. Splanchnic perfusion and sepsis. Roth BL, Nielsen TB, McKee AE, eds. Progress in clinical and biological research. New York: Alan R. Liss, 1989;299:9-17.

59. Irie H, Mori W. Fatal hepatic necrosis after shock. Acta Pathol Jpn 1986;36:363.

60. Bywaters EGL. Anatomical changes in the liver after trauma. Clin Sci 1946;6:19.

61. Fath JJ, St. Cyr JA, Konstantinides FN, et al. Alterations in amino acid clearance during ischemia predict hepatocellular ATP changes. Surgery 1985;98:396.

62. Becker W, Konstantinides F, Eyer S, et al. Plasma amino acid clearance as an indicator of hepatic function and high-energy phosphate in hepatic ischemia. Surgery 1987;102:777.

63. Schumer W, Das Gupta TK, Moss GS, et al. Effects of endotoxemia on liver cell mitochondria in man. Ann Surg 1970;171:875.

64. Mela L, Bacalzo LV Jr, Miller LD. Defective oxidative metabolism of rat liver mitochondria in hemorrhage and endotoxin shock. Am J Physiol 1971;220:571.

65. Fry DE, Silver BB, Rink RD, et al. Hepatic cellular hypoxia in murine peritonitis. Surgery 1979;85:652.

66. Asher EF, Garrison RN, Ratcliffe DJ, et al. Endotoxin, cellular function, and nutrient blood flow. Arch Surg 1983;118:454.

67. Schirmer WJ, Townsend MC, Schirmer JM, et al. Galactose elimination kinetics in sepsis: correlation of liver blood flow with function. Arch Surg 1987;122:349.

68. Machiedo GW, Hurd T, Rush BF, et al. Temporal relationship of hepatocellular dysfunction and ischemia in sepsis. Arch Surg 1988;123:424.
69. Baumgartner G, Probst P, Kraines R, et al. Kinetics of indocyanine green removal from the blood. Ann N Y Acad Sci 1970;170:134.
70. Garrison RN, Ratcliffe DJ, Fry DE. Hepatocellular function and nutrient blood flow in experimental peritonitis. Surgery 1982;92:713.
71. Asher EF, Rowe RL, Garrison RN, et al. Experimental bacteremia and hepatic nutrient blood flow. Circ Shock 1986;20:43.
72. Chaudry IH, Wichterman KA, Baue AE. Effect of sepsis on tissue adenine nucleotide levels. Surgery 1979;85:205.
73. Schirmer WJ, Schirmer JM, Naff GB, et al. Complement activation in peritonitis: association with hepatic and renal perfusion abnormalities. Am Surg 1988;53:683.
74. Schirmer WJ, Schirmer JM, Naff GB, et al. Contributions of toxic oxygen intermediaries to complement-induced reduction in effective hepatic blood flow. J Trauma 1988;28:1295.
75. Schirmer WJ, Schirmer JM, Naff GB, et al. Effects of allopurinol and ladoxamide on complement induced hepatic ischemia. J Surg Res 1988;45:28.
76. Schirmer WJ, Townsend MC, Hampton WW, et al. Galactose clearance as an estimate of effective hepatic blood flow: validation and limitations. J Surg Res 1986;41:543.
77. Gottlieb ME, Sarfeh IJ, Stratton H, et al. Hepatic perfusion and splanchnic oxygen consumption in patients postinjury. J Trauma 1983;23:836.
78. Gottlieb ME, Stratton HH, Newell JC, et al. Indocyanine green: its use as an early indicator of hepatic dysfunction following injury in man. Arch Surg 1984;119:264.
79. Dahn MS, Lange MP, Wilson RF, et al. Hepatic blood flow and splanchnic oxygen consumption measurements in clinical sepsis. Surgery 1990;107:295.
80. Dahn MS, Wilson RF, Lange P, et al. Hepatic parenchymal oxygen tension following injury and sepsis. Arch Surg 1990;125:441.
81. Quale JM, Mandel LJ, Bergasa NV, et al. Clinical significance and pathogenesis of hyperbilirubinemia associated with Staphylococcus. Am J Med 1988;85:615.
82. Carrico CJ, Meakins JL, Marchall JC, et al. Multiple-organ failure syndrome. Arch Surg 1986;121:196.
83. Becker W, Konstantinides F, Cerra F. Interactions between endotoxin, the liver, systemic hemodynamics and amino acid metabolism. Circ Shock 1987;21:301.
84. Hideko A, Ogle CK, Alexander JW, et al. Induction of hypermetabolism in guinea pigs by endotoxin infused through the portal vein. Arch Surg 1988;123:1420.
85. Marshall JC, Christou NY, Horn R, et al. The microbiology of multiple organ failure. Arch Surg 1988;123:309.
86. Mochizuki H, Trocki O, Dominioni L, et al. Mechanism of prevention of postburn hypermetabolism and catabolism by early enteral feeding. Ann Surg 1984;200:297.
87. O'Dwyer ST, Mitchie HR, Ziegler TR, et al. A single dose of endotoxin increases intestinal permeability in healthy humans. Arch Surg 1988;123:1459.
88. Schirmer WJ, Schirmer JM, Townsend MC, et al. Femur fracture with associated soft-tissue injury produces hepatic ischemia. Arch Surg 1988;123:412.
89. Seibel R, LaDuca J, Hassett JM, et al. Blunt multiple trauma (ISS—36), femur traction, and the pulmonary failure-septic state. Ann Surg 1985;202:283.
90. Amaral JF, Shearer JD, Caldwell MD. Examination of lactate metabolism in the cellular infiltrate of wounded tissue. Surg Forum 1986;37:30.
91. Morris AS, Shearer JD, Forster J, et al. The relationship of purine metabolism to the macrophage-mediated increase of high energy phosphates in skeletal muscle. J Surg Res 1986;41:339.
92. Cerra FB, Seigel JH, Border JR, et al. The hepatic failure of sepsis: cellular versus substrate. Surgery 1979;86:409.
93. Bigatello LM, Broitman SA, Fattori L, et al. Endotoxemia, encephalopathy, and mortality in cirrhotic patients. Am J Gastroenterol 1987;82:11.
94. Norton LW. Does drainage of intraabdominal pus reverse multiple organ failure? Am J Surg 1985;149:347.
95. Bunt TJ. Non-directed relaparotomy for intraabdominal sepsis: a futile procedure. Am Surg 1987;52:294.
96. Fry DE, Klamer TW, Garrison RN, et al. Atypical clostridial bacteremia. Surg Obstet Gynecol 1980;153:28.
97. Garrison RN, Fry DE, Berberich S, Polk HC Jr. Enterococcal bacteremia: clinical implications and determinants of death. Ann Surg 1982;196:43.
98. Deitch EA, Maejima K, Berg R. Effect of oral antibiotics and bacterial overgrowth on the translocation of GI tract microflora in burned rats. J Trauma 1985;25:385.
99. Bouwens L, Baekeland M, Wisse E. Cytokinetic analysis of the expanding Kupffer-cell population in rat liver. Cell Tissue Kinet 1986;19:217.
100. Alexander JW, Saito H, Trocki O, et al. The importance of lipid type in the diet after burn injury. Ann Surg 1986;204:1.
101. West MA, Keller G, Hyland B, et al. Hepatocyte function in sepsis. Kupffer cells mediate a biphasic protein synthesis response in hepatocytes after endotoxin and killed E. coli. Surgery 1985;98:388.
102. Keller G, Barke R, Harty J, et al. Decreased hepatic glutathione levels in septic shock: predisposition of hepatocytes to oxidative stress. Arch Surg 1985;120:941.
103. Morris A, Henry W, Shearer J, Caldwell M. Macrophage interaction with skeletal muscle: a potential role of macrophages in determining the energy state of healing wounds. J Trauma 1985;25:7751.
104. West MA, Keller FA, Hyland B, et al. Kupffer cell modulation of hepatocellular function in multiple systems organ failure. J Leukocyte Biol 1984;36:436.
105. Keller GA, West MA, Cerra FB, Simmons RL. Macrophage-mediated modulation of hepatic function in multiple-system failure. J Surg Res 1985;39:555.
106. Keller GA, West MA, Wilkes A, et al. Modulation of hepatocyte protein synthesis by endotoxin activated Kupffer cells II. Mediation by soluble transfer factors. Ann Surg 1985;201:429.
107. Cerra FB, Mazuski JE, Bankey PE, et al. Role of monokines in altering hepatic metabolism in sepsis. Roth BL, Nielsen TB, McKee AE, eds. Progress in clinical and biological research. New York: Alan R Liss, 1989;286:265-77.
108. Mazuski JE, Bankey PE, Carlson A, et al. Hepatocytes release factors which can modulate macrophage IL-1 secretion and proliferation. Surg Forum 1988;39:13.
109. Curran RD, Billiar TR, West MA, et al. Effect of interleukin-2 on Kupffer cell activation. Interleukin-2 primes and activates Kupffer cells to suppress hepatocyte protein synthesis in vitro. Arch Surg 1988;123:1373.
110. Mazuski JE, West MA, Towle HC, et al. Enhanced release of interleukin-1 like activity by hepatocyte:macrophage cocultures. Surg Forum 1987;38:21.
111. Coccia MT, Waxman K, Soliman MH, et al. Pentoxifylline improves survival following hemorrhagic shock. Crit Care Med 1989;17:36.
112. Doherty GM, Jensen C, Alexander HR, et al. Pentoxifylline suppression of tumor necrosis factor gene transcription. Surgery 1991;110:192.
113. Han J, Thompson P, Beutler B. Dexamethasone and pentoxifylline inhibit endotoxin-induced cachectin/tumor necrosis factor synthesis at separate points in the signaling pathway. J Exp Med 1990;172:391.
114. Endres S, Fulle HJ, Sinha B, et al. Cyclic nucleotides differentially regulate the synthesis of tumor necrosis factor-alpha and interleukin-1 beta by human mononuclear cells. Immunology 1991;72:56.
115. Strieter RM, Remick DG, Ward PA, et al. Cellular and molecular regulation of tumor necrosis factor-alpha production by pentoxifylline. Biochem Biophys Res Commun 1988;155:1230.
116. Goldberg AL, Baracos V, Rodermann P, et al. Control of protein degradation in muscle by prostaglandins, Ca^{2+}, and leukocytic pyrogen (interleukin 1). Fred Proc 1984;43:1301.
117. Smith KA. Interleukin-2: inception, impact, and implications. Science 1988;240:1169.
118. Beutler B, Cerami A. Tumor necrosis, cachexia, shock, and inflammation: a common mediator. Annu Rev Biochem 1988;57:505.
119. Miller-Graziano CL, Fink M, Wu JY, et al. Mechanisms of altered myocyte prostaglandin E2 production in severely injured patients. Arch Surg 1988;123:293.
120. Ding A, Nathan C. Analysis of nonfunctional respiratory burst in murine Kupffer cells. J Exp Med 1988;167:1154.
121. Spitzer JA, Nelson KM, Fish RE. Time course of changes in gluconeogenesis from various precursors in chronically endotoxemic rats. Metabolism 1985;34:842.
122. Cerra FB, Border JR, McMenamy RH, et al. Multiple systems organ failure. Trump BF, Crowly RA, eds. Pathophysiology of shock, anoxia, and ischemia. Baltimore: Williams and Wilkins, 1982; 254-270.
123. Harkema JM, Gorman MW, Bieber LL, et al. Metabolic interaction between skeletal muscle and liver during bacteremia. Arch Surg 1988;123:1415.
124. Cerra FB, Seigel JH, Coleman B, et al. Septic autocannibalism. Ann Surg 1980;192:570.
125. Pittiruti M, Seigel JH, Sganga G, et al. Increased dependence on leucine in posttraumatic sepsis: leucine/tryosine clearance ratio as an indicator

of hepatic impairment in septic multiple organ failure syndrome. Surgery 1985;98:378.

126. Feingold KR, Grunfeld C. Tumor necrosis factor—alpha stimulates hepatic lipogenesis in the rat in vivo. J Clin Invest 1987;80:184.

127. Ozawa K, Aoyama H, Yasuda K, et al. Metabolic abnormalities associated with postoperative organ failure. Arch Surg 1983;118:1245.

128. Cerra FB, West M, Billiar TR. Hepatic dysfunction in multiple systems organ failure. Schlag G, Redl H, eds. Progress in clinical and biological Research. New York: Alan R Liss, 1989;308:563-73.

129. Mallory TB, Sullivan ER, Burnett CH, et al. The general pathology of traumatic shock. Surgery 1950;27:629.

130. Norton L, Moore G, Eiseman B. Liver failure in the postoperative patient: the role of sepsis and immunologic deficiency. Surgery 1975;78:6.

131. Fry DE, Pearlstein L, Fulton RL, et al. Multiple system organ failure: the role of uncontrolled infection. Arch Surg 1980;115:136.

132. Strawn T, Williams HC, Flint LM Jr. The prognostic significance of serum biochemical changes following liver trauma. Am Surg 1980; 46:111.

133. Diebel LN, Robinson SL, Wilson RF, et al. Splanchnic mucosal effects of hypertonic versus isotonic resuscitation of hemorrhagic shock. Am Surg 1993;59:495.

134. Dahn MS, Lang P, Lobdell K, et al. Splanchnic and total body oxygen consumption differences in septic and injury patients. Surgery 1987;101:69.

135. Biliar TR, Bankey PE, Svingen BA, et al. Fatty acid intake and Kupffer cell function: fish oil alters eicosanoid and monokine production to endotoxin stimulation. Surgery 1988;104:343.

136. Matsubara S, Okabe K, Kiyoaki O, et al. Temporary metabolic support by extracorporeal blood therapy for liver failure after surgery. Trans Am Soc Artif Intern Organs 1988;34:266.

137. Bowyer BA, Fleming CR, Ludwig J, et al. Does longterm home parenteral nutrition in adult patients cause chronic liver disease? JPEN 1985;9:11.

138. Van Wass L, Liver CS. Early perivenular sclerosis in alcoholic fatty liver: an index of progressive liver injury. Gastroenterology 1977;73:636.

139. Baker AL, Rosenberg IH. Hepatic complications of total parenteral nutrition. Am J Med 1987;82:489.

140. Sheldon GF, Petersen SR, Sanders R. Hepatic dysfunction during hyperalimentation. Arch Surg 1978;113:504.

141. Messing B, Bories C, Kunstlinger F, et al. Does total parenteral nutrition induce gallbladder sludge formation and lithiasis? Gastroenterology 1983;84:1012.

142. Pitt HA, King W III, Mann LL, et al. Gallbladder disease in patient on long-term parenteral nutrition. Am J Surg 1983;145:106.

143. Roslyn JJ, Pitt HA, Mann LL, et al. Gallbladder disease in patients on long-term parenteral nutrition. Gastroenterology 1983;84:148.

144. Popper H. Cholestasis. Ann Rev Med 1968;19:39.

145. Rigo J, Senterre J. Is taurine essential for newborns? Biol Neonate 1977;32:73.

146. Fouin-Fortunet H, Le Quernec L, Erlinger S, et al. Hepatic alterations during total parenteral nutrition in patients with inflammatory bowel disease: a possible consequence of lithocholate toxicity. Gastroenterology 1982;82:932.

147. Reported Cirrhosis Mortality—United States, 1970-1980. MMWR 1988;33:657-659.

148. Grant PG, DuFour MC, Hartford TC. Epidemiology of alcoholic liver disease. Semin Liver Dis 1988;8:12.

149. Child CG III. The liver and portal hypertension. Philadelphia: WB Saunders, 1964.

150. Schwartz SI. Biliary tract surgery and cirrhosis: a critical combination. Surgery 1981;90:577.

151. Cryer HM, Howard DA, Garrison RN. Liver cirrhosis and biliary surgery: assessment of risk. South Med J 1985;78:138.

152. Arahna GV, Sontag SJ, Greenlee HB. Cholecystectomy in cirrhotic patients: a formidable operation. Am J Surg 1982;143:55.

153. Levine BA, Gaskill HV, Sirinek KR. Portasystemic shunting remains the

154. Garrison RN, Cryer HM, Howard DA, et al. Clarification of risk factors for abdominal operations in patients with hepatic cirrhosis. Ann Surg 1984;199:648.

155. Arahna GV, Greenlee HB. Intra-abdominal surgery in patients with advanced cirrhosis. Arch Surg 1986;121:275.

156. Tinkoff G, Rhodes M, Diamond D, et al. Cirrhosis in the trauma victim: effect on mortality rates. Ann Surg 1990;211:172.

157. Hedberg SE, Fowler DL, Ryan ELE. Injection sclerotherapy of esophageal varices using ethanolamine oleate: a pilot study. Am J Surg 1982;143:426-30.

158. Terblanche J. Injection sclerotherapy for bleeding esophageal varices. McDermott WV, ed. Surgery of the liver. Boston: Blackwell Scientific Publications, 1988; 315.

159. Chojkier M, Groszman RJ, Atterbury CE, et al. A controlled comparison of continuous intra-arterial and intravenous infusions of vasopressin in hemorrhage from oesophageal varices. Gastroenterology 1979;77:540.

160. Naeije R, Hallemans R, Mols P, et al. Effects of vasopressin and somatostation on hemodynamics and blood gases in patients with liver cirrhosis. Crit Care Med 1982;10:578.

161. Sherlock S. Hepatic encephalopathy. Sherlock S, ed. Diseases of the liver and biliary system. Boston: Blackwell Scientific Publications, 1989; 95-115.

162. Dawson AM, McLaren J, Sherlock S. Neomycin in the treatment of hepatic coma. Lancet 1957;ii:1263.

163. Morgan MH, Read AE, Speller DCE. Treatment of hepatic encephalopathy with metronidazole. Gut 1982;23:1.

164. Mortensen PB, Rasmussen HS, Hultug K. Lactulose detoxifies in vitro short-chain fatty acid production in colonic contents induced by blood: implications for hepatic coma. Gastroenterology 1988;94:750.

165. Weber FL, Banwell JG, Fresard KM, et al. Nitrogen in fecal bacterial fiber and soluble fractions of patients with cirrhosis: effects of lactulose and lactulose plus neomycin. J Lab Clin Med 1987;110:259.

166. Patil DH, Westaby D, Mahida YR, et al. Comparative modes of action of lactitol and lactulose in the treatment of hepatic encephalopathy. Gut 1987;28:255.

167. Heredia D, Caballeria J, Arroyo V, et al. Lactitol versus lactulose in the treatment of acute portal systemic encephalopathy. J Hepatol 1987;4:293.

168. Morgan MH, Hawley KM. Lactitol versus lactulose in the treatment of acute hepatic encephalopathy in cirrhotic patients: a double-blind, randomized trial. Hepatology 1987;4:236.

169. Uribe M, Campoll O, Vargas F, et al. Acidifying enemas (lactitol and lactulose) versus nonacidifying enemas (tapwater) to treat acute portal systemic encephalopathy: a double-blind, randomized clinical trial. Hepatology 1987;7:639.

170. Wilson RF, Krome R. Factors affecting prognosis in clinical shock. Ann Surg 1969;169:99.

171. Sherlock S. The haematology of liver disease. Sherlock S, ed. Diseases of the liver and biliary system, 8th ed. Boston: Blackwell Scientific Publications, 1989; 49.

172. Fisher JE, Baldessarini RJ. False neurotransmitters and hepatic failure. Lancet 1971;2:75.

173. Cerra FB, Cheung NK, Fisher JE, et al. Disease-specific amino acid infusion (F080) in hepatic encephalopathy: a prospective, randomized, double-blind, controlled trial. JPEN 1985;9:3:288.

174. Morgan MY, Jokobovits AW, James IM, et al. Successful use of bromocriptine in the treatment of chronic hepatic encephalopathy. Gastroenterology 1980;78:663.

175. Matuschak GM, Rinaldo JE, Van Theil DH, et al. Acute respiratory failure with pre-existing hepatic insufficiency is irreversible. Am Rev Respir Dis 1985;131:A135.

176. Sherlock S. Ascites. Sherlock S, ed. Diseases of the liver and biliary system, 8th ed. Boston: Blackwell Scientific Publishing, 1989; 129.

177. Flint LM. Sepsis and multiple organ failure. Moore EE, Mattox KL, Feliciano DV, eds. Trauma, 2nd ed. Norwalk: Appelton & Lange, 1991; 995-1009.

Chapter 45 Coagulation Abnormalities in Trauma

EBERHARD F. MAMMEN, M.D.

ROBERT F. WILSON, M.D.

INTRODUCTION

AXIOM Abnormally functioning hemostasis in the injured patient, unless recognized and treated promptly and appropriately, may lead not only to excessive bleeding and possible death but also to poor wound healing or thromboembolic complications.[1]

Hemostasis is designed to control blood loss and maintain blood fluidity. It involves a complex system of tissue substances, platelets, and coagulation proteins.[1] Trauma affects all of these systems and causes changes in the platelet, clotting, and fibrinolytic systems.[2,3]

Although coagulation disorders may preexist in some injured patients[4] and efforts should be made to identify such disorders, the overwhelming majority of excessive bleeding after trauma is due to damage to blood vessels that require surgical control.[2]

AXIOM Most early bleeding problems in trauma patients are due to acquired mechanical defects.

Whenever a patient develops excessive bleeding following trauma or surgery, it must be immediately determined whether the bleeding is caused by a mechanical problem—open vessels that must be sutured, tied, or coagulated—or whether it is a result of a defect in the hemostatic mechanism.

AXIOM Intraoperative and postoperative bleeding, especially when limited to the site of trauma, is usually due to inadequate surgical efforts, even when a defect is found in hemostasis tests.[5,6]

NORMAL HEMOSTASIS

Normally, hemostasis is initiated by the cooperative action of the endothelium, vasoconstrictor agents, platelets, and coagulation factors in response to a disruption of the vascular endothelial surface.[2]

Primary Hemostasis

VASOCONSTRICTION

Following trauma, injured blood vessels promptly respond with local vasoconstriction which appears to be chiefly mediated by the autonomic nervous system. This can greatly reduce blood loss from injured tissue.[6]

Thromboxane, which causes platelet aggregation and constriction of vascular smooth muscle cells, is released primarily by platelets at the site of disruption of endothelial surfaces.[7] Serotonin released by aggregating platelets in the area of injury also helps to maintain local vasoconstriction.

Epinephrine and norepinephrine can cause vasoconstriction of larger vessels. Arteries are much more efficient than veins in constricting and sealing off the injured area.

AXIOM Partial transection of a vessel, which prevents vascular occlusion by vasoconstriction, is more likely to lead to significant blood loss than is complete transection.

ENDOTHELIAL CHANGES

Endothelial cells modulate platelet reactivity via the secretion of various agents, such as prostacyclin, that not only inhibit platelet function directly but also reduce the interaction of platelets with coagulation factors and the vascular system.[3]

PLATELET ADHESION AND AGGREGATION

The exposure of collagen fibers or basement membrane in vessels initiates "platelet adhesion," which results in the deposition of a single layer of platelets at the site of injury.[1] This first step in the formation of the primary hemostatic plug requires von Willebrand factor (vWF), a protein produced by endothelial cells and found in both the vessel wall and in plasma. Platelets are nonadherent to normal endothelium, but they attach to areas of injury where the vWF binds to specific glycoprotein receptors on the platelet surface (glycoproteins Ib-IX and Ia-IIb).[8]

These initial reactions then stimulate the activation of phospholipase C, which hydrolyzes a membrane phospholipid (phosphatidyl inositol triphosphate). Products of this reaction activate protein kinase C and also increase calcium concentration in platelets. These reactions then lead to a unique series of events.

The platelets change shape and develop pseudopods. Another receptor (glycoprotein IIb-IIIa) is assembled on the platelet surface membrane, and fibrinogen and other adhesive proteins bind to this receptor causing platelet aggregation. Arachidonic acid is then liberated from membrane phospholipids and undergoes oxidation to products that include: (a) certain prostaglandins, which can serve as cofactors for collagen-induced platelet activation, and (b) thromboxane A_2, a powerful platelet activator and vasoconstrictor.

The adhesion of platelets is followed by a "release reaction" in which, among others, adenosine diphosphate (ADP) and serotonin are released from the adhered platelets. These substances stimulate platelet activation and cause aggregation of increasing numbers of platelets at the site of injury. This continuing platelet aggregation leads to the formation of a "first hemostatic plug" or "platelet plug" which facilitates "primary hemostasis" (Fig. 45–1). This is adequate to close vessels which are 50 microns or less in diameter. At this time, no fibrin can yet be demonstrated.[1] The platelets then contract and consolidate the platelet plug, further securing it to the site of injury.[3]

PROSTACYCLIN

Prostacyclin (prostaglandin I_2, PGI_2), a product of prostaglandin metabolism is produced by vascular endothelium. Prostacyclin increases platelet cyclic adenosine monophosphate (cAMP) levels by stimulating adenylate cyclase. This inhibits platelet aggregation and the release reaction;[9] prostacyclin also acts as a vasodilator, thereby helping to maintain the fluidity of blood.

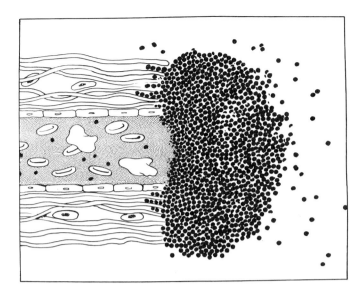

FIGURE 45–1 Schematic representation of a first hemostatic plug occluding a small blood vessel. Initially this plug is solely composed of platelets.

Secondary Hemostatic Plug

PLATELET EFFECTS

Following the adhesion and aggregation of platelets at a disrupted vessel site, the platelet surface expresses procoagulant phospholipids needed for enzyme-cofactor coagulation complexes to form. A series of enzymatic reactions is then initiated by the release of phospholipids in micellar form (platelet factor 3) from platelets.[2] Activation of procoagulant proteins results in the formation of thrombin, a proteolytic enzyme that catalyzes the formation of fibrin monomers from fibrinogen. These fibrin monomers polymerize to form a fibrin mesh which consolidates the hemostatic plug. Thrombin also stimulates platelets to release vasoactive products and adenosine 5'-diphosphate (ADP), which attract more platelets to the injured site.[2]

Coagulation proceeds because tissue thromboplastin, especially from brain, lung, liver, spleen, kidney, and placenta, as well as leukocytes and endothelial cells, powerfully activates factors VII and X to generate thrombin via the extrinsic coagulation pathway.[2]

FIBRIN FORMATION AND FIBRINOLYSIS

Hemostatic effectiveness depends on the rate of formation of the hemostatic plug as well as its structural integrity and stability.[3] Fibrin is the most important constituent of the secondary hemostatic plug, but it is subject to fibrinolytic activity, which occurs spontaneously after fibrin is formed. Fibrinolysis is usually suppressed initially by endogenous inhibitors; however, an increase of a profibrinolytic component or a deficiency of an inhibitor can result in accelerated fibrinolysis, causing premature lysis of the hemostatic plug before repair of the injured vessel is complete.[10]

CLOT COMPOSITION IN VARIOUS BLOOD VESSELS

The composition of a thrombus varies, depending on local blood flow conditions. In areas of relatively sluggish blood flow, such as large veins, where there is a long residence time for blood elements, the presence of abnormal surfaces activates clotting factors leading to a build up of procoagulants and ultimate formation of a "red thrombus."[3] This is composed of red cells trapped in fibrin strands. In regions such as peripheral arteries, where blood flow is brisk and the fluid sheer stress is greater, one is more apt to see a "white thrombus," which is predominately composed of platelets and fibrin.

ENDOTHELIAL EFFECTS

Endothelium has the capacity to express both procoagulant and anticoagulant activities and to release or inactivate agents that either promote or inhibit platelet aggregation.[11] Endothelial cells can participate actively in procoagulant reactions once coagulation is initiated with factor XIIa.[12] The presence of platelets augments these reactions.

PROCESS OF FIBRIN FORMATION

The process of fibrin formation, also referred to as "secondary hemostasis," can be divided into three phases which include: (a) the formation of activated Factor X (Factor Xa), (b) the formation of thrombin, and (c) the formation of fibrin.[1] The proteolytic cascade composing the coagulation system amplifies the response at each step. In other words, each activated (factor) enzyme tends to activate many more molecules of the next enzyme (factor), and thus an initial, small stimulus can cause a much larger response.[6] These reactions are accelerated by protein-to-protein interactions and protein-membrane surface (endothelial cell, platelet) interactions.[3] These interactions are partially responsible for the amplification of the coagulation activation process and also for its localization at the site of injury.

The coagulation process is regulated by both positive and negative feedback systems which act to control reactions (Fig. 45–2).[13] Calcium is required for the majority of coagulation reactions. This is why calcium chelating agents, such as citrate or oxalate, can be used as anticoagulants in vitro; however, they are ineffective in vivo because of their rapid metabolism.[3]

Induction of procoagulants may also occur as the result of activation of cell-mediated immune (CMI) responses.[3] Monokines, interleukin-1, and tumor necrosis factor (TNF) can induce release of tissue factor from endothelial cells, thereby initiating fibrin deposition, which is a common feature of many diseases in which CMI responses play a role. The activation of coagulation may also potentiate the inflammatory response.[14]

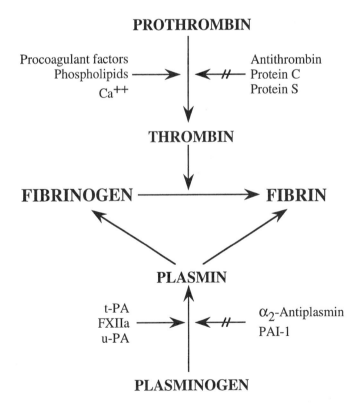

FIGURE 45–2 A simplified coagulation scheme illustrating the formation of fibrin by thrombin which is generated from prothrombin. Procoagulant factors drive this reaction, antithrombin and the protein C + S systems regulate it. Fibrinolysis is accomplished by plasmin. Its generation from plasminogen is mainly facilitated by tissue plasminogen activator (t-PA). Factor XIIa and urokinase type plasminogen activator (u-PA) play a lesser role. This reaction is controlled by α2-antiplasmin and plasminogen activator inhibitor 1 (PAI-1).[13]

Formation of Activated Factor X (Factor Xa)

The formation of activated Factor X (Xa) from Factor X can be accomplished either by the intrinsic or extrinsic coagulation pathways.

AXIOM   The intrinsic coagulation pathway, which can be monitored by activated partial thromboplastin time (APTT), begins when factor XII is activated to factor XIIa, usually on injured endothelium or platelet phospholipid surfaces.

In the intrinsic pathway, Factor XII is activated to Factor XIIa on phospholipid surfaces or collagen fibers and Factor XIIa, in turn, activates Factor XI to Factor XIa. Factor XIa then converts Factor IX to Factor IXa.[1] A complex is formed between platelet phospholipids in micellar form serving as surfaces, calcium ions serving as binders, and Factor IXa serving as the enzyme; Factor VIII:C (antihemophilic Factor A) seems to determine the reaction specificity between enzyme and substrate (Fig. 45–3).

Factor IX is produced in the liver and its synthesis, like that of prothrombin, Factor VII and Factor X, requires the presence of vitamin K. Factor VIII:C is the only clotting factor not totally synthesized in the liver.[1]

AXIOM   The extrinsic coagulation pathway, which can be monitored with prothrombin time (PT), begins when a complex of Factor VII, tissue factor, phospholipids, and calcium is formed.

The extrinsic pathway is marked by the involvement of tissue thromboplastin.[1] All forms of tissue contain a clot-promoting activity called tissue thromboplastin. Tissue thromboplastin can be separated into a protein portion (tissue factor) and a lipid portion (phospholipids).[1] Like platelet phospholipids, tissue phospholipids also seem to serve as surfaces for formation of a complex between Factor VII (enzyme), tissue factor, and calcium ions (acting as binders) (Fig. 45–4). Factor IX can also be activated by the extrinsic pathway complex to factor IXa.

AXIOM   The intrinsic and extrinsic coagulation pathways both function to activate Factor X.

Formation of Thrombin

Prothrombin is synthesized in liver parenchymal cells with the aid of vitamin K. The conversion of prothrombin to thrombin is facilitated by a complex (prothrombinase complex) formed between phospholipid micelles (acting as surfaces), calcium ions (acting as binders),

FIGURE 45–3   The generation of Factor Xa from Factor X by the intrinsic pathway of clotting (shaded area).

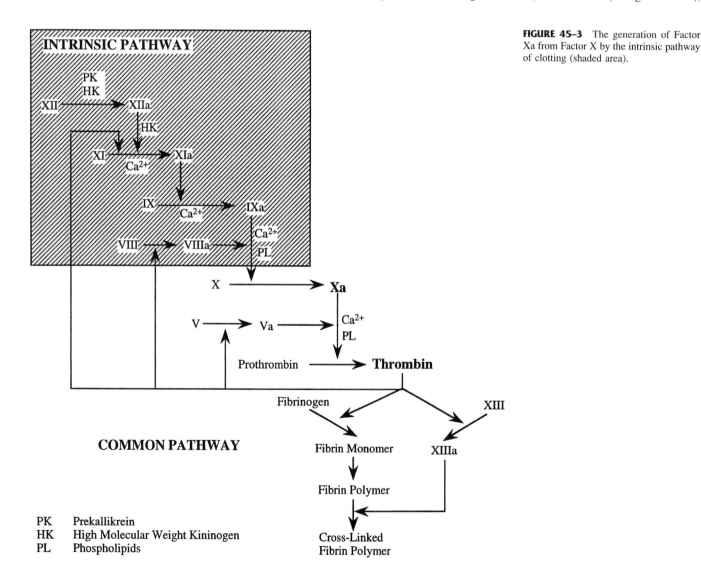

PK   Prekallikrein
HK   High Molecular Weight Kininogen
PL   Phospholipids

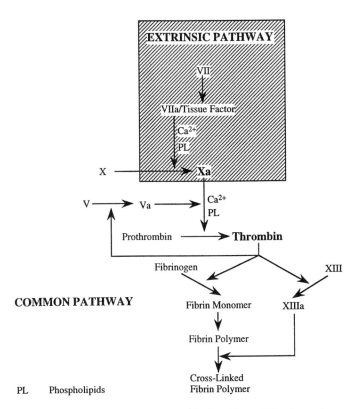

FIGURE 45–4 The formation of Factor Xa from Factor X by the extrinsic pathway of clotting (shaded area).

activated Factor X (acting as an enzyme), and Factor V (also known as Ac-globulin) which seems to determine the reaction specificity between enzyme and substrate[1] (Fig. 45–5).

AXIOM Activated Factor X, Factor V, phospholipids, and calcium form a complex that converts prothrombin to thrombin.

The entire clotting cascade (intrinsic, extrinsic, and common pathways) is illustrated in Figure 45–6.

Formation of Fibrin

Fibrin is formed from fibrinogen, a plasma protein produced by liver parenchymal cells. Normally, 200-400 mg of clottable fibrinogen is present in every 100 mL of plasma.[1] The formation of fibrin can be divided into (a) the proteolytic phase, (b) the polymerization phase, and (c) the stabilization phase.

PROTEOLYTIC PHASE. The fibrinogen molecule circulates in a dimer form and is composed of three chains called α, β, and γ. The proteolytic phase of fibrin formation is marked by the cleavage of an A and B peptide from the N-terminal end of the α and β chains, respectively, by the proteolytic enzyme, thrombin. Because fibrinogen circulates in a dimer form, a pair of A peptides and a pair of B peptides are released. The fibrinogen dimer without its fibrinopeptides A and B is called a "fibrin monomer."[1]

AXIOM After thrombin splits fibrinopeptides A and B off fibrinogen, the molecules remaining are referred to as fibrin monomers.

POLYMERIZATION PHASE. The polymerization phase is characterized by the spontaneous assembly of the fibrin monomers, whereby the three chains combine to form an end-to-end and side-to-side polymerized fibrin network.[1]

STABILIZATION PHASE. During the stabilization phase, the polymerized fibrin monomers are covalently bonded by a "fibrin stabilizing factor," which is also called activated Factor XIII.[1] Factor XIII is produced in the liver in a proenzymic form and becomes activated to its enzymatic form by thrombin.[15]

AXIOM Factor XIII is not needed to have normal PT and APTT, and no acquired, isolated Factor XIII deficiency exists.

Coagulation Inhibitors

Inappropriate activation of coagulation in blood vessels is prevented by a number of coagulation inhibitors.[3] The natural proteinase inhibitors can be subdivided into nonplasma proteinase inhibitors and plasma proteinase inhibitors. The nonplasma proteinase inhibitors block contact activation and fibrinolysis.[16] The plasma proteinase inhibitors are serine proteases which include antithrombin III and α₂-macroglobulin. These form inactive complexes with all coagulation enzymes.

Plasma proteinase inhibitors include protein C and its cofactor, protein S. Protein C is activated by thrombin when complexed with an endothelial cell surface bound receptor, called thrombomodulin. Activated protein C causes proteolytic degradation of factors Va and VIIIa. Through the destruction of these two clotting cofactors, the amount of thrombin and Factor Xa from their respective precursors is regulated. The clinical importance of antithrombin III, protein C, and protein S is attested to by the strong association between inherited deficiencies of either one of these proteins and recurrent venous thromboembolic manifestations in young individuals who do not have other risk factors for DVT.[17] These inhibitor deficiencies may also be related to the development of Warfarin-induced skin necrosis.

AXIOM Recurrent venous thromboembolic disease in young individuals without apparent predisposing factors should make one suspect an inherited deficiency of antithrombin III, protein C, or protein S.

Endothelial Cell Interactions

The endothelium plays an active role in the regulation of the coagulation mechanism.[3] Multiple anticoagulant substances, such as glycosaminoglycans, are operative on the endothelial cell surface. In the protein C/protein S pathway, endothelium provides cofactors that pro-

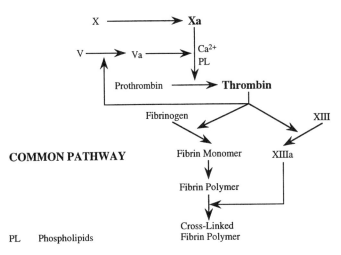

FIGURE 45–5 The generation of thrombin from prothrombin by the common pathway of clotting centering around the key enzyme, Factor Xa.

INTRINSIC PATHWAY

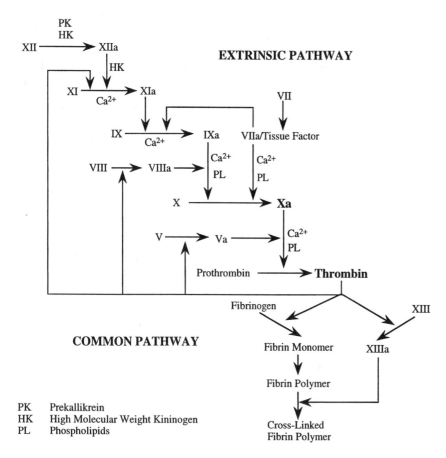

PK   Prekallikrein
HK   High Molecular Weight Kininogen
PL   Phospholipids

mote the activation of protein C and assembly of the activated protein C/protein S complex. It also synthesizes protein S.

Following exposure to cytokines and other pathologic stimuli, such as endotoxin, endothelial cell activation of clotting can occur. "Activated" endothelium can up-regulate procoagulant properties, such as tissue factor, with concomitant down-regulation of anticoagulant cofactors, such as thrombomodulin. Modulation of endothelial cell procoagulant properties by cytokines provides a mechanism linking activation of the clotting mechanism to cellular responses to various types of stress, including trauma.[11,18]

Clot Retraction

After fibrin fibers form, they begin to shorten, causing the clot to retract.[1] This fibrin shortening is due to thrombosthenin, a protein found in platelets. The actual mechanism of shortening of fibrin fibers is analogous to that involved in the shortening of actomyosin in muscle. Calcium ions and ATP must be present in both reactions. The ATP required as the energy source for clot retraction comes from platelets.[1]

Fibrinolysis

FUNCTIONS OF FIBRINOLYSIS

Clot retraction is followed by fibrinolysis, which is accomplished primarily by a proteolytic enzyme referred to as plasmin or fibrinolysin. This is formed from a precursor referred to as plasminogen. Plasminogen is produced in the liver and also is carried or produced in eosinophilic granulocytes.[6] Several plasminogen activators are recognized in tissues, particularly in the intima of blood vessels and in blood itself.[1,19]

> **AXIOM** Arrest of coagulation is mediated to some extent by the conversion of plasminogen to plasmin, a reaction that is partially controlled by activated Factor XII.

The fibrinolytic system is important in opposing any excess tendency toward blood coagulation and in maintaining the fluid characteristics of blood in the intravascular space[20] (Figure 45–7). It is also important for allowing fibroblasts to come in contact with injured tissue to repair it.

PLASMINOGEN ACTIVATORS

The two primary plasminogen activators are tissue type (t-PA) and urokinase type (u-PA) plasminogen activator. Tissue plasminogen activator is the primary physiologic activator of intravascular plasminogen.[21] t-PA is produced in endothelial cells and released by hypoxia, among other stimuli. Urokinase can be found by endothelial cells throughout the body and by epithelial cells lining various excretory ducts of the body (e.g., renal tubules, mammary ducts). Urokinase is normally found in urine, and it has been used clinically to treat thromboembolic disease.[1] Streptokinase, a bacterial product not normally found in the body, is a potent activator of plasminogen and is also used clinically to induce fibrinolysis therapeutically.[22] The ability of α_2-antiplasmin to neutralize free (nonfibrin bound) plasmin prevents inappropriate systemic activation of fibrinolysis.

> **AXIOM** Normally, no systemic plasminogen activation occurs in plasma.

When fibrin is formed, plasminogen activators and plasminogen adsorb to the fibrin surface and plasmin is generated in situ.[3] The

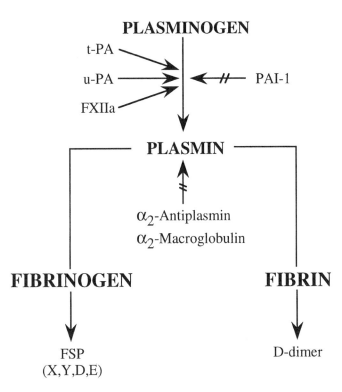

FIGURE 45–7 The fibrinolytic system centering on the generation of plasmin from plasminogen and its effects on both fibrin and fibrinogen.

formed plasmin that is complexed to fibrin is only slowly inactivated by α_2-antiplasmin, whereas plasmin that is released from digested fibrin is rapidly and irreversibly neutralized. The fibrinolytic process, thus, seems to be triggered by and confined to fibrin.

PLASMIN

The main product of the fibrinolytic pathway is plasmin, a serine protease.[3] It is a powerful proteolytic enzyme whose main target is intravascular fibrin and fibrinogen.

AXIOM Plasmin acts on a large number of proteins and, therefore, excessive fibrinolysis can produce widespread effects on a variety of systems.

Plasmin acts not only on fibrin, but it also attacks fibrinogen and Factors II, V, VIII, IX, and XI.[3] It can also degrade a number of other proteins, including adrenocorticotropic hormone (ACTH), growth hormone, and insulin. It activates Factor XII which, in turn, can trigger the coagulation, complement, and kinin systems.

FIBRIN AND FIBRINOGEN SPLIT PRODUCTS

AXIOM Digestion of fibrin and fibrinogen by plasmin leads to formation of so-called fibrin and fibrinogen split products (FSP).

Fibrin and fibrinogen are digested or broken down into fibrin and FSP.[1] The large-molecular-weight split products produced initially are called fragments X and Y or "early split products" (Figure 45–8). These can act as antithrombin and antiplatelet aggregating substances.

AXIOM Increased levels of FSP can block primary and secondary hemostasis.

FSP compete with fibrinogen for active-binding sites on the thrombin molecule, inhibit the polymerization phase of fibrin formation,

competitively inhibit thrombin, and coat the surface of platelets, thereby rendering them unaggregable. Thus, FSP, can block both primary and secondary hemostasis.[19]

AXIOM Normal thrombin clotting times plus normal fibrinogen levels exclude serious activation of the fibrinolytic system.

PLASMINOGEN ACTIVATOR INHIBITORS

Prevention of excessive fibrinolysis is largely achieved through the action of specific plasminogen activator inhibitors (PAIs) and α_2-antiplasmin. Endothelial cells produce type 1 PAI (PAI-1), the most important physiologic inhibitor of t-PA and u-PA. The synthesis of PAI-1 is affected by a variety of compounds, including endotoxin, thrombin, transforming growth factor-α, interleukin-1, and TNF-α.[23] Elevated PAI-1 levels also appear to contribute to the development of postoperative DVT.

AXIOM Disease states resulting from abnormalities in the fibrinolytic system include both hemorrhagic disorders (due to excessive fibrinolysis) and thrombosis (due to deficient or inhibited fibrinolysis).[24]

Hyperfibrinolysis can result from: (a) pharmacologic administration of activators, such as streptokinase, t-PA or u-PA, (b) increased t-PA release, or (c) defective plasmin inhibition, often because of α_2-antiplasmin deficiency. Hypofibrinolytic states can result from hereditary defects of plasminogen, increased PAI-1 levels, or from pharmacologic inhibition of fibrinolysis, such as with epsilon aminocaproic acid (EACA), tranexamic acid, or aprotinin. Laboratory evaluation of fibrinolysis to assess thrombotic disorders and bleeding includes measurements of plasminogen, plasminogen activators, plasminogen activator inhibitors, and circulating fibrinogen and cross-linked fibrin degradation products.[25]

Hyperfibrinolysis degrades increased amounts of plasma fibrinogen into degradation fragments (X, Y, D, and E). Increased degradation of cross-linked fibrin results in increased plasma levels of D-dimers.

DIAGNOSTIC PROCEDURES FOR DETECTION OF BLEEDING DISORDERS

Following trauma and prior to any type of surgery, one should eliminate the existence of a bleeding tendency.[1]

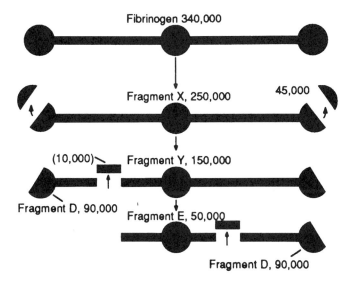

FIGURE 45–8 The proteolytic destruction of a fibrinogen molecule by plasmin yielding the various split products termed fragments X, Y, D, and E.

AXIOM In spite of recent advances in knowledge concerning the detailed biochemistry of blood coagulation, the diagnosis of hemostatic disturbances still often depends on a careful history and physical examination.

History

An accurate history obtained from the patient or from close relatives can provide clues to the existence of most congenital or previously acquired bleeding disorders.[1] Many patients with known bleeding problems wear an identification tag or have some other notification with them. Conversely, it must be recognized that many injured patients, for a variety of reasons, may not spontaneously mention an increased bleeding tendency. Therefore, it is important to ask direct questions related to bruising tendency, epistaxis, hemorrhage following minor trauma, operations or tooth extractions, melena, hematuria, joint swellings, and prolonged menstrual periods or postpartum bleeding. A family history of any bleeding tendency can also be important.

PITFALL ⊘

When a diligent effort is not made to determine whether the patient is taking drugs with anticoagulant properties, appropriate therapy may be dangerously delayed.

An effort should always be made to determine whether the injured patient has been purposefully taking anticoagulants, such as Coumadin, or especially "pain pills" containing acetylsalicylic acid, nonsteroidal antiinflammatory agents, or other compounds that may interfere with platelet function.[1] A history of excessive alcohol intake may point to hepatic dysfunction with impaired coagulation factor production.

With an accurate history, one can also differentiate, to some extent, defects in primary or secondary hemostasis.[1] Patients with primary hemostatic defects tend to give a history of oozing from cuts or incisions, bleeding from mucous membranes, or excessive bruising. In contrast, individuals with impaired secondary hemostasis due to specific coagulation factor deficiencies tend to have hemarthroses and intramuscular hematomas.

In injured patients it is important to know the severity of trauma relative to the magnitude of bleeding that followed.[1] The duration of shock, the number of blood transfusions, and the treatment with platelets and/or fresh frozen plasma (FFP) are also important.

Physical Examination

The physical examination of the patient with a possible bleeding disorder should include several observations: Is the bleeding localized or diffuse? Is it related to a traumatic or surgical lesion? Is there mucosal bleeding? Are there signs of arterial or venous thrombosis? Particular attention should also be paid to the spleen and liver. For example, the presence of an enlarged spleen in a thrombocytopenic patient suggests splenic sequestration. Hepatomegaly or other evidence of liver disease may indicate decreased factor synthesis as the etiology of prolonged PT or APTT.

When evidence of an advanced disseminated malignancy exists, acute or chronic disseminated intravascular coagulation (DIC) should be suspected as the cause of prolonged coagulation times, hypofibrinogenemia, and thrombocytopenia. Palpable purpura suggests capillary leak due to vasculitis, whereas purpura due to thrombocytopenia or platelet defects cannot usually be detected by touch. Venous telangiectasias may be seen in some patients with von Willebrand's disease (vWD), and arterial telangiectasias may be seen in liver disease. When point pressure is centrally applied to an arterial telangiectasia, the lesion fades, whereas venous telangiectasia requires confluent pressure across the entire lesion (as with a glass slide) for blanching to occur.

AXIOM Prolonged or excessive bleeding from needle puncture sites or spontaneous bleeding from mucous membranes suggests severe coagulopathy, such as DIC.

Laboratory Studies

When any evidence suggests a bleeding tendency on the basis of history or physical examination, a proper laboratory diagnosis of the underlying problem should be obtained prior to surgery, when time allows.[1] This is best done in consultation with a hematologist who has access to a laboratory that can perform sophisticated coagulation tests.

PITFALL ⊘

When only laboratory tests are used to eliminate coagulation abnormalities, mild-to-moderate disorders may be overlooked.

It must be emphasized that lack of laboratory evidence of clotting abnormalities does not necessarily correlate with lack of clinical bleeding due to clotting disorders, particularly in critically ill trauma patients.[26] Furthermore, results are not always available quickly. However, alert clinical observation plus rapidly available laboratory tests can help to direct management much more appropriately than protocols for administering FFP and platelet concentrates.[2]

The usefulness of screening coagulation tests on all patients prior to surgery is debated. In most instances, the number and type of tests that are ordered are inadequate to diagnose all possible coagulation problems.[1] Furthermore, relatively mild congenital or acquired bleeding disorders are easily overlooked by such tests because most laboratory procedures currently available are not sensitive enough.

In spite of the limitations of the laboratory diagnosis of bleeding and coagulation disorders, six screening tests (Figure 45–9) document most of the disorders likely to be involved in excess hemorrhage not due to mechanical problems.[1] Platelet counts and bleeding times screen for most of the serious quantitative and qualitative platelet abnormalities. The PT and APTT screen for all serious clotting factor deficiencies involved in the formation of thrombin. Fibrinogen determinations plus thrombin clotting times or FSP assays screen for the presence of increased fibrinolytic activity.[1] When these tests are performed by adequately trained individuals, most aspects of the hemostatic mechanisms can be screened, and any serious abnormality becomes apparent.[1,27]

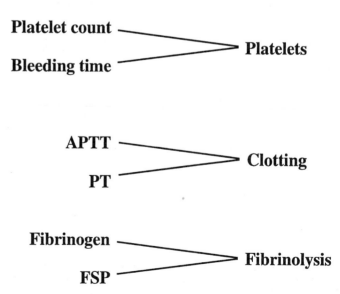

FIGURE 45–9 Six laboratory tests that allow for the quick screening of platelet and clotting function and activation of fibrinolysis.

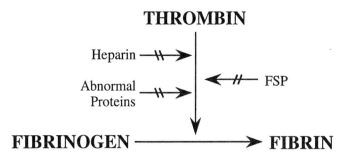

FIGURE 45–10 The principle of thrombin clotting time. Besides low-fibrinogen levels (<50 mg/dL) or functionally abnormal fibrinogen molecules (dysfibrinogenemias), FSP, heparin, and abnormal proteins influence this test.

PLATELET COUNT

A platelet count gives a quantitative assessment of the number of circulating platelets, a decrease of which is one of the most common causes for excessive surgical hemorrhage, particularly after massive transfusions.[1] Generally, a platelet count $< 100 \times 10^9$/L can increase bleeding to some degree depending on how low it is. A platelet count $< 50 \times 10^9$/L generally increases bleeding from any skin or mucosal injury. A platelet count $< 20 \times 10^9$/L may be associated with spontaneous bleeding without trauma.

BLEEDING TIME

Bleeding time (BT), preferably performed according to the procedure described by Ivy,[1] is abnormal not only in patients with thrombocytopenia, but also with many forms of thrombocytopathy, especially those that affect the formation of the first hemostatic plug. BTs should be normal when platelet counts are $> 100 \times 10^9$/L, and they are always prolonged with counts $< 50 \times 10^9$/L; however, BTs do not necessarily predict surgical bleeding.[28]

| AXIOM | Mild thrombocytopathies usually are not discovered by performing BT.[1] |

ACTIVATED PARTIAL THROMBOPLASTIN TIMES

APTT screens the activity of all coagulation factors involved in the formation of thrombin via the intrinsic and common pathways (Factors II, V, VIII, IX, X, XI, XII; Figure 45–3).[1] Only Factor VII activity is not measured by APTT. APPT, however, is not very sensitive, and the coagulation factors involved in the intrinsic pathway usually have to be reduced to $< 40\%$ of normal before the APTT is prolonged.[1] Unfortunately, excessive bleeding following trauma or during major surgical procedures can occur from relatively mild reductions in these clotting factors.

| AXIOM | Clinical coagulopathy can occur after major trauma or surgery in spite of relatively normal PT and APTT values. |

PROTHROMBIN TIMES

Prothrombin time (PT) screens the activity of all coagulation factors involved in the extrinsic and common pathway of thrombin formation (Factors II, V, VII, X; Figure 45–4), but the same lack of sensitivity of the APTT also applies to the PT. Using both the APTT and PT, however, screens for all the coagulation factors involved in thrombin formation, and any major abnormalities should become apparent with one or both tests.

| AXIOM | Normal APTT and PT effectively exclude any serious defects in the clotting system. |

FIBRINOGEN DETERMINATIONS

Fibrinogen determinations give information concerning the quantity of fibrin that can be expected to be formed. When they are > 100 mg/dL and are not associated with other defects, fibrinogen levels maintain adequate hemostasis.[1] Unfortunately, low levels of fibrinogen are usually associated with other defects, especially fibrinolysis or DIC.

THROMBIN CLOTTING TIMES

Thrombin clotting times (TCT) are most helpful in determining defects associated with the formation of fibrin from fibrinogen by thrombin (Figure 45–10).[1] TCT are abnormal when the fibrinogen level is < 50 mg/dL, when heparin is present, when abnormal plasma proteins (paraproteinemias) are present, and, most importantly, when increased quantities of FSP are present. TCT, in the absence of heparin and in the presence of > 50 mg/dL fibrinogen, is highly sensitive to the presence of increased FSP, and thus it can be a highly sensitive indicator of the presence of increased fibrinolysis.[1] If TCT were prolonged, one could request a semiquantitative split product assay or reptilase time.

OTHER TESTS

Two other screening tests that have been recommended in patients with excessive bleeding include the tube clot test and reptilase time test.[2] The tube clot test has been recommended as a rapid, easily performed screening test for coagulation abnormalities. Approximately 2-3 mL of blood are drawn into a single, clean test tube and the rate of clot formation is observed.[3] The test tube is tilted every minute or so to determine whether a clot has formed. Normal blood should clot within 10 minutes. It should then gradually retract and remain stable. Absence of clotting within 20-30 minutes indicates a major coagulopathy. Absence of retraction after a clot has formed indicates possible thrombocytopenia. When blood clots properly, but subsequently lyses rapidly (within another 5-10 minutes), excess fibrinolysis should be suspected.[3]

When systemic or local heparin has been used during clamping of a major vessel that needs repair, it may be difficult to determine whether subsequently prolonged bleeding may be due to excess residual heparin. Reptilase time, when available, can be used to differentiate hyperheparinemia from increased split products. Normal reptilase time combined with prolonged TCT is an indication of hyperheparinemia. In the presence of FSP, both tests will be prolonged.[1]

| AXIOM | When a patient with coagulopathy has a prolonged thrombin time and a normal reptilase time, excess heparin is probably present. |

CONGENITAL BLEEDING DISORDERS

Congenital Coagulation Factor Deficiencies

GENERAL CONSIDERATIONS

Congenital coagulation disorders may occasionally be the cause of pathologic bleeding in trauma patients. Because congenital disorders of coagulation usually involve a single factor, establishment of the diagnosis should theoretically not be too difficult. Plasma concentrations of the involved coagulation factors in most congenital coagulation disorders tend to be low, but accurate diagnosis still usually rests on a careful history, physical examination, and laboratory tests, especially PT and APTT, plus assay of plasma levels of specific factors.[3]

With proper diagnosis and therapy, surgical procedures can be performed on patients with congenital coagulation disorders with confi-

TABLE 45–1 **Congenital Coagulation Disorders and Their Effect on Screening Tests**

Coagulopathy	Factor Involved	Platelet Count	Bleeding Times	APTT	Prothrombin Times	Fibrinogen	Thrombin Times
Afibrinogenemia	Fibrinogen	−	−	+	+	+	+
Hypoprothrombinemia	Prothrombin	−	−	+	+	−	−
Parahemophilia	Factor V	−	−	+	+	−	−
Factor X deficiency	Factor X	−	−	+	+	−	−
Factor VII deficiency	Factor VII	−	−	−	+	−	−
Hemophilia A	Factor VIII	−	−	+	−	−	−
Hemophilia B	Factor IX	−	−	+	−	−	−
PTA deficiency	Factor XI	−	−	+	−	−	−
Hageman trait	Factor XII	−	−	+	−	−	−
Factor XIII deficiency	Factor XIII	−	−	−	−	−	−

− = Normal
+ = Abnormal

dence and with an acceptable low incidence of complications.[3] Proper hematologic management usually includes administration of a specific factor concentrate; however, in emergency situations, treatment can also be started with FFP or cryoprecipitate. In addition, meticulous intraoperative hemostasis and careful clinical and laboratory monitoring of blood coagulation during surgery and in the perioperative period are essential.

Elective surgery on patients with known congenital bleeding disorders should be performed only in centers where proper hematologic services are available.[1] This entails not only a "hemostasiologist" but also the services of a well-functioning coagulation laboratory which is capable not only of diagnosing defects but also of following the effects of specific therapeutic regimens. It must be remembered that in spite of advances in component therapy, which have unquestionably prolonged the life expectancy of many patients with congenital bleeding disorders, surgery or trauma is still the most frequent cause of death for these patients.[1] Even in cases of emergency, patients with severe congenital coagulation disorders should, whenever possible, be referred to centers specializing in the treatment of such problems.

Fortunately, most congenital bleeding disorders are diagnosed relatively early in life; however, even when no diagnosis has been established previously, a good history and physical examination usually provides clues to the problem.[1] In all patients, accurate diagnosis should be made prior to surgery, when possible.

AXIOM In many congenital coagulopathies, platelet counts and BTs are normal (Table 45–1), indicating uncomplicated formation of the first hemostatic plug.[29,30]

Congenital bleeding disorders can be divided into three major categories: (a) coagulopathies (disturbances or deficiencies in the classic clotting factors), (b) thrombocytopathies (qualitative and quantitative platelet abnormalities), and (c) telangiopathies (congenital vascular abnormalities).[1] Careful performance of the six standard screening coagulation tests noted previously generally indicates which disorder is present (Table 45–1).

HEMOPHILIAS

Pathology
Classic hemophilia, also called hemophilia A, is characterized by Factor VIII deficiency and is inherited as a sex-linked, recessive disorder. It is manifested almost exclusively in males; females are the genetic carriers. Approximately one male in 10,000 is afflicted with hemophilia A, making it one of the most common, severe, hereditary coagulation disorders.[31] Factor VIII protein complex consists of procoagulant factor VIII:C (FVIII:C) and vWF. Patients with classic hemophilia lack FVIII:C. FVIII:C deficiency in hemophiliacs may re-

sult either from low plasma factor levels or from a dysfunctional factor present in normal concentrations.

Hemophilia B (Christmas Disease), which is clinically and genetically indistinguishable from hemophilia A, occurs seven times less frequently and is caused by hereditary deficiency of Christmas factor (Factor IX).[31]

AXIOM In hemophiliacs, platelet function remains intact, allowing the first hemostatic plug to develop promptly after trauma, but excessive bleeding tends to develop after a delay that may last several hours or days.[31]

In hemophilia, fibrin formation is limited to deposition of thin strands at the wound periphery, preventing the central core of the thrombus from gaining proper consistency.[32] Because primary hemostasis is unaffected in hemophilia, the onset of abnormal bleeding is characteristically somewhat delayed. When hemorrhagic shock develops or an expanding hematoma exerts pressure on adjacent tissues or organs, bleeding may persist for several days or weeks, unless treated, because proper coagulation is needed to maintain occlusion of injured vessels.[31] For similar reasons, during surgery, these patients may not ooze excessively from small vessels, but severe bleeding can develop postoperatively.

The likelihood and severity of bleeding are primarily determined by the FVIII:C level in the plasma (Table 45–2).[29] Bleeding is unlikely in patients with FVIII:C levels > 50% of normal even after major injury or surgery. The likelihood of bleeding with FVIII:C levels < 50% is dependent on the severity of trauma. Plasma levels 25-50%, which may be present in some carriers, tend to have increased bleeding only after major trauma. Surgery or trauma may not cause significant bleeding even in patients with FVIII:C levels as low as 5-25%; however, levels 1-4% of normal predispose the

TABLE 45–2 **Relationship between Plasma Factor VIII:C Levels and Severity of Bleeding in Hemophilia***

Plasma Factor VIII:C Level (% normal)	Bleeding After Major Trauma	Bleeding After Minor Trauma	Spontaneous Bleeding
50 to 100	−	−	−
25 to 50	+	−	−
5 to 25	++	+	−
1 to 5	+++	+++	+
< 1	+++	+++	++

*The symbols used are: −, no bleeding; +, possible bleeding; ++, moderate bleeding; +++, severe bleeding.

patient to bleeding even after minor injury. Recurrent, spontaneous bleeding, usually into muscles or weight-bearing joints, generally occurs in patients with FVIII:C levels < 1%.[29]

Diagnosis

AXIOM The diagnosis of hemophilia should be suspected in males with a history of excessive bleeding since childhood.

The presence of excessive, deep-tissue bleeding after trauma or of prolonged oozing from wounds or sites of venipuncture should make one consider the possibility of a preexisting hemostatic defect.[2] Many patients with congenital bleeding disorders have identification tags that state their diagnosis and, in many cases, the mode of treatment. When reliable information cannot be obtained from the patient, relatives or friends should be questioned. Although the physical examination and the extent of bleeding relative to the magnitude of trauma may provide some important clues in the absence of a clear history of a preexisting coagulation disorder, the diagnosis is usually established by laboratory tests (Table 45–3).[30]

In hemophilia, laboratory tests typically reveal normal platelet counts, BTs, and PTs with prolonged APTT.[30] Severe trauma with prolonged shock and/or massive transfusions, however, may result in decreased platelet counts and a prolonged PT, making diagnosis more difficult. Even low FVIII:C levels, which are usually considered diagnostic of hemophilia, may be found in trauma victims who are treated with massive amounts of crystalloids and packed red blood cells. Thus, a definitive diagnosis of hemophilia may be difficult or delayed in severely injured patients. In hemodynamically stable patients in whom the diagnosis of hemophilia can be made by FVIII:C measurement, one should also look for an inhibitor as the primary cause of excessive bleeding.[1,30]

Treatment of Injury

GENERAL. Hemorrhage in hemophilia is particularly dangerous when it is intracranial, lingual, laryngeal, retropharyngeal, pericardial, or pleural. Hematomas at these sites can expand rapidly and result in lifethreatening displacement of intracranial, cervical, or thoracic organs.[31] Although these conditions require immediate Factor VIII replacement, emergency decompression of the brain or heart or establishment of airway patency may also be necessary.

AIRWAY MANAGEMENT. Airway management may be difficult in hemophiliacs because distortion of the anatomy may be caused not only by rapid accumulation of blood in the fascial planes of the neck, but also by edema secondary to venous obstruction. In addition, traumatic emergency intubation, particularly through the nose, can cause serious, continued mucosal bleeding.

INTRACRANIAL BLEEDING. Intracranial hemorrhage occurs at some time in 3-14% of hemophiliacs, is associated with a history of trauma in 45-60% of these patients, and is associated with a 25-35% mortality rate, even when treated properly.[33] Intracerebral hematoma accounts for 40% and epidural and subdural hematoma for 60% of intracranial

bleeding. Even minor head trauma can result in bleeding from small intracranial vessels; however, symptoms may not develop until 24-48 hours after injury.

AXIOM Posttraumatic intracranial bleeding in hemophiliac patients may not be significant or apparent for 24-48 hours.

The most common presenting symptoms of intracranial hemorrhage in hemophiliacs include altered sensorium, headache, emesis, and seizures. These may be accompanied by symptoms of spinal cord compression because intraspinal bleeding may also occur.[34] Management of these patients is somewhat controversial. Some surgeons believe that unless the hematoma is large or occupies the extradural space, conservative therapy with high-dose Factor VIII concentrates and frequent evaluation with CT scan are preferred.[31] They consider craniotomy only for those patients who do not improve or who deteriorate within a few hours after the start of replacement therapy.[34] Unfortunately, if this protocol is followed and is unsuccessful, the patients will have a greatly increased likelihood of having severe intracranial hypertension. Other authors, using operative indications similar to those used for nonhemophiliacs with CNS bleeding have demonstrated that the mortality rate with such therapy was 64% for patients with intracerebral hematomas but only 14% for patients with subdural or subarachnoid hemorrhage.[34]

CERVICAL SPINE ABNORMALITIES

AXIOM Hemophiliacs can have a variety of nontraumatic bony abnormalities seen on cervical spine radiography.

Patients with hemophilia may show a variety of nontraumatic roentgenographic abnormalities of the cervical spine. These include an increased atlantodens distance, endplate irregularities, and cysts within the vertebral bodies.[35] In hemophiliacs with suspected cervical spine injury, these abnormalities can make radiographic evaluation of the cervical spine extremely difficult. When doubt exists, the cervical spine should be kept immobilized until further studies can be performed.

BLEEDING INTO DEEP TISSUES. Bleeding into joints, muscles, or interfascial spaces may occur in hemophiliacs, especially those with trauma, and can result in serious complications, such as hypovolemia, peripheral neuropathies, and infection. Massive retroperitoneal bleeding may also occur; if a subsequent rupture into the peritoneal cavity were to occur, it could cause severe hypotension and/or anemia.

URINARY TRACT INJURY. Patients with hemophilia have a high incidence of urinary tract bleeding which occasionally leads to severe renal colic.[2,3] When an injured hemophiliac is to undergo emergency or elective surgery, this potential bleeding site should be examined preoperatively.

AXIOM Intraoperative positioning of hemophiliacs should be done carefully, and pressure points must be thickly padded to prevent hemorrhage.

Treatment of Congenital Coagulopathies

GENERAL GUIDELINES. General guidelines have been developed for treating patients with congenital coagulopathy who have had trauma and/or are scheduled to undergo needed surgery.[1] According to these guidelines, one should:

1. Determine the plasma level of the factor prior to surgery.
2. Exclude the presence of a possible inhibitor.
3. Infuse the factor in question and be certain that the plasma level increases appropriately.
4. Increase the concentration of the factor in plasma to its desired level immediately prior to surgery.
5. Maintain sufficient levels until wound healing is complete.

TABLE 45–3 Results of Coagulation Tests in Hemophilia A

Test	Results
Bleeding time	Normal
Platelet count	Normal
Platelet aggregation	Normal
Prothrombin time	Normal
Partial thromboplastin time	Prolonged
Factor VIII:C level	Low (diagnostic)
Factor vWF	Normal

REPLACEMENT THERAPY

Safety of Blood Products

AXIOM   Whenever a blood product is used, the risk of subsequent hepatitis and/or AIDS should be considered.

It must be kept in mind that blood and its products can carry viral contaminants; consequently, the patient and/or family should be advised of the possibility of this complication, and serial laboratory tests should be performed as needed to eliminate development of this problem.[36] Because they can also transmit AIDS, blood products used in hemophiliacs pose serious problems. Most patients who have received replacement therapy either with Factor VIII concentrates or with large amounts of cryoprecipitate have antibodies in plasma to the human immunodeficiency virus (HIV) causing AIDS.[3] It is unknown which of these antibody-positive patients will subsequently develop AIDS. Because virus-inactivated Factor VIII concentrates are now available, only these products should be used. Recently, recombinant factor concentrates have also become available.

Fresh Frozen Plasma

AXIOM   The initial treatment of excessive bleeding in hemophiliacs is volume resuscitation with blood transfusions and FFP.

Treatment of trauma patients with Factor VIII deficiency should be two-staged.[36] Initially, abnormal bleeding should be treated by immediate replacement with blood and FFP, which contains both factors VIII and IX. This will permit volume resuscitation in addition to providing factor VIII or IX. After the initial emergency has been corrected, more extensive evaluation is appropriate, including tests to determine the quantity of factor VIII or IX present in the blood. Consultation with a coagulation expert is also recommended. FFP, cryoprecipitate, or factor concentrates are given as needed to maintain factor levels at 50-100% of normal until complete healing is manifest.[29,30]

Cryoprecipitate.   When performing emergency treatment for hemophilia, cryoprecipitate can be used in situations in which the quantity of intravenous fluids must be restricted. Cryoprecipitate is prepared from single donors by a freeze-thaw technique that removes the thawed plasma before the last protein precipitate—which contains factor VIII, vWF, and fibrinogen—is dissolved.[3] Bags of cryoprecipitate are stored frozen and their contents are dissolved in 10 mL of 0.9% sodium chloride solution before use.

AXIOM   Cryoprecipitate has all of the coagulation factors present in FFP except Factors II, VII, IX, and X.

Factor VIII activity is expressed in units, and 1 unit is defined as the amount of Factor VIII in 1 mL of normal plasma. Although the amount of Factor VIII in individual cryoprecipitate bags varies somewhat (70-100 units), a bag may be assumed to contain 80 units of Factor VIII when calculating the number of bags needed for replacement therapy. Cryoprecipitate, when prepared from blood drawn in many large cities of the United States, could entail a significant risk for transmission of AIDS or hepatitis. Because they are now virus-inactivated, the use of most commercially prepared Factor VIII concentrates is considerably safer today. For this reason, these new concentrates should be given in preference to cryoprecipitate, especially in newborns and children in whom hemophilia A is newly diagnosed.

Component Therapy

WITHOUT INHIBITORS

Guidelines.   Component therapy requires an accurate diagnosis of the factor missing in the patient in order to be effective.[1] Compo-

nents used for the treatment of hemophilia A and B, the two most frequently occurring congenital coagulopathies, are expressed in units.

AXIOM   A unit of factor VIII or IX is the amount of that activity found in 1 ml of fresh plasma.

In major surgical procedures, the plasma levels of Factors VIII or IX should be raised to 50-100% of normal immediately prior to and during surgery and should be maintained at a level of at least 20-30% of normal in the postoperative period. Similar rules also apply to the other coagulation factors. The fibrinogen level should be maintained at $\geq$ 100 mg/dL at all times.

Lyophilized Factor VIII concentrates, prepared from plasma pools of up to 5000 donors, are packaged in bottles supplying 250-1000 units of Factor VIII.[3] The powder is dissolved in 10-100 mL of sterile diluent before use. Because of its convenience, lyophilized Factor VIII concentrate has received widespread use, particularly in home care programs in which patients inject themselves with concentrate at the first indication of bleeding.

Calculation of Dosage for Replacement Therapy
The Factor VIII or IX level should be raised transiently to about 0.3 units (30%) to protect against bleeding after dental extraction or to abort a beginning joint hemorrhage. The levels should exceed 0.5 units (50%) when major joint or muscular bleeding is already evident and the plasma levels should be > 1.0 unit (100%) in lifethreatening bleeding or before major surgery.[3,36] Repeated infusions at 50% of the initially calculated dose should be given every 8-12 hours to keep trough levels > 0.5 units (50%) for several days after a life-threatening bleeding episode or after surgery.

AXIOM   Generally, each unit of Factor VIII activity infused per kg of body weight should produce a 2% increase in plasma levels of Factor VIII.[1]

For Factor VIII replacement, dosage can be calculated by multiplying the patient's weight in kg by 44 and by the level in units desired. Thus, to raise the Factor VIII level of a man who weighs 68 kg (150 lb) from a level of essentially zero to a level of 1 u/mL (100%), the dosage needed would be 68 $\times$ 44 $\times$ 1 or about 3000 units.[3]

A number of other formulas have also been proposed.[37] Pool recommended that 1 unit of cryoprecipitate be given for every 6 kg of body weight initially and then 1 unit/12 kg every 12 hours for maintenance.[38] Johnson et al. recommended 3,000 units as the initial dose in average-sized adults, followed by 1,500 units every 8 hours during the first postoperative day, 1,500 units every 12 hours for the next 6 days, and then 750 units every 12 hours until wound healing is complete.[39]

AXIOM   No formula for administering blood components can substitute for careful, repeated serial laboratory and clinical observations.

Complications caused by Factor VIII concentrates can include allergic reactions, immune antibodies, and transmittal of blood-borne viruses. Consequently, virus-inactivated or recombinant Factor VIII concentrates should be the preferred concentrate for use in all patients with hemophilia A.

FACTOR VIII INHIBITORS

AXIOM   When a hemophiliac who is bleeding has a Factor VIII inhibitor, treatment is much more difficult and should be undertaken in consultation with someone experienced in such care.[1,3]

If possible, musculoskeletal bleeding in classic hemophiliacs with Factor VIII inhibitors is managed without giving Factor VIII, because it stimulates further antibody production and increases the plasma titer of antibody within 3-4 days.[40] In patients with serious bleeding and a low initial inhibitor antibody titer, a large dose of Factor VIII, calculated to overcome the inhibitor and temporarily increase plasma Factor VIII levels, may be given. When this does not control bleeding, further Factor VIII infusions are useless because of the rapid increase in antibody induced.

Prothrombin complex concentrates can be used to manage serious bleeding in patients with high titers of inhibitor. Special preparations of prothrombin complex concentrate are available, but they are very expensive. A porcine Factor VIII preparation, which is insensitive to the inhibitor, has also been used with reported good results.[40]

REPLACEMENT THERAPY FOR FACTOR IX DEFICIENCIES. In hemophilia B (Factor IX deficiency), the dose calculation for Factor IX is similar to that used for Factor VIII in hemophilia A. The half-life of Factor IX is 24 hours, and levels of 50% are desirable.[41] Each unit of Factor IX infused per kg body weight should theoretically increase levels by 1%; however, only about half the Factor IX units listed on each unit of prothrombin complex concentrate can be recovered after infusion.[3] Therefore, when prothrombin complex concentrate is given for Factor IX replacement therapy, an amount double that calculated as necessary should be given. Because prothrombin complex concentrate may also contain variable amounts of activated clotting factors, patients receiving repeated doses of Factor IX concentrate are at increased risk for developing thromboses unless heparin is added to each unit of concentrate.[41]

AXIOM In patients receiving multiple units of Factor IX concentrate, 5-10 units of heparin should be added to each milliliter of reconstituted prothrombin complex concentrate.

1-DEAMINO-8-D-ARGININE VASOPRESSIN. The drug 1-deamino-8-D-arginine vasopressin, also known as desmopressin acetate or DDAVP, is useful for treating patients with basal Factor VIII levels of 5-10% or more by mobilizing Factor VIII from endothelial stores.[42] Administration of DDAVP after minor trauma or before elective dental surgery may reduce or even obviate the need for replacement therapy. However, if hemophilia is severe, DDAVP will be ineffective.

ANTIFIBRINOLYTIC AGENTS. The antifibrinolytic agent, EACA, in doses of 2.5 g four times daily for one week can also be given to hemophiliac patients to prevent late bleeding after dental extraction or other types of oropharyngeal mucosal trauma[43] (e.g., tongue laceration); however, when prothrombin complex concentrates are given, and because they may contain activated clotting factors, EACA should not be given until 10 hours after the prothrombin complex.

OTHER COAGULATION DEFECTS

Of the various congenital coagulation factor deficiencies, only Factor XIII deficiencies have normal APTTs and PTs.[29] In all other cases, either one or both of these tests are usually abnormal.

Congenital Thrombocytopathies

The most important congenital thrombocytopathies can usually be diagnosed readily by standard screening tests[1] (Table 45–4).

VON WILLEBRAND DISEASE

Pathophysiology

Von Willebrand's disease (vWD), the most frequent congenital coagulopathy (not a true thrombocytopathy), is encountered more often than both hemophilias combined.[1] It is an autosomal-dominant bleeding disorder of variable severity with a prevalence of 30-125 per million population.[44] It results from a quantitative (type I) or qualitative (type II variants) abnormality of von Willebrand factor (vWF). This plasma protein is secreted by endothelial cells and circulates in plasma in multimers up to 14,000,000 daltons in size, and at least 21 subtypes of vWF have been identified. vWF has two known hemostatic functions: (a) large multimers of vWF are required for platelets to adhere to collagen and other biological surfaces, and (b) multimers of all sizes form complexes in plasma with Factor VIII:C. Formation of such complexes is required to maintain normal plasma Factor VIII:C levels.[44]

Diagnosis

In all congenital thrombocytopathies, except pure forms of platelet-Factor-3-release disturbances, BTs are abnormal, indicating that one of the defects present results in impaired formation of the first hemostatic plug.[1] For this reason, patients with congenital thrombocytopathies may have severe intraoperative oozing in addition to excessive postoperative hemorrhage. Bleeding manifestations in vWD are usually mild to moderate and include easy bruising, epistaxis, bleeding from small skin cuts (that may stop and start again over a period of several hours), increased menstrual bleeding (in some women), and abnormal bleeding after surgical procedures (e.g., tooth extraction and tonsillectomy).

In the laboratory, vWD is characterized by prolonged BTs from the disturbed platelet adhesion and prolonged APTTs due to an associated Factor VIII:C deficiency;[1] however, in persons with mild vWD, variations in plasma levels of Factor VIII:C may cause screening tests to be normal on some occasions. A definitive diagnosis of vWD requires measuring (a) total plasma vWF activity and antigen, and (b) the ability of the plasma to support agglutination of normal platelets by ristocetin.[45]

TABLE 45–4 *Congenital Thrombocytopathies and Their Effect on Screening Tests*

Thrombocytopathies	Function Disturbed	Platelet Count	Bleeding Times	APTT	Pro Times	Fibrinogen	Thrombin Times
Von Willebrand's syndrome	Adhesion plus occasional aggregation	−	+	+	−	−	−
Aggregation abnormalities	Aggregation	−	+	−	−	−	−
Platelet Factor 3 availability	Phospholipid release	−	−	−	−	−	−
Thrombasthenia	Aggregation and clot retraction	−	+	−	−	−	−
Thrombocytopenia	All above	+	+	−	−	−	−

− = Normal
+ = Abnormal

Treatment

The precise defect in each patient with vWD must be determined accurately in order to select the proper therapeutic regimen. Type I or type II variants of vWD, although characterized by impaired platelet adhesion, should be treated with DDAVP, FFP or cryoprecipitate and not platelet concentrates.[44] Highly purified Factor VIII concentrates do not correct the abnormal BTs of vWD.

The dosage of cryoprecipitate for treating vWD is often selected empirically and is typically 1 bag for each 10 kg of body weight every 8-12 hours just before and for several days after major surgery. Lyophilized Factor VIII concentrates should not be used as a replacement therapy for vWF because of its variable content of large multimers of vWF.[46] The serious risk of viral disease transmission with cryoprecipitate has recently directed efforts to prepare a virus-inactivated vWF concentrate.[46] Currently, virus inactivation is achieved either by pasteurization or by treating the product with solvent detergents.[47]

DDAVP is also helpful in type I vWD. Thirty minutes after intravenous administration of DDAVP in a dose of 0.3-0.4 mcg/kg one can expect a significant shortening in BTs.[48] An increase in the higher molecular weight forms of vWF in response to DDAVP also occurs. As a result, the prolonged BTs and decreased Factor VIII:C and vWF activities are frequently normalized.

About 48 hours must elapse for new endothelial stores of vWF to accumulate to permit a second injection of DDAVP to be as effective as the initial dose.[44] In some instances, DDAVP can substantially reduce the need to use plasma fractions to control or prevent bleeding. DDAVP is usually not effective in type II vWD.

OTHER CONGENITAL THROMBOCYTOPATHIES

Most thrombocytopathies produce increased capillary type bleeding; however, pure platelet Factor 3 (PF3) release disturbances may act like a coagulopathy because of the role that PF3 plays in the formation of thrombin.[49]

Most thrombocytopathies, except vWD, can be treated with platelet concentrates alone, provided the concentrates are prepared from whole blood that is < 24 hours old and provided that the platelets are used within four hours of preparation.[1] Without these precautions, concentrates may contain platelets that neither adhere to an injured vessel wall nor aggregate, thus not contributing to the formation of the first hemostatic plug. Normalization of the prolonged BTs and reduced platelet counts can serve as indicators for successful substitution therapy.

Congenital Telangiopathies

Congenital telangiopathies can be difficult to diagnose unless they are associated with prolonged BTs. Even when the diagnosis is made, congenital telangiopathies can be extremely difficult to treat.[1]

ACQUIRED BLEEDING DISORDERS

AXIOM   Acquired bleeding disorders are much more frequently encountered than those of congenital origin, particularly in adult trauma patients.[1]

Acquired bleeding disorders (Table 45–5) frequently are manifest as an overt clinical bleeding tendency prior to surgery; in most instances, the defects can be detected preoperatively by conducting a careful history and physical examination and by performing some screening tests. Some bleeding disorders, however, develop intraoperatively and/or postoperatively in patients who had no apparent hemostatic defects prior to surgery.[1]

Clotting Disorders Prior to Trauma

HEPATIC FAILURE

Liver disease (including major hepatic trauma, cirrhosis, and biliary obstruction) is a common cause of impaired coagulation.[50] Because

TABLE 45–5   Common Acquired Disorders of Hemostasis Unrelated to Surgery

Hepatic failure
Renal failure
Vitamin K deficiency
Anticoagulants
Thrombocytopenias
Vascular abnormalities
Paraproteinemias
Circulating anticoagulants

most coagulation factors, except vWF and FVIII:C, are synthesized in the liver, the blood levels of the various coagulation factors will be decreased in patients with cirrhosis, but the amount they decrease depends upon the degree of parenchymal cell damage. Vitamin-K-dependent clotting factors (Factors II, VII, IX, and X) are particularly sensitive to impaired hepatocyte function and are, therefore, often found in decreased concentrations in plasma, even in patients with mild liver diseases. Excess bleeding, however, is not apt to occur until the concentration of coagulation factors is < 10-30% of normal.

Other bleeding and clotting problems may also be encountered in cirrhosis.[50] Splenomegaly, which often develops because of the increased portal pressure present in cirrhosis, may cause thrombocytopenia; hyperbilirubinemia, which may be present, can also alter platelet function. Heparin infusions in patients with severe liver disease have been shown to increase fibrinogen levels transiently, suggesting that chronic, low-grade DIC may contribute to decreased fibrinogen. These patients may also develop hyperfibrinolysis, either of the primary type (i.e., not associated with DIC) or of the secondary type (associated with DIC).[50]

AXIOM   Severe liver disease can cause thrombocytopenia, increased fibrinolysis, and decreased production of most coagulation factors, except FVIII:C and vWF, so that a DIC-like clinical picture can be produced.

The liver is also important in clearing blood of activated metabolites of both fibrinolysis and coagulation.[50] Therefore, although the altered coagulation system in cirrhosis usually causes increased bleeding, an increased tendency toward coagulation may also be evident, producing a low-grade, consumptive coagulopathy.

Diagnosis

A strong alcohol history or clinical evidence of cirrhosis should alert one to the possibility of bleeding and clotting abnormalities due to advanced liver disease. In the laboratory, liver disease is commonly associated with low fibrinogen levels, prolonged PTs, and normal or slightly increased APTTs (Table 45–6).[50]

Vitamin-K-dependent factors are usually decreased in cirrhosis before other defects become apparent. Of these, Factor VII is most sensitive, causing prolonged PTs.[50] TCT may be prolonged due to severe hypofibrinogenemia, abnormal or dysfunctional fibrinogen molecules, or elevated FSPs. Elevated D-dimer levels suggest the presence of DIC.

Treatment

AXIOM   When coagulation tests are abnormal in patients with liver disease, little or no improvement may be evident after vitamin K injection, even after 24-48 hours.

Vitamin K therapy should be instituted for any coagulation abnormality believed to be due to liver disease, but this may not be reflected in any improvement in the PT for at least 24-48 hours.[83] Therefore, severe, acute bleeding problems in patients with liver failure should also be treated with FFP. Because Factor VII has the short-

TABLE 45–6   Laboratory Tests in Patients with Severe Liver Cirrhosis

Clotting System		Fibrinolytic System		Platelets	
PT	↑			Bleeding time	↑
APTT	↑	Plasminogen	↓	Platelet counts	↓
TCT	↑	α2-antiplasmin	↓	Adhesion	↓
		t-PA	N	Aggregation	↓
		u-PA	N		
		PAI-1	N – ↑		
Factor II, VII,					
X, IX	↓	FSP	↑		
vWF	↑	D-Dimer	↑		
Factor VIII	↑				
Other factors	↓				
Fibrinogen	↓				
Antithrombin	↓				
Protein C	↓				
Protein S	↓				

↑ = elevated or prolonged, ↓ = decreased or shortened, N = normal.
Modified from Mammen EF. Clin Lab Med 1994;14:769.

est half-life (6 hours), the least amount of FFP necessary to restore adequate levels of Factor VII is about 10 mL/kg every 6 hours.

> **AXIOM**   In patients with severe liver dysfunction, large volumes of FFP may be required to maintain normal factor levels.[3]

In addition to an initial 4-8 units of FFP, up to 2 units of additional FFP may be needed every two hours in patients with severe liver failure to maintain adequate coagulation factor levels, to normalize clotting tests, and to control excessive bleeding. When thrombocytopenia is also present, platelet concentrates may have to be given along with FFP, particularly if the patient is actively bleeding.[50]

When the volume of FFP needed would cause fluid overload, prothrombin complex concentrates (Konyne, Proplex, FEIBA) may be suitable alternatives, but their use should be undertaken with great caution because these agents have an increased risk of causing thromboembolic problems and, occasionally, even DIC.

> **AXIOM**   Although cirrhotic patients frequently have severe factor deficiencies, excessive bleeding after trauma is usually primarily because of concomitant thrombocytopenia.

When oozing persists after deficiencies in the coagulation factors and/or platelets have been corrected, intravenous DDAVP may be administered.[42] Studies have shown that the prolonged BTs frequently seen in cirrhotic patients can be improved by administration of DDAVP. In a controlled, randomized clinical study, DDAVP significantly shortened BTs in 21 cirrhotic patients.[51]

If a bleeding cirrhotic patient were found to have hypofibrinogenemia, especially with associated excessive fibrinolysis, therapy with EACA (Amicar) may be considered; however, this must be done with great care, and one must be sure that no evidence of ongoing intravascular clotting exists (i.e., D-dimers must be negative).[51]

> **AXIOM**   The use of EACA in cirrhotic patients who are bleeding excessively should be discouraged because these patients often have a consumption coagulopathy, in which case EACA would be contraindicated.[50]

RENAL FAILURE

Severe renal disease with BUN levels > 100 mg/dL can cause a reversible bleeding disorder largely related to platelet dysfunction.[3] Although no reliable correlation exists between BUN levels and bleeding tendencies, prolonged bleeding times often return to normal following dialysis.

> **AXIOM**   Increased bleeding due to a qualitative platelet problem (thrombocytopathy) can be expected in most patients with severe uremia.

The precise mechanism by which renal insufficiency causes thrombocytopathy is not known, but phenol and guanidine derivatives, which tend to be retained in uremic patients, can impair platelet aggregation and platelet adhesiveness.[52] Cryoprecipitate infusions may improve platelet function in these patients.[53] Although hemodialysis eliminates the thrombocytopathy of uremia, this procedure cannot usually be done in the presence of severe, ongoing bleeding. In such circumstances, transfusion of platelet concentrates may be necessary as an emergency; however, because these patients may develop antibodies against platelets, infusion of these concentrates must be clearly indicated. More recently, intravenous infusion of DDAVP was shown to be helpful in decreasing bleeding problems in these patients.[54] The effects of DDAVP 0.4 mcg/kg intravenously in uremic patients include shortened BTs, increased platelet retention on glass beads, and increased Factor VIII/vWF activity.

Conjugated estrogen appears to have effects like DDAVP, but the duration of its effects may be longer. In one report, the effectiveness of conjugated estrogen (Premarin®) was studied in six chronic dialysis patients with persistently prolonged BTs and histories of clinical bleeding.[55] BTs shortened in all six, and returned to normal in four. The maximal effect was noted at 2-9 days and persisted for a variable period after the medication was stopped. The doses of conjugated estrogen ranged from 10-50 mg/day.

VITAMIN K DEFICIENCY

> **AXIOM**   Vitamin K deficiency can be anticipated in patients with chronic, severe biliary tract obstruction or malabsorption.

Many of the inactive factors (proenzymes) of the coagulation system are serine proteases and contain glutamic acid residues, which provide carboxy groups to act as binding sites for calcium. Vitamin K is necessary for carboxylase to attach carboxy groups to glutamic acids. The proteins containing carboxyglutamic acid residues are, therefore, called vitamin-K-dependent factors. When they are synthesized in the absence of vitamin K, these proteins lack carboxyglutamic acid residues and, consequently, cannot bind calcium properly.[50] Oral anticoagulants (coumarin or indandione derivatives) have essentially the same effects as vitamin K deficiency.

Causes of vitamin K deficiency include inadequate dietary intake, malabsorption, lack of bile salts, obstructive jaundice, biliary fistulas, oral administration of antibiotics, and parenteral alimentation.[3] A number of newer broad-spectrum antibiotics, including cefoperozone, moxalactam, cefamandole, and ceftizoxime, can also cause a vitamin-K-dependent coagulopathy with decreased levels of Factors II, VII, IX, and X.[56] Consequently, APTT and PT will be abnormal. Other screening tests will also be normal (Table 45–7).[50]

> **AXIOM**   Coagulation defects due to pure vitamin K deficiency are partially corrected by intravenous vitamin K within 6-12 hours unless coincident liver dysfunction exists.

TABLE 45–7   Laboratory Tests in Patients with Vitamin K deficiency

PT	↑	Protein C	↓
APTT	↑	Protein S	↓
TCT	N	All other factors normal	
Factor VII	↓		
Factor X	↓		
Factor IX	↓		
Factor II	↓		

Modified from Mammen EF. Clin Lab Med 1994;14:769.

The initial treatment of vitamin K deficiency may be its administration in a dose up to 5 mg given slowly intravenously. Previous preparations of vitamin K were less purified than those used presently, and anaphylaxis and death were occasionally reported with intravenous administration of the older agents.[3] The more purified forms are less likely to cause complications, but intravenous vitamin K should be given selectively, considering this possibility.

Intramuscular vitamin K is effective when given in adequate doses (25 mg), and repeated doses of 25 mg intramuscularly for three days allows total body repletion. In acutely bleeding patients, administration of FFP generally corrects the coagulation deficit rapidly and should be given in addition to vitamin K.[50] Prothrombin complex concentrates should be used with caution because of potential thrombogenicity.

USE OF ANTICOAGULANTS

Coumarin Derivatives

Coumarin derivatives block the proper synthesis of vitamin-K-dependent coagulation factors.[50] Coumarins prolong PTs and also cause prolongation of the APTTs by reducing the levels of prothrombin (Factor II) and Factors VII, IX, and X. Coumadin has a half-life of 40 hours. Such therapy should be stopped at least 48 hours before surgery, which should be performed only when the PT has returned to within 3.0 seconds of control. In acute situations, administration of both vitamin K and FFP can rapidly reverse the effects of coumarins. Vitamin K can be given in doses of 2.5-5.0 mg intravenously or 25 mg intramuscularly. It generally takes at least 12-24 hours for intravenous vitamin K to become effective. In the meantime, ≥ 4-8 units of FFP may be required to promptly restore PTs to normal.[43]

AXIOM   Treatment of severe, active bleeding which is due either to Coumadin administration or to vitamin K deficiency should include intravenous vitamin K and at least 4-8 units of FFP.

The effect of coumarins can be potentiated by a large number of drugs (e.g., acetaminophen, heparin, phenytoin, alcohol, metronidazole, and cimetidine), and disease states (Table 45–8), such as congestive heart failure and hepatic disease.[57] Some of the drugs that inhibit the effects of Coumadin on blood coagulation include barbiturates, corticosteroids, estrogen, and alcohol. Hypothyroidism also inhibits the effects of Coumadin.

TABLE 45–8   Drugs or Disease States that Affect Warfarin Action

Potentiation
Drugs
  Androgens, chloral hydrate, chloramphenicol, clofibrate, glucagon, indomethacin, neomycin, acetaminophen, allopurinol, diazoxide, disulfiram, ethacrynic acid, heparin, 6-mercaptopurine, α-methyldopa, MAO inhibitors, nalidixic acid, sulfinpyrazone, thyroid drugs, tolbutamide, sulfa drugs, phenylbutazone, phenytoin, quinidine, salicylates, thyroxine, alcohol, anesthetics, metronidazole, and cimetidine.
Disease States
  Collagen vascular disorders, congestive heart failure, hepatitis, hyperthyroidism, vitamin-K-deficient diet, malignancy, malabsorption, and narcotic abuse.
Inhibition
Drugs
  Barbiturates, glutethimide, griseofulvin, haloperidol, corticosteroids, estrogens, meprobamate, colchicine, rifampin, tetracyclines, carbamazepine, alcohol, and cholestyramine.
Disease States
  Hereditary resistance to coumadin; hypothyroidism.

Modified from[57]

Heparin

PHYSIOLOGIC EFFECTS.   Heparin has multiple effects on hemostasis:

1. By combining with antithrombin III, it can rapidly inhibit the actions of thrombin and Factor Xa.
2. In the presence of antithrombin III, heparin can inhibit activation of Factor X. This is its most sensitive and immediate effect and is the basis for "minidose" therapy to prevent deep venous thrombosis during or after many types of surgery. Prolongation of TCT is seen before any effect on APTTs occurs.
3. In slightly larger doses, haparin can block other factors, especially Factor XIIa (enzymes) causing prolongation of the APTT.
4. In large doses, heparin can decrease platelet adhesiveness and aggregation.

Heparin has a dose-dependent mean plasma half-life of 60-90 minutes. A dose of heparin is normally almost completely cleared from the blood in 6 hours, but this time can be greatly prolonged by hepatic dysfunction, hypothermia, or shock. Twenty-five percent of administered heparin is excreted unchanged in the urine.[58]

AXIOM   Reduced plasma levels of antithrombin (because of liver disease or excessive clotting) can greatly increase the amount of heparin needed to prolong APTT.

All coagulation tests can be affected by heparin, including PTs, but APTT is usually more sensitive and thus the most frequently used test. The effect of heparin on TCT should be distinguished from other causes of coagulopathy, such as circulating FSP.

When a patient has excessive bleeding from an unknown cause and the TCT is prolonged, a reptilase time should be performed. A normal reptilase time indicates heparin effect, and a prolonged value indicates increased FSP or other reasons. Alternatively, some laboratories add toluidine blue or other heparin-removing compounds, such as protamine, to the blood sample in order to inactivate any heparin that may be present before repeating the TCT or APTT.

NEUTRALIZATION OF HEPARIN.   Because heparin is a strong, negatively charged anion, it can be neutralized with intravenous protamine sulfate, which is a strong, positively charged cation. Protamine (1.0 mg) can neutralize 100 units of heparin, which is equivalent to about 1.0 mg of heparin. The dose of protamine given should be approximately equal to the dose of heparin given, with allowance made for the half-life of heparin. For every 30 minutes after heparin has been given, the amount of protamine needed is reduced by about half.[57] Because it can have significant vasodilator and negative inotropic effects, protamine should be given slowly, and the patient should be monitored carefully to avoid hypotension or an excessive dosage of protamine which, by itself, can cause excessive bleeding. During cardiopulmonary bypass, the adequacy of the heparin dose and later reversal is often monitored by the activated clotting time (ACT). An ACT of 80-150 seconds usually indicates adequate reversal of the heparin effect.

HEPARIN-INDUCED THROMBOCYTOPENIA.   One of the important side effects of heparin is heparin-induced thrombocytopenia (HIT) syndrome which can be severe in up to 6% of patients; occasionally, it can cause paradoxical arterial thromboses. The likelihood of HIT is independent of the route of administration; however, the source of heparin does affect the frequency of this problem.[59] Thrombocytopenia is seen more frequently with bovine lung heparin than with porcine intestinal mucosa heparin.

AXIOM   Platelet counts should be carefully monitored whenever heparin is given.

A 30% decrease in platelet count within 24 hours of starting heparin or the development of arterial vascular occlusion while on heparin is suggestive of HIT. This usually occurs about 6-12 days after the initiation of heparin therapy, but it may occur at any time throughout the course of its use, particularly with repeated courses of heparin. Platelet-associated immunoglobulin has been implicated as the cause of heparin-induced thrombocytopenia. Although severe forms of HIT and particularly the thrombotic complications are believed to be immune-mediated, the immunoglobulin is not a universal finding. Patients with heparin-induced thrombocytopenia should avoid a similar type (bovine lung or porcine intestine) of heparin when retreatment is required and certain low-molecular weight (LMW) heparins may be considered as an alternative.[60]

AXIOM When a patient requiring anticoagulation develops HIT syndrome, oral anticoagulants should be begun and heparin stopped immediately.

Drug-induced Thrombocytopathy

AXIOM Thrombocytopathy can be confirmed by in vitro tests or by finding a prolonged BT in spite of a platelet count > 100 × 10⁹/L.

Many drugs can interfere with platelet function (Table 45–9). Some drugs that are more frequent causes of thrombocytopathy include chemotherapeutic agents, thiazide diuretics, alcohol, estrogen, antibiotics (especially sulfas), quinidine, quinine, methyldopa, and gold salts.[61] The most common drugs that block platelet function, however, are probably the prostaglandin inhibitors, particularly aspirin, indomethacin, and other nonsteroidal antiinflammatory drugs (NSAID).[62]

AXIOM Aspirin causes permanent impaired function of all platelets exposed to it (up to 10-12 days).

Aspirin blocks prostaglandin metabolism in the platelet by permanently acetylating cyclooxygenase. Affected platelets remain dysfunctional throughout their 10-12-day lifespan after exposure to aspirin.[62] By acetylating platelet surface proteins, aspirin also interferes with platelet adhesion to collagen.[2] As little as 80 mg of aspirin can depress platelet aggregation and prolong BTs for at least 72 hours. Simultaneous alcohol ingestion can have a profound potentiating effect on platelet dysfunction caused by aspirin. NSAIDs, such as ibuprofen have a similar, but reversible, effect (for about 6-12 hours) on platelet aggregation; however, emergency surgery may not allow enough time for spontaneous reversal of the thrombocytopathy.[62]

Patients who have ingested aspirin or NSAIDs within 72 hours of surgery should probably have BTs performed. If the BT is abnormal, the urgency of surgery dictates whether delay is advisable until BT returns to normal; DDAVP often can normalize prolonged BT caused by renal disease or aspirin.

AXIOM Platelet transfusions are indicated in patients who develop abnormal bleeding due to thrombocytopenia or thrombocytopathy during emergency major surgery.[2]

TABLE 45–9 *Commonly Used Medications Associated with Clinically Significant Disorders of Hemostasis*

Aspirin
Phenylbutazone
Indomethacin
Dipyridamole
Sulfinpyrazone
Dextran
Hydroxyethyl starch
Heparin
Dicumarol and warfarin

From[2]

Thrombolytic Agents

Streptokinase, urokinase, and tissue-type plasminogen activator (t-PA) can be administered directly into the circulation to accelerate the conversion of plasminogen to plasmin so as to produce lysis of unwanted, fresh fibrin clots.[63] Most patients receiving these agents are hospitalized, but occasionally patients with severe, accidental trauma develop extensive, lifethreatening thromboses that may not be readily treated surgically. Following trauma isolated to the extremities > 10-14 days earlier, these agents may be used occasionally to treat acute, severe pulmonary embolism.

AXIOM The use of thrombolytic agents is generally contraindicated in patients with recent trauma or fresh surgical wounds.

THROMBOCYTOPENIAS

Pathophysiology

Normal platelet counts range from 150-400 × 10⁹/L. A platelet count of 100 × 10⁹/L is safe for almost all types of surgery. A platelet count of < 100 × 10⁹/L, however, which is defined as thrombocytopenia often prolongs BT, depending on how low the platelet count is. With platelet counts of 50-100 × 10⁹/L, slightly increased bleeding may occur after injury or surgery, but spontaneous bleeding is uncommon. Patients with platelet counts of 30-50 × 10⁹/L generally do not display major hemorrhagic diathesis as long as the platelets present are normal; however, spontaneous bleeding should be anticipated with sudden reductions in platelet count to < 10-20 × 10⁹/L.[3]

AXIOM Platelet counts < 20 × 10⁹/L can cause moderate-to-severe spontaneous bleeding.

Severe platelet defects often lead to spontaneous bleeding into the skin, manifested by petechiae, purpura, or confluent ecchymoses. Thrombocytopenia can also cause spontaneous mucosal bleeding (such as epistaxis or GI, GU, or vaginal bleeding) or excessive bleeding after trauma or surgery. Heavy GI bleeding and bleeding into the central nervous system may occasionally be life-threatening manifestations of a severe thrombocytopenia.

AXIOM Thrombocytopenia does not usually cause massive bleeding into tissues or joints.

Etiology

Thrombocytopenia may be due to decreased platelet production in the bone marrow or increased peripheral platelet destruction. Decreased platelet production may be caused by drugs, chemicals, or myeloproliferative diseases, while increased peripheral destruction may result from consumption, splenomegaly, autoantibodies, isoantibodies, anaphylactic reactions, drugs, and some infections.

A large number of drugs can cause thrombocytopenia.[61] Some of the more frequent causative agents include quinidine, sulfa preparations, oral antidiabetic agents, gold salts, rifampin, and heparin. Other important points in the history that may be associated with thrombocytopenia include recent blood transfusions (e.g., posttransfusion purpura), heavy alcohol consumption (causing alcohol-induced thrombocytopenia), and symptoms of underlying immunologic disease (e.g., arthralgia, Raynaud's phenomenon, unexplained fever, etc.).[61]

Patients with malignancies frequently have chronic DIC with thrombocytopenia which may get much worse during or after surgery. Patients with burns may develop excessive bleeding for a variety of reasons, including DIC, reduced concentrations of coagulation factors due to protein loss, thrombocytopenia due to increased consumption, and thrombocytopathy related to antibiotics.

The most frequent cause of excessive bleeding after open heart surgery is thrombocytopenia combined with thrombocytopathy. Platelets are consumed during bypass, and many of the drugs given can impair the function of those that remain in the circulation.[64] Hyperfibrinolysis and heparin rebound are also possible, but they are relatively uncommon causes of excess bleeding after cardiopulmonary bypass.

Diagnosis

The presence or absence of fever is important in developing a differential diagnosis for the etiology of thrombocytopenia. Fever is usually present in thrombocytopenia due to infection, active systemic lupus erythematosus (SLE) or in thrombotic thrombocytopenic purpura (TTP); however, fever is usually absent in idiopathic thrombocytopenic purpura (ITP) and drug-related thrombocytopenias.[3]

The size of the spleen on physical examination may also be important diagnostically. The spleen is not palpably enlarged in most thrombocytopenias caused by increased platelet destruction (such as with DIC, ITP, drug-related immune thrombocytopenias, or TTP), whereas it usually is palpably enlarged in patients with thrombocytopenia secondary to increased splenic sequestration of platelets, and it is often enlarged in patients with thrombocytopenia due to lymphoma or myeloproliferative disorders.

Peripheral blood count is an important diagnostic test not only to establish the presence and severity of thrombocytopenia, but also to gather clues to its cause.[3] Platelet size should be noted; an increased proportion of large (young) platelets (determined by scanning the blood smear or by measuring mean platelet volume with an electronic blood counter) suggests compensatory increased platelet production and early release from the marrow into the bloodstream. An increased proportion of large platelets is often found in thrombocytopenias secondary to increased destruction or utilization of platelets.

Thrombocytopenia can cause disturbed primary hemostasis, defective secondary hemostasis (due to the unavailability of platelet Factor 3), and impaired clot retraction.[1] In general, thrombocytopenia does not cause a bleeding disorder when $30\text{-}50 \times 10^9/L$ or more normally functioning platelets are present; however, BT is routinely prolonged in severe thrombocytopenia or thrombocytopathy of any cause. Bone marrow aspirate may also be helpful for determining the cause of thrombocytopenia.

PITFALL ⊘

One should not assume that patients with platelet counts > $50 \times 10^9/L$ cannot have bleeding due to platelet problems.

Treatment

Management of thrombocytopenia secondary to decreased platelet production is directed toward attempting to correct its cause (e.g., to induce remission in acute leukemia).[3] Platelet concentrates can be given to increase the platelet count temporarily; however, repeated platelet transfusions can cause increased production of platelet autoantibodies, which can greatly reduce the life expectancy of subsequently transfused platelets. When rapid correction of bone marrow failure is not expected, platelet transfusions are usually reserved for treatment of active bleeding. Corticosteroids have not proved beneficial in the management of patients with thrombocytopenia secondary to bone marrow failure.[3]

AXIOM One should avoid transfusing platelets in patients with thrombocytopenia associated with autoantibodies unless the patient is bleeding significantly.

VASCULAR ABNORMALITIES

Vascular factors can act to reduce blood flow at a site of trauma by: (a) local vasoconstriction, and (b) compression by blood extravasated into surrounding tissues.[3] Bleeding disorders are rarely secondary to vessel-wall abnormalities; however, severe infections, such as meningococcemia, typhoid fever, and subacute bacterial endocarditis, can cause abnormal platelet function, coagulation defects, vascular defects, and hemorrhage. Severe vitamin C deficiency can lead to petechial hemorrhages. Excessive endogenous or exogenous steroids can cause breakdown of small blood vessels. In Henoch-Schönlein purpura, senile purpura, and hereditary hemorrhagic telangiectasia, the blood vessels are fragile and tissues throughout the body can bruise or bleed excessively with little or no trauma.[61]

PARAPROTEINEMIAS

Diseases, such as Waldenström macroglobulinemia, cryoglobulinemia, multiple myeloma, and hypergammaglobulinemia, which cause the formation of abnormal proteins, occasionally result in defects in primary and secondary hemostasis.[1] Coating of platelets by abnormal proteins may interfere with aggregation and cause prolonged BT. Secondary hemostasis may also be impaired on the basis of abnormal fibrin formation due to disturbed polymerization of fibrin monomers.[1] Paraproteinemias can also cause abnormal TCT and, when the defect is severe, the APTT and PT may also be abnormal. Therapy is difficult, but platelet concentrates, FFP, and/or purified fibrinogen, when available, may be helpful during bleeding episodes or after trauma.[61]

CIRCULATING ANTICOAGULANTS

Immune antibodies against coagulation factors can be found in patients who have been treated for congenital coagulopathies and in previously healthy individuals after blood or plasma transfusions.[52] Most of these antibodies are directed against Factor VIII:C, but other clotting factors, including vWF, may also be inhibited by immune antibodies. Because of the severity and complexity of the problem of immune antibodies against clotting factors, these patients should, when possible, be referred to centers experienced in their management.[1]

Intra- or Postoperatively Acquired Bleeding Disorders

PITFALL ⊘

If it is assumed that excessive bleeding after trauma or during surgery is due to a coagulation abnormality, attempts to obtain good local hemostasis are apt to be less vigorous.

Occasionally, severe hemostatic defects develop during or immediately following surgery in patients with no known prior bleeding problem or hemostatic defect (Table 45–10);[1] however, in such circumstances, excessive hemorrhage, especially when limited to the operative site, is usually due to open vessels and should be corrected surgically by suturing, ligation, or coagulation of open vessels.

TABLE 45–10 Bleeding in the Trauma Patient[3]

Problem	Treatment
Mechanical bleeding	Emergency operation
Massive transfusion	Correct pH, rewarm, resuscitate Platelet infusion Fresh frozen plasma (?) DDAVP, cryoprecipitate
Transfusion reaction	Stop transfusion Volume load, mannitol, HCO_3
Disseminated intravascular coagulation	Correct cause, resuscitate Platelets, FFP, cryoprecipitate
Hepatic or renal disease	Careful supportive care DDAVP, cryoprecipitate, platelets, FFP
Anticoagulant	Stop drug, reverse drug Vitamin K, protamine
Congenital coagulopathy	Replace specific factors Beware of inhibitors

TRAUMA AND ITS EFFECT ON COAGULATION

Trauma in General

Platelets and damaged tissue release procoagulatory substances, such as thromboxane, epinephrine, and serotonin, which can contribute to local vasoconstriction.[65] With the widespread distribution of tissue thromboplastin in the body, one would expect tissue trauma to accelerate clotting. Acidosis and ischemia also tend to shorten clotting times; however, all of these processes tend to consume coagulation factors and thereby cause subsequent increased bleeding. Thus, it is not surprising that patients with only mild-to-moderate injury usually have normal PT and APTT findings; however, in more severely injured patients, PT and APTT are often prolonged and usually take at least 4-6 hours to return to normal.[3]

The extent of soft-tissue damage in animals can often be directly correlated with the degree of depression of fibrinogen levels during the first six hours after trauma.[65] This is usually followed by a rebound hyperfibrinogenemia. Trauma to both femurs in dogs causes consumption of coagulation factors and increased fibrinolytic activity. Because these changes can be prevented by administration of heparin, it is clear that coagulation is taking place. This is followed in 24 hours by inhibition of fibrinolysis and a rebound increase in fibrinogen levels. This biphasic change is often seen in trauma, and is usually manifested by an initial decrease in plasma levels of fibrinogen and other clotting factors which is then followed by sustained hyperfibrinogenemia. Clinical studies in injured humans indicate the same type of response.[66,67]

The extent of these coagulation abnormalities appears to increase with the severity of injury.[2] For example, the levels of the two most important inhibitors of coagulation, antithrombin III and α_2-antiplasmin, are lowest in patients with the most severe injuries.[68,69] Patients with ISS scores > 25 also tend to develop significant immune and coagulation abnormalities.

Factors II, V, VII, and X are generally 70-90% of normal after trauma.[2] Factor VIII:C and vWF are usually also decreased to some extent. The decrease in vWF may contribute to increased bleeding after major injury or surgery because DDAVP, which increases plasma levels of vWF, has been shown to reduce blood loss in this situation.[70]

In studies of deaths following injury, patients with the most severe injuries almost invariably had the most abnormal coagulation studies.[2] Up to 50% of the patients with the most severe injuries had signs of abnormal bleeding with oozing from multiple sites and hematoma formation not associated with vascular injury. The most frequently abnormal test is often the PT. In one series, 97% of patients had abnormal PTs, 72% had abnormal platelet counts, and 70% had abnormal APTTs.[66] The greatest degree of coagulation abnormality tended to occur in patients with head injury, followed by those with gunshot wounds, blunt trauma, and stab wounds to other tissues. Patients with the most severe coagulation defects after trauma also tended to develop more organ dysfunction and stay in the ICU for longer periods of time. After severe, multiple trauma, marked changes in the serum lipid profile can also occur, and it has been suggested that these changes may be associated with inhibition of fibrinolysis.[71]

Blood levels of the plasma antiproteases, especially antithrombin III, decrease with trauma because of increased activation of the clotting system, and the extent of the decrease usually correlates with the severity of the injuries.[68,69] The resulting low antithrombin levels cause an increased tendency for thrombosis and intravascular coagulation which can further increase the tendency for multiple organ failure (MOF).

> **AXIOM** Severe antithrombin deficiencies in sepsis increase the tendency for DIC and MOF.

Trauma and sepsis can also activate Factor XII through the effect of high-molecular-weight kininogen.[72] Factor XIIa, in turn, can activate the coagulation, kinin, complement, and fibrinolytic systems. Plasmin-generated fragments of Factor XIIa can convert prekallikrein to kallikrein which, in turn, can convert kininogens to kinins (including bradykinin and myocardial depressant factor). They also activate complement C1, C3, and C5. Factor XIIa fragments may also act as substitutes for Factor D in the alternate complement pathway.

In addition to increasing plasma levels of FSPs, major injuries also cause platelet counts to decrease.[73] In survivors, these parameters normalize in the first few days following injury. In contrast, in patients who eventually die, these factors are more abnormal initially, and they tend to become even more abnormal over the next several days prior to death.

> **AXIOM** High and progressively increasing levels of FSP after trauma are a poor prognostic sign.

Plasminogen concentrations are often depressed immediately after major injury, indicating increased fibrinolysis, but they quickly return to normal, often within 24 hours, in patients with less severe injuries.[74] With most severe injuries, fibrinolytic activity and fibrinogen levels may not return to normal until five or more days after injury, even when the hospital course is otherwise uncomplicated.[67]

Patients with septic or traumatic shock may show severe and sustained reductions in plasma levels of coagulation factors because of increased consumption and a decreased ability to produce clotting factors.[71,75] Much of the response in trauma results from utilization of platelets and clotting factors for hemostasis at sites of injury.

Hypercoagulability immediately after trauma may be caused by a number of mechanisms.[2] As already noted, many tissues contain thromboplastin, which is released into the bloodstream when tissue injury occurs.[66] Epinephrine released during stress also decreases clotting times.[76] As noted earlier, this initial hypercoagulability can cause increased consumption of platelets and coagulation factors, and this can then cause hypocoagulability. It has recently been demonstrated that surgery itself activates the hemostasis system in vivo and the extent of this activation is dependent on the severity of trauma inflicted during the procedure.[77]

Head Injury

> **AXIOM** The brain has the highest tissue thromboplastin concentration of any of the body's organs.[78]

Release of thromboplastin into the bloodstream initiates coagulation and, consequently, brain injury may cause a greatly increased tendency for intravascular coagulation. Head injury lowers PAI-1 levels and increases plasma levels of fibrinopeptide A (FpA) and fibrinopeptide B (FpB).[3] As with other types of trauma, fibrinogen and antithrombin III levels are moderately decreased for several days.[78] DIC is not unusual after primary brain damage and is associated with extremely high FpA and FpB levels and low PAI-1 levels and platelet counts.

> **AXIOM** Severe derangements of clotting can occur after major head injuries due to initiation of widespread intravascular coagulation.

Head-injured patients in general have increased consumption of coagulation factors and lower platelet counts than do patients with extracranial trauma.[66] Head injury can also cause a dramatic catecholamine release from the adrenals, and this can cause a variety of complications, including hypercoagulability, arrhythmias, hypertension, and myocardial necrosis.[79] Although this response is believed to be primarily from activation of the adrenal medulla, stimulation of the anterior hypothalamus can induce hypercoagulability in adrenalectomized animals, suggesting that other mediators can also be involved.[2]

Causes of Nonmechanical Posttraumatic Bleeding

THROMBOCYTOPENIA

Studies from Harborview Medical Center by Reed et al. suggested that thrombocytopenia and platelet dysfunction are the major causes of microvascular (nonmechanical) bleeding (MVB) after massive transfusions.[80] A prospective, randomized, double-blind clinical study compared the prophylactic effects of 6 units of platelet concentrates versus 2 units of FFP administered with every 12 units of modified whole blood in patients undergoing massive transfusions (12 or more units in 12 hours). Three of 17 patients who received platelet transfusions and three of 16 patients who received FFP developed MVB. Regression lines of the platelet counts versus the units of blood during massive transfusions were essentially the same in those who were transfused with platelets and those who were not. Only one patient had MVB that appeared to be due to dilutional thrombocytopenia.

> **AXIOM** Prophylactic administration of FFP or platelets does not appear to be warranted routinely in patients receiving massive blood transfusions.[80,81]

Two types of platelet concentrates are available: (a) single unit, random-donor platelet concentrate is produced from a single unit of blood within six hours of collection, (b) multiple unit, single-donor platelet concentrate is removed by mechanical apheresis from one donor. Each collection has as many platelets as 6-10 single units. This product may be obtained from the patient's family members or from donors of known HLA-type to yield HLA-matched platelets.[3]

Some general indications for platelet transfusion include:

1. Platelet counts $< 20 \times 10^9$/L.
2. Patients who are actively bleeding or who are going to surgery and have platelet counts $< 50\text{-}60 \times 10^9$/L.
3. Patients who are actively bleeding and have had a precipitous decrease in platelet counts.
4. Patients with BTs longer than 15 minutes (regardless of the platelet count) who are actively bleeding or are about to undergo a surgical procedure.
5. Patients who have required more than 10 units of blood during a major operation and have nonmechanical bleeding.
6. Children whose transfused blood volume exceeds their normal blood volume and have non-mechanical bleeding.
7. Patients whose time on the pump for open-heart surgery has exceeded 2 hours.
8. Open-heart surgery on pediatric patients weighing < 20 kg.

In general, platelet transfusions are contraindicated in patients with a diagnosis of TTP, posttransfusion purpura (PTP), or HIT.

> **AXIOM** In addition to observing the hemostatic response after platelet transfusions, platelet counts should be performed at 1, 12, and 24 hours.[3]

Depending on the clinical situation, the platelet count at 1 hour should have increased by at least 5×10^9/L (usually 10×10^9/L) for each unit of platelets transfused. Less than that expected increase suggests that the patient may have antibodies to platelets. If the patient is rapidly consuming platelets because of bleeding, sepsis, or DIC, the platelet count will be much lower at 12 and 24 hours.[3]

REDUCED CLOTTING FACTORS

Fresh Frozen Plasma

Protocols for control of bleeding in patients with congenital clotting factor deficiencies have been determined accurately; however, the same precision cannot be expected when dealing with patients who have shock or sepsis, have received multiple blood transfusions, and/or are actively bleeding.[2]

FFP has been advocated by some as a resuscitation fluid in patients with head injury to prevent the development of abnormal coagulation.[3] Although several studies have demonstrated that patients with traumatic brain injury have a tendency to develop DIC because of the massive release of tissue thromboplastin, review of 149 head-injured patients with Glasgow Coma Scale Scores of 9 or less showed no difference between patients receiving FFP and those who did not.[81]

DDAVP

DDAVP may be especially useful in patients with isolated prolongation of BT with normal platelet counts, platelet aggregation, and coagulation parameters (including vWF) and without evidence of liver or kidney disease or exposure to antiplatelet agents.[3] Uremia is one of the established indications for the use of DDAVP because it often dramatically shortens the BT and controls hemorrhage.[3] Hepatic cirrhosis and acquired platelet dysfunctions are other indications for its use. It can be given intravenously, intranasally, or subcutaneously. BT often improves within 30 minutes following a DDAVP infusion, resulting in either satisfactory arrest of acute bleeding or good control of subsequent hemostasis during surgery.[82] However, the compound is often ineffective in patients with thrombocytopenia or congenital platelet dysfunction.[83]

Recent studies have confirmed that low levels of vWF associated with increased bleeding after injury or surgery may be increased by administration of DDAVP. In a report by Salzman et al., 70 patients undergoing major cardiac surgery received either a placebo or DDAVP.[84] The treated patients had significantly less postoperative blood loss. Other controlled clinical trials have also shown that DDAVP can improve abnormal BTs and reduce transfusion requirements following cardiopulmonary bypass surgery.[85] It also appears that the subcutaneous route of administration for DDAVP (mainly in the concentrated pharmaceutical formulation) can be particularly useful in treating mild Factor VIII:C deficiencies, even on self and home-treatment bases.[82]

DDAVP has a pronounced effect on coagulation and fibrinolytic parameters, causing a fourfold increase in vWF and an almost twofold increase in t-PA.[3] It also increases protein C concentrations. The increased Factor VIII:C levels are associated with a significant shortening in APTT. DDAVP also shortens BT in most patients.[86]

In 37 patients with prolonged BT, where thrombocytopenia, vWD, or deficiency of other coagulation factors could be excluded, the effect of a DDAVP-infusion (0.2 mcg/kg) together with the antifibrinolytic agent tranexamic acid (10 mg/kg) normalized BTs in 27 patients and partially corrected BTs in three others.[87] Among the patients in whom DDAVP was effective, this drug was later successfully used as an alternative to blood products in eight patients during and after surgery or delivery.

Side effects with DDAVP are usually transient and minor (i.e., facial flushing, conjunctival erythema, increases in heart rate, or mild headache can occur transiently during infusion).[85] DDAVP should be given with caution to patients with atherosclerosis because of reports of thrombosis.[83] It has also been found that DDAVP infusion may exacerbate the hypercoagulable state observed in surgical patients without preventing the postoperative fibrinolytic shutdown.[86] Although it is said to have 2000 times the antidiuretic effect that natural arginine vasopressin has, DDAVP seems to have caused few clinical problems in this regard.

HYPOTHERMIA

> **AXIOM** Hypothermia is one of the most common causes of altered coagulation in trauma.[3]

Shock, alcohol intoxication, massive fluid and blood infusions, exposure to cold, and prolonged surgery predispose trauma patients to hypothermia.[2] Trauma patients most apt to develop bleeding problems are those who are most seriously injured and most hypothermic. In one study, hemorrhage accounted for 90% of deaths occurring within 48 hours of abdominal injury, and at least half of those deaths were associated with a coagulopathy.[88]

The effects of decreased body temperature on clotting function result from several mechanisms, including: (a) altered platelet number, morphology, function, and sequestration, (b) increased fibrinolysis, and (c) retardation of enzyme systems involved in the initiation and propagation of clot formation.[89] These changes are reversible upon rewarming. Hypothermia may also induce DIC by producing cell injury and subsequent thromboplastin release and by causing tissue hypoxia because of a depressed cardiac output.[2] Hypothermia has also been associated with hepatic dysfunction and increased blood citrate levels following massive transfusions.

In patients with nonmechanical bleeding associated with severe hypothermia, the best course to follow is to pack the bleeding areas as needed, and complete only those portions of the surgical procedure that are absolutely necessary. The patient is then taken to ICU and rewarmed as rapidly as possible, administering FFP, platelets and other blood products as necessary.

DEXTRAN AND HYDROXYETHYL STARCH

AXIOM Administration of large volumes of dextran or HES can cause a bleeding tendency.

In centers where colloids are given to resuscitate patients from severe trauma, the use of dextran or hydroxyethyl starch (HES), particularly in large volumes, may contribute to an increased bleeding tendency. Of the many effects that dextran can have on hemostasis, perhaps the most important is its binding on platelet surfaces and thus causing defective platelet aggregation.[2] When administered to replace blood losses, large volumes of dextran (> 20 ml/kg) can also increase bleeding by causing dilution of fibrinogen and other coagulation factors.[90] Dilutional coagulopathy may also occur after HES when more than 20 mL/kg is given in any 24-hour period. Lesser quantities of HES can cause prolongation of PT and APTT, but they seldom cause excessive clinical bleeding. HES has also been shown to deplete coagulant proteins by shifting them into the interstitial space.[91]

MASSIVE TRANSFUSIONS

AXIOM The safest blood or blood product transfusion is the one not given.[1]

Diagnosis of Bleeding and Clotting Abnormalities

TYPICAL FINDINGS

AXIOM Hemostatic defects typically seen with massive blood transfusions include thrombocytopenia, thrombocytopathy, decreased Factors V and VIII, and elevated FSP.

Bleeding diathesis associated with massive blood transfusions is primarily due to thrombocytopathy, but thrombocytopenia, decreased clotting factors, and increased fibrinolytic activity may occur.[1] Occasionally, because of shock and the massive tissue trauma that are also present, DIC may further complicate the situation.

AXIOM In spite of associated bleeding and coagulation abnormalities, the most frequent cause of excessive blood loss in patients receiving massive transfusions is inadequate surgical control of open vessels.[5]

Even when a coagulopathy is diagnosed clinically and by laboratory studies, one should make an effort to find and control major bleeding sites. Discontinuing surgery while large vessels are still bleeding in the hope that local pressure and correction of the bleeding and clotting deficits and core temperature will control the blood loss are often fruitless.

AXIOM The major cause of nonmechanical bleeding during or after massive transfusions is thrombocytopathy.[5,80]

Although the number of platelets may not change significantly after 24-48 hours of storage in the blood bank, the ability of platelets to form a first hemostatic plug is greatly impaired.[1] Blood that is older than 48 hours essentially has no effective platelets. As more of the patient's own blood is lost and replaced with platelet-deficient bank blood, fewer platelets can be used to form the first hemostatic plug, which is necessary for controlling bleeding from small-diameter vessels.

AXIOM During massive transfusions, the patient's blood increasingly acquires the characteristics of bank blood.[1]

Blood stored in a blood bank undergoes a number of important changes in its hemostatic constituents, resulting in decreased levels of Factor V, Factor VIII:C, fibrinogen, and platelets; however, fibrinolysis also tends to be increased.[1] The gradual decrease in the concentration of fibrinogen in stored blood is due to increased fibrinolytic activity as evidenced by increased levels of FSPs which, in themselves, can cause increased bleeding.[1]

Factor V and Factor VIII:C are often referred to as "labile factors" because they lose their biological activity rapidly during storage, and after 21 days > 10% of their original activity remains. Indeed, about 50% of the activity of Factor V is lost within the first six days of storage.

It has been suggested that little relationship exists between the levels of coagulation factors and the amount of bleeding that occurs following massive transfusions.[80] These studies also suggested that platelets are the key components in the nonmechanical bleeding that develops following massive transfusions.

DISCREPANCIES BETWEEN STUDIES. Substantial differences in results of coagulation tests have been encountered in different studies of abnormal bleeding occurring during or following massive transfusion.[92]

Differences in Components Given. Studies in which packed red blood cells were transfused[92,93] cannot be readily compared with older studies that used whole blood[94] or modified whole blood in which only the platelets and/or cryoprecipitate were removed.[95]

Timing of Clotting Studies. Because the timing of coagulation tests during clinical investigations of transfused patients is generally arbitrary (e.g., after every 10 units of blood), normal oscillatory patterns in coagulation may be unwittingly superimposed on the results obtained, so that some studies demonstrated significant coagulation changes and others did not.[2]

Presence of Shock. The duration and severity of shock and the timing of the volume replacement and coagulation studies are perhaps the most important cause of the discrepancies between results in various series.[2] Some studies reported neither the impact of the duration of hemorrhage and shock on coagulation, nor the effectiveness of resuscitation, as judged by other clinical indicators. Many clinical studies showed that abnormal bleeding developed while the patients were in shock.[91] In contrast, studies of normovolemic hemodilution demonstrated only mild alterations in factor levels and platelet counts,[96] indicating that effective maintenance of blood volume has an important impact on subsequent clotting function.

Thus, although administration of massive blood transfusions and accompanying fluids may temporarily dilute clotting factors, severe, prolonged shock appears to be the major factor causing depression of coagulation factors. Shock can not only cause consumption of platelets and coagulation factors, but it can also decrease coagulation factor production.[93] It also reduces mobilization of coagulation factors from tissue spaces.[92]

Treatment of Nonmechanical Bleeding After Massive Transfusion

PLATELETS. Although abnormal bleeding after massive transfusions is believed to be primarily due to dilutional thrombocytopenia, the changes in platelet counts are extremely variable.[93] The level of thrombocytopenia below which abnormal bleeding occurs has been described as 50×10^9/L,[94] 65×10^9/L,[95] 70×10^9/L,[97] and 100×10^9/L;[98] however, one study demonstrated no difference between the platelet counts of patients who bled abnormally and those who did not.[91] Other studies ascribed the excessive bleeding after trauma and/or massive transfusions to multiple causes.[96]

One prospective, randomized clinical study was performed to investigate the value of prophylactic platelet transfusions in patients receiving massive blood transfusions.[80] Particular attention was paid to the volumes of various fluids and blood products administered, and patients received either platelet concentrates or an equivalent volume of FFP. It was found that no difference in platelet counts or in the incidence of bleeding existed between the two groups. The decrease in platelet numbers seen during and after massive blood transfusions is usually less than that predicted from appropriate washout equations. This implies that many individuals receiving massive transfusions are capable of rapidly mobilizing reserves of platelets.

Because splanchnic perfusion must be preserved to enable platelets sequestered in the spleen to enter the circulation, rapidly restoring and maintaining an adequate blood volume during resuscitation can be extremely important.[2] In a report by Miller et al., in which dilutional thrombocytopenia was identified as the major cause of bleeding after massive transfusions, "transfusion of 3 to 4 units of fresh blood resulted in marked increases in platelet counts."[95] This increase could partially be explained by the number of platelets present in the blood transfused[94] but was more consistent with platelet mobilization resulting from effective restoration of splanchnic blood flow. Other studies, in which fresh blood was given in a similar fashion, did not result in an increased platelet count; however, the patients were still in shock.[94]

A 1987 concensus conference[99] recommended that patients receiving massive blood transfusions be given platelet transfusions when:

1. The platelet count is $< 20 \times 10^9$/L.
2. Diffuse bleeding (oozing) occurs during or after massive transfusions.
3. The platelet count is $< 50 \times 10^9$/L in an actively bleeding patient.
4. The BT is longer than 15 minutes in a patient who is actively bleeding.

To be most effective, platelet transfusions should not be administered until the surgical bleeding has been controlled, otherwise they can be rapidly lost from the bleeding vessels.[2] Because each unit of platelet concentrate increases the platelet concentration in blood by 5-10×10^9/L, at least 6 units should be transfused to obtain a proper therapeutic effect.

Some evidence has suggested that platelet adhesion to vascular endothelium and platelet aggregation are both decreased in anemic patients, especially patients in renal failure.[2] Thus, low hematocrit values that are considered adequate for tissue oxygenation may be inadequate for hemostasis in patients with decreased or defective platelets.[98]

FRESH FROZEN PLASMA. Although no indication for prophylactic FFP administration exists when whole blood is given during massive transfusions to trauma patients,[102-103] patients who receive packed red blood cells may require FFP after each 1.5-2 blood volumes replacement; however, even in these patients, prophylactic administration of FFP, which contains all of the coagulation factors (Table 45–11), appears unwarranted unless nonsurgical bleeding (oozing) occurs and is believed to be caused by factor deficiency. In such patients, 4-8 units of FFP should be administered rapidly to correct coagulation abnormalities and bleeding.[100] Although this approach seems rational, no data is available to support it.

In one of the few objective studies in this area, Martin et al. studied the efficacy of supplemental FFP therapy after massive packed red blood cell (PRBC) treatment of hemorrhagic shock in 22 dogs.[101] Ten dogs were randomized to receive FFP, balanced electrolyte solution (BES), and PRBC, whereas 12 dogs received just BES and PRBC. All coagulation factor activities decreased with shock and decreased further with resuscitation in both groups. Factor II (a procoagulant) and AT III (an anticoagulant) decreased significantly less after resuscitation in the FFP dogs; otherwise, no postresuscitation differences were seen.

AUTOTRANSFUSION

The concern over AIDS and other blood-borne diseases has led to increasing use of autotransfusion of shed blood. Blood donated preoperatively and retransfused intra- or postoperatively obviously is associated with little risk, provided the blood was collected and stored properly and has not been stored for more than three weeks.

Intraoperatively shed blood or blood collected postoperatively from body cavities or drains is either washed in a cell saver or transfused without washing. Shed blood that is carefully washed and administered is relatively safe. Autotransfusion of nonwashed, shed blood, especially in large volumes (> 1000 mL), may be associated with a number of problems.[102] Shed blood is mostly clotted, and the clots have often lysed, so that serum rather than plasma is recovered. Transfusion of this "serum" can be associated with an activation of the hemostasis system, and cases of DIC have occurred when large quantities of shed blood have been autotransfused.

Studies of intracavity blood lost in trauma patients have demonstrated that the amount of anticoagulant needed may be less than in bleeding problems in nontrauma patients. In one series, blood was collected at thoracotomy or laparotomy without any form of anticoagulation and the blood had markedly elevated PT, APTT, and TCT levels. Fibrinogen was found to be essentially absent and FSPs were markedly elevated.[102]

TABLE 45–11 *Presence of Clotting Factors in Blood and Blood Components*

	Factors									
	I	II	V	VII	VIII	IX	X	XI	XII	XIII
Fresh whole blood	+	+	+	+	+	+	+	+	+	+
Bank blood (<5 days old)	+	+	−	+	−	+	+	+	+	+
Fresh frozen plasma	+	+	+	+	+	+	+	+	+	+
Cohn Fraction I	+	−	+?	−	+?	−	−	−	−	+
Cryoprecipitate	+	−	+	−	+	−	−	−	+	+
Factor VIII concentrates	−	−	−	−	+	−	−	+	+	+
Factor IX concentrates	−	+	−	+	−	+	+	−	−	−
Fibrinogen concentrates	+	−	+?	−	+?	−	−	−	−	+

It has been the impression of our surgical staff at Detroit Receiving Hospital that the use of autotransfused blood in trauma patients requiring massive transfusions increases the tendency to develop a severe coagulopathy, and as a consequence, autotransfusion tends to be avoided in such patients.

DISSEMINATED INTRAVASCULAR COAGULATION

Pathophysiology

In DIC, generalized activation of prothrombin to thrombin occurs with conversion of fibrinogen to fibrin.[103] However, diffuse thrombus deposition is not consistently found at autopsy in patients with clinical evidence of DIC, probably because of a concomitantly accelerated fibrinolysis.[104] In this process, consumption of fibrinogen, prothrombin, platelets, Factor V, and Factor VIII occurs. As these factors are "consumed," their concentration in the blood decreases below those needed for normal hemostasis, and a breakdown in the hemostatic mechanism results, hence the name "consumption coagulopathy."[1]

AXIOM Consumption coagulopathy is not a disease, per se, but it is a major complication of underlying disease.[1]

Experimental studies have shown that rapid injection of thrombin leads to local thrombosis.[3] Slower infusions tend to cause disseminated vessel thrombi, especially in the kidneys and adrenals, and hypofibrinogenemia. The reticuloendothelial system, particularly the liver, can generally remove fibrin and activated coagulation factors from the circulation rapidly. Consequently, suppression of reticuloendothelial system function increases the susceptibility to DIC.[105]

DIC can present in one of three forms: (a) generalized intravascular activation of the clotting system with simultaneous activation of the fibrinolytic system (secondary fibrinolysis), (b) DIC without activation of the fibrinolytic system, and (c) activation of the fibrinolytic system without intravascular clotting (primary fibrinolysis).[1]

Intravascular coagulation with secondary fibrinolysis is the most frequent type of DIC. DIC without secondary fibrinolysis is rare and has the poorest prognosis because fibrin, which is formed in DIC, is deposited in the microcirculation, causing occlusion of nutrient capillaries with resultant organ dysfunction and MOF.[1]

One of the main defenses against this diffuse intravascular coagulation is fibrinolysis. Damage to organs, such as the placenta, lung, or liver, tends to release activators of the fibrinolytic system (t-PA). Severe hypoxia, as encountered during shock or improper anesthesia, is also recognized as a powerful stimulus for activation of plasminogen to plasmin. Some organs, such as the prostate gland, pancreas and lungs, contain proteases that can directly activate plasminogen and thus cause fibrinolysis.

The degradation products of fibrin and fibrinogen acted upon by plasmin are called fibrinogen degradation products (FDPs) or FSPs.[1] These split products inhibit continuing coagulation of blood by delaying polymerization of fibrin monomers, resulting in prolonged TCT.[103,105] FSPs may also interpose themselves between fibrin monomers, causing a weak fibrin clot to form. Platelet aggregation is also blocked. When a fibrin thrombus is formed, plasmin is normally adsorbed onto the fibrin strands and there, free-from inhibitors, such as α_2-antiplasmin, it is able to digest fibrin.

Etiology

A wide variety of conditions may cause or predispose a patient to develop DIC (Table 45–12). All types of tissue damage or necrosis, such as shock, sepsis, trauma, malignancy, or burns, can release thromboplastic substances (tissue factor) that may cause DIC.[106-107] Septic shock may cause intravascular platelet aggregation and tissue-factor release (the human equivalent of the generalized Shwartzman reaction).[1] Other causes of DIC include: (a) antibody-antigen interactions associated with severe anaphylactoid reactions due to drug or antitoxin hypersensitivity, and (b) hyperacute rejection of transplanted organs.[105] All of these processes may cause intravascular platelet ag-

TABLE 45–12 **Major Predisposing Conditions Associated with Disseminated Intravascular Coagulation**

Shock
Hypothermia
Hyperthermia
Major blood type incompatibility
Massive transfusion
Autotransfusion
Hepatic cirrhosis
Liver injury
Head injury
Near-drowning
Burns
Inhalation injury
Pulmonary embolism
Fat embolism
Air embolism
Acute renal failure
Pregnancy

gregation. Severe acidosis may also cause intravascular platelet breakdown, thus explaining the presence of DIC in some nonseptic shock conditions.[108]

The body's defense mechanisms, especially the RES, can inhibit the development of DIC. Impairment of the RES due to poor liver function or prolonged shock can contribute greatly to the development of DIC when appropriate stimuli are present.[108] This probably explains the frequently increased incidence of DIC during hepatic coma or liver transplantation.[109] Other causes of DIC associated with a generalized stimulus to clotting include snake envenomation, Rocky Mountain spotted fever, and anaphylaxis.[3] Hemolysis, which may occur with a mismatched blood transfusion, may also cause DIC.[110]

Severe, nonspecific stress to the entire organism may also initiate consumptive coagulopathy. For example, increased catecholamines stimulate coagulation and vasoconstriction which causes slowing of peripheral blood flow and allows clotting to take place. Reduced blood flow through the splanchnic bed also impairs the function of the RES, which is responsible for clearance of circulating tissue debris, fibrin, bacteria, and other material that may otherwise promote microthrombosis.[103,105]

Diagnosis

Acute DIC is usually diagnosed by demonstrating: (a) the presence of a predisposing condition, (b) clinical evidence of excessive bleeding and/or microthrombosis, and (c) demonstration of laboratory changes consistent with consumptive coagulopathy. Every disease leading to tissue-factor release may potentially lead to consumption coagulopathy. Therefore, sepsis, shock, and transfusion of mismatched blood, can lead to DIC. Massive trauma, malignancy, abruptio placentae, amniotic fluid embolism, etc, are also problems that can lead to consumption coagulopathy. Whether they will or will not depends on the body's defense capabilities, the amount of stimulus, and the length of time it is present.

Clinically, patients with DIC often have diffuse bleeding from multiple sites.[1] When bleeding occurs from previously dry areas, and from other sites, such as needle punctures, Foley catheter, nasogastric tube, or tracheostomy, a major breakdown in the hemostatic mechanism must be considered.

PITFALL ⊘

Assuming that excessive intraoperative or postoperative bleeding is due to a coagulopathy rather than to a surgically correctable cause.

Diffuse bleeding from venipunctures, membranes, and wound sites characteristic of DIC should not be confused with inadequately controlled surgical bleeding.[2] Astute clinical observation can be as important as laboratory results and usually yields information more rapidly. The reliability of the diagnosis may become clouded in situations in which coagulation studies are performed too soon after the patient has received a large volume of crystalloids during resuscitation.[96] Appropriate component therapy in a bleeding patient should not be withheld in order to clarify the diagnosis.

When DIC is suspected, but no apparent bleeding occurs, close observation of renal function can be helpful. Bilateral renal cortical necrosis is probably the best known pathologic finding in DIC.[1] Renal failure with anuria which cannot be explained on the basis of hypotension is often an early sign of DIC, even before a generalized bleeding tendency becomes apparent.[1]

AXIOM   Coagulation tests are extremely important if an accurate diagnosis of consumption coagulopathy is to be made early.[1]

The laboratory diagnosis of DIC usually requires a minimum of four tests: fibrinogen levels, platelet counts, FSP, and D-dimer levels. Fibrinogen and platelets decrease because they are consumed, while FSP and D-dimer levels increase. FSP levels reflect the effects of plasmin on fibrinogen and fibrin. D-dimers are fragments derived from lysis of cross-linked fibrin and, therefore, increased D-dimer levels indicate that increased clotting has occurred.

Before the development of an assay for D-dimers, one had to measure fibrin monomers to detect increased clotting. Because D-dimer assays were more accurate, the monomer tests were largely abandoned. More recently, however, highly accurate and reliable fibrin monomer assays have been developed that could replace D-dimer assays or be added to the tests used to detect DIC. The presence of fibrin monomers indicates that thrombin has cleaved fibrinogen. Thus, monomers suggest the presence of thrombin but not plasmin.

The APTT and PT should be prolonged in DIC due to the consumption of constituents needed for coagulation. In patients with a primary, generalized intravascular fibrinolysis, one would expect decreased fibrinogen levels, elevated FSP, and normal D-dimers and monomer levels. The platelet count usually is also normal because plasmin has no effect on platelets.

AXIOM   Obtaining relatively normal values for bleeding and clotting studies does not completely eliminate the presence of early or mild DIC.

The most reliable tests for making the diagnosis of DIC and following the effects of therapy are: (a) increased FSP, monomers, and D-dimers, (b) decreased antithrombin III, (c) reduced platelet count, and (d) prolonged TCT. It is advisable to check fibrinogen levels and platelet counts frequently in patients with conditions that predispose to DIC in order to detect the process as early as possible and hopefully at a time when clinical bleeding is not yet present.

Although fibrinogen levels may be helpful in determining the activity and severity of intravascular coagulation, they can be extremely variable because they reflect the balance between synthesis and consumption.[3] During severe stress, the hepatic synthesis of fibrinogen may be increased tenfold. The half-life of fibrinogen in normal individuals is approximately 100 hours, and thrombin is believed to account for < 2% of its normal metabolism. In the absence of other serious illnesses, intermediate products of the conversion of fibrinogen to fibrin are removed from the circulating bloodstream by the reticuloendothelial system. Consequently, it may be necessary to repeat lab studies every one to two hours during the acute process to detect the progressive decreases in fibrinogen levels and platelet counts that would be expected with DIC.[1]

Although differentiating between the three forms of consumption coagulopathy may be difficult at times, accurate diagnosis is essential for proper treatment.[1] Platelet counts, fibrinogen levels, and assays for FSP and D-dimers can be helpful. Primary fibrinolysis is generally associated with a normal platelet count, low fibrinogens levels, elevated FSPs, and negative monomers and D-dimers; however, the platelet count may decrease as increased quantities for blood and fluid

are given; consequently, this criterion is valid only early in the syndrome. (Table 45–13).

The most common form of DIC (clotting plus fibrinolysis) is characterized by low platelet counts and fibrinogen levels and by elevated FSPs, monomers, and D-dimers concentrations. Rare patients with primary clotting (little or no fibrinolysis) have low platelet counts and fibrinogen levels, but negative FSP and D-dimers. The fibrin monomers test, however, would be positive (Table 45–13).

The transformation of fibrinogen to a fibrin polymer generates fibrin monomers as an intermediary step. They present in soluble form in the plasma and can also form soluble complexes with FSP. The generation of soluble fibrin monomer and fibrin complexes occurs only when the clotting process is proceeding normally and is thus termed the paracoagulation process.[103] Primary fibrinolysis (or fibrinogenolysis) generates FSP but not soluble fibrin monomers.

Recently, several monoclonal antibodies recognizing the unique fibrin degradation fragments known as D-dimer (DD) were made available for routine laboratory use.[111,112] Fragment DD, along with high molecular weight (HMW) complexes, is generated by plasmin lysis of cross-linked fibrin clots. In contrast to the FSP fragments X, Y, D, and E, which are generated by the lysis of fibrinogen and noncross-linked fibrin, the presence of D-dimers documents that both thrombin generation with cross-linking of fibrin clots via thrombin activation of Factor XIII and plasmin generation (fibrinolysis) have occurred. Detection of D-dimers, therefore, offers a unique advantage over other laboratory tests for DIC because it addresses both dimensions of DIC.[111]

Other molecular markers, including the thrombin-antithrombin-III complex (TAT), and plasmin α_2-plasmin inhibitor complex (PIC), have also been used for the diagnosis of hemostatic disorders.[112] Recent studies of DIC using polyclonal antibodies confirmed the prevalence of D-dimers[113] and showed that increased plasma levels of TAT[114] indicated thrombin generation during coagulation. They also showed that increased levels of plasmin-α_2-antiplasmin complex[115] indicated plasmin generation during fibrinolysis.

PITFALL ⊘

When blood for coagulation tests is drawn from an indwelling arterial or venous catheter, any heparin flush in the line can produce erroneous results.

Prolonged TCT often indicates the presence of FSPs; however, because heparin, even in minute quantities, also prolongs the TCT, drawing blood samples from a line that has been flushed with a heparin solution may jeopardize the accuracy of this test.[1]

An early diagnosis of a major hemostatic breakdown can occasionally be made in the operating room by a simple, whole-blood clotting test. About 2-3 mL of blood is placed in each of two test tubes without addition of an anticoagulant; they are observed for clotting by tipping one of the tubes every 30-60 seconds.[1] If no clot forms spontaneously within 30 minutes, an abnormality is present and thrombin should be added. When a clot still does not form, the patient probably has very low fibrinogen levels. When a clot forms either spontaneously or after the addition of thrombin, one looks at the quantity of clot formed. In hypofibrinogenemia, only a small blood clot forms. One also observes how well the clot persists because rapid dissolution of the clot may be an indicator of accelerated fibrinolysis.

TABLE 45–13   *Laboratory Tests in the Three Forms of DIC*

Test	Clotting and Lysis	Clotting	Lysis
Fibrinogen	↓	↓	↓
Platelets	↓	↓	N-↓
FDP	+	−	+
Monomers	+	+	−
D-dimer	+	−	−

Treatment of DIC

Patients with consumption coagulopathy are endangered by two basic events: (a) exsanguination due to the consumption coagulopathy, and (b) deposition of fibrin in the microvasculature leading to irreparable organ damage.[103] The bleeding problem is present in all forms of DIC, but excess intravascular fibrin deposition occurs only in those forms where fibrinolysis is absent or insufficiently present. Generally, a patient who has secondary fibrinolysis with FSP levels of > 40 mcg/mL or more is not likely to deposit fibrin, while a patient with FSP levels < 10 mcg/mL serum probably will.

PROPHYLAXIS. Antithrombin and protein C levels are lower than normal in DIC[3] and antithrombin prophylaxis may be efficacious in conditions of impending DIC, such as gram-negative septicemia or endotoxemia.[116] FFP and cryoprecipitate are sources of antithrombin and can help to correct the low AT III levels seen with shock, sepsis, or major trauma.[68,69] Optimal substitution can be obtained by using antithrombin concentrates, where available.

CORRECTION OF THE PRIMARY PROCESS

AXIOM   The best way to treat consumption coagulopathy is to eliminate the underlying disease process.

Abruptio placentae serves as an appropriate example because at the moment the uterus is evacuated, either spontaneously or by cesarean section, the trigger for DIC is removed and consumption coagulopathy ceases. Rapid and aggressive treatment of shock or sepsis is also crucial to reduce both the immediate morbidity and the secondary mortality from organ failure. As many as 53% of patients with acute DIC have evidence of renal microvascular thrombosis,[116] and the combination of acute oliguric renal failure and traumatic or septic shock carries an extremely high mortality.[2] DIC has also been implicated as a cause of adult respiratory distress syndrome,[105,116] although this association is not as obvious as previously believed.

If the source of the trigger mechanism in a patient with DIC (with or without secondary fibrinolysis) were eliminated promptly, then massive replacement of the lost blood and clotting factors with FFP and platelet concentrates usually would restore normal hemostasis.[1] Generally, secondary fibrinolysis also ends when intravascular clotting is arrested.

REPLACEMENT OF PLATELETS AND COAGULATION FACTORS. Although many authors stress that treatment of the underlying etiology is the only therapy necessary to arrest DIC, patients who are injured, bleeding, and require emergency surgery need vigorous replacement therapy with blood, FFP, and platelets to reverse bleeding diathesis.[2] In addition, administering these blood products helps to expand the intravascular volume. Maintaining an adequate intravascular volume is extremely helpful because a major inciting factor of DIC in trauma patients is inadequate tissue perfusion. Because it also replaces depleted antithrombin, the most important endogenous anticoagulant substance, the replenishment of FFP helps to control the hypercoagulable state.[116]

The degree to which endogenous compensation is capable of restoring adequate levels of coagulation factors and platelets to the circulation varies with the individual patient and with the rapidity of the evolution of DIC. Underlying, unsuspected hypercoagulability also may predispose patients to the development of DIC when inciting stress arises.[103] Replacement of coagulation factors and platelets should be guided by the clinical response to therapy and by the laboratory findings, especially TCT.[1]

HEPARIN

AXIOM   Heparin treatment is imperative in patients who have DIC without adequate fibrinolysis, and the earlier it is initiated, the better the prognosis.

Extensive studies have demonstrated that heparin therapy can help to reverse the DIC process;[105,116,117] however, systemic heparinization of the most common form of DIC (clotting plus lysis) has been abandoned. In addition, lost factors should be replaced with FFP and platelets by concentrates if needed. Although heparin has been used successfully in some postsurgical patients, many clinicians are unwilling to risk starting anticoagulant therapy, even at low doses, in a patient who is already bleeding excessively.

In patients with DIC without fibrinolysis, administration of platelets or FFP without heparin may result in more fibrin deposition, unless the intravascular clotting is blocked by anticoagulant therapy.[1]

AXIOM   If the primary process is not corrected in DIC and if little or no fibrinolysis is present, administration of FFP and platelets will only increase the deposition of intravascular fibrin.

DIC can generally be interrupted in an adult by rapidly administering 3000-5000 units of heparin intravenously as a loading dose, followed by 15,000-30,000 units given by continuous intravenous infusion over the next 24 hours.[1] Any bleeding that is already present will obviously not be arrested by heparin, but within hours one will usually be able to measure an increase in fibrinogen levels and platelet counts. This restoration of the hemostatic mechanisms should be aided by infusion of FFP with platelet concentrates. Generally, fibrinolysis subsides when intravascular clotting has been successfully blocked, and drugs to specifically inhibit the fibrinolytic system are rarely required.[1]

Some clinicians advocate the use of low-dose heparin (5000-7000 units subcutaneously b.i.d.) for patients with DIC.[105,116] Heparin, when complexed with antithrombin III, makes an antithrombin III molecule 1000-fold more active. It is assumed that the "activation" of antithrombin III will counteract the activation of the clotting system and thus minimize DIC. We have seen good results with this treatment modality in patients with chronic DIC, and patients with disseminated malignancies are especially likely to benefit from this treatment.

ANTITHROMBIN III CONCENTRATES. The rationale for using heparin in the treatment of DIC arose from the knowledge that the clotting system is systemically activated leading to the generation of clotting enzymes and subsequent consumption of these factors. As the clotting enymes are generated, physiologic inhibitors (antithrombin III, protein C) attempt to neutralize them. This leads to the consumption of these inhibitors. As plasma levels decrease, more clotting ensues so that a positive feedback loop develops which ultimately contributes to the death of the patient. Heparin administration was designed to interrupt this cycle. Unfortunately, heparin can significantly increase the bleeding tendency of these patients, thereby exacerbating the blood loss.

This dilemma led to the concept of administering the physiologic inhibitors of the clotting system to the patients, thereby boosting the patients' own defense system. FFP contains both antithrombin III and protein C, but large volumes are needed to increase plasma levels of antithrombin III and protein C. In the meantime, antithrombin III concentrates have been developed and are commerically available in many countries, and protein C concentrates are being developed.

Available antithrombin III concentrates are highly purified and pasteurized which make viral contamination highly unlikely.[118] Many animal models have been used to demonstrate the efficacy of these concentrates.[119,120] The outcome has generally been positive in that DIC could be interrupted, and in many models mortality could be reduced.

Similar positive results have been found when patients with DIC were treated with antithrombin III concentrates.[121-122] Most studies, however, are only case reports. No benefits were found when antithrombin III concentrates were administered during liver transplantation.[123]

There are a few larger trials that have tested the efficacy of these concentrates in patients in septic shock.[124-126] In one study, a major improvement in clinical signs of sepsis and a major reduction in mortality was found in patients treated with antithrombin III when compared with controls.[124] The addition of heparin to one group of patients did not improve outcome but it did increase clinical bleeding. In a second study, nonsurgical septic patients were treated with antithrombin III concentrates and a major improvement in the laboratory parameters of DIC and in survival were found.[125] The third and most recent study was a double-blind, placebo-controlled trial.[126] Antithrombin III therapy markedly improved the laboratory parameters of DIC in septic patients. DIC was cured in 64% of treated patients on day 2 versus 11% of controls (P < 0.01). The mortality rate decreased from 50% (9 of 18) in controls to 28% (4 of 14) of treated patients, but the difference did not reach statistical significance (P = 0.22).

Both animal and human studies seem to suggest that DIC can be greatly improved by replacing the lost antithrombin III with an appropriate concentrate; however, DIC is only one of the major metabolic derangements in septic patients.[127] A single therapeutic approach to a multifaceted problem will likely not yield a fully desirable outcome.[128] Early intervention seems to be the key to successful management.

ANTIFIBRINOLYTIC DRUGS

PITFALL ⊘

When antifibrinolytic drugs are used to treat fibrinolysis secondary to DIC, intravascular clotting may proceed at a much more dangerous rate.

Antifibrinolytic therapy with EACA or aprotinin should be considered only for patients in whom the diagnosis of primary fibrinolysis is properly established beyond any doubt.[1] Although this is very difficult to accomplish, in most instances the differentiation between DIC and primary fibrinolysis is less important than was believed previously because it is rare.[117] Primary fibrinolysis is generally associated with prostatic carcinoma and liver failure, but it can occasionally occur in trauma patients during massive blood transfusions.[2] The best laboratory test for the differentiation of primary versus secondary fibrinolysis is the D-dimer assay. In primary fibrinolysis, D-dimers levels are repeatedly negative. The treatment of primary fibrinolysis involves correction of the underlying process and administration of EACA (5 g bolus followed by 1 g/hour) and blood products.[117]

The indiscriminate use of EACA in consumption coagulopathy must be strongly discouraged because it may accentuate rather than reverse the tendency to occlude nutrient capillaries in vital organs.[1] When any doubt exists as to the type of fibrinolysis present in a patient, heparinization is recommended prior to antifibrinolytic therapy.[117]

AXIOM Antifibrinolytic therapy generally should not be given to patients with DIC unless it is given in conjunction with heparin.

FIBRIN GLUE/FIBRIN GEL. A recently introduced technique of applying fibrin glue to bleeding surfaces or intraparenchymal lesions can often control coagulopathy-induced intraoperative bleeding from solid organs.[2] The commercial material usually includes four components: (a) highly concentrated fibrinogen, (b) trypsin inhibitor (aprotinin), (c) dried thrombin, and (d) calcium chloride. Preliminary results suggest that fibrin glue achieves remarkable local hemostasis and may be lifesaving in some patients with localized bleeding from coagulation disorders, including DIC.[129] Fibrin gel, which is formed by adding thrombin and calcium to cryoprecipitate, can be used in a similar manner.

ALBUMIN RESUSCITATION

The type of resuscitation used in trauma patients may profoundly affect the coagulation status.[3] In a series of 94 patients reported by Johnson et al., 46 patients received supplemental albumin, which raised total protein concentrations from 5.8 to 6.4 gm/dl and raised albumin levels from 2.9 to 4.2 g/dL.[130] Patients receiving large quantities of albumin required more transfusions (7.1 vs 3.8 units) and more plasma (455 vs 317 ml). Administration of large amounts of albumin also correlated with a significant decrease in fibrinogen levels (238 vs 405 mg/dL) and a greater prolongation of the PT over controls (2.6 vs 1.4 seconds). The APTT was prolonged and the platelet count was decreased in all albumin-treated patients, but these changes were not significant.[133]

Other studies by the same group demonstrated that albumin resuscitation in an experimental model leads to decreased coagulation activity and coagulation protein content.[131] In a study of 20 splenectomized dogs that were resuscitated from hemorrhagic shock either with lactated Ringer's solution at 20 mL/kg or with 5% albumin, albumin resuscitation significantly reduced the mean coagulation activity with fibrinogen levels decreasing from 423 to 274 mg/dL, Factor VIII:C decreasing from 64% to 42% of normal, and prothrombin decreasing from 195% to 141%. The levels of fibrinogen, antithrombin III, and Factor VII also progressively decreased in the animals resuscitated with albumin. Levels of Factor VIII:C remained within normal limits suggesting that the albumin effect may be active on the liver rather than on the vascular endothelium that produces Factor VIII:C.[115]

⊘ **FREQUENT ERRORS**

In the Management of Coagulation Abnormalities in Injured Patients

1. *Assuming that excessive intraoperative or postoperative bleeding is due to a coagulation abnormality rather than realizing that such bleeding is often due to inadequate surgical efforts to obtain hemostasis.*
2. *Failing to obtain appropriate coagulation tests as soon as possible in patients with possible coagulation abnormalities.*
3. *Assuming that a clinical coagulation disorder cannot be present when coagulation tests are normal.*
4. *Failing to obtain an adequate history concerning drugs with possible anticoagulant effects in preoperative patients or in patients who are bleeding excessively.*
5. *Attempting to manage patients with known congenital or unusual bleeding disorders in a hospital with an inadequate coagulation laboratory.*
6. *Assuming that a platelet count $> 50 \times 10^9/L$ eliminates a bleeding disorder due to platelet deficiencies.*
7. *Drawing blood for coagulation tests from indwelling venous or arterial catheters, particularly when catheters have been flushed with heparin.*
8. *Failing to provide adequate quantities of FFP and platelets to patients who have developed a coagulopathy after massive transfusions.*
9. *Using antifibrinolytic drugs without heparin in patients who may have fibrinolysis secondary to DIC.*

▼▼▼▼▼▼▼▼▼▼▼▼▼▼▼▼▼▼▼▼▼▼▼▼▼▼▼▼▼▼

SUMMARY POINTS

1. Abnormally functioning hemostatic mechanisms in the injured patient, unless recognized and treated promptly and appropriately, may lead not only to excessive bleeding and possible death but also to poor wound healing or thromboembolic complications.

2. Most early bleeding problems in trauma patients are due to acquired mechanical defects.

3. Intraoperative and postoperative bleeding, especially when limited to the site of trauma, is usually due to inadequate surgical efforts, even when a defect is found in the bleeding or clotting tests.

4. Partial transection of a vessel, which prevents vascular occlusion by vasoconstriction, is more likely to lead to significant blood loss than to complete transection.

5. The intrinsic coagulation pathway, which can be monitored by APTT, begins when Factor XII is activated to Factor XIIa, usually on platelet phospholipid surfaces or nonphysiologic surfaces.

6. The extrinsic coagulation pathway, which can be monitored with PT, begins when a complex of Factor VII, tissue thromboplastin, and calcium is formed.

7. The intrinsic and extrinsic coagulation pathways both function to activate Factor X.

8. Activated Factor X, Factor V, phospholipids, and calcium ions form a complex that converts prothrombin to thrombin.

9. After thrombin splits fibrinopeptides A and B off fibrinogen, the molecules remaining are referred to as fibrin monomers.

10. Factor XIII is not needed to have a normal PT and APTT, and no acquired, isolated Factor XIII deficiency exists.

11. Recurrent venous thromboembolic disease in young individuals without apparent predisposing factors should make one suspect an inherited deficiency of antithrombin III, protein C, or protein S.

12. Arrest of coagulation is, to some extent, mediated by the conversion of plasminogen to plasmin, a reaction that is partially controlled by activated Factor XII.

13. Normally no systemic plasminogen activation occurs in plasma.

14. Plasmin acts on a wide variety of proteins and, therefore, excessive fibrinolysis can produce widespread effects on a variety of systems.

15. Digestion of fibrin and fibrinogen by plasmin leads to formation of so-called FSP.

16. Increased levels of FSP can block primary and secondary hemostasis.

17. Normal TCT and normal fibrinogen levels exclude a serious activation of the fibrinolytic system.

18. Disease states resulting from abnormalities in the fibrinolytic system include both hemorrhagic disorders (due to excessive fibrinolysis) and thrombosis (due to deficient inhibited fibrinolysis).

19. In spite of recent advances in knowledge concerning the detailed biochemistry of blood coagulation, the diagnosis of hemostatic disturbances still often depends on a careful history and physical examination.

20. When a diligent effort is not made to determine whether the patient is taking drugs with anticoagulant properties, appropriate therapy may be dangerously delayed.

21. Prolonged or excessive bleeding from needle puncture sites or spontaneous bleeding from mucous membranes suggests severe coagulopathy, such as DIC.

22. When laboratory tests are used to eliminate coagulation abnormalities, mild- to-moderate disorders may be overlooked.

23. When a patient is bleeding in the postoperative period and the six standard screening tests are normal, the bleeding is probably due to a mechanical problem that needs surgical correction.

24. Mild thrombocytopathies usually are not discovered by performing BT.

25. Clinical coagulopathy can occur after major trauma or surgery in spite of relatively normal PT and APTT values.

26. Normal APTT and PT effectively exclude any serious defects in the clotting system.

27. When a patient with coagulopathy has a prolonged thrombin time and a normal reptilase time, excess heparin is probably present.

28. In many congenital coagulopathies, platelet counts and BTs are normal, indicating uncomplicated formation of the first hemostatic plug.

29. In hemophiliacs, platelet function remains intact, allowing the vascular plug to develop promptly after trauma but excessive bleeding tends to develop after a delay which may last several hours or days.

30. The diagnosis of hemophilia should be suspected in males with a history of excessive bleeding since childhood.

31. Posttraumatic intracranial bleeding in hemophiliac patients may not be significant or apparent for 24-48 hours.

32. Hemophiliacs can have a variety of nontraumatic bony abnormalities seen on cervical spine radiography.

33. Intraoperative positioning of hemophiliacs should be done carefully, and pressure points must be thickly padded to prevent hemorrhage.

34. Whenever a blood product is used, the risk of subsequent hepatitis and/or AIDS should be considered.

35. The initial treatment of excessive bleeding in hemophiliacs is volume resuscitation with blood transfusions and FFP.

36. Cryoprecipitate has all of the coagulation factors present in FFP except Factors II, VII, IX, and X.

37. A unit of Factor VIII or IX is the amount of that activity found in 1 mL of fresh plasma.

38. Generally, each unit of Factor VIII activity infused per kg of body weight should produce a 2% increase in the plasma levels of Factor VIII.

39. No formula for administering blood components can substitute for careful, repeated serial laboratory and clinical observations.

40. When a hemophiliac who is bleeding has a Factor VIII inhibitor, treatment is much more difficult and should be undertaken in consultation with someone experienced in such care.

41. In patients receiving multiple units of Factor IX concentrate, 5-10 units of heparin should be added to each milliliter of reconstituted prothrombin complex concentrate.

42. Acquired bleeding disorders are much more frequently encountered than those of congenital origin, particularly in adult trauma patients.

43. Severe liver disease can cause thrombocytopenia, increased fibrinolysis, and decreased production of most coagulation factors, except Factor VIII:C and vWF, so that a DIC-like clinical picture can be produced.

44. When coagulation tests are abnormal in patients with liver disease, little or no improvement may occur after vitamin K injection, even after 24-48 hours.

45. In patients with severe liver dysfunction, large volumes of FFP may be required to maintain normal factor levels.

46. Cirrhotic patients frequently have severe factor deficiencies; however, when they bleed excessively after trauma, it is usually primarily because of concomitant thrombocytopenia.

47. The use of EACA (Amicar) in cirrhotic patients who are bleeding excessively should be discouraged because these patients often have consumption coagulopathy, in which case Amicar would be contraindicated.

48. Increased bleeding due to a qualitative platelet problem (thrombocytopathy) can be expected in most patients with severe uremia.

49. Vitamin K deficiency can be anticipated in patients with chronic, severe biliary tract obstruction or malabsorption.

50. Coagulation defects due to pure vitamin K deficiencies are partially corrected by intravenous vitamin K within 6-12 hours unless coincident liver dysfunction is present.

51. Treatment of severe, active bleeding, which is due either to coumadin administration or to vitamin K deficiency, should include intravenous vitamin K and at least 4-8 units of FFP.

52. Reduced plasma levels of antithrombin (because of liver disease or excessive clotting) can greatly increase the amount of heparin needed to prolong APTT or ACT to therapeutic levels.

53. Platelet counts should be carefully monitored whenever heparin is given.

54. If a patient requiring anticoagulation were to develop HIT syndrome, oral anticoagulants should be begun and heparin immediately discontinued.

55. Thrombocytopathy can be confirmed by in vitro tests or by finding a prolonged BT in spite of a platelet count $> 100 \times 10^9$/L.

56. Aspirin causes permanently impaired function of all platelets exposed to it (up to 10-12 days).

57. Platelet transfusions are indicated in patients who develop abnormal bleeding due to thrombocytopenia or thrombocytopathy during emergency major surgery.

58. The use of thrombolytic agents is generally contraindicated in patients with recent trauma or fresh surgical wounds.

59. Platelet counts $< 10 \times 10^9$/L frequently cause moderate-to-severe spontaneous bleeding.

60. Thrombocytopenia does not usually cause massive bleeding into tissues or joints.

61. One should not assume that patients with platelet counts $> 50 \times 10^9$/L cannot have bleeding due to a platelet problem.

62. One should avoid transfusing platelets in patients with thrombocytopenia associated with autoantibodies unless the patient is bleeding significantly.

63. If it were assumed that excessive bleeding after trauma or during surgery were due to a coagulation abnormality, attempts to obtain good, local hemostasis would apt to be less vigorous.

64. Severe antithrombin deficiencies in sepsis can increase the tendency for DIC and MOF.

65. High and progressively increasing levels of FSP after trauma are a poor prognostic sign.

66. Brain has the highest tissue thromboplastin concentration of any of the body's organs.

67. Severe derangements of clotting can occur after major head injuries due to initiation of widespread intravascular coagulation.

68. Prophylactic administration of FFP or platelets does not appear to be warranted as a routine measure in patients receiving massive blood transfusions.

69. In addition to observing the hemostatic response after platelet transfusions, platelet counts should be performed after 1, 12, and 24 hours.

70. Hypothermia is one of the most common causes of altered coagulation in trauma.

71. Administration of large volumes of dextran or HES can cause a bleeding tendency.

72. The safest unit of blood or blood product transfused is the one not given.

73. Hemostatic defects typically seen with massive blood transfusions include: thrombocytopenia, thrombocytopathy, decreased Factors V and VIII, and elevated FSP.

74. In spite of the associated bleeding and coagulation abnormalities, the most frequent cause of excessive blood loss in patients receiving massive transfusions is inadequate surgical control of open vessels.

75. The major cause of nonmechanical bleeding during or after massive transfusions is thrombocytopathy.

76. During massive transfusions, the patient's blood increasingly acquires the characteristic of bank blood.

77. Consumption coagulopathy is not a disease, per se, but it is a major complication of an underlying disease.

78. One should not assume that excessive intraoperative or postoperative bleeding is due to a coagulopathy rather than a surgically correctable cause.

79. Coagulation tests are extremely important when an accurate diagnosis of a consumption coagulopathy (DIC) is to be made.

80. Obtaining relatively normal values for bleeding and clotting studies does not eliminate the presence of early or mild DIC.

81. When blood for coagulation tests is drawn from an indwelling arterial or venous catheter, any heparin flush in the line can produce erroneous results.

82. Heparin treatment is imperative in patients who have DIC without adequate fibrinolysis, and the earlier it is initiated, the better the prognosis.

83. When the primary process is not corrected in DIC and when little or no fibrinolysis occurs, administration of FFP and platelets only increases the deposition of intravascular fibrin.

84. When antifibrinolytic drugs are used to treat fibrinolysis secondary to DIC, intravascular clotting may proceed at a much more dangerous rate.

▲▲▲▲▲▲▲▲▲▲▲▲▲▲▲▲▲▲▲▲▲▲▲▲▲▲▲▲▲▲▲▲▲▲▲▲▲

REFERENCES

1. Mammen EF. Coagulation abnormalities in trauma. Walt AJ, Wilson RF, eds. Management of trauma: pitfalls and practice. Philadelphia: Lee & Febiger, 1975; 566-587.
2. Kahn RC. Coagulation abnormalities and their management in the injured. Capan LM, Miller SM, Turndorf H, eds. Trauma: anesthesia and intensive care. Philadelphia: JB Lippincott, 1991; 207-217.
3. Rutledge R, Sheldon GF. Bleeding and coagulation problems. Moore EE, Mattox KL, Feliciano, eds. Trauma, 2nd ed. Norwalk: Appleton & Lange, 1991; 891-908.
4. Ordog GJ, Wasserberger J, Balasubramanium S. Coagulation abnormalities in traumatic shock. Ann Emerg Med 1985;14:650.
5. Wilson RF, Dulchavsky SA, Soullier G, Beckman B. Problems with 20 or more blood transfusions in 24 hours. Am Surg 1987;53:410.
6. Bick RL, Murano G. Physiology of hemostasis. Bick RL, Bennett JM, Brynes RK, et al., eds. Hematology: clinical and laboratory practice, vol 2. St. Louis: Mosby 1993; 1285-1308.
7. Nilsson IM. Coagulation and fibrinolysis. Scand J Gastroenterol Suppl 1987;137:11.
8. Bach RR. Initiation of coagulation by tissue factor. CRC Crit Rev Biochem 1988;23:339.
9. Harker LA, Fuster V. Pharmacology of platelet inhibitors. J Am Coll Cardiol 1986;8:21B.
10. Aoki N. Hemostasis associated with abnormalities of fibrinolysis. Sough Blood Rev 1989;3:11.
11. Stern DM, Kaiser E, Nawroth PP. Regulation of the coagulation system by vascular endothelial cells. Haemostasis 1988;18:202.
12. Stern D, Nawroth P, Handley D, Kisiel W. An endothelial cell-dependent pathway of coagulation. Proc Natl Acad Sci USA 1985;82:2523.
13. Guillin MC, Bezeaud A. General mechanisms of coagulation and their physiological inhibition I. General mechanisms of blood coagulation. Pathol Biol 1985;33:847.
14. Ryan J, Geczy C. Coagulation and the expression of cell mediated immunity. Immunol Cell Biol 1987;65:127.
15. Finlayson JS. Crosslinking of fibrin. Semin Thromb Hemost 1974; 1:33.
16. Bikfalvi A, Beress L. Natural proteinase inhibitors: blood coagulation inhibition and evolutionary relationships. Comp Biochem Physiol B 1987;87:435.
17. Mammen EF, Fujii Y. Hypercoagulable states. Lab Med 1989;20:611.
18. Shih GC, Hajjar KA. Plasminogen activator assembly on the human endothelial cell. Proc Soc Exp Biol Med 1994;202:258.
19. Pacques EP. Recent advances in the biochemistry of the fibrinolytic system. Behring Inst Mitt 1988;82:68.
20. Rosenberg R, Rosenberg J. Natural anticoagulant mechanisms. J Clin Invest 1984;74:1.
21. Bachman F, Kruithof I. Tissue plasminogen activator: chemical and physiology aspects. Semin Thromb Hemost 1984;10:6.
22. Benedict CR, Mueller S, Anderson HV, Willerson JT. Thrombolytic therapy: a state of the art review. Hosp Pract 1992;43:61.
23. Sorensen JV. Levels of fibrinolytic activators and inhibitors in plasma after severe trauma. Blood Coagul Fibrinolysis 1994;5:43.
24. Collen D, Lijnen HR. The fibrinolytic system in man. CRC Crit Rev Oncol Hematol 1986;4:249.
25. Francis CW, Marder VJ. Physiologic regulation and pathologic disorders and fibrinolysis. Human Pathol 1987;18:263.
26. Phillips TF, Soulier G, Wilson RF. Outcome of massive transfusion exceeding two blood volumes in trauma and emergency surgery. J Trauma 1987;27:903.
27. Giddings JC, Peake IR. Laboratory support in the diagnosis of coagulation disorders. Clin Haematol 1985;14:571.
28. Lind SE. The bleeding time does not predict surgical bleeding. Blood 1991;77:2547.
29. Mammen EF. Congential coagulation protein disorders. Bick RL, Bennett JM, Brynes RK, et al., eds. Hematology: clinical and laboratory practice, vol 2. St. Louis: Mosby, 1993; 1391-1420.
30. Mammen EF. Laboratory evaluation of congential coagulation protein disorders. Bick RL, Bennett JM, Bryns RK, et al., eds. Hematology: clinical and laboratory practice, vol 2. St. Louis: Mosby, 1993; 1421-1433.
31. Jandl JH. Disorders of coagulation. Jandl JH, ed. Blood: textbook of hematology. Boston: Little, Brown, 1987; 1095.
32. Sixma JJ, Van Den Berg A. The haemostatic plug in haemophilia A: a morphological study of haemostatic plug formation in bleeding from skin wounds of patients with severe haemophilia A. Br J Haematol 1984; 58:741.

33. Andes WA, Wulff K, Smith WB. Head trauma in hemophilia: a prospective study. Arch Intern Med 1984;144:1981.

34. Martinowitz U, Heim M, Tadmor R, et al. Intracranial hemorrhage in patients with hemophilia. Neurosurgery 1986;18:538.

35. Romeyn RL, Herkowitz HN. The cervical spine in hemophilia. Clin Orthop 1986;210:113.

36. Cox Gill J. Therapy of factor VIII deficiency. Semin Thromb Hemost 1993;19:1.

37. Rizza CR, Biggs R. Treatment of congenital deficiencies of factor VIII and factor IX. Thromb Diath Haemorrh 1969;34(Suppl):73.

38. Pool JG. Cryoprecipitated factor VIII concentrate. Thromb Diath Haemorrh 1969;35(Suppl):35.

39. Johnson AJ, Karpatkin MH, Newman J. Clinical investigation of intermediate and high-purity antihaemophilic factor VIII concentrates. Br J Haemat 1971;21:21.

40. Macik BG. Treatment of factor VIII inhibitors: products and strategies. Semin Thromb Hemost 1993;19:13.

41. Thompson AR. Factor IX concentrates for clinical use. Semin Thromb Hemost 1993;19:25.

42. Mannucci PM. Desmopressin: a nontransfusional form of treatment for congenital and acquired bleeding disorders. Blood 1988;72:1449.

43. Walsh PN, Rizza CR, Matthews J, et al. Epsilon-amino caproic acid therapy for dental extractions in haemophilia and Christmas disease: a double-blind controlled trial. Br J Haematol 1971;20:463.

44. Ruggeri ZM, Zimmerman TS. von Willebrand factor and von Willebrand disease. Blood 1987;70:895.

45. Zimmerman TS, Ruggeri ZM. Laboratory diagnosis of von Willebrand disease. Bick RL, Bennett JM, Brynes RN, et al., eds. Hematology: clinical and laboratory practice, vol 2. St. Louis: Mosby 1993; 1441-1447.

46. Scott JP, Montgomery RR. Therapy of von Willebrand disease. Semin Thromb Hemost 1993;19:37.

47. Furlan M, Lämmle B, Aeberhard A, et al. Virus-inactivated factor VIII concentrate prevents postoperative bleeding in a patient with von Willebrand disease. Transfusion 1988;28:489.

48. Castaman G, Rodeghiero F, DiBona E, Ruggeri Z. Clinical effectiveness of desmopressin in a case of acquired von Willebrand's syndrome associated with benign monoclonal gammopathy. Blut 1989;58:211.

49. George JN, Shattie SJ. The clinical importance of acquired abnormalities of platelet function. N Engl J Med 1991;324:27.

50. Mammen EF. Coagulation abnormalities in liver disease. Hematol Oncol Clin North Am 1992;6:1247.

51. Mannucci PM, Vincente V, Vianello L, et al. Controlled trial of desmopressin in liver cirrhosis and other conditions associated with prolonged bleeding time. Blood 1986;67:1148.

52. Mammen EF. Acquired coagulation protein disorders. Bick RL, Bennett JM, Brynes RD, et al., eds. Hematology: clinical and laboratory practice, vol 2. St. Louis: Mosby, 1993; 1449-1462.

53. Janson PA, Jubelirer SJ, Weinstein MJ. Treatment of the bleeding tendency in uremia with cryoprecipitate. N Engl J Med 1980;303:1318.

54. Watson AJ, Keogh JA. 1-Deamino-8-D-arginine vasopressin as a therapy for the bleeding diathesis of renal failure. Am J Nephrol 1984;4:49.

55. Liu YK, Kosfeld RE, Marcum SG. Treatment of uraemic bleeding with conjugated oestrogen. Lancet 1984;2:887.

56. Clark J, Hochman R, Rolla AR, et al. Coagulopathy associated with the use of cephalosporin or maxalactam antibiotics in acute and chronic renal failure. Clin Exp Dial Apheresis 7:177, 1983.

57. Nanfro JJ. Anticoagulants in critical care medicine. Chernow B, ed. The pharmacologic/approach in the critically ill patient, 2nd ed. Baltimore: Williams & Wilkins, 1988; 511-535.

58. Hirsh J, Dalen JE, Deykin D, Poller L. Heparin: mechanism of action, pharmacokinetics, dosing considerations, monitoring, efficacy, and safety. Chest 1992;102(Suppl):337S.

59. Kelton J, Levine M. Heparin-induced thrombocytopenia. Am J Med 1986;12:59.

60. Chong BH, Ismail F, Cada J, et al. Heparin-induced thrombocytopenia: studies with a low molecular weight heparinoid, ORG 10172. Blood 1989;73:1592.

61. Nanfro JJ. Anticoagulants in critical care medicine. Chernow B, ed. The pharmacologic approach to the critically ill patient, 3rd ed. Baltimore: Williams & Wilkins, 1994; 666-684.

62. Moncada S. Archidonic acid metabolites and the interactions between platelets and blood vessel walls. N Engl J Med 1979;300:1142.

63. Benedict CR, Mueller S, Anderson HV, et al. Thrombolytic therapy: a state of the art review. Hosp Pract 1992;15:61.

64. Woodman RC, Harber LA. Bleeding complications associated with cardiopulmonary bypass. Blood 1990;76:1680.

65. Miller WR, Willson JT, Elliot TS. Blood changes in the dog following trauma. Angiology 1959;10:375.

66. Attar S, Boyd D, Layne E, et al. Alterations in coagulation and fibrinolytic mechanisms in acute trauma. J Trauma 1969;9:939.

67. Harrigan C, Lucas CE, Ledgerwood AM. The effect of hemorrhagic shock on the clotting cascade in injured patients. J Trauma 1989;29:1416.

68. Wilson RF, Mammen EF, Robson MC, et al. Antithrombin, prekallikrein, and fibronectin levels in surgical patients. Arch Surg 1986;121:635-640.

69. Wilson RF, Farag A, Mammen EF, Fujii Y. Sepsis and antithrombin III, prekallikrein and fibronectin levels in surgical patients. Am Surg 1989;55:450-456.

70. Kobrinsky NL, Letts RM, Patel LR, et al. 1-Deamino-8-arginine vasopressin (desmopressin) decreases operative blood loss in patients having Harrington rod spinal fusion surgery. Ann Intern Med 1987;107:446.

71. Garcia Frade LJ, Landin L, Garcia Avello A, et al. PAI and D-D dimer levels are related to severity of injury in trauma patients. Fibrinolysis 1991;5:253.

72. Meier H, Pierce J. Activation and function of human Hageman factor. J Clin Invest 1977;60:18.

73. Hewson J. Massive transfusion panel discussion. Can Anaesth Soc J 1985;32:239.

74. Aasen A, Kierulf P, Vaage J, et al. Determination of components of the plasma proteolytic enzyme systems gives information of prognostic value in patients with multiple trauma. Adv Exp Med Biol 1983;156:1037.

75. Bagge L, Haglund O, Wallin R, et al. Differences in coagulation and fibrinolysis after traumatic and septic shock in man. Scand J Clin Lab Invest 1989;49:63.

76. Friedman M, Uhley HN. Role of the adrenal in hastening blood coagulation after exposure to stress. Am J Physiol 1959;197:205.

77. Kambayashyi J, Sakon M, Yokota M, et al. Activation of coagulation and fibrinolysis during surgery, analyzed by molecular markers. Thromb Res 1990;60:157.

78. Touho H, Harakawa K, Hino A, et al. Relationship between abnormalities of coagulation and fibrinolysis and postoperative intracranial hemorrhage in head injury. Neurosurgery 1986;19:523.

79. Evans DE, Alta WA, Shtasky SA, et al. Cardiac arrhythmias resulting from experimental head injury. J Neurosurg 1976;45:609.

80. Reed RL, Ciavarella D, Heimbach DM, et al. Prophylactic platelet administration during massive transfusion. A prospective randomized double-blind clinical study. Ann Surg 1986;203:40.

81. Winter JP. Early fresh frozen plasma prophylaxis of abnormal coagulation parameters in the severely head injured patient is not effective. Ann Emerg Med 1989;18:553.

82. Salva KM, Kim H, Nahum K, Fallot PL. DDAVP in the treatment of bleeding disorders. Pharmacotherapy 1988;8:94.

83. Mannucci PM, Vicente V, Viannelle L, et al. Controlled trial of desmopressin in liver cirrhosis and other conditions associated with a prolonged bleeding time. Blood 1986;67:1148.

84. Salzman EW, Weinstein MJ, Weintaub RM, et al. Treatment with desmopressin acetate to reduce blood loss after cardiac surgery, a double-blind randomized trial. N Engl J Med 1986;314:1402.

85. Kohler M, Harris A. Pharmacokinetics and hematological effects of desmopressin. Curr J Clin Pharmacol 1988;35:281.

86. Melissari E, Scully MF, Paes T, et al. The influence of DDAVP infusion on the coagulation and fibrinolytic response to surgery. Thromb Haemost 1986;55:54.

87. Schulman S, Johnson H, Egberg N, Blombäck M. DDAVP-induced correction of prolonged bleeding time in patients with congenital platelet function defects. Thromb Res 1987;45:165.

88. Patt A, McCroskey BL, Moore EE. Hypothermia induced coagulopathy in trauma. Surg Clin North Am 1988;68:775.

89. Yoshihara H, Yamamoto T, Mihara H. Changes in coagulation and fibrinolysis occurring in dogs during hypothermia. Thromb Res 1985;37:503.

90. Halonen P, Linko K, Myllyla G. A study of haemostasis following the use of high doses of hydroxyethyl starch and dextran in major laparotomies. Acta Anaesthesiol Scand 1987;31:320.

91. Lucas CE, Denis R, Ledgerwood AM, Grabow D. The effects of Hespan on serum and lymphatic albumin, globulin, and coagulant protein. Ann Surg 1988;207:416.

92. Henson JR, Neame PB, Kumar N, et al. Coagulopathy related to dilution and hypotension during massive transfusion. Crit Care Med 1985;13:387.

93. Benson RE, Ishister JP. Massive blood transfusion. Anaesth Crit Care 1980;8:152.

94. Krevans JR, Jackson DP. Hemorrhagic disorders following massive whole blood transfusions. JAMA 1955;159:171.

95. Miller RD, Robbins TO, Tong MJ, et al. Coagulation defects associated with massive blood transfusions. Ann Surg 1971;174:794.

96. Laks H, Handin RI, Martin V, et al. The effects of acute normovolemic hemodilution on coagulation and blood utilization in major surgery. J Surg Res 1976;20:225.

97. Cavins JA, Farber S, Roy AJ. Transfusions of fresh platelet concentrates to adult patients with thrombocytopenia. Transfusion 1968;8:24.

98. Voorhees AB, Elliot HE. Surgical experiences with thrombocytopenic patients. Ann NY Acad Sci 1964;115:1.

99. Consensus conference. Fresh frozen plasma: indications and risks. JAMA 1985;253:551.

100. Braumstein AH, Oberman HA. Transfusion of plasma components. Transfusion 1984;24:281.

101. Martin DJ, Lucas CE, Ledgerwood AM, et al. Fresh frozen plasma supplement to massive red blood cell transfusion. Ann Surg 1985;202:505.

102. Broadie TA. Clotting competence of intracavity blood in trauma victims. Ann Emerg Med 1981;10:127.

103. Mueller-Berghaus G. Pathophysiologic and biochemical events in disseminated intravascular coagulation: dysregulation of procoagulant and antiocoagulant pathways. Semin Thromb Hemost 1989;15:58.

104. Mammen E, Miyakawa T, Phillips T, et al. Human antithrombin concentrates and experimental disseminated intravascular coagulation. Semin Thromb Hemost 1985;22:373.

105. Bick RL. Disseminated intravascular coagulation and related syndromes. Semin Thromb Hemost 1988;14:299.

106. McManus, WF, Eurenius K, Pruitt BA. Disseminated intravascular coagulation in burned patients. J Trauma 1973;13:416.

107. Fisher D, Yawn D, Crawford E. Preoperative disseminated intravascular coagulation associated with aortic aneurysms. Arch Surg 1983;118:1252.

108. Broersma RJ, Bullemer GD, Mammen EF. Acidosis induced disseminated intravascular microthrombosis and its dissolution by streptokinase. Thromb Diath Haemorrh 1970;24:55.

109. Porte J. Coagulation and fibrinolysis in orthotopic liver transplantation: current views and insights. Semin Thromb Hemost 1993;19:191.

110. McKenna P, Scheinman H. Transient coagulation abnormalities after incompatible blood transfusion. Crit Care Med 1975;3:8.

111. Carr JM, McKinner M, McDonagh J. Diagnosis of disseminated intravascular coagulation. Am J Clin Pathol 1989;91:280-287.

112. Koyama T, Kakishita E, Nakai Y, Okamoto E. Significance of hemostatic molecular markers during disseminated intravascular coagulation in patients with liver cirrhosis treated by endoscopic embolization for esophageal varices. Am J Hematol 1991;38:90-94.

113. Elms MJ, Bunce IH, Bundensen PG, et al. Rapid detection of cross-linked fibrin degradation products in plasma using monoclonal antibody-coated latex particles. Am J Clin Pathol 1986;85:360-364.

114. Hoek JA, Aturk A, Cate JW, et al. Laboratory and clinical evaluation of an assay of thrombin-antithrombin III complexes in plasma. Clin Chem 1988;34:2058-2062.

115. Holvoet P, Boer A, Verstreken M, Collen D. An enzyme-linked immunosorbent assay (ELISA) for the measurement of plasmino-alpha$_2$-antiplasmin complex in human plasma—application to the detection of in vivo activation of fibrinolytic system. Thromb Haemost 1986;56:124-127.

116. Bick RL. Disseminated intravascular coagulation: a clinical/laboratory study of 48 patients. Ann NY Acad Sci 1981;370:843.

117. Kazmier FJ, Bowie EJW, Hagedorn AB, et al. Treatment of intravascular coagulation and fibrinolysis (ICF) syndromes. Mayo Clin Proc 1974;49:665.

118. Vinazzer H. Therapeutic use of antithrombin III in shock and disseminated intravascular coagulation. Semin Thromb Hemost 1989;15:347.

119. Gomez C, Parao JA, Rocha E. Effect of heparin and/or antithrombin III in a model of disseminated intravascular coagulation induced by endotoxin in rabbits. Sangre 1992;37:5.

120. Dickneite G, Paques EP. Reduction of mortality with antithrombin III in speticemic rats: a study of Klebsiella pneumoniae induced sepsis. Thromb Haemost 1993;69:98.

121. Del Principe D, Pietrantoni R, Menichelli A, et al. Therapy with antithrombin III in burned children—pilot study. Haematologica 1990;75(Suppl 2):33.

122. Langley PG, Hughes RD, Forbes A, et al. Controlled trial of antithrombin III supplementation in fulminant hepatic failure. J Hepatol 1993;17:326.

123. Coccheri S, Palarett G. Antithrombin III replacement in orthotopic liver transplantation. Semin Thromb Hemost 1993;19:268.

124. Blauhut B, Necek S, Vinazzer H, Bergman H. Substitution therapy with an antithrombin III concentrate in shock and DIC. Thromb Res 1982;27:271.

125. Seitz R, Egbring R. Patients in septic shock: antithrombin III supplementation. Biomed Progr 1992;5:27.

126. Fourrier F, Chopin C, Huart JJ, et al. Double-blind, placebo-controlled trial of antithrombin III concentrates in septic shock with disseminated intravascular coagulation. Chest 1993;104:882.

127. Bone RC. Sepsis and coagulation: an important link. Chest 1992;191:594.

128. Mammen EF. Perspectives for the future. Intensive Care Med 1993;19:S29.

129. Kram HB, Nathan RC, Stafford FJ, et al. Fibrin glue achieves hemostasis in patients with coagulation disorders. Arch Surg 1989;124:385.

130. Johnson SD, Lucas CE, Gerrick SJ, et al. Altered coagulation after albumin supplements for treatment of oligemic shock. Arch Surg 1979;114:379.

131. Leibold WC, Lucas CE, Ledgerwood AM, et al. Effect of albumin resuscitation on canine coagulation activity and content. Ann Surg 1983;198:630.

Chapter 46 Organ Procurement from Trauma Victims

ROBERT D. ALLABEN, M.D.
ROBERT F. WILSON, M.D.

NEED FOR ORGAN DONORS

AXIOM The main obstacle to the transplantation of organs at this time is donor availability.

Refinements in organ preservation, surgical technique, and immunosuppression with cyclosporine and other new drugs have made transplantation of solid organs increasingly more successful.[1-8] Organs and tissue currently being transplanted include blood, kidneys, hearts, heart valves, veins, livers, lungs, skin, pancreas, bone, cornea, and intestines. Available statistics from the United Network of Organ Sharing (UNOS) indicated that over 10,931 kidney transplants, 2299 heart transplants, 3442 liver transplants, and 771 pancreas transplants, were performed in 1993.[4,5] The number of centers performing liver and heart transplantation has more than tripled since 1980.[9,10]

With terminal liver or cardiac disease, the patient has little long-term options other than transplantation. Major strides have been made in the field of artificial cardiac support, but these are best viewed currently as bridges to transplantation rather than permanent substitutes.[1]

Although patients with chronic renal failure can be maintained on dialysis, the quality of life is superior for patients with a functioning renal transplant. Furthermore, the cost of long-term hemodialysis is billions of dollars yearly. If many of the patients on chronic dialysis could undergo renal transplantation, millions of dollars would be saved yearly. The cost of a liver transplant averages $267,000 and a kidney transplant $150,000.[4,5,11] However, the major expenditure for solid organ transplantation occurs during the initial year after transplantation, with the expense in subsequent years primarily for medication.

Despite these remarkable advances, 2000-3000 patients still die annually awaiting organ transplantation (Table 46-1). The desperate need for organ donations is also reflected by the large number of individuals awaiting transplantation of various organs according to data supplied by the UNOS (Table 46-2).

CHARACTERISTICS OF ORGAN DONORS

AXIOM Young, previously healthy individuals who have suffered isolated lethal head injuries or intracranial bleeding from vascular anomalies are generally the best candidates for organ donation.

In 1994, in the state of Michigan, the Transplantation Society of Michigan was notified of 478 potential organ donors. Of these, 186 actually became organ donors. Of the 186 organ donors for that year, 94 (50%) were victims of trauma (Table 46-3). For that reason, hospital emergency rooms are important sites where the initial identification of potential organ donors should occur. The possibility of a trauma victim becoming brain-dead and thereby becoming a potential organ donor should be kept in mind by paramedical personnel and emergency room nurses and physicians. One should consider the possibility of patients becoming organ donors when it is likely that they will die of: (a) isolated head injuries, (b) intracranial bleeding from a vascular anomaly, or (c) suffocation or drowning.

Severe head injury is the cause of death in 56-77% of organ donors, and subarachnoid hemorrhage and brain tumor comprise the second most common cause of death in the donor group.[12] Other donors die from drug overdose and anoxic brain injuries from various causes.

Individuals caring for such victims should be alert to the usual criteria of brain death and remember that any brain-dead individual is a potential organ donor. Any individual who is dead on arrival (DOA) or died in the emergency department (DIE) may also become a donor of various tissues.

OBTAINING ORGAN DONORS

AXIOM The major factor responsible for the shortage of donor organs is lack of donor referrals.

Approximately 4% of all deaths result in potentially suitable donors; however, less than 12-15% of these actually donate organs.[11,13] Up to 70-80% of families of potential organ donors will agree to organ donation when approached properly.[14] Because they do not think to offer organ donation during the sudden terminal illness of a family member, most families must be informed and given the opportunity. The Uniform Anatomical Gift Act was passed to serve as a solution to this issue.[15] Most states now also require that hospitals offer organ donation to the families of dying or brain-dead patients.[11] Several authorities have advocated the concept of "presumed consent".[2] Laws incorporating this consent would state that unless people have explicitly indicated that they do not want their organs donated, it is assumed that they do; transplant surgeons then may proceed with the procurement of organs. Such laws are already in effect in several European countries.

AXIOM The referral of an organ or tissue donor begins with recognition by physicians, nurses, or other individuals that a particular patient may be a suitable donor for organs or tissues.

When an individual is identified as a potential donor, even before criteria for brain death have been met, the Organ Procurement Organization serving the area should be notified. They can provide invaluable support in the care of organ donors and assist in obtaining permission for donation after the patient is declared brain dead. The telephone number of the Organ Procurement Organization should be readily available in all emergency room and critical care units. The referral of the potential organ donor may be expedited by providing the patient's height, weight, age, medical history, diagnosis, hemodynamic data, urinalysis, serum creatinine levels, culture results, and ABO blood group. The transplant coordinators may then begin evaluation of the suitability of the potential donor.

GENERAL CRITERIA FOR ACCEPTANCE OF DONORS

Criteria for acceptance of individuals as organ donors vary from organ to organ. The criteria have gradually broadened over the past several years as the techniques of organ retrieval and immunosuppression have improved and also because of the increasing number of

TABLE 46–1 Analysis of Reported Deaths in Patients Awaiting Organ Transplant

Year	Organ	No. Patients	No. Deaths Reported	Death Rate (No. Deaths/ No. Patients)
1993	Kidney	33,538	1275	3.8%
	Kidney + pancreas	1747	59	3.4%
	Pancreas	299	3	1.0%
	Liver	7040	558	7.9%
	Intestine	58	3	5.2%
	Heart	6269	762	12.2%
	Heart + lung	332	51	15.4%
	Lung	2180	252	11.6%
	Overall	50,135	2887	5.8%

(From: Data compiled by UNOS Research Department as of January 27, 1994.)

individuals awaiting transplantation. Donors of eyes, skin, bone, and other tissues need not be heartbeating cadavers at retrieval.

AXIOM Even when they do not meet criteria for whole-organ transplantation, patients frequently are suitable donors for skin, cornea, or bone.

Criteria for Donors in General

As noted previously, the ideal candidate for solid-organ donation is a previously healthy patient who has had irreversible brain injury due to head trauma, subarachnoid hemorrhage, drug overdose, primary brain tumors, or cerebral ischemia. In the past, age was a major criterion for potential organ donors. Recent data has indicated that the traditional age limits can be extended, and the chronologic age of donors is less important than their physiologic age.[12,16]

General exclusion criteria for organ donation include acute, untreated, or uncontrolled infections, positive serology for the HIV antigen, active tuberculosis, malignancies other than brain or skin, trauma or disease involving the organs considered for donation, prolonged hypotension, or severe diabetes mellitus, hypertension, or peripheral vascular disease[12,16] (Table 46–4). The suitability of potential donors with appropriately treated bacterial infection should be individually evaluated by the transplantation team.

Thoracic Organ Donors

The donor for heart or lung transplantion should not have evidence of preexisting severe valvular or coronary artery disease by history or examination.[1] The presence of pathologic Q-waves contraindicates use of the heart for transplantation. Systolic BP should be maintained at > 90 mm Hg with < 10 ug/kg/minute of dopamine. When question of cardiac suitability exists, echocardiography may be of value.

Lung donors must not have histories of chronic lung disease, such as tuberculosis, asthma, heavy smoking, severe parenchymal injury, pneumothorax, or pulmonary aspiration. Indices of lung dysfunction that are relative contraindications include a Pao_2/Fio_2 ratio < 250, peak airway pressures > 30 cm H_2O, tracheobronchitis or chest radiographic findings consistent with pneumonia, persistent atelectasis, or marked pulmonary contusion.

Abdominal Organ Donors

The potential donor of abdominal organs must be free of abdominal sepsis or direct injury to the abdominal organs considered for transplantation. Serum creatinine values > 177 umol/L (> 1.8 mg/dL) are usually predictive of poor graft function after transplantation.[12] However, the trend of these values may be just as important as the actual levels.

Patients with severe, chronic hepatic disease are obviously excluded as liver donors. However, patients with abnormal liver function tests should be individualized. Elevated transaminase levels may be due to a prior period of hypoperfusion. When levels of transaminase are only mildly to moderately elevated and are declining, the liver may be suitable for transplantation. The only contraindications to use of the pancreas for transplantation include direct injury or diabetes mellitus.

ESTABLISHING BRAIN DEATH

Until 1977, death had traditionally been defined by both the medical and the legal professions as cessation of cardiovascular and respiratory function. However, with current advances in critical care, cardiac and pulmonary function may be maintained for long periods despite the absence of brain function.[18] Consequently, criteria by which to define death as complete and irreversible cessation of brain and brain stem function have been derived.[14,19-23]

The general criteria for determination of brain death require documentation that: (a) cerebral and brain stem functions are absent, (b) the condition is irreversible, which requires that the cause(s) of the condition be known, and (3) cessation of all brain function persists after an appropriate period of observation and adequate trial of therapy.[19,24]

AXIOM The ultimate determination of brain death of a potential donor remains the clinical responsibility of the attending physician.

Specific criteria for brain death have been independently developed by several different groups to assist the attending physician with this determination.[19-24] Despite some variations in these guidelines, all require a detailed neurologic evaluation, and many also require electroencephalography (EEG); however, obtaining a flat EEG in an ICU environment with all its electrical and monitoring apparatus can be extremely difficult. When no brain function is found, a repeated confirmatory neurologic examination must be performed again after 6-12 hours. In some centers, a second examination is not performed. Furthermore, if a radioisotope or other study were to show no blood flow to brain, no other confirmatory test would be required.

AXIOM Brain death should be pronounced as soon as possible after it occurs.

"Brain death is not a chronic state".[1] Cardiac arrest usually occurs within 72 hours of the occurrence of brain death of a potential donor unless special efforts are taken to maintain adequate cardiopulmonary function.

The guidelines used at the Presbyterian University Hospital in Pittsburgh have been a model for many other centers to assist in determining brain death[1] (Table 46–5).

TABLE 46–2 Number of Patients on Waiting Lists, by Organ (1987 to 1990)

As of December 31st	1987	1988	1989	1990
Heart	699	1,032	1,324	1,796
Heart-lung	155	205	240	226
Kidney	12,099	13,944	16,363	17,955
Liver	454	617	830	1,248
Lung	16	70	94	309
Pancreas	63	164	322	474
Total	13,396	16,032	19,173	22,008

(From: United Network for Organ Sharing)

TABLE 46–3   Cause of Death in Organ Donors

	Year											
	1988		1989		1990		1991		1992		1993	
Cause of Death	N	%	N	%	N	%	N	%	N	%	N	%
Motor Vehicle	1382	33.9	1181	29.5	1216	27.0	1151	25.4	967	21.5	1030	21.3
Gunshot/Stab	625	15.3	672	16.8	745	16.5	811	17.9	833	18.5	863	17.8
Cerebrovascular	1132	27.8	1223	30.5	1464	32.5	1536	33.9	1624	36.2	1767	36.5
Head Trauma	411	10.1	439	11.0	525	11.6	470	10.4	512	11.4	546	11.3
Asphyxiation	111	2.7	119	3.0	139	3.1	146	3.2	106	2.4	129	2.7
Drowning	49	1.2	47	1.2	51	1.1	38	0.8	46	1.0	51	1.1
Drug Intoxication	54	1.3	37	0.9	32	0.7	32	0.7	36	0.8	24	0.5
Cardiovascular	94	2.3	80	2.0	80	1.8	80	1.8	82	1.8	98	2.0
Other	217	5.3	211	5.3	258	5.7	261	5.8	285	6.3	327	6.8
not reported	8		7		5		5		30		10	
Total	4083	100.0	4016	100.0	4515	100.0	4530	100.0	4521	100.0	4845	100.0

(From: UNOS OPTN data as of August 1, 1994.)
Percentages are column percentages and do not include "Not Report" cases.

Each institution must develop its own specific criteria for brain death. Sample criteria are available in the literature and may also be obtained from one's local Organ Procurement Organization. When these criteria are met, one can assure relatives that no instance of recovery of such patients has occurred.[1] Testing for these brain-death criteria in potential organ donors should be carried out by a physician or physicians who have no involvement in the proposed transplantation. Although physicians doing such testing are usually neurologists or neurosurgeons, any physician can certify brain death by using approved criteria.

When the possibility of drug effect or uncertainty concerning the nature of the intracranial pathology exists, four-vessel cerebral angiography, radionuclide cerebral imaging, or xenon-CT cerebral blood flow scan may be necessary to establish the absence of cerebral circulation.[19] Spinal cord reflexes are irrelevant in the diagnosis of brain death and, therefore, are not routinely tested.[12]

PITFALL ⊘

Not considering a brain-dead patient for organ donation because it is a "medical examiner's case."

Almost all medical examiners' cases can be used as organ or tissue donors. The medical examiner needs to be knowledgeable about donation and should be invited to witness the harvesting of donor organs. In cases where they have jurisdiction, permission of medical examiners is not required for the death certification process; however, the medical examiner's permission and consent of the next of kin are required for removal of organs for transplantation.

When any uncertainty exists regarding a patient's eligibility as an organ donor at brain death, early contact should be made with the local Organ Procurement Organization. It then will answer questions, directly assist with the management of the potential organ donor, arrange donation and procurement, account for all expenses incurred, and reimburse the hospital in which the donation was performed for expenses involved with tests to prove brain death, efforts to sustain the patient after brain death, transportation costs, and actual organ procurement.[1]

Consent for Organ Donation

The Uniform Anatomical Gift Act (UAGA) was enacted in all states to standardize methods for organ donation.[15] The uniform donor card allows adults to donate all or parts of their bodies after death for research, education, or transplantation. Victims may carry uniform donor cards, which are legal documents, but consent should also be obtained from next of kin prior to organ donation.

Consent for organ donation from the next of kin may be obtained according to the following priority list: spouse, adult son or daughter, either parent, sibling, guardian, or any other authorized person.[1] The organs being donated are listed individually, and it is stated that the donation(s) is (are) for the purpose of transplantation. After the closest available next of kin has signed this form and it has been witnessed, organ procurement may proceed. Consent may also be obtained by telephone or telegram; however, every effort should be made to talk in-person to the relative giving consent and to obtain permission in writing.

PRERETRIEVAL PATIENT MANAGEMENT

Management Prior to Brain Death

AXIOM   Consideration of patients as potential organ donors should not interfere with the treatment of their injuries or diseases.

TABLE 46–4   Donor Criteria for Various Organ Harvesting

General Criteria
 No cancer, except primary skin or brain
 No systemic infections
 No hepatitis
 No history of tuberculosis or syphilis
 No history of recent intravenous drug abuse
 No prolonged episodes of hypotension or asystole
 No acute or chronic renal failure
Criteria for Specific Organs
 Serum creatinine under 1.8 mg/dL (K), BUN < 20 mg/dL (K)
 No established hypertension (K)
 No evidence of urinary tract infection by urinalysis (K)
 No evidence of diabetes mellitus or abnormal pancreatic function (P)
 No visible infiltrate or evidence of trauma on chest radiography (Lu, H/L)
 Donor arterial oxygen tension exceeding 250 mm Hg on 100% O_2 (Lu, H/L)
 Normal ECG and cardiac function; no evidence of cardiovascular disease (H, H/L)
 Sputum obtained by bronchoscopy is free of organisms as demonstrated by Gram stain (Lu, H/L)
 Normal liver function tests (Li)

K = kidney, P = pancreas, Lu = lung, H = heart, H/L = combined heart-lung, Li = liver

TABLE 46–5 Guidelines Used at Presbyterian University Hospital in Pittsburgh for Determining Brain Death

1. Deep coma of an etiology that is established and sufficient to explain the irreversible loss of function of brain. This must be documented in the absence of hypothermia, central nervous system depressant drugs, hypovolemia, hypoxemia, or hypotension.
2. Spontaneous movement, decerebrate and decorticate posturing, and cranial reflexes must be absent.
3. Response to painful stimuli, such as supraorbital pressure or pinprick, is absent.
4. Cranial nerve reflexes are absent and this includes:
    a. Nonreactive pupils
    b. No corneal reflexes
    c. No oculocephalic reflex
    d. No oculovestibular reflex
    e. No response to upper and lower airway suctioning
5. EEG is recorded at full gain for 30 minutes, with and without auditory stimulation. This test is often utilized as a confirmatory test between the two clinical examinations.
6. Lack of function of the vagus nerve nuclei is inferred from lack of an increase in heart rate after intravenous atropine sulfate (0.04 mg/kg).

Even when a patient has been identified as potential organ donor, treatment should be given in the most appropriate way to aid in recovery. This includes maintenance of a normal or slightly increased blood volume, BP, cardiac output, oxygenation, and urine output. However, efforts to control cerebral edema may have included restriction of fluids. Under such circumstances, at the time that brain death is pronounced, the patient may have moderate-to-severe dehydration with oliguria and elevated creatinine levels. The patient may also be on dopamine or other forms of cardiovascular support.

A careful, continuing search for evidence of infection must be made. In addition to carefully monitoring the patient and his core temperature and white blood cell count, one should obtain daily chest radiography, daily sputum smears and cultures, and urine cultures.

Postbrain-death Management

AXIOM   After pronouncement of brain death, oxygenation and perfusion should be optimally maintained until the donor surgery is complete.

It is essential that, following the pronouncement of brain death, the potential donor be rapidly hydrated with appropriate solutions so that BP and blood volume can be maintained at levels that allow normal perfusion of vital organs and urinary output of at least 1.0-1.5 mL/kg/hour. The risk of acute tubular necrosis increases if the donor's systolic BP has been < 80-90 mm Hg.[12] Experimental data also suggests that this level is critical for hepatic graft function.[12,25]

Central venous pressure measurements should be utilized to evaluate right-heart filling pressures. In some instances, pulmonary artery wedge pressure (PAWP) catheter to determine left-heart filling pressures and cardiac output may be helpful. When BP cannot be maintained without a PAWP > 15 mm Hg or vasoactive drugs, dopamine and/or dobutamine in doses that do not exceed 10 mcg/kg/minute may improve BP and/or cardiac output without causing dangerous degrees of vasoconstriction.

AXIOM   Vasoconstrictor drugs should be avoided or only used in low doses in brain-dead potential organ donors.

Patients requiring <10 mcg/kg/minute dopamine at organ retrieval do not provide ideal organs for transplantation. However, in almost all instances, with appropriate rehydration, such support can be withdrawn and over a period of hours, the solid vascularized organs can become appropriate for transplantation.[1]

If a patient has a cardiac arrest before or after pronouncement of brain death, he or she should be rapidly resuscitated, using internal cardiac massage if needed. External cardiac massage for more than a few minutes generally excludes a patient from becoming a heart or lung donor. Cardiac arrest or severe hypotension for more than 15 minutes also contraindicates intrathoracic and intraabdominal organ donation.

Core temperature should be monitored constantly and the patient maintained as normothermic as possible. A warming blanket and warmed fluids and inhaled gases are used as needed to maintain core temperatures > 35°C.

Prior to being pronounced brain dead, patients with severe brain injury are usually kept at a $Paco_2$ of about 25-30 mm Hg to reduce intracranial pressure (ICP). After brain death has been declared, $Paco_2$ can be gradually normalized, but a normal or slightly alkalemic pH should be maintained.[12,16] Pao_2 should be maintained at 80-100 mm Hg using the lowest Fio_2 possible and < 10 cm H_2O PEEP. Patients with neurogenic pulmonary edema should be monitored with a pulmonary artery catheter and efforts made to reduce the PAWP to < 12-15 mm Hg.

AXIOM   Diabetes insipidus in brain-dead potential organ donors should be corrected with aqueous pitressin or desmopressin (DDAVP) as soon as possible.

With brain injury, especially involving the hypothalamus and/or posterior pituitary gland, diabetes insipidus may occur. The resultant output of large volumes of urine with a low-specific gravity can be extremely difficult to replace properly. Therefore, if the urinary output exceeds 200 mL/hour and the patient is not overloaded with fluid, consideration should be given to the administration of aqueous pitressin (10 units subcutaneously) or DDAVP. Pitressin in oil should not be used. Aqueous pitressin is metabolized relatively rapidly, but pitressin in oil may cause severe, prolonged oliguria and should not be used.

Proper electrolyte and acid-base balance is important. Hyponatremia or hypernatremia, hypocalcemia, hypokalemia, hypomagnesemia, hypophosphatemia, and hyperglycemia are common in brain-dead patients and should be frequently monitored and corrected as soon as possible.

In addition to electrolyte and glucose determinations, other tests that should be obtained by the hospital or transplantation personnel include: ABO blood group, BUN, serum creatinine, urinalysis, HIV, HTLV, CMV, hepatitis surface antigens, and blood and urine cultures. Other tests for specific organs include liver function tests on potential liver donors, ECG on potential heart donors, and blood gases and chest radiography on potential lung donors.[1]

Prevention of and monitoring for infection is critical. The results of all predonation cultures should be known. In addition, cultures of blood, urine, sputum, and flush solutions should be drawn 30 minutes before organs are removed. To help prevent bacteremia from intravenous lines, a first-generation cephalosporin is usually given immediately before organ retrieval begins.

The presence of any systemic infection is usually a contraindication to solid organ donation; however, the patient who has had a prior systemic infection may be a candidate for organ donation if the infection was eliminated prior to donor surgery.

AXIOM   Proper preoperative management of organ donors plays a critical role in determining the successful outcome of organ transplantation.

Even when no other organs or tissues can be donated, the corneas can often be used. Consequently, continuing eye care is essential. Continuous lubrication of the corneas is critical to ensure their usefulness in transplantation. Taping the lids shut may also help.

BLOOD AND TISSUE TYPING

Before moving the patient to the operating room, blood is drawn for tissue typing and stored at room temperature. Tissue typing for all solid organs is similar, but is generally not utilized in heart, liver, and pancreas donors.[1] Even in cadaveric renal transplantation, the utility of HLA matching is controversial becauses the presence of common antigens does little to indicate chromosome similarity between recipient and donor or modify rejection rates.[26-28]

AXIOM Predonation HLA matching is not required for cadaveric organ donation.

Matching is based primarily on ABO compatibility, the absence of a lymphocytotoxic cross-match, and an appropriate-sized match of donor and recipient organ. In renal transplantation, the presence of preformed cytotoxic antibodies in the recipient's serum has been associated with a high risk of hyperacute rejection.[27] The percent reactive antibody (PRA) is used as a more immediate indication of possible acute rejection.[1] At the start of the initial evaluation of potential recipients, their serum is screened against a random control panel of donor lymphocytes. If the PRA is < 15%, the probability of a lymphocytotoxic mismatch is small. If the PRA is > 15%, a prospective, lymphocytotoxic crossmatch is pursued.[29] However, when the urgency for heart or liver transplantation is great, the operation may proceed despite a positive PRA.

Operation

PITFALL ⊘

A junior surgeon should not be assigned to multiorgan donation surgery.

Multiple organ cadaveric procurement (e.g., heart, liver, kidneys) takes approximately 2-3 hours and is technically demanding.[30] At least two surgeons should participate in multiorgan procurement operations. The organ procurement operation should be delegated to highly trained surgeons with interest and expertise in transplantation surgery and organ retrieval.[2]

Although the anesthesiologist or anesthetist and operating room nurses are provided by the host hospital, the organ procurement team brings any unusual equipment, which may include sterile ice, cardioplegia solution, cannulae, and containers and plastic bags for the organs.

Removal of the pancreas, liver, or heart requires meticulous dissection and ischemia of these organs is poorly tolerated.[1] In the event of early cardiovascular collapse, the aorta can be quickly cannulated and the kidneys perfused and cooled. Under these circumstances, the kidneys are usually the only solid organs that can be donated.

The general surgical principles for organ procurement include wide exposure, dissection of each organ while the heart still beats, and placement of cannulae for in situ cold perfusion using various solutions.[6-8] The use of these solutions has dramatically extended the ex vivo preservation of liver, kidney, and pancreas grafts, often for more than 24 hours.

CURRENT STATUS OF TRANSPLANTATION

In addition to the current shortage of donors, continuing major problems include limited cold ischemia times for heart and lung transplantation.[1] The advent of cyclosporine, however, has changed the entire scope of the field of transplantation.[31-35] Recent reports from the University of Pittsburgh suggest that FK506, a new immunosuppressive agent, may hold even greater promise in the future.[36] The development of a flushing solution at the University of Wisconsin also has had a significant impact on the transplantation of livers and kidneys.[6-8]

OKT3, a monoclonal antibody, has been utilized to treat established rejection in all types of solid-organ grafts.[3] It continues to be

evaluated as part of prophylactic immunosuppression protocols. Monoclonal antibodies with even greater specificity are also being tested.

Recent results of kidney transplantation in cyclosporine-treated patients indicated patient and graft survival rates at 2 years of 95% and 85%, respectively, and the results of transplantation in diabetic patients is now identical to that seen in nondiabetics.[37] Similar advances have been made in heart transplantation. With triple immunosuppression (azathiaprine, cyclospine and prednisone), the one-year graft survival rate is 92%.[38] The one-year survival for lung transplantation, primarily in patients with advanced pulmonary vascular disease, is 71%.[39-41]

The one-year patient survival for liver transplantation is now about 80%.[9,42,43] This is largely due to improved immunosuppression, advances in operative techniques and organ preservation, and aggressive retransplantation.[44] Intraoperative venovenous bypass without heparinization can also facilitate control of hemorrhage during liver transplantation.[9]

Pancreas transplantation has recently yielded a one-year graft survival rate of 70-75%.[45,46] Intestinal transplantation, although still experimental in some centers, is being performed with increasing frequency and improved results.[1]

PITFALL ⊘

Donation of corneas, skin, bone, and/or heart valves should be considered, even when organ donation is not possible.

Skin banks have become increasingly important to burn centers for early burn coverage in patients with large burns and limited donor sites. An increasing number of bone banks have also been developed for bone graft transplantation. These grafts may be used in orthopedic reconstruction of trauma patients or reconstruction of patients after radical procedures for oncologic disease. Corneal transplantation has been highly successful for many years and should be pursued even with families who are reluctant to donate solid organs.

⊘ **FREQUENT ERRORS**

In Organ Procurement from Trauma Victims

1. *Not considering every trauma victim to be a possible donor of organs or tissues.*
2. *Failing to optimally support a potential organ donor so as to make the tissue or organs more suitable for donation.*
3. *Failing to promptly notify the local donor procurement agency of the presence of a potential organ donor.*
4. *Failing to actively pursue the diagnose of organ failure and/or infection in a potential organ donor.*

▼▼▼▼▼▼▼▼▼▼▼▼▼▼▼▼▼▼▼▼▼▼▼▼▼▼▼▼▼

SUMMARY POINTS

1.   The main obstacle to the transplantation of organs at this time is donor availability.
2.   Young, previously healthy individuals who have suffered isolated, lethal head injury or intracranial bleeding from a vascular anomaly are generally the best candidates for organ donation.
3.   The major factor responsible for the shortage of donor organs is lack of donor referrals.
4.   The referral of an organ or tissue donor begins with recognition by a physician, nurses, or other individuals that a particular patient may be a suitable donor for organs or tissues.
5.   Even when patients do not meet criteria for whole-organ transplantation, they are frequently suitable donors for skin, cornea, or bone.

6. The ultimate determination of brain death of a potential donor remains the clinical responsibility of the attending physician.

7. Brain death should be pronounced as soon as possible after it occurs.

8. One should not assume that a brain-dead patient is not eligible for organ donation because it is a "medical examiner's case."

9. Consideration of patients as potential organ donors should not interfere with the treatment of their injuries or diseases.

10. After pronouncement of brain death, oxygenation and perfusion should be optimally maintained until donor surgery is complete.

11. Vasoconstrictor drugs should be avoided or only used in low doses in brain-dead, potential organ donors.

12. Diabetes insipidus in brain-dead potential organ donors should be corrected with aquous pitressin or DDAVP as soon as possible.

13. Proper preoperative management of organ donors plays a critical role in determining the successful outcome of organ transplantation.

14. Predonation HLA matching is not essential for cadaveric organ donation.

15. A junior surgeon should not be assigned to multiorgan donation surgery.

16. Corneal, skin, or bone donation should be considered, even when organ donation is not possible.

▲▲▲▲▲▲▲▲▲▲▲▲▲▲▲▲▲▲▲▲▲▲▲▲▲▲▲▲▲▲▲

REFERENCES

1. Peitzman AB, Webster MN, Gordon RD. Organ procurement and transplantation. Moore EE, Feliciano DV, Mattox KL, eds. Trauma, 2nd ed. Appleton & Lange, 1991; 797-804.
2. Starzl TE, Miller CM, Rapaport FT. Organ procurement. In: American college of surgeons care of the surgical patient 2. Elective care, vol. 1. 1988; 1.
3. Norman DJ. An overview of the use of the monoclonal antibody OKT3 in renal transplantation. Transplant Proc 1988;20:1248.
4. Miller J. Transplantation. Am Coll Surg Bull 1988;73:40.
5. Cosimi AB. Transplantation. Am Coll Surg Bull 1989;74:41.
6. Belzer FO, Southard JH. Principles of solid-organ preservation by cold storage. Transplant 1988;45:673.
7. Todo S, Nery J, Yanaga K, et al. Extended preservation of human liver grafts with UW solution. JAMA 1989;261:711.
8. Sollinger HW, Vernon WB, D'Alessandro AM, et al. Combined liver and pancreas procurement with Belzer-UW solution. Surgery 1989;106:685.
9. Starzl TE. The status of liver transplantation. Am Coll Surg Bull 1985;70:8.
10. Starzl TE, Iwatsuki S, et al. Orthotopic liver transplantation in 1984. Transplantation 1985;17:250.
11. Evans RW, Manninen DL, Garrison LP Jr, et al. Donor availability as the primary determinant of the future of heart transplantation. JAMA 1989;255:1892.
12. Darby JM, Stein K, Grenvik A, et al. Approach to management of the heart-beating "brain dead" organ donor. JAMA 1989;261:222.
13. Kolata G. Organ shortage clouds new transplant era. Science 1983;221:32.
14. Stuart FP. Progress in legal definition of brain death and consent to remove cadaver organs. Surgery 1977;891:68.
15. Lee PP, Kissner P. Organ donation and the Uniform Anatomical Gift Act. Surgery 1986;100:867.
16. Soifer BE, Gelb AW. The multiple organ donor: identification and management. Ann Intern Med 1989;110:814.
17. Cederna J, Toledo-Pereyra LH. Multiple organ harvesting. Contemp Surg 1984;25:15.
18. Parisi JE, Kim RC, et al. Brain death with prolonged somatic survival. N Engl J Med 1982;306:14.
19. Grenvik A. Brain death and permanently lost consciousness. Shoemaker WC, Thompson WL, Holbrook PR, eds. Textbook of critical care. Philadelphia: WB Saunders, 1984; 968.
20. Guidelines for the determination of death. Report of the medical consultants on the diagnosis of death to the President's commission for the study of ethical problems in medicine and biomedical and behavioral research. JAMA 1981;246:2184.
21. A collaborative study: an appraisal of the criteria of cerebral death. A summary statement. JAMA 1977;237:982.
22. Overcast TD, Evans RW, et al. Problems in the identification of potential organ donors. Misconceptions and fallacies associated with donor cards. JAMA 1984;251:1559.
23. Veith FJ, Fein JM, et al. Brain death I. A status report of medical and ethical considerations. JAMA 1977;238:1651.
24. Pittsburgh Transplantation Foundation. Postmortem organ procurement protocol. 1985.
25. Busittil RW, Goldstein LI, et al. Liver transplantation today. Ann Intern Med 1986;104:377.
26. Salvatierra O. The current status of renal transplantation. Am Coll Surg Bull 1985;70:2.
27. Cerilli J, Newhouse YG, et al. The significance of mixed lymphocyte culture in related renal transplantation. Surgery 1980;88:631.
28. Richie RE, Johnson HK, et al. The role of HLA tissue matching in cadaveric kidney transplantation. Ann Surg 1979;189:581.
29. Hardesty RL, Griffith BP, et al. Multiple cadaveric organ procurement with emphasis on the heart. Surg Rounds 1985;8:20.
30. Starzl TE, Rowe MI, Todo S, et al. Transplantation of multiple abdominal viscera. JAMA 1989;261:1449.
31. Starzl TE, Weil R III, et al. The use of cyclosporin A and prednisone in cadaver kidney transplantation. Surg Gynecol Obstet 1980;151:17.
32. Calne RY. The use of cyclosporin A in clinical organ grafting. Ann Surg 1982;196:330.
33. Griffith BP, Hardesty RL, et al. Cardiac transplantation with cyclosporin A and prednisone. Ann Surg 1982;196:324.
34. Calne RY, Wead AJ. Cyclosporin in cadaveric renal transplantation: 3-year follow up of a European multicentre trial. Lancet 1985;2:549.
35. The Canadian Multicentre Transplant Study Group. A randomized clinical trial of cyclosporin in cadaveric renal transplantation. N Engl J Med 1983;309:809.
36. Starzl TE, Todo S, Tzakis AG, et al. Liver transplantation. Am Coll Surg Bull 1985;70:11.
37. Sutherland DER. Transplantation. Am Coll Surg Bull 1986;71:49.
38. Reitz BA. The current practice of heart transplantation. Am Coll Surg Bull 1985;70:11.
39. Dawkins KD, Jamieson SW, Hunt SA. Long term results, hemodynamics, and complications after combined heart and lung transplantation. Circulation 1985;71:919.
40. Jamieson SW, Stinson EB, Oyer PE, et al. Heart-lung transplantation for irreversible pulmonary hypertension. Ann Thorac Surg 1984;38:554.
41. Jamieson SW, Dawkins KD, Burke C. Late results of combined heart-lung transplantation. Transplant Proc 1985;17:212.
42. Starzl TE, Iwatsuki S, et al. Factors in the development of liver transplantation. Transplant Proc 1985;17:107.
43. Gordon RD, Teperman L, Iwatsuki S, et al. Orthotopic liver transplantation. Schwartz SI, Ellis H, eds. Maingot's abdominal surgery, 9th ed. Norwalk: Appleton & Lange, 1989; 1291.
44. Shaw BW Jr, Gordon RD, Iwatsuki S. Hepatic retransplantation. Transplant Proc 1985;17:264.
45. Sutherland DER, Kendall DM. Pancreas transplantation registry report and a commentary. West J Med 1985;143:845.
46. Toledo-Pereyra LH, Mittal VK. Segmental pancreatic transplantation. Arch Surg 1982;117:505.

Chapter 47 Negligence and the Trauma Surgeon

IRWIN K. ROSENBERG, M.D., J.D.

The likelihood of a medical malpractice action against trauma surgeons has become a fact of their professional and personal lives. To argue the question of whether there has been a real or only apparent increase in the number of medical malpractice cases and the size of the judgments awarded does not alter the fact. It would be equally unproductive to explore the issue of fault and to lay the blame on lawyers, judges, juries, legislators, or physicians themselves. However, many of the situations that cause malpractice claims can be avoided or modified and litigation averted. Lawsuits which cannot be prevented are handled most effectively when the physician understands the legal basis forming the framework within which malpractice cases evolve through discovery and settlement, mediation, or final adjudication. Patients who have suffered an injury present special problems; if they were to become litigants against the physician or the hospital, the claims of these patients often would arise from unique circumstances during treatment.

The patient/physician relationship has changed in the past two decades. The perception of medicine as a humanitarian "calling" and one of community service has been altered by the rise of commercialism and the prevalence of litigation in nearly every facet of our lives. Medicine has had no special privilege in our litigious society.

TORTS

The special aspect of the law that addresses matters like medical malpractice is called the law of torts. The standard of behavior used in tort law is that of the "reasonable and prudent man." In medical malpractice the standard is how the "reasonable and prudent physician" (sometimes described as the "duly careful member of the profession") would have acted under the same circumstances.

Medical malpractice is a special form of legal wrong known as a tort. The definition of a tort is unsatisfactory despite a host of attempts to define it by legal scholars from every era;[1] when one is too specific, the definition becomes inaccurate, and without specificity it remains so inclusive that it becomes of little value. A useful concept is that a tort is a breach of a civil duty, other than a contractual one, which gives rise to damages and is entitled to compensation in a court of law. The different kinds of duties and individuals to whom the duty is owed constitute the law of torts, a creature of common law. Common law is the body of jurisprudence that has arisen as a result of prior decisions of the courts, and is to be distinguished from law that derives from statutes, which are created by a legislative body. Criminal law is entirely statutory.

TORTS AND CRIME

AXIOM A tort is a legal wrong that is not a crime or a breach of contract.

A tort is not a crime. The difference lies in the interests affected, the legal remedies provided, and whether the offense is defined by statute. A crime is an offense against society in general, represented by the government. A division of the executive branch is responsible for instituting legal action in the form of a prosecution, the aims of which are to punish, deter similar action by others, to reform the individual so as to avoid a future offense, or to separate the offender from the rest of society. No attempt is made to compensate an injured party who may have been the victim of the crime; the only role of the victim of the crime is as a witness against the accused. Although the media often portray the dismissal of a criminal case as occurring because the victim "dropped the charges" against the accused, in actuality only the government has the prerogative of not pursuing a criminal action. However, from a pragmatic point of view, if the victim were the only witness to the crime, no case could be made to prosecute without that testimony.

A tort, as contrasted with a crime, is an offense charged in a civil action brought by one party (the plaintiff) against another (the defendant) for the purpose of receiving a monetary award. Society decides the norms of behavior that determine what conduct is tortious. The government is not a party to such an action except in its role of providing a judicial system. Any judgment awarded is in the form of money damages; no other award can be made in tort. Medical malpractice involves a special case of the tort referred to as negligence. Other torts are libel, slander, defamation, product liability, breach of privacy rights, interference with economic advantage, trespass, nuisance, wrongful death, false imprisonment, assault and battery, and intentional infliction of emotional distress. Some of these torts are acts against a person and others are against property. Some are intentional torts and others are not. It is worth noting that many insurance polices for medical malpractice specifically exclude coverage against claims arising from behavior of physicians that falls under the rubric of intentional tort. Battery, defined as "unwanted touching," is the most frequent example of an intentional tort charged against a physician.

Although by definition an intentional tort requires that the defendant must *intend* to commit the tort with which he is charged, it is not necessary for the plaintiff to prove the mental state of intent. Because individuals are ordinarily held by law to be responsible for their actions, the burden of proof shifts to defendants to prove diminished responsibility or some other explanation for the tort.

An offense may be both a crime and actionable in a civil court as a tort. In most instances the decision in one action is not admissible as evidence in the other. The crime is prosecuted by the state against the perpetrator, and the tort claim is brought by the injured party. Crimes are defined by statute and torts are construed by past decisions of courts in that jurisdiction (usually a state). The term "injury" is used in law to refer to any wrong or damage done to another, either in their rights, person, reputation, or property.

TORTS VERSUS BREACH OF CONTRACT

A lawsuit charging that a tort was committed must be distinguished from one claiming breach of contract. Again, the distinction lies in whose interests are concerned. A contract is between parties who have made promises to each other, such as a promise to pay in return for performance of some kind. The parties to the contract must enter into it willingly, without unfair advantage being taken (as defined by common law), and they are then bound by its terms. In tort law the interests protected are those agreed upon by society and imposed by law to protect those affected by the actions of the defendant(s). That duty may be toward another individual or class of individuals. The protected interests, whether in person or property, are based on social policy and not the will of the parties. The degree of protection, what is protected, who has the duty, and whom it affects, are constantly evolving with the common law.

Although major areas of agreement and similarities exist, each jurisdiction (state) determines what behavior is "reasonable and prudent" under given circumstances, to whom a duty is owed, and under what circumstances it is established. If a tort case were heard in a federal court, (e.g., when parties are from different states), the court would use the common law that has developed in the state in which the tort occurred and attempt to decide it as it would have been decided in the courts of that state.

AXIOM A tort is distinguished from crime and breach of contract by examining whose interests were affected, and whether they were established by the common law or the legislature.

Contract obligations are the result of the agreement of the parties making the promises and extend only to the parties to the contract. The measure of damages in litigation charging breach of contract is limited to that "reasonably within the contemplation of the parties" when the contract was made,[2] but in tort law the damage awards may be broader and include punitive damages, which are not available in a contract action. A patient who claims that a result was guaranteed by his physician or hospital may sue in a contract action. Because most states now require that any claim of guarantee must be proved in writing, such claims are seldom successful unless the physician is so foolish as to provide a written guarantee.

NEGLIGENCE

A claim that the physician has committed malpractice is the same thing as saying that he is responsible for the tort of negligence in the professional setting. The meaning of "negligence" in the legal sense is not equivalent to the state of mind of carelessness. The plaintiff must prove specific elements in order to build a prima facie case of negligence:

1. A duty recognized by law on the part of the acting party (the defendant) towards the plaintiff. (An interested observer, for example, cannot sue a physician claiming malpractice against a third party. The physician had no duty toward the observer, only toward the patient. It is true even if the third party were paying the bill; the duty would be only to the patient).
2. A failure by the acting party to comply with a certain standard of conduct, frequently referred to as the "standard of care."
3. A close causal relationship between an action (or failure to act) and any injury that results. The legal term for this is "proximate cause." For example, if a duty existed and a breach of that duty (or standard of care) occurred, but any injury sustained was not related to the breach, no liability exists.
4. "Injury" in its legal sense must occur; an action for breach of the standard of conduct that does not cause an injury, or threatens only future harm, is not legally sufficient.

AXIOM The tort of negligence requires proof of (a) existence of a duty, (b) breach of that duty, (c) proximate cause, and (d) injury.

DUTY

Duty involves the relationship between the plaintiff and defendant at the time the alleged injury arose. Once its existence is established, its nature is constant: to conform with the standard of conduct required to fulfill that duty. In the malpractice setting, the plaintiff is the patient (or surviving relative) and the defendant is the physician and/or hospital. This duty requires that the conduct of the actor (defendant) conforms to a standard of reasonableness. It often includes an expectation of control of the conduct of third parties (agents) towards the plaintiff. This may require the use of reasonable care to prevent negligent conduct by such third parties and to protect the plaintiff from reasonably anticipated injuries, such as personal attacks

by others or thefts of property. It is through an agency relationship that a hospital becomes liable for the acts of a nurse or employed physician. As to those practicing in a hospital who are not employees, that subject is called "ostensible agency," and may be the basis under certain circumstances for proving liability against the hospital as well as the practicing physician.[3]

AXIOM The standard of behavior in tort is that of the reasonably prudent physician.

A physician is ordinarily under no obligation to treat a patient unless he has accepted the patient for treatment. But the acceptance may be a "constructive" one (construed by law after interpretation of the facts of the case). A self-employed physician is ordinarily under no legal duty to treat anyone. This includes emergencies in which the physician is on the scene. Many physicians and some professional societies have taken a different *moral* position from this, but that does not change the physician's *legal* obligation to treat only those patients accepted for treatment. Once they agree to treat patients, physicians must render care.

When physicians are not self-employed, their obligations may be determined by agreements made with their employers as to who, when, and where treatment is obligated. If the physician were serving a tour of duty in an emergency room for example, and that facility were open to everyone, it may be construed that the physician had accepted any patient requesting treatment. Refusal to treat under those circumstances would cause substantial liability should an adverse result ("injury") stem from the refusal. Any action toward the patient consisting of affirmative conduct that may represent professional care will be constructively viewed as acceptance of a duty to treat. The administration of medication for pain, or the starting of an intravenous line may be taken as such affirmation or acceptance for treatment. The physician cannot, in such an instance, discontinue care of the patient without assuring the continuity of competent care. If the care were less than adequate, the physician may be held responsible for unreasonable actions.

A charitable setting or one with a third-party payor has no effect on the legal relationship between patient and physician. The source of payment is irrelevant once a physician/patient relationship is established.[4] In some hospitals a concerted effort is made to avoid admitting certain categories of seriously ill patients in order to avoid intensive care when the insurance coverage is marginal. Whether treating the patient in the emergency room is "acceptance for treatment" and carries the same obligation to assure diagnostic and therapeutic completeness as a hospital admission, varies with the particular jurisdiction in which a physician is practicing. In one outstanding example it was held that examining a child in the emergency room for suspected appendicitis was "equivalent" to hospital admission and complete care and follow-up were incumbent on the examining physician. This is the law in a minority of jurisdictions at present. But one must beware of the liability of failure to admit patients to the hospital whose medical conditions warrant such admission, or of transfers from the emergency room of patients needing further care when indications for discharge or transfer are partially for economic reasons. The physician must continually evaluate whether an unreasonable risk of harm exists to the patient and whether that risk is foreseeable. If the patient were accepted for care in the emergency room, the physician would have a duty to act "reasonably" in discharging or transferring the patient, as well as in providing treatment.

PATIENT ABANDONMENT

The abandonment of a patient is a particular kind of breach of duty. Serving a tour of duty in an emergency facility has some special features that distinguish it from the usual physician/patient encounter. The facility in which the patient is examined, the emergency room, signals a willingness to provide treatment; when a patient who presents for treatment in such a facility is refused treatment, a compelling reason must exist. If a patient would be better served in another facility, the acceptance into that institution must first be assured, the patient must not be at increased risk by the transfer, and the patient or guardian must understand the reasons and concur in the transfer. Most often, the charge of abandonment is brought by asserting that the physician withdrew from the relationship at a critical juncture without reasonable notice and, therefore, the patient did not have an opportunity to obtain alternative care.

Forms of abandonment include premature discharge from the hospital or inappropriate transfer to another facility; if it is deemed "foreseeable by the reasonably competent physician" that worsening of the patient's condition could result, considerable risk of liability exists. When the decision to transfer or discharge is based partially or wholly on economic reasons, and when the plaintiff can convince a jury that injury occurred as a result of the transfer or discharge, the likelihood of an award against the physician is high.

The appearance on the medical scene of diagnostic related groups (DRG) has had an unexpected influence on medical malpractice claims. The level of reimbursement to hospitals has been more tightly regulated by this approach to payment of costs to hospitals than ever before. It has forced hospitals to balance the use of expensive care and diagnostic procedures against the likelihood that denying that care or study will be considered a violation of the standard of care. The stage is set by the regulations that assign hospital payment according to disease entity. For it to be fully reimbursed for the care of a patient with a given DRG, the hospital must provide care until the patient is discharged from the facility. When it is apparent that certain groups of patients are likely to exceed the hospital stay prescribed for that entity, or when it is later obvious that a given patient will have a complicated course and is certain to exceed the length of stay allowed, it is in the hospital's interest to (a) deny admission to patients of that group, (b) discharge the patient (and gain full payment), or (c) transfer the patient to another facility and recoup a per diem with "supplemental payments" because of increased complexity. However, if the reason for transfer was that facilities were inadequate at the transferring institution, no supplemental benefits would be added to the per diem. Therefore, to be fully compensated for costly cases, the hospital must either continue care until discharge (the earlier the better)—even when hospital facilities are inadequate—or transfer the patient to another institution for reasons other than the existence of inadequate facilities.

Regulations like these may place the interests of the physician in conflict with those of the hospital. Both society and the patient expect that the interests of the patient will never be compromised. DRG regulations impose a time and money framework on patient care as never before. When they are not in agreement with the administration as to the medical advisability of transfers or discharges, physicians must utilize all available means to protest the decision and to document their lack of acquiescence. In a recent case, a denial of a physician's request to allow the patient to remain hospitalized was not enough to relieve the doctor of liability. He did not appeal the ruling, a mechanism for which was provided in the hospital regulations.

> **PITFALL** ⊘
>
> *Premature discharge or inappropriate transfer of a patient constitutes abandonment.*

Another effect of cost-containment efforts of hospitals alters the patient/physician relationship by forcing the physician to assume the role of hospital advocate.[20] When a given procedure offers only marginal benefit to a patient, such as an expensive modality that is rarely diagnostic in the given circumstances, the physician may be encouraged by the hospital to: (a) not order it, (b) not mention it, or (c) dissuade the patient from accepting it. If these choices were made partially or wholly for economic reasons, the physician would be exposed to liability because the best interests of the patient would not be served. The issue of which procedures offer only a "marginal" benefit and the lack of data to support the answers to such questions do not dispute the fact that liability exposure is increased by the taint of economic motives for allocation of scarce medical resources.

> **PITFALL** ⊘
>
> *Cost containment is not a defense to a charge of negligent failure to diagnose or treat.*

GOOD SAMARITAN

In most states the care rendered by a physician at the scene of a medical emergency has some protection from litigation, although many of the statutes (nicknamed Good Samaritan laws) providing for such exemption are untested or have had limited interpretation by the courts. Tort law in the United States generally does not require a bystander to voluntarily come to the aid of anyone in distress unless some other obligation toward that person exists. If, for example, the danger or harm were caused by the observer, or if the party in distress were a legal dependent or invited guest of the observer, a duty would exist to aid the victim.

Observers in this country, therefore, need not place themselves in positions of danger. For example, an expert swimmer with a rope and boat available is not required to go to the aid of someone drowning; no legal responsibility exists. That is equally true of physicians. (In many European nations an observer is required to provide aid to an endangered or injured party provided it does not expose the rescuer to unreasonable danger.) In order to encourage bystanders to aid those injured or endangered, statutes have been passed in most states that exempt a volunteer, medical professional, or lay person from liability in such a setting. But the statutes in each jurisdiction should be carefully examined for contingencies that may negate the protection. In nearly all the statutes, once care is undertaken it cannot be abandoned until transferred to competent hands. The definition of "competent hands" is arguable. Nearly all statutes are also rendered inapplicable if the physician were to send a bill for services or establish a consensual professional relationship at the accident scene.

> **PITFALL** ⊘
>
> *Do not assume that good samaritan laws will protect negligent action at the scene of an accident.*

CONSENT

Informed Consent

Duty and informed consent are intimately related. The early decisions considered informed consent similar to the granting of consent for treatment; when the consent was not deemed to be "informed," a battery has occurred. More recently the legal interpretation of informed consent has been in the context of duty, it being the physician's duty to obtain a consent which is "informed" and, therefore, negligence if that duty was breached.[13] The nature and extent of the disclosure necessary to make consent informed is a matter in most states of expert testimony because the jury cannot be expected to know this from their own life experiences. Courts in general recognize that what must be disclosed is a problem of weighing the patient's emotional stability against the need to know facts that may be material to the granting of consent.[14]

The frequency and seriousness of a possible complication must be weighed against the likely outcome were the offered procedure to be refused. No agreement, however, exists as to how infrequent or unimportant a complication must be before the physician need not disclose it. When it could be material in affecting a *prudent patient's* decision, in some jurisdictions it must be disclosed (i.e., prudent patient standard).[15] In most states, however, the standard is what the *reasonable physician* would have disclosed under the same circumstances as based on expert testimony (i.e., prudent physician standard). In a small minority of states the standard is based on what the *particular patient* would have needed to know in order to make a reasoned decision (i.e., particular patient standard).[16]

The patient-oriented standard of disclosure does not depend on what a physician may consider pertinent, and the risk of malpractice claims based on failure to obtain informed consent is increased by these standards.

It should be apparent that the change in how informed consent is viewed has shifted the law from the tort of battery to that of negligence. The advantage of this to the plaintiff should be clear; malpractice insurance coverage is primarily, and often solely, for the tort of negligence. The opportunity to collect on a judgment against the physician is considerably greater if insurance is available to pay any judgment.

> **PITFALL** ⊘
>
> *The disclosure necessary to comply with the requirement of obtaining "informed consent" depends on the standard used in that jurisdiction. The practicing physician must learn what the standard is in his or her state.*

BATTERY

Implicit in any discussion of whether a duty has been undertaken by the physician is the obverse: has consent been given by the patient? When an individual is treated or even examined by a physician without permission—an "impermissible touching"—it is a tort called battery. Battery is a different tort than negligence and is excluded from coverage in many medical malpractice policies as an "intentional tort." Policies should be carefully examined for such exclusions.

> **AXIOM** Consent is permission freely given. It is a state of mind, not a printed form.

A necessary element for a prima facie case of battery is absence of consent. Consent in a medical milieu is simply a willingness to undergo treatment. It is a state of mind. A signed consent form is merely *evidence* that consent was given; it goes toward proof that consent was freely given but is not the consent itself. Because the workings of the mind are known only by words or actions, when a patient says, "Go ahead, doc; whatever you say is okay with me", the patient will not be able to deny granting consent. The patient may claim that the statement was never made, but when evidence confirms that consent was obtained, absence of a written document is irrelevant. When a patient silently offers an arm for an injection, consent has been given;[5] however, if the patient extended the arm for an injection and instead got an incision, consent was not given.

> **PITFALL** ⊘
>
> *Extending an operative procedure beyond that understood by the patient is battery.*

If a patient were not capable of the necessary state of mind to give willing consent (e.g., mental confusion, unconsciousness, intoxication, or incompetency), even written consent would not protect the physician from a charge of battery.[6] When doubt exists as to the mental ability of the patient to understand the treatment alternatives and the risks of nontreatment, treatment may be undertaken when a court order is obtained, or when consent is given by a legally competent guardian. In an emergency situation, a court order is often impractical. To proceed without such an order and without proper consent leaves the physician unprotected against the charge of having committed a battery.

When the emergency threatens the life or limb of the patient, the requirement of consent is usually waived and it is regarded as "implied."[7] It may be better to conceive of this as a limited privilege; physicians have reason to believe that patients, could they understand the situation, would consent to treatment. This "consent," of course, is to allow the physician to act and is not a consent to be injured. If an improper operation were performed, such as the amputation of an uninjured extremity, no "implied consent" or privilege to cause injury would exist. Nor is the privilege one which allows an operation

to be extended beyond the proper conduct for care of the emergency. Even if one could argue that a given procedural extension (e.g., removing a gallbladder containing stones, or an appendix containing a carcinoid) was medically indicated in the course of treating a gunshot wound of the abdomen, the physician could be charged with battery. In this tort, one need not show that harm resulted only that the "touching" (removal of gallbladder or appendix) was without permission. Even punitive damages may be assessed. Good intentions are not necessarily an adequate defense against such a charge, although a blanket consent allowing the surgeon to perform procedures considered to be indicated at the time may help to justify actions.

It is important to remember that the tort of battery is not negated by performing a medically-indicated procedure when consent was not freely granted. Surgeons may not be defended against a charge of battery if the malpractice policy excludes coverage of intentional torts.

> **AXIOM** Battery is impermissible touching. No injury needs to be shown.

In an operation being performed for acute appendicitis a surgeon found it necessary to perform a hysterectomy and salpingo-oophorectomy for what were called "unanticipated conditions." The physician was found liable for unauthorized extension of the operative procedure. The patient's husband was next door to the operating room and the court found that there was no excuse for not seeking permission from the spouse.[8] In this case, the court would have accepted the husband's consent as "substituted judgment" during the "incompetency" (due to anesthesia) of his wife. The patient had signed a form authorizing the physician to "administer such treatment . . . as found necessary to perform this operation which is advisable in the treatment of this patient." The court found this wording so ambiguous as to be without meaning. Many consent forms have similar nearly illiterate clauses.

CONSENT WITH MINORS

When the patient is a minor, consent of the legal guardian is usually required. When the situation is an emergency that threatens life or limb and legal consent cannot be obtained within a reasonable period, the same rules apply as in an adult patient unable to give consent because of unconsciousness or incompetency. However, if the legal guardian were to refuse treatment deemed necessary by the physician, *refusal may not be conclusive*. Many states have statutes that authorize juvenile or family courts to order medical or surgical procedures; these can often be obtained in a matter of an hour with a bedside visit and consultation between judge and medical authorities. As the United Sates Supreme Court said: "Parents may be free to become martyrs themselves. But it does not follow that they are free, in identical circumstances, to make martyrs of their children before they reach the age of full and legal discretion when they can make that choice themselves".[9] Recent cases, including parents who had religious objections to treatment of their children by a physician, affirmed this ruling. In many jurisdictions a physician is *expected* to seek a court order requiring that the necessary procedures be undertaken despite parental objections.

> **PITFALL** ⊘
>
> *Refusal of permission by the legal guardian to operate upon a minor may not be conclusive. When life or limb is in jeopardy a court order should be sought.*

RELIGIOUS RESTRAINTS ON MEDICAL CARE

Most adults are entitled to refuse any recommended procedure when they are legally and intellectually competent; much of the litigation on this subject relates to the refusal of blood transfusions for religious reasons. In general, a physician is not held liable for the death of a patient who refuses to undergo transfusion after repeated warnings of the potential consequences. However, when a physician performs an operative procedure under such restriction, a dilemma may arise: if a transfusion were given because it was deemed to be "medically necessary" despite the lack of permission, the physician would be liable on charges of battery; if the patient were to die from blood loss, he could be charged with negligence, not because he failed to give the transfusion but because he operated in a negligent fashion so as to induce an inordinate amount of blood loss.

The plaintiff only needs a credible expert who will state that this operation, unless performed negligently, does not require blood transfusion. It is not surprising that some hospitals have made it a policy that if the rejection of advice (that a blood transfusion may be necessary) conflicts with accepted medical practice, the patient should be advised to seek care elsewhere. The physicians are instructed to transfer the patient to a place where this restriction is acceptable (unless such transfer jeopardizes the welfare of the patient).

The Boards of Trustees of these institutions clearly state that it is against hospital policy for a physician to agree to such restraints on medical care and that the board expects the physician to transfer such patients elsewhere. This is not often possible in the emergency setting. The legal affairs department of the institution often becomes involved; if transfer would jeopardize the welfare of the patient, a court order should be sought, after which successful litigation against the physician would be unlikely.

> **AXIOM** To undertake an operative procedure without permission to administer blood products places the physician in a legal dilemma.

In cases in which a pregnant woman or a single parent with dependent children refuses therapy that would avert an illness threatening the fetus or the lives of the children, the courts have traditionally invoked the legal doctrine of *parens patriae*. The court may order treatment to protect dependent minors or a fetus from the religious convictions of parents that, in the view of the court, are not in the best interests of the children. It ignores the right to refuse therapy by legally competent adults because of the "compelling" interests of society in the fetus or dependent children. In a recent case, which received considerable publicity in the press, a pregnant woman dying with advanced cancer had a cesarean section performed against her wishes in an attempt to salvage a very premature fetus. Mother and child died a few days later.

STANDARD OF CARE

In order to define duty and its breach one must specify the behavior to be expected under given circumstances. Few instances exist in medicine in which all authorities would agree on behavior that would be considered appropriate. Yet, in medical malpractice cases, this "standard of care" is an essential part of the proof of the case. When the duty to provide a given standard of care cannot be defined, how can one prove that the duty has been breached? The jury cannot be expected to know from their own knowledge what constitutes a deficiency in professional care. Almost all medical malpractice cases require the testimony of experts as witnesses. The exceptions to this rule are those in which a jury need have no special knowledge to perceive that negligence occurred, as in an operation on the wrong organ or extremity, a sponge inadvertently left in the abdomen, or a foreign body allowed to fall into the trachea during intubation. Because a physician is expected to use the skill and care common to the profession, an error in judgment or an adverse result is not enough to show a lack of necessary care.[10]

Physicians caring for the injured or acutely ill patient know that there is agreement on a "standard of care" in only the simplest of cases. The standard of care applicable in a given medical malpractice case is established by a group of nonprofessionals, the jury, who decides on the basis of which expert testimony is more persuasive. The physician's best defense is to document the evolution of the problem, pursuit of changing symptoms and signs, consideration of ab-

normal data, and alternatives that were considered, rejected, or accepted and the reasons for that decision. With that kind of documentation, preferably including references to the supporting literature, the defendant's expert witness should be most persuasive in convincing the jury that the care rendered was the best standard of care. The documentation of mindless observations in serial notes *ad nauseum* is not what is meant by careful record keeping.

Physicians do not guarantee the results of treatment; when proper courses are open to "reasonable" doubt, they should not be liable for honest errors of judgment, provided that such errors are the kind that any physician with the same degree of training might make when caring for a similar patient.[11] The criterion is that, to the extent physicians properly evaluate all pros and cons of situations and then make intelligent, informed decisions for which they have been trained, physicians should not be liable for injuries resulting from honest errors of judgment.

> **PITFALL** ⊘
>
> ***Reasonable possibilities in the differential diagnosis must be pursued. Failure to do so will not be excusable as "errors of judgment."***

The standard of care is determined by the jury. The matter is placed before the jury as a question of whether the skill and judgment exercised was that commonly possessed by members of the profession in good standing with the same level of training. The standard to which a physician is held cannot be the average level of care, or half of physicians would not conform to the standard. It must, therefore, be the minimum level of performance of members in good standing.[12]

> **AXIOM** The standard of care used in the courts is the *minimal* level of performance by members in good standing in the profession who have a comparable degree of training.

PROXIMATE CAUSE

The legal concept of "proximate cause" is hopelessly confused. It is best defined here as the necessary causation for the tort of negligence, or as conduct that was a "substantial factor" in causing an event. Causation is an essential part of the proof, but it is not the determinant of liability; all the other elements must also be proved. Because the conduct of the defendant must be a "substantial factor" in causing the plaintiff's injury, it follows that if other causes were additionally shown to be contributory it would not relieve the defendant of liability. This reasoning is the basis for the principle of joint and several liability. The conduct in question includes *all* things contributing to the result, either acts of commission or omission, so that failure to do the necessary thing is as culpable as doing that deemed improper.

> **AXIOM** Proximate cause exists when an action or inaction is "substantially" responsible for the injury that results.

The concept of proximate cause is critical in the proof of the tort of negligence. If an event were going to happen whether or not the defendant intervened, then the defendant would not be a "substantial factor" in bringing about the result. It does not matter that the defendant had a duty toward the plaintiff, or that the duty was breached by a violation of the "standard of care." When the action that was a breach—the violation of the standard of care—was not a *substantial factor* in causing the injury that the plaintiff suffered, then no malpractice has occurred. If a sponge were inadvertently left in the abdomen and the patient then died of a myocardial infarction that was properly managed, no malpractice charge could be sustained unless the plaintiff could show that the retained sponge was a material and substantial factor in the death.

DEFENSIVE MEDICINE

"Defensive medicine" may be defined as the attempt to amass an unassailable record of diagnostic studies in anticipation of future litigation. The continued application of this approach, when pursued by most physicians, unfortunately becomes incorporated into the standard of care whether it is the "best" medical practice or not. In other words, when everyone else does it, we have to do it too!

At present, the legal system makes no allowance for cost allocation of scarce medical resources.[17] The relationship between physician and patient is conceived of as an individual one and does not acknowledge the need for such apportionment. The law requires that the risk and discomfort of a procedure must be weighed against possible benefit, *but not its cost.* A defense that claims that a procedure was too expensive to use for the patient or, even worse, for the group to which the patient belongs, will not be accepted by a judge or jury.

When restrictions on the use of scarce or expensive modalities are formally instituted by the hospital or its staff, however, those regulations may serve as evidence of the constraints within which the physician was forced to operate and help to limit liability. The publication by the hospital staff of a protocol, providing specific examples in which a scarce or expensive test should or should not be used, may serve as evidence of the standard of care in that institution. But medical standards at the specialty level of practice still exist and are not local standards but national ones. Physicians are obligated to employ their best judgment; when they believe a procedure is indicated for the patient, despite restrictions placed upon its use, physicians must lodge vigorous protests and utilize all available appeal procedures before they can claim that the matter was beyond their control.

Some courts have held, after testimony of plaintiff's experts, that failure to utilize any and all means available that may have aided the diagnosis or treatment of a patient is a violation of the standard of care. This approach fuels the argument of those who favor the practice of defensive medicine. It is naturally much easier to testify in retrospect that a given modality would have aided in the diagnosis or treatment. The question is more properly phrased: "Would the reasonably competent physician, faced with this problem in this patient, have chosen to use that diagnostic or therapeutic modality?" If a diagnostic modality were not available in one facility, but has become a component of the standard of care, it may become necessary to transfer a patient to another facility that has such capability. When this can be accomplished without jeopardizing the welfare of the patient, the required standard of care is satisfied. A hospital that has made no effort to facilitate arrangements for such an exigency exposes itself to considerable liability, and the physicians practicing there many need to show what efforts they have made to change the policy or to obtain the diagnostic modality. Examples of this include a cranial CT scan in closed-head injury or arteriography following trauma.

Critics of the defensive posture taken by many physicians, especially in the excessive use of radiographic and laboratory studies, lay a portion of the blame on the teachers in academic centers. Costs in academic centers have tended to be much higher than those in community hospitals, and this may be at least partially attributable to an overzealous use of these diagnostic tools. These academicians, it is said, stress the laboratory approach to diagnosis and inculcate this attitude in the residents emerging from their programs. These physicians imbued with a strong laboratory orientation, it is argued, then practice "defensive medicine" in the community.

A study by the American Medical Association in 1983 stated that 40% of its respondents admitted to ordering additional tests and 27% to giving additional treatment at least partially because of a perceived threat of litigation.[18] But it is worth recalling that physicians are innocent of negligence as long as, in the opinion of the "respected minority" of practicing members in good standing in the field, they acted within the broad range of conduct consistent with the level of knowledge and skill generally possessed by similar professionals under comparable circumstances.[19] The legal system is, in essence, condoning and respecting a certain level of uncertainty as part of medical practice. But many physicians are uncomfortable with an uncertainty level capable of reduction, even if the reduction would not change prognostication or therapeutic alternatives.

> **AXIOM** The accumulation of unessential data may reduce the amount of discomfort a physician has with an uncertain diagnosis, but is not in the best interest of the patient.

Contrary to popular medical opinion, the existence of a particular diagnostic or therapeutic technology does not create a requirement to use that tool indiscriminately. One must instead answer the question as to whether the decision that is being made is consistent with the practice of professional peers and serves the best interests of the patient. Definitive answers to this serious problem do not exist and the best legal advice is to fully investigate all likely diagnoses using modalities that are medically "appropriate." All decisions must be clearly in the best interest of the patient.

INJURY

In the tort of negligence, the term "injury" means any harm that occurs as a result of the failure to fulfill one's duty. That usually means, in the instance of medical malpractice, physical injury caused or contributed to by negligence. Money damages awarded are influenced by the nature and extent of the injury and the implications of the injury for the plaintiff and dependents. If the injury was death, the claim is preserved in the form of a wrongful death action brought by the survivors.

Economic damages are calculated by the earnings that are lost to the patient or survivors as a result of disability or death, and are based on life expectancy data, anticipated inflation rates, and probable salary predicted for the patient's field of endeavor. Noneconomic damages are based on such things as pain, suffering, and lost companionship. Punitive damages may be assessed in circumstances that the jury considers egregious.

> *PROLONGATION OF LIFE*
> *Vex not his ghost; O, let him pass! he hates him*
> *That would upon the rock of this tough world*
> *Stretch him out longer.*[19]

The definition of death has been revised in most jurisdictions, but not all have accepted the wording of the Uniform Death Act. This model statute, adopted by many legislatures verbatim, defines death in terms of the irreversibility of circulatory and respiratory function or the irreversibility of function of the entire brain including the brain stem. When organs are used for subsequent transplantation, "death" requires confirmation by another and independent physician; neither physician may be involved in the procedure or care of the organ recipient. All physicians in a given jurisdiction must learn the definition of death accepted in the state in which they are practicing whether it is defined in statutes by the legislature or in the common law.

> **PITFALL** ⊘
>
> *For physicians to be unfamiliar with the definition of death in their jurisdiction is to invite litigation.*

It is a common practice in some busy emergency rooms to use patients arriving too late for resuscitation as "models" on which inexperienced personnel may practice resuscitation techniques, such as endotracheal intubation and insertion of central venous lines. In this litigious climate it is foolhardy to continue that practice, despite laudatory goals and the advantages such models may offer. This caution is issued without considering the moral issues raised by such procedures and the brutalization of attitudes they may engender.

CONCLUSION

No foolproof way exists to assure that litigation can be avoided. It is nearly a certainty that physicians will have contact with the legal system, as either witness or litigant, during their professional lives. The more that is known about the system and the principles that guide it, the better physicians can defend themselves. Better understanding can more effectively bring about reform. Some physicians approach the necessary discovery procedures and testimony with arrogance, which serves them poorly with the jury and judge. Others react with denial, hoping that the case will disappear if they have as little to do with it as possible; they are of little help in their own defense. Active participation with legal counsel in developing the best approach for an effective defense and in choosing credible experts is essential.

Tort reform legislation has had a salutary effect in some jurisdictions, and alternatives to the tort system have been explored in others. In the meantime, physicians must protect themselves with knowledge and continue to practice the best level of medical care. In the final analysis, that is the best defense to a charge of professional negligence.

▼▼▼▼▼▼▼▼▼▼▼▼▼▼▼▼▼▼▼▼▼▼▼▼▼▼▼▼▼▼

SUMMARY POINTS

1. A tort is a legal wrong that is not a crime or a breach of contract.

2. A tort is distinguished from crime and breach of contract by examining whose interests were affected, and whether they were established by the common law or the legislature.

3. The tort of negligence requires proof of: (a) existence of a duty, (b) breach of that duty, (c) proximate cause, and (d) injury.

4. The standard of behavior in tort is that of the reasonably prudent physician.

5. Premature discharge or inappropriate transfer of a patient can constitute abandonment.

6. Cost containment is not a defense to a charge of negligent failure to diagnose or treat.

7. Do not assume that good samaritan laws protect negligent action at the scene of an accident.

8. The disclosure necessary to comply with the requirement of obtaining "informed consent" depends on the standard used in the jurisdiction. The practicing physician must learn what the standard is.

9. Consent is permission freely given. It is a state of mind, not a printed form.

10. Extending an operative procedure beyond that understood by the patient is a battery.

11. Battery is impermissible touching. No injury need be shown.

12. Refusal of permission by the legal guardian to operate upon a minor may not be conclusive. When life or limb is in jeopardy a court order should be sought.

13. To undertake an operative procedure without permission to administer blood products places the physician in a legal dilemma.

14. Reasonable possibilities in the differential diagnosis must be pursued. Failure to do so will not be excusable as "errors of judgement."

15. The standard of care used in the courts is the *minimal* level of performance by members in good standing in the profession who have comparable degrees of training.

16. Proximate cause exists when an action or inaction is "substantially" responsible for the injury that results.

17. The accumulation of unessential data may reduce the amount of discomfort a physician has with an uncertain diagnosis, but is not in the best interest of the patient.

18. For the physician to be unfamiliar with the definition of death in his jurisdiction is to invite litigation.

▲▲▲▲▲▲▲▲▲▲▲▲▲▲▲▲▲▲▲▲▲▲▲▲▲▲▲▲▲▲▲▲

REFERENCES

1. Miles. Digest of English civil law, Book II. 1910; xiv, xv.
2. Bauer. Consequential damages in contract. 80 U.Pa.L.Rev. 687, 1932.
3. McPherson V. Tamiami Trail Tours Inc., 383 F.2d 527 (5th Cir. 1967).
4. Le Juene Road Hospital Inc. v. Watson, 171 So.2d 202 (Fla. App. 1965).
5. O'Brien v. Cunard, 154 Mass. 272, 1891.
6. Bolton v. Stewart, 191 S.W.2d 798, (Tex. Civ. App. 1945).
7. Luka v. Lowrie, 171 Mich. 122, 1912.
8. Rogers v. Lumberman's Mutual Casualty Co., 119 So.2d 649 (La. App. 1960).
9. Prince v. Commonwealth, 321 U.S. 158 (1943).
10. Hoffman v. Naslund, 274 Minn. 521, 1966.
11. Loudon v. Scott, 58 Mont. 65, 1920.
12. Sim v. Weeks, 7 Cal. App. 2d 28, 1935.
13. Natanson v. Kline, 186 Kan. 393, on rehearing 187 Kan. 186, 1960.
14. Plant, An analysis of "informed consent", 36 Ford. L. Rev. 639 (1968).
15. Canterbury v. Spence, 464 F.2d 772 (D.C. Cir. 1972) cert. den. 409 US. 1064 (1972).
16. Scott v. Bradford, 606 P.2d 554 (Okla. 1979).
17. Marsh. Health care cost containment and the duty to treat. J Leg Med 1985;6:157.
18. Amer. Med. News, 27 (15):25, April 20, 1984.
19. King JH. The law of medical malpractice. St. Paul: West Publishing Co., 1977.
20. Morreim EH. Cost containment and the standard of medical care, 75 Cal. L. Rev. 5, 1987.
21. Shakespeare W. King Lear, Act V, iii.

SUGGESTED READING

1. Prosser WL. Law of torts, 4th ed. St. Paul: West Publishing Co., 1971.
2. Marsh FH. Health care cost containment and the duty to treat. J Leg Med 1985;6:157.
3. Morreim EH. Cost constraints as a malpractice defense. Hastings Center Report 1988;18:5.
4. Charfoos L. The medical malpractice case: a handbook, 2nd ed. Englewood Cliffs: Prentice-Hall, 1977.
5. Holder AR. Medical malpractice law. New York: Wiley, 1975.

INDEX

Q

Quadriplegia, functional levels of, 208, 209t
Quinidine, for cardiac resuscitability, 38
Quinine, addiction to, 164

R

Rabies, treatment, 856
Radial artery, anatomy of, 738, 742f
Radial nerve, anatomy of, 737, 742f
  injuries of, neuropathies associated with, 752
Radiation, as factor in wound healing, 73
Radiation therapy, in injured pregnant women, 631-632
Radiography, in eye trauma examination, 231
  in heart injuries, 344, 353
  in intrathoracic great vessel injury, blunt injuries, 375-376, 375f-377f, 375t
    penetrating injuries, 363-364
  in laryngotracheal injuries, 298-299
  in maxillofacial trauma patients, 256-257, 256f
  in musculoskeletal trauma diagnosis, 643
  in neck-injured patients, 274-275
  plain film, in acute trauma, 105
    of great vessels, 116-117, 117f
Radioisotope scans, in abdominal injury evaluation, 417
  in septic patients, 842
Radioisotope scintiscan, in splenic injuries, 481-482, 481f
Radiological studies. *See also* X-ray(s)
  in abdominal vascular injuries, 556-557
  in acute trauma, 105-127. *See also specific modalities, e.g.,*
      Ultrasonography
    abdomen, 119-121
    anesthesia during, 107
    ankles, 123, 124f
    brain, 108-109
    chest, 112-119. *See also under* Chest
    child abuse, 124
    clinical indications, 107
    consultation and preparation for, 107
    cost-effectiveness, 124
    errors in, 125
    extremities, 122-124
    face, 109, 109f
    facilities for, 105, 106f
      for unstable patients, 105
    failure of diagnosis, 124
    femoral neck, 122-123, 123f
    forearm, 122
    general considerations, 108
    knees, 123
    lower leg, 122
    neck, 112
    patient history prior to, 107
    pelvis, 121-122
    personnel for, 107
    physical examination prior to, 107
    planning for, 107-108
    prerequisites for effective examinations, 107-108
    reports following, 108
    skull, 108
    spine, 109-112, 110f-112f
    urinary tract, 122
    vascular injuries, 123-124
    wrist, 122
  in acute trauma recovery, 124
  in ARDS diagnosis, 880, 880f, 881f
  in child abuse, 124
  in colon and rectal injuries, 539
  in diaphragmatic injuries, 437-441, 437f-439f
  in esophageal injuries, 391

  in fat embolism syndrome, 707
  in hand injury evaluation, 744
  in heart failure, 921, 921f
  in injured pregnant women, 631-632
  in pelvic fractures, 583-585, 584f-586f
  in renal injuries, 602-604, 603f
  in septic patients, 842
Radiology, medicolegal aspects of, 107
Radionuclide angiography (RNA), following heart injuries, 354-355
  in heart failure, 921
Radionuclide imaging, in acute trauma, 105
  in diaphragmatic injuries, 440
  in renal injuries, 604
  in vascular injury evaluation, 715
Radius, distal, fractures of, 651-652
  head of, fractures of, 651
    subluxation of, in children, 668
  shaft of, fractures of, 651
Rajpal, S.C., in colon and rectal injuries, 535
Rambdohr, in stomach injuries, 497
Ramus(i), ichial, fractures of, treatment, 594
  pubic, fractures of, treatment, 594
Rape, in nonpregnant women, 622
Rectum, injuries to, 534-553, 546-551
  anal sphincter wounds, 548
  associated injuries, 538, 547
  blunt trauma, 537-538
  clinical examination in, 538
  complications, 549
  contrast studies in, 539
  CT in, 539
  diagnosis, 538-540, 547
  diagnostic peritoneal lavage in, 539
  endoscopy in, 538-539
  foreign bodies, management, 548
  gunshot wounds, 536, 536t
  historical perspectives, 534-535
  iatrogenic injuries, 536-537
  impalement injuries, 548
  impalements in, 536-537
  incidence, 546
  in infants and children, treatment, 139
  laparoscopy in, 539
  laparotomy in, 539-540
  mechanisms of, 535-538, 536t, 537t
  mortality rates, 548-549, 549t, 550t
  outcome following, 548-549, 549t, 550t
  pathophysiology, 535-538, 536t, 537t
  pelvic fractures and, 593
  penetrating trauma, 535-537, 536t, 537t
  perineal wounds, 548
  radiological examination in, 539
  significance of, 546
  stab wounds, 536, 536t
  treatment, 547-548, 547f
    anal detachment repair, 548
    cleansing of distal rectum, 547-548
    diverting colostomy, 547, 547f
    errors in, 551
    presacral drainage, 548, 550f
    rectal repair, 547
  posttraumatic complications, 977
Red blood cells (RBCs), frozen, for transfusion, 59
  packed, for transfusion, 59
  preservation of, techniques, 59
  viability of, decreased, strorage of blood and, 61
  washed, for transfusion, 59
Reflex(es), baroreceptor, in heart failure, 916
Refractive lesions, 226
Regional trauma systems, concept behind, 1
Rehabilitation, following spinal cord injuries, objectives, 217
  following trauma-related surgery in the elderly, 156